MW00396417

Principles of Molecular Diagnostics and Personalized Cancer Medicine

Principles of Molecular Diagnostics and Personalized Cancer Medicine

EDITORS

Dongfeng Tan, MD

Professor
Department of Pathology and Laboratory Medicine, and
Department of Gastrointestinal Medical Oncology
The University of Texas MD Anderson Cancer Center
Houston, Texas

Henry T. Lynch, MD

Chairman
Preventive Medicine and Public Health
Professor of Medicine
Director
Creighton Hereditary Cancer Center
Creighton University School of Medicine
Omaha, Nebraska

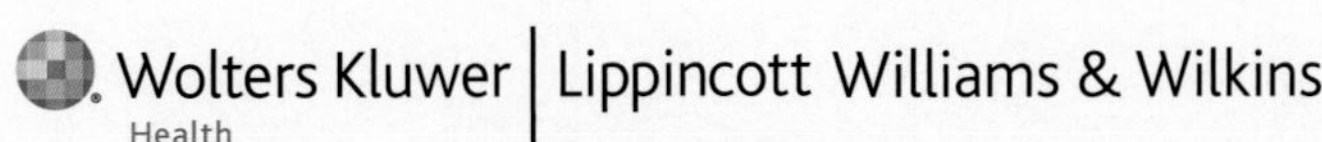

Philadelphia • Baltimore • New York • London
Buenos Aires • Hong Kong • Sydney • Tokyo

Senior Executive Editor: Jonathan W. Pine, Jr.
Senior Product Manager: Emilie Moyer
Senior Manufacturing Manager: Benjamin Rivera
Production Product Manager: David Orzechowski
Design Coordinator: Joan Wendt
Production Service: Integra Software Services

Two Commerce Square
2001 Market Street
Philadelphia, PA 19103

Printed in the People's Republic of China

Library of Congress Cataloging-in-Publication Data

Principles of molecular diagnostics and personalized cancer medicine / editors, Dongfeng Tan, Henry T. Lynch.
p. ; cm.
Includes bibliographical references.
ISBN 978-1-4511-3197-0
I. Tan, Dongfeng. II. Lynch, Henry T.
[DNLM: 1. Neoplasms—diagnosis. 2. Neoplasms—therapy. 3. Individualized Medicine—methods.
4. Medical Oncology—methods. 5. Molecular Diagnostic Techniques.
6. Molecular Targeted Therapy. QZ 241]
616.99'4—dc23

2012029838

The authors, editors, and publisher have exerted every effort to ensure that drug selection and dosage set forth in this text are in accordance with current recommendations and practice at the time of publication. However, in view of ongoing research, changes in government regulations, and the constant flow of information relating to drug therapy and drug reactions, the reader is urged to check the package insert for each drug for any change in indications and dosage and for added warnings and precautions. This is particularly important when the recommended agent is a new or infrequently employed drug.

Some drugs and medical devices presented in the publication have Food and Drug Administration (FDA) clearance for limited use in restricted research settings. It is the responsibility of the health care provider to ascertain the FDA status of each drug or device planned for use in their clinical practice.

To purchase additional copies of this book, call our customer service department at (800) 638-3030 or fax orders to (301) 223-2320. International customers should call (301) 223-2300.

Visit Lippincott Williams & Wilkins on the Internet: at LWW.com. Lippincott Williams & Wilkins customer service representatives are available from 8:30 am to 6 pm, EST.

10 9 8 7 6 5 4 3 2 1

CCS1112

This book is dedicated to my wife **Hong (Helen) Zou**, *my daughters* **Connie** *and* **Christina**, *my mother* **Shubao Tang**, *and my late father* **Jiaqi Tan**

Dongfeng Tan, MD, FCAP

I dedicate this book to my late wife, **Jane**, *who worked with me on all of my research. Despite this ongoing commitment, she remained a devoted mother to our three children and a loving and beloved wife throughout our more than sixty years of marriage.*

Henry T. Lynch, MD

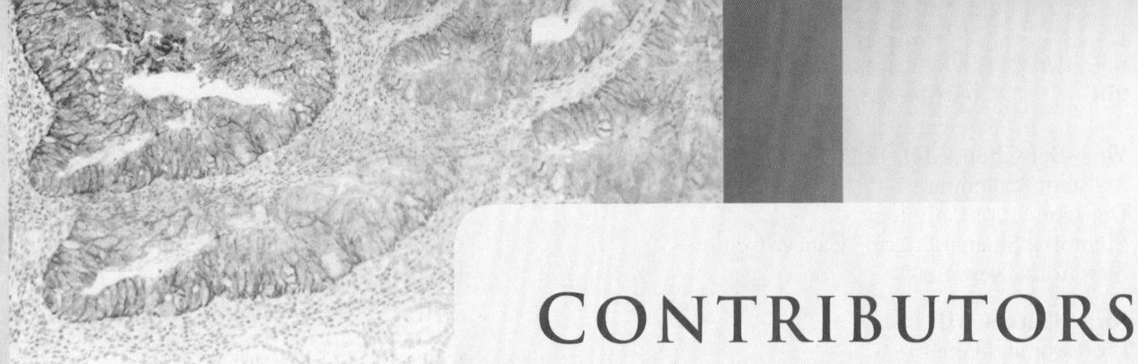

CONTRIBUTORS

Daniel Abate-Daga, PhD
Fellow
Surgery Branch
National Cancer Institute
Bethesda, Maryland

Hikmat A. Al-Ahmadie, MD
Assistant Attending
Department of Pathology
Memorial Sloan-Kettering Cancer Center
New York, New York

Scott J. Antonia, MD, PhD
Chair
Department of Thoracic Oncology
Co-Leader
Immunology Program
Senior Member
H. Lee Moffitt Cancer Center
Professor
University of South Florida Oncologic Sciences
Tampa, Florida

Christina M. Bagby, DO
Department of Pathology
The Johns Hopkins University School of Medicine
Department of Gynecologic Pathology
The Johns Hopkins Hospital
Baltimore, Maryland

Madhuri Bajaj, MD
Karmanos Cancer Institute
Wayne State University School of Medicine
Detroit, Michigan

Ryan P. Bender, PhD, FACMG
Director
Department of Molecular Diagnostics
Caris Life Sciences
Phoenix, Arizona

Pavan Kumar Bhamidipati, MD
Assistant Professor
Department of Leukemia
The University of Texas MD Anderson Cancer Center
Houston, Texas

David G. Bostwick, MD, MBA
Chief Medical Officer
Bostwick Laboratories, Inc.
Glen Allen, Virginia

Robert E. Brown, MD
Professor and Harvey S. Rosenberg Endowed Chair
Department of Pathology and Laboratory Medicine
The University of Texas Medical School at Houston
Houston, Texas

Jamie J. Buryanek, MD
Assistant Professor
Department of Pathology and Laboratory Medicine
The University of Texas Medical School at Houston
Houston, Texas

George A. Calin, MD, PhD
Associate Professor
Center for RNA Interference and Non-Coding RNAs
Graduate School of Biomedical Sciences
Department of Experimental Therapeutics
The University of Texas MD Anderson Cancer Center
Houston, Texas

Michael A. Carducci, MD
AEGON Professor in Prostate Cancer Research
Co-Director, Prostate Cancer Program
The Sidney Kimmel Comprehensive Cancer Center
The Johns Hopkins Hospital
Baltimore, Maryland

Lea Carrington, MS, MBA, MT(ASCP)
Associate Director, Hematology
FDA/CDRH/OIVD/DIHD
Silver Spring, Maryland

Maria Chan, PhD
Division Director
Division of Immunology and Hematology Devices
FDA/CDRH/OIVD/DIHD
Silver Spring, Maryland

Yao Chang, PhD
Associate Investigator
Institute of Infectious Diseases and Vaccinology
National Health Research Institutes
Zhunan, Taiwan

Ying-Bei Chen, MD, PhD
Assistant Attending
Department of Pathology
Memorial Sloan-Kettering Cancer Center
New York, New York

Jorge Cortes, MD
Professor and Chief
Department of Leukemia
The University of Texas MD Anderson Cancer Center
Houston, Texas

C. Lance Cowey, MD
Medical Oncologist
Baylor Sammons Cancer Center
Dallas, Texas

Garrett M. Dancik, PhD
Post-Doctoral Researcher
Department of Surgery
University of Colorado
Aurora, Colorado

Chau Dang, MD
Associate Attending Physician
Memorial Sloan-Kettering Cancer Center
New York, New York

John De Groot, MD
Department of Neurosurgery
The University of Texas MD Anderson Cancer Center
Houston, Texas

George Deeb, MD
Assistant Professor of Oncology
Director of Hematopathology
Associate Director of Flow and Image Cytometry Laboratory
Department of Pathology
Roswell Park Cancer Institute
Buffalo, New York

Amit Deorukhkar, PhD
Instructor
Department of Radiation Oncology-Research
The University of Texas MD Anderson Cancer Center
Houston, Texas

Sadhna Dhingra, MBBS, MD
Fellow, Surgical Pathology
Department of Pathology and Genomic Medicine
The Methodist Hospital
Houston, Texas

Richard R. Drake, MD, PhD
Professor
Cell and Molecular Pharmacology/Hollings Cancer Center
Medical University of South Carolina
Charleston, South Carolina

Michael C. Dugan, MD
President
MCDXI Medical Diagnostics International
Chief Medical Advisor
bioTheranostics, Inc.
San Diego, California

S. Gail Eckhardt, MD
Professor, Stapp Harlow Chair in Cancer Research
Department of Medicine
University of Colorado Anschutz Medical Campus
Aurora, Colorado

Adel El-Naggar, MD, PhD
Professor of Pathology and Head and Neck Surgery
Department of Pathology and Head and Neck Surgery
The University of Texas MD Anderson Cancer Center
Houston, Texas

Jeannelyn S. Estrella, MD
Department of Pathology
The University of Texas MD Anderson Cancer Center
Houston, Texas

Melissa L. Fishel, PhD
Research Assistant Professor
Herman B Wells Center for Pediatric Research
Indianapolis, Indiana

Keith T. Flaherty, MD
Associate Professor
Department of Medicine
Harvard Medical School
Director of Developmental Therapeutics
Department of Cancer Center
Massachusetts General Hospital
Boston, Massachusetts

Gregory N. Fuller, MD, PhD
Professor and Chief
Section of Neuropathology
The University of Texas MD Anderson Cancer Center
Houston, Texas

Jeana Garris, MD
Department of Gastrointestinal Oncology
The University of Texas MD Anderson Cancer Center
Houston, Texas

David Geller, MD
Department of Othopedic Surgery
Montefiore Medical Center
The Children's Hospital at Montefiore
The Albert Einstein College of Medicine
Bronx, New York

Anatole Ghazalpour, PhD, FACMG
Associate Director
Department of Molecular Diagnostics
Caris Life Sciences
Phoenix, Arizona

Jonathan Gill, MD
Department of Pediatrics
Montefiore Medical Center
The Children's Hospital at Montefiore
The Albert Einstein College of Medicine
Bronx, New York

Christopher D. Gocke, MD
Associate Professor
Department of Pathology and Oncology
School of Medicine
The Johns Hopkins University
Interim Director
Division of Molecular Pathology
Department of Pathology
The Johns Hopkins Hospital
Baltimore, Maryland

Kathryn A. Gold, MD
Department of Medical Oncology
The University of Texas MD Anderson Cancer Center
Houston, Texas

David W. Goodrich, PhD
Professor of Oncology
Pharmacology and Therapeutics
Roswell Park Cancer Institute
Buffalo, New York

Richard Gorlick, MD
Vice Chairman, Pediatrics
Department of Pediatrics
Montefiore Medical Center
The Children's Hospital at Montefiore
The Albert Einstein College of Medicine
Bronx, New York

Axel Grothey, MD
Professor and Consultant
Department of Medical Oncology
Mayo Clinic
Rochester, Minnesota

James L. Gulley, MD, PhD
Senior Investigator
Medical Oncology Branch
Center for Cancer Research
Deputy Chief
Laboratory of Tumor Immunology and Biology
National Cancer Institute
National Institutes of Health
Bethesda, Maryland

Kun Guo, MD, PhD
Assistant Professor
Department of Hepatobiliary and Pancreas Surgery
The First Affiliated Hospital of Xi'an Jiaotong University
Xi'an, China

Hiroshi Harada, PhD
Group Leader and Lecturer
Group of Radiation and Tumor Biology
Career-Path Promotion Unit for Young Life Scientist
Kyoto University
Kyoto, Japan

Elisabeth I. Heath, MD
Associate Professor of Oncology
Department of Oncology
Wayne State University School of Medicine
Director, Prostate Cancer Research
Karmanos Cancer Institute
Detroit, Michigan

David G. Hicks, MD
Professor
Pathology and Laboratory Medicine
University of Rochester Medical Center
Rochester, New York

Whitney A. High, MD, JD, MEng
Associate Professor
Department of Dermatology & Pathology
Vice Chair of Clinical Affairs
Department of Dermatology
Director
Dermatopathology Laboratory
Department of Dermatology
University of Colorado School of Medicine
Denver, Colorado

Masahiro Hiraoka, MD, PhD
Professor
Department of Radiation Oncology and Image-Applied Therapy
Kyoto University Graduate School of Medicine
Chairman and Professor
Radiation Oncology
Kyoto University Hospital
Kyoto, Japan

Jiang Hongchi, MD
Member of the Standing Committee
Chinese Society of Surgery
Chinese Medical Association
Beijing, China
Chief
Department of General Surgery
The First Affiliated Hospital of Harbin Medical University
Harbin, China

Yun-Fu Hu, PhD
Associate Director
Immunology
FDA/CDRH/OIVD/DIHD
Silver Spring, Maryland

Joleen M. Hubbard, MD
Assistant Professor and Senior Associate Consultant
Department of Medical Oncology
Mayo Clinic
Rochester, Minnesota

Clifford Hudis, MD
Chief
Breast Cancer Medicine Service
Attending
Department of Medicine
Memorial Sloan-Kettering Cancer Center
Professor of Medicine
Weill Cornell Medical College
New York, New York

Kristin Huntoon, MD, PhD
Molecular Pathogenesis Unit
Surgical Neurology Branch
National Institute of Neurological Disorders and Stroke
National Institutes of Health
Bethesda, Maryland

Thomas E. Hutson, DO
Director
Genitourinary Oncology Program
Baylor Sammons Cancer Center
Dallas, Texas

Yuichi Ishikawa, MD, PhD
Vice Director
The Cancer Institute
Member and Chief
Division of Pathology
The Cancer Institute
Director
Department of Pathology
The Cancer Institute Hospital
Japanese Foundation for Cancer Research
Tokyo, Japan

Elias Jabbour, MD
Associate Professor
Department of Leukemia
The University of Texas MD Anderson Cancer Center
Houston, Texas

Milind Javle, MD
Associate Professor
Attending Physician
Gastrointestinal Medical Oncology
The University of Texas MD Anderson Cancer Center
Houston, Texas

Komal Jhaveri, MD
New York University Cancer Institute
New York, New York

Dan Jones, MD, PhD
Medical Director
Quest Diagnostics
Nichols Institute
Chantilly, Virginia

Ahmed O. Kaseb, MD
Medical Oncology
The University of Texas MD Anderson Cancer Center
Houston, Texas

Lev M. Kats, BSc (Hons), PhD
Harvard Medical School
Research Fellow
Medicine/Division of Genetics
Beth Israel Deaconess Medical Center
Boston, Massachusetts

Mark R. Kelley, PhD
Betty and Earl Herr Professor
Pediatric Oncology Research
Professor
Departments of Pediatrics, Biochemistry & Molecular Biology and Pharmacology & Toxicology
Associate Director
Herman B Wells Center for Pediatric Research
Associate Director of Basic Science Research
Indiana University Simon Cancer Center
Indianapolis, Indiana

Yoon Jun Kim, MD, PhD
Department of Internal Medicine
Liver Research Institute
Seoul National University College of Medicine
Seoul, Korea

Joseph W. Kim, MD
Medical Oncology Fellow
Medical Oncology Branch
Laboratory of Tumor Immunology and Biology
Clinical Fellow
Medical Oncology Branch
National Cancer Institute
National Institutes of Health
Bethesda, Maryland

Edward S. Kim, MD
Department of Medical Oncology
The University of Texas MD Anderson Cancer Center
Houston, Texas

Sunil Krishnan, MD
Associate Professor
Department of Radiation Oncology
The University of Texas MD Anderson Cancer Center
Houston, Texas

Robert J. Kurman, MD
Richard W. TeLinde Distinguished Professor of Gynecologic Pathology
Departments of Gynecology, Obstetrics, Pathology and Oncology
The Johns Hopkins University School of Medicine
Director of Gynecologic Pathology
Department of Gynecologic Pathology
The Johns Hopkins Hospital
Baltimore, Maryland

Stephen Lanspa, MD
Professor of Medicine
Department of Preventive Medicine
Creighton University School of Medicine
Omaha, Nebraska

Joel A. Lefferts, PhD, HCLD
Assistant Professor of Pathology
Assistant Director, Molecular Pathology
Department of Pathology
Dartmouth-Hitchcock Medical Center
Lebanon, New Hampshire

Stephen Leong, MD
Assistant Professor
Department of Medicine
University of Colorado Anschutz Medical Campus
Aurora, Colorado

Chun Li, PhD
Professor
Experimental Diagnostic Imaging
The University of Texas MD Anderson Cancer Center
Houston, Texas

John W. Linford, MD
Medical Oncology
The University of Texas MD Anderson Cancer Center
Houston, Texas

Mikhail Lisovsky, MD, PhD
Geisel School of Medicine at Dartmouth
Hanover, New Hampshire

Gary Lu, MD, FACMG
Director of Clinical Cytogenetics
Department of Hematopathology
The University of Texas MD Anderson Cancer Center
Houston, Texas

Henry T. Lynch, MD
Chairman
Preventive Medicine and Public Health
Professor of Medicine
Director
Creighton Hereditary Cancer Center
Creighton University School of Medicine
Omaha, Nebraska

Jane F. Lynch, BSN
Professor of Medicine
Department of Preventive Medicine
Creighton University School of Medicine
Omaha, Nebraska

Anirban Maitra, MBBS
Professor of Pathology and Oncology
The Sol Goldman Pancreatic Cancer Research Center
Affiliate Faculty
Department of Chemical and Biomolecular Engineering
Affiliate Faculty
McKusick-Nathans Institute of Genetic Medicine
The Johns Hopkins University School of Medicine
Baltimore, Maryland

Elizabeth Mansfield, PhD
Director
Personalized Medicine Staff
FDA/CDRH/OIVD/DIHD
Silver Spring, Maryland

Lainie P. Martin, MD
Assistant Professor
Attending Physician
Department of Medical Oncology
Fox Chase Cancer Center
Philadelphia, Pennsylvania

Osamu Matsubara, MD
Department of Pathology
National Defense Medical College
Saitama, Japan

Matthew J. McGinniss, PhD
Senior Director
Department of Molecular Diagnostics
Caris Life Sciences
Phoenix, Arizona

Marco Dal Molin, MD
Post-Doctoral Fellow
Department of Pathology
The Sol Goldman Pancreatic Cancer Center
The Johns Hopkins University School of Medicine
Baltimore, Maryland

Richard A. Morgan, PhD
Staff Scientist
Surgery Branch
National Cancer Institute
Bethesda, Maryland

Markus Morkel, MD, PhD
Research Group Leader
Department of Developmental Genetics
Max-Planck-Institute for Molecular Genetics Scientist
Laboratory of Molecular Tumor Pathology
Charité Universitätsmedizin Berlin
Berlin, Germany

John C. Morris, MD
Professor
Division of Hematology-Oncology
Department of Medicine
University of Cincinnati
Director
Experimental Therapeutics
Thoracic Cancer and Head and Neck Cancer Programs
Division of Hematology-Oncology
Department of Medicine
University of Cincinnati Barrett Cancer Center
Cincinnati, Ohio

Brian J. Morrison, PhD
Post-Doctoral Fellow
Division of Hematology-Oncology
Department of Medicine
Vontz Center for Molecular Studies
University of Cincinnati
Cincinnati, Ohio

Ronald Myint, MD
Department of Medical Oncology
The University of Texas MD Anderson Cancer Center
Houston, Texas

Marina Nikiforova, MD
Associate Professor of Pathology
Director
Molecular Anatomic Pathology Laboratory
Division of Molecular Anatomic Pathology
Department of Pathology
University of Pittsburgh School of Medicine
Pittsburgh, Pennsylvania

Julius O. Nyalwidhe, PhD
Assistant Professor
Department of Microbiology and Molecular Cell Biology
Leroy T. Canoles Cancer Research Center
Eastern Virginia Medical School
Norfolk, Virginia

Adriana Olar, MD
Neuropathology Fellow
Department of Pathology and Genomic Medicine
The Methodist Hospital
Houston, Texas

Andre M. Oliveira, MD, PhD
Associate Professor and Consultant
Department of Laboratory Medicine
Mayo Clinic Rochester
Rochester, Minnesota

Naohide Oue, MD, PhD
Associate Professor
Department of Molecular Pathology
Hiroshima University Institute of Biomedical & Health Sciences
Hiroshima, Japan

Qiulu Pan, MD
Science Director
Department of Molecular Oncology
Quest Diagnostics Nichole Institute
Chantilly, Virginia

Pier Paolo Pandolfi, MD, PhD
George C. Reisman Professor of Medicine and Professor of Pathology
Harvard Medical School
Boston, Massachusetts

Reena Philip, PhD
Deputy Division Director
FDA/CDRH/OIVD/DIHD
Silver Spring, Maryland

Jennifer Picarsic, MD
Assistant Professor
Department of Pathology
University of Pittsburgh
Faculty
Department of Pediatric Pathology
Children's Hospital of Pittsburgh of UPMC
Pittsburgh, Pennsylvania

Mary C. Pinder-Schenck, MD
Assistant Professor
Department of Oncologic Sciences
University of South Florida
Assistant Member
Department of Thoracic Oncology
H. Lee Moffitt Cancer Center
Tampa, Florida

Todd M. Pitts, MS
Research Instructor
Department of Medicine
University of Colorado Anschutz Medical Campus
Aurora, Colorado

Laura B. Pitzonka, BS
Pre-Doctoral Fellow
Pharmacology and Therapeutics
Roswell Park Cancer Institute
Buffalo, New York

Markus Reschke, PhD
Harvard Medical School
Research Fellow
Medicine/Division of Genetics
Beth Israel Deaconess Medical Center
Boston, Massachusetts

Victor E. Reuter, MD
Professor of Pathology
Department of Pathology
Weill Medical College of Cornell University
Vice Chairman
Department of Pathology
Memorial Sloan-Kettering Cancer Center
New York, New York

Miguel Reyes-Múgica, MD
Professor
Department of Pathology
University of Pittsburgh
Faculty
Department of Pediatric Pathology
Children's Hospital of Pittsburgh of UPMC
Pittsburgh, Pennsylvania

Keila Rivera-Roman, MD
Assistant Professor
Pathology and Laboratory Medicine
Medical Sciences Campus
University of Puerto Rico
San Juan, Puerto Rico

Manuel Salto-Tellez, MD, FRCPath
Chair of Molecular Pathology
Queens University Belfast & Belfast Health and Social Care Trust
Belfast, Ireland

Daniel J. Sargent, PhD
Division of Biomedical Statistics and Informatics
Mayo Clinic
Rochester, Minnesota

Russell J. Schilder, MD
Professor
Chief, Gynecologic Medical Oncology
Department of Medical Oncology
Thomas Jefferson University
Philadelphia, Pennsylvania

Oliver J. Semmes, PhD
Professor
Department of Microbiology and Molecular Cell Biology
Eastern Virginia Medical School
Norfolk, Virginia

Kazuhiro Sentani, MD, PhD
Assistant Professor
Department of Molecular Pathology
Hiroshima University Institute of Biomedical & Health Sciences
Hiroshima, Japan

Maitri Y. Shah, MS, BPharm
Graduate School of Biomedical Sciences
Department of Experimental Therapeutics
The University of Texas MD Anderson Cancer Center
Houston, Texas

A. Dean Sherry, PhD
Professor of Chemistry
University of Texas at Dallas
Richardson, Texas
Director
Advanced Imaging Research Center
Professor of Radiology
University of Texas Southwestern Medical Center
Dallas, Texas

Qian Shi, PhD
Division of Biomedical Statistics and Informatics
Mayo Clinic
Rochester, Minnesota

le-Ming Shih, MD, PhD
Professor
Department of Pathology
The Johns Hopkins University School of Medicine
Department of Gynecologic Pathology
The Johns Hopkins Hospital
Baltimore, Maryland

Charles Dwo-Yuan Sia, PhD
Investigator
Institute of Infectious Diseases and Vaccinology
National Health Research Institutes
Zhunan, Taiwan

Peter Silberstein, MD
Internal Medicine Department
Creighton University School of Medicine
Omaha, Nebraska

Frank A. Sinicrope, MD
Professor of Medicine and Oncology
Department of Medicine
Mayo Clinic and Mayo Cancer Center
Rochester, Minnesota

Heath Skinner, MD, PhD
Assistant Professor
Department of Radiation Oncology
The University of Texas MD Anderson Cancer Center
Houston, Texas

Carrie L. Snyder, MSN
Professor of Medicine
Department of Preventive Medicine
Creighton University School of Medicine
Omaha, Nebraska

Jason C. Steel, PhD
Research Assistant Professor
Division of Hematology-Oncology
Department of Internal Medicine
Vontz Center for Molecular Studies
University of Cincinnati
Cincinnati, Ohio

Ih-Jen Su, MD, PhD
Distinguished Investigator and Professor
Institute of Infectious Diseases and Vaccinology
National Health Research Institutes
Zhunan, Taiwan

Andrea Suárez, MD, PhD
Department of Dermatology
Weill Cornell Medical College
Dermatology Resident
New York Presbyterian Hospital
New York, New York

Xiankai Sun, PhD
Assistant Professor
Radiology & Advanced Imaging Research
University of Texas Southwestern Medical Center
Dallas, Texas

Laura J. Tafe, MD
Assistant Professor of Pathology
Assistant Director, Molecular Pathology
Department of Pathology
Dartmouth-Hitchcock Medical Center
Lebanon, New Hampshire

Aik-Choon Tan, PhD
Assistant Professor
Department of Medicine
University of Colorado Anschutz Medical Campus
Aurora, Colorado

Dongfeng Tan, MD
Professor
Department of Pathology and Laboratory Medicine, and Department of Gastrointestinal Medical Oncology
The University of Texas MD Anderson Cancer Center
Houston, Texas

Ping Tang, MD, PhD
Professor
Pathology and Laboratory Medicine
University of Rochester Medical Center
Rochester, New York

John J. Tentler, PhD
Associate Professor
Department of Medicine
Anschutz Medical Campus
University of Colorado
Aurora, Colorado

Brett J. Theeler, MD
Major, United States Army Medical Corps
Neurology
Walter Reed National Military Medical Center
Bethesda, Maryland

Dan Theodorescu, MD, PhD
Director
University of Colorado Cancer Center
University of Colorado
Attending Urologic Oncologist
Department of Surgery
University of Colorado Hospital
Aurora, Colorado

Jorge Torres-Mora, MD
Fellow Bone and Soft Tissue Pathology
Department of Laboratory Medicine and Petrology
Mayo Clinic Rochester
Rochester, Minnesota

Yingfei Wei, PhD
CEO
Elixirin Corporation
San Francisco, California

Qingyi Wei, MD, PhD
Professor
Department of Epidemiology
The University of Texas MD Anderson Cancer Center
Houston, Texas

Hyun Goo Woo, MD, PhD
Department of Physiology
Ajou University School of Medicine
Suwon, Korea

Yunkou Wu, PhD
Assistant Instructor
Advanced Imaging Research Center
University of Texas Southwestern Medical Center
Dallas, Texas

Keping Xie, MD, PhD
Professor
Gastrointestinal Medical Oncology
The University of Texas MD Anderson Cancer Center
Houston, Texas

YingWei Xue, MD
Professor
Department of Oncological Surgery
Harbin Medical University
Director
Department of Gastrointestinal Surgery
The Third Affiliated Hospital of Harbin Medical University
Harbin, China

Bin Yang, MD, PhD, FCAP
Associate Professor
Pathology and Laboratory Medicine Institute
Cleveland Clinic
Cleveland, Ohio

James C. Yao, MD
Associate Professor and Deputy Chairman
Gastrointestinal Medical Oncology
The University of Texas MD Anderson Cancer Center
Houston, Texas

Wataru Yasui, MD, PhD
Professor
Department of Molecular Pathology
Hiroshima University
Hiroshima, Japan

C. Cameron Yin, MD, PhD
Associate Professor
Department of Hematopathology
The University of Texas MD Anderson Cancer Center
Houston, Texas

Seung Kew Yoon, MD, PhD
Professor
Department of Internal Medicine
The Catholic University of Korea
Seoul, Republic of Korea

Harry H. Yoon, MD, PhD
Professor of Medicine and Oncology
Department of Medicine
Mayo Clinic and Mayo Cancer Center
Rochester, Minnesota

Michio Yoshimura, PhD
Assistant Professor
Department of Radiation Oncology and Image-Applied Therapy
Graduate School of Medicine
Kyoto University
Assistant Professor
Radiation Oncology
Kyoto University Hospital
Kyoto, Japan

Grace Yu, PhD
Assistant Investigator
Institute of Infectious Diseases and Vaccinology
National Health Research Institutes
Zhunan, Taiwan

Guo-Liang Yu, PhD
President and CEO
Epitomics, Inc.
San Francisco, California

XueFeng Yu, MD
Associate Professor
Department of Oncological Surgery
Harbin Medical University
Department of Gastrointestinal Surgery
The Third Affiliated Hospital of Harbin Medical University
Harbin, China

W.K. Alfred Yung, MD, PhD
Professor and Chair
Department of Neuro-Oncology
The University of Texas MD Anderson Cancer Center
Houston, Texas

Shengle Zhang, MD, PhD
Associate Professor
Department of Pathology
State University of New York Upstate Medical University
Attending Pathologist
Director of Anatomic Molecular Pathology Laboratories
Department of Pathology
State University of New York Upstate Medical University Hospital
Syracuse, New York

Yanqiao Zhang, MD, PhD
Professor and Chief
Department of Gastrointestinal Medical Oncology
Tumor Hospital
Harbin Medical University
Harbin, China

Qing Zhao, MD, PhD
Assistant Professor
Pathology and Laboratory Medicine
Boston Medical Center
Boston University School of Medicine
Boston, Massachusetts

Zhengping Zhuang, MD, PhD
Head, Molecular Pathogenesis Unit
Surgical Neurology Branch
National Institute of Neurological Disorders and Stroke
National Institutes of Health
Bethesda, Maryland

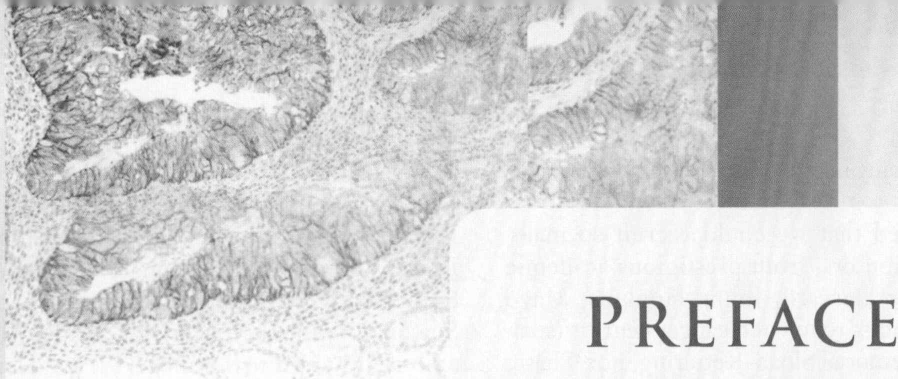

PREFACE

Personalized medicine, in concert with targeted oncologic therapy, has become one of the most active, rapidly advancing, and clinically challenging pursuits in cancer treatment. A major concern for molecular geneticists and clinicians must be to focus upon prioritizing those issues that are most important for research and targeted management in these most prolific days of cancer medicine. In no area of medicine is this more apparent than in cancer medicine, where arrays of specific genetic alterations have been used to manage various types of malignancies. The discoveries that form our understanding of cancer have substantially accelerated over the past decade. These emerging findings have significantly affected the traditional practice of oncology and have resulted in a subspecialized multidisciplinary approach to patient care that incorporates personalized therapies such as targeted molecular therapy, prognosis, risk assessment, and prevention, all of which are primarily based on molecular diagnostics and imaging.

This book, written by a cadre of renowned experts in cancer research, pathology, clinical trials, molecular diagnostics, personalized therapy, bioinformatics, and federal regulations, provides broad, comprehensive perspectives on the current trends in molecular diagnosis of cancer and personalized cancer medicine. It updates readers on recently acquired knowledge and emphasizes new uses for that knowledge in the changing landscape of specialized multidisciplinary care and personalized medicine.

The book consists of 7 sections and 70 chapters. Although the chapters follow a sequence from pathogenesis to therapy, each chapter stands alone in its treatment of the subject matter. Section I updates readers on general cancer biology and genetics and provides a basis for the more specialized sections that follow. Cancer cell proliferation, signal transduction pathways, cancer stem cells, and the interaction between genetics and environmental factors in carcinogenesis are emphasized. Section II is devoted to molecular technologies, including the popular polymerase chain reaction technique, single nucleotide polymorphisms, whole-genome assessments, and next-generation sequencing. Section III provides rich information on molecular imaging and screening, genetic counseling, minimal residual disease detection, circulating tumor cell tests, molecular cancer prognosis assessment, regulatory perspectives on genetic tests, quality assurance and standardization of molecular diagnostics, and the use of biostatistics and bioinformatics in molecular tests and personalized cancer medicine.

Section IV focuses on molecular diagnostics of common malignancies. Detailed information is provided on the use of molecular methods in clinical cancer assessment. Section V reviews and updates information on the molecular basis of cancer therapy and emphasizes critical molecules as special treatment targets, particularly genes/DNA, RNA, proteins/antibodies, and nanoparticles. Section VI covers personalized targeted therapy for the most common human malignancies. The goal of such therapy is to deliver the right drug to the right patient at the right time at the right dose. This effort requires the integration of information from the DNA, RNA, and protein levels with predictors of treatment response to particular therapies. Novel therapeutic agents against specific genetic, molecular, and antigenic targets are discussed, as is the process for deciding whether to use these agents (for example, the need to determine whether specific *KRAS*, and *BRAF* mutations are present in colorectal cancer before treating it with EGFR antagonists). The book concludes with Section VII, which covers the future of molecular pathology and personalized medicine in cancer management. Clearly, over the next 10 years, we will have the opportunity to clinically evaluate a number of novel biological and chemical agents that target specific molecular irregularities in malignant cells.

This textbook assists pathologists, oncologists, other clinicians, and basic scientists and provides a basis for interactions among all professionals involved in multidisciplinary cancer care. It also provides timely information that is necessary for continued medical education. As such, this book is invaluable to practicing physicians at all levels of experience who need to keep up with advances to provide molecular diagnoses and to deliver personalized treatment. Moreover, the information presented in this book should supply a basis upon which research investigators can evaluate new approaches to molecular diagnostics and targeted therapy, allowing them to understand and critically assess the many new products of the biotechnology revolution.

We are delighted that we could recruit so many extraordinary contributors, from prestigious academic institutions (such as Harvard, Johns Hopkins, Mayo Clinic and Max-Planck), renowned cancer centers (such as MD Anderson, Memorial Sloan-Kettering, Fox Chase, and Roswell Park), well-established diagnostic companies (such as Quest and Bostwick), and governmental regulatory agencies (such as FDA, NCI and NIH), who have actively exemplified their areas of expertise in the book. We are very grateful for their dedicated commitment. In addition, we acknowledge the critical review of relevant chapters and the useful comments and suggestions of Zachary Bohannan, Russell Broaddus, Sarah J. Bronson, Dawn Chalaire, Suzanne Cheng, Lei Du, Jill Delsigne, Stephanie Deming, Kathryn Hale, Elizabeth Hess, Shilpa Jain, Luanne Jorewicz, Tamara Locke, Joseph Munch, Donald Norwood, John Palma, Sunita Patterson, Amelia Scholtz, Karen Stuyck, Ann Sutton, Bryan Tutt, Markeda Wade, Maryam Zenali, among others. Furthermore, we have been graciously assisted and encouraged by the professionals of our publishers, such as Jonathan Pine, a senior executive editor at Lippincott Williams & Wilkins, Emilie Moyer and Jennifer Kowalak, the book's project managers, David Orzechowski and Lydia Shinoj, and others.

Dongfeng Tan, MD

Henry T. Lynch, MD

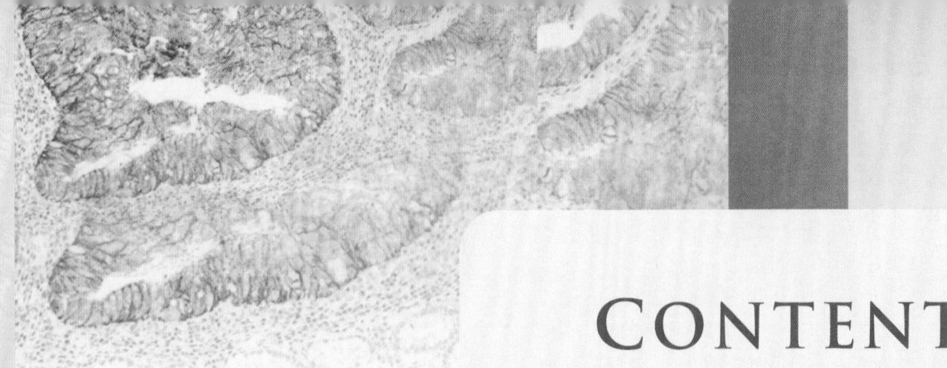

CONTENTS

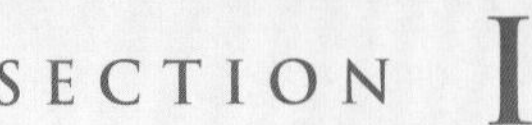

Introduction of Cancer Biology and Cancer Genetics

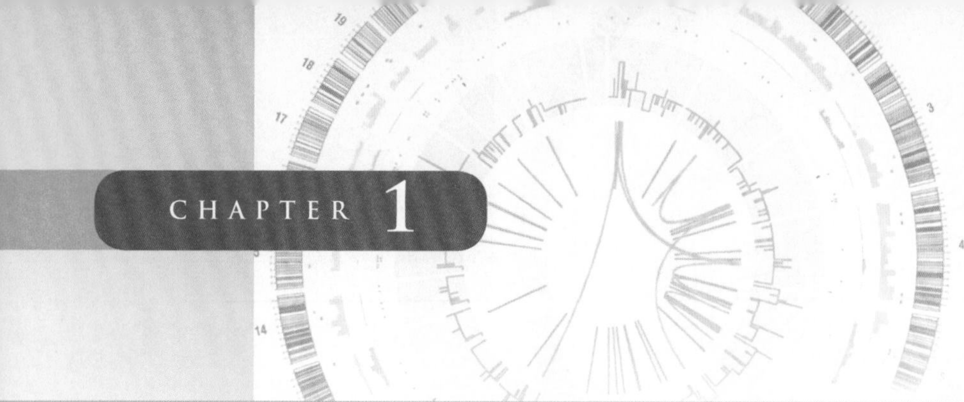

Cell Proliferation and Apoptosis

Laura B. Pitzonka and David W. Goodrich

INTRODUCTION

A cell's birth and its death are both governed by exquisite, genetically programmed regulatory pathways. These pathways specify when and where cells are added or subtracted during normal development and tissue homeostasis. Defects in these pathways can lead to abnormal cell accumulation, a defining characteristic of cancer since its first written description in ancient Egypt.[1] More recently, we have refined our understanding of the key biological capabilities of cancer cells that distinguish them from normal cells. These "hallmarks of cancer" include maintaining proliferative signaling, subverting growth suppressors, achieving replicative immortality, preventing programmed apoptotic cell death, becoming invasive, destabilizing the genome to increase phenotypic variation, and recruiting host cells to facilitate tumor growth and spread.[2] Five of these seven hallmarks are directly related to the regulatory systems that control cell proliferation and apoptosis.

Abnormal cell accumulation is not just a key criterion for cancer diagnosis. The progressively increasing number and spread of cancer cells is what ultimately compromises a patients' health. Indeed, the goal of most current cancer therapies is to reduce cancer cell numbers and to prevent their further expansion. Cell accumulation is also fundamental to tumorigenesis for another, more subtle reason. Cancer is a progressive disease that develops through multiple stages. Each stage is associated with characteristic molecular, genetic, and cellular changes that specify the acquisition of increasingly malignant phenotypes.[3,4] Progression from one stage to the next is driven by an evolutionary process of spontaneous genetic variation and selection. Cancer cell variants that acquire malignant properties increase in number due to their competitive advantage. Eventually, through multiple rounds of variation, selection, and expansion, cancer cells evolve from early benign neoplasia to lethal cancer. Without continuous cell proliferation and survival, this evolutionary process cannot occur.

Both cancer cells and normal cells utilize the same general molecular toolbox to orchestrate cell proliferation and apoptosis. The cancer cell differs from its normal counterpart in that the normal stringency of regulation is relaxed, allowing cancer cells to survive and proliferate when normal cells do not. However, these differences are subtle. Most current therapies that target rapidly proliferating cancer cells also kill rapidly dividing normal cells, typically accounting for the dose-limiting toxicities associated with such therapy. A deeper understanding of how cell proliferation and apoptosis are regulated differently in cancer cells and in normal cells is required to develop new diagnostic and therapeutic strategies that are more selective for cancer cells. Subsequent chapters in this book detail many efforts to leverage new discoveries for the development of improved therapies and diagnostic indicators. The goals of this chapter are to provide a brief introduction to the fundamental molecular pathways that define our current understanding of cell proliferation and apoptosis, to summarize how these pathways are altered in cancer, and to provide selected examples of newer areas of research relevant to cell proliferation and apoptosis.

CELL PROLIFERATION

For most multicellular organisms, including humans, cells possess an intrinsic proliferative capacity that is in vast excess of that required to meet the needs of normal development and homeostasis. For example, human cells of the gut epithelium can divide more than once or twice a day in vivo. A cell dividing exponentially at this rate would generate the trillions of cells necessary to produce a human body in less than a month. Thus, the proliferative capacity of cells is not rate limiting. Rather, highly regulated mechanisms have evolved to restrain this excess proliferative capacity to appropriate times and places. It is this excess proliferative capacity that provides the biological foundation upon which a cancer cell is built. The key in understanding cancer cell proliferation, then, is to characterize the mechanisms that are normally used to restrain the proliferative capacity of cells and to understand how these mechanisms fail during the development of cancer.

The cell division cycle is divided into four phases called G1 (gap 1), S (synthesis), G2 (gap 2), and M (mitosis). DNA replication occurs during S phase. For a typical cell cultured in vitro, this takes about 8 hours and is invariant under normal conditions. Fully replicated chromosomes are segregated to each of the two daughter nuclei by the process of mitosis during M phase. M phase takes about 1 hour. Cytokinesis, the division of the mother cell into two daughter cells, occurs after the chromosomes are properly segregated in M phase. G1 phase precedes S phase, whereas G2 phase precedes M phase. G1 and G2 phases are required for the synthesis of cellular constituents needed to support the following phase and ultimately to accumulate sufficient biomass to produce two viable daughter cells. In mammalian cells, the length of G2 phase is about 2 hours. The length of G1 phase is highly variable and can range from a few minutes to several days or longer. In human cells, the varying length of G1 phase accounts for most of the differences in cell cycle times observed in different biological contexts. Cells can also exit the cell cycle permanently or for extended periods of time. In this situation, cells are in a metabolically active but nonproliferative state that is often referred to as G0. It should be noted that the vast majority of cells in the adult human body are not actively dividing and exist in a G0-like state. Proliferation is typically confined to a small fraction of stem or progenitor cells that are necessary to maintain homeostasis in tissues that naturally turnover. Thus, cell proliferation is regulated not so much by the speed at which the cell division cycle occurs, but rather by the number of cells that are actively participating in a cell division cycle.

Successful cell division requires an ordered and unidirectional transition from one cell cycle phase to the next. The cell cycle is precisely ordered because certain events must be completed before others are begun. Starting mitosis before the completion of DNA replication, for example, would prevent daughter cells from each receiving a complete copy of the genome. The ordering of typical biochemical pathways is accomplished by the substrate–product relationship. The product of one reaction serves as the substrate for the next. The rate of the first reaction, therefore, limits that of the next. Cell cycle regulation is different in that it is controlled by a separate regulatory system that is linked to, but largely independent of, the biochemical reactions that carry out the actual work of cell division. This regulatory system enforces a series of checkpoints, allowing progression to the next cell cycle phase only after completion of the current phase.

Two classes of checkpoints exist, intrinsic and extrinsic. Intrinsic checkpoints govern the order and fidelity of cell cycle events that occur within actively dividing cells. Errors in intrinsic checkpoints like those governing mitosis, for example, can lead to abnormal chromosome segregation and aneuploidy that is characteristic of virtually all cancers. Conversely, extrinsic checkpoints integrate information from the surrounding environment to determine if it is appropriate for a cell to proliferate. Deregulation of extrinsic checkpoints involving growth factor, nutrient, or differentiation signaling can be detrimental to a cell. Such defects may convince a cell that it is appropriate to divide when, in fact, it is not. A detailed discussion of the many varieties of cell cycle checkpoints that operate in normal cells is beyond the scope of this section. Rather, the core cell cycle regulatory machinery that is shared by these checkpoints will be summarized and how this core regulatory machinery is altered in cancer will be described. Examples of cell cycle regulation linked to the emerging research areas of cell growth control and cellular energetics will also be briefly discussed.

The Core Cell Cycle Regulatory System

The core machinery that drives transitions through the various stages of the cell division cycle is composed of a series of serine or threonine kinases known as cyclin-dependent kinases (CDKs). Transit of cell cycle checkpoints and progression from one phase to the next ultimately require the activation of different CDKs. These enzymes are extremely well-conserved throughout evolution to such an extent that CDKs from human cells can functionally substitute for the relevant enzymes in unicellular yeasts, species separated by a billion years of evolutionary time. Since activation of CDKs is the central and rate-limiting event in cell cycle transitions, it is not surprising that their activity is carefully regulated at multiple levels. At one level, the CDK enzymes require a cyclin regulatory subunit for activity, and cyclins are expressed only at particular stages of the cell cycle. A given catalytic subunit, therefore, remains inactive until a relevant cyclin is synthesized. While a cyclin regulatory subunit is required for activity, it is not sufficient. A series of phosphorylation and dephosphorylation events on the cyclin/CDK complex are also required for robust activity. Phosphorylation by the CDK-activating kinase (CAK) increases cyclin/CDK activity. CAK is itself a CDK composed of cyclin H and CDK7. Phosphorylation at other sites suppresses CDK activity by blocking access to its adenosine triphosphate (ATP) binding site. Dephosphorylation of these sites, typically by phosphatases of the *CDC25* family, activates cyclin/CDK activity and is probably rate limiting for triggering cell cycle transitions.

Another level of regulation is the presence of a diverse family of protein inhibitors known as CDK inhibitors (CKIs) that can inhibit CDK activity or block their activation. Two general classes of CKIs have been described. One class is broad spectrum as they inhibit multiple CDKs, and this class includes p21CIP1, p27KIP1, and p57KIP2. The other class is specific for cyclin D/CDK4 or cyclin D/CDK6 enzymes and includes p16INK4, p15INK4B, p18INK4C, and p19INK4D. The synthesis, degradation, and activity of these CKIs are regulated by both intrinsic and extrinsic checkpoints. For example, cell cycle regulation by cell–cell contact or transforming growth factor β is mediated by increased levels of p27KIP1 that inhibit CDK activity, thus preventing cell cycle progression.

Once activated, the CDKs that drive the transition into a particular cell cycle phase often need to be deactivated before completion of that phase and transition to the ensuing phase. For example, the CDKs required for initiation of mitosis also prevent exit from mitosis and entry into G1 phase. Thus, an additional level of CDK regulation involves their specific degradation in a precise order. It is now generally understood that ubiquitin-mediated proteolysis is responsible for this regulation. Hence, synthesis, posttranslational modification, and programmed degradation all contribute to the regulation of CDK activity.

This CDK-based regulatory system is utilized by most intrinsic checkpoints to ensure the proper ordering and fidelity of key cell cycle events such as DNA replication and mitosis. The same basic regulatory system is also used by checkpoints that govern responses to cellular stress. For example, DNA damage initiates a response in normal cells that includes cell cycle withdrawal and transcriptional induction of DNA repair genes. Cell cycle withdrawal is presumably induced to allow time for damage repair prior to resumption of DNA replication or mitosis. However, cell cycle withdrawal can be permanent. This unique stress-induced, permanently arrested cell cycle state is called cellular senescence. Senescent cells are distinguishable from G0-arrested cells both morphologically and molecularly. Interestingly, oncogenic stress in the form of inappropriate mitogenic signaling or loss of normal growth restraints can also induce senescence. Thus, cells have a built-in fail-safe mechanism that can be triggered to prevent cell proliferation when errors in normal cell cycle regulation are sensed. The abrogation of such fail-safe mechanisms is a hallmark of cancer.

One key fail-safe pathway is centered on the *TP53* tumor suppressor gene. *TP53* plays an important role in the regulation of cell cycle, senescence, and apoptosis in response to a variety of stresses including oncogenic stress and damaged DNA. *TP53* protein (p53) functions as a sequence-specific, DNA-binding transcription factor. In normal cells, a particular stress will induce an increase in p53 levels by inhibiting its normally rapid degradation. p53 is targeted for ubiquitin-dependent proteolysis by association with the *MDM2* protein. This association is inhibited by the phosphorylation of p53 at specific amino-terminal residues. Phosphorylation of p53 at these residues is triggered by stress-responsive kinases like ATM. ATM signaling blocks p53 degradation, allowing p53 to activate the transcription of its target genes. p53 influences the expression of many genes, but for the purposes of this discussion one key example is the CKI p21CIP1. As discussed above, p21CIP1 is a CKI that can inhibit the activity of multiple CDKs. Thus, stress generates a signal that can activate p53 by posttranslational modification. Increased p53 upregulates CKIs that inhibit CDK activity and halt cell cycle progression (Fig. 1.1).

The majority of cells in the human body are not actively participating in the cell cycle. In the adult, proliferation is confined to small populations of cells that are responsible for tissue homeostasis. The remaining differentiated cells are actively metabolizing, but not proliferating. Thus, cell accumulation is primarily controlled by a binary, on–off cell cycle switch. The on–off switches that control exit from or reentry into the cell cycle are influenced by extrinsic checkpoints that integrate information from both the environment and within the cell to determine whether cell proliferation is appropriate. This information is then relayed to the core CDK-based cell cycle regulatory system that

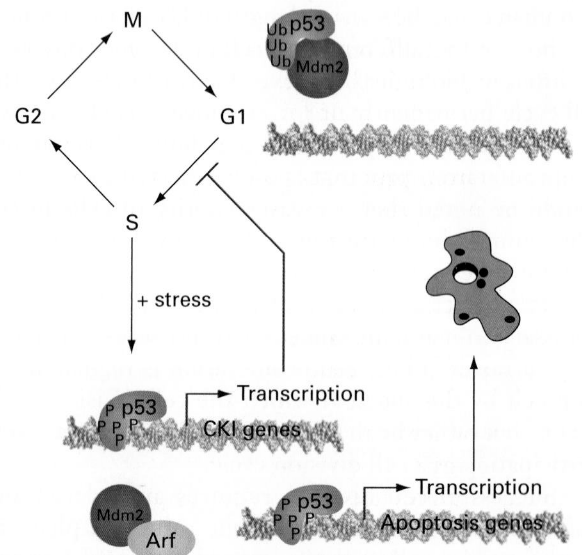

FIGURE 1–1 *TP53* regulates cell proliferation and apoptosis in response to stress. The figure depicts the basic *TP53*-mediated regulatory switch that governs cell fate in response to stress. TP53 encodes a sequence-specific DNA-binding transcription factor (p53) that can activate numerous genes involved in cell proliferation and apoptosis. In normal unstressed cells, p53 is unstable as it is targeted for ubiquitin-dependent proteolytic degradation by the Mdm2 family of proteins. Thus, p53-mediated gene expression is low. In the presence of a variety of different stresses, stress response kinases like ATM phosphorylate TP53 and/or induce p19Arf, both of which have the end result of preventing the p53/Mdm2 interaction. This stabilizes p53, allowing it to activate gene expression that can block cell cycle progression or induce apoptosis.

executes the go or no go decision. The cell cycle is not free running. Extrinsic checkpoints are enforced in each subsequent G1 phase. Since extrinsic checkpoints are continuously enforced, cell accumulation requires persistent mitogenic signaling.

How do extracellular growth factors impinge on the core CDK cell cycle regulatory system? Growth factors function as ligands for specific receptors, and ligand/receptor interaction triggers signaling cascades within the cell. These signaling cascades are typically constructed of sequentially activated protein kinases, often with significant cross-talk and feedback between them. Phosphorylation mediated by these signaling kinase networks can influence each of the major regulatory mechanisms used to control CDK activity. For example, G0 cells are devoid of significant CDK activity because their levels of cyclin expression are low. However, upon mitogenic growth factor signaling, signaling kinases phosphorylate transcription factors to activate expression of D-type cyclins throughout G1 phase. Extracellular signaling can also have the opposite effect of switching cell proliferation off. High-density cell–cell contact or transforming growth factor β, for example, upregulates the levels of CKIs like p27KIP1 to diminish CDK activity and ultimately facilitate exit from the cell cycle.

Once CDKs are activated, how do they actually cause the transition from one cell cycle phase to the next? Surprisingly, the answer to this question is not very well understood. All relevant CDK substrates have probably not been identified, but one important substrate is the product of the retinoblastoma tumor suppressor gene (*RB1*) and the other members of its gene family (*RBL1* and *RBL2*). *RB1* is widely expressed and is known to constrain cells from progressing through the cell cycle by repressing the expression of genes necessary for cell cycle events.[5] *RB1* protein (pRb) binds with the E2F transcription factors. There are at least eight structurally related E2F transcription factors, five of which (*E2F1-5*) interact with the *RB1* gene family proteins. When bound to E2Fs, pRb is able to negatively regulate transcription of E2F target genes by at least two different mechanisms. One is by inhibiting the activity of the E2F transcriptional activation domain. The other is by recruiting chromatin-modifying activities like histone deacetylases to promoters bound by the pRb/E2F complex. These chromatin-modifying activities typically alter chromatin to a more closed state that represses gene transcription. E2Fs regulate many genes important for the cell cycle like cyclins, dihydrofolate reductase, DNA polymerase, and thymidine kinase. Thus, by blocking E2F transcriptional activation and actively silencing the expression of E2F target genes, pRb restrains cell proliferation. Upon phosphorylation of pRb by CDKs, the pRb/E2F interaction is disrupted, thus liberating E2F to activate the expression of cell cycle genes. It is also important to note that like p53, pRb is critical for enforcing cellular senescence in response to a number of stresses including oncogenic signaling. The *RB1* regulatory pathway constitutes one binary, on–off cell cycle switch (Fig. 1.2).[6]

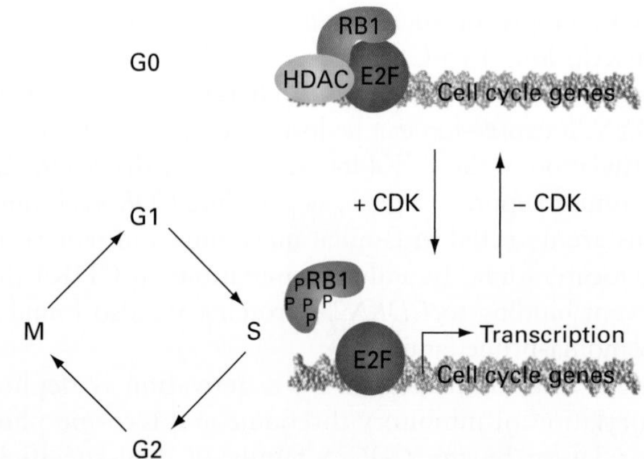

FIGURE 1–2 The *RB1* pathway regulates cell proliferation in response to extrinsic and intrinsic signaling. The figure shows the basic *RB1* protein (pRb)–mediated cell cycle switch that integrates information from both extrinsic and intrinsic signaling pathways to determine whether a cell should commit to a round of cell division. In G0 cells, pRb is in complex with E2F transcription factors, and this interaction blocks the ability of E2Fs to activate transcription by recruiting chromatin-modifying factors like histone deacetylases to the promoter. Upon upregulation of cyclin-dependent kinase (CDK) activity in response to various signaling pathways, pRb is phosphorylated and the pRb/E2F interaction is disrupted. Liberation of E2F causes increased expression of genes required for the cell division cycle. Decreases in CDK activity due to growth-suppressive signaling flip the switch in the other direction, encouraging exit from the cell cycle. As pRb is dephosphorylated during M phase, the switch is reset every cycle.

Cancer-Associated Defects in the Core Cell Cycle Regulatory System

Due to the complexity of CDK regulation, many different types of molecular alterations can cause abnormal CDK activation during tumorigenesis. The overexpression of cyclin D1 has been observed in many human cancers due to gene amplification or translocation of the cyclin D1 gene (*CCND1*). The *CCND1* gene is amplified in a wide variety of human cancers including small cell lung tumors (10%), primary breast cancers (13%), bladder cancer (15%), esophageal carcinoma (34%), and squamous cell carcinoma of the head and neck (43%).[7] Chromosome translocations involving *CCND1* have been observed in parathyroid adenoma and mantle cell lymphomas.[8] As *CCND1* protein is an important growth factor–responsive cyclin, deregulated expression may drive CDK activity in the absence of appropriate growth factors.

CDK activation can also occur by inactivation of CKIs. Genetic mutation of CKI genes is observed frequently in human cancer. Loss of a CKI removes an inhibitor that normally constrains CDK activity, thereby providing a proliferative stimulus. For example, the INK4 locus is contained within chromosomal region 9p21, a region frequently lost in human cancers.[9] The DNA at this locus is also frequently methylated in some tumor types, including bladder cancer and leukemia. Extensive

DNA methylation silences gene expression by inhibiting transcription. Two CKIs are encoded within the INK4 locus, *CDKN2A* and *CDKN2B*. Therefore, *CDKN2A* and *CDKN2B* expression can be lost in tumors due to loss or methylation of the INK4 locus. It is likely that *CDKN2A* is a tumor suppressor gene, as germline *CDKN2A* mutations are detected in familial melanoma and pancreatic adenocarcinoma. In addition, mutations in CDK4 that prevent binding to *CDKN2A* proteins are also found in melanoma-prone families.

An important step in CDK activation is dephosphorylation of inhibitory threonine and tyrosine phosphorylation by the *CDC25* family of dual-specificity phosphatases. In vitro, *CDC25* family members are potential oncogenes, as their overexpression can cooperate with *RB1* loss or *HRAS* activation to induce oncogenic transformation of primary cells. Inappropriately high levels of *CDC25* may provide an oncogenic stimulus by activating CDK activity. Overexpression of *CDC25* genes has been detected in numerous human cancers,[10] and *CDC25A* may be a direct transcriptional target for other oncogenes like *MYC*.

RB1 is the prototypical tumor suppressor gene. Its mutational inactivation causes the hereditary pediatric cancer retinoblastoma. *RB1* mutations have also been observed with varying frequency in nearly every human cancer where it has been examined.[11,12] In some cancers, such as osteosarcoma and small cell lung cancer, the frequency of *RB1* mutation can exceed 90%. In other cancer types, *RB1* mutation is very rare. However, there are multiple ways by which *RB1* can be inactivated. Viral proteins like human papillomavirus E7 protein, which is often associated with cervical cancer, are known to bind pRb and inhibit its function. Upstream regulators within the *RB1* pathway, such as CDKs and CKIs, are also frequently altered in human cancer. Most clinically prevalent human cancers like carcinoma of the breast, prostate, or lung show some defect in this larger *RB1* pathway at frequencies exceeding 70%.

TP53 is the most frequently mutated gene in human cancer.[13] Germline *TP53* mutation causes the cancer-prone Li-Fraumeni syndrome. Loss of *TP53* is expected to abrogate various checkpoints that monitor cell damage and stress, including DNA or chromosome damage. Loss of these checkpoints not only allows incipient cancer cells to proliferate under conditions where they normally would not but also increases genomic instability. Increased genomic instability accelerates the accumulation of genetic mutations that drive cancer progression. Other members of the *TP53* pathway are also altered in human cancer. One example is *MDM2*. Overexpression of *MDM2*, sometimes mediated by gene amplification, is frequently observed in human cancer.[14] Excessive *MDM2* protein causes rapid degradation and inactivation of p53. p53 is also regulated by the p19ARF protein. p19ARF protein binds MDM2 to prevent MDM2 from targeting p53 for degradation. Thus, p19ARF loss destabilizes p53. p19ARF is encoded within the INK4 locus that is frequently lost in human cancer. Loss of this locus, therefore, can compromise both the *RB1* and *TP53* checkpoint pathways.

Cell Growth Control through PI3K/Akt/mTOR Signaling

Much of our current understanding of the cell cycle is focused on regulation of DNA replication and mitosis. However, cells must do considerably more than replicate and segregate their genome in order to proliferate. The biomass of the cell must be approximately doubled to support the generation of two viable daughter cells. For rapidly proliferating cancer cells, the amount of time and energy devoted to generating sufficient biomass far exceeds that devoted to DNA replication and mitosis. Multiple extrinsic and intrinsic cellular signals regulate biomass production (i.e., cell growth), and cell growth status is in turn linked to the core cell cycle regulatory system. Beginning in G1 phase, cells increase in size as they increase their biomass in preparation for DNA replication and cell division. To increase in size, cells promote anabolic processes such as protein, lipid, and carbohydrate synthesis.[15,16] Many cellular signaling pathways converge on the major protein kinase mTOR (mammalian target of rapamycin) to regulate these processes. mTOR is a serine/threonine protein kinase of the phosphatidylinositol 3-kinase (PI3K)/protein kinase B (Akt) pathway that is activated in response to growth, nutrient, and energy signals for protein synthesis.[17-19] Efficient protein synthesis is a key requirement for cell growth. Therefore, the integration of these signals on mTOR demonstrates the significant role mTOR and its associated networks play in regulating cell growth and proliferation.

mTOR exists as two functionally distinct complexes that coexist in cells and are conserved from yeast to humans. The complexes are mTOR complex 1 (mTORC1) and mTOR complex 2 (mTORC2).[20] The two complexes are distinguished by their sensitivity to rapamycin. mTORC1 is very sensitive to inhibition by rapamycin, whereas mTORC2 is insensitive.[21] Much of what has been learned about mTOR function has come from studies utilizing rapamycin. Therefore, mTORC1 is the best characterized of the two complexes and will be the focus of further discussion. For more information regarding mTORC2, see a recent review by Alessi et al.[22]

mTORC1 is comprised of mTOR, Raptor (regulatory associated protein of mTOR), and LST8 (lethal with SEC18 protein), and it has mTORC1 has two well-characterized downstream targets, S6K1/S6K2 (S6 kinases 1 and 2, collectively referred to as S6K) and 4E-BP1/4E-BP2 (eukaryotic translation initiation factor 4E binding proteins 1 and 2, collectively referred to as 4E-BP). mTORC1 activates S6K and inhibits 4E-BP via phosphorylation. Active S6K phosphorylates downstream targets, such as ribosomal S6 protein and

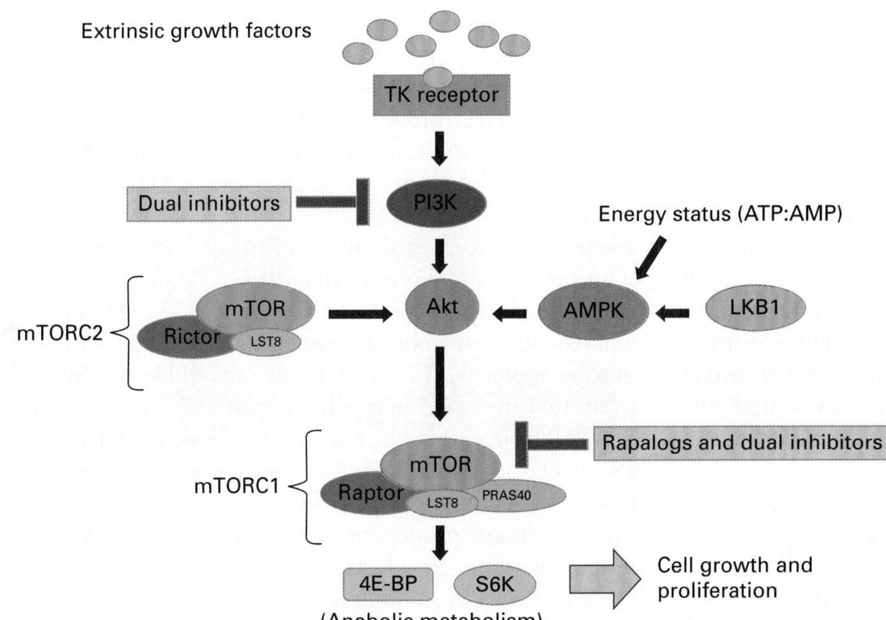

FIGURE 1–3 mTOR signaling regulates anabolic metabolism for cell growth. Extrinsic growth factors bind growth factor receptors and activate the phosphatidylinositol 3-kinase (PI3K)/ protein kinase B (Akt) signaling pathway, while energy status (the AMP/ATP ratio) modulates AMPK activity. These two antagonistic pathways regulate mTORC1 activity, which mediates the phosphorylation of 4E-BP and S6K. mTORC2 is thought to act on Akt upstream of mTORC1. mTORC1 is typically hyperactive in cancer due to upstream mutations. First-generation mTOR inhibitors (Rapalogs) inhibit mTORC1 activity by inducing an allosteric chance in the protein. Second-generation inhibitors (dual inhibitors) target the kinase domain of both PI3K and mTORC1.

eIF4B (eukaryotic translation initiation factor 4B) to trigger mRNA translation, while inhibition of 4E-BP promotes cap-dependent translation due to the release of 4E-BP from eIF4E (eukaryotic translation initiation factor 4E) at the 5′ 7-methyl-GTP cap of mRNAs.[23] The resulting increase in mRNA translation via mTORC1 signaling increases protein synthesis and thus cell growth (Fig. 1.3).

mTORC1 signaling has also been shown to regulate nuclear accumulation of the transcription factor sterol regulatory element-binding protein 1 (SREBP-1), which is important for lipid synthesis. Although the mechanism of SREBP-1 activation is not clear, it is known that SREBP-1 targets lipogenic genes such as acetyl-CoA carboxylase (ACC), fatty acid synthase (FASN), stearoyl-CoA desaturase 1 (SCD-1), and glucokinase (GK). SREBP-1 activity is required for cell growth as demonstrated in a study by Porstmann et al.,[24] which shows that SREBP-1 depletion restricts mammalian cell growth and *Drosophila* size. This suggests that one way the PI3K/Akt/ mTOR pathway regulates cell size is by promoting lipid biosynthesis.

Given the importance of the mTOR pathway in cell growth control, it is not surprising that components of this pathway are disrupted in cancer. Interestingly, mutations in mTOR itself have yet to be reported in cancer. Aberrant mTORC1 signaling in cancer is caused by deregulation of upstream effectors that lead to mTORC1 hyperactivation.[25,26] Activators of mTORC1 include Akt, a serine/threonine kinase involved in glucose metabolism, cell proliferation, and apoptosis, and PI3K, an enzyme that interacts with IRS-1 (insulin receptor substrate) and regulates cell growth, proliferation, and differentiation. Inhibitors of mTORC1 include two tumor suppressor proteins, phosphatase and tensin homolog (*PTEN*) and liver kinase B1 (*LKB1*). *PTEN* inhibits Akt activity, whereas LKB1 is a serine/threonine kinase that has growth-suppressing effects via the activation of multiple downstream kinases that then act on mTORC1. PI3K and Akt are often mutated, amplified, or overexpressed in cancer,[25] whereas *PTEN* and *LKB1* are lost in many tumors types.[27,28]

Targeting mTOR signaling is an active area of therapeutic development. Rapamycin is the first mTOR inhibitor to have been described and it functions by inducing an allosteric change in mTOR that inhibits its activity.[29] Rapamycin does not inhibit mTORC2; however, the downregulation of mTORC1's kinase activity is enough to inhibit cell growth and proliferation.[17,20,26] Multiple first-generation rapamycin-derivative mTOR inhibitors have been developed. These are termed "rapalogs." Two rapalogs in particular have shown successful antitumor effects in the clinic. Everolimus and temsirolimus are approved for the treatment of renal cell carcinoma, and temsirolimus is also approved for the treatment of mantle cell lymphoma.[17]

Unfortunately, tumors can develop resistance to these first-generation mTOR inhibitors. First-generation rapalogs induce an intrinsic negative feedback loop that activates Akt upstream of mTOR and eventually overrides mTORC1 inhibition. To address this issue, second-generation inhibitors that directly target the kinase domain of mTOR have been developed.[30-32] These competitive modulators also inhibit P13K since PI3K and mTOR have high sequence homology within their respective catalytic clefts.[33] Unlike rapalogs, second-generation dual inhibitors inhibit 4E-BP1 phosphorylation and cap-dependent translation. Inhibition of 4E-BP1 phosphorylation causes eIF4E hyperactivation, which induces apoptosis.[34]

Second-generation PI3K/mTOR dual inhibitors potently block the proliferation of many different cancer cell lines via cell cycle arrest and/or apoptosis[35,36] and increase the efficacy of other genotoxic therapies when used in combination.[37,38] Such combination therapy thus blocks cell proliferation at two fundamental levels, cell division and cell growth. Multiple second-generation PI3K/mTOR inhibitors are in early stage clinical trials. AZD8055, AZD2014, OSI-027, and INK-128 have broad antitumor cytostatic activity and have demonstrated efficacy against a range of solid tumors and hematological malignancies.[39-41]

Cellular Energetics Regulate Proliferation

To grow and proliferate, cells must rapidly generate energy, or ATP. ATP is used by dividing cells to fuel the synthesis of proteins, nucleic acids, and fatty acids. ATP production also regulates cellular redox status to prevent reactive oxygen species from accumulating in cells, potentially damaging cellular membranes and proteins and causing cell death. Normal cells use glucose for the generation of ATP and macromolecule synthesis as glucose provides the carbon, oxygen, and hydrogen for anabolic processes.[42]

To generate ATP from glucose under normal aerobic conditions, cells use glycolysis and oxidative phosphorylation. Glycolysis is a series of reactions that metabolize glucose to pyruvate in the cell cytoplasm and yield a net of 2 ATP per glucose molecule and produce the cofactor nicotinamide adenine dinucleotide (NADH). Pyruvate produced during glycolysis moves into the mitochondrial matrix where it enters the tricarboxylic acid (TCA) cycle. The TCA cycle uses pyruvate to drive a series of reactions that donate electrons via NADH and FADH2 to a linked set of protein complexes in the inner mitochondrial membrane called the electron transport chain. Electrons flow from NADH and FADH2 to oxygen to establish a proton gradient across the inner mitochondrial membrane. This proton gradient is used to drive ATP production via oxidative phosphorylation. Utilization of the TCA cycle and oxidative phosphorylation yields a net of 36 ATP per glucose molecule (Fig. 1.4). Under anaerobic conditions, pyruvate is not used in the TCA cycle and is instead converted into lactic acid by lactate dehydrogenase in a process termed anaerobic glycolysis. Since pyruvate is not used in the TCA cycle and no oxidative phosphorylation follows, a cell only produces a net yield of 2 ATP per glucose under anaerobic glycolysis.

Most cells in an adult organism are not actively proliferating. In this case, cells produce ATP mainly via glycolysis and oxidative phosphorylation. However, cellular metabolism is significantly altered in cancer, and this altered metabolism helps maintain the high rate of proliferation in cancer cells. Additionally, this altered metabolic state helps cancer cells evade checkpoints that normally block proliferation under the stressful metabolic conditions typically encountered during tumorigenesis. The altered metabolic phenotype observed in cancer cells is called the Warburg effect[43] and is characterized by a shift in ATP production from oxidative phosphorylation to glycolysis even under aerobic conditions (termed aerobic glycolysis). Instead of metabolizing glucose through the mitochondria by oxidative phosphorylation, which produces 36 ATP, cancer cells convert most incoming glucose

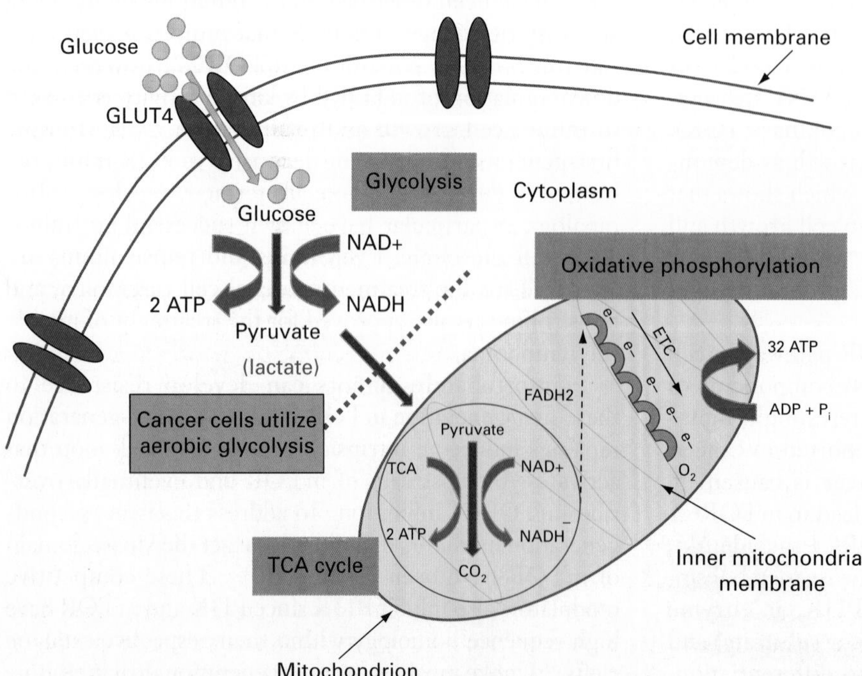

FIGURE 1–4 Cell metabolism differs in normal and cancer cells. In normal cells, glycolysis metabolizes glucose to pyruvate in the cytoplasm to yield a net of 2 ATP per glucose molecule. Pyruvate produced during glycolysis enters the tricarboxylic acid (TCA), which drives a series of reactions and establishes a proton gradient in the inner mitochondrial membrane. The electron transport chain (ETC) utilizes the proton gradient to produce 36 ATP via oxidative phosphorylation. Cancer cells metabolize glycolysis to lactate to produce ATP, even in an oxygenated environment. This aerobic glycolysis promotes cancer cell growth by providing energy and cofactors that support anabolic pathways.

into lactate using aerobic glycolysis. Since aerobic glycolysis produces a net yield of only 2 ATP per glucose molecule, cancer cells must increase their uptake of glucose to meet their energetic needs. Supporting this, most tumor cells overexpress the glucose receptor, GLUT4.[44] Aerobic glycolysis occurs in many solid human tumors and is easily noted in the clinic. High glucose uptake in tumors can be visualized using positron emission tomography scanning of the tumors with radiolabeled 2-deoxyglucose.

The shift to less efficient aerobic glycolysis in cancer cells seems paradoxical, but the metabolic changes associated with aerobic glycolysis extend beyond ATP production. The NADH produced in aerobic glycolysis reduces NADP+ to produce nicotinamide adenine dinucleotide phosphate, a cofactor required in many enzymatic reactions involved in the synthesis of proteins, membranes, and nucleic acids. Cancer cells appear to sacrifice efficient energy production in favor of increased production of cofactors required for biomass synthesis. Supporting this is the fact that the activation of pathways regulating cell metabolism often accompanies the activation of pathways that regulate cell growth. The integration of growth and proliferation signals with the regulation of cell metabolism is crucial for cell survival. In multicellular organisms, cells survive because they sense their environment and signal for appropriate levels of growth and proliferation depending on nutrient conditions. If nutrients and ATP are plentiful, the presence of growth factors activates various extracellular and intracellular signals to promote cell growth and proliferation.

PI3K signaling through Akt and mTOR is one major signaling pathway activated under nutrient-rich conditions. If ATP becomes depleted, cellular signaling will inhibit the PI3K pathway and stimulate the uptake of nutrients to decrease ATP expenditure, while promoting ATP production. A delicate process of checks and balances exists. One of the main signaling nodes regulating this balance, coupling energetic pathways to cellular growth and proliferation pathways, is AMPK (5′ AMP-activated protein kinase). AMPK is an enzyme that plays a key role in maintaining energy homeostasis in cells by sensing the ratio of AMP:ATP. It's signaling converges antagonistically with the PI3K pathway as AMPK inhibits mTOR activity. When a high cellular AMP:ATP ratio exists (signifying a decrease in energy), AMPK is activated by a conformational change that exposes its active site. The upstream serine/threonine signaling kinase, LKB1, phosphorylates AMPK at Thr-172, causing activation. Once activated, AMPK increases cellular energy levels by stimulating catabolic, energy-producing pathways (i.e., fatty acid oxidation, the uptake of glucose, and mitochondrial biogenesis) and inhibiting anabolic, energy-consuming pathways (i.e., the synthesis of fatty acids, glycogen, and proteins).[45,46] When the AMP:ATP ratio becomes low again, the conformation change in AMPK is reversed. Decreased AMPK activity allows mTOR signaling to resume and anabolic pathways to predominate for cell growth.

Multiple diseases are associated with deregulated cellular metabolism and AMPK function.[47] In cancer, it is very clear that coordination of deregulated cell metabolism, growth, and proliferation is crucial for tumorigenesis. Alterations in the PI3K/mTOR and LKB1/AMPK signaling pathways ensure anabolic processes are favored to support cell proliferation, while alterations in cell metabolism (the Warburg effect) ensure cancer cells can produce enough ATP and essential cofactors in their often oxygen-deprived tumor microenvironment. The altered metabolism of cancer cells has received significant attention for antitumor therapy. Various glycolytic and glucose uptake inhibitors are used in the treatment of cancer.[48]

APOPTOSIS

Apoptosis is an organized, genetically programmed form of cell death that is essential for normal development and tissue homeostasis.[49] It has been estimated that 50 to 70 billion cells perish via apoptosis each day in the average adult. The scale of cell turnover can be appreciated by the calculation that each individual will produce and eradicate a mass of cells equal to their entire body weight over the course of a year. Thus, the regulation of both apoptosis and cell proliferation is essential for normal physiology. Like defects in cell cycle control, abnormal regulation of apoptosis can lead to extended cell survival, cell accumulation, and neoplastic transformation. As cancer cells treated with chemotherapy, radiation, or immunotherapy often die by apoptotic cell death, defects in apoptotic pathways can also confer resistance to therapy.

Apoptotic cell death is discernible at the physiological, cellular, and molecular levels from necrotic forms of cell death that occur in response to acute cell injury. During necrotic cell death, cells and organelles expand and rupture, spilling their contents into the surrounding microenvironment and triggering inflammatory and immune responses that can be detrimental to the host. Further, the body does not efficiently remove necrotic cells, potentially leading to a variety of obstructive conditions and widespread tissue damage. Apoptosis, on the other hand, is characterized by rapid shrinkage of the cell, maintenance of organelle integrity, chromatin condensation, and DNA fragmentation. The condensing cell is ultimately segregated into vesicles termed apoptotic bodies that are removed by phagocytosis. This process minimizes exposure of the microenvironment to the contents of the dying cell. Thus, apoptotic cell death typically does not trigger inflammatory or immune responses and has minimal effects on overall tissue structure and function.

In a general sense, the regulation of apoptosis is analogous to the regulation of the cell cycle. In both cases, disparate signaling pathways engage a core regulatory apparatus that ultimately commits a cell to its particular fate. In both cases, commitment coincides with activation of a family of related enzymes. Cell cycle regulation is mediated by CDK activation, while apoptosis is triggered by caspase activation. A final analogy is that both CDKs and caspases can be activated by either intrinsic or extrinsic signaling. Many environmental, pharmacologic, or physiologic stimuli can trigger apoptosis. A thorough discussion of these is beyond the scope of this chapter. Rather, we will focus on the core apoptotic regulatory system based on caspase activation.

The Core Apoptotic Regulatory System

The core regulatory machinery that commits cells to death and executes the molecular and cellular changes of apoptosis is composed of the caspase family of proteases. The HUGO gene nomenclature committee currently recognizes 12 caspase genes in humans, only some of which are involved in the regulation of apoptosis. Apoptotic caspases are conserved throughout evolution and exist in a wide variety of multicellular organisms, including nematodes, insects, and mammals. Even unicellular yeasts have caspase-like activity that plays a role in an apoptosis-like form of cell death. Caspases are cysteine-dependent proteases that have the unique property of cleaving substrates after aspartic acid residues.[50] They are expressed as inactive zymogens that require proteolytic processing for activation. Active caspases possess the ability to process their own zymogen form. This can lead to a self-perpetuating chain reaction of increasing caspase activity.

Caspases can be grouped into three subfamilies based on their protease site specificities. The group I or ICE subfamily of caspases (CASP1,4-5) prefers the tetrapeptide sequence WEHD and is believed to function mainly in inflammation. Group II caspases (CASP2-3,7) have specificity for the DEXD amino acid motif. Group III caspases (CASP6,8,9-10) prefer the (I/L/V)EXD motif. Group II and group III caspases are the primary caspases activated during apoptosis. Apoptotic caspases can be divided further into two subcategories, initiator or execution caspases. Initiator caspases (CASP2,8-10) directly receive the intrinsic or extrinsic death signals. Initiator caspases, in turn, activate downstream effector caspases by proteolytic processing of their zymogen form. Once activated, effector caspases (CASP3,6-7) mediate the cleavage of other protein substrates to facilitate the cellular and molecular demolition of the cell.

The activation of initiator caspases can occur through extrinsic, receptor-mediated signaling. Ligand binding to death receptors of the tumor necrosis factor (TNF) superfamily, including TNF, FAS, and TRAIL, causes receptor clustering. Clustered receptors recruit various proteins to their intercellular cytoplasmic domains through characteristic protein–protein interaction motifs like the death domain. Recruitment of these proteins leads to the formation of the death-inducing signaling complex that is responsible for activation of initiator CASP8. CASP8, in turn, activates effector caspases, committing the cell to apoptotic cell death.

Activation of initiator caspases can also occur through an intrinsic, mitochondrial-mediated process. Rather than ligand–receptor interaction, the key event in this pathway is permeabilization of the mitochondrial outer membrane (MOMP). This has two effects. One, mitochondrial transmembrane potential is lost, which arrests the bioenergetic function of the organelle. Second, various pro-apoptotic proteins like cytochrome c and Smac/DIABLO are released from the mitochondrial intermembrane space into the cytosol. These proteins cause caspase activation by two different mechanisms. Cytochrome c induces oligomerization of APAF1 and formation of the apoptosome complex containing APAF1, cytochrome c, and initiator CASP9. CASP9 is active within the apoptosome, leading to subsequent activation of effector caspases. Smac/DIABLO, on the other hand, facilitates caspase activation by binding to and blocking the activity of naturally occurring caspase inhibitors called IAPs (inhibitor of apoptosis proteins). Eight mammalian IAPs that function in the regulation of apoptosis are currently known. IAPs bind directly to caspases through their characteristic BIR (baculoviral IAP repeat) domain. IAP/caspase interactions can have a number of consequences. For example, the IAP XIAP can block the catalytic activity of activated effector caspases, can prevent the activation of effector caspases by inhibiting the apoptosome, or can target caspases for proteasome-dependent degradation. While the receptor and mitochondrial pathways of caspase activation are separate, there is considerable cross-talk between the two. For example, receptor-mediated caspase activation can also trigger the mitochondrial pathway, further amplifying the resulting caspase activation cascade.

How does intrinsic apoptotic signaling cause MOMP? The *BCL2* family proteins are important regulators of this process.[51,52] The members of this protein family contain various combinations of four important structural motifs common to the family, the *BCL2* homology domains BH1, BH2, BH3, and BH4. These motifs specify protein interactions between members of the *BCL2* family and with other cellular proteins. Two members of this family, BAX and BAK, are redundant pro-apoptotic effectors of MOMP and contain BH1-3 domains. These proteins can cause MOMP through creation of large holes in the outer mitochondrial membrane similar to lipidic pores.[53,54] MOMP is antagonized by anti-apoptotic members of the *BCL2* protein family such as BCL-2, BCL-xL, and MCL-1 that uniquely contain BH4 motifs in addition to BH1-3 motifs. These anti-apoptotic proteins dock with the mitochondrial outer membrane and interact with a number of mitochondrial proteins, including BAX and BAK, to prevent MOMP. The final group of *BCL2* family proteins like BIM, BAD, PUMA, and NOXA contain only BH3 domains. These proteins can heterodimerize with the anti-apoptotic *BCL2* family proteins and neutralize their activity. *BCL2* proteins are subject to various posttranslational modifications that affect their stability and their interactions with other proteins.[55] Thus, intrinsic signaling pathways influence the relative concentrations of pro-apoptotic and anti-apoptotic *BCL2* family proteins and their posttranslational modifications to regulate apoptotic cell death.

Caspase Substrates

Caspases target hundreds of different protein substrates within cells for limited and controlled proteolysis.[56,57] This proteolysis serves a number of related functions. One, it provides a regulatory function, particularly during apoptotic signaling itself. As discussed above, one of the primary substrates of active caspases is the inactive zymogen forms of the caspases themselves. Two, caspase proteolysis effects the structural changes necessary to dismantle the cell. These structural changes are often associated with the morphological alterations characteristic of apoptotic cells including membrane blebbing, organelle fragmentation, and chromatin condensation. Three, caspase proteolysis serves to stop housekeeping functions in the cell such as RNA transcription and protein translation. Four, caspase proteolysis alters the immunogenicity of cellular components to minimize immune and inflammatory responses. Finally, caspase proteolysis marks apoptotic cells for removal and facilitates phagocytosis.

The structural changes occurring within apoptotic cells are profound. For example, numerous components of the cytoskeleton are targeted by caspases, including the actin microfilament network, microtubular proteins, and intermediate filament proteins. Several components of focal adhesion sites, cell–cell adherens junctions, cadherin junctions, and desmosomes are caspase substrates. Proteolytic cleavage of such substrates likely contributes to the retraction, rounding, and membrane blebbing characteristic of apoptotic cells. Another characteristic of apoptotic cells is the fragmentation of organelles like the Golgi apparatus. Caspase proteolysis contributes to these processes as well. For example, caspase cleavage of the Golgi stacking protein GRASP65 is necessary for rapid Golgi breakdown.[58] Key proteins involved in transcription and translation are also targeted by caspases, presumably to shut down these cellular processes during cell death. These proteins include a large number of transcription factors (e.g., SP1, NFkBp65, NFATc1), translation factors (e.g., eIF3, eIF4E), and ribosomal proteins (e.g., RPP0, p70S6K).

One of the most obvious and distinctive features of apoptotic cell death is the condensation and eventual fragmentation of the nucleus and the DNA. Nuclear condensation and fragmentation is associated with the disintegration of the nuclear lamina, a process facilitated by caspase proteolysis of the nuclear lamins.[59] Nuclear fragmentation is also caused by reorganization of the actin cytoskeleton. ROCK1 kinase activity can reorganize the actin–myosin network, and caspase cleavage constitutively activates ROCK1. The nuclear envelope is attached to the actin cytoskeleton, so as the cytoskeleton is reorganized by activated ROCK1 the nuclear envelope is pulled apart and fragmented.[60] Fragmentation of genomic DNA into a regularly sized ladder of fragments is one of the defining molecular features of apoptotic cell death.[61] This fragmentation is mediated by caspase-activated DNase (CAD). In normal cells, CAD is found in an inactive complex with ICAD (inhibitor of CAD). Caspases target ICAD for proteolysis, freeing CAD to fragment the DNA.[62,63]

An important physiological feature of apoptotic cell death is that dying cells are efficiently removed by phagocytosis. Caspase-mediated proteolysis facilitates this process as well. For example, apoptotic cells can secrete or release molecules that attract phagocytes. One example is the release of the chemoattractant lipid lysophosphatidylcholine in a CASP3-dependent manner.[64] Lysophosphatidylcholine is generated by iPLA2 (Ca^{2+}-independent phospholipase A2)-mediated hydrolysis of membrane phosphatidylcholine. iPLA2 is activated by CASP3-mediated cleavage. Apoptotic cells are also marked for phagocytosis. One such mark is the membrane phospholipid phosphatidylserine. Phosphatidylserine is normally restricted to the inner leaflet of the plasma membrane. In apoptotic cells, this phospholipid is translocated to the outer membrane leaflet where it can be recognized by phagocytes.[65] Translocation of phosphatidylserine is a caspase-dependent process.[66] The oxidized low-density lipoproteins, calreticulin, ICAM3, annexin-1, and integrins are other molecules that have been implicated in targeting apoptotic cells for phagocytosis. All of these are exposed on apoptotic bodies or apoptotic cells, but only some of them are exposed in a caspase-dependent manner.

Defects in the Core Apoptotic Regulatory System Observed in Cancer

The prevention of programmed cell death is a hallmark of cancer as demonstrated by the accumulation of molecular alterations that compromise the normal regulation of apoptosis in cancer. These alterations typically decrease the sensitivity of incipient cancer cells to specific apoptotic pathways that would normally be engaged in the context of tumor initiation and progression. Paradoxically, cancer cells may actually be more sensitive to other apoptotic pathways than normal cells, a fact that current chemotherapy often relies on for a favorable therapeutic index. For overall tumor expansion, it is only necessary that cell death occurs at a lower frequency than cell division. The molecular alterations in the apoptotic regulatory system that occur in cancer can be grouped into three categories, upregulation of core anti-apoptotic genes, downregulation of core pro-apoptotic genes, and derangement of the upstream signaling pathways that engage the core apoptotic regulatory system.

The upregulation of anti-apoptotic genes not only facilitates the survival and expansion of incipient cancer cells but may also compromise the effectiveness of cancer therapy. Upregulation of *BCL2* family members is a common occurrence in human cancer,[67] and *BCL2* itself was one of the first human oncogenes to be discovered.[68] IAP genes are also mutated, amplified, or upregulated in human cancer.[69] The oncogenic potential of excessive *BCL2* or IAP family genes has been extensively documented in both in vitro and animal experimental systems. Due to their prominent role in oncogenesis, developing inhibitors of *BC-2* or IAP family proteins is an active area of therapeutic development.

As the balance of pro-apoptotic and anti-apoptotic regulators is critical for establishing the sensitivity of cells to programmed cell death, downregulation of pro-apoptotic regulatory genes is also frequently observed in human cancer. The pro-apoptotic BCL-2 family genes have been observed to suffer loss-of-function mutations or downregulation in some types of cancer. These changes are typically associated with poor prognosis because they potentially limit the effectiveness of cytotoxic therapy.[70,71] Receptor-mediated apoptotic pathways are also targeted for alterations in cancer. Death receptors like CD95 or TRAIL can be downregulated or mutated so they no longer bind their ligands efficiently, or they no longer effectively transmit the signal generated by ligand binding.[72]

A classic example of the disruption of upstream apoptotic signaling pathways during tumorigenesis is the *TP53* gene. *TP53* is the most frequently mutated gene in human cancer, and it primarily functions as a central stress response effector. *TP53* induces cell cycle arrest or apoptosis in response to a wide variety of stresses that occur during tumorigenesis including DNA damage, oncogenic signaling, hypoxia, and biosynthetic stress. At the molecular level, *TP53* protein functions as a transcription factor to elicit these cellular changes. Some pro-apoptotic regulatory genes whose expression is increased by *TP53* include *BAX*, *CD95*, *NOXA*, and *PUMA*.[73] Therefore, the loss of *TP53* function in incipient cancer cells increases their survival and proliferation during the stressful process of tumorigenesis.

CONCLUSION

The inappropriate accumulation and spread of cancer cells is the defining and life-threatening feature of this disease. It is the ability of cancer cells to evolve and adapt to adverse environmental conditions, including those intentionally imposed by therapy, that makes cancer so difficult to treat effectively. The regulation of cell proliferation and apoptosis is central to the acquisition of these core hallmarks of the cancer cell. Cells are endowed with a proliferative capacity that far exceeds that necessary for normal development and homeostasis. Over eons of evolutionary time, we have evolved elaborate means to harness and restrain this proliferative capacity so that cell proliferation and cell death occur only at select times and places. It is the breakdown of these ordered regulatory systems that allows the inherent proliferative capacity of cells to reveal themselves in the form of cancer.

By the time a typical patient is diagnosed with cancer, multiple regulatory pathways have already been compromised. As we have summarized in this chapter, the core regulatory systems that control the cell cycle, cell growth, cellular energetics, and apoptosis all change and co-evolve during cancer progression. It is very difficult to envision the therapeutic reconstruction of all these regulatory pathways that would be necessary to restore normalcy on the cancer cell. The genie is out of the bottle. However, the evolutionary process that allows incipient cancer cells to acquire its lethal malignant properties also potentially saddles them with unique vulnerabilities. By targeting these unique vulnerabilities, we can reverse cancer cell accumulation while sparing normal cells. Subsequent chapters in this book detail the discovery of such vulnerabilities and the efforts to develop these discoveries into useful tools for the diagnosis and treatment of cancer.

REFERENCES

1. Olszewski MM. Concepts of cancer from antiquity to the nineteenth century. *Univ Tor Med J.* 2010;87:181-186.
2. Hanahan D, Weinberg RA. Hallmarks of cancer: the next generation. *Cell.* 2011;144:646-674.
3. Weinstein IB. The origins of human cancer: molecular mechanisms of carcinogenesis and their implications for cancer prevention and treatment—twenty-seventh G.H.A. Clowes memorial award lecture. *Cancer Res.* 1988;48:4135-4143.
4. Fearon ER, Vogelstein B. A genetic model for colorectal tumorigenesis. *Cell.* 1990;61:759-767.
5. Chinnam M, Goodrich DW. RB1, development, and cancer. *Curr Top Dev Biol.* 2011;94:129-169.
6. Yao G, Lee TJ, Mori S, et al. A bistable Rb-E2F switch underlies the restriction point. *Nat Cell Biol.* 2008;10:476-482.
7. Sherr CJ. The Pezcoller lecture: cancer cell cycles revisited. *Cancer Res.* 2000;60:3689-3695.
8. Motokura T, Bloom T, Kim HG, et al. A novel cyclin encoded by a bcl1-linked candidate oncogene. *Nature.* 1991;350:512-515.
9. Kamb A. Cyclin-dependent kinase inhibitors and human cancer. *Curr Top Microbiol Immunol.* 1998;227:139-148.
10. Boutros R, Lobjois V, Ducommun B. CDC25 phosphatases in cancer cells: key players? Good targets? *Nat Rev Cancer.* 2007;7:495-507.
11. Burkhart DL, Sage J. Cellular mechanisms of tumour suppression by the retinoblastoma gene. *Nat Rev Cancer.* 2008;8:671-682.
12. Malumbres M, Barbacid M. To cycle or not to cycle: a critical decision in cancer. *Nat Rev Cancer.* 2001;1:222-231.
13. Prives C, Hall PA. The p53 pathway. *J Pathol.* 1999;187:112-126.
14. Rayburn E, Zhang R, He J, Wang H. MDM2 and human malignancies: expression, clinical pathology, prognostic markers, and implications for chemotherapy. *Curr Cancer Drug Targets.* 2005;5:27-41.
15. Lempiainen H, Shore D. Growth control and ribosome biogenesis. *Curr Opin Cell Biol.* 2009;21:855-863.
16. Tapon N, Moberg KH, Hariharan IK. The coupling of cell growth to the cell cycle. *Curr Opin Cell Biol.* 2001;13:731-737.
17. Dancey J. mTOR signaling and drug development in cancer. *Nat Rev Clin Oncol.* 2010;7:209-219.
18. Steelman LS, Chappell WH, Abrams SL, et al. Roles of the Raf/MEK/ERK and PI3K/PTEN/Akt/mTOR pathways in controlling growth and sensitivity to therapy-implications for cancer and aging. *Aging (Albany, NY).* 2011;3:192-222.
19. Tomasoni R, Mondino A. The tuberous sclerosis complex: balancing proliferation and survival. *Biochem Soc Trans.* 2011;39:466-471.
20. Garcia-Echeverria C. Blocking the mTOR pathway: a drug discovery perspective. *Biochem Soc Trans.* 2011;39:451-455.

21. Huang J, Manning BD. The TSC1-TSC2 complex: a molecular switchboard controlling cell growth. *Biochem J*. 2008;412:179-190.
22. Alessi DR, Pearce LR, Garcia-Martinez JM. New insights into mTOR signaling: mTORC2 and beyond. *Sci Signal*. 2009;2:pe27.
23. Bracho-Valdes I, Moreno-Alvarez P, Valencia-Martinez I, Robles-Molina E, Chavez-Vargas L, Vazquez-Prado J. mTORC1- and mTORC2-interacting proteins keep their multifunctional partners focused. *IUBMB Life*. 2011;63:880-898.
24. Porstmann T, Santos CR, Griffiths B, et al. SREBP activity is regulated by mTORC1 and contributes to Akt-dependent cell growth. *Cell Metab*. 2008;8:224-236.
25. Fresno Vara JA, Casado E, de Castro J, Cejas P, Belda-Iniesta C, Gonzalez-Baron M. PI3K/Akt signalling pathway and cancer. *Cancer Treat Rev*. 2004;30:193-204.
26. Hennessy BT, Smith DL, Ram PT, Lu Y, Mills GB. Exploiting the PI3K/AKT pathway for cancer drug discovery. *Nat Rev Drug Discov*. 2005;4:988-1004.
27. Mehenni H, Lin-Marq N, Buchet-Poyau K, et al. LKB1 interacts with and phosphorylates PTEN: a functional link between two proteins involved in cancer predisposing syndromes. *Hum Mol Genet*. 2005;14:2209-2219.
28. Shorning BY, Clarke AR. LKB1 loss of function studied in vivo. *FEBS Lett*. 2011;585:958-966.
29. Choi J, Chen J, Schreiber SL, Clardy J. Structure of the FKBP12-rapamycin complex interacting with the binding domain of human FRAP. *Science*. 1996;273:239-242.
30. Garcia-Echeverria C. Allosteric and ATP-competitive kinase inhibitors of mTOR for cancer treatment. *Bioorg Med Chem Lett*. 2010;20:4308-4312.
31. Vilar E, Perez-Garcia J, Tabernero J. Pushing the envelope in the mTOR pathway: the second generation of inhibitors. *Mol Cancer Ther*. 2011;10:395-403.
32. Zhang YJ, Duan Y, Zheng XF. Targeting the mTOR kinase domain: the second generation of mTOR inhibitors. *Drug Discov Today*. 2011;16:325-331.
33. Park S, Chapuis N, Tamburini J, et al. Role of the PI3K/AKT and mTOR signaling pathways in acute myeloid leukemia. *Haematologica*. 2010;95:819-828.
34. Hsieh AC, Costa M, Zollo O, et al. Genetic dissection of the oncogenic mTOR pathway reveals druggable addiction to translational control via 4EBP-eIF4E. *Cancer Cell*. 2010;17:249-261.
35. Chresta CM, Davies BR, Hickson I, et al. AZD8055 is a potent, selective, and orally bioavailable ATP-competitive mammalian target of rapamycin kinase inhibitor with in vitro and in vivo antitumor activity. *Cancer Res*. 2010;70:288-298.
36. Sini P, James D, Chresta C, Guichard S. Simultaneous inhibition of mTORC1 and mTORC2 by mTOR kinase inhibitor AZD8055 induces autophagy and cell death in cancer cells. *Autophagy*. 2010;6:553-554.
37. Maira SM, Furet P, Stauffer F. Discovery of novel anticancer therapeutics targeting the PI3K/Akt/mTOR pathway. *Future Med Chem*. 2009;1:137-155.
38. Fasolo A, Sessa C. Current and future directions in mammalian target of rapamycin inhibitors development. *Expert Opin Investig Drugs*. 2011;20:381-394.
39. Falcon BL, Barr S, Gokhale PC, et al. Reduced VEGF production, angiogenesis, and vascular regrowth contribute to the antitumor properties of dual mTORC1/mTORC2 inhibitors. *Cancer Res*. 2011;71:1573-1583.
40. Garcia-Martinez JM, Wullschleger S, Preston G, et al. Effect of PI3K- and mTOR-specific inhibitors on spontaneous B-cell follicular lymphomas in PTEN/LKB1-deficient mice. *Br J Cancer*. 2011;104:1116-1125.
41. Marshall G, Howard Z, Dry J, et al. Benefits of mTOR kinase targeting in oncology: pre-clinical evidence with AZD8055. *Biochem Soc Trans*. 2011;39:456-459.
42. Levine AJ, Puzio-Kuter AM. The control of the metabolic switch in cancers by oncogenes and tumor suppressor genes. *Science*. 2010;330:1340-1344.
43. Warburg O. On the origin of cancer cells. *Science*. 1956;123:309-314.
44. Medina RA, Owen GI. Glucose transporters: expression, regulation and cancer. *Biol Res*. 2002;35:9-26.
45. Viollet B, Andreelli F. AMP-activated protein kinase and metabolic control. *Handb Exp Pharmacol*. 2011;203:303-330.
46. Xiao B, Sanders MJ, Underwood E, et al. Structure of mammalian AMPK and its regulation by ADP. *Nature*. 2011;472:230-233.
47. Steinberg GR, Kemp BE. AMPK in health and disease. *Physiol Rev*. 2009;89:1025-1078.
48. Pelicano H, Martin DS, Xu RH, Huang P. Glycolysis inhibition for anticancer treatment. *Oncogene*. 2006;25:4633-4646.
49. Kerr JF, Wyllie AH, Currie AR. Apoptosis: a basic biological phenomenon with wide-ranging implications in tissue kinetics. *Br J Cancer*. 1972;26:239-257.
50. Stennicke HR, Salvesen GS. Properties of the caspases. *Biochim Biophys Acta*. 1998;1387:17-31.
51. Llambi F, Green DR. Apoptosis and oncogenesis: give and take in the BCL-2 family. *Curr Opin Genet Dev*. 2011;21:12-20.
52. Indran IR, Tufo G, Pervaiz S, Brenner C. Recent advances in apoptosis, mitochondria and drug resistance in cancer cells. *Biochim Biophys Acta*. 2011;1807:735-745.
53. Terrones O, Antonsson B, Yamaguchi H, et al. Lipidic pore formation by the concerted action of proapoptotic BAX and tBID. *J Biol Chem*. 2004;279:30081-30091.
54. Schafer B, Quispe J, Choudhary V, et al. Mitochondrial outer membrane proteins assist Bid in Bax-mediated lipidic pore formation. *Mol Biol Cell*. 2009;20:2276-2285.
55. Kutuk O, Letai A. Regulation of Bcl-2 family proteins by post-translational modifications. *Curr Mol Med*. 2008;8:102-118.
56. Luthi AU, Martin SJ. The CASBAH: a searchable database of caspase substrates. *Cell Death Differ*. 2007;14:641-650.
57. Taylor RC, Cullen SP, Martin SJ. Apoptosis: controlled demolition at the cellular level. *Nat Rev Mol Cell Biol*. 2008;9:231-241.
58. Lane JD, Lucocq J, Pryde J, et al. Caspase-mediated cleavage of the stacking protein GRASP65 is required for Golgi fragmentation during apoptosis. *J Cell Biol*. 2002;156:495-509.
59. Rao L, Perez D, White E. Lamin proteolysis facilitates nuclear events during apoptosis. *J Cell Biol*. 1996;135:1441-1455.
60. Croft DR, Coleman ML, Li S, et al. Actin-myosin-based contraction is responsible for apoptotic nuclear disintegration. *J Cell Biol*. 2005;168:245-255.
61. Wyllie AH. Glucocorticoid-induced thymocyte apoptosis is associated with endogenous endonuclease activation. *Nature*. 1980;284:555-556.
62. Enari M, Sakahira H, Yokoyama H, Okawa K, Iwamatsu A, Nagata S. A caspase-activated DNase that degrades DNA during apoptosis, and its inhibitor ICAD. *Nature*. 1998;391:43-50.
63. Sakahira H, Enari M, Nagata S. Cleavage of CAD inhibitor in CAD activation and DNA degradation during apoptosis. *Nature*. 1998;391:96-99.
64. Lauber K, Bohn E, Krober SM, et al. Apoptotic cells induce migration of phagocytes via caspase-3-mediated release of a lipid attraction signal. *Cell*. 2003;113:717-730.
65. Fadok VA, Voelker DR, Campbell PA, Cohen JJ, Bratton DL, Henson PM. Exposure of phosphatidylserine on the surface of apoptotic lymphocytes triggers specific recognition and removal by macrophages. *J Immunol*. 1992;148:2207-2216.
66. Martin SJ, Finucane DM, Amarante-Mendes GP, O'Brien GA, Green DR. Phosphatidylserine externalization during CD95-induced apoptosis of cells and cytoplasts requires ICE/CED-3 protease activity. *J Biol Chem*. 1996;271:28753-28756.
67. Reed JC. Dysregulation of apoptosis in cancer. *J Clin Oncol*. 1999;17:2941-2953.
68. Tsujimoto Y, Finger LR, Yunis J, Nowell PC, Croce CM. Cloning of the chromosome breakpoint of neoplastic B cells with the t(14;18) chromosome translocation. *Science*. 1984;226:1097-1099.
69. LaCasse EC, Mahoney DJ, Cheung HH, Plenchette S, Baird S, Korneluk RG. IAP-targeted therapies for cancer. *Oncogene*. 2008;27:6252-6275.
70. Schuyer M, van der Burg ME, Henzen-Logmans SC, et al. Reduced expression of BAX is associated with poor prognosis in patients with epithelial ovarian cancer: a multifactorial analysis of TP53, p21, BAX and BCL-2. *Br J Cancer*. 2001;85:1359-1367.
71. Sinicrope FA, Rego RL, Okumura K, et al. Prognostic impact of bim, puma, and noxa expression in human colon carcinomas. *Clin Cancer Res*. 2008;14:5810-5818.
72. Tschopp J, Martinon F, Hofmann K. Apoptosis: silencing the death receptors. *Curr Biol*. 1999;9:R381-R384.
73. Zilfou JT, Lowe SW. Tumor suppressive functions of p53. *Cold Spring Harb Perspect Biol*. 2009;1:a001883.

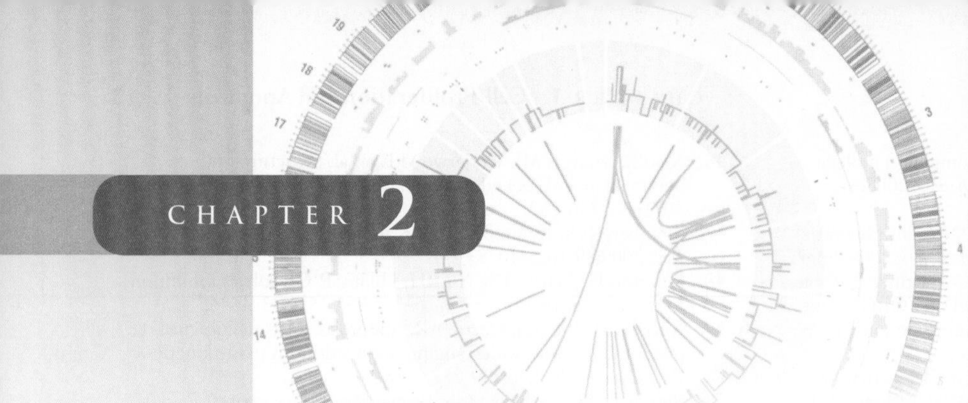

CHAPTER 2

CANCER STEM CELLS

Sadhna Dhingra and Dongfeng Tan

For the last two decades, the prevailing concept of cancer initiation has been the stochastic model. According to this model, cancers develop from normal somatic cells that acquire random mutations in oncogenes and tumor suppressor genes that result in enhanced cell proliferation, inhibition of differentiation, and clonal selection. According to this concept, each tumor cell is equally capable of forming a new tumor and the tumors are clonal in origin. However, growing evidence has created a paradigm shift from this model toward the "cancer stem cell" (CSC) concept. According to the CSC theory, cancers consist of a heterogeneous population of cells—similar to normal adult tissues—and include stem cells, transit amplifying cells, and terminally differentiated cells (mature cells). These cells form the cellular hierarchy in a tumor, and only a minority of CSCs is responsible for tumor formation and growth.

In early 2006, a working group of the American Association for Cancer Research operationally defined a CSC as a malignant cell within a tumor that has two main properties: the ability to self-renew and the ability to differentiate into heterogeneous lineages of cancer cells that comprise the tumor.[1] Self-renewal means that the stem cells have the ability to give rise to a progeny with the same proliferation potential and thereby to maintain the stem cell pool. In contrast, differentiation leads to the maturation and formation of heterogeneous cellular subsets with more specialized functions and less proliferative potential. Xenotransplantation assays have demonstrated that only a specific subset of cells within a tumor is able to generate a phenocopy of the original tumor cells when introduced into immunodeficient mice. These assays serve as the gold standard for demonstrating the "stemness" of cancer cells.

CSCs fuel tumor growth by asymmetric cell division. Each stem cell divides, producing one identical quiescent daughter stem cell and one transient amplifier cell. The majority of this transient amplifier cells and the bulk of the tumor cells are susceptible to current chemotherapeutic regimens.

A characteristic feature of self-renewing cells is increased telomerase activity. This enzyme ensures that the length of telomeres remains constant after cell division. Thus, these cells are not subject to the aging effect and maintain an infinite replication potential. In contrast, as normal tissue stem cells differentiate, they lose their potential to self-renew, probably due to loss of telomerase activity. However, CSCs in tumors demonstrate telomerase activation and stabilization and are necessary for tumor progression.[2]

CSCs themselves have unique properties that make them different from the rest of the tumor cell population. For example, they have very low proliferation potential, which allows them to elude traditional radiotherapy and chemotherapy regimens, which are designed to target rapidly multiplying cells. Also, they have a very efficient system to pump out drugs, making them highly resistant to most conventional therapies. Current therapies might therefore affect the bulk of a tumor but spare the CSCs, which are responsible for tumor recurrence and metastasis. Quiescent CSCs that have drifted to distant sites through interacting with the new microenvironment could be responsible for the development of metastatic tumors long after curative surgical treatment of primary cancers. Thus, there is a need for novel therapeutic targets directed toward CSCs and the stem cell microenvironment.

EVOLUTION OF THE CSC CONCEPT

The quest to understand cancer pathogenesis dates back to Grecian times. The first known theory of carcinogenesis was proposed by Hippocrates, Celsius, and Galen, who based their hypothesis that cancer is caused by excess of black bile on the humoral nature of disease.[3] The concept of stem cells as a precursor of cancer was not introduced until the mid-1800s, when Rudolph Virchow, the "father of pathology," observed that certain cancers, such as teratocarcinoma, showed morphologic resemblance to a developing fetus.[4] In 1867, Julius Cohnheim formally proposed the "embryonic rest hypothesis" for cancers on the basis of Virchow's observations and the fact that both embryonic rests and tumors have an inherent capacity for proliferation and differentiation. Cohnheim hypothesized that tumors develop from residual embryonic rests and not from adult tissues.[5] This theory formed the basis of the modern CSC concept, but it lost importance soon after because the hypothesis was not supported by results from experimental investigations.

Parallel to the development of the embryonal rest theory, another hypothesis pertaining to the clonal evolution of cancers was rapidly gaining favor among scientists. Heralded by Percival Potts, this new theory was based on the observation of increased testicular cancer in chimney sweepers, which linked environmental exposure to cancer, and on Peyton Rous' experiments that established a link between virus and tumors.[6] In 1971, Alfred G. Knudson proposed the "two-hit" hypothesis for cancer, which explained the basis for both hereditary and non-hereditary cancers.[7] Five years later, Peter C. Nowell proposed the multistep model of carcinogenesis, which states that the progression of cancer occurs through a serial, stepwise acquisition of genetic mutations and the sequential selection of more aggressive clones.[8]

In the last half of the 19th century and for much of the 20th century, the "embryonal rest" theory of carcinogenesis took a backseat and the theory of clonal evolution of cancers prevailed. Interest in stem cell biology was revived in the 1960s, when James E. Till and Ernest A. McCulloch definitively demonstrated the existence of hematopoietic stem cells (HSCs) in their experiments on lethally irradiated mice.[9] In a series of landmark experiments, Gordon Barry Pierce observed that teratocarcinomas contain multipotent stem cells that are also found in embryoid bodies in tumors.[10] His observations resurrected the "embryonic rest" theory of carcinogenesis, and he went on to propose the early CSC concept: "Carcinoma is a caricature of the normal process of tissue renewal."[11] According to this concept, cancers arose due to maturation arrest of stem cells. Thus in cancers, as opposed to normal tissues, a stem cell produces many more malignant stem cells than they differentiate.

In the late 20th century, crucial technological advances in laboratory medicine led to the development of radiolabeling techniques with autoradiography, commercial fluorescence-activated cell sorting (FACS), well-validated cell surface markers, the mouse xenograft assay, and high-speed multiparameter flow cytometry for HSCs. Combined with easy accessibility of the bone marrow for ex vivo analysis, these developments helped research on hematological malignancies to flourish. In their study on human acute myeloid leukemia (AML), John Dick and colleagues provided the first direct evidence of a minority stem cell population in leukemias, which they referred to as "leukemia-initiating cells"[12] and which are now known as leukemia stem cells. They subsequently demonstrated that human AML originated from HSCs.[13] These landmark studies by John Dick and colleagues were followed by multiple reports by other researchers that provided evidence of a hierarchical organization of hematological malignancies and an origin from stem cells.[14,15]

Evidence of the existence of stem cells in solid tumors was introduced by Michael Clarke and Peter Dirks. In a landmark paper in 2003, Clarke and colleagues reported cellular heterogeneity in breast cancers.[16] Applying the stem cell concept to solid tumors, they demonstrated in a xenograft assay that as few as 100 cells with $CD44^{+}$/$CD24^{-/low}$ phenotype based on cell surface marker expression showed tumor-initiating properties. Other cell populations with an alternate phenotype were not found to be tumorigenic. Each time the tumorigenic cells were serially passaged, some of the cells produced new tumors containing $CD44^{+}/CD24^{-/low}$ tumorigenic cells as well as other, more differentiated cells. At about the same time, Peter Dirks and colleagues identified CD133-positive CSCs in human tumors.[17] This publication was followed by a deluge of reports by additional researchers on CSCs in other solid tumors, such as cancers of the colon, liver, lung, and prostate.[18-21] Most of those studies used xenotransplantation assays to show that small populations of cells identified by specific markers were able to regenerate cancers when transplanted into immunodeficient mice in a variable time period and that these transplanted tumors displayed cellular heterogeneity similar to that of the primary tumor.

ORIGIN OF CSCS

CSCs are thought to originate from transformation of normal tissue stem cells or of the more differentiated cell population. The more differentiated cells could be tissue progenitor cells or they could be differentiated malignant cells in a tumor that dedifferentiate secondary to a mutagenic event or immune response and acquire stem cell–like properties. In solid organ tumors, acquisition of the CSC phenotype occurs through epithelial-to-mesenchymal transition (EMT).

To understand the origin of cancer from tissue stem cells, it is imperative to comprehend the differences between adult tissue stem cells (mesenchymal or epithelial or hematopoietic), progenitor cells, and CSCs. Adult tissue stem cells are quiescent cells with very low proliferation rates, which undergo mitotic division to produce two similar daughter stem cells or daughter cells that differentiate and mature to resemble adult tissues. Like CSCs, adult stem cells have the properties of self-renewal and differentiation and they replenish the cell population of the mature organ in which they reside. Progenitor cells are more differentiated than normal adult tissue stem cells, and they are committed to form a specific differentiated cell. They possess the differentiation property but have limited capacity to self-renew, unlike the adult tissue stem cells that can divide indefinitely. As described by Wicha et al.[22] and Ratajczak et al.,[23] CSCs share many properties with adult tissue stem cells such as self-renewal, differentiation, long telomeres, active telomerase expression, increased ATP-binding cassette (ABC) membrane transporter activity, and the secretion of several growth factors, cytokines, and angiopoietic factors. They also share similar pathways of self-renewal at the molecular level (Wnt, Sonic hedgehog [Shh], and Notch signaling pathways) and activation of anti-apoptotic pathways. They respond to similar motomorphogens such as stromal cell–derived factor 1 (SDF-1) and hepatocyte growth factor (HGF)/scatter factor, which regulate trafficking of normal stem cells and promote the metastasis of corresponding CSCs. Because they also express similar surface receptors (CXCR4, Sca-1, CD133, c-kit, c-met), similar markers can be used to distinguish between them.

Recent evidence has shown that both adult tissue stem cells and progenitor cells have the ability to transform into CSCs. In most cancers, a mutation in these cells appears to be the initiating event that leads to their transformation. Subsequent multiple hits by oncogenic mutations lead to accumulation of mutations over a period of time, and this is followed by unregulated expansion of CSCs. The strongest evidence of HSCs being the origin of CSCs comes from studies of Dick and colleagues on human AML. They found that the cells responsible for leukemia initiation in non-obese, diabetic mice with severe combined immunodeficiency (NOD/SCID) had the $CD34^+CD38^-$ immunophenotype exclusively, which was similar to that of HSCs.[13] Jamieson et al.[24] showed that progenitor cells acquired self-renewal properties in the blast crisis phase of chronic myeloid leukemia. In the chronic phase of this disease, the BCR-ABL mutation affected HSCs in a way that caused aberrant stem cell differentiation and survival and eventually led to production of an expanded progenitor population that aberrantly acquired self-renewal properties, resulting in leukemic stem cell transformation and blast crisis. Similarly, Cozzio et al.[25] demonstrated that transduction of the MLL-ENL fusion gene into HSCs and more differentiated granulocyte progenitors resulted in leukemic transformation.

Similarly, for solid tumors it has been theorized that CSCs can originate from either organ-specific tissue stem cells or tissue progenitor cells. The expression of markers of normal tissue stem cells (e.g., CD133, nestin, c-kit, SOX 2, OCT 4, Musashi-1) in primary tumors or cultured cell lines indicates that these tumors are derived from normal tissue stem cells.[17,26-28] Dontu et al.[29] proposed that mammary carcinogenesis results from the transformation of normal tissue stem cells or progenitor cells that leads to the well-recognized phenotypic diversity and clinical heterogeneity in biological behavior.

Another recent concept is that CSCs originate from bone marrow–derived "mesenchymal stem cells" in solid tumors. Bone marrow–derived stem cells (BMDCs) are a heterogeneous group of cells that include both HSCs and mesenchymal stem cells. HSCs give rise to formed elements in blood, whereas mesenchymal stem cells give rise to adipocytes, chondrocytes, osteocytes, and the marrow mesenchyme that form the microenvironment for HSCs. The *Helicobacter*-induced gastric cancer model is an ideal model for demonstrating the origin of CSCs from BMDCs. Using the *H. felis*/C57BL/6 mouse model of gastric cancer, in 2004, Houghton et al.[30] demonstrated that chronic infection with *Helicobacter* promoted chronic tissue inflammation that led to the engraftment of gastric glands with BMDCs over time, which was followed by intraepithelial dysplasia and invasive cancer. Later, in 2009, Cao et al.[31] reported isolating BMDCs from 13 of 20 human gastric cancer tissues. The rat model of Barrett metaplasia is another example of BMDCs serving as the origin of cancer.[32] This phenomenon of origin of tumors from BMDCs has also been noticed for some malignancies arising in solid organ transplant recipients: donor BMDCs have been shown to give rise to Kaposi sarcoma and skin carcinoma.[33]

The phenomenon of EMT is also known to induce the CSC phenotype in solid tumors.[34] EMT involves a complex series of molecular events that lead to loss of the epithelial cell phenotype and acquisition of the mesenchymal phenotype by tumor cells. This transition occurs through loss of E-cadherin (CDH1)–dependent cell contacts between contiguous cells. As a result, the cells lose cell-to-cell adhesion properties and acquire myofibroblast-like characteristics. Phenotypically, this transition is evidenced by decreased expression of epithelial cytokeratins, loss of E-cadherin, and acquisition of mesenchymal markers such as vimentin, smooth muscle actin, fibronectin, and N-cadherin expression. EMT is also an early process of metastasis and is associated with poor clinical outcomes. Experimental studies performed on non-tumorigenic immortalized human mammary epithelial cell lines have demonstrated transformation to the mesenchymal phenotype on exposure to the transcription factors *snail*, *twist*, or tumor growth factor-β1 and also acquisition of the $CD44^{high}/CD24^{low}$ CSC profile. These mesenchymal-type epithelial cells were shown to generate 30 times more mammospheres than vector control cells did, suggesting that EMT generates CSCs from differentiated mammary epithelial cells.[35] In colorectal, pancreatic, and other tumors, it has similarly been shown that tumor cells at the tumor–host interface express both EMT-associated genes and stemness-associated genes.[34]

CSC ASSAYS

The availability of sensitive and specific technologies for isolating and enriching CSCs is vital for oncological stem cell research. The primary challenge to studying CSCs is their paucity in tumors: on the basis of cell surface marker expression, they comprise less than 5% of the total tumor cell population.[36] In vitro assays are based on the differentiation potential of CSCs and are useful for isolating and characterizing these cells. These assays include FACS, magnetic bead–activated cell sorting, immunohistochemical (IHC) analysis for cell surface markers, and tumor sphere–forming assays. The selection and isolation of potential CSCs in tumors with the use of FACS and IHC analysis, followed by in vitro sphere-forming assays or in vivo xenotransplantation studies, have greatly enhanced our understanding of CSC biology.

The most widely used method for isolating and enriching CSCs is flow cytometry (FACS or magnetic bead–activated cell sorting). Using this technique, the CSC population can be quantified, isolated, and analyzed by the expression of cell surface markers derived from the characterization of normal stem cells. This technique can be used for both hematopoietic malignancies and solid tumors. Bonnet and Dick[13] were among the first researchers to apply flow cytometry to identify and sort leukemic CSCs that showed the $CD34^+/CD38^-$ phenotype according to cell surface marker expression. Since then, this technique has been widely used in a variety of hematopoietic and solid tumors, such as breast CSCs with the $CD44^+/CD24^-$ phenotype and pancreatic tumor-initiating cells with $CD44^+/CD24^+/EpCAM^+$ surface marker expression.

Detection of "side population" cells by FACS is another method of CSC enrichment. In normal tissues, the side population cells express high levels of stem-like genes and are multipotent with potential for multilineage differentiation and thus behave in a manner similar to CSCs.[37] Side population cells have been identified in a variety of cancer cell lines, and they have been found to comprise between 1% and 20% of the total cell population. Detection of side population cells is based on the principle that adult stem cells express high levels of proteins in the ABC transporter family that are responsible for the expulsion of foreign materials, including Hoechst 33342 dye, from the cell.[38]

Flow cytometry is not without disadvantages. Its major limitation is that it requires analysis of a sufficient number of dyscohesive cells to obtain a statistically significant numbers of CSCs, which are rare in tumors. This technique works well for hematological malignancies, but it can be difficult to obtain disaggregated cells from solid tumors. Another disadvantage of FACS is its inability to discriminate between true labeling and nonspecific staining of cell markers. The use of IHC analysis to identify CSCs can overcome some of the barriers of FACS. IHC analysis is a simple, reproducible technique that identifies CSCs by cell marker protein expression on archival tissues such as formalin-fixed, paraffin-embedded tissues or frozen tissues. Microscopic evaluation of the tissue architecture, cellular localization, and intensity of cell marker staining can help differentiate true-positive CSCs from false labeling.

Flow cytometry and IHC analysis use cell markers to sort and isolate cells of interest. The term "cell marker" implies protein expression that helps identify a particular phenotype. These are often cluster of differentiation (CD) markers, such as CD133, and other markers that reflect functional attributes, such as cell adhesion molecules, cytoprotective enzymes (e.g., aldehyde dehydrogenase [ALDH]), and drug efflux pumps (e.g., ABC transporters). CSC markers are cell surface antigens that are expressed in both normal tissue stem cells and CSCs. Some markers are shared by CSCs of various origins, whereas others are specific for the tumor type. Table 2.1 illustrates commonly used CSC immunomarkers in solid and hematopoietic malignancies. The combination of cell surface markers determines the immunophenotypic profile of the organ-specific CSCs. Some examples of multimarker CSC immunophenotypic profiles in various cancers are described in Table 2.2.

As yet, there is no consensus about the "best" marker for identifying CSCs in any particular cancer. None of the markers used to isolate stem cells in various normal and cancerous tissues is expressed exclusively by stem cells. For example, the well-known stem cell marker CD44 is also an intercellular adhesion molecule and is expressed in a wide variety of non–stem cells in tumors and in normal tissues and organs, such as gastric tissue and gastric adenocarcinoma (Fig. 2.1).[39] For clinical selection of cases that would respond to targeted therapy, robust immunomarkers that characterize CSCs are needed. Although useful for characterizing CSCs by cell surface marker expression, flow cytometry and IHC analysis do not allow for functional characterization of CSCs, which is better assessed by in vitro colony-forming unit, tumor sphere–forming, or in vivo xenotransplantation assays.

In vitro assays such as colony-forming unit and sphere-forming assays are useful surrogates for xenotransplantation studies and have been used to identify and enrich CSCs.[40-42] The colony-forming unit assay involves plating freshly dissociated cancer cells in low densities onto a semisolid matrix such as Matrigel. After several weeks, epithelial colonies adherent to the matrix are formed, which are then counted with the use of a dissecting microscope. This assay has not been widely used for quantification of progenitor cells, presumably because of the difficulty in obtaining accurate colony counts through different focal planes.[43]

The sphere-forming assay is based on the fact that the growth of cancer cells cultured at low density in semiliquid, serum-free, non-adherent medium rich in fibroblast

TABLE 2–1 Common Putative CSC Immunomarkers Used for Identification and Enrichment of CSCs in Solid and Hematopoietic Tumors

	CSC Immunomarkers
Solid Tumors[a]	
Breast cancer	CD24, CD44, CD133, ALDH1, EpCAM, OCT 4
Colorectal cancer	CD44, CD133, CD166, ALDH1, EphB, EpCAM
Brain tumor(glioma, medulloblastoma)	CD15, CD133, Olig2, nestin
Melanoma	CD133, CD166, CD271, ABCB5
Pancreatic cancer	CD44, CD24, CD133, ALDH, EpCAM, nestin
Ovarian cancer	CD24, CD44, CD117, CD133, OCT 4, Nanog, ABCG2, ALDH
Head and neck cancer	CD44, CD133, ALDH, BMI-1
Prostate cancer	CD44, CD49f, CD133, CD166, BMI-1, β-catenin, Smo, TRA-1-160, CD151, OCT 4
Endometrial carcinoma	CD133, Musashi-1, Notch-1
Hepatobiliary	CD44, CD90, CD133, ABCG2, ALDH, EpCAM
Ewing sarcoma	CD44, CD133, ALDH
Lung cancer	ABCG2, CD44, CD133, CD166, ALDH, GLDC
Gastric carcinoma	CD44, nestin
Osteosarcoma	CD133, ALDH, OCT 4
Retinoblastoma	CD133, CD44, ABCG2, MCM2,
Hematopoietic Malignancies	
Acute myeloid leukemia	CD34, CD38, ALDH, CD44
Acute T-lymphoblastic leukemia	CD 34, CD90, CD110
Acute B-lymphoblastic leukemia	CD133, CD19, CD38, CD34

[a]Cancer stem cell studies are still in "infant" phase. Different investigators claim different markers, and many cancer stem cell markers are to be confirmed by strict stem cell analysis criteria.
ALDH, aldehyde dehydrogenase; CSC, cancer stem cell.

growth factor and epidermal growth factor results in the formation of tumor spheres within a few weeks. Tumor spheres are a clonal population derived from a single tumor cell that possesses the properties of self-renewal and differentiation. The tumor-initiating cells are identified and isolated from these spheres using FACS and stem cell surface markers such as CD133. Serial culture of CD133-positive cells results in secondary and tertiary tumor spheres, with phenotypes similar to that of the primary spheres. Studies in the neural field have demonstrated that the stem cell content in this assay is variable and depends on the stage of culture: the content is very high in the initial stages of culture and then declines until the next subculturing step is carried out. This pattern is thought to be due to cellular differentiation into mature cells over time.[41] Similarly, in their experimental

TABLE 2–2 Immunophenotype Profiles of Cancer Stem Cells in Common Malignancies

		Immunophenotypic Profile
Solid Tumors		
	Breast cancer	$EpCAM^{+}CD44^{+}CD24^{-/low}$
	Colorectal cancer	$EpCAM^{high}CD44^{+}CD166^{+}$
	Melanoma	$CD133^{+}CD166^{+}$
	Pancreatic cancer	$CD44^{+}CD24^{+}EpCAM^{+}$
	Prostate cancer	$CD44^{+}\alpha2\beta1^{high}CD133^{+}$
	Hepatocellular carcinoma	$CD133^{+}CD44^{+}$
Hematopoietic Tumors		
	Acute myeloid leukemia	$CD34^{+}CD38^{-}$
	Acute T-lymphoblastic leukemia	$CD\ 34^{+}CD90^{+}CD110^{+}$, $CD34^{+}CD7^{+}$
	Acute childhood B-lymphoblastic leukemia	$CD34^{+}CD19^{+}CD38^{-}$, $CD34^{+}CD19^{+}CD38^{+}$

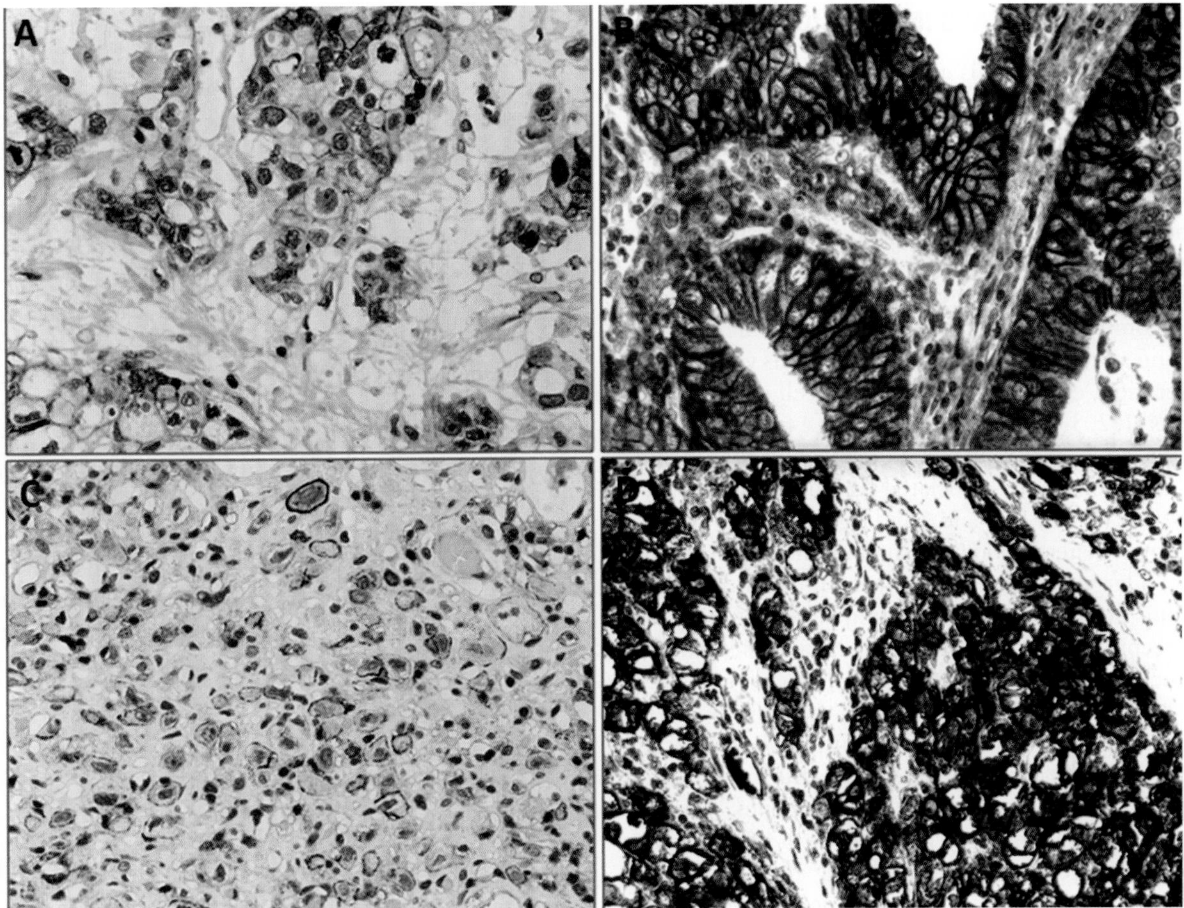

FIGURE 2–1 Membranous CD44 expression. **A:** Gastric adenocarcinoma, intestinal subtype, CSC of immunoexpression < 50. **B:** Gastric adenocarcinoma, intestinal subtype, CSC > 50. **C:** Gastric adenocarcinoma, diffuse subtype, CSC < 50. **D:** Gastric adenocarcinoma, diffuse subtype, CSC > 50. Immunoperoxidase, ×400 (A, B, C, D). CSC, cancer stem cell.

study using mammosphere assays, Moraes et al.[44] demonstrated that regenerative stem cells represent only 15% to 33% of the total cell population in mammospheres and that the remaining cells are downstream progenitor cells with no proliferative potential. Assays using tumor sphere formation have been an important experimental tool for CSC research. However, this assay does not help distinguish between the regenerative potential of multipotent stem cells and that of more differentiated progenitor cells.[44]

In vivo tumorigenic assessment requires the use of immunocompromised mice, particularly SCID mice, which lack both T cells and B cells. SCID mice can be crossed with NOD mice, which lack natural killer cell activity and have other immune deficiencies such as defects in macrophage activity and complement activation. Potential stem cells purified from tumors are xenografted into SCID/NOD IL2Rγ^{null} mice (currently, it is the best recipient for CSC study).[45] These mice are then examined at various times for tumor formation. Potential stem cells from tumors produced in these mice are further identified and isolated using FACS and cell markers. Those cells are then transplanted into a second recipient animal. Multiple serial transplantation leading to the sustained formation of tumors that recapitulate the phenotype of the original tumor is evidence of the self-renewal and differentiation of CSCs. In vivo assays are the only means that can demonstrate both these essential properties of CSCs. This is the most robust assay for detecting CSCs. The drawbacks of the assay are that it is expensive, time consuming, and labor intensive and that it cannot be applied to high-throughput screening studies.

Other techniques for identifying CSCs include labeling retention assays, which use bromodeoxyuridine as a label.[1] This method is based on the assumption that normal cells and CSCs are quiescent and do not enter the cell cycle for long periods and hence that they retain the labeled state for an extended period. However, this assumption cannot be applied universally: not all stem cells retain a label, and not all label-retaining cells are stem cells. Moreover, as with other stem cell detection assays, this particular test has to be coupled with a functional assay to demonstrate the cell renewal and differentiation properties of the labeled cells and to accurately characterize cells as CSCs.

SIGNALING PATHWAYS IN CSC BIOLOGY

Normal tissue stem cells and CSCs share certain signaling pathways. Transformation of a normal tissue stem cell into a CSC occurs due to accumulation of multiple genetic alterations, epigenetic changes, and deregulation of signaling pathways. The key signaling pathways that have been the focus of research are Notch, Shh, and Wnt/β-catenin pathways.

The Notch signaling cascade is important for cell-to-cell communication. It regulates embryonic development and adult maintenance of homeostasis via stem cell proliferation, cell differentiation, and cell death. Notch proteins (1, 2, 3, and 4) are members of a transmembrane receptor family that bind five Notch ligands that include other cell membrane–associated ligands, such as Delta-like ligands (DLL) 1, 3, and 4 and jagged ligands 1 and 2. The Notch genes encode transmembrane receptors that include a large extracellular domain and an intracellular signaling domain. Notch signaling is activated by ligand–receptor interaction, which leads to the secretion of γ-secretase that in turn causes the release and translocation of the intracellular domain into the nucleus. There the intracellular domain interacts with the core-binding factor 1 transcription factor and causes the upregulation of human embryonic stem (*Hes*) target genes. The *Hes* family of genes is involved in cell growth and differentiation. The effects of Notch signaling are complex and vary depending on the cell type. For example, Notch signaling can promote the proliferation, survival, and differentiation of T-cell precursors, whereas it inhibits the growth of and induces apoptosis in B-cell precursors.[46] Similarly, Notch can be oncogenic in some solid tumors (e.g., medulloblastoma, osteosarcoma, Ewing sarcoma, and breast adenocarcinoma) but induce growth arrest in other solid tumors (e.g., small cell lung cancer, basal cell carcinoma [BCC]).[46] Moreover, another role of Notch is its tumor suppressor function.[47]

Wnt proteins consist of 19 highly conserved glycoproteins that regulate cell-to-cell interaction during various stages of embryogenesis. The signaling of these proteins acts to regulate the development of a variety of organ systems, including the cardiovascular, central nervous system, renal, lung, and hematopoietic systems. In adults, Wnt signaling has a key role in the regulation of tissue self-renewal, particularly in intestinal crypts, hair follicles, and bone growth plates. Wnt proteins serve as ligands for the Frizzled (Fz) transmembrane receptor, and through canonical signaling they lead to accumulation of β-catenin in the nucleus, which ultimately leads to transcriptional upregulation of Wnt target genes. In epithelial tumors such as colon cancer and breast cancer, the interactions between tumor cells and the microenvironment (e.g., tumor-infiltrating inflammatory cells, myofibroblasts, and other stromal cells) can locally affect the intracellular canonical Wnt signaling and differentially trigger stemness, cell proliferation, EMT, and invasive behavior.

Hedgehog (Hh) signaling plays an important role in embryonic development and is responsible for maintenance of the stem cell population in adults. The pathway is initiated by binding of the Hh ligand to Patched (Ptc), which is a 12-transmembrane protein receptor. Ptc acts as an inhibitor of the receptor smoothened (Smo), a 7-transmembrane protein related to the Fz family of Wnt receptors and to other 7-transmembrane G-protein-coupled receptors. In the presence of Hh, the Hh–Ptc complex causes Smo activation, which leads to activation of the Gli family of zinc-finger transcription factors. In vertebrates, there are three Gli proteins: Gli1 serves to activate Hh target genes, Gli2 acts as both an activator and a repressor, and Gli3 acts as a repressor of target-gene transcription. Hh signaling seems to depend on the relative balance of the Gli activator and repressor forms.[48] Hh pathway mutation with constitutive activation leading to tumorigenesis is a well-recognized phenomenon in BCC and medulloblastoma. Inappropriate activation of this pathway has also been observed for a variety of other human cancers, including brain, gastrointestinal, lung, breast, and prostate cancers. This pathway has also been shown to regulate the proliferation of CSCs and to increase tumor invasiveness.[49]

Stem Cell Niche

"Stem cell niche" refers to the existence of stem cells in non-epithelial stromal tissue that form the unique microenvironment. By definition, "niche" is a habitat supplying the factors necessary for the existence of an organism.[50] Functionally, a niche is characterized by its persistence on removal of stem cells and the ability to reacquire and maintain introduced stem cells.[51] Normal stem cells rely on this microenvironment to maintain their stemness. Similarly, CSCs reside in a supportive functional microenvironment, called the CSC niche, which is essential for their survival. This concept was first proposed by Schofield[52] in 1978, when he described that in the hematopoietic system a stem cell is essentially a fixed tissue cell in association with other cells that determine its behavior. He further stated that maturation of a stem cell is prevented and, as a result, its continued proliferation as a stem cell is assured. Unless they can occupy a similar stem cell niche, its progeny are first-generation colony-forming cells that proliferate and mature to acquire a high probability of differentiation.

The cellular composition of a niche includes a variety of stromal cells such as mesenchymal and immune cells, a vascular network, soluble factors, extracellular matrix components, and tumor-associated fibroblasts. A complex interplay between CSCs and the niche regulates the stemness, proliferation, and apoptosis resistance of stem cells. CSCs interact with the niche via adhesion molecules and paracrine factors. The niche provides a permissive environment for the CSCs to self-renew, give rise to more differentiated cells, and at the same time maintain their undifferentiated state. It protects the CSCs from genotoxic insults and contributes to their propensity for enhanced chemoresistance or radioresistance. The niche facilitates tumor progression by causing dedifferentiation of non-CSCs in the tumor and by inducing EMT. It also plays a role in metastasis through the formation of a pre-metastatic niche. Various signaling pathways have been identified within several mammalian adult niches, including Activin/Nodal, Akt/PTEN, JAK/STAT, PI3K, tumor growth factor-β, Wnt, bone morphogenetic proteins (BMPs), fibroblast growth factor, Hh, Notch, and cell signaling pathways. These pathways control stem cell renewal and regulate the lineage in different systems.

Experimental studies with *Drosophila*, *Caenorhabditis elegans*, and mammals have greatly enhanced our understanding of the interaction of stem cells with non-epithelial stromal cells. The best characterized somatic stem cell niches are the ones that support the germline stem cells (GSCs) in the ovaries and testes of the fruit fly *Drosophila*.[53,54] In both organs, GSCs exist in a specific region anchored to non-dividing somatic support cells (niche cells) that provide the microenvironment and control the asymmetric cell division of GSCs. The GSCs physically anchor to niche cells, and during cell division they orient their mitotic spindles with respect to the niche such that the daughter cell that maintains contact with the niche cell retains the characteristics of the GSC. The other daughter cell loses physical adherence to the niche cells and undergoes differentiation. It is the physical dissociation from niche cells that allows activation of differentiation genes and causes differentiation to occur. Xie and Spradling[55] showed that GSCs need a signal mediated by decapentaplegic, a member of the tumor growth factor-β superfamily, to remain adhered to niche cells and to control the frequency of cell division. The niche cells are a source of cell signaling molecules, such as Hh, wingless, and armadillo, which have been suggested to be involved in the regulation of GSCs and the maintenance of their stem cell state.[56]

Niches for mammalian adult stem cells have been well characterized in a variety of tissues, such as the hematopoietic system and gastrointestinal tract, skin, and neural tissues. Normally, the niche maintains stem cells in a quiescent state by providing signals that inhibit cell proliferation and growth. Stem cells become activated to divide and proliferate in response to proliferating signals from the niche. Thus, a homeostatic regulation of proliferation and antiproliferation signals maintains balanced control of stem cell proliferation. Deregulation of signaling pathways in the niches may lead to conversion into a microenvironment that favors uncontrolled proliferation and expansion of a stem cell population that has accumulated intrinsic mutations over a period of time.

The bone marrow niche is perhaps one of the best described stem cell niche. Bone marrow contains two well-characterized HSC niches: the osteoblastic/endosteal niche and the vascular niche.[57] Higher oxygen levels are found in the vascular niche, which is found along the endothelial cells of sinusoidal blood vessels, than in the osteoblastic niche, thus favoring cell cycle progression in the vascular niche. HSCs in the osteoblastic niche are in a quiescent microenvironment, whereas the vascular niche favors HSC proliferation and further differentiation.[58] According to a hypothetical model of hematopoiesis, HSCs are in a G0 state in the osteoblastic niche. The cells move to the vascular niche under conditions of regional hypoxia to undergo differentiation and to provide peripheral blood with the necessary supply of mature blood cells.[54] Once mature blood cells are no longer needed, the HSCs return to the osteoblastic niche in the G0 phase. The signaling molecules involved in the maintenance of the HSC pool include Wnt, BMP, jagged 1/Notch, angiopoietin-1/Tie 2, thrombopoietin, and osteopontin in the osteoblastic niche and CXCR4, CXCL12, and VCAM-1 in the vascular niche.[54] In leukemias, the leukemic CSCs compete with resident HSCs for normal osteoblastic and vascular niches, as they have similar maintenance requirements. As a result, the HSCs decrease in number and are replaced by leukemic CSCs. For example, for both AML and chronic myeloid leukemia, experimental evidence has shown that CD44 is essential for the homing and engraftment of CSCs to the niche.[59,60] CD44-expressing leukemic cells adhere to the niche and bond to the hyaluronic acid expressed on the surface of sinusoidal endothelial cells or to endosteum in bone marrow. This step is crucial for the maintenance of leukemic CSCs.

Experimental evidence suggests that neural stem cells occupy specialized niches in the subventricular zone of the lateral ventricle and in the subgranular zone of the hippocampus. The stem cells are thought to exist in close association with blood vessels. Secretion of cytokines such as vascular endothelial growth factor (VEGF), erythropoietin, and brain-derived neutrophilic factor supports and maintains the relationship of stem cells with endothelial cells.[48] Brain tumors have been shown to have stem cell niches. Studies have demonstrated that tumor cells that express stem cell markers CD133 and nestin are localized to perivascular zones.[61]

Skin, which undergoes continuous sloughing and self-renewal, has three stem cell niches: the interfollicular epidermis (IFE), the sebaceous gland, and the hair follicle. The IFE contains epidermal stem cells located throughout the basal layer and organized as epidermal-proliferating units with a stem cell in the center surrounded by its progeny. Definitive markers to identify IFE stem cells have not been defined, but on the basis of their location within the basal layer, it is thought that the local microenvironment supports and sustains the epidermal-proliferating units.[62] The second specialized niche exists at the periphery of sebaceous gland, where stem cells differentiate into lipid-producing cells. Cell signaling pathways involving c-myc and Rac1 play critical roles in the maintenance of both epidermal and sebaceous stem cell niches. The third specialized niche is the hair follicle. The IFE extends downward to form the outer root sheath of the hair, which contains a specialized region known as the "bulge" that contains both epidermal and non-epidermal stem cells (e.g., neural crest stem cells). The Wnt/β-catenin signaling pathway is the best characterized cell signaling pathway implicated in the regulation of bulge stem cells. Wnt signaling has been reported to play a role in promoting stem cell activation and expansion in the skin.

The skin malignancies that are best known to originate from stem cell niches include BCC and malignant melanoma. BCC is a slowly growing, locally invasive skin cancer that arises in sun-exposed parts of the epidermis. Most BCCs show constitutive activation of the Shh signaling pathway due to loss of heterozygosity of Ptc or activating mutations in the SmoM2 gene. Experimental studies on mice using clonal analysis have demonstrated that BCC originates from resident progenitor cells of the IFE and the upper infundibulum.[63] Malignant melanoma is an aggressive skin neoplasm. The existence of stem cells in melanomas was first demonstrated in 2005 with the use of tumor sphere–forming assays. Subsequently, melanoma stem cells were identified using the surface markers CD133 and nestin. Recently, melanoma stem cells were identified based on their expression of the ABC transporter and the ABCB5 chemotherapy resistance protein. $ABCB5^+$ melanoma cells evade tumor immunity through the downregulation of major histocompatibility complex class 1, inhibition of interleukin-2, and induction of tolerance to T cells and thus play a role in tumor progression.[48,64]

In the gastrointestinal tract, the stem cell compartment varies according to location. In the stomach, stem cells reside in the neck or isthmus region of the gastric gland. In the small intestine, the compartment is believed to be at the base of the crypts of Leiberkühn, at cell position 4 to 5 from the bottom of the crypt. In the large intestine, the cells are presumed to be located mid-crypt in the ascending colon region and at the crypt base in the descending colon region. Generally, it is believed that there are 4 to 6 stem cells in the stem cell compartment.[65] At all these sites, the stem cells are surrounded by a niche composed of mesenchymal cells and extracellular substrates, which provide an optimal microenvironment for stem cells to give rise to differentiated progeny. Intestinal subepithelial myofibroblasts are specialized mesenchymal cells that form a protective fenestrated sheath around gastric glands and crypts and that extend throughout the lamina propria to merge with the pericytes of blood vessels. These cells are thought to play an important role in epithelial proliferation and differentiation through epithelial–mesenchymal interactions. An important inherent characteristic of niche is "niche succession," which refers to the clonal dominance of a single crypt by progeny of a single stem cell through clonal succession. Using CpG methylation patterns to identify the stem cell niche, Shibata and colleagues[66] provided great insight into the mechanisms of niche succession. The crypt methylation pattern revealed loss of clonal heterogeneity in crypts, providing evidence of niche succession. Mathematical modeling suggested that approximately every 8.2 years, all stem cell lineages within a crypt niche, except for one, become extinct. This stochastic extinction of stem cell lineages results in the loss of most mutations, but some random mutations may become randomly fixed as a result of niche succession and cause tumor progression.

The Wnt signaling pathway is a prominent molecular pathway that maintains the fate of stem cells by controlling their proliferation, differentiation, and apoptosis along the crypt-villus axis. Intestinal subepithelial myofibroblasts in the stem cell niche produce Wnt ligands, which together with BMP antagonists are involved in the preservation of the stem cell pool. The adenoma polyposis coli (APC) gene is located on chromosome 5q21 and its protein product binds and downregulates β-catenin and inhibits the Wnt signaling pathway. APC gene mutation is an early event in the transition of healthy mucosa toward colon carcinoma that results in the stabilization and nuclear translocation of β-catenin, leading to transcriptional upregulation of genes that control cell proliferation and differentiation.[67] Thus, APC plays a vital role in regulating Wnt signaling, and inactivation of the APC gene provides stem cells with a selective growth advantage by allowing unregulated activation of Wnt signaling, which leads to colon carcinogenesis. APC gene mutations are seen in sporadic colon cancers and in familial adenomatous polyposis. Other major alternative pathogenetic mechanisms in colon cancer involve mutations in proto-oncogenes, such as *K-ras*, and microsatellite instability, which is associated with defective DNA mismatch repair genes and is seen in colon cancers of patients with hereditary non-polyposis coli.[68]

Niche and EMT: The niche also plays a vital role in inducing tumor cell dedifferentiation and EMT. During EMT, epithelial cells lose cell-to-cell adhesion properties and acquire a mesenchymal-like phenotype along with stem cell properties. EMT is an early process in the invasion-metastasis phenomenon. Intestinal subepithelial myofibroblasts in the niche secrete HGF, causing dedifferentiation of non-tumorigenic tumor cells into more immature cells by reactivating the Wnt pathway. These dedifferentiated cancer cells display CSC properties. Hypoxia in the tumor microenvironment also promotes the stem cell phenotype in the non–stem cell population, and it causes expansion of the existing stem cell pool through the upregulation of stem cell factors such as OCT 4, NANOG, and c-MYC. One mechanism of hypoxia-induced dedifferentiation is the activation of the Wnt signaling pathway via glycogen synthase kinase 3β, which leads to induction of the key EMT-inducing transcription factor snail.[67]

Niche and metastasis: The local microenvironment at the metastatic sites is in a dynamic state and undergoes many changes secondary to cytokines from primary tumors and metastatic tumor cells. In many solid tumors, the presence of an increased proportion of CSCs in both circulating tumor cells and at established sites of metastasis suggests that CSCs have an increased propensity to metastasize and populate the metastatic sites as compared with differentiated tumor cells. In hypoxic conditions, the oncogene mesenchymal-to-epithelial transition factor is upregulated in CSCs. The mesenchymal-to-epithelial transition factor binds to HGF in the extracellular matrix and leads to enhanced transcription of plasminogen activator inhibitor type 1 and cyclooxygenase-2, both of which enhance coagulation and lead to formation of a fibrin nest. The fibrin nest induces vasculogenesis, serving as a CSC niche and supporting the homing of circulating CSCs.[54]

Another pathogenetic mechanism that mediates the homing of CSCs to metastatic sites is the expression of SDF-1 (also called CXCL12, a cytokine belonging to the CXC family). The SDF-1 receptor CXCR4 is expressed on CSCs in many primary solid tumors.[69] CXCR4 expression mediates the homing of CSCs to metastatic sites that express high levels of SDF-1, such as liver and bone marrow. Antibody blocking of CXCR4 expressed by tumor cells and SDF-1 expression by niche stromal cells could be a possible therapeutic option. Besides being the most common site of hematological malignancy, bone marrow is a ubiquitous site of metastasis for many solid tumors. The bone marrow niche, especially the osteoblastic niche, is a fertile location for the homing and engraftment of non-hematopoietic tumor cells such as prostate cancer, breast cancer, and multiple solid tumor cells. The bone metastasis of prostate cancer is supported by urokinase-type plasminogen activator or prostate-specific antigen secreted by prostate cancer cells that alter the bone microenvironment to enhance osteoblast proliferation.[70] In osteolytic solid tumor metastasis, the RANK ligand is produced by activated osteoblasts and stromal cells, leading to increased osteoclast activity. Growth factors, such as tumor growth factor-β released from resorbing bone, act in a paracrine manner to enhance tumor growth.[48] VEGF receptor 1^+ hematopoietic progenitor cells are activated by cytokines released from the primary tumor and travel to sites of future metastasis. It is thought that these cells change the local microenvironment to make it favorable for metastasis.

Stem Cells and Therapeutic Resistance

CSCs represent approximately 0.1% to 10% of all tumor cells, depending on the system and cancer type.[45] Current cancer chemotherapeutic drugs are aimed at targeting actively proliferating tumor cells by blocking DNA synthesis or inhibiting the cell cycle. CSCs are unaffected by currently available drugs because these are quiescent cells and because the depletion of proliferating tumor cells secondary to conventional chemotherapy leads to natural selection of CSCs, which are responsible for tumor relapse. Specific membrane proteins have been associated with CSC drug resistance. Highly expressed in normal stem cells, ABC drug transporters are membrane efflux pumps that protect against xenobiotic molecules as they expel the drugs, thereby reducing the concentration of the drugs within the cells. Expression of multiple drug resistance transporters such as ABCB1 (also called P-glycoprotein) and ABCG2 (breast carcinoma resistance protein 1) has been reported to be associated with chemoresistance.[68] Blocking the function of surface-expressed drug pumps may be an option in conjunction with CSC chemotherapy. CSCs also overexpress enzymes such as ALDH1, which makes the cells resistant to cyclophosphamide.[71] Akt signaling activity is thought to mediate resistance in hepatocellular CSCs, indicating upregulation in the survival pathway.[72] Overexpression of anti-apoptotic proteins in CSCs, such as BCL-2 and survivin, leads to apoptosis resistance and thereby contributes to chemoresistance.[73]

CSCs are resistant to radiotherapy as well, because of their properties of slower cell cycling, lower proliferation rate, and increased expression of DNA repair and anti-apoptosis genes. Gliomas treated with radiotherapy show residual tumors that are enriched for fraction of tumor cells expressing CD133. The radioresistance of $CD133^+$ glioma cells has been attributed to higher activation of DNA repair pathways, such as those involving DNA checkpoint kinases (chk).[74] Chk-1 and Chk-2 proteins play a role in the execution of the checkpoint response to cell cycle delay or arrest and this elicits the repair of the DNA damage. Small-molecule inhibition of chk-1 or chk-2 kinases could make CSCs more sensitive to radiation. In colorectal cancer, the maternal embryonic leucine zipper kinase has been thought to be associated with radioresistance.[75] Diehn et al.[76] reported that a low level of reactive oxygen species contributes to the radioresistance of breast CSCs. Notch pathway defects have also been reported to be related to radioresistance.[77] Thus, tumors enriched with CSCs display resistance against chemotherapy or radiotherapy and confer a bad prognosis. There is a need to develop new approaches to target these cells.

NEW THERAPIES TARGETING STEM CELLS

Therapies targeting CSCs could be designed in multiple ways. CSC differentiation could be induced, the cells could be eliminated by inhibiting the maintenance of the stem cell state, or the CSC niche could be targeted.

Differentiation Therapy

Therapies targeted to induce the differentiation of CSCs is a promising approach, as it reduces tumor progression by causing these cells to lose their self-renewal property and leads to depletion of the CSC pool. Differentiation-inducing agents such as retinoids, BMP, and histone deacetylase inhibitors hold promise for clinical use as an adjunct to conventional chemotherapy or radiotherapy for solid tumors. Vitamin A and its analogues (retinoids) are potent modulators of differentiation and can reverse the malignant progression through signal modulations mediated by nuclear retinoid receptors. Clinical use of all-*trans* retinoic acid in acute promyelocytic leukemia is a popular example of differentiation therapy, which leads to frequent remission by inducing differentiation of promyelocytes. In vitro experiments have shown that the use of all-*trans* retinoic acid for gliomas can induce differentiation of stem-like glioma cells, thus inducing therapy-sensitizing effects (including chemotherapy and radiotherapy), impairment of angiogenic cytokine secretion, and disruption of stem-like glioma cell motility.[78] BMPs are crucial growth factors that regulate the proliferation and apoptosis of neural stem cells and promote differentiation. Piccirillo et al.[79] reported that exposure of mice to BMPs, particularly BMP4, led to a significant reduction in CSCs in gliomas through the canonical activation of the BMP receptor and the Smad signaling cascade. This exposure significantly reduced the proliferation potential and increased the expression of markers of neural differentiation. Thus, BMP has therapeutic potential as a differentiation-inducing agent for CSCs.

Some cancer cells are prevented from entering the differentiation pathway partly because of abnormal chromatin modification enzymes. Histone deacetylases are enzymes involved in the remodeling of chromatin by deacetylating the lysine residues of core nucleosomal histones and causing compaction of the DNA/histone complex. This compaction blocks gene transcription and inhibits differentiation, providing a rationale for developing inhibitors of histone deacetylase. Suberoylanilide hydroxamic acid (SAHA), an FDA-approved inhibitor of this enzyme, is used for treating cutaneous T-cell lymphoma. Experimental studies have shown that SAHA induces profound antiproliferative activity by causing tumor cells to undergo cell cycle arrest and differentiation that is dependent on the presence of SAHA.[80]

Inhibition of Maintenance of the Stem Cell State by Targeting Signaling Pathways

The critical dependence of CSCs on self-renewal makes their regulatory signaling pathways an obvious focus for developing experimental therapeutic agents. Investigational agents targeting CSC signal pathways (Fig. 2.2), including the Notch, Hh, and Wnt, are currently in late preclinical development stages; some are in early phase I or II testing with human subjects.[81]

Inhibition of the Notch pathway by γ-synthetase inhibitors is in an early phase of clinical trials. Two of these agents (RO4929097 [Roche] and MK0752 [Merck]) are in phase I testing after evaluation of a variety of

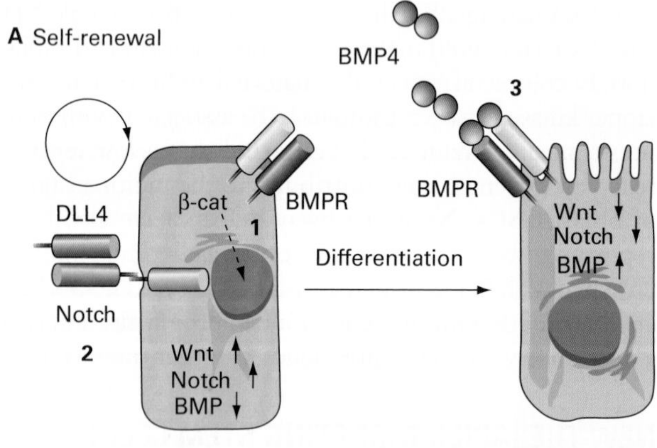

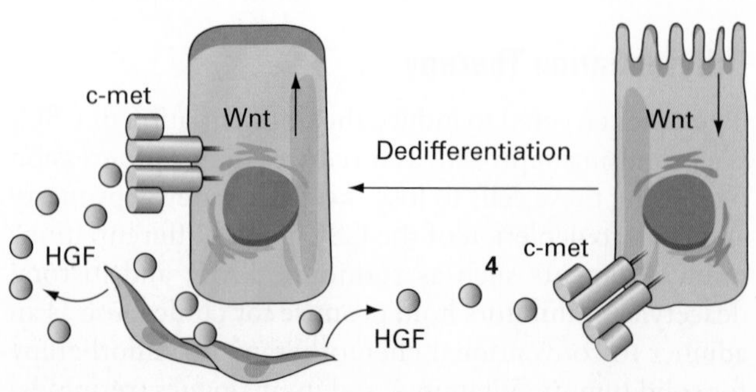

FIGURE 2–2 CSC signal pathways and potential therapeutic significance. **A:** Signals that help to maintain CSCs include Notch and Wnt. DLL4 stimulates Notch receptors on neighboring cells and, together with β-catenin, directs an immature transcription profile that promotes self-renewal. BMP4 counteracts this self-renewal activity by binding to BMP receptors on CSCs, thereby interfering with Wnt signaling and subsequently promoting differentiation. **B:** Colon CSCs in vivo are found intimately associated with HGF-producing myofibroblasts. HGF maintains colon CSCs in a stem cell state and prevents differentiation. HGF produced by myofibroblasts can also upregulate the Wnt cascade in more differentiated tumor cells, thereby reinstalling CSC features (dedifferentiation). These signals that govern CSC behavior have therapeutic potential. Some possibilities to interfere with the self-renewal capacities of CSCs exist. These include (1) inhibitors of the Wnt pathway that prevent β-catenin–dependent transcription; (2) Notch inhibitors, preventing either the ligand from interacting with the receptor or the activation of the receptor (γ-secretase inhibitors), which are currently under evaluation; (3) BMPR agonists that activate differentiation programs and could be used to target CSCs; and (4) inhibitors of the receptor kinase c-met that could modulate the interaction between stromal cells and CSCs to prevent dedifferentiation. BMP, bone morphogenetic proteins; CSC, cancer stem cell; HGF, hepatocyte growth factor.

schedules to determine safe and tolerable administration regimens.[46] Experimental evidence supports the use of γ-synthetase inhibitors for glioblastoma.[82] It also has therapeutic potential in tumors for which Notch has an important oncogenic role in pathogenesis, such as T-acute lymphoblastic leukemia, medulloblastoma, osteosarcoma, Ewing sarcoma, breast adenocarcinoma, melanoma, and prostate, pancreatic, and ovarian carcinomas.[45] However, the use of γ-synthetase inhibitors is associated with significant gut toxicity and goblet cell metaplasia. The endothelial Notch ligand DLL4 has recently emerged as a critical regulator of tumor angiogenesis. Blockade of DLL4-Notch signaling in tumors has been shown to result in inhibitory effects on tumor growth due to the dysregulation of angiogenesis.[83] Anti-DLL4 agents are in phase I clinical development.

The Wnt signaling pathway can be inhibited in a number of ways by targets that act at different levels of the pathway. One such potential therapeutic agent is the Dickkopf (Dkk1) protein, which prevents formation of the Fz–Wnt–LRP6 complex by binding to low-density lipoprotein receptor–related protein 6 (LRP6). Another approach has been the development of small molecules that inhibit Wnt signaling.[84] These small molecules can be a membrane-bound acyltransferase that inhibits synthesis of Wnt by inhibiting the activity of porcupine or they can promote the destruction of β-catenin by inhibiting the enzyme tankyrase, which normally destroys the scaffold protein ankyrin. In addition, the small molecule ICG-001 (Institute for Chemical Genomics) was reported to selectively inhibit Wnt/β-catenin signaling by interrupting β-catenin binding to cyclic AMP-response element-binding protein.[85] ICG-001 treatment of colon carcinoma cell lines resulted in apoptosis but spared normal colonic epithelial cells.[45] Furthermore, several compounds are being tested preclinically to target the PDZ domain of Disheveled, a key protein in the Wnt signaling pathway that links extracellular signals and downstream signals and may be able to inhibit both non-canonical and canonical Wnt signaling pathways.[86]

Most drugs that inhibit the Hh pathway are targeted against the signaling molecule Smo, which lies downstream of the Hh receptor Patched 1 (PTCH1). Cyclopamine was the first drug that was developed against Smo. Since then, several small molecules which are Smo antagonists have been developed that have a higher potency than cyclopamine. GDC-0449 (Genentech) is one such drug that has shown promising results among patients with advanced BCC or medulloblastoma.[87,88] Other Hh pathway inhibitors are in various phases of clinical trials. These include IPI-926 (Infinity Pharmaceuticals), a cyclopamine-derived inhibitor of the Hh pathway, and Smo inhibitors PF-04449913 (Pfizer) and LDE225 (Novartis).[46] Understanding the mechanism of activation of the Hh pathway is helpful in selecting appropriate therapy. In BCC and medulloblastoma, the Hh pathway is constitutively activated due to somatic mutation in the signaling pathway. Such tumors respond to Hh inhibitors alone. However, patients with tumors that are not mutation driven and show aberrant activation of Hh signaling due to paracrine deregulation of signaling may benefit from the use of Hh inhibitors in conjunction with cytotoxic chemotherapy.[47]

Targeting the CSC Niche

Therapeutic targeting of CSC niches is a potential option, as it provides various targets such as the niche vasculature, osteoblasts and osteoclasts, and signaling molecules that promote CSC homing and proliferation. The vascular niche supports CSCs by supplying nutrients and oxygen. This niche is maintained by tumor angiogenesis that, in turn, depends on VEGF upregulation. Oxygen tension is a key regulator of VEGF expression, predominantly via hypoxia-inducible factor. Under hypoxic conditions, hypoxia-inducible factor translocates to the nucleus and binds to hypoxia response elements, thereby initiating transcription of the VEGF gene that initiates tumor angiogenesis.[89]

Therapeutic targeting of angiogenesis has been a major focus of clinical and translational research, which has led to the development of many clinically approved anti-angiogenic agents (e.g., bevacizumab, sorafenib, sunitinib, temesirolimus, and everolimus). The anti-VEGF drug bevacizumab is a monoclonal antibody that is approved by the FDA for use in multiple solid tumors (e.g., metastatic colorectal cancer, metastatic renal cell cancer, non–small cell lung cancer, metastatic HER2-negative breast cancer, and glioblastoma).[48] Ritter et al.[90] demonstrated with in vitro studies that VEGF along with fibroblast growth factor 2 secreted by breast cancer cells is a chemoattractant for stromal BMDCs and that inhibition of VEGF decreases the migration of mesenchymal stem cells toward breast cancer. These findings suggest that anti-VEGF drugs can alter the microenvironment to inhibit the induction of mesenchymal stem cells into breast cancer. Similarly, animal studies of malignant glioma have demonstrated that inclusion of anti-VEGF antibody in the therapeutic regimen, along with cytotoxic drugs, decreased the number of residual CSCs surviving chemotherapy.[91] Thalidomide and thalidomide-derived immunomodulatory drugs such as lenalidomide are anti-angiogenic drugs clinically approved for treatment of multiple myeloma. Jakubikova et al.[92] showed that lenalidomide targeted side population cells and decreased their numbers in multiple myeloma. In addition, the proteasome inhibitor bortezomib is an FDA-approved front-line treatment of multiple myeloma. This agent induces osteoblast differentiation from osteoblastic precursors and mesenchymal stem cells via multiple signaling pathways, such as modulation of bone transcription factor runt-related transcription factor 2 and the β-catenin/T-cell factor signaling pathway.[93,94] Other options include antibody blocking of molecules that promote homing of CSCs.

These molecules include CD44 and CXCR4, which are expressed by tumor cells, and SDF-1 (CXCL12), which is expressed by niche stromal cells.

Other Potential Targets of CSCs

Certain cell surface markers, such as CD44, are desirable antigen targets for immunotherapy. Anti-CD44 antibody therapy represents an important anti-CSC approach. Experimental studies of AML have shown that the anti-CD44 antibodies H90 and A3D8 promote terminal differentiation of AML blasts and induce apoptosis.[95,96]

ALDH1, an enzyme known for alcohol metabolism, is also involved in drug resistance. It is involved in the metabolism of chemotherapeutic drugs such as cyclophosphamide and cisplatin. It also metabolizes retinol to retinoic acid, a key molecule involved in cell differentiation. ALDH1 is recognized as a CSC marker and is expressed in a variety of tumors, including those of the breast, prostate, liver, and colon. Expression of ALDH1 is correlated with poor prognosis in breast cancer.[97] A strong correlation between ALDH1 expression and HER2 overexpression has been observed, which suggests that HER2 may play a role in breast cancer by regulating the CSC population.[98] Treatment of HER2-expressing breast cancers with the HER2 inhibitor trastuzumab as adjuvant therapy has proven to be clinically effective for these tumors.

The presence of ABC transporters is another protective mechanism of stem cells that has been implicated in drug resistance. The transporters are efflux pumps that extrude chemotherapeutic drugs or xenobiotic toxins, thus mediating chemoresistance. Antibody inhibition of the ABC transporters is another potential therapeutic target for CSCs.

CONCLUSIONS

The "cancer stem cell hypothesis," as a basis of oncogenesis, has been a focus of research in the last two decades. A large amount of experimental evidence supports this hypothesis, yet some unanswered questions make it a controversial topic among cancer biologists. The popular controversial issues relate to the origin of CSCs, the application of data generated from current animal models to humans, and the number of CSCs present in a tumor. A formal proof that CSCs can only originate from normal tissue stem cells has yet to be obtained. Hence, some cancer biologists prefer to refer to these cells as "tumor-initiating cells" or "tumor-propagating cells" vis-à-vis CSCs. The evidence of CSCs' existence comes from experimental studies in which they have been isolated from human cancer cell lines transplanted into immunocompromised mice. However, several aspects of this theory and the xenotransplantation assay methods are questionable. Further improvements in methods, such as humanized mouse models, are needed to clearly elucidate CSCs' proposed role in tumorigenesis. In addition, better characterization of cell surface markers is needed to identify CSCs.

For believers, the postulated CSC model explains a long-standing problem of tumor eradication by chemotherapy. Conventional chemotherapy helps eradicate the tumor, leading to initial clinical and pathological remission. However, this is sometimes followed by recurrence and metastasis, with more aggressive and chemoresistant phenotypes, resulting in increased mortality. Thus, therapies that target CSCs hold promise. However, a theoretical risk exists that bystander normal tissue stem cells will be eradicated during CSC-targeted treatment. Future studies focused on identifying CSCs' unique expression profiles and functional properties will allow the development of targeted drugs that are not toxic to normal tissue stem cells. Alternative therapeutic approaches include targeting the molecular pathways or the microenvironment.

Finally, whether all stem cells in a tumor or in different tumors are the same is unknown. Leukemic studies have shown that CSCs are heterogeneous in their self-renewal kinetics and have different cell surface marker phenotypes in different tumors.[99] This heterogeneity underscores the importance of personalized medicine in cancer patients.

REFERENCES

1. Clarke MF, Dick JE, Dirks PB, et al. Cancer stem cells—perspectives on current status and future directions: AACR Workshop on cancer stem cells. *Cancer Res*. 2006;66(19):9339-9344.
2. Kim NW, Piatyszek MA, Prowse KR, et al. Specific association of human telomerase activity with immortal cells and cancer. *Science*. 1994;266(5193):2011-2015.
3. Sell S. On the stem cell origin of cancer. *Am J Pathol*. 2010;176(6):2584-2594.
4. Virchow R. Editorial. *Virchows Arch Pathol Anat Physiol Klin Med*. 1855;8:23-54.
5. Houghton JM, Morozov A, Smirnova I, Wang TC. Stem cells and cancer. *Semin Cancer Biol*. 2007;17:191-205.
6. Classics of oncology: Peyton Rous (1879–1970). *CA Cancer J Clin*. January-February 1972;22(1):21-22.
7. Knudson AG. Mutation and cancer: statistical study of retinoblastoma. *Proc Natl Acad Sci U S A*. 1971;68(4):820-823.
8. Nowell PC. The clonal evolution of tumor cell populations. *Science*. 1976;194:23-28.
9. Till JE, McCulloch EA. A direct measurement of the radiation sensitivity of normal mouse bone marrow mouse cells. *Radiat Res*. 1961;14:213-222.
10. Kliensmith LJ, Pierce GB Jr. Multipotentiality of single embryonal carcinoma cells. *Cancer Res*. 1964;24:1544-1551.
11. Pierce GB, Speers WC. Tumors as caricatures of the process of tissue renewal: prospects for therapy by directing differentiation. *Cancer Res*. 1988;48:1996-2004.
12. Lapidot T, Sirard C, Vormoor J, et al. A cell initiating human acute myeloid leukaemia after transplantation into SCID mice. *Nature*. 1994;367(6464):645-648.
13. Bonnet D, Dick JE. Human acute myeloid leukemia is organized as a hierarchy that originates from a primitive hematopoietic cell. *Nat Med*. 1997;3(7):730-737.
14. Fialkow PJ, Singer JW, Raskind WH, et al. Clonal development, stem-cell differentiation, and clinical remissions in acute non-lymphocytic leukemia. *N Engl J Med*. August 1987;317(8):468-473.
15. Najfeld V, Zucker-Franklin D, Adamson J, Singer J, Troy K, Fialkow PJ. Evidence for clonal development and stem cell origin of M7 megakaryocytic leukemia. *Leukemia*. 1988;2(6):351-357.

16. Al-Hajj M, Wicha MS, Benito-Hernandez A, Morrison SJ, Clarke MF. Prospective identification of tumorigenic breast cancer cells. *Proc Natl Acad Sci U S A*. 2003;100(7):3983-3988.
17. Singh SK, Hawkins C, Clarke ID, et al. Identification of human brain tumour initiating cells. *Nature*. 2004;432(7015):396-401.
18. Dalerba P, Dylla SJ, Park IK, et al. Phenotypic characterization of human colorectal cancer stem cells. *Proc Natl Acad Sci U S A*. 2007;104(24):10158-10163.
19. Liu LL, Fu D, Ma Y, Shen X. The power and the promise of liver cancer stem cell markers. *Stem Cells Dev*. December 2011;20(12): 2023-2030.
20. Kim CF, Jackson EL, Woolfenden AE, et al. Identification of bronchioalveolar stem cells in normal lung and lung cancer. *Cell*. 2005;121(6):823-835.
21. Lawson DA, Xin L, Lukacs R, Xu Q, Cheng D, Witte ON. Prostate stem cells and prostate cancer. *Cold Spring Harb Symp Quant Biol*. 2005;70:187-196.
22. Wicha S, Suling Liu, Dontu G. Cancer stem cells: an old idea—a paradigm shift. *Cancer Res*. 2006;66:1883-1890.
23. Ratajczak MZ, Kucia M, Dobrowolska H, Wanzeck J, Reca R, Ratajczak J. Emerging concept of cancer as a stem cell disorder. *Cent Eur J Biol*. 2006;1(1):73-87.
24. Jamieson CH, Ailles LE, Dylla SJ. Granulocyte macrophage progenitors as candidate leukemic stem cells in blast crisis. *N Engl J Med. 2004*;351:657-667.
25. Cozzio A, Passegué E, Ayton PM, Karsunky H, Cleary ML, Weissman IL. Similar MLL-associated leukemias arising from self-*renewing stem* cells and short-lived myeloid progenitors. *Genes Dev*. 2003;17(24):3029-3035.
26. Ricci-Vitiani L, Lombardi DG, Pilozzi E, et al. Identification and expansion of human colon-cancer-initiating cells. *Nature*. 2007;445(7123):111-115.
27. Collins AT, Berry PA, Hyde C, Stower MJ, Maitland NJ. Prospective identification of tumorigenic prostate cancer stem cells. *Cancer Res*. 2005;65(23):10946-10951.
28. Hemmati HD, Nakano I, Lazareff JA, et al. Cancerous stem cells can arise from pediatric brain tumors. *Proc Natl Acad Sci U S A*. 2003;100(25):15178-15183.
29. Dontu G, El-Ashry D, Wicha MS. Breast cancer, stem/progenitor cells and the estrogen receptor. *Trends Endocrinol Metab*. 2004; 15(5):193-197.
30. Houghton J, Stoicov C, Nomura S, et al. Gastric cancer originating from bone marrow-derived cells. *Science*. 2004; 306(5701):1568-1571.
31. Cao H, Xu W, Qian H, et al. Mesenchymal stem cell-like cells derived from human gastric cancer tissues. *Cancer Lett*. February 2009;274(1):61-71.
32. Hutchinson L, Stenstrom B, Chen D, et al. Human Barrett's adenocarcinoma of the esophagus, associated myofibroblasts, and endothelium can arise from bone marrow-derived cells after allogeneic stem cell transplant. *Stem Cells Dev*. 2011;20(1): 11-17.
33. Avital I, Moreira AL, Klimstra DS, et al. Donor-derived human bone marrow cells contribute to solid organ cancers developing after bone marrow transplantation. *Stem Cells*. 2007;25(11):2903-2909.
34. Hollier BG, Evans K, Mani SA. The epithelial-to-mesenchymal transition and cancer stem cells: a coalition against cancer therapies. *J Mammary Gland Biol Neoplasia*. 2009;14(1): 29-43.
35. Mani SA, Guo W, Liao MJ, et al. The epithelial-mesenchymal transition generates cells with properties of stem cells. *Cell*. 2008;133(4):704-715.
36. Li C, Heidt DG, Dalerba P, et al. Identification of pancreatic cancer stem cells. *Cancer Res*. 2007;67:1030-1037.
37. Wu C, Alman BA. Side population cells in human cancers. *Cancer Lett*. 2008;268(1):1-9.
38. Williams A, Datar R, Cote R. Technologies and methods used for detection, enrichment and characterization of cancer stem cells. *Natl Med J India*. 2010;23(6):346-350.
39. Dhingra S, Feng W, Brown RE, et al. Clinicopathologic significance of putative stem cell markers, CD44 and nestin, in gastric adenocarcinoma. *Int J Clin Exp Pathol*. 2011;4(8):733-741.
40. Song Z, Yue W, Wei B, et al. Sonic hedgehog pathway is essential for maintenance of cancer stem-like cells in human gastric cancer. *PLoS One*. 2011;6(3):e17687.
41. Vescovi AL, Galli R, Reynolds BA. Brain tumour stem cells. *Nat Rev Cancer*. 2006;6(6):425-436.
42. Lenkiewicz M, Li N, Singh SK. Culture and isolation of brain tumor initiating cells. *Curr Protoc Stem Cell Biol*. 2009;chap 3: unit 3.3.
43. Stingl J. Detection and analysis of mammary gland stem cells. *J Pathol*. 2009; 217:229-241.
44. Moraes RC, Zhang X, Harrington N, et al. Constitutive activation of smoothened (SMO) in mammary glands of transgenic mice leads to increased proliferation, altered differentiation and ductal dysplasia. *Development*. 2007;134(6):1231-1242.
45. Quintana E, Shackleton M, Sabel MS, et al. Efficient tumour formation by single human melanoma cells. *Nature*. December 2008;456(7222):593-598.
46. Zweidler-McKay PA. Notch signaling in pediatric malignancies. *Curr Oncol Rep*. 2008;10(6):459-468.
47. Klinakis A, Lobry C, Abdel-Wahab O, et al. A novel tumour-suppressor function for the Notch pathway in myeloid leukaemia. *Nature*. May 2011;473(7346):230-233.
48. Takebe N, Harris PJ, Warren RQ, Ivy SP. Targeting cancer stem cells by inhibiting Wnt, Notch, and Hedgehog pathways. *Nat Rev Clin Oncol*. 2011;8(2):97-106.
49. Gupta S, Takebe N, Lorusso P. Targeting the Hedgehog pathway in cancer. *Ther Adv Med Oncol*. 2010;2(4):237-250.
50. Burness ML, Sipkins DA. The stem cell niche in health and malignancy. *Semin Cancer Biol*. 2010;20(2):107-115.
51. Spradling A, Drummond-Barbosa D, Kai T. Stem cells find their niche. *Nature*. 2001;414:98-104.
52. Schofield R. The relationship between the spleen colony-forming cell and the haemopoietic stem cell. *Blood Cells*. 1978;4:7-25.
53. Deng W, Lin H. Spectrosomes and fusomes anchor mitotic spindles during asymmetric germ cell divisions and facilitate the formation of a polarized microtubule array for oocyte specification in Drosophila. *Dev Biol*. 1997;189(1):79-94.
54. Decotto E, Spradling AC. The Drosophila ovarian and testis stem cell niches: similar somatic stem cells and signals. *Dev Cell*. 2005;9(4):501-510.
55. Xie T, Spradling AC. A niche maintaining germ line stem cells in the Drosophila ovary. *Science*. 2000;290(5490):328-330.
56. Iwasaki H, Suda T. Cancer stem cells and their niche. *Cancer Sci*. 2009;100(7):1166-1172.
57. Ding L, Saunders TL, Enikolopov G, Morrison SJ. Endothelial and perivascular cells maintain haematopoietic stem cells. *Nature*. January 2012;481(7382):457-462.
58. Li L, Neaves WB. Normal stem cells and cancer stem cells: the niche matters. *Cancer Res*. May 2006;66(9):4553-4557.
59. Krause DS, Lazarides K, von Andrian UH, Van Etten RA. Requirement for CD44 in homing and engraftment of BCR-ABL-expressing leukemic stem cells. *Nat Med*. 2006;12(10):1175-1180.
60. Bendall LJ, Kirkness J, Hutchinson A, et al. Antibodies to CD44 enhance adhesion of normal CD34+ cells and acute myeloblastic but not lymphoblastic leukaemia cells to bone marrow stroma. *Br J Haematol*. 1997;98(4):828-837.
61. Calabrese C, Poppleton H, Kocak M, et al. A perivascular niche for brain tumor stem cells. *Cancer Cell*. 2007;11(1):69-82.
62. Braun KM, Prowse DM. Distinct epidermal stem cell compartments are maintained by independent niche microenvironments. *Stem Cell Rev*. 2006;2(3):221-231.
63. Youssef KK, Van Keymeulen A, Lapouge G, et al. Identification of the cell lineage at the origin of basal cell carcinoma. *Nat Cell Biol*. 2010;12(3):299-305.
64. Girouard SD, Murphy GF. Melanoma stem cells: not rare, but well done. *Lab Invest*. May 2011;91(5):647-664.
65. Brittan M, Wright NA. Gastrointestinal stem cells. *J Pathol*. 2002;197:492-509.
66. Kim KM, Shibata D. Methylation reveals a niche: stem cell succession in human colon crypts. *Oncogene*. 2002;21(35): 5441-5449.
67. Borovski T, De Sousa E Melo F, Vermeulen L, Medema JP. Cancer stem cell niche: the place to be. *Cancer Res*. 2011;71(3):634-639.
68. Leedham SJ, Thliveris AT, Halberg RB, Newton MA, Wright NA. Gastrointestinal stem cells and cancer: bridging the molecular gap. *Stem Cell Rev*. 2005;1(3):233-241.

69. Ehtesham M, Mapara KY, Stevenson CB, Thompson RC. R4 mediates the proliferation of glioblastoma progenitor cells. *Cancer Lett*. 2009;274(2):305-312.
70. Logothetis CJ, Lin SH. Osteoblasts in prostate cancer metastasis to bone. *Nature Rev*. 2005;5:21-28.
71. Soltanian S, Matin MM. Cancer stem cells and cancer therapy. *Tumour Biol*. 2011;32(3):425-440.
72. Chuthapisith S, Eremin J, El-Sheemey M, Eremin O. Breast cancer chemoresistance: emerging importance of cancer stem cells. *Surg Oncol*. 2010;19(1):27-32.
73. Van Stijn A, van der Pol MA, Kok A, et al. Differences between the CD34+ and CD34- blast compartments in apoptosis resistance in acute myeloid leukemia. *Haematologica*. 2003;88(5): 497-508.
74. Bao S, Wu Q, McLendon RE, et al. Glioma stem cells promote radioresistance by preferential activation of the DNA damage response. *Nature*. 2006;444(7120):756-760.
75. Choi S, Ku JL. Resistance of colorectal cancer cells to radiation and 5-FU is associated with MELK expression. *Biochem Biophys Res Commun*. 2011;412(2):207-213.
76. Diehn M, Cho RW, Lobo NA, et al. Association of reactive oxygen species levels and radioresistance in cancer stem cells. *Nature*. 2009;458(7239):780-783.
77. Wang J, Wakeman TP, Lathia JD, et al. Notch promotes radioresistance of glioma stem cells. *Stem Cells*. 2010;28(1):17-28.
78. Campos B, Wan F, Farhadi M, et al. Differentiation therapy exerts antitumor effects on stem-like glioma cells. *Clin Cancer Res*. 2010;16(10):2715-2728.
79. Piccirillo SG, Reynolds BA, Zanetti N, et al. Bone morphogenetic proteins inhibit the tumorigenic potential of human brain tumour-initiating cells. *Nature*. 2006;444(7120):761-765.
80. Munster PN, Troso-Sandoval T, Rosen N, Rifkind R, Marks PA, Richon VM. The histone deacetylase inhibitor suberoylanilide hydroxamic acid induces differentiation of human breast cancer cells. *Cancer Res*. 2001;61(23):8492-8497.
81. Medema JP, Vermeulen L. Microenvironmental regulation of stem cells in intestinal homeostasis and cancer. *Nature*. 2011;474:318-326.
82. Chen J, Kesari S, Rooney C, et al. Inhibition of Notch signaling blocks growth of glioblastoma cell lines and tumor neurospheres. *Genes Cancer*. August 2010;1(8):822-835.
83. Kuhnert F, Kirshner JR, Thurston G. Dll4-Notch signaling as a therapeutic target in tumor angiogenesis. *Vasc Cell*. 2011;3(1):20.
84. Chen B, Dodge ME, Tang W, et al. Small molecule-mediated disruption of Wnt-dependent signaling in tissue regeneration and cancer. *Nat Chem Biol*. 2009;5(2):100-107.
85. Emami KH, Nguyen C, Ma H, et al. A small molecule inhibitor of beta-catenin/CREB-binding protein transcription [corrected]. *Proc Natl Acad Sci U S A*. 2004;101(34):12682-12687.
86. Alison MR, Lim SM, Nicholson LJ. Cancer stem cells: problems for therapy? *J Pathol*. 2011;223(2):147-161.
87. Von Hoff DD, LoRusso PM, Rudin CM, et al. Inhibition of the hedgehog pathway in advanced basal-cell carcinoma. *N Engl J Med*. 2009;361(12):1164-1172.
88. Rudin CM, Hann CL, Laterra J, et al. Treatment of medulloblastoma with hedgehog pathway inhibitor GDC-0449. *N Engl J Med*. 2009;361(12):1173-1178.
89. Fan F, Schimming A, Jaeger D, Podar K. Targeting the tumor microenvironment: focus on angiogenesis. *J Oncol*. 2012;2012: 281261.
90. Ritter E, Perry A, Yu J, Wang T, Tang L, Bieberich E. Breast cancer cell-derived fibroblast growth factor 2 and vascular endothelial growth factor are chemoattractants for bone marrow stromal stem cells. *Ann Surg*. February 2008;247(2): 310-314.
91. Folkins C, Man S, Xu P, Shaked Y, Hicklin DJ, Kerbel RS. Anticancer therapies combining antiangiogenic and tumor cell cytotoxic effects reduce the tumor stem-like cell fraction in glioma xenograft tumors. *Cancer Res*. April 2007;67(8): 3560-3564.
92. Jakubikova J, Adamia S, Kost-Alimova M, et al. Lenalidomide targets clonogenic side population in multiple myeloma: pathophysiologic and clinical implications. *Blood*. April 2011;117(17):4409-4419.
93. Mukherjee S, Raje N, Schoonmaker JA, et al. Pharmacologic targeting of a stem/progenitor population in vivo is associated with enhanced bone regeneration in mice. *J Clin Invest*. February 2008;118(2):491-504.
94. Qiang YW, Hu B, Chen Y, et al. Bortezomib induces osteoblast differentiation via Wnt-independent activation of beta-catenin/TCF signaling. *Blood*. April 2009;113(18):4319-4330.
95. Gadhoum Z, Delaunay J, Maquarre E, et al. The effect of anti-CD44 monoclonal antibodies on differentiation and proliferation of human acute myeloid leukemia cells. *Leuk Lymphoma*. 2004;45(8):1501-1510.
96. Charrad RS, Gadhoum Z, Qi J, et al. Effects of anti-CD44 monoclonal antibodies on differentiation and apoptosis of human myeloid leukemia cell lines. *Blood*. 2002;99(1):290-299.
97. Ginestier C, Hur MH, Charafe-Jauffret E, et al. ALDH1 is a marker of normal and malignant human mammary stem cells and a predictor of poor clinical outcome. *Cell Stem Cell*. 2007;1(5):555-567.
98. Korkaya H, Paulson A, Iovino F, Wicha MS. HER2 regulates the mammary stem/progenitor cell population driving tumorigenesis and invasion. *Oncogene*. 2008;27(47):6120-6130.
99. Shackleton M, Quintana E, Fearon ER, Morrison SJ. Heterogeneity in cancer: cancer stem cells versus clonal evolution. *Cell*. 2009;138(5):822-829.

CHAPTER 3

CELL SIGNAL TRANSDUCTION

Markus Morkel

INTRODUCTION

Cell signal transduction molecules transmit extracellular or intracellular information in order to initiate an appropriate cellular response. Extracellular information is generally presented in the form of signaling molecules, i.e., growth factor ligands, which can bind to corresponding receptors displayed on the surface or contained within the cytoplasm of the signal-receiving cell. Autocrine, paracrine and endocrine signals originate from within the signal-receiving cell, from a neighboring cell, or from a remote source, respectively.

In general, binding of a ligand to its cognate receptor initiates a cellular response that is specific for the type of the receptor and often involves alteration of the activities of enzymes and other signaling molecules, which interact in order to change conformation, subcellular localization, covalent modification, stability, concentration, or integrity. A series of signaling molecules that commonly relay specific signals are referred to as cell signaling pathways or cell signaling cascades; however, such pathways rarely display a linear relationship between the signal-initiating ligand/receptor pair and the cellular response generated. Activities of signaling pathways are almost invariably amplified or impaired by molecular interactions within the pathway or between interlaced pathways (i.e., by pathway cross-talk). Feedback inhibition is a widely used mechanism to attenuate signal transduction during sustained ligand/receptor interaction. Ultimately, signaling pathways converge on transcription factors (TFs) that control the activity of sets of target genes or on other cellular regulators that are independent of transcription. Different cell types will respond to an equivalent signal in alternate manners, since the quality of response is determined by the presence and the concentrations of specific receptors, signaling molecules, and TFs. In addition, the epigenetic status of the genome within the cell may command the utilization of specific sets of target genes.

In the untransformed cell, the integrity of the signal transduction apparatus ensures an appropriate cellular response to extracellular and intracellular cues, resulting in precise regulation of cellular responses such as proliferation, differentiation, morphology, metabolism, and apoptosis. Strict regulation of these processes ensures tissue homeostasis and organ integrity. In the tumor cell, however, mutations in genes coding for signal transducers and TFs can alter the normal cellular signal transduction and response. Such mutations can be either inherited, resulting in tumor predisposition, or somatic (i.e., arise through spontaneous events in the tumor-initiating cell), resulting in the formation of sporadic cancers. Often, a combination of both inherited and sporadic somatic mutations is required to inactivate both functional alleles of a recessive tumor suppressor.[1] In addition, large-scale genomic copy number alterations (i.e., deletion or amplification of parts of the genome) and disturbed epigenetic control (i.e., hypo- and hypermethylation of genomic DNA or alterations in the histone code) contribute to the untimely expression or loss of signal transducers or TFs. This ultimately results in inappropriate modulation of target gene activity in tumor cells. As a consequence of these alterations in signaling networks, cell and tissue homeostasis are gradually compromised during tumor progression (for seminal reviews, see references 2-4).

This chapter catalogs common pathways and themes in normal signal transduction, while the subsequent chapters on oncogenes and tumor suppressors focus on common aberrations found in tumor cells. The functions of many genes implicated in cell signal transduction have been studied in mice and other model organisms. Due to space constraints, only selected informative mouse models are referenced in this chapter; further in-depth information on all mutants can be obtained via the Mouse Genome Informatics database (http://www.informatics.jax.org/).

CELL SIGNALING PATHWAYS

Receptor Tyrosine Kinase Signaling

Receptor tyrosine kinases (RTKs) comprise a superfamily of transmembrane receptors that regulate almost every aspect of cellular activity and of superordinate function during organ development and homeostasis (Figs. 3.1 and 3.2).[5] RTK signals are crucial for controlling cell proliferation, for maintaining the balance between cell adhesion and motility, for proper cell positioning within an organ, and for regulating cellular differentiation. RTKs are composed of an N-terminal extracellular growth factor–binding domain and a C-terminal intracellular tyrosine kinase domain. The extracellular growth factor–binding domain shows family-specific architecture and often contains diverse structural repeat elements, including for instance cadherin domains, leucine-rich domains, and fibronectin-like domains, which are the basis for specificity of the ligand–receptor interaction. The intracellular C-terminal cytoplasmic receptor domain has intrinsic tyrosine kinase activity. Binding of a growth factor ligand to an RTK induces receptor dimerization and/or conformational changes and invariably leads to autophosphorylation of tyrosine residues on the intracellular domain. Phosphorylated tyrosine residues are interpreted via cytoplasmic adaptor molecules such as GRB/SOS proteins, which link RTKs to downstream signaling cascades. The approximately 20 families of RTKs contain among them the epidermal growth factor (EGF), fibroblast growth factor (FGF), hepatocyte growth factor (HGF), vascular endothelial growth factor (VEGF), and platelet-derived growth factor receptors and Ephrin receptors.

EGF signals are transduced by four receptors encoded by the *EGFR/HER1*, *ERBB2/HER2/NEU*, *ERBB3*, and *ERBB4* genes, all of which provide essential proliferative and morphogenetic cues during development and adult organ homeostasis. Gene deletion studies in the mouse have shown that loss of *Egfr* results in the malformation of multiple epithelia during embryonic development.[6,7] Oncogenic deregulation of EGF signals by overexpression or mutation of receptors is a frequent event in the initiation and progression of many tumors, for instance in ERBB2-positive mammary carcinoma,[8] and studies in

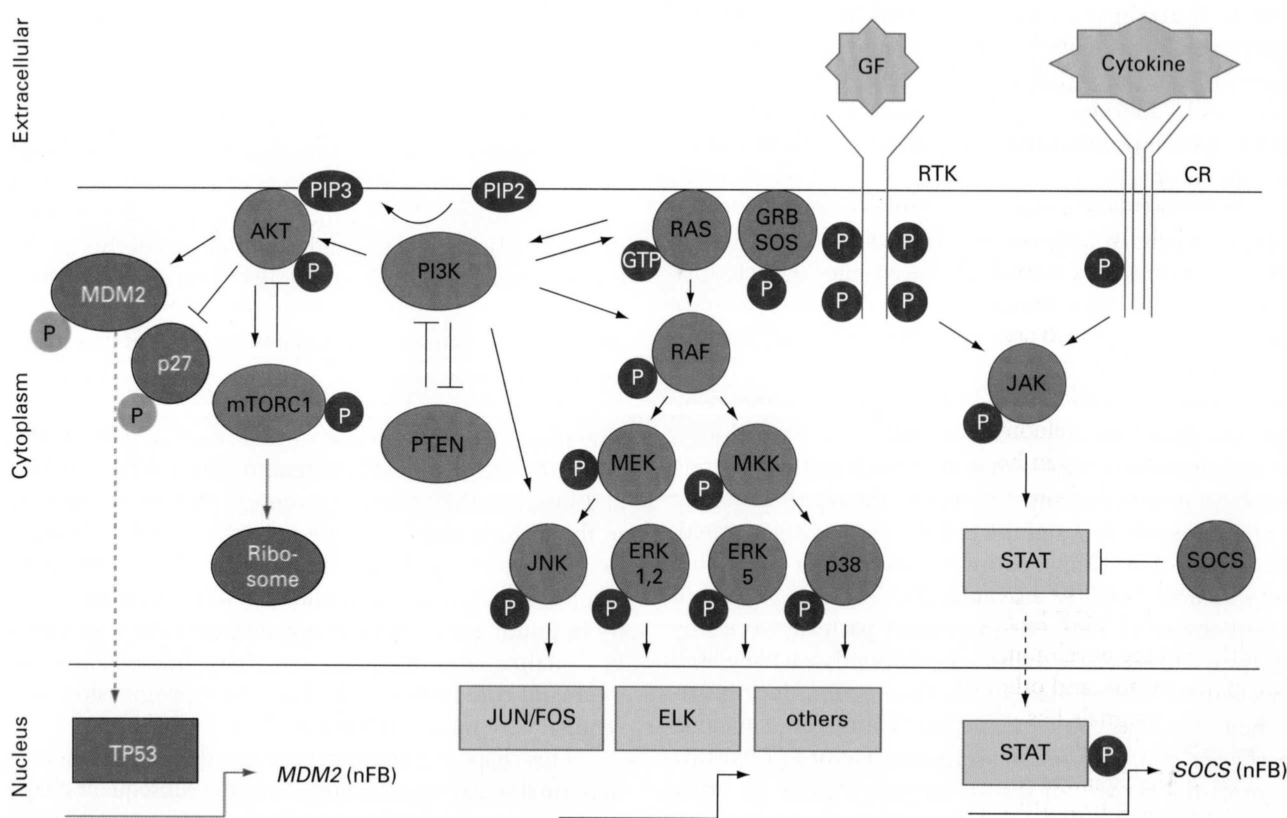

FIGURE 3–1 Key players and molecular interactions in the RTK, MAPK, PI3K, and JAK/STAT pathways. CR: Cytokine receptor. Common color scheme for all figures: Ligands are in yellow; transmembrane receptors in red; signal transducers in blue; hormones in purple; TFs in green. Key interactions peripheral to the core pathway are in brown or in light colors. Full arrows: molecular interactions; dashed arrows: translocations. Key covalent modifications or small signaling molecules are indicated by dark blue circles: P, phosphorylation; GTP, guanosine triphosphate binding; Ubi, ubiquitinylation. Only target genes that constitute negative feedback (nFB) loops are given. For further information and abbreviations, see main text and references therein.

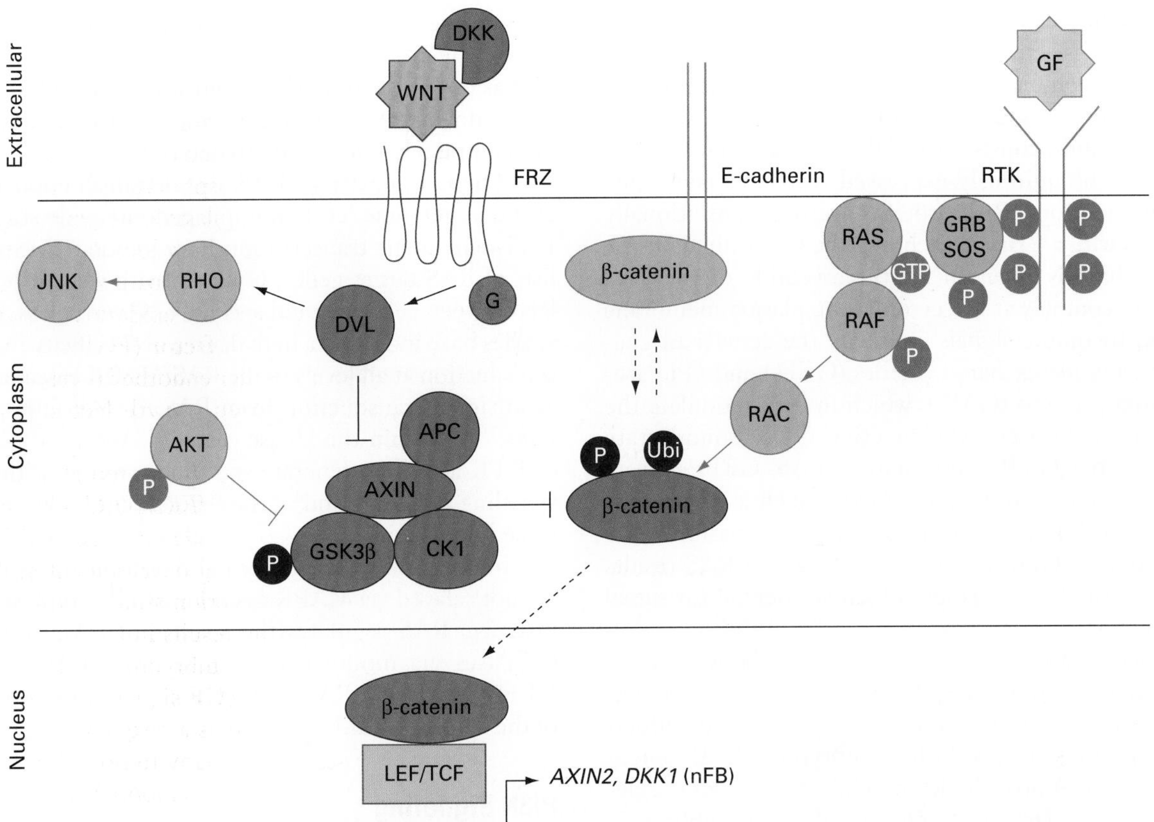

FIGURE 3–2 Key players and molecular interactions in the canonical Wnt signaling cascade. For symbol references, see Fig. 3.1. The target genes *AXIN2* and *DKK1* constitute negative feedback loops. For a more complete list of pathway components, target genes, and references, see http://www.stanford.edu/group/nusselab/cgi-bin/wnt/. For further information and molecule abbreviations, see main text and references therein.

mice have shown that mutations are causative for tumor formation.[9,10]

FGF signaling is initiated by the binding of FGF ligands (a family comprising of 22 ligands in mouse and man) to one of four cognate FGF receptors in either an autocrine or paracrine manner. FGF receptors have various splice forms, which are able to mediate the signal with different ligand specificities. FGF signals mainly regulate cell motility, proliferation, and differentiation during early embryonic development, as well as during organogenesis and adult organ homeostasis. Deletion studies in the mouse have indicated that the first requirement for FGF signals is in the development of embryonic mesoderm, as inactivation of *Fgf8*, or the gene coding for its high-affinity receptor *Fgfr3*, results in the disruption of gastrulation.[11,12] FGF ligands and receptors have further functions in the development of the skeleton, vasculature, intestine, gonads, and other organs, and untimely activation of FGF signals has often been implicated in cancer development.[13]

HGF, the ligand of the MET receptor, initiates a proliferative and cell motility signal, which is essential for embryonic development and wound healing. HGF/MET signals regulate muscle cell precursor migration during embryonic development, and activated MET signals have been shown to confer migratory, i.e., prometastatic, traits to tumor cells.[14]

VEGFs comprise a family of five ligands, which initiate signals via VEGF receptors, a family of three receptors with multiple isoforms. VEGFs often act in a paracrine manner to regulate the proliferation of adjacent endothelial cells, and thus provide key angiogenic and vasculogenic signals during development, in the adult and in disease[15]; however, they have many functions beyond regulation of vascularization.

Due to their key roles in initiating signals essential for proliferation, motility, differentiation, and apoptosis, many RTKs and their downstream signal transducers are among the prime targets for selective antitumor drug development. Generally, RTK signals activate complex downstream transduction cascades. Among these, the mitogen-activated protein kinase (MAPK) and the phosphatidylinositol 3-kinase (PI3K) cascades are prominent; however, RTK signal transduction can also result in the activation or repression of a multitude of other signaling pathways.

MAPK Signaling

The multiple branches of the intracellular MAPK cascades represent central signaling relays for RTK signals (see Fig. 3.1). Generally, specific phosphorylation of tyrosine residues located at the intracellular domain of RTKs initiates the phosphorylation and activation of an adaptor complex composed of GRB and SOS proteins, which induces activity of small GTPases associated with the adaptor complex. An important cytoplasmic family of GTPases for transduction of RTK signals is the RAS (*Ra*t *s*arcoma) family, consisting of HRAS, NRAS, and KRAS, which are ubiquitously expressed, yet have cell type–specific functions. RAS proteins are posttranslationally modified with a farnesyl anchor at the C-terminal CAAX motif, which is essential for the assembly of the RAS signaling complex at the cytoplasmic plasma membrane surface. Incoming signals modulate the activity of guanine nucleotide exchange factors (GEFs) and GTPase-activating proteins (GAPs), which in turn modulate the equilibrium between the inactive GDP-bound state and the active GTP-bound state of RAS. GEFs activate signal transmission, whereas GAPs, such as the tumor suppressor NF1, inactivate signal transmission. The conversion of GDP-bound to GTP-bound RAS results in a conformational change, which is essential for signal transduction.

There is a high degree of specificity between individual members of the RAS GTPase family. For instance, deletion of *Kras* in the mouse compromises proliferation of various tissues during embryonic development and leads to embryonic death, while homozygous deletion of *Nras* or *Hras* does not cause abnormal embryonic development or apparent adult phenotypes.[16] Due to their central, and limiting, roles in MAPK signal transduction, RAS proteins underlie the formation of multiple human heritable diseases[17] and are important proto-oncogenes. Oncogenic forms arise mainly by mutations that inhibit the intrinsic GTPase function and thus interfere with their return to the inactive conformation.[18] A large body of evidence has been collected that substantiates a causative role for *RAS* oncogenes in the formation and progression of many types of cancer.[19] Indeed, activating mutations in the *KRAS*, *HRAS*, and *NRAS* genes are the most frequent mutations found in human solid tumors and also cause tumors when introduced into the mouse.[20,21]

MAP kinase cascades are classically comprised of three serially ordered cytoplasmic kinases encoded by the *MAP3K*, *MAP2K*, and *MAPK* genes belonging, for instance, to the *RAF*, *MEK*, and *ERK* families. RAF kinases directly interact with RAS GTPases.[22] During mouse embryonic development, RAF kinases, encoded by the *Araf*, *Braf*, and *Craf* genes, are essential for the formation of a large number of tissues, including those arising from endothelial, hematopoietic, and neural lineages. Mice, which are compound-mutant for multiple *RAF* family genes, generally show more severe and earlier embryonic phenotypes as compared with single mutants, indicating functional overlap between RAF proteins. Mutated forms of *RAF* genes are also frequently found in tumors, usually in a mutually exclusive manner from mutated *RAS* oncogenes. Major MAPK cascades downstream of RAF and RAS are the ERK1/2, ERK5, JNK, and p38 cascades. Activities of MAPK cascades converge on multiple TFs, for instance JUN and FOS (which constitute the transcriptional-activating AP1 complex), as well as on ELK, SRF, MYC, and many others.[19] TF networks downstream of MAPK cascades are complex and not completely understood to date.

The complexity of RAS signal transduction recurs at the target gene level; multiple genome-wide studies of RAS-dependent transcription have generated extensive lists of RAS target genes, however, with very little overlap between cell types and species.[23] Nevertheless, recent studies have indicated a high degree of specificity in signal transduction at all levels of the RAS/MAPK cascade, such as in signal transduction from RAS to RAF family proteins,[24] or within the kinase cascades. Yet, how patterns of RTK activities generate specific responses within the signaling networks and in the regulation of TFs remains to be fully elucidated.

Importantly, RAS proteins also transduce signals that are not relayed via MAPK cascades to TF complexes. For instance, RAS regulates the activity of RAL and RAC GTPases via modulation of RAL- and RAC-specific GEFs.[25] RAL and RAC play central roles in remodeling of the cytoskeleton.[26]

PI3K Signaling

Another key signaling cascade downstream of RTKs and RAS,[27] as well as other receptors (such as G-protein-coupled receptors), is the PI3K signaling cascade, which regulates proliferation, metabolism, and cell survival (see Fig. 3.1).[28] PI3K complexes, along with the lipid phosphatase phosphatase and tensin homologue deleted on chromosome ten (PTEN), integrate multiple signals to modulate the conversion of the phosphatidylinositol phosphate PIP2 to PIP3 (phosphatidylinositol (3,4,5)-triphosphate) at the cell membrane. The second messenger PIP3 then activates downstream substrates, among which is the AKT kinase. AKT phosphorylates and inhibits key pro-apoptotic proteins, such as BAD and the p53 feedback inhibitor MDM2.[29,30] Consequently, AKT provides an important cell survival (anti-apoptotic) signal. The mammalian target of the immunosuppressant drug rapamycin (mTOR) is an important AKT substrate, which is able to control AKT activity by negative feedback.[31] Other AKT substrates are able to activate the cell cycle, increase glucose catabolism, and activate protein translation.

In the mouse, deletion of *Pten* or components of the PI3K complex, such as *Pik3ca*, results in embryonic lethality, with affected embryos displaying differentiation and apoptosis defects. Mice heterozygous for *Pten* develop multiple neoplasms as adults. A comparable *PTEN* haplodeficiency underlies human familial neoplastic diseases including Cowden syndrome.[32] Deletion of any of the AKT kinase genes *Akt1*, *Akt2*, or *Akt3* in the mouse results in viable offspring; however, these mice have several developmental defects and/or pathological phenotypes, suggesting imperfect control of cellular proliferation and apoptosis.

AKT-dependent as well as AKT-independent PI3K signals play important roles in tumor progression.[33] Likewise, PIP3-dependent and PIP3-independent functions have been described for PTEN, partly mediated by modulation of its subcellular localization. For instance, nuclear PTEN can interact and modulate activity of the TF p53.[34] In colon and other cancers, the PI3K/PTEN/AKT cascade is often found to be deregulated through mutations, for instance, those found in *PIK3CA* or *AKT*.[35,36]

JAK-STAT Signaling

A common event downstream of multiple receptors, including the cytokine receptors (such as interferon and interleukin receptors) and RTKs (such as EGFR), is the activation of Janus kinase (JAK)/signal transducer and activator of transcription (STAT) signaling (see Fig. 3.1). Ligand binding to such receptors leads to receptor dimerization or oligomerization, bringing bound JAK kinases in close approximation with one another. The resulting tyrosine transphosphorylation of JAKs allows STAT binding. STAT proteins are both TFs and JAK substrates. Single phosphorylation of STATs leads to dimerization, followed by nuclear transport and accumulation of STATs, where they bind to promoters of specific sets of target genes. Dephosphorylation of STATs by specific phosphatases and activities of the suppressor of cytokine signaling (SOCS) class of feedback inhibitors attenuates STAT signaling.[37,38] In mice, deletion of any of the three *Jak* genes results in defects in the hematopoietic, immune, and/or nervous system development, due to failure of cytokine signaling. Deletion of *Jak1* or *Jak2* is lethal, whereas *Jak3*-deficient mice have a severe combined immunodeficiency phenotype. Deletion of individual *Stat* genes results in diverse growth and differentiation defects and, in the case of *Stat1*, to an increase in tumor susceptibility.

Wnt Signaling

Wnt ligands comprise a large family of glycoproteins that control proliferation, stem cell–like properties, and cellular differentiation during gastrulation, organ development, and adult organ homeostasis. Wnt signaling can occur via the canonical Wnt/β-catenin pathway (Fig. 3.2) or via non-canonical pathways. In canonical Wnt signaling, extracellular Wnt morphogens bind to Frizzled receptors, which are transmembrane G-protein-coupled receptors. Signaling strength and specificity are, in many instances, modulated by co-ligands, such as R-Spondin (RSPO), co-receptors, such as the low-density lipoprotein receptors LRP5/6 and the G-protein-coupled receptors LGR4/5, as well as extracellular inhibitors, such as Dickkopf (DKK) and Frizbee (FRZB) proteins. Intracellularly, Wnt signals are transduced via the Dishevelled (DVL) family of phosphoproteins to the so-called β-catenin destruction complex, consisting of the CK1 and GSK3β kinases, AXIN1/2, and the adenomatous polyposis coli (APC) protein. Canonical Wnt signaling results in the inactivation of the β-catenin destruction complex and subsequent stabilization and nuclear translocation of β-catenin in a process that requires the RHO family GTPase RAC1.[39] In the nucleus, stabilized β-catenin is a co-activator of the LEF/TCF family of TFs, ultimately activating sets of target genes involved in cell cycle progression, stem cell maintenance, and/or cellular differentiation. Well-known Wnt target genes include *CCND1* and *MYC*, which control the cell cycle and cellular metabolism.[40,41] β-Catenin-mediated activation of the Wnt signal inhibitor genes *DKK1* and *AXIN2* provides negative feedback regulation. Non-canonical Wnt signal transduction cascades, such as the planar cell polarity pathway and Wnt-Ca^{2+} signaling via PLC, are also present in a cell context–dependent manner, but will not be discussed further here.[42]

Deletion of *Ctnnb1*, the gene coding for β-catenin, or of *Wnt3* in the mouse results in lack of mesoderm formation and thus arrest of development during gastrulation.[43,44] Deletion of other Wnt signaling components, as well as conditional knockout of *Ctnnb1* in various tissues, has led to the identification of roles for Wnt/β-catenin signals in the formation and/or maintenance of virtually all organs.[45] For instance, in the intestinal epithelium, Wnt signals induce several transcriptional programs essential for stem cell maintenance, cell proliferation, and differentiation into the Paneth cell lineage.[46] Experimental abrogation of intestinal Wnt signals consequently results in loss of stem cells, crypts, and intestinal epithelium.[47] In line with the key physiological role of Wnt in the control of the intestinal stem cell compartment, β-catenin hyperactivation, e.g., by mutational inactivation of *APC* or mutational activation of *CTNNB1*, results in hyperproliferation and intestinal tumor formation in mice.[48,49] Indeed, loss of heterozygosity of APC underlies the initiation of the majority of human colon cancers; therefore, this gene has been dubbed the "gatekeeper" of intestinal tumor formation.[50] Recent studies have indicated that β-catenin activity is further deregulated during colon cancer progression by stromal growth factor signals and KRAS activation.[51,52] It is important to note that β-catenin is not only the central signal transducer of the canonical Wnt signaling pathway but also a component of epithelial adherens junctions. Therefore, Wnt signals may not only indirectly, i.e., via transcriptional regulation, but also directly impinge on the structural integrity of epithelia.

Notch Signaling

Notch signals are also frequently involved in stem cell maintenance and the control of cellular differentiation (Fig. 3.3). Generally, Notch signals are transmitted between neighboring cells, since they require cell–cell

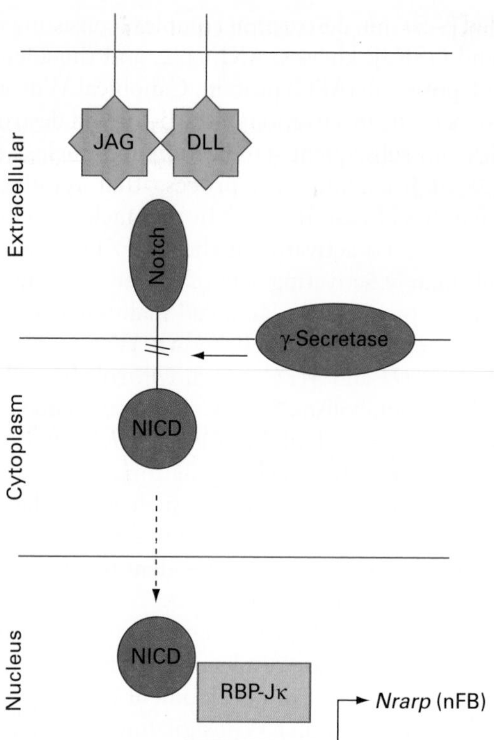

FIGURE 3–3 Key players in the Notch signaling cascade. For symbol references, see Fig. 3.1. For further information and molecule abbreviations, see main text and references therein.

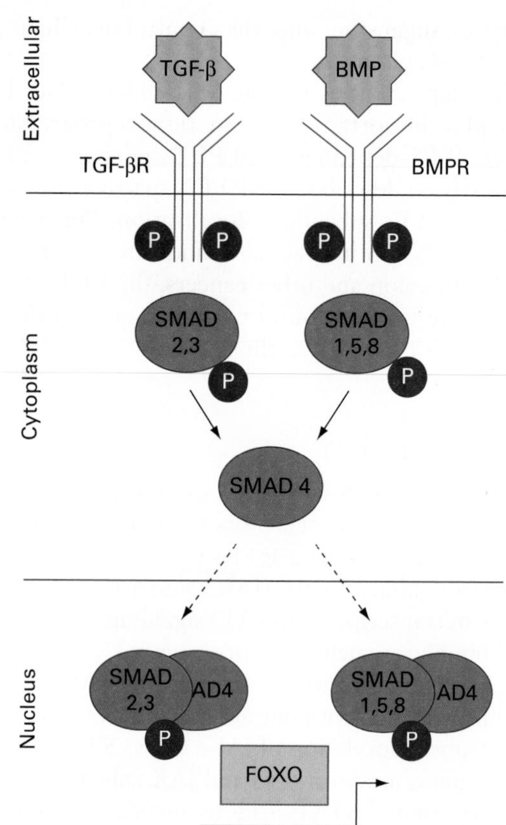

FIGURE 3–4 Key players in the TGF-β and BMP signaling cascades. For symbol references, see Fig. 3.1. For further information and molecule abbreviations, see main text and references therein.

interaction between the membrane-bound Delta (DLL) or Jagged (JAG) ligands and the (likewise membrane-bound) Notch receptor. Ligand binding to the receptor results in Notch receptor cleavage by γ-secretase or ADAM family proteases and the consequent release of the intracellular Notch intracellular domain (NICD). In the nucleus, the NICD acts as a co-activator for CSL/RBP-Jκ TF complexes, leading to the activation of general or tissue-specific target genes, such as *HES*, *HEY*, *NRARP*, and *MYC*. Since reception of the signal by the receptor-expressing cell generally results in inactivation of genes coding for Notch ligands, the pathway often acts in a "boundary-sharpening" manner between neighboring tissue compartments, for instance for somite formation during embryonic body axis elongation, or in the specification of neural tissue.[53] Gene knockout of *Notch1* in the mouse results in defects in somitogenesis and vasculature formation, while *Notch2* mutants display defects in neural and other tissues. In cooperation with Wnt, Notch signals control the stem cell compartment in the intestine and in other tissues. Due to its key role in specifying and maintaining stem cell compartments, the role of the Notch signaling pathway during tumor progression has recently received much attention.[54,55]

TGF-β Superfamily Signaling

Originally described as a novel growth factor that cooperated with EGF in cellular transformation, the transforming growth factor-β (TGF-β) family has been recognized as one of the fundamental controllers of cellular proliferation, differentiation, and apoptosis in embryogenesis and adult organ homeostasis (Fig. 3.4).[56] The TGF-β superfamily comprises TGF-β, growth and differentiation factor (GDF), and bone morphogenetic protein (BMP) ligands, which bind to cognate receptors that harbor serine–threonine kinase activity. Tetramerized receptors (composed of type I and type II receptor dimers) phosphorylate intracellular signal transducers termed SMADs. SMAD2 and SMAD3 transduce TGF-β and GDF signals, while SMAD1, SMAD5, and SMAD8 transduce BMP signals. These receptor-regulated SMADs (collectively termed R-SMADs) all dimerize with the common partner SMAD4 upon phosphorylation and shuttle to the nucleus, where they interact with various TF complexes, for example, FOXO factors. TGF-β signals in the mouse, for instance, through the ligand encoded by *Nodal*, play key roles in mesoderm and endoderm formation, as well as in specification of the embryonic anterior–posterior and left–right body axes. BMP signals likewise play roles in embryonic axis and mesoderm formation and have central roles in the formation of bones and neural tissue. Signals from the TGF-β family have complex and often opposing roles in the homeostasis of many organs in the adult, and misregulation of these signals can contribute to progression or suppression of many forms of cancer. For instance, in mammary cancer, TGF-β signals are mostly prometastatic, while in colon cancer TGF-β and BMP signals are instead tumor suppressive.[57]

Signaling by Nuclear Receptors

Nuclear receptors are zinc finger–containing TFs, whose activity is directly regulated through binding of an intracellular ligand (Fig. 3.5). Among the ligands for nuclear receptors are derivatives of vitamin D, vitamin A, estrogen, androgens, and glucocorticoids. In addition, many receptors with as yet unknown ligand specificity exist (termed orphan receptors). Upon ligand binding, nuclear receptors activate specific gene expression programs to control aspects of embryonic development, cell and organ metabolism, and immune functions. In line with this, mice deficient for certain nuclear receptors are resistant to the activity of the hormone ligand. For instance, male mice deficient for the androgen receptor gene (*Ar*) have neither male nor female reproductive organs. Mice deficient for the vitamin D receptor gene (*Vdr*) or retinoic acid receptor genes *Rara* and *Rarg* (either individually or in combination) display female or male sterility, respectively, in addition to other developmental defects that lead to low postnatal survival. An important example of nuclear receptor signaling in cancer is the progression of prostate cancer from androgen-sensitive to androgen-refractory disease. The former can be treated by androgen-deprivation therapy, while the latter is resistant to this form of therapy and incurable in most cases.[58]

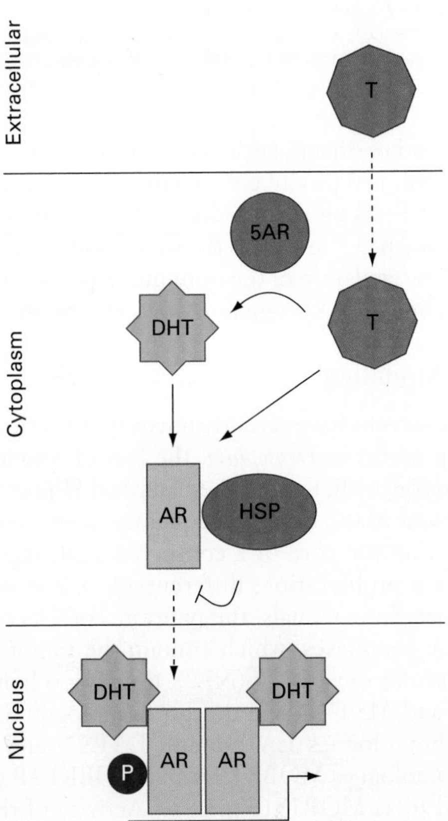

FIGURE 3–5 Androgen signaling as an archetype for the type I nuclear receptor signaling pathway. Testosterone (T) is intracellularly modified to dihydrotestosterone (DHT) by 5-alpha reductase (5AR), which exhibits greater receptor binding affinity than T. In the absence of ligand, the androgen receptor is bound and inactivated in the cytoplasm by heat shock proteins (HSP). For symbol references, see Fig. 3.1. For further information and molecule abbreviations, see main text and references therein.

Hedgehog Signaling

The Hedgehog signaling pathway controls many processes that contribute to embryonic organ development and adult organ homeostasis by regulating cell proliferation, stemness, and differentiation (Fig. 3.6). Hedgehog ligand production, modification, cleavage, and secretion are tightly regulated in the signal-emanating cell. Once secreted, Hedgehog ligands, such as SHH, build morphogen gradients. Secreted Hedgehog ligands bind to a receptor complex composed primarily of the 12-pass transmembrane receptor Patched (PTCH) and the G-protein-coupled receptor Smoothened (SMO). As a result, SMO is released from repression by PTCH and is able to release constitutive inactivation of the GLI family of transcriptional regulators. This is achieved by inactivation of the SUFU protease, which, in the absence of Hedgehog ligand binding, processes transcription-activating GLI factors into a shorter repressive form (GLI-R). As a net result, Hedgehog signals

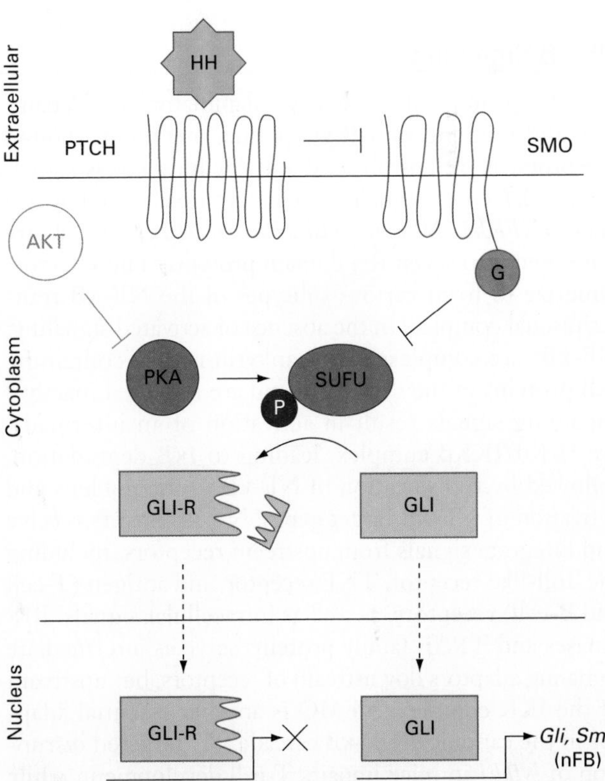

FIGURE 3–6 Key players in the Hedgehog signaling cascade. For symbol references, see Fig. 3.1. For further information and molecule abbreviations, see main text and references therein.

activate GLI-dependent genes. *SHH* and *GLI* genes themselves are among the GLI target genes, providing yet another level of regulation within the pathway. First discovered as a morphogenetic pathway in the fruit fly, many components of the Hedgehog pathway have been shown to be essential for proper tissue and organ formation in vertebrates.[59] During mouse development, deletion of any of the three mammalian ligands (termed Sonic [*Shh*], Indian [*Ihh*], and Desert [*Dhh*] Hedgehog) disrupts various morphogenetic processes. Heterozygous *Shh* mutants have shortened digits and other skeletal anomalies, while homozygous mutants die prenatally with more severe phenotypes. Deletion of *Ihh* likewise disrupts formation of the skeletal and nervous system, while deletion of *Dhh* causes skeletal and genital malformations. Similar to this, mutants for individual *Gli* genes or for *Smo* display skeletal, neural, and other developmental defects. Mutations in Hedgehog signaling components and deregulation of Hedgehog signaling also play important roles in cancer initiation and development; for instance, mutations in *PTCH* (leading to constitutive Smoothened signaling) underlie basal cell carcinoma syndromes and medulloblastoma. In this setting, as well as in normal tissue generation, Hedgehog also cross-talks with canonical Wnt/β-catenin signals.[60,61] Upregulation of Hedgehog ligand production is observed in several human cancers, such as brain, prostate, pancreas, and lung, and likely augments tumor growth through autocrine (tumor–tumor) and paracrine (tumor–stroma) signaling mechanisms.

NF-κB Signaling

NF-κB signaling integrates key inflammatory, DNA damage, and immune signals via plasma membrane–bound receptors, as well as physical and chemical stress signals (Fig. 3.7). Central signaling mediators are encoded by five genes (*NFKB1*, *NFKB2*, *REL*, *RELA*, *RELB*), which are translated into seven Rel domain proteins. These factors dimerize to form various subtypes of the NF-κB transcriptional complex. In the absence of activated signaling, NF-κBs are complexed with ankyrin repeat–containing IκB proteins in the cytoplasm and are rendered inactive. Incoming signals result in activation of an intermediate IKKα/IKKβ complex, leading to IκB degradation, followed by translocation of NF-κB to the nucleus and activation of NF-κB target genes. NF-κB factors receive and integrate signals from upstream receptors, including the Toll-like receptor, TNF receptor, and antigen (T-cell and B-cell) receptors, as well as intracellular signals. RIP kinases and TRAF family proteins serve as intermediate signaling adaptors downstream of receptors, but upstream of the IKK complex. NEMO is another essential adaptor in the canonical NF-κB cascade.[62,63] Targeted disruption of *Nfkb1* in mice impairs T-cell development, while *Rela* or *Nemo*-deficient mouse embryos die due to massive hepatic apoptosis. Development and maintenance of

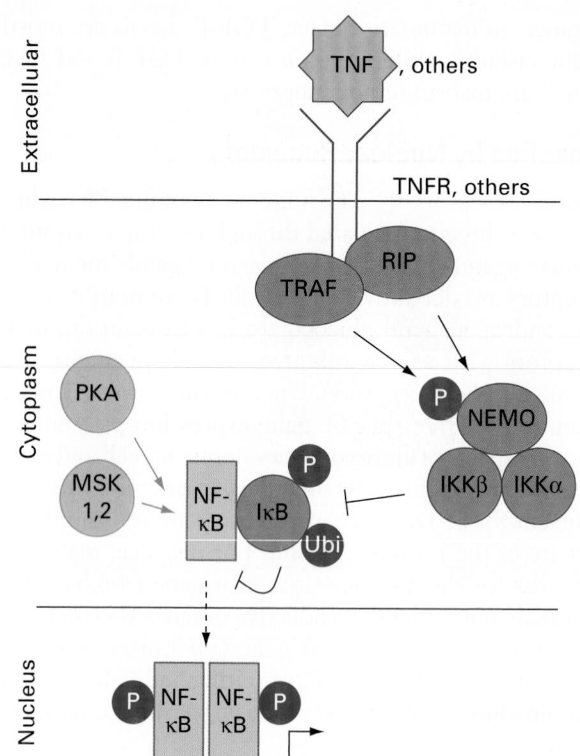

FIGURE 3–7 Key players in the NF-κB signaling cascade. For symbol references, see Fig. 1. For further information and molecule abbreviations, see main text and references therein.

multiple other organs, such as epidermis, spleen, and skeletal system, is typically compromised in mice with deletions of NF-κB signal transducers. Competition between NF-κB and p53,[64] as well as the well-documented roles for NF-κB in regulation of the immune response and inflammation, links NF-κB signaling to cancer progression.

Hippo Signaling

Genetic screens have recently uncovered a series of interacting proteins in *Drosophila*, the loss of which induced tissue overgrowth. Four of these, termed Hippo, Salvador, Warts, and Mats, have subsequently been identified as constituting the core of a conserved signaling pathway regulating proliferation, differentiation, and ultimately organ size. In mammals, the pathway consists of a series of kinase complexes, which contain the tumor suppressor Neurofibromatosis 2 (NF2), the Hippo homologues MST1 and MST2, the Salvador homologue SAV1, the Warts homologues LATS1 and LATS2, and the two Mats homologues MOBKL1A and MOBKL1B (together referred to as MOB1) (Fig.3.8).[65] Activity of the kinase complexes ultimately leads to phosphorylation and inactivation of the transcriptional co-activators YAP and TAZ. In a phosphorylated state, YAP and TAZ are bound in the cytoplasm to 14-3-3 proteins, while in a non-phosphorylated state they localize to the nucleus and activate a number of TFs, among these the TEAD1-4 factors.

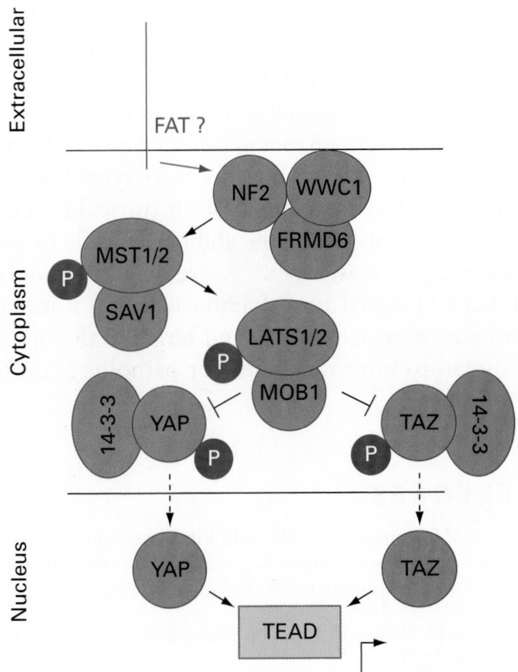

FIGURE 3–8 Key players in the mammalian Hippo pathway. For symbol references, see Fig. 3.1. For further information and molecule abbreviations, see main text and references therein.

Several studies in mice have demonstrated a conserved role for Hippo signals as central regulators of cell proliferation, differentiation, contact inhibition, and regulation of organ size. Liver-specific deletion of *Sav1*, *Mst1*, or *Mst2* in the mouse increased organ size and led to the formation of hepatocellular carcinoma. Overexpression of *Yap* in the liver induced a similar phenotype. These and other studies implicated components of the kinase complexes as tumor suppressors, while YAP and TAZ are considered oncogenes. Double *Yap/Taz* knockout mice die at the 16-cell morula stage, indicating that Hippo signals play a fundamental role from the start of cellular interactions. There is very little information available to date surrounding how Hippo signaling receives and integrates information. Recent papers have, however, reported cross-talk between Hippo and proliferative signals such as MAPK and STAT signals, morphogenetic pathways such as Wnt and Hedgehog,[66,67] and cell adhesion complexes. In Drosophila, atypical FAT-type cadherins are major upstream receptors for mediating contact inhibition; however, their mammalian homologues have not yet been studied in detail. Due to the identification of the known tumor suppressor NF2 as a component of the Hippo signaling cascade, and of YAP or TAZ overexpression in a variety of human tumors, the Hippo pathway has emerged as a focus point for recent tumor research. Indeed, animal and cell culture studies have recently linked Hippo signals via TAZ and YAP to anchorage-independent growth, invasiveness, epithelial-to-mesenchymal transition (EMT), and regulation of tumor stemness.[65,68]

CELLULAR RESPONSES

Signaling pathways, such as those sketched above, converge on cellular effectors that change cellular characteristics, such as the rates of proliferation and apoptosis or decisions to differentiate. In the process, gene expression profiles, protein repertoires, states of neighboring signaling pathways, epigenetic profiles, cellular metabolism, and contacts with surrounding cells are modified. To achieve this, signaling cascades ultimately control TFs, which activate and/or repress sets of target genes. Alternatively, some signal transducers can directly impinge on cellular activities in the absence of de novo transcription, for instance, by direct modulation of components of the cytoskeleton or cell adhesion complexes or by regulation of actuators of the cell cycle machinery. An important immediate response to certain signals is the induction of apoptosis, i.e., programmed cell death (for details, see Chapter 1). Most signals are, however, interpreted by inducing changes in RNA transcription.

The human genome encodes more than 1,500 TFs, which integrate signals in the nucleus to regulate cellular transcription of protein-coding mRNAs and diverse classes of non-coding RNAs.[69] TFs are overrepresented among proto-oncogenes, and mutations in TF genes are causative for a large proportion of heritable diseases. Activities of TFs are often regulated by ligand binding (e.g., nuclear receptors, see above), covalent modifications followed by nuclear translocation (e.g., STATs), complex formation with co-factors (e.g., β-catenin as a co-factor of LEF/TCF in Wnt signaling), or release from inhibitory complexes (e.g., IκB regulation of NF-κB). While major aspects of the human TF network have not been studied in detail to date, a small number of TFs have received a fair amount of attention due to their essential roles in the regulation of gene expression programs.

p53 (encoded by the *TP53* gene) integrates cellular stress responses such as DNA damage, hypoxia, oncogene activation, and loss of cell adhesion.[70] In unstressed cells, p53 stability and activity is restricted by the ubiquitin ligase MDM2. The *MDM2* gene, in turn, is a transcriptional target of p53, thereby constituting a negative feedback loop that controls p53 activity.[71] Upon cellular stress, MDM2 activity is restrained and p53 stabilized, either to induce cell cycle arrest allowing for genome repair or to activate apoptosis or senescence programs to eliminate the cell. Activated p53 has many (>100) target genes. In line with its central role in coordinating the cellular stress response, loss of *Tp53* causes early-onset tumors in multiple tissues in the mouse.[72] In contrast, mice with a hyperactive *Tp53* mutation are protected from tumors, but display phenotypes indicative of early aging.[73]

Snail (SNAI1) and SLUG belong to a family of zinc finger TFs that repress the expression of epithelial-specific genes in mesenchymal lineages, for instance *CHD1* that codes for the epithelial cell adhesion molecule E-cadherin. In many cell types, Snail family TFs can be activated by certain combinations of RTK, TGF-β, and Wnt signals. The collective activities of these factors can, therefore, result in the repression of epithelial and the induction of mesenchymal cellular traits—processes collectively known as epithelial-to-mesenchymal transition.[74] Coordinated induction of EMT is essential for proper embryonic development, for instance, during formation of mesoderm in the embryonic primitive streak during gastrulation. In the adult, complete or partial EMT is mostly associated with pathological conditions. For instance, loss of E-cadherin-based cell adhesion and the induction of cell motility are fundamental processes in tumor metastasis.

E2F and DP factors form heterodimers that bind to promoters of cell cycle–regulated genes and thereby control entry into the S-phase of the cell cycle. E2F/DP complexes activate cell cycle–specific genes, while trimeric complexes of E2F/DP and one of the so-called pocket proteins RB, p107, and p130 function as transcriptional repressors. Pocket protein activity, in turn, is controlled by cyclins and cyclin-dependent kinases. Since deregulation of cell cycle control is a key feature of many, if not all, tumors, genes coding for the cell cycle machinery upstream of E2F/DP are enriched for oncogenes and tumor suppressors, such as the oncogenes *CCND1* and *CDK4* and the tumor suppressors *RB* and *CDKN2A*(p16)/*INK4A*.[75,76] However, aside from mutations in the immediate cell cycle machinery, many of the signaling pathways described in the previous section target cell cycle regulators to exert their effects, among these the RTK, Wnt, and TGF-β signals.

MYC is a helix-loop-helix TF, which integrates many cellular signals to adapt proliferation and metabolism by binding to a multitude of genomic sites.[77] MYC is therefore a potent oncogene. The *MYC* gene is a transcriptional target of multiple pro-proliferative signaling pathways such as Wnt, JAK/STAT, and MAPK. Recent research has also identified TF-independent roles for MYC, such as in the direct regulation of protein synthesis.[78]

The hypoxia-inducible factor-1a (HIF1a) plays a key role in adapting cells to their environment. HIF1a is activated as part of the hypoxic and other stress responses and in turn induces the transcription of genes that control angiogenesis and cellular metabolism. Under normal oxygen conditions, HIF1a is targeted by the Von Hippel–Lindau tumor suppressor (VHL) complex and thereby earmarked for degradation. Under hypoxic conditions, e.g., in a growing tumor, HIF1a avoids VHL-mediated degradation and is stabilized. Activation of HIF1a target genes, such as *VEGF*, induces the formation of vasculature and therefore allows for growth of the tumor beyond limits set by existing blood vessels.[79]

In summary, cellular signaling cascades and TF activities control cellular activities during embryonic development and in adult body homeostasis. Oncogenic deregulation of signal transduction is, however, not compatible with cellular homeostasis, but bestows cancer cells with a selective advantage, leading to clonal expansion of subsets of cells within the tumor. Common effects of oncogenic signals are, therefore, acceleration of the cell cycle (leading to clonal expansion), repression of the apoptotic response (enhancing cell survival), induction of angiogenesis (providing nutrients and oxygen), as well as modification of cellular metabolism (providing energy) or morphology (providing the ability to invade neighboring tissues and metastasize).[80] As we begin to understand differences of signal transduction between normal and tumor cells, new diagnostics and targeted therapies can be designed to improve molecular pathology and treatment of cancer.

REFERENCES

1. Berger AH, Knudson AG, Pandolfi PP. A continuum model for tumour suppression. *Nature*. August 2011;476(7359):163-169.
2. Hunter T. Oncoprotein networks. *Cell*. February 1997;88(3):333-346.
3. Hanahan D, Weinberg RA. The hallmarks of cancer. *Cell*. January 2000;100(1):57-70.
4. Hanahan D, Weinberg RA. Hallmarks of cancer: the next generation. *Cell*. March 2011;144(5):646-674.
5. Lemmon MA, Schlessinger J. Cell signaling by receptor tyrosine kinases. *Cell*. June 2010;141(7):1117-1134.
6. Threadgill DW, Dlugosz AA, Hansen LA, et al. Targeted disruption of mouse EGF receptor: effect of genetic background on mutant phenotype. *Science*. July 1995;269(5221): 230-234.
7. Miettinen PJ, Berger JE, Meneses J, et al. Epithelial immaturity and multiorgan failure in mice lacking epidermal growth factor receptor. *Nature*. July 1995;376(6538):337-341.
8. Hynes NE, MacDonald G. ErbB receptors and signaling pathways in cancer. *Curr Opin Cell Biol*. April 2009;21(2):177-184.
9. Ji H, Li D, Chen L, et al. The impact of human EGFR kinase domain mutations on lung tumorigenesis and in vivo sensitivity to EGFR-targeted therapies. *Cancer Cell*. June 2006;9(6):485-495.
10. Arteaga CL. EGF receptor mutations in lung cancer: from humans to mice and maybe back to humans. *Cancer Cell*. June 2006;9(6):421-423.
11. Meyers EN, Lewandoski M, Martin GR. An Fgf8 mutant allelic series generated by Cre- and Flp-mediated recombination. *Nat Genet*. February 1998;18(2):136-141.
12. Ciruna B, Rossant J. FGF signaling regulates mesoderm cell fate specification and morphogenetic movement at the primitive streak. *Dev Cell*. July 2001;1(1):37-49.
13. Turner N, Grose R. Fibroblast growth factor signalling: from development to cancer. *Nat Rev Cancer*. February 2010;10(2):116-129.
14. Birchmeier C, Birchmeier W, Gherardi E, Vande Woude GF. Met, metastasis, motility and more. *Nat Rev Mol Cell Biol*. December 2003;4(12):915-925.
15. Ellis LM, Hicklin DJ. VEGF-targeted therapy: mechanisms of anti-tumour activity. *Nat Rev Cancer*. August 2008;8(8):579-591.
16. Johnson L, Greenbaum D, Cichowski K, et al. K-ras is an essential gene in the mouse with partial functional overlap with N-ras. *Genes Dev*. October 1997;11(19):2468-2481.
17. Schubbert S, Zenker M, Rowe SL, et al. Germline KRAS mutations cause Noonan syndrome. *Nat Genet*. March 2006;38(3):331-336.
18. Scheffzek K, Ahmadian MR, Kabsch W, et al. The Ras-RasGAP complex: structural basis for GTPase activation and its loss in oncogenic Ras mutants. *Science*. July 1997;277(5324):333-338.
19. Malumbres M, Barbacid M. RAS oncogenes: the first 30 years. *Nat Rev Cancer*. June 2003;3(6):459-465.
20. Haigis KM, Kendall KR, Wang Y, et al. Differential effects of oncogenic K-Ras and N-Ras on proliferation, differentiation and tumor progression in the colon. *Nat Genet*. May 2008;40(5): 600-608.

21. Johnson L, Mercer K, Greenbaum D, et al. Somatic activation of the K-ras oncogene causes early onset lung cancer in mice. *Nature*. April 2001;410(6832):1111-1116.
22. Moodie SA, Willumsen BM, Weber MJ, Wolfman A. Complexes of Ras.GTP with Raf-1 and mitogen-activated protein kinase kinase. *Science*. June 1993;260(5114):1658-1661.
23. Schäfer R, Sers C. RAS oncogene-mediated deregulation of the transcriptome: from molecular signature to function. *Adv Enzyme Regul*. 2011;51(1):126-136.
24. Blasco RB, Francoz S, Santamaría D, et al. c-Raf, but not B-Raf, is essential for development of K-Ras oncogene-driven non-small cell lung carcinoma. *Cancer Cell*. May 2011;19(5):652-663.
25. Vial E, Sahai E, Marshall CJ. ERK-MAPK signaling coordinately regulates activity of Rac1 and RhoA for tumor cell motility. *Cancer Cell*. July 2003;4(1):67-79.
26. Narumiya S, Tanji M, Ishizaki T. Rho signaling, ROCK and mDia1, in transformation, metastasis and invasion. *Cancer Metastasis Rev*. June 2009;28(1-2):65-76.
27. Kauffmann-Zeh A, Rodriguez-Viciana P, Ulrich E, et al. Suppression of c-Myc-induced apoptosis by Ras signalling through PI(3)K and PKB. *Nature*. February 1997;385(6616): 544-548.
28. Carracedo A, Pandolfi PP. The PTEN-PI3K pathway: of feedbacks and cross-talks. *Oncogene*. September 2008;27(41): 5527-5541.
29. del Peso L, González-García M, Page C, Herrera R, Nuñez G. Interleukin-3-induced phosphorylation of BAD through the protein kinase Akt. *Science*. October 1997;278(5338):687-689.
30. Mayo LD, Donner DB. A phosphatidylinositol 3-kinase/ Akt pathway promotes translocation of Mdm2 from the cytoplasm to the nucleus. *Proc Natl Acad Sci U S A*. September 2001;98(20):11598-11603.
31. Guertin DA, Sabatini DM. Defining the role of mTOR in cancer. *Cancer Cell*. July 2007;12(1):9-22.
32. Eng C. PTEN: one gene, many syndromes. *Hum Mutat*. September 2003;22(3):183-198.
33. Vasudevan KM, Barbie DA, Davies MA, et al. AKT-independent signaling downstream of oncogenic PIK3CA mutations in human cancer. *Cancer Cell*. July 2009;16(1):21-32.
34. Li AG, Piluso LG, Cai X, Wei G, Sellers WR, Liu X. Mechanistic insights into maintenance of high p53 acetylation by PTEN. *Mol Cell*. August 2006;23(4):575-587.
35. Parsons DW, Wang T-L, Samuels Y, et al. Colorectal cancer: mutations in a signalling pathway. *Nature*. August 2005;436(7052):792.
36. Sjöblom T, Jones S, Wood LD, et al. The consensus coding sequences of human breast and colorectal cancers. *Science*. October 2006;314(5797):268-274.
37. Levy DE, Darnell JE. Stats: transcriptional control and biological impact. *Nat Rev Mol Cell Biol*. September 2002;3(9):651-662.
38. Murray PJ. The JAK-STAT signaling pathway: input and output integration. *J Immunol*. March 2007;178(5):2623-2629.
39. Wu X, Tu X, Joeng KS, Hilton MJ, Williams DA, Long F. Rac1 activation controls nuclear localization of beta-catenin during canonical Wnt signaling. *Cell*. April 2008;133(2):340-353.
40. He TC, Sparks AB, Rago C, et al. Identification of c-MYC as a target of the APC pathway. *Science*. September 1998;281(5382): 1509-1512.
41. Tetsu O, McCormick F. Beta-catenin regulates expression of cyclin D1 in colon carcinoma cells. *Nature*. April 1999;398(6726):422-426.
42. Huelsken J, Birchmeier W. New aspects of Wnt signaling pathways in higher vertebrates. *Curr Opin Genet Dev*. September 2001;11(5):547-553.
43. Huelsken J, Vogel R, Brinkmann V, Erdmann B, Birchmeier C, Birchmeier W. Requirement for beta-catenin in anterior-posterior axis formation in mice. *J Cell Biol*. February 2000;148(3): 567-578.
44. Barrow JR, Thomas KR, Boussadia-Zahui O, et al. Ectodermal Wnt3/beta-catenin signaling is required for the establishment and maintenance of the apical ectodermal ridge. *Genes Dev*. February 2003;17(3):394-409.
45. Grigoryan T, Wend P, Klaus A, Birchmeier W. Deciphering the function of canonical Wnt signals in development and disease: conditional loss- and gain-of-function mutations of beta-catenin in mice. *Genes Dev*. September 2008;22(17):2308-2341.
46. van der Flier LG, Clevers H. Stem cells, self-renewal, and differentiation in the intestinal epithelium. *Annu Rev Physiol*. 2009;71:241-260.
47. van de Wetering M, Sancho E, Verweij C, et al. The beta-catenin/ TCF-4 complex imposes a crypt progenitor phenotype on colorectal cancer cells. *Cell*. November 2002;111(2):241-250.
48. Harada N, Tamai Y, Ishikawa T, et al. Intestinal polyposis in mice with a dominant stable mutation of the beta-catenin gene. *EMBO J*. November 1999;18(21):5931-5942.
49. Moser AR, Dove WF, Roth KA, Gordon JI. The Min (multiple intestinal neoplasia) mutation: its effect on gut epithelial cell differentiation and interaction with a modifier system. *J Cell Biol*. March 1992;116(6):1517-1526.
50. Fearon ER, Vogelstein B. A genetic model for colorectal tumorigenesis. *Cell*. June 1990;61(5):759-767.
51. Vermeulen L, De Sousa E Melo F, van der Heijden M, et al. Wnt activity defines colon cancer stem cells and is regulated by the microenvironment. *Nat Cell Biol*. May 2010;12(5):468-476.
52. Phelps RA, Chidester S, Dehghanizadeh S, et al. A two-step model for colon adenoma initiation and progression caused by APC loss. *Cell*. May 2009;137(4):623-634.
53. Pourquié O. Vertebrate segmentation: from cyclic gene networks to scoliosis. *Cell*. May 2011;145(5):650-663.
54. Polyak K, Weinberg RA. Transitions between epithelial and mesenchymal states: acquisition of malignant and stem cell traits. *Nat Rev Cancer*. April 2009;9(4):265-273.
55. Ranganathan P, Weaver KL, Capobianco AJ. Notch signalling in solid tumours: a little bit of everything but not all the time. *Nat Rev Cancer*. May 2011;11(5):338-351.
56. Waite KA, Eng C. From developmental disorder to heritable cancer: it's all in the BMP/TGF-beta family. *Nat Rev Genet*. October 2003;4(10):763-773.
57. Padua D, Massagué J. Roles of TGFbeta in metastasis. *Cell Res*. January 2009;19(1):89-102.
58. Massard C, Fizazi K. Targeting continued androgen receptor signaling in prostate cancer. *Clin Cancer Res*. June 2011;17(12): 3876-3883.
59. Marini KD, Payne BJ, Watkins DN, Martelotto LG. Mechanisms of Hedgehog signalling in cancer. *Growth Factors*. December 2011;29(6):221-234.
60. Yang SH, Andl T, Grachtchouk V, et al. Pathological responses to oncogenic Hedgehog signaling in skin are dependent on canonical Wnt/beta3-catenin signaling. *Nat Genet*. September 2008;40(9):1130-1135.
61. Shin K, Lee J, Guo N, et al. Hedgehog/Wnt feedback supports regenerative proliferation of epithelial stem cells in bladder. *Nature*. April 2011;472(7341):110-114.
62. Oeckinghaus A, Hayden MS, Ghosh S. Crosstalk in NF-κB signaling pathways. *Nat Immunol*. August 2011;12(8):695-708.
63. Hayden MS, Ghosh S. Shared principles in NF-kappaB signaling. *Cell*. February 2008;132(3):344-362.
64. Webster GA, Perkins ND. Transcriptional cross talk between NF-kappaB and p53. *Mol Cell Biol*. May 1999;19(5): 3485-3495.
65. Pan D. The hippo signaling pathway in development and cancer. *Dev Cell*. October 2010;19(4):491-505.
66. Varelas X, Miller BW, Sopko R, et al. The Hippo pathway regulates Wnt/beta-catenin signaling. *Dev Cell*. April 2010;18(4): 579-591.
67. Fernandez-L A, Northcott PA, Dalton J, et al. YAP1 is amplified and up-regulated in hedgehog-associated medulloblastomas and mediates Sonic hedgehog-driven neural precursor proliferation. *Genes Dev*. December 2009;23(23):2729-2741.
68. Cordenonsi M, Zanconato F, Azzolin L, et al. The hippo transducer TAZ confers cancer stem cell-related traits on breast cancer cells. *Cell*. November 2011;147(4):759-772.
69. Vaquerizas JM, Kummerfeld SK, Teichmann SA, Luscombe NM. A census of human transcription factors: function, expression and evolution. *Nat Rev Genet*. April 2009;10(4):252-263.
70. Levine AJ, Oren M. The first 30 years of p53: growing ever more complex. *Nat Rev Cancer*. October 2009;9(10):749-758.
71. Wu X, Bayle HJ, Olson D, Levine AJ. The p53-mdm-2 autoregulatory feedback loop. *Genes Dev*. May 1993;7:1126-1132.
72. Donehower LA, Harvey M, Slagle BL, et al. Mice deficient for p53 are developmentally normal but susceptible to spontaneous tumours. *Nature*. March 1992;356(6366):215-221.

73. Tyner SD, Venkatachalam S, Choi J, et al. p53 mutant mice that display early ageing-associated phenotypes. *Nature*. January 2002;415(6867):45-53.
74. Peinado H, Olmeda D, Cano A. Snail, Zeb and bHLH factors in tumour progression: an alliance against the epithelial phenotype? *Nat Rev Cancer*. May 2007; 7(6):415-428.
75. Polager S, Ginsberg D. p53 and E2f: partners in life and death. *Nat Rev Cancer*. October 2009;9(10):738-748.
76. Chen H-Z, Tsai S-Y, Leone G. Emerging roles of E2Fs in cancer: an exit from cell cycle control. *Nat Rev Cancer*. November 2009;9(11):785-797.
77. Soucek L, Evan GI. The ups and downs of Myc biology. *Curr Opin Genet Dev*. February 2010;20(1):91-95.
78. Cole MD, Cowling VH. Transcription-independent functions of MYC: regulation of translation and DNA replication. *Nat Rev Mol Cell Biol*. October 2008;9(10): 810-815.
79. Dewhirst MW, Cao Y, Moeller B. Cycling hypoxia and free radicals regulate angiogenesis and radiotherapy response. *Nat Rev Cancer*. June 2008;8(6):425-437.
80. Vogelstein B, Kinzler KW. Cancer genes and the pathways they control. *Nat Med*. August 2004;10(8):789-799.

CHAPTER 4

ONCOGENES

Sadhna Dhingra and Dongfeng Tan

INTRODUCTION

Oncogenes are altered genes that are implicated in the pathogenesis of cancers. Carcinogenesis is a multistep process that almost always requires alteration in both proto-oncogenes and tumor suppressor genes. Proto-oncogenes are normal, innocuous counterparts of oncogenes in a cell that help regulate normal cell growth and development through encoded proteins such as growth factors, growth factor receptors, signal transducers, and cell cycle proteins. When these proto-oncogenes get altered or activated by spontaneous or exogenous mutagenic factors such as viruses, chemicals, or radiation, they transform to oncogenes. These oncogenes produce oncoproteins, which are encoded protein products that serve functions similar to those served by their normal counterparts but are devoid of internal regulatory control. These oncoproteins act on various cellular pathways and cause the cell to escape from the normal cell cycle. Gradual accumulation of multiple oncogenetic mutations over a period of time results in transformed cells with dysregulated autonomous cell growth and malignant transformation.

Proto-oncogene activation to form oncogenes may occur as a result of gene amplification, point mutation, or chromosomal translocation. The *ERBB2* oncogene is an example of gene amplification and has been reported in breast, lung, and oral cancers.[1] The *ras* family genes (H-ras, K-ras, and N-ras) are mutation-dependent oncogenes and have been reported in a variety of cancers such as pancreatic and colon cancers.[2] Burkitt lymphoma and chronic myelogenous leukemia are classic examples of cancers associated with translocation-dependent activation of oncogenes.[3] Normal cell proliferation typically follows a sequence of events that starts with the binding of a growth factor to its specific receptor on the cell membrane. The activation of the growth factor receptor leads to the activation of signal-transducing proteins on the inside of the cell membrane followed by the transmission of the transduced signal through the cytosol to the nucleus via second messengers. In the nucleus, the activation of transcriptional proteins initiates transcription and leads to the cell's progression into the cell cycle.

The database of clinically relevant oncogenes is rapidly expanding. Since oncogenes and oncoproteins are mutated counterparts of normal genes and encoded proteins, they can be broadly grouped, based on their roles in cell proliferation pathways, into three categories: those that initiate signaling at the cell surface (e.g., growth factors and growth factor receptors), those that are part of intracellular signal transduction pathways (e.g., guanosine triphosphate [GTP]–binding proteins, nonreceptor tyrosine kinases, RAS signaling proteins, and WNT signaling proteins), and those that function at the nuclear level (e.g., transcriptional activators, cyclins, and cyclin-dependent kinases).

Oncogenes can be detected at the DNA, RNA, or protein levels using various techniques such as restriction enzyme analysis, polymerase chain reaction, Southern blotting, Northern blotting, in situ hybridization, and monoclonal antibodies. This detection ability has resulted in the widespread use of oncogenes as tumor biomarkers. The molecular detection of oncogenes serves as an important armamentarium for oncologists in patient care, as it provides diagnostic and prognostic information about tumors and also detects therapeutic targets in certain tumors. A detailed description of all oncogenes is beyond the scope of this chapter, since they are discussed throughout this book. We briefly review certain clinically significant oncogenes.

ONCOGENES ASSOCIATED WITH EPIDERMAL GROWTH FACTOR RECEPTOR SUPERFAMILY

C-erbB-2

One of the four components of the human epidermal growth factor receptor (HER) superfamily is HER2 (aka Her2/neu or C-erbB-2) protein, a 185-kDa transmembrane growth factor receptor–like protein that is encoded by the C-erbB-2 gene located on chromosome 17q21. Historically, the *neu* gene was described in the early 1980s in glioblastomas induced in adult rats after they were exposed to the carcinogen *N*-ethyl-*N*-nitrosourea.[4] Around the same time, it was shown that the *v-erB* oncogene was derived from *c-erB-2*, a cellular gene encoding for epidermal growth factor receptor (EGFR).[5] Later it was learned that *c-erB-2* is the human counterpart of the *neu* oncogene and encodes the HER2 protein. A wide variety of cancers such as those of the breast,[6] stomach,[7] lung (non–small cell lung cancer),[8] and urinary bladder[9] show *ERBB2* gene amplification and HER2 protein overexpression. HER2 overexpression and amplification are associated with aggressive disease and unfavorable prognosis. This protein is expressed in 25% to 30% of all breast cancers.[10] HER2 overexpression is detected by immunohistochemistry with membranous staining using monoclonal or polyclonal antibodies to HER2.

Overexpression of Her2 causes increased cell proliferation, metastasis, and angiogenesis and decreased apoptosis. The EGFR superfamily is composed of four closely related type 1 transmembrane tyrosine kinase receptors (HER1 or EGFR, HER2, HER3, and HER4), and their activation, overexpression, and signal transduction occur as a result of receptor dimerization, either as homodimerization (between two molecules of the same receptor) or as heterodimerization (between different receptors). The formation of HER2–HER3 heterodimers leads to the activation of the phosphatidylinositol 3-kinase (PI3K)/protein kinase B (Akt)/mammalian target of rapamycin (mTOR) pathway, which further facilitates angiogenesis, cell proliferation, and anti-apoptotic activity.[11]

HER2 overexpression and amplification are unique to tumoral tissue and thus provide an attractive therapeutic target. The current anti-HER2 therapeutic approaches approved by the US Food and Drug Administration (FDA) for clinical use include monoclonal antibodies and small-molecule tyrosine kinase inhibitors (TKIs).[12] Trastuzumab is a recombinant humanized IgG1 monoclonal antibody against the extracellular juxtamembrane domain of the transmembrane HER2 receptor. The antibody binding leads to the inhibition of downstream signaling pathways, cell cycle arrest, and a reduction in angiogenesis. Therefore, in patients with breast tumors in which HER2 is amplified, trastuzumab increases survival rates when combined with chemotherapeutic drugs. Small-molecule TKIs inhibit the kinase activity of HER2 receptors, which leads to the inhibition of the ras/raf1/MAPK and PI3K/Akt pathways and subsequently to decreased cellular proliferation and increased apoptosis.[12] Lapatinib is the potent adenosine triphosphate (ATP)–competitive inhibitor of the HER2 and EGFR tyrosine kinase domains and is known to improve prognosis in patients with HER2-amplified breast cancers when used in combination with chemotherapy. It has also been reported to produce a modest response in the treatment of brain metastases.[13] Clinical trials are also under way for pertuzumab, which is another promising humanized monoclonal antibody that binds to domain II of HER2 and blocks receptor dimerization. It can be used in combination with trastuzumab and/or chemotherapy and has been shown in clinical trials to be effective in patients whose disease has progressed while receiving trastuzumab.[11]

Additionally, trastuzumab has shown promising overall survival benefit in patients with HER2-positive gastroesophageal junction cancers or gastric adenocarcinomas, according to the results of trastuzumab for gastric cancer (ToGA) clinical trial, which is the first multicenter randomized phase III trial investigating the efficacy and outcome of targeted therapies in gastric cancer in combination with platinum-based chemotherapy in a subset of patients with HER2-positive tumors.[14] These results mandate routine HER2 testing of gastric cancers and gastroesophageal cancers to select the subset of patients who could benefit from the combination of trastuzumab and chemotherapy. Clinical trials are ongoing to determine the efficacy of lapatinib in HER2-overexpressing esophageal and gastric cancers.[7] Numerous other promising HER2-targeted drugs are in developmental phases.

EGFR

EGFR is the HER1/erbB1 component of the HER superfamily. These receptors contain an extracellular domain, a transmembrane domain, and an intracytoplasmic domain with tyrosine kinase activity that is required for signal transduction. Inactivated EGFR exists in a monomeric form. Activation occurs by binding of ligands such as epidermal growth factor (EGF) and transforming growth factor-β (TGF-β). This binding leads to the dimerization of the EGFR receptor (either homodimerization or heterodimerization) and the activation of intrinsic kinase activity, which causes tyrosine autophosphorylation or transphosphorylation. The tyrosine phosphorylation leads to the transduction of downstream signaling pathways through the recruitment and activation of adaptor and transducer proteins. The downstream signaling pathways affected include the PI3K/Akt/mTOR, RAS/RAF/MAPK, and JAK/STAT cascades. The PI3K/Akt/mTOR pathway causes the downregulation of cell cycle inhibitor p27, leading to increased cell proliferation and the upregulation of vascular endothelial growth factor (VEGF), which causes increased angiogenesis.

Dysregulation of the EGFR signaling pathway in carcinogenesis has been well established and is associated with aggressive disease and poor outcomes.[15] Aberrant activation of EGFR can be ligand dependent or ligand independent. Ligands that activate EGFR include EGF, TGF-β, and heparin-binding EGFR-like growth factor.[16] Ligand-dependent activation of EGFR is seen in ovarian epithelial carcinoma.[17] Ligand-independent signaling pathway activation occurs as a result of EGFR gene mutations and amplifications. The EGFR gene is the cellular homologue of the v-erbB oncogene originally identified in avian erythroblastosis viruses. Gain-of-function mutations of the EGFR gene at exons 19 and 21 are associated with the development of lung adenocarcinoma.[18] EGFR gene amplification and rearrangements have been reported in glial neoplasms. Certain gene rearrangements, such as frame deletions spanning exons 2 to 7, lead to the formation of the truncated variant of the receptor (EGFRvIII), which lacks the extracellular domain to bind ligands; however, EGFRvIII is constitutively active and drives glioma growth.[19] Cancers of the breast, colon, and head and neck have been reported to show varying numbers of dinucleotide repeats in intron 1 of EGFR, and the number of repeats is inversely proportional to receptor overexpression.[20] Another method of enhanced signaling of the EGFR pathway is heterodimerization with other members of the EGFR family, particularly cross-talk with HER2 and HER3 heterodimers.[21] EGFR-HER2 heterodimers leading to co-expression of HER2 and EGFR are associated with poor prognosis in patients with breast tumors.[22]

In the recent past, the EGFR pathway has been a focus of intense research for the development of targeted cancer therapies. Like HER2 antagonists, EGFR antagonists include small-molecule TKIs and monoclonal antibodies. These have been approved by the FDA for the treatment of advanced or metastatic cancers of lung (non–small cell type), colorectum, pancreas, and breast and squamous cell carcinoma of the head and neck.[16,23] Clinical trials are being conducted to determine the efficacy of gefitinib and erlotinib in the treatment of advanced ovarian cancers,[24] high-grade gliomas,[25] and advanced prostate cancers.[26]

Gefitinib and erlotinib are the two reversible small-molecule TKIs that competitively bind the ATP pocket located in the intracellular receptor domain, thus blocking the receptor tyrosine kinase phosphorylation. EGFR-TKIs are oral drugs that are usually well tolerated by patients and have mild and reversible skin and gastrointestinal side effects. In locally advanced or metastatic lung adenocarcinoma, activating somatic mutations in exons 18 to 21 of the tyrosine kinase domain of EGFR has been shown to be a positive predictor of response to small-molecule EGFR-TKI treatment.[27] Lapatinib is a small-molecule inhibitor of both EGFR and HER2 that is used in combination with capecitabine or letrozole in patients whose HER2-positive breast cancer has not responded to other chemotherapy regimens.

Cetuximab and panitumumab are two anti-EGFR humanized monoclonal antibodies of the IgG1 subclass that reduce EGFR activity either by binding to and blocking the extracellular EGF ligand binding or by causing the internalization and destruction of EGFR. This reduces the number of receptors available on the surface, which further decreases or inhibits receptor dimerization and tyrosine phosphorylation, thereby preventing downstream signaling and growth stimulation. These humanized antibodies also facilitate antibody-directed cancer cell killing by the immune system.[24] Cetuximab is approved by the FDA for the treatment of locally advanced or metastatic squamous cell carcinoma of the head and neck. A subset of patients with treatment-resistant metastatic colorectal carcinoma have had improved clinical outcomes with cetuximab or panitumumab either alone or in combination with chemotherapy.[23]

With the exception of non–small cell lung cancers with activating EGFR mutations, current EGFR-targeted therapies have shown only modest clinical response against most cancers. Most patients show an initial response to EGFR-TKIs but eventually acquire resistance. Among the multiple mechanisms that contribute to resistance are EGFR resistance mutations (T790M point mutation at exon 20 of the *EGFR* gene), KRAS mutations, mesenchymal-to-epithelial transition factor amplification, and the activation of other signaling pathways such as VEGF and insulin-like growth factor-1.[28] Newer drugs are being developed to overcome resistance to EGFR antagonists.

ONCOGENES IN SIGNALING PATHWAYS

Strict regulation of cell signaling pathways maintains tissue homeostasis and organ integrity. In cancer cell, mutations in oncogenes coding for signal transducers and transcription factors can alter the normal cellular signal transduction and response, leading to carcinogenesis (Fig. 4.1). Many important oncogenes involve varied cell signaling pathways, such as RAS/RAF/MAPK pathway and PI3K/AKT/mTOR pathway. Therefore, most novel targeted therapies are aimed at these major signaling pathways. For instance, sunitinib's antitumor effect is due to its inhibitory activity of multiple tyrosine kinase receptors, resulting in the inactivation of RAS/RAF/ERK signaling. We briefly discuss oncogenes in RAS/RAF/ERK pathway. For more information regarding oncogenes in cell signaling pathways, the reader is advised to refer to the relevant chapters in the book.

RAS Genes

Mutations of the *ras* gene are the single most common abnormality of dominant oncogenes in human cancers. About 33% of all human cancers contain RAS point mutations, resulting in activated RAS.[29] The clinical implications of *ras* activation in tumors vary. In some tumors,

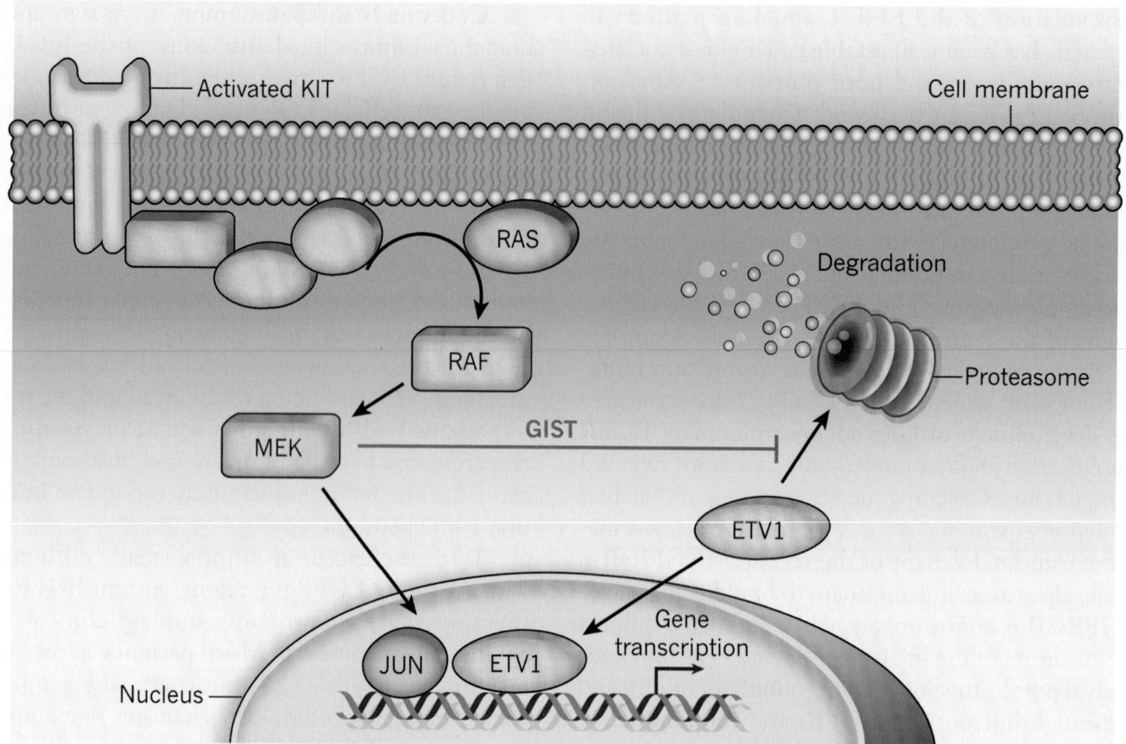

FIGURE 4–1 Activation of the receptor tyrosine kinase KIT triggers the RAS/RAF/MEK pathway. This pathway ultimately results in changes in gene transcription mediated by activating specific transcription factors such as JUN. The transcription factor ETV1 acts downstream of the RAS/RAF/MEK pathway and can directly regulate gene expression. It is found that ETV1 is essential for KIT-mediated development of gastrointestinal stromal tumors (GISTs). Normally, proteasomal degradation of ETV1 leads to a decrease in ETV1-dependent gene transcription. In GIST, signaling from mutant KIT leads to increased activity of MEK, which then blocks ETV1 degradation. The combination of MEK activation and developmental expression of ETV1 produces the gene expression profile that is characteristic of GIST. (Michael C Heinrich, Christopher L Corless. *Nature*. 2010;467(7317):796-797, with copyright permission.)

such as lung and colorectal cancers, K-ras mutations are associated with worse prognosis; whereas in others, such as bladder cancers and leukemias, there is no correlation between *ras* mutation and the clinical aggressiveness of the disease.

The *ras* gene encodes three small GTP-binding proteins, N-RAS, H-RAS, and K-RAS. K-RAS has two alternative splice variants, K-RAS4A and K-RAS4B.[30] The RAS proteins are localized at the inner (cytoplasmic) aspect of the plasma membrane, and they switch back and forth between an activated, signal-transmitting form and an inactive, quiescent state due to alternative binding with GTP and guanosine diphosphate (GDP). This transition is regulated by guanine nucleotide exchange factors that promote formation of GTP and by GTPase-activating proteins, which cause hydrolysis of GTP and convert active GTP-bound RAS to inactive GDP-bound RAS. Thus, through their rapid hydrolysis of GTP to GDP, GTPase-activating proteins keep a check on uncontrolled signal transduction by RAS. The regulation of RAS by GTPases is the most important mechanism that is altered as a result of mutations in the *ras* gene.[30] The activation of RAS mainly affects the raf/MEK/ERK kinase downstream signaling pathway, which in turn activates Ets, a family of nuclear transcription factors.[31] Other downstream signaling pathways, such as PI3K/Akt/serine–threonine kinase, are also activated by RAS, and their activation leads to the activation of the nuclear transcription factor NF-κB. RAS exerts direct control on the cell cycle through cyclins and cyclin-dependent kinases, which regulate the passage of cells from G0 to S phase. Additionally, RAS regulation gets disturbed as a result of alterations in other signaling components, such as receptor tyrosine kinases. In many cancers, overexpression of EGFR is frequently associated with activated ras and ras-mediated signaling, resulting from activated EGFR tyrosine kinase activity.[31]

The incidence of *ras* gene mutations varies among different cancers; however, certain carcinomas such as colon, pancreas, and thyroid cancers contain a high incidence of *ras* gene mutations. Mutated *ras* genes drive carcinogenesis by increasing cell proliferation, suppressing apoptosis, remodeling the cellular microenvironment, and facilitating immune evasion and metastasis. These multiple roles make RAS a viable therapeutic target. Potential anti-Ras treatment strategies target various aspects of the signaling pathway. These targets may be associated with the plasma membrane (farnesyltransferase inhibitors), downstream signaling (Raf and MEK protein kinase inhibitors), autocrine growth factor signaling (EGF receptor inhibitors), or gene expression (H-ras and c-raf-1 inhibitors).[31] These are currently being evaluated in clinical trials.

K-ras has gained clinical importance in recent years due to the FDA recommendation for testing colorectal tumors for KRAS mutations before the initiation of EGFR-targeted therapy in patients with metastatic colorectal cancer. The KRAS oncoprotein is a central downstream transducer of EGFR signaling. Mutations of the K-ras oncogene result in the constitutive activation of EGFR and are predictors of resistance to EGFR-targeted therapy in colorectal cancers. The response rates to the anti-EGFR monoclonal antibodies cetuximab and panitumumab, which are approved by the FDA for the treatment of metastatic colorectal cancer, are limited to a subset of patients, and studies have shown that presence of KRAS mutations is the predominant mechanism of resistance to EGFR therapy.[32] The majority (about 85%) of KRAS mutations in colorectal carcinoma occur in exon 2 at codons 12 and 13, and a minority occur in exons 3 and 4 (codons 61, 117, and 146).[33] This is the basis of the FDA recommendation for testing for KRAS exon 2 mutations in surgical specimens of colorectal cancers in patients with advanced disease.

BRAF Oncogene

The BRAF oncogene is located on chromosome 7q34, encodes a serine–threonine kinase, and is the principal downstream effector of the RAS/RAF/MAPK signaling pathway. Mutations in the BRAF oncogene are most commonly seen in melanomas; however, other cancers—such as acute leukemia, lymphoma, and cancers of the lung, thyroid, and colon—may also show these mutations.[34] This oncogene has achieved clinical importance due to its diagnostic and pathogenetic value in colorectal carcinoma and its potential to predict refractoriness to EGFR-targeted therapy for metastatic colorectal cancers. The BRAF oncogene can be mutated anywhere along its sequence; however, the most common activating mutation occurs in exon 15 at codon 600 and is popularly called BRAF V600E. Molecular analysis of this mutation has diagnostic implications in colorectal cancers, as approximately 90% of sporadic microsatellite instability–high colorectal cancers show this mutation. Colorectal carcinomas that arise in patients with Lynch syndrome almost never show this mutation.[35] Thus, the workup for this mutation helps to differentiate the two entities. Testing for the BRAF mutation is also indicated in metastatic colorectal carcinomas that are negative for KRAS mutation and are being considered for EGFR-targeted treatment. This is based on studies that show that the presence of BRAF mutations in such cases predicts tumor refractoriness or low response rates to EGFR-targeted therapy with monoclonal antibodies such as cetuximab.[36] Knowledge of BRAF gene mutation also provides some prognostic information, as the presence of the BRAF V600E mutation is associated with a poor outcome in microsatellite-stable colorectal carcinoma.[35]

In conclusion, this review provides a brief overview of certain oncogenes and their clinical relevance in oncology. Extensive research over the past two decades has led to major breakthroughs in our understanding of the role of oncogenes in carcinogenesis and the development of targeted anticancer drugs that act on signaling pathways. However, our understanding is yet incomplete, as these therapeutic agents have shown a variable clinical response. This is perhaps because each cancer is driven by multiple oncogenic events leading to multiple activated signaling pathways that form a complex network through cross-talk, presenting a major challenge for the development of treatment strategies.

REFERENCES

1. Pillai R. Oncogenes and oncoproteins as tumor markers. *Eur J Surg Oncol.* 1992;18(5):417-424.
2. Spandidos DA. Mechanism of carcinogenesis: the role of oncogenes, transcriptional enhancers and growth factors. *Anticancer Res.* 1985;5(5):485-498.
3. Wong-Staal F. The oncogene and its potential role in carcinogenesis. *Arch Toxicol Suppl.* 1985;8:61-72.
4. Maguire HC Jr, Greene MI. The neu (c-erbB-2) oncogene. *Semin Oncol.* 1989;16(2):148-155.
5. Pastan I. c-erbB-2 and human cancer. *Jpn J Cancer Res.* October 1993;84(10):inside front cover.
6. Perren TJ. c-erbB-2 oncogene as a prognostic marker in breast cancer. *Br J Cancer.* 1991;63(3):328-332.
7. Kaur A, Dasanu CA. Targeting the HER2 pathway for the therapy of lower esophageal and gastric adenocarcinoma. *Expert Opin Pharmacother.* 2011;12(16):2493-2503.
8. Takenaka M, Hanagiri T, Shinohara S, et al. The prognostic significance of HER2 overexpression in non-small cell lung cancer. *Anticancer Res.* 2011;31(12):4631-4636.
9. Fleischmann A, Rotzer D, Seiler R, Studer UE, Thalmann GN. Her2 amplification is significantly more frequent in lymph node metastases from urothelial bladder cancer than in the primary tumours. *Eur Urol.* 2011;60(2):350-357.
10. De Potter CR. The neu-oncogene: more than a prognostic indicator? *Hum Pathol.* 1994;25(12):1264-1268.
11. Gradishar WJ. HER2 therapy—an abundance of riches. *N Engl J Med.* 2012;366(2):176-178.
12. Baselga J. Treatment of HER2-overexpressing breast cancer. *Ann Oncol.* 2010;21(suppl 7):vii36-vii40.
13. Lin NU, Diéras V, Paul D, et al. Multicenter phase II study of lapatinib in patients with brain metastases from HER2-positive breast cancer. *Clin Cancer Res.* 2009;15(4):1452-1459.
14. Bang YJ, Van Cutsem E, Feyereislova A, et al.; ToGA Trial Investigators. Trastuzumab in combination with chemotherapy versus chemotherapy alone for treatment of HER2-positive advanced gastric or gastro-oesophageal junction cancer (ToGA): a phase 3, open-label, randomised controlled trial. *Lancet.* 2010;376(9742):687-697.
15. Lemmon MA, Schlessinger J. Cell signaling by receptor tyrosine kinases. *Cell.* 2010;141:1117-1134.
16. Han W, Lo HW. Landscape of EGFR signaling network in human cancers: biology and therapeutic response in relation to receptor subcellular locations. *Cancer Lett.* January 2012. [E-pub ahead of print].
17. Alberti C, Pinciroli P, Valeri B, et al. Ligand-dependent EGFR activation induces the co-expression of IL-6 and PAI-1 via the NFkB pathway in advanced-stage epithelial ovarian cancer. *Oncogene.* December 2011. [E-pub ahead of print].
18. Dienstmann R, De Dosso S, Felip E, Tabernero J. Drug development to overcome resistance to EGFR inhibitors in lung and colorectal cancer. *Mol Oncol.* 2012;6(1):15-26.

19. Wong AJ, Ruppert JM, Bigner SH, et al. Structural alterations of the epidermal growth factor receptor gene in human gliomas. *Proc Natl Acad Sci U S A*. 1992;89(7):2965-2969.
20. Brandt B, Meyer-Staeckling S, Schmidt H, Agelopoulos K, Buerger H. Mechanisms of egfr gene transcription modulation: relationship to cancer risk and therapy response. *Clin Cancer Res*. 2006;12(24):7252-7260.
21. Rosell R, Taron M, Reguart N, Isla D, Moran T. Epidermal growth factor receptor activation: how exon 19 and 21 mutations changed our understanding of the pathway. *Clin Cancer Res*. 2006;12(24):7222-7231.
22. Balz LM, Bartkowiak K, Andreas A, et al. The interplay of HER2/HER3/PI3K and EGFR/HER2/PLC-γ1 signalling in breast cancer cell migration and dissemination. *J Pathol*. January 2012. [E-pub ahead of print].
23. Vecchione L, Jacobs B, Normanno N, Ciardiello F, Tejpar S. EGFR-targeted therapy. *Exp Cell Res*. 2011;317(19):2765-2771.
24. Haldar K, Gaitskell K, Bryant A, Nicum S, Kehoe S, Morrison J. Epidermal growth factor receptor blockers for the treatment of ovarian cancer. *Cochrane Database Syst Rev*. October 2011;(10):CD007927.
25. Voelzke WR, Petty WJ, Lesser GJ. Targeting the epidermal growth factor receptor in high-grade astrocytomas. *Curr Treat Options Oncol*. 2008;9(1):23-31.
26. Blackledge G, Averbuch S, Kay A, Barton J. Anti-EGF receptor therapy. *Prostate Cancer Prostatic Dis*. 2000;3(4):296-302.
27. Dacic S. Molecular diagnostics of lung carcinomas. *Arch Pathol Lab Med*. 2011;135(5):622-629.
28. Giaccone G, Wang Y. Strategies for overcoming resistance to EGFR family tyrosine kinase inhibitors. *Cancer Treat Rev*. 2011;37(6):456-464.
29. Baines AT, Xu D, Der CJ. Inhibition of Ras for cancer treatment: the search continues. *Future Med Chem*. 2011; 3(14):1787-1808.
30. Pylayeva-Gupta Y, Grabocka E, Bar-Sagi D. RAS oncogenes: weaving a tumorigenic web. *Nat Rev Cancer*. 2011;11(11): 761-774.
31. Cox AD, Der CJ. Ras family signaling: therapeutic targeting. *Cancer Biol Ther*. 2002;1(6):599-606.
32. Lièvre A, Bachet JB, Le Corre D, et al. KRAS mutation status is predictive of response to cetuximab therapy in colorectal cancer. *Cancer Res*. 2006;66(8):3992-3995.
33. Grossmann AH, Samowitz WS. Epidermal growth factor receptor pathway mutations and colorectal cancer therapy. *Arch Pathol Lab Med*. 2011;135(10):1278-1282.
34. Nissan MH, Solit DB. The "SWOT" of BRAF inhibition in melanoma: RAF inhibitors, MEK inhibitors or both? *Curr Oncol Rep*. 2011;13(6):479-487.
35. Sharma SG, Gulley ML. BRAF mutation testing in colorectal cancer. *Arch Pathol Lab Med*. 2010;134(8):1225-1228.
36. De Roock W, Claes B, Bernasconi D, et al. Effects of KRAS, BRAF, NRAS, and PIK3CA mutations on the efficacy of cetuximab plus chemotherapy in chemotherapy-refractory metastatic colorectal cancer: a retrospective consortium analysis. Lancet Oncol. August 2010;11(8):753-762. PMID: 20619739.

CHAPTER 5

Tumor Suppressor Genes

Markus Reschke, Lev M. Kats, and Pier Paolo Pandolfi

INTRODUCTION

Over the past 25 years, it has become increasingly clear that cancer is a genetic disease and that mutations in the genome are both the cause and consequence of cancer progression. We now know that cancer develops through a complex multistep process whereby through a series of sequential genetic alterations, that are either inherited or acquired somatically, premalignant cells attain properties that are necessary or favorable for uncontrolled proliferation. There are two classes of genes that are altered in cancer: oncogenes and tumor suppressor genes (TSGs). Although many definitions and numerous criteria have been proposed over the years, in essence oncogenes are those genes that are hyperactivated to drive transformation, whereas TSGs are those that are inactivated to drive transformation.[1-3]

Historically, oncogenes were the first to be discovered, originally through studies of retroviruses and transformed cells. Oncogenes were subsequently shown to be aberrant forms of normal cellular genes, the so-called proto-oncogenes that are abnormally activated in human cancer through point mutation, gene amplification, or genomic rearrangement.[4] Genetically, oncogenes behave in a dominant fashion (with some exceptions), with only one of the two alleles being altered. Oncogenes are only briefly mentioned in this chapter, but are reviewed in detail elsewhere in this book.

The discovery of oncogenes sparked the hypothesis that just as some genes favor malignant transformation, there must be others that oppose it (Table 5.1). This hypothesis turned out to be correct, with the first TSG being proposed in 1971 by Alfred Knudson following his groundbreaking work on retinoblastoma.[5] Based on Knudson's observations, researchers for a long time thought that both alleles of a TSG must be fully inactivated before an effect is manifested and therefore mutations in TSGs are recessive. We know now that although the Retinoblastoma (*RB*) TSG follows the so-called two-hit model of cancer susceptibility, this is not the case for all TSGs, and in some cases, loss of a single allele or even partial inactivation (e.g., by transcriptional silencing) can be sufficient to promote tumorigenesis.[6,7] Cancer cells vary from their nonmalignant counterparts with respect to numerous capabilities, including their ability to respond to positive and negative growth signals, repair their DNA, balance ATP production with macromolecular synthesis, and avoid programmed cell death[1,2]; thus, it is perhaps not surprising that TSGs perform a wide variety of biological functions (Fig. 5.1). In this introductory chapter, we provide an overview of TSGs as well as the emerging concept of a continuum model of tumor suppression. In addition, we discuss the potential for modulating TSGs in human cancer therapy.

BIOLOGICAL FUNCTIONS OF TSGs

Apoptosis, Senescence, and Regulation of Cell Cycle

One of the most fundamental properties of cancer cells is their ability to resist cell death, circumvent growth-suppressive mechanisms, and continue to divide in the face of anti-proliferative signals.[1-3] In order to maintain homeostasis between the many cell types throughout development and adulthood, multicellular organisms have evolved complex pathways to limit unwanted cellular replication. Normal cells possess a myriad of abnormality sensors that detect both intrinsic (originating inside the cell) and extrinsic (originating outside the cell) signals and

M. Reschke and L.M. Kats contributed equally

TABLE 5–1 Examples of Tumor Suppressor Genes That Are Inactivated in Human Cancer Susceptibility (CS) Syndromes and/or Sporadic Cancer. Whether or Not These Genes Display Haplo-insufficient Properties Is Indicated

Gene	CS Syndrome	Sporadic Cancers	Haplo-insufficient (Y/N)
p53	Li-Fraumeni syndrome	Multiple tumor types	Y
RB	Retinoblastoma	Multiple tumor types	N
PTEN	Cowden syndrome	Multiple tumor types	Y
APC	Familial adenomatous polyposis	Colorectal cancer	Y
BRCA1/2	Familial breast and ovarian cancer	Breast cancer, ovarian cancer	N
VHL	Von Hippel-Lindau syndrome	Renal cell carcinoma	N
TSC1/2	Tuberous sclerosis	Renal cell carcinoma	Y
SMAD4	Juvenile polyposis	Pancreatic cancer, colon cancer	Y
NF1	Neurofibromatosis	Sarcomas, gliomas	Y
INK4a	Melanoma	Many tumor types	Y
PTCH	Basal cell nevus syndrome	Medulloblastoma, retinoblastoma	Y
NPM	None known	Myelodysplastic syndrome, leukemia, lymphomas	Y
$p27^{kip1}$	Multiple endocrine neoplasia syndrome	Breast cancer, leukemia, colon cancer	Y
DOK2	None known	Lung cancer	Y

maintain tight control over the cell's growth and division cycle. If excessive DNA damage, an imbalance in metabolite pools, or an unexpected spike in proliferative cues are detected, cells can activate molecular programs that result in one of three outcomes: (1) a temporary block in cell cycle progression; (2) cellular senescence—permanent cell cycle arrest associated with characteristic morphological changes; or (3) apoptosis—programmed cell death. All cancer cells must somehow overcome these mechanisms if they are to become fully malignant.[1-3]

Two "classical" TSGs that are among the most frequently inactivated genes in human cancer are *TP53* (*p53*)[8] and Retinoblastoma 1 (*RB*).[9] The proteins encoded by these genes form critical nodes in the overlapping and partially redundant circuits that control cell survival and replication decisions. Originally discovered due to their loss or mutation in familial and sporadic cancers, their status as TSGs has been firmly confirmed by biochemical and genetic studies in both human cell lines and mouse models. Invariably, proper activation of *p53* or *RB* acts as a powerful brake on cellular replication, and conversely, their inactivation favors growth and transformation.

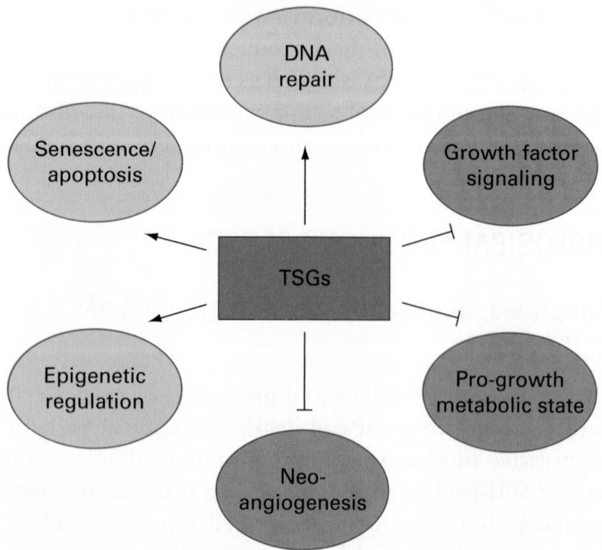

FIGURE 5–1 Biological functions of tumor suppressor genes (TSGs). TSGs perform a wide variety of biological functions. In general, TSGs facilitate those processes that maintain homeostasis (green) and oppose those processes that favor growth and replication (red). Note, however, that the effects of TSGs can be highly context dependent, as discussed throughout the text.

The molecular mechanisms of *p53* and *RB* function are closely related yet distinct. Both proteins are regulated and activated by a wide variety of input signals and function essentially by regulating transcription of key target genes. The output of *p53* is highly dependent on the cellular context and the nature and duration of the stress signal, but most often results in expression of the powerful cell cycle blocker *p21* and/or the apoptosis triggers PUMA and NOXA.[8] In contrast, the best characterized target of *RB* is the family of E2F transcription factors that coordinate expression of genes necessary for DNA synthesis and replication. RB physically interacts with E2Fs and, when bound at E2F-responsive loci, represses gene expression, thereby blocking the cell from entering the S (synthesis) phase of the cell cycle.[9]

Although direct mutation or loss of *p53* and *RB* is the most common way of circumventing the canonical antiproliferative response, some cancers instead choose to inactivate key players that are either upstream or downstream of *p53/RB*. The *INK4a/ARF* locus encodes two distinct and structurally unrelated proteins that block inactivation of *RB* and *p53* by their respective negative regulators, CDK4/CDK6 and MDM2. Intriguingly, the two genes possess distinct first exons but share downstream exons that are translated in alternative reading frames (the organization is conserved between humans and mice).[10] While the evolutionary significance of linking the two TSGs in a single locus is unclear, it creates an Achilles' heel for transformation since a single genetic hit can simultaneously compromise both *RB* and *p53* function.

Regulation of Ligand-Dependent Signaling

The growth, division, and differentiation of normal cells are linked to external cues that are tightly regulated by individual tissue microenvironments through the release of various growth factors, cytokines, and hormones. In the absence of these positive signals, cells usually remain quiescent and in some cases may even undergo apoptosis. Cancer cells, on the other hand, abrogate the requirement for such signals, enabling them to set their own replicative pace.

Growth factor signaling is mediated by branched circuits that convey the flow of information from the membrane to the nucleus. The cascade is initiated by the binding of various ligands to transmembrane receptors that typically contain intracellular tyrosine kinase motifs. Once activated, they emit signals to downstream targets that control cellular programs such as protein translation, cell division, and energy metabolism. At the same time, negative feedback loops act to dampen the signal to ensure that the output is temporally limited and thus wholly dependent on the continued presence of the extracellular trigger. While many cancers hyperactivate signaling pathways via mutations that result in ligand-independent constitutive activation of various components (such mutations are considered to be oncogenic rather than tumor suppressive because they result in a gain of function), we now know that inactivation of negative mechanisms can be an equally potent transforming event.

The prototypical tumor suppressor in this category is the lipid phosphatase PTEN, which opposes the highly oncogenic pro-growth and pro-survival PI3K/AKT signaling pathway.[11,12] Once activated by extracellular signals, the lipid kinase PI3K phosphorylates the membrane phospholipid phosphatidylinositol (3,4)-bisphosphate (PIP2) to generate phosphatidylinositol (3,4,5)-trisphosphate (PIP3). PIP3 in turn recruits AKT to the membrane, where it becomes phosphorylated by its activating kinases, PDK1 (at threonine 308) and mTORC2 (at serine 473). From there, the signal becomes highly branched and multifaceted, as activated AKT phosphorylates its downstream targets involved in cell growth and survival, glucose import, and protein translation. PTEN dephosphorylates PIP3 to PIP2, thereby directly undoing the work of activated PI3K and limiting the flux through the pathway. Transcriptional silencing, loss-of-function mutations, or complete loss of the *PTEN* gene is frequent in many types of cancer and has been shown to drive transformation and tumorigenesis in vitro and in vivo.

There are many other notable examples of TSGs that in one way or another regulate membrane signaling; however, it is important to note that the effects of deregulation of these pathways on cancer progression are highly context dependent. Excessive proliferation can trigger senescence or result in premature terminal differentiation, a dead end for premalignant cells. Some signaling cascades, such as Notch, can be both oncogenic (hyperactivated in T-cell acute lymphoblastic leukemia) and tumor suppressive (inactivated in chronic myelomonocytic leukemia), even within the same tissue[13,14]; others, such as transforming growth factor (TGF)-β, can oppose transformation at early stages of disease, but favor progression and metastasis at later stages[15]; and yet others, such as DCC, may promote growth and behave as an oncogene in the presence of their cognate ligand or alternatively promote apoptosis and act as a tumor suppressor if the ligand is absent.[16] Deregulation of growth factor signaling in cancer remains an intense area of research, and has, and will continue to present attractive targets for development of novel therapeutics.

DNA Repair and Maintenance of Genome Integrity

The multistep acquisitions of genetic changes that disable TSGs and activate oncogenes depend in a large part on an increased level of genomic instability. It is generally thought that a cell must sustain at least four, but probably more, mutations to become transformed, and given the remarkable accuracy of DNA replication in eukaryotic organisms, mutations that disable cellular systems involved in sensing and repairing damaged DNA provide a big selective advantage for cancer cells.[1,2] Consistent with this notion, individuals that inherit mutations in various components of the DNA damage response are predisposed to cancer, as exemplified by *BRCA1* and *BRCA2* in familial breast and ovarian cancer. Indeed, many TSGs have been catalogued whose inactivation in one way or another drives the genomic instability that fuels cancer progression. Among them are MLH1 and MSH2 (frequently mutated or silenced in familial and sporadic colorectal cancer)—essential components of the mismatch repair system that detects and corrects individual nucleotide substitutions; the Fanconi anemia complex that facilitates resolution of DNA cross-links; and the ATM kinase that is triggered by DNA double-strand breaks and in turn drives activation of DNA repair and cell cycle checkpoints.[17]

No discussion of DNA damage would be complete without mentioning p53 whose central role in maintaining genome integrity has led to its moniker "the guardian of the genome."[8] DNA damage sensors such as ATM/ATR, in addition to recruiting proteins involved directly in DNA repair, also activate *p53*, which rapidly puts a halt to any further replicative activity. If the input suggests that the damage can be repaired, the arrest induced by *p53* is only temporary. On the other hand, if the damage is too great, to ensure that genetic errors are not propagated, *p53* can activate senescence or apoptosis as discussed above. Thus, loss of *p53* function significantly compromises the ability of cells to fix genetic errors, even if the other components of the DNA damage machinery remain intact.

Another apparatus that is increasingly being recognized for its role in cancer and aging is that which controls telomere stability.[18] In mammalian cells, telomeres are complex nucleoprotein structures that protect and replicate the ends of chromosomes. In most human cells, telomeres become progressively shorter with every cell division, eventually reaching a critical point that triggers *p53*-mediated senescence. Even if this response can be overcome, continued replication eventually leads to crisis, a cellular phase marked by overwhelming genome disorganization and eventual death of the cell. Paradoxically, telomere dysfunction can both aid and limit cancer progression, genetically behaving as a tumor suppressor in some settings and an oncogene in others. At early stages of the transformation process, telomere erosion can lead to chromosomal rearrangements and aneuploidy, particularly in the absence of a functional p53 response (which would otherwise recognize naked chromosome ends as a classical DNA double-stranded break). In advanced tumors, however, telomerase activity is frequently reactivated in order to allow the rapidly dividing cells to avoid crisis and thus attain replicative immortality. Notably, TERT, the central enzymatic component of telomerase, has recently been implicated in other non-telomere–related oncogenic pathways, further underlying the importance of this protein in cancer.[19]

Angiogenesis

The requirement for ample nutrients and oxygen, as well as removal of waste products, means that growing solid tumors must establish an adequate blood supply. In order to do so, many cancers frequently activate the so-called angiogenic switch, inducing the normally quiescent vasculature to sprout new connections in a process termed neo-angiogenesis.[20] At the molecular level, this process is controlled by the HIF (hypoxia-inducible factor) family of transcription factors, which coordinate the expression of various endothelial and hematopoietic growth factors including VEGF (vascular endothelial growth factor) and PDGF (platelet-derived growth factor). HIF activity is in turn controlled by specialized oxygen-responsive propyl hydroxylases and the VHL E3 ubiquitin ligase, which, under conditions of normoxia (normal oxygen concentration), marks HIFα subunits for degradation by the proteasome. Loss of *VHL* function leads to constitutive HIF activation and consequently favors angiogenesis. The *VHL* gene is thus an important TSG antagonizing the angiogenic switch, and it has been shown that *VHL* is a frequent target of inactivating events in many types of cancer, particularly those with a high vascular component.[21,22]

Metabolism

More than 50 years ago, Otto Warburg made the observation that cancer cells reprogram their energy metabolism.[23] Over the past decade, this observation has been substantiated and expanded, and the genetic events that trigger this metabolic switch are now being uncovered. The difference between "normal" glucose metabolism and the "Warburg" metabolism (also known as oxidative glycolysis) is essentially as follows: in the presence of oxygen, normal (differentiated) cells use pyruvate generated from glycolysis to drive the TCA cycle in the mitochondria; in contrast, cancer cells (and rapidly proliferating normal cells) instead prefer to redirect pyruvate, and other glycolytic intermediates, into anabolic pathways. Although less efficient in terms of ATP production (cancer cells typically compensate by increasing their glucose uptake), Warburg metabolism allows for the rapid generation of macromolecules required for cell growth.[24] Notably, at least two enzymes in the TCA cycle, SDH (succinate dehydrogenase) and FH (fumarate hydratase), are bona fide TSGs. Inactivation of *SDH* and *FH* stabilizes HIFα subunits, triggering a pseudo-hypoxia response characterized by increased glycolysis.[25] Additionally, loss of a number of other TSGs including *PTEN* and *p53* has also been shown to favor metabolic rewiring by various mechanisms.[12,26]

Epigenetic Regulators, miRNAs, and ceRNAs

Regulation of gene expression in eukaryotic cells is an extremely complex process that is controlled at many different levels, both before and after transcription. While transcription factors that bind specific DNA sequences and facilitate or hinder the recruitment of RNA polymerase to particular loci have long been known for their role in cancer, other mechanisms such as those that control the state of chromatin, DNA methylation, and RNA stability are now increasingly being recognized as TSGs or oncogenes.

The TET gene family encodes three proteins, TET1-3, that catalyze the hydroxylation of the methylated nucleotide 5-methylcytosine (5mC) to 5-hydroxymethylcytosine (5hmC).[27] 5mC is a crucial epigenetic mark and if deregulated leads to genome-wide inappropriate gene silencing and activation. 5hmC appears to facilitate DNA demethylation by both passive (during DNA replication) and active (independent of DNA replication) mechanisms. Notably, the *TET2* gene is frequently inactivated in myeloid malignancies, and its role as a TSG in the hematopoietic system has been confirmed by a series of mouse modeling studies.[28,29]

Control of gene expression by small non-coding RNA molecules is ubiquitous in mammalian cells and can also be deregulated in cancer. microRNAs are ~22 nucleotide RNA molecules that guide the RNA-induced silencing complex (RISC) to microRNA response elements (MREs) on target transcripts, usually resulting in degradation of the transcript or inhibition of its translation. Importantly, recent evidence suggests that miRNAs are part of a larger regulatory framework that potentially includes virtually all RNA molecules in the genome. RNAs that share an MRE for the same miRNA can compete for miRNA binding and consequently directly regulate each other in conditions where the miRNA concentration is a limiting factor. This previously unappreciated phenomenon, which has been termed ceRNA (competing endogenous RNA), can apply to both protein-coding and non-coding transcripts.[30] The discovery that miRNAs such as *Let-7* and ceRNAs such as *PTENP1* (a transcribed pseudogene), *ZEB2*, *CNOT6L*, and *VAPA* have tumor-suppressive properties is expanding the search for new TSGs into unchartered areas of the human genome.[31-34]

HAPLO-INSUFFICIENCY AND CANCER

From a genetic perspective, a gene is said to be haplo-insufficient if loss of a single allele is enough to at least partially abrogate gene function. The question of whether TSGs can be haplo-insufficient is not merely a theoretical one, but has important implications for cancer diagnosis and treatment, as we will discuss later. In order to fully appreciate our current understanding of dose-dependent effects of TSGs, it is useful to consider it from a historical perspective.

As we alluded to earlier, the story began 40 years ago, when Alfred Knudson first formulated his revolutionary "two-hit model" of cancer (Fig. 5.2).[5] Knudson undertook a statistical analysis of sporadic and familial cases of retinoblastoma (a cancer of the eye) and hypothesized that tumor development can only be initiated when both alleles of a TSG are fully inactivated. This hypothesis was based on the observations that familial retinoblastoma is inherited in a dominant manner, frequently affects both eyes, and occurs early in life, whereas sporadic disease occurs later in life and typically affects only one eye. Knudson postulated that in familial cases, cancer predisposition occurs through an inherited heterozygous mutation and that a subsequent second hit, which is acquired somatically, is required for tumor development. Since the probability that an individual with the inherited allele would ultimately develop disease due to a second hit was almost 100%, the disease phenotype manifested in a dominant manner. At the time it was not clear whether the two mutations required for tumorigenesis occur in the same gene or in different genes, but it was theorized that the second allele of the inherited disease gene could be the target of inactivation or deletion. Indeed, the discovery of the RB and the subsequent verification that both alleles of RB are frequently mutated in retinoblastoma patients confirmed Knudson's hypothesis and established RB as the first recognized TSG.[35]

Following Knudson's landmark study, other researchers began to search for TSGs by using genetic analyses on various types of inherited and sporadic cancers. One strategy was to examine tumors for deleted chromosomal regions and then to confirm that the second allele of the putative TSG was also mutated or deleted. Overall, these studies were tremendously successful and led to the discovery of numerous TSGs including *p53*,[36] *VHL*,[37] *APC*,[38] and *BRCA1/2*.[39] However, as more and more cancers were analyzed, it became apparent that not all genes that are recurrently lost in cancer follow the "two-hit model." Additionally, as the technology to target genes in mice

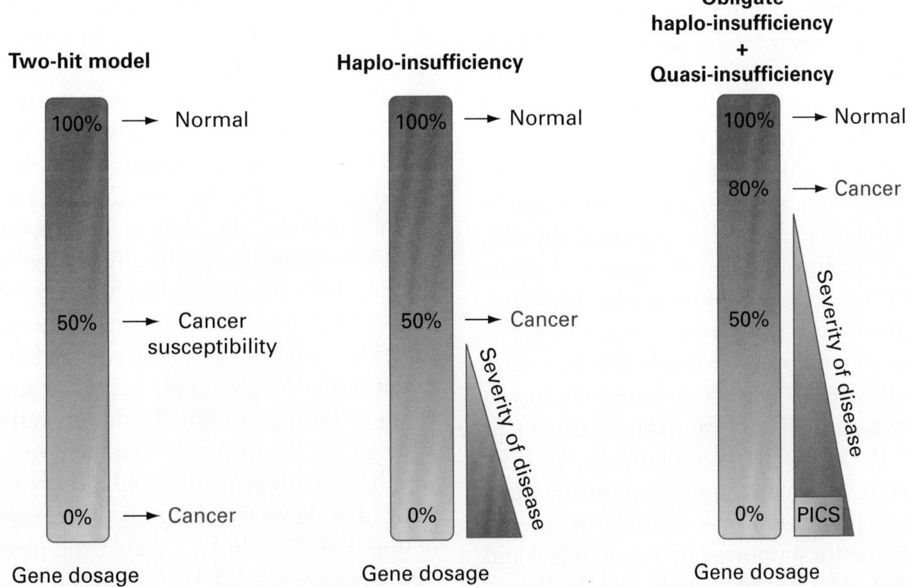

FIGURE 5–2 Current paradigms of tumor suppression. Tumor suppressor genes (TSGs) can be broadly classified into three categories. The first category follows the two-hit model proposed by Alfred Knudson where heterozygous deletion of a TSG confers cancer susceptibility and complete deletion is required for tumor formation (e.g., *Rb*, left panel). The second category is haplo-insufficient TSGs (e.g., *p53*, middle panel). Here, the inactivation of a single allele is sufficient to induce tumorigenesis. Further reduction in the dose of a haplo-insufficient TSG dictates the severity of the disease. The third category is obligate haplo-insufficient TSGs (e.g., *PTEN*, right panel). In this category, heterozygous loss is paradoxically more tumorigenic than homozygous loss. Complete inactivation can trigger a powerful senescence response (in the case of *PTEN* loss termed PICS) that opposes cancer progression. (Adapted from Berger AH, Knudson AG, Pandolfi PP. *Nature*. 2011 Aug 10;476(7359):163-9.)

became available, mouse models of cancer increasingly pointed to the existence of other mechanisms of tumor suppression.[40,41]

The earliest identified examples of haplo-insufficient TSGs were observed in patients suffering from Li-Fraumeni syndrome.[42] Analysis of the *p53* locus in these individuals revealed that although both alleles of *p53* were commonly mutated or lost, in some cases, only one allele was affected. This led to the hypothesis that the inactivation of a single *p53* allele could be sufficient to drive disease development (see Fig. 5.2). Definitive proof subsequently came from the analysis of transgenic mouse models. *p53* knockout mice are viable and fertile, but promptly develop a variety of tumors that ultimately lead to death of the animals.[43] *p53* heterozygous mice have a longer life span than *p53* null mice, but importantly have a significantly shorter life expectancy than wild-type control animals. Detailed morphological and histological analysis of *p53* heterozygotes showed that they also develop tumors in many different tissues. Importantly, many of these tumors do not show alteration of the remaining *p53* allele, particularly in older animals (curiously tumors in younger animals typically display loss of heterozygosity (LOH) at the *p53* locus).[40] At the same time, similar findings were also reported for the cell cycle inhibitor p27.[41]

Two recent important additions to the haplo-insufficiency hypothesis are the concepts of quasi-insufficiency—partial loss (<50%) of TSG activity is sufficient to initiate tumorigenesis—and obligate haplo-insufficiency—only partial loss, and not total loss of TSG activity, can initiate tumorigenesis (see Fig. 5.2).[6,7] One TSG that demonstrates both quasi-insufficient and haplo-insufficient properties is *PTEN*. As for other TSGs like RB and *p53*, germ-line mutations in *PTEN* cause an inherited human cancer predisposition syndrome called Cowden syndrome. *PTEN* knockout animals die during early embryonic development, whereas *PTEN* heterozygous animals develop autoimmunity and multiple tumors in different organs including the prostate, thyroid, and endometrium. Similar to the heterozygous *p53* situation, not all *PTEN* heterozygous tumors display LOH.[11,12] Interestingly, recent studies using conditional and hypomorphic *PTEN* transgenic mouse models where *PTEN* level varied from 0% to 80% demonstrated that even a subtle 20% reduction in *PTEN* can lead to cancer in particular organs.[44] Paradoxically, complete loss of *PTEN* in the mouse prostate appears to oppose tumorigenesis rather than increase it. In vivo observations of disease latency and penetrance are supported by biochemical and mechanistic evidence. The loss of a single *PTEN* allele is sufficient to hyperactivate the PI3K–AKT signaling pathway and thus confer a proliferative and survival advantage to cells. Conversely, total abolition of *PTEN* expression leads to induction of *p19*^{Arf}, *p53*, and *p21*, triggering a powerful fail-safe senescence mechanism (termed *PTEN* loss–induced cellular senescence or PICS). Concomitant deletion of *p53* in *PTEN*-deficient prostates bypasses PICS and results in aggressive cancer.[45]

For some genes, loss of a single allele may only be sufficient when combined with certain other genetic events. This situation, which has been termed compound haplo-insufficiency, is exemplified by 5q-syndrome, a disease that manifests as myeloid dysplasia in affected patients and is characterized by loss of the q-arm of one copy of chromosome 5.[46] Despite extensive efforts, no corresponding mutation or deletion on the other copy of chromosome 5 could be identified in these patients, strongly suggesting that loss of only one allele of a gene, combined with loss of single alleles of other genes on 5q, could lead to transformation. Interestingly, in some cases compound haplo-insufficiency may be "asymmetric," where the phenotype of one gene is potentiated by the loss of another, but not vice versa.[47]

The evidence from studies of *p53*, *PTEN*, and other haplo-insufficient TSGs (see Table 5.1) recently led Berger et al. to propose that TSGs can behave in a dose-dependent manner—the so-called continuum model of tumor suppression (see Fig. 5.2).[6] The implication of this model is that events that do not result in genomic loss of a particular TSG, but nonetheless (partially) influence its expression at the transcriptional or translational level, can contribute to oncogenic transformation. Importantly, the function of TSGs that have not been completely lost can potentially be restored, thus offering potential strategies for therapeutic intervention.

TARGETING TSGs FOR CANCER THERAPY

Most current anticancer treatments do not target specific pathways that are deregulated in cancer cells, but instead focus on pathways that are largely common to rapidly dividing cells. However, because many normal cells in the body are also proliferating, it is often difficult or impossible to use these treatments to suppress the cancer without harming the patient. The current hope in cancer research is that by fully defining the genetic landscape of cancer, we will be able to generate specifically tailored targeted therapies that are both more effective and less toxic. Traditionally, cancer drug discovery has largely concentrated on gain-of-function mutations in oncogenes rather than inactivating mutations in TSGs, simply because it appeared to be easier to do so both conceptually and operationally. While this strategy has led to the development of a number of drugs that have made it to the clinic, there is an accumulating body of evidence that suggests that reactivating or even targeting TSGs could be a viable complementary approach in many cases (Fig. 5.3). This is particularly true for those TSGs that display haplo-insufficient properties.

Reactivation of TSG Function

Since the discovery that *p53* is an extremely powerful tumor suppressor, researchers have sought to restore its function in tumors in order to reestablish its anticancer

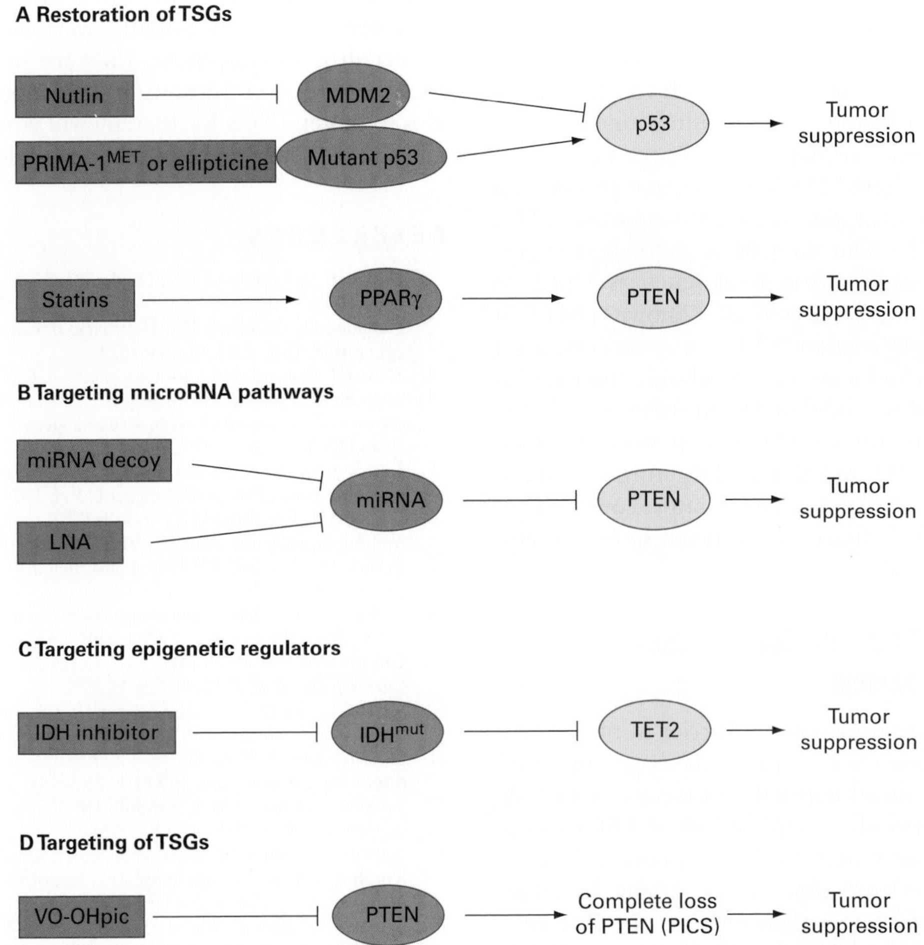

FIGURE 5–3 Strategies that aim to modulate tumor suppressor gene (TSG) function for cancer therapy. **A:** TSG function can be restored using small molecule inhibitors. p53 can be stabilized at the protein level by inhibiting its negative regulator MDM2 using Nutlins. The wild-type activity of a mutant p53 protein can be restored by PRIMA-1^{MET} or ellipticine. Statins can enhance the levels of *PTEN* through peroxisome proliferator–activated receptor (PPAR)γ signaling. **B:** Targeting microRNA pathways: Oncogenic microRNAs that suppress TSGs can be inhibited through microRNA decoys or locked nucleic acids (LNAs). **C:** The tumor-suppressive epigenetic regulator TET2 is inhibited by mutant IDH enzymes. Inhibition of mutant IDH can oppose tumorigenesis by restoring TET2 function. **D:** Inhibition of obligate haplo-insufficient TSGs (e.g., PTEN activity is blocked by VO-OHpic) can elicit a potent senescence response (PICS) that leads to tumor suppression. (Adapted in part from Nardella C, Clohessy JG, Alimonti A, et al., *Nat Rev Cancer.* 2011;11:503-511.)

properties. Expression of *p53* in human cancer cell lines using an adenovirus-based delivery system inhibits cell proliferation and survival,[48] and importantly, restoration of *p53* activity in established tumors leads to tumor regression in genetically engineered mouse models.[49,50] Several strategies to reactivate the *p53* pathway have been proposed. In cases where *p53* is mutated, it may be possible to use small molecules like Prima-1^{MET} or ellipticine that can bind to the mutant protein, inducing a structural change that restores its wild-type tumor-suppressive function.[51,52] In situations where *p53* expression is partially lost, but at least one wild-type allele of the gene remains, it may be possible to increase p53 protein by antagonizing its negative regulator Mdm2. Mdm2 is an E3 ubiquitin ligase that targets p53 for degradation by the proteasome. Nutlins are small molecule inhibitors that block the interaction between Mdm2 and p53, thereby stabilizing p53 protein and function (Fig. 5.3A). Preliminary evidence demonstrates that Nutlins are able to reactivate the p53 pathway and inhibit cancer cell proliferation in vivo.[53]

Another TSG the restoration of which may benefit cancer patients is *PTEN*. As in the case of *p53*, *PTEN* is often inactivated in cancer by mechanisms that do not involve genomic loss. Statins are small molecules that increase PTEN levels through peroxisome proliferator–activated receptor (PPAR)γ signaling and could be used to treat tumors with lowered expression of PTEN (see Fig. 5.3A).[54] The *PTEN* gene is under the control of a powerful microRNA network that is aberrantly upregulated in some cancers.[55] Antagonizing these microRNAs using microRNA decoys or the novel technology of locked nucleic acids (Fig. 5.3B)[56] has been suggested as a strategy to reestablish *PTEN* function.

In recent years, it has become apparent that epigenetic factors are widely involved in tumorigenesis. Dysfunction of enzymes that directly or indirectly modify DNA and histones can simultaneously inactivate multiple TSGs. In particular, cancer cells commonly display an altered DNA methylation profile that leads to transcriptional silencing of, among others, *Rb1*, *VHL*, and *BRCA1*.[57] One epigenetic factor that is currently being targeted for drug development is *TET2*. As discussed previously, *TET2* is itself a known TSG that regulates DNA methylation.[58,59] In some cancers, most notably acute myeloid leukemia and glioblastoma multiforme, *TET2* activity is inhibited by the onco-metabolite 2-hydroxyglutarate produced by mutations in the metabolic enzymes IDH1 and IDH2. Targeting of mutant IDH enzymes by small molecule inhibitors could lead to restoration of TET2 function and result in tumor suppression (Fig. 5.3C).[60]

Suppression of TSG Function to Induce Fail-Safe Mechanisms

Cellular senescence is a powerful barrier to tumor progression and consequently "pro-senescence therapy" is emerging as a novel approach to treat cancer.[61] As we discussed previously, complete loss of TSGs can in some cases trigger senescence, and, provocatively, it may be possible to treat some cancer patients by inhibiting TSG function rather than restoring it. One gene that is a potential candidate for this strategy is *PTEN*. Partial loss of *PTEN* is a frequent early event in cancer. In the presence of a competent *p53* response, *PTEN* loss induces PICS and targeting *PTEN* using the small molecule inhibitor VO-OHpic was recently shown to induce PICS in vitro and in vivo (Fig. 5.3D).[62] Using VO-OHpic on early tumors with partially abrogated *PTEN* expression and at least one unmodified *p53* allele may yet prove to be a successful therapeutic strategy. Additionally, VO-OHpic may synergize with p53-enhancing drugs (e.g., Nutlins), which are able to further elevate the senescence response even in a situation where the p53 pathway is fully intact.[62]

CONCLUDING REMARKS

Over the past 30 years, we have gained tremendous insights into the genetics of cancer. Initially using cytogenetic analysis and techniques such as restriction fragment length polymorphism, and more recently with high-throughput sequencing technology, researches have probed the cancer genome and catalogued many alterations in TSGs and oncogenes. The challenge now is to understand the functional meaning of this genetic information—as the genetic information is per se meaningless in the absence of genetic annotation—and to translate our understanding of the molecular events that lead to cellular transformation into novel therapeutic strategies. Although TSGs were initially overlooked as targets for cancer drug development, they are now beginning to receive more careful attention. Undoubtedly, new strategies to target TSGs for therapy will continue to emerge and will in the future benefit cancer patients.

REFERENCES

1. Hanahan D, Weinberg RA. The hallmarks of cancer. *Cell.* 2000;100:57-70.
2. Hanahan D, Weinberg RA. Hallmarks of cancer: the next generation. *Cell.* 2011;144:646-674.
3. Sherr CJ. Principles of tumor suppression. *Cell.* 2004;116:235-246.
4. Stehelin D, Varmus HE, Bishop JM, et al. DNA related to the transforming gene(s) of avian sarcoma viruses is present in normal avian DNA. *Nature.* 1976;260:170-173.
5. Knudson AG Jr. Mutation and cancer: statistical study of retinoblastoma. *Proc Natl Acad Sci U S A.* 1971;68:820-823.
6. Berger AH, Knudson AG, Pandolfi PP. A continuum model for tumour suppression. *Nature.* 2011;476:163-169.
7. Berger AH, Pandolfi PP. Haplo-insufficiency: a driving force in cancer. *J Pathol.* 2011;223:137-146.
8. Zilfou JT, Lowe SW. Tumor suppressive functions of p53. *Cold Spring Harb Perspect Biol.* 2009;1:a001883.
9. Chinnam M, Goodrich DW. RB1, development, and cancer. *Curr Top Dev Biol.* 2011;94:129-169.
10. Sherr CJ. The INK4a/ARF network in tumour suppression. *Nat Rev Mol Cell Biol.* 2001;2:731-737.
11. Di Cristofano A, Pandolfi PP. The multiple roles of PTEN in tumor suppression. *Cell.* 2000;100:387-390.
12. Salmena L, Carracedo A, Pandolfi PP. Tenets of PTEN tumor suppression. *Cell.* 2008;133:403-414.
13. Aster JC, Blacklow SC, Pear WS. Notch signalling in T-cell lymphoblastic leukaemia/lymphoma and other haematological malignancies. *J Pathol.* 2011;223:262-273.
14. Klinakis A, Lobry C, Abdel-Wahab O, et al. A novel tumour-suppressor function for the Notch pathway in myeloid leukaemia. *Nature.* 2011;473:230-233.
15. Ikushima H, Miyazono K. TGFbeta signalling: a complex web in cancer progression. *Nat Rev Cancer.* 2010;10:415-424.
16. Carvalho AL, Chuang A, Jiang WW, et al. Deleted in colorectal cancer is a putative conditional tumor-suppressor gene inactivated by promoter hypermethylation in head and neck squamous cell carcinoma. *Cancer Res.* 2006;66:9401-9407.
17. Negrini S, Gorgoulis VG, Halazonetis TD. Genomic instability—an evolving hallmark of cancer. *Nat Rev Mol Cell Biol.* 2010;11:220-228.
18. Artandi SE, DePinho RA. Telomeres and telomerase in cancer. *Carcinogenesis.* 2010;31:9-18.
19. Park JI, Venteicher AS, Hong JY, et al. Telomerase modulates Wnt signalling by association with target gene chromatin. *Nature.* 2009;460:66-72.
20. Baeriswyl V, Christofori G. The angiogenic switch in carcinogenesis. *Semin Cancer Biol.* 2009;19:329-337.
21. Poon E, Harris AL, Ashcroft M. Targeting the hypoxia-inducible factor (HIF) pathway in cancer. *Expert Rev Mol Med.* 2009;11:e26.
22. Gossage L, Eisen T. Alterations in VHL as potential biomarkers in renal-cell carcinoma. *Nat Rev Clin Oncol.* 2010;7:277-288.
23. Warburg O. On respiratory impairment in cancer cells. *Science.* 1956;124:269-270.
24. Vander Heiden MG. Targeting cancer metabolism: a therapeutic window opens. *Nat Rev Drug Discov.* 2011;10:671-684.
25. King A, Selak MA, Gottlieb E. Succinate dehydrogenase and fumarate hydratase: linking mitochondrial dysfunction and cancer. *Oncogene.* 2006;25:4675-4682.
26. Vousden KH. Alternative fuel—another role for p53 in the regulation of metabolism. *Proc Natl Acad Sci U S A.* 2010;107:7117-7118.
27. Cimmino L, Abdel-Wahab O, Levine RL, et al. TET family proteins and their role in stem cell differentiation and transformation. *Cell Stem Cell.* 2011;9:193-204.

28. Moran-Crusio K, Reavie L, Shih A, et al. Tet2 loss leads to increased hematopoietic stem cell self-renewal and myeloid transformation. *Cancer Cell*. 2011;20:11-24.
29. Quivoron C, Couronne L, Della Valle V, et al. TET2 inactivation results in pleiotropic hematopoietic abnormalities in mouse and is a recurrent event during human lymphomagenesis. *Cancer Cell*. 2011;20:25-38.
30. Salmena L, Poliseno L, Tay Y, et al. A ceRNA hypothesis: the Rosetta Stone of a hidden RNA language? *Cell*. 2011;146:353-358.
31. Bussing I, Slack FJ, Grosshans H. let-7 microRNAs in development, stem cells and cancer. *Trends Mol Med*. 2008;14:400-409.
32. Karreth FA, Tay Y, Perna D, et al. In vivo identification of tumor-suppressive PTEN ceRNAs in an oncogenic BRAF-induced mouse model of melanoma. *Cell*. 2011;147:382-395.
33. Poliseno L, Salmena L, Zhang J, et al. A coding-independent function of gene and pseudogene mRNAs regulates tumour biology. *Nature*. 2010;465:1033-1038.
34. Tay Y, Kats L, Salmena L, et al. Coding-independent regulation of the tumor suppressor PTEN by competing endogenous mRNAs. *Cell*. 2011;147:344-357.
35. Friend SH, Bernards R, Rogelj S, et al. A human DNA segment with properties of the gene that predisposes to retinoblastoma and osteosarcoma. *Nature*. 1986;323:643-646.
36. Baker SJ, Fearon ER, Nigro JM, et al. Chromosome 17 deletions and p53 gene mutations in colorectal carcinomas. *Science*. 1989;244:217-221.
37. Tory K, Brauch H, Linehan M, et al. Specific genetic change in tumors associated with von Hippel-Lindau disease. *J Natl Cancer Inst*. 1989;81:1097-1101.
38. Levy DB, Smith KJ, Beazer-Barclay Y, et al. Inactivation of both APC alleles in human and mouse tumors. *Cancer Res*. 1994;54:5953-5958.
39. Gudmundsson J, Johannesdottir G, Bergthorsson JT, et al. Different tumor types from BRCA2 carriers show wild-type chromosome deletions on 13q12-q13. *Cancer Res*. 1995;55:4830-4832.
40. Venkatachalam S, Shi YP, Jones SN, et al. Retention of wild-type p53 in tumors from p53 heterozygous mice: reduction of p53 dosage can promote cancer formation. *EMBO J*. 1998;17:4657-4667.
41. Fero ML, Randel E, Gurley KE, et al. The murine gene p27Kip1 is haplo-insufficient for tumour suppression. *Nature*. 1998;396:177-180.
42. Malkin D, Li FP, Strong LC, et al. Germ line p53 mutations in a familial syndrome of breast cancer, sarcomas, and other neoplasms. *Science*. 1990;250:1233-1238.
43. Jacks T, Remington L, Williams BO, et al. Tumor spectrum analysis in p53-mutant mice. *Curr Biol*. 1994;4:1-7.
44. Alimonti A, Carracedo A, Clohessy JG, et al. Subtle variations in Pten dose determine cancer susceptibility. *Nat Genet*. 2010;42:454-458.
45. Chen Z, Trotman LC, Shaffer D, et al. Crucial role of p53-dependent cellular senescence in suppression of Pten-deficient tumorigenesis. *Nature*. 2005;436:725-730.
46. Ebert BL. Deletion 5q in myelodysplastic syndrome: a paradigm for the study of hemizygous deletions in cancer. *Leukemia*. 2009;23:1252-1256.
47. Ma L, Teruya-Feldstein J, Behrendt N, et al. Genetic analysis of Pten and Tsc2 functional interactions in the mouse reveals asymmetrical haploinsufficiency in tumor suppression. *Genes Dev*. 2005;19:1779-1786.
48. Chada S, Menander KB, Bocangel D, et al. Cancer targeting using tumor suppressor genes. *Front Biosci*. 2008;13:1959-1967.
49. Ventura A, Kirsch DG, McLaughlin ME, et al. Restoration of p53 function leads to tumour regression in vivo. *Nature*. 2007;445:661-665.
50. Xue W, Zender L, Miething C, et al. Senescence and tumour clearance is triggered by p53 restoration in murine liver carcinomas. *Nature*. 2007;445:656-660.
51. Bykov VJ, Issaeva N, Shilov A, et al. Restoration of the tumor suppressor function to mutant p53 by a low-molecular-weight compound. *Nat Med*. 2002;8:282-288.
52. Peng Y, Li C, Chen L, et al. Rescue of mutant p53 transcription function by ellipticine. *Oncogene*. 2003;22:4478-4487.
53. Vassilev LT, Vu BT, Graves B, et al. In vivo activation of the p53 pathway by small-molecule antagonists of MDM2. *Science*. 2004;303:844-848.
54. Teresi RE, Planchon SM, Waite KA, et al. Regulation of the PTEN promoter by statins and SREBP. *Hum Mol Genet*. 2008;17:919-928.
55. Poliseno L, Salmena L, Riccardi L, et al. Identification of the miR-106b~25 microRNA cluster as a proto-oncogenic PTEN-targeting intron that cooperates with its host gene MCM7 in transformation. *Sci Signal*. 2010;3:ra29.
56. Lanford RE, Hildebrandt-Eriksen ES, Petri A, et al. Therapeutic silencing of microRNA-122 in primates with chronic hepatitis C virus infection. *Science*. 2010;327:198-201.
57. Esteller M. Cancer epigenetics for the 21st century: what's next? *Genes Cancer*. 2011;2:604-606.
58. Ko M, Huang Y, Jankowska AM, et al. Impaired hydroxylation of 5-methylcytosine in myeloid cancers with mutant TET2. *Nature*. 2010;468:839-843.
59. Tahiliani M, Koh KP, Shen Y, et al. Conversion of 5-methylcytosine to 5-hydroxymethylcytosine in mammalian DNA by MLL partner TET1. *Science*. 2009;324:930-935.
60. Dang L, Jin S, Su SM. IDH mutations in glioma and acute myeloid leukemia. *Trends Mol Med*. 2010;16:387-397.
61. Nardella C, Clohessy JG, Alimonti A, et al. Pro-senescence therapy for cancer treatment. *Nat Rev Cancer*. 2011;11:503-511.
62. Alimonti A, Nardella C, Chen Z, et al. A novel type of cellular senescence that can be enhanced in mouse models and human tumor xenografts to suppress prostate tumorigenesis. *J Clin Invest*. 2010;120:681-693.

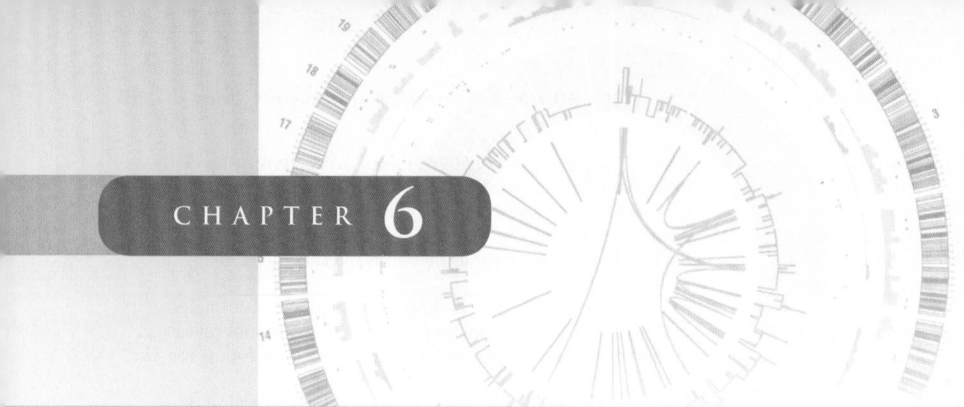

CHAPTER 6

Viruses and Human Cancers: Pathogenesis and Therapeutic Implication

Ih-Jen Su, Yao Chang, Grace Yu, and Charles Dwo-Yuan Sia

BACKGROUND

Viruses can contribute to the development of several human cancers.[1] Among them, malignant lymphoma is the human cancer most frequently associated with oncogenic viruses.[2,3] The association of viruses with human cancers can be traced back to 1960 when Denis Burkitt first noted the prevalence of a unique tumor involving the jaw and/or abdomen of African children.[2] The African Burkitt lymphoma (BL) was later identified to be closely associated with Epstein-Barr virus (EBV). Following BL, EBV was later found to be associated with nasopharyngeal carcinoma (NPC), which is most prevalent in Hong Kong Cantonese.[4] EBV was later found to cause post-transplant lymphoproliferative disorders,[5] Hodgkin lymphoma (HL),[6] and T-cell and nasal NK/T-cell lymphoma.[7,8] The ubiquitous EBV has been linked to a spectrum of epithelial malignancies and the smooth muscle tumor in acquired immunodeficiency syndrome (AIDS) patients,[9] raising the possibility of a passenger role for EBV with these malignancies. Other members of DNA viruses were later found to be associated with human cancers (Table 6.1). The hepatitis B virus (HBV) was established to cause hepatocellular carcinoma (HCC), representing the first example of human virus–associated cancer controllable by vaccination.[10,11] Human papillomaviruses (HPVs) were found to be associated with cervical cancer and recently head and neck cancers[12,13] and is the second human cancer potentially controllable by vaccination. The vaccination program in the control of virus-associated human cancers represents a big success in the battle against human cancers. In 2000, Kaposi sarcoma herpes virus (KSHV) or human herpes virus (HHV-8) was found to cause Kaposi sarcoma in either human immunodeficiency virus (HIV)–positive or HIV-negative individuals.[14,15] Besides DNA viruses, RNA viruses were later found to be associated with adult T-cell lymphoma/leukemia (ATLL) in southern Japan and the Caribbean regions.[16,17] In 1988, hepatitis C virus (HCV) was found to be the cause of non-A, non-B hepatitis and was closely related to the development of HCC.[18,19] Overall, the virus-associated cancers account for about 15% of human cancers, but are much prevalent in the Asia-Pacific regions.[1] Although several other viruses such as polyomaviruses, herpes simplex virus, and adenovirus can exert transforming properties, the linkage to human cancers is loose and will not be discussed in this review.

THE FATE OF VIRUS-INFECTED CELLS

The characteristic clinical and histopathologic features of virus-associated cancers can be explained by the biology of virus–host interaction in virus-infected cells as shown in Fig. 6.1. Once the viruses infect the host cells, three major virus–host interactions will occur. In principle, the virus will try to manipulate the host machinery in favor of virus replication. The host cells, however, try to control the virus replication via the type I interferon regulatory system.[20,21] On the other hand, the host proteasomal degradation system will be activated to process the viral proteins through endoplasmic reticulum (ER) and assemble with HLA molecule to present to the Golgi apparatus and finally target the viral antigenic epitope with restricted HLA on the cell membrane. A cytotoxic T-cell (CTL) response to attack the virus-infected cells will then be initiated.[22,23] However, the virus is smart

TABLE 6–1 A List of Oncogenic Viruses, Virus-Associated Human Cancers, and the Candidate Oncoproteins

Viruses	Human Cancers	Viral Oncoproteins
(A) DNA viruses		
Epstein-Barr virus	Burkitt, Hodgkin, NPC, NK/T, PTLD, DLBCL	LMP-1, LMP2A
Hepatitis B virus	Hepatocellular carcinoma	HBx, pre-S mutants
Papilloma virus	Cervical cancers	E6, E7
Kaposi sarcoma herpes virus (HHV-8)	Kaposi sarcoma, effusion lymphoma	K9, Kaposin (K12), v IL-6
? Polyoma virus	Merkel cell carcinoma	T antigens
(B) RNA viruses		
HTLV-1	Adult T lymphoma	Tax
Hepatitis C virus	Hepatoma, lymphoma	Core protein

DLBCL, diffuse large B-cell lymphoma; HHV-8, human herpes virus; HTLV-1, human T-cell leukemia virus type 1; NPC, nasopharyngeal carcinoma; PTLD, post-transplant lymphoproliferative disorder.

enough to manipulate the transport system or the HLA molecules to escape from CTL immune attack. Besides the conventional CTL response, a complex interaction of the inflammatory components such as the regulatory T cells, inflammatory cytokines, PD-1/PDl ligand, and macrophages has been recently found to interplay and accounts for the local immunosuppression and the final development of virus-associated cancers.[24-26] If surviving from the CTL attack, the virus-infected cells will activate the second biologic machinery, the ER stress response, proteasomal ubiquitination degradation, and the autophagy system to handle the excess viral antigens.[27-29] An ER stress-related, inflammatory response will also be induced and proinflammatory cytokines are released. If the ER stress is not properly resolved, the apoptosis machinery will be activated and the virus-infected cells will then be removed by the scavenger macrophages.[30,31] However, if the virus-infected cells survive from the ER stress response, the viral proteins may accumulate in the ER and initiate the third biologic event or the sustained ER stress response. The sustained ER stress condition in chronic virus infection will result in DNA damage through oxidative intermediate (ROS) formation.[32,33] The DNA repair system will then be activated. If the DNA repair system fails, then chromosomal abnormalities or aneuploidy will ensue,[34,35] explaining the complex chromosomal abnormalities of virus-associated solid cancers in chronic virus infection. The virus-infected cells showing chromosomal abnormality and genomic instability will start to proliferate and become transformed and proliferated, resulting in the full-blown development of virus-associated cancers.

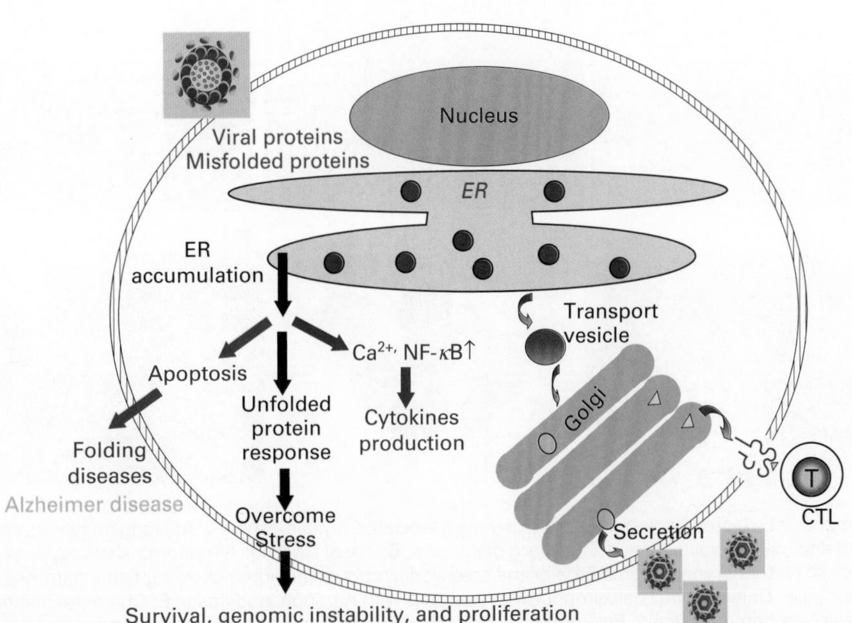

FIGURE 6–1 Diagram showing the fate of virus-infected cells. Basically, there are three major events occurring in the virus-infected cells.

FACTORS ASSOCIATED WITH THE DURATION OF TUMOR DEVELOPMENT AFTER VIRUS INFECTION

The virus-associated human cancers can affect children or adults. The duration from infection to tumor development ranges from months to years in post-transplant lymphoma and BL. The NPC, cervical cancers, and ATLL can occur in young adults 30 to 50 years of age, and at least two to three decades are required from the initial virus infection to tumor development. The HBV-related HCC, however, can affect a wide spectrum of age groups such as 5- to 10-year-old children, young adults, and elderly adults, suggesting that multiple biologic and immunologic events are involved in different individuals.[36,37] The HCV-related HCC usually pursues a long course of initiation and HCC usually develops at the seventh decade. The affected age of different virus-associated cancers provides informative knowledge to understand the underlying mechanism of viral tumorigenesis. BL has a consistent chromosomal translocation involving IgH and c-myc oncogene.[38] Although the nasal NK/T-cell lymphoma has a recurrent chromosomal deletion of the 6q25 region,[39] no specific oncogene or tumor suppressor gene has been identified yet. The same is true for human T-cell leukemia virus type 1 (HTLV-1)–associated ATL and no consistent chromosomal translocation or mutation has been identified so far. In solid tumors such as HCC, NPC, or cervical cancers, the chromosomal abnormalities are usually complex and no specific mutations are identified.[40,41] In general, tumors exhibiting a unique oncogene activation like BL tend to have a short duration of tumor development starting from virus infection. In this case, the viral oncoproteins may drive the subsequent oncogene activation or interact with the host proteins, rapidly leading to the tumor formation in a direct manner. However, for tumors that lack specific chromosomal abnormalities, viruses may play an indirect, stress-induced role in initiating inflammation, DNA damage, and aneuploidy. The aneuploidy will drive genomic instability and finally evolve into tumor formation, usually several decades after virus infection. These two entirely different patterns of viral tumorigenesis suggest that different mechanisms of viral tumorigenesis are involved.

TWO MAJOR HISTOPATHOLOGIC FEATURES REFLECT THE UNDERLYING IMMUNOPATHOGENESIS AND STRESS-RELATED DNA DAMAGE AND GENOMIC INSTABILITY

The virus-associated human cancers usually present with unique clinicopathologic features such as the paraneoplastic syndrome and drug resistance, either de novo or after chemotherapy.[42,43] These clinical features are related to the activation of nuclear factor κB (NF-κB) signals that make virus-infected cells resistant to chemotherapy and secrete cascades of proinflammatory cytokines.[44,45] The histopathology of virus-associated human cancers exhibits two characteristic features (Fig. 6.2). The most well-known feature is the rich inflammatory background as observed in HL and NPC or the so-called lymphoepithelioma. Current studies have revealed a complex interplay of CD4 FoxP3 regulatory T cells (Treg), CD8 T cells, cytokines and chemokines, the expression

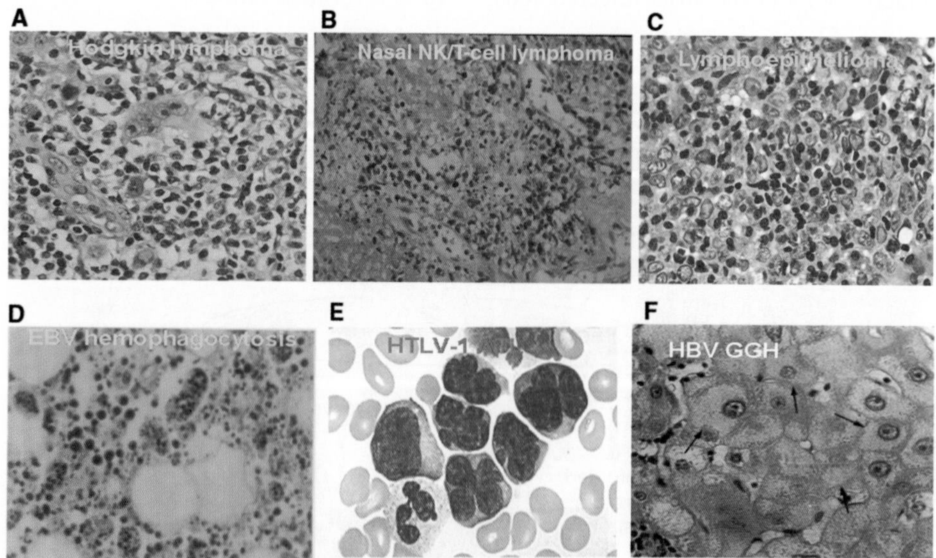

FIGURE 6–2 The characteristic histopathologic features of virus-associated human cancers. **A:** Hodgkin lymphoma showing rich inflammatory background and multinucleated Reed-Sternberg giant cells. **B:** Nasal NK/T-cell lymphoma showing angiocentricity and inflammatory background. **C:** Nasopharyngeal carcinoma or the so-called lymphoepithelioma showing rich inflammatory cells admixed with the undifferentiated tumor cells. **D:** Nasal NK/T-cell lymphoma presenting with hemophagocytosis. **E:** Characteristic flower- or clover-shaped nuclei of HTLV-1 adult T-cell lymphoma/leukemia. **F:** Ground glass hepatocytes (arrows) showing glassy appearance of the cytoplasm in chronic HBV infection.

of PD-1/PD-1 ligand, and tumor-associated macrophages (TAMs) in the inflammatory milieu of tumor tissues.[46-48] In EBV-associated NK/T- or T-cell lymphoma, macrophage activation with hemophagocytosis is frequently observed and usually indicates an ominous prognosis.[49,50] One unexpected development previously neglected by the pathologists is the role of macrophages in tumor tissues. TAM is now recognized to play an important role in tumor progression and prognosis through the secretion of proinflammatory cytokines, leading to local immunosuppression and to support the growth of tumor cells.[51,52] The second histopathologic feature of virus-associated human cancers is the characteristic nuclear morphology such as the Reed-Sternberg (RS) giant cells in HL[53] and the "clover-shaped" or flower-shaped nuclei in HTLV-1+ ATLL.[54] These nuclear morphologic changes are related to the disturbed mitotic spindle machinery induced by viral oncoproteins through direct interaction with host proteins in cell cycle regulation such as cyclins or the ER or oxidative stress–induced DNA damage and genomic instability.[55,56] Besides the characteristic nuclear morphology, the hepatocytes of chronic HBV infection frequently exhibit characteristic glassy or so-called ground glass hepatocytes (GGHs), a phenomenon associated with ER stress response induced by the overloaded or malfolded HBV surface antigens.[57,58] These characteristic histopathologic features reflect the underlying molecular, immunologic, and cell biology of virus-infected tumor cells. The recent advances in cell biology and immunology have clarified part of the pathogenesis and mechanism underlying the clinical and histopathologic features of virus-associated human cancers. However, much remains to be clarified in the future.

In the following sections, we will explore specifically the underlying pathogenesis of the two histopathologic features in individual virus-associated human cancer, with specific emphasis on EBV-associated human cancers and HBV-related liver cancers. Implications for tumor immunotherapy and therapy based on the immunopathogenesis and mechanism will be briefly discussed.

EBV AND HUMAN CANCERS: HL AS A PROTOTYPE MODEL TO EXPLORE THE INTERACTION BETWEEN VIRUS AND HOST CELLS

EBV establishes successful lifelong persistence in healthy carriers. Since many EBV proteins have oncogenic potential and can be the targets recognized by the host immune system, the virus stays peacefully with the host by restraining viral replication and expression of latency program of viral proteins. However, aberrant reactivation of EBV from the latent phase into the replicative (lytic) phase is frequently linked to the development or progression of EBV-associated cancers, among which NPC is a typical example. Serologic studies indicate that such viral reactivation is not only a cancer risk factor but also a significant marker for diagnosis, prognosis, and tumor recurrence.[59,60] The EBV latent membrane protein 1 (LMP1) is a well-documented oncoprotein generally detected in tissues of HL and NPC but only rarely in normal tissues.[61,62]

HL is the prototype of EBV-associated cancers that exhibit the two characteristic histopathologic features: the rich inflammatory background and the unique RS giant cells.[63,64] The malignant, multinucleated RS cells represent a histologic hallmark of HL, but the RS cells occupy only a small proportion of the cell component in the tumor tissues. By contrast, the reactive inflammatory cells, including lymphocytes, eosinophils, neutrophils, plasma cells, and macrophages, constitute the majority of HL tumor mass. Like local inflammation, many cytokines and chemokines are detected in HL, including interleukin (IL)-5, IL-6, IL-10, transforming growth factor (TGF)-β, granulocyte/macrophage colony stimulating factor (GM-CSF), and TNF-β.[65,66] These cytokines may mediate complex cross-talk between malignant cells and inflammatory infiltrates, and these chronic events may support tumor cell proliferation, progression, and survival. Production of the inflammatory cytokines and chemokines in HL results from constitutive activation of some transcription factors, such as NF-κB and STATs, in both tumor cells and stromal cells.[65,66] EBV LMP1 is the viral oncoprotein that activates the transcription factors, resulting in cytokine secretion and upregulation of growth factor receptors such as CD30, CD40, and C-MET in RS cells.[67,68]

The second EBV-associated cancer that exhibits a rich inflammatory background and characteristic nuclear morphology of tumor cells is the NPC or "lymphoepithelioma" because histologically it shows an inflammation-like microenvironment. Most of the infiltrating lymphocytes in the tumors are CD3+ T cells with variable CD4/CD8 composition, while B cells, monocytes, granulocytes, and other stromal cells are also present therein.[69] In contrast to their conventional antitumor functions, these infiltrating immune cells are considered to facilitate NPC progression in several ways. For example, inflammatory cytokines produced by the immune cells may serve as growth factors for tumor cells, while cell-to-cell interaction through membrane-bound CD40 and CD40 ligand may be another way in which T cells promote survival of NPC cells. Accumulating evidence supports the idea. LMP1 and Zta are two viral inducers of chemokines in NPC cells, contributing to intensive infiltration of immune cells. While Zta majorly upregulates IL-8, LMP1 induces a broader spectrum of chemokines that attract T cells.[70,71] LMP1 and Zta may also contribute to the establishment of an inflammation-like microenvironment through upregulation of other cytokines (such as IL-6) and transcription factors (such as NF-κB or Egr-1).[72] Distinct from other head and neck carcinomas, NPC is also featured by the tumor cells with the undifferentiated or poorly differentiated phenotype. A subcategory of NPC with spindle-shaped nuclei, suggesting the epithelial-to-mesenchymal transition (EMT), exhibits high metastatic potential.[73] The lymphoepithelioma-like carcinomas can also emerge at various anatomic sites apart from the nasopharynx, including the salivary gland, lung, stomach, and thymus.[74] Interestingly, many lymphoepithelioma-type cancers are also consistently associated with EBV infection, suggesting that EBV is a common etiologic factor causing the histopathologic characteristics of nuclear "undifferentiation" or EMT phenomenon. Reduction of epithelial differentiation and induction of EMT change can be caused by two EBV latent proteins, LMP1 and LMP2A.[73,75] Thus, EBV plays a pivotal role in the pathomorphogenesis of lymphoepitheliomas.

Cellular stresses caused by extrinsic stimuli or intrinsic events are important inducers of EBV reactivation or viral oncogenes, explaining the high incidence of NPC in Hong Kong Cantonese boat men. For example, oxidative stress and DNA-damaging agents have been shown to induce the expression program of EBV lytic genes.[76] EBV reactivation can also be triggered by some chemical carcinogens that have been implicated as risk factors of EBV-associated cancers such as NPC and BL.[77] The cooperation of EBV lytic infection and carcinogens synergistically increases oxidative stress, genomic instability, and malignant phenotypes of NPC cells, which is an integral link of environmental factors to EBV-associated cancers. As well as the exogenous stimuli, some endogenous stresses play regulatory roles in EBV gene expression. ER stress frequently occurs in hypoxia, inflammation, or solid tumors, resulting from accumulation of misfolded proteins and perturbation of ER homeostasis.[78] ER stress induces EBV reactivation in B lymphocytes, while upregulating the viral oncoprotein LMP1 in NPC cells.[79] XBP-1, a transcription factor activated under ER stress, is critical for expression of the EBV genes.[79] On the other hand, LMP1 expression in HL cells can be induced by some cytokines produced under inflammatory stress.[80] Cellular stresses can also be the downstream effects caused by EBV proteins. For instance, an EBV nuclear protein EBNA1 increases oxidative stress that enhances genomic instability.[81] Expression of LMP1 can induce ER stress in B lymphocytes, which serves as a mechanism sustaining LMP1 expression.[82] In response to ER stress, cells may activate either cytoprotective pathways to recover from the stress or cytotoxic pathways to suicide under the stress. Interestingly, LMP1-induced ER stress preferentially activates the cytoprotective pathways and attenuates the cytotoxic pathways in HL cells, thus promoting survival of tumor cells. Moreover, our recent study also suggests that EBV LMP1 is one of the candidate molecules to induce the multinuclear morphology of RS cells. Although the mechanism of the LMP1-induced cytologic change has not been fully confirmed, our study showed that LMP1 could increase cytoplasmic localization of cyclin A, and the cytoplasmic cyclin A promotes the multinucleation of HL cells.[83,84] Distinct from the cytoplasmic localization of cyclin A in RS cells, the mononuclear Hodgkin cells consistently express nuclear cyclin A. EBV-positive HL cells consistently express large amounts of EBV LMP-1 in the cytoplasm. The accumulation of these viral oncoprotein LMP-1 will induce ER stress response. The RS cells of HL express strong ER stress survival proteins XBP-1 and GRP78, but not the apoptotic ER stress proteins CHOP and ASK1.[85] Although EBV may account for the characteristic histopathologic features of HL, the same histopathologic features in EBV-negative HL suggest that other unidentified pathogens or a similar mechanism exists. Therefore, cellular stresses seem to be coupled with EBV-associated cancers in several ways. Initially, the stresses may dysregulate the "silent program" of EBV, triggering aberrant EBV reactivation and oncogene expression. Subsequently, the viral oncoproteins may induce cellular stresses and adapt them for some events of oncogenesis, especially for genomic instability and cell survival. Furthermore, the feedback cross-talk between viral oncoproteins and cellular stresses forms a driving force that forwards host cells toward malignant phenotypes. Blockage of critical stress pathways is a possible approach to inhibit both expression and effects of EBV oncoproteins. For example, XBP-1 is not only an inducer of LMP1 but also involved in the survival pathways under ER stress, serving as an attractive therapeutic target for EBV-associated cancers.

HBV AND HCC DEVELOPMENT: STRESS-DEPENDENT AND STRESS-INDEPENDENT CELL PROLIFERATION, DNA DAMAGE, AND GENOMIC INSTABILITY

HCC is one of the most common malignancies around the world, ranking fifth in men and seventh in women, with more than half of the cases occurring in Asia. The high incidence of HCC in Asia largely reflects the prevalence of chronic HBV infection in over 8% of the population.[86] The nationwide massive vaccination program has been extremely successful in high-incidence areas, such as Taiwan, and the incidence of chronic HBV infection and HBV-related HCC has been largely reduced upon vaccination.[87] However, there are more than 350 million individuals who remain chronically infected by HBV, and its late complications still account for approximately 1 million deaths per year worldwide. Besides antivirals, the development of ideal agents for targeted therapy or chemoprevention is in high demand.

The pathogenesis of HBV-mediated tumorigenesis can be largely attributed to the lifelong battle between the virus and the host immune response. For chronic carriers, persistent HBV infection induces a weak adaptive immune response with inefficient T-cell responses or immune tolerance and therefore fails to eliminate HBV in the host. Albeit incapable of complete viral clearance, the immune-mediated damages and the subsequent regeneration in the liver contribute significantly to the progression to liver cirrhosis and HCC.[88] In addition, viral factors including insertional mutagenesis of the viral genome and the expression of viral oncoproteins such as HBx and pre-S mutant large surface proteins also play a role in the advanced stage of tumorigenesis.[89-91] Thus, it is likely that the interplay between virus and host factors contributes synergistically to activate oncogenic pathways that subsequently lead to hepatocyte transformation.

HBV is a small DNA virus and has a partially double-stranded circular genome consisting of only four open-reading frames, encoding the viral envelop/ surface, nucleocapsid, polymerase with a reverse transcriptase activity, and X proteins. The surface gene is further divided into three continued coding regions (pre-S1, pre-S2, and S regions) with two internal start codons (pre-S2 and S ATG).[92] All three regions together encode the hepatitis B large surface proteins (LHBs), and this gene product is essential for both virus assembly and infectivity. Among the viral products, two viral proteins, the X protein (HBx) and the LHB protein with internal deletions over the pre-S region, are now considered viral oncoproteins and tumor promoters.[93,94] HBx and pre-S mutants have shown to exert their effects on the cell cycle, cell growth, and apoptosis by interfering cellular signaling pathways and gene transcriptions.[58,93] Their roles in tumorigenesis were further supported by the development of advanced liver diseases and HCC in transgenic mice.[95,96]

HBx protein consists of 154 amino acids with a molecular weight of 17 kDa. The multifunctional property of HBx exerted in both in vitro and transgenic mice strongly argues that HBx contributes directly or, at least, functions as a cofactor in hepatocarcinogenesis.[97] HBx itself is a promising gene transactivator that can activate a variety of viral and cellular promoters and proto-oncogenes such as c-jun, c-fos, and c-myc.[98] In addition, HBx also activates transcription factors such as NF-κB, activator protein-1 (AP-1), and activating transcription factor (ATF)/cAMP-responsive element binding transcription factor (CREB) in the nucleus.[99-101] In addition, the expression of HBx in HepG2 cells renders resistance to Fas ligand–mediated apoptosis through activating the SAPK–Janus kinase (JAK) pathway.[102] HBx also interacts directly with p53 and thus represses p53-mediated gene transcription.[103] Albeit HBx interferes with numerical signal pathways in the in vitro model of cell culture, its clinical and pathological relevance remains controversial. The detection of HBx in the liver has been really challenging due to the few antibodies available for immunohistochemical staining. Thus, the role of HBx in HBV-mediated hepatocarcinogenesis remains to be elucidated.

Besides HBx, the large surface antigens with internal deletions over either pre-S1 (pre-S1 mutant) or pre-S2 (pre-S2 mutant) regions have been linked to advanced stages of liver disease and HCC, indicating a contributing role of pre-S mutants in hepatocarcinogenesis.[58,104] The presence of pre-S mutants in serum has been reported to be a predictive marker of advanced liver disease and HCC.[105] The pre-S mutants were found to accumulate in the ER of hepatocytes, causing the characteristic glassy or ground glass hepatocytes.[106,107] There are two different types of GGHs: the singular-distributed type I GGHs containing pre-S1 mutants and the clonally proliferated type II GGHs harboring pre-S2 mutants.[108] Notably, type II GGHs consistently cluster in groups and occur at the advanced stages of virus replication and are associated with cirrhosis and HCC. Therefore, type II GGHs are now considered as preneoplastic lesions in the liver.[58] The accumulation of these pre-S mutants in ER has been demonstrated to induce ER stress response due to the accumulation of malfolded viral products in the ER.[57] To cope with HBV-induced ER stress, hepatocytes express stronger levels of ER chaperone proteins (GRP78 and GRP94), cyclooxygenase-2 (COX-2), and vascular endothelial growth factor A (VEGF-A) to sustain their survival.[108-110] The activation of ER stress further promotes calcium release from the ER, leading to the increase in oxidative stress intermediates and subsequent oxidative DNA damages.[96] Based on studies on the biologic nature of pre-S1 and pre-S2 mutants, we consider it highly plausible that a stronger ER stress in type I GGHs may render cell death or growth arrest, but a milder but sustained ER stress in type II GGHs may confer growth advantages by generating resistance to more stringent conditions. Genomic instability is generally a prerequisite for carcinogenesis in most cancer development. Sustained ER stress induced by pre-S2 mutant LHBs has been shown to induce strong oxidative DNA damages in the in vitro culture cell lines, in type II GGHs from HCC patients, and in pre-S2 mutant transgenic mice, suggesting that pre-S2 LHB itself is genotoxic. Our recent investigations reveal that ER stress signal is involved in the induction of cytoplasmic cyclin A, which subsequently contributes to aberrant centrosome overduplication and hence hepatocyte aneuploidy (Wang and Su et al., manuscript in preparation). The sustained stress-induced DNA damage and chromosomal abnormalities can explain the complex chromosomal changes in HBV-related HCC. The oncogenic potential of the pre-S2 mutant LHBs can be attributed not only to the induction of a sustained ER stress but also to its functions in gene transactivation. In addition, the pre-S2 mutant LHB binds directly to c-Jun activation domain-binding protein 1 (JAB1), renders its nuclear translocation, and subsequently targets $p27^{Kip1}$ to proteasome-dependent degradation.[111] This will in turn activate cyclin-dependent kinase-2 (Cdk2) and result in hyperphosphorylation in retinoblastoma (Rb) and hence in the expression of cyclin A and cell cycle progression. Additionally, mTOR signals can be induced to become activated by pre-S mutant LHBs, which can feedback suppress the synthesis of surface antigens during the disease progression.[110,112] Therefore, controlling the genotoxic damages by HBV oncoproteins during chronic HBV infection may be a useful approach for HCC chemoprevention in the future.

HCV INFECTION AND CANCER FORMATION: INFLAMMATION-DRIVEN MECHANISMS FOR TUMOR DEVELOPMENT

HCV, identified in 1989,[113] was a positive sense RNA virus responsible for the majority of non-A, non-B hepatitis cases before its identification. The World Health Organization (WHO) estimates that 130 to 170 million people were exposed to contaminated blood and chronically infected with HCV worldwide. HCV establishes chronic infection in 80% of HCV-infected patients and causes inflammation-associated diseases including liver fibrosis, cirrhosis (10% to 30%), and cancer (1% to 3%) two to three decades after infection.[114] Hepatocyte is the major cell type supporting HCV replication, and HCC is the main cancer type associated with HCV infection.

There are two characteristic features of HCV-related hepatitis. The first feature is the infiltration of lymphocytes in the lobules and portal tracts, suggesting that inflammation is an important driving force for the pathogenesis of HCC development in HCV-infected patients.[115] The second feature is the frequent fatty change or steatosis of hepatocytes in more than 60% of the liver biopsies.[116] These histopathologic features are not unique to HCV infection as they are also commonly present in HBV infection or autoimmune hepatitis. So far, no pathognomonic feature has been identified from HCV(+) liver biopsy and the main diagnosis for HCV infection is based on seroconversion and HCV RNA detection in the serum and liver. HCV-associated HCC usually develops in the context of fibrosis and cirrhosis,[116] suggesting an important role of the host response to HCV-associated HCC. These histological features identified from HCV(+) liver biopsy suggest that inflammation plays a dominant role in HCV-associated pathology.

It has been shown that HCV has evolved several strategies to escape immune clearance and thereby establish chronic infection.[117] One important feature for HCV to establish chronic infection is that HCV NS3/4A protease can cleave host adapt proteins and block the activation of innate immunity.[118] In order to control HCV-associated disease progression, elimination of virus replication and modulation of immune response might be two critical targets for HCV treatment.

HPV AND CERVICAL CANCER: INTERACTION BETWEEN VIRAL AND CELLULAR PROTEINS AND THE IMMUNOMODULATION

HPV can infect epithelial cells of the anogenital region and cause benign and malignant lesions. More than 60 HPV genotypes have been identified.[119] Some types (HPV 16 and HPV 18) of HPV infection of the anogenital region present a high risk of malignant transformation, whereas infections by other types (HPV 6 and HPV 11) have a low risk of malignant transformation and result in benign papillomatous lesions.[120,121] The distribution of high-risk HPV genotypes in different geographic regions is varied and constitutes a big challenge to HPV vaccination.[122]

The difference between the high-risk and the low-risk HPVs is closely related to their expression of two viral oncoproteins, the *E6* and *E7*. Specific cellular proteins bind efficiently to the HPV *E6* and *E7* oncoproteins of high-risk types of HPV.[123] The *E6* oncoprotein binds to the p53 protein,[124] promoting the degradation of p53. The *E7* oncoprotein binds to the retinoblastoma gene (*Rb*).[125] Both viral oncoproteins play roles in the regulation of mitotic cell cycle progression. Interference with these functions may lead to chromosomal instability and aneuploidy. The interaction of high-risk E6 and E7 proteins with cellular factors may be important for the malignant progression of HPV-infected epithelial cells. However, viral E6 and E7 gene expression is necessary but not sufficient for the final development of malignant growth. Other cellular factors, such as cooperation with other ras oncoproteins, or the environmental factors such as growth factors or cytokines may influence the malignant progression of HPV-infected cells and will lead to the final emergence of malignancy.

As compared with EBV-associated HL and NPC, HPV-associated cervical cancers exhibit less histopathologic features of virus-associated cancers. However, recent studies have also indicated that Treg cells characterized by their ability to suppress the effector activity of antigen-specific lymphocytes are also involved in the local immunosuppression of HPV-related cervical cancer.[126] This is evident through the findings that $CD4^+FOXP3^+$ T cells generated against the viral E6 and E7 capsid proteins with regulatory property could be detected in cervical tissues and tumor-draining lymph nodes of subjects with cervical cancer.[127] T cells with undetectable FOXP3, but which exhibit regulatory function, have also been reported to be found in individuals with oncogenic HPV-induced disease.[128] Treg cells through interaction with cervical cancer cells have been suggested to acquire great suppressive activity.[126] Within the context of these findings, targeting Treg cell–mediated immunosuppression becomes key in the development of immune intervention strategies against HPV-induced cervical cancer.

OTHER VIRUS-ASSOCIATED HUMAN CANCERS

HTLV-1–Associated ATLL

The discovery of HTLV-1 in ATLL is a turning point in the well-established tumorigenicity of retroviruses in animals. ATLL is prevalent in the coastal regions of southern Japan, in the Caribbean, and in regions of central Africa.[16,17] The latency period between primary infection and lymphomagenesis is several decades. It is estimated that only 1 out of 25 to 30 infected individuals will eventually develop ATLL. The HTLV-1 DNA is consistently present in lymphoma/leukemic cells in a clonally integrated pattern, indicating its causal role in ATLL tumorigenesis. However, because of the long latency, only a minor percentage of infected individuals develop ATLL. Moreover, the candidate viral oncoprotein Tax, a transcriptional regulator, is not expressed in the indolent stage of pre-leukemic cells.[129] Both facts suggest that other promotion factors exist, consistent with at least the "two-hit" hypothesis in tumorigenesis. The 40-kDa tax protein can initiate an aberrant activation of IL-2 autocrine loop through activation of NF-κB signals.[130] ATLL cells constitutively express CD25 and resemble CD25+CD4+ regulatory T cells, expressing FoxP3.[131] HTLV-1 also encodes an antisense transcript, the HTLV-1 bZIP factor (HBZ), which can upregulate FoxP3.[132] Both mechanisms are considered to be key mechanisms in HTLV-1 tumorigenesis.

The characteristic clover- or flower-shaped nuclei of ATLL is still a mystery. Whether the sustained expression of HTLV-1 Tax in T cells will cause ER stress and result in the abnormal nuclear morphology as described above still needs to be explored.

KSHV/HHV-8 and Human Cancers

Although Kaposi sarcoma has been presumed to be caused by viruses for a long time, it was not until 2000 when Yen Chang discovered the linkage to Kaposi sarcoma virus (KSHV/HHV-8) in HIV/AIDS patients.[133] This virus was later found to be consistently present in non-HIV Kaposi sarcoma,[134] indicating an etiologic role for KSHV/HHV-8 in Kaposi sarcoma. This virus was later demonstrated to be associated with effusion large B-cell lymphoma.[135] The occurrence of this virus-associated cancer predominantly in AIDS and non-AIDS patients is in some way similar to EBV-associated cancers. So far, there are few papers addressing the difference in gene expression of HHV-8 in AIDS-related and non-AIDS–related cancers as that reported in EBV-associated cancers. However, the peculiar association of this virus with Kaposi sarcoma and the unique manifestation of effusion-type B-cell lymphoma indicate that HHV-8 drives an autocrine pathway of specific growth factors such as VEGF (Kaposi sarcoma) and may modify the adhesion membrane protein (effusion lymphoma). Other biologic behaviors imposed by this virus remain to be clarified in the future.

IMMUNOTHERAPY FOR VIRUS-ASSOCIATED CANCERS

The apparent infiltration of immune cells and expression of viral antigens in virus-associated human cancers suggest that virus-associated human cancers will be the most ideal target for tumor immunotherapy. The concept of anti-EBV immunotherapy encounters a big problem that the tumors of NPC and HL are shielded by strong local immunosuppressive effects, which block the transfer of peripheral antivirus immunity into the tumor tissues.[136] Although some of the intratumoral T cells exhibit activated phenotypes, their proliferation and cytotoxic activity are actually impaired.[137] Therefore, the tumor microenvironment mimics chronic virus infection where antivirus lymphocytes are "exhausted" and unresponsive to immune stimulation. Notably, the impairment of local immunity also affects the clinical outcome of conventional anticancer therapies, as the exhaustion level of intratumoral CD8 T cells predicts a poor prognosis of NPC.[138]

There are multiple potent mechanisms contributing to the local immune suppression in NPC and HL. Suppressive cytokines such as IL-10 and TGF-β are elevated in the tumors,[139] produced from malignant or stromal cells. Regulatory T cells are also prevalently present in NPC and HL, acting as major suppressive immune cells therein. Meanwhile, tumor cells or infiltrates can produce other inhibitory factors such as Fas ligand, gelectin-9, or PD-L1, causing cytotoxic or exhaustion effects in T cells.[140] It remains unclear how these suppressive mechanisms work together and which factor is pivotal to the inhibitory effects on intratumoral lymphocytes, but EBV seems to play a critical role driving the immunosuppressive tumor microenvironment. For example, EBV EBNA1 upregulates chemokines that preferentially recruit regulatory T cells.[141] IL-10 and TGF-β can be induced by several EBV gene products (LMP1, Zta, and EBER) in B cells.[142] LMP1 can also upregulate PD-L1 expression in HL.[143] In addition, Zta promotes the expression of several immune modulators from NPC cells, which bias monocytes into suppressive cells producing IL-10.[144] To remove or overcome these suppressive effects is an important direction toward the success of immunotherapy of NPC or HL.

Besides EBV-associated cancers, attempts to develop therapeutic HPV vaccines for cervical cancers have been extensive. Several prototypic HPV therapeutic vaccines comprising the E7 oncogenic protein of HPV 16, or E7 fused to the E6 oncogenic protein, or the viral L2/L1 capsids that are delivered in protein/adjuvant formulation have been tested in patients with cervical intraepithelial neoplasia (CIN). However, results obtained from these clinical trials were not entirely satisfactory, as judged by the poor T-cell responses that were detected in many of the test subjects.[145] The succinct interpretation of these results would be the immunosuppressive state of the patients as T cells of a large number of them were found to be unresponsive to viral E6 and E7 protein stimulation in vitro.[146] Currently, primary HPV 16 and HPV 18 infection can be partially prevented by vaccination with the virus-like Gardasil and Cervarix vaccines marketed by Merck & Co and GSK (GlaxoSmithKline) Biologicals, respectively. Both of these vaccines elicit virus-neutralizing antibody responses to protect against the development of CIN caused by HPV 16 and HPV 18. So far, available data collected from clinical trials conducted in different countries show that the vaccines have efficacy in the 64% to 71%

range.[147] These findings imply that the current prophylactic HPV vaccines are unable to confer cross-protection in subjects infected or coinfected with other oncogenic HPV(s). Despite the Gardasil and Cervarix vaccines providing protection to HPV-naïve women from infection by HPV 16 and HPV 18, respectively, they lack therapeutic effect. Therefore, the development of an effective immune intervention strategy against HPV-induced CIN is an unmet medical need that has to be pursued to provide help to the vast number of women infected with HPV.

Effective immunotherapy for virus-associated human cancers, like the prophylactic HBV and HPV vaccines, is always a forever challenging topic in the therapy of human cancers. From the preclinical and clinical findings gathered up to now, we learn that targeting the preexisting virus-specific Treg cells in patients before they are administered with immunogenic epitope-based vaccine that preferentially induces antiviral effector T cells, but not Treg cells, is the appropriate approach to take. Further clarification of the local immunosuppression in tumor tissues will provide us a better strategy to reach success of tumor immunotherapy for human cancers.

NF-κB SIGNAL PATHWAY REPRESENTS POTENTIAL THERAPEUTIC AND CHEMOPREVENTIVE TARGET IN VIRUS-ASSOCIATED CANCERS

Up to now, there has been a consistent activation of NF-κB signals in virus-associated human cancers, which raises the potential of targeting the NF-κB pathway as therapeutic and chemopreventive therapy in virus-associated human cancers.[148,149] In EBV-associated NPC, HL, and nasal NK/T-cell lymphoma, NF-κB signal is consistently activated and represents a major mechanism of virus-induced tumorigenesis.[150] The commercial availability of inhibitors for NF-κB signals may represent a potential drug, either used alone or in combination with chemotherapeutic agents, for trials in virus-associated cancers to suppress the proinflammatory cytokine release and to reduce the drug resistance, besides the inhibition of tumor growth. The involvement of stress and inflammation conditions in the development of virus-associated cancers provides the strategy to adopt chemopreventive agents or natural products to prevent or reduce tumor formation in high-risk individuals. Current studies suggest that natural products that exhibit pleiotropic effects and few side effects are ideal chemopreventive agents, among which the agonists of peroxisome proliferator–activated receptors (PPARs) represent the most promising candidates.[151,152] The PPAR signaling pathway shows pleiotropic effects to regulate the lipid and glucose metabolism; the anti-stress and anti-inflammatory effects through NF-κB, AP-I, and Stats pathway; and the anti-proliferation effects of many cancers.[153,154] Furthermore, most of the currently studied chemopreventive agents such as resveratrol, curcumin, and unsaturated fatty acids in fish oils, vegetables, and fruits all exhibited high PPAR agonistic activities.[155,156] Clinical trials to apply these natural products exhibiting PPAR agonists, either alone or in combination, in chemoprevention for high-risk HCC patients to avoid tumor recurrence after surgery are now under study.

ACKNOWLEDGMENTS

This program project received support from the National Health Research Institutes, the Excellence Center Project of the Department of Education (National Cheng Kung University), and the National Science Council, Taiwan. Thanks are also given to Lily Hui-Ching Wang and Shu-Jen Liu for their discussion on the manuscript.

REFERENCES

1. Parkin DM. The global health burden of infection-associated cancers in the year 2002. *Int J Cancer*. 2006;118:3030-3044.
2. Burkitt D. A sarcoma involving the jaws in African children. *Br J Surg*. 1958;46:218-223.
3. Epstein MA, Achong BG, Barr YM. Virus particles in cultured lymphoblasts from Burkitt's lymphoma. *Lancet*. 1964;1:702-703.
4. Henle G, Henle W. Epstein-Barr virus-specific IgA serum antibodies as an outstanding feature of nasopharyngeal carcinoma. *Int J Cancer*. 1976;17:1-7.
5 Paya CV, Fung JJ, Nalesnik MA, et al. Epstein-Barr virus-induced posttransplant lymphoproliferative disorders. ASTS/ASTP EBV-PTLD Task Force and The Mayo Clinic Organized International Consensus Development Meeting. *Transplantation*. 1999;68:1517-1525.
6. Flavell KJ, Murray PG. Hodgkin's disease and the Epstein-Barr virus. *Mol Pathol*. 2000;53:262-269.
7. Su IJ, Hsieh HC, Lin KH, et al. Aggressive peripheral T cell lymphoma containing Epstein-Barr viral DNA: A clinicopathologic and molecular analysis. *Blood*. 1991,77:799-808.
8. Harabuchi Y, Yamanaka N, Kataura A, et al. Epstein-Barr virus in nasal T-cell lymphomas in patients with lethal midline granuloma. *Lancet*. 1990;335:128-130.
9. McClain KL, Leach CT, Jenson HB, et al. Association of Epstein-Barr virus with leiomyosarcomas in children with AIDS. *N Engl J Med*. 1995;332:12-18.
10. Beasley RP, Hwang LY, Lin CC, Chien CS. Hepatocellular carcinoma and hepatitis B virus. A prospective study of 22 707 men in Taiwan. *Lancet*. 1981;2:1129-1133.
11. Beasley RP, Hwang LY, Stevens CE, et al. Efficacy of hepatitis B immune globulin for prevention of perinatal transmission of the hepatitis B virus carrier state: final report of a randomized double-blind, placebo-controlled trial. *Hepatology*. 1983;3:135-141.
12. zur Hausen H. Human papillomaviruses and their possible role in squamous cell carcinomas. *Curr Top Microbiol Immunol*. 1977;78:1-30.
13. Mork J, Lie AK, Glattre E, et al. Human papillomavirus infection as a risk factor for squamous-cell carcinoma of the head and neck. *N Engl J Med*. 2001;344:1125-1131.
14. Jacobson LP, Jenkins FJ, Springer G, et al. Interaction of human immunodeficiency virus type 1 and human herpesvirus type 8 infections on the incidence of Kaposi's sarcoma. *J Infect Dis*. 2000;181:1940-1949.
15. Wang QJ, Jenkins FJ, Jacobson LP, et al. CD8+ cytotoxic T lymphocyte responses to lytic proteins of human herpes virus 8 in human immunodeficiency virus type 1-infected and -uninfected individuals. *J Infect Dis*. 2000;182:928-932.
16. Hinuma Y, Komoda H, Chosa T, et al. Antibodies to adult T-cell leukemia-virus-associated antigen (ATLA) in sera from patients with ATL and controls in Japan: a nation-wide sero-epidemiologic study. *Int J Cancer*. 1982;29:631-635.
17. Blattner WA, Kalyanaraman VS, Robert-Guroff M, et al. The human type-C retrovirus, HTLV, in Blacks from the Caribbean region, and relationship to adult T-cell leukemia/lymphoma. *Int J Cancer*. 1982;30:257-264.

18. Sakamoto M, Hirohashi S, Tsuda H, et al. Increasing incidence of hepatocellular carcinoma possibly associated with non-A, non-B hepatitis in Japan, disclosed by hepatitis B virus DNA analysis of surgically resected cases. *Cancer Res*. 1988;48:7294-7297.
19. Saito I, Miyamura T, Ohbayashi A, et al. Hepatitis C virus infection is associated with the development of hepatocellular carcinoma. *Proc Natl Acad Sci U S A*. 1990;87:6547-6549.
20. Perry AK, Chen G, Zheng D, Tang H, Cheng G. The host type I interferon response to viral and bacterial infections. *Cell Res*. 2005;15:407-422.
21. Stark GR, Kerr IM, Williams BR, Silverman RH, Schreiber RD. How cells respond to interferons. *Annu Rev Biochem*. 1998;67:227-264.
22. Soghoian DZ, Streeck H. Cytolytic CD4(+) T cells in viral immunity. *Expert Rev Vaccines*. 2010;9:1453-1463.
23. Martorelli D, Muraro E, Merlo A, Turrini R, Rosato A, Dolcetti R. Role of CD4+ cytotoxic T lymphocytes in the control of viral diseases and cancer. *Int Rev Immunol*. 2010;29:371-402.
24. Keynan Y, Card CM, McLaren PJ, Dawood MR, Kasper K, Fowke KR. The role of regulatory T cells in chronic and acute viral infections. *Clin Infect Dis*. 2008;46:1046-1052.
25. Jin HT, Ahmed R, Okazaki T. Role of PD-1 in regulating T-cell immunity. *Curr Top Microbiol Immunol*. 2011;350:17-37.
26. bol S, Halstead SB. How innate immune mechanisms contribute to antibody-enhanced viral infections. *Clin Vaccine Immunol*. 2010;17:1829-1835.
27. Levine B, Mizushima N, Virgin HW. Autophagy in immunity and inflammation. *Nature*. 2011;469:323-335.
28. Gao G, Luo H. The ubiquitin-proteasome pathway in viral infections. *Can J Physiol Pharmacol*. 2006;84:5-14.
29. Shoji-Kawata S, Levine B. Autophagy, antiviral immunity, and viral countermeasures. *Biochim Biophys Acta*. 2009;1793:1478-1484.
30. Kepp O, Senovilla L, Galluzzi L, et al. Viral subversion of immunogenic cell death. *Cell Cycle*. 2009;8:860-869.
31. Devitt A, Marshall LJ. The innate immune system and the clearance of apoptotic cells. *J Leukoc Biol*. 2011;90:447-457.
32. Malhotra JD, Kaufman RJ. Endoplasmic reticulum stress and oxidative stress: a vicious cycle or a double-edged sword? *Antioxid Redox Signal*. 2007;9:2277-2293.
33. Gregersen N, Bross P. Protein misfolding and cellular stress: an overview. *Methods Mol Biol*. 2010;648:3-23.
34. Thompson SL, Bakhoum SF, Compton DA. Mechanisms of chromosomal instability. *Curr Biol*. 2010;20:R285-R295.
35. Merlo LM, Wang LS, Pepper JW, Rabinovitch PS, Maley CC. Polyploidy, aneuploidy and the evolution of cancer. *Adv Exp Med Biol*. 2010;676:1-13.
36. Liu CJ, Kao JH. Hepatitis B virus-related hepatocellular carcinoma: epidemiology and pathogenic role of viral factors. *J Chin Med Assoc*. 2007;70:141-145.
37. Lee CM, Lu SN, Changchien CS, et al. Age, gender, and local geographic variations of viral etiology of hepatocellular carcinoma in a hyperendemic area for hepatitis B virus infection. *Cancer*. 1999;86:1143-1150.
38. Zimonjic DB, Keck-Waggoner C, Popescu NC. Novel genomic imbalances and chromosome translocations involving c-myc gene in Burkitt's lymphoma. *Leukemia*. 2001;15:1582-1588.
39. Sun HS, Su IJ, Lin YC, Chen JS, Fang SY. A 2.6 Mb interval on chromosome 6q25.2-q25.3 is commonly deleted in human nasal natural killer/T-cell lymphoma. *Br J Haematol*. 2003;122:590-599.
40. Albertson DG, Collins C, McCormick F, Gray JW. Chromosome aberrations in solid tumors. *Nat Genet*. 2003;34:369-376.
41. Kakati S, Sandberg AA. Chromosomes in solid tumors. *Virchows Arch B Cell Pathol*. 1978;29:129-137.
42. Schreiber RD, Old LJ, Smyth MJ. Cancer immunoediting: integrating immunity's roles in cancer suppression and promotion. *Science*. 2011;331:1565-1570.
43. Tsuruo T, Naito M, Tomida A, et al. Molecular targeting therapy of cancer: drug resistance, apoptosis and survival signal. *Cancer Sci*. 2003;94:15-21.
44. Yamamoto Y, Gaynor RB. Role of the NF-kappaB pathway in the pathogenesis of human disease states. *Curr Mol Med*. 2001;1:287-296.
45. Baldwin AS. Control of oncogenesis and cancer therapy resistance by the transcription factor NF-kappaB. *J Clin Invest*. 2001;107:241-246.
46. Gorgun G, Anderson KC. Intrinsic modulation of lymphocyte function by stromal cell network: advance in therapeutic targeting of cancer. *Immunotherapy*. 2011;3:1253-1264.
47. Palucka AK, Ueno H, Fay JW, Banchereau J. Taming cancer by inducing immunity via dendritic cells. *Immunol Rev*. 2007;220: 129-150.
48. Aldinucci D, Gloghini A, Pinto A, De Filippi R, Carbone A. The classical Hodgkin's lymphoma microenvironment and its role in promoting tumour growth and immune escape. *J Pathol*. 2010;221:248-263.
49. Imashuku S, Hibi S, Ohara T, et al. Effective control of Epstein-Barr virus-related hemophagocytic lymphohistiocytosis with immunochemotherapy. Histiocyte Society. *Blood*. 1999;93:1869-1874.
50. Su IJ, Chen RL, Lin DT, Lin KS, Chen CC. Epstein-Barr virus (EBV) infects T lymphocytes in childhood EBV-associated hemophagocytic syndrome in Taiwan. *Am J Pathol*. 1994;144: 1219-1225.
51. Mantovani A, Schioppa T, Porta C, Allavena P, Sica A. Role of tumor-associated macrophages in tumor progression and invasion. *Cancer Metastasis Rev*. 2006;25:315-322.
52. Allavena P, Sica A, Solinas G, Porta C, Mantovani A. The inflammatory micro-environment in tumor progression: the role of tumor-associated macrophages. *Crit Rev Oncol Hematol*. 2008;66: 1-9.
53. Weiss LM, Movahed LA, Warnke RA, Sklar J. Detection of Epstein-Barr viral genomes in Reed-Sternberg cells of Hodgkin's disease. *N Engl J Med*. 1989;320:502-506.
54. Jeon HJ, Lee MJ, Jeong YK, Lee DM, Oh YK, Kim CW. Adult T cell leukemia/lymphoma with lymphopenia in a Korean. *J Korean Med Sci*. 2000;15:233-239.
55. Kehn K, Berro R, de la Fuente C, et al. Mechanisms of HTLV-1 transformation. *Front Biosci*. 2004;9:2347-2372.
56. Matsuoka M, Jeang KT. Human T-cell leukaemia virus type 1 (HTLV-1) infectivity and cellular transformation. *Nat Rev Cancer*. 2007;7:270-280.
57. Wang HC, Huang W, Lai MD, Su IJ. Hepatitis B virus pre-S mutants, endoplasmic reticulum stress and hepatocarcinogenesis. *Cancer Sci*. 2006;97:683-688.
58. Su IJ, Wang HC, Wu HC, Huang WY. Ground glass hepatocytes contain pre-S mutants and represent preneoplastic lesions in chronic hepatitis B virus infection. *J Gastroenterol Hepatol*. 2008;23:1169-1174.
59. Chien YC, Chen JY, Liu MY, et al. Serologic markers of Epstein-Barr virus infection and nasopharyngeal carcinoma in Taiwanese men. *N Engl J Med*. 2001;345:1877-1882.
60. de-Vathaire F, Sancho-Garnier H, de-The H, et al. Prognostic value of EBV markers in the clinical management of nasopharyngeal carcinoma (NPC): a multicenter follow-up study. *Int J Cancer*. 1988;42:176-181.
61. Brooks L, Yao QY, Rickinson AB, Young LS. Epstein-Barr virus latent gene transcription in nasopharyngeal carcinoma cells: coexpression of EBNA1, LMP1, and LMP2 transcripts. *J Virol*. 1992;66:2689-2697.
62. Herbst H, Dallenbach F, Hummel M, et al. Epstein-Barr virus latent membrane protein expression in Hodgkin and Reed-Sternberg cells. *Proc Natl Acad Sci U S A*. 1991;88: 4766-4770.
63. Diehl V, Thomas RK, Re D. Part II: Hodgkin's lymphoma—diagnosis and treatment. *Lancet Oncol*. 2004;5:19-26.
64. Re D, Thomas RK, Behringer K, Diehl V. From Hodgkin disease to Hodgkin lymphoma: biologic insights and therapeutic potential. *Blood*. 2005;105:4553-4560.
65. Khan G. Epstein-Barr virus, cytokines, and inflammation: a cocktail for the pathogenesis of Hodgkin's lymphoma? *Exp Hematol*. 2006;34:399-406.
66. Skinnider BF, Mak TW. The role of cytokines in classical Hodgkin lymphoma. *Blood*. 2002;99:4283-4297.
67. Soni V, Cahir-McFarland E, Kieff E. LMP1 TRAFficking activates growth and survival pathways. *Adv Exp Med Biol*. 2007;597:173-187.
68. Horie R, Watanabe T, Morishita Y, et al. Ligand-independent signaling by overexpressed CD30 drives NF-kappaB activation in Hodgkin-Reed-Sternberg cells. *Oncogene*. 2002;21:2493-2503.
69. Huang YT, Sheen TS, Chen CL, et al. Profile of cytokine expression in nasopharyngeal carcinomas: a distinct expression

of interleukin 1 in tumor and CD4+ T cells. *Cancer Res.* 1999;59:1599-1605.
70. Hsu M, Wu SY, Chang SS, et al. Epstein-Barr virus lytic transactivator Zta enhances chemotactic activity through induction of interleukin-8 in nasopharyngeal carcinoma cells. *J Virol.* 2008;82:3679-3688.
71. Lai HC, Hsiao JR, Chen CW, et al. Endogenous latent membrane protein 1 in Epstein-Barr virus-infected nasopharyngeal carcinoma cells attracts T lymphocytes through upregulation of multiple chemokines. *Virology.* 2010;405:464-473.
72. Chang Y, Lee HH, Chen YT, et al. Induction of the early growth response 1 gene by Epstein-Barr virus lytic transactivator Zta. *J Virol.* 2006;80:7748-7755.
73. Horikawa T, Yang J, Kondo S, et al. Twist and epithelial-mesenchymal transition are induced by the EBV oncoprotein latent membrane protein 1 and are associated with metastatic nasopharyngeal carcinoma. *Cancer Res.* 2007;67:1970-1978.
74. Iezzoni JC, Gaffey MJ, Weiss LM. The role of Epstein-Barr virus in lymphoepithelioma-like carcinomas. *Am J Clin Pathol.* 1995;103:308-315.
75. Kong QL, Hu LJ, Cao JY, et al. Epstein-Barr virus-encoded LMP2A induces an epithelial-mesenchymal transition and increases the number of side population stem-like cancer cells in nasopharyngeal carcinoma. *PLoS Pathog.* 2010;6:e1000940.
76. Lassoued S, Gargouri B, El Feki Ael F, Attia H, Van Pelt J. Transcription of the Epstein-Barr virus lytic cycle activator BZLF-1 during oxidative stress induction. *Biol Trace Elem Res.* 2010;137:13-22.
77. Huang SY, Fang CY, Tsai CH, et al. N-methyl-N'-nitro-N-nitrosoguanidine induces and cooperates with 12-O-tetradecanoylphorbol-1,3-acetate/sodium butyrate to enhance Epstein-Barr virus reactivation and genome instability in nasopharyngeal carcinoma cells. *Chem Biol Interact.* 2010;188:623-634.
78. Zhao L, Ackerman SL. Endoplasmic reticulum stress in health and disease. *Curr Opin Cell Biol.* 2006;18:444-452.
79. Hsiao JR, Chang KC, Chen CW, et al. Endoplasmic reticulum stress triggers XBP-1-mediated up-regulation of an EBV oncoprotein in nasopharyngeal carcinoma. *Cancer Res.* 2009;69:4461-4467.
80. Kis LL, Takahara M, Nagy N, Klein G, Klein E. Cytokine mediated induction of the major Epstein-Barr virus (EBV)-encoded transforming protein, LMP-1. *Immunol Lett.* 2006;104: 83-88.
81. Gruhne B, Sompallae R, Marescotti D, Kamranvar SA, Gastaldello S, Masucci MG. The Epstein-Barr virus nuclear antigen-1 promotes genomic instability via induction of reactive oxygen species. *Proc Natl Acad Sci U S A.* 2009;106:2313-2318.
82. Lee DY, Sugden B. The LMP1 oncogene of EBV activates PERK and the unfolded protein response to drive its own synthesis. *Blood.* 2008;111:2280-2289.
83. Chang KC, Chang Y, Jones D, Su IJ. Aberrant expression of cyclin A correlates with morphogenesis of Reed-Sternberg cells in Hodgkin lymphoma. *Am J Clin Pathol.* 2009;132:50-59.
84. Knecht H, McQuain C, Martin J, et al. Expression of the LMP1 oncoprotein in the EBV negative Hodgkin's disease cell line L-428 is associated with Reed-Sternberg cell morphology. *Oncogene.* 1996;13:947-953.
85. Chang KC, Chen PC, Chen YP, Chang Y, Su IJ. Dominant expression of survival signals of endoplasmic reticulum stress response in Hodgkin lymphoma. *Cancer Sci.* 2011;102:275-281.
86. Merican I, Guan R, Amarapuka D, et al. Chronic hepatitis B virus infection in Asian countries. *J Gastroenterol Hepatol.* 2000;15:1356-1361.
87. Chien YC, Jan CF, Kuo HS, Chen CJ. Nationwide hepatitis B vaccination program in Taiwan: effectiveness in the 20 years after it was launched. *Epidemiol Rev.* 2006;28:126-135.
88. Chisari FV, Ferrari C. Hepatitis B virus immunopathogenesis. *Annu Rev Immunol.* 1995;13:29-60.
89. Bonilla Guerrero R, Roberts LR. The role of hepatitis B virus integrations in the pathogenesis of human hepatocellular carcinoma. *J Hepatol.* 2005;42:760-777.
90. Liu XH, Lin J, Zhang SH, et al. COOH-terminal deletion of HBx gene is a frequent event in HBV-associated hepatocellular carcinoma. *World J Gastroenterol.* 2008;14:1346-1352.
91. Hildt E, Hofschneider PH. The PreS2 activators of the hepatitis B virus: activators of tumour promoter pathways. *Recent Results Cancer Res.* 1998;154:315-329.
92. Burda MR, Gunther S, Dandri M, Will H, Petersen J. Structural and functional heterogeneity of naturally occurring hepatitis B virus variants. *Antiviral Res.* 2001;52:125-138.
93. Tan A, Yeh SH, Liu CJ, Cheung C, Chen PJ. Viral hepatocarcinogenesis: from infection to cancer. *Liver Int.* 2008;28:175-188.
94. Lin CL, Kao JH. Hepatitis B viral factors and clinical outcomes of chronic hepatitis B. *J Biomed Sci.* 2008;15:137-145.
95. Kim CM, Koike K, Saito I, Miyamura T, Jay G. HBx gene of hepatitis B virus induces liver cancer in transgenic mice. *Nature.* 1991;351:317-320.
96. Hsieh YH, Su IJ, Wang HC, et al. Pre-S mutant surface antigens in chronic hepatitis B virus infection induce oxidative stress and DNA damage. *Carcinogenesis.* 2004;25:2023-2032.
97. Park NH, Song IH, Chung YH. Chronic hepatitis B in hepatocarcinogenesis. *Postgrad Med J.* 2006;82:507-515.
98. Benn J, Su F, Doria M, Schneider RJ. Hepatitis B virus HBx protein induces transcription factor AP-1 by activation of extracellular signal-regulated and c-Jun N-terminal mitogen-activated protein kinases. *J Virol.* 1996;70:4978-4985.
99. Lucito R, Schneider RJ. Hepatitis B virus X protein activates transcription factor NF-kappa B without a requirement for protein kinase C. *J Virol.* 1992;66:983-991.
100. Benn J, Schneider RJ. Hepatitis B virus HBx protein activates Ras-GTP complex formation and establishes a Ras, Raf, MAP kinase signaling cascade. *Proc Natl Acad Sci U S A.* 1994;91:10350-10354.
101. Maguire HF, Hoeffler JP, Siddiqui A. HBV X protein alters the DNA binding specificity of CREB and ATF-2 by protein-protein interactions. *Science.* 1991;252:842-844.
102. Lee YH, Yun Y. HBx protein of hepatitis B virus activates Jak1-STAT signaling. *J Biol Chem.* 1998;273:25510-25515.
103. Truant R, Antunovic J, Greenblatt J, Prives C, Cromlish JA. Direct interaction of the hepatitis B virus HBx protein with p53 leads to inhibition by HBx of p53 response element-directed transactivation. *J Virol.* 1995;69:1851-1859.
104. Tsai HW, Lin YJ, Lin PW, et al. A clustered ground-glass hepatocyte pattern represents a new prognostic marker for the recurrence of hepatocellular carcinoma after surgery. *Cancer.* 2011;117:2951-2960.
105. Chen CH, Hung CH, Lee CM, et al. Pre-S deletion and complex mutations of hepatitis B virus related to advanced liver disease in HBeAg-negative patients. *Gastroenterology.* 2007;133:1466-1474.
106. Cohen C. "Ground-glass" hepatocytes. *S Afr Med J.* 1975;49:1401-1403.
107. Su IJ, Lai MY, Hsu HC, et al. Diverse virological, histopathological and prognostic implications of seroconversion from hepatitis B e antigen to anti-HBe in chronic hepatitis B virus infection. *J Hepatol.* 1986;3:182-189.
108. Wang HC, Wu HC, Chen CF, Fausto N, Lei HY, Su IJ. Different types of ground glass hepatocytes in chronic hepatitis B virus infection contain specific pre-S mutants that may induce endoplasmic reticulum stress. *Am J Pathol.* 2003;163: 2441-2449.
109. Hung JH, Su IJ, Lei HY, et al. Endoplasmic reticulum stress stimulates the expression of cyclooxygenase-2 through activation of NF-kappaB and pp38 mitogen-activated protein kinase. *J Biol Chem.* 2004;279:46384-46392.
110. Yang JC, Teng CF, Wu HC, et al. Enhanced expression of vascular endothelial growth factor-A in ground glass hepatocytes and its implication in hepatitis B virus hepatocarcinogenesis. *Hepatology.* 2009;49:1962-1971.
111. Hsieh YH, Su IJ, Wang HC, et al. Hepatitis B virus pre-S2 mutant surface antigen induces degradation of cyclin-dependent kinase inhibitor p27Kip1 through c-Jun activation domain-binding protein 1. *Mol Cancer Res.* 2007;5:1063-1072.
112. Teng CF, Wu HC, Tsai HW, Shiah HS, Huang W, Su IJ. Novel feedback inhibition of surface antigen synthesis by mammalian target of rapamycin (mTOR) signal and its implication for hepatitis B virus tumorigenesis and therapy. *Hepatology.* 2011;54:1199-1207.

113. Houghton M. The long and winding road leading to the identification of the hepatitis C virus. *J Hepatol.* 2009;51:939-948.
114. Perz JF, Armstrong GL, Farrington LA, Hutin YJ, Bell BP. The contributions of hepatitis B virus and hepatitis C virus infections to cirrhosis and primary liver cancer worldwide. *J Hepatol.* 2006;45:529-538.
115. Napoli J, Bishop GA, McGuinness PH, Painter DM, McCaughan GW. Progressive liver injury in chronic hepatitis C infection correlates with increased intrahepatic expression of Th1-associated cytokines. *Hepatology.* 1996;24:759-765.
116. Hourigan LF, Macdonald GA, Purdie D, et al. Fibrosis in chronic hepatitis C correlates significantly with body mass index and steatosis. *Hepatology.* 1999;29:1215-1219.
117. Rosenberg W. Mechanisms of immune escape in viral hepatitis. *Gut.* 1999;44:759-764.
118. Foy E, Li K, Wang C, et al. Regulation of interferon regulatory factor-3 by the hepatitis C virus serine protease. *Science.* 2003;300:1145-1148.
119. de Villiers EM, Fauquet C, Broker TR, Bernard HU, zur Hausen H. Classification of papillomaviruses. *Virology.* 2004;324:17-27.
120. Munoz N, Bosch FX, de Sanjose S, et al. Epidemiologic classification of human papillomavirus types associated with cervical cancer. *N Engl J Med.* 2003;348:518-527.
121. Lacey CJ, Lowndes CM, Shah KV. Chapter 4: burden and management of non-cancerous HPV-related conditions: HPV-6/11 disease. *Vaccine.* 2006;24(suppl 3):S3/35-41.
122. Smith JS, Lindsay L, Hoots B, et al. Human papillomavirus type distribution in invasive cervical cancer and high-grade cervical lesions: a meta-analysis update. *Int J Cancer.* 2007;121:621-632.
123. Munger K, Howley PM. Human papillomavirus immortalization and transformation functions. *Virus Res.* 2002;89:213-228.
124. Huibregtse JM, Scheffner M, Howley PM. A cellular protein mediates association of p53 with the E6 oncoprotein of human papillomavirus types 16 or 18. *EMBO J.* 1991;10:4129-4135.
125. Dyson N, Howley PM, Munger K, Harlow E. The human papilloma virus-16 E7 oncoprotein is able to bind to the retinoblastoma gene product. *Science.* 1989;243:934-937.
126. van der Burg SH, Piersma SJ, de Jong A, et al. Association of cervical cancer with the presence of CD4+ regulatory T cells specific for human papillomavirus antigens. *Proc Natl Acad Sci U S A.* 2007;104:12087-12092.
127. Bhat P, Mattarollo SR, Gosmann C, Frazer IH, Leggatt GR. Regulation of immune responses to HPV infection and during HPV-directed immunotherapy. *Immunol Rev.* 2011;239:85-98.
128. Heusinkveld M, Welters MJ, van Poelgeest MI, et al. The detection of circulating human papillomavirus-specific T cells is associated with improved survival of patients with deeply infiltrating tumors. *Int J Cancer.* 2011;128:379-389.
129. Barbeau B, Mesnard JM. Does the HBZ gene represent a new potential target for the treatment of adult T-cell leukemia? *Int Rev Immunol.* 2007;26:283-304.
130. Li M, Siekevitz M. A cis element required for induction of the interleukin 2 enhancer by human T-cell leukemia virus type I binds a novel Tax-inducible nuclear protein. *Mol Cell Biol.* 1993;13:6490-6500.
131. Karube K, Ohshima K, Tsuchiya T, et al. Expression of FoxP3, a key molecule in CD4CD25 regulatory T cells, in adult T-cell leukaemia/lymphoma cells. *Br J Haematol.* 2004;126:81-84.
132. Zhao T, Satou Y, Sugata K, et al. HTLV-1 bZIP factor enhances TGF-beta signaling through p300 coactivator. *Blood.* 2011;118:1865-1876.
133. Chang Y, Cesarman E, Pessin MS, et al. Identification of herpesvirus-like DNA sequences in AIDS-associated Kaposi's sarcoma. *Science.* 1994;266:1865-1869.
134. Su IJ, Hsu YS, Chang YC, Wang IW. Herpesvirus-like DNA sequence in Kaposi's sarcoma from AIDS and non-AIDS patients in Taiwan. *Lancet.* 1995;345:722-723.
135. Jarrett RF. Viruses and lymphoma/leukaemia. *J Pathol.* 2006;208:176-186.
136. Stewart TJ, Abrams SI. How tumours escape mass destruction. *Oncogene.* 2008;27:5894-5903.
137. Keir ME, Butte MJ, Freeman GJ, Sharpe AH. PD-1 and its ligands in tolerance and immunity. *Annu Rev Immunol.* 2008;26:677-704.
138. Chuang HC, Lay JD, Chuang SE, Hsieh WC, Chang Y, Su IJ. Epstein-Barr virus (EBV) latent membrane protein-1 down-regulates tumor necrosis factor-alpha (TNF-alpha) receptor-1 and confers resistance to TNF-alpha-induced apoptosis in T cells: implication for the progression to T-cell lymphoma in EBV-associated hemophagocytic syndrome. *Am J Pathol.* 2007;170:1607-1617.
139. Stearns ME, Garcia FU, Fudge K, Rhim J, Wang M. Role of interleukin 10 and transforming growth factor beta1 in the angiogenesis and metastasis of human prostate primary tumor lines from orthotopic implants in severe combined immunodeficiency mice. *Clin Cancer Res.* 1999;5:711-720.
140. Hsu MC, Hsiao JR, Chang KC, et al. Increase of programmed death-1-expressing intratumoral CD8 T cells predicts a poor prognosis for nasopharyngeal carcinoma. *Mod Pathol.* 2010;23:1393-1403.
141. Voo KS, Peng G, Guo Z, et al. Functional characterization of EBV-encoded nuclear antigen 1-specific CD4+ helper and regulatory T cells elicited by in vitro peptide stimulation. *Cancer Res.* 2005;65:1577-1586.
142. Ruf IK, Rhyne PW, Yang C, Cleveland JL, Sample JT. Epstein-Barr virus small RNAs potentiate tumorigenicity of Burkitt lymphoma cells independently of an effect on apoptosis. *J Virol.* 2000;74:10223-10228.
143. Yamamoto R, Nishikori M, Kitawaki T, et al. PD-1-PD-1 ligand interaction contributes to immunosuppressive microenvironment of Hodgkin lymphoma. *Blood.* 2008;111: 3220-3224.
144. Lee CH, Yeh TH, Lai HC, et al. Epstein-Barr virus Zta-induced immunomodulators from nasopharyngeal carcinoma cells upregulate interleukin-10 production from monocytes. *J Virol.* 2011;85:7333-7342.
145. Wherry EJ, Blattman JN, Ahmed R. Low CD8 T-cell proliferative potential and high viral load limit the effectiveness of therapeutic vaccination. *J Virol.* 2005;79:8960-8968.
146. Matsumoto K, Leggatt GR, Zhong J, et al. Impaired antigen presentation and effectiveness of combined active/passive immunotherapy for epithelial tumors. *J Natl Cancer Inst.* 2004;96:1611-1619.
147. Kreimer AR, Gonzalez P, Katki HA, et al. Efficacy of a bivalent HPV 16/18 vaccine against anal HPV 16/18 infection among young women: a nested analysis within the Costa Rica Vaccine Trial. *Lancet Oncol.* 2011;12:862-870.
148. Xiao G, Fu J. NF-kappaB and cancer: a paradigm of Yin-Yang. *Am J Cancer Res.* 2011;1:192-221.
149. Kim HJ, Hawke N, Baldwin AS. NF-kappaB and IKK as therapeutic targets in cancer. *Cell Death Differ.* 2006;13:738-747.
150. Chuang HC, Lay JD, Hsieh WC, Su IJ. Pathogenesis and mechanism of disease progression from hemophagocytic lymphohistiocytosis to Epstein-Barr virus-associated T-cell lymphoma: nuclear factor-kappa B pathway as a potential therapeutic target. *Cancer Sci.* 2007;98:1281-1287.
151. Sporn MB, Suh N, Mangelsdorf DJ. Prospects for prevention and treatment of cancer with selective PPARgamma modulators (SPARMs). *Trends Mol Med.* 2001;7:395-400.
152. Sertznig P, Seifert M, Tilgen W, Reichrath J. Present concepts and future outlook: function of peroxisome proliferator-activated receptors (PPARs) for pathogenesis, progression, and therapy of cancer. *J Cell Physiol.* 2007;212:1-12.
153. Reuter S, Gupta SC, Chaturvedi MM, Aggarwal BB. Oxidative stress, inflammation, and cancer: how are they linked? *Free Radic Biol Med.* 2010;49:1603-1616.
154. Qi C, Zhu Y, Reddy JK. Peroxisome proliferator-activated receptors, coactivators, and downstream targets. *Cell Biochem Biophys.* 2000;32(Spring):187-204.
155. Aggarwal BB, Takada Y, Oommen OV. From chemoprevention to chemotherapy: common targets and common goals. *Expert Opin Investig Drugs.* 2004;13:1327-1338.
156. Plat J, Mensink RP. Food components and immune function. *Curr Opin Lipidol.* 2005;16:31-37.

SECTION II

Molecular Techniques

CHAPTER 7

INTRODUCTION TO MOLECULAR TECHNIQUES AND INSTRUMENTATION

Shengle Zhang and Dongfeng Tan

INTRODUCTION

Rapid development of molecular technology and its application in oncology have revealed numerous genetic alterations in carcinoma, sarcoma, and lymphoma/leukemia. The identification of these alterations is invaluable not only for studying carcinogenesis but also for diagnosing cancer, assessing prognosis, and predicting therapeutic response as molecular biomarkers. Identification of these alterations can also aid in the design of new drugs. The technique used to study these alterations depends on the type of molecule being queried. DNA and RNA molecules are usually analyzed by polymerase chain reaction (PCR), fluorescence in situ hybridization (FISH), microarray, or DNA sequencing, while proteins are analyzed by immunohistochemical (IHC) analysis, flow cytometry, or proteomic techniques. Because molecular tests are usually complicated, time consuming, and costly, it is important to select the appropriate method before developing a test. The clinical utility of the assay should be considered first, e.g., Will the results of the assay significantly alter the patient's treatment? In addition, the following factors should be considered: (1) type of genetic alteration being studied (e.g., amplification, mutation, deletion, and translocation) and detection methods; (2) clinical sensitivity and specificity of the assay if it is used for diagnosis; (3) accuracy (analytic specificity), precision (reproducibility), and detection limit (analytic sensitivity); (4) simplicity of the assay, which is usually associated with high precision and low cost; and (5) type of tissues available, e.g., paraffin-embedded versus fresh tissue. See Table 7.1 for a summary of commonly used molecular techniques and their clinical uses. In the following paragraphs, we will describe how these molecular techniques are implemented in the clinic, from sample collection to data analysis.

TUMOR SPECIMENS

Carcinomas, sarcomas, and lymphomas are usually biopsied, excised, or aspirated for histologic evaluation. Thus, most of the available tissue types are formalin-fixed paraffin-embedded (FFPE) tissues, cytological smears, or cell blocks. For hematopoietic neoplasms, bone marrow biopsies and peripheral blood samples are usually used.

Formalin-Fixed Paraffin-Embedded Tissue

FFPE tissue is the most commonly available source of solid tumor tissue in pathology labs. DNA stored in paraffin blocks at room temperature is a stable and easy-to-use source for molecular assays, including PCR, FISH, and DNA sequencing. However, because RNA is single stranded, it is less stable than double-stranded DNA and often digested by endogenous and exogenous RNAses before tissue fixation or degraded in natural environment after tissue fixation. Thus, immediate fixation after removing the tissue from the patient is critical for preserving the RNA. In general, reverse transcription (RT)-PCR with an amplicon larger than 200 base pairs (bp) may not give a satisfactory result using FFPE tissue. Some commercial RNA stabilizing agents, such as RNA*later* (Ambion Inc., Austin, TX), can be useful for preserving the RNA in the tissue. Freshly frozen tissue, stored at less than –20°C, is a suitable source for both DNA and RNA, but is not routinely available in most pathology labs.[1]

TABLE 7–1 Commonly Used Molecular Methods for the Detection of DNA, RNA, and Proteins

Molecular Targets	Cytogenetics	PCR (DNA)	RT-PCR (RNA)	FISH	DNA/RNA microarray	Array CGH	Sanger sequencing	Next-generation sequencing	Mass spectrometry	Flow cytometry	Immunohistochemical analysis
DNA											
Deletion/insertion	X	X		X	X	X	X	X			
Amplification	X	X		X	X	X					
Point mutation/SNP		X			X		X	X	X		
Gene fusion (translocation)	X	X		X	X		X	X			
Ploidy/polysomy	X	X		X	X	X		X	X	X	
Hypermethylation		X						X			
Genome		X			X		X	X			
RNA											
mRNA level			X	X	X			X			
Gene fusion (translocation)			X	X			X	X			
miRNA/siRNA			X		X			X			
Transcriptome			X		X		X	X			
Protein											
Expression level									X	X	X
Amino acid changes									X	X	X

Another obstacle in the use of FFPE tissue is the decalcification of bone-containing tissue, which is a routine procedure in pathology labs. The conventional decalcifier RDO (hydrochloric acid) can significantly degrade RNA and DNA, making PCR and FISH assays difficult.[2] The decalcifier ethylenediaminetetraacetic acid (EDTA), by contrast, may protect DNA during tissue extraction, but the procedure takes a longer time (more than 24 hours).[3] A recent study showed that rapid decalcification (half an hour) with Nitrical (Decal Chemical Corp, Tallman, NY) can preserve DNA to a certain degree, but not RNA, allowing satisfactory results in FISH and PCR assays.[2]

Cytological Smears and Cell Blocks

In general, cytological smears contain fewer cells than excised tissue or biopsy samples. However, cells in smears are usually a good source of DNA/RNA, since (1) smears are regularly fixed in alcohol or air-dried immediately after sampling, preserving the DNA/RNA and (2) tumor cells are usually found in clusters and thus are easier to isolate from adjacent non-tumor cells. The smears are an even better tissue source for FISH assays, since the cells are left intact without truncation. Cytological cell blocks can be used for DNA/RNA isolation as well, but these are not usually as good as smears owing to a higher percentage of non-tumor cells or debris in the sample.

Bone Marrow Aspirates and Peripheral Blood Samples

Bone marrow aspirates and peripheral blood samples are commonly used for evaluation of leukemia/lymphoma. Anticoagulants are usually used during the samplings. Heparin is an unacceptable anticoagulant for collecting samples for PCR, as it inhibits DNA polymerase. However, EDTA and acid citrate dextrose are acceptable anticoagulants for molecular tests. Another obstacle in using blood samples is that hemoglobin associated with hemolysis in the samples may interfere with PCR, especially RT-PCR.[4]

NUCLEIC ACID ISOLATION

Nucleic acids are generally isolated by liquid-phase or solid-phase extraction.[5] Phenol-chloroform extraction, the most commonly used liquid-phase method, is being decreasingly used for clinical samples, as it is a time-consuming and complex method that generates low yields. Compared with the liquid-phase method, the solid-phase method is easier to perform, is more reproducible, can be adapted to small tissue samples, and can be automated. This method is based on the principle of DNA/RNA adsorption to silica in the presence of chaotropic salts, such as guanidine thiocyanate and alcohol. A silica-impregnated filter in a plastic column is the most commonly used format. After cell lysis and protein digestion, the nucleic acid is precipitated with alcohol and applied to the silica-impregnated filter, which binds the nucleic acids but not the cellular debris in the solution. The bound DNA/RNA is usually washed and subsequently eluted with nuclease-free water.

During DNA/RNA isolation, the percentage of tumor cells in the sample should be considered. Tumor cells in clinical samples are always mixed with non-tumor stromal cells, such as fibroblasts and inflammatory cells. Different molecular assays require different minimal percent tumor cellularity. For example, *KRAS* mutation analysis by Sanger DNA sequencing requires a minimum of 20% tumor cellularity, while pyrosequencing requires at least 5%. In samples with lower percent cellularity, microdissection by the manual or laser capture technique or a modified PCR procedure (such as co-amplification at lower denaturation temperature [COLD]-PCR) should be applied.[6]

DETECTION OF NUCLEIC ACIDS

Southern and Northern blotting with radioactive isotope or fluorescently labeled probes has been used to analyze DNA and RNA for decades. However, these techniques are decreasingly employed in clinical labs, as they are time consuming and labor consuming and require large amounts of DNA/RNA. Target and signal amplification of DNA/RNA are the two main techniques currently used for molecular diagnostic analysis of tumors.[7] PCR, ligase chain reaction, transcription-based amplification system, and strand displacement amplification are examples of target amplification, while branched DNA, hybrid capture, and invasive signal amplification are examples of signal amplification.[7,8] In situ hybridization (FISH or chromogenic ISH [CISH]) is another important technique used in molecular oncology, as it is performed in the context of tumor morphology. Nowadays, the most commonly used molecular techniques for clinical samples are PCR- and ISH-based assays. In addition, DNA/RNA microarrays, after years of preclinical validation, have started to be used in clinical practice. Next-generation sequencing (NGS), a group of new and powerful molecular tools, has not yet been used clinically, but will be before long owing to its high accuracy, ability to be performed on a large scale, and relatively low cost.

Polymerase Chain Reaction

PCR is a molecular technique used to amplify the number of copies of a specific region of DNA to facilitate analysis of genetic alterations. A basic PCR setup requires the following components: (1) a DNA template, which is the target sequence to be amplified; (2) a pair of primers, which are complementary to the ends of the sense and antisense strands of the DNA target; (3) DNA polymerase with a temperature optimum at around 70°C; (4) deoxynucleotide triphosphates (dNTPs), the building blocks for

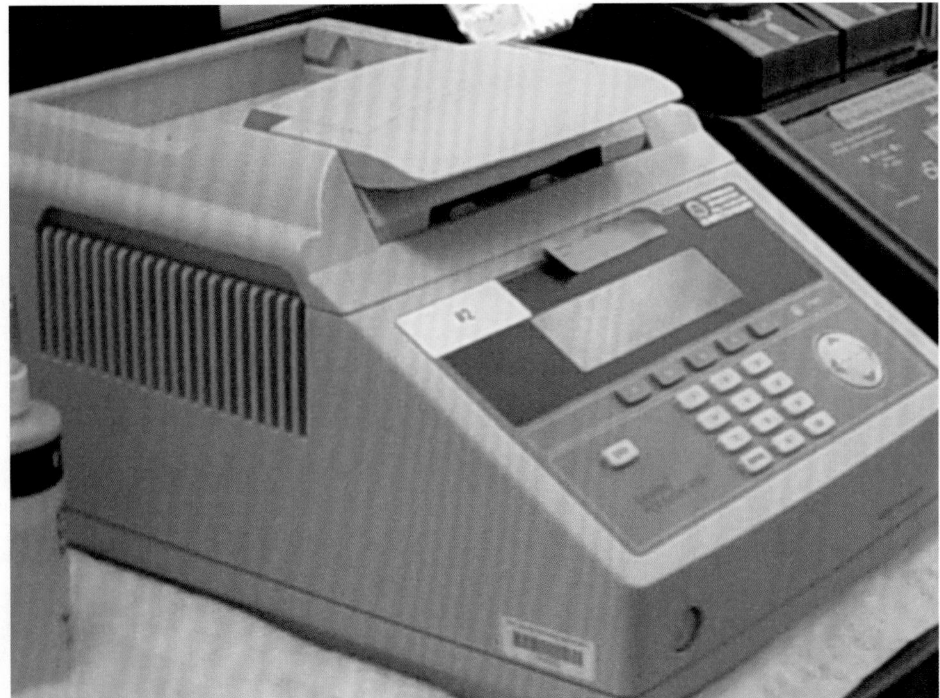

FIGURE 7–1 A photograph of the GeneAMP PCR System 9700 designed for medium- to high-throughput DNA and RNA applications, with 60-well to dual 384-well formats and variable cycling speeds (https://products.appliedbiosystems.com).

DNA synthesis; and (5) a buffered solution with a suitable chemical environment for DNA polymerase.[8,9]

PCR is commonly carried out in a reaction volume of 25 to 50 µl in a thermal cycler, i.e., "PCR instrument." Various PCR instruments from different manufacturers are commercially available (see http://www.labcompare.com/General-Laboratory-Equipment/211-DNA-Thermal-Cycler-PCR-Instrument). The GeneAmp PCR System 9700 is one of the most commonly used thermal cyclers in clinical labs (Fig. 7.1). The thermal cycler heats and cools the reaction tubes to achieve the temperatures required at each step of the reaction. Typical steps are as follows: (1) a DNA denaturation step at 94°C to 98°C for 20 to 30 seconds to yield single-stranded DNA through melting; (2) an annealing step at 50°C to 65°C for 20 to 40 seconds to allow annealing of primers to the single-stranded DNA template. Typically, the annealing temperature is 3°C to 5°C below the melting temperature of the primers used; (3) an extension step at 72°C to 75°C, which is the optimal temperature for most DNA polymerases, for synthesis of new DNA. The extension time depends on the DNA polymerase used and the length of DNA target to be amplified, but is usually 1 minute; (4) a final elongation cycle, usually at 72°C for 10 minutes, to ensure that the single-stranded DNA is fully extended; and (5) a final hold cycle at 4°C to 15°C for short-term storage.[8,9]

The PCR products, also called amplicons, are usually further analyzed by electrophoresis, hybridization, enzyme digestion, and DNA sequencing. DNA electrophoresis is used to separate the DNA fragments by size using a viscous medium, such as agarose or polyacrylamide gel. Agarose is usually used for longer DNA molecules, while polyacrylamide gel is used for shorter molecules and when higher resolution is necessary. After electrophoresis, the DNA fragments are stained with a fluorescent dye, such as ethidium bromide, and are visualized under ultraviolet light.[8,9] Capillary electrophoresis using a 310/3100 Genetic Analyzer (Applied Biosystems, Carlsbad, CA) has much higher resolution and can detect differences in size as small as three bases (Fig. 7.2). Amplicons analyzed by capillary electrophoresis are usually generated with primers prelabeled with a fluorescent dye. The amplicons can also be analyzed with probes through hybridization, such as dot/blot hybridization.[7] To detect point mutations, amplicons can be digested by restriction endonucleases, as the mutations often either create or destroy a restriction site.[7] This method has been used to detect an *EGFR* point mutation that creates an endonuclease restriction site that is not present in the wild-type sequence (Fig. 7.3).[10] Amplicons can also be used for DNA sequencing analysis, such as Sanger sequencing and pyrosequencing.[7]

PCR has broad applications in revealing tumor genetic alterations and can be used to detect DNA deletions/insertions, point mutations, including single nucleotide polymorphisms, amplifications, gene fusions, and hypermethylation.[7] The analytic sensitivity of PCR is usually high, with a capability of detecting trace DNA from as few as 100 cells. The analytical specificity of PCR is also high when the proper primers are used. DNA sequencing of the amplicon is usually not necessary for confirmation,

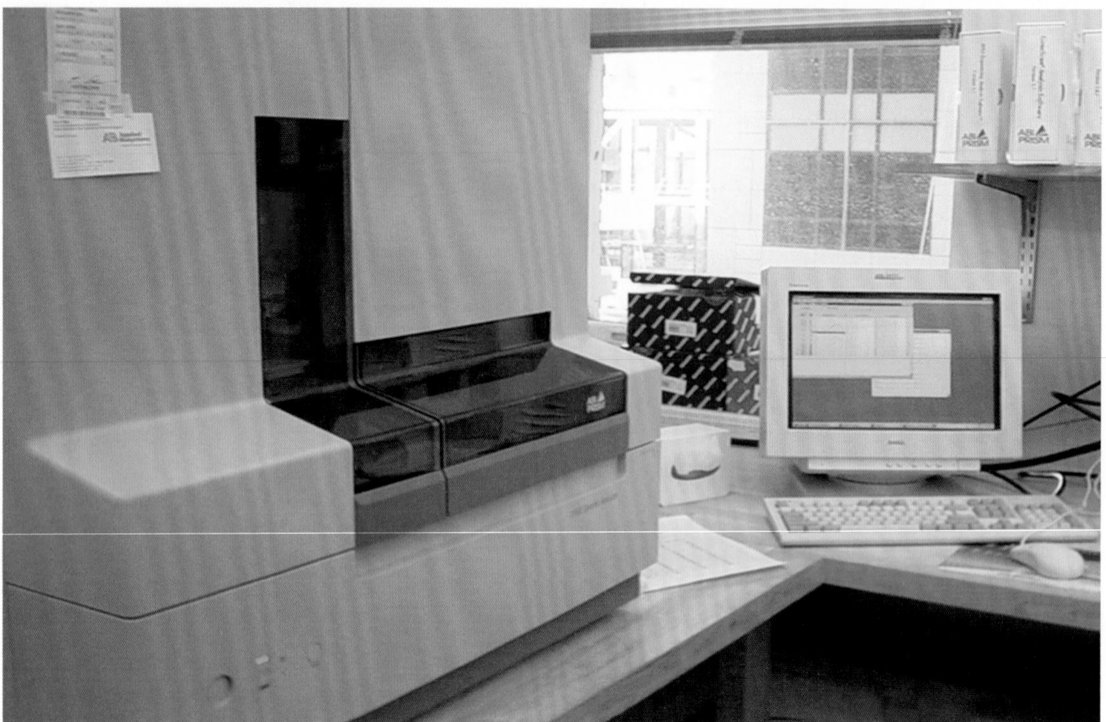

FIGURE 7–2 A photograph of the ABI Prism 3100 Genetic Analyzer with a capillary electrophoresis and fluorescent detection system used for DNA fragmentation and sequencing (http://www.appliedbiosystems.com).

unless an unexpected or indistinct band is present in the electrophoresis.

There are different types of PCR that are useful in certain situations.[7,11] For example, nested PCR is a highly sensitive qualitative assay in which the initial amplicon is reamplified with a new set of primers intrinsic to the first. Multiplex PCR uses two or more pairs of primers targeting different DNAs in the same reaction mix. Two types of PCR are especially useful in molecular oncology. The first is the tumor clonality assay. In normal female cells, one of the two X chromosomes is inactivated with an approximately equal chance, but in neoplastic cells

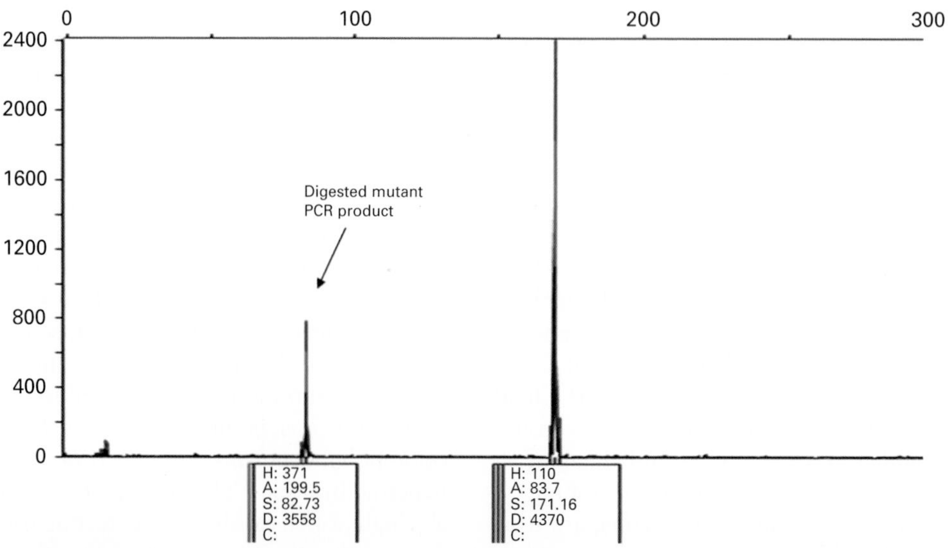

FIGURE 7–3 DNA fragmentation analysis of an *EGFR* gene point mutation (L858R) using capillary electrophoresis with the ABI 310 Genetic Analyzer. The 83-bp PCR product indicates a new Sau96I restriction site that was created by the point mutation (L858R).

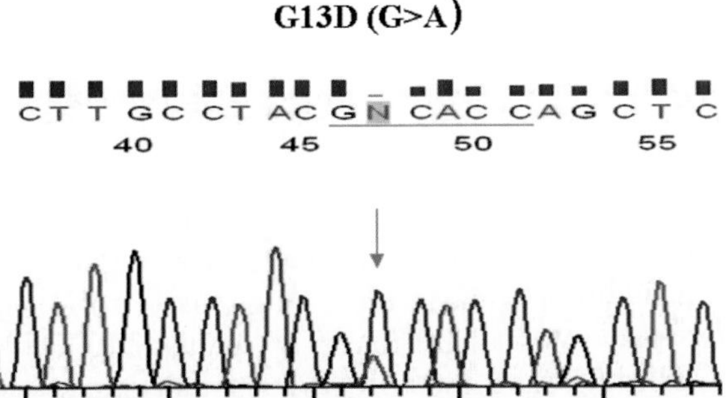

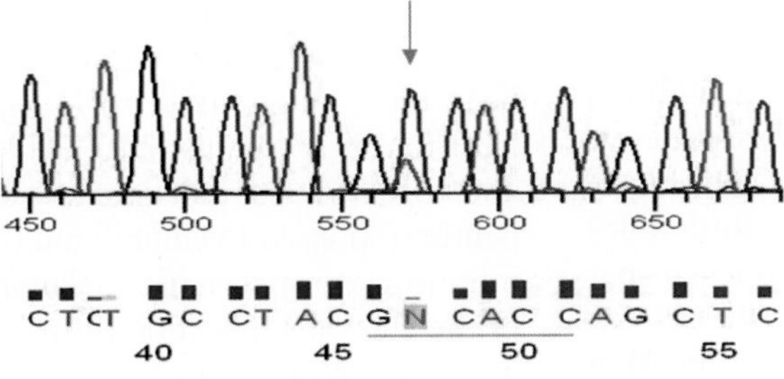

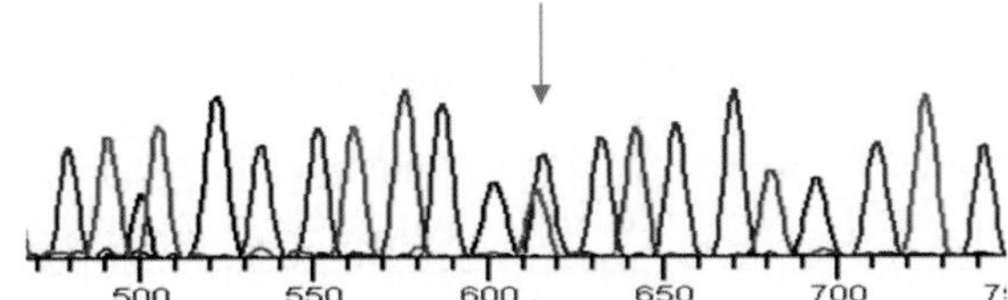

FIGURE 7–4 DNA sequencing showing amplification of a selected *KRAS* gene mutant (G13D) by COLD-PCR. The mutant/wild-type ratio is significantly increased with COLD-PCR (*arrows*).

both are either inactivated (methylated) or activated (unmethylated) owing to clonality. For example, analysis of the methylation status of endonuclease sites (HpaII and HhaI) in the human androgen receptor gene can be used to detect the status of clonality.[11,12] The second type of PCR is COLD-PCR. This is based on the fact that G/C to A/T mutations decrease the melting temperature of the DNA. Therefore, using a lower denaturation temperature in the assay can preferentially amplify the mutant DNA, especially when the mutants are a minority of the alleles. A good example of an application of COLD-PCR is the detection of *KRAS* mutations in colon and lung cancers.[6] The wild-type *KRAS* gene has the sequence GGT and GGC at codons 12 and 13, respectively. Because G to A/T mutations account for approximately 93% of all possible *KRAS* mutations, the test sensitivity of COLD-PCR compared with regular PCR can be increased by 80% in those samples with a lower mutant to wild-type ratio (Fig. 7.4).

Contamination in PCR assays is not unusual in the clinical molecular lab, and thus, the technician should be extremely cautious. Carryover contamination of PCR products is the most common and serious issue. Thus, every step in the process, including DNA isolation, the PCR reaction, electrophoresis, and product handling, should strictly follow standard procedures.[7,11] Another type of contamination is crossover contamination occurring between samples. This type of contamination is less common and easier to clean up. One of the chemical methods used to reduce the chance of contamination is to substitute deoxyuridine triphosphate for deoxythymidine triphosphate in the reaction mix, which results in incorporation of uridine in place of thymidine in the amplicon. PCR products with a uridine base can be digested by uracil-*N*-glycosylase before a new round of PCR, preventing carryover contamination.[13]

Reverse Transcription-PCR

In RT-PCR, RNA is first reverse-transcribed into complementary DNA (cDNA) using reverse transcriptase, and then the cDNA is amplified by conventional PCR or real-time PCR. RT-PCR is used to detect mRNA expression, gene fusions, and RNA viruses. An example of the successful use of RT-PCR in the clinic is the US Food and Drug Administration (FDA)–approved Onco*type* DX kit (Genomic Health, Inc. Redwood City, CA), which detects the expression of a 21-gene panel of RNAs to quantify the likelihood of breast cancer recurrence and predict the likely benefit from certain types of chemotherapy (http://www.oncotypedx.com). In addition, RT-PCR has been extensively used to detect gene fusions associated with chromosomal translocations.[7,11] The advantage of RT-PCR over regular PCR for detecting gene fusions is the simplicity of the primer design. Because the gene fusions associated with the translocation occur predominantly in intron areas with variable fusion points, multiple primers need to be designed for the different fusion regions for regular PCR. In RT-PCR, however, the primers are designed to target the two fusion exons only, since the intron areas are excised during the splicing process.[7,11] Therefore, RT-PCR is a more practical approach than regular PCR for detecting gene fusions. It is important to note that if FFPE tissue is used as the RNA source, the size of the amplicon should be less than 150 bp due to RNA degradation. Rapid amplification of cDNA ends (RACE) is a special type of RT-PCR that can be used to obtain a full-length mRNA sequence when only one translocation partner of the fusion transcript is known.[11] This method was successfully applied to identify the *ERG* gene, a translocation partner of *TMPRSS2* gene, in prostate cancer.[14]

Real-Time PCR

Real-time PCR allows the investigator to monitor the progress of the PCR with quantification in "real time." In addition, the entire assay is performed in a closed system with no requirement for amplicon separation by electrophoresis, as seen in regular PCR.[7,11] Instrumentation for real-time PCR includes a fluorescent detector in addition to a PCR thermocycler. In the reaction, a fluorescent dye or fluorescently labeled probe is required in addition to primers. SYBR Green, a dye that can bind to double-stranded DNA, is commonly used. Several sequence-specific fluorescently labeled probes (also called fluorescent reporters) have been developed, including the TaqMan probe (Applied Biosystems, Carlsbad, CA), a molecular beacons probe (Cepheid, Inc., Sunnyvale, CA), and a fluorescence resonance energy transfer probe (Invitrogen, Inc., Carlsbad, CA). In real-time PCR, the amount of amplicon is correlated with the fluorescence intensity and can be calculated with an appropriate standard control. Either DNA or RNA molecules can be detected with real-time PCR. When real-time PCR is used for RNA detection, it is called real-time RT-PCR or RT^2-PCR. Real-time PCR can detect most genetic alterations that regular PCR or RT-PCR does, including point mutations or single nucleotide polymorphisms, deletions, gene fusions, and amplifications. Detection and quantification of the *BCR-ABL* gene fusion is an example of an application of real-time RT-PCR (Fig. 7.5). Compared with regular PCR, real-time PCR has the following advantages: (1) it is quantitative; (2) the assay is performed in a closed system with a reduced chance of carryover or crossover contamination; (3) the assay can be performed quickly with no need for electrophoresis (a few hours); and (4) a probe is used to detect the product, which provides double confirmation. However, a disadvantage is that the size of the amplicon is not detected with real-time PCR. Because of its advantages over regular PCR, real-time PCR has been increasingly used in clinical molecular diagnostic labs. Recently (August 2011), the FDA-approved Cobas 4800 BRAF V600 mutation assay for predicting the therapeutic response of vemurafenib (serine–threonine kinase inhibitor) on metastatic melanoma is another example of the clinical application of real-time PCR (http://www.molecular.roche.com).

Fluorescence In Situ Hybridization

FISH uses fluorescently tagged DNA probes to identify nucleotide sequences of interest and is usually performed on FFPE tissues or cytological specimens.[15] FISH assays for DNA can be used to detect aneuploidy, chromosomal/interstitial deletions, gene amplifications, and translocations. FISH probes for DNA may target a locus (gene), centromere, or entire chromosome (painting) using different fluorescent colors, such as red, green, gold, and aqua. FISH probes may also target RNA, usually mRNA. A fluorescent microscope with different color filters is required to view the FISH slides. The typical procedure for FISH of DNA in paraffin-embedded tissue sections (3 to 5 μm thick) includes (1) deparaffinization with xylene and ethanol; (2) target retrieval with a microwave,

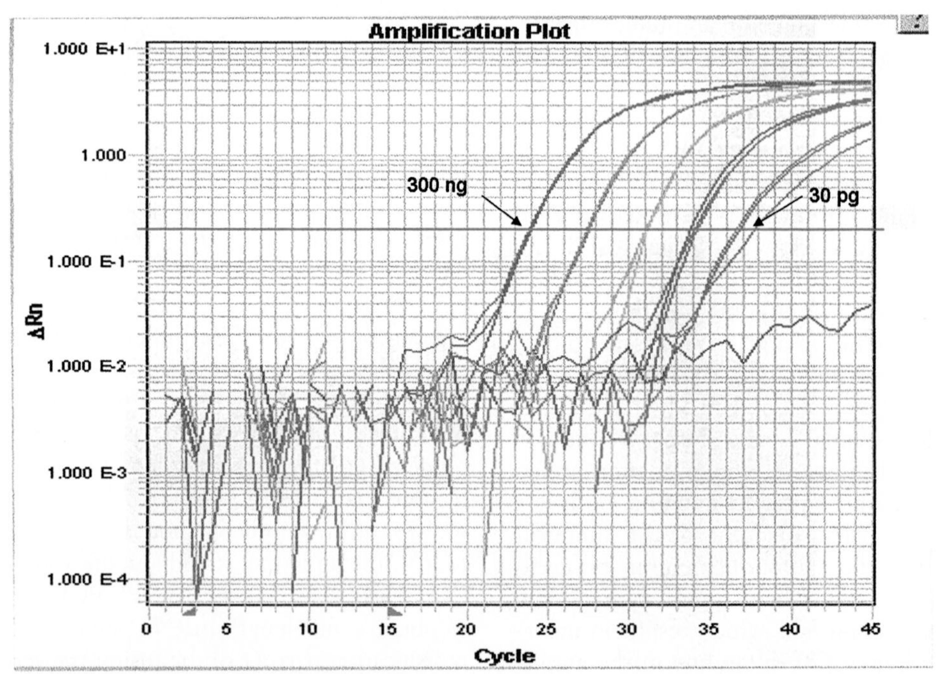

FIGURE 7–5 Real-time RT-PCR for analysis of the *BCR-ABL* gene fusion with the ABI 7900HT Real-Time PCR system (http://www3.appliedbiosystems.com). The test can be performed with as little as 30 pg of RNA (final dilution curve).

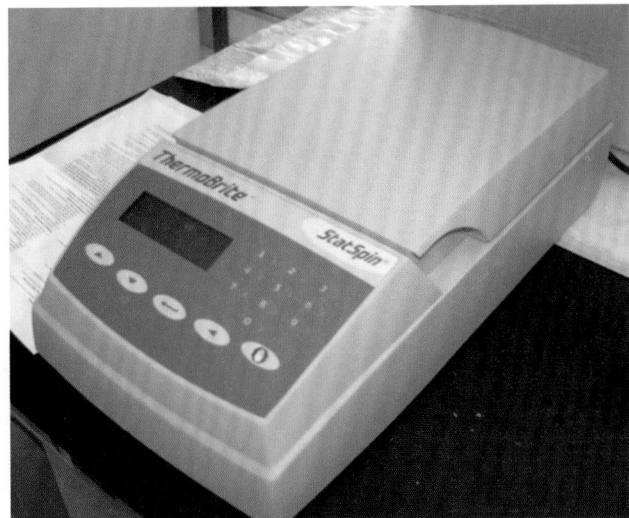

FIGURE 7–6 ThermoBrite (Abbott Molecular, Des Plaines, IL) is a programmable system for DNA denaturation and hybridization. Up to 12 FISH slides can be processed at the same time (http://www.abbottmolecular.com/static/cms_workspace/ThermoBrite_Sell_Sheet.pdf).

heat, or citrate buffer if necessary; (3) protein digestion with proteinases; (4) application of the FISH probe, (5) DNA denaturation at 73°C for 5 minutes, followed by hybridization of the FISH probe at 37°C overnight, using the ThermoBrite system (Fig. 7.6); (6) unbound probe washed out and nuclei counterstained with DAPI; and (7) the fluorescent signal visualized by fluorescent microscopy.[16] Compared with the PCR method, FISH, which is performed in tissues, has the following advantages: (1) it is a morphology-based test. Although cells in FISH slides viewed under a fluorescent microscope are not as clear as those in hematoxylin and eosin–stained slides viewed under a light microscope, the size and shape of the nuclei can be easily identified with DAPI stain. (2) A small number of cells are needed. In most FISH assays, only 100 to 200 cells of interest are counted. (3) FISH is easier to perform. No DNA/RNA isolation or complicated instrumentation is required. (4) Carryover contamination is not an issue. However, FISH assays cannot be used to detect minor genetic alterations, such as point mutations, since the probes are generally larger than 30 kb and, thus, FISH is a low-resolution assay. Further, the turnaround time is usually longer than that for PCR owing to the overnight hybridization step that is required.

FISH assays for DNA have been extensively used in diagnosing and predicting disease prognosis and therapeutic response for a variety of tumors. The PathVysion HER-2 DNA Probe Kit is an FDA-approved assay for predicting prognosis and therapeutic response to Herceptin (trastuzumab) in patients with breast cancer. The PathVysion kit consists of two labeled DNA probes: the LSI HER2 (c-erbB2) probe labeled with SpectrumOrange spans the *HER2* gene and the CEP17 probe labeled with SpectrumGreen hybridizes to alpha-satellite DNA located at the centromere of chromosome 17 and is used as a control (http://www.abbottmolecular.com/products/oncology/fish/breast-cancer-pathvysion.html). The average signal ratio of *HER2* to CEP17 of 20 interphase nuclei is then quantified using the following criteria: a signal ratio less than 1.8 is negative; more than 2.2, positive; and between 1.8 and 2.2, equivocal (Fig. 7.7). If the signal ratio is equivocal, then an additional 20 nuclei need to be evaluated. However, a ratio of 2.0 or greater indicates that the patient is eligible for Herceptin treatment.[17]

The UroVysion Bladder Cancer Kit is another FDA-approved FISH assay used to detect aneuploidy for chromosomes 3, 7, and 17 and loss of the 9p21 locus in urine specimens from patients with hematuria. The UroVysion kit consists of three alpha-satellite repeat sequence (centromeric region) probes (CEP3 labeled with SpectrumRed, CEP7 labeled with SpectrumGreen, and CEP17 labeled with SpectrumAqua) and a locus-specific probe for the *p16* gene at 9p21. The presence of one or more numeric chromosomal abnormalities in the UroVysion assay is suggestive of tumor

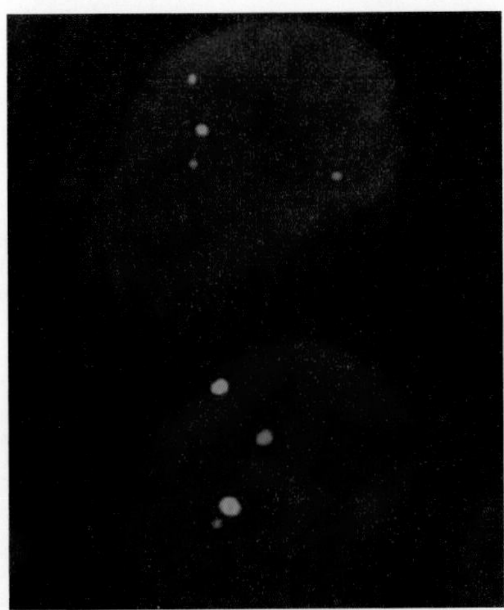

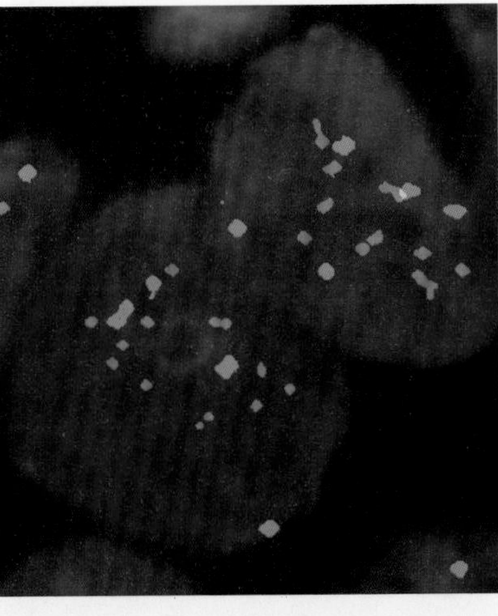

FIGURE 7–7 FISH analysis of the *HER2* gene in breast cancer using PathVysion probes. The left photo shows no gene amplification in tumor cells, while the right photo shows amplification (HER2/CEP17 > 2.2).

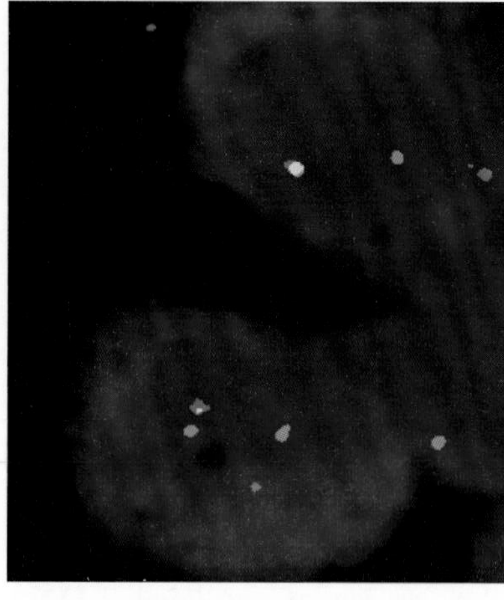

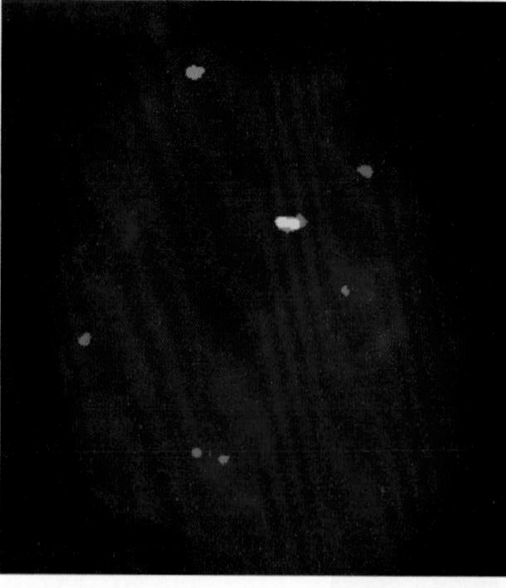

FIGURE 7–8 FISH analysis of the *ALK* gene rearrangement in non–small cell lung cancer using Vysis ALK probes. The left photo shows the tumor cell(s) with *ALK* gene break-apart (green and red signal separation), while the right photo shows the ALK gene 5′ deletion (green signal loss) plus break-apart.

recurrence in patients with a history of urothelial carcinoma (http://www.abbottmolecular.com/products/oncology/fish/bladder-cancer-urovysion.html).

Other kits include the Vysis CLL FISH Probe Kit, which is an FDA-approved assay for the subclassification and prognosis of chronic lymphocytic leukemia that detects deletions of LSI TP53, LSI ATM, and LSI D13S319 and gain of D12Z3 (http://www.abbottmolecular.com/us/aboutus/press-releases/fda-clears-fish-panel-for-leukemia.html). Recently, a Vysis ALK rearrangement FISH probe kit has been approved by the FDA for analyzing *ALK* genetic alterations in non–small cell lung cancer (NSCLC) to predict therapeutic response to crizotinib (http://www.abbottmolecular.com/us/products/oncology/fish/lung-cancer/vysis-lsi-alk-dual-color-break-apart-rearrangement-probe.html). The probes can detect both *ALK* gene break-apart and 5′ deletions, two rearrangements seen in a small subset of NSCLC (Fig. 7.8).

A number of FISH probes can be used as analyte-specific reagents (ASRs) to identify and quantitate genetic alterations in neoplasms. Several of these ASRs are commercially available from Abbott Molecular (http://www.abbottmolecular.com/us/technologies/fish.html). The Vysis LSI EGFR SpectrumOrange/CEP7 SpectrumGreen probe is an ASR for analyzing *EGFR* gene amplification or high polysomy in a variety of neoplasms, including NSCLC, colon adenocarcinoma, and glioblastoma multiforme (GBM).[18-20] *EGFR* amplification, defined as a ratio of *EGFR* to CEP7 ≥ 2.0, can be seen in approximately 20% of GBMs[19] but is rare in NSCLC and colon cancer. High *EGFR* gene copy numbers in NSCLC and colon cancer are mostly associated with high polysomy of chromosome 7 and not amplification (Fig. 7.9). The cutoff value of the assay is different for different tumors. For example, high polysomy is designated as ≥4 *EGFR* gene copies in ≥40% tumor cells in NSCLC,[18] while there is an average of ≥3 *EGFR* gene copies per nucleus in colon adenocarcinoma.[20,21] The Vysis 1p36/1q25 and 19q13/19p13 FISH Probe Kit is an ASR for detecting a 1p/19q deletion in oligodendroglioma. The 1p/19q deletion can be identified in 80% oligodendrogliomas and is associated with better prognosis and higher sensitivity to certain chemotherapies.[22] Although the 1p/19q deletion is not specific for oligodendroglioma and can be identified in 10% of astrocytomas or glioblastomas, it is frequently used to facilitate the diagnosis of oligodendroglioma.

FISH with break-apart probes is an indirect but good method for the detection of chromosomal translocation.

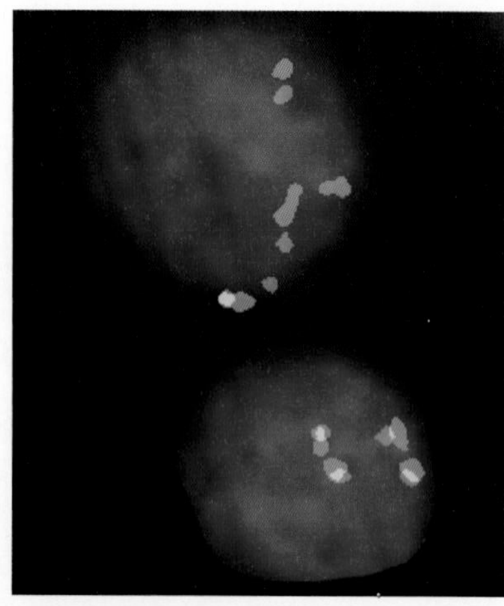

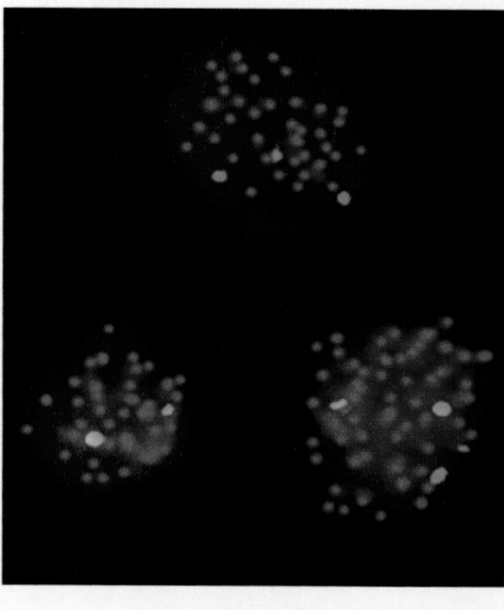

FIGURE 7–9 FISH analysis of *EGFR* gene copy number using Vysis LSI EGFR probes. The left photo shows lung adenocarcinoma cells with *EGFR* high polysomy (EGFR and CEP7 ≥ 4), while the right photo shows glioblastoma multiforme cells with *EGFR* gene amplification (EGFR/CEP7 ratio ≥ 2).

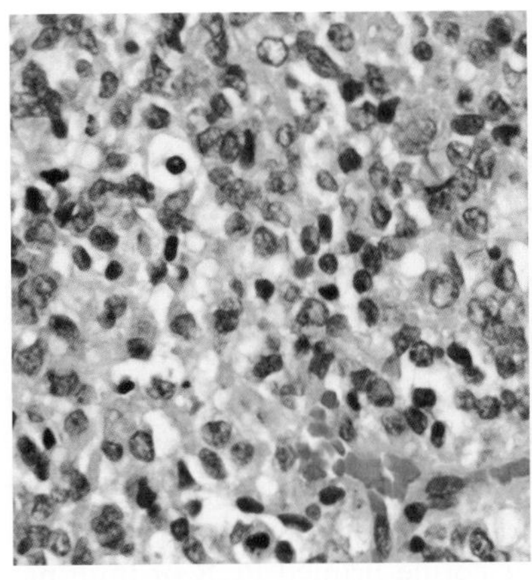

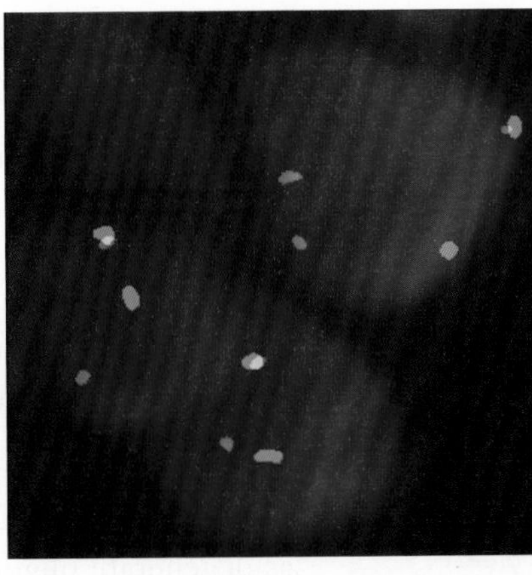

FIGURE 7–10 FISH analysis of the *SS18 (SYT)* gene rearrangement using Vysis SYT break-apart probes. The left photo shows a metastatic synovial sarcoma of the lung, which was poorly differentiated and difficult to diagnosis (hematoxylin and eosin stain). The right photo shows the *SS18* gene break-apart (separation of green and red signals), a diagnostic molecular feature of synovial sarcoma.

Whenever a translocation between chromosomes occurs, the relevant genes at each chromosome will have a breakpoint. Detection of one gene breakpoint can be used as a surrogate test for chromosomal translocation. For example, the *SS18–SSX1/2* gene fusion associated with the t(X;18)(p11;q11) translocation can be identified in over 90% of synovial sarcomas. Detection of the *SS18 (SYT)* gene breakpoint showed excellent sensitivity and specificity (Fig. 7.10). The *EWS* gene break-apart test for Ewing tumor/Primitive neuroectodermal tumor (PNET), however, is less specific, since other sarcomas, such as clear cell sarcoma, extraskeletal myxoid chondrosarcoma, and desmoplastic small round cell tumors, carry the *EWS* gene–associated translocation as well.

Another type of FISH probe used to detect translocations is a dual-color, dual-fusion probe, which is more specific for gene fusion/translocation. The LSI IGH/CCND1 Dual-Color Dual-Fusion Translocation Probe (http://www.abbottmolecular.com/products/oncology.html), for example, is used to detect t(11;14)(q13;q32), a characteristic genetic alteration in mantle cell lymphoma, with excellent specificity and sensitivity (Fig. 7.11). The synthetic oligonucleotide probe (a 25mer to 35mer) can be labeled with fluorochromes (Oligo-FISH) to detect DNA with better resolution, brighter signals, shorter turnaround time, and lower manufacturing costs compared with conventional FISH.[23] FISH-based assays can also be used for RNA or microRNA detection; although not used clinically yet, they have great potential for clinical applications.[24,25]

Chromogenic In Situ Hybridization

CISH, like FISH, is a process in which a labeled complementary DNA/RNA strand is used to localize a specific DNA/RNA sequence in a tissue specimen. Instead of the fluorescent labeling used in FISH, CISH uses a peroxidase or alkaline phosphatase reaction to covert a chromogen, diaminobenzidine or phosphate, to a colored product visible under a bright-field microscope. Typically, after hybridization with a DNA or RNA probe labeled with digoxigenin, an antibody against digoxigenin is applied followed by a second antibody labeled with peroxidase or alkaline phosphatase.[26] CISH, like FISH, may be used to evaluate gene amplification, gene deletion, and altered chromosome number. CISH has been successfully used to detect *N-myc* amplification in neuroblastoma.[26] Since differences between colored products is not as evident as in the FISH method, CISH is usually not ideal for evaluating genetic alterations that require two or more colored signals, such as for gene break-apart rearrangements. Recently, the FDA has approved a dual-color CISH assay developed by Ventana (Tucson, AZ) for identifying *HER2* gene amplification. This assay enables visualization of the *HER2* and Chr17 centromere by co-hybridization of the *HER2* and Chr17 centromere probes

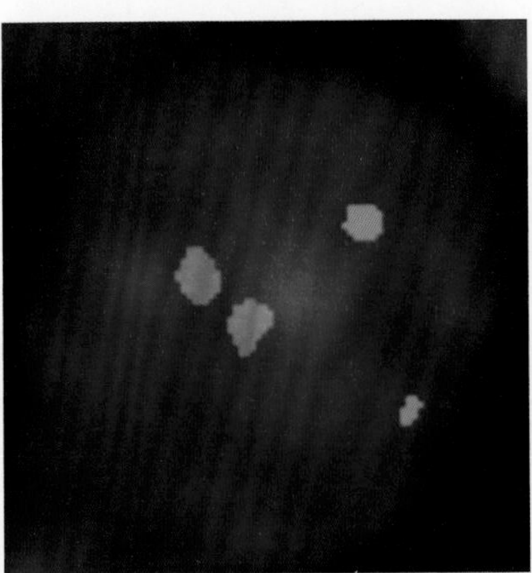

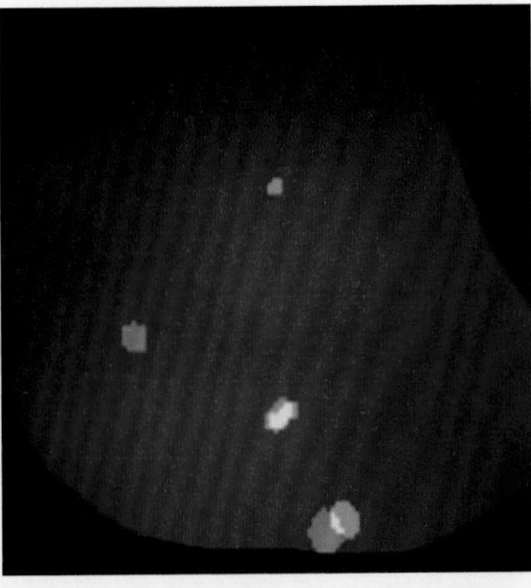

FIGURE 7–11 FISH analysis of the *IGH-CCND1* gene fusion using the Vysis IgH/CCND1 dual-color, dual-fusion probes. The left photo shows a normal lymphocyte (two red and two green signals), while the right photo shows a mantle cell lymphoma cell with the *IgH-CCND1* gene fusion (one red, one green, and two "yellow" fused signals).

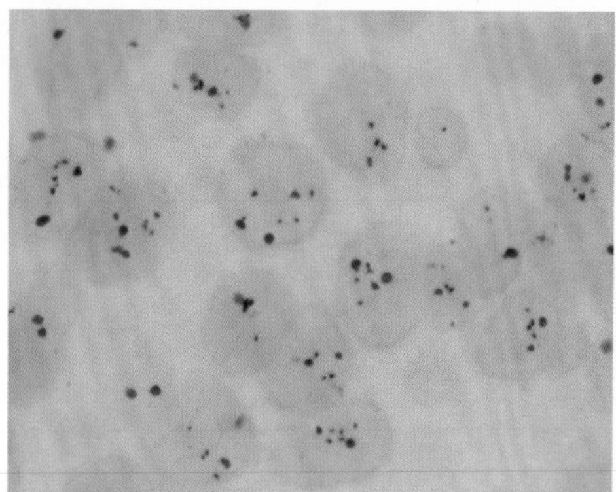

FIGURE 7–12 CISH analysis of the *HER2* gene in breast cancer using VENTANA INFORM *HER2* dual *ISH* probe cocktails. Black dots represent the *HER2* gene signals, while the red dots represent the Chr17 signals, which serve as a control.

on the same slide. *HER2* is detected by a dinitrophenyl-labeled probe and visualized with the *ultra*View silver in situ hybridization dinitrophenyl kit, and the Chr 17 centromere is targeted with a digoxigenin-labeled probe and detected with the *ultra*View Red ISH digoxigenin kit (Fig. 7.12; http://www.ventanamed.com/documents/INFORM_HER2_Dual_ISH_F&B_brochure.pdf). The results for *HER2* using the CISH kit are similar to those from the PathVysion FISH kit.[27]

Compared with FISH, CISH has the following advantages: (1) clearer cell morphology, (2) only a regular light microscopy is required, (3) the signal can be preserved long term, and (4) the assay can be automated with a regular instrument used for IHC analysis. CISH with a multiple color detection system, such as the dual-color ISH assay for *HER2*, will significantly expand its clinical application. CISH can also be used to evaluate mRNA expression in paraffin-embedded tumor tissue and has great potential for future clinical application.[28]

Comparative Genomic Hybridization and Array CGH

Comparative Genomic Hybridization (CGH) is a technique that bridges the gap between molecular genetics and cytogenetics. In CGH, DNA from a tumor sample and DNA from a paired normal control are amplified separately using a whole-genome amplification approach such as degenerate oligonucleotide-primed PCR or multiple displacement amplification.[29,30] Subsequently, the amplified tumor DNA and the amplified normal control DNA are labeled with different fluorochromes, for example, red for tumor DNA and green for normal control DNA. In standard CGH, the mixed, labeled DNA is allowed to compete to hybridize to metaphase chromosomes.

Copy number variants create a major source of genetic variation among individuals. Array CGH (aCGH) is a variant of CGH and is a powerful method used to detect and compare the copy numbers of DNA sequences at high resolution.[31] In aCGH, after labeling, the two DNA samples are mixed together and allowed to compete to hybridize to an array platform containing small pieces of chromosome. aCGH uses a chip of DNA (usually bacterial artificial chromosomes [BACs]) affixed to a microscope slide. Each BAC clone corresponds to a specific part of a chromosome, and computer software analyzes the ratio of red to green fluorescence on each spot, which corresponds to a loss or gain of that region (Fig. 7.13). aCGH

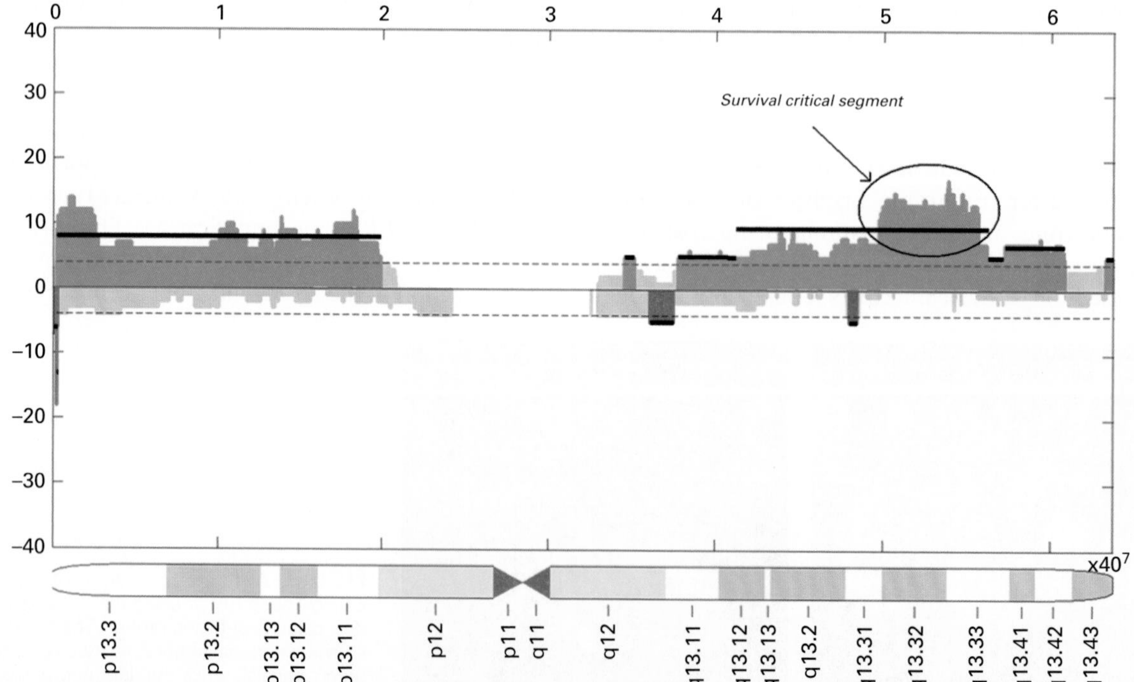

FIGURE 7–13 Gene amplifications (DNA gain) are in green and gene deletions (DNA loss) are in red. Results of the 244K oligonucleotide Agilent array demonstrating gene amplification at one locus (19q13.3), which has association with patients' survival.

is now widely used in hematopoietic and solid tumor diagnosis, tumor classification, and assessment of tumor prognosis.[32] For example, disease-predisposing germ-line mutations in cancer susceptibility genes (e.g., *BRCA1* and *MSH2*) may consist of large genomic rearrangements, including deletions and duplications, that are challenging to detect and characterize using standard PCR-based mutation screening methods (e.g., semi-quantitative multiplex PCR and multiplex ligation–dependent probe amplification). Such rearrangements range in size from single exons up to hundreds of kilobases of sequence. Custom-designed aCGH arrays focused on only a few target regions (*zoom-in aCGH*) may circumvent this drawback. Benefits of zoom-in aCGH include the ability to target almost any region in the genome and unbiased coverage of exonic and intronic sequence, which facilitates convenient design of primers for sequence determination of the breakpoints.[32] An example of aCGH evaluating gastric cancer is illustrated in Fig. 7.14.

Like any technique, aCGH has disadvantages and limitations. It cannot detect polyploidies, such as triploidies, as they cause no imbalance in the total DNA content. In addition, aCGH cannot detect balanced translocations or inversions as the total amount of DNA in the test sample is the same as in the control sample. aCGH systems also cannot detect changes in DNA sequences (point mutations, intragenic insertions or deletions, triplet repeat expansion, etc.) or gains or losses in regions of the genome not covered by the array.

DNA/RNA Microarray

DNA microarray, also known as gene chip or DNA chip, is a technique used to simultaneously detect the expression of thousands of genes (RNA) or sequencing alterations (DNA), including single nucleotide polymorphisms of a genome.[33,34] A collection of short DNA sequences or probes is attached to a solid surface for hybridization with the target cDNA or cRNA.[33,35,36] aCGH, as mentioned in the previous paragraph, is a type of DNA microarray, which detects genomic copy number variations at a higher resolution than chromosome-based CGH.[30] The probe-target hybridization can be quantified by measuring the relative abundance of fluorophore-labeled targets.[33,34] In Affymetrix microarrays, the probes are synthesized and then attached to a solid surface, such as glass or silicon, through a covalent bond by surface engineering.[34] The Illumina platform uses microscopic beads instead of a large solid support (http://www.illumina.com/technology/dasl_assay.ilmn). Alternatively, microarrays can be constructed by direct synthesis of oligonucleotide probes on solid surfaces.[33]

Microarray technology has been used not only in basic research but also in patient management. Two microarray-based assays have so far been approved by the FDA for clinical application. The first is MammaPrint (Agendia BV, The Netherlands), a microarray-based assay designed to individualize treatment for patients with breast cancer. It is offered as a prognostic test for women under the age of 61 years with lymph node–negative breast cancer. The assay can detect a 70-gene expression profile involving genes that regulate cell proliferation and invasion, metastasis, stromal integrity, and angiogenesis.[37] The second is the AmpliChip CYP450 Test (Roche Diagnostics, Pleasanton, CA), a microarray-based assay that analyzes the CYP2D6 and CYP2C19 genotypes of the cytochrome P450 gene, which allows doctors to select the most effective medicine with the least side effects. It uses a DNA microarray from Affymetrix (GeneChip) to classify individuals as having one of two CYP2C19 phenotypes by testing three alleles and one of four CYP2D6 phenotypes by testing 27 alleles.[38]

Although microarray technology is a powerful tool for gene expression and genotype analysis, its reliability

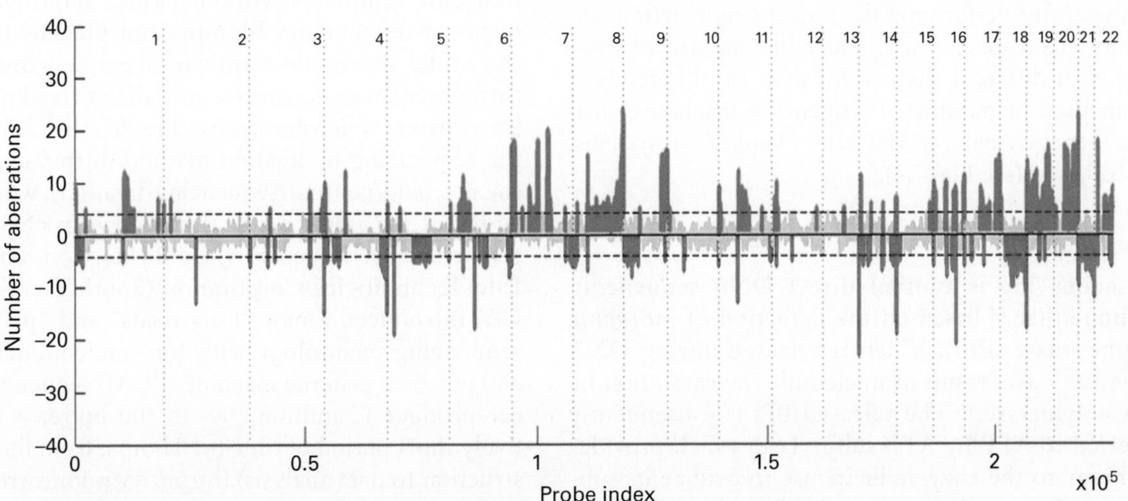

FIGURE 7–14 Global abnormalities of gene amplification and deletion using 244K array comparative genomic hybridization (aCGH). Green signal corresponds to gene amplification. Red signal corresponds to gene deletion.

and reproducibility have been questioned.[39] The results of microarray are sometimes significantly different between platforms and labs. Even using the same tissue and platform, the reproducibility between assays has been low.[40] This irreproducibility could be associated with the uniqueness of the arrays, variability between different persons, and the statistical methods used. The first "standard" set for microarray analysis was the "minimum information about a microarray experiment (MIAME)" outlined by the Microarray Gene Expression Data Society.[40] The intent of the MIAME standards was to provide enough experimental details to allow other researchers or technologists to reproduce published microarray-based results.[41] Acceptable reproducibility can be achieved by using appropriate controls and following strict procedures and standards for microarrays.[41] Microarray techniques are expected to be applied more and more in clinical practice in the near future.[42]

Direct DNA Sequencing and NGS

Sanger DNA Sequencing

The most commonly used direct DNA sequencing method is Sanger DNA sequencing, an enzymatic technique developed by Sanger et al.[43] It utilizes an oligonucleotide primer that is extended by DNA polymerase in the presence of deoxynucleotide triphosphates (dNTPs). The key principle of the Sanger method is the use of 2′,3′-dideoxynucleotide triphosphates (ddNTPs) as DNA chain terminators in addition to 2′-dNTPs.[44] After a ddNTP is incorporated into an elongating DNA chain, further extension is impossible owing to the absence of the 3′-hydroxyl group in the ddNTP, which prevents the formation of a phosphodiester bond with the succeeding dNTP. The chain-termination method requires a single-stranded DNA template, a primer, a DNA polymerase, normal dNTPs, and ddNTPs that terminate DNA strand elongation. Each type of ddNTP (ddATP, ddGTP, ddCTP, or ddTTP) is labeled with a different fluorescent dye. After performing the sequencing reaction and capillary electrophoresis, a ladder-like pattern of fragments with different fluorescent dyes can be detected and analyzed by automated sequencing machines, such as the Genetic Analyzer 310/3100 (Applied Biosystems, Carlsbad, CA) (see Fig. 7.4).

Pyrosequencing

Pyrosequencing is another direct DNA sequencing technique that is based on the detection of inorganic pyrophosphate (PPi), which is released during DNA synthesis[45,46] as a result of nucleotide incorporation by DNA polymerase.[47] The released PPi is subsequently converted to ATP by ATP sulfurylase, which provides the energy to the enzyme luciferase to oxidize its substrate luciferin and generate visible light. The light emitted is proportional to the number of incorporated nucleotides. Because the quantity of added nucleotide is known, the sequence of the template can be determined. Compared with Sanger sequencing, pyrosequencing can be done more quickly and is less expensive. But this technique has not been used for genome sequencing due to limitations in the read length (300 to 500 nucleotides).[47]

Next-Generation Sequencing

In recent years, a massively parallel sequencing platform, called next-generation sequencing, has been developed. It can simultaneously sequence 100,000 DNA fragments and has dramatically changed the landscape of genetic studies. RNA-Seq for transcriptomes, Chip-Seq for DNA–protein interactions, and CNV-Seq for large genome nucleotide variations are examples of the intriguing new applications of NGS.[48] Several NGS platforms have been developed by different manufacturers. The first of these instruments was the Roche 454 Genome Sequencer (GS) introduced in 2004, which was able to simultaneously sequence 100,000 DNA fragments with a read length greater than 100 bp (http://www.454.com/). The current model GS FLX Titanium is capable of more than 1 million reads in excess of 400 bp. The Illumina Genome Analyzer was introduced in 2006 and is capable of generating tens of millions of 32-bp reads (http://www.illumina.com/). The Illumina GAIIx can produce 200 million 75- to 100-bp reads, while the Sequencing by Oligonucleotide Ligation and Detection (SOLiD) by Applied Biosystems can produce 400 million 50-bp reads (http://www3.appliedbiosystems.com). The True Single Molecule Sequencing (tSMS) by Helicos BioSciences can produce 400 million 25- to 35-bp reads (http://www.helicosbio.com). Except for the Helicos tSMS, all platforms use clonally amplified templates that are amplified using either emulsion PCR (Roche 454 and SOLiD) or solid-phase amplification (Illumina). Helicos tSMS uses single DNA or RNA molecule templates without clonal amplification. In terms of sequencing, Illumina and Helicos tSMS use the cyclic reversible termination sequencing method (http://seqanswers.com/forums/showthread.php?t=21; http://www.helicosbio.com). The SOLiD system uses the sequencing by ligation method (http://sequencing.soe.ucsc.edu/content/sequencing-ligation), while Roche 454 uses pyrosequencing (http://www.roche-applied-science.com). Recently (July 2011), Ion Torrent by Life Technologies Corporation (South San Francisco, CA) introduced a new "long reads" and "paired-end" sequencing technology with Ion semiconductor chips and personal genome machine (PGM) sequencer, which can produce 12 million 200- to 500-bp reads in a relatively short period of time (~10 hours, from library construction to data analysis) (http://www.iontorrent.com). See Chapter 9 for more details of using RNA-Seq for transcriptome analysis.

DETECTION OF GENE PRODUCTS—PROTEINS

Proteomics

Proteins, the functional end products of genes, ultimately control the entire spectrum of biological processes. Likewise, changes in protein structure, expression levels, molecular interactions, and subcellular localization modulate critical cellular functions. Searching for specific tumor markers has long been a dream of researchers and clinicians and has been carried out for decades, mainly using biochemical and immunologic methods, such as protein electrophoresis, Western blotting, and monoclonal antibody techniques. Some tumor-associated biomarkers, such as alpha-fetoprotein for hepatocellular carcinoma and beta-HCG for choriocarcinoma, were discovered and used for tumor screening, disease diagnosis, and follow-up testing. Recently, the field of proteomics, the large-scale study of a complete set of proteins, has offered powerful tools to identify novel proteins and their structures and functions. Elucidating the full protein content of a cell, tissue, or organism under defined conditions is the central mandate of the field of proteomics. Proteomics consists of a group of methods, including two-dimensional electrophoresis and liquid chromatography for protein separation, high-performance liquid chromatography, spectroscopy, mass spectrometry, and antibody microarray.[49,50] Proteomics has been rapidly and extensively employed to explore tumor biomarkers in a variety of carcinomas with promising results and is expected to be applied more in the clinical setting before long.[51-54]

Currently, mass spectrometry is arguably the most important and powerful technology for proteomics.[55] Mass spectrometry, a technique used to measure the mass-to-charge ratio of gas phase ions, has been utilized as a diagnostic tool in clinical labs for several decades. It was initially used to measure micromolecules, such as lipids and carbohydrates. In the past decade, effective ionization of macromolecules, such as proteins and nucleic acids, together with significant improvements in the detection sensitivity and analytical capabilities of mass spectrometry instrumentation has led to increased adoption of mass spectrometry–based methods in cancer detection and diagnosis.[56]

The use of mass spectrometry for the detection and quantitation of clinically relevant proteins has certain theoretical advantages over classic immunoassays. One of the major advantages of mass spectrometry is its direct measurement of an analyte versus indirect assessment via antibodies or molecular affinity probes; mass spectrometry avoids the problem of cross-reactivity of immunoassays. The direct measurement by mass spectrometry of modifications that add mass to an analyte also allows for better assessment of adduct formation, chemical modification, and degradation of proteins. Mass spectrometry is well suited for measuring both single and multiple posttranslational modifications.[57] Furthermore, analysis by mass spectrometry provides structural information not captured by immunoassays. Detailed information on the principles and applications of mass spectrometry in cancer management can be found in Chapter 11.

IHC Analysis

IHC, the analysis of protein expression in cells based on antibody recognition, has been used in routine pathologic practice for decades and plays a critical role in tumor diagnosis and prognosis and prediction of therapeutic response. Many tumor-associated proteins with clinical utility have been identified. For example, p53 and AMACR have been used to distinguish between benign and malignancy in a variety of tissue types.[58,59] DNA mismatch repair proteins (hMLH-1, hMSH-2, hMSH-6, and PMS2) and Her2/neu have been used for disease prognosis and prediction of therapeutic response in colon and breast cancer, respectively.[17,60] Further, recent developments in gene expression profiling have facilitated the discovery of novel protein biomarkers, such as ERG for prostate cancer and TLE for synovial sarcoma.[61,62] Compared with DNA/RNA testing methods, IHC is a morphology-based assay and is easier to perform. In addition, a new wave of development is beginning with current increases in the knowledge of gene expression profiling and proteomics. Drawbacks of IHC are that it is only semi-quantitative; the results show higher variability than other methods, and, sometimes, nonspecific antibody reactions (see Chapter 10 for more details).

Flow Cytometry

Flow cytometry is another powerful method used to detect protein expression on a cell surface. It can simultaneously measure cell size, granularity, and fluorescence intensity as the cells flow in a fluid stream through a beam of light in a detection system.[63,64] Fluorescently labeled antibodies are usually used to reveal the expression of a variety of antigens or biomarkers on the cell surface. Thousands of cells with different colored fluorescent labels can be analyzed in a minute using flow cytometry,[65] and it is especially suitable for the evaluation of individual cells in diseases such as lymphomas and leukemia.[66] Flow cytometry has become an indispensable tool for diagnosing and classifying of lymphoma and leukemia (see Chapter 14 of this book for more details).[67,68]

CONCLUSION

Knowledge of molecular oncology and advanced molecular techniques have initiated and improved the development of molecular diagnostics and personalized cancer medicine. Since multiple genetic alterations usually occur in cancers, such as in the pathways of apoptosis, AKT, p53, EGF, MMPs, and VEGF (http://www.abcam.com/ps/pdf/cancer/cancer_poster_840x552.pdf), detection of several genetic alterations in a single test is becoming a trend for establishing future assays. PCR array, DNA/RNA microarray, and, especially, NGS platforms will play a key role in these approaches. Life Technologies Corporation (South San Francisco, CA) has recently introduced the Ion AmpliSeq Cancer Panel which, using Ion semiconductor chips and PGM sequencer, can generate 190 amplicons in a single tube, covering 739 known mutations in 46 tumor suppressor genes or oncogenes including *EGFR*, *KRAS*, and *BRAF*. This panel assay can be completed in 1 day (3.5 hours for constructing library, 4 hours for preparing template, 1.5 hours for running sequence, and 1 hour for analyzing data) with as low as 10 ng DNA input from FFPE samples. Although many new molecular techniques emerge every year, it is important to select the most appropriate, rather than latest, methods for setting up clinical assays. As mentioned in the beginning of this chapter, selection of assays or methods depends largely on clinical needs, assay's performances, tissue availability, and cost-effectiveness.

REFERENCES

1. Zehnbauer BA. Clinical testing of patient's specimens. In: Pfeifer JD, ed. *Molecular Genetic Testing in Surgical Pathology*. Philadelphia, PA: Lippincott Williams & Wilkins; 2006:171-185.
2. Mead KA, Tull J, Drotar N, et al. Decalcification with Nitrical® can preserve DNA/RNA for *in situ* hybridization and proteins for immunohistochemistry in formalin-fixed paraffin embedded tissues. *Mod Pathol*. 2011;24(S1):452A.
3. Wickham CL, Boyce M, Joyner MV, et al. Amplification of PCR products in excess of 600 base pairs using DNA extracted from decalcified, paraffin wax embedded bone marrow trephine biopsies. *Mol Pathol*. 2000;53:19-23.
4. Haverstick DM, Groszbach AR. Specimen collection and processing. In: Bruns DE, ed. *Fundamentals of Molecular Diagnostics*. St. Louis, MO: Saunders; 2007:25-37.
5. Lo YMD, Chiu RWK. Nucleic acid isolation. In: Bruns DE, ed. *Fundamentals of Molecular Diagnostics*. St. Louis, MO: Saunders/Elsevier; 2007:39-45.
6. Zuo Z, Chen SS, Chandra PK, et al. Application of COLD-PCR for improved detection of *KRAS* mutations in clinical samples. *Mod Pathol*. 2009;22:1023-1031.
7. Wittwer CT, Kusukawa N. Nucleic acid techniques. In: Bruns DE, ed. *Fundamentals of Molecular Diagnostics*. St. Louis, MO: Saunders/Elsevier; 2007:45-79.
8. Smith Zagone MJ, Pulliam JF, Farkas DH. Molecular pathology methods. In: Leonard DGB, ed. *Molecular Pathology in Clinical Practice*. New York, NY: Springer; 2007:15-40.
9. Frayling IM, Payne DA, Highsmith WE, et al. Molecular diagnostic technologies. In: Coleman WB, Gregory J, eds. *Molecular Diagnostics for Clinical Laboratorian*. 2nd ed. Totowa, NJ: Humana Press; 2005:65-149.
10. Pan Q, Pao W, Ladanyi M. Rapid polymerase chain reaction-based detection of epidermal growth factor receptor gene mutations in lung adenocarcinomas. *J Mol Diagn*. 2005;7:396-403.
11. Pfeifer JD. Polymerase chain reaction. In: Pfeifer JD, ed. *Molecular Genetic Testing in Surgical Pathology*. Philadelphia, PA: Lippincott Williams & Wilkins; 2006:86-110.
12. Allen RC, Zoghbi HY, Moseley AB, et al. Methylation of HpaII and HhaI sites near the polymorphic CAG repeat in the human androgen-receptor gene correlated with X chromosome activation. *Am J Hum Genet*. 1992;51:1229-1239.
13. Longo MC, Berninger MD, Hartley JL. Use of uracil DNA glycosylase to control carry-over contamination in polymerase chain reaction. *Gene*. 1990;93:125-128.
14. Tomlins SA, Rhodes DR, Perner S, et al. Recurrent fusion of *TMPRSS2* and ETS transcription factor genes in prostate cancer. *Science*. 2005;310:644-648.
15. Perry A. Fluorescence *in situ* hybridization. In: Pfeifer JD, ed. *Molecular Genetic Testing in Surgical Pathology*. Philadelphia, PA: Lippincott Williams & Wilkins; 2006:72-85.
16. Mehra S, de la Roza G, Tull J, et al. Detection of *FOXO1(FKHR)* gene break-apart by fluorescence in situ hybridization (FISH) in formalin fixed paraffin embedded alveolar rhabdomyosarcomas and its clinicopathological correlation. *Diagn Mol Pathol*. 2008;17:14-20.
17. Wolff AC, Hammond ME, Schwartz JN, et al. American Society of Clinical Oncology/College of American Pathologists guideline recommendations for human epidermal growth factor receptor 2 testing in breast cancer. *J Clin Oncol*. 2007;25:118-145.
18. Cappuzzo F, Hirsch FR, Rossi E, et al. Epidermal growth factor receptor gene and protein and Gefitinib sensitivity in non-small-cell lung cancer. *J Natl Cancer Inst*. 2005;97:643-655.
19. Reardon DA, Quinn JA, Vredenburgh JJ, et al. Phase 1 trial of Gefitinib plus sirolimus in adults with recurrent malignant glioma. *Clin Cancer Res*. 2006;12:860-868.
20. Cappuzzo F, Finocchiaro G, Rossi E, et al. EGFR FISH assay predicts for response to cetuximab in chemotherapy refractory colorectal cancer patients. *Ann Oncol*. 2008;19:717-723.
21. Moroni M, Veronese S, Benvenuti S, et al. Gene copy number for epidermal growth factor receptor (EGFR) and clinical response to antiEGFR treatment in colorectal cancer: a cohort study. *Lancet Oncol*. 2005;6:279-286.
22. Smith JS, Perry A, Borell TJ, et al. Alterations of chromosome arms 1p and 19q as predictors of survival in oligodendrogliomas, astrocytomas, and mixed oligoastrocytomas. *J Clin Oncol*. 2000;18:636-645.
23. Aurich-Costa J, Keenan P, Zamechek L, et al. Oligo fluorescence in situ hybridization (Oligo-FISH), a new strategy for enumerating chromosomes in interphase nuclei. *Fertil Steril*. 2007;88:86-89.
24. Raj A, van den Bogaard P, Rifkin SA, et al. Imaging individual mRNA molecules using multiple singly labelled probes. *Nat Methods*. 2008;5:877-879.
25. Deo M, Yu J-Y, Chung K-H, et al. Detection of mammalian microRNA expression by in situ hybridization with RNA oligonucleotides. *Dev Dyn*. 2006;235:2538-2548.
26. Bhargava R, Oppenheimer O, Gerald W, et al. Identification of MYCN gene amplification in neuroblastoma using chromogenic in situ hybridization (CISH): an alternative and practical method. *Diagn Mol Pathol*. 2005;14(2):72-76.
27. Bartlett JMS, Campbell FM, Ibrahim M, et al. A UK NEQAS ISH multicenter ring study using the Ventana *HER2* dual-color ISH assay. *Am J Clin Pathol*. 2011;135:157-162.
28. Ting DT, Lipson D, Paul S, et al. Aberrant overexpression of satellite repeats in pancreatic and other epithelial cancers. *Science*. 2011;331:593-595.
29. Vanneste E, Voet T, Le Caignec C, et al. Chromosome instability is common in human cleavage-stage embryos. *Nat Med*. 2009;15:577-583.
30. Shinawi M, Cheung S-W. The array CGH and its clinical applications. *Drug Discov Today*. 2008;18:760-770.
31. Kallioniemi A, Kallioniemi OP, Sudan D. Comparative genomic hybridisation for molecular cytogenetic analysis of solid tumours. *Science*. 1992;258:818-821.
32. Staaf J, Borg A. Zoom-in array comparative genomic hybridization (aCGH) to detect germline rearrangements in cancer susceptibility genes. *Methods Mol Biol*. 2010;653:221-235.
33. Bilitewaki U. DNA microarray: an introduction to the technology. *Methods Mol Biol*. 2009;509:1-11.
34. Auer H, Newsom DL, Kornacker K. Expression profiling using Affymetrix GeneChip microarrays. *Methods Mol Biol*. 2009;509:35-46.
35. Brown P, Botstein D. Exploring the new world of the genome with DNA microarrays. *Nat Genet*. 1999;21:33-37.
36. Heller MJ. DNA microarray technology: devices, systems, and applications. *Annu Rev Biomed Eng*. 2002;4:129-152.
37. Slodkowska EA, Ross JS. MammaPrint 70-gene signature: another milestone in personalized medical care for breast cancer patients. *Expert Rev Mol Diagn*. 2009;9:417-422.
38. de Leon J, Susce MT, Murray-Carmichael E. The AmpliChip CYP450 genotyping test: integrating a new clinical tool. *Mol Diagn Ther*. 2006;10:135-151.

39. Wang Y, Barbacioru C, Hyland F, et al. Large scale real-time PCR validation on gene expression measurements from two commercial long-oligonucleotide microarrays. *BMC Genomics.* 2006;7:59.
40. Brazma A, Hingamp P, Quackenbush J, et al. Minimum information about a microarray experiment (MIAME)—toward standards for microarray data. *Nat Genet.* 2001;29:365-371.
41. Enkemann SA. Standards affecting the consistency of gene expression arrays in clinical applications. *Cancer Epidemiol Biomarkers Prev.* 2010;19:1000-1003.
42. Weihua Tang W, Zhiyuan Hu Z, Muallem H, et al. Quality assurance of RNA expression profiling in clinical laboratories. *J Mol Diagn.* 2012;14:1-11.
43. Sanger F, Nicklen S, Coulsen AR. DNA sequencing with chain-terminating inhibitors. *Biotechnology.* 1992;24:104-108.
44. Pfeifer JD. DNA sequence analysis. In: Pfeifer JD, ed. *Molecular Genetic Testing in Surgical Pathology.* Philadelphia, PA: Lippincott Williams & Wilkins; 2006:123-139.
45. Ronaghi M, Uhlén M, Nyrén P. A sequencing method based on real-time pyrophosphate. *Science.* 1998;281:363-365.
46. Nyrén P. The history of pyrosequencing. *Methods Mol Biol.* 2007;373:1-14.
47. Ronaghi M. Pyrosequencing sheds light on DNA sequencing. *Genome Res.* 2001;11:3-11.
48. Costa V, Angelini C, De Feis I, et al. Uncovering the complexity of transcriptomes with RNA-Seq. *J Biomed Biotechnol.* 2010;2010:1-19.
49. Westermeier R, Marouga R. Protein detection methods in proteomics research. *Biosci Rep.* 2005;25:19-32.
50. Goncalves A, Bertucci F. Clinical application of proteomics in breast cancer: state of the art and perspectives. *Med Princ Pract.* 2011;20:4-18.
51. Buxbaum JL, Eloubeidi MA. Molecular and clinical markers of pancreas cancer. *JOP.* 2010;11:536-544.
52. Boja E, Rodriguez H. The path to clinical proteomics research: integration of proteomics, genomics, clinical laboratory and regulatory science. *Korean J Lab Med.* 2011;31:61-71.
53. Abu-Asab MS, Chaouchi M, Alesci S, et al. Biomarkers in the age of omics: time for a systems biology approach. *Omics.* 2011;15:105-112.
54. Masuda T, Miyoshi E. Cancer biomarkers for hepatocellular carcinomas: from traditional markers to recent topics. *Clin Chem Lab Med.* 2011;49:959-966.
55. Bouras G, Nakanishi T, Fujita Y, et al. Identification of β-tubulin as a common immunogen in gastrointestinal malignancy by mass spectrometry of colorectal cancer proteome: implications for early disease detection. *Anal Bioanal Chem.* 2012. [Epub ahead of print].
56. Wehr AY, Hwang WT, Blair IA, et al. Relative quantification of serum proteins from pancreatic ductal adenocarcinoma patients by stable isotope dilution liquid chromatography-mass spectrometry. *J Proteome Res.* 2012. [Epub ahead of print]. doi:10.1021/pr201011f.
57. Chen YT, Chen HW, Domanski D, et al. Multiplexed quantification of 63 proteins in human urine by multiple reaction monitoring-based mass spectrometry for discovery of potential bladder cancer biomarkers. *J Proteomics.* 2012. [Epub ahead of print].
58. Yaziji, H, Massarani-Wafai R, Gujrati M, et al. Role of p53 immunohistochemistry in differentiating reactive gliosis from malignant astrocytic lesions. *Am J Surg Pathol.* 1996;20:1086-1090.
59. Evans AJ. α-Methylacyl CoA racemase (P504S): overview and potential uses in diagnostic pathology as applied to prostate needle biopsies. *J Clin Pathol.* 2003;56:892-897.
60. Lanza G, Gafa R, Maestri I, et al. Immunohistochemical pattern of MLH1/MSH2 expression is related to clinical and pathological features in colorectal adenocarcinomas with microsatellite instability. *Mol Pathol.* 2002;15:741-749.
61. Miettinen M, Wang ZF, Paetau A, et al. ERG transcription factor as an immunohistochemical marker for vascular endothelial tumors and prostatic carcinoma. *Am J Surg Pathol.* 2011;35:432-441.
62. Terry J, Tsuyoshi Saito T, Subramanian S, et al. TLE1 as a diagnostic immunohistochemical marker for synovial sarcoma emerging from gene expression profiling studies. *Am J Surg Pathol.* 2007;31:240-246.
63. Villas BH. Flow cytometry: an overview. *Cell Vis.* 1998;5:56-61.
64. Jennings CD, Foon KA. Recent advances in flow cytometry: application to the diagnosis of hematologic malignancy. *Blood.* 1997;90:2863-2892.
65. Wood B. 9-Color and 10-color flow cytometry in the clinical laboratory. *Arch Pathol Lab Med.* 2006;130:680-690.
66. Craig FE, Foon KA. Flow cytometric immunophenotyping for hematologic neoplasms. *Blood.* 2008;111:3941-3967.
67. Stetler-Stevenson M, Davis B, Wood B, et al. 2006 Bethesda International Consensus conference on flow cytometry immunophenotyping of hematolymphoid neoplasia. *Cytometry B Clin Cytom.* 2007;72B:S3.
68. Calvo KR, McCoy CS, Stetler-stevenson M. Flow cytometry immunophenotyping of hematolymphoid neoplasia. *Methods Mol Biol.* 2011;699:295-316.

CHAPTER 8

Transcriptome Analysis

Shengle Zhang

INTRODUCTION

The transcriptome is the set of all RNA molecules in given cells, including coding messenger RNA (mRNA) and noncoding RNAs, such as ribosomal RNA (rRNA), transfer RNA (tRNA), microRNA (miRNA), and small interfering RNA (siRNA).[1,2] Approximately 25,000 genes in mammalian genomes are transcribed to mRNA and further translated to proteins to carry out various biologic functions, such as cell proliferation and differentiation.[3] rRNA, a component of the ribosome, assembles polypeptides or proteins from amino acids. tRNA carries amino acids to the ribosome for polymerization into a polypeptide. miRNA and siRNA are relatively new classes of noncoding RNAs, which play important roles in cell regulation.[4,5] miRNAs are a group of 18- to 25-nucleotide RNAs that serve as posttranscriptional regulators by binding to complementary sites on mRNA.[6] siRNAs are a group of 20- to 25-nucleotide double-stranded RNA molecules that interfere with the expression of specific genes.[5] Another new class of noncoding RNAs, intergenic RNAs, has recently been discovered, but their regulatory function has not yet been defined.[2]

Transcriptome analysis usually refers to a study of mRNA expression.[3,7] However, with expanding knowledge of regulatory RNAs, transcriptome analysis has been extended to the analysis of miRNAs and siRNAs.[8-10] In addition, the emerging technique of next-generation sequencing (NGS), which detects not only levels of RNAs but also their sequences, has revealed many novel mutations, altered splice sites, and gene fusions in carcinomas.[11-14] The techniques available for transcriptome analysis include microarray, large-scale real-time reverse-transcription (RT)-polymerase chain reaction (PCR), large-scale tag-based sequencing, and RNA-Seq (NGS). The features of each technique are summarized in Table 8.1. We describe each technique in detail in the following paragraphs.

TRANSCRIPTOME ANALYSIS OF mRNA

Since the 1970s, Northern blotting has been used for quantitation of mRNA. With this method, RNA is transferred from an agarose gel to diazobenzyloxymethyl-paper and gene-specific DNA probes are hybridized to the RNA. This time-consuming method can only be used to analyze one or a few gene transcripts and therefore is rarely used nowadays.[15] A newer method, tag-based sequencing, which originated from serial analysis of gene expression (SAGE) in the early 1990s,[16] has evolved and greatly contributed to transcriptome analysis.[17,18] In the mid-1990s, DNA/RNA microarray technology, which can measure the expression of 30,000 to 40,000 mRNAs per assay, was developed.[3,15] In recent years, large-scale real-time RT-PCR has been used to measure the expression of over 1,000 mRNAs with reliable results.[19] In 2006, the first transcriptome was sequenced using NGS (454/Roche). Since then, several other NGS platforms with higher efficiency have been developed, including the Illumina Genome Analyzer, ABI SOLiD, and HeliScope.[20] We introduce and compare the microarray, tag-based sequencing, large-scale RT-PCR, and NGS techniques below.

mRNA Transcriptome Analysis by Microarray

Analyzing the mRNA transcriptome by microarray is also called gene expression profiling. Microarrays are composed of microchips or microbeads, which are made

TABLE 8-1 Technologies Used in Transcriptome Analysis

Features	Microarray	Real-Time RT-PCR	Tag-Based Sequencing	RNA-Seq
Principle	Hybridization	RT-PCR	Sanger sequencing	"Next-generation" sequencing
Detection of unknown RNA sequence	No	No	Yes	Yes
Resolution	Probe-based	Primer-based	Single base	Single base
Sensitivity	Low	High	High	High
Specificity	Low	High	High	High
Quantification	Relative measure	Absolute measure	Absolute measure	Absolute measure
Precision (reproducibility)	Low	High	High	High
Dynamic range	Low	High	Not practical	High
Throughput	High	Moderate	Low	High
Cost (relative)	Moderate	Moderate	High	Low

from a solid surface, such as glass, plastic, or silicon, with thousands of DNA probes corresponding to known genes.[21] The key principle is hybridization between two complementary DNA (cDNA) strands, i.e., probe and sample DNA, which occurs through the formation of hydrogen bonds. Before hybridization, the mRNA should be transcribed to cDNA by reverse transcriptase using polythymidine as a "universal" primer to target the polyadenosine tail of mRNA, or some other sequence-specific primers. Nonspecifically bound DNA is removed by washing, and the specifically bound DNA labeled with a fluorescent dye generates a signal that can be detected with a scanner and analyzed by computer software (http://www.vbi.vt.edu/index.php/core_laboratory_facility/affymetrix_technology_description).[21]

Multiple microarray platforms are available with different designs based on (1) the types of probes used, e.g., short- or long-oligonucleotides on chips or beads; (2) how the probes are attached, e.g., spotting, in situ polymerization, or microbeads; and (3) the probe labeling method.[7] Microarrays from Applied Biosystems (AB; Foster City, CA) are made with 60-mer oligonucleotide probes on nylon microchips using the contact spotting method.[19] The AB Human Genome Microarray contains 31,700 probes representing 27,868 individual human genes.[19] The Affymetrix (Santa Clara, CA) and Agilent (Palo Alto, CA) platforms use in situ photolithographic synthesis with 25-mer and 60-mer oligonucleotide probes, respectively.[3,19] This technique uses light and light-sensitive masking agents to build a designed DNA sequence on a silica surface (http://www.dkfz.de/gpcf/24.html). In situ–synthesized arrays are suitable for applications using over 10,000 probes, such as in genome-wide analysis.[7] The Agilent Whole Human Genome Oligo Microarray contains 44,000 probes representing 41,000 genes/transcripts. The Affymetrix GeneChip Human Genome U133 plus 2.0 Array contains 54,000 probes representing over 47,000 genes/transcripts (http://media.affymetrix.com/support/technical/datasheets/hgu133arrays_datasheet.pdf). The BeadArray platform provided by Illumina (San Diego, CA) uses bead-based technology. Three micrometer silica beads are assembled in microwells of either fiber optic bundles or planar silica slides. The beads have a uniform spacing of ~5.7 μm when randomly assembled on one of these two substrates. Each bead is covered with hundreds of thousands of copies of a specific oligonucleotide that acts as the capture sequence (http://www.illumina.com/technology/beadarray_technology.ilmn). Each bead array of the Sentrix Array Matrix represents up to 1,624 unique bead types containing different probe sequences.[22] After a hybridization-based procedure, including cDNA-mediated annealing, selection, extension, and ligation (DASL), the captured sequences can be identified by correlating bead types and the specific oligonucleotide probes attached.[22,23] Because the probe groups span only about 50 bases, the bead array platform is capable of detecting partially degraded RNA (at levels as little as 50 ng), which is commonly seen in formalin-fixed, paraffin-embedded samples.[24,25] The Whole-Genome DASL HT Assay with the whole-genome probe set on Illumina's BeadChips can provide large-scale (>47,000 gene targets) and reproducible expression profiles with formalin-fixed, paraffin-embedded samples (http://www.illumina.com/technology/dasl_assay.ilmn). The Affymetrix and Agilent microarrays, however, require RNA from snap-frozen tissue or fresh tissues stored in RNARetain solution to generate satisfactory results.

Microarrays have been used extensively to study mRNA expression in tumors. However, measuring the upregulation or downregulation of mRNA expression by microarray is only a preliminary step, as often the expression of dozens of mRNAs or more is altered.[21] Thus, RT-PCR or immunohistochemical (IHC) analysis, if the antibodies are available, is necessary to verify the results from the microarrays. For example, we measured mRNA expression in a group of gastric carcinomas using Affymetrix GeneChip Human Genome U133 arrays. At least 40 mRNAs were upregulated compared with the corresponding normal gastric mucosae (Fig. 8.1). Among them, Claudin 3 and Claudin 4 were increased by 80- and 22-fold, respectively, in the intestinal type of

Fragment Name		Known Gene Name	Fragment ID	Sequence Clusters Cluster Cyto Map Cyto Band	Sequence Clusters Cluster Accession	Affy Fragment (Chip)	nl gas muc gr(8)vs ca gas	Direction (nl gas muc gr(8) ca gas	Change Pvalue (nl gas muc gr(8) vs ca gas	Limit (nl gas muc gr(8) vs ca)	Conf Limit Direction (nl gas muc gr(8))	95% Conf Limit (nl gas muc gr(8) vs ca gas)	Lower 95% Conf Limit Direction (nl gas muc gr(8) vs ca)
37892_at	...	collagen, type XI, alpha 1	108420	1p21	Hs.82772	108420(28)	17.85	Up	0.00001	37.06	Up	8.60	Up
201428_at	...	claudin 4	232092	7q11.23	Hs.5372	232092(28)	21.98	Up	0.00350	81.88	Up	5.90	Up
202790_at	...	claudin 7	233454	17p13	Hs.278562	233454(28)	17.11	Up	0.00564	78.12	Up	3.75	Up
202859_x_at	...	interleukin 8	233523	4q13-q21	Hs.624	233523(28)	18.97	Up	0.06543	553.48	Up	1.54	Down
203691_at	...	protease inhibitor 3, skin-derived (SKALP)	234353	20q12-q13	Hs.112341	234353(28)	19.29	Up	0.01805	152.47	Up	2.44	Up
203828_s_at	...	natural killer cell transcript 4	234490	16p13.3	Hs.943	234490(28)	10.76	Up	0.00104	33.24	Up	3.48	Up
203953_s_at	...	claudin 3	234615	7q11.23	Hs.25640	234615(28)	79.59	Up	0.05313	7270.12	Up	1.15	Down
203954_x_at	...	claudin 3	234616	7q11.23	Hs.25640	234616(28)	23.01	Up	0.05961	677.27	Up	1.28	Down
204259_at	...	matrix metalloproteinase 7 (matrilysin, uterine)	234921	11q21-q22	Hs.2256	234921(28)	10.60	Up	0.08346	227.78	Up	2.03	Down
205043_at	...	cystic fibrosis transmembrane conductance r...	235705	7q31.2	Hs.663	235705(28)	25.42	Up	0.00120	98.33	Up	6.57	Up
205242_at	...	chemokine (C-X-C motif) ligand 13 (B-cell ch...	235904	4q21	Hs.100431	235904(28)	10.94	Up	0.12622	441.96	Up	3.69	Down
205261_at	...	progastricsin (pepsinogen C)	235923	6p21.3-p21...	Hs.1867	235923(28)	29.94	Down	0.26368	411.01	Up	368552.01	Down
205470_s_at	...	kallikrein 11	236132	19q13.3-q1...	Hs.57771	236132(28)	12.12	Down	0.08544	2.24	Up	328.93	Down
205476_at	...	chemokine (C-C motif) ligand 20	236138	2q33-q37	Hs.75498	236138(28)	46.09	Up	0.00080	204.23	Up	10.40	Up
205890_s_at	...	ubiquitin D	236552	6p21.3	Hs.44532	236552(28)	17.26	Up	0.01465	124.73	Up	2.39	Up
205979_at	...	secretoglobin, family 2A, member 1	236641	11q13	Hs.97644	236641(28)	11.61	Down	0.26409	72.00	Up	9700.35	Down
206224_at	...	cystatin SN	236885	20p11.21	Hs.123114	236885(28)	10.17	Up	0.17233	1045.38	Up	10.10	Down
206262_at	...	alcohol dehydrogenase 1C (class 1), gamma...	236923	4q21-q23	Hs.2523	236923(28)	10.10	Down	0.21259	19.36	Up	1973.55	Down
206334_at	...	lipase, gastric	236995	10q23.31	Hs.159177	236995(28)	71.65	Down	0.23133	605.23	Up	3106957.37	Down
206391_at	...	retinoic acid receptor responder (tazarotene i...	237052	3q25.32	Hs.82547	237052(28)	15.12	Up	0.11919	993.89	Up	4.35	Down
206392_s_at	...	retinoic acid receptor responder (tazarotene i...	237053	3q25.32	Hs.82547	237053(28)	25.24	Up	0.08056	1396.67	Up	2.19	Down
206560_s_at	...	melanoma inhibitory activity	237221	19q13.32-q...	Hs.279651	237221(28)	14.61	Up	0.26117	15925....	Up	74.58	Down
207033_at	...	gastric intrinsic factor (vitamin B synthesis)	237694	11q13	Hs.110014	237694(28)	38.62	Down	0.10104	5.61	Up	8373.48	Down
207037_at	...	tumor necrosis factor receptor sUperfamily, ...	237698	18q22.1	Hs.114676	237698(28)	10.22	Up	0.00047	26.36	Up	3.96	Up
207139_at	...	ATPase, H+/K+ exchanging, alpha polypeptide	237800	19q13.1	Hs.36992	237800(28)	44.78	Down	0.01182	5.93	Down	338.33	Down
207430_s_at	...	microseminoprotein, beta-	238087	10q11.2	Hs.433392	238087(28)	17.02	Down	0.29868	327.45	Up	94835.32	Down
207546_at	...	ATPase, H+/K+ exchanging, beta polypeptide	238202	13q34	Hs.813	238202(28)	47.95	Down	0.03619	1.73	Down	1331.57	Down
207714_s_at	...	serine (or cysteine) proteinase inhibitor, cl...	238370	11	Hs.241579	238370(28)	14.86	Up	0.00015	31.65	Up	6.98	Up
207981_s_at	...	estrogen-related receptor gamma	238627	1q41	Hs.151017	238627(28)	12.03	Down	0.00946	3.04	Down	47.60	Down
208063_s_at	...	calpain 9 (nCL-4)	238707	1q42.11-q4...	Hs.113292	238707(28)	19.98	Down	0.09940	3.88	Up	1547.82	Down
209462_at	...	amyloid beta (A4) precursor-like protein 1	240090	19q13.1	Hs.74565	240090(28)	13.74	Down	0.00249	4.38	Down	43.10	Down
209875_s_at	...	secreted phosphoprotein 1 (osteopontin, bon...	240496	4q21-q25	Hs.313	240496(28)	13.36	Up	0.01335	52.90	Up	3.37	Up
210068_s_at	...	aquaporin 4	240688	18q11.2-q1...	Hs.288650	240688(28)	13.55	Down	0.00002	6.80	Down	26.96	Down
210119_at	...	potassium inwardly-rectifying channel, subfa...	240738	21q22.2	Hs.17287	240738(28)	14.02	Down	0.15762	10.06	Up	1977.92	Down
210297_s_at	...	microseminoprotein, beta-	240912	10q11.2	Hs.433392	240912(28)	10.83	Down	0.36907	583.70	Up	68465.00	Down
210375_at	...	prostaglandin E receptor 3 (subtype EP3)	240988	1p31.2	Hs.170917	240988(28)	12.01	Down	0.06668	1.45	Up	208.58	Down
210511_s_at	...	inhibin, beta A (activin A, activin AB alpha poly...	241116	7p15-p13	Hs.727	241116(28)	24.27	Up	0.00052	57.89	Up	10.18	Up
210906_x_at	...	aquaporin 4	241488	18q11.2-q1...	Hs.288650	241488(28)	14.55	Down	0.07626	1.89	Up	400.18	Down
211379_x_at	...	UDP-Gal:betaGlcNAc beta 1,3-galactosyltran...	241930	3q25	Hs.267695	241930(28)	11.33	Down	0.13597	5.91	Up	757.71	Down

FIGURE 8–1 Example of preliminary gene expression data from an Affymetrix microarray. The gene expression profiling was generated based on the average of three intestinal-type gastric cancers and eight normal corresponding mucosae. More than 40 genes were found to be upregulated in the tumors. Upregulation was defined as having at least 10-fold higher mRNA levels than the levels in normal mucosae.

TABLE 8-2 Claudin mRNA Expression Measured by Affymetrix Microarray in Intestinal-Type Gastric Carcinoma[a]

Gene Name	Fragment ID	Chromosome	Access No.	Fold Change	Regulation	*P* Value
Claudin 3	234615	7q11.23	Hs.25640	79.59	Up	0.05313
Claudin 4	232092	7q11.23	Hs.5372	21.98	Up	0.0035
Claudin 7	233454	17p13	Hs.278562	17.11	Up	0.00564

[a]Data were generated based on an average of three gastric cancers and eight normal gastric mucosae.

gastric cancer and by 99- and 13-fold in the diffuse type of gastric cancer (Tables 8.2 and 8.3). The overexpression of the Claudins in gastric cancer was confirmed by IHC using commercially available antibodies against the Claudins (Zymed Laboratory Inc.; South San Francisco, CA; Fig. 8.2A and B). We also found that Claudins were overexpressed in dysplasia and intestinal metaplasia of the esophagus.[26] In addition, many other mRNAs that were found to be upregulated by the microarray analysis should also be validated, as they may encode novel tumor-associated biomarkers.

The microarray technique is a powerful tool that is widely used to search for biomarkers in a variety of neoplasms.[7,13,27] Expression profiles revealed by microarray have had significant impacts on molecular oncology and its clinical application. One example of the successful clinical application of the microarray technique is MammaPrint, a US Food and Drug Administration–cleared assay capable of testing 70 relevant genes in breast cancer using the Agilent platform (http://www.agendia.com/pages/mammaprint/21.php). It provides additional prognostic information beyond what clinical and pathological features currently offer.[28] Another exciting example of the successful uses of gene expression analysis is the discovery of *TMPRSS2* gene–associated fusions, which are caused by translocation or deletion, in prostate cancer.[29] This discovery showed that gene fusions occur not only in lymphoma and sarcoma but also in carcinoma.

Although microarray technology is an effective tool for analyzing gene expression on a genome-wide scale, its reliability, compatibility, and standardization have been questioned.[19] mRNA expression profiles are sometimes dramatically different between microarray platforms, between laboratories, and using different analytical methods. Even using the same tissue and platform at one institution, the reproducibility between assays has been low.[15,30] This poor reproducibility has been blamed on the uniqueness of the arrays, the variability among users, and the differences in the data processing.[30] For those reasons, the Microarray Gene Expression Data Society outlined the "minimum information about a microarray experiment (MIAME)," one of the first standards established for microarray experimentation.[30] The intent of the MIAME standards was to provide enough experimental details to allow other researchers or technologists to reproduce published microarray-based results.[30] Recent experimentation has shown promising results, indicating that reproducible data can be achieved through the use of appropriate controls, strict procedures, and standards for microarray assays.[15]

mRNA Transcriptome Analysis by Tag-Based Sanger Sequencing

An expressed sequence tag (EST) is a short piece of cDNA that is complementary to a portion of a specific mRNA and acts as a "tag" for a unique gene transcript. Approximately 66 million ESTs are now available in public databases, such as GenBank, and can be mapped to specific chromosome locations using physical mapping techniques. Because these short tags allow the unequivocal identification of transcripts or genomic regions, high-throughput tag-based sequencing can provide a transcriptome- or genome-wide database through analysis with computer software.[18] SAGE is one such technique that uses short sequence tags in mRNA expression profiling.[16] Several other tag-based sequencing methods that take advantage of the high-throughput nature of SAGE have also been developed, including cap analysis of gene expression (CAGE), *trans*-spliced exon-coupled RNA

TABLE 8-3 Claudin mRNA Expression Measured by Affymetrix Microarray in Diffuse-Type Gastric Carcinoma[a]

Gene Name	Fragment ID	Chromosome	Access No.	Fold Change	Regulation	*P* Value
Claudin 3	234615	7q11.23	Hs.25640	98.66	Up	0.01487
Claudin 4	232092	7q11.23	Hs.5372	13.4	Up	0.00747
Claudin 7	233454	17p13	Hs.278562	15.16	Up	0.0002

[a]Data were generated based on an average of three gastric cancers and eight normal gastric mucosae.

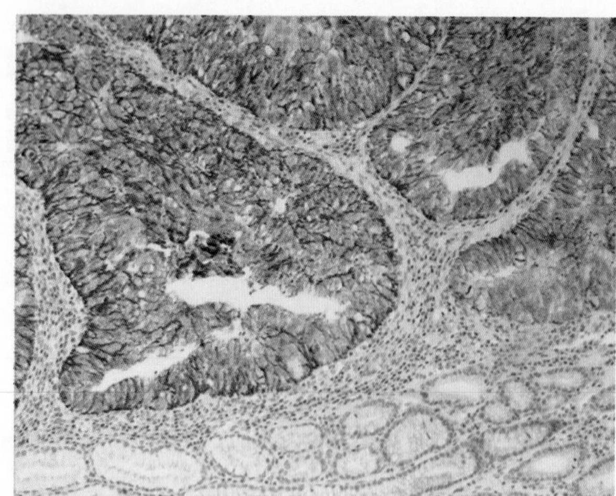

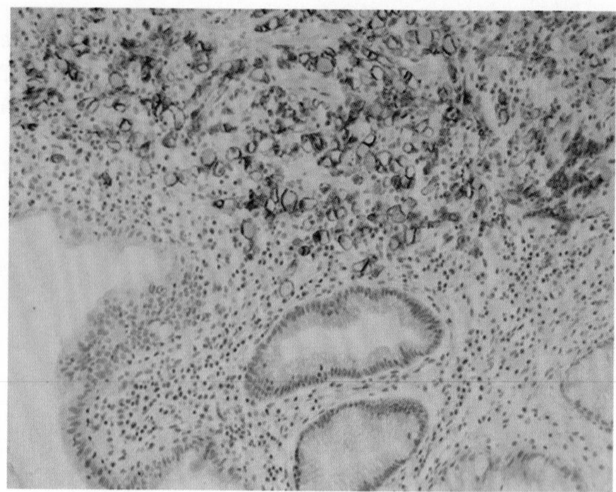

FIGURE 8–2 **A:** Validation of Claudin 4 overexpression in intestinal-type gastric cancer by immunohistochemical analysis. The tumor cells show strong membrane staining, while the adjacent normal epithelia remain unstained. **B:** Validation of Claudin 4 overexpression in diffuse-type gastric cancer by immunohistochemical analysis. The tumor cells show strong membrane staining, while the adjacent normal epithelia remain unstained.

end determination (TEC-RED), and 5′-SAGE.[18] CAGE expressing profiling is particularly suitable for investigating the transcriptional regulatory network that drives gene expression and regulatory noncoding RNAs.[31] It has been estimated, however, that tag-based sequencing detects only about 60% of transcripts in cells.[1] Compared with the microarray method, tag-based Sanger sequencing can detect unknown transcripts and has single-base resolution with "absolute" quantification of gene expression and low background noise. Tag-based sequencing has been widely used to search for tumor biomarkers in carcinomas of the stomach, ovary, and breast.[11,32,33] The cost, however, is higher than the other methods mentioned in this chapter.

mRNA Transcriptome Analysis by Large-Scale Real-Time RT-PCR

Analysis of gene expression by large-scale real-time RT-PCR is often referred to as the "gold standard" owing to its detection sensitivity, sequence specificity, large dynamic range, and high precision.[19,34] RT-PCR or real-time RT-PCR was first employed to verify the expression of selected mRNAs identified by microarray analysis. However, it has been extended to gene expression profiling owing to its expanding capability to be performed on a large scale. The most commonly used platform for real-time PCR–based gene expression profiling is the TaqMan Gene Expression Array (Applied Biosystems). This platform allows genome-wide gene expression analysis using a comprehensive collection of primer and probe sets (>700,000), and more than 2,000 mRNAs can be measured on a single chip of the microfluidic dynamic array (http://www.ncbi.nlm.nih.gov/projects/genome/probe/doc/ProjTaqMan.shtml).[34] The assay consists of two sequence-specific primers and a TaqMan minor groove–binding probe with a fluorescent reporter dye and a quencher moiety attached. The assay utilizes the 5′-nuclease activity of AmpliTaq Gold DNA polymerase to hydrolyze a target-specific probe bound to its target amplicon during PCR.[19] The primer set and the TaqMan probe provide two levels of sequence specificity. This method has been increasingly used in the search for tumor biomarkers, for example, in hepatocellular carcinoma,[35] melanoma,[36] and transitional cell carcinoma of the bladder.[37]

mRNA Transcriptome Analysis by RNA Sequencing

In recent years, a massively parallel NGS sequencing platform has been developed. It can simultaneously sequence thousands of DNA fragments, a capability that has dramatically changed the landscape of genetic studies.[38] RNA-Seq for transcriptome analysis, Chip-Seq for analyzing DNA–protein interactions, and CNV-Seq for analyzing large genome nucleotide variations are intriguing applications of NGS.[2] RNA-Seq, a sequencing-based method, is perhaps the most attractive of these methods because it enables transcriptome analysis. Several RNA-Seq platforms are available from different manufacturers. The first of these instruments was the Roche 454 Genome Sequencer (GS) introduced in 2004 (http://www.454.com/), which can simultaneously sequence 100,000 DNA fragments with a read length greater than 100 base pairs (bp). The current model GS FLX Titanium offers more than 1 million reads in excess of 400 bp. The Illumina Genome Analyzer (GA) (http://www.illumina.com) was introduced in 2006 and can generate tens of millions of 32-bp reads. The Illumina GAIIx can produce 200 million 75- to 100-bp reads. Currently, the Sequencing by Oligonucleotide Ligation and Detection (SOLiD) system from Applied Biosystems (http://www.appliedbiosystems.com) can produce 400 million 50-bp reads, and Helicos' true Single Molecule Sequencing (tSMS; http://www.helicosbio.com) can produce 400 million 25- to 35-bp reads.

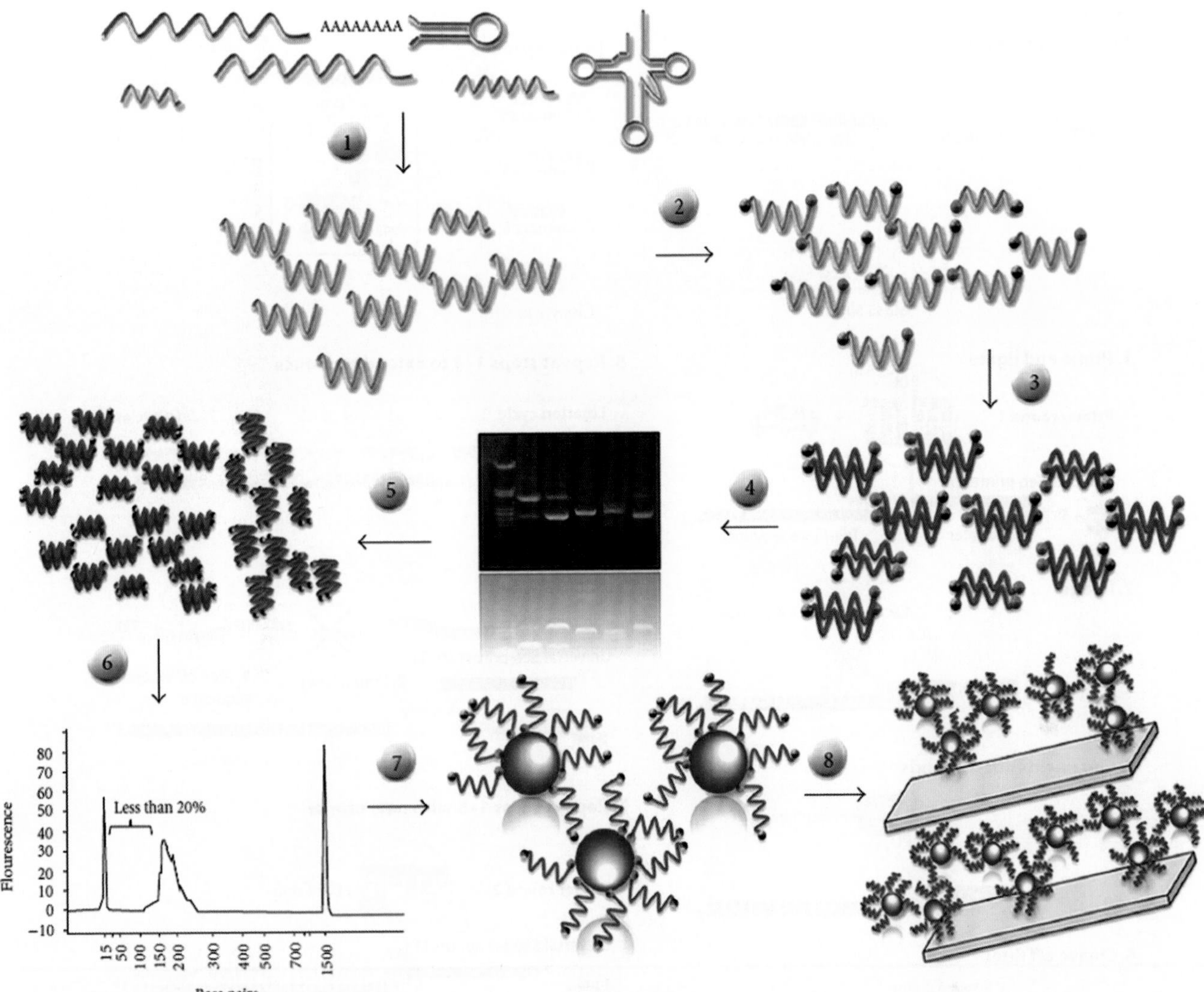

FIGURE 8–3 Schematic of a workflow for library preparation and clonal amplification in RNA-Seq experiments on the SOLiD platform. A total RNA sample after depletion of rRNA containing both polyadenosine and non-polyadenosine mRNA, tRNAs, miRNAs, and small noncoding RNAs is depicted. Ribo-depleted total RNA is fragmented **(1)**, ligated to specific adaptor sequences **(2)**, and retro-transcribed **(3)**. The resulting cDNA is size-selected by gel electrophoresis **(4)**, and cDNAs are PCR amplified **(5)**. The size distribution is then evaluated **(6)**. Emulsion PCR with one cDNA fragment per bead is used for the clonal amplification of cDNA libraries **(7)**. In the final step, purified and enriched beads are deposited onto glass slides **(8)** ready to be sequenced by ligation. (Adapted from an open access article, Costa V, Angelini C, De Feis I, et al., *J Biomed Biotechnol.* 2010;2010:1-19.)

Although there are several different platforms, some aspects of the assays are the same. For example, most of these platforms require RNA isolation and cDNA preparation. Except for the Helicos tSMS, all platforms use clonally amplified templates using either emulsion PCR (Roche 454 and SOLiD) or solid-phase amplification (Illumina). Figure 8.3 shows an example of DNA library preparation and clonal amplification using the SOLiD platform.[2] Helicos' tSMS uses single DNA or RNA templates without clonal amplification. In terms of sequencing methods, the Illumina platform and Helicos tSMS use the cyclic reversible termination method (http://seqanswers.com/forums/showthread.php?t=21; http://www.helicosbio.com/Portals/0/Documents/Helicos%20tSMS%20Technology%20Primer.pdf). The SOLiD system uses sequencing by ligation (http://sequencing.soe.ucsc.edu/content/sequencing-ligation), while Roche 454 uses pyrosequencing (http://www.roche-applied-science.com/publications/multimedia/genome_sequencer/flx_presentation/wbt.htm). Figure 8.4 shows an example of NGS with a SOLiD platform.[38] Recently (July 2011), Ion Torrent by Life Technologies Corporation (South San Francisco, CA) introduced a new "long reads" and "paired-end" sequencing technology with Ion semiconductor chips and Personal Genome Machine (PGM) sequencer, which can produce 12 million 200- to 500-bp reads in a relatively short period of time (~10 hours, from library construction to data analysis). This PGM sequencer can be used for RNA profiling study in combination with Ion Total RNA-Seq Kit (http://www.iontorrent.com).

RNA-Seq has several advantages over the hybridization-based, PCR-based, or tag sequencing–based

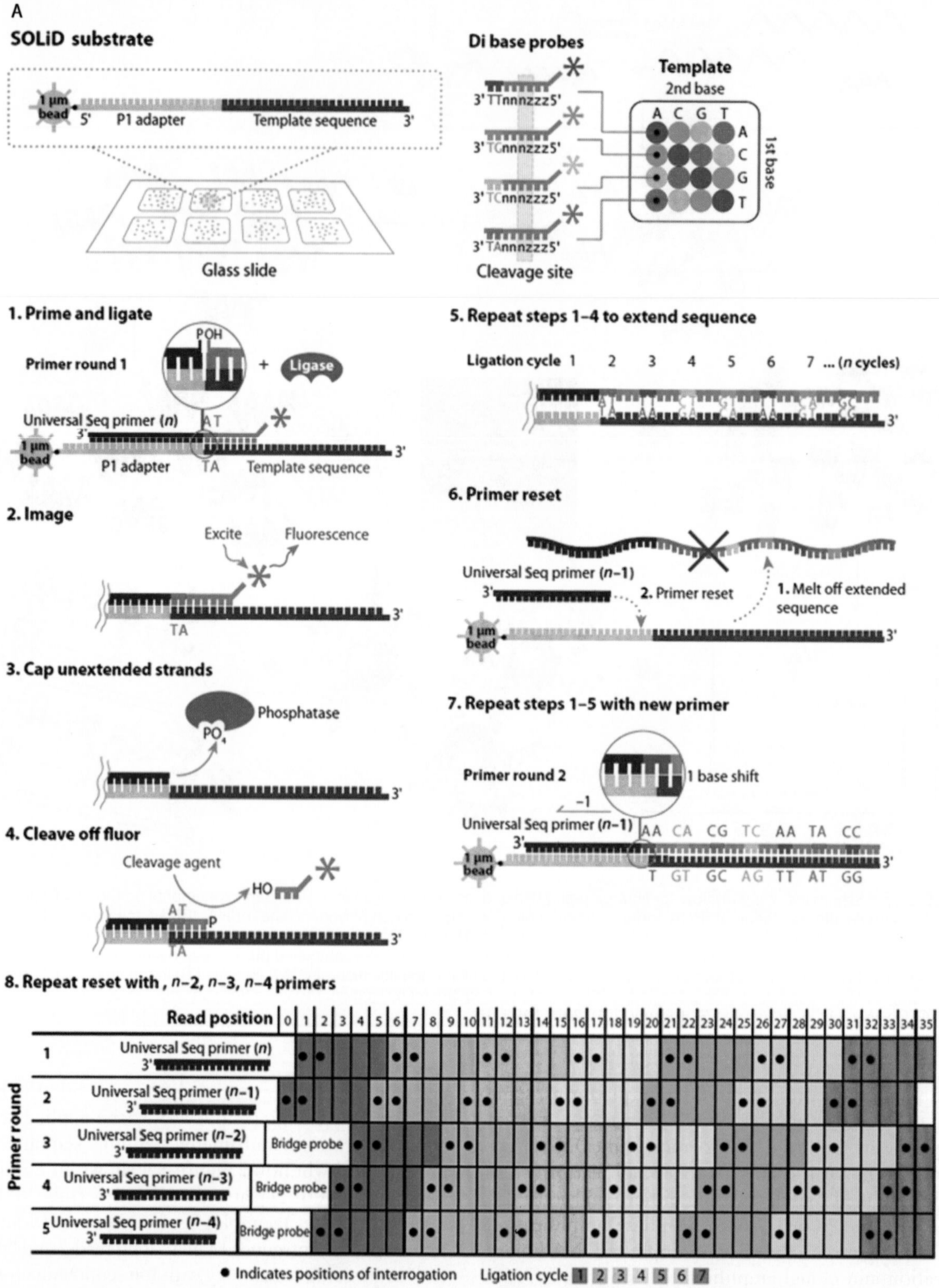

FIGURE 8–4 **A:** The ligase-mediated sequencing approach using the Applied Biosystems SOLiD sequencer. In a manner similar to Roche/454 emulsion PCR amplification, DNA fragments for SOLiD sequencing are amplified on the surfaces of 1 μm magnetic beads to provide sufficient signal during the sequencing reactions, which are then deposited onto a flow cell slide. Ligase-mediated sequencing begins by annealing a primer to the shared adapter sequences on each amplified fragment and then DNA ligase is provided along with specific fluorescently labeled octamers, whose 4th and 5th bases are encoded by the attached fluorescent group. Each ligation step is followed by fluorescence detection, after which a regeneration step removes bases from the ligated octamer (including the fluorescent group) and concomitantly prepares the extended primer for another round of ligation. **B:** Principles of two-base encoding. Because each fluorescent group on a ligated octamer identifies a two-base combination, the resulting sequence reads can be screened for base-calling errors vs. true polymorphisms or single-base deletions by aligning the individual reads to a known high-quality reference sequence. (Adapted with permission from Mardis ER, *Annu Rev Genomics Hum Genet.* 2008;9:387-402.)

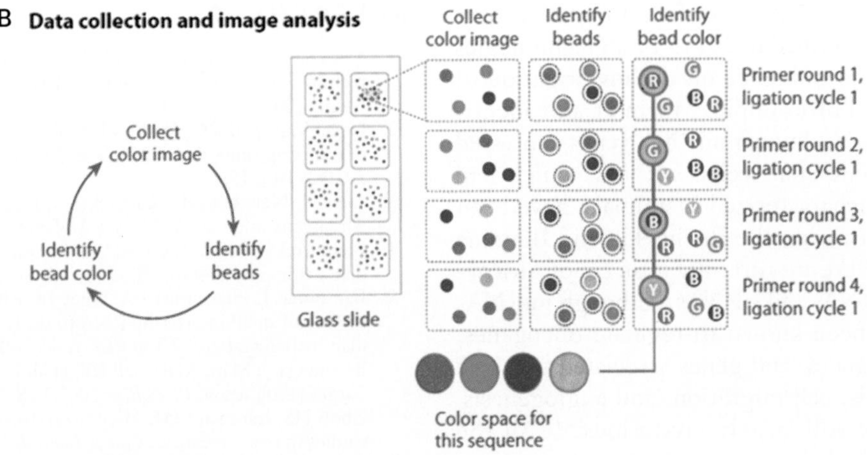

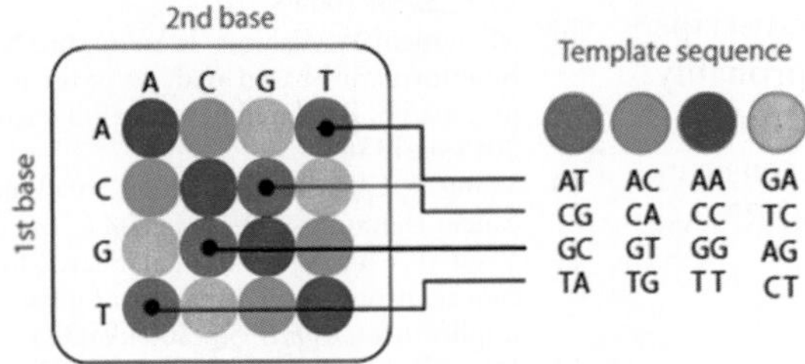

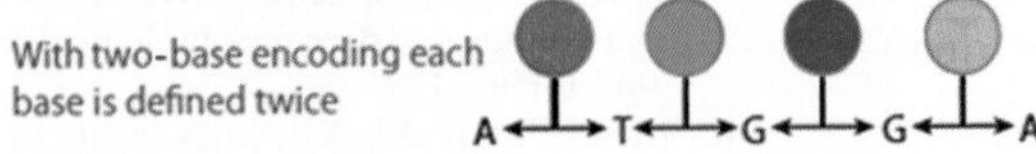

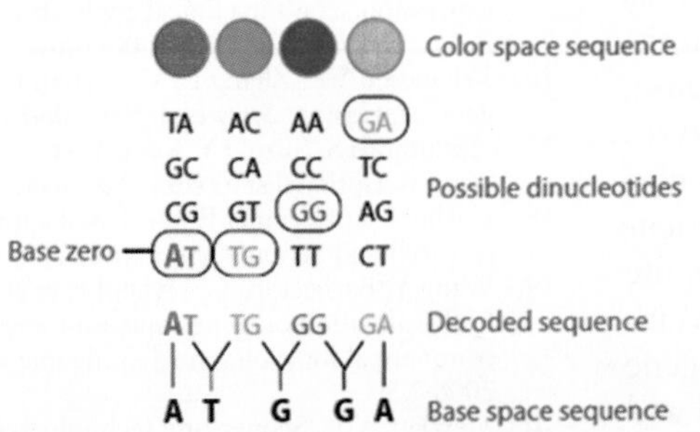

FIGURE 8–4 (Continued)

techniques. (1) It gives a comprehensive view of the transcriptome, as it measures mRNAs, noncoding RNAs, and small RNAs; (2) novel sequences, including mutations, altered splicing sites, and gene fusions, can be detected, since prior DNA sequence knowledge is not required for assay design; and (3) the assay can be performed with very high throughput and in a quantitative manner at a lower cost than other methods.[2,12] RNA-Seq has been extensively used to search for altered gene expression, mutations, splicing, and gene fusions in a variety of neoplasms and shows promise as a powerful tool for identifying more tumor biomarkers and new therapeutic strategies in the future.[2,14,39,40]

TRANSCRIPTOME ANALYSIS OF miRNA AND siRNA

miRNAs and siRNAs are two important classes of RNAs that regulate gene expression. They are the most studied noncoding RNAs.[4] Both miRNAs and siRNAs are very attractive molecules for scientists, oncologists, and pathologist because they can be used not only as tumor biomarkers in molecular diagnostics and classification but also as agents for anticancer therapies.[41-43] In addition, miRNAs and siRNAs are small molecules that are stable in paraffin-embedded tissue, the most widely available tissue source in anatomic pathology. While approximately 500 miRNAs were found in 2007,[4] over 30,000 have been identified in 2011.[9] NGS technologies have had a profound influence on the investigation of noncoding RNAs. For example, Morin et al.[44] identified 104 novel and 334 known miRNA genes expressed in human embryonic stem cells. siRNAs, which had been previously uncharacterized in animals, have been explored extensively using the Roche 454 and Illumina NGS platforms.[45,46] We are currently in an era of "discovery" regarding miRNAs and siRNAs. Although miRNAs and siRNAs have been known to regulate oncogenes, tumor suppressor genes, and genes associated with the cell cycle, apoptosis, cell migration, and angiogenesis, their functions are still largely mysterious.[4,47] All the techniques mentioned above, i.e., microarray, real-time PCR, tag-based sequencing, and RNA-Seq, have been successfully used to investigate the miRNA transcriptome in various carcinomas.[48,49] RNA-Seq is probably the most powerful tool used to date for small nuclear RNA transcriptome analysis because of its high sensitivity and specificity, capability of discovering novel RNAs, and relatively low cost.[2,9]

PERSPECTIVE

Transcriptome analyses using a variety of techniques are powerful approaches to qualitatively and/or quantitatively reveal altered mRNA expression, splice sites, gene fusions, and regulatory RNAs in carcinomas, sarcomas, and lymphomas. The findings from these studies are not only valuable for understanding carcinogenesis but can also be used as biomarkers for tumor diagnosis, disease prognosis, prediction of therapeutic response, and molecular classification. Transcriptome analyses can also identify molecular targets for the design of new therapeutic agents. Gene fusions in tumors are particularly valuable as biomarkers, since they are usually quite tumor specific and occur with high frequency.[48,50] With conventional cytogenetic metaphase analysis, many gene fusions in lymphomas and sarcomas were identified and effectively used for tumor diagnosis, disease prognosis, and minimal residual disease monitoring, for example, *BCR-ABL* in chronic myelogenous leukemia and *SS18-SSX* in synovial sarcoma.[48,50] However, metaphase analysis in carcinomas of epithelial origin, such as lung and breast cancers, has been unsatisfactory owing to difficulty in the culture of epithelial carcinoma cells. Microarrays were also used to identify *TMPRSS2* overexpression in prostate cancer, which led to the subsequent discovery of the *TMPRSS2*-associated fusion, which has become a very useful biomarker for prostate cancer.[29,51] With the more powerful RNA-Seq technique for transcriptome analysis, more gene fusions in other carcinomas are expected to be identified in the near future and translated into clinical applications, including molecular diagnostics and individualized cancer therapy.

REFERENCES

1. Morzova O, Hirst M, Marra MA. Applications of new sequencing technologies for transcriptome analysis. *Annu Rev Genomics Hum Genet.* 2009;10:135-151.
2. Costa V, Angelini C, De Feis I, et al. Uncovering the complexity of transcriptomes with RNA-Seq. *J Biomed Biotechnol.* 2010;2010:1-19.
3. Auer H, Newsom DL, Kornacker K. Expression profiling using Affymetrix microarray. *Methods Mol Biol.* 2009;509:35-46.
4. Blenkiron C, Miska EA. miRNAs in cancer: approaches, aetiology, diagnostics and therapy. *Hum Mol Genet.* 2007;16:R106-R133.
5. Bantounas I, Phylactoul LA, Uney JB. RNA interference and the use of small interfering RNA to study gene function in mammalian systems. *J Mol Endocrinol.* 2004;33:545-557.
6. Brennecke J, Stark A, Russell RB, et al. Principles of MicroRNA-Target recognition. *PLoS Biol.* 2005;3:e85(404-418).
7. Chon HS, Lancaster JM. Microarray-based gene expression studies in ovarian cancer. *Cancer Control.* 2011;18:8-15.
8. Slaby O, Svoboda M, Michalek J, et al. MicroRNAs in colorectal cancer: translation of molecular biology into clinical application. *Mol Cancer.* 2009;8:102.
9. Mizuguchi Y, Mishima T, Yokomuro S, et al. Sequencing and bioinformatics-based analyses of the microRNA transcriptome in hepatitis B-related hepatocellular carcinoma. *PLoS One.* 2011;6:e15304.
10. Wang X, Chen Y, Ren J, et al. Small interfering RNA for effective cancer therapies. *Mini Rev Med Chem.* 2011;11:114-124.
11. Yasui W, Oue N, Ito R, et al. Search for new biomarkers of gastric cancer through serial analysis of gene expression and its clinical implications. *Cancer Sci.* 2004;95:385-392.
12. Wang Z, Gerstein M, Snyder M. RNA-Seq: a revolutionary tool for transcriptomics. *Nat Rev Genet.* 2009;10:57-63.
13. Stroncek DF, Jin P, Wang E, et al. Global transcriptional analysis for biomarker discovery and validation in cancer and hematological malignancy biologic therapies. *Mol Diagn Ther.* 2009;13:181-193.
14. Tuch BB, Laborde RR, Xu X, et al. Tumor transcriptome sequencing reveals allelic expression imbalances associated with copy number alterations. *PLoS One.* 2010;5:e9317.
15. Enkemann SA. Standards affecting the consistency of gene expression arrays in clinical applications. *Cancer Epidemiol Biomarkers Prev.* 2010;19:1000-1003.
16. Velculescu VE, Zhang L, Vogelstein B, et al. Serial analysis of gene expression. *Sciences.* 1995;270:484-487.
17. Hashimoto S, Suzuki Y, Kasai Y, et al. 5′-end SAGE for analysis of transcriptional start sites. *Nat Biotechnol.* 2004;22:1146-1149.
18. Harbers M, Carninci P. Tag-based approaches for transcriptome research and genome annotation. *Nat Methods.* 2005;2:495-502.
19. Wang Y, Barbacioru C, Hyland F, et al. Large scale real-time PCR validation on gene expression measurements from two commercial long-oligonucleotide microarrays. *BMC Genomics.* 2006;7:59.
20. Metzker, ML. Sequencing technologies—the next generation. *Nat Rev Genet.* 2010;11:31-46.
21. Watson MA. Microarrays. In: Pfeifer JD, ed. *Molecular Genetic Testing in Surgical Pathology.* Philadelphia, PA: Lippincott Williams & Wilkins; 2006:152-170.
22. Chen R, Fan J-B, Campbell D, et al. High-throughput SNP genotyping on universal bead arrays. *Mutation Res.* 2005;573: 70-82.
23. Gunderson KL, Kruglyak S, Graige MS, et al. Decoding randomly ordered DNA arrays. *Genome Res.* 2004;14:870-877.
24. Hoshida Y, Villanueva A, Kobayashi M, et al. Gene expression in fixed tissues and outcome in hepatocellular carcinoma. *N Engl J Med.* 2008;359:1995-2004.
25. Chien J, Fan JB, Bell DA, et al. Analysis of gene expression in stage I serous tumors identifies critical pathways altered in ovarian cancers. *Gynecol Oncol.* 2009;114:3-11.
26. Montgomery E, Mamelak AJ, Gibson M, et al. Overexpression of claudin proteins in esophageal adenocarcinoma and its precursor lesion. *Appl Immunohistochem Mol Morphol.* 2006;14:24-30.
27. Goodison S, Sun Y, Urquidi V. Derivation of cancer diagnostic and prognostic signature from gene expression data. *Bioanalysis.* 2010;2:855-862.

28. Kim C, Taniyama Y, Paik S. Gene-expression-based and predictive markers for breast cancer—a primer for practicing pathologists. *Arch Pathol Lab Med.* 2009;133:855-859.
29. Tomlins SA, Rhodes DR, Perner S, et al. Recurrent fusion of TMPRSS2 and ETS transcription factor genes in prostate cancer. *Science.* 2005;310:644-648.
30. Brazma A, Hingamp P, Quackenbush J, et al. Minimum information about a microarray experiment (MIAME)—toward standards for microarray data. *Nat Genet.* 2001;29:365-371.
31. de Hoon M, Hayashizaki Y. Deep cap analysis gene expression (CAGE): genome-wide identification of promoters, quantification of their expression, and network inference. *BioTechniques.* 2008;44:627-632.
32. Hough CD, Sherman-Baust CA, Pizer ES, et al. Large-scale serial analysis of gene expression reveals genes differentially expressed in ovarian cancer. *Cancer Res.* 2000;60:6281-6287.
33. Abba MC, Drake JA, Hawkins KA, et al. Transcriptomic changes in human breast cancer progression as determined by serial analysis of gene expression. *Breast Cancer Res.* 2004;6:R499-R513.
34. Spurgeon SL, Jones RC, Ramakrishnan R. High throughput gene expression measurement with real time PCR in a microfluidic dynamic array. *PloS One.* 2008;3:e1662.
35. Paradis V, Bieche I, Dargere D, et al. Molecular profiling of hepatocellular carcinomas (HCC) using a large-scale real-time RT-PCR approach. *Am J Pathol.* 2003;163:733-741.
36. Ju J, Rastell L, Malyanker UM, et al. The melanoma vascular mimicry phenotype defined in gene expression and microsome sequencing analysis. *Cancer Genomics Proteomics.* 2004;1:355-362.
37. Pignot G, Bieche I, Vacher S, et al. Large-scale real-time reverse transcription-PCR approach of angiogenic pathways in human transitional cell carcinoma of the bladder: identification of VEGFA as a major independent prognostic marker. *Eur Urol.* 2009;56:678-688.
38. Mardis ER. Next-generation DNA sequencing methods. *Annu Rev Genomics Hum Genet.* 2008;9:387-402.
39. McPherson A, Hormozdiari F, Zayed A, et al. deFuse: an algorithm for gene fusion discovery in tumor RNA-Seq data. *PLoS Comput Biol.* 2011;7:e1001138.
40. Berger MF, Levin JZ, Vijayendran K, et al. Integrative analysis of the melanoma transcriptome. *Genome Res.* 2010;20:413-427.
41. Duchaine TF, Slack FJ. RNA interference and micro-RNA–oriented therapy in cancer: rationales, promises, and challenges. *Curr Oncol.* 2009;16:61-66.
42. Ryther RCC, Flynt AS, Phillips III, et al. siRNA therapeutics: big potential from small RNAs. *Gene Ther.* 2005;12:5-11.
43. Bishop JA, Benjamin H, Cholakh H, et al. Accurate classification of non-small cell lung carcinoma using a novel microRNA-based approach. *Clin Cancer Res.* 2010;16:610-619.
44. Morin RD, O'Connor MD, Griffith M, et al. Application of massively parallel sequencing to microRNA profiling and discovery in human embryonic stem cells. *Genome Res.* 2008;18:610-621.
45. Ghildiyal M, Seitz H, Horwich MD, et al. Endogenous siRNAs derived from transposons and mRNAs in Drosophila somatic cells. *Science.* 2008;320:1077-1081.
46. Watanabe T, Totoki Y, Toyoda A, et al. Endogenous siRNAs from naturally formed dsRNAs regulate transcripts in mouse oocytes. *Nature.* 2008;453:539-543.
47. Krol J, Loedige I, Filipowicz W. The widespread regulation of microRNA biogenesis, function and decay. *Nat Rev Genet.* 2010;11:597-610.
48. Kaul KL. Solid tumors. In: Leonard DGB, ed. *Molecular Pathology in Clinical Practice.* New York, NY: Springer; 2006:269-313.
49. Szczyrba J, Loprich E, Wach S, et al. The microRNA profile of prostate carcinoma obtained by deep sequencing. *Mol Cancer Res.* 2010;8:529-538.
50. Bagg A. Neoplastic hematopathology. In: Leonard DGB, ed. *Molecular Pathology in Clinical Practice.* New York, NY: Springer; 2006:321-383.
51. Zhang S, Pavlovitz B, Tull J, et al. Detection of *TMPRSS2* gene deletions and translocations in carcinoma, intraepithelial neoplasia and normal epithelium of the prostate by direct fluorescence *in situ* hybridization. *Diagn Mol Pathol.* 2010;19:151-156.

CHAPTER 9

IMMUNOHISTOCHEMISTRY

Jeannelyn S. Estrella

A number of antibodies have been developed for immunohistochemical analysis to complement and/or serve as surrogate markers for genetic alterations with diagnostic, prognostic, and predictive value because immunohistochemistry has several advantages. Immunohistochemistry is relatively fast and inexpensive, is widely available, and is routinely performed on archival formalin-fixed, paraffin-embedded tissue. Moreover, the staining pattern can be correlated with tumor morphology by light microscopy, overcoming frequent challenges such as inadequate material and non-tumoral contamination encountered in molecular analyses.

C-KIT/CD117

V-kit Hardy-Zuckerman 4 feline sarcoma viral oncogene homolog (KIT) encodes a type 3 transmembrane receptor[1] for mast/stem cell growth factor,[2] c-kit, a proto-oncogene which plays an important role in differentiation of hematopoietic progenitors,[3] mast cells,[4] primary melanocytes and germ cells,[5] and interstitial cells of Cajal.[6] Germ-line mutations lead to piebaldism, an autosomal dominant disease characterized by absence of pigment in patches of skin and hair on the forehead, ventral chest, and abdomen and extremities.[7] Somatic mutations lead to mastocytosis,[8,9] acute myeloid leukemia,[10] and seminomas/dysgerminomas.[11] Gastrointestinal stromal tumors (GISTs) arise from both germ-line and somatic mutations of the *KIT* gene.[12-14] Immunohistochemical staining for c-kit, using antibodies assigned to the 117 cluster designation antigen group (CD117), is widely used to detect *KIT* mutations, especially in the diagnosis of GISTs; however, not all CD117-positive tumors harbor *KIT* mutations.[15]

DNA MISMATCH REPAIR PROTEINS AND MICROSATELLITE INSTABILITY

Microsatellite instability (MSI) is the clonal change in the number of DNA nucleotide repeat sequences (microsatellites) in the genome[16] and is caused by mutational inactivation of genes involved in DNA repair, namely *MLH-1*, *PMS-2*, *MSH-2*, and *MSH-6*. The proteins encoded by these DNA mismatch repair genes function as heterodimers, MLH-1 associates with PMS-2 while MSH-2 associates with MSH-6.[17] Germ-line mutations in these genes lead to hereditary nonpolyposis colorectal cancer, also known as Lynch syndrome.[18-24] Biallelic methylation of the *MLH-1* promoter that inactivates the gene,[25] frequently accompanied by *BRAF* mutations,[26] is responsible for most of the sporadic colorectal carcinomas that harbor MSI.

The Bethesda guidelines[27,28] have standardized the detection of MSI by polymerase chain reaction (PCR) and have made this analysis a reliable and reproducible method of MSI testing. Immunohistochemistry for the four DNA mismatch repair proteins has similar specificity and sensitivity[29] and has the advantage of pinpointing the culprit gene. For example, tumors with (a) complete loss of PMS-2 with preserved nuclear expression of MLH-1, MSH-2, and MSH-6; (b) complete loss of MSH-2 and MSH-6 nuclear expression together with preserved nuclear expression of MLH-1 and PMS-2; and (c) complete loss of MSH-6 with preserved nuclear expression of MSH-2, MLH-1, and PMS-2 are most likely associated with Lynch syndrome and harbor germ-line mutations of the *PMS-2*, *MSH-2*, and *MSH-6* genes, respectively. Gene mutational analysis can, therefore, be targeted to the specific gene. In cases with both MLH-1 and PMS-2 complete loss of nuclear expression, *MLH-1* promoter methylation test with or without *BRAF* gene mutational analysis can be performed to exclude Lynch syndrome without resorting to MLH-1 gene mutational analysis.[29]

It has been well established that MSI status also has prognostic value in colorectal carcinoma, as patients with microsatellite instability-high (MSI-H) tumors have better prognosis than those with microsatellite stable tumors.[30] Its role as a predictive marker, however, is controversial. A recent meta-analysis showed that patients with MSI-H tumors do not benefit from fluorouracil-based adjuvant chemotherapy.[31] Other studies have reported increased survival in patients with MSI-H tumors when topoisomerase I inhibitor, irinotecan, was added to their chemotherapy regimen.[32,33] Prospective, randomized clinical trials are needed to elucidate the most appropriate treatment regimen for patients with MSI-H colorectal carcinoma.

EGFR

Epidermal growth factor receptor (EGFR) encodes a cell surface transmembrane glycoprotein that binds to epidermal growth factor,[34] which in turn induces receptor dimerization and tyrosine autophosphorylation[35] and leads to cell proliferation.[36,37] EGFR mutations[38,39] and amplification[40] have been associated with non–small cell lung carcinoma and have predictive value in this setting. It has been well established that patients with non–small cell lung carcinoma with EGFR gene alterations respond to EGFR tyrosine kinase inhibitors gefitinib[39,41-45] and erlotinib.[46-48] EGFR protein expression by immunohistochemistry is associated with gene amplification[40,49,50]; however, it does not correlate with *EGFR* mutations[51-53] nor does it correlate with responsiveness to gefitinib[54,55] and erlotinib.[48,56]

FLI-1

Friend leukemia virus integration 1 (FLI1) is a small locus in chromosome 11 (11q23-q24)[57] that is a common viral integration site in the mouse genome and a member of the *ets* family of proto-oncogenes involved in sequence-specific DNA binding leading to transcription activation.[58] *FLI1* is implicated in a variety of chromosomal translocations associated with peripheral neuroectodermal tumors (Ewing sarcoma and neuroepithelioma)[59] and viral-induced leukemias.[60] Overexpression of the FLI-1 protein, demonstrated by strong nuclear immunoreactivity, may be diagnostic for Ewing sarcoma/primitive neuroectodermal tumor when combined with characteristic morphology, CD99 immunopositivity, and absence of immunoreactivity for lymphoblastic, epithelial, and myogenic markers.[15] However, a wide variety of tumors also exhibit immunoreactivity for FLI-1, including lymphoblastic lymphoma, melanoma, synovial sarcoma, and some carcinomas and vascular tumors.[15]

HER-2/*NEU*

V-erb-b2 erythroblastic leukemia viral oncogene homolog 2 (ERBB2) is the official name provided by the HUGO Gene Nomenclature Committee for HER-2/*neu*, an oncogene that encodes a member of the EGFR family of receptor tyrosine kinases involved in kinase-mediated activation of downstream signaling pathways such as those involving mitogen-activated protein kinase (MAPK) and phosphatidylinositol 3-kinase (PI3K),[61,62] which regulate proliferation, migration, differentiation, and apoptosis.[63] HER-2/*neu* gene amplification is found in a wide variety of carcinomas and in glioblastomas. In carcinomas of the breast,[64,65] bladder,[66] colorectum,[67] endometrium,[68,69] ovary,[70] stomach,[71] prostate,[72] and salivary gland,[73] HER-2/*neu* gene amplification has been associated with poor prognosis. In breast carcinomas, wherein HER-2/*neu* has been studied the most, its status is also a predictive marker for several systemic therapies.[74]

HER-2/*neu* overexpression detected by immunohistochemistry has been shown to correlate with HER-2/*neu* gene amplification by fluorescence in situ hybridization (FISH), provided that certain guidelines are met. For breast carcinomas, positive staining is defined as homogenous, strong, circumferential membranous labeling (Fig. 9.1A) in greater than 30% of invasive tumor.[74] For gastroesophageal and gastric carcinomas, positive staining is defined as moderate to strong circumferential or basolateral membranous labeling (Fig. 9.1B) in greater than 10% of invasive tumor.[75]

IDH1

Isocitrate dehydrogenase 1 (NADPH), soluble (IDH1) encodes a protein found in the cytoplasm and peroxisomes, isocitrate dehydrogenase, which catalyzes the NADPH-dependent oxidative decarboxylation of isocitrate to 2-oxoglutarate.[76] The majority of *IDH1* mutations occur at codon 132 with a substitution of arginine to histidine (R132H).[77] The resultant mutant IDH1 catalyzes the NADPH-dependent reduction of alpha-ketoglutarate to *R*(–)-2-hydroxyglutarate (2HG).[77] In turn, 2HG has been shown to inhibit histone demethylation required for terminal differentiation of lineage-specific progenitor cells.[78] *IDH1* mutations have been identified in acute myeloid leukemia and myelodysplastic syndromes/myeloproliferative neoplasms,[79-82] chondrosarcoma,[83] glioma,[84,85] and cholangiocarcinoma.[86] In diffuse low-grade (WHO grade II) gliomas, *IDH1* mutation status identifies a distinct subgroup of tumors in that the *IDH1* wild-type tumors were located in the frontotemporoinsular region, exhibited an infiltrative pattern on magnetic resonance imaging, lacked p53 expression and 1p19q deletion, and had a dismal outcome.[85] Although DNA sequencing or PCR- and restriction endonuclease–based detection[87] of *IDH1* mutations is available, immunohistochemistry specifically targeting IDH protein containing the R132H mutation has been developed, with a sensitivity of 94% and a specificity of 100% (Fig. 9.2).[88]

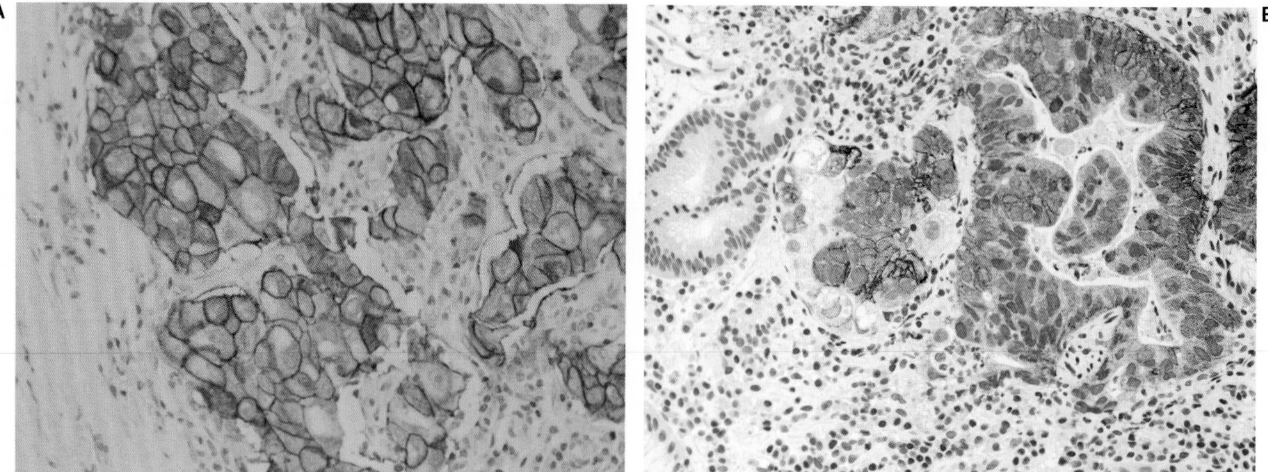

FIGURE 9–1 HER-2/*neu* immunohistochemistry. **A:** Homogenous, strong, circumferential membranous staining in breast carcinoma (×200). **B:** Moderate basolateral membranous labeling in gastric carcinoma (×200).

p53

Tumor protein p53 (TP53), described in 1979 as the first tumor suppressor gene identified, is involved in important cellular processes such as DNA damage response, apoptosis, and cell cycle regulation.[89] Somatic *TP53* gene alterations are found in a wide variety of malignancies while germline mutations are associated with Li-Fraumeni and Li-Fraumeni–like syndromes, leading to early-onset cancers. Missense mutations lead to protein accumulation owing to increased half-life and can be detected by immunohistochemistry; however, nonsense and frameshift mutations that lead to loss of protein expression cannot be detected by immunohistochemistry.[90] Inasmuch, p53 overexpression by immunohistochemistry only modestly correlates with *TP53* mutation status. However, strong and diffuse staining for p53 is used in practice to identify precursor lesions of serous carcinoma of the gynecologic tract, adenocarcinoma of gallbladder, squamous cell carcinoma of head and neck, and urothelial carcinoma of bladder.[15]

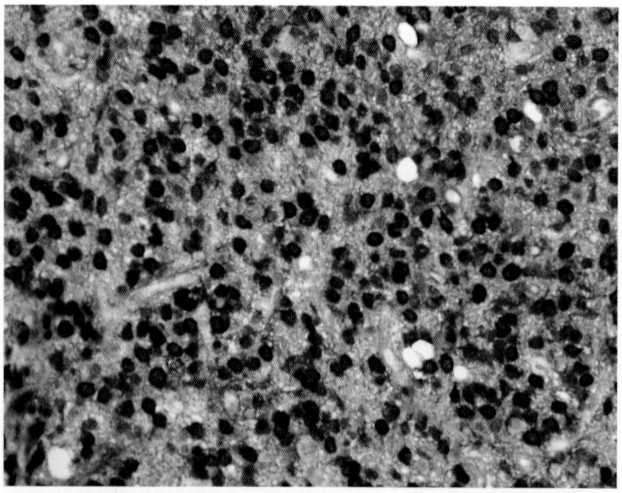

FIGURE 9–2 IDH1 immunohistochemistry. **A:** Diffuse glioma harboring *IDH1* mutation shows strong cytoplasmic staining in tumor cells in contrast to the absent staining in endothelial cells, perivascular lymphocytes, and residual glial cells. Courtesy of Dr. Gregory Fuller.

PTEN

Phosphatase and tensin homolog (PTEN) is a tumor suppressor gene located on chromosomal sub-band 10q23.3[91] and encodes a dual-specificity protein tyrosine phosphatase[92] that dephosphorylates phosphatidylinositol-3,4,5-trisphosphate (PIP3),[93] thus downregulating the PI3K/Akt pathway[94,95] and mediating cell cycle arrest and apoptosis.[96] Germ-line mutations in the *PTEN* gene was first described in Cowden syndrome, an autosomal dominant disease characterized by multiple hamartomas and carcinomas of the breast, thyroid, and uterus,[97,98] and also accounts for Bannayan-Riley-Ruvalcaba,[99] Proteus,[100,101] and Proteus-like[100,102] syndromes. Somatic aberrations in *PTEN* have been identified in brain, breast, colon (Fig. 9.3), kidney, prostate, skin, and uterine cancers.[91,92,103-105] Furthermore, loss of PTEN expression has been shown to have prognostic and predictive value. Loss of PTEN expression has been associated with poor outcome in breast,[106] endometrial,[103] and prostate[107] carcinomas. Loss of PTEN expression has also been shown to confer resistance to trastuzumab in breast cancer patients,[108] cetuximab in metastatic colorectal cancer patients,[109] and erlotinib in lung cancer patients.[110]

Immunohistochemical analysis has been shown to be a highly specific and sensitive surrogate test for *PTEN* mutations.[107,111] Moreover, immunohistochemistry identifies tumors with epigenetic alterations such as promoter hypermethylation, inactivating *PTEN* with resultant loss of protein expression. PTEN localizes to both cytoplasmic

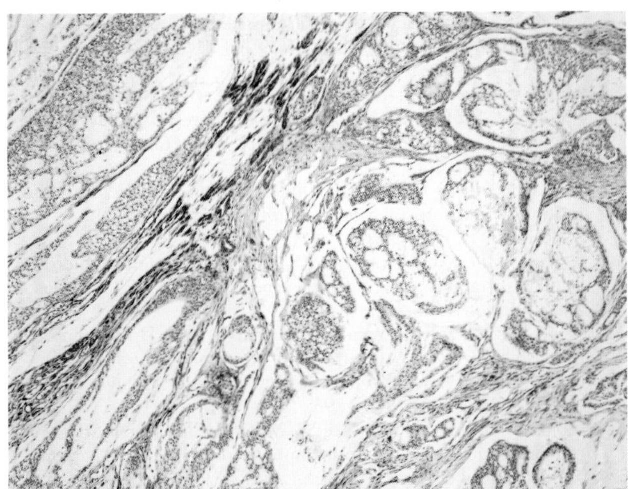

FIGURE 9–3 PTEN immunohistochemistry. Mucinous carcinoma of colon with loss of PTEN expression. There is retained nuclear and cytoplasmic expression in stromal cells which serve as internal control (×100).

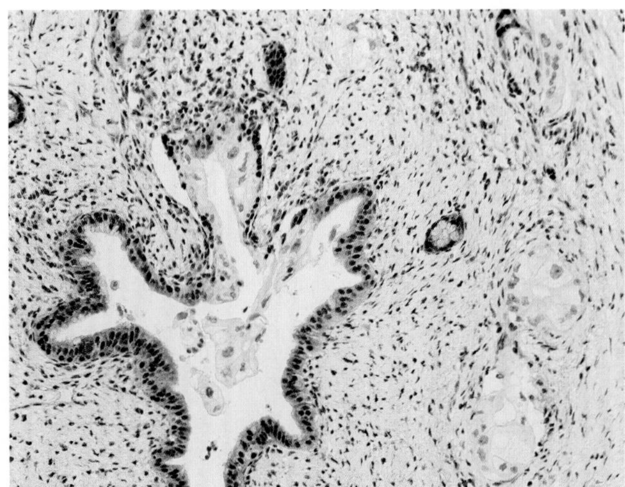

FIGURE 9–4 SMAD4 immunohistochemistry. Pancreatic ductal adenocarcinoma with loss of SMAD4 expression in tumor cells, including tumor cells colonizing a benign duct. There is retained nuclear and cytoplasmic expression in benign ducts and stromal cells (×100).

and nuclear compartments and is ubiquitously present in stromal cells such as vascular endothelial cells, which may serve as internal positive control. The literature, however, is plagued by a widely variable scoring system for loss of PTEN expression. In two validation studies for PTEN immunohistochemistry,[107,111] a binary scoring system with a 10% cutoff was employed. In addition, Lotan et al. considered markedly reduced staining, as compared with stromal cells, to be a negative result.[107]

SMAD4/DPC4

SMAD family member 4 (SMAD4, DPC4, MADH4) is a member of the Smad family of signal transduction proteins that regulate transcription of target genes involved in cell proliferation and differentiation, in response to transforming growth factor beta (TGF-β) signaling.[112] Germ-line mutations in the *SMAD4* gene are associated with juvenile polyposis syndrome, an autosomal dominant disease characterized by multiple hamartomatous polyps in the gastrointestinal (GI) tract and increased risk of GI tract malignancy.[113,114] Somatic inactivation of *SMAD4*, either by homozygous deletion (30%) or by inactivating mutation coupled with loss of heterozygosity (20%), occurs in pancreatic adenocarcinoma[115] and has been shown to confer worse prognosis.[116] Moreover, patients with extensive metastatic tumor burden, but not with locally advanced disease without metastasis, have tumors that are significantly more likely to demonstrate *SMAD4* gene inactivation.[117]

In both germ-line and somatic mutations of the *SMAD4* gene, protein expression by immunohistochemistry has been shown to mirror gene status, wherein inactivation of *SMAD4* results in loss of nuclear protein expression in the lesional tissue (Fig. 9.4).[118,119]

TFE3

Transcription factor binding to IGHM enhancer 3 (TFE3) is a member of the microphthalmia transcription factor/transcription factor E (MiTF-TFE) family of basic helix-loop-helix leucine zipper transcription factors,[120] which activates transcription of genes involved in TGF-β signaling pathway.[121,122] Chromosomal translocation of *TFE3* with various fusion partners has been described in alveolar soft part sarcoma,[123] a subset of renal cell carcinomas[124-127] and perivascular epithelioid cell neoplasms (PEComas).[128] These tumors that harbor the *TFE3* translocations show strong nuclear immunoreactivity with TFE3 antibody.[129]

In summary, immunohistochemistry is a useful tool in evaluating mutations, amplifications, chromosomal translocations, and epigenetic alterations of genes with diagnostic, prognostic, and predictive values. Immunohistochemistry overcomes problems frequently encountered in molecular analyses such as availability, cost, and use of formalin-fixed, paraffin-embedded archival material. Certain limitations, however, are innately tied to immunohistochemical analysis, the most important being nonspecific reactivity.

REFERENCES

1. Yarden Y, Kuang WJ, Yang-Feng T, et al. Human proto-oncogene c-kit: a new cell surface receptor tyrosine kinase for an unidentified ligand. *EMBO J.* 1987;6(11):3341-3351.
2. Williams DE, Eisenman J, Baird A, et al. Identification of a ligand for the c-kit proto-oncogene. *Cell.* 1990;63(1):167-174.
3. André C, d'Auriol L, Lacombe C, et al. c-kit mRNA expression in human and murine hematopoietic cell lines. *Oncogene.* 1989;4(8):1047-1049.
4. Nocka K, Majumder S, Chabot B, et al. Expression of c-kit gene products in known cellular targets of W mutations in normal and W mutant mice—evidence for an impaired c-kit kinase in mutant mice. *Genes Dev.* 1989;3(6):816-826.

5. Geissler EN, Ryan MA, Housman DE. The dominant-white spotting (W) locus of the mouse encodes the c-kit proto-oncogene. *Cell.* 1988;55(1):185-192.
6. Huizinga JD, Thuneberg L, Klüppel M, et al. W/kit gene required for interstitial cells of Cajal and for intestinal pacemaker activity. *Nature.* 1995;373(6512):347-349.
7. Giebel LB, Spritz RA. Mutation of the KIT (mast/stem cell growth factor receptor) protooncogene in human piebaldism. *Proc Natl Acad Sci U S A.* 1991;88(19):8696-8699.
8. Longley BJ, Tyrrell L, Lu SZ, et al. Somatic c-KIT activating mutation in urticaria pigmentosa and aggressive mastocytosis: establishment of clonality in a human mast cell neoplasm. *Nat Genet.* 1996;12(3):312-314.
9. Longley BJ Jr, Metcalfe DD, Tharp M, et al. Activating and dominant inactivating c-KIT catalytic domain mutations in distinct clinical forms of human mastocytosis. *Proc Natl Acad Sci U S A.* 1999;96(4):1609-1614.
10. Wang C, Curtis JE, Geissler EN, et al. The expression of the proto-oncogene C-kit in the blast cells of acute myeloblastic leukemia. *Leukemia.* 1989;3(10):699-702.
11. Tian Q, Frierson HF Jr, Krystal GW, et al. Activating c-kit gene mutations in human germ cell tumors. *Am J Pathol.* 1999;154(6):1643-1647.
12. Hirota S, Isozaki K, Moriyama Y, et al. Gain-of-function mutations of c-kit in human gastrointestinal stromal tumors. *Science.* 1998;279(5350):577-580.
13. Nishida T, Hirota S, Taniguchi M, et al. Familial gastrointestinal stromal tumours with germline mutation of the KIT gene. *Nat Genet.* 1998;19(4):323-324.
14. Andersson J, Sjögren H, Meis-Kindblom JM, et al. The complexity of KIT gene mutations and chromosome rearrangements and their clinical correlation in gastrointestinal stromal (pacemaker cell) tumors. *Am J Pathol.* 2002;160(1):15-22.
15. Dabbs DJ. *Diagnostic Immunohistochemistry: Theranostic and Genomic Applications.* 3rd ed. Philadelphia, PA: Saunders/Elsevier; 2010:xviii, 941p.
16. Thibodeau SN, Bren G, Schaid D. Microsatellite instability in cancer of the proximal colon. *Science.* 1993;260(5109):816-819.
17. Boland CR, Koi M, Chang DK, et al. The biochemical basis of microsatellite instability and abnormal immunohistochemistry and clinical behavior in Lynch syndrome: from bench to bedside. *Fam Cancer.* 2008;7(1):41-52.
18. Bronner CE, Baker SM, Morrison PT, et al. Mutation in the DNA mismatch repair gene homologue hMLH1 is associated with hereditary non-polyposis colon cancer. *Nature.* 1994;368(6468):258-261.
19. Fishel R, Lescoe MK, Rao MR, et al. The human mutator gene homolog MSH2 and its association with hereditary nonpolyposis colon cancer. *Cell.* 1993;75(5):1027-1038.
20. Leach FS, Nicolaides NC, Papadopoulos N, et al. Mutations of a mutS homolog in hereditary nonpolyposis colorectal cancer. *Cell.* 1993;75(6):1215-1225.
21. Lindblom A, Tannergård P, Werelius B, et al. Genetic mapping of a second locus predisposing to hereditary non-polyposis colon cancer. *Nat Genet.* 1993;5(3):279-282.
22. Nicolaides NC, Papadopoulos N, Liu B, et al. Mutations of two PMS homologues in hereditary nonpolyposis colon cancer. *Nature.* 1994;371(6492):75-80.
23. Papadopoulos N, Nicolaides NC, Wei YF, et al. Mutation of a mutL homolog in hereditary colon cancer. *Science.* 1994;263(5153):1625-1629.
24. Peltomäki P, Lothe RA, Aaltonen LA, et al. Microsatellite instability is associated with tumors that characterize the hereditary non-polyposis colorectal carcinoma syndrome. *Cancer Res.* 1993;53(24):5853-5855.
25. Kane MF, Loda M, Gaida GM, et al. Methylation of the hMLH1 promoter correlates with lack of expression of hMLH1 in sporadic colon tumors and mismatch repair-defective human tumor cell lines. *Cancer Res.* 1997;57(5):808-811.
26. Deng G, Bell I, Crawley S, et al. BRAF mutation is frequently present in sporadic colorectal cancer with methylated hMLH1, but not in hereditary nonpolyposis colorectal cancer. *Clin Cancer Res.* 2004;10(1 pt 1):191-195.
27. Boland CR, Thibodeau SN, Hamilton SR, et al. A National Cancer Institute Workshop on Microsatellite Instability for cancer detection and familial predisposition: development of international criteria for the determination of microsatellite instability in colorectal cancer. *Cancer Res.* 1998;58(22):5248-5257.
28. Umar A, Boland CR, Terdiman JP, et al. Revised Bethesda Guidelines for hereditary nonpolyposis colorectal cancer (Lynch syndrome) and microsatellite instability. *J Natl Cancer Inst.* 2004;96(4):261-268.
29. de la Chapelle A, Hampel H. Clinical relevance of microsatellite instability in colorectal cancer. *J Clin Oncol.* 2010;28(20):3380-3387.
30. Popat S, Hubner R, Houlston RS. Systematic review of microsatellite instability and colorectal cancer prognosis. *J Clin Oncol.* 2005;23(3):609-618.
31. Des Guetz G, Schischmanoff O, Nicolas P, et al. Does microsatellite instability predict the efficacy of adjuvant chemotherapy in colorectal cancer? A systematic review with meta-analysis. *Eur J Cancer.* 2009;45(10):1890-1896.
32. Fallik D, Borrini F, Boige V, et al. Microsatellite instability is a predictive factor of the tumor response to irinotecan in patients with advanced colorectal cancer. *Cancer Res.* 2003;63(18):5738-5744.
33. Bertagnolli MM, Niedzwiecki D, Compton CC, et al. Microsatellite instability predicts improved response to adjuvant therapy with irinotecan, fluorouracil, and leucovorin in stage III colon cancer: Cancer and Leukemia Group B Protocol 89803. *J Clin Oncol.* 2009;27(11):1814-1821.
34. Chen WS, Lazar CS, Lund KA, et al. Functional independence of the epidermal growth factor receptor from a domain required for ligand-induced internalization and calcium regulation. *Cell.* 1989;59(1):33-43.
35. Van Patten SM, Heisermann GJ, Cheng HC, et al. Tyrosine kinase catalyzed phosphorylation and inactivation of the inhibitor protein of the cAMP-dependent protein kinase. *J Biol Chem.* 1987;262(7):3398-3403.
36. Wang SC, Nakajima Y, Yu YL, et al. Tyrosine phosphorylation controls PCNA function through protein stability. *Nat Cell Biol.* 2006;8(12):1359-1368.
37. Andl CD, Mizushima T, Nakagawa H, et al. Epidermal growth factor receptor mediates increased cell proliferation, migration, and aggregation in esophageal keratinocytes in vitro and in vivo. *J Biol Chem.* 2003;278(3):1824-1830.
38. Kosaka T, Yatabe Y, Endoh H, et al. Mutations of the epidermal growth factor receptor gene in lung cancer: biological and clinical implications. *Cancer Res.* 2004;64(24):8919-8923.
39. Marchetti A, Martella C, Felicioni L, et al. EGFR mutations in non-small-cell lung cancer: analysis of a large series of cases and development of a rapid and sensitive method for diagnostic screening with potential implications on pharmacologic treatment. *J Clin Oncol.* 2005;23(4):857-865.
40. Hirsch FR, Varella-Garcia M, Bunn PA Jr, et al. Epidermal growth factor receptor in non-small-cell lung carcinomas: correlation between gene copy number and protein expression and impact on prognosis. *J Clin Oncol.* 2003;21(20):3798-3807.
41. Lynch TJ, Bell DW, Sordella R, et al. Activating mutations in the epidermal growth factor receptor underlying responsiveness of non-small-cell lung cancer to gefitinib. *N Engl J Med.* 2004;350(21):2129-2139.
42. Paez JG, Jänne PA, Lee JC, et al. EGFR mutations in lung cancer: correlation with clinical response to gefitinib therapy. *Science.* 2004;304(5676):1497-1500.
43. Mitsudomi T, Kosaka T, Endoh H, et al. Mutations of the epidermal growth factor receptor gene predict prolonged survival after gefitinib treatment in patients with non-small-cell lung cancer with postoperative recurrence. *J Clin Oncol.* 2005;23(11):2513-2520.
44. Han SW, Kim TY, Hwang PG, et al. Predictive and prognostic impact of epidermal growth factor receptor mutation in non-small-cell lung cancer patients treated with gefitinib. *J Clin Oncol.* 2005;23(11):2493-2501.
45. Bell DW, Lynch TJ, Haserlat SM, et al. Epidermal growth factor receptor mutations and gene amplification in non-small-cell lung cancer: molecular analysis of the IDEAL/INTACT gefitinib trials. *J Clin Oncol.* 2005;23(31):8081-8092.
46. Perez-Soler R. Phase II clinical trial data with the epidermal growth factor receptor tyrosine kinase inhibitor erlotinib (OSI-774) in non-small-cell lung cancer. *Clin Lung Cancer.* 2004;6 (suppl 1):S20-S23.

47. Miller VA, Riely GJ, Zakowski MF, et al. Molecular characteristics of bronchioloalveolar carcinoma and adenocarcinoma, bronchioloalveolar carcinoma subtype, predict response to erlotinib. *J Clin Oncol*. 2008;26(9):1472-1478.
48. Tsao MS, Sakurada A, Cutz JC, et al. Erlotinib in lung cancer—molecular and clinical predictors of outcome. *N Engl J Med*. 2005;353(2):133-144.
49. Jeon YK, Sung SW, Chung JH, et al. Clinicopathologic features and prognostic implications of epidermal growth factor receptor (EGFR) gene copy number and protein expression in non-small cell lung cancer. *Lung Cancer*. 2006;54(3):387-398.
50. Dacic S, Flanagan M, Cieply K, et al. Significance of EGFR protein expression and gene amplification in non-small cell lung carcinoma. *Am J Clin Pathol*. 2006;125(6):860-865.
51. Suzuki S, Dobashi Y, Sakurai H, et al. Protein overexpression and gene amplification of epidermal growth factor receptor in nonsmall cell lung carcinomas. An immunohistochemical and fluorescence in situ hybridization study. *Cancer*. 2005;103(6):1265-1273.
52. Li AR, Chitale D, Riely GJ, et al. EGFR mutations in lung adenocarcinomas: clinical testing experience and relationship to EGFR gene copy number and immunohistochemical expression. *J Mol Diagn*. 2008;10(3):242-248.
53. Pinter F, Papay J, Almasi A, et al. Epidermal growth factor receptor (EGFR) high gene copy number and activating mutations in lung adenocarcinomas are not consistently accompanied by positivity for EGFR protein by standard immunohistochemistry. *J Mol Diagn*. 2008;10(2):160-168.
54. Cappuzzo F, Hirsch FR, Rossi E, et al. Epidermal growth factor receptor gene and protein and gefitinib sensitivity in non-small-cell lung cancer. *J Natl Cancer Inst*. 2005;97(9):643-655.
55. Parra HS, Cavina R, Latteri F, et al. Analysis of epidermal growth factor receptor expression as a predictive factor for response to gefitinib ("Iressa", ZD1839) in non-small-cell lung cancer. *Br J Cancer*. 2004;91(2):208-212.
56. Brugger W, Triller N, Blasinska-Morawiec M, et al. Prospective molecular marker analyses of EGFR and KRAS from a randomized, placebo-controlled study of erlotinib maintenance therapy in advanced non-small-cell lung cancer. *J Clin Oncol*. 2011;29(31):4113-4120.
57. Baud V, Lipinski M, Rassart E, et al. The human homolog of the mouse common viral integration region, FLI1, maps to 11q23-q24. *Genomics*. 1991;11(1):223-224.
58. Ben-David Y, Giddens EB, Letwin K, et al. Erythroleukemia induction by Friend murine leukemia virus: insertional activation of a new member of the ets gene family, Fli-1, closely linked to c-ets-1. *Genes Dev*. 1991;5(6):908-918.
59. Bonin G, Scamps C, Turc-Carel C, et al. Chimeric EWS-FLI1 transcript in a Ewing cell line with a complex t(11;22;14) translocation. *Cancer Res*. 1993;53(16):3655-3657.
60. Truong AH, Ben-David Y. The role of Fli-1 in normal cell function and malignant transformation. *Oncogene*. 2000;19(55): 6482-6489.
61. Wallasch C, Weiss FU, Niederfellner G, et al. Heregulin-dependent regulation of HER2/neu oncogenic signaling by heterodimerization with HER3. *EMBO J*. 1995;14(17):4267-4275.
62. Le XF, Lammayot A, Gold D, et al. Genes affecting the cell cycle, growth, maintenance, and drug sensitivity are preferentially regulated by anti-HER2 antibody through phosphatidylinositol 3-kinase-AKT signaling. *J Biol Chem*. 2005;280(3):2092-2104.
63. Citri A, Yarden Y. EGF-ERBB signalling: towards the systems level. *Nat Rev Mol Cell Biol*. 2006;7(7):505-516.
64. Borg A, Tandon AK, Sigurdsson H, et al. HER-2/neu amplification predicts poor survival in node-positive breast cancer. *Cancer Res*. 1990;50(14):4332-4337.
65. Tandon AK, Clark GM, Chamness GC, et al. HER-2/neu oncogene protein and prognosis in breast cancer. *J Clin Oncol*. 1989;7(8):1120-1128.
66. Fleischmann A, Rotzer D, Seiler R, et al. Her2 amplification is significantly more frequent in lymph node metastases from urothelial bladder cancer than in the primary tumours. *Eur Urol*. 2011;60(2):350-357.
67. Park DI, Kang MS, Oh SJ, et al. HER-2/neu overexpression is an independent prognostic factor in colorectal cancer. *Int J Colorectal Dis*. 2007;22(5):491-497.
68. Santin AD, Bellone S, Van Stedum S, et al. Amplification of c-erbB2 oncogene: a major prognostic indicator in uterine serous papillary carcinoma. *Cancer*. 2005;104(7):1391-1397.
69. Hetzel DJ, Wilson TO, Keeney GL, et al. HER-2/neu expression: a major prognostic factor in endometrial cancer. *Gynecol Oncol*. 1992;47(2):179-185.
70. Slamon DJ, Godolphin W, Jones LA, et al. Studies of the HER-2/neu proto-oncogene in human breast and ovarian cancer. *Science*. 1989;244(4905):707-712.
71. Begnami MD, Fukuda E, Fregnani JH, et al. Prognostic implications of altered human epidermal growth factor receptors (HERs) in gastric carcinomas: HER2 and HER3 are predictors of poor outcome. *J Clin Oncol*. 2011;29(22):3030-3036.
72. Neto AS, Tobias-Machado M, Wroclawski ML, et al. Her-2/neu expression in prostate adenocarcinoma: a systematic review and meta-analysis. *J Urol*. 2010;184(3):842-850.
73. Press MF, Pike MC, Hung G, et al. Amplification and overexpression of HER-2/neu in carcinomas of the salivary gland: correlation with poor prognosis. *Cancer Res*. 1994;54(21):5675-5682.
74. Wolff AC, Hammond ME, Schwartz JN, et al. American Society of Clinical Oncology/College of American Pathologists guideline recommendations for human epidermal growth factor receptor 2 testing in breast cancer. *J Clin Oncol*. 2007;25(1):118-145.
75. Hofmann M, Stoss O, Shi D, et al. Assessment of a HER2 scoring system for gastric cancer: results from a validation study. *Histopathology*. 2008;52(7):797-805.
76. Geisbrecht, BV, Gould SJ. The human PICD gene encodes a cytoplasmic and peroxisomal NADP(+)-dependent isocitrate dehydrogenase. *J Biol Chem*. 1999;274(43):30527-30533.
77. Dang L, White DW, Gross S, et al. Cancer-associated IDH1 mutations produce 2-hydroxyglutarate. *Nature*. 2009;462(7274): 739-744.
78. Lu C, Ward PS, Kapoor GS, et al. IDH mutation impairs histone demethylation and results in a block to cell differentiation. *Nature*. 2012;483(7390):474-478.
79. Abbas S, Lugthart S, Kavelaars FG, et al. Acquired mutations in the genes encoding IDH1 and IDH2 both are recurrent aberrations in acute myeloid leukemia: prevalence and prognostic value. *Blood*. 2010;116(12):2122-2126.
80. Ho PA, Alonzo TA, Kopecky KJ, et al. Molecular alterations of the IDH1 gene in AML: a Children's Oncology Group and Southwest Oncology Group study. *Leukemia*. 2010;24(5):909-913.
81. Green A, Beer P. Somatic mutations of IDH1 and IDH2 in the leukemic transformation of myeloproliferative neoplasms. *N Engl J Med*. 2010;362(4):369-370.
82. Abdel-Wahab O, Manshouri T, Patel J, et al. Genetic analysis of transforming events that convert chronic myeloproliferative neoplasms to leukemias. *Cancer Res*. 2010;70(2):447-452.
83. Amary MF, Bacsi K, Maggiani F, et al. IDH1 and IDH2 mutations are frequent events in central chondrosarcoma and central and periosteal chondromas but not in other mesenchymal tumours. *J Pathol*. 2011;224(3):334-343.
84. Yan H, Parsons DW, Jin G, et al. IDH1 and IDH2 mutations in gliomas. *N Engl J Med*. 2009;360(8):765-773.
85. Metellus P, Coulibaly B, Colin C, et al. Absence of IDH mutation identifies a novel radiologic and molecular subtype of WHO grade II gliomas with dismal prognosis. *Acta Neuropathol*. 2010;120(6):719-729.
86. Borger DR, Tanabe KK, Fan KC, et al. Frequent mutation of isocitrate dehydrogenase (IDH)1 and IDH2 in cholangiocarcinoma identified through broad-based tumor genotyping. *Oncologist*. 2012;17(1):72-79.
87. Meyer J, Pusch S, Balss J, et al. PCR- and restriction endonuclease-based detection of IDH1 mutations. *Brain Pathol*. 2010;20(2):298-300.
88. Capper D, Weissert S, Balss J, et al. Characterization of R132H mutation-specific IDH1 antibody binding in brain tumors. *Brain Pathol*. 2010;20(1):245-254.
89. Vogelstein B, Lane D, Levine AJ. Surfing the p53 network. *Nature*. 2000;408(6810):307-310.
90. Greenblatt MS, Bennett WP, Hollstein M, et al. Mutations in the p53 tumor suppressor gene: clues to cancer etiology and molecular pathogenesis. *Cancer Res*. 1994;54(18):4855-4878.
91. Steck PA, Pershouse MA, Jasser SA, et al. Identification of a candidate tumour suppressor gene, MMAC1, at chromosome 10q23.3 that is mutated in multiple advanced cancers. *Nat Genet*. 1997;15(4):356-362.
92. Li J, Yen C, Liaw D, et al. PTEN, a putative protein tyrosine phosphatase gene mutated in human brain, breast, and prostate cancer. *Science*. 1997;275(5308):1943-1947.

93. Maehama T, Dixon JE. The tumor suppressor, PTEN/MMAC1, dephosphorylates the lipid second messenger, phosphatidylinositol 3,4,5-trisphosphate. *J Biol Chem*. 1998;273(22):13375-13378.
94. Li J, Simpson L, Takahashi M, et al. The PTEN/MMAC1 tumor suppressor induces cell death that is rescued by the AKT/protein kinase B oncogene. *Cancer Res*. 1998;58(24): 5667-5672.
95. Stambolic V, Suzuki A, de la Pompa JL, et al. Negative regulation of PKB/Akt-dependent cell survival by the tumor suppressor PTEN. *Cell*. 1998;95(1):29-39.
96. Myers MP, Pass I, Batty IH, et al. The lipid phosphatase activity of PTEN is critical for its tumor suppressor function. *Proc Natl Acad Sci U S A*. 1998;95(23):13513-13518.
97. Eng C. Will the real Cowden syndrome please stand up: revised diagnostic criteria. *J Med Genet*. 2000;37(11):828-830.
98. Liaw D, Marsh DJ, Li J, et al. Germline mutations of the PTEN gene in Cowden disease, an inherited breast and thyroid cancer syndrome. *Nat Genet*. 1997;16(1):64-67.
99. Marsh DJ, Dahia PL, Zheng Z, et al. Germline mutations in PTEN are present in Bannayan-Zonana syndrome. *Nat Genet*. 1997;16(4):333-334.
100. Zhou X, Hampel H, Thiele H, et al. Association of germline mutation in the PTEN tumour suppressor gene and Proteus and Proteus-like syndromes. *Lancet*. 2001;358(9277): 210-211.
101. Levine RA, Forest T, Smith C. Tumor suppressor PTEN is mutated in canine osteosarcoma cell lines and tumors. *Vet Pathol*. 2002;39(3):372-378.
102. Zhou XP, Marsh DJ, Hampel H, et al. Germline and germline mosaic PTEN mutations associated with a Proteus-like syndrome of hemihypertrophy, lower limb asymmetry, arteriovenous malformations and lipomatosis. *Hum Mol Genet*. 2000;9(5):765-768.
103. Salvesen HB, Stefansson I, Kalvenes MB, et al. Loss of PTEN expression is associated with metastatic disease in patients with endometrial carcinoma. *Cancer*. 2002;94(8):2185-2191.
104. Zhou XP, Loukola A, Salovaara R, et al. PTEN mutational spectra, expression levels, and subcellular localization in microsatellite stable and unstable colorectal cancers. *Am J Pathol*. 2002;161(2):439-447.
105. Birck A, Ahrenkiel V, Zeuthen J, et al. Mutation and allelic loss of the PTEN/MMAC1 gene in primary and metastatic melanoma biopsies. *J Invest Dermatol*. 2000;114(2):277-280.
106. Depowski PL, Rosenthal SI, Ross JS. Loss of expression of the PTEN gene protein product is associated with poor outcome in breast cancer. *Mod Pathol*. 2001;14(7):672-676.
107. Lotan TL, Gurel B, Sutcliffe S, et al. PTEN protein loss by immunostaining: analytic validation and prognostic indicator for a high risk surgical cohort of prostate cancer patients. *Clin Cancer Res*. 2011;17(20):6563-6573.
108. Nagata Y, Lan KH, Zhou X, et al. PTEN activation contributes to tumor inhibition by trastuzumab, and loss of PTEN predicts trastuzumab resistance in patients. *Cancer Cell*. 2004;6(2):117-127.
109. Frattini M, Saletti P, Romagnani E, et al. PTEN loss of expression predicts cetuximab efficacy in metastatic colorectal cancer patients. *Br J Cancer*. 2007;97(8):1139-1145.
110. Sos ML, Koker M, Weir BA, et al. PTEN loss contributes to erlotinib resistance in EGFR-mutant lung cancer by activation of Akt and EGFR. *Cancer Res*. 2009;69(8):3256-3261.
111. Sangale Z, Prass C, Carlson A, et al. A robust immunohistochemical assay for detecting PTEN expression in human tumors. *Appl Immunohistochem Mol Morphol*. 2011;19(2):173-183.
112. Liu F, Pouponnot C, Massague J. Dual role of the Smad4/DPC4 tumor suppressor in TGFbeta-inducible transcriptional complexes. *Genes Dev*. 1997;11(23):3157-3167.
113. Howe JR, Mitros FA, Summers RW. The risk of gastrointestinal carcinoma in familial juvenile polyposis. *Ann Surg Oncol*. 1998;5(8):751-756.
114. Howe JR, Roth S, Ringold JC, et al. Mutations in the SMAD4/DPC4 gene in juvenile polyposis. *Science*. 1998;280(5366): 1086-1088.
115. Hahn SA, Schutte M, Hoque AT, et al. DPC4, a candidate tumor suppressor gene at human chromosome 18q21.1. *Science*. 1996;271(5247):350-353.
116. Blackford A, Serrano OK, Wolfgang CL, et al. SMAD4 gene mutations are associated with poor prognosis in pancreatic cancer. *Clin Cancer Res*. 2009;15(14):4674-4679.
117. Iacobuzio-Donahue CA, Fu B, Yachida S, et al. DPC4 gene status of the primary carcinoma correlates with patterns of failure in patients with pancreatic cancer. *J Clin Oncol*. 2009;27(11):1806-1813.
118. Langeveld D, van Hattem WA, de Leng WW, et al. SMAD4 immunohistochemistry reflects genetic status in juvenile polyposis syndrome. *Clin Cancer Res*. 2010;16(16):4126-4134.
119. Wilentz RE, Su GH, Dai JL, et al. Immunohistochemical labeling for dpc4 mirrors genetic status in pancreatic adenocarcinomas: a new marker of DPC4 inactivation. *Am J Pathol*. 2000;156(1):37-43.
120. Beckmann H, Su LK, Kadesch T. TFE3: a helix-loop-helix protein that activates transcription through the immunoglobulin enhancer muE3 motif. *Genes Dev*. 1990;4(2):167-179.
121. Hua X, Liu X, Ansari DO, et al. Synergistic cooperation of TFE3 and smad proteins in TGF-beta-induced transcription of the plasminogen activator inhibitor-1 gene. *Genes Dev*. 1998;12(19):3084-3095.
122. Hua X, Miller ZA, Benchabane H, et al. Synergism between transcription factors TFE3 and Smad3 in transforming growth factor-beta-induced transcription of the Smad7 gene. *J Biol Chem*. 2000;275(43):33205-33208.
123. Ladanyi M, Lui MY, Antonescu CR, et al. The der(17)t(X;17)(p11;q25) of human alveolar soft part sarcoma fuses the TFE3 transcription factor gene to ASPL, a novel gene at 17q25. *Oncogene*. 2001;20(1):48-57.
124. Sidhar SK, Clark J, Gill S, et al. The t(X;1)(p11.2;q21.2) translocation in papillary renal cell carcinoma fuses a novel gene PRCC to the TFE3 transcription factor gene. *Hum Mol Genet*. 1996;5(9):1333-1338.
125. Weterman MA, Wilbrink M, Geurts van Kessel A. Fusion of the transcription factor TFE3 gene to a novel gene, PRCC, in t(X;1)(p11;q21)-positive papillary renal cell carcinomas. *Proc Natl Acad Sci U S A*. 1996;93(26):15294-15298.
126. Heimann P, El Housni H, Ogur G, et al. Fusion of a novel gene, RCC17, to the TFE3 gene in t(X;17)(p11.2;q25.3)-bearing papillary renal cell carcinomas. *Cancer Res*. 2001;61(10):4130-4135.
127. Argani P, Antonescu CR, Illei PB, et al. Primary renal neoplasms with the ASPL-TFE3 gene fusion of alveolar soft part sarcoma: a distinctive tumor entity previously included among renal cell carcinomas of children and adolescents. *Am J Pathol*. 2001;159(1):179-192.
128. Argani P, Aulmann S, Illei PB, et al. A distinctive subset of PEComas harbors TFE3 gene fusions. *Am J Surg Pathol*. 2010;34(10):1395-1406.
129. Argani P, Lal P, Hutchinson B, et al. Aberrant nuclear immunoreactivity for TFE3 in neoplasms with TFE3 gene fusions: a sensitive and specific immunohistochemical assay. *Am J Surg Pathol*. 2003;27(6):750-761.

CHAPTER 10

CANCER GENOMIC SEQUENCING

Yingfei Wei and Guo-Liang Yu

INTRODUCTION

Cancer is often associated with genetic abnormalities, either in inherited forms or caused by somatic mutations. DNA, which is the genetic material that ultimately encodes proteins, consists of four nucleotide bases: adenine (A), guanine (G), cytosine (C), and thymine (T). The order of the nucleotide bases in a DNA molecule is known as the DNA "sequence." This sequence, in turn, determines the sequence of amino acids, which are the building blocks of proteins. The methods and technologies that are used to determine the order of nucleotides are commonly referred to as DNA sequencing.

The first DNA sequences were obtained in the early 1970s using laborious methods based on two-dimensional gel electrophoresis. Following the development of dye-based sequencing methods with automated analysis, the DNA sequencing process became simpler and orders of magnitude faster. The high speed of sequencing attained with modern DNA sequencing technology has been instrumental in the sequencing of the human genome.

Knowledge of DNA sequences has become indispensable for basic biological research and is increasingly important in numerous applied fields, such as molecular diagnostics, drug discovery, forensic biology, and environmental sciences. Sequencing of the DNA of cancers has been making a profound impact on the understanding, diagnosis, and treatment of these malignancies.

DNA SEQUENCING TECHNOLOGIES

First Generation

The initial DNA sequencing technologies were developed in academic laboratories in the 1970s. Allan Maxam and Walter Gilbert developed a method based on chemical modification and subsequent cleavage of DNA at specific nucleotide bases.[1] Although this method has the advantage of using purified DNA directly, it is no longer used today due to its technical complexity, extensive use of hazardous chemicals, and difficulty in scaling up.[2]

The chain-termination method developed by Sanger and coworkers about the same time soon became the method of choice for its reliability and scalability.[3,4] Most of the modern technologies used in sequencing the human genome are based on this method. It requires a single-stranded DNA template, a DNA polymerase, a DNA primer, the normal deoxynucleotide triphosphates (dNTPs), and dideoxyNTPs (ddNTPs) that terminate DNA strand elongation.

In the traditional Sanger method, the DNA samples are divided into four biochemical reactions, each containing all four of the standard dNTPs (dATP, dGTP, dCTP, and dTTP), DNA primer, and DNA polymerase. To each reaction is added only one of the four chain-terminating nucleotides (ddATP, ddGTP, ddCTP, or ddTTP). The ddNTPs lack the 3′-OH group required for the formation of a phosphodiester bond between two nucleotides, thus terminating the DNA strand and creating DNA fragments of various lengths. One of the components (primer, dNTP, or ddNTP) is radioactively or fluorescently labeled. The newly synthesized and labeled DNA fragments from each reaction are thermally or chemically denatured and then separated by electrophoresis with a resolution of just one nucleotide. The DNA bands are visualized by autoradiography X-ray film or gel image. Finally, the DNA sequence is determined by counting the bands on lanes corresponding to each ddNTP. Figure 10.1 illustrates the Sanger DNA sequencing process.

Using four differently colored fluorescent dyes to label the ddNTPs allows all four biochemical reactions to take place simultaneously, thereby increasing the

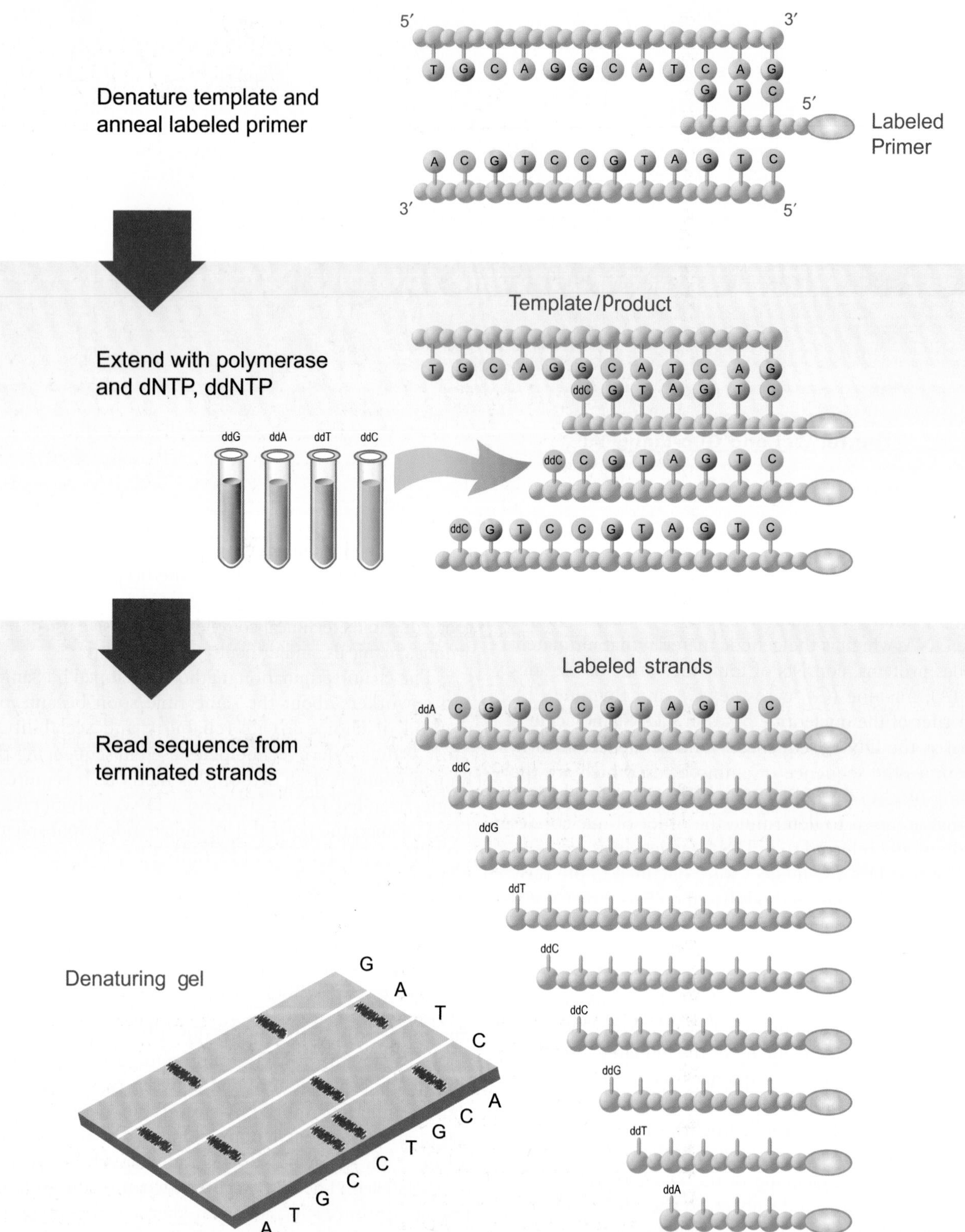

FIGURE 10–1 Sanger DNA sequencing. The traditional Sanger sequencing involves denaturing of the DNA template, annealing labeled primer, and extending the newly synthesized DNA with DNA polymerase and dNTPs. The synthesis is terminated with ddNTPs in each corresponding reaction. The resulting DNA fragments are separated by gel electrophoresis with a resolution of one nucleotide.

efficiency of this method by fourfold. Thus, only one sequencing reaction is needed for each DNA sequence, allowing faster and more economical data analysis.[5,6] Modern high-throughput automated DNA sequencing technology is based on this technique.

Based on these advances in technology, the first generation of automated DNA sequencers was developed and marketed by Applied Biosystems, Inc. The machines were used primarily for the first sequencing of the human genome. These automated DNA sequencers can sequence up to 384 DNA samples in a single run and operate up to 24 runs a day. With these first-generation machines, overlapping sequences of small DNA fragments (typically less than 500 bases) are generated. The overlapping sequences are then assembled by computers to reveal the entire genome sequence.

A common approach to generating fragments consists of cleaving the genomic DNA with restriction enzymes or shearing large DNA fragments into smaller ones. The fragmented DNA is cloned into a plasmid vector and amplified in *Escherichia coli* bacteria. The number of clones must be large enough to cover all DNA fragments multiple times to ensure that the overlapping sequence can be obtained to cover the whole genome, chromosome (an organized structure of DNA and proteins), or targeted sequencing region. Plasmids containing small DNA fragments purified from individual bacterial colonies are subjected to sequencing reactions using fluorescent dye–labeled chemicals. DNA sequencers use capillary electrophoresis to separate the fragments by size and an optical image system to detect and record the fluorescent dyes. The results are displayed as fluorescent peak trace chromatograms that are typically 200 to 400 bases long. The data are processed through an automated data analyzer and sequence assembly.[7,8]

A common challenge of DNA sequencing on first-generation machines is the poor quality of the first 20 to 40 bases of the sequence. In addition, the quality of sequencing traces deteriorates after 500 to 700 bases. Software has been developed to help with base culling and trimming, but manual curation of sequences is still unavoidable with these machines.

Second Generation

Sequencing the first human genome took 13 years and cost almost US $3 billion. A number of alternative sequencing technologies have been generated during the past decade that simplify the sequencing process, improve accuracy, increase throughput, and reduce cost. These alternative approaches can be grouped into four categories[9]: microelectrophoretic methods,[10] sequencing by hybridization,[11] real-time sequencing of single molecules,[12,13] and cyclic array sequencing.[14,15]

The most advanced and commercially available second-generation DNA sequencing platforms are based on cyclic array parallel sequencing.[9,16,17] These platforms include Roche's 454,[15,18] Illumina's genome analyzer,[19] Applied Biosystem's SOLiD,[14,20] and HeliScope's single-molecule sequencer.[21,22] These platforms avoid using vector cloning and *E. coli* amplification for DNA template preparation, as is the case in the traditional DNA sequencers. Instead, the DNA library is generated by random fragmentation of DNA followed by in vitro linking of common adaptor sequences. Amplified pieces of DNA, called amplicons, are generated by in situ colonies of DNA,[23] emulsion polymerase chain reaction (PCR),[24] or bridge PCR.[25,26] In all cases, the PCR amplicons derived from any given DNA molecule from an organism end up spatially clustered on the genome (Fig. 10.2).

The cyclic array sequencing process consists of alternating cycles of enzyme-driven biochemistry and image-based data collection. The platforms rely on DNA synthesis driven by ligase[27,28] or polymerase.[29,30] Fluorescently labeled nucleotide bases are incorporated into the newly synthesized DNA by the enzymes, and data are acquired by imaging the full array of each cycle. Figure 10.3 illustrates the DNA sequencing process employed by the Roche, Illumina, Applied Biosystem, and HeliScope systems. Each of these platforms has its advantages and limitations compared with conventional Sanger sequencing approaches. In general, cyclic array–based sequencers greatly increase throughput and sensitivity and significantly reduce costs. The major disadvantages are shorter read length and lower accuracy. However, those weaknesses are offset by higher throughput capability; oversampling (sequencing a large excess of DNA sequences in the targeted region); and advanced bioinformatics-based digital data collection, processing, and assembly software. Table 10.1 summarizes the key features and cost comparison of each platform.

GENOMIC SEQUENCING

High-throughput DNA sequencing technologies enabled the completion of the Human Genome Project, which was started in 1990. After 13 years of collective effort from 18 countries, the 3 billion base pairs of the human genome sequence were finally decoded in 2003.[31] From the information on the complete sequence, scientists identified more than 15,000 full-length human genes and 3.7 million mapped human single-nucleotide polymorphisms. The complete genome sequence of many model organisms was obtained during the same period, including those of *E. coli*, *Saccharomyces cerevisiae*, *Caenorhabditis elegans*, *Drosophila melanogaster*, and laboratory mice and rats. According to the Genome OnLine Database,[32] by the end of October 2011, there were 2,971 genome projects completed worldwide, including 166 for eukaryotes, 2,658 for bacteria, and 147 for Archaea.

The rapid progress of genome research and a glimpse into its potential applications has attracted capital investment in the development and commercialization of molecular medicine, alternative energy, environmental

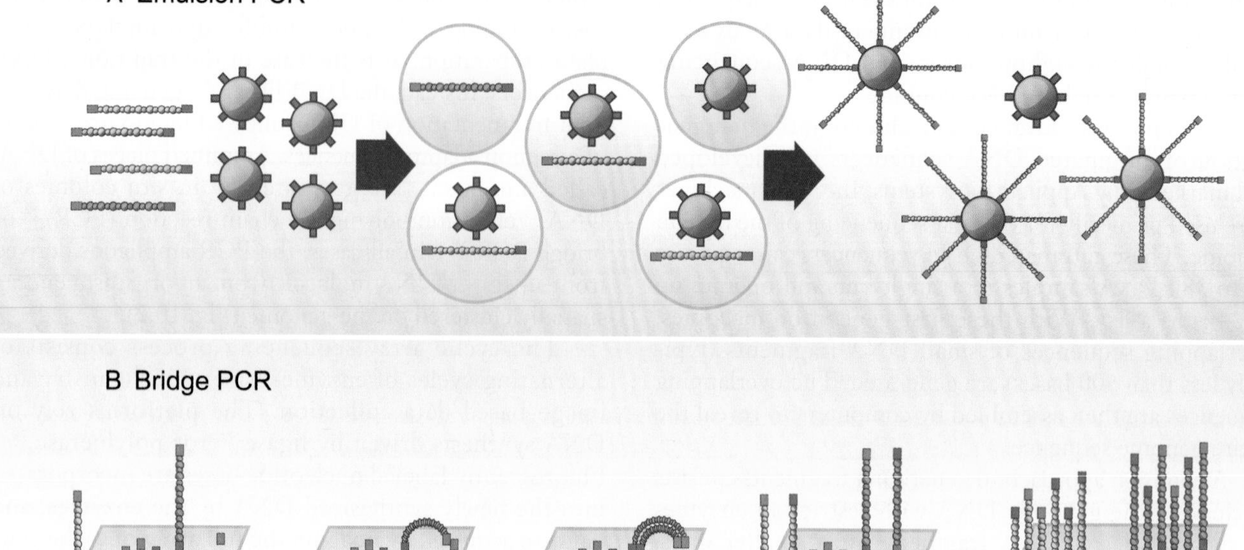

FIGURE 10–2 **A:** Clonal DNA amplification. Emulsion polymerase chain reaction (PCR) is the basis for 454 and SOLiD sequencing platforms to amplify the DNA template. Briefly, an in vitro constructed single-strand shotgun library flanked by adaptors on each end (shown as gold and green) is amplified by PCR in the context of water–oil emulsion. Microbeads attached with one of the PCR primers on the surface (via the 5′-end) are also included in the reaction. The template concentration is controlled such that most bead-containing compartments have no or one template molecule present in each emulsion. PCR amplicons are captured on the surface of the beads, and for each bead several million copies of the amplicons are produced. After the emulsion is broken, clonally amplified DNA template on the surface of each bead can be subjected for sequencing. **B:** Bridge PCR is the basis for Illumina sequencing platform. Briefly, the same adaptor-flanked shotgun library is amplified by PCR, but this time both primers are densely attached to the surface of a solid substrate, such as a microtiter dish. As a result, the amplification products are clustered around the original template from the library.

science, bioarchaeology, anthropology, evolution, and agriculture. New technologies and instrumentation in high-throughput DNA sequencing have further fueled the advancement of basic life sciences and commercialization of genomic-based products. The impact of genomic sequencing on cancer research has been significant and long lasting. Figure 10.4 summarizes the major developmental milestones of DNA sequencing.

Technologies promoted by the Human Genome Project and the information revealed from sequencing profoundly affected the advancement of biological and clinical research. The benefits have included improved earlier detection of genetic predispositions, diagnosis, determination of disease status, and prognosis. The availability of the human genome sequence has also helped significantly with rational drug design, discovery of new disease targets, gene therapy, pharmacogenomics, personalized medicine, and development of new therapies.

CANCER GENOME SEQUENCING

The cancer genome is characterized by its frequent complex structural aberrations of the chromosome, including point mutations, copy number alterations, and chromosomal rearrangements. Therefore, analysis of the cancer genome structure and DNA sequence can provide insights into cancer biology, diagnosis, and effective therapeutics for disease intervention. The recent advancements in massive parallel sequencing (that is, second-generation sequencing) have provided powerful tools to uncover, with higher efficiency and resolution, underlying chromosomal alterations as well as specific gene mutations in various cancer types.

Second-generation sequencing can be applied to DNA or RNA targeted to the whole genome or the transcriptome (the set of all RNA molecules of an organism), respectively, and to the analysis of structural changes, point mutations, gene expression, and chromosomal conformation.[33] The structural variation in the cancer genome has been studied using the paired-end reads technique, in which the sequence is read out from each end of paired DNA fragments. In this approach, paired-end reads from the cancer chromosome region or the whole-cancer genome are aligned with a normal DNA sequence and examined algorithmically to identify putative structure variations.[34]

Since the adult acute myeloid leukemia genome sequence was first reported in 2008,[35] at least five cancer genomes have been completely sequenced together with normal genomes. The results have revealed large

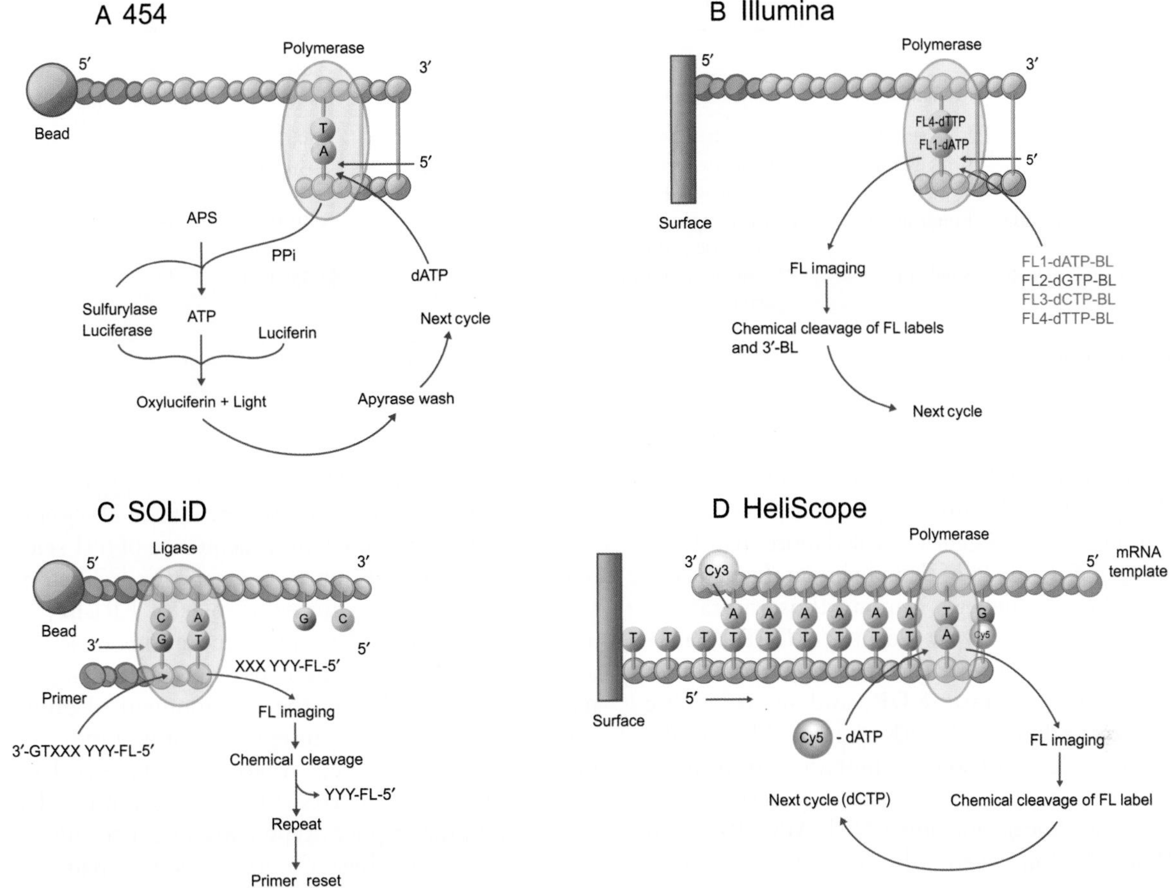

FIGURE 10–3 **A:** Process of second-generation DNA sequencing technologies. 454 DNA pyrosequencing. Clonally amplified DNA fragments on the surface of microbeads (see Fig. 10.2A for details) are deposited on a picotiter plate for sequencing with one DNA capture bead in each well. Each well is preloaded with enzymes necessary for pyrophosphate detection (sulfurylase and luciferase). Each cycle consists of adding one nucleotide to the plate at a time followed by substrates (adenosine 5′ phosphosulfate and luciferin). If the nucleotide has its complementary nucleotide to bind in the DNA extension, light will be released and detected by the instrument. Based on the light and the nucleotide added to the plate, the sequence in each reaction well can be determined. **B:** Illumina DNA sequencing. To initiate e™ach sequencing cycle, all four specifically labeled reversible terminators (FL-dNTPs-BL) are added to each flow cell with DNA polymerase. The fluorescence image captures the signal and determines the sequence based on the specific fluorescence emission. After that, 5′-FL and 3′-BL are chemically removed and the next sequencing cycle is initiated. **C:** SOLiD DNA sequencing. The uniqueness of SOLiD sequencing technology is that it ligates two nucleotides at a time to generate a sequence signal. Similar to 454, the fragments of the DNA library are amplified by emulsion polymerase chain reaction (PCR). The key for SOLiD technology is the use of an 8-mer oligo as probe, which is fluorescence labeled at the 5′-end, has a built-in cleavage site (between position XXX– and –YYY), and includes two nucleotides at the 3′-end. After ligation and imaging, the last three nucleotides and fluorescence dyes are cleaved, leaving a 5-mer oligo attached to the template. This sequencing cycle is repeated a few times before the system is reset by melting away the extended fragments and re-annealing the template to a new primer, with one base shift toward the bead, followed by new ligation cycles (see http://www.appliedgene.com/sequencing_3.html for a detailed explanation). To read the complete sequencing, five rounds of primer annealing are necessary. **D:** With the HeliScope sequencing platform, there is no clonal amplification step involved. Single nucleic acid molecules are sequenced directly. Poly-A-tailed template molecules are captured by hybridization to surface-tethered poly-T oligomers to yield an array of primed single-molecule sequencing templates. Templates are labeled with Cy3 at the 3′-end so that imaging can correlate the subset of the templates used to the sequencing read. Each cycle consists of polymerase-driven incorporation of a single species of Cy5-labeled nucleotide, followed by fluorescence imaging and chemical cleavage of the label.

variations in the types of cancer DNA aberrations, which include point mutations, insertions, deletions, amplifications, and chromosomal rearrangements. Whole-genome sequencing has allowed the detection of genomic alterations that had not been observable using previous methods, such as somatic mutations of non-coding or unannotated regions. Physical coverage, which is important for detecting rearrangements, can be controlled by changing the size of the DNA fragment between the paired reads. In addition, increasing the distance between the paired reads leads to higher physical coverage and less sequence coverage, and therefore to a lower cost.[35]

Targeted DNA Sequencing

In contrast to whole-cancer genome sequencing, targeted sequencing has the advantage of increased sequence coverage for the DNA regions of interest at lower cost and

TABLE 10–1 Comparison of Second-Generation DNA Sequencing Technologies

Platform	Amplification	Sequencing by Synthesis	Cost Per Megabase Pair	Cost Per Instrument	Read length (bp)	Reference
Roche 454	Emulsion PCR	Polymerase (pyrosequencing)	~$60	$500,000	250	18
Illumina genome analyzer	Bridge PCR	Polymerase (reversible terminators)	~$2	$430,000	36	19
Applied Biosystem SOLiD	Emulsion PCR	Ligase (octamers with two-base ending)	~$2	$591,000	35	20
HeliScope single-molecule sequencer	Single molecule	Polymerase (asynchronous extension)	~$1	$1,350,000	30	21,22

PCR, polymerase chain reaction.

higher throughput. Studies carried out by Ding et al.,[36] who used targeted DNA sequencing, on 188 human lung adenocarcinomas and 623 genes revealed more than 1,000 somatic mutations, with 26 of them being mutated at significantly higher frequencies. Among those mutations were epidermal growth factor receptor (EGFR) homologue ERBB4, ephrin receptor EPHA3, vascular endothelial growth factor receptor KDR, and neurotrophic tyrosine receptor kinase (NTRK) genes. The results also provided evidence of somatic mutations in primary lung adenocarcinoma for several tumor suppressor genes involved in other cancers, including NF1, APC, RB1, and ATM.[36] These findings shed light on several important signaling pathways involved in lung adenocarcinoma and have suggested new molecular targets for treatment.

At the same time, the Cancer Genome Atlas Research Network published an article reporting their integrative analysis of DNA copy number, gene expression, and DNA methylation aberrations in 206 glioblastomas as well as the nucleotide sequence of 601 selected genes in 91 matched tumor–normal pairs.[37] Their analysis provided insights into the roles of ERBB2, NF1, and TP53; uncovered frequent mutations of PIK3R1; and provided a comprehensive view of the signaling pathways altered during the development of glioblastoma. Furthermore, the integration of mutation, DNA methylation, and clinical treatment data revealed the connection between MGMT promoter methylation and hypermutator phenotype consequent to mismatch repair deficiency. These observations have had important potential clinical implications for glioblastoma diagnosis and treatment.[37]

In addition to high-throughput sequencing, both the lung adenocarcinoma and glioblastoma studies used

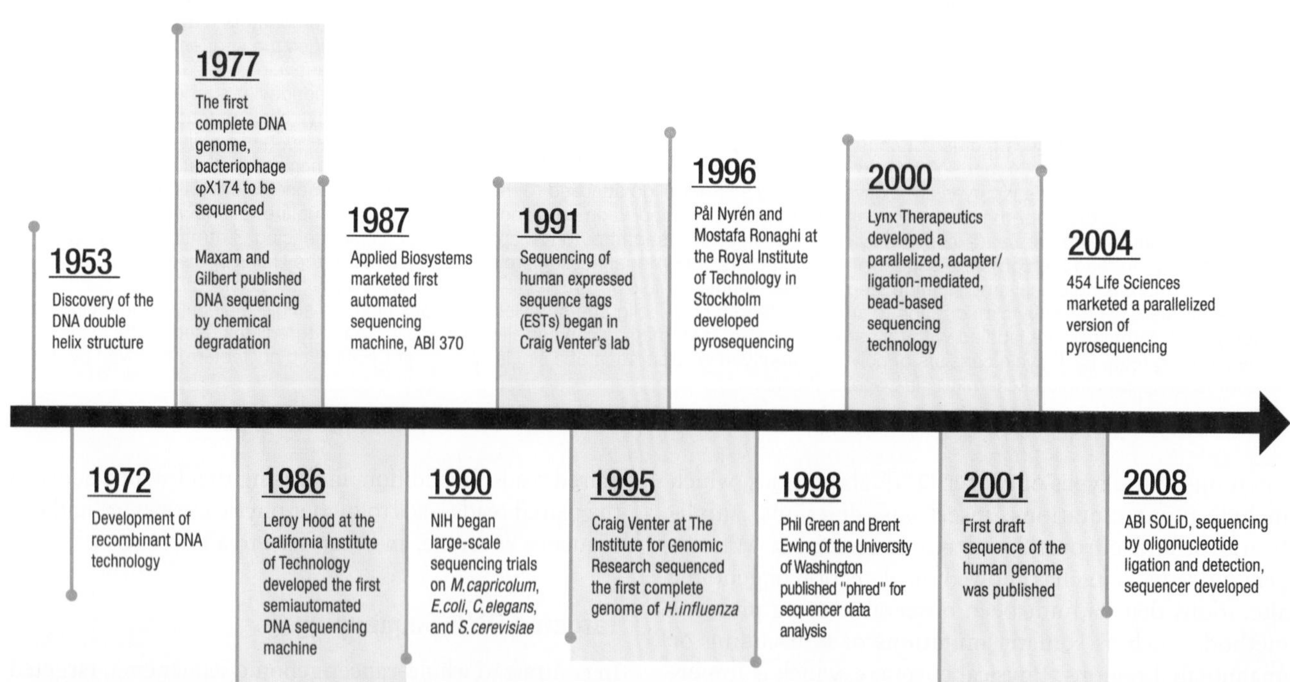

FIGURE 10–4 Major developmental milestones of DNA sequencing.

high-density single-nucleotide polymorphism microarray, gene expression, and quantitative PCR. This combined approach has been effectively applied to many other cancer genomic studies as well.[38-40]

In addition to analyzing targeted cancer genes, Sobreira and colleagues described their efforts in targeted breakpoint capture followed by second-generation sequencing. The researchers took this new approach to determine the precise structural characterization of translocation breakpoints and related chromosomal aberrations.[41]

Transcriptome Characterization

Transcriptome characterization involves the sequencing of RNA extracted from cells. This approach provides comprehensive data sets from which correlations to known genomic changes can be studied. This information can be used to detect alternative splice isoforms and fusion transcripts.[42] Furthermore, RNA sequencing can provide evidence leading to the discovery of genes that had not been annotated due to a lack of expressed sequence tags or were missed in silicon prediction.[43,44] It also allows analysis of gene expression profiles and is particularly powerful for identifying low-abundant transcripts.[45] The study of messenger RNA and microRNAs in particular and their roles in regulating the expression of specific genes in normal cells and cancer cells is rapidly expanding our knowledge in this aspect of biology.[46]

APPLICATION OF CANCER GENOME SEQUENCING

Early Discovery of Cancer Genes

BRCA1 and BRCA2

BRCA genes are tumor suppressor genes that produce proteins involved in DNA repair. Predisposing mutations in BRCA1 and BRCA2 genes have been associated with a high incidence of familial early-onset breast and ovarian cancers.[47-49] After the BRCA1 and BRCA2 genes were mapped to chromosome 17q in 1990[50,51] and chromosome 13q in 1994,[52] respectively, intense efforts to isolate them were made. Combining the complementary DNA library screening with hybrid-selected sequences and PCR approaches, the full-length BRCA1 and BRCA2 genes (encoding 1,863 and 3,418 amino acid proteins, respectively) were obtained by scientists from Myriad Genetics in 1994 and 1995.[48,49] Genetic testing of these two genes at an early age for women with a family history of breast cancer combined with prophylactic intervention significantly reduces the risk of breast cancer.[53]

HNPCC Genes

Hereditary nonpolyposis colorectal cancer (HNPCC) is an inherited condition carrying a high risk of colon and other cancers. HNPCC genes are involved in DNA mismatch repair, predominantly genes MSH2, MLH1, and MSH6, which account for approximately 80%, 30%, and 7% to 10% of these cancer cases, respectively. Similar to the case of BRCA genes, the cloning of genes MSH2 and MLH1 was facilitated by genomic sequencing.[54-56] Mutations in these genes have been observed in HNPCC kindreds.[57,58] Genetic testing of the HNPCC genes is now commercially available.

Cancer Biomarkers

Cancer biomarkers include diagnostic markers, prognostic markers, and predictive markers. Most cancer biomarkers are targeted to expressed cancer genes, such as tumor suppressors, oncogenes, and secreted proteins in plasma. The reliability of a biomarker is directly associated with its sensitivity and specificity. In a recent review, Kulasingam and Diamandis summarized the current tumor biomarkers and the strategies for tumor biomarker discovery through the use of emerging technologies.[59]

Understanding specific DNA sequence aberrations for individual cancer types and individual patients may help guide future diagnosis and treatment. The second-generation sequencing approaches have greatly facilitated the study of personalized tumor biomarkers. Leary and colleagues developed the personalized analysis of rearrangement ends (PARE) method, which can identify translocations in solid tumors from cancer patients' plasma samples.[60] Their findings support the notion that cancer genomes house a spectrum of genetic alterations, many of which are unique to the individual tumor. More validation and lower cost are required for this approach to become common clinical practice.

Cancer Therapeutics

One of the most important goals of molecular analysis of patients and their tumors is to inform clinical decision making. The availability of specific DNA sequence information has allowed the development of several diagnostic and prognostic tests that help drive clinical decisions in cancer treatment. Moreover, once a cancer marker has been correlated to the cause versus result of a disease, it can be used as the direct target for cancer therapy development.

Perhaps the best examples are clinical tests that guide the use of gefitinib or erlotinib for treating non–small cell lung cancer (NSCLC) with EGFR mutations and the treatment of HER2/Neu-positive breast cancer with trastuzumab. In the case of EGFR inhibitors gefitinib and erlotinib, treatment significantly enhances survival among NSCLC patients whose tumors carry EGFR mutations but has no benefit for patients with tumors with normal EGFR.[61-63] This realization has significantly improved the efficacy of NSCLC treatment and has reduced unnecessary cost and destruction to patients. Other examples include the testing of cytochrome P450 polymorphisms, which affect the metabolism of drugs (such as tamoxifen), and guidance of chronic myelogenous leukemia treatment with imatinib through testing for the Bcr-Abl mutation, which encodes for a mutant protein that drives cancer cell proliferation.[64]

DNA mutations and rearrangements are unique to cancer cells, giving rise to very specific markers. However, complete testing for each patient would require sequencing billions of DNA nucleotide bases and is prohibitively costly, even with second-generation sequencing platforms. Vogelstein and colleagues explored another possible marker of cancerous cells, that of mitochondrial DNA.[65] They found that more than 80% of cancers have mutations in the DNA of their mitochondria. These changes are easy to identify through complete sequencing because the mitochondrial DNA genome is much smaller (~16,000 base pairs) than the cell nucleus genome. Vogelstein's group have developed a method that could be used to monitor the progress of cancer treatment: massively parallel sequencing of a patient's mitochondrial DNA on a sequencing-by-synthesis platform.[65] As more advanced DNA sequencing technology becomes available and affordable, this approach will likely emerge as a powerful guide in clinical cancer treatment.

Cancer Drug Resistance

One of the main causes of failure in the treatment of cancer is the development of drug resistance by the cancer cells. The resistance can be due to a patient's health status, protein mutations that existed prior to treatment, or acquisition through the selective pressure exerted by treatment with anticancer drugs. The cancer multidrug resistance gene, which is also known as p-glycoprotein, has long been known to affect patients across a broad spectrum of cancers.[66] Several discoveries in recent years have demonstrated that patients carry specific gene structures or gene expression abnormalities that contribute to the disease's resistance to therapeutic treatment.

In a study of acquired drug resistance among patients with NSCLC treated with cetuximab, Yonesaka and colleagues found that activation of ERBB2 signaling and cetuximab resistance were strongly correlated.[67] In another study, Li and colleagues reported that amplification of the LAPTM4B and YWHAZ genes contributed to chemotherapy resistance and recurrence of breast cancer.[68]

In all these cases, an integrated genomics approach, including DNA sequencing, was applied to identify and analyze the targeted region of interest and its role in cancer drug resistance.

SUMMARY

The development and commercialization of high-throughput DNA sequencing technology over the past decade have significantly enhanced cancer research, diagnosis, and treatment. With the continuing advances in sequencing technologies and data analysis capabilities, the genome landscape of more and more cancer types will be unveiled.

One of the critical challenges is to develop cost-effective systems that allow for functional characterization of mutations and other sequence anomalies in a systematic and high-throughput manner. The broad availability of such systems will provide clues to candidate genes in carcinogenesis or metastasis, thereby establishing their role in targeted therapy development as well as in diagnosis and prognosis.[69,70] Sequencing technology will play an increasingly important role in facilitating the understanding of cancer genetics and mechanisms, thereby leading to better disease prevention, detection, and clinical intervention.

REFERENCES

1. Maxam AM, Gilbert W. A new method for sequencing DNA. *Proc Natl Acad Sci U S A*. 1977;74(2):560-564.
2. Pesole G, Saccone C. *Handbook of Comparative Genomics: Principles and Methodology*. New York, NY: Wiley-Liss; 2003:133.
3. Sanger F, Coulson AR. A rapid method for determining sequences in DNA by primed synthesis with DNA polymerase. *J Mol Biol*. 1975;94(3):441-448.
4. Sanger F, Nicklen S, Coulson AR. DNA sequencing with chain-terminating inhibitors. *Proc Natl Acad Sci U S A*. 1977; 74(12):5463-5467.
5. Smith LM, Sanders JZ, Kaiser RJ, et al. Fluorescence detection in automated DNA sequence analysis. *Nature*. 1986; 321(6071):674-679.
6. Smith LM, Fung S, Hunkapiller MW, Hunkapiller TJ, Hood LE. The synthesis of oligonucleotides containing an aliphatic amino group at the 5' terminus: synthesis of fluorescent DNA primers for use in DNA sequence analysis. *Nucleic Acids Res*. 1985;13(7):2399-2412.
7. Swerdlow H, Wu SL, Harke H, Dovichi NJ. Capillary gel electrophoresis for DNA sequencing. Laser-induced fluorescence detection with the sheath flow cuvette. *J Chromatogr*. 1990;516:61-67.
8. Hunkapiller T, Kaiser RJ, Koop BF, Hood L. Large-scale and automated DNA sequence determination. *Science*. 1991;254:59-67.
9. Shendure J, Ji H. Next-generation DNA sequencing. *Nat Biotechnol*. 2008;26:1135-1145.
10. Blazej RG, Kumaresan P, Mathies RA. Microfabricated bioprocessor for integrated nanoliter-scale Sanger DNA sequencing. *Proc Natl Acad Sci U S A*. 2006;103:7240-7245.
11. Gresham D, Dunham MJ, Botstein D. Comparing whole genomes using DNA microarrays. *Nat Rev Genet*. 2008;9:291-302.
12. Soni GV, Meller A. Progress toward ultrafast DNA sequencing using solid-state nanopores. *Clin Chem*. 2007;53:1996-2001.
13. Healy K. Nanopore-based single-molecule DNA analysis. *Nanomedicine*. 2005;2:459-481.
14. Shendure J, Porreca GP, Reppas NB, et al. Accurate multiplex polony sequencing of an evolved bacterial genome. *Science*. 2005;309:1728-1732.
15. Margulies M, Egholm M, Altman WE, et al. Genome sequencing in microfabricated high-density picolitre reactors. *Nature*. 2005;437:376-380.
16. Mardis ER. The impact of next-generation sequencing technology on genetics. *Cell*. 2007;24(3):133-141.
17. Mardis ER. A decade's perspective on DNA sequencing technology. *Nature*. 2011;470:198-203.
18. Green RE, Krause J, Ptak SE, et al. Analysis of one million base pairs of Neanderthal DNA. *Nature*. 2006;444:330-336.
19. Mardis ER. Next-generation DNA sequencing methods. *Annu Rev Genomics Hum Genet*. 2008;9:387-402.
20. McKernan KJ, Peckham HE, Costa GL, et al. Sequence and structural variation in a human genome uncovered by short-read, massively parallel ligation sequencing using two-base encoding. *Genome Res*. 2009;19(9):1527-1541.
21. Braslavsky I, Hebert B, Kartalov E, Quake SR. Sequence information can be obtained from single DNA molecules. *Proc Natl Acad Sci U S A*. 2003;100:3960-3964.

22. Harris TD, Buzby PR, Babcock H, et al. Single-molecule DNA sequencing of a viral genome. *Science.* 2008;320:106-109.
23. Mitra RD, Church GM. In situ localized amplification and contact replication of many individual DNA molecules. *Nucleic Acids Res.* 1999;27(24):e34-e39.
24. Dressman D, Yan H, Traverso G, Kinzler KW, Vogelstein B. Transforming single DNA molecules into fluorescent magnetic particles for detection and enumeration of genetic variations. *Proc Natl Acad Sci U S A.* 2003;100:8817-8822.
25. Adessi C, Matton G, Ayala G, et al. Solid phase DNA amplification: characterization of primer attachment and amplification mechanisms. *Nucleic Acids Res.* 2000;28(20):e87.
26. Fedurco M, Romieu A, Williams S, et al. BTA, a novel reagent for DNA attachment on glass and efficient generation of solid-phase amplified DNA colonies. *Nucleic Acids Res.* 2006;34:e22.
27. Valouev A, Ichikawa J, Tonthat T, et al. A high-resolution, nucleosome position map of *C elegans* reveals a lack of universal sequence-dictated positioning. *Genome Res.* 2008;18(7):1051-1063.
28. Brenner S, Johnson M, Bridgham J, et al. Gene expression analysis by massively parallel signature sequencing (MPSS) on microbead arrays. *Nat Biotechnol.* 2000;18:630-634.
29. Mitra RD, Shendure J, Olejnik J, et al. Fluorescent in situ sequencing on polymerase colonies. *Anal Biochem.* 2003;320:55-65.
30. Turcatti G, Romieu A, Fedurco M, Tairi AP. A new class of cleavable fluorescent nucleotides: synthesis and optimization as reversible terminators for DNA sequencing by synthesis. *Nucleic Acids Res.* 2008;36:e25.
31. Collins FS, Morgan M, Patrinos A. Human Genome Project: lessons from large-scale biology. *Science.* 2003;300:286-290.
32. GOLD. http://genomesonline.org. Accessed October 2011.
33. Mardis ER, Wilson RK. Cancer genome sequencing: a review. *Hum Mol Genet.* 2009;18(2):R163-R168.
34. Korbel JO, Urban AE, Affourtit JP, et al. Paired-end mapping reveals extensive structural variation in the human genome. *Science.* 2007;318:420-426.
35. Meyerson M, Gabriel S, Getz G. Advances in understanding cancer genomes through second-generation sequencing. *Nat Genet.* 2010;11:685-696.
36. Ding L, Getz G, Wheeler DA, et al. Somatic mutations affect key pathways in lung adenocarcinoma. *Nature.* 2008;455:1069-1075.
37. The Cancer Genome Atlas Consortium. Comprehensive genomic characterization defines human glioblastoma genes and core pathways. *Nature.* 2008;455:1061-1068.
38. Weir BA, Woo MS, Getz G, et al. Characterizing the cancer genome in lung adenocarcinoma. *Nature.* 2007;450: 893-898.
39. Chiang DY, Getz G, Jaffe DB, et al. High-resolution mapping of copy-number alterations with massively parallel sequencing. *Nat Methods.* 2009;6:99-103.
40. Wood LD, Parsons DW, Jones S, et al. The genomic landscapes of human breast and colorectal cancers. *Science.* 2007;318:1108-1113.
41. Sobreira NLM, Gnanakkan V, Walsh M, et al. Characterization of complex chromosomal rearrangements by targeted capture and next-generation sequencing. *Genome Res.* 2011;21:1720-1727.
42. Trapnell C, Pachter L, Salzberg SL. TopHat: discovering splice junctions with RNA-Seq. *Bioinformatics.* 2009;25:1105-1111.
43. Sultan M, Schulz MH, Richard H, et al. A global view of gene activity and alternative splicing by deep sequencing of the human transcriptome. *Science.* 2008;321:956-960.
44. Mortazavi A, Williams BA, McCue K, et al. Mapping and quantifying mammalian transcriptomes by RNA-Seq. *Nat Methods.* 2008;5:621-628.
45. Morrissy AS, Morin RD, Delaney A, et al. Next-generation tag sequencing for cancer gene expression profiling. *Genome Res.* 2009:19:1825-1835.
46. He L, He X, Lowe SW, Hannon GJ. microRNAs join the p53 network—another piece in the tumour-suppression puzzle. *Nat Rev Cancer.* 2007;7:819-822.
47. Easton DF, Bishop DT, Ford D, et al. Genetic linkage analysis in familial breast and ovarian cancer: results from 214 families. *Am J Hum Genet.* 1993;52:678-701.
48. Miki Y, Swensen J, Shattuck-Eidens D, et al. A strong candidate for the breast and ovarian cancer susceptibility gene *BRCA1*. *Science.* 1994;266:66-71.
49. Wooster R, Bignell G, Lancaster L, et al. Identification of the breast cancer susceptibility gene *BRCA2*. *Nature.* 1995;378:789-792.
50. Hall JM, Lee MK, Newman B, et al. Linkage of early-onset familial breast cancer to chromosome 17q21. *Science.* 1990; 250:1684-1689.
51. Narod SA, Feunteun J, Lynch H, et al. Familial breast-ovarian cancer locus *on* chromosome 17q12-q23. *Lancet.* 1991;338:82-83.
52. Wooster R, Neuhausen SL, Mangion J, et al. Localization of a breast cancer susceptibility gene, BRCA2, to chromosome 13q12-13. *Science.* 1994;265:2088-2090.
53. Kurian AW, Sigal BM, Plevritis SK. Survival analysis of cancer risk reduction strategies for *BRCA1/2* mutation carriers. *J Clin Oncol.* 2010;28(2):222-231.
54. Fishel R, Lescoe M, Rao M, et al. The human mutator gene homolog MSH2 and its association with hereditary nonpolyposis colon cancer. *Cell.* 1993;75(5):1027-1038.
55. Nicolaides NC, Papadopoulos N, Liu B, et al. Mutations of two PMS homologues in hereditary nonpolyposis colon cancer. *Nature.* 1994;371(6492):75-80.
56. Papadopoulos N, Nicolaides N, Wei Y, et al. Mutation of a mutL homolog in hereditary colon cancer. *Science.* 1994; 263(5153):1625-1629.
57. Wijnen J, Khan PM, Vasen H, et al. Majority of hMLH1 mutations responsible for hereditary nonpolyposis colorectal cancer cluster at the exonic region 15-16. *Am J Hum Genet.* 1996;58(2):300-307.
58. Liu T. Mutational screening of hMLH1 and hMSH2 that confer inherited colorectal cancer susceptibility using denature gradient gel electrophoresis (DGGE). *Methods Mol Biol.* 2010;653:193-205.
59. Kulasingam V, Diamandis EP. Strategies for discovering novel cancer biomarkers through utilization of emerging technologies. *Nat Clin Pract Oncol.* 2008;5:588-599.
60. Leary RJ, Kinde I, Diehl F, et al. Development of personalized tumor biomarkers using massively parallel sequencing. *Sci Transl Med.* 2010;2(20):20.
61. Mitsudomi T, Morita S, Yatabe Y, et al. Gefitinib versus cisplatin plus docetaxel in patients with non-small-cell lung cancer harbouring mutations of the epidermal growth factor receptor (WJTOG3405): an open label, randomized phase 3 trial. *Lancet Oncol.* 2009;11:121-128.
62. Mok TS, Wu Y-L, Thongprasert S, et al. Gefitinib or carboplatin–paclitaxel in pulmonary adenocarcinoma. *N Engl J Med.* 2009; 361:947-957.
63. Rosell R, Moran T, Queralt C, et al. Screening for epidermal growth factor receptor mutations in lung cancer. *N Engl J Med.* 2009;361:958-967.
64. Harris T. Does large scale DNA sequencing of patient and tumor DNA yet provide clinically actionable information? *Discov Med.* 2010;10(51):144-150.
65. He Y, Wu J, Dressman DC, et al. Heteroplasmic mitochondrial DNA mutations in normal and tumour cells. *Nature.* 2010;464:610-614.
66. Cancer multidrug resistance. *Nat Biotechnol.* 2000;18: IT18-IT20.
67. Yobesaka K, Zejnullahu K, Okamoto I, et al. Activation of ERBB2 signaling causes resistance to the EGFR-directed therapeutic antibody cetuximab. *Sci Transl Med.* 2011;3(99):99.
68. Li Y, Zou L, Li Q, et al. Amplification of LAPTM4B and YWHAZ contributes to chemotherapy resistance and recurrence of breast cancer. *Nat Med.* 2010;16:214-218.
69. Luo B, Cheung HW, Subramanian A, et al. Highly parallel identification of essential genes in cancer cells. *Proc Natl Acad Sci U S A.* 2008;105:20380-20385.
70. Scott KL, Kabbarah O, Liang MC, et al. GOLPH3 modulates mTOR signalling and rapamycin sensitivity in cancer. *Nature.* 2009;459:1085-1090.

CHAPTER 11

MASS SPECTROMETRY: PRINCIPLES AND APPLICATIONS IN CANCER DIAGNOSIS AND MANAGEMENT

Oliver J. Semmes, Richard R. Drake, and Julius O. Nyalwidhe

INTRODUCTION

Over the last two decades, there has been an increasing use of mass spectrometry (MS) technology applied to the clinical analysis of biomolecules, from a variety of fluid or tissue sources. Mass spectrometers excel at precise determination of the masses of biomolecules to the atomic level, which allows for the identification and quantitation of multiple analytes in complex mixtures. There have been revolutionary improvements in detection sensitivity and analytical capabilities of instrumentation, fueling the application of MS-based methods to cancer and other diseases research. The applications have largely been developed in university-based research institutions but are being increasingly adopted in clinical laboratories and clinical diagnostic settings. This chapter provides an overview of the principles of MS and the types of instrumentation being utilized in the context of current clinical applications to cancer. The application of these approaches to the analysis of biomolecules (proteins, nucleic acids, lipids, carbohydrates, small molecule metabolites, and drugs) will be summarized, with a perspective on how MS is expected to impact cancer diagnosis and detection in the immediate future.

AN OVERVIEW OF MS

MS has been utilized as a diagnostic tool in clinical laboratories for several decades. MS instruments are composed of three main components, namely the ionization source, the analyzer, and the detector. Basically, MS measures the mass-to-charge (m/z) ratio of gas phase ions. The ion source converts analyte molecules into gas phase ions, the ionized analytes are separated in the mass analyzer based on their m/z ratio, and the detector records the abundance of the ions at each m/z value. Initially, MS instrumentation was mainly coupled with gas chromatography (GC/MS) and utilized for the identification and quantitation of small molecules. Getting a sample into the gas phase and ionizing it caused unpredictable fragmentation of large biomolecules rendering analysis beyond the ability of early MS adopters. Over the last few decades, novel innovations have resulted in the development of alternative methodologies that have been used to effectively ionize macromolecules such as proteins and nucleic acids. With the application of these new "soft" ionization methods, namely matrix-assisted laser desorption ionization (MALDI)[1,2] and electrospray ionization (ESI),[3] the integrity of the analyte is preserved thus allowing mass analysis with accuracy. These ionization innovations made biological molecules readily amenable to MS and consequently garnered the 2002 Nobel Prize in Chemistry for John Fenn, Koichi Tanaka, and Kurt Wuthrich. The introduction of MS to biology has driven the further development of high performance, robust MS instrumentation that has increased the power of MS-based approaches in the identification and characterization of biomolecules.

To date, significant progress has been made in identifying tumor characteristics of various cancers through advances in molecular biology technologies. This has been driven by the discovery of tumor-related aberrations that affect nucleic acids at genomic, transcriptional, and posttranscriptional levels. Differences between cellular states are reflected in changes in gene expression that are recognizable at the level of both the transcript (mRNA) and translated proteins. As the functional end product of genes, proteins ultimately control all biological processes. Likewise, changes in protein structure, expression levels, molecular interactions, and events that determine subcellular localization will modulate critical cellular functions. The number of proteins produced by the cells is significantly higher than the number of genes because proteins vary in their stability and are affected by posttranscriptional and posttranslational changes, such as splicing of mRNA, gene fusions, and protein posttranslational modifications. Understanding the full protein content of a cell, tissue, or organism under defined conditions is the central mandate to the field of proteomics.[4] Currently, MS is arguably the most important and powerful technologies for proteomics.[5] Further developments of technology and methodology in the field of MS in recent years have provided improved and novel strategies for both global and targeted understanding of protein function. Some of these MS technologies and methodologies are discussed in the following section.

MS IONIZATION METHODS

All MS techniques rely upon the formation and manipulation of ions in an electrical/magnetic field. The ions of interest are positively charged particles subject to sequential ionization physics. Ionization is thus a critical step to MS analysis that is achieved via several methodologies. Figure 11.1 represents schematic diagrams summarizing the two main ionization methods that are discussed in the following sections.

Matrix-Assisted Laser Desorption/Ionization Mass Spectrometry

Historically, the first attempts to use light as a mass spectrometric ionization method for organic molecules date back to the 1970s.[6-8] These earlier methods on laser desorption of organic ions were restricted to molecular masses < 2,000 Da since molecules with higher masses needed higher irradiances (laser power/area) for ion

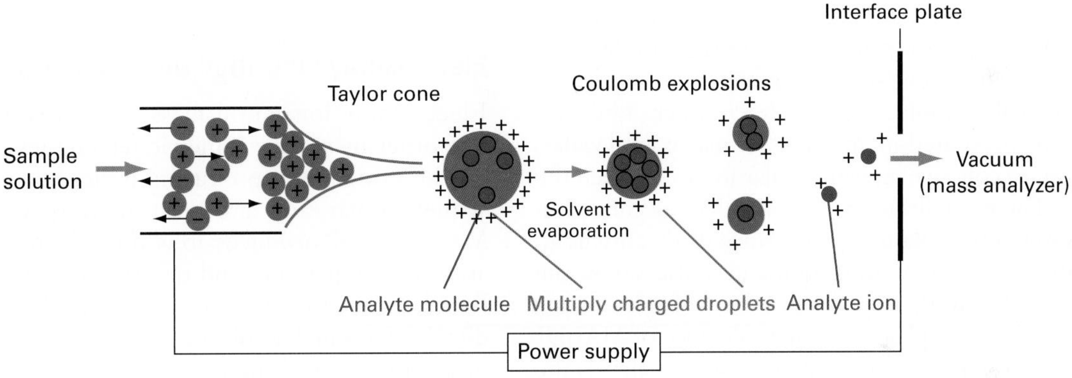

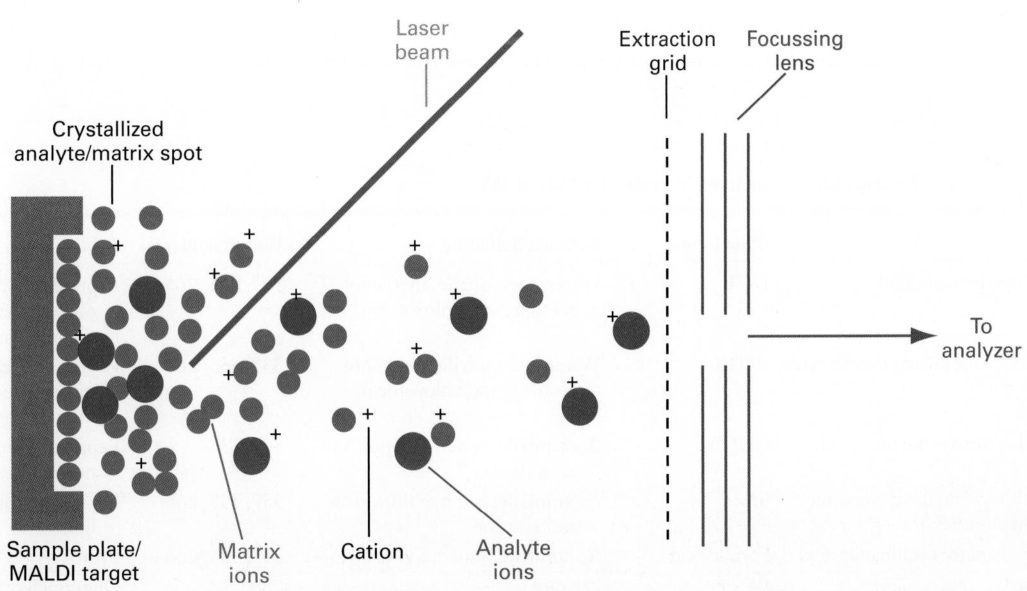

FIGURE 11–1 Schematic of ionization process in matrix-assisted laser desorption ionization (MALDI) (*upper*) and electrospray ionization (ESI) (*lower*).

production. The higher laser power invariably resulted in the fragmentation and destruction of larger organic molecules. The destruction of these large molecules was postulated to be due to the transfer of energy into photodissociation channels. The fact observed in earlier studies that "soft" desorption of molecular ions was efficient only in highly absorbing species provided the impetus to search for chemical matrix formulations that would enable the uniform analysis of high mass macromolecules. In MALDI, the analyte is homogeneously mixed and crystallized on a metallic target with a matrix solution consisting of small, highly absorbing molecular species. Irradiation of matrix-coated sample with laser enables desorption and ionization of the molecules regardless of their individual absorption characteristics.[1,2] Matrix is postulated to serve three main functions during the ionization process. The first function of matrix is the effective absorption and transfer of energy from laser light into the crystalline system. This induces a spontaneous phase transition of a portion of the sample into gaseous species and the analyte molecules desorb together with matrix molecules with limited internal excitation and fragmentation. There are different models that have been proposed for the mechanism of desorption and these are discussed in detail in available literature. The second function of matrix serves to isolate analyte molecules from each other. The analytes are incorporated in an excess of matrix molecules, which reduce cohesive intermolecular forces between the analytes. The crystallization process, which occurs upon evaporation of the volatile organic solvents that are used, is essential for efficient ionization and it also serves the purpose of cleaning the analyte by removing contaminants. This partly explains the high tolerance of MALDI to most contaminants. The final function of matrix is the ionization of the analyte. To date, the active role of the matrix in the ionization of analytes during the MALDI process has not been fully elucidated. It is postulated that the matrix molecules are actively involved after their photoexcitation or photoionization and subsequent transfer of protons to the analyte. The discovery of new matrices and determination of their modes of action in ionization is still a subject of ongoing research. The choice of matrix to be used in a MALDI experiment is dependent on the wavelength of the laser to be used and the class and solubility of the analyte. Laser ion sources in use for MALDI may differ in some technical details, but all comprise some common features including the use of pulse durations of 1 to 200 ns. The most commonly used lasers are nitrogen lasers emitting at 337 nm or Nd-YAG lasers whose emission wavelength of 1,064 nm has been transferred to 355 or 266 nm by frequency tripling or quadrupling using nonlinear optical crystals. For the required irradiances in the range of 10^6 to 10^7 W/cm^2, the laser beams are focused to values between 30 and 500 μM by suitable optical lenses. The ions formed in the source after irradiation are accelerated in a two-stage acceleration system employing pulsed ion extraction. After leaving the ion source, all ions have the same nominal kinetic energy (see Fig. 11.1). Table 11.1 summarizes a list of the most commonly used matrix substances, their physical properties, and their applications.

Electrospray Ionization Mass Spectrometry

Electrospray ionization mass spectrometry (ESI-MS) like other mass spectrometric techniques is also based on the principle of producing molecular ions for subsequent separation and mass analysis. In contrast to MALDI, ESI produces ions directly from liquids at atmospheric pressure and the MS is readily coupled to liquid chromatography (LC) systems. The analytes are dissolved in suitable solvents, e.g., a mixture of methanol or acetonitrile (or other volatile organics) and acidified water. The analyte solution is infused into fused silica at a constant flow rate and introduced to a "source" where intact analyte molecules in gaseous phase free of solvent or other solute molecules are produced and directed to the analyzer and detector. During the ESI process,

TABLE 11-1 The Most Commonly Used Matrices for MALDI MS

Matrix	Other Names	Solvents/Solubility	Wavelength (nm)	Applications
2,5-Dihydroxybenzoic acid	DHB	Water, acetonitrile, methanol, acetone, and chloroform	337, 355, 266	Peptides, nucleotides, oligonucleotides, and oligosaccharides
DHB + 10% 5-methoxy salicylic acid	sDHB	Water, acetonitrile, methanol, acetone, and chloroform	337, 355, 266	Peptides, nucleotides, oligonucleotides, and oligosaccharides
α-Cyano-4-hydroxycinnamic acid	CHCA	Acetonitrile, water, ethanol, and acetone	337, 355	Peptides, lipids, and nucleotides
3,5-Dimethoxy-4-hydroxycinnamic acid (sinapinic acid)	SA	Acetonitrile, water, chloroform, and acetone	337, 355, 266	Peptides, proteins, and lipids
4-Hydroxy-3-methoxycinnamic acid	Ferulic acid	Acetonitrile, water, and propanol	337, 355, 266	Proteins
Picolinic acid	PA	Ethanol	266	Oligonucleotides
3-Hydroxy picolinic acid	HPA	Ethanol	337, 355	Oligonucleotides

a spray of fine, highly charged droplets is created at atmospheric pressure in the presence of a high electric field (>2 kV). There are different types of sources, the simplest consisting of a metallic capillary tip at elevated voltage relative to a counter electrode and the interface plate which has a small orifice where the ions are guided into the mass spectrometer.

The process of ionization in ESI has been the subject of investigation and debate.[9,10] It is postulated that the electric field between the capillary tip and the interface plate induces a charge on the surface of the emerging liquid, dispersing it by Coulomb forces into a fine spray of charged droplets (see Fig. 11.1). These droplets carry an excess of charge and are attracted to the inlet of the mass spectrometer that is at a lower potential. In some sources, a countercurrent flow of dry gas ("nitrogen curtain") is used to assist evaporation thus reducing the diameter of the droplets. The reduction in size increases the charged density on the surface of the droplets until the so-called Rayleigh limit is reached. At this point, the Coulomb repulsion and the surface tension are of the same order. This introduces instability resulting into the "Coulomb explosion" that tears the droplet apart, producing numerous smaller charged droplets that undergo the same process repeatedly. The final result is the production of minute droplets with diameters in the nanometer range. Due to their small size, the charge density and radius of curvature at the droplet surface produce an electric field strong enough to finally desorb the analyte ions into gaseous state and are introduced into the analyzer.

COMMONLY USED MASS ANALYZERS

Mass analyzers are the central component of MS instruments. In almost all applications, the key parameters for analysis are sensitivity, resolution, mass accuracy, and the ability to generate information-rich tandem (MS^n) spectra. Currently, five types of mass analyzers are commonly used for biomedical research. Quadrupole (Q), ion trap (quadrupole ion trap, QIT; linear ion trap, LIT; or linear trap quadrupole, LTQ), time-of-flight (TOF), Fourier transform ion cyclotron resonance (FTICR), and the Orbitrap mass analyzer. These analyzers vary in their physical principles and analytical performance. They can be used independently as standalone instruments or combined in "hybrid" instruments designed to combine the capabilities of different mass analyzers. These configurations include Q–Q–Q, Q–Q–LIT, Q–Q–TOF, Q–TOF, TOF–TOF, and LTQ–FTICR. The characteristics and capabilities of the instrument setups are summarized in Table 11.2 and their features have been extensively reviewed.[11,12]

TOF Analyzers

In TOF analysis, the m/z of an ion is determined by measuring their flight time. After the acceleration of the ions in the ion source to a fixed kinetic energy, they pass a field-free drift tube with a velocity proportional to $(m_i/z_i)^{-1/2}$ (m_i/z_i is the mass-to-charge ratio of a given ion species). Due to their mass-dependent velocity, ions are separated during their flight. A detector at the end of the flight tube produces a signal for each ion species. In reflector TOF instruments, the ions are accelerated and separated along a flight tube before being turned around in a reflector, which compensates for slight differences in kinetic energy, and then impinged on a detector that amplifies and counts arriving ions. TOF–TOF analyzers—these instruments incorporate a collision cell between two TOF sections. Ions of specified m/z ratio are selected in the first TOF section, fragmented in the collision cell, and the masses of the fragments are separated in the second TOF section before detection.

Quadrupole Analyzers

Quadrupoles select by time-varying electric fields between four parallel rods in which opposite electrodes are connected. To one pair of electrodes is applied a potential of $U + V \cos \omega t$, where U is a DC voltage and V is the peak amplitude of an RF (radio frequency) voltage at the frequency $\omega = 2\pi\nu$. To the other pair of electrodes a potential of the same amplitude is applied, but the polarity of the DC voltage is reversed and the RF voltage is shifted in phase by 180°. Ions injected from the source parallel to the rods in the quadrupole undergo transverse oscillation caused by the perpendicular DC and RF voltages applied to the rods. With the proper selection of U and V, ions of a given m/z ratio will have stable trajectories and will ultimately emerge the quadrupole toward the detector (resonant ions). Ions with other values of m/z ratio will have unstable oscillations that increase in amplitude until they collide with the rods, thus not been transmitted (nonresonant ions). In Q–q–Q instruments ions of a particular m/z are selected in a quadrupole (Q1), fragmented in second quadrupole which is a collision cell (q2), and the fragments separated in the third quadrupole (Q3) before the detector.

Ion Trap Analyzers

Ions created by ESI are focused using an octupole transmission system into the ion trap. Ions may be gated into the trap through the use of a pulsing lens or through a combination of RF potentials applied to the ring electrode. The pulsed transmission of ions into the trap differentiates ion traps from "beam" instruments such as quadrupoles where ions continually enter the mass analyzer. The trap acts as a storage device for the confinement of gaseous ions in the absence of solvent. The confining capacity of the trap arises from the formation of a trapping potential when appropriate potentials are applied to the electrodes of the trap. The time during which ions are allowed into the trap is optimized to maximize signal while minimizing *space–charge* effects. Space–charge occurs when excess ions in the trap cause a distortion of the electrical fields resulting in an overall reduction in performance. The ion trap is typically filled with helium

TABLE 11-2 Comparison of Performance Characteristics of Commonly Used Mass Spectrometers for Proteomics

Instrument	Mass Resolution	Mass Accuracy (ppm)	Sensitivity	*m/z* Range	Scan Rate	Dynamic Range	MS/MS Capability	Ion Source	Main Applications
QIT	1,000[a]	100–1,000	Picomole	50–2,000 200–4,000	Moderate	1E3	MS^n [d]	ESI	Protein identification of low complex samples. PTM identification
LTQ	2,000[a]	100–500	Picomole	50–2,000 200–4,000	Fast	1E4	MS^n [d]	ESI	High-throughput, large-scale protein identification from complex peptide mixtures by online LC–MS^n, PTM identification
Q–q–Q	1,000	100–1,000	Attomole to femtomole	10–4,000	Moderate	6E6	MS/MS	ESI	Quantification in SRM mode, PTM detection in precursor ion and neutral loss scanning modes
Q–q–LIT	2,000[a]	100–500	Femtomole	5–2,800	Fast	4E6	MS^n [d]	ESI	Quantification in SRM mode, PTM detection in precursor ion and neutral loss scanning modes
TOF	10,000–20,000	10–20[b]; <5[c]	Femtomole	No upper limit	Fast	1E4	n/a[e]	MALDI	Protein identification from in-gel digestion of gel separated protein bands by PMF
TOF–TOF	10,000–20,000	10–20[b]; <5[c]	Femtomole	No upper limit	Fast	1E4	MS/MS	MALDI	Protein identification from in-gel digestion of gel separated protein bands by PMF or sequence tagging via CID MS/MS
Q–q–TOF	10,000–20,000	10–20[b]; <5[c]	Femtomole	No upper limit	Moderate to fast	1E4	MS/MS	MALDI ESI	Protein identification from complex peptide mixtures; intact protein analysis; PTM identification
FTICR	50,000–750,000	<2	Femtomole	50–2,000 200–4,000	Slow	1E3	MS^n [d]	MALDI ESI	Top–down proteomics; high mass accuracy PTM characterization
LTQ–Orbitrap	30,000–100,000	<5	Femtomole	50–2,000 200–4,000	Moderate to fast	4E3	MS^n [d]	MALDI ESI	Top–down proteomics; high mass accuracy PTM characterization; protein identification from complex peptide mixtures; quantification

[a]Mass resolution achieved at normal scan rate; higher resolution achievable at a lower scan rate.

[b]With external calibration.

[c]With internal calibration.

[d]$n > 2$, up to 13.

[e]Fragmentation achievable by post source decay.

MS/MS, tandem mass spectrometry; *m/z*, mass-to-charge; QIT, quadrupole ion trap; ESI, electrospray ionization; LTQ, linear trap quadrupole; Q-q-Q, triple quadrupole; SRM, single reaction monitoring; Q-q-LIT, double quadrupole ion trap; PMF, peptide mass fingerprinting; Q-q-TOF, double quadrupole time of flight MS, mass spectrometry; PTM, posttranslational modification; LC, liquid chromatography; TOF, time-of-flight; MALDI, matrix-assisted laser desorption ionization; CID, collision-induced dissociation; FTICR, Fourier transform ion cyclotron resonance.

Adapted from Hans X, Aslanian A and Yates JR. Mass spectrometry for proteomics. Curr. Opin. Chem. Biol. 2008;12:483-90.

to a pressure of about 1 mtorr. Collisions with helium dampen the kinetic energy of the ions and serve to quickly focus trajectories toward the center of the ion trap, enabling trapping of injected ions.[13,14] Trapped ions are further focused toward the center of the trap through the use of an oscillating potential, called the *fundamental rf*, applied to the ring electrode. An ion will be stably trapped depending upon the values of the mass and charge of the ion, the size of the ion trap (r), the oscillating frequency of the fundamental rf (w), and the amplitude of the voltage on the ring electrode (V). Analytes with a specific m/z can be selected and detected by varying these parameters. Alternatively, an analyte can be selected and fragmented before scanning out the daughter ions to generate a tandem mass spectrum.

FTICR Analyzers

Fourier transform mass spectrometry (FTMS) performs mass measurements with very high resolution and accuracy. FTMS is based on the ion cyclotron resonance (ICR) principle. After ionization the ions are trapped in an ICR cell, which is situated in the homogeneous region of a magnet (a permanent magnet, electromagnet, or superconducting magnet). Common ICR cells are cubic, orthorhombic, or cylindrical with measurements of several centimeters. In the cubic and orthorhombic cells, one opposing pair of plates is oriented orthogonal to the direction of the magnetic field lines and two pairs of plates lie parallel to the field. The plates that are perpendicular to the field are the trapping plates. One opposing pair that is oriented parallel to the field is used for ion excitation (transmitter plates) and the other pair is used for ion detection (receiver plates). In the strong magnetic field, ions of the same charge and velocity are constrained to move in circular orbits forming an "ion packet" after excitation. Each "ion packet" emits an RF signal to the receiver plates at its characteristic cyclotron frequency.[15,16] A positive ion packet coming closer to the receiver plates attracts electrons in the external circuit and induces a so-called image current. This signal causes a small AC voltage to develop, which is amplified and registered as transient. The amplitude of the transient is proportional to the number of ions in the cell. The ions remain in the analyzer cell after detection (non-destructive detection) and can be analyzed in further experiments (e.g., by tandem mass spectrometry [MS/MS]). In an FTMS, usually all ions of different m/z are excited and detected simultaneously (multichannel analysis). A composite transit signal is obtained that represents a "time-domain" spectrum, i.e., the signal intensity is recorded against time.

Orbitrap Analyzer

This new mass analyzer that incorporates novel instrumentation technology was invented by Makarov in 1999.[17] In the Orbitrap, ions are trapped and orbit around a central spindle-like electrode and oscillate harmonically along its axis with a frequency characteristic of their m/z values, inducing an image current in the outer electrodes that is Fourier transformed into the time domain producing mass spectra.

COMMONLY USED FRAGMENTATION METHODS

MS/MS is a key technique for the identification and characterization of biomolecules. An efficient, non-processive, fragmentation process is essential to tandem MS approaches. There are various MS fragmentation technologies each with specific mechanisms resulting in different fragmentation products.

Collision-Induced Dissociation

Collision-induced dissociation (CID) is the most widely used MS/MS technique for most applications.[18] In this fragmentation technique using proteins/peptides as an example, it is observed that their positively charged ions are internally heated by multiple collisions with inert gas atoms (e.g., argon). This leads to peptide backbone fragmentation of the amide (C–N) bond resulting in a series of b- and y-fragment ions. The fragmentation technique is not very efficient in generating sequence information of peptides larger than 15 amino acids and intact proteins. It also has the inherent limitations of inducing internal fragmentation and neutral loses of small molecules such as water, ammonia, and labile posttranslational modifications, e.g., phosphorylation. This is attributed to the slow-heating energetic feature that is associated with this method.

Electron Capture Dissociation

Electron capture dissociation (ECD)—in this method developed in 1998, the capture of a thermal electron by a multiply protonated peptide/protein cation induces backbone fragmentation at the N–Cα bond to produce c- and z-type fragment ions.[19,20] ECD provides more extensive fragmentation resulting in richer MS/MS spectra and better sequence coverage and the preservation of labile posttranslational modifications.[21,22] This fragmentation technique is a powerful tool for top-down analysis of intact proteins.[23] The main limitation on the use of ECD is the high cost and sophistication of FTICR instruments.

Electron Transfer Dissociation

Electron transfer dissociation (ETD)—in this process developed in 2004, the electrons transfer from radical anions with low electron affinity to multiply protonated peptide cations initiating backbone fragmentation to produce c- and z-ion series.[24,25] ETD MS/MS provides superior sequence coverage for small- to medium-sized peptides and is highly complementary to conventional CID for proteome identification applications.[26,27] ETD is useful in the analysis of large peptides and intact proteins with a sequential ion/ion reaction, proton transfer/charge reduction (PTR), by which the ETD-produced multiply charged fragments are de-protonated with even-electron anions resulting in singly and doubly charged ions.[28] This allows for sequence analysis of 15 to 40 amino acids at both N- and C-terminus of the protein. ETD is currently being utilized in the analysis of labile posttranslational modification analyses such as phosphorylation and glycosylation.[29,30]

MS DETECTORS

Electron multipliers and channel electron multipliers are used universally for detecting ions that are generated at the source and analyzed in MS instruments. Transmitted ions with specific *m/z* ratio are deflected into the collector of a detector. When an ion strikes the collector, an electron cascade is triggered and the resulting signal after amplification is sent to the data acquisition computer for conversion into mass chromatograms/spectra.

CLINICAL APPLICATION OF MS

The use of MS for the detection/quantitation of clinically relevant molecules has certain theoretical advantages over classic immunoassays and/or indirect chemical tests. Much of the advantage derives from the direct measurement of an analyte versus the indirect assessment via antibodies or molecular affinity probes. By definition, direct assays are inherently more specific and provide an expanded analytical range that can be devoid of common immunoassay characteristics. Immunoassay issues of cross-reactivity, the "hook" or prozone, and matrix effects are all eliminated when the analyte is directly measured. Overcoming each of these common assay maladies eliminates either extra steps or additional reagents that routinely add significant costs and challenges to robustness of current immunoassays. In addition, multiplexed analysis of analytes, another problem for immunoassay platforms, can reach near unlimited complexity when MS is employed.

Analysis by MS also provides structural information not captured in immunoassays. There is no requirement for robust epitope presentation and both specific and variable molecular structures can be analyzed. MS is adept at measuring both single and multiple posttranslational modifications. For instance, immediately adjacent phosphorylation sites can be quantitated for all possible modification combinations. The direct measurement by MS of modifications that add mass to an analyte will also allow for better assessment of adduct formation, chemical modification, and degradation of proteins.

Rapid analytical times, especially for targeted mass ranges, coupled with multiplexed analysis, promise that mature MS-based clinical assays will be faster than most immunoassays. This increased speed comes with reduced processing steps and elimination of ncubation/reaction times prior to analysis. Furthermore, the absence of expensive immunoreagents and/or secondary signal amplification steps will likely realize significant cost savings per assay. As a system MS clinical tests have few barriers to adoption into clinical laboratories.

CURRENT CLINICAL APPLICATIONS OF MS FOR PEPTIDE/PROTEIN ANALYSIS

Currently, routine incorporation of MS in clinical tests for cancer is still rare, generally involving the incorporation of assays that detect co-factorial events such as endocrine/metabolism tests into the cancer diagnostic workflow. In anticipation of increased future demand for MS in the clinic, Waters launched the clinic-ready MassTrak system that has received FDA approval as a medical device. Other mass spectrometer manufacturers, such as Bruker and Shimadzu, are following suit. We summarize below several areas in the spectrum of cancer care where MS-based assays are near clinic ready.

Detection of Opportunistic Infections in Immunosuppressed Cancer Patients

Aggressive chemotherapies associated with the treatment of hematologic cancers are associated with development of immunosuppression. Indeed one of the most common complications associated with the treatment of patients with hematologic cancers is opportunistic infections.[31] Immunosuppressed environments can give rise to invasive bacterial, yeast, and viral infections. A first-line defense in the treatment of these infections is initial identification of the invasive species as treatment strategy depends on species-specific drug susceptibility. Infection with *Aspergillus* should be treated differently than infection with *Candida*. Furthermore, species-specific resistance/sensitivity profiles can be quite distinct necessitating identification of the species or stain level. Serology and subculture approaches are standard clinical methodologies for the identification of infections. However, maturing approaches to detection and quantitation of infectious agents using well-defined MALDI–TOF processes allow for the accurate identification of yeast and bacterial species. The approach depends upon a species/strain-specific expression pattern derived from either whole organism lysates or chemo-physical selective extracts. The methodology can be very rapid, cost effective, and highly specific.[32,33] The instrumentation cost is moderate and reagents cost extremely low pushing overall assay cost well below standard culture-based assays. In addition, a single run can often provide a view of the infectious population with simultaneous identification of multiple species.

Quantitating Exposure to Carcinogens via Albumin Adduct Formation

The dietary mycotoxin aflatoxin B1 is a known liver carcinogen and exposure to aflatoxin B1 is a prominent risk factor in Asian populations.[34] Mutagenesis by aflatoxin B1 occurs via DNA guanine adducts formation. Coincidently, AFB1 also catalyzes albumin adducts, the quantitation of which is a direct indicator of AFB1 exposure. LC–MS/MS methods that incorporate quantitation by isotope dilution can be used to measure AFB1–albumin adducts. The resulting assay is both a measure of exposure to AFB1 and a biomarker for risk of development of hepatocellular carcinoma. In the appropriate population, such a test could prove useful in liver cancer prognosis.

Detection of Parathyroid Gland Tumors

The production of parathyroid hormone (PTH) is intimately linked to the functional status of the parathyroid gland and increased levels are associated with a variety of disease states, including the presence of parathyroid gland tumors. Exceptionally high level of PTH is a strong indicator of glandular tumors. During normal production of PTH, a 115-amino acid precursor is processed to a 90-amino acid pro-PTH and subsequently into the mature 84-amino acid bioactive peptide.[35] As is often the case with posttranslational processing of peptides, numerous isoforms with unknown biological potential have been observed and there is growing evidence that these alternative isoforms may serve as better disease biomarkers either alone or in multiplex. Although current immunoassays can distinguish between some of the isoforms, these are multifactorial assays that are not able to specifically measure each and/or the ratios of all PTH isoforms. Furthermore, most of the isoforms display undefined cross-reactivity and inter-reactivity, which can lead to imprecise quantitation via standard immunoassay. Mass spectrometry immunoassays (MSIAs) using an antibody to full length PTH and detection with MALDI–TOF as well as stable isotope multiple reaction monitoring approach using triple quadrupole LC–MS/MS methods have been developed that can effectively distinguish and simultaneously measure multiple PTH isoforms.[36] The use of these approaches provides greater specificity and accuracy at dramatically reduced costs and is likely to replace current immunoassays used in the clinic.

Measurement of Thyroglobulin for Determination of Thyroid Cancer Recurrence

Thyroglobulin (Tg) is specifically expressed in the thyroid. Much the way rising levels of prostate-specific antigen are used to monitor recurrence of prostate cancer, following removal of the thyroid, rising Tg signals the recurrence of thyroid cancer.[37] The removal of the thyroid should coincide with low levels of this thyroid-specific protein and thus post-surgery assessment is an important clinical test for recurrence. Although there is an effective immunoassay available for the detection and semiquantitation of Tg, this measurement mode has been impaired by masking of immunodetection by patient-derived anti-thyroglobulin (TgAb). To circumvent the Tg masking by patient-derived TgAb clinical laboratories are looking to LC–MS/MS method for analysis of tryptic fragments of Tg that can provide direct quantitation of total Tg.[38] Again the accuracy, specificity, and lowered costs are strong factors that should drive clinical utility of the mature assay.

FUTURE APPLICATIONS OF MS ANALYSIS OF PROTEIN/PEPTIDE IN THE CLINICAL LABORATORY

Pathology assessments are largely based upon morphology. For instance, the pathologic evaluation of prostate biopsies and prostatectomy specimens has discrete morphological scoring objectives. The Gleason score (GS) system is based exclusively on the architectural pattern of the glands of the prostate tumor.[39,40] GS is one of the most powerful predictors of disease progression for patients with prostrate cancer. However, the predictive value of this system, as with most systems for tumor grading, is greatest in tumors of low (GS4/5) and high (GS8/10) grades. Differences in survival between patients with GS6 and GS7 tumors show clearly that this category of tumors, which is the majority, requires further risk stratification.[41-44] It is believed that these decisions could be best solved with more accurate molecular characterization of the individual's biological samples. In fact, the emerging field of morphoproteomics[45-48] attempts to assemble whole system networks to develop sophisticated approaches, beyond histopathology, that reflect the true heterogeneity of a cancer.

Imaging Mass Spectrometry

Imaging mass spectrometry (IMS), in which MS analysis is rasterized across whole tissue sections, seems well suited to integration within a pathology workflow. There have been many studies that tout the potential for this technique to reveal molecular details that can be mapped to tissue morphology.[45-49] For example, our laboratory employed IMS to specifically map the expression of an endogenous peptide fragment of MEKK2 to prostate tumor.[49] IMS is also amenable to MSIA in which the expression of endogenous tissue molecules can be targeted by antibodies conjugated to ionizable probes.[50,51] In fact, we have recently shown that this tissue-based MSIA can be extended to specific glycan content. We used as probes a class of boronolectin specifically engineered to target the expression of the cancer antigen Sialo-Lewis X.[52] One of the scientific goals of this area of research is multiplexed multimodal mapping of clinical tissue samples to reveal expression patterns that contribute to clinical decision-making. Such mapping efforts go beyond diagnostics/prognostic applications into potential near-real-time assessment of drug delivery and determination of surgical margins.

Desorption Electrospray Ionization

The development of atmospheric desorption approaches such as desorption electrospray ionization (DESI) allows for rapid analysis of unfixed tissues and fluids, a move that brings such methods closer to the clinical operating arena.[53,54] One example of the more interesting developments in this area is the fabrication of a DESI source into a scalpel with the concept of direct analysis of surgically derived ions.[55,56] Clearly, as innovative as these approaches are there is still significant proof-of-concept studies needed. These include both discovery of robust biomarkers of tumor margins as well as demonstration that "molecular" margins are associated with better outcomes than traditional measures of tumor margin.

Reaction Monitoring

Multiple reaction monitoring (MRM) has clearly become the de rigueur for development of protein/peptide-based clinical assays.[57,58] MRM-based methods are poised to replace most chemical tests and immunoassays in the clinic assuming they can demonstrate robust specificity at reduced costs. There have been several recent demonstrations of robust assays that are capable of accurately measuring as many as 40 individual biomarkers[59] with demonstrable reproducibility between laboratories.[60,61] In fact, the clinical laboratories with an eye toward adoption of MRM-MS are focusing on the front-end steps to produce standard operating procedures that retain sufficient sensitivity and specificity prior to MS.

Successful transition of MRM-MS to the clinic can be accelerated through discovery of structural aspects of proteins/peptides that are traditional elusive to standard clinical approaches. For instance, the development and implementation of immunoassays for specific posttranslational modification of proteins have been problematic. We and others have employed modern MRM-MS strategies to comprehensively map and quantitate protein posttranslational modification.[62] The method works well with no front-end preparation for abundant proteins and there are efforts underway to catalog methodologies for MRM-MS analysis of such proteins.[63] However, it is necessary to employ an enrichment step for most low abundance proteins and the effectiveness of these approaches will surely be the threshold for development of clinically useful assays of lower abundance cancer biomarkers. MRM-MS is also effective for the quantification of specific protein glycosylation events, a capability that opens the door for utility of protein-conjugated glycans as biomarkers. The inherent value of such an assay is that there are no antibodies that assess sialic acid in this context and no methods for quantitation that are rapid and robust.[64] It is a realistic expectation that MRM-MS will become a routine clinical assay format.

APPLICATION OF MS TO THE DETECTION OF OTHER BIOMOLECULES

MS techniques are just as applicable to other biomolecules relevant to cancer research, including the analysis of lipids, carbohydrates, nucleic acids, and small molecule/drug metabolites. In general, the same separation and ionization configurations (i.e., MALDI and electrospray) described in the preceding sections are applicable to the analysis of these biomolecules, with specific method modifications (like ETD) introduced based on the chemical properties of the target molecules. In the following paragraphs, how MS is being applied for each of the listed biomolecule classes will be summarized.

Metabolomics and Drug Metabolites

Metabolomics can be broadly described as the measure of the concentration and distribution of endogenous physiological and xenobiotic low-molecular-weight compounds in a tissue or fluids.[65] The majority of endogenous metabolites represent metabolic intermediates and final products of cellular reactions (amino acids, organic acids, carbohydrates, and lipids), as well as their respective catabolic products. The molecular weights of these metabolites are generally in the 100 to 1,200 Da mass ranges, sizes that can be ideal for many MS-based evaluations. In relation to other "omics" approaches, the measure of these metabolic changes in physiologically relevant samples could serve as indicators of altered molecular function like cancer and thus reflect the cumulative effects of altered gene regulation and protein function.[65,66] An additional advantage to the approach is the more finite number of metabolic target molecules relative to the much larger numbers of transcripts and proteins. For analysis of drug metabolites, and particularly for most cancer chemotherapeutic molecules, MS is an ideal approach due to relatively defined nature of drugs and their respective metabolites.

Using MS and nuclear magnetic resonance methods, cumulative metabolomic analyses of tumors have described elevated levels of glycolytic enzymes/metabolism and glutamine utilization (e.g., the Warburg effect[67,68] and increased levels of choline phospholipids[65,69]). These types of changes in tumors, although well described, have been difficult to exploit for diagnostics due to the individual metabolic differences of each organ and how tumors affect specific metabolism, with many changes in lipid, amino acid, citric acid cycle, and nucleotides. The metabolome is also a "moving target" and can vary greatly with each meal, level of physical activity, and therapeutic treatments. Despite these limitations, the abundance of metabolites and relatively low target numbers (thousands) compared with proteins and gene transcripts make these attractive targets for MS-based assays. While global profiling approaches for metabolites are available commercially from companies like Metabolon and in academic research centers, the majority of the cancer metabolome is being characterized by individual laboratories that focus on specific intermediate pathway metabolites and drug metabolism pathways. This broad pipeline has not only spurred interest in employing MS for these approaches but also hindered development of specific metabolic laboratory diagnostic assays due to wide differences in sample procurement, metabolite extraction, sample processing, and instrumentation.[70]

This is also reflected in the MS approaches being taken. Global profiling approaches rely on the use of LC–ESI-MS/MS instruments, increasingly Orbitrap/FTICR-type platforms that allow multidimensional fractionations of complex metabolomes. There are several recent examples of large-scale analysis of the metabolome of tissues and fluids associated with prostate cancer.[66,71] For targeted analysis of smaller defined numbers of metabolites (~5 to 10), or single metabolites, triple quadrupole instruments and MRM methods are the best current options. Analysis of steroid compounds[72] and drug metabolites of tamoxifen[73] is an example of the use of this approach in relation to cancer research. A similar approach is used to monitor dietary intervention compounds, i.e., soy isoflavones.[74] In general, these types of specific analyses are performed in individual laboratories and specialized centers. In the clinical laboratory, in relation to cancer, determination of vitamin D levels in serum and concentration determinations of immunosuppressive drugs are the only metabolite analysis performed routinely in many hospital and commercial diagnostic centers.[70] While there still remains a large gap in moving some of the more specialized analyses into the realm of routine clinical diagnostics for cancer, continued refinements in MS instrumentation, analysis software, and assay development will likely serve to rapidly close this gap.

Phospholipids and Sphingolipids

Lipids in cellular membranes are major determinants of cellular structure and functional activity, and modulations in their composition can have significant impact on carcinogenesis and therapeutic response. Lipids are composed of two main structural classes, namely glycerol phospholipids and sphingosine phospholipids. Diversity in structure is derived from the composition of polar head groups (choline, ethanolamine, serine, and inositol) linked via phosphate to the glycerol or sphingosine backbone and a range of fatty acid molecules of 14 to 22 carbons with different levels of saturated double bonds. For MS analysis, long-established tissue extraction and subcellular fractionation methods are utilized to enrich and separate the hydrophobic lipid compartments from the more hydrophilic cellular components. Following extraction, the lipids can be further fractionated by multiple MS approaches.[75,76] One of these methods, termed shotgun lipidomics, involves direct analysis of the entire lipid extract using multidimensional separations prior to ESI-MS/MS analysis. Extracts can also be readily analyzed by MALDI–TOF profiling with dihydroxybenzoic acid matrix. Ionization is also affected by the saturation and fatty-acid chain length of the lipids and is a function of the total lipid concentration. For any MS approach, ion suppression caused by the most abundant phospholipid species (e.g., phosphatidylcholine) is a major factor in hindering analysis of lower abundant species and frequently necessitates multiple fractionation schemes or specialized extraction methods to enrich specific lipid structural subclasses.[81] Displacement of sodium and potassium counterions is also a consideration, generally done by inclusion of ammonia or lipid-soluble amines.

Bioactive sphingolipids, which include ceramide, glucosylceramide, sphingosine, and sphingosine-1-phosphate, are known effectors of cell proliferation, inflammation, growth arrest, apoptosis, and metastasis in many types of cancers.[77,78] Ceramide, for example, is an important regulator of tumor cell death following exposure to stress stimuli.[77-79] It has been reported that decreases/absence of intracellular ceramide results in resistance to cell death signals[80] and conversely, restoration of intracellular ceramide can cause cancer cells to be resensitized to stress stimuli.[81] Being able to reproducibly measure ceramide metabolites and other lipids thus offers significant diagnostic targets across many cancer types, many of which have not been extensively explored.[82] Individual research laboratories have reported extensive quantitative sphingolipid assays using triple quadrupole instrumentation.[83] The optimization of methods and quantitative analysis aspects of this approach position this platform closer to a direct clinical assay capability.

Carbohydrates and Glycosylation

In this era of different "omics" designations, the study of the role of sugars/carbohydrates and glycoprotein/glycolipid species in cancer research can fall into many categories. Metabolomics encompasses the analysis of sugars involved in energy metabolism, proteomics covers many of the analyses associated with glycoproteins, and likewise lipidomics covers glycolipid species. Specific analysis of glycosylation changes associated with cancer generally focuses on asparagine-linked (N-linked) and serine/threonine-linked (O-linked) glycoproteins from tissues and body fluids. The majority of current FDA-approved tumor markers are glycoproteins or glycan antigens, and it is well documented that malignant transformation and cancer progression result in fundamental changes in the glycosylation patterns of cell surface and secreted glycoproteins.[84-86] Hence, this specific section addresses the MS methods applied to the analysis of the glycan species attached to glycoproteins.

The most common types of structural glycosylation changes associated with cancer include alterations in the levels of different sugar moieties like fucose,[87] sialic acid,[88] polylactosamine or β1,6-GlcNAc branching[89] in N-linked structures. There are also several structural motifs identified as tumor antigen structures, which include Tn and STn antigens[90] in O-linked structures, blood group–related carbohydrate antigens,[91] or Lewis antigens (i.e., sialyl-LeX, sialyl-LeA, and LeY)[85,92,93] in either N-linked or O-linked structures. In trying to analyze these types of glycan changes by MS methods, a decision must be made prior to the experiment on whether to analyze only the glycan moieties, which must be released from the peptide/protein carrier, or the glycopeptides directly. Either approach has different procedures associated with them and which ones to use depend largely on the type of MS platform to be used, which can be electrospray ion trap, MALDI, and triple quadrupole configurations.[94]

An inherent challenge for analyzing complex mixtures of glycopeptides is that the higher collision energies required for efficient peptide fragmentation destroy the sugar constituents. Conversely, lower collision energies that fragment the carbohydrates efficiently do not fragment the peptide components. Thus, many experimental factors are associated with the MS analysis of glycans and glycopeptides.[95] The complete structural analysis of most glycan structures is feasible by multiple MS approaches singly and in combination. Definitive structural determinations that include anomeric linkages between constituent sugars require significant amounts of material and multiple methodologies to accomplish.[96] While potentially important to cancer biology, these approaches are not amenable to diagnostic assay development. In this regard, glycopeptide-based approaches using triple quadrupole MS, and newer fragmentation options like high-energy collisional dissociation (HCD) and ETD, are emerging as the methods most amenable to future clinical assay development.

The analysis of glycoproteins for carbohydrate compositions generally requires digestion with proteases to generate complex mixtures of peptides and glycopeptides. These mixtures can still be effectively evaluated with collision-induced fragmentation approaches that rely on identifying specific diagnostic fragment ions in the MS mode (without precursor selection) or MS/MS mode (with precursor selection). The most common marker ions derived from glycopeptides in CID are oxonium ions of *m/z* 204 (*N*-acetylhexosamine), *m/z* 366 (hexose + *N*-acetylhexosamine), and *m/z* 292 (sialic acid). In particular, the marker ion at *m/z* 204 has been shown to be indicative for both *N*-glycans and *O*-glycans.[94] Scanning for these diagnostic fragment ions has been classically performed on triple quadrupole mass spectrometers in the precursor-ion scanning mode. Incorporation of the more refined fragmentation patterns following ETD and HCD methods offers the potential to develop deconvolution software programs that can accurately identify both structural details of peptide and glycan constituents. For glycan analysis related to cancer diagnostics, there remains a great need for standardization of sample preparation techniques, optimization of clinical sample choices, and improvements in MS and software analysis workflows.

Oligonucleotides

There is a long history of the application of MALDI-TOF-MS in the analysis of single-nucleotide polymorphisms (SNPs), cytosine methylation, oligonucleotides for quality control purposes, and other applications involving polymerase chain reaction–amplified products.[97-100] In relation to cancer diagnostics and other related applications, this is still an area of promise and emerging research strategies. Two main structural factors hinder oligonucleotide analysis by MALDI–TOF: the depurination of bases after protonation and the large net negative charge of the sugar–phosphate backbones for sodium and potassium counterions.[97] These factors significantly affect peak resolution and cumulatively limit the size of DNA oligomers to be analyzed to no more than 50 bases. Solutions like use of ammonium salts to block counterion affinities[101] and chemical modifications have addressed the major issues. Multiplexed targeting of specific SNP sequences is currently the most prevalent use of the approach with well-defined methodologies,[102] and commercial platforms exist for these types of studies via Sequenom and Bruker Daltonics. As the immense amount of cancer genetic data becomes vetted to more refined groups of target sequences, it is likely that MALDI–TOF-based SNP and methylation analytical assays will become more widely available.

PERCEIVED BOTTLENECKS TO CLINICAL IMPLEMENTATION OF MS

The discovery rate for biomarkers, for which validation has demonstrated strong clinical utility, is quite slow. This limitation to biomarker development is obviously not circumvented by MS, as it is not a technological barrier but rather a process deficiency. The discovery of biomarkers uniquely accessed by MS will assist in the movement of MS-based methods to the clinic and ultimately the clinical validation of novel MS-based biomarker assays will usher through clinical acceptance of the methodology. The validation pipeline and approval process for antibodies is proven and tested whereas many aspects of MS-based assays are either being developed or being evaluated in clinical laboratories.

Significant hurdles in the development pipeline for MS-based diagnostic assays are standardization of sample acquisition and processing. Just as was done for clinical immunoassays, MS-based approaches will need to become kits with process standards, quality control steps, portability reference standards, normalization protocols, and all other associated elements of robust clinical assays. Pipeline standards for sample collection, front-end processing to either enrich or "cleanup" the analytes, and throughput improvements are all required. Imaginative and simple solutions to clinical sample acquisition are being examined for inclusion into MS assay workflows. For instance, ionization directly from sterile wooden tips (commonly used in the clinic) saturated with sample is likely to facilitate acquisition of a wide range of patient samples.[103] Likewise because of the heavy reliance of MRM on immune-based enrichment of protein targets, stable rapid solid-phase immunoassay platforms are being integrated into the workflow. For instance, carcinoembryonic antigen (CEA) is a well-established and important cancer biomarker for which a recent nanoparticle-based immunoassay chip combined with a plasma MS readout was described.[104] This system's promise lies in the replacement of current CEA assays with one that is cheaper, faster, and more reproducible. Ultimately, MS-based diagnostic assays for cancer biomarkers will move forward when and if they fill a clinically relevant need. This need can be as easily driven by cost and performance as by the novelty of the biomarker.

REFERENCES

1. Karas M, Hillenkamp F. Laser desorption ionization of proteins with molecular masses exceeding 10,000 daltons. *Anal Chem.* 1988;60:2299-2301.
2. Wada Y, Tamura J, Musselman BD, Kassel DB, Sakurai T, Matsuo T. Electrospray ionization mass spectra of hemoglobin and transferrin by a magnetic sector mass spectrometer. Comparison with theoretical isotopic distributions. *Rapid Commun Mass Spectrom.* January 1992;6(1):9-13.
3. Fenn JB, Mann M, Meng CK, Wong SF, Whitehouse CM. Electrospray ionization for mass spectrometry of large biomolecules. *Science.* 1989;246:64-71.
4. Anderson NL, Anderson NG. Proteome and proteomics: new technologies, new concepts, and new words. *Electrophoresis.* 1998;19:1853-1861.
5. Aebersold R, Mann M. Element-coded affinity tags for peptides and proteins. *Nature.* 2003;422:198-207.
6. Meuzelaar HL, Kistemaker PG, Posthumus MA. Recent advances in pyrolysis mass spectrometry of complex biological materials. *Biomed Mass Spectrom.* October 1974;1(5):312-319.
7. Fenselau C, Liberato DJ, Yergey JA, Cotter RJ, Yergey AL. Comparison of thermospray and fast atom bombardment mass spectrometry as solution-dependent ionization techniques. *Anal Chem.* December 1984;56(14):2759-2762.
8. Hardin ED, Vestal ML. Direct comparison of secondary ion and laser desorption mass spectrometry on bioorganic molecules in a moving belt liquid chromatography/mass spectrometry system. *Anal Chem.* 1981;53:1492-1497.
9. Alexander AJ, Kebarle P, Fuciarelli AF, Raleigh JA. Characterization of radiation-induced damage to polyadenylic acid using high-performance liquid chromatography/tandem mass spectrometry. *Anal Chem.* October 1987;59(20): 2484-2491.
10. Smith RD, Wahl JH, Light-Wahl KJ, Winger BE. New developments in microscale separations and mass spectrometry for biomonitoring: capillary electrophoresis and electrospray ionization mass spectrometry. *J Toxicol Environ Health.* October-November 1993;40(2-3):147-158.
11. Yates JR. Mass spectral analysis in proteomics. *Annu Rev Biophys Biomol Struct.* 2004;33:297-316.
12. Domon B, Aebersold R. Mass spectrometry and protein analysis. *Science.* 2006;312:212-217.
13. Liu J, Cooks RG, Ouyang Z. Biological tissue diagnostics using needle biopsy and spray ionization mass spectrometry. *Anal Chem.* December 2011;83(24):9221-9225.
14. Comisarow MB, Marshall AG. The early development of Fourier transform ion cyclotron resonance (FT-ICR) spectroscopy. *J Mass Spectrom.* 1996;31:581-585.
15. Mize TH, Amster IJ. Broad-band ion accumulation with an internal source MALDI-FTICR-MS. *Anal Chem.* December 2000;72(24):5886-5891.
16. Scigelova M, Hornshaw M, Giannakopulos A, Makarov A. Fourier transform mass spectrometry. *Mol Cell Proteomics.* 2011;10:9431-9438.
17. Makarov A. Electrostatic axially harmonic orbital trapping: a high-performance technique of mass analysis. *Anal Chem.* 2000;72:1156-1162.
18. Johnson RS, Martin SA, Biemann K, Stults JT, Watson JT. Novel fragmentation process of peptides by collision-induced decomposition in a tandem mass spectrometer: differentiation of leucine and isoleucine. *Anal Chem.* 1987;59:2621-2625.
19. McLafferty FW, Kelleher NL, Begley TP, Fridriksson EK, Zubarev RA, Horn DM. Two-dimensional mass spectrometry of biomolecules at the subfemtomole level. *Curr Opin Chem Biol.* October 1998;2(5):571-578. Review.
20. Zubarev R. Protein primary structure using orthogonal fragmentation techniques in Fourier transform mass spectrometry. *Expert Rev Proteomics.* 2006;3(2):251-261.
21. Shi SD, Hemling ME, Carr SA, Horn DM, Lindh I, McLafferty FW. Phosphopeptide/phosphoprotein mapping by electron capture dissociation mass spectrometry. *Anal Chem.* 2001;73:19-22.
22. Zabrouskov V, Whitelegge JP. Increased coverage in the transmembrane domain with activated-ion electron capture dissociation for top–down Fourier-transform mass spectrometry of integral membrane proteins. *J Proteome Res.* 2007;6: 2205-2210.
23. Ge Y, Lawhorn BG, ElNaggar M, et al. Top down characterization of larger proteins (45 kDa) by electron capture dissociation mass spectrometry. *J Am Chem Soc.* 2002;124:672-678.
24. Syka JEP, Coon JJ, Schroeder MJ, Shabanowitz J, Hunt DF. Peptide and protein sequence analysis by electron transfer dissociation mass spectrometry. *Proc Natl Acad Sci U S A.* 2004;101:9528-9533.
25. Pitteri SJ, Chrisman PA, Hogan JM, McLuckey SA. Electron transfer ion/ion reactions in a three-dimensional quadrupole ion trap: reactions of doubly and triply protonated peptides with $SO_2^{\bullet-}$. *Anal Chem.* 2005;77:1831-1839.
26. Good DM, Wirtala M, McAlister GC, Coon JJ. Performance characteristics of electron transfer dissociation mass spectrometry. *Mol Cell Proteomics.* 2007;6:1942-1951.
27. Coon JJ, Ueberheide B, Syka JEP, et al. Protein identification using sequential ion/ion reactions and tandem mass spectrometry. *Proc Natl Acad Sci U S A.* 2005;102:9463-9468.
28. Chi A, Bai DL, Geer LY, Shabanowitz J, Hunt DF. Analysis of intact proteins on a chromatographic time scale by electron transfer dissociation tandem mass spectrometry. *Int J Mass Spectrom.* 2007;259:197-203.
29. Chi A, Huttenhower C, Geer LY, et al. Analysis of phosphorylation sites on proteins from *Saccharomyces cerevisiae* by electron transfer dissociation (ETD) mass spectrometry. *Proc Natl Acad Sci U S A.* 2007;104:2193-2198.
30. Catalina MI, Koeleman CAM, Deelder AM, Wuhrer M. Electron transfer dissociation of *N*-glycopeptides: loss of the entire *N*-glycosylated asparagine side chain. *Rapid Commun Mass Spectrom.* 2007;21:1053-1061.
31. O'Brien MM, Donaldson SS, Balise RR, Whittemore AS, Link MP. Second malignant neoplasms in survivors of pediatric Hodgkin's lymphoma treated with low-dose radiation and chemotherapy. *J Clin Oncol.* 2010;28:1232-1239.
32. Bader O, Weig M, Taverne-Ghadwal L, Lugert R, Gross U, Kuhns M. Improved clinical laboratory identification of human pathogenic yeasts by matrix-assisted laser desorption ionization time-of-flight mass spectrometry. *Clin Microbiol Infect.* 2011;17:1359-1365.
33. De Carolis E, Posteraro B, Lass-Flörl C, et al. Species identification of *Aspergillus*, *Fusarium* and *Mucorales* with direct surface analysis by matrix-assisted laser desorption ionization time-of-flight mass spectrometry. *Clin Microbiol Infect.* 2011; 18:475-484.
34. Kensler TW, Qian G-S, Chen J-G, Groopman JD. Translational strategies for cancer prevention in liver. *Nat Rev Cancer.* 2003;3:321-329.
35. Kumar V, Barnidge DR, Chen L-S, et al. Quantification of serum 1–84 parathyroid hormone in patients with hyperparathyroidism by immunocapture in situ digestion liquid chromatography–tandem mass spectrometry. *Clin Chem.* 2010;56:306-313.
36. Bystrom CE. The analysis of native proteins and peptides in the clinical lab using mass spectrometry. *Clin Lab Med.* 2011;31:397-405.
37. Pelttari H, Välimäki MJ, Löyttyniemi E, Schalin-Jäntti C. Post-ablative serum thyroglobulin is an independent predictor of recurrence in low-risk differentiated thyroid carcinoma: a 16-year follow-up study. *Eur J Endocrinol.* 2010;163:757-763.
38. Hoofnagle AN, Becker JO, Wener MH, Heinecke JW. Quantification of thyroglobulin, a low-abundance serum protein, by immunoaffinity peptide enrichment and tandem mass spectrometry. *Clin Chem.* 2008;54:1796-1804.

39. Egevad L. Recent trends in Gleason grading of prostate cancer: I. Pattern interpretation. *Anal Quant Cytol Histol*. 2008;30: 190-198.
40. Egevad L. Recent trends in Gleason grading of prostate cancer. II. Prognosis, reproducibility and reporting. *Anal Quant Cytol Histol*. 2008;30:254-260.
41. Freedland SJ. Screening, risk assessment, and the approach to therapy in patients with prostate cancer. *Cancer*. 2011;117: 1123-1135.
42. Pinthus JH, Witkos M, Fleshner NE, et al. Prostate cancers scored as Gleason 6 on prostate biopsy are frequently Gleason 7 tumors at radical prostatectomy: implication on outcome. *J Urol*. 2006;176:979-984; discussion 984.
43. Kattan MW, Potters L, Blasko JC, et al. Pretreatment nomogram for predicting freedom from recurrence after permanent prostate brachytherapy in prostate cancer. *Urology*. 2001;58:393-399.
44. Lughezzani G, Briganti A, Karakiewicz PI, et al. Predictive and prognostic models in radical prostatectomy candidates: a critical analysis of the literature. *Eur Urol*. 2010;58:687-700.
45. Liu J, Brown RE. Morphoproteomics demonstrates activation of mammalian target of rapamycin pathway in papillary thyroid carcinomas with nuclear translocation of MTOR in aggressive histological variants. *Mod Pathol*. 2011;24:1553-1559.
46. Brown RE. Morphoproteomics: exposing protein circuitries in tumors to identify potential therapeutic targets in cancer patients. *Expert Rev Proteomics*. 2005;2:337-348.
47. Tan D. Morphoproteomics: a novel approach to identify potential therapeutic targets in cancer patients. *Int J Clin Exp Pathol*. 2008;1:331-332.
48. Brown RE. Morphogenomics and morphoproteomics: a role for anatomic pathology in personalized medicine. *Arch Pathol Lab Med*. 2009;133:568-579.
49. Cazares LH, Troyer D, Mendrinos S, et al. Imaging mass spectrometry of a specific fragment of mitogen-activated protein kinase/extracellular signal-regulated kinase kinase kinase 2 discriminates cancer from uninvolved prostate tissue. *Clin Cancer Res*. 2009;15:5541-5551.
50. Lemaire R, Stauber J, Wisztorski M, et al. Tag-mass: specific molecular imaging of transcriptome and proteome by mass spectrometry based on photocleavable tag. *J Proteome Res*. 2007;6:2057-2067.
51. Thiery G, Shchepinov MS, Southern EM, et al. Multiplex target protein imaging in tissue sections by mass spectrometry—TAMSIM. *Rapid Commun Mass Spectrom*. 2007;21:823-829.
52. Dai C, Cazares LH, Wang L, et al. Using boronolectin in MALDI-MS imaging for the histological analysis of cancer tissue expressing the sialyl Lewis X antigen. *Chem Commun (Camb)*. 2011;47:10338-10340.
53. Cooks RG, Manicke NE, Dill AL, et al. New ionization methods and miniature mass spectrometers for biomedicine: DESI imaging for cancer diagnostics and paper spray ionization for therapeutic drug monitoring. *Faraday Discuss*. 2011;149:247-267; discussion 333-356.
54. Eberlin LS, Liu X, Ferreira CR, Santagata S, Agar NYR, Cooks RG. Desorption electrospray ionization then MALDI mass spectrometry imaging of lipid and protein distributions in single tissue sections. *Anal Chem*. 2011;83:8366-8371.
55. Schäfer K-C, Szaniszló T, Günther S, et al. In situ, real-time identification of biological tissues by ultraviolet and infrared laser desorption ionization mass spectrometry. *Anal Chem*. 2011;83:1632-1640.
56. Schäfer K-C, Balog J, Szaniszló T, et al. Real time analysis of brain tissue by direct combination of ultrasonic surgical aspiration and sonic spray mass spectrometry. *Anal Chem*. 2011;83:7729-7735.
57. Grebe SK, Singh RJ. LC–MS/MS in the clinical laboratory—where to from here? *Clin Biochem Rev*. 2011;32:5-31.
58. Strathmann FG, Hoofnagle AN. Current and future applications of mass spectrometry to the clinical laboratory. *Am J Clin Pathol*. 2011;136:609-616.
59. Rezeli M, Végvári A, Fehniger TE, Laurell T, Marko-Varga G. Moving towards high density clinical signature studies with a human proteome catalogue developing multiplexing mass spectrometry assay panels. *J Clin Bioinforma*. 2011;1:7.
60. Addona TA, Abbatiello SE, Schilling B, et al. Multi-site assessment of the precision and reproducibility of multiple reaction monitoring-based measurements of proteins in plasma. *Nat Biotechnol*. 2009;27:633-641.
61. Whiteaker JR, Zhao L, Abbatiello SE, et al. Evaluation of large scale quantitative proteomic assay development using peptide affinity-based mass spectrometry. *Mol Cell Proteomics*. 2011;10:M110.005645.
62. Guo X, Ward MD, Tiedebohl JB, Oden YM, Nyalwidhe JO, Semmes OJ. Interdependent phosphorylation within the kinase domain T-loop regulates CHK2 activity. *J Biol Chem*. 2010;285:33348-33357.
63. Domanski D, Smith DS, Miller CA, et al. High-flow multiplexed MRM-based analysis of proteins in human plasma without depletion or enrichment. *Clin Lab Med*. 2011;31:371-384.
64. Zhao Y, Jia W, Wang J, Ying W, Zhang Y, Qian X. Fragmentation and site-specific quantification of core fucosylated glycoprotein by multiple reaction monitoring-mass spectrometry. *Anal Chem*. 2011;83:8802-8809.
65. Spratlin JL, Serkova NJ, Eckhardt SG. Clinical applications of metabolomics in oncology: a review. *Clin Cancer Res*. 2009;15:431-440.
66. Trock BJ. Application of metabolomics to prostate cancer. *Urol Oncol*. 2011;29:572-581.
67. Koppenol WH, Bounds PL, Dang CV. Otto Warburg's contributions to current concepts of cancer metabolism. *Nat Rev Cancer*. 2011;11:325-337.
68. Vander Heiden MG, Cantley LC, Thompson CB. Understanding the Warburg effect: the metabolic requirements of cell proliferation. *Science*. 2009;324:1029-1033.
69. Griffin JL, Shockcor JP. Metabolic profiles of cancer cells. *Nat Rev Cancer*. 2004;4:551-561.
70. Grant RP. High throughput automated LC–MS/MS analysis of endogenous small molecule biomarkers. *Clin Lab Med*. 2011;31:429-441.
71. Sreekumar A, Poisson LM, Rajendiran TM, et al. Metabolomic profiles delineate potential role for sarcosine in prostate cancer progression. *Nature*. 2009;457:910-914.
72. Kushnir MM, Rockwood AL, Roberts WL, Yue B, Bergquist J, Meikle AW. Liquid chromatography tandem mass spectrometry for analysis of steroids in clinical laboratories. *Clin Biochem*. 2011;44:77-88.
73. Teunissen SF, Rosing H, Seoane MD, et al. Investigational study of tamoxifen phase I metabolites using chromatographic and spectroscopic analytical techniques. *J Pharm Biomed Anal*. 2011;55:518-526.
74. Twaddle NC, Churchwell MI, Doerge DR. High-throughput quantification of soy isoflavones in human and rodent blood using liquid chromatography with electrospray mass spectrometry and tandem mass spectrometry detection. *J Chromatogr B Analyt Technol Biomed Life Sci*. 2002;777:139-145.
75. Wolf C, Quinn PJ. Lipidomics: practical aspects and applications. *Prog Lipid Res*. 2008;47:15-36.
76. Lee JY, Min HK, Moon MH. Simultaneous profiling of lysophospholipids and phospholipids from human plasma by nanoflow liquid chromatography–tandem mass spectrometry. *Anal Bioanal Chem*. 2011;400:2953-2961.
77. Ogretmen B, Hannun Y. Biologically active sphingolipids in cancer pathogenesis and treatment. *Nat Rev Cancer*. 2004;4: 604-616.
78. Liu X, Cheng JC, Turner LS, et al. Acid ceramidase upregulation in prostate cancer: role in tumor development and implications for therapy. *Expert Opin Ther Targets*. 2009;13:1449-1458.
79. Spiegel S, Milstien S. Functions of the multifaceted family of sphingosine kinases and some close relatives. *J Biol Chem*. 2007;282:2125-2129.
80. Bonnaud S, Niaudet C, Pottier G, et al. Sphingosine-1-phosphate protects proliferating endothelial cells from ceramide-induced apoptosis but not from DNA damage-induced mitotic death. *Cancer Res*. 2007;67:1803-1811.
81. Samsel L, Zaidel G, Drumgoole HM, et al. The ceramide analog, B13, induces apoptosis in prostate cancer cell lines and inhibits tumor growth in prostate cancer xenografts. *Prostate*. 2004;58:382-393.
82. Haynes CA, Allegood JC, Park H, Sullards MC. Sphingolipidomics: methods for the comprehensive analysis of sphingolipids. *J Chromatogr B Analyt Technol Biomed Life Sci*. 2009;877:2696-2708.

83. Bielawski J, Pierce JS, Snider J, Rembiesa B, Szulc ZM, Bielawska A. Comprehensive quantitative analysis of bioactive sphingolipids by high-performance liquid chromatography–tandem mass spectrometry. *Methods Mol Biol.* 2009;579:443-467.
84. Yang L, Nyalwidhe JO, Guo S, Drake RR, Semmes OJ. Targeted identification of metastasis-associated cell-surface sialoglycoproteins in prostate cancer. *Mol Cell Proteomics.* 2011;10:M110.007294.
85. Drake PM, Cho W, Li B, et al. Sweetening the pot: adding glycosylation to the biomarker discovery equation. *Clin Chem.* 2010;56:223-236.
86. Meany DL, Chan DW. Aberrant glycosylation associated with enzymes as cancer biomarkers. *Clin Proteomics.* 2011;8:7.
87. Mehta A, Block TM. Fucosylated glycoproteins as markers of liver disease. *Dis Markers.* 2008;25:259-265.
88. Varki NM, Varki A. Diversity in cell surface sialic acid presentations: implications for biology and disease. *Lab Invest.* 2007;87:851-857.
89. Lau KS, Dennis JW. *N*-Glycans in cancer progression. *Glycobiology.* 2008;18:750-760.
90. Itzkowitz SH, Yuan M, Montgomery CK, et al. Expression of Tn, sialosyl-Tn, and T antigens in human colon cancer. *Cancer Res.* 1989;49:197-204.
91. Ichikawa D, Handa K. Histo-blood group A/B antigen deletion/reduction vs. continuous expression in human tumor cells as correlated with their malignancy. *Int J Cancer.* 1998;76(2):284-289.
92. Nakamori S, Kameyama M, Imaoka S, et al. Increased expression of sialyl Lewisx antigen correlates with poor survival in patients with colorectal carcinoma: clinicopathological and immunohistochemical study. *Cancer Res.* 1993;53:3632-3637.
93. Ugorski M, Laskowska A. Sialyl Lewis(a): a tumor-associated carbohydrate antigen involved in adhesion and metastatic potential of cancer cells. *Acta Biochim Pol.* 2002;49:303-311.
94. Wuhrer M, Catalina MI, Deelder AM, Hokke CH. Glycoproteomics based on tandem mass spectrometry of glycopeptides. *J Chromatogr B Analyt Technol Biomed Life Sci.* 2007;849:115-128.
95. Wuhrer M, Deelder AM, van der Burgt YEM. Mass spectrometric glycan rearrangements. *Mass Spectrom Rev.* 2011;30:664-680.
96. Stumpo KA, Reinhold VN. The *N*-glycome of human plasma. *J Proteome Res.* 2010;9:4823-4830.
97. Gut IG. DNA analysis by MALDI-TOF mass spectrometry. *Hum Mutat.* 2004;23:437-441.
98. Corona G, Toffoli G. High throughput screening of genetic polymorphisms by matrix-assisted laser desorption ionization time-of-flight mass spectrometry. *Comb Chem High Throughput Screen.* 2004;7:707-725.
99. Jurinke C, Denissenko M, Oeth P, Ehrich M, van den Boom D, Cantor C. A single nucleotide polymorphism based approach for the identification and characterization of gene expression modulation using MassARRAY. *Mutat Res-Fund Mol M.* 2005;573:83-95.
100. Ding C, Cantor CR. A high-throughput gene expression analysis technique using competitive PCR and matrix-assisted laser desorption ionization time-of-flight MS. *Proc Natl Acad Sci U S A.* 2003;100:3059-3064.
101. Pieles U, Zürcher W, Schär M, Moser HE. Matrix-assisted laser desorption ionization time-of-flight mass spectrometry: a powerful tool for the mass and sequence analysis of natural and modified oligonucleotides. *Nucleic Acids Res.* 1993;21:3191-3196.
102. Sauer S, Reinhardt R, Lehrach H, Gut IG. Single-nucleotide polymorphisms: analysis by mass spectrometry. *Nat Protoc.* 2006;1:1761-1771.
103. Hu B, So P-K, Chen H, Yao Z-P. Electrospray ionization using wooden tips. *Anal Chem.* 2011;83:8201-8207.
104. Chen B, Hu B, Jiang P, He M, Peng H, Zhang X. Nanoparticle labelling-based magnetic immunoassay on chip combined with electrothermal vaporization-inductively coupled plasma mass spectrometry for the determination of carcinoembryonic antigen in human serum. *Analyst.* 2011;136:3934-3942.

CHAPTER 12

CANCER PROTEOMICS

Kristin Huntoon and Zhengping Zhuang

INTRODUCTION

In the post-genomic era of science, the capacity to discover new molecular targets for therapy, biomarkers for early detection, and cutoff points for therapeutic interventions rests in the field of proteomics. Since most biological functions are orchestrated and catalyzed by proteins, designing novel therapeutic interventions that target these molecules with the aid of proteomics could lead to major insights. Moreover, in patients with cancer, patient-specific targeted therapies are the gold standard to which clinicians strive, and proteomics can enable the design and optimization of such therapies by direct analysis of patients' tumor tissue or even their blood. Proteomics can be used to identify biomarkers that not only aid in diagnosis but also assist in clinical management by allowing for the early detection of clinically silent lesions, by better defining subtypes of disease, and by predicting or monitoring response to treatment.[1-3] Furthermore, proteomics has the potential to resolve many long-standing basic questions about the mechanisms and pathogenesis of highly heterogeneous and complex diseases such as cancer.

The rapid pace of developments in the field of proteomics has largely been associated with advancements in comprehensive sequence databases, instrumentation, techniques, methodologies, and integrative software. The term *proteome* was first coined by Wilkins and Williams to describe the protein complement of the genome of a cell in the mid-1990s.[4] As we understand it now, the proteome has a greater scope, offering complementary information not only about the genome but also about the epigenome and transcriptome, making it an attractive collection of data encompassing various levels of interacting material. In general, the term *proteomics* describes "any large scale protein-based systematic analysis of the entire proteome or a defined sub-proteome from a cell, tissue, or entire organism."[5] Although the genome is the entire set of genetic instructions, the proteome is orders of magnitude more complex than the genome because the proteome includes processes such as splicing, posttranslational modifications, protein degradation, acetylation, and phosphorylation that are associated with drug perturbations and disease. Furthermore, differences in protein abundance within the cell vary greatly, and the difficulty encountered in identifying less abundant proteins remains a challenge.

Unlike the genome, the proteome is dynamic. The proteome exerts temporal and spatial control in response to cellular or environmental factors. This makes the study of proteomics the gateway to functional genomics and ultimately to functional biology. Due to the reasons already listed, researchers typically use the tools of proteomics to study the proteome of a given sample under well-defined conditions, and the results are compared with another condition, species, tumor, or stage. Functional correlations can be drawn in determining not only the identity and quantity of the protein but also the amount of protein modification, interaction, and subcellular localization. Such functional correlations complicate protein analysis. In addition, perfecting the separation of proteins on the basis of localization, addressing the intrinsic hydrophobic and hydrophilic nature of protein, and maintaining protein stability are all part of balancing the convoluted conditions that have been defined over time and continue to be improved upon.

The advances that are the product of proteomics have yielded new diagnostic techniques and therapeutic targets of disease and have offered a more comprehensive insight into biological processes. With further maturation and optimization of the current technology and additional incentivized tools, new platforms of proteomics will continue to drive dramatic advances in biological and disease processes.

SAMPLE PREPARATION/SELECTIVE TISSUE DISSECTION

To ensure that a quality sample is obtained for analysis, maintaining the purity of the initial specimen is absolutely necessary. This is especially true in tissue samples, for which a selective dissection is required to limit any heterogeneity or contamination of tissue from other structures, cell lineages, or disease. Tissue biopsy specimens are plagued by the fact that they contain many different cell types, particularly in diseases states in which the sample may contain a small number of abnormal cells in close proximity to a large area of healthy unaffected tissue. Some of the techniques currently used in sample preparation are subcellular fraction, selective tissue microdissection, and laser capture microdissection (discussed later in this section).

Fine needle microdissection is another sectioning technique that is gaining in popularity. The technique, which increases the integrity of the protein sample, is rather simple. Specifically, after histological examination, areas of interest are identified and microdissected with a microdissector under the microscope using tissue margins as a guide for the purity of the sample. These samples can be preserved and microdissected with various fixative methods, including paraffin embedding and fresh freezing.[6,7]

Laser capture microdissection allows the selective dissection of tissue with a laser that activates a transfer film to adhere to specific cells of interest that have been identified in a specimen by microscopy. This method allows for greater specificity by limiting the collection of any undesirable tissue or cell.[8,9] A shortcoming of this technique results from the denaturation of proteins, and thus the quantity of pure sample may be lacking. The laser microdissection technique provides more accurate targeting and easier operation than existing needle microdissection techniques do, especially when genetic analyses such as chromosomal analysis or loss of heterozygosity analysis are being performed.[8]

Isolation of subcellular compartments requires both mechanical and chemical disruption of the cell in order to isolate a particular fraction of high-yield material devoid of contaminating structures. Lysing of the cells with ultracentrifugation, along with centrifugation at various speeds and in several different density solutions, permits characteristic separation of various organelles while preserving the natural conformation of the protein of interest.[10] However, this labor-intensive technique requires large volumes of specimen, which is often impractical, especially in clinical settings.[11]

Taking these concepts one step forward is the process of analyzing slices of tissues directly with a coupled mass spectrometry (MS), a process termed *in situ proteomics*. Since spatial distribution is maintained, this process allows for the comparison of specific molecules and proteins without the loss of the pathologic architecture for further comparisons to be extrapolated. The sections are frozen and immobilized onto a matrix (sinapinic acid)-assisted laser desorption/ionization–time-of-flight (MALDI-TOF) target plate. A matrix solution containing H_2O/acetonitrile/trifluoroacetic acid is applied to the tissue surface to generate a homogeneous crystal field, which contains co-crystallized proteins. An initial survey scan profile is taken with data acquisition randomly across the section, generating a "molecular image" for every point that is descriptive of the specific molecules in that particular point in the tissue.[12]

In addition to preventing contamination of tissue or cells, other concerns in sample preparation include protecting the protein from proteases, retaining the original posttranslational modifications, and preventing solubilization of all proteins in the tissue sample. Methylation, acetylation, and phosphorylation can be inferred by the observation of common mass shifts (+14, +42, +80, respectively).[13] Mass shifts due to glycosylation are much more difficult to determine because these shifts involve more than several hundred daltons and a combination of sugar residues, the most common being GalNAc and GlcNAc, resulting in an increase of up to 203 Da.[14] Most of these items may be optimized with the use of specific buffers, conditions, and processing, but care should be taken to ensure that the protein(s) remains in its full, processed, natural in vivo state.

SEPARATION AND DETECTION METHODS

There are two typical proteomic approaches that utilize a mixture of common technologies. In the first approach, proteins are isolated in highly concentrated urea buffer and then undergo separation by 2D gel electrophoresis. Protein can be visualized by Coomassie, silver, or fluorescence stain, which enables detailed analysis of any spots of interest. These so-called spots of interest are defined primarily by differential proteomics, i.e., an absent or present spot compared with stage, differentiation, treatment, age, cell type, etc., between two or more samples. These spots of interest are excised from the gel and digested with trypsin; the resulting peptide residues are eluted, extracted, and purified from the gel. The peptide residues are analyzed by using mass spectrometer(s), and the data that are generated are compared with a host of trypsin digests of peptide sequences derived in silico from RNA/DNA sequences and protein databases. If a generated peptide contains a certain level of similarity to a peptide sequence obtained in the database, the identity of the protein can be determined.

The second proteomic approach again involves isolating the protein in a concentrated urea buffer. In this case, however, digestion with trypsin occurs before any separation. An extensive mixture of peptides is separated into 7 to 12 fractions according to their respective charge when placed in an acidic environment with the use of a high-pressure/performance liquid chromatography (HPLC) column. After the charge separation, each fraction is subjected to a reverse-phase separation, according to the hydrophobic properties of the fraction in the buffers of changing polarities. This separation is performed in such a way that temporal elutions from the HPLC are directly analyzed by an in-line mass spectrometer, in which the more hydrophobic elutions are retained and are the last eluted. In addition, HPLC is commonly applied before MS to enrich the protein of interest. As with the first approach, the peptides are compared with an in silico–derived database of peptide sequences to determine the identity of the precursor protein.

Traditionally, almost all proteomic analysis was gel-based in the separation of either intact or digested forms of protein, primarily due to the fact that gels allow for highly reproducible, well-defined protein separation with sensitive detection. High-resolution 2D gel electrophoresis—a two-step separation process involving both isoelectrical focusing (IEF) and sodium dodecyl sulfate–polyacrylamide gel electrophoresis (SDS-PAGE)—is applied. IEF separates proteins on the basis of various charges, allowing the detection of differing peptides and proteins as well as charge isoforms of the same protein, thus deciphering phosphorylated versus unphosphorylated protein. The pH gradient to separate the proteins can be performed by either a mobile or an immobile pH gradient. In the mobile gradient, the protein sample is applied to a glass tube that has various ampholytes buffering an SDS-PAGE gel. Once an electrical current is applied, the proteins migrate according to their pK_a, with the acidic substances migrating fastest toward the anode (+ pole) and the basic substances migrating in the opposite direction. Immobilized pH gradients are much more robust and stable. Here, the gradient is determined by a mixture of immobilines that covalently attach to acrylamide, making the system much more reproducible.

SDS-PAGE separation is a guiding principle of proteomics. SDS denatures the 3D structure of the proteins, and the polyacrylamide acts as a mesh to further separate the proteins on the basis of size, i.e., molecular weight (number of amino acids). With use of a standard marker of defined size, the apparent weight can be determined on the basis of the extent of migration corresponding to the marker proteins. When SDS-PAGE is used in 2D gel electrophoresis after IEF, equilibration from a urea-based buffer system to an SDS buffer system must be performed to maintain the proper oxidation state of each residue.

On completion of the 2D gel electrophoresis, visualization of the resolved proteins/peptides may be performed. However, due to the nature of the gel, fixation is required to ensure that the proteins maintain their position and do not diffuse. Staining can be accomplished with multiple agents, including Coomassie, silver, zinc, or fluorescent protein stain; radioactive detection strategies can be used as well. The techniques that are used depend on gel thickness, spot or band size, amount of protein detectable, and other variables. The pitfalls and advantages of each staining agent, the final use of the stained proteins, and the information that the user wants to obtain all need to be carefully considered (Fig. 12.1).

Regardless of the staining method used, 2D gel images need to be digitized for further analyses. With more than 2,000 spots per gel and multiple different samples to compare, even a well-trained eye could miss key spots of interest. There are various methods for digitizing gels, but many researchers use a phosphorimager or flatbed scanner. Once the 2D gel image is digitized, software can be used to construct a normalized *x*- and *y*-axis grid system for comparing the 2D pattern of spots and determining spots of interest in the samples.

MASS SPECTROSCOPY

One of the core technologies that is a cornerstone of proteomics is MS. The guiding principle of spectrometry is that molecules can be ionized and separated on the basis of their intrinsic mass-to-charge ratio. Collectively, the results yield information that can be used to determine the molecular weight and structure. The rationale for this technology is that each amino acid has a distinctive molecular weight, which in turn gives each peptide a

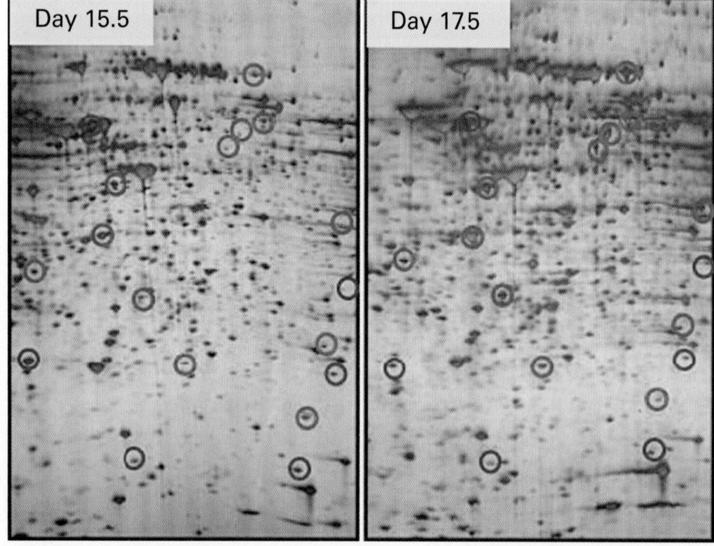

FIGURE 12–1 Two-dimensional gel electrophoresis of microdissected embryo liver tissue comparing Day 12.5 and Day 17.5. The red circles denote protein that increases in intensity in the Day 17.5 sample, whereas the blue circles denote protein that decreases in intensity in the Day 17.5 sample compared with the Day 12.5 tissue.

characteristic molecular weight. This information is then used to decipher the sequence of amino acids in a peptide or protein. This technology can also aid in elucidating protein complex formation, including posttranscriptional modifications, enzyme–substrate binding, and antigen–antibody or orphan–receptor interactions.

Two major types of devices are commonly used for ionization in proteomics—electrospray ionization (ESI) and MALDI. The coupling of ESI with liquid chromatography/HPLC has revolutionized the separation and identification of proteins and peptides, although a recent version of ESI, called *nanospray ionization* because of its smaller volume of liquid and smaller ionized droplets, is gaining in popularity. Instead of a flow system, MALDI is a solid-state technique in which a laser vaporizes a mixture of sample and matrix that has been spotted and dried on a metal target plate, making the re-analysis of previous samples a trial task. However, one advantage of ESI over MALDI is its ability to analyze larger proteins.[15] This gel-free separation—sometimes referred to as *hyphenated technology*—has become the mainstay in the proteomics field since early 2000.

The determination of the molecular mass of peptides can be made either by proteolysis, called "bottom-up" spectroscopy, or by measurement of intact proteins, called "top-down" spectroscopy. Neither of these methods is mutually exclusive; in reality, they are quite complementary, helping to form a complete picture of the protein. The bottom-up approach is the traditional methodology, first digesting specific enzymes to produce 5 to 20 amino acid fragments. The top-down method begins with intact protein that is fragmented in a high-energy collision. The fragments and remaining intact protein are matched piecewise to known sequences in a database until the identity of the protein is obtained.

BIOINFORMATICS

Proteomics projects have produced enormous quantities of digital information, and researchers are swamped by data-dense digital results. An analytical bottleneck of countless mass spectra, gel images, and chromatograms makes it challenging to decipher meaningful conclusions. One of the initiatives to resolve the multiple MS output formats is the Human Proteome Organization (HUPO) Proteomics Standards Initiative (PSI), which designed mzZL, a single data format.[16] Similarly, standard libraries and databases are being established to harness the information in countless protein fragments. For example, the PRoteomics IDEntifications database (PRIDE, http://www.ebi.ac.uk/pride) at the European Bioinformatics Institute contains 60 species, more than 2.5 million protein identifications, and 11.5 million peptides.[17]

A network needs to be established for all of the proteomics data, especially for diseases such as cancer, which involve perturbations of multiple cross-talking pathways.[1] PROTEOME-3D is one such systematic analysis platform that includes a user-friendly, customized, queryable database of published identified proteins, along with graphical tools to represent the entire proteome landscape, the ability to trend data gathered from multiple large-scale experiments, and an interactive interface to identify and analyze networks and pathways.[18]

PROTEIN CHIP

The field of large-scale high-throughput biology via microarrays has resulted in a new era of technology development and a plethora of analyzable data.[19] This format enables rapid and straightforward parallel detection and side-by-side analyses of countless elements.[20,21] Proteins are more challenging than DNA to prepare for the microarray format, and protein functionality is often dependent on the state of the protein (such as posttranslational modifications, partnership with other proteins, protein subcellular localization, and reversible covalent modifications [e.g., phosphorylation]). The information gathered from these analyses is crucial to understanding many basic cellular events mediating complex processes and those causing disease.[22-25]

With recent advances in protein microarrays, more than 100 proteins and even the entire proteome can be analyzed.[22,23,26-28] Various other formats have seen similar advances, including tissue arrays,[29] living cell arrays,[30,31] peptide arrays,[32-35] antibody/antigen arrays,[36,37] protein arrays,[20,38-41] carbohydrate arrays,[42,43] and small molecule arrays.[40]

In general, there are two major divisions of protein microarrays, analytical and functional. Analytical microarrays are constructed with a high density of their respective reagent, i.e., the antigens or antibody that will be used to detect proteins in a mixture. Functional microarrays are designed by immobilizing large numbers of defined proteins on their surface. Identification of novel drug targets and biochemical activities can easily be addressed with such protein microarrays (Fig. 12.2). In general, protein chips are a simplified, predesigned, rapid-analysis format for relatively less complicated protein samples.

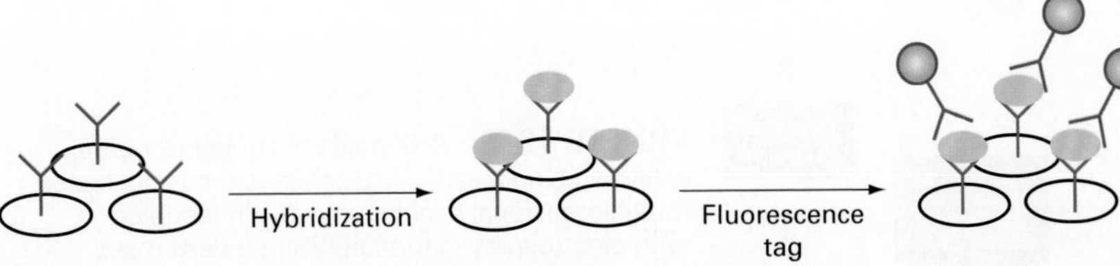

FIGURE 12–2 Schematic of proteomic analysis using a protein chip with antibody-coupled matrix.

SHOTGUN SEQUENCING

Shotgun proteomics is analogous to shotgun sequencing of DNA, in which the material being sequenced is fragmented, and segments that are obtained are aligned according to commonalities until a master sequence is reached. In proteomics, fragments are the product of proteases (such as trypsin). The peptides that are yielded are further separated by 2D chromatography, at which point the peptides are eluted into a tandem mass spectrometer for computational analysis. The introduction of the multidimensional protein identification technology (MudPIT) was essentially the first effective large-scale shotgun proteomics analysis tool.[44-46] This microcapillary column not only has the capacity to identify complex protein mixtures but is also able to detect and identify membrane and low-abundance proteins.[45]

ANALYSIS OF MS/PROTEOMIC DATA

The integration of the proteomics community is essential for the advancement of biomedical research. One example is the Human Protein Atlas, a resource for major relevant research on cancer biomarkers (http://www.proteinatlas.org). This virtual pictorial atlas displays protein expression as immunohistological images of sections obtained from human tissues. In addition, these microscopic view images contain samples from widely used and characterized cell lines, cells from patients with leukemia or lymphoma, and cells from correlative normal cell lines and individuals. In its newest version, this atlas includes information on 15,598 antibodies and contains a total of 9,103,793 images.

An additional resource is the in vitro diagnostic multivariate index assay (IVDMIA), designed by the US Food and Drug Administration to aid in multiplex analysis and complex diagnostic algorithms. IVDMIAs harness multiple molecular and nonmolecular markers to produce a diagnostic, prognostic, and/or predictive index for patients. IVDMIAs seek to answer clinical problems that are not sufficiently addressed by current diagnostic testing by simultaneously taking advantage of multiple peptides, antibodies, and genetic markers; the combination or algorithm used is not intuitively obvious and is frequently proprietary.[47] This crossroad of prognostic index and proteomics is vital for diagnosis and early intervention in diseases such as cancer.

CAPILLARY ISOELECTRIC FOCUSING

One of the drawbacks to many of the current technologies is the extraction of low concentrations of the analyte after multiple rounds of purification, making MS measurements difficult to interpret or obtain. One advancement has been electrokinetic focusing and high resolving power in the capillary isoelectric focusing (CIEF)–based multidimensional separation platform (Fig. 12.3). CIEF obtains high-resolution separation-based differences not only on pK but also on evenly distributing doubly charged peptides over the entire pH gradient by increasing the number of CIEF fractions.[48-52]

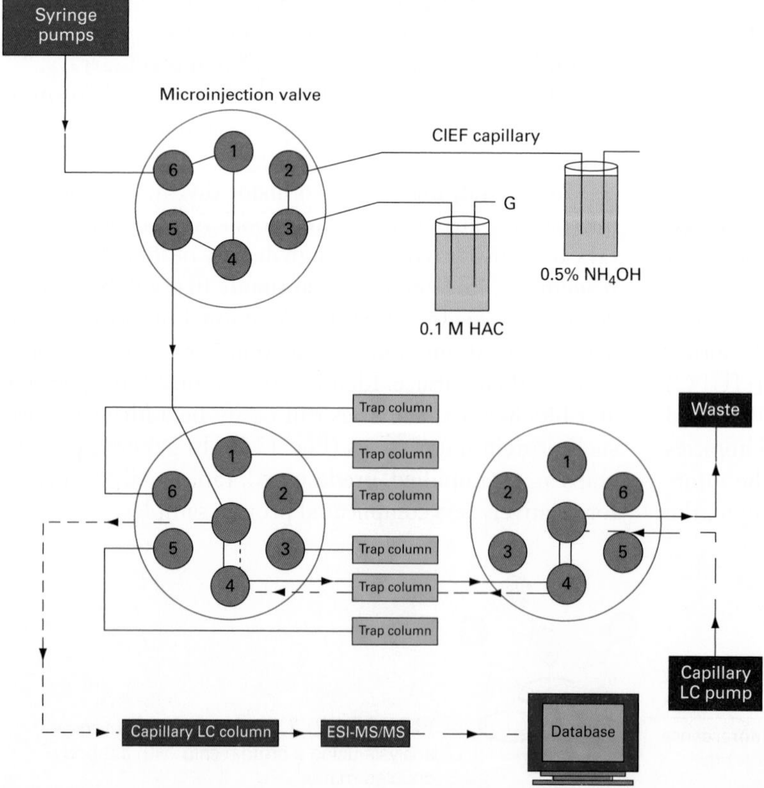

FIGURE 12–3 Schematic of liquid proteome analysis using a capillary isoelectric focusing–based multidimensional separation platform coupled with electrospray ionization (ESI)-tandem mass spectrometry (MS).

The existing proteomic analysis based on traditional analytic methodologies lacks a fair proportion of small and membrane proteins that are critical targets for therapies.[53,54] This may be due to the fact that solubilization in many existing protein-isolation methods—especially solubilization of enriched membrane factions—is based on detergents,[55-58] organic solvents,[59-62] and organic acids,[45,46] which subsequently proteolytically digest and cleave the protein of interest before analysis. Two-dimensional PAGE has had limited success as well, due to first separation—the isoelectric focusing of the protein—promoting the tendency of membrane proteins to precipitate because of their inherent hydrophobic nature.[45,46,53,55,59,63-65] However, when CIEF is coupled with nano reversed-phase liquid chromatography (nanoRPLC) separations, researchers have identified further enhancement of membrane proteins.[48]

PROTEOMICS: BEYOND THE BENCH

It is hoped that proteomics can reach the bedside in the form of clinical proteomics, an interdisciplinary field of clinical science, protein biochemistry, physical analysis of biomolecules, and computer science. The goal of this collaborative effort across fields is to translate basic scientific knowledge into effective clinical applications for patient treatment.[66] Ideally, particularly in the field of oncology, the discovery of biomarkers that are readily accessible through the circulating blood and are selectively overexpressed in pathological tissues has become a major research objective. Owing to the performance of MS technology,[67] current high-throughput proteomic analysis allows for the identification of a high number of proteins that are differentially expressed in cancerous tissues. The focus is on the group of proteins that are necessarily located either at the exterior face of the plasma membrane or in the extracellular matrix. Indisputably, this set of molecules has a high potential to serve as an innovative tool for effective imaging and targeted cancer therapy approaches. In this attractive therapeutic concept, specific cancer proteins are reached by intravenously administered ligands that are coupled to cytotoxic therapies, whether it is a drug, another protein, excitable reagent, etc.[68] In this way, such compounds would be able to induce cancer destruction while sparing normal tissues, the ultimate quest for oncologists and cancer researchers.

REFERENCES

1. Pitteri S, Hanash S. A systems approach to the proteomic identification of novel cancer biomarkers. *Dis Markers.* 2010;28(4):233-239.
2. Hanash SM, Pitteri SJ, Faca VM. Mining the plasma proteome for cancer biomarkers. *Nature.* 2008;452(7187):571-579.
3. Dunn MJ. PROTEOMICS: ten years in the field. *Proteomics.* 2010;10(1):1-3.
4. Wilkins MR, Pasquali C, Appel RD, et al. From proteins to proteomes: large scale protein identification by two-dimensional electrophoresis and amino acid analysis. *Nat Biotechnol.* 1996;14(1):61-65.
5. Speicher D. Gel-based proteome analysis. In: Coligan JE, Ploegh HL, Speicher DW, Wingfield PT, eds. *Current Protocols in Protein Science.* New York, NY: Wiley; 2003:22.20.21-22.20.22.
6. Chuaqui R, Vargas MP, Castiglioni T, et al. Detection of heterozygosity loss in microdissected fine needle aspiration specimens of breast carcinoma. *Acta Cytol.* 1996;40(4):642-648.
7. Emmert-Buck MR, Roth MJ, Zhuang Z, et al. Increased gelatinase A (MMP-2) and cathepsin B activity in invasive tumor regions of human colon cancer samples. *Am J Pathol.* 1994;145(6):1285-1290.
8. Emmert-Buck MR, Chuaqui RF, Zhuang Z, et al. Laser capture microdissection. *Science.* 1996;274(5289):998-1001.
9. Banks RE, Dunn MJ, Forbes MA, et al. The potential use of laser capture microdissection to selectively obtain distinct populations of cells for proteomic analysis—preliminary findings. *Electrophoresis.* 1999;20(4-5):689-700.
10. Duclos S, Desjardins M. Organelle proteomics. *Methods Mol Biol.* 2011;753:117-128.
11. van den Heuvel LP, Farhoud MH, Wevers RA, et al. Proteomics and neuromuscular diseases: theoretical concept and first results. *Ann Clin Biochem.* 2003;40(pt 1):9-15.
12. Chaurand P, Schwartz SA, Caprioli RM. Imaging mass spectrometry: a new tool to investigate the spatial organization of peptides and proteins in mammalian tissue sections. *Curr Opin Chem Biol.* 2002;6(5):676-681.
13. Galasinski SC, Louie DF, Gloor KK, et al. Global regulation of post-translational modifications on core histones. *J Biol Chem.* 2002;277(4):2579-2588.
14. Vosseller K, Wells L, Hart GW. Nucleocytoplasmic O-glycosylation: O-GlcNAc and functional proteomics. *Biochimie.* 2001;83(7):575-581.
15. Domon B, Aebersold R. Mass spectrometry and protein analysis. *Science.* 2006;312(5771):212-217.
16. Martens L, Chambers M, Sturm M, et al. mzML—a community standard for mass spectrometry data. *Mol Cell Proteomics.* 2011;10(1):R110 000133.
17. Vizcaino JA, Côté R, Reisinger F, et al. The Proteomics Identifications database: 2010 update. *Nucleic Acids Res.* 2010;38(Database issue):D736-D742.
18. Lundgren DH, Eng J, Wright ME, et al. PROTEOME-3D: an interactive bioinformatics tool for large-scale data exploration and knowledge discovery. *Mol Cell Proteomics.* 2003;2(11):1164-1176.
19. Zhu H, Snyder M. Protein chip technology. *Curr Opin Chem Biol.* 2003;7(1):55-63.
20. Zhu H, Bilgin M, Bangham R, et al. Global analysis of protein activities using proteome chips. *Science.* 2001;293(5537): 2101-2105.
21. Yanagida M. Functional proteomics; current achievements. *J Chromatogr B Analyt Technol Biomed Life Sci.* 2002;771(1-2):89-106.
22. Haab BB. Advances in protein microarray technology for protein expression and interaction profiling. *Curr Opin Drug Discov Devel.* 2001;4(1):116-123.
23. Cahill DJ. Protein and antibody arrays and their medical applications. *J Immunol Methods.* 2001;250(1-2):81-91.
24. Templin MF, Stoll D, Schrenk M, et al. Protein microarray technology. *Trends Biotechnol.* 2002;20(4):160-166.
25. Zhu H, Snyder M. Protein arrays and microarrays. *Curr Opin Chem Biol.* 2001;5(1):40-45.
26. Stoll D, Templin MF, Schrenk M, et al. Protein microarray technology. *Front Biosci.* 2002;7:c13-c32.
27. Zhu H, Snyder M. "Omic" approaches for unraveling signaling networks. *Curr Opin Cell Biol.* 2002;14(2):173-179.
28. Lueking A, Horn M, Eickhoff H, et al. Protein microarrays for gene expression and antibody screening. *Anal Biochem.* 1999;270(1):103-111.
29. Kononen J, Bubendorf L, Kallioniemi A, et al. Tissue microarrays for high-throughput molecular profiling of tumor specimens. *Nat Med.* 1998;4(7):844-847.
30. Uetz P, Giot L, Cagney G, et al. A comprehensive analysis of protein-protein interactions in *Saccharomyces cerevisiae*. *Nature.* 2000;403(6770):623-627.
31. Ross-Macdonald P, Coelho PS, Roemer T, et al. Large-scale analysis of the yeast genome by transposon tagging and gene disruption. *Nature.* 1999;402(6760):413-418.

32. Fodor SP, Read JL, Pirrung MC, et al. Light-directed, spatially addressable parallel chemical synthesis. *Science*. 1991;251(4995):767-773.
33. Walter G, Büssow K, Cahill D, et al. Protein arrays for gene expression and molecular interaction screening. *Curr Opin Microbiol*. 2000;3(3):298-302.
34. Emili AQ, Cagney G. Large-scale functional analysis using peptide or protein arrays. *Nat Biotechnol*. 2000;18(4):393-397.
35. Houseman BT, Huh JH, Kron SJ, et al. Peptide chips for the quantitative evaluation of protein kinase activity. *Nat Biotechnol*. 2002;20(3):270-274.
36. Haab BB, Dunham MJ, Brown PO. Protein microarrays for highly parallel detection and quantitation of specific proteins and antibodies in complex solutions. *Genome Biol*. 2001;2(2):RESEARCH0004.
37. Joos TO, Schrenk M, Hopfl P, et al. A microarray enzyme-linked immunosorbent assay for autoimmune diagnostics. *Electrophoresis*. 2000;21(13):2641-2650.
38. Arenkov P, Kukhtin A, Gemmell A, et al. Protein microchips: use for immunoassay and enzymatic reactions. *Anal Biochem*. 2000;278(2):123-131.
39. Ge H. UPA, a universal protein array system for quantitative detection of protein-protein, protein-DNA, protein-RNA and protein-ligand interactions. *Nucleic Acids Res*. 2000;28(2):e3.
40. MacBeath G, Schreiber SL. Printing proteins as microarrays for high-throughput function determination. *Science*. 2000;289(5485):1760-1763.
41. Zhu H, Klemic JF, Chang S, et al. Analysis of yeast protein kinases using protein chips. *Nat Genet*. 2000;26(3):283-289.
42. Wang D, Liu S, Trummer BJ, et al. Carbohydrate microarrays for the recognition of cross-reactive molecular markers of microbes and host cells. *Nat Biotechnol*. 2002;20(3):275-281.
43. Houseman BT, Mrksich M. Carbohydrate arrays for the evaluation of protein binding and enzymatic modification. *Chem Biol*. 2002;9(4):443-454.
44. Link AJ, Eng J, Schieltz DM, et al. Direct analysis of protein complexes using mass spectrometry. *Nat Biotechnol*. 1999;17(7):676-682.
45. Washburn MP, Wolters D, Yates JR 3rd. Large-scale analysis of the yeast proteome by multidimensional protein identification technology. *Nat Biotechnol*. 2001;19(3):242-247.
46. Wolters DA, Washburn MP, Yates JR 3rd. An automated multidimensional protein identification technology for shotgun proteomics. *Anal Chem*. 2001;73(23):5683-5690.
47. Zhang Z, Chan DW. The road from discovery to clinical diagnostics: lessons learned from the first FDA-cleared in vitro diagnostic multivariate index assay of proteomic biomarkers. *Cancer Epidemiol Biomarkers Prev*. 2010;19(12):2995-2999.
48. Eisenhofer G, Huynh TT, Elkahloun A, et al. Differential expression of the regulated catecholamine secretory pathway in different hereditary forms of pheochromocytoma. *Am J Physiol Endocrinol Metab*. 2008;295(5):E1223-E1233.
49. Guo T, Wang W, Rudnick PA, et al. Proteome analysis of microdissected formalin-fixed and paraffin-embedded tissue specimens. *J Histochem Cytochem*. 2007;55(7):763-772.
50. Li J, Yin C, Okamoto H, et al. Identification of a novel proliferation-related protein, WHSC1 4a, in human gliomas. *Neuro Oncol*. 2008;10(1):45-51.
51. Wang W, Guo T, Rudnick PA, et al. Membrane proteome analysis of microdissected ovarian tumor tissues using capillary isoelectric focusing/reversed-phase liquid chromatography-tandem MS. *Anal Chem*. 2007;79(3):1002-1009.
52. Wang Y, Rudnick PA, Evans EL, et al. Proteome analysis of microdissected tumor tissue using a capillary isoelectric focusing-based multidimensional separation platform coupled with ESI-tandem MS. *Anal Chem*. 2005;77(20):6549-6556.
53. Wu CC, MacCoss MJ, Howell KE, et al. A method for the comprehensive proteomic analysis of membrane proteins. *Nat Biotechnol*. 2003;21(5):532-538.
54. Wu CC, Yates JR 3rd. The application of mass spectrometry to membrane proteomics. *Nat Biotechnol*. 2003;21(3):262-267.
55. Wei J, Sun J, Yu W, et al. Global proteome discovery using an online three-dimensional LC-MS/MS. *J Proteome Res*. 2005;4(3):801-808.
56. Han DK, Eng J, Zhou H, et al. Quantitative profiling of differentiation-induced microsomal proteins using isotope-coded affinity tags and mass spectrometry. *Nat Biotechnol*. 2001;19(10):946-951.
57. Hixson KK, Rodriguez N, Camp DG, et al. Evaluation of enzymatic digestion and liquid chromatography-mass spectrometry peptide mapping of the integral membrane protein bacteriorhodopsin. *Electrophoresis*. 2002;23(18):3224-3232.
58. Ruth MC, Old WM, Emrick MA, et al. Analysis of membrane proteins from human chronic myelogenous leukemia cells: comparison of extraction methods for multidimensional LC-MS/MS. *J Proteome Res*. 2006;5(3):709-719.
59. Blonder J, Hale ML, Lucas DA, et al. Proteomic analysis of detergent-resistant membrane rafts. *Electrophoresis*. 2004;25(9):1307-1318.
60. Blonder J, Goshe MB, Moore RJ, et al. Enrichment of integral membrane proteins for proteomic analysis using liquid chromatography-tandem mass spectrometry. *J Proteome Res*. 2002;1(4):351-360.
61. Goshe MB, Blonder J, Smith RD. Affinity labeling of highly hydrophobic integral membrane proteins for proteome-wide analysis. *J Proteome Res*. 2003;2(2):153-161.
62. Wang H, Qian WJ, Mottaz HM, et al. Development and evaluation of a micro- and nanoscale proteomic sample preparation method. *J Proteome Res*. 2005;4(6):2397-2403.
63. Pedersen SK, Harry JL, Sebastian L, et al. Unseen proteome: mining below the tip of the iceberg to find low abundance and membrane proteins. *J Proteome Res*. 2003;2(3):303-311.
64. Schirmer EC, Florens L, Guan T, et al. Nuclear membrane proteins with potential disease links found by subtractive proteomics. *Science*. 2003;301(5638):1380-1382.
65. Nielsen PA, Olsen JV, Podtelejnikov AV, et al. Proteomic mapping of brain plasma membrane proteins. *Mol Cell Proteomics*. 2005;4(4):402-408.
66. Celis JE, Moreira JM. Clinical proteomics. *Mol Cell Proteomics*. 2008;7(10):1779.
67. Schirle M, Bantscheff M, Kuster B. Mass spectrometry-based proteomics in preclinical drug discovery. *Chem Biol*. January 2012;19(1):72-84.
68. Geiger T, Wehner A, Schaab C, et al. Comparative proteomic analysis of eleven common cell lines reveals ubiquitous but varying expression of most proteins. *Mol Cell Proteomics*. January 2012. [Epub ahead of print].

CHAPTER 13

Morphoproteomics

Robert E. Brown and Jamie J. Buryanek

BACKGROUND AND DEFINITION

Completion of the human genome project inarguably provided a foundation for personalized medicine. Subsequently, the role of microRNAs in modifying the translation of genomic signals into effector proteins has been recognized. The microenvironment of the cell has been found to be increasingly important in potentially creating epigenetic modifications of the cell through endogenous toxicants such as reactive oxygen species and free radicals.[1,2] Thus, genetic, epigenetic, transcriptional, post-transcriptional, and translational events, coupled with posttranslational modifications of proteins, ultimately lead to functional protein expressions (proteomics) that define the biology of a cell. The influence of the microenvironment on the cell and of the cell on its microenvironment is also conveyed to a large extent by proteins, peptides, and the by-products of their actions.

Morphoproteomics combines morphology and proteomics to provide insight and context for the abnormal biology in lesional tissues and in particular tumors.[3-5] Specifically, bright-field microscopy and immunohistochemistry allow for the detection of protein analytes in both tumoral and companionate stromal and endothelial cells with respect to their quantification in each component using a visual estimation of the intensity of their chromogenic signal and/or the percentage of tumor cells with nuclear immunopositivity in the case of cell cycle–related analytes, by automated cellular imaging; their site of tissue/subcellular compartmentalization; and an assessment of their state of molecular activation to include compartmental translocation, phosphorylation on putative sites of activation, and correlative, functional grouping. In the process, morphoproteomics uncovers opportunities for therapeutic interventions customized for the individual patient (personalized medicine).

This chapter illustrates the application of morphoproteomics in the identification of protein analytes in tumors for purposes of defining the biology of the tumor; identifying therapeutic targets in tumors and developing combinatorial strategies customized for the individual patient; detecting cancer stem cells and that population of tumor cells with stemness characteristics and/or showing epithelial–mesenchymal transition with therapeutic implications; and sequentially monitoring recurrent tumors for signatures of resistance and adaptive mechanisms, again with recommendations for therapeutic intervention. A schematic providing a visual depiction of the integration of morphology and proteomics (morphoproteomics) as a means of defining the biology of a tumor, its potential interactions with the microenvironment, and the phenomenon of stemness/epithelial–mesenchymal transition is contained in Figure 13.1.

MORPHOPROTEOMICS: APPLICATIONS IN DEFINING THE BIOLOGY OF THE TUMOR AND ITS MICROENVIRONMENT

Signal transduction pathways involved in protein synthesis, promoting growth of the tumor, ensuring survival through their antiapoptotic-, angiogenic-, and chemoresistance-inducing actions, and facilitating invasive and metastatic potential help define the biology of an individual patient's tumor. The process of selecting the protein analytes for inclusion in this application involves a computer-assisted search of the National Library of Medicine's MEDLINE database and reliance on profiles from our library of archival morphoproteomic cases with a similar tumoral phenotype. Table 13.1 provides a categorical summary of such pathways and corresponding

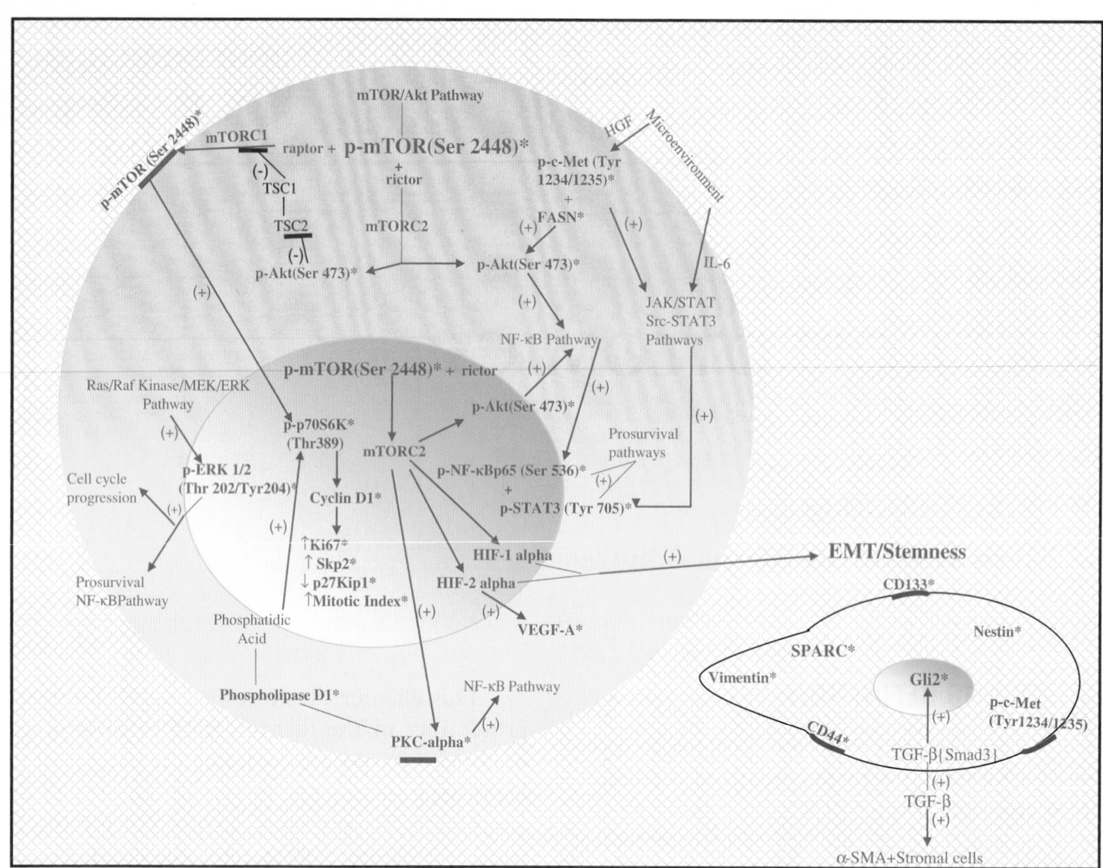

FIGURE 13–1 Schematic depiction of the application of morphoproteomics in the assessment of the activation of signal transduction pathways of convergence using phosphospecific probes, when applicable, subcellular compartmentalization of protein analytes, and correlative expression of downstream effectors. Additionally, it connects such signaling, along with a potential role of the tumoral microenvironment, to the phenomenon of epithelial–mesenchymal transition/stemness in a subpopulation of tumor cells and outlines the identification of such cells by morphoproteomics. Notably, the protein analytes that are in bold and indicated by an asterisk (*) in the different subcellular compartments are among those assessable by morphoproteomic analysis. References from the scientific literature supporting their associations, downstream effects, and role in EMT/stemness have been cited in the text (vide infra). Abbreviations: mTOR (mammalian target of rapamycin); phosphorylated (p)-mTOR (Ser[serine] 2448); mTORC1, mTORC2 (mammalian target of rapamycin complex 1 and 2, respectively); p-Akt (protein kinase B) phosphorylated on Ser(serine)473; TSC1/TSC2 (tuberous sclerosis complex 1 and 2); p-p70S6K (kinase) phosphorylated on Thr (threonine)389; Skp (S-phase kinase–associated protein)2; MEK (mitogen-activated protein kinase/extracellular signal-regulated kinase kinase); p-ERK (extracellular signal-regulated kinase) phosphorylated on Thr (threonine)202/Tyr(tyrosine)204; IL (interleukin)-6; JAK/STAT (Janus kinases/signal transducer and activator of transcription); HGF (hepatocyte growth factor); p-c-Met (mesenchymal–epithelial transition kinase) phosphorylated on Tyr (tyrosines)1234/1235; FASN (fatty acid synthase); p-NF-kappa B (nuclear factor kappa B)p65 phosphorylated on Ser (serine) 536; HIF-2 alpha (hypoxia-inducible factor-2 alpha); VEGF-A (vascular endothelial growth factor-isoform A); PKC (protein kinase C)-alpha; EMT (epithelial–mesenchymal transition); CD (cluster of differentiation); SPARC (secreted protein acidic and rich in cysteine); alpha-SMA (smooth muscle actin); TGF (transforming growth factor)-beta; Gli (glioma-associated oncogene)2 protein.

protein analytes assessable by morphoproteomic analysis that could serve as therapeutic targets.

Bright-field microscopy also allows for the assessment of the tumoral microenvironment in each case to include the presence or absence of a desmoplastic and/or myxoid stroma and the tumor's vascular network. Moreover, a probe for alpha-smooth muscle actin, a surrogate marker of transforming growth factor (TGF)-β, can also help define the stromal cells and the cytokine milieu associated with the tumor and its microenvironment. Such a finding together with nuclear glioma-associated oncogene 2 (Gli2) protein expression in the tumor would support TGF-β{Smad3} signaling and epithelial–mesenchymal transition in the right context and could direct therapy accordingly. The expression of chemotherapy-enhancing and anti-angiogenic–facilitating proteins such as secreted protein acidic and rich in cysteine (SPARC; osteonectin) can also be assessed by morphoproteomics. These are summarized in Table 13.1 and illustrated in Figure 13.2.

MORPHOPROTEOMICS: APPLICATIONS IN IDENTIFYING THERAPEUTIC TARGETS IN TUMORS AND DEVELOPING COMBINATORIAL STRATEGIES CUSTOMIZED FOR THE INDIVIDUAL PATIENT

In addition to morphoproteomic profiling of relatively rare tumoral phenotypes, we have developed, in collaboration with our clinical colleagues, morphoproteomic-guided algorithms for the treatment of more common tumoral types. The following is an example of such an

TABLE 13–1 Biologic Tumoral Profiling Using Morphoproteomic Analysis by Immunohistochemistry

Molecular Pathway	Corresponding Protein Analyte
Upstream Signal Transducers	
Human epidermal growth factor receptor	HER-2/neu
Epidermal growth factor receptor (EGFR)	EGFRvIII/EGFR
Estrogen receptor signaling	ER-alpha
Mesenchymal–epithelial transition (Met) receptor (HGF receptor)	Phosphorylated (p)-c-Met (Tyr1234/1235)
Protein kinase C (PKC) alpha	cPKC-α
Phospholipase D	Phospholipase D1
	Phospholipase D2
	p-p70S6K (Thr389) [nuclear]
Pathways of Convergence of Upstream Signaling	
Ras/Raf kinase/extracellular signal-regulated kinase (ERK)	p-ERK1/2 (Thr202/Tyr204)
mTORC1 (raptor+mTOR)	p-mTOR (Ser2448) [cytoplasmic plasmalemmal]
	p-p70S6K (Thr389) [nuclear]
mTORC2 (rictor +mTOR)	p-mTOR (Ser2448) [nuclear]
	p-Akt (Ser473) [nuclear]
Signal transducer and activator of transcription	p-STAT3 (Tyr705)
Nuclear Cell Cycle–Related Analytes	
G1, S, G2, and M phases	Ki-67
Cyclin-dependent kinase activators	Cyclin D1
	S-phase kinase–associated protein (Skp)2
Cyclin-dependent kinase inhibitors	p53 (facilitator as mutant/inactivated form)
	p27Kip1
	p16INK4a
Repair enzymes	Topoisomerase II alpha
Tumorigenic/Chemoresistance Factors	
p38 mitogen-activated protein kinase	p-p38MAPK (Thr180/Tyr182)
Signal transducer and activator of transcription 3	p-STAT3 (Tyr705)
Nuclear factor (NF) kappa B	p-NF-kappaBp65 (Ser536)
Antiapoptotic protein, Bcl-2	Bcl-2
Multidrug-resistant pump (MDR_1)	P-glycoprotein
Estrogen receptor (ER) signaling (medulloblastoma)	ER-beta
Heat shock protein chaperone system	Hsp90
Cyclooxygenase-2	COX-2
Fatty acid synthase	FASN
Excision repair cross-complementation group 1 (platinum resistance)	ERCC1
CD44 (platinum resistance)	CD44
Angiogenic Factors	
Vascular endothelial growth factor (VEGF) signaling pathway	VEGF-A (tumoral)
	p-ERK1/2 (endothelial)
Tumoral Stem Cell/Epithelial–Mesenchymal Transition Markers	
Stemness	CD44 (in the right context)
	ALDH1
Neural precursor lineage	CD56
	CD133
	Nestin
Tumor-propagating (progenitor) lineage	CD15 (medulloblastoma)
Sonic Hedgehog indicators	CD15 (medulloblastoma)
	ER-beta (medulloblastoma)
	Glioma-associated oncogene protein (Gli2) [nuclear]

(*Continued*)

TABLE 13–1 Biologic Tumoral Profiling Using Morphoproteomic Analysis by Immunohistochemistry (*Continued*)

Molecular Pathway	Corresponding Protein Analyte
Epithelial–mesenchymal transition indicators	Vimentin (acquired positive expression)/E-cadherin (loss [low or negative expression])/beta catenin (cytoplasmic and/or nuclear translocation)
	Gli2 (TGF-beta{Smad3} signaling in the right context [e.g., supported by alpha-smooth muscle actin + stromal cells in tumoral microenvironment])
Differentiation-Associated/Proapoptotic/Chemotherapy and Antiangiogenic Facilitating Pathways	
Tumor necrosis factor–related apoptosis-inducing ligand	TRAIL-R1 (DR4)
Melatonin receptor 1a	MTR-1A
ER signaling (astrocytic lineage tumors)	ER-beta
Secreted protein acidic and rich in cysteine (osteonectin)	SPARC (facilitates uptake of nab-paclitaxel in tumor cells and intratumoral endothelial cells)
Peroxisome proliferator–activated receptor gamma	PPAR gamma

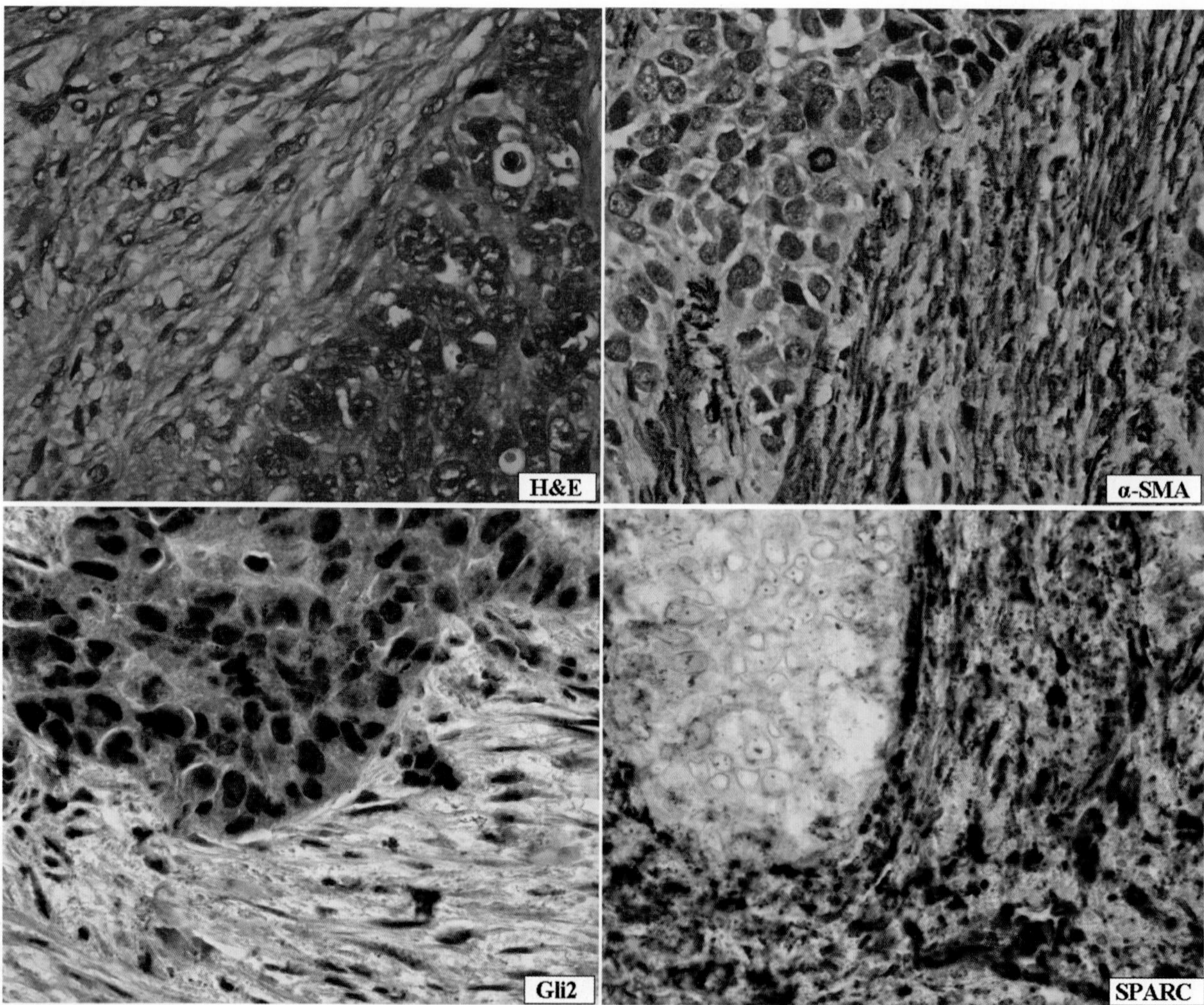

FIGURE 13–2 High-grade uterine "carcinosarcoma" with depiction of infiltrating carcinomatous component and adjacent desmoplastic stroma (H&E, upper left frame). Brown (diaminobenzidine, DAB) chromogenic signal for alpha-smooth muscle actin expression confirms the myofibroblastic nature of the stroma (upper right frame) and together with companionate nuclear signal for glioma-associated oncogene 2 (Gli2) protein (lower left frame) suggests an intratumoral cytokine milieu of transforming growth factor (TGF)-β and the presence of TGF-β{Smad3} signaling in the tumor cells.[6-9] SPARC (osteonectin) expression, primarily in the tumoral stroma (lower right frame), provides a therapeutic option to use nanoparticle albumin-bound paclitaxel as an antitumorigenic agent.[10,11] Parenthetically, paclitaxel also interferes with TGF-β{Smad3} signaling by stabilizing tubulin and sequestering Smad3 protein (original magnification of digital images ×400).[12,13]

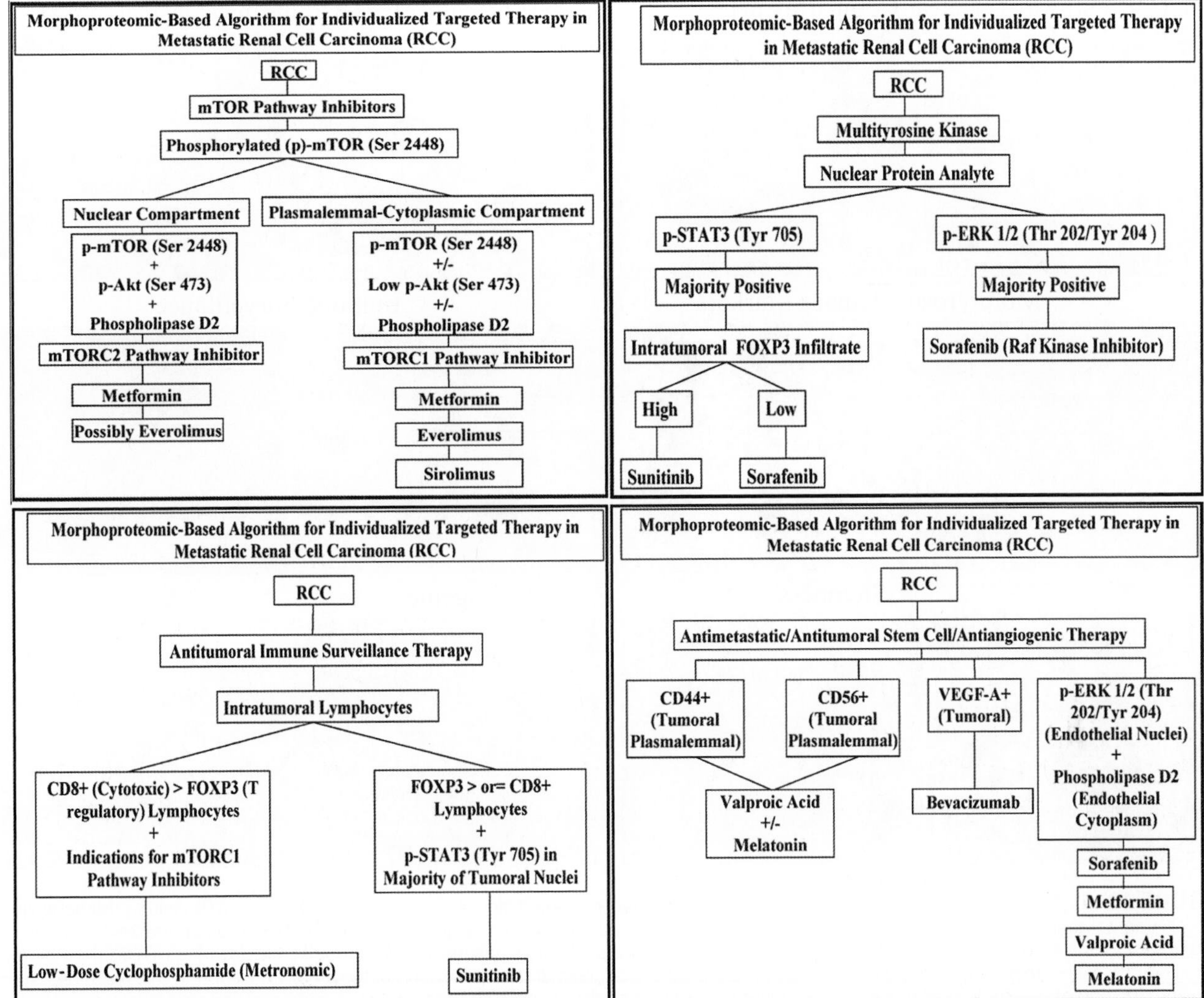

FIGURE 13–3 This morphoproteomic-based algorithmic approach is accompanied by a full narrative report on each patient's specimen with supporting references from the preclinical and clinical scientific literature. It also provides for the combinatorial application of multiple agents in the treatment of recurrent and metastatic renal cell carcinoma. The final decision on the use of one or more agents rests with the judgment of the patient's oncologist in the context of the clinical status of the patient.

algorithmic approach for recurrent and metastatic conventional renal cell carcinoma that takes into account the application of the National Cancer Institute (NCI)–approved therapies and off-label use of other agents (standard medications and nutraceuticals) in a therapeutic salvage mode for those patients who have failed conventional therapies and have recurrent disease. The composite algorithm and the corresponding morphoproteomic images are illustrated in Figures 13.3 and 13.4.

This application has resulted in the morphoproteomic profiling of over 40 metastatic renal cell carcinomas to date, with documentation of the patients' clinical and radiographic responses to such therapies. Preliminary outcomes data using this algorithmic approach in renal cell carcinoma have been presented and published in abstract form in conjunction with the 2010 ASCO Annual Meeting[29] and are the subject of a comprehensive manuscript in preparation. Similarly, collaborative studies in patients with conventionally treated but recurrent pediatric tumors in the central nervous system have shown responses to morphoproteomic-guided targeted therapy.[30]

MORPHOPROTEOMICS: APPLICATIONS IN DETECTING CANCER STEM CELLS AND EPITHELIAL–MESENCHYMAL TRANSITION WITH THERAPEUTIC IMPLICATIONS

There is a shifting paradigm in tumorigenesis, specifically with regard to the role of cancer stem cells, the acquisition of stemness characteristics and of epithelial–mesenchymal transition in the chemoradioresistance of a tumoral subpopulation, and in promoting metastatic and recurrent disease in a distant site in collaboration with the microenvironment and adaptation of the tumor's biology.[31,32] The identification of circulating tumor cells

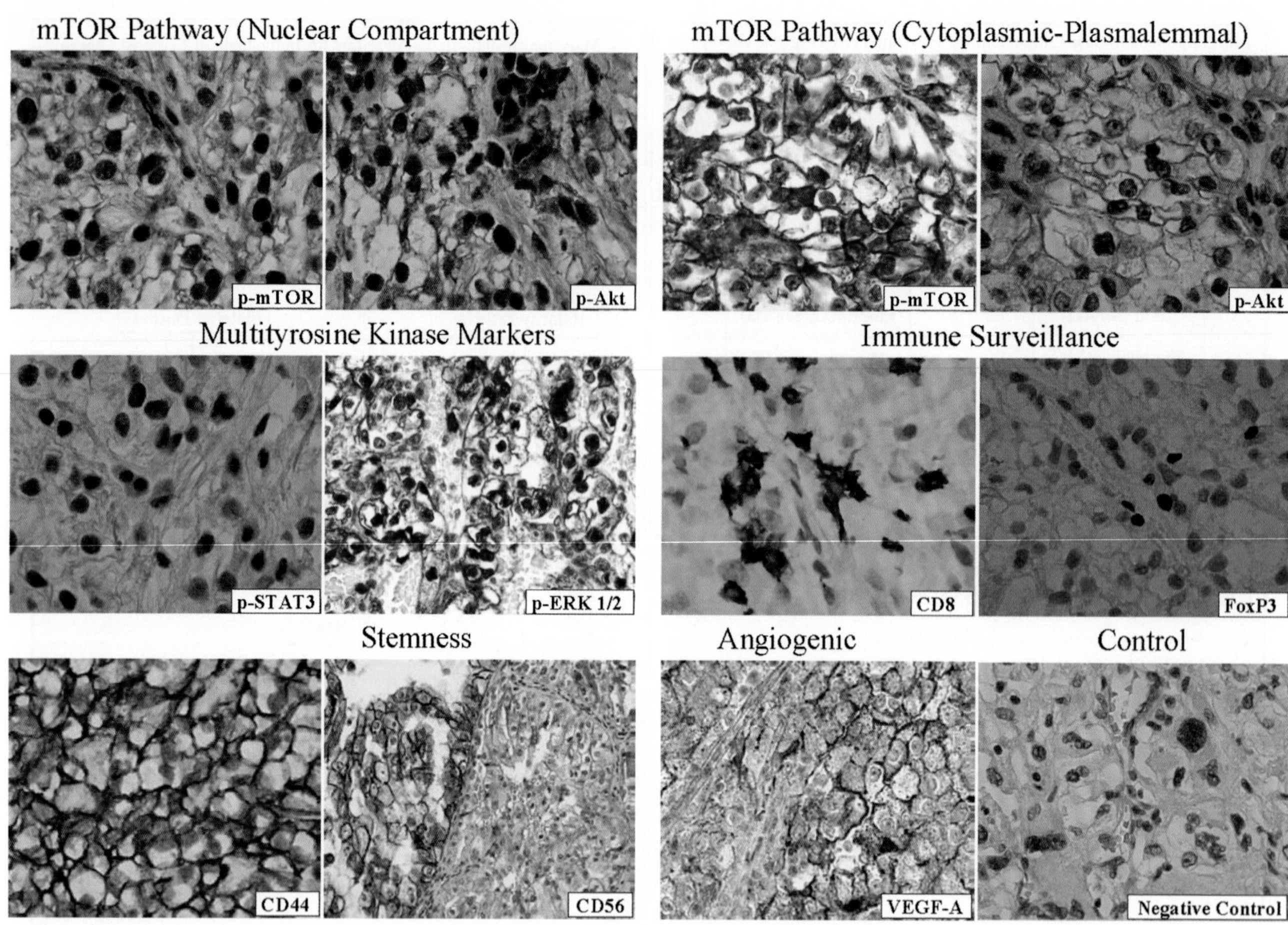

FIGURE 13–4 Digital images corresponding to the morphoproteomic-based algorithmic approach (see Fig. 13.3) include the subcellular compartmentalization of the chromogenic signal for phosphorylated (p)-mammalian target of rapamycin (mTOR) on serine 2448 and for p-Akt (Ser473) in predominantly nuclear (favoring mTORC2 pathway signaling) vs. plasmalemmal-cytoplasmic (favoring mTORC1 pathway signaling)[14-18]; assessment of the nuclear expression (translocation) of p-signal transducer and activator of transcription 3 (STAT3) on tyrosine 705 and of p-extracellular signal-regulated kinase (ERK)1/2 on threonine 202/tyrosine 204 in consideration of the selection of multityrosine kinase inhibitors such as sorafenib vs. sunitinib[19-21]; intratumoral lymphocyte enumeration using immunohistochemical probes to detect antitumoral CD8+ cytotoxic T lymphocytes and FoxP3+ T regulatory cells implicated in suppression of host antitumoral immune surveillance in consideration of sunitinib vs. sorafenib therapy[22,23]; stemness markers including plasmalemmal CD44 and CD56 (NCAM) expression[24-27]; angiogenic protein analytes such as vascular endothelial growth factor (VEGF)-A, the target for bevacizumab[28]; and finally, a negative control runs with each specimen (original magnifications ×200 for digital images p-ERK 1/2, CD56, and VEGF-A and ×400 for the remainder).

with stemness characteristics and in the case of epithelial tumors (carcinomas) of mesenchymal markers and a composite phenotype[33] lend credence to this phenomenon.

Morphoproteomics has application in identifying the component of cancer stem cells/tumoral progenitor cells and their microanatomical location such as the perivascular niche[4] and in defining those stemness and epithelial–mesenchymal characteristics that could enable collaboration with the microenvironment in promoting migration and metastasis. The current thinking with regard to reversing this process and dealing with the microenvironment includes promoting differentiation into a more benign phenotype and reversing the epithelial–mesenchymal transition (promoting mesenchymal to epithelial transition); keeping the tumor cells in a quiescent (non-proliferative) state; modifying the microenvironment to interrupt signal transduction pathways that might be serving to provide paracrine stimulation for growth and further epithelial–mesenchymal transition; and depriving the tumoral stem cells and those with stemness characteristics of their perivascular niche and reducing their migratory and metastatic potential.[32,34]

Most importantly, there is a growing body of evidence that both the acquisition of stemness characteristics and of epithelial–mesenchymal transition in cancer and the associated metastatic potential and chemoresistance are related to hypoxia and hypoxia-inducible factors (HIFs).[35-38] Specifically, HIF-2 alpha appears to be a consistent initiator of both processes in response to hypoxia[39-43] and is apparently dependent on mTORC2 signaling.[44] TGF-β{Smad3} signaling also appears to be a major player in the epithelial–mesenchymal transition of malignant tumors.[45] Morphoproteomics is capable of assessing the concomitants of both HIF-2 alpha and TGF-β{Smad3} signaling in the context of the histopathologic features and markers of epithelial–mesenchymal transition and stemness in cancer (see Table 13.1; Figs. 13.1 and 13.5).

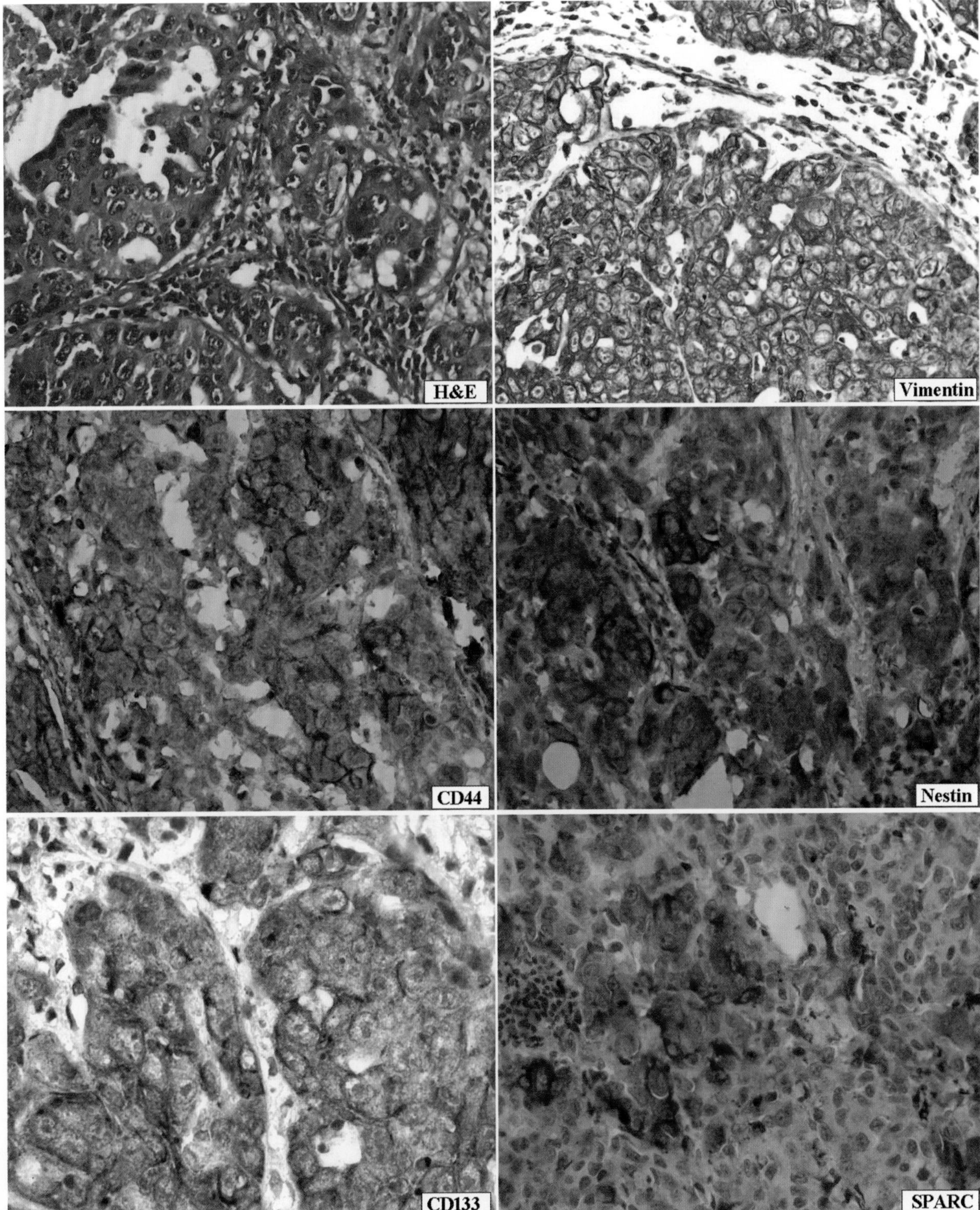

FIGURE 13–5 Digital images of a triple-negative breast carcinoma to include representative hematoxylin–eosin (H&E); vimentin immunopositivity consistent with some degree of epithelial–mesenchymal transition[46]; and subsets of CD44+ (plasmalemmal), nestin+, CD133+ (plasmalemmal), and secreted protein acidic and rich in cysteine (SPARC)+ tumor cells consistent with stemness characteristics (original magnifications ×200 for digital images of vimentin, CD44, nestin, and SPARC; ×400 for H&E; and ×600 for CD133).[47-50]

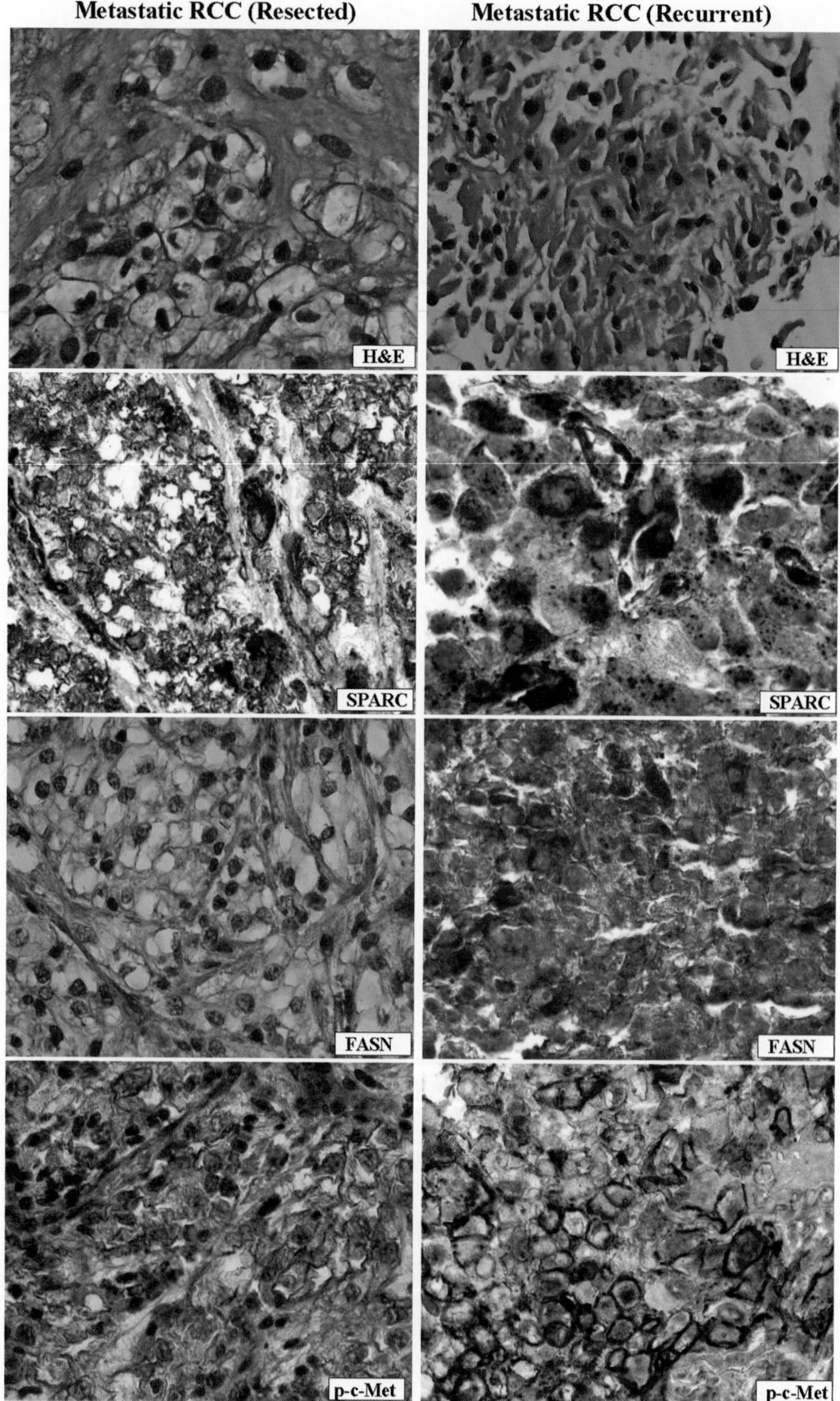

FIGURE 13–6 Metastatic renal cell carcinomas in the same patient from the right lower lobe and left lung resected and biopsied, respectively, to illustrate resistance signatures and therapeutic opportunities revealed by morphoproteomic analysis to include transition from a classic conventional clear cell renal cell carcinoma histopathology in the resected metastasis (upper left hand frame) to a more eosinophilic with occasional spindle cell morphology in the recurrent specimen (upper right hand frame) in H&E sections; expression of secreted protein acidic and rich in cysteine (SPARC) in both specimens indicative of epithelial–mesenchymal transition (EMT)/stemness, unusual for classic clear cell renal cell carcinoma not undergoing EMT[52,53]; and relative overexpression of the fatty acid synthase (FASN)/c-Met pathway in the recurrent specimen. The latter is consistent with increased stemness and epithelial–mesenchymal transition and a role for a hypoxic microenvironment via hypoxia-inducible factor (HIF)-1 alpha in inducing this phenomenon.[34,54-57] It also raises the option of using an inhibitor of FASN such as metformin[58] in combination with a c-Met tyrosine kinase inhibitor such as crizotinib,[59] along with inhibitors of the mTORC2 pathway and HIF-1 alpha and HIF-2 alpha (original magnification ×600 for H&E upper left hand frame and SPARC right hand frame; ×400 for all remaining frames).

MORPHOPROTEOMICS: APPLICATIONS IN MONITORING RECURRENT TUMORS FOR SIGNATURES OF RESISTANCE WITH THERAPEUTIC IMPLICATIONS

Morphoproteomics has application in assessing the response and resistance signatures in certain tumors. For example, in the Ewing family of tumors, we have been able to provide morphoproteomic correlates of response and resistance signatures to anti-insulin-like growth factor-1 receptor (IGF-1R) therapy and combinatorial therapy with anti-IGF-1R and temsirolimus.[51] Parenthetically, in other tumoral types in which morphoproteomics has been applied, we have detected the translocation of the constitutively activated, phosphorylated (p)-IGF-1R into the cytoplasmic and nuclear subcellular compartments, which could also render this activated molecule relatively inaccessible to the inhibitory action of targeted antibody therapy. More recently, we have identified and characterized a subset of recurrent and resistant metastatic renal cell carcinomas using morphoproteomic analysis. Such resistance appears to be associated with exaggerated epithelial–mesenchymal transition.

The morphoproteomic findings include microanatomical evidence of variable transition states from a clear cell morphology to a sarcomatoid appearance and the acquisition of SPARC expression and variable expression of phosphorylated (p)-c-Met (Tyr1234/1235). In the context of the tumoral microenvironment, morphoproteomics also provides therapeutic options to moderate the influence of the microenvironment on such an exaggerated state of epithelial–mesenchymal transition, to subdue the proliferative state of the tumor cells, and to essentially reverse the process. The morphoproteomic markers common to this process in this resistant and recurrent subset with therapeutic options are illustrated in Figure 13.6 (see also Fig. 13.1; vide supra).

SUMMARY

Morphoproteomics provides a mechanism by which the pathologist can help define the biology of an individual patient's tumor in the context of its microenvironment and enables the pathologist, in collaboration with the clinical oncologist, to design algorithmic approaches to morphoproteomic-guided targeted therapy for various tumoral phenotypes. Moreover, morphoproteomics has application in identifying stemness and epithelial–mesenchymal transition states that might predict tumoral metastasis and the propensity for recurrent disease, along with the opportunity of selecting therapeutic agents that deal with these tumoral subpopulations and signal transduction processes responsible for their initiation. Sequential monitoring of tumor specimens from the same patient using this approach also uncovers response and resistance signatures amenable to therapeutic intervention. Finally, morphoproteomics offers the patient whose tumor has failed conventional therapy or for which there is no therapeutic protocol hope in the development of therapeutic strategies customized and targeted for that individual patient's tumor (personalized medicine).

ACKNOWLEDGMENTS

The authors wish to thank Ms. Bheravi Patel for help with the manuscript and for graphic support and Ms. Pamela K Johnston, HT (ASCP), for her technical expertise.

REFERENCES

1. Ziech D, Franco R, Pappa A, Panayiotidis MI. Reactive oxygen species (ROS)–induced genetic and epigenetic alterations in human carcinogenesis. *Mutat Res.* 2011;711(1-2):167-173.
2. Giannoni E, Parri M, Chiarugi P. Emt and oxidative stress: a bidirectional interplay affecting tumour malignancy. *Antioxid Redox Signal.* November 2011. 2012: 16(11): 1248-1263.
3. Brown RE. Morphoproteomics: exposing protein circuitries in tumors to identify potential therapeutic targets in cancer patients. *Expert Rev Proteomics.* 2005;2:337-348.
4. Brown RE. Morphogenomics and morphoproteomics: a role for anatomic pathology in personalized medicine. *Arch Pathol Lab Med.* 2009;133:568-579.
5. Tan D. Morphoproteomics: a novel approach to identify potential therapeutic targets in cancer patients. *Int J Clin Exp Pathol.* 2008;1:331-332.
6. Aoyagi-Ikeda K, Maeno T, Matsui H, et al. Notch induces myofibroblast differentiation of alveolar epithelial cells via transforming growth factor-{beta}-Smad3 pathway. *Am J Respir Cell Mol Biol.* July 2011;45(1):136-144.
7. Javelaud D, Alexaki VI, Dennler S, et al. TGF-beta/SMAD/GLI2 signaling axis in cancer progression and metastasis. *Cancer Res.* September 2011;71(17):5606-5610.
8. Dennler S, Andre J, Alexaki I, et al. Induction of sonic hedgehog mediators by transforming growth factor-beta: Smad3-dependent activation of Gli2 and Gli1 expression in vitro and in vivo. *Cancer Res.* 2007;67(14):6981-6986.
9. Lin M, Guo LM, Liu H, et al. Nuclear accumulation of glioma-associated oncogene 2 protein and enhanced expression of forkhead-box transcription factor M1 protein in human hepatocellular carcinoma. *Histol Histopathol.* 2010;25(10):1269-1275.
10. Gradishar WJ. Albumin-bound paclitaxel: a next-generation taxane. *Expert Opin Pharmacother.* 2006;7(8):1041-1053.
11. Desai NP, Trieu V, Hwang LY, et al. Improved effectiveness of nanoparticle albumin-bound (nab) paclitaxel versus polysorbate-based docetaxel in multiple xenografts as a function of HER2 and SPARC status. *Anticancer Drugs.* 2008;19(9):899-909.
12. Zhang D, Sun L, Xian W, et al. Low-dose paclitaxel ameliorates renal fibrosis in rat UUO model by inhibition of TGF-beta/Smad activity. *Lab Invest.* 2010;90(3):436-447.
13. Gong K, Xing D, Li P, et al. cGMP inhibits TGF-{beta} signaling by sequestering Smad3 with CYTOSOLIC {beta}2-tubulin in pulmonary artery smooth muscle cells. *Mol Endocrinol.* 2011;25(10):1794-1803.
14. Rosner M, Hengstschlager M. Cytoplasmic and nuclear distribution of the protein complexes mTORC1 and mTORC2: rapamycin triggers dephosphorylation and delocalization of the mTORC2 components rictor and sin1. *Hum Mol Genet.* 2008;17(19):2934-2948.
15. Hresko RC, Mueckler M. mTOR.RICTOR is the Ser473 kinase for Akt/protein kinase B in 3T3-L1 adipocytes. *J Biol Chem.* 2005;280(49):40406-40416.
16. Huang J, Manning BD. A complex interplay between Akt, TSC2 and the two mTOR complexes. *Biochem Soc Trans.* 2009;37:217-222.
17. Dhingra S, Rodriguez ME, Shen Q, et al. Constitutive activation with overexpression of the mTORC2-phospholipase D1 pathway in uterine leiomyosarcoma and STUMP: morphoproteomic analysis with therapeutic implications. *Int J Clin Exp Pathol.* 2010;4(2):134-146.

18. Shen Q, Stanton ML, Feng W, et al. Morphoproteomic analysis reveals an overexpressed and constitutively activated phospholipase D1-mTORC2 pathway in endometrial carcinoma. *Int J Clin Exp Pathol.* 2010;4(1):13-21.
19. Chen KF, Tai WT, Huang JW, et al. Sorafenib derivatives induce apoptosis through inhibition of STAT3 independent of Raf. *Eur J Med Chem.* 2011;46(7):2845-2851.
20. Adnane L, Trail PA, Taylor I, et al. Sorafenib (BAY 43-9006, Nexavar), a dual-action inhibitor that targets RAF/MEK/ERK pathway in tumor cells and tyrosine kinases VEGFR/PDGFR in tumor vasculature. *Methods Enzymol.* 2006;407:597-612.
21. Bai L, Yang JC, Ok JH, et al. Simultaneous targeting of Src kinase and receptor tyrosine kinase results in synergistic inhibition of renal cell carcinoma proliferation and migration. *Int J Cancer.* July 2011. 2012:130(11):2693-2702.
22. Finke JH, Rini B, Ireland J, et al. Sunitinib reverses type-1 immune suppression and decreases T-regulatory cells in renal cell carcinoma patients. *Clin Cancer Res.* 2008;14(20):6674-6682.
23. Busse A, Asemissen AM, Nonnenmacher A, et al. Immunomodulatory effects of sorafenib on peripheral immune effector cells in metastatic renal cell carcinoma. *Eur J Cancer.* 2011;47(5): 690-696.
24. Loo D, Beltejar C, Hooley J, et al. Primary and multipassage culture of human fetal kidney epithelial progenitor cells. *Methods Cell Biol.* 2008;86:241-255.
25. Terpe HJ, Storkel S, Zimmer U, et al. Expression of CD44 isoforms in renal cell tumors. Positive correlation to tumor differentiation. *Am J Pathol.* 1996;148(2):453-463.
26. Metsuyanim S, Harari-Steinberg O, Buzhor E, et al. Expression of stem cell markers in the human fetal kidney. *PLoS One.* 2009;4(8):e6709.
27. Pode-Shakked N, Metsuyanim S, Rom-Gross E, et al. Developmental tumourigenesis: NCAM as a putative marker for the malignant renal stem/progenitor cell population. *J Cell Mol Med.* 2009;13(B):1792-1808.
28. Ferrara N, Hillan KJ, Gerber HP, et al. Discovery and development of bevacizumab, an anti-VEGF antibody for treating cancer. *Nat Rev Drug Discov.* 2004;3(5):391-400.
29. Doshi GK, Buryanek J, Brown RE, et al. Adaptive targeted therapy in metastatic renal cell carcinoma: using morphoproteomics to guide treatment selection. *J Clin Oncol* (2010 ASCO Annual Meeting Proceedings (Post-Meeting Edition)). 2010;28(15 suppl) (May 20 supplement):e15069.
30. Wolff JE, Brown RE, Buryanek J, et al. Preliminary experience with personalized and targeted therapy for pediatric brain tumors. *Pediatr Blood Cancer.* 2012:59 (1):27-33.
31. Alison MR, Murphy G, Leedham S. Stem cells and cancer: a deadly mix. *Cell Tissue Res.* 2008;331(1):109-124.
32. Tang C, Ang BT, Pervaiz S. Cancer stem cell: target for anticancer therapy. *FASEB J.* 2007;21(14):3777-3785.
33. Armstrong AJ, Marengo MS, Oltean S, et al. Circulating tumor cells from patients with advanced prostate and breast cancer display both epithelial and mesenchymal markers. *Mol Cancer Res.* 2011;9(8):997-1007.
34. Chaffer CL, Weinberg RA. A perspective on cancer cell metastasis. *Science.* 2011;331(6024):1559-1564.
35. Li Z, Rich JN. Hypoxia and hypoxia inducible factors in cancer stem cell maintenance. *Curr Top Microbiol Immunol.* 2010;345: 21-30.
36. Haase VH. Oxygen regulates epithelial-to-mesenchymal transition: insights into molecular mechanisms and relevance to disease. *Kidney Int.* 2009;76(5):492-499.
37. Hill RP, Marie-Egyptienne DT, Hedley DW. Cancer stem cells, hypoxia and metastasis. *Semin Radiat Oncol.* 2009;19(2):106-111.
38. Maugeri-Sacca M, Vigneri P, De Maria R. Cancer stem cells and chemosensitivity. *Clin Cancer Res.* 2011;17(15):4942-4947.
39. Heddleston JM, Li Z, McLendon RE, Hjelmeland AB, Rich JN. The hypoxic microenvironment maintains glioblastoma stem cells and promotes reprogramming towards a cancer stem cell phenotype. *Cell Cycle.* 2009;8(20):3274-3284.
40. Li Z, Bao S, Wu Q, et al. Hypoxia-inducible factors regulate tumorigenic capacity of glioma stem cells. *Cancer Cell.* 2009;15(6):501-513.
41. Seidel S, Garvalov BK, Wirta V, et al. A hypoxic niche regulates glioblastoma stem cells through hypoxia inducible factor 2 alpha. *Brain.* 2010;133:983-995.
42. Wang X, Schneider A. HIF-2alpha-mediated activation of the epidermal growth factor receptor potentiates head and neck cancer cell migration in response to hypoxia. *Carcinogenesis.* 2010;31(7):1202-1210.
43. Gordan JD, Bertout JA, Hu CJ, Diehl JA, Simon MC. HIF-2alpha promotes hypoxic cell proliferation by enhancing c-myc transcriptional activity. *Cancer Cell.* 2007;11(4):335-347.
44. Toschi A, Lee E, Gadir N, Ohh M, Foster DA. Differential dependence of hypoxia-inducible factors 1 alpha and 2 alpha on mTORC1 and mTORC2. *J Biol Chem.* 2008;283(50):34495-34499.
45. Do TV, Kubba LA, Du H, Sturgis CD, Woodruff TK. Transforming growth factor-beta1, transforming growth factor-beta2, and transforming growth factor-beta3 enhance ovarian cancer metastatic potential by inducing a Smad3-dependent epithelial-to-mesenchymal transition. *Mol Cancer Res.* 2008;6(5):695-705.
46. Sethi S, Sarkar FH, Ahmed Q, et al. Molecular markers of epithelial-to-mesenchymal transition are associated with tumor aggressiveness in breast carcinoma. *Transl Oncol.* 2011;4(4): 222-226.
47. Gupta PB, Onder TT, Jiang G, et al. Identification of selective inhibitors of cancer stem cells by high-throughput screening. *Cell.* 2009;138(4):645-659.
48. Parry S, Savage K, Marchio C, et al. Nestin is expressed in basal-like and triple negative breast cancers. *J Clin Pathol.* 2008;61(9):1045-1050.
49. Liu J, Brown RE. Immunohistochemical detection of epithelial mesenchymal transition associated with stemness phenotype in anaplastic thyroid carcinoma. *Int J Clin Exp Pathol.* 2010;3(8):755-762.
50. Zhao P, Lu Y, Jiang X, et al. Clinicopathological significance and prognostic value of CD133 expression in triple-negative breast carcinoma. *Cancer Sci.* 2011;102(5):1107-1111.
51. Subbiah V, Naing A, Brown RE, et al. Targeted morphoproteomic profiling of Ewing's sarcoma treated with insulin-like growth factor 1 receptor (IGF1R) inhibitors: response/resistance signatures. *PLoS One.* 2011;6(4):e18424.
52. Sakai N, Baba M, Nagasima Y, et al. SPARC expression in primary human renal cell carcinoma: upregulation of SPARC in sarcomatoid renal carcinoma. *Hum Pathol.* 2001;32(10): 1064-1070.
53. Conant JL, Peng Z, Evans MF, et al. Sarcomatoid renal cell carcinoma is an example of epithelial-mesenchymal transition. *J Clin Pathol.* October. 2011;64 (12):1088-1092.
54. Hung CM, Kuo DH, Chou CH, et al. Osthole suppresses hepatocyte growth factor (HGF)-induced epithelial-mesenchymal transition via repression of the c-Met/Akt/mTOR pathway in human breast cancer cells. *J Agric Food Chem.* 2011;59(17):9683-9690.
55. Ide T, Kitajima Y, Miyoshi A, et al. The hypoxic environment in tumor-stromal cells accelerates pancreatic cancer progression via the activation of paracrine hepatocyte growth factor/c-Met signaling. *Ann Surg Oncol.* 2007;14(9):2600-2607.
56. Eckerich C, Zapf S, Fillbrandt R, Loges S, Westphal M, Lamszus K. Hypoxia can induce c-Met expression in glioma cells and enhance SF/HGF-induced cell migration. *Int J Cancer.* 2007;121(2):276-283.
57. Chen HH, Su WC, Lin PW, Guo HR, Lee WY. Hypoxia-inducible factor-1alpha correlates with MET and metastasis in node-negative breast cancer. *Breast Cancer Res Treat.* 2007;103(2):167-175.
58. Algire C, Amrein L, Zakikhani M, et al. Metformin blocks the stimulative effect of a high-energy diet on colon carcinoma growth in vivo and is associated with reduced expression of fatty acid synthase. *Endocr Relat Cancer.* 2010;17(2):351-360.
59. Ou SH, Kwak EL, Siwak-Tapp C, et al. Activity of crizotinib (PF02341066), a dual mesenchymal-epithelial transition (MET) and anaplastic lymphoma kinase (ALK) inhibitor, in a non-small cell lung cancer patient with de novo MET amplification. *J Thorac Oncol.* 2011;6(5):942-946.

CHAPTER 14

Flow Cytometry

George Deeb

INTRODUCTION

The applications of flow cytometry are widely used in cancer diagnostics and scientific research and more noticeably in those related to hematolymphoid neoplasms. The role of flow cytometry assessment has become essential in aiding the multimodality approach of diagnosing, classifying, and monitoring the clinical course of hematolymphoid neoplasms. This chapter attempts to generally discuss the major roles of flow cytometry in cancer diagnostics and specifically focus on hematolymphoid neoplasms. The roles of flow cytometry in the diagnostic workup and management of hematolymphoid neoplasms include, but are not restricted to, determining the lineage, maturity, and neoplastic nature, aiding the differential diagnosis, defining the tumor-associated aberrant immunophenotypes, detecting minimal residual disease (MRD), predicting the genotype by defining surrogate phenotypes, and defining prognostic markers and therapeutic targets. Moreover, in the advent of advanced molecular genetic technologies, flow cytometry may have a significant role in purifying the immunophenotypically characterized tumor cells, with the aim of dissecting their genetic aberrations and therefore contributing further to personalized cancer therapy.

THE PRINCIPLES OF FLOW CYTOMETRY

Flow cytometry analyzes cells in single cell suspension that pass (flow) individually through incident laser light. Different types of data are eventually collected upon the passage of each individual cell through the beam of the laser; the collected data result from the scattered light and the emitted fluorescence.[1] The collected data encompass physical and fluorescent characteristics of the analyzed cells. The physical characteristics are obtained from the scattered light that is detected by differently localized photodetectors that are aligned along the axis (forward scatter) or perpendicular to the axis (side scatter) of the laser beam. The forward scatter and side scatter provide information regarding the cell diameter (size) and cytoplasmic complexity (intracytoplasmic organelles and granularity), respectively. These physical characteristics of the analyzed cells are utilized in separating the cells into distinct populations based on their size and cytoplasmic complexity. The fluorescent characteristics of the cells of interest are obtained upon exciting the fluorochromes that are attached to the cells via antibodies or bound to the DNA. The fluorescent characteristics are utilized to determine the type of the cells or to assess their DNA content.[2,3] The fluorochromes attached to the cells are conjugated to monoclonal antibodies directed against antigens that may have membranous, intracytoplasmic, or intra-nuclear localizations. Multiple fluorochromes, ranging from 3 to 10 or more, could be assessed on a single cell in typical flow cytometry analysis.[2,4] The collected data are stored digitally and analyzed computationally using different types of analyzing software that generate single-dimensional or multidimensional plots (dot plots).[3] The dot plots depict the collected multiparametric data and the number of fluorochromes in addition to forward scatter and side scatter parameters[2] for each cell in the analyzed sample. Hence, the analysis is designated multiparameter flow cytometry (MFC).

The recent advances in MFC allow rapid, powerful, and efficient characterization of samples with variable cellular compositions and complexity such as blood and bone marrow.[5,6] The capability of analyzing expeditiously tens of thousands to millions of cells and the high throughput of the technology make it an essential ancillary study in the current clinical practice of diagnostic neoplastic hematology. MFC is principally beneficial in establishing the neoplastic nature, classifying, and assessing the prognostications of the hematolymphoid neoplasms.[7,8]

THE ROLES OF FLOW CYTOMETRY IN THE DIAGNOSTIC WORKUP AND MANAGEMENT OF HEMATOLYMPHOID NEOPLASMS

An integrated multimodality approach to the diagnosis and classification of hematolymphoid neoplasms has been proven essential to achieve the most appropriate classification according to the recent World Health Organization (WHO) classification of tumors of hematopoietic and lymphoid tissues.[9] Achieving the most appropriate classification is critical for planning therapy and predicting the clinical outcome.[10] The multimodality diagnostic approach encompasses morphologic, immunophenotypic, cytogenetic, and molecular evaluation of different types of tissue samples involved by the disease under assessment. Among these modalities, coupling of morphologic and immunophenotypic evaluation is the first step needed to triage the appropriate cytogenetic and molecular testing thereafter.[11] The immunophenotypic evaluation is commonly carried out by immunohistochemistry, which is performed on tissue sections, and/or by MFC, which is performed on cell suspensions of different types of specimens. MFC is routinely used to determine the lineage and differentiation, the maturity (immature vs. mature), the clonality or the neoplastic nature (whenever it is applicable), the antigen expression patterns (including specific immunophenotypic characteristics, Table 14.1, and occasionally prognostic markers relevant to certain neoplasms), and the MRD of the hematolymphoid neoplasms.[3,7,12] Based on the international consensus recommendations on the flow cytometric immunophenotyping analysis of hematolymphoid neoplasia (Bethesda 2006),[13-15] MFC is recommended to be used in several medical indications including cytopenia (mainly involving two or more lineages), leukocytosis, morphologic identification of abnormal cells in the evaluated specimen, monoclonal gammopathies and abnormal plasma cell proliferation, and organomegaly or neoplastic tissue masses. Considering all the above, MFC has been proven indispensable in working up hematolymphoid neoplasms.[5,7]

Determining the Lineage and Maturity of Hematolymphoid Neoplasms

The hematopoietic cells express variable patterns of antigens throughout their differentiation, lineage commitment, and cell maturation evolving into terminally mature functional cells.[31] The antigen expression patterns of the normal hematopoietic cells have been studied by MFC.[32,33] The antigen expression patterns are detected by monoclonal antibodies that target majorly surface antigens; these antibodies are designated cluster designation (CD) according to the International Workshop on Human Leukocyte Differentiation Antigens. The eighth workshop identified 339 CDs.[34]

Defining the antigen expression patterns by assessing expression of surface CDs and intracellular markers is crucial in the immunophenotypic classification of the neoplastic cells by assigning the most accurate lineage, maturation stage, and aberrant immunophenotypic features compared with their postulated normal counterparts.[7] The WHO classification of hematopoietic and lymphoid neoplasms is divided broadly according to the neoplastic cell lineage into myeloid, lymphoid (B- or T-lineage), and histiocytic and according to the neoplastic cell maturation into immature (acute leukemia) and mature (chronic leukemia and lymphoma).[9]

Lineage assignment usually dictates the therapeutic modalities of the hematolymphoid neoplasms since the chemotherapeutic approach to acute leukemia, as an example, is essentially different between those of myeloid and lymphoid lineages.[35,36] In the modern integrated hematopathology practice, lineage assignment is often established based on detecting the expression of lineage-specific markers by MFC in addition to the morphologic and genetic findings.[24]. Based merely on MFC, there are lineage-specific markers and lineage-associated markers used for lineage assignment according to WHO classification.[9] The markers that are lineage-specific and sufficient for lineage assignment themselves are cytoplasmic myeloperoxidase for myeloid lineage and surface CD3 or cytoplasmic CD3 (epsilon chain) for T-lineage.[16] Determination of the monocytic differentiation of the myeloid lineage and the B-lineage is based on the combination of two or more lineage-specific and associated markers. Finally, simultaneous expression of markers sufficient in establishing more than one lineage could assign mixed-lineage phenotype (B/myeloid or T/myeloid) to acute leukemia, which is rarely encountered.[24,25]

In addition to assigning lineage, the developmental stage or maturation of the hematolymphoid neoplasms is also very critical in dictating the appropriate therapy. It is well established in clinical practice that the treatment of immature neoplasms (acute leukemia) is essentially different from that of the mature myeloproliferative and lymphoproliferative neoplasms. MFC determines the maturation stages by highlighting sets of flow cytometric characteristics that are usually associated with immature state of the neoplastic cells in comparison with the maturation patterns of their postulated normal counterparts. The immature immunophenotypic characteristics detected by MFC generally include, but are not restricted to, expression of surface markers, individually or in variable combinations, such as CD34 and CD117, and intracellular markers such as terminal deoxynucleotidyl transferase (TdT). In addition, the immature neoplastic cells usually exhibit absence or weak expression of surface CD45 in comparison with the bright expression of this marker as exhibited by normal reactive lymphocytes. It is noteworthy that the immaturity status is not restricted to

TABLE 14–1 Multiparameter Flow Cytometry (MFC) Immunophenotypic Characteristics of Selected Hematolymphoid Neoplastic Entities According to the World Health Organization (WHO) Classification of Tumors of Hematopoietic and Lymphoid Tissue[9]

WHO Entities	MFC Characteristics	Comments and References
Mastocytosis	Aberrant expression of CD2 and CD25	These markers are expressed by neoplastic mast cells and are absent in the benign counterparts[7,9]
Myelodysplastic syndrome (MDS)	Aberrant expression of lymphoid antigens by the myeloid immature cells (myeloblasts) such as CD7 and CD56 and immunophenotypic abnormalities of mature myeloid cells such as decreased side scatter value of neutrophils (decreased granularity)	These are few immunophenotypic features out of several that could be encountered in global assessment of MDS by MFC[16,17]
Acute myeloid leukemia (AML), all subtypes	Expression of myeloid lineage–specific and associated markers such as cytoplasmic myeloperoxidase, CD13, and CD33 and immature/early markers such as CD34 and CD117	The MFC expression patterns are variable in AML due to the diversity of combination of markers and their intensity of expression. In addition, there are immunophenotypic features characteristic of monocytic (e.g., CD11c, CD14, and CD64), erythroid (e.g., glycophorin-A, CD36, and bright CD71), and megakaryocytic (e.g., CD41, CD42, and CD61) differentiations[7,9,12,18]
AML with t(8;21)(q22;q22) [*AML1-ETO*]	Aberrant expression of CD19 and/or CD56 is commonly encountered	Ossenkoppele et al.[16]; Hrusak and Porwit-MacDonald[19]; Yang et al.[20]
AML (promyelocytic) with t(15;17)(q22;q12) [*PML-RARA*]	High autofluorescence intensity in comparison with other types of AML and lacking CD34 and/or HLA-DR expression	Ossenkoppele et al.[16]; Di Noto et al.[21]; Hayden et al.[22]; Dong et al.[23]
AML (megakaryoblastic) with t(1;22)(p13;q13) [*RBM15-MKL1*]	Expression of variable combination of CD41, CD42, and/or CD61 and lacking expression of CD34, CD45, and HLA-DR	Expression of markers associated with megakaryocytic differentiation[9,11,12]
AML with mutated *NPM1* (provisional entity)	Lacking expression of CD34 and weak or absent expression of HLA-DR	Ossenkoppele et al.[16]
Mixed phenotype acute leukemia	The simultaneous expression of markers sufficient in establishing more than one lineage such as B or T and myeloid (mixed phenotype B/myeloid or T/myeloid acute leukemia)	Swerdlow et al.[9]; Weinberg and Arber[24]; Matutes et al.[25]
B and T lymphoblastic leukemia/lymphoma	Expression of lymphoid lineage–specific and associated markers such as CD19, CD20, CD22, and CD79a for B-lineage and cytoplasmic (epsilon) and uncommonly surface CD3 for T-lineage, immature markers such as CD34 and terminal deoxynucleotidyl transferase (TdT) and others such as CD10	Occasional aberrant expression of myeloid-associated antigens such as CD13 and/or CD33[3,6,11,12,18,26]
Chronic lymphocytic leukemia/small lymphocytic lymphoma	Co-expression of CD5 and CD23 in addition to weak expression of CD20 and surface light chain immunoglobulin. Expression of ZAP70 and to a lesser extent CD38 is an independent prognosticator	An overlap of immunophenotypic features between chronic lymphocytic leukemia and mantle cell lymphoma was reported[3,5,7,27,28]
Mantle cell lymphoma	Co-expression of CD19 and CD5 and bright expression of CD20 and surface light chain immunoglobulin	de Tute[3]; Jennings and Foon[5]; Craig and Foon[7]; Morice et al.[28]
Follicular lymphoma	Co-expression of CD20 and CD10	de Tute[3]; Jennings and Foon[5]; Craig and Foon[7]; Morice et al.[28]
Hairy cell leukemia	Bright expression of CD20, CD22, CD11c, and CD123 with co-expression of CD25 and CD103	de Tute[3]; Venkataraman et al.[29]; Stetler-Stevenson and Tembhare[30]
Plasma cell myeloma	Usually this neoplasm lacks CD19 and CD45 expression, occasionally aberrantly expresses CD56 and CD117, and exhibits restricted expression of cytoplasmic kappa or lambda light chain immunoglobulin	Lacking of CD19 and CD45 expression and aberrant expression of CD56 and CD117 are MFC characteristics of neoplastic plasma cells in comparison with their benign counterparts[7,12]
T-cell large granular lymphocytic leukemia	Commonly CD8 positive with variable expression of CD16, CD56, and CD57	de Tute[3]; Craig and Foon[7]; Calvo et al.[12]
Adult T-cell leukemia/lymphoma	Commonly CD4 positive with bright expression of CD25	Usually associated with human T-lymphotropic virus 1 (HTLV-1) infection[7,12]
Sezary syndrome	Commonly CD4 positive with common loss of CD7 and CD26 expression	de Tute[3]; Craig and Foon[7]; Calvo et al.[12]
NK-cell lymphoproliferative neoplasm	Variable expression of CD2, CD7, CD8, CD16, CD56, and/or CD57 and lacking of surface CD3 expression	Restricted expression of killer cell immunoglobulin receptors[7,12]

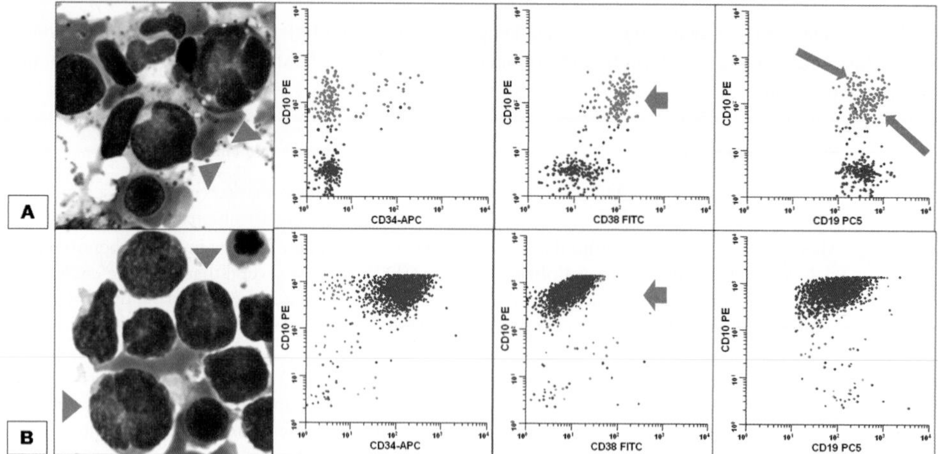

FIGURE 14–1 Multiparameter flow cytometry (MFC) analyses depicting some of the principles utilized to identify the neoplastic cell population. Bone marrow aspirate smears and MFC analyses of bone marrow samples, from two different patients, with benign B-precursors (hematogones) **(A)** and B lymphoblastic leukemia **(B)**. It is difficult to differentiate between the neoplastic lymphoblasts (**B**, *arrow heads*) and their postulated normal counterpart (hematogones) (**A**, *arrow heads*) based merely on the cytomorphologic evaluation as shown in the bone marrow aspirate smears (**A** and **B**). Based on MFC analyses, the hematogones exhibit spectrum of maturation encompassing distinct early and intermediate/late subpopulations (**A**, *long arrows*) and homogenous CD38 expression (**A**, *short arrow*); in contrast, the neoplastic B lymphoblasts show distinct tight population and noticeable underexpression of CD38 (**B**, *short arrow*). The microscopic photomicrographs are those of bone marrow aspirate smears corresponding to the MFC analyses, Wright-Giemsa stain, ×1000. The dot plots are those of four-color MFC analyses. PE, phycoerythrin; APC, allophycocyanin; FITC, fluorescein isothiocyanate; PC5, phycoerythrin-cyanine 5.1.

these markers since not all cases of acute leukemia express CD34 or TdT.[5,7] Other findings are usually helpful in this situation including morphologic correlation such as the blastic cytomorphologic features and/or certain genetic abnormalities that are commonly associated with specific subtypes of acute leukemia. On the other side of the maturation spectrum, there are immunophenotypic markers usually associated with maturity such as bright expression of CD20 and CD45 or expression of surface light chain immunoglobulin in B-lineage neoplasms in the absence of CD34 and TdT expression. Overall, these assignments should be entertained cautiously and should be correlated with morphologic and genetic findings whenever available since some acute leukemia cases may exhibit aberrant antigen expression such as unusual expression of surface light chain immunoglobulin by rare cases of B lymphoblastic leukemia.[37]

Determining the Presumptive and Definite Neoplastic Nature of Hematolymphoid Neoplasms

In addition to establishing the cell lineage and maturity status, MFC is also critically helpful in establishing the neoplastic nature of the disease and in differentiating it from reactive hematolymphoid processes that may mimic neoplasia. The neoplastic nature could be postulated based on aberrant antigen expressions that deviate from those of presumptive normal counterpart cells seen in the same tissue type such as underexpression, overexpression, or asynchronous expression of lineage-associated antigens or aberrant expression of cross-lineage antigens. As an example, detecting the underexpression of CD38, overexpression of CD10, and aberrant myeloid marker expression (CD13 and/or CD33) on the neoplastic cells of B lymphoblastic leukemia was shown to be helpful in differentiating them from benign B-lineage precursors (hematogones), which are their postulated normal counterparts in the bone marrow (Fig. 14.1 A and B).[26,38] Also, the MFC may represent indirect evidence of clonality and therefore neoplastic nature by detecting restricted expression of kappa or lambda light chain immunoglobulin by mature B-lineage lymphoproliferative neoplasms.[3,7] Detection of restricted light chain immunoglobulin expression is consistent with the presence of monotypic B-lineage population that is usually associated with genetic monoclonality within the right histomorphologic and clinical context and with careful attention to the reported occasional association of restricted light chain expression with some reactive lymphoproliferations.[7] The loss of expression of pan-T-cell markers such as CD3, CD2, CD5, and/or CD7 may suggest evidence of neoplasia in mature T-cell lymphoproliferative neoplasms.[6,7] Similar to restricted expression of light chain in B-lineage neoplasms, restricted expression of one of the T-cell receptor V-β subtypes may be consistent with genetic monoclonality in mature T-cell lymphoproliferative neoplasms in the right clinicopathologic context.[7]

Aiding the Differential Diagnosis of Hematolymphoid Neoplasms

Upon assigning the lineage and maturation stage of the neoplastic hematolymphoid cells and further supporting the neoplastic nature of these cells, additional immunophenotypic characteristics may provide a strong presumptive evidence of the classification of the hematolymphoid neoplasm or narrow down the differential diagnostic possibilities that could be further refined and confirmed by morphologic and/or genetic findings. The differential diagnosis of mature small-cell-size lymphocytic neoplasms includes certain classes with commonly encountered immunophenotypic characteristics such as 1) the co-expression of CD5 and CD23 in addition to weak expression of CD20 and surface light chain immunoglobulin in chronic lymphocytic leukemia (CLL), 2) co-expression of CD19 and CD5 and bright expression of CD20 and surface light chain immunoglobulin in mantle cell lymphoma, and 3) co-expression of CD20 and CD10 in follicle center cell lymphoma such as follicular lymphoma.[5,7] An overlap of immunophenotypic features between these neoplasms was reported,[3] and the aforementioned immunophenotypic characteristics are not restricted to certain entity. Careful comprehensive correlation with morphology and genetics should be entertained whenever possible for definitive classification.

Defining the Tumor-Associated Aberrant Immunophenotypes and Detecting MRD of Hematolymphoid Neoplasms

It is always beneficial to comprehensively determine the unique morphologic, genetic, and aberrant immunophenotypic characteristics of the neoplastic cells in the pre-therapeutic samples. These tumor-unique characteristics are essential for detecting residual neoplastic cells in the post-treatment follow-up samples, which aids in assessing the response to therapy and the clinical management. The response to therapy may include overt persistent disease, MRD, or post-remission early or overtly recurrent disease (relapse). This is mainly critical in the management of patients with acute leukemia; the acute leukemic cells usually exhibit unique aberrant antigen expression patterns,[39,40] which are characterized by MFC and could be labeled leukemia-associated aberrant immunophenotypes (LAIPs).[41,42] MFC critically aids in characterizing the LAIPs by identifying the specific antigen expression patterns of the population of interest that deviate from the expected normal patterns by asynchronous expression of lineage-associated antigens related to different maturational stages, variations in the intensities of expression (underexpression or overexpression) of the lineage-associated antigens, or aberrant expression of cross-lineage antigens (lineage infidelity).[39,43] Several issues should be considered regarding the LAIPs: (1) the neoplastic leukemic cells may lack specific LAIPs,[43] (2) LAPIs are usually disease- and patient-specific and should be determined individually for each patient as there is no universal marker that could be used to follow up the acute leukemic cells, (3) LAIPs may change in follow-up and relapse samples (Fig. 14.2),[44,45] and (4) the detection of LAIPs may be occasionally related to the clones of the antibodies and the conjugated fluorochromes that may affect the detection of the aberrant antigen and its intensity of expression.[41] For the LAIPs to be beneficial in the detection of MRD, the markers that constitute useful LAIPs should be distinctly identified as trans-lineage markers, stable throughout the disease follow-ups and expressed by the majority of the neoplastic leukemic cells.[41] The detection of MRD by MFC has been proven to be prognostically independent in acute myeloid leukemia (AML). Quantifying the frequency of residual leukemic cells may predict relapse, the duration of remission, and the overall survival[39] and may potentially contribute, in conjunction with traditional prognosticators such as cytogenetic and molecular parameters, to better planning of therapeutic approach for good versus high-risk AML patients.[42] Overall, flow cytometry is more sensitive and specific than morphologic inspection in detecting MRD in acute leukemia.[46] MFC has also the advantages of being independent from the specific genetic abnormalities and applicable to the majority of acute leukemia, mainly AML, as the majority of the leukemic cell populations harbor aberrant immunophenotypes.[40] MFC has also been predictive of clinical prognosis in pediatric and adult acute lymphoblastic leukemia.[47,48] Additionally, pediatric patients with MRD detected by MFC prior to allogeneic hematopoietic cell transplant encountered poorer clinical course.[49]

The utility of MFC in detecting MRD is not limited to acute leukemia but extends to other hematolymphoid neoplasms applying the same principle of detecting very low frequencies of the neoplastic cells that may exhibit unique aberrant immunophenotypic features facilitating such detection. Despite the inherent underestimation of the tumor burden of the plasma cell myeloma in the bone marrow samples obtained for MFC analysis due to sampling variation, hemodilution, red blood cell lysing, and fragility of the neoplastic cells,[50] several studies showed the importance of detection of MRD in plasma cell myeloma by MFC as the detection of MED is shown to be clinically significant in predicting overall survival at the time of diagnosis.[51] In addition, it was shown in a retrospective study that patients who had significant residual neoplastic plasma cells detected by MFC prior to autologous stem cell transplant had shorter progression-free survival.[52]

The MFC has the ability to overcome sample- and technical-related challenges in estimating the quantity of the neoplastic plasma cells in the bone marrow samples since it is capable of analyzing simultaneously several cellular components and characterizing the neoplastic and the remaining benign cellular populations present in the bone marrow sample. In an attempt to factor for the analysis-inherent issues, such as hemodilution, which preclude an accurate assessment of the burden of plasma cell neoplasm in the bone marrow samples, Frebet et al.[50] studied the ratio of neoplastic plasma cells over the CD34-positive precursors to standardize the MFC analysis for quantifying plasma cells.

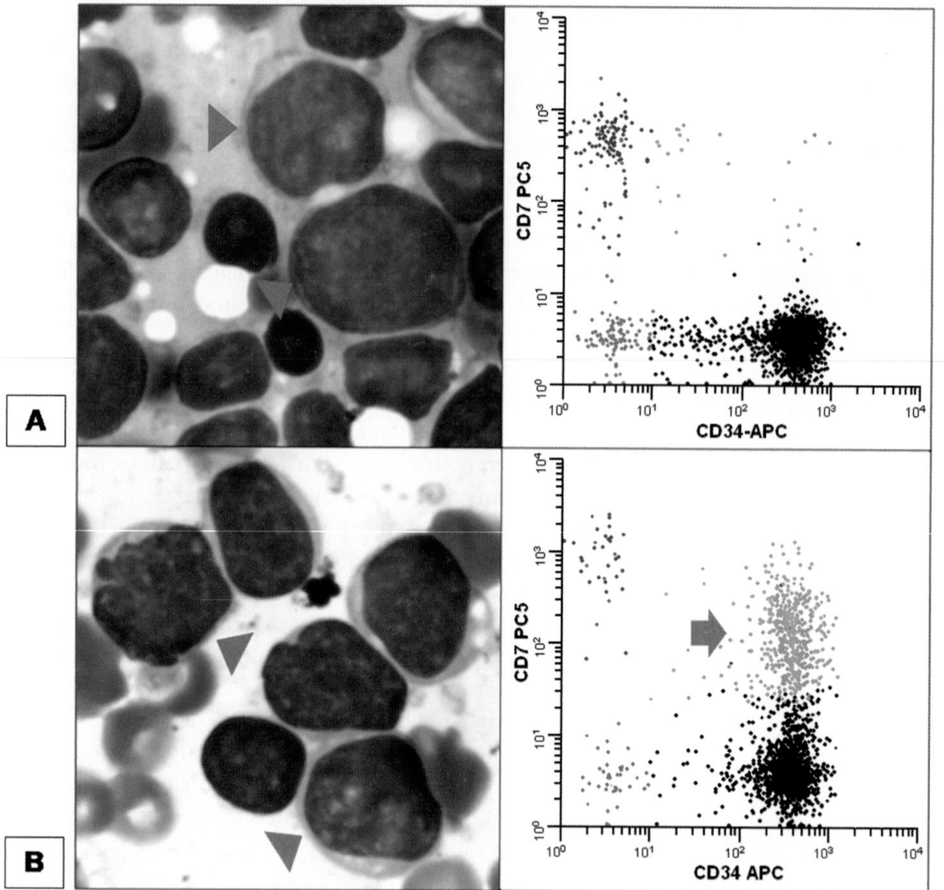

FIGURE 14–2 Multiparameter flow cytometry (MFC) analyses illustrating occasional immunophenotypic changes of the neoplastic cell population between primary diagnosis and relapse. Bone marrow aspirate smears and MFC analyses of bone marrow samples from a patient with relapsed acute myeloid leukemia (AML) post-allogeneic peripheral blood stem cell transplant. **(A)** Primary diagnostic AML and **(B)** post-transplant relapsed AML. The myeloblasts in both samples have similar cytomorphologic features (**A** and **B**, *arrow heads*) and identical cytogenetic abnormalities but newly detected CD7 expression (*arrow*) in post-transplant AML. The microscopic photomicrographs are those of bone marrow aspirate smears corresponding to the MFC analyses, Wright-Giemsa stain, ×1000. The dot plots are those of four-color MFC analyses. APC, allophycocyanin; PC5, phycoerythrin-cyanine 5.1.

Predicting the Genotype of Hematolymphoid Neoplasms

MFC has a significantly shorter turnaround time than cytogenetic and molecular diagnostic analyses. In conjunction with morphologic assessment, MFC could prompt the appropriate workup including triaging the most relevant confirmatory genetic testing.[11] MFC could aid in this process by detecting immunophenotypic characteristics that are commonly reported to be associated with certain genetic abnormalities. MFC has the ability to predict what should be confirmed thereafter by appropriate genetic testing. For example, predicting immunophenotypic features could be seen in AML with t(8;21)(q22;q22) [*AML1-ETO*][19,20] and in AML (acute promyelocytic leukemia) with t(15;17)(q22;q12) [*PML-RARA*].[21] This prediction is very critical when targeted therapy, all-*trans* retinoic acid (ATRA), is recommended to be immediately initiated based on the morphologic suspicion of AML with t(15;17)(q22;q12).[21] In such instances, MFC findings further support the morphologic impression awaiting definite genetic confirmation of *PML-RARA* translocation/fusion. Aberrant expression of CD19, a pan-B-lineage marker, is frequently encountered on the myeloblasts of AML with t(8;21)(q22;q22),[19] and aberrant expression of CD56 (neural cell adhesion molecule 1; *NCAM1*) may indicate worse prognosis in this overall good risk group of AML (Fig. 14.3).[20] More interestingly, AML with t(15;17)(q22;q12) commonly encounters immunophenotypic characteristics that exhibit high autofluorescence intensity in comparison with other types of AML[22] and lack expression of CD34 and/or HLA-DR.[21-23]

It is always intriguing when MFC immunophenotyping of the hematolymphoid neoplasms is able to detect surrogate phenotypic features for clinically relevant genetic abnormality. As discussed above, this concept is fully utilized in AML, but it may be occasionally encountered in the lymphoproliferative neoplasms. Some of the independent prognostic markers of the clinical behavior of CLL include the mutational status of the immunoglobulin heavy chain gene (IGHV), genetic abnormalities detected by FISH, and expression of CD38 and ZAP70 (zeta-chain(TCR)–associated protein kinase 70 kDa).[27] The expression of CD38 and ZAP70 could be routinely assessed by MFC in all types of leukemia. ZAP70 was mainly shown to be a surrogate for CLL with unmutated IGHV and, therefore, may predict the genotype.[53-56]

Defining Prognostic Markers and Therapeutic Targets of Hematolymphoid Neoplasms

As previously discussed, MFC is a robust technology to characterize the immunophenotypes of the neoplastic hematolymphoid cells and their specific discriminatory

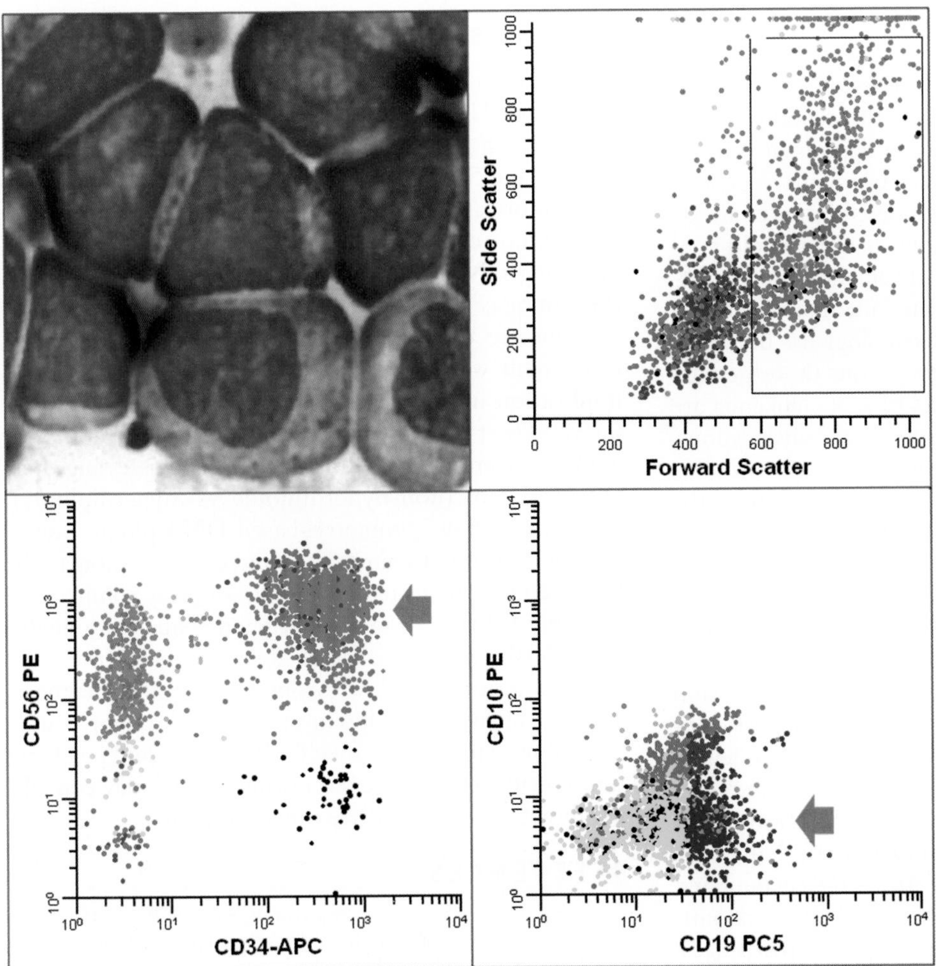

FIGURE 14–3 Multiparameter flow cytometry (MFC) analysis identifying aberrant expression patterns that may suggest certain genetic abnormalities. Bone marrow aspirate smear and MFC analysis of bone marrow sample from patient with acute myeloid leukemia (AML) with t(8;21)(q22;q22) [*AML1-ETO*]. The myeloblasts express aberrant CD19 and CD56 (*arrows*), which are common aberrancies seen in this type of AML. The microscopic photomicrograph is of bone marrow aspirate smear corresponding to the MFC analysis, Wright-Giemsa stain, ×1000. The dot plots are those of four-color MFC analyses. PE, phycoerythrin; APC, allophycocyanin; PC5, phycoerythrin-cyanine 5.1.

markers that may help detect MRD and occasionally predict the associated genetic abnormalities (the genotypes). The aforementioned utility is based mainly on multiple characteristics/markers; however, individual marker expression detected by MFC may also be a prognosticator by itself. Expression of CD56 was shown to have worse effects on the disease-free survival and overall survival of patients with AML with t(8;21)(q22;q22)[20] and predict worse outcomes in patients with AML with t(15;17)(q22;q12) despite targeted therapy and regardless of the white blood cell count.[21]

There are few markers detected by flow cytometry that are shown to carry independent prognostic indications in mature lymphoid neoplasms that include CLL. The expression of CD38 and ZAP70 was proven to be a poorer predictor of time needed from diagnosis to therapy and survival.[53,54]

Detecting certain target antigens has become crucial for immunotherapy for hematolymphoid neoplasms. Targeted immunotherapy is an essential therapeutic modality for primary or refractory lymphoproliferative neoplasms. Humanized monoclonal antibody targeting CD20 surface marker (anti-CD20, rituximab) expressed by the lymphoproliferative neoplasm cells has further improved patients' survival in mature B-cell non-Hodgkin lymphoma.[57] Detecting the expression of the targeted antigens by MFC is critical for the therapeutic planning of the hematolymphoid neoplasm that is treated with targeted immunotherapy. MFC is routinely available in most clinical laboratories, amenable to test various types of samples, and capable of multiparametric assessment of the cells of interest. Examples of markers that may be detected by flow cytometry and amenable to targeted therapy include CD20 for the treatment of CD20-positive low-grade and high-grade mature B-cell lymphoproliferative neoplasms,[58,59] CD52 by anti-CD52 (alemtuzumab) for CLL and T-cell lymphoproliferative neoplasms,[60] and CD80 by anti-CD80 (galiximab), which is still under investigation for the treatment of refractory follicular lymphoma.[61,62]

Detecting Recurrent Fusion Proteins in Leukemia

The cytogenetic abnormalities detected during the initial diagnostic workup of adult AML are the most relevant prognostic factors that predict complete remission and survival.[63] The recurrent genetic abnormalities became the foundation of the most recent WHO classification of de novo AML.[9] Expeditious confirmation of AML with t(15;17)(q22;q12), one of the listed AML with recurrent genetic abnormalities, is very critical in the clinical management since there is an effective targeted therapy, ATRA, that is available for this type of AML.[21] Routine clinical MFC analysis has the ability to predict genotype based on traditional immunophenotyping by detecting certain characteristics that may be surrogate for the genotype; these findings should always be confirmed by appropriate genetic testing. Therefore, utilizing the flow cytometry capability in detecting proteins (antigens) translated from the fusion genes of the recurrent genetic abnormalities could contribute significantly to the acute leukemia diagnosis, classification, and therefore appropriate initiation of therapy. Recently, flow cytometry–based technology has been able to detect fusion proteins resulting from these genetic abnormalities.[64,65] Certain subtypes of acute leukemia are characterized genetically by chromosomal translocations, resulting in fusion genes that were proven to have a significant role in their leukemogenesis. Dekking et al. from the EuroFlow Consortium[65] developed a flow cytometric assay to detect the common fusion proteins in acute leukemia and chronic myelogenous leukemia utilizing bead-bound fluorochrome-conjugated fusion protein–capturing antibodies. This assay could be performed routinely in the clinical flow cytometry laboratory. The assay targeted several fusion proteins including *BCR-ABL1* encountered in B lymphoblastic leukemia/lymphoma and chronic myelogenous leukemia with t(9;22)(q34;q11.2), *TEL-AML1* encountered in B lymphoblastic leukemia/lymphoma with t(12;21)(p13;q22), *E2A-PBX1* encountered in B lymphoblastic leukemia/lymphoma with t(1;19)(q23;p13.3), *MLL-AF4* encountered in AML with t(9;11)(p22;q23), *CBFB-MYH11* encountered in AML with inv(16)(p13.1q22)/t(16;16)(p13.1;q22), *AML1-ETO* encountered in AML with t(8;21)(q22;q22), and *PML-RARA* encountered in AML with t(15;17)(q22;q12). It seems very innovative and efficient to utilize flow cytometry to correlate simultaneously with the immunophenotypic and genetic findings.

OTHER APPLICATIONS OF FLOW CYTOMETRY

Coupling Phenotype with Morphology (Imaging Flow Cytometry)

The traditional flow cytometry analysis is performed on cells in suspension that are dissociated from their tissue samples and therefore are not amenable to cytomorphologic assessment. Coupling of flow cytometry with the cytomorphologic evaluation may further empower the traditional flow cytometry analysis. The imaging flow cytometry has the ability of coupling the high-throughput multiparametric flow cytometry analysis with the capability of the fluorescent microscopy by capturing digital images for acquired events.[66,67] Maguire et al.[66] depicted the utility of imaging flow cytometry (ImageStream platform, Amnis Corporation, Seattle, WA) in detecting the nuclear translocation of p65 component of NF-κB (nuclear factor of kappa light polypeptide gene enhancer in B cells 1) in leukemic cell lines treated with daunorubicin in variably heterogeneous samples.

DNA Analysis and Tumor Cell Sorting

There are other applications of flow cytometry that have been utilized in cancer diagnosis, management, and scientific research, such as assessing the DNA analysis (DNA content and S-phase fraction)[68] of solid and hematopoietic tumors and identifying and quantifying circulating solid tumor cells[68,69] and endothelial progenitor cells.[70] Assessing DNA content, mainly assessing the ploidy of the tumor cells, has been shown recently to still have relevance to cancer management and research. Ploidy assessment was proven to have significant prognostic implication in plasma cell myeloma as shown recently by Mateos et al.[71]; the authors utilized the capability of MFC for identifying the plasma cells and assessing their DNA content (non-hyperdiploidy vs. hyperdiploidy). In addition, flow cytometry–based DNA ploidy assessment was utilized to purify the pancreatic carcinoma cells from heterogeneous tissue samples for array comparative genomic hybridization and targeted sequencing analyses.[72] Furthermore, the future is promising for the powerful applications of flow cytometry in cancer diagnosis and management by coupling the high-throughput utility of flow cytometry in specifically sorting and purifying tumor cells to the molecular testing[72,73] that may contribute directly to individualize cancer therapy.

REFERENCES

1. Tung JW, Heydari K, Tirouvanziam R, Sahaf B, Parks DR, Herzenberg LA. Modern flow cytometry: a practical approach. *Clin Lab Med*. 2007;27:453-468, v.
2. Dunphy CH. *Integrated Hematopathology: Morphology and FCI with IHC*. Chicago, IL: American Society for Clinical Pathology; 2010:xi, 323 p.
3. de Tute RM. Flow cytometry and its use in the diagnosis and management of mature lymphoid malignancies. *Histopathology*. 2011;58:90-105.
4. Wood B. 9-color and 10-color flow cytometry in the clinical laboratory. *Arch Pathol Lab Med*. 2006;130:680-690.
5. Jennings CD, Foon KA. Recent advances in flow cytometry: application to the diagnosis of hematologic malignancy. *Blood*. 1997;90:2863-2892.
6. Martinez A, Aymerich M, Castillo M, et al. Routine use of immunophenotype by flow cytometry in tissues with suspected hematological malignancies. *Cytometry B Clin Cytom*. 2003;56:8-15.
7. Craig FE, Foon KA. Flow cytometric immunophenotyping for hematologic neoplasms. *Blood*. 2008;111:3941-3967.
8. Vardiman JW, Thiele J, Arber DA, et al. The 2008 revision of the World Health Organization (WHO) classification of myeloid neoplasms and acute leukemia: rationale and important changes. *Blood*. 2009;114:937-951.
9. Swerdlow SH, International Agency for Research on Cancer, World Health Organization. *WHO Classification of Tumours of Haematopoietic and Lymphoid Tissues*. 4th ed. Lyon, France: International Agency for Research on Cancer; 2008:439 p.
10. Haferlach T, Bacher U, Kern W, Schnittger S, Haferlach C. Diagnostic pathways in acute leukemias: a proposal for a multimodal approach. *Ann Hematol*. 2007;86:311-327.
11. Peters JM, Ansari MQ. Multiparameter flow cytometry in the diagnosis and management of acute leukemia. *Arch Pathol Lab Med*. 2011;135:44-54.
12. Calvo KR, McCoy CS, Stetler-Stevenson M. Flow cytometry immunophenotyping of hematolymphoid neoplasia. *Methods Mol Biol*. 2011;699:295-316.
13. Wilson WH. International consensus recommendations on the flow cytometric immunophenotypic analysis of

hematolymphoid neoplasia. *Cytometry B Clin Cytom*. 2007;72 (suppl 1):S2.

14. Davis BH, Holden JT, Bene MC, et al. 2006 Bethesda International Consensus recommendations on the flow cytometric immunophenotypic analysis of hematolymphoid neoplasia: medical indications. *Cytometry B Clin Cytom*. 2007;72(suppl 1):S5-S13.
15. Wood BL, Arroz M, Barnett D, et al. 2006 Bethesda International Consensus recommendations on the immunophenotypic analysis of hematolymphoid neoplasia by flow cytometry: optimal reagents and reporting for the flow cytometric diagnosis of hematopoietic neoplasia. *Cytometry B Clin Cytom*. 2007;72(suppl 1):S14-S22.
16. Ossenkoppele GJ, van de Loosdrecht AA, Schuurhuis GJ. Review of the relevance of aberrant antigen expression by flow cytometry in myeloid neoplasms. *Br J Haematol*. May 2011;153(4):421-436.
17. Chu SC, Wang TF, Li CC, et al. Flow cytometric scoring system as a diagnostic and prognostic tool in myelodysplastic syndromes. *Leuk Res*. 2011;35:868-873.
18. Jennings CD, Foon KA. Flow cytometry: recent advances in diagnosis and monitoring of leukemia. *Cancer Invest*. 1997;15: 384-399.
19. Hrusak O, Porwit-MacDonald A. Antigen expression patterns reflecting genotype of acute leukemias. *Leukemia*. 2002;16: 1233-1258.
20. Yang DH, Lee JJ, Mun YC, et al. Predictable prognostic factor of CD56 expression in patients with acute myeloid leukemia with t(8:21) after high dose cytarabine or allogeneic hematopoietic stem cell transplantation. *Am J Hematol*. 2007;82:1-5.
21. Di Noto R, Mirabelli P, Del Vecchio L. Flow cytometry analysis of acute promyelocytic leukemia: the power of "surface hematology". *Leukemia*. 2007;21:4-8.
22. Hayden PJ, O'Connell NM, O'Brien DA, O'Rourke P, Lawlor E, Browne PV. The value of autofluorescence as a diagnostic feature of acute promyelocytic leukemia. *Haematologica*. 2006;91:417-418.
23. Dong HY, Kung JX, Bhardwaj V, McGill J. Flow cytometry rapidly identifies all acute promyelocytic leukemias with high specificity independent of underlying cytogenetic abnormalities. *Am J Clin Pathol*. 2011;135:76-84.
24. Weinberg OK, Arber DA. Mixed-phenotype acute leukemia: historical overview and a new definition. *Leukemia*. 2010;24: 1844-1851.
25. Matutes E, Pickl WF, Van't Veer M, et al. Mixed-phenotype acute leukemia: clinical and laboratory features and outcome in 100 patients defined according to the WHO 2008 classification. *Blood*. 2011;117:3163-3171.
26. Seegmiller AC, Kroft SH, Karandikar NJ, McKenna RW. Characterization of immunophenotypic aberrancies in 200 cases of B acute lymphoblastic leukemia. *Am J Clin Pathol*. 2009;132: 940-949.
27. Shanafelt TD. Predicting clinical outcome in CLL: how and why. *Hematology (Am Soc Hematol Educ Program)*. 2009:421-429.
28. Morice WG, Kurtin PJ, Hodnefield JM, et al. Predictive value of blood and bone marrow flow cytometry in B-cell lymphoma classification: comparative analysis of flow cytometry and tissue biopsy in 252 patients. *Mayo Clin Proc*. 2008;83:776-785.
29. Venkataraman G, Aguhar C, Kreitman RJ, Yuan CM, Stetler-Stevenson M. Characteristic CD103 and CD123 expression pattern defines hairy cell leukemia: usefulness of CD123 and CD103 in the diagnosis of mature B-cell lymphoproliferative disorders. *Am J Clin Pathol*. 2011;136:625-630.
30. Stetler-Stevenson M, Tembhare PR. Diagnosis of hairy cell leukemia by flow cytometry. *Leuk Lymphoma*. 2011;52(suppl 2): 11-13.
31. Wood BL. Myeloid malignancies: myelodysplastic syndromes, myeloproliferative disorders, and acute myeloid leukemia. *Clin Lab Med*. 2007;27:551-575, vii.
32. van Lochem EG, van der Velden VH, Wind HK, te Marvelde JG, Westerdaal NA, van Dongen JJ. Immunophenotypic differentiation patterns of normal hematopoiesis in human bone marrow: reference patterns for age-related changes and disease-induced shifts. *Cytometry B Clin Cytom*. 2004;60:1-13.
33. Kussick SJ, Wood BL. Using 4-color flow cytometry to identify abnormal myeloid populations. *Arch Pathol Lab Med*. 2003;127:1140-1147.
34. Carey JL, McCoy JP, Keren DF. *Flow Cytometry in Clinical Diagnosis*. 4th ed. Chicago, IL: American Society for Clinical Pathology; 2007:xv, 384 p.
35. Casasnovas RO, Slimane FK, Garand R, et al. Immunological classification of acute myeloblastic leukemias: relevance to patient outcome. *Leukemia*. 2003;17:515-527.
36. Qadir M, Barcos M, Stewart CC, Sait SN, Ford LA, Baer MR. Routine immunophenotyping in acute leukemia: role in lineage assignment and reassignment. *Cytometry B Clin Cytom*. 2006;70:329-334.
37. Kansal R, Deeb G, Barcos M, et al. Precursor B lymphoblastic leukemia with surface light chain immunoglobulin restriction: a report of 15 patients. *Am J Clin Pathol*. 2004;121:512-555.
38. McKenna RW, Asplund SL, Kroft SH. Immunophenotypic analysis of hematogones (B-lymphocyte precursors) and neoplastic lymphoblasts by 4-color flow cytometry. *Leuk Lymphoma*. 2004;45:277-285.
39. San Miguel JF, Martinez A, Macedo A, et al. Immunophenotyping investigation of minimal residual disease is a useful approach for predicting relapse in acute myeloid leukemia patients. *Blood*. 1997;90:2465-2470.
40. Baer MR. Detection of minimal residual disease in acute myeloid leukemia. *Curr Oncol Rep*. 2002;4:398-402.
41. Freeman SD, Jovanovic JV, Grimwade D. Development of minimal residual disease-directed therapy in acute myeloid leukemia. *Semin Oncol*. 2008;35:388-400.
42. Buccisano F, Maurillo L, Spagnoli A, et al. Cytogenetic and molecular diagnostic characterization combined to postconsolidation minimal residual disease assessment by flow cytometry improves risk stratification in adult acute myeloid leukemia. *Blood*. 2010;116:2295-2303.
43. Kern W, Haferlach C, Haferlach T, Schnittger S. Monitoring of minimal residual disease in acute myeloid leukemia. *Cancer*. 2008;112:4-16.
44. Baer MR, Stewart CC, Dodge RK, et al. High frequency of immunophenotype changes in acute myeloid leukemia at relapse: implications for residual disease detection (Cancer and Leukemia Group B Study 8361). *Blood*. 2001;97:3574-3580.
45. Voskova D, Schoch C, Schnittger S, Hiddemann W, Haferlach T, Kern W. Stability of leukemia-associated aberrant immunophenotypes in patients with acute myeloid leukemia between diagnosis and relapse: comparison with cytomorphologic, cytogenetic, and molecular genetic findings. *Cytometry B Clin Cytom*. 2004;62:25-38.
46. Grimwade D, Vyas P, Freeman S. Assessment of minimal residual disease in acute myeloid leukemia. *Curr Opin Oncol*. 2010;22:656-663.
47. Campana D. Minimal residual disease in acute lymphoblastic leukemia. *Hematology (Am Soc Hematol Educ Program)*. 2010;2010:7-12.
48. Kikuchi M, Tanaka J, Kondo T, et al. Clinical significance of minimal residual disease in adult acute lymphoblastic leukemia. *Int J Hematol*. October 2010;92(3):481-489.
49. Foster JH, Hawkins DS, Loken MR, Wells DA, Thomson B. Minimal residual disease detected prior to hematopoietic cell transplantation. *Pediatr Blood Cancer*. July 2011;57(1):163-165.
50. Frebet E, Abraham J, Genevieve F, et al. A GEIL flow cytometry consensus proposal for quantification of plasma cells: application to differential diagnosis between MGUS and myeloma. *Cytometry B Clin Cytom*. May 2011;80(3):176-185.
51. Paiva B, Vidriales MB, Perez JJ, et al. Multiparameter flow cytometry quantification of bone marrow plasma cells at diagnosis provides more prognostic information than morphological assessment in myeloma patients. *Haematologica*. 2009;94:1599-1602.
52. Liu H, Yuan C, Heinerich J, et al. Flow cytometric minimal residual disease monitoring in patients with multiple myeloma undergoing autologous stem cell transplantation: a retrospective study. *Leuk Lymphoma*. 2008;49:306-314.
53. Crespo M, Bosch F, Villamor N, et al. ZAP-70 expression as a surrogate for immunoglobulin-variable-region mutations in chronic lymphocytic leukemia. *N Engl J Med*. 2003;348: 1764-1775.
54. Del Giudice I, Morilla A, Osuji N, et al. Zeta-chain associated protein 70 and CD38 combined predict the time to first treatment in patients with chronic lymphocytic leukemia. *Cancer*. 2005;104:2124-2132.
55. Sheikholeslami MR, Jilani I, Keating M, et al. Variations in the detection of ZAP-70 in chronic lymphocytic leukemia:

comparison with IgV(H) mutation analysis. *Cytometry B Clin Cytom*. 2006;70:270-275.
56. Hamblin TJ. Prognostic markers in chronic lymphocytic leukaemia. *Best Pract Res Clin Haematol*. 2007;20:455-468.
57. Hamilton A, Gallipoli P, Nicholson E, Holyoake TL. Targeted therapy in haematological malignancies. *J Pathol*. 2010;220:404-418.
58. Freedman A. Follicular lymphoma: 2011 update on diagnosis and management. *Am J Hematol*. 2011;86:768-775.
59. Pfreundschuh M, Kuhnt E, Trumper L, et al. CHOP-like chemotherapy with or without rituximab in young patients with good-prognosis diffuse large-B-cell lymphoma: 6-year results of an open-label randomised study of the MabThera International Trial (MInT) Group. *Lancet Oncol*. 2011;12:1013-1022.
60. Boyd K, Dearden CE. Alemtuzumab in the treatment of chronic lymphocytic lymphoma. *Expert Rev Anticancer Ther*. 2008;8:525-533.
61. Czuczman MS, Thall A, Witzig TE, et al. Phase I/II study of galiximab, an anti-CD80 antibody, for relapsed or refractory follicular lymphoma. *J Clin Oncol*. 2005;23:4390-4398.
62. Leonard JP, Friedberg JW, Younes A, et al. A phase I/II study of galiximab (an anti-CD80 monoclonal antibody) in combination with rituximab for relapsed or refractory, follicular lymphoma. *Ann Oncol*. 2007;18:1216-1223.
63. Grimwade D, Walker H, Oliver F, et al. The importance of diagnostic cytogenetics on outcome in AML: analysis of 1,612 patients entered into the MRC AML 10 trial. The Medical Research Council Adult and Children's Leukaemia Working Parties. *Blood*. 1998;92:2322-2333.
64. Weerkamp F, Dekking E, Ng YY, et al. Flow cytometric immunobead assay for the detection of BCR-ABL fusion proteins in leukemia patients. *Leukemia*. 2009;23:1106-1117.
65. Dekking E, van der Velden VH, Bottcher S, et al. Detection of fusion genes at the protein level in leukemia patients via the flow cytometric immunobead assay. *Best Pract Res Clin Haematol*. 2010;23:333-345.
66. Maguire O, Collins C, O'Loughlin K, Miecznikowski J, Minderman H. Quantifying nuclear p65 as a parameter for NF-kappaB activation: correlation between ImageStream cytometry, microscopy, and Western blot. *Cytometry A*. 2011;79:461-469.
67. Grimwade L, Gudgin E, Bloxham D, Scott MA, Erber WN. PML protein analysis using imaging flow cytometry. *J Clin Pathol*. 2011;64:447-450.
68. Krueger SA, Wilson GD. Flow cytometric DNA analysis of human cancers and cell lines. *Methods Mol Biol*. 2011;731: 359-370.
69. Sun YF, Yang XR, Zhou J, Qiu SJ, Fan J, Xu Y. Circulating tumor cells: advances in detection methods, biological issues, and clinical relevance. *J Cancer Res Clin Oncol*. 2011;137:1151-1173.
70. Morita R, Sato K, Nakano M, et al. Endothelial progenitor cells are associated with response to chemotherapy in human non-small-cell lung cancer. *J Cancer Res Clin Oncol*. 2011;137: 1849-1857.
71. Mateos MV, Gutierrez NC, Martin-Ramos ML, et al. Outcome according to cytogenetic abnormalities and DNA ploidy in myeloma patients receiving short induction with weekly bortezomib followed by maintenance. *Blood*. 2011;118: 4547-4553.
72. Ruiz C, Lenkiewicz E, Evers L, et al. Advancing a clinically relevant perspective of the clonal nature of cancer. *Proc Natl Acad Sci U S A*. 2011;108:12054-12059.
73. Obro NF, Madsen HO, Ryder LP, Andersen MK, Schmiegelow K, Marquart HV. Approaches for cytogenetic and molecular analyses of small flow-sorted cell populations from childhood leukemia bone marrow samples. *J Immunol Methods*. 2011;369:69-73.

CHAPTER 15

CANCER CYTOGENOMICS

Gary Lu

INTRODUCTION

Cancer cytogenomics arose with the development of a series of array-based technologies using comparative genomic hybridization (CGH) and single nucleotide polymorphism (SNP) analysis and their application to clinical cancer genetics.[1] Cytogenomic abnormalities are biomarkers that can be detected by one of three methods: routine karyotyping, fluorescence in situ hybridization (FISH), and the one using either array CGH (aCGH) or SNP. Before the most recent next-generation sequencing technologies to characterize cancer genome become commonplace, these three methods in combination are now able to provide important insights into accurately identifying and precisely defining cytogenomic abnormalities and create new clinical cancer cytogenomic databases. With the continuing improvement and maturation of array-based methods for identifying balanced translocation, new abnormalities, and their clinical correlations, clinical cancer cytogenomics will be of great use to clinicians for cancer diagnosis, prognosis, and treatment, especially in the rapidly developing field of personalized therapy. In addition, the genome-wide human SNP array, which features more than 1.8 million markers of genetic variation, including both SNPs and probes for the detection of copy number variation and other genetic abnormalities such as acquired uniparental disomy and loss of heterozygosity, has significantly increased the overall power of genetic detection in cancer cytogenomics.[2]

FISH analysis can selectively identify acquired cancer-related cytogenomic changes in interphase cells and confirm masked chromosomal translocations in metaphase cells. However, FISH is informative only for the specific cytogenomic abnormalities that are targeted by the probes used. Current array-based methods can detect a much wider range of abnormalities at much higher resolution,[3] although most of the abnormalities thus identified still need to be analyzed and stratified before their clinical significance is clear. It is expected that the use of karyotyping will decrease to a certain level in the future and that FISH, with its specific targets, and array-based methods, with their wide spectrum of detection, will complement each other. Thus, this chapter mainly focuses on FISH in clinical cancer cytogenomics.

PRINCIPLES AND CLINICAL LABORATORY APPLICATION

Principles

Fluorescence In Situ Hybridization

FISH is used to detect or confirm abnormalities in any of 24 human chromosomes. It is a biomarker-targeting test, and therefore its application to clinical cancer cytogenomics is limited to those biomarkers that have specifically targeted probes available. Briefly, the sample DNA in chromosomes or nuclei is first denatured and then treated with a fluorescently labeled probe of interest, which binds only to those parts of the chromosome or nucleus with which it shows a high degree of sequence complementarity. The probe then hybridizes with the sample DNA at the target site as the DNA re-anneals back into a double helix. Sites where the fluorescent probe has bound to the chromosome or nuclei are identified by fluorescence microscopy.[4] The FISH probes can be labeled with different colors of fluorescent dye to distinguish different markers. Cells do not have to be actively dividing for FISH analysis to be effective.

FISH probes are often derived from fragments of human genomic DNA that have been isolated, purified, and amplified. The human genome is much larger than the stretch that can be directly sequenced, and thus it is

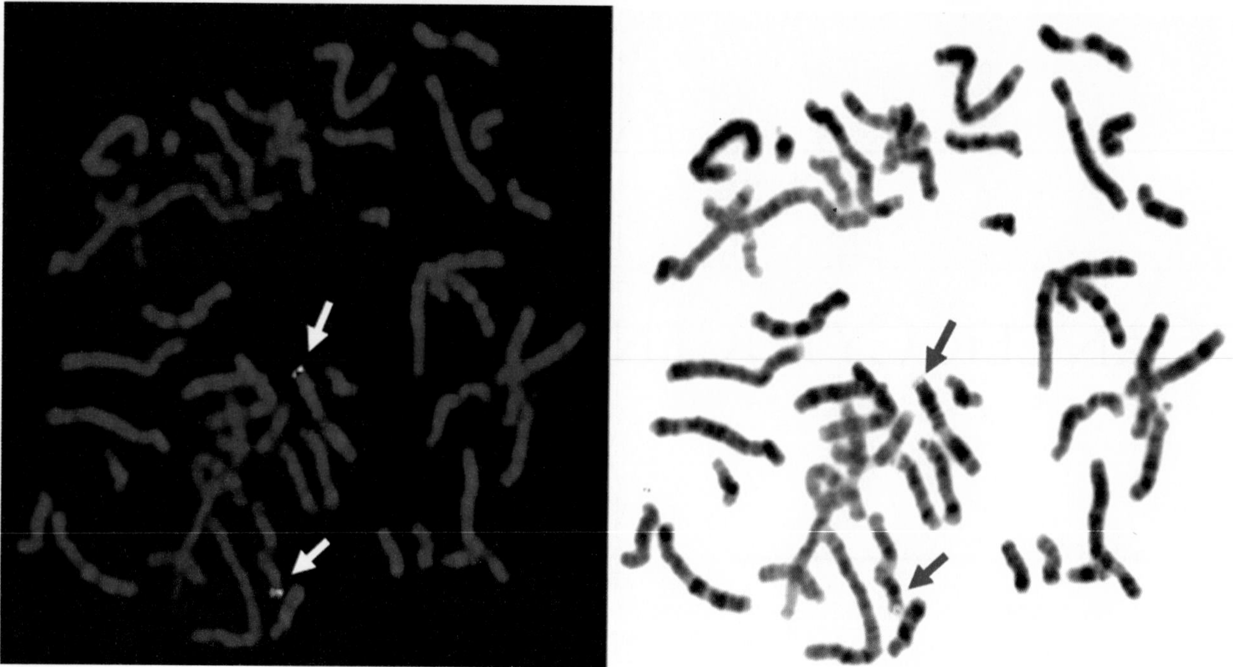

FIGURE 15–1 Home-brewed fluorescence in situ hybridization probes for 11p15/*NUP98*.

necessary to cut the whole genome into fragments to make FISH probes.[4] These fragments are put in order by breaking down a copy of each fragment into much smaller fragments using sequence-specific endonucleases. To preserve these small fragments with their individual DNA sequences, the fragments are added into bacteria populations that are continually replicating. Each clonal population of bacteria that maintains a single artificial chromosome is called a bacterial artificial chromosome (BAC), which can be grown, extracted, and labeled. BAC clones are the basis for most FISH probes. FISH probes can be "home-brewed" using the following major steps: (1) inoculate Luria-Bertani broth with a bacterial clone; (2) extract BAC clone DNA; (3) perform fluorescent labeling using the nick translation kit; and (4) precipitate the probe with Cot1 DNA. FISH probes that were home-brewed in the author's research laboratory at the University of Texas MD Anderson Cancer Center to identify 11p15/*NUP98* rearrangement commonly associated with myeloid neoplasms are shown in Figure 15.1.[5]

Array Comparative Genomic Hybridization

The method of aCGH is a combination of CGH and microarray. This method combines CGH with high-throughput microarrays to simultaneously analyze up to thousands of discrete regions of the human genome and identify unbalanced cytogenomic abnormalities. This method also combines the locus-specific nature of FISH with the global genome view of high-resolution chromosomes; thus, it represents the integration of traditional and molecular cytogenetic techniques.

The principles of aCGH are basically similar to those of FISH.[6] The basic methodology for aCGH analysis includes the following: (1) **Genomic DNA extraction.** Two types of DNA are used: test DNA from a sample (such as leukemic blood, bone marrow, tumor tissue, and body fluid) from a patient and normal reference DNA from a normal control. (2) **DNA labeling**. The test DNA is then labeled with a fluorescent dye of a specific color (e.g., Cy5/red), while DNA from a reference sample (normal female) is labeled with a dye of a different color (e.g., Cy3/green). (3) **Microarray DNA hybridization**. The test genomic DNA and reference DNA are denatured to single strands, mixed together, and then applied to a microarray slide. When applied to the slide, the DNAs attempt to hybridize with the arrayed single-strand probes. (4) **Scanning and data analysis.** Digital imaging systems are used to capture and quantify the relative fluorescence intensities of the labeled DNA probes that have hybridized to each target. Using computer software, the fluorescence ratio of the test and reference hybridization signals is determined at different positions along the genome, and it provides information on the relative copy number of sequences in the test genome as compared with the normal genome, thus detecting submicroscopic chromosomal deletions and duplications.

Types of Probes

Fluorescence In Situ Hybridization

There are three types of FISH probe and each type has its own application. **Locus-specific probes** bind to a particular region of a chromosome or nucleus. This type of probe is useful for identifying changes in a specific locus or gene, such as translocation, deletion, and amplification. **Centromeric repeat probes** are generated from repetitive sequences found in the centromere region of each chromosome and are usually used to identify changes in the number of chromosomes. Combined with a locus-specific probe, they can also be used to determine whether genetic material is missing from a particular chromosome.

Whole-chromosome probes are actually collections of smaller probes, each of which binds to a different sequence along the length of a given chromosome, and which together cover the entire chromosome. Whole-chromosome probes are particularly useful for examining unknown material attached to a given chromosome or a chromosome marker whose original chromosome is unknown. This is called whole-chromosome painting.

The size of the FISH probe varies significantly depending on the locus targeted and the techniques and materials used to design the probe. They range from as small as 1,500 bp to as large as several hundred thousand base pairs. Large probes hybridize to less specific targets than small probes. The probe must be long enough to hybridize specifically with its target but not so long as to impede the hybridization process. The overlap of hybridization defines the resolution of detectable features.

Array Comparative Genomic Hybridization

The two probes most commonly used for aCGH to detect cancer cytogenomic abnormalities are BAC **clone probe** and **oligonucleotide probe**. Both types of probes have advantages and disadvantages. BAC clones, which are usually 80 to 200 kb, may miss alterations smaller than the size of a clone but are less likely to detect alterations of unclear clinical significance, whereas oligonucleotides, which are much smaller probes, usually 25 to 85 bp, may detect small alterations that would not be seen using a BAC microarray; however, oligonucleotide arrays are more likely to detect small alterations of unclear clinical significance. SNP is able to detect loss of heterozygosity and uniparental disomy.[7]

Clinical Cancer Diagnostic Laboratory Application

Fluorescence In Situ Hybridization

FISH has proven to be a powerful tool for detecting cytogenomic abnormalities in both constitutional diseases and cancers. Tissues used for FISH studies vary depending on the clinical setting. In cancer cytogenomics, tissue samples used are usually peripheral blood (e.g., leukemic blood), bone marrow (aspirate or core), lymph nodes, paraffin-embedded tissue (i.e., pathologic slides), or body fluids such as pleural fluid. FISH on paraffin-embedded tissue is challenging because processing conditions for different cases and for different FISH probes vary (Table 15.1).

TABLE 15-1 FISH Protocol for Paraffin-Embedded Tissue Slides

Deparaffinizing slides

1. Bake the slide(s) overnight at 60°C.
2. Immerse slide(s) in a coplin jar containing CitriSolv for 5 min at room temperature.
3. Repeat step 2 twice using fresh CitriSolv each time. Air-dry slide(s).
4. Dehydrate slide(s) in 100% EtOH for 1 min at room temperature. Repeat once with fresh 100% EtOH. Air-dry slide(s).

Slide pretreatment

1. Prewarm a coplin jar containing 50 mL of pretreatment solution to 80°C in a water bath.
2. Immerse slide(s) in the pretreatment solution for 10 min.
3. Rinse slide(s) in a coplin jar of purified water for 3 min at room temperature.

Protease treatment

1. Remove slide(s) from the coplin jar and remove excess water by blotting the edges of the slides on a paper towel.
2. Prewarm a coplin jar with sufficient protease solution to 37°C in a water bath. It is important to make sure the temperature does not exceed 37°C, which would inactivate the protease.
3. Immerse slide(s) in the protease solution for 15 min.
4. Rinse slide(s) in a coplin jar of purified water for 3 min. Air-dry slide(s).

Dehydration

1. Dehydrate slide(s) in a series of 70%, 85%, and 100% EtOH.
2. Air-dry slide(s).

Hybridization

Preparation of the probes

1. Apply the appropriate probe mixture(s) to slide(s), apply coverslip, and seal with rubber cement.
2. Place slide(s) in a ThemoBrite machine and denature at 73°C for 3 min.
3. Incubate slide(s) at 37°C overnight in a ThemoBrite machine or humidified chamber.

Posthybridization wash

1. Prewarm a coplin jar of 2 × SSC/0.3% NP-40 in a 73°C water bath for at least 30 min.
2. Prepare another jar of 2 × SSC/0.3% NP-30 and leave at room temperature. Remove rubber cement and coverslip from the slide(s).
3. Immerse slide(s) in prewarmed 2 × SSC/0.3% NP-40 at 73°C and agitate for 1–3 s. Remove slide(s) after 2 min.
4. Transfer slide(s) to the second coplin jar of 2 × SSC/0.3% NP-40 at room temperature. Agitate for 1–3 s. Remove slide(s) after 1 min and air-dry slide(s) in the dark.
5. Counterstain slide(s) with DAPI.

FISH, fluorescence in situ hybridization; min, minute(s); s, second(s).

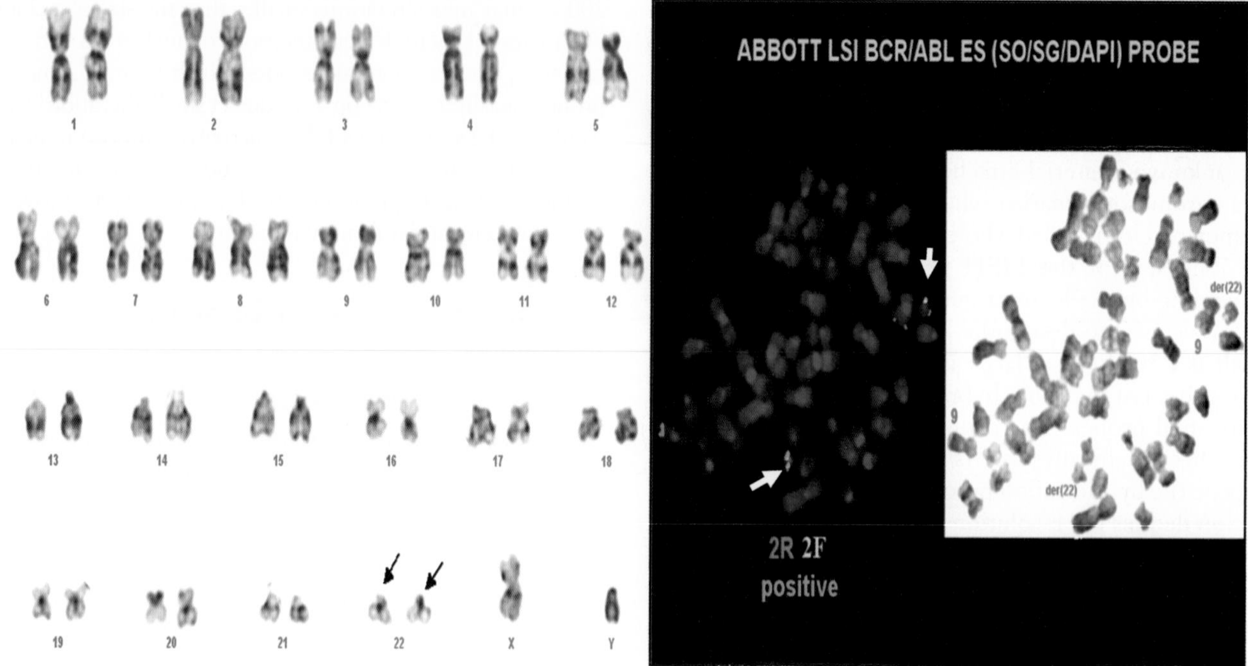

FIGURE 15–2 Cryptic t(9;22)(q34;q11.2) in chronic myelogenous leukemia (CML). The normal-looking karyotype (*left*) was from a 65-y-old man newly diagnosed with CML. Reverse transcription polymerase chain reaction analysis to detect the b3a2 *BCR/ABL* fusion transcript coding for the 210-kDa *BCR/ABL* protein revealed 100% BCR to ABL transcription. Concurrent fluorescence in situ hybridization mapback confirmed the presence of cryptic t(9;22)(q34;q11.2) *(right)*.

Array Comparative Genomic Hybridization

Laboratory step-by-step protocol for aCGH or SNP is variable depending on different platforms and can be provided by manufacturers. Sample types for aCGH or SNP are similar to those for FISH. However, because of the relative low sensitivity, achieving good quality and quantity of DNA from samples is one of the important steps for aCGH or SNP.

DETECTION OF CYTOGENOMIC ABNORMALITIES IN CANCER

FISH is a sensitive method for detecting cytogenomic abnormalities associated with cancers. The cytogenomic abnormalities detected by FISH are of diagnostic, predictive or prognostic, and/or therapeutic significance. The incorporation of FISH has added significant value to cancer patient care. FISH is routinely used in conjunction with other cytogenomic analysis, currently karyotyping or chromosomal analysis, although array-based methods or SNP arrays are expected to replace part of these in the future. In certain types of cancers, however, FISH demonstrates its advantage over chromosomal analysis in that the cancer cells grow poorly in culture, often resulting in a low metaphase index or culture failure. Other advantages of FISH include its ability to specify complex chromosomal abnormalities using whole-chromosome painting probes and identify cryptic rearrangements that cannot be detected by karyotyping (Fig. 15.2). FISH is also widely employed for diagnosis, prognosis, or treatment application in certain types of solid tumors with specific cytogenomic abnormalities and is especially useful in the rapidly developing field of personalized therapy.

aCGH or SNP has been widely used in prenatal or postnatal diagnosis, especially for such conditions as developmental delay, mental retardation, multiple congenital anomalies, autism, dysmorphism, and abnormal ultrasound findings. Several submicroscopic genomic deletion or genomic duplication syndromes have been defined by aCGH, including 1p36 deletion syndrome (Fig. 15.3).[8] Recent studies using aCGH have shed light on clinical cancer cytogenomics including hematological malignancies and solid tumors, mainly myelodysplastic syndrome (MDS), multiple myeloma, chronic lymphocytic leukemia (CLL), oligodendroglial tumors, or glioblastomas.[9-13] Due to the high resolution, the clinical significance of most of the smaller abnormalities detected so far by aCGH or SNP is still unknown. However, when the new technologies are further developed and become more matured, thus the clinical significance of the newly detected abnormalities is known, aCGH or SNP would be applied more to a certain level in clinical cancer cytogenomics.

Chronic Myelogenous Leukemia

Chronic myelogenous leukemia (CML) is a myeloproliferative neoplasm originating from a clonal, pluripotent hematopoietic stem cell demonstrating the *BCR/ABL1* fusion gene resulting from t(9;22)(q34;q11.2) (Fig. 15.4). CML is used as a prototype for the development of cancer cytogenomics because of the correlation of t(9;22)(q34;q11.2) with the disease's pathogenesis and the success of imatinib mesylate as the front-line therapy for the disease.[14,15] t(9;22)(q34;q11.2) was the first cytogenomic marker specifically associated with cancer.[16]

t(9;22)(q34;q11.2), in conjunction with other cytogenomic abnormalities, drives the course of CML through

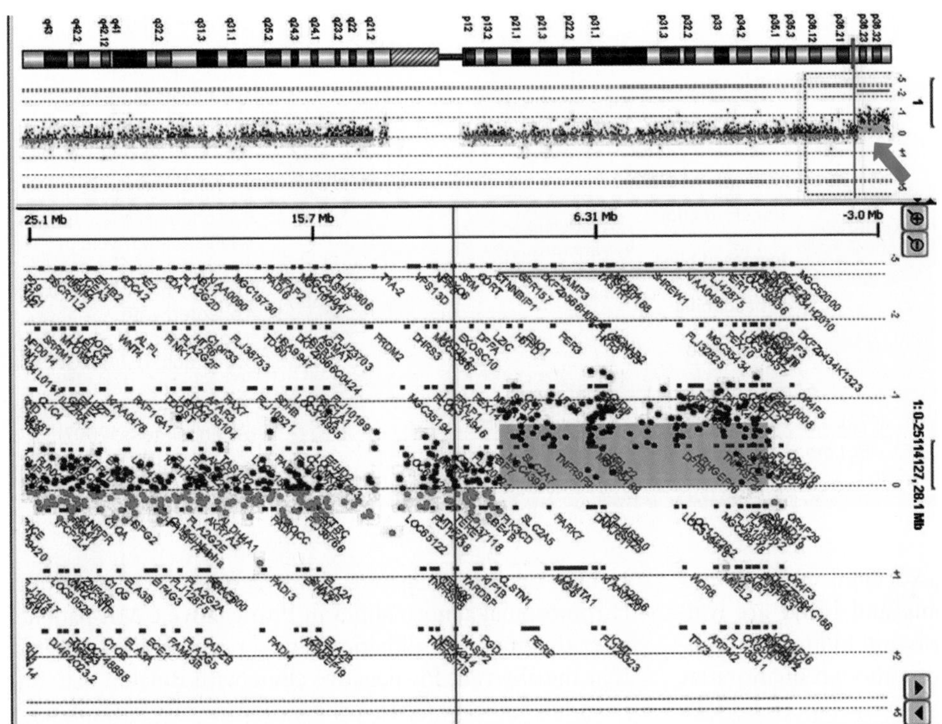

FIGURE 15–3 1p36 deletion by array comparative genomic hybridization in a patient with 1p36 deletion syndrome. Microarray analysis shows a loss of the short arm of chromosome 1 at band p36.3 *(arrow)*. The loss is about 1 Mb in size.

three different phases,[17] as illustrated in Figure 15.5. With the discovery of the *BCR/ABL1* fusion gene and the subsequent development of the effective tyrosine kinase inhibitors, such as the current front-line drug, imatinib mesylate, for patients in chronic phase, the prognosis of CML has improved remarkably over the past decade, and it is expected that the disease will be curable with future improvement of this small-molecule tyrosine kinase inhibitor.

Typically, t(9;22)(q34;q11.2) is present and easily identified in most patients with CML, although its variants involving different chromosomes are also possible (Fig. 15.6A). Such variants are often associated with less response to therapy, probably owing to the involvement of additional genes.[18] Results of cytogenomic analyses by both karyotyping and FISH are an important part of criteria to define clinical response to imatinib for disease progression or overall survival according to the International Randomized Study of Interferon versus STI571 (IRIS). Cytogenetic response has been classically defined based on the results of evaluation of a minimum of 20 bone marrow metaphase cells: partial cytogenetic response is defined when 1 to 35% Philadelphia chromosome (Ph)-positive (Ph$^+$) metaphases are detected while complete cytogenetic response is defined when 0% Ph$^+$ metaphases are present. Therefore, karyotyping and/or FISH remains routine in CML follow-up. In addition, cytogenomic abnormality can be a marker for therapy resistance. *ASS* gene, mapped next to *ABL1*, is deleted in some patients with CML,[19,20] and the *ASS* deletion is considered to be associated with therapy resistance in a subset of CML patients. The *ASS* deletion can be detected by FISH using a three-color probe that includes aqua for the *ASS* gene (Fig. 15.6B). Amplification of the

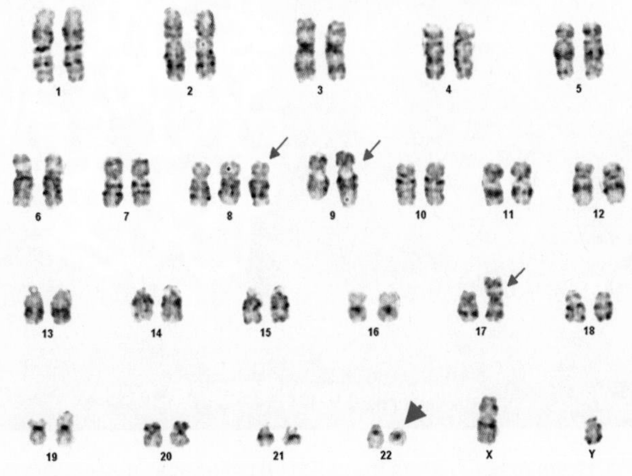

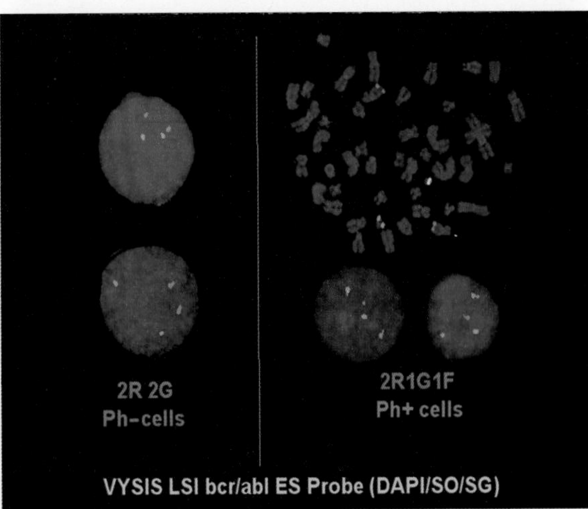

FIGURE 15–4 A typical t(9;22)(q34;q11.2) with +8 and i(17)(q10) *(left)* from a patient with chronic myelogenous leukemia in blast crisis. Fluorescence in situ hybridization was positive for *BCR/ABL1* rearrangement (*right*).

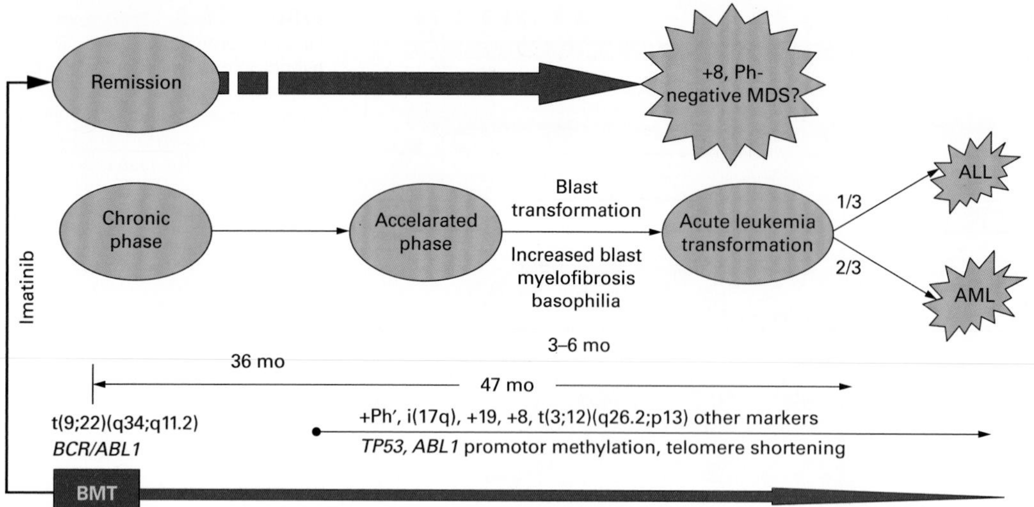

FIGURE 15–5 Cytogenomic changes associated with chronic myelogenous leukemia development and progression. MDS, myelodysplastic syndrome; ALL, acute lymphoblastic leukemia; AML, acute myeloid leukemia; BMT, bone marrow transplantation. (Adapted with modification from Lu G, Xu X, eds. *Clinical Genetic Counseling*. Beijing: Beijing University Medical Science Press; 2007).

BCR/ABL1 fusion gene is also associated with therapy resistance.[21] Currently, karyotyping and FISH are routinely performed in CML diagnosis and follow-up monitoring during and after treatment, although quantitative reverse transcription polymerase chain reaction (RT-PCR) has greater sensitivity in detecting *BCR/ABL1* rearrangement, especially in cases of minimal residual disease. For unknown reasons, probably because of cell selection, however, FISH results are positive in some cases of CML that are negative for *BCR/ABL1* according to RT-PCR.

The presence of clonal cytogenomic abnormalities, including trisomy 8 (the most frequent), monosomy 7, and trisomy 6, in Ph-negative CML patients after treatment with imatinib has been studied.[22-25] The incidence, etiology, and prognosis of these abnormalities remain unclear, and therefore their clinical significance is still controversial, although the emergence of an imatinib-correlated MDS has been reported.[23] Clonal del(20q), identified as a divergent change or a new separate clone, is one of the structural chromosomal abnormalities in Ph-negative CML patients after treatment with imatinib, but a recent study indicated that the aberrant Ph-negative clone with isolated del(20q) does not indicate CML progression or myelodysplasia.[26] To illustrate the clinical significance of such cytogenomic clones in treated Ph-negative CML cases, however, more studies with large cohorts are needed. Routine karyotyping and FISH analysis after treatment for CML to monitor for the presence of abnormal clones is appropriate.

Acute Myeloid Leukemia

The World Health Organization has designated several different classes of acute myeloid leukemia (AML) on the basis of clinical characteristics, pathogenesis, and recurrent cytogenomic abnormalities (Table 15.2).[27] The most common categories, with recurrent cytogenomic abnormalities

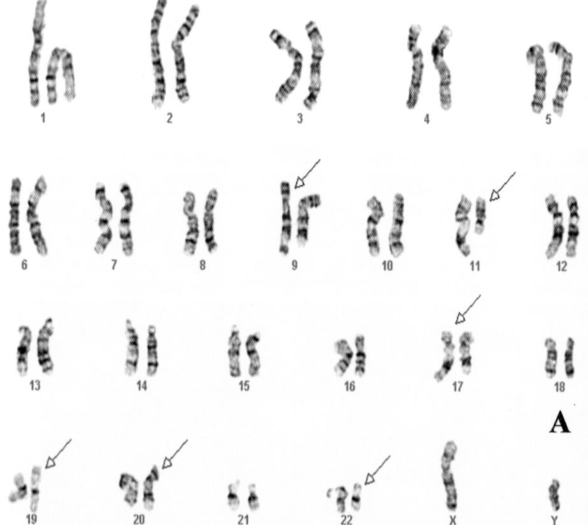

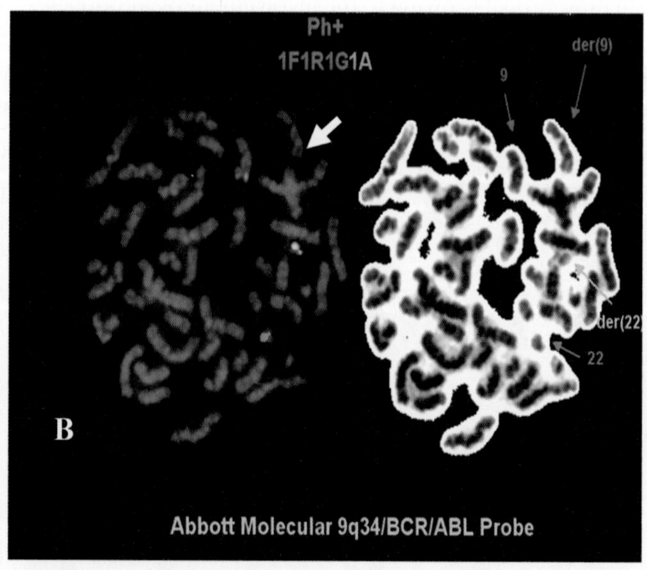

FIGURE 15–6 **A:** A karyotype with a six-way translocation t(9;22;19;11;17;20) (q34;q11.2;p13.3;q13;q21;q11.2) from a chronic myelogenous leukemia (CML) patient. **B:** *ASS* deletion in a case of t(9;22)(q34;q11.2)-positive CML; an aqua signal is missing on the der(9) t(9;22) (*white arrow*). (Panel B courtesy of Lina Wu at The University of Texas MD Anderson Cancer Center. Panel A adapted from Lu G, Xu X, eds. *Clinical Genetic Counseling*. Beijing: Beijing University Medical Science Press; 2007.)

TABLE 15–2 Specific Cytogenomic Abnormalities in Acute Myeloid Leukemia

World Health Organization Classification by Cytogenomic Abnormality	Genes and Cancer Genetics	Major Clinical Features	Major Morphologic Features	Prognosis
AML with t(8;21)(q22;q22)	*RUNX1/RUNX1T1* 1. *RUNX1* encodes core-binding factor subunit alpha, which is essential for hematopoiesis 2. Often with del(9q) and loss of X or Y 3. *KRAS* or *NRAS* mutations in ~30% of pediatric patients	Myeloid sarcomas may be present at diagnosis with low blast count (<20%) in bone marrow	1. Large blasts showing abundant granular cytoplasm with perinuclear clearing and large orange-pink granules 2. Auer rods 3. Small blasts predominantly in peripheral blood	1. Good response to chemotherapy with high complete remission rate and long-term disease-free survival when treated with high-dose cytarabine in consolidation phase 2. Adverse factors: CD56+, *KIT* mutations
AML with t(15;17)(q24;q21)[a]	*PML/RARA* 1. *PML* (promyelocytic leukemia gene) is a nuclear regulatory factor gene, whereas *RARA* is a retinoic acid receptor alpha gene 2. Present in almost all acute promyelocytic leukemia patients, with a few demonstrating cryptic t(15;17) or variant translocations involving 17q21/*RARA* 3. Often with secondary +8 (10–15% of patients) 4. *FLT3* mutations in up to 45% of patients, most commonly *FLT3-ITD*, which is associated with increased white blood cell count	Typically associated with disseminated intravascular coagulation and very high leukocyte count with rapid doubling time in hypogranular acute promyelocytic leukemia	1. Hypergranular type: irregular and greatly variable nuclear size and shape, often kidney shaped or bilobed; densely packed or coalescent large granules, bundles of Auer rods (faggot cells) in cytoplasm; strong myeloperoxidase staining; leukemic promyelocytes occasionally present in peripheral blood 2. Hypogranular type: apparent paucity or even absence of granules, predominantly bilobed nuclear shape; faggot cells may be identified; strong myeloperoxidase reaction	1. Particularly sensitive to treatment with all-trans retinoic acid 2. Best prognosis among specific cytogenetic AMLs 3. Less favorable prognosis in CD56+ cases
AML with inv(16)(p13.1q22) or t(16;16)(p13.1;q22)	*CBFB/MYH11* 1. inv(16) is the most common 2. *MYH11* encodes for a smooth muscle myosin heavy chain, whereas *CBFB* encodes for the core-binding factor beta subunit 2. The *Cbfb/Myh11* product impairs gene transcription involved by enhancers of T cells, cytokine genes, and others 3. Fluorescence in situ hybridization and reverse transcription polymerase chain reaction are often necessary to confirm the subtle change of inv(16) 4. +22 is the most common second change and a clue for inv(16) in some cases	Myeloid sarcomas found at initial diagnosis or at relapse, or may be the only evidence of relapse in some cases	1. Variable number of abnormal eosinophils at all stages of maturation, involving the immature eosinophilic granules mainly at promyelocytes and myelocytes but not present at later stages of eosinophil maturation 2. Large purple-violet color eosinophilic granules in immature eosinophils, and even dense enough to obscure the cell morphology 3. Occasionally lacks abnormal eosinophilia 4. Some patients have blast counts of less than 20% in bone marrow	1. Longer remissions when treated with high-dose cytarabine in the consolidation phase 2. Higher relapse and worse survival in *KIT*-positive cases 3. Improved outcome in cases with +22
AML with 11q23 abnormalities [t(9;11)(p22;q23)]	*MLLT3/MLL* 1. The *Mllt3/Mll* fusion protein impairs gene transcription regulation via chromatin modeling 2. Secondary +8 is common but appears not to influence survival	1. May present disseminated intravascular coagulation and extramedullary sarcomas and/or tissue infiltration	1. Demonstrates predominant monoblasts and promonocytes 2. Large monoblasts with abundant cytoplasm containing round nuclei with delicate lacy chromatin, moderate to intense basophilic and scattered azurophilic granules, and one or more large prominent nucleolus	1. Intermediate survival 2. Patients with <20% blasts must be closely monitored for AML development

(Continued)

TABLE 15–2 Specific Cytogenomic Abnormalities in Acute Myeloid Leukemia (Continued)

World Health Organization Classification by Cytogenomic Abnormality	Genes and Cancer Genetics	Major Clinical Features	Major Morphologic Features	Prognosis
		2. Strongly associated with acute monocytic and myelomonocytic leukemia	3. Promonocytes with irregular and delicate nuclear folds 4. Positive nonspecific esterase stain in both monoblasts and promonocytes	
AML with t(6;9)(p23;q34)	*DEK/NUP214* 1. The *Dek/Nup214* fusion protein aberrantly impairs transcription and alters nuclear transport 2. Commonly associated with *FLT3* mutations in up to 70% of pediatric patients and 80% of adult patients	1. Usually presents with anemia, thrombocytopenia, and pancytopenia 2. Generally lower white blood cell count (12 × 10^9/L) than other AML types	1. Most commonly of maturation and monocytic morphology 2. High basophil count in 44–62% of cases 3. Often granulocytic and erythroid dysplasia 4. Auer rods present in about one-third of cases 5. Myeloperoxidase positive; positive or negative for esterase stain	1. Generally poor 2. Elevated white blood cell count predictive of shorter overall survival and increased blast count in bone marrow associated with shorter disease-free survival 3. Stem cell transplantation predictive of better survival 4. Patients with <20% blasts must be closely monitored for AML development
AML with inv(3)(q21q26.2) or t(3;3)(q21;q26.2)	*RPN1/EVI1* 1. *Rpn1/Evi1* product may result in increased cell proliferation and impaired cell differentiation 2. −7 is the most common second change, followed by del(5q) 3. May be an acquired change in aggressive phase of chronic myelogenous leukemia	1. Most commonly presents with anemia and a normal platelet count 2. Marked thrombocythemia in up to 22% of cases 3. Hepatosplenomegaly in a subset of patients, but uncommon for lymphadenopathy	1. Giant and hypogranular platelets with anemia 2. Increased blast count with normal or increased small atypical monolobed or bilobed megakaryocytes 3. Blast count less than 20% at diagnosis in a subset of cases, including cases with features of chronic myelomonocytic leukemia 4. Multilineage dysplasia frequently found in small, hypolobed megakaryocytes	1. Aggressive, with short overall survival times 2. Patients with <20% blasts must be closely monitored for AML development
AML with t(1;22)(p13;q13)	*RBM15/MKL1* 1. *RBM15* encodes RNA recognition motifs and a Spen paralog and ortholog C-terminal domain, whereas *MKL1* encodes a DNA-binding motif involved in chromatin organization 2. The *Rbm15/Mkl1* product may modulate chromatin organization, *HOX*-induced differentiation, and extracellular signaling pathways 3. Usually present as an isolated change	1. Restricted to de novo AML in infants and children <3 y (median, 4 mo) 2. Marked organomegaly, in particular hepatosplenomegaly 3. Often thrombocytopenia	1. Similar to the findings in acute megakaryoblastic leukemia, demonstrating a heteromorphous population of megakaryoblasts, with micromegakaryocytes common 2. Negative Sudan black B and myeloperoxidase staining 3. Blast count <20% in a subset of cases owing to secondary bone marrow fibrosis	1. Controversial prognosis, may be poor or respond well to intensive AML chemotherapy with long disease-free survival times 2. Patients with <20% blasts must be tested for bone marrow fibrosis

AML, acute myeloid leukemia.

[a]Variant t(15;17)(q24;q21) includes t(11;17)(q23;q21), t(11;17)(q13;q21), t(5;17)(q23;q21), and t(17;17)(q11.2;q21).

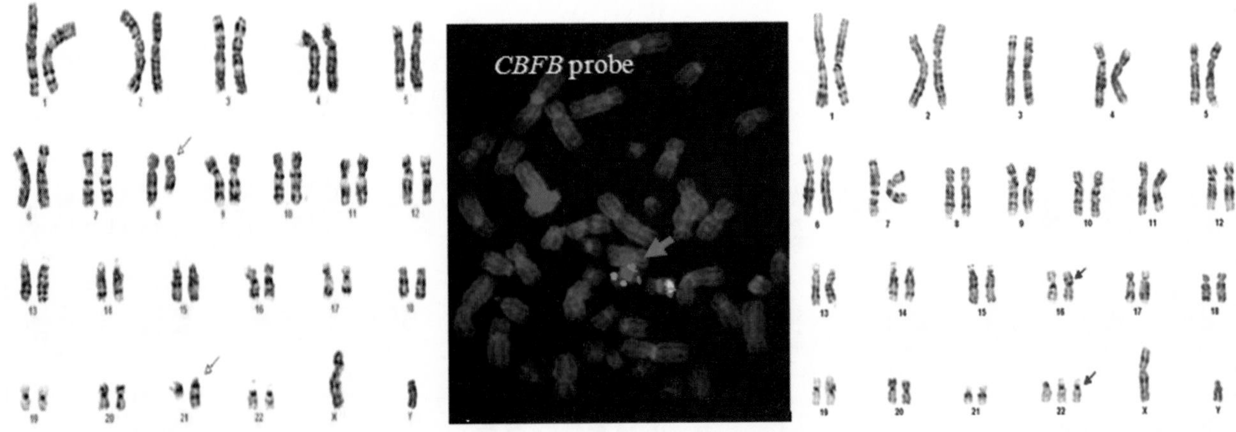

FIGURE 15–7 t(8;21)(q22;q22) (*left*), inv(16)(p13.1q22) (*right*), and the inv(16) was confirmed by FISH using *CBFB* probe (*middle*). (The left karyotype is adapted from Lu G, Xu X, eds. *Clinical Genetic Counseling*. Beijing: Beijing University Medical Science Press; 2007).

(most often translocations) that involve specific gene rearrangements and demonstrate characteristic morphologic and immunophenotypic features, are AML with t(8;21)(q22;q22)/*RUNX1-RUNX1T1* (Fig. 15.7); AML with inv(16)(p13.1q22) (Fig. 15.7) or t(16;16)(p13.1q22)/*CBFB-MYH11*; and AML with t(15;17)(q24;q21)/*PML-RARA* (also called acute promyelocytic leukemia [APL]) (Fig. 15.8).

FISH probes for the recurrent translocations are available and can be used in combination with morphologic, immunophenotypic, and molecular findings for accurate and timely diagnosis of AML. APL is also considered a prototype of AML for the development of cancer cytogenomics because of the association of the promyelocytic leukemia *(PML)/RARA* fusion gene, which results from t(15;17)(q24;q21), with disease pathogenesis and its therapy. The *PML* gene is a nuclear regulatory factor gene, whereas the *RARA* gene encodes retinoic acid receptor alpha.[28-31] t(15;17)(q24;q21) results in a *PML/RARA* fusion gene whose protein product is responsible for the APL phenotype. t(15;17)(q24;q21) can be detected in about 90% of APL patients; the remaining 10% of cases of APL result from variants involving different gene partners.[28] FISH using the dual-color, dual-fusion *PML/RARA* translocation probe or the break apart *RARA* probe is the standard test for timely APL diagnosis (Fig. 15.8).

APL is frequently associated with bleeding caused by disseminated intravascular coagulation. Thus, because of the urgent need for accurate diagnosis and prompt

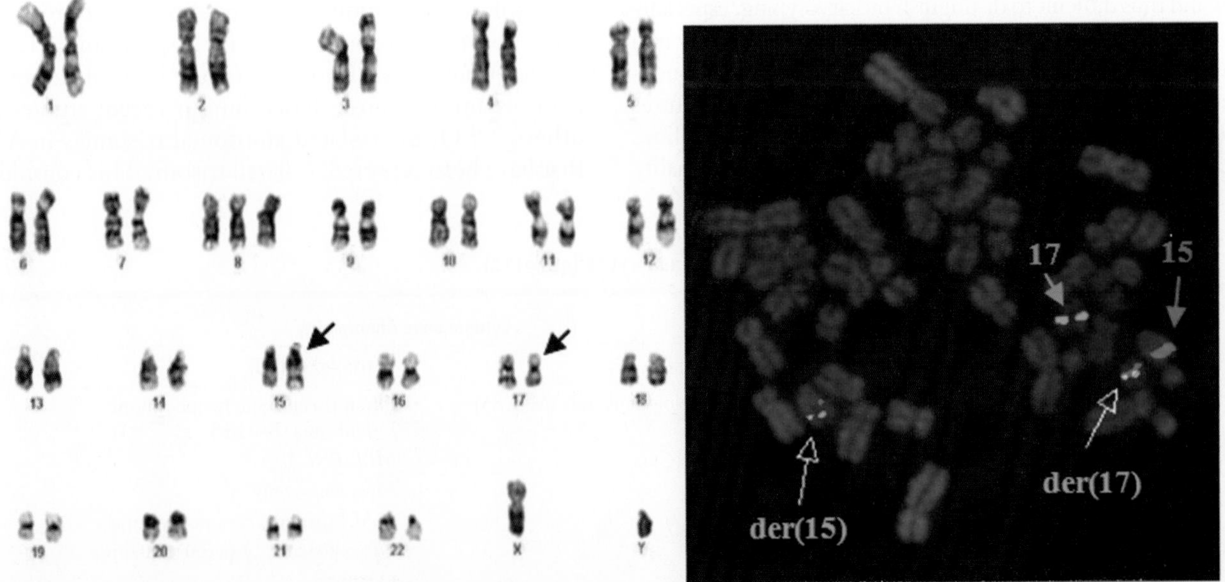

FIGURE 15–8 Karyotype with a t(15;17)(q24;q21) (*left*) and a fluorescence in situ hybridization (FISH) mapback (*right*). FISH using the dual-color, dual-fusion *PML/RARA* translocation probe reveals two fusion signal patterns and one red and one green signal pattern (*right*). (The karyotype is adapted from Lu G, Xu X, eds. *Clinical Genetic Counseling*. Beijing: Beijing University Medical Science Press; 2007.)

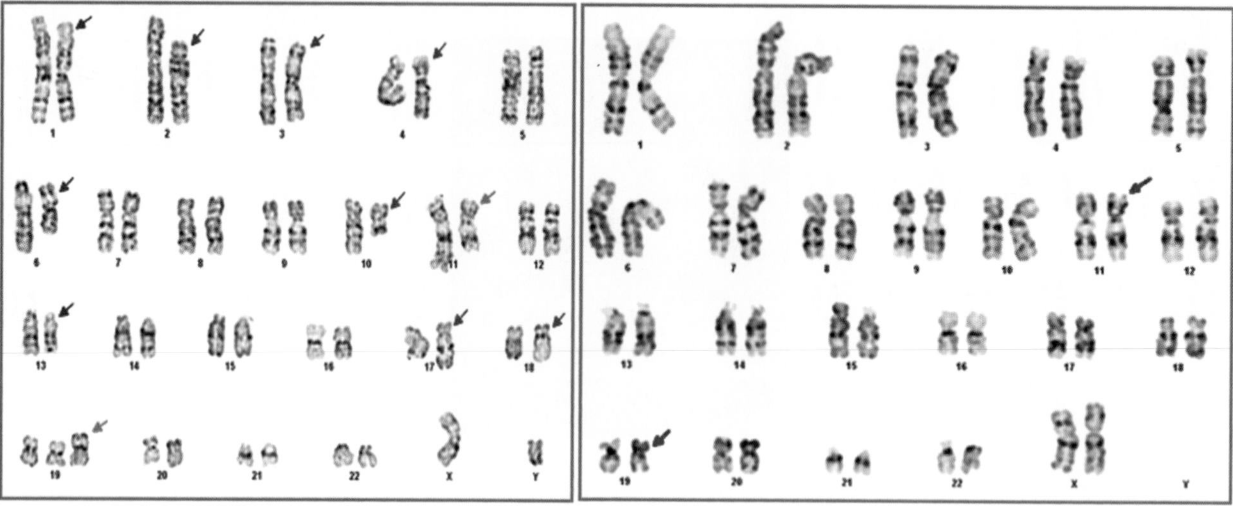

FIGURE 15–9 Karyotype t(11;19)(q23;p13.3) *(left)* and t(11;19)(q23;q13.1) *(right)*. The left karyotype is from a 5-mo-old male infant diagnosed with B-cell acute lymphoblastic leukemia who died 7 mo after diagnosis. The right karyotype is from a 60-y-old woman diagnosed with acute myeloid leukemia in 2011, whose disease relapsed in 8 mo.

treatment for APL patients, FISH results should be available within 24 hours. Once a positive result is reported, treatment can begin immediately to prevent disseminated intravascular coagulation and to target the disease itself. Therapeutic management for APL includes retinoic acid and arsenic trioxide. Both agents directly target *PML/RARA*-mediated transcriptional repression and protein stability, inducing to various extents promyelocyte differentiation and clinical remission of APL. Retinoic acid targets the *RARA* moiety of the fusion, whereas arsenic trioxide targets its *PML* part.[29,31]

Some cytogenomic abnormalities associated with AML are difficult for inexperienced persons to identify. For example, t(11;19)(q23;p13.1) and t(11;19)(q23;p13.3) are very similar and thus difficult to distinguish by karyotyping, especially in samples with suboptimal chromosome morphology and banding resolution (Fig. 15.9). Because of the different oncogenes involved and thus different clinicopathologic features seen between patients with the two different abnormalities (Table 15.3),[32,33] accurate identification of the abnormality is clinically important and usually needs to be confirmed by FISH analysis in combination with karyotyping.

For timely detection of cytogenomic abnormalities in new cases of acute leukemia, strict guidelines and protocols for detection of chromosomal abnormalities should be established and consistently followed in clinical cytogenomic laboratories.[34] This ensures the accuracy of AML diagnoses, including for cases with inconclusive conventional karyotyping results, which can actually harbor uncommon but clinically significant cytogenomic abnormalities such as heterogeneously staining regions (Fig. 15.10A) and double minutes (Fig. 15.10B), which are the most common markers associated with therapy resistance and poor prognosis in cancer.[35]

Isolated trisomies of autosomal chromosomes, including chromosomes 4, 8, 11, 13, 14, and 21, may define groups of AML patients on the basis of pathologic features and prognoses based on our recent studies and others.[36-42] Of the isolated autosomal trisomies in AML that have been reported, isolated trisomy 11 is considered

TABLE 15–3 Comparison between t(11;19)(q23;p13.1) and t(11;19)(q23;p13.3)

Clinical Features	Cytogenomic Abnormality	
	t(11;19)(q23;p13.1)	t(11;19)(q23;p13.3)
Leukemia	Often acute myeloid leukemia (M4/M5)	Often B-cell acute lymphoblastic leukemia (B-ALL)
Gene involved	*MLL/ELL*	*MLL/ENL*
Congenital	Rare	Most commonly
Sex ratio	1:1	B-ALL patients commonly female
Age at diagnosis	Often adult	Often pediatric, especially infantile
Central nervous system involvement	Less common	Common
Organomegaly	In ~50% of cases	Uncommon
Prognosis	Very poor (median overall survival 6 months)	Very poor (median overall survival <1 year)
Treatment	Stem cell transplantation required	Stem cell transplantation required

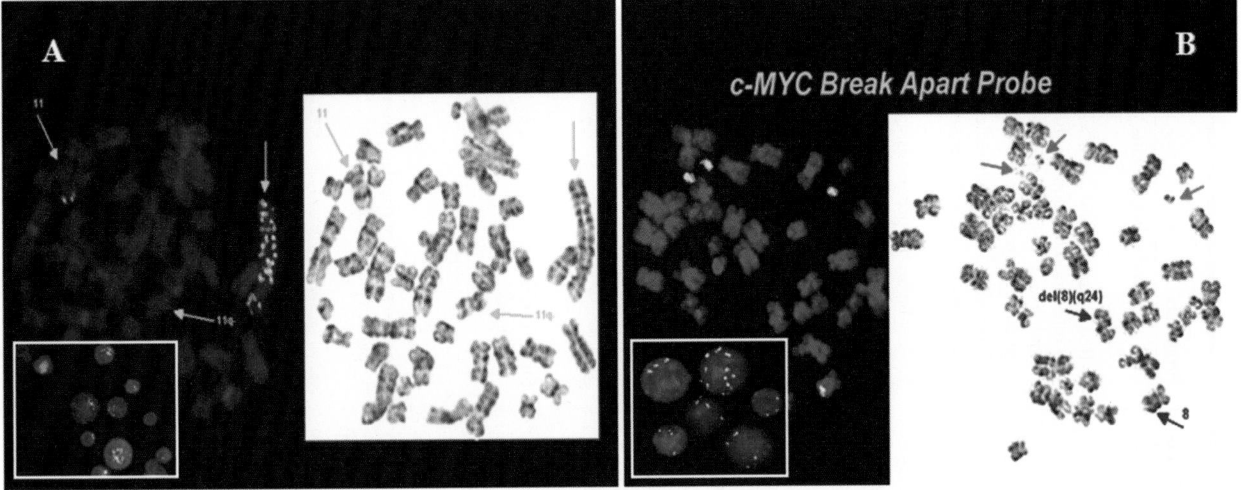

FIGURE 15–10 Fluorescence in situ hybridization (FISH) mapback for *MYC* amplification and *MLL* gene amplification. *MLL* amplification was detected in an abnormal chromosome 4 demonstrating heterogeneously staining regions in a patient with relapsed acute myeloid leukemia and refractory to therapy (**A**). FISH mapback using *MYC* probe onto double minutes in a metaphase from an acute myeloid leukemia patient who was refractory to therapy (**B**).

the most adverse marker of disease progression and prognosis. AML patients with isolated trisomy 11 usually have short disease-free survival and overall survival times even when treated with high doses of chemotherapy, and MDS with isolated trisomy 11 tends to progress to AML quickly, usually in a median of 5 months.[36,37] FISH follow-up to monitor disease progression is necessary for patients with previously detected isolated trisomy 11 or any other isolated trisomy.

Patients with an isolated isochromosome 17q, i(17)(q10), may also represent a subgroup of AML. As in our recent studies, myeloid neoplasms with isolated i(17)(q10) demonstrate distinctive morphologic features, including multilineage dysplasia and concurrent myeloproliferative features; have a high risk of leukemic transformation; and harbor wild-type *TP53*.[43] Both transformed and de novo AML with isolated i(17)(q10) usually require stem cell transplantation because of their aggressive disease progression. FISH with a *TP53* probe is a reliable follow-up test for monitoring disease progression in patients with previously detected isolated i(17)(q10).

Pediatric B-Cell Acute Lymphoblastic Leukemia

Precursor lymphoid neoplasms are primarily pediatric malignancies; 75% of cases occur in children younger than 6 years. Precursor B-cell acute lymphoblastic leukemia (B-ALL) accounts for approximately 85% of cases that present as ALL.[44-48] The accuracy and timeliness of diagnosis and treatment for pediatric B-ALL affect prognosis. For children with leukemia, the earlier the treatment starts, the better the prognosis and the longer the disease-free survival. Several characteristic cytogenomic abnormalities have been associated with pediatric B-ALL (Table 15.4).[27] Abnormalities of t(9;22)(q34;q11.2)/*BCR-ABL1* or t(4;11)(q21;q23)/*MLL-AF1* or near-haploidy/low hypodiploidy indicate high-risk disease, whereas t(12;21)(p13;q22)/*ETV6-RUNX1* and high hyperdiploidy are considered characteristics of relatively low-risk disease. Patients with t(9;22)(q34;q11.2), t(4;11)(q21;q23), or complex karyotypes are transplantation candidates, and allogeneic transplantation remains the best option for treatment.

Because of the low metaphase index, suboptimal chromosomal morphology, and low level of chromosome banding in B-ALL cases, FISH analysis with a pediatric B-ALL probe panel has become a routine test for pediatric B-ALL patients. FISH analysis should be performed in suspected pediatric B-ALL cases, and selected FISH probes are used by some institutions that have specific therapy protocols. Currently, FISH probes for pediatric B-ALL include CEP4, CEP10, and CEP17 for gain of chromosomes 4, 10, and 17, respectively; *BCR/ABL1* for t(9;22)(q34;q11.2), which results in the *BCR/ABL1* fusion gene that encodes a 190-kDa protein; *ETV6-RUNX1* for t(12;21)(p13;q22); and *p16* for del(9)(p21). The probe for *MLL* rearrangements can also be used. Integration of pediatric probe panel FISH with routine karyotyping significantly increases the detection rate of cytogenomic abnormalities to greater than 75% (Fig. 15.11).[44,48]

Near-haploid B-ALL (Fig. 15.12) is one of the most important types of pediatric B-ALL because of its poor prognosis; however, its identification by standard karyotyping is difficult. Endoreduplication doubles the number of chromosomes in some near-haploid B-ALL patients, resulting in an additional near-diploid or a hyperdiploid clone, making the diagnosis easy to miss and thus leading to inappropriate treatment.[48] Structural abnormalities providing a clue to the differentiation of near-haploid from hyperdiploid, which is usually associated with a favorable prognosis, are uncommon in the near-haploid karyotype.

An isochromosome for the long arm of chromosome 21 with 21q22 duplication, named iAMP21, has

TABLE 15-4 Common Recurrent Cytogenomic Abnormalities Associated with Pediatric B-Cell Acute Lymphoblastic Leukemia

Cytogenomic Abnormality	Genes and Cancer Genetics	Major Clinical Features[a]	Major Morphologic Features[b]	Prognosis
t(9;22)(q34;q11.2)	*BCR/ABL1* 1. Produces a 190 kDa fusion protein in most pediatric patients and about 50% of adult patients 2. May present with other abnormalities	1. More common in adults than in children 2. Similar clinical features to those seen in other patients with B-ALL in adults but most pediatric cases are high risk 3. May demonstrate organ involvement but lymphomatous involvement is rare	No distinguishing features from other types of B-ALL	1. Worse than other patients with B-ALL 2. Better prognosis if age is >10 y, white blood cell count is high, and disease responds to therapy in pediatric patients 3. Imatinib used in adult patients may improve early event-free survival
t(12;21)(p13;q22)	*ETV6/RUNX1(TEL/AML1)* 1. *Runx1/Etv6* product negatively acts on the function of the transcription *RUNX1*, which is considered an early lesion in leukemogenesis 2. *ETV6-RUNX1* rearrangement is necessary but not sufficient for the development of leukemia	1. Accounts for about 25% of pediatric B-ALL, not seen in infants 2. Similar clinical features to those seen in other B-ALL patients	No distinguishing features from other types of B-ALL	1. Very favorable prognosis with cures in >90% of pediatric patients 2. Less favorable prognosis in patients older than 10 y and with high white blood cell count, but still better than in other B-ALL patients
t(1;19)(q23;p13.3)	*E2A/PBX1* 1. The protein that is encoded by the chimeric gene *E2A/PBX1* mainly functions as a transcriptional activator in oncogenesis 2. Loss of der(1)t(1;19) in some cases 3. Variant translocation t(17;19)(q22;p13.3) involving *E2A/HLF* in rare cases associated with dismal prognosis	Typical B-cell precursor ALL clinical features	1. No distinguishing features from other types of B-ALL 2. Blasts with characteristic expression of CD10, CD19, and cytoplasmic μ heavy chain	1. Intermediate risk, with overall survival worse than t(12;21)(p13;q22) or hyperdiploid pediatric B-cell ALL 2. Increased risk of central nervous system relapse in some cases
t(5;14)(q31;q32)	*IL3/IGH* 1. *IL3/IGH* rearrangement results in constitutive *IL3* overexpression 2. Often detected by routine karyotyping	1. In both pediatric and adult patients 2. Similar clinical features to those seen in other B-ALL patients 3. May present asymptomatically and with low blast count	1. Increase in circulating eosinophils 2. No other distinguishing features from other types of B-ALL	Similar to that of other B-ALL patients
t(4;11)(q21;q23)	*MLL/AF4* 1. *AF4* is one of a very large number of translocation partners (19p13.3/ENL in T-cell acute lymphoblastic leukemia, 9p22/AF9 in acute myeloid leukemia) with *MLL* 2. Frequently associated with *FLT3* overexpression	1. Most common in infants <1 y of age 2. Often very high white blood cell count (>100 × 10^9/L) and high incidence of central nervous system involvement at presentation 3. May have organ involvement, but pure lymphomatous presentation is rare	No distinguishing features from other types of B-ALL; mixed B-lymphoid/myeloid in some cases	Poor prognosis, particularly in infant patients <6 mo of age

iAMP21	*RUNX1* 1. Chromosome 21 instability leading to 21q22 intrachromosomal amplification 2. Gene amplification in a 5.1 Mb region including *RUNX1*, miR-802, and several genes mapping to the Down syndrome critical region 3. As a primary genetic event in tumorigenesis	1. Common or pre–B-ALL 2. Older age (median 9 y) 3. Threefold increase in relapse risk	1. A new distinct subgroup of childhood B-cell precursor acute lymphoblastic leukemia 2. A lower white cell count (median 3.9), otherwise no distinguishing features from other types of B-ALL so far	1. Dismal outcome if treated with standard therapy 2. Significantly inferior median event-free (29%) and overall survival (71%) at 5 y 3. Preferred bone marrow transplantation in first remission
Hypodiploid	1. Chromosome numerical change from 45 to near-haploid 2. Nonspecific structural abnormalities may be seen in nonnear-haploid cases 3. Near diploid or hyperdiploid may be seen in a minor population owing to endoreduplication	1. In both pediatric and adult patients but near-haploid limited to pediatric patients 2. Similar clinical features to those seen in other B-ALL patients	No distinguishing features from other types of B-ALL	1. Poor prognosis 2. A better prognosis in patients with 44–45 chromosomes, worst prognosis in near-haploid cases
Hyperdiploid	1. Non-random gain of chromosomes, with 21, X, 14, and 4 most common and 1, 2, and 3 least common 2. Usually no structural changes	1. Common in pediatric patients, accounting for about 25% of B-ALL patients 2. Not in infants and rare in adults 3. Similar clinical features to those seen in other B-ALL patients	No distinguishing features from other types of B-ALL	Simultaneous trisomies for chromosomes 4, 10, and 17 associated with the best prognosis

B-ALL, B-cell acute lymphoblastic leukemia; y, years.

[a]Common clinical features in B-ALL: bone marrow failure (thrombocytopenia and/or anemia and/or neutropenia) at presentation or in the disease course; variable leukocyte count; frequent lymphadenopathy, hepatomegaly, and splenomegaly; bone pain and arthralgias

[b]Common morphologic features: circulating blasts with bone marrow packed with immature lymphoid cells..

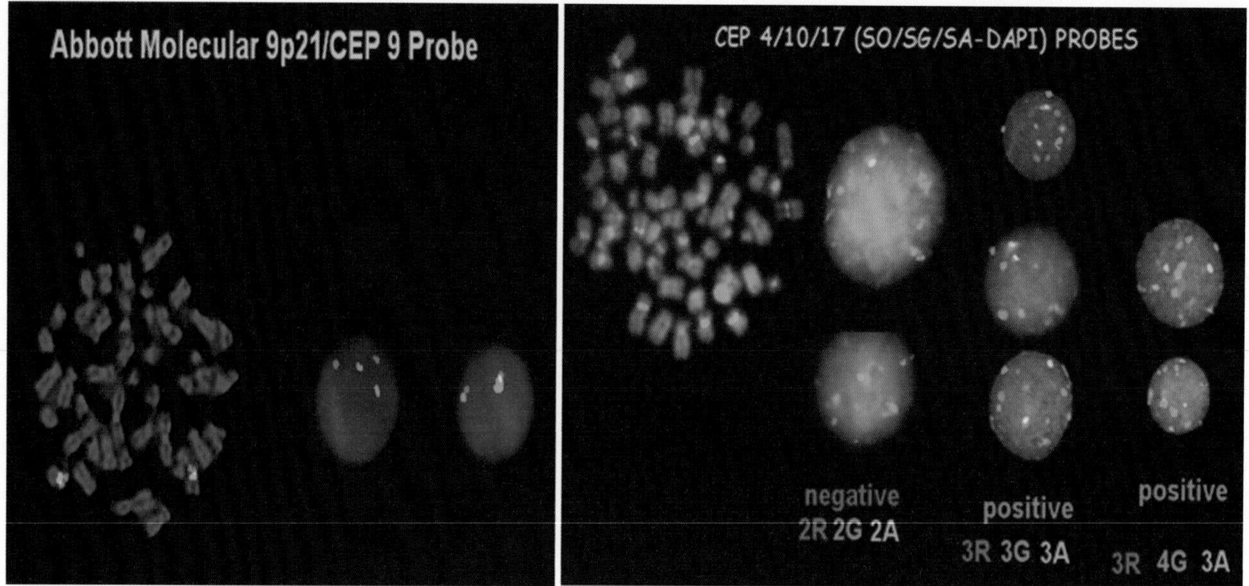

FIGURE 15–11 Partial pediatric B-cell acute lymphoblastic leukemia (B-ALL) fluorescence in situ hybridization (FISH) probe panel. FISH using a partial B-ALL probe panel in a 6-year-old B-ALL patient showed negative for del(9p21) (*red*), but revealed trisomies for chromosomes 4 (*red*), 10 (*green*), and 17 (aqua).

recently been shown to define a subset of pediatric B-ALL patients. This unique cytogenomic abnormality is associated with an increased risk of both early and late relapse, and it can lead to an unfavorable outcome when patients are treated with standard therapy because of the effect of *RUNX1* amplification.[45] FISH is currently the most reliable method for detecting this abnormality (Fig. 15.13).

B-Cell Lymphoma with Recurrent Cytogenomic Abnormalities

Although morphology and immunophenotype are sufficient for the diagnosis of most lymphomas, cytogenomic tests are still an important component for an accurate diagnosis. Characteristic chromosomal translocations are often revealed in lymphomas, and they mostly involve the mature B-cell lineage; an exception is t(2;5)(p23;q35), which involves the *ALK* gene mapped to chromosome 2p23 and is associated with T-cell-type anaplastic large-cell lymphoma. A recent study revealed t(6;7)(p25.3;q23.3), which results in *RFA7H/DUSP22* rearrangement and is commonly associated with *ALK*-negative anaplastic large-cell lymphoma.[49] The characteristic translocations in B-cell lymphomas include t(11;14)(q13;q32), resulting in *IgH/CCND1* associated with mantle cell lymphoma; t(8;14)(q24;q32), resulting in *IgH/MCY* and its variants associated with Burkitt lymphoma; t(14;18)(q32;q22), resulting in *IgH/BCL2* and associated with follicular lymphoma; and t(11;18)(q21;q21), resulting in the *API2/MALT1* fusion transcript lined with low-grade extranodal marginal zone B-cell lymphoma of mucosa-associated lymphoid tissue (MALT lymphoma).[50-56]

t(11;18)(q21;q21) can be seen in about 15% of MALT lymphomas, and several other less common translocations involving 18q21/*MALT* have been reported in

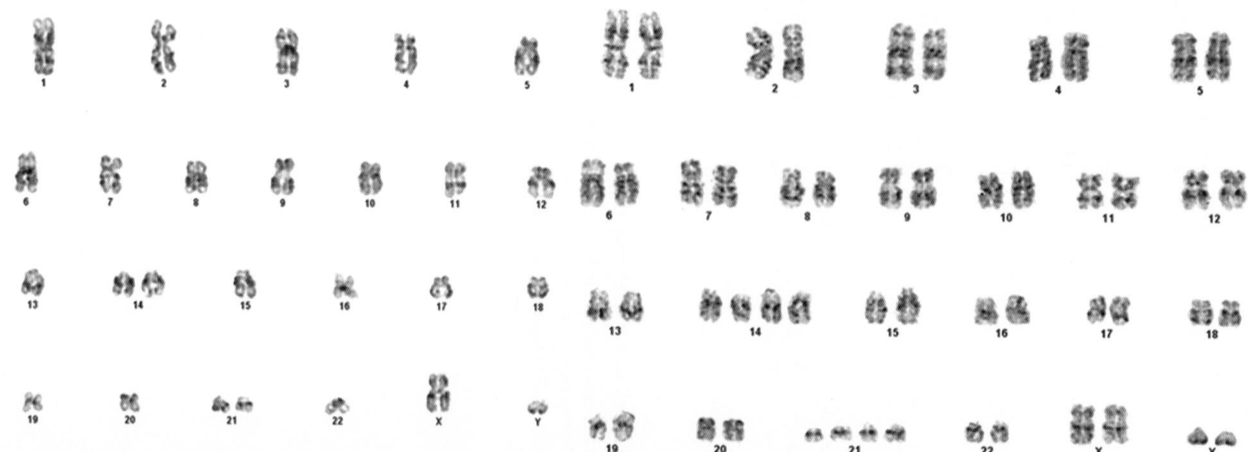

FIGURE 15–12 Near-haploid karyotype of a pediatric patient with B-cell acute lymphoblastic leukemia. The haploid cell (*left*) underwent endoreduplication and resulted in the hyperdiploid karyotype (*right*). (Adapted from Zhou Y, Medeiros LJ, Lu G, Ramos-Bueso C. Pediatric B-cell acute lymphoblastic leukemia, Review. Am J Clin Pathol. 2012)

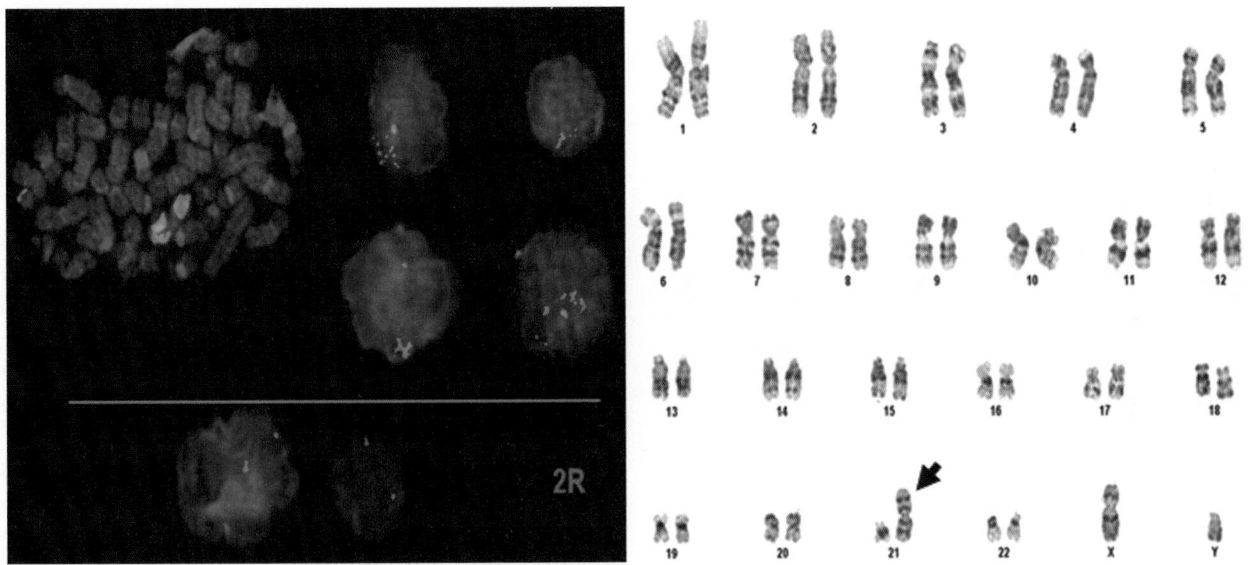

FIGURE 15–13 Isochromosome iAMP21 with *RUNX1* amplification. iAMP21 was detected in a pediatric patient with B-cell acute lymphoblastic leukemia. An add-on fluorescence in situ hybridization study with the *RUNX1* probe revealed *RUNX1* amplification. (Adapted from Zhou Y, Medeiros LJ, Lu G, Ramos-Bueso C. Pediatric B-cell acute lymphoblastic leukemia, Review. Am J Clin Pathol. 2012)

this disease.[56] These include t(14;18)(q32;q21), t(1;14)(p22;q32), and t(3;14)(p14.1;q32), which result in overexpression of *MALT1*, *BCL10*, and *FOXP1*, respectively, in about 10%, 5%, and 10% of MALT lymphoma cases, respectively. t(1;14)(p22;q32) is usually associated with advanced stage in MALT lymphomas. These translocations can be seen at various frequencies in various sites, including the stomach, skin, salivary gland, intestine, lung, and ocular adnexae. t(11;18) can be seen in the intestine, stomach, and lung at frequencies of 13%, 24%, and 43%, respectively; t(14;18) is seen in the salivary gland, skin, and ocular adnexae at frequencies of 12%, 14%, and 24%, respectively; and t(1;14) seen in the salivary gland, lung, and intestine at frequencies of 2%, 7%, and 12%, respectively.[56]

FISH probes are available for the detection of gene rearrangements resulting from the translocations in lymphomas. Because of the paradigm for frequent *IgH* rearrangements, FISH with an *IgH* probe can be a primary assay for B-cell lymphoma cases that show no disease-specific morphology or immunophenotype. Additional attention should be paid to the development of therapy-related MDS and/or AML (tMDS/tAML) in treated lymphoma patients, usually 3 to 5 years after therapy.[57] Secondary changes can be detected during the patient's treatment; they may be present as clonal evolution changes together with the primary cytogenomic abnormalities associated with the specific lymphoma (Fig. 15.14).

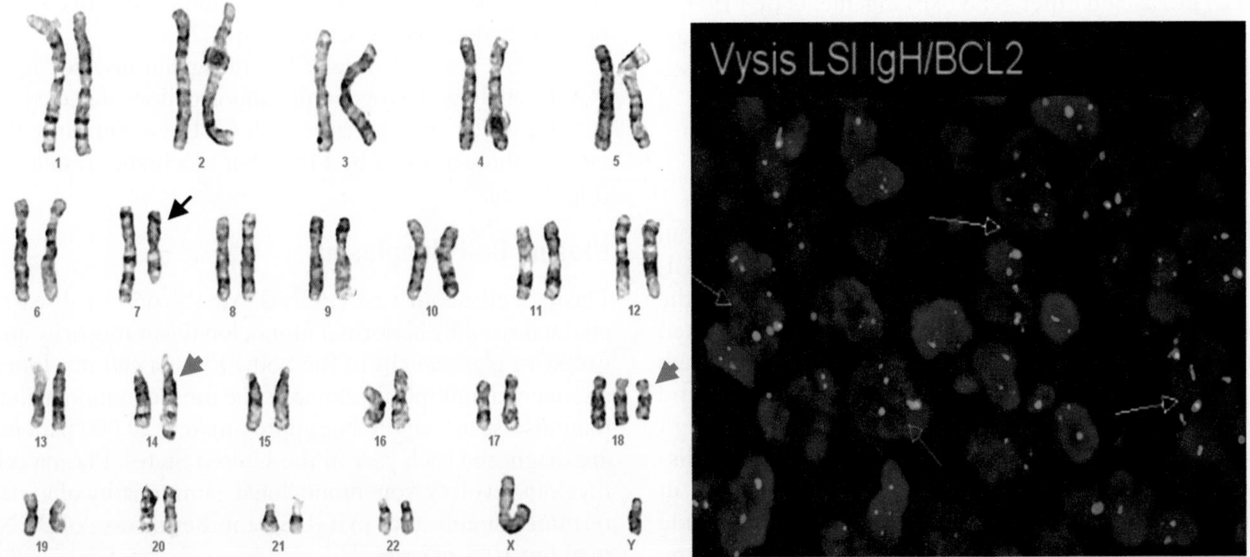

FIGURE 15–14 Clonal evolution in a patient with follicular lymphoma. An additional del(7q) was observed in 4 of the 20 cells analyzed in a follow-up bone marrow sample from a male patient 63 mo after therapy. Fluorescence in situ hybridization on a paraffin-embedded slide showed *IgH/BCL2* rearrangement.

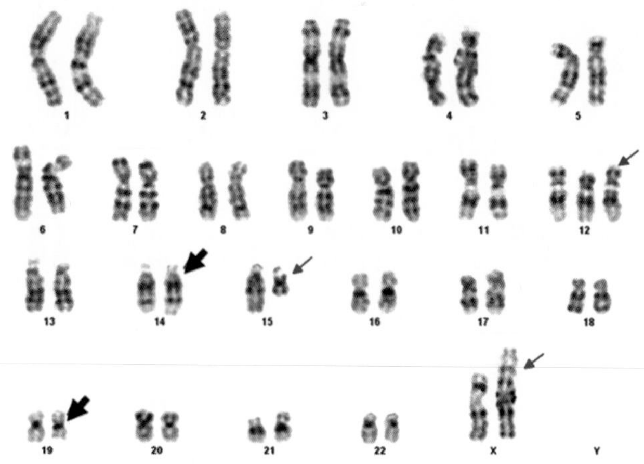

FIGURE 15–15 t(14;19)(q32;q13.2) in chronic lymphocytic leukemia (CLL). The karyotype is from a female CLL patient who had t(14;19)(q32;q13.2) (*big black arrows*) in addition to trisomy 12 and t(X;15)(p22.1;q22) (*small blue arrows*).

Double-hit lymphoma (DHL), a rare type of lymphoma that is associated with an extremely unfavorable prognosis, demonstrates concurrent chromosomal translocations mainly involving *BCL2* and *MYC*. It is one of the aggressive B-cell lymphomas. *BCL2* rearrangement is thought to precede *MYC* events in DHL lymphomagenesis. Most DHL cases are de novo or following follicular lymphoma.[58] Other oncogenes besides *BCL2* and *MYC* are also involved at a lower frequency, including *BCL3*, *BCL6*, and *CCND1*; therefore, *BCL6*(+)/*MYC*(+) DHL, *BCL2*(+)/*BCL6*(+)/*MYC*(+) triple-hit lymphomas, and *CCND1*(+)/*MYC*(+) DHL have been named.[58,59] Because of the poor prognosis in DHL and because there are currently no other reliable diagnostic tools to identify DHL, it is appropriate to test all diffuse large B-cell and related lymphomas that demonstrate *BCL2* rearrangement but do not confirm typical Burkitt lymphoma morphology for *MYC*, *BCL2*, and other gene rearrangements by FISH to identify DHL. A recent study indicates that *MYC* rearrangement or high *MYC* activity in B-cell lymphomas is an independent negative prognostic factor, regardless of any other genetic abnormalities present.[60]

Chronic Lymphocytic Leukemia

The course of chronic lymphocytic leukemia (CLL) can vary from indolent disease to rapid progression, and CLL response to chemotherapy is limited. In addition to the biochemical markers whose high levels are correlated with shorter time from diagnosis to progression, such as CD38, unmutated IgV(H), beta 2-microglobulin, and ZAP-70, new prognostic markers developed through cytogenomic technology that are associated with disease prognosis and/or progression have been found in the majority of patients with CLL.[61-64] These include del(17p13/*TP53*), del(11q22/*ATM*), del(13q14), trisomy 12, and del(6q21-24).[64] del(13q)/-13 is usually considered a favorable prognostic marker, whereas del(17p13/*TP53*) and mutations of the *TP53* gene are the most unfavorable markers. del(17p13/*TP53*) is usually associated with an aggressive clinical course and short overall survival, and therefore it should be evaluated in patients being considered for treatment with novel agents and/or allogeneic stem cell transplantation. del(11q22/*ATM*) can be found in about one-third of CLL patients, and it is associated with significantly shorter median progression-free survival times than those seen in other CLL patients. Patients with del(11q22/*ATM*) often require treatment with an alkylating agent in addition to a nucleoside analog and rituximab, whereas patients with trisomy 12 or del(6q21-24) are classified into an intermediate-risk cytogenomic group.[64,65]

FISH using a CLL probe panel has become a prognostic monitoring tool for disease progression in CLL patients, and it has also become a post-therapy monitoring tool. The probes used in the panel typically include LSI-*ATM*, LSI-*TP53*, CEP12, LSI-D13S319, and LSI-*LAMP*. del(17p13/*TP53*) is one of the most important indicators for multiagent chemoimmunotherapy in CLL, and the therapy choice includes fludarabine, lenalidomide, high-dose glucocorticoid regimens, and phosphatidylinositol 3-kinase inhibitor CAL-101.[66] FISH using LSI-*TP53* probe should be performed in any of relapsed CLL cases. Recently, FISH using a dual-color, break apart *IgH* probe has been proposed for selected CLL patients on the basis of findings that rearrangements involving the *IgH* locus are of clinical significance.[67] For example, studies have defined patients with a subtle translocation, t(14;19)(q32;q13.2), which results in *IgH/BCL3* rearrangement (Fig. 15.15), as a subgroup of CLL because of the associated atypical cell morphology and phenotype, lymphocytosis, frequent lymphadenopathy, young age at diagnosis (median 50 to 60 years), male predominance, and aggressive disease course.[68-70] Because of the subtlety of this translocation and low mitotic index, FISH is currently the best choice for confirmation in patients with a previously detected t(14;19)(q32;q13.2).

CLL is currently one of few malignant diseases using aCGH analysis. Cytogenomic abnormalities detected by aCGH, which are associated with CLL, are currently the same as those assessed by FISH, but at a higher resolution (Fig. 15.16).

Plasma Cell Neoplasms

Plasma cell neoplasms (PCNs) are a group of diseases characterized by abnormal monoclonal gammopathy and excessive plasma cells in the body. Plasma cell myeloma, also named multiple myeloma, is the most common malignant disease among PCNs; approximately 20,000 patients are diagnosed each year in the United States. Plasma cell myeloma evolves from monoclonal gammopathy of undetermined significance (MGUS), another disease of PCN, in about 10% of cases.[71,72]

Cytogenomic abnormalities in plasma cells play an important role in PCN pathogenesis and progression;

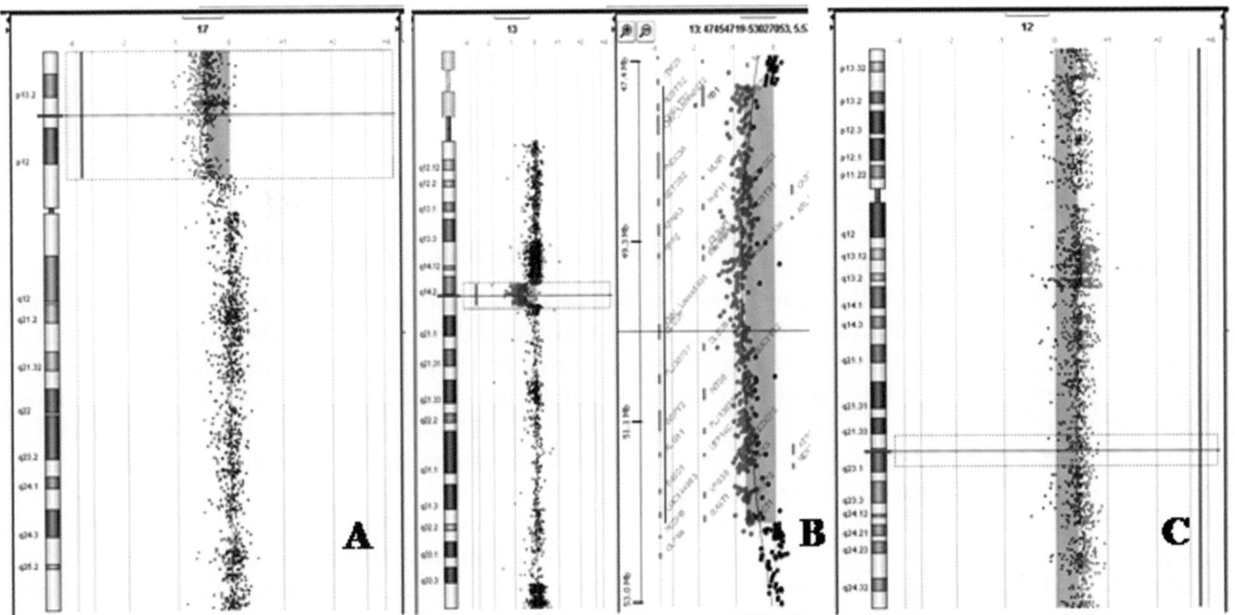

FIGURE 15–16 Cytogenomic abnormalities identified by array comparative genomic hybridization in a B-cell chronic lymphocytic leukemia patient. The abnormalities include del(17p) **(A)**, del(13q) **(B)**, and trisomy 12 **(C)**. The deleted segment in del(17p) covers most of the short arm of chromosome 17, whereas about 5.57 Mb nucleotides including the *RB1* gene are deleted at 13q14.2.

therefore, identifying cytogenomic abnormalities would improve treatment planning. It has been proposed that at least three cytogenomic pathways are commonly associated with PCN development, including (1) the aneuploidy pathway, (2) the *IgH* pathway, and (3) the del(13q)/-13 pathway[71,72]. These three pathways usually coexist and interact during PCN development and disease progression.[73]

Almost all MGUS cases are aneuploid, showing chromosome gains typically in the odd-numbered chromosomes (Fig. 15.17).[71] *IgH* rearrangements in the *IgH* pathway occur in as many as 65% of patients with PCN. These rearrangements affect more than a dozen other genes, most commonly *CCND1-XT*, *FGFR3*, *MAF*, *CCND3*, and *MAFB* in chromosomes 11, 4, 16, 6, and 20, respectively[74,75]; other affected genes are still unknown. *IgH* translocations are believed to be both primary and secondary genetic events in the development of PCNs. Interstitial del(13q)/-13 has been observed in as many as 70% of plasma cell myeloma cases and is an indicator of disease progression.[71,75-78]

In general, patients with t(11;14)(q13;q32) as the sole abnormality or as part of a complex karyotype without

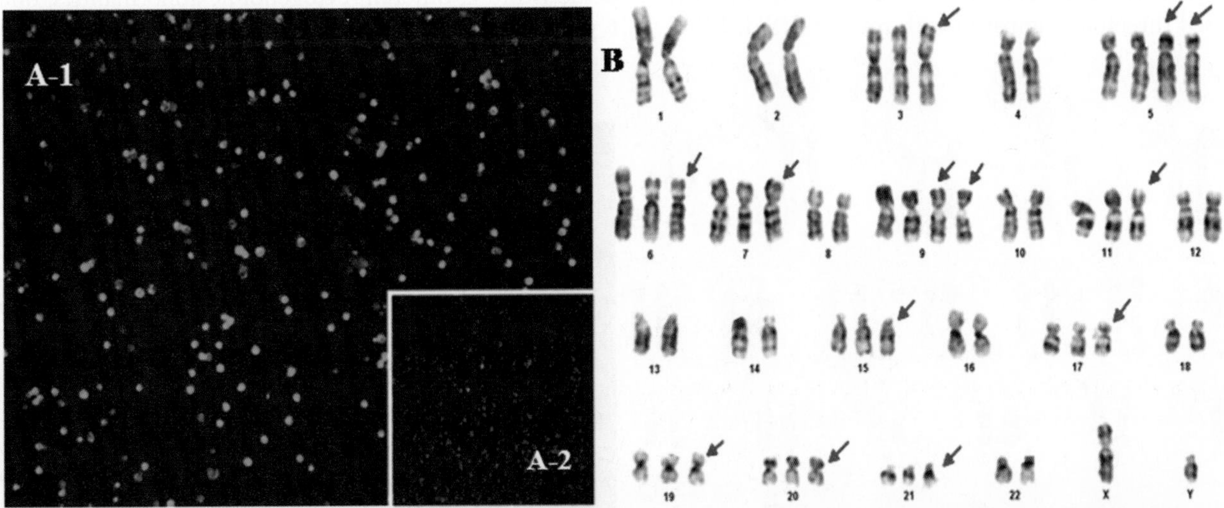

FIGURE 15–17 Hyperdiploid and CD138-labeled plasma cells. Plasma cell enrichment (PCE) resulted in significantly increased plasma cell density (**A**-1) compared with density in plasma cells that were not subjected to PCE (**A**-2); thus, PCE allows increased detection of cytogenomic abnormalities, including hyperdiploid (**B**). (Adapted from Lu G, et al. Plasma cell enrichment enhances detection of high-risk cytogenomic abnormalities by FISH and improves risk stratification of patients with plasma cell neoplasms. Arch Pathol & Lab Med. 2012)

high-risk cytogenomic abnormalities are considered to be in the standard-risk group, whereas patients with t(4;14)(p16;q32) or t(14;16)(q32;q23), alone or in combination with hypodiploidy, are considered to be in the high-risk group.[71,76,79] The presence of an *MYC* rearrangement resulting from t(8;14)(q24.1;q32) or one of its variants can indicate progression to late-stage plasma cell myeloma.[80,81] del(1p21/*CDC14C*) and 1q21/*CKS1B* gain in chromosome 1, usually considered markers associated with disease progression in PCNs, are seen in as many as 45% of plasma cell myeloma patients. The presence of 1q21/*CKS1B* gain indicates the need for more intensive chemotherapy.[82-84] It has been recently reported that 1q21/*CKS1B* gain has an adverse effect on progression-free and overall survival times in plasma cell myeloma patients treated with bortezomib,[85] and del(17p13/*TP53*) is considered the most unfavorable marker.[86,87]

Interphase FISH has proven to be a powerful assay in the detection of cytogenomic abnormalities; therefore, accurate and sensitive methods for detecting cytogenomic abnormalities by interphase FISH in PCNs are in demand.[87] Plasma cell count and plasma cell density are important factors involved in the detection of cytogenomic abnormalities by FISH.[88] The technique of plasma cell enrichment can increase plasma cell density in samples for cytogenomic study (Fig. 15.17), which thus significantly increases the sensitivity of FISH in detecting cytogenomic abnormalities.[89] Studies of interphase FISH on plasma cell–enriched samples from PCN patients in combination with follow-up clinicopathologic analysis after plasma cell enrichment, recently performed in the author's research laboratory at MD Anderson Cancer Center, allowed the accurate detection of high-risk cytogenomic abnormalities in patients who had minimal residual disease or whose disease was in remission. Detection rate of high-risk cytogenomic abnormalities significantly increased threefold compared with routine FISH. FISH probe panel for high-risk cytogenomic abnormalities in PCNs usually includes probes for *IgH* rearrangements, *IgH/FGFR3*, *IgH/MAF*, *IgH/CCND1-XT*, del(17p13/*TP53*), del(13q/*RB1*), and 1q21/*CKS1B* gain. The subtle translocation t(4;14)(p16;q32) almost always needs to be confirmed by FISH (Fig. 15.18).

Therapy-Related Myeloid Neoplasms

Therapy-related myeloid neoplasms comprise mainly tMDS and tAML. tMDS and tAML occur in about 10% of treated lymphoma patients in the 3 to 15 years after autologous stem cell transplantation after chemotherapy and/or radiation therapy. This risk is lower than that in patients with breast cancer, multiple myeloma, or a germ cell tumor.[90-93]

Prognosis in tMDS and tAML is usually poor, and therefore timely diagnosis is critical. It is not uncommon, however, for a secondary clone of cytogenomic abnormalities (Table 15.5) associated with tMDS or tAML to be detected before evidence of morphologic anomalies in bone marrow is found. It is also not uncommon for the secondary clone commonly associated with tMDS and tAML, such as del(5q)/-5, del(7q)/-7, or 11q23 rearrangements (detected by karyotyping), to be present in a single cell in the sample. FISH analysis is thus appropriate in such cases to confirm the presence of the abnormal clone. Therefore, close follow-up monitoring by FISH and karyotyping for the occurrence of secondary cytogenomic abnormalities in treated cancer patients has become routine; cytogenomic abnormalities detected should be timely informed to pathologists and/or oncologists for cases with discordant findings by concurrent bone marrow morphologic evaluation and flow cytometric analysis.

It has been proposed that there are two types of tMDS/tAML, each associated with a certain therapy, demonstrating different cytogenomic abnormalities: one type is related to alkylating drugs and radiation, and the

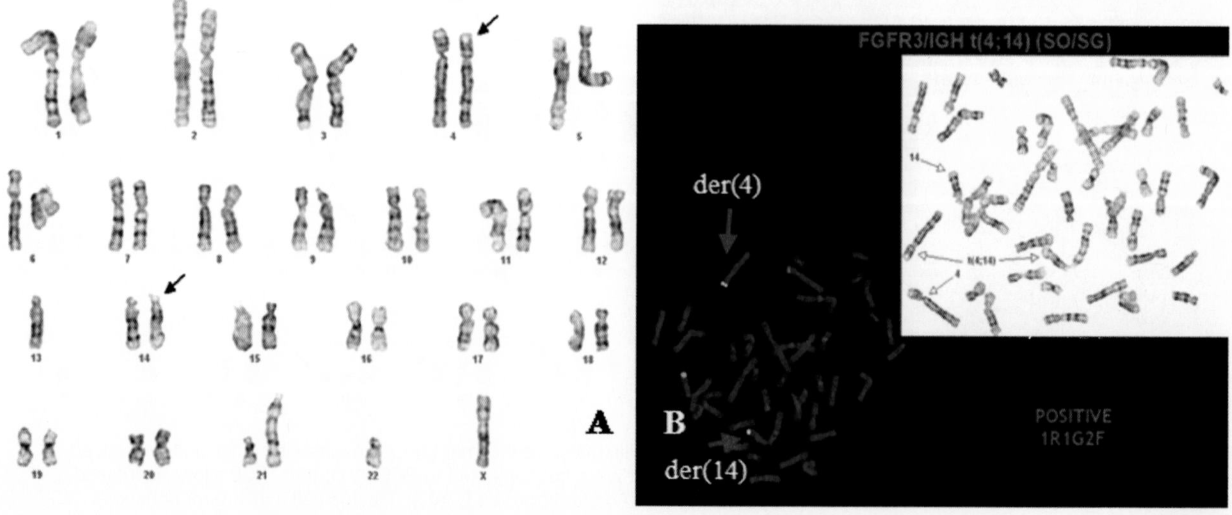

FIGURE 15–18 t(4;14)(p16;q32) (**A**, *arrows*) confirmed by fluorescence in situ hybridization mapback using *IgH/FGFR3* probes (**B**).

TABLE 15-5 Common Cytogenomic Abnormalities in Therapy-Related Myelodysplastic Syndrome and Acute Myeloid Leukemia

Abnormality	Occurrence	Genes Involved
-7/del(7q)	Up to 55%	*ASNS, PLANH1, EPO, MET*
-5/del(5q)	Up to 55%	*EGR1, IRF1, CSF1R*
11q23 rearrangements	High, accounting for 5–10% of all 11q23/*MLL* rearrangements observed in leukemia	*MLL*
21q22 rearrangements	15%	*RUNX1*
t(8;21)(q22;q22)	9%	*RUNX1/RUNX1T1*
inv(16)(p13;q22)	9%	*CBFB/MYH11*
t(3;21)(q26;q22)	3%	*RUNX1/EVI1*
t(15;17)(q24;q21)	2%	*PML/RARA*
del(17p13)	Accounts for about 25% of all del(17p) observed in leukemia	*TP53*
t(9;22)(q34;q11.2)	2%	*BCR/ABL1*
12p rearrangements	4%	*ETV6*
11p15 rearrangements	3–5%	*NUP98*

Adapted with modification from Lu G, Xu X, eds. *Clinical Genetic Counseling*. Beijing: Beijing University Medical Science Press; 2007.

other type is related to DNA topoisomerase II inhibitors (Table15.6; Fig. 15.19).[92,93] Alkylating drugs are usually used as part of a combination, and exposure to prednimustine, mechlorethamine, or procarbazine is associated with an increased risk of developing tMDS or tAML. Epipodophyllotoxins, etoposide, teniposide, and anthracyclines are the DNA topoisomerase II inhibitors most often associated with tMDS or tAML.[92]

Solid Tumors and Targeted Therapy

Cytogenomic abnormalities in solid tumors are also of diagnostic, prognostic, and therapeutic significance. Because of the difficulty of detecting cytogenomic abnormalities in metaphase cancer cells in cultures, and because of the need for prompt diagnosis and treatment for some types of tumors, such as glioma associated with del(1p36/19q13), FISH analysis of tumor cells is by far the most reliable test in cancer cytogenomics for solid tumors.

FISH analysis of solid tumors should be closely integrated with cytopathologic evaluation to ensure that the FISH probe is applied to the correct sections of the slide, which are usually ascertained by a pathologist. Slide sections with a single layer of tumor cells are the best selection for FISH analysis. FISH results from solid tumors must be interpreted on the basis of the guidelines proposed by the appropriate clinical organization, such as the American Society of Clinical Oncology (ASCO) and the College of American Pathologists (CAP).[94,95] For example, criteria to define positive results of *HER2* amplification in breast cancer have been established on the basis of the ratio of *HER2*/CEP17 as <1.80 for normal, 1.80 to 2.20 for equivocal level, and >2.20 for amplification. Results at the equivocal level should be further analyzed and interpreted in combination with findings from immunohistochemical study and clinical information. Different guidelines are used for specific probes associated with different tumors. Solid tumor tissue sample types used in FISH include formalin-fixed, paraffin-embedded, unstained slides, fine-needle aspirate specimens, cytospin or cytologic touch preparations from body fluids. The tissue sample can be fresh or frozen.

Several cytogenomic abnormalities have been found to be specifically associated with different solid tumors, particularly in sarcomas. Primary abnormalities, usually present as the sole change, are usually reciprocal

TABLE 15-6 Clinical Features of Therapy-Related Myelodysplastic Syndrome and Acute Myeloid Leukemia Resulting from Treatment with Alkylating Agents and Radiation or from DNA Topoisomerase II Inhibitors

Clinical Feature	Alkylating Agents/Radiation	DNA Topoisomerase II Inhibitor
Antecedent phase (myelodysplastic syndrome)	Often	Rare
Major morphologic features	Isolated cytopenia/pancytopenia, trilineage dysplasia	Monocytic and/or myelomonocytic components
Latency	5–8 years	2–3 years
Most common cytogenomic changes	-5/del(5q), -7/del(7q)	Rearrangements involving 11q23/*MLL*
Prognosis	Unfavorable	Unfavorable

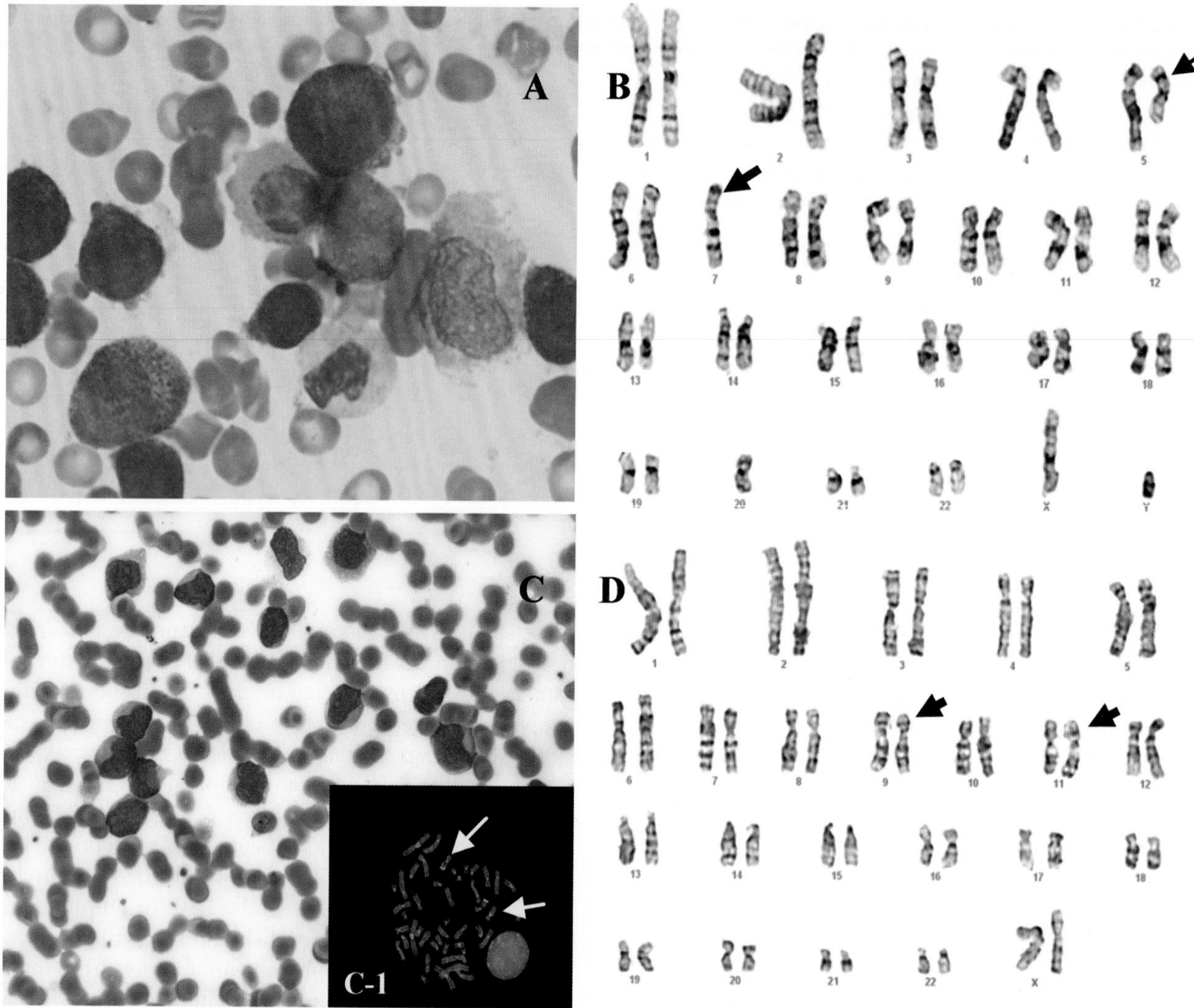

FIGURE 15–19 Del(5q)/-7 and *MLL* rearrangement in therapy-related myelodysplastic syndrome and acute myeloid leukemia (tMDS/tAML). **A** and **B:** Pathologic sample and karyotype from a 70-y-old man with a history of non-Hodgkin lymphoma, who was treated with alkylating agents and radiation for 26 mo before achieving remission. Flow cytometric analysis revealed 3% blasts, which suggests tMDS; bone marrow morphologic evaluation confirmed tMDS, showing increased megakaryocytes with small hypolobed forms and 16% ringed sideroblasts; del(5q) and -7 were detected in a bone marrow aspirate sample (B); tAML was diagnosed 4 mo thereafter. **C** and **D:** Pathologic sample and karyotype from a 67-y-old woman whose breast cancer had been treated with an epipodophyllotoxin for 18 mo, who presented with recent weakness and anemia. Flow cytometric analysis revealed 58% myeloblasts confirmed by bone marrow evaluation (C) leading to a diagnosis of tAML. A clone with t(9;11)(p22;q23) (D) involving the *MLL* gene confirmed by FISH mapback (C-1). (Panels B and D are adapted from Lu G, Xu X, eds. *Clinical Genetic Counseling*. Beijing: Beijing University Medical Science Press; 2007.)

translocations producing chimeric or fusion genes (Table 15.7). The primary abnormalities are believed to play an important role in the earliest stages of tumor initiation. For example, in alveolar rhabdomyosarcoma, which is an aggressive neoplasm, specific t(2;13)(q35;q14) or t(1;13)(p36;q14) results in *PAX3/FOXO1* and *PAX7/FOXO1* fusion genes in approximately 80% of cases. FISH study using dual-color break apart probe is a routine test to identify *FOXO1* rearrangement. *FOXO1* amplification can also be detected in some cases (Fig. 15.20).[96,97] The presence of t(11;22)(q24;q12) or t(21;22)(q22;q12), (Fig. 15.21) resulting in *EWSR1* rearrangement, routinely detected by FISH, is associated with Ewing sarcoma and is used for its differential diagnosis from other small round blue cell neoplasms.[98,99] Loss of heterozygosity involving 1p36 and 19q13 is a common cytogenomic alteration in brain tumors, particularly anaplastic oligodendroglioma (Fig. 15.22). Loss of 1p36/19q13 has been associated with chemosensitivity, extended response to chemotherapy, and extended survival.

HER2 gene is amplified (Fig. 15-23) in about 25% of breast cancers. *HER2* amplification is responsible for its protein overexpression and is associated with poor outcome in node-negative breast cancer. It is thus used as a therapeutic marker for personalized therapy with trastuzumab, an anti-*HER2* antibody.[100-102] About 20% of gastric adenocarcinoma also show *HER2* amplification.[103] Other tumors that show *HER2* amplification include ovarian carcinomas, salivary gland carcinomas,

TABLE 15-7 Cytogenomic Abnormality Detected by Fluorescence In Situ Hybridization Used for Solid Tumor Diagnosis

Cytogenomic Abnormality	Tumor
del(1p36/19q13)	Brain tumor
2p24.1/*N-MYC* amplification	Neuroblastoma
12q13.3/*CHOP* rearrangement, i.e., t(12;16)(q13;p11.2)	Myxoid liposarcoma
13q14.1/*FOXO1 (FKHR)* rearrangement, i.e., t(2;13)(q35;q14)	Alveolar rhabdomyosarcoma
16p11.2/*FUS* rearrangement	Low-grade fibromyxoid sarcoma and myxoid liposarcoma
18q11.2/*SYT* rearrangement, i.e., t(X;18)(p11.2;q11.2)	Synovial sarcoma
22q12.2/*EWSR1* rearrangement, i.e., t(11;22)(q24;q12) or t(21;22)(q22;q12)	Ewing sarcoma
2p23/*ALK* rearrangement, i.e., t(2;5)(p23;q35)	Anaplastic large-cell lymphoma
UroVysion panel [+3, +7, +17, del(9p21/*p16*)]	Bladder cancer
+7, +17	Papillary renal cell carcinoma
del(3)(p25.3/*VHL*)	Clear cell renal carcinoma
12p13/*ETV6 Gain* or *ETV6* amplification	Germ cell tumors
6p24.3/*RREB1* gain, 6q23/*MYB* loss, 11q13/*CCND1* gain	Melanoma

endometrial carcinomas as well as non–small cell lung cancers at variable rates. Trastuzumab and lapatinib (a *HER* tyrosine kinase inhibitor) are effective at prolonging survival in *HER2*-positive patients with breast cancer or carcinoma of the stomach or gastroesophageal junction.[100,103] Therefore, *HER2* FISH is now a routine test for all primary breast cancer patients using ASCO–CAP guidelines.

Detection of *EGFR* amplification (Fig. 15.23), *c-MET* amplification, and *ALK* as well as *ROS1* rearrangements is of therapeutic importance in non–small cell lung cancer.[104-109] Patients with *EGFR* mutations respond dramatically to *EGFR* tyrosine kinase inhibitors such as gefitinib or erlotinib, resulting in longer progression-free survival.[104,106] Crizotinib was recently approved as the targeting agent for patients with non–small cell lung cancer demonstrating *ALK* as well as *ROS1* rearrangements.[108,109] Because the *ALK* rearrangement, which occurs in about 3% to 5% of patients with non–small cell lung cancer, results from a small inversion in the 2p23 region of the short arm of chromosome 2, the length of the dual-color break apart FISH pattern for a positive result is smaller (Fig. 15.24A) than that resulting from translocation between two different chromosomes in other tumors. Therefore, protocol and guidelines should be established for FISH analysis for this unique pattern. Because the target area of the drug

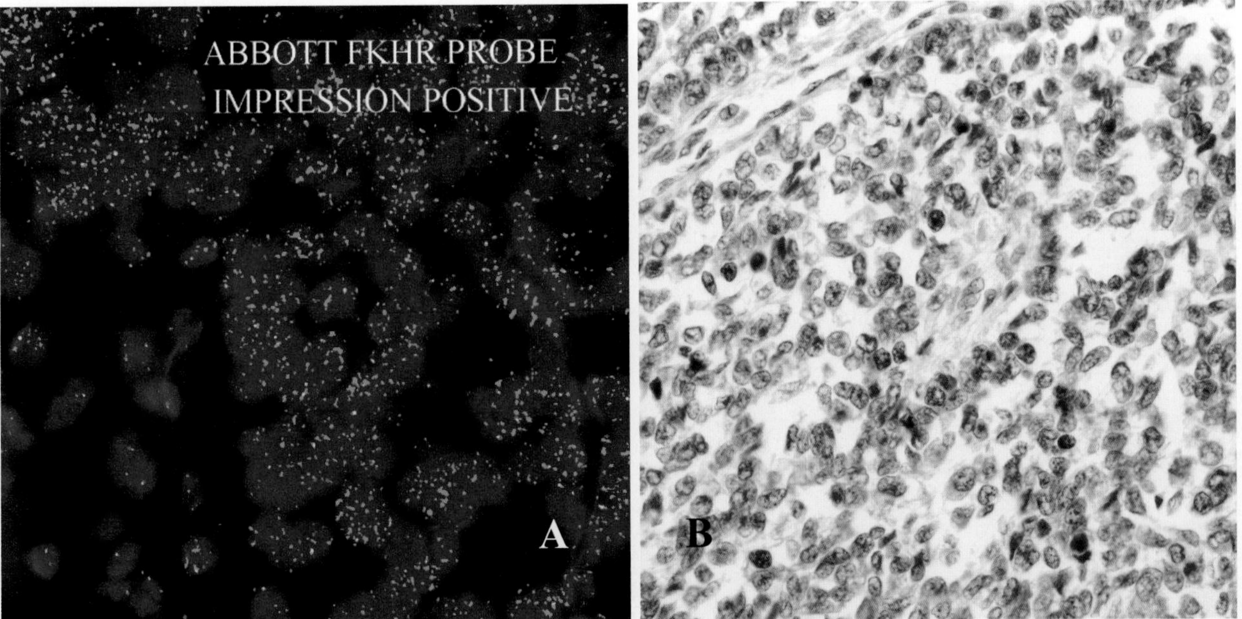

FIGURE 15–20 *FOXO1 (FKHR)* amplification in rhabdomyosarcoma. A rhabdomyosarcoma sample from an 8-y-old child was analyzed at The University of Texas MD Anderson Cancer Center by fluorescence in situ hybridization, which showed *FOXO1* rearrangement with 3′*FOXO1* amplification **(A)**, and by immunohistochemical stain with *FOXO1* antibody, which was positive (×100) **(B)**.

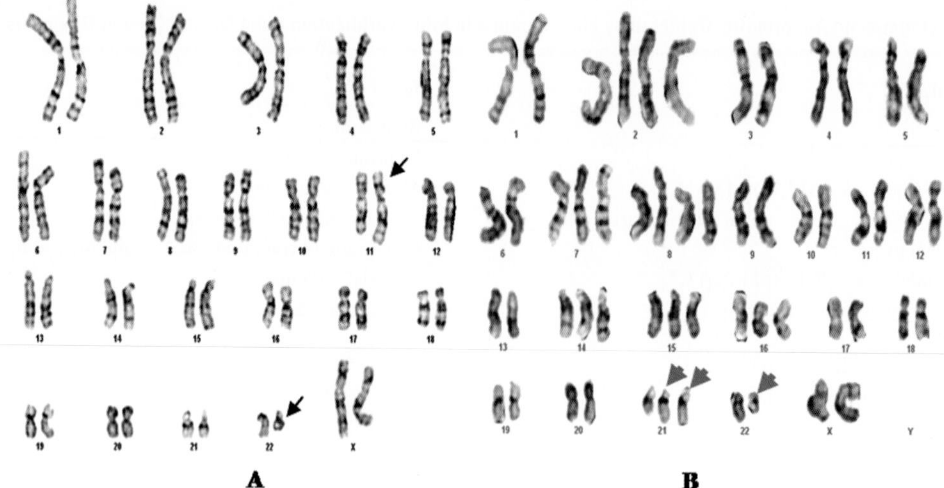

FIGURE 15–21 Karyotypes showing t(11;22)(q24;q12) **(A)** and t(21;22)(q22;q12) **(B)** in Ewing sarcoma.

crizotinib is located within the area targeted by the red probe, the current signal enumeration rules for positive *ALK* rearrangement mainly include (1) the presence of at least one set of red (3′-, or telomeric end) and green (5′- or centromeric end) signals that are two or more signal diameters apart; (2) the presence of a single red signal without a corresponding green signal in addition to fused and/or broken apart signals. Probe validation is a critical step before the test can be applied in clinical patient care.

Several other important diagnostic FISH tests for solid tumors have been routinely used, including UroVysion for bladder cancer. FISH analysis has proven to be superior to urine cytologic analysis, regardless of the tumor stage and grade, although FISH was shown to be slightly less specific than cytology.[110] UroVysion is a multitarget FISH assay that detects aneuploidy of chromosomes 3, 7, and 17 and loss of 9p21/*p16*. The chromosome enumeration probe of CEP3 is labeled in spectrumRed, that of CEP7 in spectrumGreen, that of CEP17 in spectrumAqua, and that of locus-specific identifier 9p21/*p16* in its own color (Fig. 15.24B). UroVysion is currently approved by the U.S. Food and Drug Administration for the detection of urothelial carcinoma in patients with hematuria and for surveillance of patients with bladder cancer. Usually, criteria to define positive results are multiple gain of chromosomes 3, 7, or 17 in 4 or more than 4 cells; loss of 9p21/*p16* in 12 or more than 12 cells; isolated trisomy 3, 7, or 17 in more than 10% of

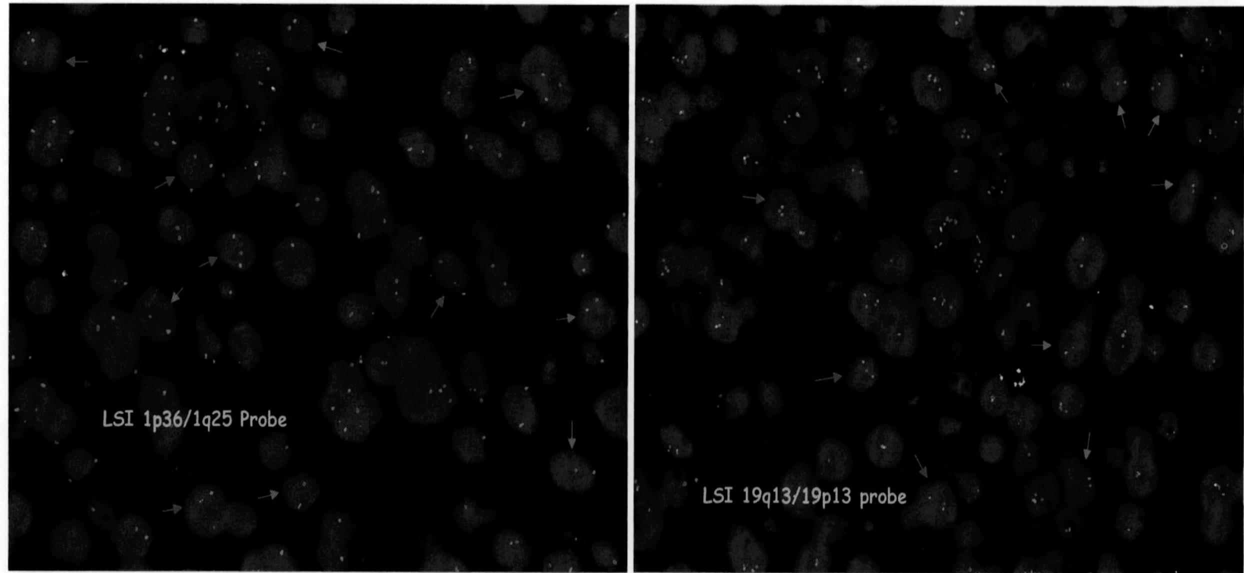

FIGURE 15–22 1p36/19q13 deletions. The fluorescence in situ hybridization (FISH) images are from a 34-y-old patient with left frontal anaplastic astrocytoma. The patient had a long-standing history of right-sided hearing loss and dizziness with left-sided headaches. FISH on interphase cells revealed del(1p36)/del(19q13) (*red arrows*).

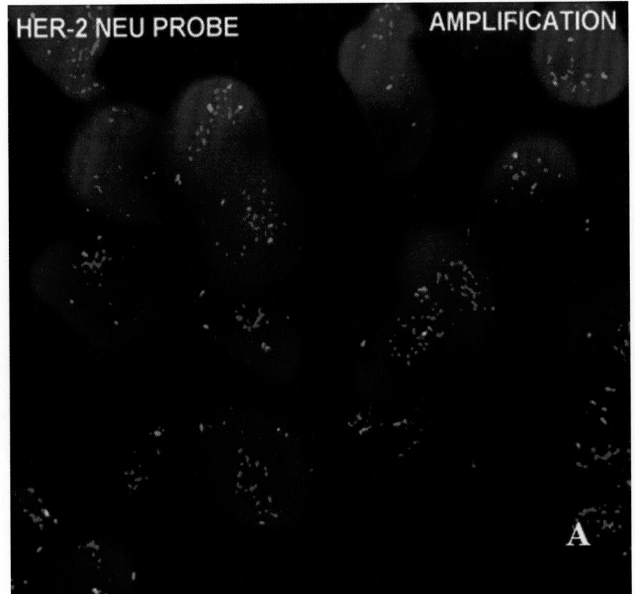

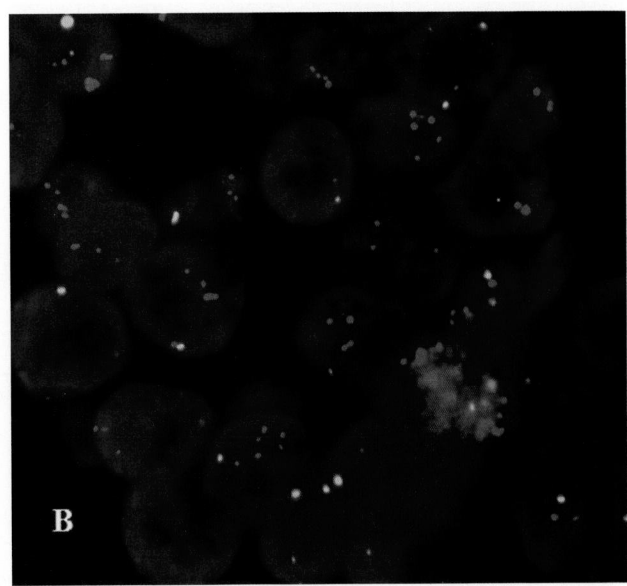

FIGURE 15–23 Fluorescence in situ hybridization showing *HER2* amplification in breast cancer **(A)** and *EGFR* amplification in non–small cell lung cancer **(B)**.

cells analyzed. The clinical utility of urine-based tumor markers remains useful but it was not well established and their use had not been recommended by guideline panels. Other cytogenomic abnormalities commonly detected by FISH associated with solid tumors include gain or amplification of 12p13/*ETV6* in germ cell tumors[111] and gain of 6p24.3/*RREB1* or 11q13/*CCND1*, or 6q23/*MYB* loss in melanoma.[112]

FISH analysis is also useful for the diagnosis and personalized therapy analysis of myeloid and lymphoid neoplasms with eosinophilia and abnormalities of platelet-derived growth factor receptor, alpha (*PDGFRA*), platelet-derived growth factor receptor, beta (*PDGFRB*), and fibroblast growth factor receptor 1 (*FGFR1*). *PDGFRA* rearrangement resulting in *FIP1L1-PDGFRA* fusion at the 4q12 region is an excellent example and is mainly seen in chronic hypereosinophilic syndrome/chronic eosinophilic leukemia. The *PDGFRA* rearrangement can also be observed in some AML cases (Fig. 15.25A). Tumors with *PDGRFA* and *PDGFRB* rearrangements respond to therapy with imatinib mesylate.[113,114] However, no established tyrosine kinase inhibitor therapy by far exists for myeloproliferative neoplasms with *FGFR1* rearrangement.

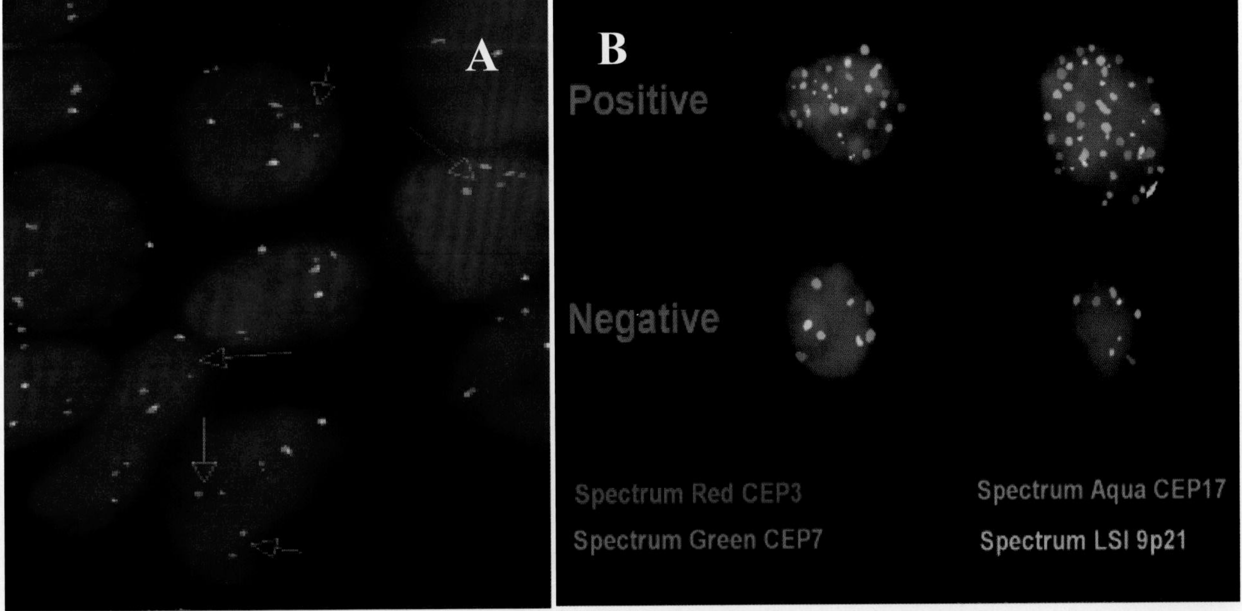

FIGURE 15–24 FISH results for *ALK* rearrangement and UroVysion. FISH study revealed *ALK* rearrangement in a patient with lung adenosarcoma **(A)**, aneuploidy for chromosomes 3, 7, and 17 in bladder cancer **(B)**.

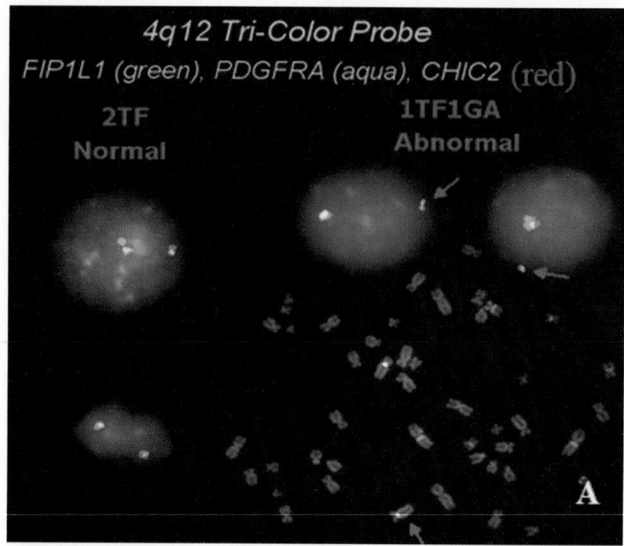

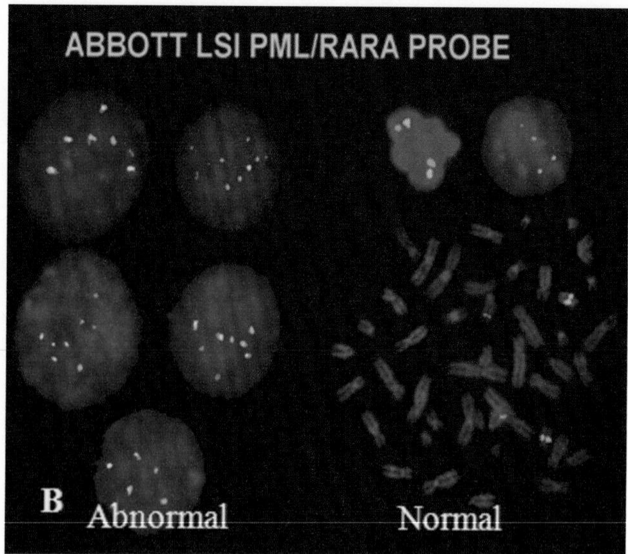

FIGURE 15–25 *PDGFRA* rearrangement and *PML/RARA* amplification. Image **A** shows *PDGFRA* rearrangement resulted from *CHIC2* deletion confirmed by FISH in a patient diagnosed with acute myeloid leukemia showing eosinophilia. Image **B** shows multiple copies of chimeric *PML/RARA* in a patient with acute promyelocytic leukemia who was refractory to therapy with retinoic acid and arsenic trioxide.

CONCLUSION

FISH currently remains a routine and reliable clinical cytogenomic test in cancer. Cancer cytogenomic abnormalities can be detected by FISH for various clinical utility at different stages of disease course: (1) prevention, (2) diagnosis, (3) prognosis, (4) therapeutics, (5) progression (including metastases), (6) remission, (7) residual disease, (8) therapy-related secondary malignancies, (9) relapse, and (10) chemoresistance (Fig. 15.26). Recent studies have shed light on the association of cytogenomic abnormalities targeted by FISH with cancer prevention, metastases, and therapy resistance. Studies on melanoma have set a model of cancer prevention based on the findings of the correlation of ultraviolet exposure with melanoma and the discovery of melanoma susceptibility genes such as *CDKN2A* and *CDK4*,[115] whereas others have demonstrated that 3q26/*TERC* amplification would be a good potential marker for cancer prevention in cervical cancers.[116,117] Cytogenomic abnormalities associated with cancer metastases have been studied, including amplification of *LAMP3*, *PROX1*, and *PRKAA1* for subsequent development of lymph node metastases in patients with cervical cancer,[118] *HER2* amplification in lymph node metastases from urothelial bladder cancer,[119] and *CCND1* gene numerical aberration for occult cervical lymph node metastasis in TNM stage I and II squamous cell carcinoma of the oral cavity.[120] With the use of more new effective therapeutic drugs or personalized therapies, and thus the cancer patient's longer overall survival, like the isolated trisomy 8 clone in Ph-negative treated CML patients, new cytogenomic abnormalities associated with drug-correlated myeloproliferative neoplasms are also expected. Finally, like heterogeneously staining regions and double minutes detected in both therapy-resistant hematologic malignancies and solid tumors, gene amplification (such as *BCR/ABL1* amplification in therapy-resistant CML and *PML/RARA* amplification in refractory APL) (Fig. 15.25B), other cytogenomic markers associated with therapy resistance, or refractory therapy would also be expected. It is expected that with the more comprehensive development of cancer genomic medicine and new technologies such as aCGH, SNP, and eventually next-generation whole-genome sequencing, additional new cytogenomic markers detectable by FISH for clinical cancer cytogenomics will be furnished.[121] Therefore, integrated with tumor cell morphology evaluation, immunophenotypic analysis, and gene mutation study, the demand for clinical cancer cytogenomic FISH will remain strong in the future.

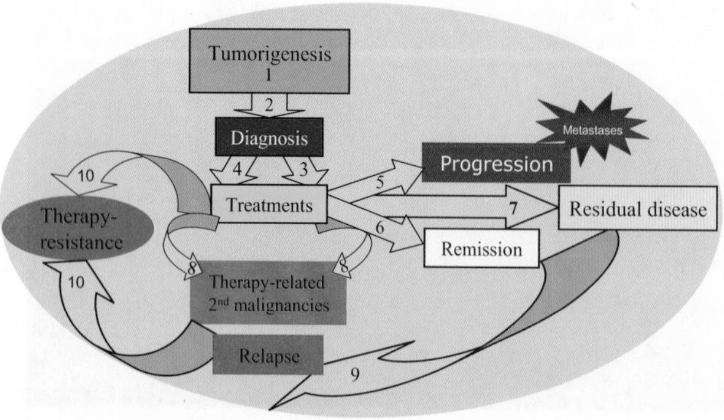

FIGURE 15–26 Ten FISH routes in clinical cancer cytogenomics.

REFERENCES

1. Bernheim A. Cytogenomics of cancers: from chromosome to sequence. *Mol Oncol.* 2010;4:309-322.
2. Heid IM, Jackson AU, Randall JC, et al. Meta-analysis identifies 13 new loci associated with waist-hip ratio and reveals sexual dimorphism in the genetic basis of fat distribution. *Nat Genet.* 2010;42:949-960.
3. Barrett MT, Scheffer A, Ben-Dor A, et al. Comparative genomic hybridization using oligonucleotide microarrays and total genomic DNA. *Proc Natl Acad Sci U S A.* 2004;101:17765-17770.
4. Liehr T. Application of yeast artificial chromosomes in fluorescence in situ hybridization. *Methods Mol Biol.* 2006;349:175-186.
5. Hollink IH, van den Heuvel-Eibrink MM, Arentsen-Peters ST, et al. NUP98/NSD1 characterizes a novel poor prognostic group in acute myeloid leukemia with a distinct HOX gene expression pattern. *Blood.* 2011;118:3645-3656.
6. Lucito R, Healy J, Alexander J, et al. Representational oligonucleotide microarray analysis: a high-resolution method to detect genome copy number variation. *Genome Res.* 2003;13: 2291-2305.
7. Shaffer LG, Bejjani BA, Torchia B, Kirkpatrick S, Coppinger J, Ballif BC. The identification of microdeletion syndromes and other chromosome abnormalities: cytogenetic methods of the past, new technologies for the future. *Am J Med Genet.* 2007;145:335-345.
8. Gajecka M, Mackay KL, Shaffer LG. Monosomy 1p36 deletion syndrome. *Am J Med Genet C Semin Med Genet.* 2007;145C: 346-356.
9. Kolquist KA, Schultz RA, Furrow A, et al. Microarray-based comparative genomic hybridization of cancer targets reveals novel, recurrent genetic aberrations in the myelodysplastic syndromes. *Cancer Genet.* 2011;204:603-628.
10. Sargent R, Jones D, Abruzzo LV, et al. Customized oligonucleotide array-based comparative genomic hybridization as a clinical assay for genomic profiling of chronic lymphocytic leukemia. *J Mol Diagn.* 2009;11:25-34.
11. Kreisel F, Kulkarni S, Kerns RT, et al. High resolution array comparative genomic hybridization identifies copy number alterations in diffuse large B-cell lymphoma that predict response to immuno-chemotherapy. *Cancer Genet.* 2011;204:129-137.
12. Sharma S, Free A, Mei Y, Peiper SC, Wang Z, Cowell JK. Distinct molecular signatures in pediatric infratentorial glioblastomas defined by aCGH. *Exp Mol Pathol.* 2010;89: 169-174.
13. Idbaih A, Kouwenhoven M, Jeuken J, et al. Chromosome 1p loss evaluation in anaplastic oligodendrogliomas. *Neuropathology.* 2008;28:440-443.
14. Soverini S, Hochhaus A, Nicolini FE, et al. BCR-ABL kinase domain mutation analysis in chronic myeloid leukemia patients treated with tyrosine kinase inhibitors: recommendations from an expert panel on behalf of European Leukemia Net. *Blood.* 2011;118:1208-1215.
15. Breccia M, Efficace F, Alimena G. Imatinib treatment in chronic myelogenous leukemia: what have we learned so far? *Cancer Lett.* 2011;300:115-121.
16. Nowell PC, Hungerford DA. A minute chromosome in human chronic granulocytic leukemia. *Science.* 1960;132:149.
17. Lu G, Xu M, eds. *Clinical Genetic Counseling.* Beijing: Beijing University Medical Sciences Press; 2009.
18. Tan J, Cang S, Seiter K, et al. t(3;9;22) 3-way chromosome translocation in chronic myeloid leukemia is associated with poor prognosis. *Cancer Invest.* 2009;27:718-722.
19. Smoley SA, Brockman SR, Paternoster SF, Meyer RG, Dewald GW. A novel tricolor, dual-fusion fluorescence in situ hybridization method to detect BCR/ABL fusion in cells with t(9;22)(q34;q11.2) associated with deletion of DNA on the derivative chromosome 9 in chronic myelocytic leukemia. *Cancer Genet Cytogenet.* 2004;148:1-6.
20. Storlazzi CT, Specchia G, Anelli L, et al. Breakpoint characterization of der(9) deletions in chronic myeloid leukemia patients. *Genes Chromosomes Cancer.* 2002;35:271-276.
21. Gorre ME, Mohammed M, Ellwood K, et al. Clinical resistance to STI-571 cancer therapy caused by BCR-ABL gene mutation or amplification. *Science.* 2001;293:876-880.
22. Feldman E, Najfeld V, Schuster M, Roboz G, Chadburn A, Silver RT. The emergence of Ph-, trisomy 8+ cells in patients with chronic myeloid leukemia treated with imatinib mesylate. *Exp Hematol.* 2003;31:702-707.
23. Karimata K, Masuko M, Ushiki T, et al. Myelodysplastic syndrome with Ph negative monosomy 7 chromosome following transient bone marrow dysplasia during imatinib treatment for chronic myeloid leukemia. *Intern Med.* 2011;50:481-485.
24. Larsson N, Billström R, Lilljebjörn H, et al. Genetic analysis of dasatinib-treated chronic myeloid leukemia rapidly developing into acute myeloid leukemia with monosomy 7 in Philadelphia-negative cells. *Cancer Genet Cytogenet.* 2010;199:89-95.
25. Zámecníkova A, Al Bahar S, Ramesh P. Trisomy 6 in a CML patient receiving imatinib mesylate therapy. *Leuk Res.* 2008;32:1454-1457.
26. Sun J, Yin CC, Cui W, Chen SS, Medeiros LJ, Lu G. Chromosome 20q deletion: a recurrent cytogenetic abnormality in patients with chronic myelogenous leukemia in remission. *Am J Clin Pathol.* 2011;35:391-397.
27. Swerdlow SH, Campo E, Harris NL, et al., eds. *WHO Classification of Tumours of Haematopoietic and Lymphoid Tissues.* 4th ed. Lyon: International Agency for Research on Cancer; 2008.
28. Mattson JC. Acute promyelocytic leukemia. From morphology to molecular lesions. *Clin Lab Med.* 2000;20:83-103.
29. Lallemand-Breitenbach V, de Thé H. PML nuclear bodies. *Cold Spring Harb Perspect Biol.* 2010;2:a000661.
30. Nagai S, Takahashi T, Kurokawa M. The impact of molecularly targeted therapies upon the understanding of leukemogenesis and the role of hematopoietic stem cell transplantation in acute promyelocytic leukemia. *Curr Stem Cell Res Ther.* 2010;5:372-378.
31. Chen Z, Tong JH, Dong S, Zhu J, Wang ZY, Chen SJ. Retinoic acid regulatory pathways, chromosomal translocations, and acute promyelocytic leukemia. *Genes Chromosomes Cancer.* 1996;15:147-156.
32. Rubnitz JE, Raimondi SC, Tong X, et al. Favorable impact of the t(9;11) in childhood acute myeloid leukemia. *J Clin Oncol.* 2002;20:2302-2309.
33. Moorman AV, Hagemeijer A, Charrin C, Rieder H, Secker-Walker LM. The translocations, t(11;19)(q23;p13.1) and t(11;19)(q23;p13.3): a cytogenetic and clinical profile of 53 patients. European 11q23 Workshop participants. *Leukemia.* 1998;12:805-810.
34. Mascarello JT, Hirsch B, Kearney HM, et al.; Working Group of the American College of Medical Genetics Laboratory Quality Assurance Committee. Section E9 of the American College of Medical Genetics technical standards and guidelines: fluorescence in situ hybridization. *Genet Med.* 2011;13:667-675.
35. Bae SY, Kim JS, Han EA, et al. Concurrent MYC and MLL amplification on dmin and hsr in acute myeloid leukemia. *Leuk Lymphoma.* 2008;49:1823-1825.
36. Alseraye FM, Zuo Z, Bueso-Ramos C, Wang S, Medeiros LJ, Lu G. Trisomy 11 as an isolated abnormality in acute myeloid leukemia is associated with unfavorable prognosis but not with an NPM1 or KIT mutation. *Int J Clin Exp Pathol.* 2011;4:371-377.
37. Wang SA, Jabbar K, Lu G, et al. Trisomy 11 in myelodysplastic syndromes defines a unique group of disease with aggressive clinicopathologic features. *Leukemia.* 2010;24:740-747.
38. Silva FP, Lind A, Brouwer-Mandema G, Valk PJ, Giphart-Gassler M. Trisomy 13 correlates with RUNX1 mutation and increased FLT3 expression in AML-M0 patients. *Haematologica.* 2007;92:123-126.
39. Gupta V, Minden MD, Yi QL, Brandwein J, Chun K. Prognostic significance of trisomy 4 as the sole cytogenetic abnormality in acute myeloid leukemia. *Leuk Res.* 2003;27:983-991.
40. Bains A , Lu G, Yao H, Luthra R, Medeiros LJ, Sargent RL. Molecular and clinicopathologic characterization of AML with isolated trisomy 4. *Am J Clin Pathol.* 2012;137:387-394.
41. Cui W, Bueso-Ramos CE, Sun J, Chen S, Muddasani R, Lu G. Trisomy 14 as a sole chromosome abnormality is associated with older age, heterogeneous groups of myeloid tumors and a wide spectrum of disease progression. *J Biomed Biotechnol.* 2010;2010:365318.
42. Paulsson K, Säll T, Fioretos T, Mitelman F, Johansson B. The incidence of trisomy 8 as a sole chromosomal aberration in myeloid malignancies varies in relation to gender, age, prior iatrogenic genotoxic exposure, and morphology. *Cancer Genet Cytogenet.* 2001;130:160-165.

43. Kanagal-Shamanna R, Bueso-Ramos CE, Barkoh B, et al. Myeloid neoplasms with isolated isochromosome 17q represent a clinicopathologic entity associated with myelodysplastic/myeloproliferative features, a high risk of leukemic transformation, and wild-type TP53. *Cancer*. 2011. doi:10.1002/cncr.26537.
44. Onciu M. Acute lymphoblastic leukemia. *Hematol Oncol Clin North Am*. 2009;23:655-674.
45. Rand V, Parker H, Russell LJ, et al. Genomic characterization implicates iAMP21 as a likely primary genetic event in childhood B-cell precursor acute lymphoblastic leukemia. *Blood*. 2011;117:6848-6855.
46. Harrison CJ, Haas O, Harbott J, et al.; Biology and Diagnosis Committee of International Berlin-Frankfürt-Münster study group. Detection of prognostically relevant genetic abnormalities in childhood B-cell precursor acute lymphoblastic leukaemia: recommendations from the Biology and Diagnosis Committee of the International Berlin-Frankfürt-Münster study group. *Br J Haematol*. 2010;151:132-142.
47. Aburawi HE, Biloglav A, Johansson B, Paulsson K. Cytogenetic and molecular genetic characterization of the "high hyperdiploid" B-cell precursor acute lymphoblastic leukaemia cell line MHH-CALL-2 reveals a near-haploid origin. *Br J Haematol*. 2011;154:275-277.
48. Kebriaei P, Anastasi J, Larson RA. Acute lymphoblastic leukaemia: diagnosis and classification. *Best Pract Res Clin Haematol*. 2002;15(4):597-621.
49. Feldman AL, Dogan A, Smith DI, et al. Discovery of recurrent t(6;7)(p25.3;q32.3) translocations in ALK-negative anaplastic large cell lymphomas by massively parallel genomic sequencing. *Blood*. 2011;117:915-919.
50. Freedman A. Follicular lymphoma: 2011 update on diagnosis and management. *Am J Hematol*. 2011;86:768-775.
51. Pileri SA, Agostinelli C, Sabattini E, et al. Lymphoma classification: the quiet after the storm. *Semin Diagn Pathol*. 2011;28:113-123.
52. Inghirami G, Pileri SA; European T-Cell Lymphoma Study Group. Anaplastic large-cell lymphoma. *Semin Diagn Pathol*. 2011;28:190-201.
53. Du MQ. MALT lymphoma: many roads lead to nuclear factor- b activation. *Histopathology*. 2011;58:26-38. doi:10.1111/j.1365-2559.2010.03699.x.
54. Zullo A, Hassan C, Andriani A, et al. Primary low-grade and high-grade gastric MALT-lymphoma presentation. *J Clin Gastroenterol*. 2010;44:340-344.
55. Sagaert X, De Wolf-Peeters C, Noels H, Baens M. The pathogenesis of MALT lymphomas: where do we stand? *Leukemia*. 2007;21:389-396.
56. Streubel B, Simonitsch-Klupp I, Müllauer L, et al. Variable frequencies of MALT lymphoma-associated genetic aberrations in MALT lymphomas of different sites. *Leukemia*. 2004;18:1722-1726.
57. Larson RA. Etiology and management of therapy-related myeloid leukemia. *Hematology (Am Soc Hematol Educ Program)*. 2007;1:453-459.
58. Aukema SM, Siebert R, Schuuring E, et al. Double-hit B-cell lymphomas. *Blood*. 2011;117:2319-2331.
59. Smith SM, Anastasi J, Cohen KS, Godley LA. The impact of MYC expression in lymphoma biology: beyond Burkitt lymphoma. *Blood Cells Mol Dis*. 2010;45:317-323.
60. Schrader A, Bentink S, Spang R, et al. High myc activity is an independent negative prognostic factor for diffuse large B cell lymphomas. *Int J Cancer*. 2011. doi:10.1002/ijc.26423.
61. Van Bockstaele F, Janssens A, Piette A, et al. Kolmogorov-Smirnov statistical test for analysis of ZAP-70 expression in B-CLL, compared with quantitative PCR and IgV(H) mutation status. *Cytometry B Clin Cytom*. 2006;70:302-308.
62. Caporaso N, Goldin L, Plass C, et al. Chronic lymphocytic leukaemia genetics overview. *Br J Haematol*. 2007;139:630-634.
63. Murashige N, Kami M, Takaue Y. ZAP-70 in chronic lymphocytic leukemia. *N Engl J Med*. 2003;349:506-507.
64. Döhner H, Stilgenbauer S, Benner A, et al. Genomic aberrations and survival in chronic lymphocytic leukemia. *N Engl J Med*. 2000;343:1910-1916.
65. Parker TL, Strout MP. Chronic lymphocytic leukemia: prognostic factors and impact on treatment. *Discov Med*. 2011;57:115-123.
66. Brown JR. The treatment of relapsed refractory chronic lymphocytic leukemia. Hematology Am Soc Hematol Educ Program. 2011:2011:110-118. Review.
67. Lu G, Kong Y, Yue C. Genetic and immunophenotypic profile of IGH@ rearrangement detected by fluorescence in situ hybridization in 149 cases of B-cell chronic lymphocytic leukemia. *Cancer Genet Cytogenet*. 2010;196:56-63.
68. Huh YO, Abruzzo LV, Rassidakis GZ, et al. The t(14;19)(q32;q13)-positive small B-cell leukaemia: a clinicopathologic and cytogenetic study of seven cases. *Br J Haematol*. 2007;136:220-228.
69. Huh YO, Schweighofer CD, Ketterling RP, et al. Chronic lymphocytic leukemia with t(14;19)(q32;q13) is characterized by atypical morphologic and immunophenotypic features and distinctive genetic features. *Am J Clin Pathol*. 2011;135:686-696.
70. Michaux L, Dierlamm J, Wlodarska I, Bours V, Van den Berghe H, Hagemeijer A. t(14;19)/BCL3 rearrangements in lymphoproliferative disorders: a review of 23 cases. *Cancer Genet Cytogenet*. 1997;94:36-43.
71. Liebisch P, Dohner H. Cytogenetics and molecular cytogenetics in multiple myeloma. *Eur J Cancer*. 2006;42:1520-1596.
72. Rasillo A, Tabernero MD, Sánchez ML, et al. Fluorescence in situ hybridization analysis of aneuploidization patterns in monoclonal gammopathy of undetermined significance versus multiple myeloma and plasma cell leukemia. *Cancer*. 2003;97:601-609.
73. Avery TP, Shah ND, Fu W, et al. Multiple myeloma and other plasma cell myeloma. In: Kantarjian HM, Wolff RA, Koller CA, eds. *The MD Anderson Manual of Medical Oncology*. 2nd ed. New York, NY: McGraw-Hill; 2011.
74. Bergsagel PL, Kuehl WM. Chromosome translocations in multiple myeloma. *Oncogene*. 2001;20:5611-5622.
75. Kaufmann H, Ackermann J, Baldia C, et al. Both IGH translocations and chromosome 13q deletions are early events in monoclonal gammopathy of undetermined significance and do not evolve during transition to multiple myeloma. *Leukemia*. 2004;18:1879-1882.
76. Fonseca R, Bergsagel PL, Drach J, et al. International Myeloma Working Group molecular classification of multiple myeloma: spotlight review. *Leukemia*. 2009;23:2210-2221.
77. Avet-Loiseau H, Li JY, Morineau N, et al. Monosomy 13 is associated with the transition of monoclonal gammopathy of undetermined significance to multiple myeloma. Intergroupe Francophone du Myelome. *Blood*. 1999;94:2583-2589.
78. Fonseca R, Oken MM, Harrington D, et al. Deletions of chromosome 13 in multiple myeloma identified by interphase FISH usually denote large deletions of the q arm or monosomy. *Leukemia*. 2001;15:981-986.
79. Sawyer JR. The prognostic significance of cytogenetics and molecular profiling in multiple myeloma. *Cancer Genet*. 2011;204:3-12.
80. Chiecchio L, Dagrada GP, White HE, et al. Frequent upregulation of MYC in plasma cell leukemia. *Genes Chromosomes Cancer*. 2009;48:624-636.
81. Chng WJ, Huang GF, Chung TH, et al. Clinical and biological implications of MYC activation: a common difference between MGUS and newly diagnosed multiple myeloma. *Leukemia*. 2011;25:1026-1035.
82. Chang H, Qi X, Jiang A, Xu W, Young T, Reece D. 1p21 deletions are strongly associated with 1q21 gains and are an independent adverse prognostic factor for the outcome of high-dose chemotherapy in patients with multiple myeloma. *Bone Marrow Transplant*. 2010;45:117-121.
83. Chang H, Ning Y, Qi X, Yeung J, Xu W. Chromosome 1p21 deletion is a novel prognostic marker in patients with multiple myeloma. *Br J Haematol*. 2007;139:51-54.
84. Nemec P, Zemanova Z, Greslikova H, et al. Gain of 1q21 is an unfavorable genetic prognostic factor for multiple myeloma patients treated with high-dose chemotherapy. *Biol Blood Marrow Transplant*. 2010;16:548-554.
85. Chang H, Trieu Y, Qi X, Jiang NN, Xu W, Reece D. Impact of cytogenetics in patients with relapsed or refractory multiple myeloma treated with bortezomib: adverse effect of 1q21 gains. *Leuk Res*. 2011;35:95-98.
86. Boyd KD, Ross FM, Tapper WJ, et al.; NCRI Haematology Oncology Studies Group. The clinical impact and molecular biology of del(17p) in multiple myeloma treated with conventional or thalidomide-based therapy. *Genes Chromosomes Cancer*. 2011;50:765-774.

87. Rajkumar SV. Multiple myeloma: 2011 update on diagnosis, risk-stratification, and management. *Am J Hematol.* 2011;86:57-65.
88. Lu G, Zhang XX, You J, Chen W. Assessment of bone marrow plasma cells by flow cytometric and fluorescence in situ hybridization evaluations in 244 cases of plasma cell neoplasms. *Int J Lab Hematol.* 2011;3:545-550.
89. Pozdnyakova O, Crowley-Larsen P, Zota V, Wang SA, Miron PM. Interphase FISH in plasma cell dyscrasia: increase in abnormality detection with plasma cell enrichment. *Cancer Genet Cytogenet.* 2009;189:112-117.
90. Hake CR, Graubert TA, Fenske TS. Does autologous transplantation directly increase the risk of secondary leukemia in lymphoma patients? *Bone Marrow Transplant.* 2007;39:59-70.
91. Sill H, Olipitz W, Zebisch A, Schulz E, Wölfler A. Therapy-related myeloid neoplasms: pathobiology and clinical characteristics. *Br J Pharmacol.* 2011;162:792-805.
92. Pedersen-Bjergaard J, Andersen MK, Andersen MT, Christiansen DH. Genetics of therapy-related myelodysplasia and acute myeloid leukemia. *Leukemia.* 2008;22:240-248.
93. Lu G. Clinical cytogenetic diagnosis of therapy-related acute myeloid leukemia. *Beijing Da Xue Xue Bao.* 2005;37:10-13.
94. Cooley LD, Mascarello JT, Hirsch B, et al.; Working Group of the American College of Medical Genetics (ACMG) Laboratory Quality Assurance Committee. Section E6.5 of the ACMG technical standards and guidelines: chromosome studies for solid tumor abnormalities. *Genet Med.* 2009;11:890-897.
95. Nakhleh RE, Grimm EE, Idowu MO, Souers RJ, Fitzgibbons PL. Laboratory compliance with the American Society of Clinical Oncology/College of American Pathologists guidelines for human epidermal growth factor receptor 2 testing: a College of American Pathologists survey of 757 laboratories. *Arch Pathol Lab Med.* 2010;134:728-734.
96. Liu J, Guzman MA, Pezanowski D, et al. FOXO1-FGFR1 fusion and amplification in a solid variant of alveolar rhabdomyosarcoma. *Mod Pathol.* 2011;24:1327-1335.
97. Downs-Kelly E, Shehata BM, López-Terrada D, et al. The utility of FOXO1 fluorescence in situ hybridization (FISH) in formalin-fixed paraffin-embedded specimens in the diagnosis of alveolar rhabdomyosarcoma. *Diagn Mol Pathol.* 2009;18:138-143.
98. Toomey EC, Schiffman JD, Lessnick SL. Recent advances in the molecular pathogenesis of Ewing's sarcoma. *Oncogene.* 2010;29(32):4504-4516.
99. Balamuth NJ, Womer RB. Ewing's sarcoma. *Lancet Oncol.* 2010;11:184-192.
100. Galanina N, Bossuyt V, Harris LN. Molecular predictors of response to therapy for breast cancer. *Cancer J.* 2011;17:96-103.
101. Baselga J. Treatment of HER2-overexpressing breast cancer. *Ann Oncol.* 2010;suppl 7:vii36-vii40.
102. Cantaloni C, Tonini R E, Eccher C, et al. Diagnostic value of automated Her2 evaluation in breast cancer: a study on 272 equivocal (score 2+) Her2 immunoreactive cases using an FDA approved system. *Appl Immunohistochem Mol Morphol.* 2011;19:306-312.
103. Albarello L, Pecciarini L, Doglioni C. HER2 testing in gastric cancer. *Adv Anat Pathol.* 2011;18:53-59.
104. Vecchione L, Jacobs B, Normanno N, Ciardiello F, Tejpar S. EGFR-targeted therapy. *Exp Cell Res.* 2011;317:2765-2771.
105. Mok TS. Personalized medicine in lung cancer: what we need to know. *Nat Rev Clin Oncol.* 2011;8:661-668.
106. Salgia R, Hensing T, Campbell N, et al. Personalized treatment of lung cancer. *Semin Oncol.* 2011;38:274-283.
107. Salgia R. Role of c-Met in cancer: emphasis on lung cancer. *Semin Oncol.* 2009;36(suppl 1):S52-S58.
108. Tiseo M, Gelsomino F, Bartolotti M, et al. Anaplastic lymphoma kinase as a new target for the treatment of non-small-cell lung cancer. *Expert Rev Anticancer Ther.* 2011;11:1677-1687.
109. Bergethon K, Shaw AT, Ou SH, et al. ROS1 rearrangements define a unique molecular class of lung cancers. *J Clin Oncol.* 2012:30:863-870.
110. Caraway NP, Khanna A, Fernandez RL, et al. Fluorescence in situ hybridization for detecting urothelial carcinoma: a clinicopathologic study. *Cancer Cytopathol.* 2010;118: 259-268.
111. Rodriguez S, Jafer O, Goker H, et al. Expression profile of genes from 12p in testicular germ cell tumors of adolescents and adults associated with i(12p) and amplification at 12p11.2-p12.1. *Oncogene.* 2003;22:1880-1891.
112. Gerami P, Zembowicz A. Update on fluorescence in situ hybridization in melanoma: state of the art. *Arch Pathol Lab Med.* 2011;135:830-837.
113. La Starza R, Specchia G, Cuneo A, et al. The hypereosinophilic syndrome: fluorescence in situ hybridization detects the del(4)(q12)-FIP1L1/PDGFRA but not genomic rearrangements of other tyrosine kinases. *Haematologica.* 2005;90:596-601.
114. Pardanani A, Brockman SR, Paternoster SF, et al. FIP1L1-PDGFRA fusion: prevalence and clinicopathologic correlates in 89 consecutive patients with moderate to severe eosinophilia. *Blood.* 2004;104:3038-3045.
115. Chin Lynda. The genetics of malignant melanoma: lessons from mouse and man. *Nat Rev Cancer.* August 2003;3(8): 559-570.
116. Heselmeyer K, Schröck E, du Manoir S, et al. Gain of chromosome 3q defines the transition from severe dysplasia to invasive carcinoma of the uterine cervix. *Proc Natl Acad Sci U S A.* 1996;93:479-484.
117. Andersson S, Sowjanya P, Wangsa D, et al. Detection of genomic amplification of the human telomerase gene TERC, a potential marker for triage of women with HPV-positive, abnormal Pap smears. *Am J Pathol.* 2009;175:1831-1847.
118. Wangsa D, Heselmeyer-Haddad K, Ried P, et al. Fluorescence in situ hybridization markers for prediction of cervical lymph node metastases. *Am J Pathol.* 2009;175:2637-2645.
119. Fleischmann A, Rotzer D, Seiler R, Studer UE, Thalmann GN. Her2 amplification is significantly more frequent in lymph node metastases from urothelial bladder cancer than in the primary tumours. *Eur Urol.* 2011;60:350-357.
120. Myo K, Uzawa N, Miyamoto R, Sonoda I, Yuki Y, Amagasa T. Cyclin D1 gene numerical aberration is a predictive marker for occult cervical lymph node metastasis in TNM Stage I and II squamous cell carcinoma of the oral cavity. *Cancer.* 2005;104:2709-2716.
121. Chung CC, Chanock SJ. Current status of genome-wide association studies in cancer. *Hum Genet.* 2011;130:59-78.

CHAPTER 16

DNA HYPERMETHYLATION IN CANCER

Bin Yang

INTRODUCTION

Genetics is the study of information inherited on the basis of DNA sequence. In contrast, epigenetics is the study of reversible changes in gene function that can be inherited and occur without any change in the DNA sequence. One example of an epigenetic change is DNA methylation, which can induce various gene expression patterns in a tissue-specific and developmental-stage-specific manner. DNA methylation occurs throughout the genome and involves the addition of a methyl group to the cytosine ring of a CpG dinucleotide. The methylation process is catalyzed by an enzyme called DNA methyltransferase (DNMT) and results in the formation of methyl cytosines. DNA methylation within a promoter region is associated with silencing of the affiliated gene. Methylation patterns are established during development and are normally maintained throughout the life of an individual. Thus, DNA methylation is a key regulator of gene transcription and genomic stability, and inappropriately altered DNA methylation patterns are frequently detected as epigenetic changes in human cancer. According to Knudson's two-hit theory of tumorigenesis,[1] disruption of the function of a tumor suppressor gene requires a complete loss of function of both copies of the involved gene. Chromosomal analysis has determined that the first hit often takes the form of a loss of heterozygosity. However, the mode of inactivation of the second allele is not always understood. Traditionally, it has been believed that the second hit can be carried out genetically by point mutations, that is, germline mutation in familial cancers or somatic mutation in non-inherited tumors. It has been debated for decades whether the initiation and progression of cancer can also be caused by epigenetic changes, such as DNA methylation, that are not caused by alterations in the primary DNA sequence.[2-5] Recent molecular studies have demonstrated that gene inactivation can, in fact, occur by aberrant DNA methylation.[6] It is now established that not only are epigenetic changes as frequent as genetic changes in cancers, but that both genetic and epigenetic processes are also intricately related to tumorigenesis.

EPIGENETIC CONTROL OF GENE EXPRESSION IN NORMAL CELLS

Epigenetics is defined as a heritable change in gene expression without an alteration in the DNA sequence. Among epigenetic changes, DNA methylation is the major alteration that takes place during aging, embryogenesis, and carcinogenesis. All cells in the body are descendants of a fertilized egg and in almost all cases contain the same set of genes. However, there is great diversity in normal cell types that carry out a variety of specific functions. These specific properties are, for the most part, determined by activating expression or repression of sets of genes by epigenetic controls. Such epigenetic events reprogram the cell's gene expression to control differentiation in normal development. Therefore, cell differentiation requires cell type–specific silencing of some genes and activation of others.

The major change that leads to gene silencing during embryogenesis and development is DNA methylation at CpG sites.[7] This form of methylation prevents the binding of transcription factors to CpG dinucleotides in gene promoter regions. In mammals, patterns of DNA methylation are species and tissue specific. Ablation of DNA methylation stops development (embryogenesis), activates apoptosis, and is usually lethal. Aberrant patterns of DNA methylations can result in malignant transformation of cells. One of the best examples of the tight control of gene expression through epigenetic mechanisms involving methylation-based gene silencing is the inactivation of the X chromosome in females. Recent studies also indicated that DNA methylation is a primary mechanism for silencing primordial germ cell genes in both germ cell and somatic cell lineages. In sum, epigenetic changes are responsible for X chromosome inactivation in females, chromatin structure stability, genome integrity, modulation of tissue-specific gene expression, embryonic development, and genomic imprinting.

The epigenetic methylation of DNA has other functions. It permanently silences the large amount of "junk" DNA, such as repetitive sequences, that has entered our genome throughout the course of evolution, mostly by viral transfection. It is estimated that 45% of the human genome consists of viral transposons, endogenous retroviruses, and repeat sequences that are capable of transpositions and that subsequently cause instability and inappropriate expression of local genes if not kept in check by strong silencing mechanisms. Epigenetic changes play critical roles in controlling host–viral interactions in several DNA virus infections. For example, latency versus episomal expression in Epstein-Barr virus infection is linked to several human neoplasms and is tightly controlled through host cell DNA methylation. Methylation in regulatory and L1 open reading frame regions in human papillomavirus (HPV)-16 and HPV-18 is implicated in promoting the switch from an episomal to an integrated state of HPV DNA in infected cervical epithelial cells. These are just a few of the many strategies that involve epigenetic regulation that have evolved for viral–host interaction.

DNA METHYLATION, CHROMATIN STRUCTURE, AND GENE EXPRESSION

DNA methylation, chromatin remodeling, and gene silencing are closely interconnected.[8,9] For example, early studies revealed that high levels of CpG methylation coincide with heterochromatic regions and that hypomethylation or demethylation is associated with euchromatin formation. In human cells, histones undergo many posttranslational modifications, such as methylation, phosphorylation, ubiquitination, and ribosylation. Among the histone modifications implicated in gene silencing, the best characterized to date are histone deacetylation and methylation of histone H3 at lysine 9. Aberrant epigenetic silencing of tumor suppressor genes by promoter DNA hypermethylation and histone deacetylation plays an important role in the pathogenesis of some cancers. It is increasingly clear that histone deacetylation and methylation of histone H3 at lysine 9 work hand in hand with DNA methylation to repress transcription. DNA hypermethylation is often coupled with histone deacetylation and unmethylated CpG island chromatin is enriched in hyperacetylated histones. Chromatin modification provides the other major epigenetic mechanism of gene silencing by rendering methylated promoter regions completely inaccessible for transcription.

The potential reversibility of epigenetic abnormalities has promoted the development of pharmacologic inhibitors of DNA methylation and histone deacetylation as possible anticancer therapeutics. Recent preclinical studies of DNMT and histone deacetylase inhibitors have yielded encouraging results, especially against hematologic malignancies.

DNA METHYLATION IN CANCER

DNA methylation, which has recently been investigated extensively, has been studied in various human diseases, including cancer, and the analysis of DNA methylation has detected useful biomarkers for diagnosing cancer, monitoring treatment effects, and predicting cancer prognosis.

Two Major Methylation Alterations in Cancer Cells

Although the underlying mechanisms are still largely unknown, recent studies have shown that two major changes in methylation status occur during carcinogenesis: regional promoter hypermethylation and genome-wide hypomethylation. The most studied alteration of DNA methylation in cancer is the aberrant hypermethylation of CpG islands surrounding promoter regions.[10] These methylation changes are critical to transcriptional silencing of the involved genes. DNA methylation of genes tends to occur primarily in promoter regions that contain CpG islands, defined as 1.0-kb stretches of DNA that contain the CpG sequence at a higher frequency than the rest of the genome. Methylation of CpG islands in the promoter region silences gene expression and is a normal event that regulates gene expression, particularly during embryogenesis. However, when aberrant DNA methylation of tumor suppressor genes occurs in tumors, it is implicated in neoplastic transformation. Although hypermethylation of the promoter regions of tumor suppressor genes is one of the hallmarks of cancer cells, genome-wide hypomethylation was recognized many years ago in tumors using methylation-sensitive restriction digestion and Southern blot analysis. Malignant cells may have 20% to 40% less methylation at CpG islands genome-wide than their normal counterparts. This form of hypomethylation mostly occurs at the coding regions and introns of genes.

Both decreases and increases in DNA methylation are a frequent characteristic of a wide variety of cancers. There is often more hypomethylation than hypermethylation of DNA during carcinogenesis, leading to a net decrease in the genomic 5-methylcytosine content. Although the exact methylation changes between different cancers of the same type are not the same, there are cancer type–specific differences in the frequency of hypermethylation or hypomethylation of certain genomic sequences. These opposite types of DNA methylation changes appear to be mostly independent of one another, although they may arise because of a similar abnormality, leading to long-lasting epigenetic instability in cancers. While the transcription-silencing role of DNA hypermethylation at promoters of many tumor suppressor genes is clear, the biological effects of cancer-linked hypomethylation of genomic DNA are less well understood. Evidence suggests that DNA hypomethylation functions in direct or indirect control of transcription and in destabilizing chromosomal integrity. Recent studies of cancer-linked DNA hypomethylation indicate that changes to DNA methylation during tumorigenesis and tumor progression have a previously underestimated plasticity and dynamic nature.

Multiple Gene Methylation Is a Hallmark of Cancer Cells

Genomic screening of 98 different primary human tumors has revealed that each tumor contains, on average, about 600 aberrantly methylated CpG islands out of approximately 45,000 CpG islands in the genome. Genes frequently mutated in cancers, such as p15, p16, and APC, can be silenced through promoter methylation as well, although many of the methylated CpG islands are present in genomic regions containing genes that have not yet been identified but may play an important role in tumorigenesis. To date, most studies have focused on aberrant CpG island methylation status in less than 100 relatively well-characterized candidate tumor suppressor genes in the most common human cancers, such as colon, lung, breast, and prostate cancers. These tumor suppressor genes are key elements involved in major signaling pathways, including but not limited to the p53, Wnt/β-catenin, pRb, AKT/PKB, JAK/STAT, and Ras/RAF/MAPK pathways. Aberrant methylation is also involved in regulating many cellular and biological functions, such as cell cycle control, genome stability, DNA repair, apoptosis, angiogenesis, invasion, and metastasis. Therefore, DNA promoter methylation can silence the expression of specific target genes and, in doing so, disrupt the fundamental pathways that are thought to lead to cancer. The current evidence suggests that concurrent methylation of multiple CpG islands is a hallmark of a vast majority, if not all, of human cancers. This epigenetic hallmark in cancer cells can be used as a potential molecular biomarker for the accurate detection of cancer cells in pathologic specimens.

Methylation in Cancer Is Tissue and Stage Specific

Aberrant DNA methylation has been demonstrated in almost all kinds of tumors, from epithelial carcinomas to mesenchymal sarcomas and from melanoma to hematopoietic malignancies. The aberrant methylation of genes that suppress tumorigenesis occurs early in tumor development and increases progressively, eventually contributing to the malignant phenotype.[11] On the basis of published DNA methylation profiles in various tumors, similar patterns of CpG island methylation are shared by different tumor types. However, methylation of CpG islands can be quantitatively different in individual tumors within a tumor type and may be non-random and tumor type and stage specific. Studies have clearly shown that late-stage cancers tend to harbor more aberrant methylation of CpG islands of candidate tumor suppressor genes compared with early tumor precursors. Consistent with the concept of multistep tumorigenesis, incremental accumulation of multiple epigenetic alterations has been observed during the progression from cancer precursors to late-stage frankly invasive cancer in many types of human cancers.

DNA Methylation and Cancer Classification

The most common clinical application for DNA methylation testing in colorectal cancer is as part of the workup of hereditary non-polyposis colorectal cancer (HNPCC, or Lynch syndrome). Tumors resulting from HNPCC can be distinguished from most cases of the microsatellite instability (MSI)–high (H) subset of sporadic colorectal cancers by the absence of methylation of the *MLH1* promoter, which characterizes most cases of sporadic MSI-H colorectal cancer. However, assessment of *MLH1* methylation by itself is probably not adequate to distinguish between all sporadic and all HNPCC-associated MSI-H cancers because methylation of *MLH1* can be seen as a "second hit" in individuals with a germline *MLH1* mutation. The CpG island methylator phenotype (CIMP), defined as widespread promoter CpG island methylation, has been established as a unique epigenetic phenotype in colorectal cancer. CIMP is correlated with *MLH1* methylation and is independent of MSI status. CIMP-positive colorectal tumors have a distinct clinical, pathologic, and molecular profile. Typically, they are associated with older age, right side ascending colon, female gender, poor differentiation, *BRAF* mutations, wild-type *p53*, Wnt/β-catenin pathway activation, and stable chromosomes. Particularly, CIMP status may help distinguish between sporadic and HNPCC-related tumors with MSI, because most sporadic MSI-H colon cancers exhibit CIMP, whereas most HNPCC-associated cancers do not. Determination of CIMP status may also be useful in evaluating the prognosis of colon cancer. A relationship between CIMP and the poor prognosis of microsatellite-stable (MSS) colon cancers has recently been reported.[12] It has also been shown that MSS tumors with *BRAF* mutations are usually heavily methylated. Therefore, it is possible that the relationship between worse prognosis and *BRAF* mutation is actually a relationship between poor prognosis and high levels of methylation (CIMP) in these colon cancers.

DNA Methylation and Tumor Progression

It has been demonstrated that epigenetic events are involved in initiation phase and early stage of tumorigenesis since promoter methylation has been frequently seen in precancer stage or cancer precursors in several human neoplasms.[13] The stepwise progression to esophageal adenocarcinoma involves an initial stage of intestinal metaplasia (Barrett esophagus) followed by low-grade and high-grade dysplasia and finally adenocarcinoma. A recent study of promoter methylation of 10 candidate genes (*HPP1*, *RUNX3*, *RIZ1*, *CRBP1*, *3-OST-2*, *APC*, *TIMP3*, *P16*, *MGMT*, *P14*) using methylation-specific polymerase chain reaction (MSP) revealed that hypermethylation of *P16*, *RUNX3*, and *HPP1* in Barrett esophagus or low-grade dysplasia may represent independent risk factors for further progression to high-grade dysplasia or adenocarcinoma.[14]

The progression from cervical intraepithelial neoplasia to invasive squamous cell carcinoma requires additional genetic and epigenetic alterations that have not been characterized fully. This morphologically well-characterized progressive model of cervical tumorigenesis provides a great platform in studying epigenetic alterations at the early stage of malignant transformation. A recent study examined aberrant promoter methylation of 15 tumor suppressor genes using a multiplex, nested-MSP approach in 11 high-grade squamous intraepithelial lesions (HSILs), 17 low-grade squamous intraepithelial lesions (LSILs), and 11 normal cervical tissues from liquid-based cervical cytology samples.[15] Aberrant promoter methylation of *DAPK1* and *CADM1* (IGSF4) occurred at a high frequency in HSILs and was absent in LSILs and normal cervix. DNA methylation profiling will likely add a new dimension to the application of molecular biomarkers for the prediction of disease progression and for risk assessment in cervical squamous lesions.

DNA Methylation Profiling as a Biomarker in Cancer Detection

As stated earlier, methylation of multiple candidate tumor suppressor genes is a hallmark of cancer cells in comparison with their normal counterparts. Thus, molecular changes associated with epigenetic gene silencing may serve as potential markers for risk assessment, early diagnosis, and prognostication. Molecular signatures of cancer cells can be used to improve cancer detection and the assessment of cancer risk. Hypermethylation of the promoter region of cancer-related genes provides some of the most promising markers for cancer diagnosis. DNA-based markers have advantages because of the inherent stability of DNA compared with RNA and some proteins. Also, the constant patterns of abnormal CpG island methylation at the promoter region in genes of interest allow a simpler detection strategy than is possible for many of the common mutations in cancer. Such mutations, even for the same tumor type, can differ widely from patient to patient in their position within the gene. In contrast, for any given gene, a single assay for the detection of promoter methylation abnormalities will work in virtually all patients and all types of cancers. Another possible advantage to the use of hypermethylation as a marker for cancer diagnosis is the evidence from recent studies indicating that specific methylation profiles exist in different types of cancer. Utilizing specific methylation profiles will be helpful in differentiating one cancer type from another, particularly in certain clinical settings, such as the differential diagnosis of whether a liver nodule is a primary tumor or a metastatic lesion. Finally, although methylation of individual tumor suppressor genes occasionally can be seen in benign processes, methylation of multiple tumor suppressor genes is a hallmark in malignant neoplasms. Therefore, concurrent methylation of a panel of candidate tumor suppressor genes can be applied as surrogate biomarkers in the detection of malignancy in clinical samples.

Aberrant CpG island methylation has been used as a molecular tool for the detection of cancer cells in a variety of tissue and cytologic samples. Liquid-based cytology samples, such as body fluids and fine needle aspiration biopsy (FNAB) samples, provide excellent materials for PCR-based methylation assays because cells are not fixed in formalin. A recent study demonstrated that MSP detected aberrant promoter methylation in the sputum of patients with lung cancer up to 3 years before clinicopathological detection of tumors in smokers. Similar approaches have also been applied to bronchial and breast ductal lavage, cervical smears, urine, peritoneal washings, and FNAB specimens. In some patients, dying tumor cells can release fragments of genomic DNA, which can be used as biomarkers for the diagnosis of cancer. Using MSP, it is possible to detect methylated genes released from tumors in the serum of patients. In some studies, there has been a very good correlation between the detection of the methylated gene in serum and the methylation of the identical gene in the primary tumor. This approach has the potential to be used for early diagnosis of cancer and to monitor response to chemotherapy.

Because of its often occult location, cholangiocarcinoma's early detection is paramount in improving clinical management and the patient's survival. Yang et al. have shown that MSP analysis of the promoter methylation of a panel of CpG islands is a sensitive and accurate method in detection of cholangiocarcinoma in cytologic specimens. Using a panel of 12 tumor suppressor genes, they reported that DNA methylation profiles accurately differentiated malignant cells from reactive cells in biliary brushings.[16] Similarly, Watanabe et al. found that aberrant methylation of *SFRP1* (SARP2) occurred in 79% of pancreatic carcinomas and 56% of malignant intraductal papillary mucinous neoplasms but was rarely seen in pancreatic specimens from patients with chronic pancreatitis and from healthy controls.[17] Hypermethylation of *SFRP1* in pancreatic juice thus may be a highly sensitive and useful marker in differentiating pancreatic carcinoma from chronic pancreatitis.

DNA Methylation as a Target for Cancer Chemoprevention and Treatment

The fundamental difference between genetic alterations and epigenetic changes is that the former are irreversible and the latter are potentially reversible. The potential reversibility of epigenetic changes in neoplasia presents new opportunities for the clinical treatment of cancer. This fact has drawn great attention from clinicians and pharmaceutical professionals searching for agents that can reverse abnormal DNA methylation and inhibit DNA hypermethylation as potential tumor therapies. The potent and specific inhibitor of DNA methylation decitabine reactivates most of the silenced tumor suppressor genes in cancer cells. This result provides the rationale for further investigation into the potential of this demethylating agent as a cancer treatment. Because it is unlikely that a single agent has the potential to cure malignant disease because of the rapid development of drug resistance to single-drug therapy, the interaction of decitabine with other agents that enhance its antineoplastic activity is also being investigated. The discovery of the "cross-talk" between DNA methylation and chromatin remodeling pathways has also provided a novel opportunity for therapeutic intervention. Gene silencing by aberrant methylation and histone deacetylation can be reversed by combining DNA methylation and histone acetylation inhibitors. An alternative approach would be to inhibit DNA methylation by targeting DNMT. Inhibition of the function of DNMT1 and DNMT3b using small interfering RNAs dramatically enhanced the chemosensitivity of ovarian cancer cells to cisplatin-based chemotherapy. It seems certain that ongoing analyses of epigenetic changes in cancers will play an important role not only in early detection of cancer but also in refining therapeutic strategies and in monitoring chemotherapeutic responses.

DNA Methylation as a Prognostic or Predictive Biomarker

Another potential application of the assessment of CpG island hypermethylation involves using the function of the silenced genes to gauge prognosis. Glioblastoma is the most common brain tumor and is notoriously chemoresistant. Recent epigenetic studies have identified a marker that seems to strongly predict a patient's tumor chemosensitivity. Alkylating agents, such as temozolomide, are the primary form of glioblastoma chemotherapy and injure DNA, which results in apoptotic cell death. O^6-methylguanine–DNA methyltransferase (MGMT) is an enzyme that can repair the DNA damage caused by this agent. Methylation of the promoter of *MGMT* turns off transcription of the gene, reducing the intracellular level of MGMT and thereby inhibiting the repair mechanism. In principle, therefore, interference with MGMT should enhance the antitumor effect of alkylating agents. Investigators have found that the prognosis is better for patients who have tumors in which there is methylation of the *MGMT* promoter than for patients who have tumors without methylation at this locus.[18] Furthermore, almost all of the benefit of adding temozolomide to radiotherapy occurs within subgroups of patients who have this promoter methylated. Therefore, detection of *MGMT* promoter methylation in biopsy samples from glioblastoma patients may be a useful epigenetic tool for predicting a patient's sensitivity to alkylating agents such as temozolomide. Similar studies have been carried out in other cancers. For instance, loss of BRCA1 protein expression, either by mutation or by BRCA1 promoter methylation, is associated with increased platinum-based chemosensitivity and favorable overall survival after complete resection of sporadic ovarian cancer.[19] Methylation of RASSF1A promoter is frequently seen in many cancers including lung cancer. It has been shown that patients with non–small cell carcinoma who harbor methylation of RASSF1A promoter have twice much longer survival than those without RASSF1a methylation (34 months vs. 13 months) treated with gemcitabine.[20] Although these studies provide exciting hope for clinical utility of epigenetic biomarkers in the prediction of chemosensitivity and

TABLE 16–1 Epigenetic Changes Differ from Genetic Alterations

Epigenetic Control in Normal Cells
- involved in embryonic development and cell differentiation
- involved in genomic imprinting
- involved in inactivation of X chromosome in female
- involved in silencing of intragenomic parasitic DNA elements, such as transposons
DNA Methylation, Histone Deacetylation, and Chromatin Structure
- *Euchromatin* state often associates with DNA promoter hypomethylation, histone acetylation, and activation of genes
- *Heterochromatin* state frequently associates with DNA promoter hypermethylation, histone deacetylation, and silencing of genes
Difference between Epigenetics and Genetics
- *Genetics* studies the makeup of nucleic acids and the alteration of DNA sequence, such as point mutation and deletion. *Epigenetics* studies the function and modifications that are "above and beyond" the DNA sequence, such as DNA methylation, histone acetylation, and microRNA
- Both genetic and epigenetic changes are inheritable
- Genetic alterations, such as mutation and deletion, are often irreversible, whereas epigenetic change is usually *reversible*

TABLE 16-2 Epigenetic Alterations in Cancer and Other Human Disorders

Epigenetic Changes in Cancer Cells
- Hypermethylation of DNA promoter regions of a set of genes, mostly candidate tumor suppressor genes, is the hallmark of tumorigenesis
- Genome-wide hypomethylation, mainly at the coding sequences and repetitive introns
- DNA methylation is closely linked to chromatin structure and histone deacetylation
- DNA methylation is linked to microRNA changes
Clinical Significance of Detection of DNA Methylation Profiling in Cancer Cells
- Biomarkers for risk assessment of development of diseases
- Biomarkers for early detection of cancer cells and its precursors
- Molecular reclassification of neoplasm based on combined genetic and epigenetic alterations
- Biomarkers for chemosensitivity and chemoresistance
- Epigenetic-based pharmacogenomics to demethylate target genes and reverse tumor phenotype
- Prognostic indicator for surveillance of cancer treatment and monitoring recurrence

prognosis, larger studies must be performed to determine the clinical applicability of such findings, but the results suggest that the relatively easy and rapid detection of hypermethylated CpG islands of specific genes may prove to be clinically valuable.

SUMMARY

Epigenetic changes occur frequently during tumor development. The major change is aberrant DNA methylation, which typically silences the expression of genes that suppress tumorigenesis. Aberrant DNA methylation profiling is a promising ancillary molecular tool in the early and accurate detection of cancer cells in clinical samples. In addition, aberrant DNA methylation profiling may be a useful molecular biomarker in predicting the chemoresponsiveness or prognosis of patients with cancer. Finally, epigenetic changes are potential targets for therapeutic intervention using inhibitors of DNA methylation.

REFERENCES

1. Knudson AG Jr. The genetic predisposition to cancer. *Birth Defects Orig Artic Ser*. 1989;25:15-27.
2. Feinberg AP, Vogelstein B. Hypomethylation distinguishes genes of some human cancers from their normal counterparts. *Nature*. 1983;301:89-92.
3. Jones PA, Baylin SB. The fundamental role of epigenetic events in cancer. *Nat Rev Genet*. 2002;3:415-428.
4. Baylin SB, Herman JG. DNA hypermethylation in tumorigenesis: epigenetics joins genetics. *Trends Genet*. 2000;16:168-174.
5. Costello JF, Fruhwald MC, Smiraglia DJ, et al. Aberrant CpG-island methylation has non-random and tumour-type-specific patterns. *Nat Genet*. 2000;24:132-138.
6. Herman JG, Graff JR, Myohanen S, Nelkin BD, Baylin SB. Methylation-specific PCR: a novel PCR assay for methylation status of CpG islands. *Proc Natl Acad Sci U S A*. 1996;93:9821-9826.
7. Yang B, Guo M, Herman JG, Clark DP. Aberrant promoter methylation profiles of tumor suppressor genes in hepatocellular carcinoma. *Am J Pathol*. 2003;163:1101-1107.
8. Evron E, Dooley WC, Umbricht CB, et al. Detection of breast cancer cells in ductal lavage fluid by methylation-specific PCR. *Lancet*. 2001;357:1335-1336.
9. Esteller M, Sanchez-Cespedes M, Rosell R, Sidransky D, Baylin SB, Herman JG. Detection of aberrant promoter hypermethylation of tumor suppressor genes in serum DNA from non-small cell lung cancer patients. *Cancer Res*. 1999;59:67-70.
10. Erhlich M. Cancer-linked DNA hypomethylation and its relationship to DNA hypermethylation. *Curr Top Microbiol Immunol*. 2006;310:251-274.
11. De Bustos C, Ramos E, Young JM, et al. Tissue-specific variation in DNA methylation levels along human chromosome 1. *Epigenetics Chromatin*. 2009;2:7.
12. Issa J-P. Colon cancer: it's CIN or CIMP. *Clin Cancer Res*. 2008;14:5939.
13. Kaz AM, Wong CJ, Luo Y, et al. DNA methylation profiling in Barrett's esophagus and esophageal adenocarcinoma reveals unique methylation signatures and molecular subclasses. *Epigenetics*. 2011;6:1403-1412.
14. Schulmann K, Sterian A, Berki A, et al. Inactivation of p16, RUNX3, and HPP1 occurs early in Barrett's-associated neoplastic progression and predicts progression risk. *Oncogene*. 2005;24:4138-4148.
15. Gustafson KS, Furth EE, Heitjan DF, Fansler ZB, Clark DP. DNA methylation profiling of cervical squamous intraepithelial lesions using liquid-based cytology specimens: an approach that utilizes receiver-operating characteristic analysis. *Cancer*. 2004;102(4):259-268.
16. Yang B, House MG, Guo M, Herman JG, Clark DP. Promoter methylation profiles of tumor suppressor genes in intrahepatic and extrahepatic cholangiocarcinoma. *Mod Pathol*. 2005;18(3):412-420.
17. Watanabe H, Okada G, Ohtsubo K, et al. Aberrant methylation of secreted apoptosis-related protein 2 (SARP2) in pure pancreatic juice in diagnosis of pancreatic neoplasms. *Pancreas*. 2006;32(4):382-389.
18. Hegi ME, Diserens AC, Gorlia T, et al. MGMT gene silencing and benefit from temozolomide in glioblastoma. *N Engl J Med*. 2005;352(10):997-1003.
19. Swisher EM, Gonzalez RM, Taniguchi T, et al. Methylation and protein expression of DNA repair genes: association with chemotherapy exposure and survival in sporadic ovarian and peritoneal carcinomas. *Mol Cancer*. 2009;8:48.
20. Fischer JR, Ohnmacht U, Rieger N, et al. Prognostic significance of RASSF1A promoter methylation on survival of non-small cell lung cancer patients treated with gemcitabine. *Lung Cancer*. 2007;56(1):115-123.

CHAPTER 17

SINGLE NUCLEOTIDE POLYMORPHISMS

Qingyi Wei

INTRODUCTION

In the long journey of evolution, organisms develop and grow into a variety of species by changing their genetic makeup in response to constant environmental pressure. One of the important genetic changes in this great adaptation to the daunting war between the organisms and the environment is single nucleotide polymorphism (SNP) (http://www.ncbi.nlm.nih.gov/projects/SNP/) that exists in all living organisms, including humans. Today, the amount of information about genetic variation in humans has been exploding, thanks to the Human Genome Project (http://www.ornl.gov/sci/techresources/Human_Genome/home.shtml), which has identified approximately 20,000 to 25,000 genes in the human genome. This has led to subsequent efforts such as the Environmental Genome Project (http://www.niehs.nih.gov/research/supported/programs/egp/), the HapMap project (http://hapmap.ncbi.nlm.nih.gov/), the 1000 Genome Project (http://www.1000genomes.org/), and several other unique or derived online databases. Currently, many other online tools also provide us an easy access to such huge data resources for ongoing and future research.

TYPES OF SNPs

SNP is a detectable and heritable variation in the DNA sequence in the form of a single nucleotide (i.e., A, T, C, or G) that is located anywhere in the genome sequence in every cell. Therefore, by definition, a given SNP leads to different genotypes, three genotypes to be more exact, among individuals or a given population. Relative to a germline mutation, which can also occur very soon after fertilization of the germ cells and is often rare (minor allele frequency [MAF] < 1%) but often functional with a known phenotype or a disease manifestation, an SNP is relatively common, occurring in at least 1% of the general population. Such a genetic variation in the form of SNPs accounts for about 90% of all human genetic variations, equivalent to every 100 to 300 bases along the three-billion-base human genome (http://www.ornl.gov/sci/techresources/Human_Genome/home.shtml). Based on the locations and functional relevance of a change in the nucleotides of the genome, SNPs have been categorized into several types for the purpose of clarity in research or their roles in the development of diseases. For effective, scientific communication that helps identify the same SNP in publications, each of the SNPs has been given a unique reference SNP ID number (rs#), when it was first discovered and reported to the databases for archiving SNPs.

The types of SNP include, but are not limited to, coding and non-coding SNPs, according to their physical locations in the coding (including non-synonymous sites) and non-coding regions (or untranslated region, UTR) of the gene, respectively; non-synonymous and synonymous SNPs, depending on whether a change of the nucleotide in DNA causing a change in RNA codon may or may not lead to a change in the amino acid of the protein, respectively; and tagging and non-tagging SNPs, when they are selected based on their linkage disequilibrium (LD, at least $r^2 > 0.8$) with other SNPs to maximize genotyping efficiency. For example, a well-known SNP in the *TP53* 72 codon SNP (rs1042522) is a coding or non-synonymous SNP of the human p53 tumor suppressor gene, because it causes a G or C residue change (c.7579472G>C) at a position that leads to either an amino acid arginine (CGC) or proline (CCC) at the 72 codon (Arg72Pro). The *TP53* 72 codon SNP is not a tagging SNP, however, because it is not in high LD with other SNPs in the same gene, as specified by the HapMap database (http://hapmap.ncbi.nlm.nih.gov/) and detected by SNPInfo (http://www.

niehs.nih.gov/snpinfo). More definition of an SNP can be found at http://www.dnabaser.com/articles/SNP/SNP-single-nucleotide-polymorphism.html.

SIGNIFICANCE OF SNPs

It was initially estimated that there were more than 10 million SNPs in the human genome (http://www.ornl.gov/sci/techresources/Human_Genome/project/about.shtml), some of which can be common or rare, that have determined various phenotypes, including height, weight, hair color, eye color, and skin color. More importantly, these SNPs may be responsible for various degrees of response to environmental exposure and medical treatment, which would have a great impact on disease course and life expectancy in humans. However, the scale and the complexity of SNPs in humans and their potential in disease diagnosis, treatment, and prevention were not fully understood and appreciated until the completion of the Human Genome Project. When the common disease–common variant hypothesis[1] was popular among scientists and SNP chips were invented so that one can interrogate the genotypes of up to millions of SNPs, investigators started to concentrate their research efforts in performing genome-wide association studies (GWASs) on various diseases,[2] including cancer, wherein common disease-causing alleles or variants are expected to be identified and also used to identify populations at high risk for developing diseases.[3] As of June 2011, 1,449 genome-wide associations have been identified for common variants in studies of 237 traits at $P \leq 5 \times 10^{-8}$ (http://www.genome.gov/multimedia/illustrations/GWAS_2011_2.pdf). Based on these data, the strength of the associations with an odds ratio of >2 is likely for those SNPs that are potentially functional, if they are located in non-synonymous sites, promoters (1 or 5 kb), 5′-UTRs, or 3′-UTRs.[4] However, GWASs have missed many unknown rare variants that are mostly likely to be functional. It appears possible that such rare variants will be identified for these traits in the years to come, as the direct sequencing efforts become increasingly affordable and popular.[5]

SNP DATABASE

The Human Genome Project reveals that SNPs are the most common genetic variations in the genome, which occur about once every 1,200 bp.[6] Thus, there are more than 10 millions of SNPs in the human genome, and this number could be increased to more than 15 million when the 1000 Genome Project is completed.[7] In the meantime, GWAS has identified thousands of disease susceptibility loci, and many remain to be identified in the upcoming direct sequencing studies, which are potential targets for disease prevention in personalized risk assessment and for treatment in personalized medicine. The challenge is to continuously identify the unreported disease-causing SNPs for additional studies on risk of developing human diseases. Compilation of SNP information is very important for post-GWAS association and genetic studies, population genetics and bioinformatics studies, and evolutionary and systems biology research as well as for positional cloning and physical mapping projects.

Several SNP databases have been developed, including the dbSNP database from the National Center for Biotechnology Information (NCBI) (http://www.ncbi.nlm.nih.gov/projects/SNP/), the SNPedia database from a hybrid organization (http://www.snpedia.com/index.php/SNPedia), the OMIM database for the association between polymorphisms and diseases (http://www.ncbi.nlm.nih.gov/omim), the Human Gene Mutation Database that provides gene mutations causing or associated with human inherited diseases and functional SNPs (http://www.hgmd.org/), and GWAS Central (http://www.gwascentral.org/index), a database for the integration and comparative interrogation of GWAS datasets. The dbSNP database is the most frequently used, many SNPs of which have been validated in the HapMap database in the form of SNP frequencies, genotypes, and haplotypes (Fig. 17.1) that can be accessed from the widely used Haploview program.[8] The HapMap also contains a genome browser for finding the SNPs of interest within the database. SNPInfo is a web-based SNP selection tool, by which investigators can specify genes or linkage regions and select SNPs for further functional validation based on GWAS results, LD, and predicted functional characteristics of both coding and non-coding SNPs.[9]

METHODS OF DETECTING SNP GENOTYPES

Several genotyping methods are available, including either low throughput with polymerase chain reaction (PCR)–based assays using manually designed primers or high throughput using commercially available service with the most updated genotyping platforms. For good and efficient PCR-based genotyping assays, the good quality of the DNA is key to success. Genomic DNA is preferred in performing PCR-based genotyping assay, mostly extracted from the blood samples by using blood DNA mini kits. Before performing genotyping assay, the DNA purity and concentration should be determined by spectrophotometer measurement of absorbance at 260 and 280 nm and stored at −20°C until used. The following are some often used genotyping methods in interrogating an individual genotype.

PCR–Single-Strand Conformation Polymorphism

The single-strand conformation polymorphism (SSCP) method detects some conformational difference of single-stranded nucleotide sequences of identical length as induced by differences in the sequences harboring an SNP or mutation. This method can distinguish the sequences by means of gel electrophoresis that separates the different conformations of the DNA molecules as a result of having or not having a particular SNP or mutation.[10] This method

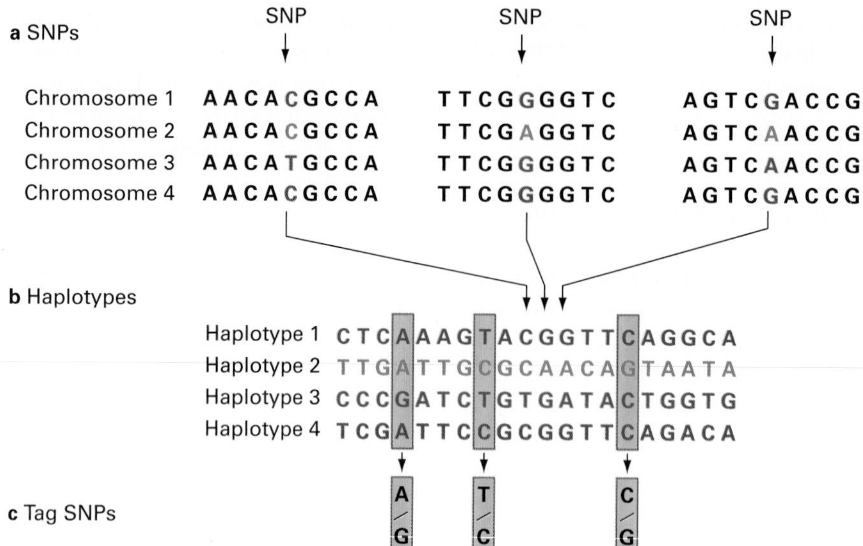

FIGURE 17–1 Construction of haplotypes by the known single nucleotide polymorphisms (SNPs) and corresponding tagSNPs (http://hapmap.ncbi.nlm.nih.gov/whatishapmap.html).

was often used in the early days of mutation research, in which the main purpose was to identify novel mutations. Later on, when SNPs became a focus of research, the SSCP method was also often used in association studies to detect known SNPs that did not have a restriction site suitable for the PCR-restriction fragment length polymorphism (RFLP). For example, the *CCND1* has a splicing polymorphism (rs9344) at nucleotide 870 (870G>A), codon 242, in exon 4, which was not matched with any available restriction enzyme in the sequence. By using the primers 5′-TACTACCGCCTCACACGCTTCC-3′ (sense) and 5′-TTGGCACCAGCCTCGGCATTTC-3′ (antisense), the PCR products contain a 138-bp fragment. These fragments can be amplified in PCR mixture, and the PCRs can be performed by incubating the fragments and reaction mixture. For SSCP analysis, the PCR mixture is loaded on a mutation detection enhancement gel for electrophoresis. After electrophoresis, the gels are dried and imaged by exposure to X-ray film. The band shift patterns were visualized by autoradiography. Based on these band shift patterns, subjects are divided into groups for the three *CCND1* genotypes, GG, GA, and AA.[11] This method works for the known SNPs to be genotyped in a low-throughput manner, whose sequences do not contain a restriction site, although it is also good for detecting unknown variants or mutations in the DNA fragments of interest.

PCR–Restriction Fragment Length Polymorphism

Because a recognized restriction site in a DNA fragment can be detected by a corresponding restriction enzyme, such a restriction enzyme can be used to distinguish the polymorphic site.[12] This is the most popular genotyping method used in association studies at a time when SNPs were discovered and regarded as important risk factors for cancer. This is particularly true when the Human Genome Project has discovered millions of SNPs that had never been reported before. Here is an example to illustrate the use of the PCR-RFLP method in an association study. For example, the *TNFAIP2* rs8126 T>C polymorphism contains a sequence change that can be recognized by the restriction enzyme *Apa*I. Therefore, the following sequences of the primers can be used in the genotyping assay: 5′-GGGGCCGGCTCTCTTGGGCC-3′ and 5′-CACACGTACAAAGACCTTGGGCATCC-3′. These primers generated PCR products of 105 and 108 bp that can be digested by a restriction enzyme *Apa*I to identify genotypes for the rs8126 T>C. For validation, which is often necessary, particularly when an artificial mutation is introduced to create a restriction site, the genotypes of rs8126 T>C can also be confirmed by direct sequencing.[13] This method only works well for the known SNPs to be genotyped in a low-throughput manner, whose sequences do contain a restriction site. However, this method could not be used to detect unknown variants or mutations in the DNA fragments of interest as the SSCP does.

TaqMan Assay

The TaqMan assays are provided by Applied Biosystems (ABI) with in-house designed probes that consist of a fluorophore covalently attached to the 5′-end of the oligonucleotide probe and a quencher at the 3′-end. With an ABI PRISM 7700 Sequence Detection System, this PCR-based assay is performed with laser scanning technology. The mechanism of this assay system is to excite fluorescent dyes present in the specially designed TaqMan probes using several different fluorophores (e.g., 6-carboxyfluorescein, acronym: FAM, or tetrachlorofluorescein, acronym: TET) and quenchers (e.g., tetramethylrhodamine, acronym: TAMRA, or dihydrocyclopyrroloindole tripeptide minor groove binder, acronym: MGB). The system includes a built-in thermal cycler, a laser to induce fluorescence, a CCD (charge-coupled device) detector, real-time sequence detection software, and TaqMan reagents for the fluorogenic 5′ nuclease assay. The cycle-by-cycle detection of the increase in the amount of PCR product is quantified in real time as the special probes, "reporter dye," fluoresces, when the "quencher" is removed from the fragment during the PCR extension cycle.[14]

This method is quite robust for the known SNPs to be genotyped in a median-throughput manner but not good for unknown variants in the DNA fragments of interest. This method is very effective and reliable for validating the top-hit SNPs identified in GWAS.

SNPlex

SNPlex is a platform for SNP genotyping developed and provided also by ABI. Using capillary electrophoresis, this assay can be performed on ABI's popular 3730xl DNA analyzers, in which up to 48 SNPs by design can be genotyped in a single reaction after a successful design from submitted SNPs from customers.[15] In this assay, the design rate is critical for the users who apply the assay of the sets of SNPs they selected for their studies (Fig. 17.2). Briefly, the design of a panel of SNP sets for SNPlex is a paid service from ABI, in which the design rate is critical for the customized panel, relying much on the sequences around the SNP. In general, the SNPlex assay for SNP sets containing TaqMan assay–validated SNPs has a satisfying design rate, often >90%. However, the successful rate of calling the genotypes can be influenced by the quality of DNA. Usually, genotype calling fails for the following reasons[15]: (i) the SNP may be within a repeat sequence found many times in the genome; (ii) the SNP sequence may contain a second SNP near the first; and (iii) the SNP context sequence may contain one or more sequences of low complexity. For customer-supplied SNP sets containing confirmed dbSNPs, according to the company, the design rate is usually between 80% and 85%. The most common causes of failed assay designs are multiple genome hits and nucleotide compositions that conflict with the assay design rules, and another factor negatively impacting the design rate is a low number of submitted SNPs.[15] Therefore, SNPlex, although economical by design, did not always fit the needs of the investigators, because some selected SNPs may or may not be able to be included in the panel of the assays, and once included in the panel, not all SNPs will have a genotyping calling, which often needs to be made up by other genotyping methods, including the TaqMan assays.

GoldenGate

The Illumina GoldenGate genotyping assay is another median-throughput genotyping platform, a paid service provided by Illumina, Inc. This assay is a flexible, preoptimized assay, using a discriminatory DNA polymerase and ligase to interrogate the genotypes. In general, this assay can detect 96, or from 384 to 3,072 SNP loci simultaneously (Fig. 17.3). According to the company's web site introduction (http://www.illumina.com/technology/goldengate_genotyping_assay.ilmn), the protocol can be performed manually or can be easily automated with LIMS and the AutoLoader 2, in which a streamlined workflow allows a single technician to generate over 300,000 genotypes in just six hands-on hours. This assay utilizes the iScan system or BeadArray Reader with standard panels for humans and mice, and in addition, its custom panels

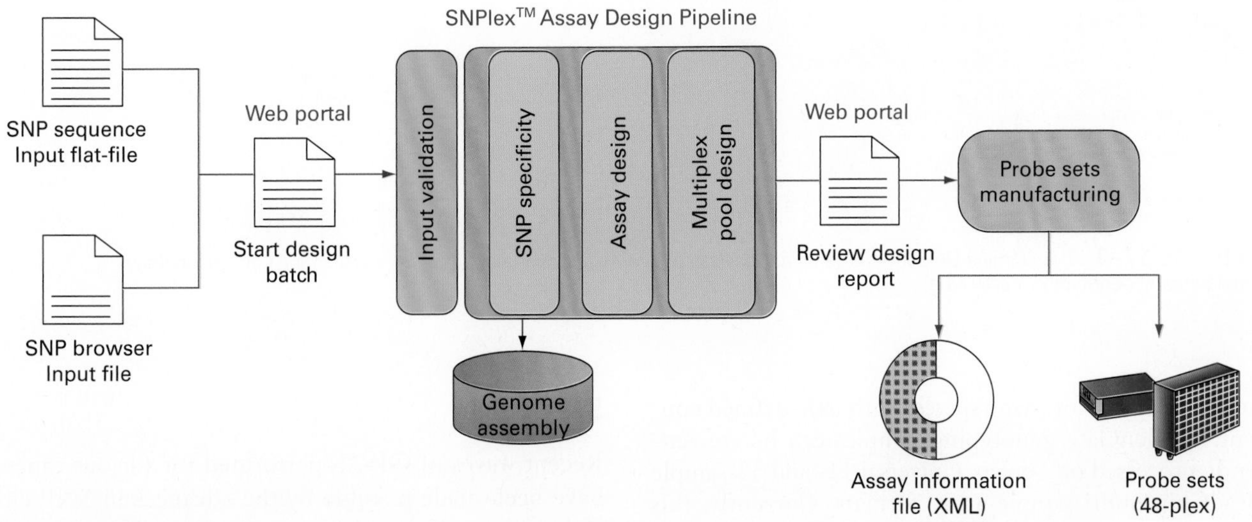

FIGURE 17–2 User-defined SNPlex system assays are designed by means of a proprietary assay design pipeline, which can be accessed through the Applied Biosystems' web site.[15]

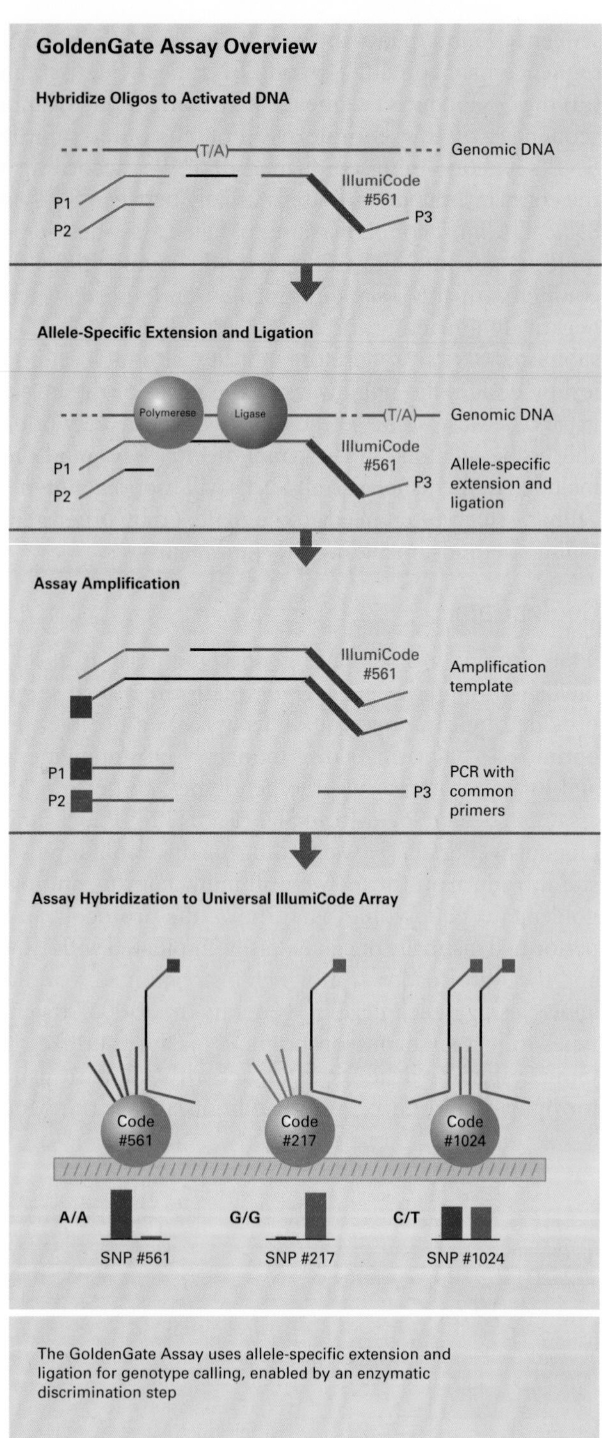

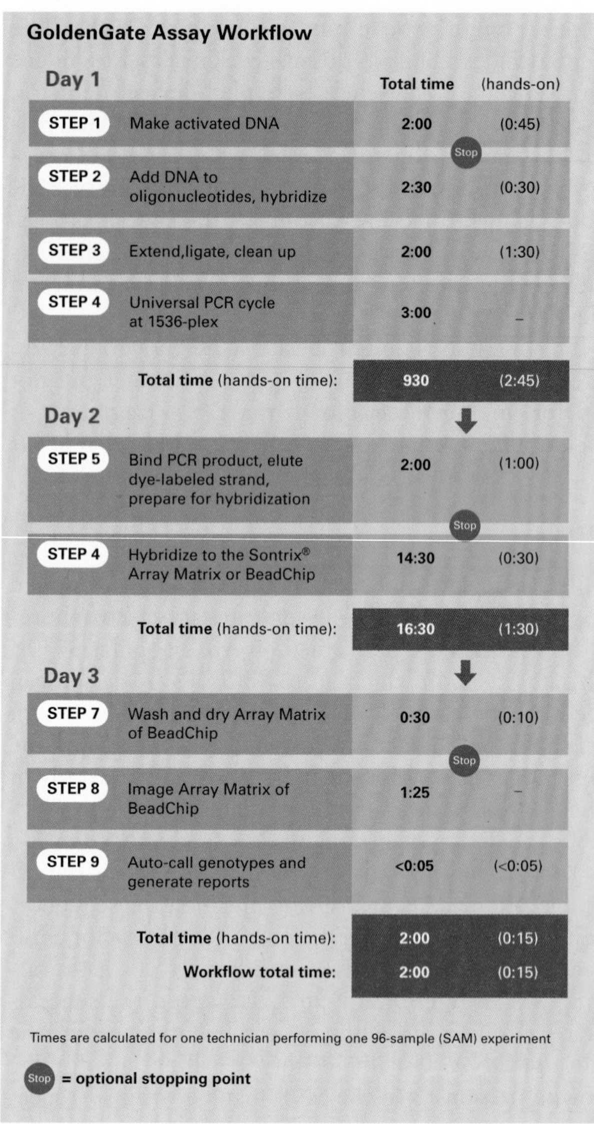

FIGURE 17–3 The Illumina GoldenGate genotyping assay overview and workflow (http://www.illumina.com/technology/goldengate_genotyping_assay.ilmn).

can be designed for many species with user-defined content. GoldenGate genotyping samples can be conveniently processed on Sentrix Universal 12- and 32-sample BeadChip multi-sample array formats. Currently, this platform is ideal for post-GWAS replications up to 3,072 SNP loci for validation for the top-hit SNPs identified in GWAS.

SNP Chips

Recent waves of GWAS performed for various cancers have been made possible by the advances in SNP chip technologies. Two major companies have dominated the market: Illumina and Affymetrix. Starting from an early 100K chip up to that of 4.3 million markers, Illumina has made a great progress in SNP chip invention and application to GWAS. The genotyping is processed by the iScan system that is a cutting-edge, dedicated array scanner. The latest Illumina Omni5 chip (http://www.illumina.com/applications/gwas.ilmn) contains 4.3 million markers, with room for an additional 500,000 markers to be added by the customers (Fig. 17.4). This chip uses SNPs with MAF > 1.0 selected from the 1000 Genomes Project with population coverage percentage of variation capture ($r^2 > 0.8$) of 87% for Caucasians, 77% for Asians, and 56% for Yorubans. In contrast, the most current and popular chip made by Affymetrix is SNP Array 6.0, which contains 1,852,426 markers, including 906,600 SNPs and 945,826 copy number variations (CNVs), using the GenoChip Scanner 3000 for processing and genotyping.

By design, the chips used in GWAS only help investigate the common (MAF > 0.10) SNPs in association with diseases, including cancer. Since 2005, GWAS reports in major journals have been sharply increasing, having identified 1,449 significant (at $P < 5 \times 10^8$) loci for 237 traits (Fig. 17.5). However, disease association with rare SNPs or other single nucleotide variants (SNVs), such as insertions and deletions, will have to rely on direct sequencing of the whole genome.

Whole-Genome Sequencing

The next-generation sequencing technologies have been much advanced to provide the promise of sequencing the whole genome at an affordable price, although currently exomic sequencing is more popular because of the affordable price. As an example, the first report of a small cell lung cancer genome revealed complex mutation signatures of tobacco exposure (Fig. 17.6).[16] The whole-genome sequencing of normal tissues will no doubt further increase the number of SNVs we have ever known, particularly for those rare SNPs that are likely to be disease causing. In fact, some cancer hospitals are beginning to use whole-genome sequencing approach to provide diagnosis for those patients who may benefit from the sequencing results, because they may not have other available tools for their diagnosis (http://www.nature.com/news/2010/100914/full/news.2010.465.html).

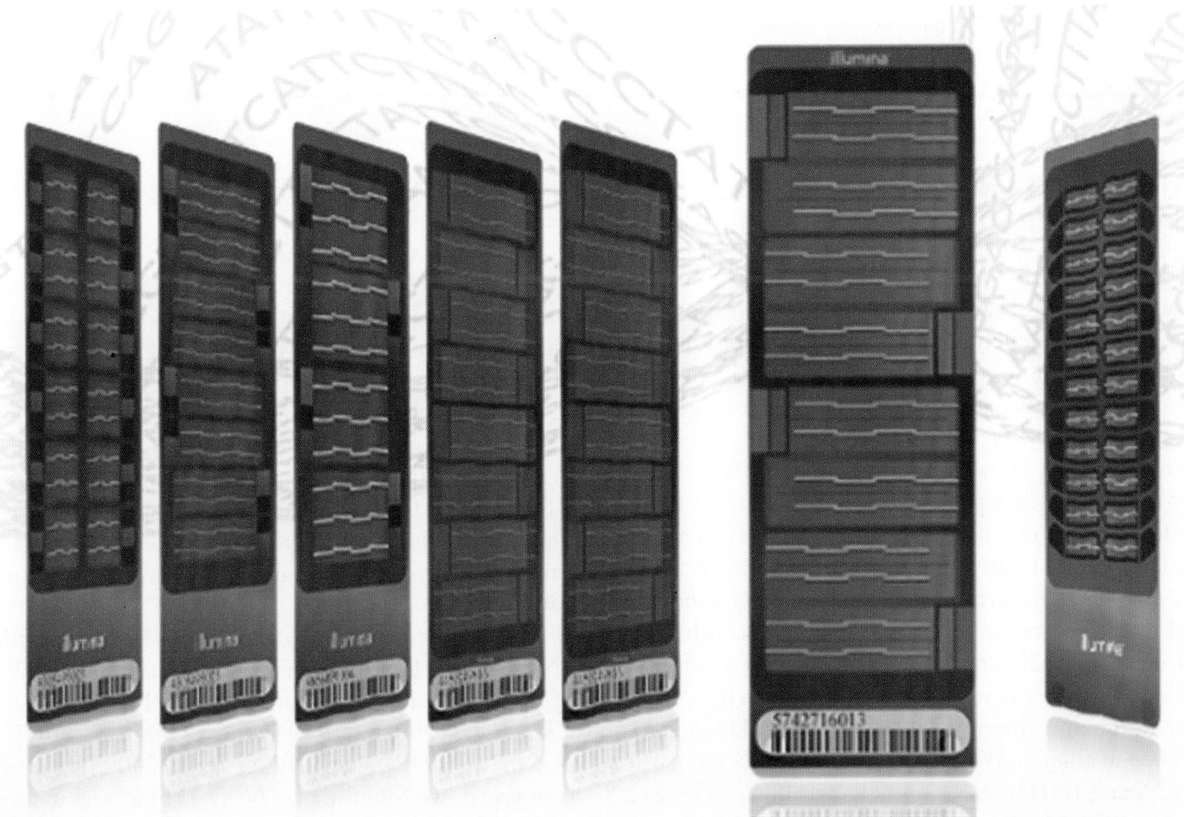

FIGURE 17–4 The new Illumina Omni5 capturing variation down to 1% minor allele frequency (MAF), with more than 4.3 million high-value markers and room for 500K customized SNPs (NHGRI GWAS Catalog; http://www.illumina.com/applications/gwas.ilmn).

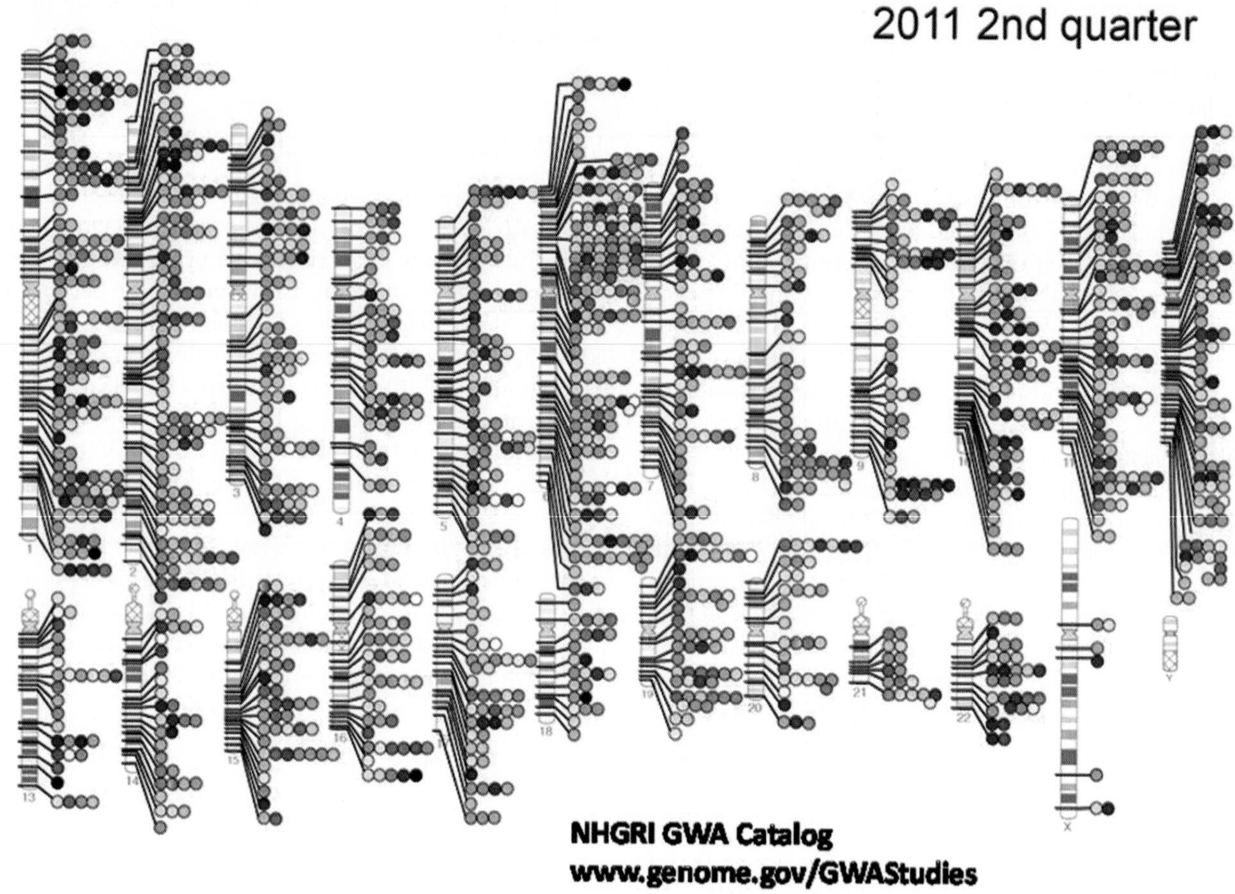

FIGURE 17–5 Published genome-wide association studies through June 2011; 1,449 published GWA at $P \leq 5 \times 10^{-8}$ for 237 traits (http://www.genome.gov/gwastudies/).

APPLICATION OF SNPs IN CLINICAL RESEARCH TOWARD PERSONALIZED CANCER MEDICINE

It is a known fact that patients' genetic background contributes to the risk of cancer and their various response to cancer therapies, namely chemotherapy and radiotherapy, which lead to variation in patients' survival. It is of great interest for the physicians to understand the roles genetic factors play in patients' treatment response.

For example, it is important to identify reliable biologic markers that predict the risk of normal tissue damage by radio(chemo)therapy before treatment. To this end, we investigated the association between SNPs in the transforming growth factor 1 (*TGFβ1*) gene and risk of radiation pneumonitis (RP) in patients with non–small cell lung cancer (NSCLC).[17] In this study, we included 164 patients with NSCLC treated with definitive radio(chemo)therapy, whose genomic DNA samples were available. We genotyped three SNPs of the *TGFβ1* gene (rs1800469:C-509T, rs1800471:G915C, and rs1982073:T869C) by the PCR-RFLP method. The genotype data were analyzed by Kaplan-Meier cumulative probability for the risk of grade ≥ 3 RP and Cox proportional hazards analyses for the effect of *TGFβ1* genotypes on such risk.

In this patient population, radiation doses ranging from 60 to 70 Gy (median ± 63 Gy) in 30 to 58 fractions were given to 96.3% of patients and platinum-based chemotherapy was given to 89.6% of the patients; the proportion of patients who developed grade ≥ 3 RP was 22.0%. However, we found in multivariate analysis that CT/CC genotypes of *TGFβ1* rs1982073:T869C was associated with a statistically significantly lower risk of RP grade ≥ 2 ($P = 0.007$), compared with the TT genotype, after adjustment of Karnofsky performance status, smoking status, pulmonary function, and dosimetric parameters.

In another study, we explored whether functional SNPs of base excision repair genes can predict RP.[18] Out of the selected SNPs of *ADPRT* (rs1136410 [V762A]), *XRCC1* (rs1799782 [R194W], rs25489 [R280H], and rs25487 [Q399R]), and *APEX1* (rs1130409 [D148E]) we genotyped, we found that *APEX1* D148E was associated with increased hazard of developing grade ≥ 2 RP in an allele dose–response manner (Trend tests: $P = 0.001$). These studies suggest that SNPs of genes involved in some

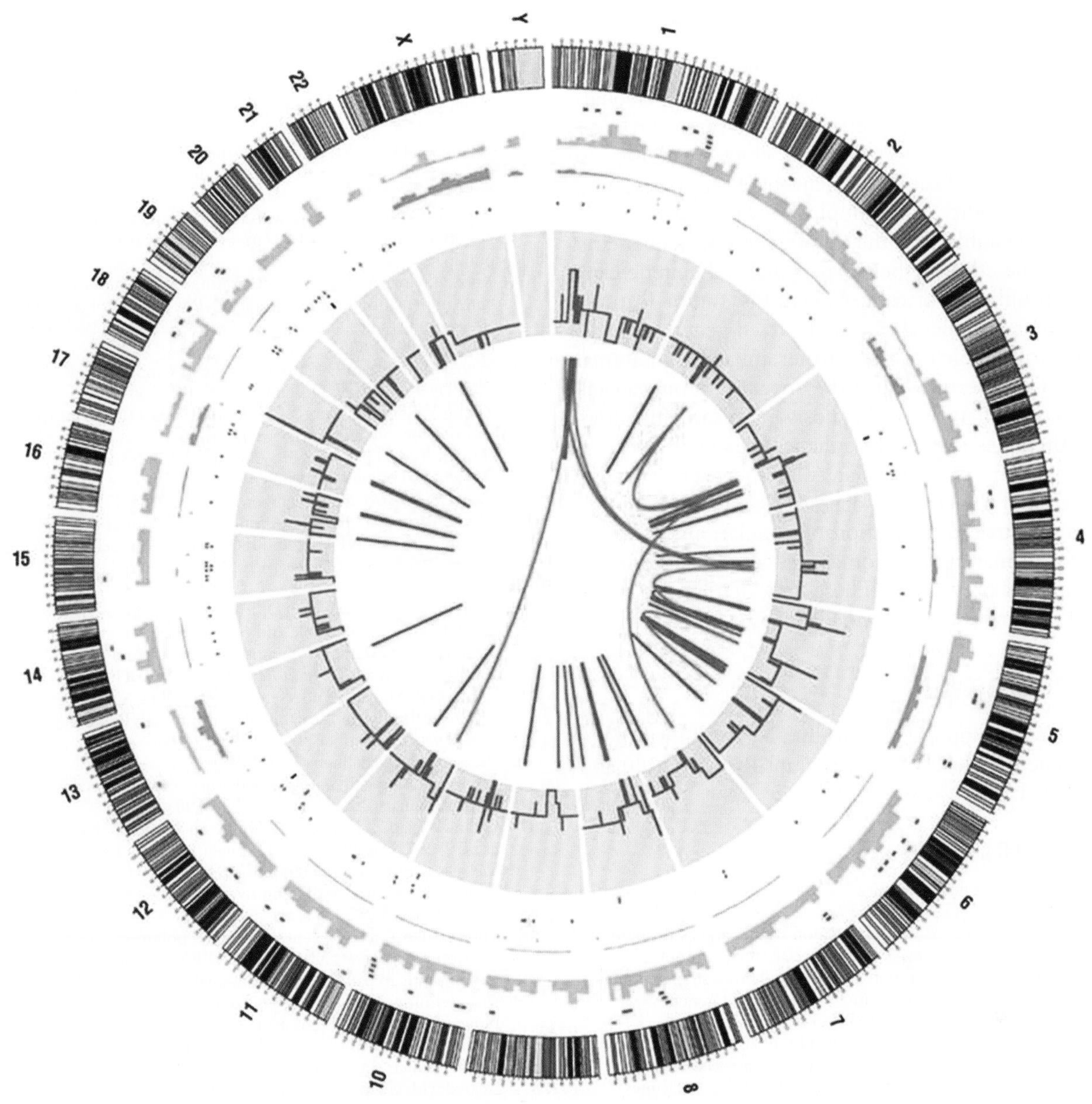

FIGURE 17–6 The compendium of somatic mutations in a small cell lung cancer genome. Figurative representation of the catalog of somatic mutations in the genome of NCI-H209. Chromosome ideograms are shown around the outer ring and are oriented pter-qter in a clockwise direction with centromeres indicated in red. Other tracks contain somatic alterations: validated insertions (light green rectangles); validated deletions (dark green rectangles); heterozygous (light orange bars) and homozygous (dark orange bars) substitutions shown by density per 10 Mb; coding substitutions (colored squares; silent in gray, missense in purple, nonsense in red, and splice site in black); copy number (blue lines); validated intrachromosomal rearrangements (green lines); validated interchromosomal rearrangements (purple lines).[16]

biological pathways, such as growth factors and DNA repair, may be biomarkers for susceptibility to RP in lung cancer patients who received definitive radiotherapy. Such biomarkers, once validated in prospective studies, will help with personalized therapy, an important part of personalized cancer medicine.

It is conceivable that there are some genetic factors that may have an effect on the response to chemotherapies. Indeed, in one of our published studies, we investigated the role of *TNFRSF1B* +676 T>G polymorphism in the survival of NSCLC patients treated with chemoradiotherapy.[19] We have shown that patients with the *TNFRSF1B* +676 GG genotype had a significantly better overall survival compared with patients with the TT genotype. Further stepwise multivariate Cox regression analysis showed that the *TNFRSF1B* +676 GG genotype was an independent prognosis predictor in this NSCLC patient cohort, in the presence of node status and tumor stage. These data suggest a possible role of *TNFRSF1B* +676 T>G (rs1061622) in the prognosis of NSCLC. Further large and functional studies are needed to confirm our findings.

CONCLUSIONS

With the advances in genotyping technologies, much of the genetic studies of cancer is now heading to personalized cancer medicine. For etiological research, progress has been made in GWAS using SNP chips, in addition to pathway-based and candidate gene–based SNP research, with the possibility of developing risk prediction models. It is inevitable that the whole-genome sequencing will push the edge further to personalized genetic cancer risk profiling. For cancer diagnosis, tumor features at a genome-wide level can be depicted genetically and epigenetically, which can be further enhanced in animal models. These features open the door to not only a cancer genetic signature for diagnosis but also many alternative therapies that could enhance treatment efficacy, targeted therapies in particular. All of these achievements in research of the etiology, diagnosis, and treatment will lead to effective identification of populations at risk to allow for primary prevention as well as earlier diagnosis for secondary prevention. These indicate that the prime time of personalized cancer medicine is coming soon.

ACKNOWLEDGMENT

This work was supported in part by a National Institute of Environmental Health Sciences grant R01 ES11740 and R01 CA 131274.

REFERENCES

1. Lander ES. The new genomics: global views of biology. *Science*. October 1996;274(5287):536-539.
2. Manolio TA. Genome-wide association studies and assessment of the risk of disease. *N Engl J Med*. July 2010;363(2):166-176.
3. Stranger BE, Stahl EA, Raj T. Progress and promise of genome-wide association studies for human complex trait genetics. *Genetics*. February 2011;187(2):367-383.
4. Hindorff LA, Sethupathy P, Junkins HA, et al. Potential etiologic and functional implications of genome-wide association loci for human diseases and traits. *Proc Natl Acad Sci U S A*. June 2009;106(23):9362-9367.
5. Meyerson M, Gabriel S, Getz G. Advances in understanding cancer genomes through second-generation sequencing. *Nat Rev Genet*. October 2010;11(10):685-696.
6. Sherry ST, Ward MH, Kholodov M, et al. dbSNP: the NCBI database of genetic variation. *Nucleic Acids Res*. January 2001;29(1):308-311.
7. Zhang W, Dolan ME. Impact of the 1000 genomes project on the next wave of pharmacogenomic discovery. *Pharmacogenomics*. February 2010;11(2):249-256.
8. Barrett JC. Haploview: visualization and analysis of SNP genotype data. *Cold Spring Harb Protoc*. October 2009;2009(10):pdb.ip71.
9. Xu Z, Taylor JA. SNPinfo: integrating GWAS and candidate gene information into functional SNP selection for genetic association studies. *Nucleic Acids Res*. July 2009;37(Web Server issue):W600-W605.
10. Weber JL. Human DNA polymorphisms and methods of analysis. *Curr Opin Biotechnol*. December 1990;1(2):166-171.
11. Zheng Y, Shen H, Sturgis EM, et al. Cyclin D1 polymorphism and risk for squamous cell carcinoma of the head and neck: a case-control study. *Carcinogenesis*. August 2001;22(8):1195-1199.
12. Weber JL. Human DNA polymorphisms and methods of analysis. *Curr Opin Biotechnol*. December 1990;1(2):166-171.
13. Liu Z, Wei S, Ma H, et al. A functional variant at the miR-184 binding site in TNFAIP2 and risk of squamous cell carcinoma of the head and neck. *Carcinogenesis*. November 2011;32(11):1668-1674.
14. De la Vega FM, Lazaruk KD, Rhodes MD, Wenz MH. Assessment of two flexible and compatible SNP genotyping platforms: TaqMan SNP Genotyping Assays and the SNPlex Genotyping System. *Mutat Res*. June 2005;573(1-2):111-135.
15. Tobler AR, Short S, Andersen MR, et al. The SNPlex genotyping system: a flexible and scalable platform for SNP genotyping. *Biomol Tech*. December 2005;16(4):398-406.
16. Pleasance ED, Stephens PJ, O'Meara S, et al. A small-cell lung cancer genome with complex signatures of tobacco exposure. *Nature*. January 2010;463(7278):184-190.
17. 'Yuan X, Liao Z, Liu Z, et al. Single nucleotide polymorphism at rs1982073:T869C of the TGFbeta 1 gene is associated with the risk of radiation pneumonitis in patients with non-small-cell lung cancer treated with definitive radiotherapy. *J Clin Oncol*. July 2009;27(20):3370-3378.
18. Yin M, Liao Z, Liu Z, et al. Functional polymorphisms of base excision repair genes XRCC1 and APEX1 predict risk of radiation pneumonitis in patients with non-small cell lung cancer treated with definitive radiation therapy. *Int J Radiat Oncol Biol Phys*. November 2011;81(3):e67-e73.
19. Guan X, Liao Z, Ma H, et al. TNFRSF1B +676 T>G polymorphism predicts survival of non-small cell lung cancer patients treated with chemoradiotherapy. *BMC Cancer*. October 2011;11:447.

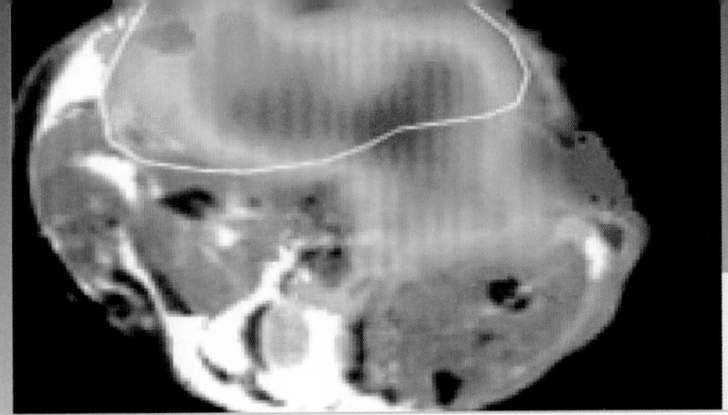

SECTION III

Molecular Tests and Cancer Management

CHAPTER 18

Overview of Molecular Tests and Personalized Cancer Medicine

Manuel Salto-Tellez

Cancer is a heterogeneous disease. Indeed, many experts will argue that the term cancer encompasses more than 100 different diseases, which share common characteristics such as local invasion, distant spread, and the potential to cause death and, at the same time, have different sites of origin, biological backgrounds, and sensitivities to therapeutic intervention.[1] Thus, the disparity in the evolution of outcomes in different cancer types over the last few decades is not surprising. For instance, while we have witnessed a considerable improvement in testicular and breast cancer, with 5-year survival rates moving from 57% and 60% to 96% and 90%, respectively, other common cancer types (such as lung or colon) have experienced little improvement over the same time period.[2,3]

This intrinsic heterogeneity does not only affect cancer as a whole. Within specific forms of cancer, we know that some subtypes have a morphomolecular profile that makes them more amenable to curative interventions, while others gain little improvement with our currently available drugs. This is well epitomized in the field of chronic myeloid leukemia, in which the majority of patients are expected to obtain a favorable outcome with standard-dose imatinib, but a third of patients do not achieve the desired effect and must be considered resistant.[4]

The realization of this extraordinary heterogeneity, and the need to define clear cancer subtypes with targeted therapies capable of predicting improvements in outcome and at the same time exclude those patients in whom response is highly unlikely, is at the heart of personalized medicine in cancer.

THE MOLECULAR BASIS OF DISEASE AS THE DRIVER FOR PERSONALIZED MEDICINE

In 1998, more than 45 years after the discovery of the DNA helix, reported in 1953,[5] the impact of molecular biology in the practice of medicine in general, and cancer in particular, was very limited. At that time, the director of the National Cancer Institute challenged "the scientific community to harness the power of comprehensive molecular analysis technologies to make the classification of tumors vastly more informative." This challenge aimed to change "the basis of tumor classification from morphological to molecular characteristics."[3] More than a decade after the "director's challenge," the modern world of personalized medicine and molecular diagnostics could be illustrated by the "bottle and the glass" paradigm depicted in Figure 18.1. While for many cancer types the glass is almost empty, for some there is already enough "fluid" to change the traditional standard of care with the means of molecular information.

Section IV of this book will provide a systematic review of the principles of molecular diagnostics and personalized medicine applied to the commonest malignancies, focusing on those cancers where "there is some fluid in the glass." In this chapter, our aim is to provide a broad set of definitions to frame this discussion and, based on specific examples of current tests, to illustrate some of the strengths, weaknesses, and opportunities derived from our current knowledge and understanding. As personalized medicine and molecular diagnostics are clearly interlinked, it is important to understand the latter to be able to perceive the specific weight of the former.

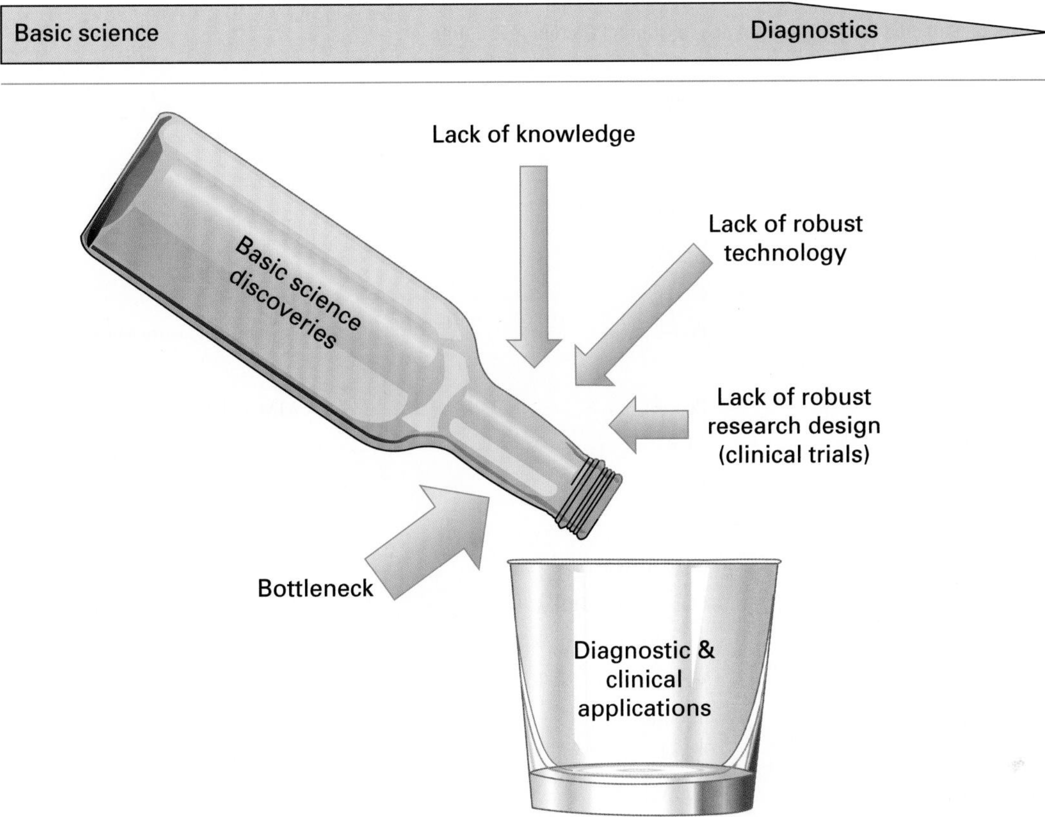

FIGURE 18–1 Illustration of the natural flow of knowledge from basic science discoveries to diagnostic/clinical applications and the recurrent arguments explaining why this has not happened as promptly as it should have, including a "lack of knowledge of the true meaning of certain biomarkers," a "lack of robust technology to implement these biomarkers in the diagnostic setting," or a "lack of robust clinical trial design to generate sufficient evidence for the use of biomarkers routinely."

MOLECULAR DIAGNOSTICS: THREE LEVELS OF TESTING

Molecular diagnostics is the application of molecular biology techniques and our knowledge of the molecular basis of disease for diagnostic, prognostic, and/or therapeutic purposes. When this molecular diagnostic approach is applied to the materials usually diagnosed by anatomic pathologists and cytopathologists, the terms "Molecular Surgical Pathology" or "Molecular Cytopathology" apply.[6,7] Most of the molecular testing of cancer is performed on formalin-fixed, paraffin-embedded (FFPE) tissue and, as such, fall into the realm of "Molecular Surgical Pathology." Exceptions to this rule are the molecular diagnostics of leukemias or the application of molecular diagnostics to circulating malignant cells.

Cancer molecular tests can be divided into three main types, namely diagnostic, genetic, and therapeutic. *Diagnostic* tests are used because pathologists have difficulties in placing the right diagnostic label to the individual patient. This is why classically we test for sarcoma[8] or lymphoma[9] translocations, because the detection of a specific fusion product is pathognomonic of a specific disease subgroup, which, in some instances, also carries a prognostic and/or therapeutic dimension. *Genetic* tests are performed in FFPE materials to confirm or exclude an inherited origin to the cancer. The prototype, available in molecular diagnostic laboratories for more than a decade, is the analysis of microsatellite instability in the context of the diagnosis of hereditary non-polyposis colorectal cancer. *Therapeutic* tests are at the core of the so-called therapeutic pathology or personalized medicine. Oncologists now have an increasing *armamentarium* of antibodies and small molecule inhibitors, able to target specific key genes and pathways in oncogenesis (Table 18.1).[10]

This revolution in oncology is also deeply transforming the way we practice molecular testing and, therefore, the way modern pathology is carried out. Indeed, there are at least six solid tumors, where the genotype of specific single biomarkers indicates which patients are more likely to respond to which therapy (Fig. 18.2).

PERSONALIZED MEDICINE: SINGLE VERSUS MULTIPLE BIOMARKERS

The examples of personalized medicine discussed in this chapter so far, and the majority of those described in Section IV, represent single biomarkers associated with the response of individual drugs. The pattern of biomarker discovery in this case is relatively simple: the primary site of activity of a drug is known (or, at least, the main

TABLE 18–1 Selected Target Therapeutics in Clinical Oncology Practice

Targeted Therapeutics	Target	Tumor
Antibodies		
Bevacizumab	VEGF	Breast Ca/CRC/NSCLC
Cetuximab	EGFR/KRAS	CRC and HN Ca
Panitumumab	EGFR	CRC
Rituximab	CD20	B-cell lymphoma
Trastuzumab	Her-2	Breast Ca/Gastric cancer
Small molecule inhibitors		
Bortezomib	Proteasome	MM and MCL
Crizotinib	ALK	NSCLC
Erlotinib	EGFR	NSCLC/pancreatic cancer
Gefitinib	EGFR	NSCLC
Imatinib	c-kit/BCR-ABL	GIST/CML
Lapatinib	Her-2 and EGFR	Breast Ca
Sorafenib	VEGFR/PDGFR/RAF	HCC and RCC
Sunitinib	VEGFR/PDGFR/RET	GIST and RCC
Temsirolimus	mTOR	RCC
Vemurafenib	BRAF	Melanoma
Vorinostat/Bortezomib	HDAC	Cutaneous TCL

Breast Ca, breast cancer; CRC, colorectal cancer; NSCLC, non–small cell lung carcinoma; HN Ca, head and neck cancer; MM, multiple myeloma; MCL, mantle cell lymphoma; GIST, gastrointestinal stromal tumor; CML, chronic myeloid leukemia; HCC, hepatocellular carcinoma; RCC, renal cell carcinoma; TCL, T-cell lymphoma.

biological pathway), and the members of this pathway are then analyzed at three main levels to establish a relation between therapeutic intervention and therapeutic response. These levels cut across the main dogma of molecular biology and include DNA (usually by mutation analysis), RNA (mostly in the form of single gene copy number by fluorescence in situ hybridization [FISH]), and protein (with immunohistochemistry [IHC] representing the most cost-effective manner of detection).

The other end of the spectrum is the application of large gene expression signatures for prognostication and patient stratification. The advent of microarray-based profiling, targeting thousands of messenger RNA transcripts in a single experiment, has facilitated the identification of prognostic and potentially therapeutic subclasses. For example, three profiles have shown prognostic ability in early-stage breast cancer: MammaPrint, a 70-gene profile; Oncotype DX, a 21-gene score for recurrence; and a 76-gene outcome, the Rotterdam signature.[11-13] In colon cancer, two recent studies have established gene expression assays to predict prognosis/recurrence in stage II disease.[14,15] A 133-gene signature in acute myeloid leukemia carries prognostic value.[16] Although these molecular classifications provide very promising stratifications for new treatments, two main criticisms have been exercised to date, namely that (a) the incorporation of gene expression signatures into routine clinical practice should be confirmed beforehand by suitably powered, randomized, controlled trials[17] and (b) these are, primarily, single-laboratory tests that do not seem to be robust enough to be widely distributed in accredited laboratories.

In between a single biomarker and the analysis of the gene expression of thousands of genes, the testing of several single biomarkers up front is becoming a pattern for novel clinical trials. The BATTLE trial arguably represents the best known model to date.[18] The phase 1 of this trial involved the stratification of patients in 4 therapeutic arms based on the analysis of 11 biomarkers involved in 4 non–small cell lung carcinoma (NSCLC) molecular pathways: DNA mutation analysis of *EGFR*, *KRAS*, and *BRAF*; FISH-detected copy number of *EGFR* and *Cyclin D1* copy number; and protein expression of VEGF, VEGFR, three RXR receptors and Cyclin D1 by IHC. This trial illustrates a series of important aspects of future personalized medicine, namely (a) the need to stratify with biomarkers associated with known therapeutic responses; (b) the need to sample cancers for therapeutic decision making, which may be independent from the "diagnostic sampling"; and (c) the difficulty of translating single biomarkers into a

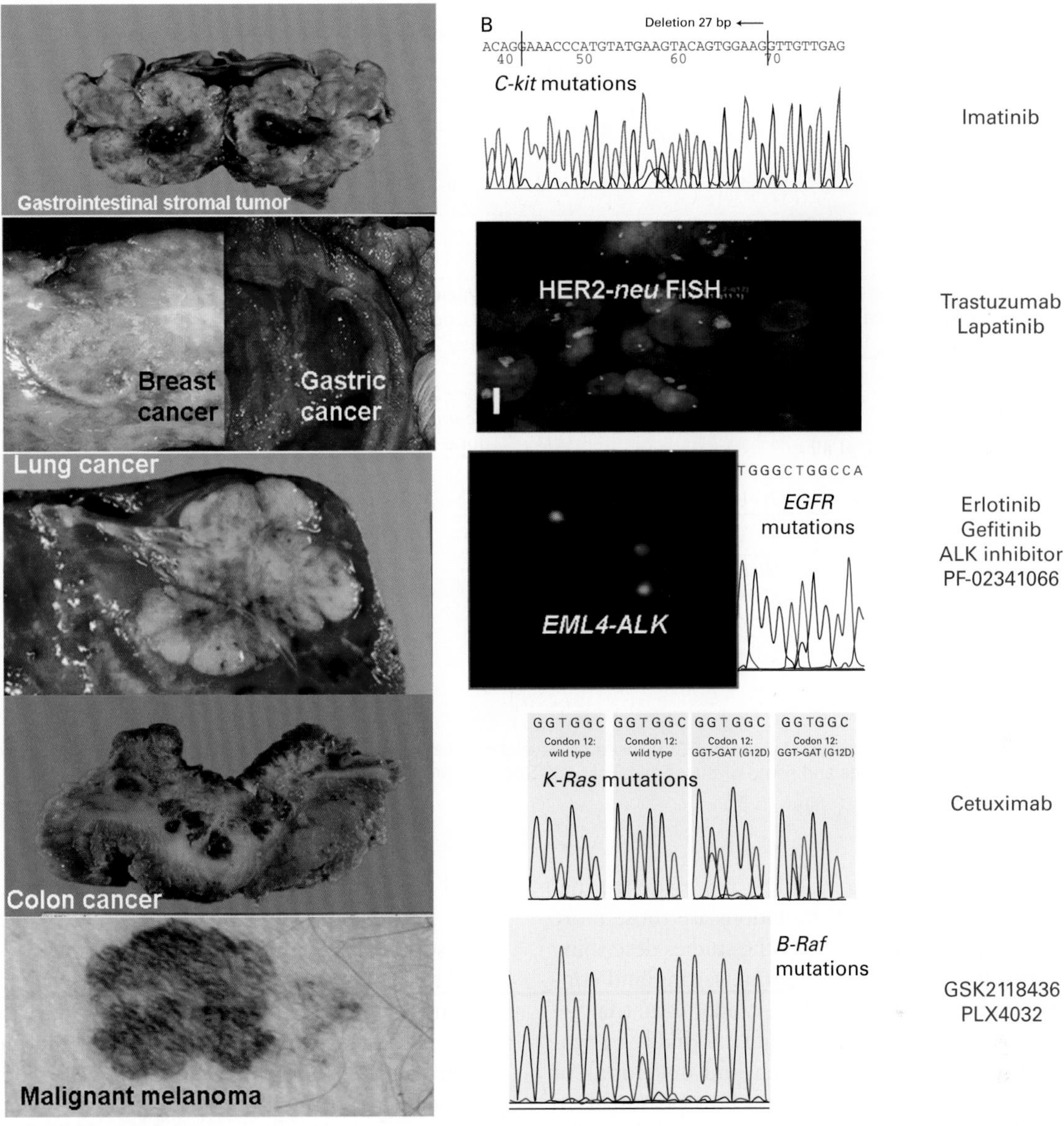

FIGURE 18–2 Morphological, molecular, and therapeutic dimensions of oncologic personalized medicine.

single technology platform, when these biomarkers cut across DNA, RNA, and protein.

TIME FRAMES FOR PERSONALIZED MEDICINE DISCOVERY TO DATE

What are the time frames for bringing a new anticancer drug as standard of care? This has definitely changed in the course of time. Let us take the small molecule inhibitors gefitinib and erlotinib as examples. The main time frames for the development of the drugs, and the characterization of epidermal growth factor receptor (EGFR) as a biomarker, are as follows.

In 1964, Stanley Cohen, American biochemist and Nobel Prize Laureate in Physiology and Medicine (1986), isolated and characterized a salivary gland protein that could stimulate the proliferation of epithelial cells and was thus named epidermal growth factor or EGF.[19] In the 1970s, Graham Carpenter discovered the specific *binding receptors* for EGF on target cells, or *EGFR*, a 170-kDa membrane protein that increased the incorporation of 32-phosphorus in response to EGF treatment of A431 epidermoid carcinoma cells.[20] In 1984, Ullrich et al. isolated, cloned, characterized, and genetically sequenced *EGFR* from normal placenta and A431 tumor cells, postulating that modification of proteins by phosphorylation on tyrosine residues might be a critical step in tumorigenesis.[21]

After those 20 years, it took another 20 years to establish gefitinib and erlotinib as bona fide treatment options and *EGFR* mutation analysis as the necessary companion biomarker. This is depicted in Figure 18.3 and involved the description of the presence of the EGFR in lung cancer (1987)[22]; the evidence that blocking the receptor slows malignant cell growth[23]; the production of the first small

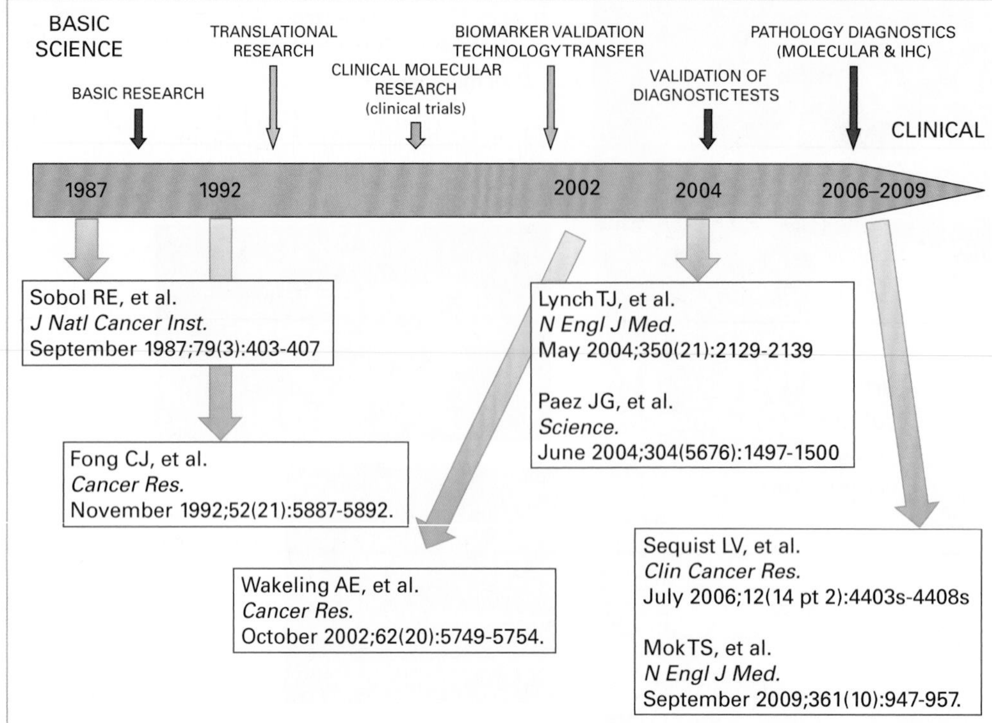

FIGURE 18–3 Pathway of the last 20 years of EGFR research development following the classic pipeline from basic science to clinical applications, including time frames and some of the seminal papers. See text for more detailed explanation and full references.

molecule inhibitor targeting EGFR[24]; the evidence that those lung cancers with EGFR mutations are those more likely to respond to the drug[25,26]; and the studies describing the use of this biomarker in the routine setting and confirming this evidence in a prospective, randomized trial.[27,28]

This process is obviously too long and likely to represent a suboptimal use of research and development resources and is key to understanding how personalized medicine is likely to change the time frames of drug discovery and the significant resources associated with it.

TIME FRAMES FOR PERSONALIZED MEDICINE DISCOVERY: THE FUTURE

The overall annual costs of cancer measured in pure economic terms, namely direct medical expenses and lost productivity, are increasing at an exponential rate: in 2008 it was estimated to be $228 billion in the United States alone and £18.3 billion in the United Kingdom.[29,30] It is estimated that the bulk of this cost is related to the huge development costs for cancer medicines. In a seminal paper on the subject, Sullivan et al. indicate that "Several drivers of cost, such as over-use, rapid expansion, and shortening life cycles of cancer technologies (such as medicines and imaging modalities), and the lack of suitable clinical research and integrated health economic studies, have converged with more defensive medical practice, a less informed regulatory system, a lack of evidence-based sociopolitical debate, and a declining degree of fairness for all patients with cancer."[31] Of all the funding spent in drug development, it is the phase 3 trial component that carries, by far, the greatest expense and also the highest chance of failure.[32]

This situation, which for many is clearly unsustainable in the long term, may be palliated (at least in part) by the advent of personalized medicine and biomarker-driven drug development. A very recent example has been provided by crizotinib, the development of which—from publication of the discovery of the ALK fusion gene in NSCLC to Food and Drug Administration (FDA) approval in just 4 years—presents a clear contrast with the EGFR paradigm highlighted before. The FDA approval of crizotinib is based on data from a phase 2 study[33] and a part 2 expansion cohort of a phase 1 study.[34] The approval of the drug and its biomarker before ongoing phase 3 trials have ended is a clear indication of the effect that a companion diagnostic predictor of therapeutic response (i.e., personalized medicine) has in the streamline, simplification, and savings of time and resources related to drug development.

TUMOR SAMPLING AND PERSONALIZED MEDICINE

Modern diagnostics is experiencing a *small sample revolution*: biopsy needles are getting smaller, imaging experts are more likely to obtain minute samples of tissue from anatomical areas unreachable to date with minimally invasive procedures, and, as a result, pathologists are required to provide more information with less material. This conundrum needs to be solved in three different ways:

(a) Clear protocols to make the most of diagnostic materials. The main example is the evolution that the value of cytopathology samples has experienced in the context of molecular diagnostics,[35] from opinions that rendered this material second rate for molecular testing to the routine use of fine-needle aspiration materials or pleural effusions for *EGFR* mutation analysis.[36]

(b) Protocols to obtain a *therapeutic* sample after a *diagnostic* sample when needed. The advantage of this approach was clearly established by the BATTLE trial described above.

(c) Sampling of more accessible body components, such as peripheral blood and, in particular, the detection of circulating tumor cells,[37] exosomes, and free nucleic acids.[38,39] Although there is no unequivocal evidence that any of these modalities alone can substitute more traditional molecular test approaches, it is likely that technical developments will make them more reliable and reproducible for future diagnostics.

COMMON DRUGS AND TESTS IN PERSONALIZED MEDICINE: LESSONS FROM THE PAST TO UNDERSTAND THE FUTURE

The tests mentioned in this section will be discussed in detail in subsequent chapters. Hereby, we would like to analyze aspects of these tests that draw important lessons to understand important aspects of personalized medicine as a whole.

HER2/neu and the Need for Better Testing

Of all the available examples, perhaps HER2/neu (ERBB2 or v-erb-b2 erythroblastic leukemia viral oncogene homolog 2, neuro/glioblastoma derived oncogene homolog [avian]) testing and subsequent treatment of breast cancer with drugs such as trastuzumab or lapatinib is the archetype of personalized medicine.

Traditionally, international diagnostic and therapeutic guidelines have allowed both immunohistochemical and genomic approaches to HER2/neu testing.[40] Because of the broad availability and higher affordability of IHC, these guidelines essentially support the approach of using IHC as the first line of HER2/neu status detection. Unfortunately, when the HER2/neu testing performance of general laboratories in busy and not-so-specialized local or community hospitals is analyzed, serious discrepancies start to emerge.[41] This discrepancy clearly affects patient treatment in a proportion of patients: up to 15% of patients could be overtreated, while 5% of patients may be undertreated.[42-44] This is due to both technical and IHC interpretative issues. Thus, the current status of HER2/neu testing is suboptimal and calls for more stringent rules in relation to who should interpret the test, where should the test be performed, and which is the best technical platform for the analysis,[45] particularly now that the Her2/neu–trastuzumab paradigm is also applicable to gastric cancer.[46]

EGFR Testing and the Taxonomy of Cancer

Traditionally, pathologists have been the taxonomists of diseases in general and cancer in particular. When it was obvious that a molecular basis of taxonomy was more likely, in some instances, to generate cancer subtypes with stronger diagnostic, prognostic, and therapeutic value, the mood in the pathology community became rather somber.[47,48] From a closer look at the status of the classification of those cancers in which personalized medicine is a reality, it is clear that the current classification is truly morphomolecular; in other words, high-quality morphological assessment in *conditio sine qua non* for high-quality molecular diagnostics, and as a result, phenotype and genotype are not mutually exclusive in personalized medicine diagnostics, but truly complementary. Perhaps, the diagnosis of lung cancer is a good example of this change of paradigm. An analysis of the current modus operandi will let us see that:

(a) Long gone are the days in which the main diagnostic distinction was between small cell and non–small cell carcinoma of the lung. Today, the place in the morphological continuum where the pathologist places their morphological diagnosis (Fig. 18.4) may dictate future molecular testing and hence treatment.

(b) The traditional WHO classification of lung cancer is long,[49] cumbersome, and, for the most part, irrelevant in relation to therapeutic decision making. In contrast, the emerging molecular classification of lung cancer is characterized by single biomarkers, many of which are *druggable* or potentially *druggable* targets, such as EGFR, KRAS, BRAF, EML4-ALK, FGFR4, PIK3CA/MEK, or HER2/neu. Needless to say, such classification is much more objective and reproducible (as it is the product of a laboratory test, rather than the subjective interpretation of morphology) and holds much more clinical/therapeutic relevance (one could say that almost half of the lung adenocarcinomas are definable by a personalized medicine paradigm). It is, obviously, a less affordable classification, although, as it will be argued below, the current technology developments may change this characteristic as well.

KRAS/BRAF and What Represents a Good Biomarker Validation

KRAS mutation analysis is one of the most prominent tests in solid tumor molecular diagnostic analysis. Monoclonal antibody treatments such as cetuximab have been developed that target the extracellular binding domain of EGFR, thus competitively inhibiting the binding of ligand to its receptor. However, a significant proportion of EGFR-positive colorectal cancers (CRCs)

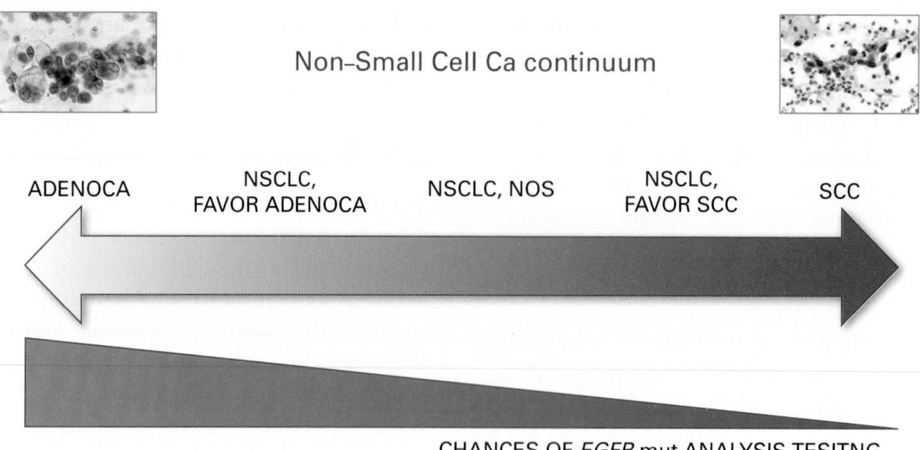

FIGURE 18–4 Illustration of morphological diagnosis of non–small cell carcinoma of the lung and likelihood of *EGFR* mutation analysis testing.

remain resistant to this therapy. One reason for resistance is that the pathway may also be activated downstream of EGFR due to mutation of the KRAS oncogene, which occurs in approximately 30% to 40% of CRCs. The overall survival benefit in patients with stage IV CRC following treatment with anti-EGFR therapies has been modest; however, when patients are stratified for KRAS mutation status, overall and progression-free survival rates are significantly improved for patients with wild-type *KRAS*.[50-55]

KRAS mutation analysis provides a good example for two key issues related to personalized medicine, namely (a) the best technology platform for molecular testing and (b) biomarker readiness for therapeutic decision making.

A large number of technologies have been postulated for *KRAS* testing,[56] which include Sanger sequencing, pyrosequencing, allelic-specific real-time polymerase chain reaction (PCR), post-PCR fluorescent melting curve analysis with specific probes and PCR clamping methods, and variations of the above. These are usually laboratory approaches published in single-test studies (or small comparative analyses). In general, there are few comprehensive, multicenter, multi-technique studies applied to a single set of clinical samples to address the reliability of individual technical approaches to molecular testing. The study by Whitehall et al. is, to our knowledge, the first one to assess the concordance of different methods for the detection of *KRAS* mutations across multiple testing sites and using the same clinical specimens.[57] Although excellent agreement between methods was observed, it was less than 100%, raising a key question in personalized medicine test validation: When is a technical approach good enough to be incorporated in a routine molecular diagnostic armamentarium? This is important because it is evident now that increased test sensitivity enhances the predictive value of personalized medicine.[58]

When is a biomarker ready for clinical use in a personalized medicine setting is another key question that can be addressed with the cetuximab/KRAS paradigm. In 2008, Di Nicolantonio et al. indicated the need of testing for *BRAF* mutation analysis to characterize a subgroup of *KRAS* wild-type patients who will respond to cetuximab treatment.[59] This finding was logical: only a proportion of wild-type KRAS CRCs will respond to cetuximab and there are other downstream members of the same pathway (BRAF, MEK, ERK/MAPK) that, conceptually, could play a role in this setting. However, subsequent studies have shown contradictory findings, and as a result, BRAF is not consolidated as a cetuximab-related biomarker.[60,61] Once again, clear multinational, multicenter studies to evaluate cost-efficiency in biomarker analysis appear to be needed as the key element in future validations.

Overall Survival and Tumor Recurrence: Personalized Medicine in the Right Context

Patients treated with cetuximab had a slightly superior overall survival rate compared with patients treated with the best supportive care, 6.1 versus 4.6 months.[62] Trastuzumab carries a median survival improvement of 25.1 versus 20.3 months in metastatic breast cancers that overexpress HER2 and 13.8 versus 11.1 months in gastric cancer.[63,46] The IPASS trial showed a clear progression-free survival advantage for gefitinib, but no overall survival advantage (apparently due to cross over). Imatinib and sunitinib have changed the outcome of patients with gastrointestinal stromal tumor and prolonged survival by manyfold, but treatment failure and tumor progression seem inevitable over time and constitute an unresolved clinical challenge.[64]

Whenever we talk about personalized medicine, two contradictory ideas evolve. On the one hand, we are improving patients' lives. On the other hand, the improvement is very modest and, in most occasions, far from curative. Issues such as tumor resistance and strategies to overcome it, and the aim to transform cancer into a chronic disease with a succession of tests and therapies, will be very much in the heart of the future development of personalized medicine.[65,66]

FUTURE CHALLENGES

Intratumor Heterogeneity

Heterogeneity is usually considered in relation to "cancer" as a whole or the subtypes that can be defined in "individual cancer types." However, there is increasing evidence that intratumor heterogeneity (or the fact that each single cancer is far from homogeneous) may be at the heart of key aspects in personalized medicine such as partial response, tumor recurrence, or drug resistance. One of the main future challenges in personalized medicine will be to integrate enough redundancy in our studies to understand the full heterogeneity of individual cancers. This will be achieved by analyzing as many different parts of the tumor as possible (*topographic heterogeneity*),[67] as many cell types as available (*histogenetic heterogeneity*),[68] as many samples from the same tumor in the course of time (*temporal heterogeneity*), and as many body compartments as possible, such as primary tumor, circulating tumor cells, and exosomes or plasma (*compartmental heterogeneity*).[69,70]

Such comprehensive analyses will require totally different approaches to the bioimaging and pathological sampling of cancers (particularly in the context of clinical trial material), will demand a much more judicious use of retrospective tissue collections, and will call for totally new protocols for systematic re-biopsy of patients within specific windows of treatment.

Well-Annotated Clinical Samples for Discovery (Biobanks)

The sustainable and clinically meaningful advancement of personalized medicine will require the restructuring of tissue procurement to become a routine part of patient care. Accordingly, tissue banking will need to evolve from its traditional research role in large academic medical centers into the everyday practice of surgical pathology. In short, all patients and patient samples will need to be treated as potential research subjects. Successful implementation of this model will require consideration of financial and ethical concerns, but, eventually, will lead to a much faster process of biomarker validation and personalized medicine implementation.[71]

New Technologies for Biomarker Discovery and Biomarker Analysis

The majority of the biomarkers applied in personalized medicine are single gene mutations, epigenetic modifications, gene translocations, or gene amplifications.[72] Many retrospective studies, as well as prospective clinical trials, are currently applying high-throughput technologies to fasten the process of discovery of biomarkers with predictive value. Indeed, the last decade has witnessed a plethora of technical developments that, beyond the known paradigm of gene expression arrays discussed before, aim to facilitate this quest.[73] Of these, next-generation and third-generation sequencing technologies are some of the most exciting tools today.[74] This technology, which is currently driving genomic research in cancer,[75] will pose one of the most challenging and interesting conundrums in practicing oncology in a few decades. Indeed, determining the suitability of whole-genome sequencing for diagnostic applications in cancer, having to determine the specific information of interest for a given patient from the large pool of data that will be available, and how to present this in "clinical reports" that are as informative as possible without each single bit of information being "therapeutically binding," is a question with ethical, legal, diagnostic, and therapeutic dimensions that will dictate the practical future of whole-genome information. As the price of whole-genome sequencing falls to "a few thousand dollars," the regulation of the clinical use of genomic information is key for the future of personalized medicine as a whole.

PERSONALIZED MEDICINE: A CHANGE OF PARADIGM THAT IS HERE TO STAY

The promise of personalized medicine provides not only numerous challenges but also a remarkable opportunity. At a time when the availability and the use of funds for cancer research is under scrutiny, personalized medicine provides a focus for cost-effective, patient-driven research. Today's pharmaceutical industry is under pressure due to major loss of revenue owing to patent expirations, increasingly cost-constrained health-care systems, and more demanding regulatory requirements. To them, personalized medicine provides the perfect environment to substantially increase the number and quality of innovative, cost-effective new medicines, without incurring unsustainable R&D costs.[76] This, which invariably would require us all to revisit the links between health care, academia, and industry, may govern the way we understand drug discovery in the years to come.

REFERENCES

1. La Thangue NB, Kerr DJ. Predictive biomarkers: a paradigm shift towards personalized cancer medicine. *Nat Rev Clin Oncol.* August 2011;8(10):587-596.
2. National Cancer Institute. SEER Cancer Statistics Review 1975–2004 [online]. http://seer.cancer.gov/csr/1975_2004/ December 2011.
3. NIH Guide: Director's Challenge towards a molecular classification of tumors 1998. http://grants.nih.gov/grants/guide/rfa-files/rfa-ca-98-027.html. Accessed July 23, 2008.
4. Breccia M, Alimena G. The current role of high-dose imatinib in chronic myeloid leukemia patients, newly diagnosed or resistant to standard dose. *Expert Opin Pharmacother.* September 2011;12(13):2075-2087.
5. Watson JD, Crick FH. Molecular structure of nucleic acids; a structure for deoxyribose nucleic acid. *Nature.* 1953;171(4356):737-738.
6. Lauwers GY, Black-Schaffer S, Salto-Tellez M. Molecular pathology in contemporary diagnostic pathology laboratory: an opinion for the active role of surgical pathologists. *Am J Surg Pathol.* 2010;34(1):115-117.
7. Salto-Tellez M, Koay ESC. Molecular diagnostic cytopathology—definitions, scope and clinical utility. *Cytopathology.* 2004;15:252-255.

8. Romeo S, Dei Tos AP. Clinical application of molecular pathology in sarcomas. *Curr Opin Oncol.* July 2011;23(4):379-384.
9. Bagg A. Molecular diagnosis in lymphoma. *Curr Hematol Rep.* July 2005;4(4):313-323.
10. Quek TPL, Yan B, Yong WP, Salto-Tellez M. Targeted therapeutics-oriented tumor classification: a paradigm shift. *Personalized Med.* 2009;6(5):465-468.
11. van 't Veer LJ, Dai H, van de Vijver MJ, et al. Gene expression profiling predicts clinical outcome of breast cancer. *Nature.* 2002;415:530-536.
12. Paik S, Shak S, Tang G, et al. A multigene assay to predict recurrence of tamoxifen-treated, node-negative breast cancer. *N Engl J Med.* 2004;351:2817-2826.
13. Wang Y, Klijn JG, Zhang Y, et al. Gene expression profiles to predict distant metastasis of lymph-node-negative primary breast cancer. *Lancet.* 2005;365:671-679.
14. Gray RG, Quirke P, Handley K, et al. Validation study of a quantitative multigene reverse transcriptase–polymerase chain reaction assay for assessment of recurrence risk in patients with stage II colon cancer. *J Clin Oncol.* doi:10.1200/JCO.2010.32.8732.
15. Kennedy RD, Bylesjo M, Kerr P, et al. Development and independent validation of a prognostic assay for stage II colon cancer using formalin-fixed paraffin-embedded tissue. *J Clin Oncol.* doi:10.1200/JCO.2011.35.4498.
16. Rosenwald A, Wright G, Chan WC, et al. The use of molecular profiling to predict survival after chemotherapy for diffuse large-B-cell lymphoma. *N Engl J Med.* 2002;346:1937-1947.
17. McDermott U, Downing JR, Stratton MR. Genomics and the continuum of cancer care. *N Engl J Med.* January 2011;364(4):340-350.
18. Kim ES, Herbst RS, Lee JJ, et al. The BATTLE trial (Biomarker-integrated Approaches of Targeted Therapy for Lung Cancer Elimination): personalizing therapy for lung cancer [abstract]. In: Proceedings of the 101th Annual Meeting of the American Association for Cancer Research; April 17–21, 2010; Washington, DC. Philadelphia (PA): AACR; 2010. Abstract nr LB-1.
19. Cohen S. Isolation and biological effects of an epidermal growth-stimulating protein. *Natl Cancer Inst Monogr.* April 1964;13:13-37.
20. Carpenter G. Regulation of epidermal growth factor (EGF) receptor activity during the modulation of protein synthesis. *J Cell Physiol.* April 1979;99(1):101-106.
21. Ullrich A, Coussens L, Hayflick JS, et al. Human epidermal growth factor receptor cDNA sequence and aberrant expression of the amplified gene in A431 epidermoid carcinoma cells. *Nature.* May-June 1984;309(5967):418-425.
22. Sobol RE, Astarita RW, Hofeditz C, et al. Epidermal growth factor receptor expression in human lung carcinomas defined by a monoclonal antibody. *J Natl Cancer Inst.* September 1987;79(3):403-407.
23. Fong CJ, Sherwood ER, Mendelsohn J, Lee C, Kozlowski JM. Epidermal growth factor receptor monoclonal antibody inhibits constitutive receptor phosphorylation, reduces autonomous growth, and sensitizes androgen-independent prostatic carcinoma cells to tumor necrosis factor alpha. *Cancer Res.* November 1992;52(21):5887-5892.
24. Wakeling AE, Guy SP, Woodburn JR, et al. ZD1839 (Iressa): an orally active inhibitor of epidermal growth factor signaling with potential for cancer therapy. *Cancer Res.* October 2002;62(20):5749-5754.
25. Paez JG, Jänne PA, Lee JC, et al. EGFR mutations in lung cancer: correlation with clinical response to gefitinib therapy. *Science.* June 2004;304(5676):1497-1500.
26. Lynch TJ, Bell DW, Sordella R, et al. Activating mutations in the epidermal growth factor receptor underlying responsiveness of non-small-cell lung cancer to gefitinib. *N Engl J Med.* May 2004;350(21):2129-2139.
27. Mok TS, Wu YL, Thongprasert S, et al. Gefitinib or carboplatin-paclitaxel in pulmonary adenocarcinoma. *N Engl J Med.* September 2009;361(10):947-957.
28. Sequist LV, Joshi VA, Jänne PA, et al. Epidermal growth factor receptor mutation testing in the care of lung cancer patients. *Clin Cancer Res.* July 2006;12(14 pt 2):4403s-4408s.
29. Yabroff KR, Warren JL, Brown ML. Costs of cancer care in the USA: a descriptive review. *Nat Clin Pract Oncol.* 2007;4:643-656.
30. Azorsa DO, Gonzales IM, Basu GD, et al. Synthetic lethal RNAi screening identifies sensitizing targets for gemcitabine therapy in pancreatic cancer. *J Transl Med.* 2009;7:43.
31. Sullivan R, Peppercorn J, Sikora K, et al. Delivering affordable cancer care in high-income countries. *Lancet Oncol.* September 2011;12(10):933-980.
32. Verweij J. Phasing out phase III trials? How much evidence do we need if the target is clearly hit? [abstract]. In: Proceedings of the AACR-NCI-EORTC International Conference on Molecular Targets and Cancer Therapeutics;{{{-4064}}} November 12–16, 2011; San Francisco, CA. Philadelphia (PA): AACR; 2011.
33. ClinicalTrials.gov. An investigational drug, crizotinib (PF-02341066), is being studied in tumors, except non-small cell lung cancer, that are positive for anaplastic lymphoma kinase (ALK). http://clinicaltrials.gov/ct2/show/NCT00932451?term=crizotinib+AND+Anaplastic+Lymphoma+Kinase&rank=5. Accessed February 22, 2011.
34. Clinicaltrials.gov. A study of oral PF-02341066, a c-Met/hepatocyte growth factor tyrosine kinase inhibitor, in patients with advanced cancer. http://clinicaltrials.gov/ct2/show/NCT00585195. Accessed February 22, 2011.
35. Eberhard DA, Giaccone G, Johnson BE; Non-Small-Cell Lung Cancer Working Group. Biomarkers of response to epidermal growth factor receptor inhibitors in Non-Small-Cell Lung Cancer Working Group: standardization for use in the clinical trial setting. *J Clin Oncol.* February 2008;26(6): 983-994.
36. Santis G, Angell R, Nickless G, et al. Screening for EGFR and KRAS mutations in endobronchial ultrasound derived transbronchial needle aspirates in non-small cell lung cancer using COLD-PCR. *PLoS One.* 2011;6(9):e25191.
37. Sun YF, Yang XR, Zhou J, Qiu SJ, Fan J, Xu Y. Circulating tumor cells: advances in detection methods, biological issues, and clinical relevance. *J Cancer Res Clin Oncol.* August 2011;137(8): 1151-1173.
38. György B, Szabó TG, Pásztói M, et al. Membrane vesicles, current state-of-the-art: emerging role of extracellular vesicles. *Cell Mol Life Sci.* August 2011;68(16):2667-2688.
39. Friel AM, Corcoran C, Crown J, O'Driscoll L. Relevance of circulating tumor cells, extracellular nucleic acids, and exosomes in breast cancer. *Breast Cancer Res Treat.* October 2010;123(3):613-625.
40. Wolff AC, Hammond ME, Schwartz JN, et al. American Society of Clinical Oncology/College of American Pathologists guideline recommendations for human epidermal growth factor receptor 2 testing in breast cancer. *J Clin Oncol.* 2007;25(1):118–145.
41. Sauter G, Lee J, Bartlett JM, Slamon DJ, Press MF. Guidelines for human epidermal growth factor receptor 2 testing: biologic and methodologic considerations. *J Clin Oncol.* 2009;27(8):1323-1333.
42. Roche PC, Suman VJ, Jenkins RB, et al. Concordance between local and central laboratory HER2 testing in the breast intergroup trial N9831. *J Natl Cancer Inst.* 2002;94(11):855-857.
43. Paik S, Bryant J, Tan-Chiu E, et al. Real-world performance of HER2 testing: national surgical adjuvant breast and bowel project experience. *J Natl Cancer Inst.* 2002;94(11):852-854.
44. Zujewski JO. "Build quality in"—HER2 testing in the real world. *J Natl Cancer Inst.* 2002;94(11):788-789.
45. Salto-Tellez M, Yau EX, Yan B, Fox SB. Where and by whom should gastric cancer HER2/neu status be assessed? Lessons from breast cancer. *Arch Pathol Lab Med.* June 2011;135(6): 693-695.
46. Bang YJ, Van Cutsem E, Feyereislova A, et al.; ToGA Trial Investigators. Trastuzumab in combination with chemotherapy versus chemotherapy alone for treatment of HER2-positive advanced gastric or gastro-oesophageal junction cancer (ToGA): a phase 3, open-label, randomised controlled trial. *Lancet.* August 2010;376(9742): 687-697.
47. Rosai J. The continuing role of morphology in the molecular age. *Mod Pathol.* 2001;14:258-260.
48. Heffner DK. The end of surgical pathology. *Ann Diagn Pathol.* 2001;5:368-373.
49. Travis WD, Brambilla E, Noguchi M, et al. International Association for the Study of Lung Cancer/American Thoracic Society/European Respiratory Society International Multidisciplinary Classification of Lung Adenocarcinoma. *J Thorac Oncol.* February 2011;6(2):244-285.

50. Amado RG, Wolf M, Peeters M, et al. Wild-type KRAS is required for panitumumab efficacy in patients with metastatic colorectal cancer. *J Clin Oncol.* 2008;26:1626-1634.
51. Jimeno A, Messersmith WA, Hirsch FR, Franklin WA, Eckhardt SG. KRAS mutations and sensitivity to epidermal growth factor receptor inhibitors in colorectal cancer: practical application of patient selection. *J Clin Oncol.* 2009;27:1130-1136.
52. Allegra CJ, Jessup JM, Somerfield MR, et al. American Society of Clinical Oncology provisional clinical opinion: testing for KRAS gene mutations in patients with metastatic colorectal carcinoma to predict response to anti-epidermal growth factor receptor monoclonal antibody therapy. *J Clin Oncol.* 2009;27: 2091-2096.
53. De Roock W, Piessevaux H, De Schutter J, et al. KRAS wild-type state predicts survival and is associated to early radiological response in metastatic colorectal cancer treated with cetuximab. *Ann Oncol.* 2008;19:508-515.
54. Lievre A, Bachet JB, Boige V, et al. KRAS mutations as an independent prognostic factor in patients with advanced colorectal cancer treated with cetuximab. *J Clin Oncol.* 2008;26: 374-379.
55. Lievre A, Bachet JB, Le Corre D, et al. KRAS mutation status is predictive of response to cetuximab therapy in colorectal cancer. *Cancer Res.* 2006;66:3992-3995.
56. Monzon FA, Ogino S, Hammond ME, Halling KC, Bloom KJ, Nikiforova MN. The role of KRAS mutation testing in the management of patients with metastatic colorectal cancer. *Arch Pathol Lab Med.* October 2009;133(10):1600-1606.
57. Whitehall V, Tran K, Umapathy A, et al. A multicenter blinded study to evaluate KRAS mutation testing methodologies in the clinical setting. *J Mol Diagn.* November 2009;11(6):543-552.
58. Molinari F, Felicioni L, Buscarino M, et al. Increased detection sensitivity for KRAS mutations enhances the prediction of anti-EGFR monoclonal antibody resistance in metastatic colorectal cancer. *Clin Cancer Res.* July 2011;17(14):4901-4914.
59. Di Nicolantonio F, Martini M, Molinari F, et al. Wild-type BRAF is required for response to panitumumab or cetuximab in metastatic colorectal cancer. *J Clin Oncol.* December 2008;26(35):5705-5712.
60. Blank PR, Moch H, Szucs TD, Schwenkglenks M. KRAS and BRAF mutation analysis in metastatic colorectal cancer: a cost-effectiveness analysis from a Swiss perspective. *Clin Cancer Res.* October 2011;17(19):6338-6346.
61. Rizzo S, Bronte G, Fanale D, et al. Prognostic vs predictive molecular biomarkers in colorectal cancer: is KRAS and BRAF wild type status required for anti-EGFR therapy? *Cancer Treat Rev.* November 2010;36(suppl 3):S56-S61.
62. Jonker DJ, O'Callaghan CJ, Karapetis CS, et al. Cetuximab for the treatment of colorectal cancer. *N Engl J Med.* November 2007;357(20):2040-2048.
63. Slamon DJ, Leyland-Jones B, Shak S, et al. Concurrent administration of anti-HER2 monoclonal antibody and first-line chemotherapy for HER2-overexpressing metastatic breast cancer. A phase III, multi- national, randomised controlled trial. *N Engl J Med* .2001;344:783-792.
64. Montemurro M, Bauer S. Treatment of gastrointestinal stromal tumor after imatinib and sunitinib. *Curr Opin Oncol.* July 2011;23(4):367-372.
65. Mehta R, Jain RK, Badve S. Personalized medicine: the road ahead. *Clin Breast Cancer.* March 2011;11(1):20-26.
66. Beijnen JH, Schellens JH. Personalized medicine in oncology: a personal view with myths and facts. *Curr Clin Pharmacol.* August 2010;5(3):141-147.
67. Lee AJ, Swanton C. Tumour heterogeneity and drug resistance: personalising cancer medicine through functional genomics. *Biochem Pharmacol. Decem*ber 2011. [Epub ahead of print].
68. Thabut D, Routray C, Lomberk G, et al. Complementary vascular and matrix regulatory pathways underlie the beneficial mechanism of action of sorafenib in liver fibrosis. *Hepatology.* August 2011;54(2):573-585.
69. Mittendorf EA, Wu Y, Scaltriti M, et al. Loss of HER2 amplification following trastuzumab-based neoadjuvant systemic therapy and survival outcomes. *Clin Cancer Res.* December 2009;15(23):7381-7388.
70. Punnoose EA, Atwal SK, Spoerke JM, et al. Molecular biomarker analyses using circulating tumor cells. *PLoS One.* September 2010;5(9):e12517.
71. McDonald SA, Watson MA, Rossi J, Becker CM, Jaques DP, Pfeifer JD. A new paradigm for biospecimen banking in the personalized medicine era. *Am J Clin Pathol.* November 2011;136(5):679-684.
72. Alymani NA, Smith MD, Williams DJ, Petty RD. Predictive biomarkers for personalised anti-cancer drug use: discovery to clinical implementation. *Eur J Cancer.* March 2010;46(5): 869-879.
73. Wistuba II, Gelovani JG, Jacoby JJ, Davis SE, Herbst RS. Methodological and practical challenges for personalized cancer therapies. *Nat Rev Clin Oncol.* March 2011;8(3):135-141.
74. Ross JS, Cronin M. Whole cancer genome sequencing by next-generation methods. *Am J Clin Pathol.* October 2011;136(4):527-539.
75. Harris TJ, McCormick F. The molecular pathology of cancer. *Nat Rev Clin Oncol.* 2010;7:251-265.
76. Paul SM, Mytelka DS, Dunwiddie CT, et al. How to improve R&D productivity: the pharmaceutical industry's grand challenge. *Nat Rev Drug Discov.* March 2010;9(3):203-214.

CHAPTER 19

Molecular Screening, Genetic Counseling, and Cancer Prevention: Lynch Syndrome as a Model

Henry T. Lynch, Carrie L. Snyder, Jane F. Lynch, Stephen Lanspa, and Peter Silberstein

INTRODUCTION

The rapidly evolving hereditary and genomic technologies for cancer risk assessment are revolutionizing cancer control through the diagnosis of hereditary cancer syndromes, their targeted therapy, and cancer screening and management, in accord with newly identified personalized medicine concepts.[1] This approach should be highly efficient. However, particularly at the community level, clinicians may not have the expertise and/or the time required to adequately provide genetic counseling, order DNA tests, and interpret their clinical and genetic/genomic findings. However, genetic counselors and/or centers of cancer genetic expertise can assist the busy clinician in this labor-intensive effort. Centers of expertise may be an academic and community-based health center partnership designed to deliver high-quality evidence-based services, a medical geneticist, and/or genetic counselor. This approach enables the dissemination of potentially effective cancer control measures in the community setting.

NUTS AND BOLTS OF DIAGNOSIS, SCREENING, AND MANAGEMENT

Family History

A comprehensive cancer family history is the linchpin in this cancer control effort; unfortunately, it has often been ignored or insufficiently recorded in patients' medical records, thus compromising the opportunity for hereditary cancer syndrome diagnosis and DNA testing, consequently limiting clinical and molecular translation of its findings to highly targeted surveillance and personalized medical management.[2] It logically follows, however, that once a hereditary cancer syndrome has been identified, at-risk family members must be the first to understand the importance of DNA testing, give signed informed consent, and appreciate fully the need to comply with targeted surveillance and management recommendations in the interest of achieving maximum cancer control benefit.

The nuts and bolts for the collection of a comprehensive cancer family history will necessarily involve the following: (1) provide the patient with detailed information about privacy and confidentiality issues, with the mentioned need for signed informed consent once all questions have been answered; (2) develop rapport with patient and his/her family members and, when possible, their family physicians; (3) construct a comprehensive family history generation by generation by asking questions that help elucidate details regarding accurate genealogy and cancer of *all* anatomic sites; (4) verify pathology of all cancer occurrences whenever possible; (5) meticulously enter these data into a hereditary cancer registry, which may be used for both clinical and research purposes.

The patient's modified nuclear pedigree (Fig. 19.1) is an excellent example of the minimal family history content that is initially required for establishing the vital data

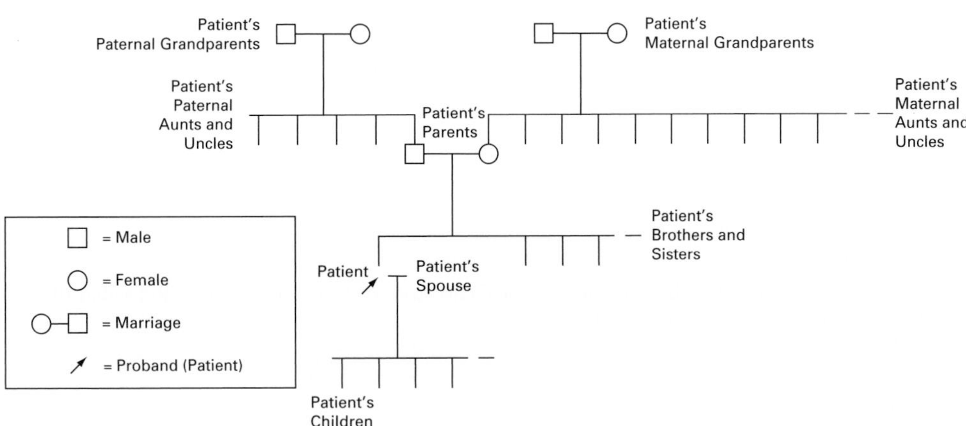

FIGURE 19–1 This portrays the patient's modified nuclear pedigree and represents the minimal amount of information often required to establish a hereditary cancer syndrome diagnosis, starting with the proband's siblings and progeny, then evaluating both maternal and paternal lineage, aunts and uncles, and both sets of grandparents, who then represent greater age with such individuals being more genetically informative, having passed through the cancer risk age. (From Lynch HT, et al. *Surv Dig Dis.* 1984;2:244-260. Reproduced with permission.)

set for the diagnosis of a family with a hereditary cancer predisposition syndrome.[3-5]

However, productive as this process might be, there nevertheless exists a litany of the following obfuscating factors that may confound this entire process: (1) unavailable medical records; (2) small family size; (3) early death of genetically informative relatives from comorbidities other than cancer; (4) failure to investigate diverse cancer types that could be integral to a hereditary cancer syndrome diagnosis, such as carcinoma of the ovary in the hereditary breast–ovarian cancer (HBOC) syndrome; (5) false paternity; (6) failure to disclose vital information because of fear of insurance and/or employment discrimination; (7) emotional distress, including fear that the family's knowledge of its cancer-prone history will potentially result in alienation of parents, progeny, and/or siblings; and (8) adoption.

Extended Pedigrees

Syndrome diagnosis, DNA testing, and cancer control can be maximized to the greatest degree possible when the pedigree is extended. This can then enable more efficient identification and appropriate disclosure of powerful information about the cancer's genotypic and phenotypic features that are part of the germline mutation's clinical expression in the family, inclusive of its penetrance. Importantly, many more high-risk family members may be identified and thereby become candidates for available targeted DNA testing, screening, and management. Such a detailed and time-consuming effort is frequently performed as part of a research program concerning the natural history and the phenotypic and genotypic heterogeneity of the hereditary syndrome.

Pedigrees Featuring Clinical Nuances of Phenotypic and Genotypic Heterogeneity

Figures 19.2–19.8 describe certain clinical genetic variations in Lynch syndrome (LS) pedigrees and portray the clinical nuances that the clinician and genetic counselor are likely to encounter when evaluating these patients/families.

Once entered into a hereditary cancer family registry, this information can be of critical long-term value to clinicians, patients, and cancer genetic researchers. The construction of such a comprehensive cancer family history should not be treated as a mere pedantic exercise, since the identification of a hereditary cancer-prone family enables a team approach with potential for highly targeted molecularly based counseling, surveillance, management, and psychological help for many at-risk family members. In the case of LS, our hereditary cancer model, Table 19.1 depicts its cardinal clinical, pathologic, and molecular genetic diagnostic features.

Figure 19.2 depicts a classical LS pedigree wherein the *MLH1* mismatch repair (MMR) mutation segregated with LS's integral cancers through four generations. Note in particular the extremely early ages of cancer onset and metachronous colorectal cancer (CRC) occurrences (III-1 and III-4), which are highly characteristic for LS and which fit the Amsterdam criteria.

Figure 19.3 is an LS pedigree wherein the proband manifested Muir-Torre syndrome's cutaneous stigmata and both he (III-2) and his son (IV-2) were carriers of the *MSH2* germline mutation. Of interest is the finding of prostate cancer in the proband and son in addition to pancreatic cancer in the proband. Noteworthy was early-onset cancer of the transverse colon and prostate in his son (IV-2), and CRC at age 35 in a second son (IV-3).

TABLE 19–1 Cardinal Features of Lynch Syndrome

- Autosomal dominant inheritance pattern seen for syndrome cancers in the family pedigree
- Earlier average age of CRC onset than in the general population:
  average age of 45 y in Lynch syndrome vs. 63 y in the general population
- Proximal (right-sided) colonic cancer predilection:
  70–85% of Lynch syndrome CRCs are proximal to the splenic flexure
- Accelerated carcinogenesis (tiny adenomas can develop into carcinomas more quickly):
  within 2–3 y in Lynch syndrome vs. 8–10 y in the general population
- High risk of additional CRCs:
  25–30% of patients having surgery for a Lynch syndrome–associated CRC will have a second primary CRC within 10 y of surgical resection if the surgery was less than a subtotal colectomy
- Increased risk for malignancy at certain extracolonic sites:
  - endometrium (40–60% lifetime risk for female mutation carriers)
  - ovary (12–15% lifetime risk for female mutation carriers)
  - stomach (higher risk in families indigenous to the Orient, reason unknown at this time)
  - small bowel
  - hepatobiliary tract
  - pancreas
  - upper uro-epithelial tract (transitional cell carcinoma of the ureter and renal pelvis)
  - prostate cancer
  - breast cancer
  - adrenal cortical carcinomas
  - brain (glioblastomas in the Turcot's syndrome variant of the Lynch syndrome)
- Sebaceous adenomas, sebaceous carcinomas, and multiple keratoacanthomas in the Muir-Torre syndrome variant of Lynch syndrome
- Pathology of CRCs is more often poorly differentiated, with an excess of mucoid and signet-cell features, a Crohn's-like reaction, and a significant excess of infiltrating lymphocytes within the tumor
- Increased survival from CRC
- The sine qua non for diagnosis of Lynch syndrome is the identification of a germline mutation in a mismatch repair gene (most commonly *MLH1*, *MSH2*, or *MSH6*) that segregates in the family: i.e., members who carry the mutation show a much higher rate of syndrome-related cancers than those who do not carry the mutation

CRC, colorectal cancer.

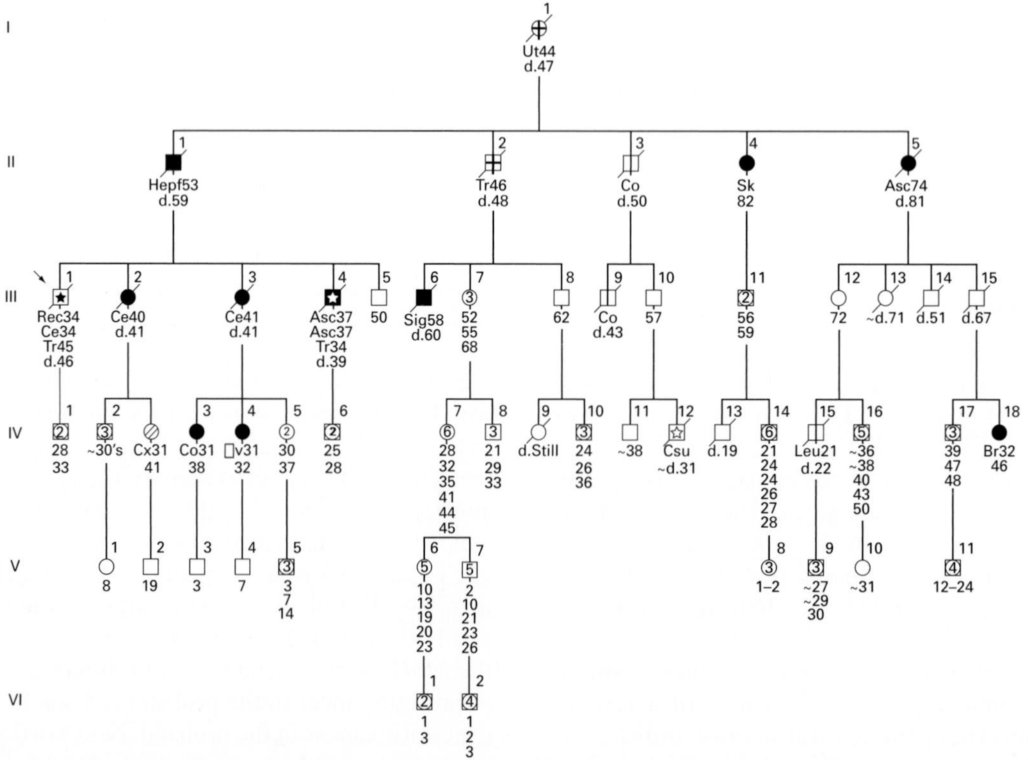

FIGURE 19–2 A classical Lynch syndrome family with verification through multiple cases with the *MLH1* mismatch repair germline mutation.

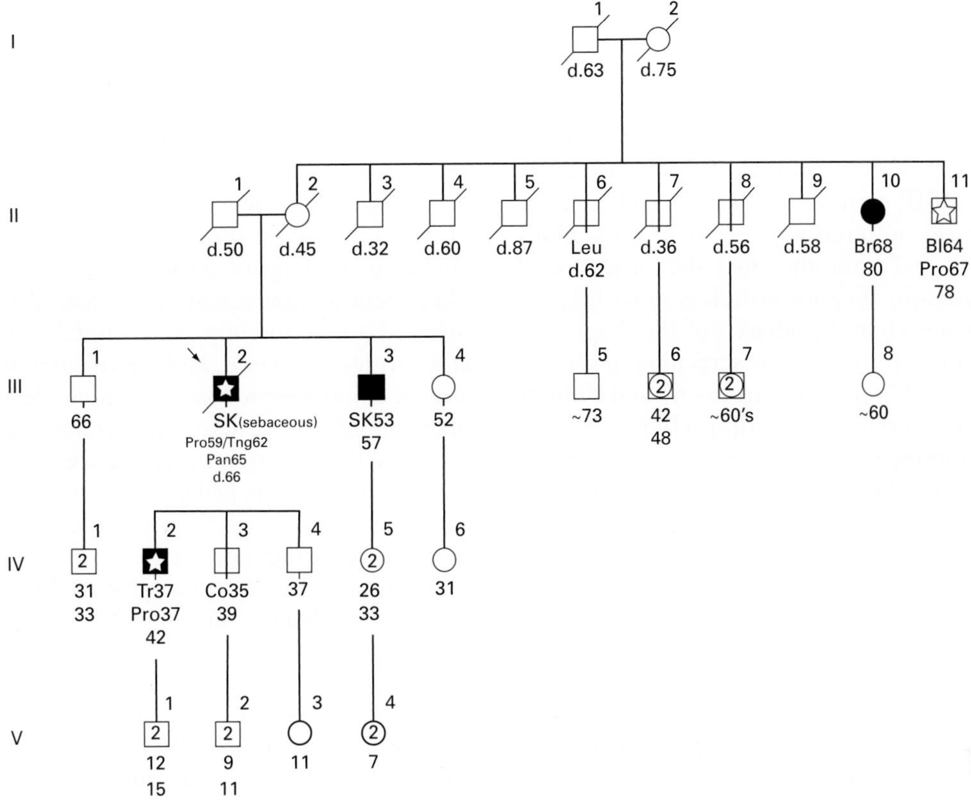

FIGURE 19–3 This is another example of the Muir-Torre variant of Lynch syndrome, with genetic confirmation by virtue of the *MSH2* mutation. Note the occurrence of prostate cancer with early onset in the proband and his son, diagnosed at age 37.

Figure 19.4 is a pedigree that contains integral LS cancers through three generations, including metachronous classic early-onset colorectal and endometrial cancer in the proband (III-1). However, three individuals (II-2, II-3, and III-1) have been tested for MMR germline mutations, but a deleterious mutation was not found. One possibility is that we may be dealing with the epithelial cell adhesion molecule (*EPCAM*)

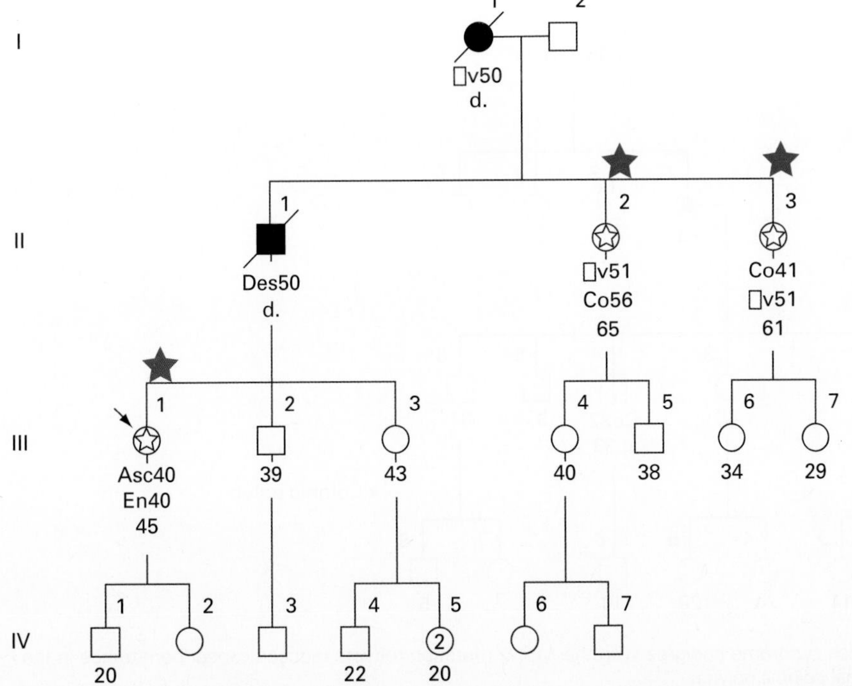

FIGURE 19–4 This is an example of a Lynch syndrome family with a classical phenotype but in which evaluations by several different highly competent laboratories have failed to identify mismatch repair mutations. Stars indicate individuals who have been tested.

gene and its LS connection.[6] While sporadic cancer or chance may be a remote possibility for this familial aggregation, we still must consider strongly that we may be dealing with a hereditary variant of LS and therein we should use the same screening and management strategies that we would use for a classical LS family with an MMR germline mutation. Such families are frequently encountered as a result of meticulous pedigree studies, and while they may defy evidence of a germline mutation, they nevertheless must be provided genetic counseling, be advised of the diagnostic limitations, and receive advice for screening and management of high-risk individuals (progeny and siblings of affected) in the interest of caution. High-risk individuals are encouraged to follow these intense screening measures while the search for a genetic mutation continues, through newly developed molecular genetic technologies.

Figure 19.5 is an LS pedigree with an *MSH2* germline mutation. The mother (III-2) of the proband (IV-1) has colonic adenomas but as yet no evidence of cancer. This finding may suggest reduced penetrance, a phenomenon that often poses a dilemma when attempting to establish a diagnosis. However, based upon her position in the pedigree, she is classified as an obligate gene carrier. It is noteworthy that III-2's father (II-1) and paternal grandmother (I-1) had colon cancer as did the proband's brother (IV-4), with their early ages of onset that fit the LS diagnosis. The mother's (III-2) absence of CRC may also be due to reduced penetrance and/or compliance with colonoscopy, with polypectomy providing primary prevention of CRC.

Figure 19.6 involves a knowledgeable dermatologist who diagnosed the Muir-Torre syndrome based on cutaneous findings of sebaceous tumors in his 34-year-old patient and immediately considered LS and recommended a colonoscopy. An early CRC was diagnosed and surgically excised, and appropriate follow-up with annual colonoscopies was recommended. This finding of carcinoma of the descending colon at age 39 was followed by DNA testing with evidence of an *MSH2* mutation. Looking at this pedigree, genetic testing would not have been considered and the proband would not have been aware of the increased risk of colon cancer if the dermatologist had not recommended the colonoscopy. Now, the proband's entire family can benefit from this knowledge.

Figure 19.7 shows a classical phenotypic setting of cancer expression consonant with an LS diagnosis. Interestingly, the proband (IV-2) was tested in the year 2000 with no mutation identified. However, her mother was tested in early 2008 with an initial finding of an

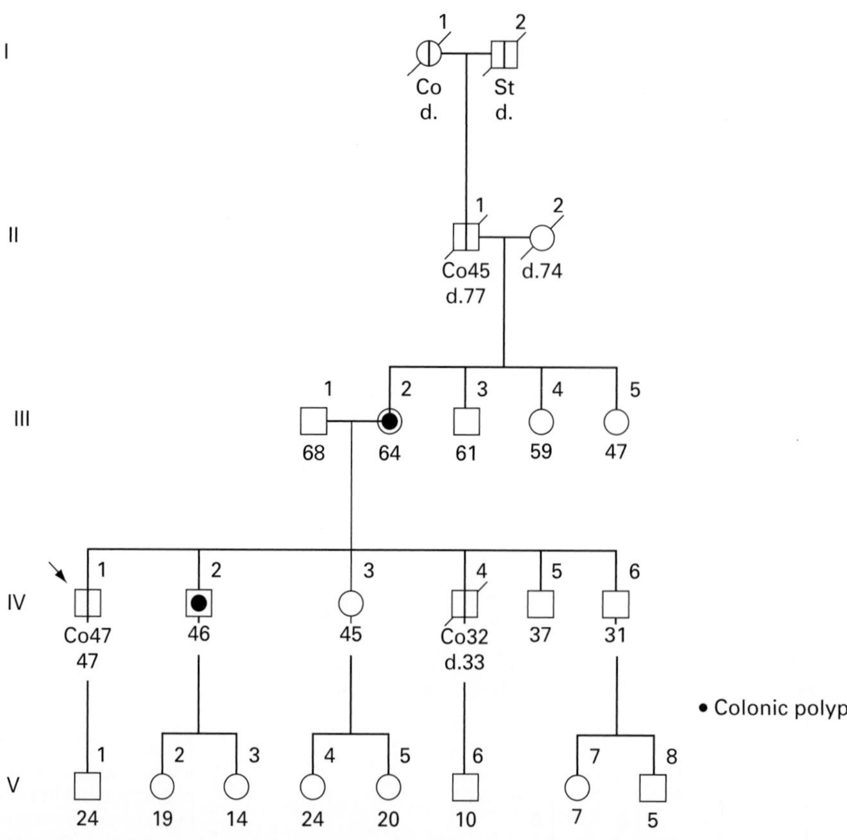

FIGURE 19–5 This example of a classical Lynch syndrome pedigree with the *MSH2* mutation reflects reduced cancer penetrance in the proband's mother. Note also a history of occasional colonic polyps.

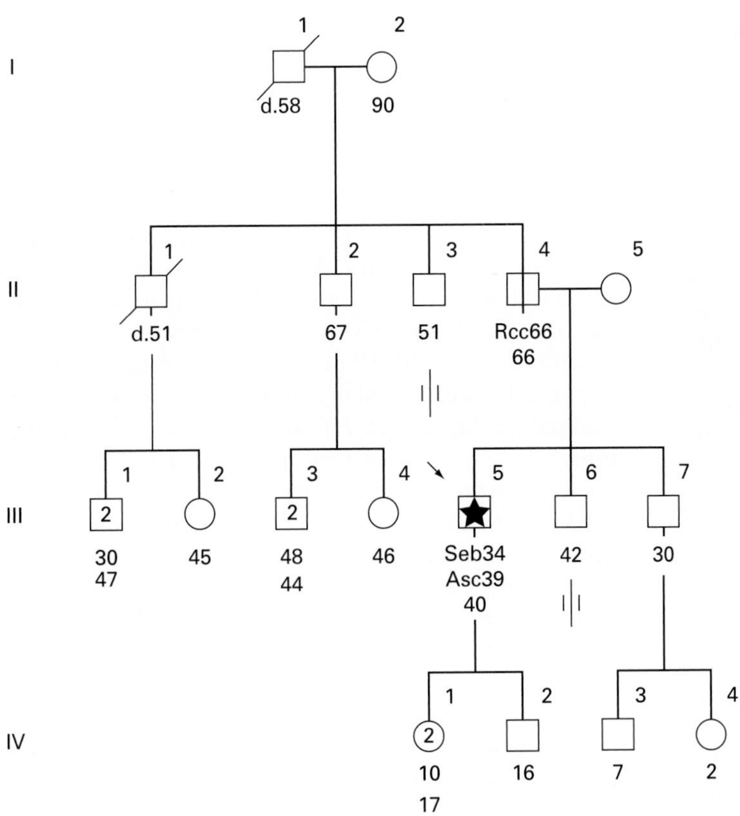

FIGURE 19–6 This is an example of a family wherein a dermatologist recognized the Muir-Torre syndrome significance of sebaceous carcinoma and recommended colonoscopy with finding of early-onset colorectal cancer. Note that the *MSH2* mutation was present in the proband.

MMR germline mutation in which the *MSH2* gene was completely deleted. In late 2008, it was discovered that a deletion in the *EPCAM* gene can cause the inactivation of *MSH2*, and it was confirmed that this is what had occurred in the mother.

EPCAM and LS

The underlying molecular defect responsible for a portion of Amsterdam criteria families without an identified MMR mutation is a mutation in the *EPCAM* gene,

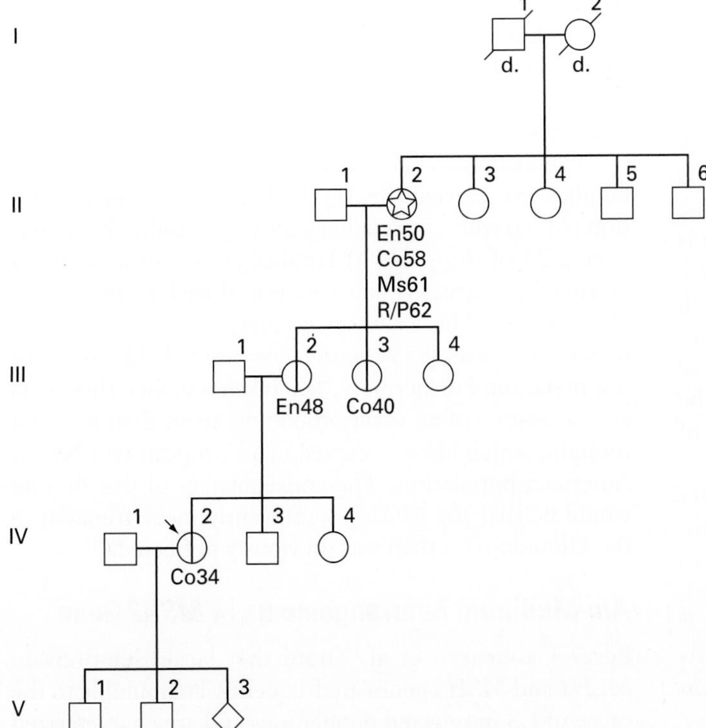

FIGURE 19–7 The proband with early-onset colorectal cancer was tested for a mismatch repair mutation in 2000 with lack of evidence for the same. However, we see that the results of her mother's test in 2008 are reported as deletion of the entire *MSH2* mismatch repair gene. Later in 2008, this was attributed to an upstream mutation on the *EPCAM* gene which silences the *MSH2* gene.

located immediately 5′ of *MSH2*.[6-8] A germline deletion removing the 3′ end of *EPCAM* results in tissue-specific methylation and silencing of the otherwise intact *MSH2* gene.

Ligtenberg et al.[6] were the first to describe a subset of families with cancer-prone phenotypes consonant with LS which included microsatellite instability (MSI) and immunohistochemistry (IHC) wherein a deletion at the 3′ end of the gene encoding EPCAM was identified. These individuals with *EPCAM* mutations harbored MSI-H and therein IHC tests showed a loss of MSH2 protein in the absence of an identifiable mutation of the *MSH2* gene.[6,7] Importantly, the *EPCAM* mutations co-segregated with the LS phenotype in approximately 19% of LS families that lacked *MLH1/MSH2* mutations.[7] *EPCAM* deletions accounted for about 2.3% of explained MSH2-deficient families.[9]

EPCAM deletions encompass its transcription termination (polyadenylation) signal, permitting transcription to proceed from *EPCAM* downstream across the intervening sequence into *MSH2*, essentially overriding the *MSH2* promoter. This results in promoter methylation and *MSH2* gene silencing. However, since expression of the *EPCAM* gene is restricted primarily to epithelial tissues, it therefore appears to be the inactivation of *MSH2* in deletion carriers. Thus, the functional impact that germline *EPCAM* deletions have on *MSH2* activity is confined to epithelial tissues, such as colonic mucosa. This in turn appears to influence the phenotypic expression associated with this type of mutation.

EPCAM deletion carriers may have phenotypic features that differ from carriers of *MSH2* mutations, namely, an almost exclusive expression of cancers in the colon and rectum, with a paucity of endometrial cancers. CRC occurs in *EPCAM* deletion–positive individuals with a frequency comparable to that of carriers of an *MSH2* mutation. Of great interest, however, is the minimal risk of endometrial cancer in individuals with some *EPCAM* deletions when compared with *MSH2* mutation carriers. Importantly, though, when the *EPCAM* gene extends into, or in close proximity to, the *MSH2* gene, the risk of endometrial cancer becomes equivalent to that with *MSH2* mutations, a higher risk than in those whose deletion is farther from *MSH2*. Determination of the precise boundaries of deletions involving *EPCAM* is likely to be of importance for personalized clinical management of these families.

We have studied an extremely large family (Fig. 19.8) containing more than 700 individuals wherein 50 individuals manifested CRC.[10] A deletion confined to *EPCAM* was identified in this highly extended kindred, which has been studied by us for more than 35 years.[10] The breadth and size of this *EPCAM*-prone family is testament to the potential impact of a single mutation event.[10]

FOUNDER MUTATIONS

American Founder Mutation of *MSH2*

Wagner et al.,[11] working on DNA from families with phenotypes consistent with LS, noted that *MSH2* and *MLH1* mutations had been found in approximately two-thirds of Amsterdam criteria–positive families and in much lower percentages of the Amsterdam criteria–negative families, thereby recognizing that a considerable proportion of such LS families were not able to be accounted for with the major MMR genes. They therefore analyzed 59 clinically well-defined families from the Creighton resource for *MSH2*, *MLH1*, and *MSH6* germline mutations. Findings showed that approximately 27% of the mutations were genomic rearrangements (12 in *MSH2* and 2 in *MLH1*), and notably the deletion encompassing exons 1 to 6 of *MSH2* was detected in seven apparently unrelated families (12% of the total cohort) and was subsequently found to be a founder mutation. This work led to the identification of a "... common North American deletion in *MSH2*, accounting for ~ 10% of [the] cohort. Genealogical, molecular, and haplotype studies showed that this deletion represents a North American founder mutation that could be traced back to the 19th century."[11]

Lynch et al.[12] provided further description of the prevalence of the large genomic deletion encompassing exons 1 to 6 of the *MSH2* gene, found to be widespread in the US population as the result of a founder effect. These investigators concluded that there was a high frequency and continent-wide geographic distribution of a cancer-predisposing founder mutation "... of the *MSH2* gene in a large, outbred (as opposed to genetically isolated) population, and the ease with which the mutation can be detected, suggest that the routine testing of individuals at risk for HNPCC [LS] in the United States should include an assay for this mutation until more is learned about its occurrence."[12]

Clendenning et al.[13] described the detection of 32 new families that carried the *MSH2* American founder mutation (AFM) wherein detailed genealogic studies have connected 27 of the 41 AFM families known to date into 7 extended pedigrees. They were traced back to around the 18th century. These authors predicted an age of approximately 500 years (95% confidence interval, 425–625) for this mutation. Furthermore, "... Taken together, these data are suggestive of an earlier founding event than was first thought, which likely occurred in a European or a Native American population. The consequences of this finding would be that the AFM is significantly more frequent in the United States than was previously predicted."[13]

Alu-Mediated Rearrangements in *MSH2* Gene

Pérez-Cabornero et al.[14] note that large deletions in *MLH1* and *MSH2* genes are frequently attributable to the cause of LS in selected populations and are characterized

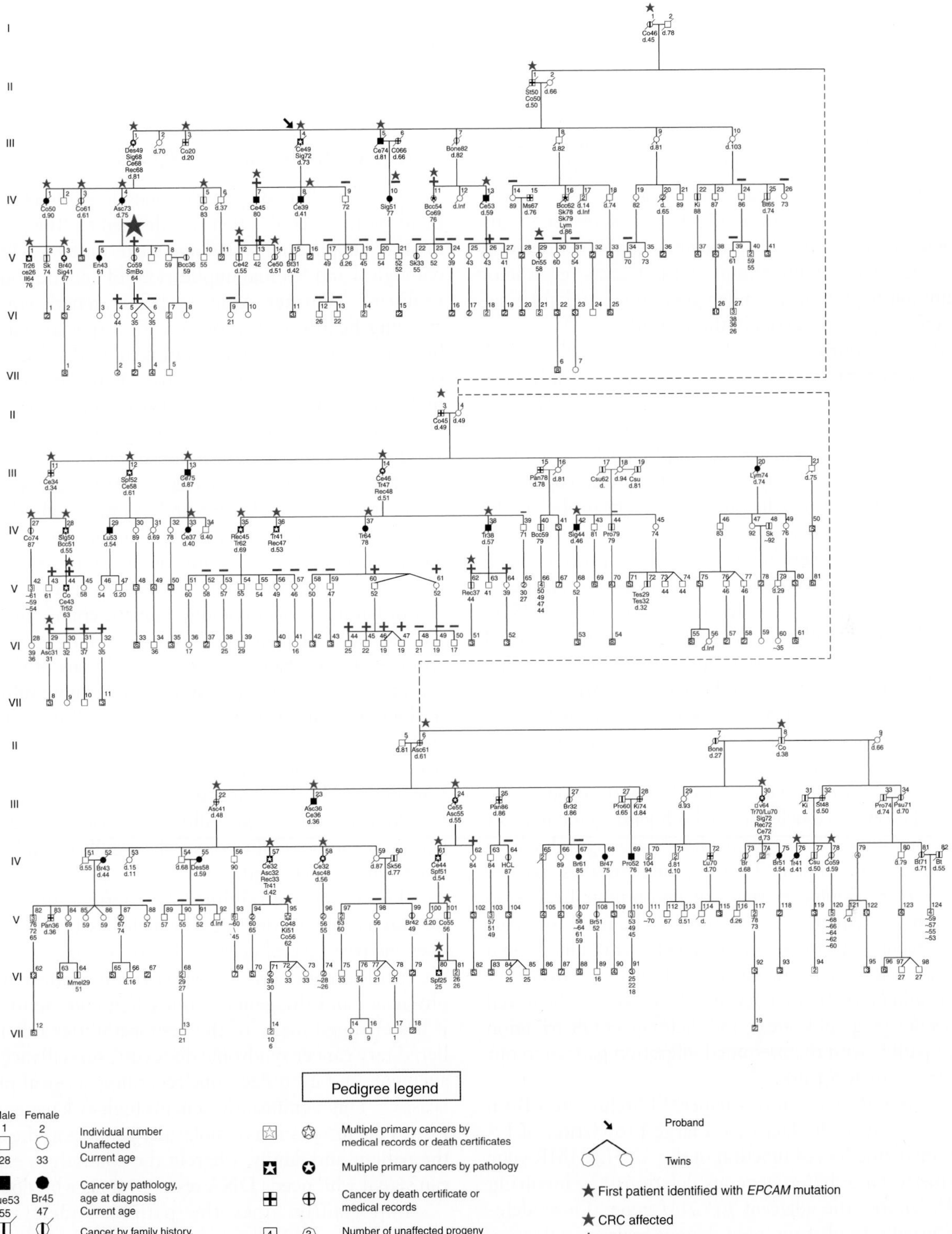

Pedigree legend

Male Female
1 2 Individual number
Unaffected
28 33 Current age

Lue53 Br45 Cancer by pathology, age at diagnosis
55 47 Current age

d.54 d.86 Cancer by family history, age at death

Multiple primary cancers by medical records or death certificates

Multiple primary cancers by pathology

Cancer by death certificate or medical records

4 3 Number of unaffected progeny (both sexes)

Proband

Twins

★ First patient identified with *EPCAM* mutation

★ CRC affected

+ *EPCAM*

FIGURE 19–8 This is an example of the recently identified *EPCAM* mutation that portrays a family with site-specific colorectal cancer (CRC). Noteworthy is the absence of extracolonic cancers including the second most common cancer in Lynch syndrome, namely endometrial carcinoma. (Published with permission from Lynch HT, et al. *Am J Gastroenterol.* 2011;106:1829-1836. Copyright © 2003 American College of Gastroenterology; published by Elsevier Science, Inc.)

by "... break point determination, haplotype analysis, and genotype-phenotype correlation ...." Their study involved 303 patients from 160 suspected LS unrelated families, all of whom were evaluated using heteroduplex analysis by capillary array electrophoresis. "... More than 16% (24 of 160) of the families had pathogenic mutations (8 *MLH1*, 15 *MSH2*, and 1 *MSH6*). Twelve of these families (50%) are carriers of a novel mutation. Seven of the 15 positive *MSH2* families (47%) are carriers of a rearrangement. The exon 7 deletion and exon 4 to 8 deletion of *MSH2* are new founder mutations. The segregation of a common haplotype, a similar phenotype, and anticipation effects were observed in these families ...."

Pérez-Cabornero et al.[14] note that as much as 15% of all pathogenic mutations in *MSH2* and *MLH1*[15] are caused by gross genomic rearrangements in MMR gene alterations, which account for traditional methods of mutation analysis. They have employed heteroduplex analytic methods, namely capillary array electrophoresis coupled with multiplex ligation-dependent probe amplification, previously described,[16] wherein numerous differing mutations were identified, a high proportion of which were rearrangements found in the *MSH2* gene. They described two founder mutations in the *MSH2* gene wherein a similar break point was identified in all of the index cases of the carrier family. They conclude that "... These mutations seem to be associated with founder effects, as a common haplotype was associated with each; besides, the normal exon 4 to 8 deletion seems to be associated with anticipation."

Pérez-Cabornero et al.[14] conclude that the exon 7 deletion and exon 4 to 8 deletion are both pathogenic founder mutations involved in causing LS in a geographic area located in central Spain. Therein, their findings indicate that "... large genomic rearrangements occur in these genes with a high frequency and emphasize the need to incorporate techniques to randomly detect them. This should facilitate the genetic diagnosis of Lynch syndrome ... The origin of *MSH2* founder rearrangement can be linked to specific geographic areas, and their current distribution is compatible with the presumed migration pattern in our country (namely Spain) ...."

In an editorial[17] on this paper,[14] Hitchins and Burn call attention to the fact that a large proportion of LS cases involving loss of function of the *MSH2* MMR gene are due to large heterogeneous deletions "... involving *MSH2* and/or the adjacent *EPCAM* gene. These deletions usually result from homologous malrecombination events between *Alu* elements, a family of short interspersed nuclear elements (SINE). Recent recognition of the extent of these deletions influences phenotypic outcome provided new impetus for fine-mapping the break points ...." Hitchins and Burn credit the work of Pérez-Cabonero et al.[14] as uncovering new evidence for *Alu*-mediated ancestral founder mutation, which they describe as the first such finding that has led to a revisitation of the role of *Alu* elements as causal factors in LS. Furthermore, they raise the question as to whether *Alu* density "... is a danger sign for genomic regions prone to rearrangement and what additional factors may be required to actuate these events remain to be discovered ...."[17]

GENETIC COUNSELING AND TESTING

Aronson,[18] in defining genetic counseling, offers the statement by Resta et al.[19] that it is defined as "the process of helping people understand and adapt to the medical psychological and familial implications of genetic conditions to disease." Further, Aronson defines genetic counselors as being health professionals with a specialized degree in genetics and counseling and who work as an integral component of a multidisciplinary team for counseling high-risk individuals who may harbor a personal or family history suspicious for a specific hereditary syndrome.

Personalized genetic counseling that includes an explanation of the disorder's natural history, DNA testing implications, risk evaluation and its impact on other family members, coupled with its recommended screening and management implications is imperative when there is discovery of a family history consonant with a hereditary or familial cancer etiology. Genetic counseling should always take place *prior* to DNA testing. This must include an in-depth coverage of the pros and cons of the DNA testing process, so that the patient can be more fully aware of the potential for discrimination regarding insurability and/or employment, which is more often a function of patients' perception than fact; other factors include emotional insecurity, fear, anxiety, apprehension, and expense, should a deleterious germline mutation be discovered, and even the possibility of survivor guilt should a negative result be identified.[3,5]

The clinical discipline of genetic counseling for hereditary cancer disorders, which has been emerging over the past several decades, has been a true blessing to the medical geneticist, cancer specialist, family practice physician, and the genetic counseling community, since it has changed many of the responsibilities inherent in hereditary cancer syndrome discovery, surveillance, management, and even decisions regarding surgical prophylaxis.[20-22] This significantly benefits high-risk patients, as it fosters the integration of molecular genetics at the level of the patient and family, wherein the counselor's expertise can signal who needs DNA testing versus who does not.[4]

Importantly, does the patient understand the intended message? The answer clearly relates to his/her health educational level, which might be limited to, for example, only the fourth- to sixth-grade level. If the counselor assumes a much higher health care literacy level, the counseling message will be wholly ineffective. It is at this level that simple models may provide an effective basis for communication when describing the clinical implications for DNA testing, coupled with hereditary cancer transmission. Such a model, for example, may involve a drawing clearly depicting the portion of the patient's own family pedigree highlighting the history of cancer, thereby making for a more personal impact of this knowledge.

DNA Testing for Pathogenic Germline Mutations

Testing for most of the known cancer-causing germline mutations is often available commercially in molecular genetic laboratories and/or on a research basis. Once such a mutation has been identified in a family, at-risk relatives can then be tested and classified with greater precision as carriers or non-carriers of the deleterious mutation.

But how can genetic testing in a genetically informative family member alter the risk status assessment of other family members? Watson et al.[23] partially answered this question by showing how the presence of cancer-associated mutations in certain family members and their close relatives could determine carrier risk status changes leading from risk uncertainty to certainty, namely to carrier or non-carrier status, even in patients' more distant relatives. These findings harbor practical clinical implications for the intrinsic application of knowledge about the importance of germline cancer-causing mutations for virtually all forms of hereditary cancer. Specifically, such risk status changes can impact cancer prevention recommendations among likely germline mutation carriers versus non-carriers, given their respective requirements for confirmatory DNA testing and heightened cancer prevention, based upon mutation findings in their relatives. In the ideal situation, a diligent family history collection, coupled with its meticulous assessment, with appropriate DNA testing, followed by its vital clinical translation, will often enable one to inform untested family members about possible changes in their carrier risk status attributed to results from mutation testing of their relatives.

Occasionally, those who undergo genetic counseling and testing for a pathogenic mutation will receive nondiagnostic or equivocal results, such as "no mutation found" or a finding of a "variant of uncertain significance." Thus, the stakes are often high for patients and families, with respect to whether inherited susceptibility can be confirmed or not. Considering the host of technical, logistic, psychosocial, and economic challenges that exist in genetic counseling and testing for hereditary cancer syndrome susceptibility, the preliminary question is, "Who needs to be tested?"[4] A related question is, "Which hereditary disorder is most likely to be present and which pathogenic germline mutation is most likely the culprit?" Perhaps due to the technical complexities of testing and counseling, these questions may at first be intimidating to many genetic counselors and clinicians, including even those who are medical geneticists.[4]

In the ideal clinical setting, the pathogenic mutation accounting for cancer susceptibility in a given family will have already been identified with confirmation in an affected family member. The discovery of a pathogenic mutation will have the highest yield through the testing of an individual in whom the disease shows an early age of onset, bilaterality, or association with other integral syndrome cancers. Therein, DNA testing should be done on such a genetically informative individual only after appropriate genetic counseling.

Ladabaum et al.[24] investigated cost-effectiveness of a Markov model to identify LS considering attention to sex, age at screening, and differential effects for probands and relatives. The target population comprised all those with newly diagnosed CRC and their relatives. The time horizon was lifetime, and the perspective was third-party payer. The outcome measures were life-years, cancer cases and deaths, and costs coupled with incremental cost-effectiveness ratios. The results considered current rates of germline testing, screening, and prophylactic surgery, which "... reduced deaths from colorectal cancer by 7% to 42% and deaths from endometrial and ovarian cancer by 1% to 6%. Among tumor-testing strategies, immunohistochemistry followed by *BRAF* mutation testing for all persons with CRC was preferred, with an incremental cost-effectiveness ratio of $36 200 per life-year gained." The authors concluded that widespread CRC testing led to LS diagnosis yielding substantial benefits at acceptable cost. This was particularly noteworthy for women with an LS mutation, enabling them to begin regular screening and consider the option of risk-reducing gynecologic surgery, with the result of cost-effectiveness of this testing which was dependent on the participation among relatives at risk for LS.

In an accompanying editorial, Burt[25] notes that the cost-effectiveness of these approaches "... was very sensitive to the number of relatives who would undergo mutation-specific testing after disease-causing mutation was found in an index case. It is interesting that success of tumor testing first has already led some institutions and health policy organizations to recommend MSI or IHC testing in all patients with colon cancer and perhaps in all women with endometrial cancer to find those who should then have genetic testing for Lynch syndrome."[26-28]

Genetic Counseling: Medical, Legal, and Ethical Considerations

Medical geneticists and genetic counselors, while more often available in many urban centers in the United States, may be rare or even nonexistent in small cities and in rural communities. Nevertheless, the extreme clinical importance of genomic findings demands that the patient receive this information in a timely manner and, at the same time, be made aware of the full need for and the medical significance of screening and management recommendations should they manifest a pathogenic mutation. Their emotional needs must be met and they must not only appreciate the impact of the finding of this deleterious mutation in them and their close relatives but, moreover, also be fully cognizant of the need to share this knowledge with close as well as distant relatives, whenever this is possible, so that its life-saving benefit may be pursued.

While this material may be highly complex, it clearly would be best handled in a patient- or family-centered setting. However, as already mentioned, such a structured genetic counseling setting may be exceedingly difficult to find for those patients scattered across the United States in rural communities, so that the second best approach may necessitate telephonic disclosure of the results. Such a study was mounted by Rice et al.[29] involving 228 female study participants who completed retrospective, self-administered mailed surveys pertinent to telephonic disclosure of their pre-test genetic counseling results, which revealed an absence of any significant problem between result disclosure methods and the outcome variables investigated. Furthermore, "... A majority (90%) of individuals who received positive results by telephone returned for follow up visits. Factors which genetic counselors believed [to have] influenced their clinical decision to offer telephone disclosure, such as history of breast cancer, a priori risk of genetic mutation and family history of known mutation were not shown to significantly impact the actual disclosure method ...." The authors concluded that such telephone disclosure of DNA test results was clinically appropriate "... when counselors utilize their clinical judgment to determine which patients are appropriate candidates."

Genetic Counseling and Testing of Children

The genetic testing of children has special considerations.[30] Specifically, it must strike a balance relevant to the child's autonomy versus the early onset of a particular hereditary disorder such as colorectal adenomas at a relatively early age and its subsequent CRC risk, as in familial adenomatous polyposis (FAP), thereby indicating the importance of early genetic testing versus diseases of later onset where the premorbid diagnostic features may only rarely occur.

In a setting in which one encounters an early-onset cancer, in those cases where children are at increased risk for early-onset disease, even when no treatment is available, the American Medical Association (AMA) suggests that the option of testing the child should be placed at the discretion of the parents.[31] Offit and Thom[30] note that the American College of Medical Genetics is perhaps more open to testing children when the balance of harms and benefits is uncertain. They also note that the American Society for Clinical Oncology (ASCO) recommends that the decision for testing of potentially affected children should take into account the availability of evidence-based risk-reduction strategies, coupled with the problem of developing a malignancy during childhood.

Discrimination Concerns: Genetic Information Nondiscrimination Act

The potential of health insurance discrimination based on genetic information remains a concern for individuals who undergo genetic testing for their cancer risk. The Genetic Information Nondiscrimination Act (GINA) was signed into law on May 21, 2008.[32,33] As summarized by the Department of Health and Human Services, GINA is a new Federal law that prohibits discrimination in health coverage and employment based on genetic information. GINA, along with the Health Insurance Portability and Accountability Act (HIPAA),[34] prohibits health insurers from requesting or requiring genetic information from an individual or their family members to use for decisions regarding coverage, rates, or preexisting conditions. This law applies to group and individual health insurers. GINA also prohibits most employers from using genetic information for hiring, firing, promotion decisions, or any other issues regarding terms of employment.

GINA does not apply to members of the US Military, to veterans obtaining health care through the Veteran's Administration, or to the Indian Health Service. It also does not include protection from genetic discrimination in life insurance, disability insurance, or long-term care insurance.

ETHICAL AND REGULATORY ISSUES IN DIRECT-TO-CONSUMER PERSONAL GENOME TESTING

Advances in molecular genetic technology and its recognition by consumers have led to genetic testing companies offering direct-to-consumer (DTC) testing through kits sold on the Internet. Pirzadeh-Miller et al.[35] discuss the pros and cons of DTC genetic testing. These authors take the position that many of the DTC tests "... are of questionable accuracy and utility and combine tests that provide mundane information about genetic traits with those for serious genetic conditions with life-threatening implications for the patient and the entire family ... Numerous studies have shown that average patients and clinicians are not well versed on even the most basic elements of genetic testing and result interpretation. It is even less likely that consumers and clinicians will understand the subtle differences between DTC companies and tests—particularly genomic profiling based on single nucleotide polymorphisms (SNPs)—which are offered by most DTC companies ...." Furthermore, these authors note that the US General Accounting Office concluded that such tests were "... 'misleading and of little or no practical use.'[36] The risk profiles provided by such companies have been described as having 'no predictive value' and may falsely alarm or reassure consumers."[37] These authors conclude that it will be important that those patients who inquire about DTC genetic testing for cancer risk "... should be cautioned that the information they receive may be inaccurate and misleading ... Potential benefit and minimization of harm can be facilitated by involvement of qualified genetics professionals to allow for appropriate test interpretation in the context of medical and family histories."[35]

Samuel et al.[38] discuss DTC personal genome testing (PGT) screening of customers' genomes with the intent of identifying single nucleotide polymorphisms

(SNPs) that may be predisposing to differing hereditary disorders, inclusive of cancer. While DTC-PGT is a relatively new program, its technology will likely show rapid expansion commensurate with consumers' desire to learn more about their genetic profile. They have provided an overview dealing with the broader ethical and regulatory issues promulgated by personal genome tests that are marketed directly to the public, all in concert with information about health risks. These authors conclude that those companies that market DTC-PGT are obligated to ensure "... balanced and understandable information to consumers and should offer only genetic tests that have been properly evaluated. The goal of regulation should be to reduce the potential harms of DTC-PGT through a range of measures that is consistent with the goals of the consumer movement and with the ethics of health professions. The best policy outcomes are likely to emerge from constructive engagement between the health professions, consumer organizations, industry and international regulatory bodies ...." We subscribe fully to this admonition. We believe that such an offering of DTC-PGT should be preceded by genetic counseling coupled with further genetic counseling once the results of the DTC-PGT become available to the patient. Clearly, the patient must be fully apprised of the full significance of a deleterious cancer-causing germline mutation prior to subscribing to testing and in follow-up genetic counseling. If positive for the test, the patient will need full disclosure of available screening and management options, should they exist; if negative for the test, they must realize that their cancer risk is in accord with general population estimates for the particular cancer and they must be told how and when screening and management is indicated.

PRACTICAL EDUCATIONAL/COUNSELING EXAMPLES

New Innovative Education Method

Manne et al.[39] studied the need for creating alternative educational messages for implementation of cancer control, particularly for CRC in LS. This involved the development of a self-administered computer-based strategy, namely, a CD-ROM intervention for educational messages directed at patients with suspected LS regarding MSI and IHC testing. Findings showed that in the education plus CD-ROM setting, there was a significant increase in knowledge about MSI and IHC tests, inclusive of greater satisfaction with the preparation for decision making relevant to testing, with a lower decisional conflict and greater decisional self-efficacy. These authors concluded that "Incorporation of new media education strategies for individuals at risk for LS may be a valuable component of the informed consent process. As clinical criteria for MSI and IHC testing continue to expand, the need for alternative educational approaches to meet this increased demand could be met by the self-administered computer-based strategy ...." Clearly, their study demonstrated that all of the high-risk patients with CRC can benefit from a computer-based multimedia intervention.[39] This is important, given the fact that some investigators are recommending expanded MSI testing for all CRC patients.[40-42] The CD could be easily adapted, should MSI testing become routine before adjuvant chemotherapy.[43] Finally, informed consent may be indicated for MSI testing,[44] although in clinical practice these recommendations remain inconsistent. However, patient knowledge is rather limited about the MSI test, particularly about its purpose and implications.[45]

Family Information Service

The Family Information Service (FIS) is an extremely valuable application of an expanded genetic counseling model enabling one to communicate effectively with a large number of family members who have gathered together as a group, particularly once a deleterious germline mutation has been identified in the family.[46] This approach to hereditary cancer education, DNA testing, and cancer control has many advantages: (1) It enables a physician, genetic counselor, or other key members of the cancer genetics team to explain fully what it means to be at increased cancer risk based upon the presence of a significant cancer family history and/or a cancer-causing germline mutation. (2) It provides an opportunity to cover highly pertinent aspects of cancer screening and management, with particular focus given to available, highly targeted cancer control approaches. (3) Through follow-up one-on-one discussions with family members, it provides an opportunity for the team to learn more about those family members in the pedigree who are in attendance at the FIS versus those who either elected not to attend or simply had no knowledge of the fact that they were even part of the pedigree and thereby at heightened hereditary cancer risk. Those individuals who did *not* attend the FIS, but who may yet be at inordinately high cancer risk, and thereby could benefit immensely from appropriate education and individual personalized counseling should be informed of the team's and/or family's willingness to assist them. Their more genetically informed close relatives in attendance at the FIS may be in a position to help in this process.[47] (4) This entire process allows for collection of patients' DNA for genetic testing following genetic counseling where the pros and cons of germline mutation testing are presented in depth so that the patient can be fully informed about all facets of DNA testing. Therein, the patient will be in the best possible position to follow his/her wishes to provide informed, signed consent. (5) It supports those high-risk family members who may otherwise be reluctant to bring forth concerns about some of the multifaceted issues involved in their cancer risk status and its assessment through DNA testing. They may be able to more freely discuss any emotionally threatening concerns that heretofore may not have been broached in a one-on-one genetic counseling session. (6) The FIS may be one of the most cost-effective and emotionally sound approaches known to the hereditary cancer educational process.

Logistics of the FIS

In preparation for the FIS, key family members will often volunteer to help inform their relatives about the objectives of the FIS, encouraging their attendance and helping to identify a meeting place such as their physician's waiting room or their local hospital's outpatient department. These FISs often take place on a weekend when such facilities are less likely to be used. Indeed, once a convenient time and place are decided, family members can set up appointments for each family member, should they wish to meet with the physician and/or genetic counselors for individualized genetic counseling. If DNA had been previously collected and results of testing are available, coupled with informed consent, they can be given their results in this very FIS setting.

DUTY TO WARN

Highly pertinent questions include what kind of counseling will be provided for a patient with a pathogenic mutation and whether that counseling should be mandatory. Does the proband have the responsibility to inform relatives about the familial mutation, even if the relatives do not want to know whether or not they carry it? If the patient is considered to be responsible for notifying family members that a parent, sibling, or other close relative has HBOC or LS, for example, what happens if the patient fails to communicate this information to his or her relatives for personal reasons? Should it instead be the responsibility of the doctor, or perhaps even the State Department of Health? Can notification be forced and, if so, under what circumstances?

These questions point out the need for criteria, and perhaps even regulations, regarding which family members to inform and how to inform them about their life-threatening clinical situation: even their legal implications, if any. Would such criteria be uniform across the country? Policies and procedures in a major city hospital may be very different from that in a rural setting. What follow-up will there be with family members who may be at risk for HBOC or LS? Whose responsibility will it be to ensure that those family members are sufficiently informed, screened, and managed, so that this cancer control effort will be readily available and affordable?[48]

Offit et al.[49] appropriately note that the physician may not have the time necessary to assume primary responsibility for identifying and counseling those who might be at inordinately high hereditary cancer risk by virtue of their membership in a high-risk family, and may find it impossible to reach all of the at-risk family members. Therein, the clinician may not have the time necessary to provide knowledge about germline mutation testing, the significance of a positive DNA test, the significance of a negative DNA test, and the appropriate screening and management opportunities for the germline mutation carriers. Thus, this enormous workload in certain situations, coupled with the attendant threat of liability for physician involvement, would discourage some physicians, including those involved in the emerging subspecialty of genetic medicine. Furthermore, a mandatory "duty to warn" could lead to apprehension and anxiety among some family members who have an intense fear of employment or insurance discrimination. Other emotionally stressful issues impacting upon the decision-making process are blaming and discrimination from other family members, and therein this might be reconciled by simply refusing participation in this process.

A violation of HIPAA as well as certain state regulations involved in overriding patients' confidentiality and genetic privacy may be in violation of certain state regulations and therein may contribute to appellate court decisions making the physician liable for failure to warn relatives of their hereditary disease risk.

Physicians involved in ethical and legal concerns about "failure to warn" have led to positions taken by the AMA and ASCO, wherein these organizations have noted that the physician's obligations (if any) "... to patients' relatives are best fulfilled by communication of familial risk to the individual undergoing testing. Such communication about familial risks should be carefully documented as part of the process of an informed consent before testing and at time of counseling ... Because the laws of Mendel will continue to apply to these new markers of genetic risk, the issues surrounding familial notification will loom even larger. The increasing availability of DNA testing will require greater emphasis on informed consent as a process of communication and education, so as to better facilitate the translation of genomic medicine to clinical practice." Clearly, these issues require more painstaking research.

Direct Contact with High-Risk Family Members

Aktan-Collan et al.,[50] in their review of the literature pertinent to the role of communication in hereditary cancer–prone families, note that informing relatives of the serious genetic condition segregating in the family may be mentally challenging and discomforting for the proband, especially when distant relatives are concerned. Because of this, probands tend to inform the nuclear family rather than more distant relatives, leaving the latter unaware of their risk status.[51] Unfortunately, our own experience indicates that the overwhelming majority of hereditary cancer–prone families identified and managed in the typical clinical setting will involve the proband and, hopefully, that individual's first-degree relatives as part of a nuclear family, but rarely the more distant potentially at-risk relatives. These relatives, if not contacted and given sufficiently detailed information about their potential high-risk status in the pedigree and its cancer control implications, may unfortunately sustain cancer-related morbidity and mortality as a consequence of failure to be tested,[52,53] effectively screened, and managed.

Aktan-Collan et al.[50] appropriately stress that identifying patients'/families' hereditary cancer predisposition has limited significance if family members are not informed, tested when appropriate, and entered into a targeted cancer prevention program. In the Aktan-Collan et al. study involving LS,[50] where cancer prevention was the ultimate goal in concert with investigating attitudes toward its psychosocial consequences, the potentially life-saving strategy of directly contacting relatives showed substantial benefit. Their study involved 286 healthy adult members of LS families, each of whom harbored a 50% risk of manifesting an LS predisposing mutation. They were contacted by letter wherein 112 participated in counseling and predictive testing. One month after the test, 73 respondents provided baseline information which was then compared with 299 corresponding subjects from the authors' previous study,[54-56] who had been approached via the proband. Findings showed that, of the 51% that consented to the study, 92% approved of the direct contact. Thirty-three percent had tried to seek information. After testing, fear of cancer increased among the mutation carriers and decreased among non-carriers but almost all participants, independent of their test results, were satisfied with their decision to participate. This was similar to a previous study utilizing the proband-mediated approach. It was concluded that relatives in these LS families became informed of the value of genetic counseling, testing, screening, and management. Furthermore, their attitudes and the psychosocial consequences were encouraging and were similar to those using the proband-mediated approach. Clearly, the authors were able to demonstrate fully the appropriateness of direct contact as an alternative method in cases such as LS, where there exists a life-threatening but nevertheless treatable disease.

Aktan-Collan et al.[50] note that the mean age of the family members contacted was appreciably higher than 25 years, the age conventionally recommended for initiating colonoscopy among mutation-positive individuals. It is, therefore, perhaps not surprising that among the 32 mutation-positive individuals, colorectal neoplasia was identified in 11 (34%) in the first post-test colonoscopy. Unfortunately, two of these patients harbored locally advanced disease. These findings clearly show the importance of providing earlier information about a family's risk status for a hereditary cancer syndrome.

Aktan-Collan et al.[50] note that this study was in part a response to their earlier experience involving their predictive genetic testing program,[54] in which some relatives who had not applied for genetic counseling developed colon cancer. Without exception, these individuals expressed disappointment that their relatives had not warned them of their risk. In addition, the previous program had confirmed high levels of satisfaction and had found no serious psychological side-effects related to testing.[54-56] These results have since been confirmed by other studies.[57-59] Aktan-Collan et al.[50] also note that active recruitment of potential high-risk patients is a novel approach that raises the ethical dilemma of respect for autonomy and privacy versus beneficence, which relates to the duty to warn. This may be the first prospective large-scale study of hereditary cancer–prone families concerned about attitudes toward a direct contact recruitment method with comparison of psychosocial responses.

Several groups have proposed that the duty to warn patients may help waive the requirement for confidentiality in cases of life-threatening disease with prevention and treatment options.[60-64] In the literature surveyed by Aktan-Collan et al.,[50] they found studies that acknowledged that in the interest of preventing harm in such conditions,[65] confidentiality may be breached. Thus, the conflict between confidentiality and the duty to warn has not been completely resolved.[50]

It is important that the physician, genetic counselors, social workers, and other key health care workers encourage probands and their key relatives to discuss the importance of DNA testing and the natural history of the hereditary cancer existing in their family with their high-risk relatives. Attention must be given to motivating factors and barriers that may exist to their undergoing such genetic testing and compassionately educating these relatives so that they can more effectively grasp the potential benefit that may be accrued to them through this knowledge and how this can foster effective cancer control measures. Thus, family members can effectively reinforce the professional knowledge they receive from their physicians and genetic counselors so that this might hopefully alter the clinical course of those cancers constituting the hereditary syndromic cancer setting to which they are exposed. In reviewing this subject, Aronson[18] has noted that the overall uptake for LS testing as a clinical example has been lower than anticipated based upon expressed interest.[66,67] She notes that a strong motivator surrounds the relief generated from uncertainty particularly through learning that an at-risk relative was found to not be a mutation carrier.[66,67] Testing may also be motivated through the need to make decisions about family planning and reproductive matters.[66]

Physicians' duty to warn individuals of their cancer risk status may arise when the patient declines to inform at-risk relatives of the hereditary disorder that is occurring in the family. Thus, we have the confounding situation impacting the genetic counselor and treating physician surrounding the legal, moral, and ethical issues relevant to their duty to "... respect the autonomy and confidentiality of their patient against the ethical principles of nonmalfeasance and beneficence for at-risk relatives."[18]

This issue of duty to warn may become emotionally laden for both the physician and the at-risk patient/family, given the potentially grave health impact inclusive of potential death due to the predisposition to cancer and its potential prevention such as prophylactic subtotal colectomy in FAP. The fear of disclosure by the family may be heavily impacted by patients' perception of insurance or employment discrimination and the attendant fear and anxiety knowing that the doctor/genetic counselor advised them in appropriate detail what the disease would mean to them should they, in fact, harbor the deleterious mutation and develop potentially diagnostic signs and symptoms consistent with the disease's natural history. Perhaps one could better understand a patient's dilemma surrounding the issue of not wanting to know test results when the disorder, such as carcinoma of the pancreas, has a severely dismal outlook from the standpoint of its inability to be detected early and its high mortality rate when identified, even under the best of circumstances. An example of a clinical non-cancer–associated model would be Huntington's disease wherein the presence of that disorder's deleterious mutation indicates its dismal natural history and medicine's inability to cure so that the end result is an untimely death.

In summing up this issue, Aronson emphasizes the need to have greater knowledge about the multiple complex ethical, legal, and psychosocial concerns surrounding genetic testing for hereditary forms of cancer wherein the role of the counselor is to explore those facts "... that are likely to motivate, deter, and cause distress in probands who wish to undergo genetic testing. Exploring these issues, assessing the risk in the family, and relaying the necessary information about the genetic syndrome and testing process, provides the tools to allow the proband to make an informed decision about genetic testing and enables the genetic counselor to best facilitate this process."[18]

Offit et al.[49] discuss the failure to warn family members about their hereditary disease risk, which has resulted in at least three malpractice suits against physicians in the United States.[68-70] They discuss the conflict that may arise pertinent to the physician's ethical obligations, if any, to warn family members of identification of a cancer gene mutation "... regarding the conflict between the physician's ethical obligations to respect the privacy of genetic information vs the potential legal liabilities resulting from the physician's failure to notify at-risk relatives. In many cases, state and federal statutes that bear on the issue of 'duty to warn' of inherited health risk are also in conflict ...." Offit et al. conclude that health care professionals harbor such responsibility to warn, but therein "... to encourage but not to coerce the sharing of genetic information in families, while respecting the boundaries imposed by the law and by the ethical practice of medicine."

Offit et al. comment on a Presidential Commission[71] that had defined conditions "... under which it would be ethically acceptable for physicians to breach confidentiality and disclose information to relatives. These conditions include (1) the high likelihood of harm if the relative were not warned, (2) the identifiability of the relative, and (3) the notion that the harm resulting from failure to disclose would outweigh the harm resulting from disclosure.[71-73] In the absence of a federally defined legal 'duty to rescue,' which exists in certain parts of Canada,[74] the health care professional's duty to warn is generally viewed as discretionary and not compulsory, ie, legally excusable and not legally mandated."

SCREENING AND MANAGEMENT

Colorectal Screening in LS

An appropriate emphasis has been given to the role of the gastroenterologist and gastrointestinal surgeon, who have been responsible for colonoscopic screening for CRC, given the fact that this is the most common cancer in LS. Due to the high rates of right-sided tumors in LS, likely showing an accelerated growth curve, colonoscopy at frequent intervals has long been the screening tool of choice. We recommend annual colonoscopy beginning at age 20 to 25 for carriers of an LS mutation. For example, in order to test the efficacy of a screening program in the Netherlands, de Jong et al.[53] compared mortality rates before and after 1990. Their study suggests a 70% decrease in CRC mortality.

The CRC screening protocol we have designed for LS must take into consideration LS's natural history, particularly its early age of onset, predilection to the proximal colon, pattern of multiple primary cancers, accelerated carcinogenesis, and improved survival compared by stage with CRC's occurrence in the general population. Therefore, considering this natural history background, we initiate colonoscopic screening between the ages of 20 and 25 and repeat it every other year through age 40 and annually thereafter, demanding an excellent cleanout for best prospects for visibility. This is an absolute necessity in order to achieve excellent visualization throughout the colon, particularly the cecum where some estimates indicate one-third of the CRCs in LS occur.

Because of the cancer risk of the upper gastrointestinal tract, we recommend upper gastroduodenoscopy or push enteroscopy to be initiated at age 30 and repeated every other year. Attention must be focused on stomach and small bowel, particularly the duodenum. Schulmann et al.[75] described 32 small bowel cancers from the German HNPCC database. Median age at diagnosis was 39 years. Fifty percent of the cancers were in the duodenum. These upper gastrointestinal recommendations are particularly apropos for individuals of Japanese, Korean, and Chinese ethnicity, especially in the Orient where gastric cancer is the second most common cancer in LS while endometrial cancer is the second most common cancer in LS in Western countries.

Stoffel et al.[76] conducted a randomized multi-center study to ascertain if chromoendoscopy was superior to intensive conventional endoscopy for detecting adenomas missed by standard colonoscopy in patients with a prior history of neoplasia. They were able to control for the potential effect of procedure time on adenoma detection rate. They found that chromoendoscopy doubled the adenoma yield after a standard colonoscopy and detected significantly more adenomas than intensive inspection exams done without using dye. Chromoendoscopy identified additional adenomas in 44% of subjects and changed management for 26% of subjects ($n = 7$) who would have been misclassified as "adenoma free" after the first standard colonoscopy.

Findings showed that 38% of adenomas found in these patients were detected on the second exams, suggesting that a single conventional colonoscopy may miss approximately one of every three adenomas present. Conventional exam missed half of the total adenomas in subjects who underwent chromoendoscopy, a much higher miss rate than the 26% to 27% for adenomas 1 to 5 mm previously reported in studies of tandem exams using conventional colonoscopy. Furthermore, these authors note that "Most of the adenomas found in our second exams were small (<5 mm) and none met definitions for advanced adenomas based on size or histology. Even so, 75% (18 of 24) of the missed adenomas were located in the right colon and 42% (10 of 24) had a flat morphology—characteristics that may be associated with a more aggressive natural history."[77-79]

Stoffel et al.[80] also evaluated the colonic adenoma miss rate among LS patients undergoing original colonoscopy. They compared the sensitivity of chromoendoscopy versus intensive inspection for identifying polyps missed by conventional colonoscopy. This included 54 subjects with LS who underwent tandem colonoscopies, all of whom initially had a conventional colonoscopy with removal of all visualized polyps. The second colonoscopy "... was randomly assigned as either pancolonic indigo carmine chromoendoscopy or standard colonoscopy with intensive inspection lasting >20 minutes. Size, histology, and number of polyps detected on each exam were recorded." After standard colonoscopy, subjects were randomized to a second exam: 28 with chromoendoscopy and 26 with intensive inspection. The mean length of time since last colonoscopy was 17.5 months. Seventeen polyps (10 adenomas and 7 hyperplastic polyps) were identified during the standard colonoscopies, while 23 additional polyps (12 adenomas and 11 hyperplastic polyps) were identified in the second exams, yielding an adenoma miss rate of 55%. Furthermore, 15 polyps (5 adenomas and 10 hyperplastic polyps) were identified in those cases who had chromoendoscopy, while 8 polyps (7 adenomas and 1 hyperplastic polyp) were identified in those who had intensive inspection. Finally, "... Chromoendoscopy was associated with more normal tissue biopsies (11 vs 5) and longer procedure times compared with intensive inspection (29.8 +/– 9.5 vs 25.3 +/– 5.8 minutes; $P = 0.04$). Controlling for age, number of previous colonoscopies, procedure time, and prior colonic resection, chromoendoscopy detected more polyps ($P = 0.04$), but adenoma detection was not significantly different compared with intensive inspection ($P = 0.27$)."[80] These authors concluded that while small adenomas are frequently missed in patients with LS, and while chromoendoscopy failed to detect more missed adenomas compared with intensive inspection, it is clear that larger trials will be required to determine optimal surveillance techniques in this LS high-risk population.

Järvinen and colleagues[52] demonstrated the benefit of colonoscopic screening in LS through a controlled clinical trial extending over 15 years. The incidence of CRC was compared in two cohorts of at-risk members of 22 LS families. CRC developed in 8 screened subjects (6%), compared with 19 controls (16%; $P = 0.014$). The CRC rate was reduced by 62% in those who were screened using colonoscopy. All CRCs in the screened group were local, causing no deaths, compared with nine deaths caused by CRC in the controls (family members who declined colonoscopy). It was concluded that CRC screening at 3-year intervals more than cuts in half the risk of CRC, prevents CRC deaths, and decreases overall mortality by about 65% in LS families. The relatively high incidence of CRC even in the screened subjects (albeit without deaths) in our opinion argues for shorter screening intervals, e.g., 1 year. For example, Vasen and colleagues[81] discovered five interval cancers in LS patients within 3½ years following a normal colonoscopy.

Edelstein et al.[82] recently confirmed the accelerated carcinogenesis in LS. In 54 patients, the cumulative risk of colorectal neoplasia was 43% by age 40 and 72% by age 80. Polyp dwell time was 33 months for advanced adenomas and 35.2 months for CRC, arguing for annual colonoscopy.

Hurlstone et al.[83] note that in LS-associated CRC, flat and diminutive adenomas occur, particularly in the proximal colon, and have a high risk of malignant transformation. Various techniques have been employed to improve the yield of small flat lesions. Chromoendoscopy with indigo carmine or methylene blue has been employed and so-called narrow band imaging (NBI) has emerged, but has yet to gain truly widespread use. Hurlstone et al.[83] studied 25 asymptomatic Amsterdam criteria I–positive (AC-I+) patients who underwent tandem or "back-to-back" colonoscopy. This included conventional colonoscopy using targeted chromoscopy followed by pan-colonic chromoscopic colonoscopy. Compared with conventional colonoscopy, pan-chromoscopy identified significantly more pedunculated adenomas ($P = 0.001$) and flat adenomas ($P = 0.004$), which heretofore may have been missed (interval cancers). It was concluded that pan-colonic chromoscopic colonoscopy improves detection of significant neoplastic lesions in LS CRC screening; it may also help stratify risk in AC-I+ patients and aid planning of colonoscopic surveillance.

Lecomte et al.[84] compared conventional colonoscopy with chromoendoscopy using indigo carmine dye sprayed onto the entire proximal colon. Findings showed that chromoendoscopy significantly increased detection of adenomas in the proximal colon from 3/33 patients to 10/33 patients ($P = 0.005$). These investigators concluded that high-resolution colonoscopy with chromoendoscopy markedly improves the detection of adenomas in patients with LS and may help in CRC prevention.

East et al.[85] have suggested that NBI colonoscopy improves the detection of flat adenomas in LS. They studied 62 patients from LS families scheduled for surveillance colonoscopy. Patients had conventional white-light colonoscopy followed by NBI. More flat adenomas versus pedunculated adenomas were found during the NBI colonoscopy (45% vs. 12%).

Subtotal Colectomy versus Limited Resection for CRC in LS

Natarajan et al.[86] investigated advantages and disadvantages of subtotal colectomy for CRC in patients with LS. Cases were patients who underwent subtotal colectomy in one of two settings, namely, no CRC diagnosis (prophylactic) or at diagnosis of initial CRC; controls for these two types of cases were, respectively, patients who either underwent no colon surgery or those who had a limited resection at the time of diagnosis of their first CRC. Results showed that event-free survival did not reach 50%, so event-free survival at 5 years was used as the parameter for comparing the two groups. Therein, "... The event-free survival for subsequent colorectal cancer, subsequent abdominal surgery, and death was 94%, 84%, and 93%, respectively, for cases and 74%, 63%, and 88% respectively, for controls. Times to subsequent colorectal cancer and subsequent abdominal surgery were significantly shorter in the control group (P <.006 and P <.04, respectively). No significant difference was identified with respect to survival between the cases and controls." The authors concluded that even in the *absence* of survival benefit between cases and controls, the increased incidence of metachronous CRC and therein increased abdominal surgeries among controls clearly fostered the use of subtotal colectomy in patients with LS.

Extracolonic Cancer Screening in LS

We must also be cognizant of the fact that a litany of extracolonic cancers are recognized components of LS. Small bowel cancer has been mentioned. Other gastrointestinal cancers associated with LS are gastric, hepatobiliary, and pancreatic adenocarcinomas. In Brazilian families with LS,[87] the most frequent extracolonic cancers are breast, endometrial, uterine cervix, and prostate. Gastric cancer was a more common tumor in men by threefold (12 of 77 extracolonic cancers) over hepatobiliary or pancreatic cancer. Only one small bowel cancer was reported among the extracolonic cancers in these men; three occurred in females. In the women from these families, gastric cancer was the most common extracolonic cancer after breast and gynecologic malignancy. No pancreas cancers were reported in the women. In the Netherlands, Capelle et al.[88] also report a significant risk of gastric cancer in LS (8.0% lifetime risk in males; 5.3% in females) and suggest screening by gastroscopy. The median age of onset of gastric cancer was 52 years (range 24 to 81 years) in a report from the French Cancer Genetics Network.[89] The risk of pancreatic cancer was reported as 3.7% up to age 70.[90] The National Comprehensive Cancer Network states there are no current recommendations for screening LS patients for pancreatic cancer.[91]

Thus, there is a need to consider screening for gastric cancer, particularly in the Orient where it is the second most common cancer in LS; the importance of small bowel cancer and pancreatic cancer; the need to involve the gynecologist for screening and management of endometrial cancer (the second most common cancer in LS in Western countries), as well as ovarian cancer; the involvement of the urologist for transitional cell carcinoma of the upper uro-epithelial tract; as well as other specialties relevant to the differing tumor spectrum in LS pedigrees. Since gastroenterologists and colorectal surgeons, as well as medical oncologists and medical geneticists, are often the physicians who may be providing counseling and recommending management of LS patients, this simply emphasizes the importance of knowledge about LS and the need to provide full care of high-risk patients.

Prophylactic Surgery and Risk Reduction for Endometrial and Ovarian Cancer in LS

Schmeler et al.[92] have shown significant risk reduction for carcinoma of the endometrium and ovary through prophylactic surgery in women at inordinately high risk for LS who have completed their families, have had genetic counseling relevant to the pros and cons of this surgery, and have signed informed consent. We found it extremely important that these patients fully understood the reduced penetrance of carcinoma of the endometrium and ovary, as well as the limitations of screening, particularly in ovarian carcinoma. Schmeler's findings were based on 61 women who had undergone prophylactic hysterectomy compared with 210 mutation-positive women who had not undergone the surgery acting as controls, and 47 women who had undergone prophylactic bilateral salpingo-oophorectomy with 223 mutation-positive women who had not undergone the surgery as controls. Those who had undergone prophylactic surgery had no manifestations of endometrial, ovarian, or primary peritoneal cancer. On the other hand, among the control group for endometrial cancer, 69 women (33%) had been diagnosed with this cancer before the end of the study; among the control group for ovarian cancer, 12 women (5%) were diagnosed with ovarian cancer during that time. These findings suggest that prophylactic hysterectomy with bilateral salpingo-oophorectomy is effective in preventing endometrial and ovarian cancer in women carrying a mutation for LS.

We must also consider the limitations in screening for the endometrium and ovaries. We therefore provide the option of prophylactic hysterectomy and bilateral salpingo-oophorectomy once the patient no longer desires more children.[92]

Satisfaction with Ovarian Cancer Risk-Reduction Strategies

Westin et al.[93] examined patients' overall satisfaction rate with ovarian periodic screening (PS) versus risk-reducing salpingo-oophorectomy (RRSO), and therein they identified factors that may influence patient satisfaction with ovarian cancer management options for reducing the risk of ovarian cancer. This study involved patients with HBOC where ovarian cancer risk is strikingly increased.

The median satisfaction with decision (SWD) scale "... was significantly higher in the RRSO group compared with the PS group ($P < .001$). *BRCA* mutation carriers had higher median SWD scores regardless of management type ($P = .01$). Low satisfaction scores were associated with high levels of uncertainty and the perception that the decision between PS and RRSO was difficult to make ($P = .001$). Satisfaction was unrelated to demographics, clinical factors, or concerns of cancer risk."

They concluded that those women who showed the highest risk of breast and ovarian cancer were satisfied with their choice of risk-reduction strategy. When decision making was difficult, the satisfaction levels were lower. It was further concluded that the decision-making process may enhance overall levels of satisfaction. They also found that more women at high risk for HBOC who had prophylactic bilateral salpingo-oophorectomy were satisfied that they went ahead with this risk-reduction strategy when compared with those who underwent PS.

But will patients' medical insurance provide appropriate coverage of this prophylactic surgery? Lynch et al.[94] provided a partial answer to this subject. This involved a 43-year-old woman from an HBOC family who showed linkage to *BRCA1* and therein was at inordinately high risk for ovarian carcinoma. However, she was initially denied insurance coverage for prophylactic oophorectomy despite strong recommendations by her gynecologist and a cancer geneticist-medical oncologist (HTL). This denial was based upon the insurance company's claim that the surgery was not medically necessary since her hereditary cancer predisposition to carcinoma of the breast and ovary was not an illness. The case was litigated, following which a summary judgment issued by the Douglas County (Nebraska) District Court ruled in favor of the denial decision of Blue Cross/Blue Shield. However, on appeal to the Nebraska Supreme Court, it was concluded that the patient did, in fact, require this prophylactic surgery. They overruled the District Court's decision for denial. Therein, this litigation provides the basis, if not a precedent, for insurance coverage of prophylactic oophorectomy for patients at high risk for HBOC and other hereditary forms of cancer.

WHAT'S NEW ON THE HORIZON? IMPLICATIONS FOR LS PATIENTS/FAMILIES

miRNAs

Balaguer et al.[95] investigated microRNAs (miRNAs), namely small noncoding transcripts which appear to harbor an important pathogenic role in carcinogenesis and which discriminate between different types of cancer. This study involved an analysis of "... genome-wide miRNA expression profiles in 54 CRC tissues [22 with Lynch syndrome, 13 with sporadic MSI due to *MLH1* methylation, 19 without MSI (or microsatellite stable, MSS)] and 20 normal colonic tissues by miRNA microarrays ...." An miRNA-based predictor was developed in order to differentiate both types of MSI by quantitative reverse transcriptase polymerase chain reaction. Importantly, results showed that a subset of nine miRNAs "... significantly discriminated between tumor and normal colonic mucosa tissues (overall error rate = 0.04). More importantly, Lynch syndrome tumors displayed a unique miRNA profile compared with sporadic MSI tumors; ... [and the investigators] developed a miRNA predictor capable of differentiating between types of MSI and an independent sample set." It was concluded that these CRC tissues manifested distinct miRNA profiles when compared with normal colonic mucosa. This is an exceedingly important molecular genetic finding, given their discovery of a unique miRNA expression profile "... that can successfully discriminate between Lynch syndrome, sporadic MSI, and sporadic MSS colorectal cancers ...." These findings are scientifically provocative and therein will play an important role for advancements in diagnosis, prognosis, and therapy that will likely evolve from these discoveries.[95]

Impact of *BRAF* Mutation

Tran et al.[96] investigated whether *BRAF* mutant CRC may be further defined by a distinct pattern of metastatic spread and therein the impact of *BRAF* mutation and MSI was examined with respect to prognosis in metastatic CRC. This involved 524 metastatic CRC patients where *BRAF* status was confirmed. Therein, 57 (11%) were identified as *BRAF* mutant tumors. These *BRAF* mutant tumors were found to be significantly associated "... with right-sided primary tumor, MSI, and poorer survival (median, 10.4 months vs 34.7 months, $P < .001$). A distinct pattern of metastatic spread was observed in *BRAF* mutant tumors, namely higher rates of peritoneal metastases (46% vs 24%, $P = .001$), distant lymph node metastases (53% vs 38%, $P = .008$), and lower rates of lung metastases (35% vs 49%, $P = .049$). In additional survival analyses, MSI tumors had significantly poorer survival compared with microsatellite stable tumors (22.1 months vs 11.1 months, $P = .017$), but this difference was not evident in the *BRAF* mutation population ...." It was therefore concluded that there exists a distinct pattern of metastatic spread in CRC which, in this investigation, "... further defines *BRAF* mutant CRC as a discrete disease subset ...."

Gene Therapy

What does the future hold for restoring the mutant gene to its favored wild-type status so that a particular hereditary disorder may be ameliorated or outright corrected? This is a frequent interest among MMR LS mutation carriers. Hemophilia in a mouse model has possibly accomplished this objective. Specifically, Li et al.[97] described the editing of the human genome as a way to "... correct disease-causing mutations is a promising approach for the treatment of genetic disorders ... [and therein] editing improves on simple gene-replacement strategies by effecting in situ correction of a mutant gene, thus restoring normal gene function under the control of endogenous regulatory elements and reducing risks associated with random insertion into the genome ...." Attention was focused on the liver, which is the major site of synthesis of plasma proteins including blood coagulation factors and which is a potential model for gene therapy for hemophilia B caused by deficiency of blood factor IX, which is encoded by the *F9* gene. Furthermore, "... Most affected individuals have circulating levels of factor IX that are below 1% of normal (5,000 ng ml^{-1}), but restoration to about 5% activity (250 ng ml^{-1}) converts severe haemophilia B to a mild form.[98] Most mutations in the *F9* gene are distributed across the coding sequences of exons 2-8 .... Thus, specific targeting of any single mutant allele would not allow complete coverage of the wide spectrum of mutations found in the human population. However, zinc finger nuclease (ZFN)-mediated targeting of a promoterless therapeutic gene fragment[99,100] (that is, a partial cDNA preceded by a splice acceptor site) into the first intron of *F9* would allow for splicing of a wild-type coding sequence within exon 1, leading to expression of functionally active factor IX and rescue of the defect caused by most mutations ...." They then investigated whether ZFNs, "... combined with a targeting vector carrying the wild-type *F9* exons 2-8 could induce gene targeting in vivo and correct a mutated *F9* in situ." Given this model, they were able to show that this approach was sufficient to correct for the prolonged clotting times in their hemophilia B mouse model and that this remained persistent even after induced liver regeneration. They concluded that "... ZFN-driven gene correction can be achieved in vivo, raising the possibility of genome editing as a viable strategy for the treatment of genetic disease."

Epigenetics and LS

Epigenetics is defined as "heritable changes in gene expression that are not due to any alteration in the DNA sequence."[101,102] One of the best described epigenetic influences involves DNA methylation. Hypermethylation of a gene promoter can result in silencing of gene expression, as has been observed in LS. Hitchins et al.[103] demonstrated that hypermethylation of one allele of *MLH1* in somatic cells throughout the body (a germline epimutation) predisposes an individual to the development of cancer in a pattern typical of LS.

Hitchins et al.[104] describe constitutional epimutations of tumor suppressor genes as those which are manifest as "... promoter methylation and transcriptional silencing of a single allele in normal somatic tissues, thereby predisposing to cancer." They describe a pedigree wherein the phenotype appears to be classical for LS, which harbors the dominant transmission of "... soma-wide highly mosaic MLH1 methylation and transcriptional repression linked to a particular genetic haplotype. The epimutation was erased in spermatozoa but reinstated in the somatic cells of the next generation. The affected haplotype harbored two single nucleotide substitutions in tandem; c.-27C>A located near the transcription initiation site and c.85G>T. The c.-27C>A variant significantly reduced transcriptional activity in reporter assays and is the probable cause of this epimutation."

Importantly, these constitutional epimutations of cancer-related genes provide an alternative mechanism for cancer causality. For example, Hitchins et al.[104] note that "... Some are caused by underlying *cis*-acting genetic alterations proximate to the affected gene and display autosomal dominant inheritance. However, the mechanistic basis for *MLH1* epimutations that are reversible between generations remains undefined. This study of a cancer-affected family with dominant inheritance of a mosaic MLH1 epimutation through generations provides evidence of a cis-genetic basis for constitutional epigenetic silencing of MLH1. The identification of a 5′UTR germline c.-27C>A variant raises the interesting possibility that promoter variants of unknown pathogenic significance within the MLH1 and other genes may confer cancer susceptibility through their association with epigenetic modifications. This finding indicates a close interaction between genotype and epigenotype in a cancer-associated gene."

Van Engeland et al.[105] reviewed recent evidence which indicates that epigenetic alterations add to the complexity of the pathogenesis of CRC, wherein they characterize a subgroup of CRCs that harbor distinct etiology and prognosis. A number of epigenetic changes were highlighted, including histone modifications, chromatic looping, miRNA expression, DNA methylation, and nucleosomal positioning. A full understanding of epigenetics and its role in CRC carcinogenesis, particularly its role in heritable cancers, is a challenge that will likely provide researchers and clinicians with insight into how best to identify and manage familial CRC cases.

Aspirin and Polyp Regression

Burn et al.[106] conducted the largest ever clinical trial in the setting of FAP and identified a trend of reduced polyp mode, both number and size, with administration of 600 mg of aspirin daily. Resistant starch did not have an effect on adenomas. Chan[107] in a perspective account of the Burn et al.[106] study notes that the role of aspirin in the clinical management of FAP patients fosters its role as a chemopreventive agent for CRC among broader populations.

An earlier study by Burn et al.[108] utilizing aspirin, conducted on a large cohort of LS patients, failed to reveal significant polyp regression. However, a recent study by Burn et al.,[109] through an extension of time in the interest of greater maturity of the study, has shown evidence for polyp regression. Specifically, Burn et al.,[109] in the CAPP2 randomized trial, assigned carriers of LS germline mutations to be randomly assigned by a two-by-two factorial design for receipt of 600 mg aspirin or aspirin placebo or 30 g resistant starch or starch placebo, for up to 4 years, with the primary endpoint being CRC occurrence. This study involved 861 participants who were assigned to aspirin or aspirin placebo with a mean follow-up of 55.7 months. Findings showed 48 participants to have developed 53 CRCs (18 of 427 randomly assigned to aspirin; 30 of 434 to aspirin placebo). Results showed that "... Poisson regression taking account of multiple primary events gave an incidence rate ratio (IRR) of 0.56 (95% CI 0.32-0.99, p = 0.05). For participants completing two years of intervention (258 aspirin, 250 aspirin placebo), per-protocol analysis yielded an HR of 0.41 (0.19-0.86, p = 0.02) and an IRR of 0.37 (0.18-0.78, p = 0.008)." It was concluded that "600 mg aspirin per day for a mean of 25 months substantially reduced cancer incidence after 55.7 months in carriers of hereditary colorectal cancer. Further studies are needed to establish the optimum dose and duration of aspirin treatment."

Other LS cancers showed an aspirin effect. Specifically, 18 participants manifested endometrial cancer, wherein 5 were randomly assigned to aspirin and 13 to aspirin placebo. Furthermore, "... in total, 38 participants developed cancer at a site other than the colorectum (additionally, two participants had colorectal and another Lynch syndrome cancer) of whom 16 were randomly assigned to aspirin and 22 to aspirin placebo .... The HR for those randomly assigned to aspirin was 0.63 (95% CI 0.34-1.19 p = 0.16 ...) and the IRR was 0.63 (95% CI 0.34-1.16 p = 0.14) compared with the aspirin placebo group ...."

The findings in this study support the hypothesis "... of a delayed effect of aspirin on colorectal cancer by showing that aspirin reduced incidence of colorectal cancer with the effect becoming apparent after 3-4 years from the start of aspirin intervention, a difference consistent with faster cancer development in those with Lynch syndrome." A second hypothesis pertains to whether LS cancers are more responsive to aspirin, a concern which remains elusive. However, in CAPP2, "... non-Lynch syndrome extracolonic cancers seemed unaffected by aspirin intervention ...."

This study raised several important questions, as follows: "(1) whether aspirin targets the minority of adenomas with the greatest malignant potential; (2) whether some Lynch syndrome colorectal cancers arise from lesions other than adenomas[110]; and (3) why do some tumours seem to be resistant to the effects of aspirin? The mechanism by which aspirin suppresses cancer development long after cessation of exposure to the drug is unclear ...."

Mcilhatton et al.[111] note that aspirin (acetylsalicylic acid [ASA]) and nitric oxide–donating ASA (NO-ASA) have been found to suppress MSI in MMR-deficient cells linked to LS, at doses 300- to 3,000-fold less than ASA. They, therefore, investigated an LS mouse model that manifests MMR-deficient intestinal tumors "... that appear pathologically identical to LS/HNPCC ... that ASA (400 mg/kg) and low-dose NO-ASA (72 mg/kg) increased life span by 18% to 21% ... ASA treatment resulted in intestinal tumors with reduced high MSI (H-MSI) and increased low MSI (L-MSI) ... Low-dose NO-ASA had minimal effect on MSI status. In contrast to previous studies, high-dose NO-ASA (720/1,500 mg/kg) treatments increased tumor burden, decreased life span, and exacerbated MSI uniquely in the LS/HNPCC mouse model ...." The authors concluded that these MMR LS mice may be "... specifically sensitive to intrinsic pharmacokinetic features of this drug ..." and therein their findings of long-term treatment with ASA may provide a chemopreventive option for LS patients and therein since low-dose NO-ASA "... shows equivalent life span increase at 10-fold lower doses than ASA, it may have the potential to significantly reduce the gastropathy associated with long-term ASA treatment."

Tan et al.,[112] noting the evidence for aspirin and nonsteroidal anti-inflammatory drugs (NSAIDs) as cancer prevention agents, investigated whether aspirin may have a protective effect in the development of pancreatic cancer, with particular attention to a potential association among aspirin, NSAID, and acetaminophen and pancreatic cancer risk wherein they used a clinic-based case–control study "... of 904 rapidly ascertained histologically or clinically documented pancreatic ductal adenocarcinoma cases, and 1,224 age- and sex-matched healthy controls ...." They did not find any relationship between non-aspirin NSAID or acetaminophen use and risk of pancreatic cancer. However, aspirin use for 1 d/mo or greater "was associated with a significantly decreased risk of pancreatic cancer (OR = 0.74, 95% CI: 0.60-0.91, P = 0.005) compared with never or less than 1 d/mo. Analysis by frequency and frequency-dosage of use categories showed reduced risk (P = 0.007 and 0.022, respectively). This inverse association was also found for those who took low-dose aspirin for heart disease prevention (PR = 0.67, 95% CI: 0.49-0.92, P = 0.013) .... These data ... suggest that aspirin use, but not non-aspirin NSAID use, is associated with lowered risk of developing pancreatic cancer." These studies show remarkable cancer prevention effects of one of the most commonly used drugs in medical practice.

5-FU, Deficient MMR, and LS

Sinicrope et al.[113] investigated the impact of 5-fluorouracil (FU)–based adjuvant therapy on recurrent variables in patients with stage II and III CRC (n = 2,141) who had defective function of the DNA MMR system. These patients were treated in randomized trials of 5-FU–based adjuvant therapy. Testing parameters involved time to recurrence (TTR), disease-free survival (DFS), and overall survival (OS). Those tumors showing deficient MMR (dMMR) were assessed by presumed germline versus sporadic origin, which included their prognostic and predictive impact. Results showed that 344 of the 2,141 (16.1%) CRCs showed dMMR. When compared with proficient MMR (pMMR) tumors, "... dMMR was associated with reduced 5-year recurrence rates (33% vs 22%; $P < .001$), delayed TTR ($P < .001$), and fewer distant recurrences (22% vs 12%; $P < .001$). In multivariable models, dMMR was independently associated with delayed TTR (hazard ratio = 0.72, 95% confidence interval = 0.56 to 0.91, $P = .005$) and improved DFS ($P = .035$) and OS ($P = .031$). In stage III cancers, 5-FU-based treatment vs surgery alone or no 5-FU was associated with reduced distant recurrence for dMMR tumors (11% vs 29%; $P = .011$) and reduced recurrence to all sites for pMMR tumors ($P < .001$) ...." *BRAF* mutation testing and gene sequencing were used to distinguish between sporadic dMMR tumors and those associated with germline mutations. The dMMR tumors with suspected germline mutations showed improved DFS after 5-FU–based treatment, in contrast to sporadic dMMR tumors where no benefit was observed ($P = 0.006$). It was concluded that there were reduced rates of tumor recurrence, delayed TTR, and improved survival rates in patients with dMMR compared with pMMR CRCs. Furthermore, 5-FU–based adjuvant treatment in dMMR stage III tumors showed distant recurrences to be reduced by 5-FU–based adjuvant treatment, but that this reduction disappeared when dMMR tumors associated with germline mutations were removed from the outcome.

But what about stage II and stage III CRCs in MMR mutation confirmed LS patients? Unfortunately, to the best of our knowledge, 5-FU–based adjuvant therapy studies have not yet been investigated in a sufficiently large number of MMR mutation confirmed LS patients manifesting stage II and stage III CRC to provide an answer to this question.

Exomes: Novel Molecular Genetic Developments

Newly developed "next-generation" DNA sequencing (NGS) technologies provide remarkable power for genomic studies.[114,115] This new molecular genetic development is of keen interest. Its power harbors the following attributes: low sequencing cost; simple sample preparation; high speed; mass production; and sequencing individual and population genomes.

This exome sequencing involves only the exome part of the genome through NGS sequencing. Mutations in the protein-coding region contribute approximately 85% of the genetic disease–causing mutations. Cost is substantially lower (currently under $2,000 per sample, compared with past expenses of approximately $5,000 to $50,000 per sample for whole genome sequencing). Further advantages are its focus on analyzing exon sequences, which is simpler than that for whole genome sequencing, and finally, information identified in affected genes can be biologically translated.

GENETICALLY BASED THERAPEUTIC DIFFERENCES IN CANCER

The veritable logarithmic advances in molecular biology, genetics, and genomics not only have led to unique carcinogenic predisposition pathways but, moreover, have also given rise to their utilization for therapeutic benefit. Currently, we have demonstration of a therapeutic cancer reduction benefit through aspirin in LS (discussed subsequently), but hopefully to expand its potential we have elected to discuss other cancer models, inclusive of breast and lung cancer, and certain novel therapeutic benefits.

PARP Inhibitors and Breast Cancer

BRCA1 and *BRCA2* mutations occur in approximately 5% of women with breast cancer and markedly increase the risk of both breast and ovarian cancers. *BRCA1* and *BRCA2* genes have a role in DNA homologous recombination repair. Patients with inherited *BRCA1* or *BRCA2* have a mutation in one of these genes. During the formation of cancer, the wild-type allele gene is also lost, causing this DNA repair mechanism to fail. Synthetic lethality has been shown in pre-clinical models to occur when BRCA-deficient cells are dependent on DNA repair mechanism of single-stranded breaks on poly(ADP-ribose) polymerase (PARP). Thus, inhibition of PARP in patients with *BRCA* mutation was postulated to have significant anti-tumor effects.

Olaparib (AZD2281) is an oral PARP inhibitor, which is not approved by the FDA. Audeh et al.[116] studied this drug in 54 metastatic breast cancer patients with *BRCA1* and *BRCA2* mutations. The patients had a median of three prior chemotherapy regimens. This regimen was very well tolerated. This phase II study was a single-arm study and utilized two different doses of olaparib. The response rate was 41% utilizing one dose and 22% with the other, with progression-free survival of 5.7 and 3.8 months, respectively. No survival data were provided nor was this drug compared with standard therapy.

O'Shaughnessy et al.[117] performed an open label phase II study in triple-negative breast cancer of gemcitabine and carboplatin with and without iniparib. There was significant increase in response rate (32% to 52%); progression-free survival (3.6 to 5.9 months), and OS (7.7 to 12.3 months). These results were promoted as a major breakthrough in cancer treatment. Unfortunately, the confirmatory randomized phase III trial[117] that was reported at the 2011 annual meeting of the American Society of Clinical Oncology did not confirm these findings. Though there was a slight significant increase in progression-free survival (4.1 to 5.1 months), there was no significant change in OS (11.1 to 11.8 months) and the trial was a negative trial. Further analysis of iniparib suggests that it may not be a true PARP inhibitor.

Breast Cancer—Platinum

Pre-clinical studies have shown that mouse and human breast cancer cell lines that lack BRCA1 or BRCA2 proteins are more susceptible to damage from chemotherapy that causes double-strand DNA breaks such as anthracyclines and platinum agents and less sensitive to micro-tubule damaging agents such as taxanes. It has been theorized that *BRCA* mutated patients may be more sensitive to chemotherapy that cause DNA damage such as platinum agents. Byrski et al.[118] evaluated 102 women who were *BRCA1* mutation positive and had neoadjuvant chemotherapy for breast cancer. Ten out of 12 women treated with cisplatinum experienced a pathological complete remission (pCR). In this non-randomized observational study, 16% of women treated with other regimens achieved a pCR.

Kriege et al.[119] evaluated retrospectively 93 *BRCA1* and 28 *BRCA2* mutated patients with metastatic breast cancer and compared them with other patients who were incorporated in the same database. The most common regimens were anthracycline based or cytoxan, methotrexate, and fluorouracil. They found that patients negative for *BRCA1* had no improvement in response compared with the matched controls. Patients with *BRCA2* had statistically improved response rate (50% to 89%); progression-free survival and OS compared with matched patients in the database. *BRCA1* patients are more frequently triple negative than are *BRCA2* patients and this might explain some of the differential response to chemotherapy. In a more recent analysis, Kriege et al.[120] evaluated the use of taxane chemotherapy in 48 *BRCA1/2* patients with metastatic breast cancer and compared them with matched controls. They found that *BRCA1/2* patients that were hormone receptor negative had a lower response rate (20% vs. 42%) than the controls, but they also found that there was no difference in response rate in the hormone receptor–positive patients.

Arun et al.,[121] in a retrospective review of MD Anderson patients treated with neoadjuvant therapy, evaluated 57 breast cancer patients who had *BRCA1* and 23 with *BRCA2* mutations. Forty-six percent of those with *BRCA1* mutations, 13% with *BRCA2*, and 22% of non-*BRCA* carriers achieved a pCR. Patients who achieved a pCR had better 5-year survival. Robson,[122] in a recent editorial, felt that there is insufficient evidence to recommend platinum treatment in patients with *BRCA* mutations.

Ovarian Cancer in *BRCA1/2* Mutation Carriers

Multiple groups have shown that patients with *BRCA1/2* mutation have prolonged survival after they develop ovarian cancer. All of these studies are retrospective and compare patients with *BRCA1/2* with patients without the mutation treated in the same setting and time period. Chetrit et al.[123] compared 213 Israeli Ashkenazi Jewish women with *BRCA1/2* to 392 women of similar ethnic background. Being a mutation carrier reduced the death rate by 28% and women with stage III or IV cancer had a 5-year survival of 38% if they had the mutation but only 25% if they did not. Cass et al.[124] evaluated 34 women with germline mutation who had ovarian cancer and compared them with 37 Jewish women who did not have the mutation. The *BRCA* mutation patients had a statistically improved survival of 91 months as compared with 54 months among the non-carriers. Boyd et al.[125] evaluated 88 patients with hereditary *BRCA* mutations and compared them with 101 Jewish women without the mutation. The *BRCA* patients had statistically improved OS as well as TTR after primary chemotherapy of 14 versus 7 months.

These findings held in most studies even after controlling for age of diagnosis, morphology, and grade of tumor. It is felt that patients with a *BRCA* mutation may have better response because they are more sensitive to platinum-based DNA damage. This has yet to be proven in a randomized trial.

Norquist et al.[126] evaluated 110 *BRCA1/2* patients with ovarian cancer. Forty-six percent of platinum-resistant ovarian cancer patients had secondary mutations in *BRCA1/2* restoring *BRCA* function while only 5% of platinum-sensitive recurrence had restoration of *BRCA* function. Sixty-seven percent of patients with prior breast cancer had a secondary mutation as compared with only 17% without a history of breast cancer. Thus, prior chemotherapy either for breast or for ovarian cancer can restore the function of *BRCA* and make ovarian cancer patients less sensitive to platinum. Since the standard of care first-line chemotherapy for all metastatic ovarian patients is platinum-based therapy, these retrospective findings have not affected choice of chemotherapy in *BRCA* mutation–negative patients.

Audeh et al.[116] evaluated 54 women with *BRCA* mutations and ovarian cancer who had received an average of three lines of previous chemotherapy and were treated with the oral PARP inhibitor olaparib. The average response rate was 12%. This oral agent in this phase II trial was given at two different dose ranges. Lee et al.[127] evaluated 26 women with *BRCA* mutations and previous exposure to platinum chemotherapy to olaparib and carboplatin. Responses were noted in 35% of these women.

Fanconi Anemia

One type of Fanconi anemia has mutations in both of the individual's *BRCA2* genes. There are six genes associated with Fanconi anemia such as *FANC* as well as *BRCA2* (*FANCD1*). Taniguchi et al.[128] showed that the *FANC-BRCA* pathway is disrupted in ovarian cancer. These ovarian cancer cell lines are sensitive to cisplatinum. Demethylation of *FANCF* (one of the Fanconi genes) which restores the activity of *FANC* results in cisplatinum resistance. Dhillon et al.[129] describe how resistance to the PARP inhibitor in ovarian cancer can occur when there are secondary mutations in *BRCA1/2* that restore the function of *BRCA1/2*. They showed that 7 of 10 patients with *BRCA1/2* mutation who developed platinum resistance developed a secondary mutation in *BRCA1/2*, presumably restoring *BRCA* function. Fong et al.[130] showed that patients that responded to PARP inhibitors in ovarian cancer were most likely those that also were platinum sensitive presumably because they were still functionally BRCA deficient. The response rate to olaparib in *BRCA* ovarian cancer patients was 69% (platinum sensitive), 45% (platinum resistant), and 23% (platinum refractory).

Non–Small Cell Lung Cancer and Survival in Platinum-Based Chemotherapy

Excision repair cross-complementation group 1 (ERCC1) plays a central role in DNA repair and, in particular, repair to the DNA damage created by platinum–DNA adducts. Olaussen et al.[131] evaluated 761 patients who had adjuvant therapy for lung cancer. Of those, 44% had absence of ERCC1. Platinum-based chemotherapy improved the survival of those patients who were ERCC1 negative but not those who had normal ERCC1. It is postulated that platinum chemotherapy is more effective in ERCC1-negative patients because they cannot repair the DNA damage that is done by cisplatinum. Olaussen et al. further showed that the survival of patients who did not have chemotherapy was longer in those who had normal levels of ERCC1. These patients have a more intact DNA repair mechanism and may have less virulent cancers.

Wu et al.[132] conducted a genome-wide scan of 307,260 SNPs in 327 advanced-stage non–small cell lung cancer (NSCLC) patients who were treated with platinum-based chemotherapy with or without radiation. Each SNP was assessed with OS by multivariable Cox proportional hazard regression analysis. Results showed that SNP rs1878022 in the chemokine-like receptor 1 (*CMKLR1*) "... was statistically significantly associated with poor overall survival in the MD Anderson discovery population (hazard ratio [HR] of death = 1.59, 95% confidence interval [CI] = 1.32 to 1.92, $P = 1.42\times10^{-6}$) in the PLATAX clinical trial (HR of death = 1.23, 95% CI = 1.00 to 1.51, $P = .05$), in the pooled Mayo Clinic and PLATAX validation (HR of death = 1.22, 95% CI = 1.06 to 1.40, $P = .005$), and in pooled analysis of all three populations (HR of death = 1.33, 95% CI = 1.19 to 1.48, $P = 5.13\times10^{-7}$). Carrying a variant genotype of rs10937823 was associated with decreased overall survival (HR of death = 1.82, 95% CI = 1.42 to 2.33, $P = 1.73\times10^{-6}$) in the pooled MD Anderson and Mayo Clinic populations but not in the PLATAX trial patient population (HR of death = 0.96, 95% CI = 0.69 to 1.35)." These findings harbor important implications for further development of personalized chemotherapy for NSCLC patients. These results are very important given the magnitude of lung cancer, which accounts for approximately 28% of the annual cancer-related burden of death in the United States. However, the 5-year survival rate is only 15%. In addition, NSCLC accounts for more than 80% of the total burden of lung cancer cases and unfortunately its diagnosis is often at a late stage. Platinum-based chemotherapy is the most important treatment option for advanced-stage NSCLC and it has been associated with improved OS. Importantly, response to platinum-based chemotherapy is quite variable, even in the presence of strikingly similar clinical manifestations. It is in this realm that SNPs have received considerable attention as predictors of OS for NSCLC patients under treatment with platinum-based chemotherapy.[133]

Wu et al.[132] have reviewed several recently published genome-wide association studies in which genetic variants influencing risk of lung cancer were identified.[134] The PLATAX validation population involved 420 NSCLC stage III and IV patients who received chemotherapy (cisplatin and docetaxel) "... within the pharmacogenomic, open-label, single-arm multicenter PLATAX trial ...."

It is noteworthy that Wu et al. note that candidate gene studies have indicated that "... genetic variation in genes within the platinum drug action pathway may be associated with response to chemotherapy.[135]... Linkage studies using lymphoblastoid cell lines from pedigrees of Caucasian individuals have indicated that approximately 47% of the variation in susceptibility to cisplatin-induced cytotoxicity is because of heritable factors.[136] These results indicate that there are unidentified genetic factors playing a major role in determining patient responses to platinum-based chemotherapeutics ... the variants identified in these previous reports were located within genes not previously considered as candidates for chemotherapy response ...." Wu et al. showed that SNP rs10937823 was statistically associated with decreased OS in the MD Anderson and Mayo Clinic populations but not associated with decreased OS in patients enrolled in the PLATAX clinical trial.

In conclusion, Wu et al. note that theirs is the first genome-wide study for the assessment of genetic factors influencing OS for advanced-stage NSCLC patients who receive platinum-based chemotherapy and therein it provides valuable information on additional biomarkers "... that can be integrated with known epidemiological, clinical, and genetic risk factors to potentially identify patients who are more likely to respond to chemotherapy, thereby helping the physician develop individualized treatment regimens."

SUMMARY

The linchpin for hereditary cancer syndrome diagnosis is the family history. Identifying cancers of all anatomic sites, whenever possible, is crucial given the fact that hereditary cancer syndromes are frequently diagnosed based upon the *pattern* of their tumor combinations. The sine qua non for such diagnoses in this day and age, thanks to advances in the molecular genetics arena, will be the presence of a diagnostic germline mutation. When present, a patient's cancer risk status can best be calculated through the knowledge of the mutation's penetrance. Genetic heterogeneity must be considered due to potential environmental interactions as well as modifier alleles and/or genetic polymorphisms. The mutation evidence in the proband will also enable at-risk family members to be tested. Genetic counseling is mandatory coupled with targeted screening and management recommendations whenever possible.

This chapter attempts to answer many of the clinical concerns that embrace the multiple facets of a patient's hereditary cancer syndrome diagnosis, screening, and management. Problem areas are addressed, inclusive of issues such as patients in extended families who may be at inordinately high risk for the particular hereditary cancer segregating among them, but who have never been educated sufficiently about this issue; some may not even know they are a bloodline part of the family. In addition, there may be a lack of physician knowledge and absence of available genetic counselors or cancer centers with hereditary cancer expertise, particularly in rural areas of the United States. Other barriers may include lack of funds or insurance coverage to defray the cost of testing, lack of records because of adoption, and loss or absence of medical records resulting in incomplete knowledge of family history; collectively, these may pose a clinically negative barrier to the counselor; and the list goes on. There is a dire need to ameliorate many of these issues, given the potential for significant reduction in patients' morbidity and mortality once a hereditary cancer syndrome diagnosis has been certified in the family.

Clearly, education will be extremely advantageous to all parties who are involved in any hereditary cancer syndrome setting.

REFERENCES

1. MacDonald DJ, Blazer KR, Weitzel JN. Extending comprehensive cancer center expertise in clinical cancer genetics and genomics to diverse communities: the power of partnership. *J Natl Compr Canc Netw*. 2010;8:615-624.
2. Guttmacher AE, Collins FS, Carmona RH. The family history—more important than ever. *N Engl J Med*. 2004;351:2333-2336.
3. Lynch HT, Snyder CL, Lynch JF, Riley BD, Rubinstein WS. Hereditary breast-ovarian cancer at the bedside: role of the medical oncologist. *J Clin Oncol*. 2003;21:740-753.
4. Lynch HT, Boland CR, Rodriguez-Bigas MA, Amos C, Lynch JF, Lynch PM. Who should be sent for genetic testing in hereditary colorectal cancer syndromes? *J Clin Oncol*. 2007;25:3534-3542.
5. Lynch HT, Marcus JN, Lynch J, Snyder CL, Rubinstein WS. Breast cancer genetics: syndromes, genes, pathology, counseling, testing, and treatment. In: Bland KI, Copeland EM III, eds. *The Breast: Comprehensive Management of Benign and Malignant Disorders*. 4th ed. Philadelphia, PA: Saunders; 2009:371-415.
6. Ligtenberg MJL, Kuiper RP, Chan TL, et al. Heritable somatic methylation and inactivation of *MSH2* in families with Lynch syndrome due to deletion of the 3′ exons of *TACSTD1*. *Nat Genet*. 2009;41:112-117.
7. Kovacs ME, Papp J, Szentirmay Z, Otto S, Olah E. Deletions removing the last exon of TACSTD1 constitute a distinct class of mutations predisposing to Lynch syndrome. *Hum Mutat*. 2009;30:197-203.
8. Kobelka CE. Silencing is not-so golden: a new model for inheritance of Lynch syndrome. *Clin Genet*. 2009;75:522-523.
9. Kuiper RP, Vissers LELM, Venkatachalam R, et al. Recurrence and variability of germline *EPCAM* deletions in Lynch syndrome. *Hum Mutat*. 2011;32:407-414.
10. Lynch H, Riegert-Johnson D, Snyder C, et al. Lynch syndrome associated extracolonic tumors are rare in two extended families with the same *EPCAM* deletion. *Am J Gastroenterol*. 2011;106:1829-1836.
11. Wagner A, Barrows A, Wijnen JT, et al. Molecular analysis of hereditary nonpolyposis colorectal cancer in the United States: high mutation detection rate among clinically selected families and characterization of an American founder genomic deletion of the *MSH2* gene. *Am J Hum Genet*. 2003;72:1088-1100. PMC1180263.
12. Lynch HT, Coronel SM, Okimoto R, et al. A founder mutation of the *MSH2* gene and hereditary nonpolyposis colorectal cancer in the United States. *JAMA*. 2004;291:718-724.
13. Clendenning M, Baze ME, Sun S, et al. Origins and prevalence of the American founder mutation of *MSH2*. *Cancer Res*. 2008;68:2145-2153.
14. Pérez-Cabornero L, Borrás Flores E, Infante Sanz M, et al. Characterization of new founder Alu-mediated rearrangements in *MSH2* gene associated with a Lynch syndrome phenotype. *Cancer Prev Res*. 2011;4:1546-1555.
15. Wang Y, Friedl W, Lamberti C, et al. Hereditary nonpolyposis colorectal cancer: frequent occurrence of large genomic deletions in MSH2 and MLH1 genes. *Int J Cancer*. 2003;103:636-641.
16. Perez-Cabornero L, Velasco E, Infante M, et al. A new strategy to screen MMR genes in Lynch syndrome: HA-CAE, MLPA and RT-PCR. *Eur J Cancer*. 2009;45:1485-1493.
17. Hitchins MP, Burn J. *Alu* in Lynch syndrome: a danger SINE? *Cancer Prev Res*. 2011;4:1527-1530.
18. Aronson M. Genetic counseling for hereditary colorectal cancer: ethical, legal, and psychosocial issues. *Surg Oncol Clin N Am*. 2009;18:669-685.
19. Resta R, Biesecker BB, Bennett RL, et al. A new definition of genetic counseling: National Society of Genetic Counselors' Task Force report. *J Genet Counsel*. 2006;15:77-83.
20. Hartmann LC, Sellers TA, Schaid DJ, et al. Efficacy of bilateral prophylactic mastectomy in BRCA1 and BRCA2 gene mutation carriers. *J Natl Cancer Inst*. 2001;93:1633-1637.
21. Rebbeck TR, Lynch HT, Neuhausen SL, et al.; for The Prevention and Observation of Surgical End Points Study Group. Prophylactic oophorectomy in carriers of *BRCA1* or *BRCA2* mutations. *N Engl J Med*. 2002;346:1616-1622.
22. Rebbeck TR, Friebel T, Lynch HT, et al. Bilateral prophylactic mastectomy reduces breast cancer risk in *BRCA1* and *BRCA2* mutation carriers: the PROSE Study Group. *J Clin Oncol*. 2004;22:1055-1062.
23. Watson P, Narod SA, Fodde R, et al. Carrier risk status changes resulting from mutation testing in hereditary nonpolyposis colorectal cancer and hereditary breast-ovarian cancer. *J Hum Genet*. 2003;40:591-596. PMC1735553.
24. Ladabaum U, Wang G, Terdiman J, et al. Strategies to identify the Lynch syndrome among patients with colorectal cancer: a cost-effectiveness analysis. *Ann Intern Med*. 2011;155:69-79.
25. Burt RW. Who should have genetic testing for Lynch syndrome? *Ann Intern Med*. 2011;155:127-128.
26. Teutsch SM, Bradley LA, Palomaki GE, Haddow JE, Piper M, Calonge N; EGAPP Working Group. The Evaluation of Genomic Applications in Practice and Prevention (EGAPP) initiative: methods of the EGAPP Working Group. *Genet Med*. 2009;11:3-14.
27. Mvundura M, Grosse SD, Hampel H, Palomaki GE. The cost-effectiveness of genetic testing strategies for Lynch syndrome among newly diagnosed patients with colorectal cancer. *Genet Med*. 2010;12:93-104.

28. Vasen HF, Möslein G, Alonso A, et al. Recommendations to improve identification of hereditary and familial colorectal cancer in Europe. *Fam Cancer*. 2010;9:109-115.
29. Rice CD, Ruschmann JG, Martin LJ, Manders JB, Miller E. Retrospective comparison of patient outcomes after in-person and telephone results disclosure counseling for BRCA1/2 genetic testing. *Fam Cancer*. 2010;9:203-212.
30. Offit K, Thom P. Ethical and legal aspects of cancer genetic testing. *Semin Oncol*. 2007;34:435-443.
31. American Medical Association. Opinion 2.138—genetic testing of children. 2007. http://www.ama-assn.org/ama/pub/physician-resources/medical-ethics/code-medical-ethics/opinion2138.page. Accessed June 24, 2011.
32. Genetic Information Nondiscrimination Act of 2007. 2007. S 358, HR 493, 110th Cong, 1st Sess.
33. Hudson KL, Holohan MK, Collins FS. Keeping pace with the times—the Genetic Information Nondiscrimination Act of 2008. *N Engl J Med*. 2008;358:2661-2663.
34. U.S. Department of Health and Human Services. HIPAA—general information. December 14, 2005. http://www.cms.hhs.gov/HIPAAGenInfo/. Accessed January 29, 2007.
35. Pirzadeh-Miller S, Bellcross C, Robinson L, Matloff ET. Direct-to-consumer genetic testing: helpful, harmful, or pure entertainment? *Community Oncol*. 2011;8:263-268.
36. U.S. Government Accounting Office. GAO report: direct-to-consumer genetic tests: misleading test results are further complicated by deceptive marketing and other questionable practices. 2010. http:www.gao.gov/products/GAO-10-847T. Accessed July 11, 2011.
37. Udesky L. The ethics of direct-to-consumer genetic testing. *Lancet*. 2011;376:1377-1378.
38. Samuel GN, Jordens CFC, Kerridge I. Direct-to-consumer personal genome testing: ethical and regulatory issues that arise from wanting to 'know' your DNA. *Intern Med J*. 2010;40:220-224.
39. Manne SL, Meropol NJ, Weinberg DS, et al. Facilitating informed decisions regarding microsatellite instability testing among high-risk individuals diagnosed with colorectal cancer. *J Clin Oncol*. 2010;28:1366-1372.
40. Hampel H, Frankel WL, Martin E, et al. Feasibility of screening for Lynch syndrome among patients with colorectal cancer. *J Clin Oncol*. 2008;26:5783-5788.
41. Evaluation of Genomic Applications in Practice and Prevention (EGAPP) Working Group. Recommendations from the EGAPP Working Group: genetic testing strategies in newly diagnosed individuals with colorectal cancer aimed at reducing morbidity and mortality from Lynch syndrome in relatives. *Genet Med*. 2009;11:35-41.
42. Hampel H, Frankel W, Panescu J, et al. Screening for Lynch syndrome (hereditary nonpolyposis colorectal cancer) among endometrial cancer patients. *Cancer Res*. 2006;66:7810-7817.
43. Ribic CM, Sargent DJ, Moore MJ, et al. Tumor microsatellite-instability status as a predictor of benefit from fluorouracil-based adjuvant chemotherapy for colon cancer. *N Engl J Med*. 2003;349:247-257.
44. Palomaki GE, McClain MR, Melillo S, Hampel HL, Thibodeau SN. EGAPP supplementary evidence review: DNA testing strategies aimed at reducing morbidity and mortality from Lynch syndrome. *Genet Med*. 2009;11:42-65.
45. Manne SL, Chung DC, Weinberg DS, et al. Knowledge and attitudes about microsatellite instability testing among high-risk individuals diagnosed with colorectal cancer. *Cancer Epidemiol Biomarkers Prev*. 2007;16:2110-2117.
46. Lynch HT. Family Information Service and hereditary cancer. *Cancer*. 2001;91:625-628.
47. Lynch HT, Snyder C, Lynch J, Ghate S, Thome S. Family information service (FIS) in a *BRCA1* extended family. *J Clin Oncol*. 2006;24:55s (Abstract).
48. Wizemann T, Berger AC; for the Institute of Medicine of the National Academies. *The Value of Genetic and Genomic Technologies Workshop Summary*. Washington, DC: The National Academies Press; 2010:873-880.
49. Offit K, Groeger E, Turner S, Wadsworth EA, Weiser MA. The "duty to warn" a patient's family members about hereditary disease risks. *JAMA*. 2004;292:1469-1473.
50. Aktan-Collan K, Haukkala A, Pylvänäinen K, et al. Direct contact in inviting high-risk members of hereditary colon cancer families to genetic counselling and DNA testing. *J Med Genet*. 2007;44:732-738.
51. Mesters I, Ausems M, Eichhorn S, Vasen H. Informing one's family about a genetic testing for hereditary non-polyposis colorectal cancer (HNPCC): a retrospective exploratory study. *Fam Cancer*. 2005;4:163-167.
52. Järvinen HJ, Aarnio M, Mustonen H, et al. Controlled 15-year trial on screening for colorectal cancer in families with hereditary nonpolyposis colorectal cancer. *Gastroenterology*. 2000;118:829-834.
53. de Jong AE, Hendriks YMC, Kleibeuker JH, et al. Decrease in mortality in Lynch syndrome families because of surveillance. *Gastroenterology*. 2006;130:665-671.
54. Aktan-Collan K, Mecklin J-K, Jarivnen HJ, et al. Predictive genetic testing for hereditary non-polyposis colorectal cancer: uptake and long-term satisfaction. *Int J Cancer (Pred Oncol)*. 2000;89:44-50.
55. Aktan-Collan K, Haukkala A, Mecklin J-P, Uutela A, Kääriäinen H. Psychological consequences of predictive genetic testing for hereditary non-polyposis colorectal cancer (HNPCC): a prospective follow-up study. *Int J Cancer*. 2001;93:608-611.
56. Aktan-Collan K, Haukkala A, Mecklin JP, Uutela A, Kaariainen H. Comprehension of cancer risk one and 12 months after predictive genetic testing for hereditary non-polyposis colorectal cancer. *J Med Genet*. 2001;38:787-792.
57. Meiser B, Collins V, Warren R, et al. Psychological impact of genetic testing for hereditary non-polyposis colorectal cancer. *Clin Genet*. 2004;66:502-511.
58. Claes E, Denayer L, Evers-Kiebooms G, et al. Predictive testing for hereditary nonpolyposis colorectal cancer: subjective perception regarding colorectal and endometrial cancer, distress, and health-related behavior at one year post-test. *Genet Test*. 2005;9:54-65.
59. Gritz ER, Peterson SK, Vernon SW, et al. Psychological impact of genetic testing for hereditary nonpolyposis colorectal cancer. *J Clin Oncol*. 2005;23:1902-1910.
60. de Wert G. Cascade screening: whose information is it anyway? *Eur J Hum Genet*. 2005;13:397-398.
61. Newson AJ, Humphries SE. Cascade testing in familial hypercholesterolaemia: how should family members be contacted? *Eur J Hum Genet*. 2005;13:401-408.
62. Godard B, Hurlimann T, Letendre M, Égalité N; INHERIT BRCAs. Guidelines for disclosing genetic information to family members: from development to use. *Fam Cancer*. 2006;5:103-116.
63. Svendsen M. Genetics and prevention: a policy in the making. *New Genet Soc*. 2006;25:51-68.
64. Tupasela A. When legal worlds collide: from research to treatment in hereditary cancer prevention. *Eur J Cancer Care (Engl)*. 2006;15:257-266.
65. Kääriäinen H, Rantanen E, Hietala M. Summary of the guidelines for genetic counselling, 2006. *Eurogentest*. 2006. http://eurogentest.org/web/files/public/unit3/summaryofguidelinesMay06.pdf. Accessed August 13, 2012.
66. Keller M, Jost R, Kadmon M, et al. Acceptance of and attitude toward genetic testing for hereditary nonpolyposis colorectal cancer: a comparison of participants and nonparticipants in genetic counseling. *Dis Colon Rectum*. 2004;47:153-162.
67. Lerman C, Hughes C, Trock BJ, et al. Genetic testing in families with hereditary nonpolyposis colon cancer. *JAMA*. 1999;281:1618-1622.
68. Pate v. Threlkel, 661 So.2d 278 (1995). 1995.
69. Safer v. Estate of Pack, 677 A.2d 1188 (NJ App), appeal denied, 683 A2d1163 (NJ 1996). 1996.
70. Molloy v Meier, Nos. C9-02-1821, C9-02-1837 (Minn 2004). 2004.
71. President's Commission for the Study of Ethical Problems in Medicine and Biomedical and Biobehavioral Research. *Screening and Counseling for Genetic Conditions: The Ethical, Social, and Legal Implications of Genetics Screening, Counseling, and Education Programs*. Washington, DC: US Government Printing Office; 1998.
72. American Society of Human Genetics. ASHG statement: professional disclosure of familial genetic information. *Am J Hum Genet*. 1998;62:474-483.
73. Andrews LB, Fullerton JE, Holtzman NA, Motulsky AG. *Assessing Genetic Risks: Implications for Health and Social Policy*. Washington, DC: National Academy Press; 1994.
74. Linden AM. *Canadian Tort Law*. 5th ed. Toronto, ON: Butterworths; 1993.

75. Schulmann K, Brasch FE, Kunstmann E, et al. HNPCC-associated small bowel cancer: clinical and molecular characteristics. *Gastroenterology*. 2005;128:590-599.
76. Stoffel EM, Turgeon DK, Stockwell DH, et al.; for Great Lakes-New England Clinical Epidemiology and Validation Center of the Early Detection Research Network. Chromoendoscopy detects more adenomas than colonoscopy using intensive inspection without dye spraying. *Cancer Prev Res*. 2008;1:507-513.
77. Butterly LF, Chase MP, Pohl H, Fiarman GS. Prevalence of clinically important histology in small adenomas. *Clin Gastroenterol Hepatol*. 2006;4:343-348.
78. O'Brien MJ, Winawer SJ, Zauber AG, et al. The National Polyp study. Patient and polyp characteristics associated with high-grade dysplasia in colorectal adenomas. *Gastroenterology*. 1990;98:371-379.
79. Soetikno RM, Kaltenbach T, Rouse RV, et al. Prevalence of non-polypoid (flat and depressed) colorectal neoplasms in asymptomatic and symptomatic adults. *JAMA*. 2008;299:1027-1035.
80. Stoffel EM, Turgeon DK, Stockwell DH, et al.; for Great Lakes-New England Clinical Epidemiology and Validation Center of the Early Detection Research Network. Missed adenomas during colonoscopic surveillance in individuals with Lynch syndrome (hereditary nonpolyposis colorectal cancer). *Cancer Prev Res*. 2008;1:470-475.
81. Vasen HFA, Nagengast FM, Khan PM. Interval cancers in hereditary non-polyposis colorectal cancer (Lynch syndrome). *Lancet*. 1995;345:1183-1184.
82. Edelstein DL, Axilbund J, Baxter M, et al. Rapid development of colorectal neoplasia in patients with Lynch syndrome. *Clin Gastroenterol Hepatol*. 2011;9:340-343.
83. Hurlstone DP, Karajeh M, Cross SS, et al. The role of high-magnification-chromoscopic colonoscopy in hereditary nonpolyposis colorectal cancer screening: a prospective "back-to-back" endoscopic study. *Am J Gastroenterol*. 2005;100:2167-2173.
84. Lecomte T, Cellier C, Meatchi T, et al. Chromoendoscopic colonoscopy for detecting preneoplastic lesions in hereditary non-polyposis colorectal cancer syndrome. *Clin Gastroenterol Hepatol*. 2005;3:897-902.
85. East JE, Suzuki N, Stavrinidis M, Guenther T, Thomas HJW, Saunders BP. Narrow band imaging for colonoscopic surveillance in hereditary non-polyposis colorectal cancer. *Gut*. 2008;57:65-70.
86. Natarajan N, Watson P, Silva-Lopez E, Lynch HT. Comparison of extended colectomy and limited resection in patients with Lynch syndrome. *Dis Colon Rectum*. 2010;53:77-82.
87. da Silva FC, de Oliveira LP, Santos EM, et al. Frequency of extracolonic tumors in Brazilian families with Lynch syndrome: analysis of a hereditary colorectal cancer institutional registry. *Fam Cancer*. 2010;9:563-570.
88. Capelle LG, van Grieken NCT, Lingsma HF, et al. Risk and epidemiological time trends of gastric cancer in Lynch syndrome carriers in the Netherlands. *Gastroenterology*. 2010;138:487-492.
89. Bonadona V, Bonaïti B, Olschwang S, et al. Cancer risks associated with germline mutations in *MLH1*, *MSH2*, *MSH6* genes in Lynch syndrome. *JAMA*. 2011;305:2304-2310.
90. Kastrinos F, Mukherjee B, Tayob N, et al. Risk of pancreatic cancer in families with Lynch syndrome. *JAMA*. 2009;302:1790-1795.
91. National Comprehensive Cancer Network. *National Comprehensive Cancer Network*. 2011. www.nccn.org. Accessed August 13, 2012.
92. Schmeler KM, Lynch HT, Chen L-M, et al. Prophylactic surgery to reduce the risk of gynecologic cancers in the Lynch syndrome. *N Engl J Med*. 2006;354:261-269.
93. Westin SN, Sun CC, Lu KH, et al. Satisfaction with ovarian carcinoma risk-reduction strategies among women at high risk for breast and ovarian carcinoma. *Cancer*. 2011;117:2659-2667.
94. Lynch HT, Severin MJ, Mooney MJ, Lynch JF. Insurance adjudication favoring prophylactic surgery in hereditary breast-ovarian cancer syndrome. *Gynecol Oncol*. 1995;57:23-26.
95. Balaguer F, Moreira L, Lozano JJ, et al. Colorectal cancers with microsatellite instability display unique miRNA profiles. *Clin Cancer Res*. 2011;17:6239-6249.
96. Tran B, Kopetz S, Tie J, et al. Impact of BRAF mutation and microsatellite instability on the pattern of metastatic spread and prognosis in metastatic colorectal cancer. *Cancer*. 2011;117:4623-4632.
97. Li H, Haurigot V, Doyon Y, et al. *In vivo* genome editing restores haemostatis in a mouse model of haemophilia. *Nature*. 2011;475:217-221.
98. Pollak ES, High KA. Hemophilia A: factor IX deficiency. In: Scriver CR, Beaudet AL, Valle D, Sly WS, eds. *The Metabolic and Molecular Bases of Inherited Disease*. New York, NY: McGraw Hill; 2001:4393-4413.
99. Umov FD, Miller JC, Lee YL, et al. Highly efficient endogenous human gene correction using designed zinc-finger nucleases. *Nature*. 2005;435:646-651.
100. Moehle EA, Rock JM, Lee YL, et al. Targeted gene addition into a specified location in the human genome using designed zinc finger nucleases. *Proc Natl Acad Sci U S A*. 2007;104:3055-3060.
101. Esteller M. Epigenetics in cancer. *N Engl J Med*. 2008;358:1148-1159.
102. Holliday R. The inheritance of epigenetic defects. *Nature*. 1983;301:89-92.
103. Hitchins MP, Wong JJL, Suthers G, et al. Inheritance of a cancer-associated *MLH1* germ-line epimutation. *N Engl J Med*. 2007;356:697-705.
104. Hitchins M, Rapkins R, Chau-To K, et al. Dominantly inherited constitutional epigenetic silencing of *MLH1* in a cancer-affected family is linked to a single nucleotide variant within the 5'UTR. *Cancer Cell*. 2011;20:200-213.
105. van Engeland M, Derks S, Smits KM, Meijer GA, Herman JG. Colorectal cancer epigenetics: complex simplicity. *J Clin Oncol*. 2011;29:1382-1391.
106. Burn J, Bishop T, Chapman PD, et al.; International CAPP Consortium. A randomized placebo-controlled prevention trial of aspirin and/or resistant starch in young people with familial adenomatous polyposis. *Cancer Prev Res*. 2011;4:655-665.
107. Chan AT. Aspirin and familial adenomatous polyposis: coming full circle. *Cancer Prev Res*. 2011;4:623-627.
108. Burn J, Bishop T, Mecklin J-P, et al.; for the CAPP2 Investigators. Effect of aspirin or resistant starch on colorectal neoplasia in the Lynch syndrome. *N Engl J Med*. 2008;359:2567-2578.
109. Burn J, Gerdes A-M, Macrae F, et al. Aspirin reduces cancer risk in carriers of hereditary colorectal cancer: the CAPP2 Randomised Controlled Trial. *Lancet*. 2011;378:2081-2087.
110. Jass JR, Walsh MD, Barker M, Simms LA, Young J, Leggett BA. Distinction between familial and sporadic forms of colorectal cancer showing DNA microsatellite instability. *Eur J Cancer*. 2002;38:858-866.
111. Mcilhatton MA, Tyler J, Kerepesi LA, et al. Aspirin and low-dose nitric oxide-donating aspirin increase life span in a Lynch syndrome mouse model. *Cancer Prev Res*. 2011;4:684-693.
112. Tan X-L, Reid Lombardo KM, Bamlet WR, et al. Aspirin, nonsteroidal anti-inflammatory drugs, acetaminophen, and pancreatic cancer risk: a clinic-based case-control study. *Cancer Prev Res*. 2011;4:1835-1841.
113. Sinicrope FA, Foster NR, Thibodeau SN, et al. DNA mismatch repair status and colon cancer recurrence and survival in clinical trials of 5-fluorouracil-based adjuvant therapy. *J Natl Cancer Inst*. 2011;103:863-875.
114. Audeh MW, Carmichael J, Penson RT, et al. Oral poly(ADP-ribose) polymerase inhibitor olaparib in patients with BRCA1 or BRCA2 mutations and recurrent ovarian cancer: a proof-of-concept trial. *Lancet*. 2010;376:245-251.
115. O'Shaughnessy J, Schwartzberg LS, Danso MA, et al. A randomized phase III study of iniparib (BSI-201) in combination with gemcitabine/carboplatin (G/C) in metastatic triple-negative breast cancer (TNBC). *J Clin Oncol*. 2011;29(May 20 suppl):1007 (Abstract).
116. Byrski T, Gronwald J, Huzarski T, et al. Pathologic complete response rates in young women with *BRCA1*-positive breast cancers after neoadjuvant chemotherapy. *J Clin Oncol*. 2010;28:375-379.
117. Kriege M, Seynaeve C, Meijers-Heijboer H, et al. Sensitivity to first-line chemotherapy for metastatic breast cancer in BRCA1 and BRCA2 mutation carriers. *J Clin Oncol*. 2009;27:3764-3771.
118. Kriege M, Jager A, Hooning MJ, et al. The efficacy of taxane chemotherapy for metastatic breast cancer in BRCA1 and BRCA2 mutation carriers. *Cancer*. 2012;118:899-907.
119. Arun B, Bayraktar S, Liu DD, et al. Response to neoadjuvant systemic therapy for breast cancer in BRCA mutation carriers and noncarriers: a single-institution experience. *J Clin Oncol*. 2011;29:3739-3746.
120. Robson ME. Should the presence of germline BRCA1/2 mutations influence treatment selection in breast cancer? *J Clin Oncol*. 2011;29:3724-3726.
121. Chetrit A, Hirsh-Yechezkel G, Ben-David Y, Lubin F, Friedman E, Sadetzki S. Effect of BRCA1/2 mutations on long-term

survival of patients with invasive ovarian cancer: the National Israeli Study of Ovarian Cancer. *J Clin Oncol.* 2008;26:20-25.

122. Cass I, Baldwin RL, Varkey T, Moslehi R, Narod SA, Karlan BY. Improved survival in women with *BRCA*-associated ovarian carcinoma. *Cancer.* 2003;97:2187-2195.
123. Boyd J, Sonoda Y, Federici MG, et al. Clinicopathologic features of BRCA-linked and sporadic ovarian cancer. *JAMA.* 2000;283:2260-2265.
124. Norquist B, Wurz KA, Pennil CC, et al. Secondary somatic mutations restoring BRCA1/2 predict chemotherapy resistance in hereditary ovarian carcinomas. *J Clin Oncol.* 2011;29:3008-3015.
125. Lee J, Annunziata CM, Minasian LM, et al. Phase I study of the PARP inhibitor olaparib (O) in combination with carboplatin (C) in BRCA1/2 mutation carriers with breast (Br) or ovarian (Ov) cancer (Ca). *J Clin Oncol.* May 2011;29(suppl):2520 (Abstract).
126. Taniguchi T, Tischkowitz M, Ameziane N, et al. Disruption of the Fanconi anemia-BRCA pathway in cisplatin-sensitive ovarian tumors. *Nat Med.* 2003;9:568-574.
127. Dhillon KK, Swisher EM, Taniguchi T. Secondary mutations of BRCA1/2 and drug resistance. *Cancer Sci.* 2011;102:663-669.
128. Fong PC, Yap TA, Boss DS, et al. Poly(ADP)-ribose polymerase inhibition: frequent durable responses in BRCA carrier ovarian cancer correlating with platinum-free interval. *J Clin Oncol.* 2011;28:2512-2519.
129. Olaussen KA, Dunant A, Fouret P, et al.; IALT Bio Investigators. DNA repair by ERCC1 in non-small-cell lung cancer and cisplatin-based adjuvant chemotherapy. *N Engl J Med.* 2006;355:983-991.
130. Wu X, Ye Y, Rosell R, et al. Genome-wide association study of survival in non-small cell lung cancer patients receiving platinum-based chemotherapy. *J Natl Cancer Inst.* 2011;103: 817-825.
131. Wu X, Lu C, Ye Y, et al. Germline genetic variations in drug action pathways predict clinical outcomes in advanced lung cancer treated with platinum-based chemotherapy. *Pharmacogenet Genomics.* 2008;18:955-965.
132. Wang Y, Broderick P, Webb E, et al. Common 5p15.33 and 6p21.33 variants influence lung cancer risk. *Nat Genet.* 2008;40:1407-1409.
133. Hildebrandt MA, Gu J, Wu X. Pharmacogenetics of platinum-based chemotherapy in NSCLC. *Expert Opin Drug Metab Toxicol.* 2009;5:745-755.
134. Dolan ME, Newbold KG, Nagasubramanian R, et al. Heritability and linkage analysis of sensitivity to cisplatin-induced cytotoxicity. *Cancer Res.* 2004;64:4353-4356.
135. Ng SB, Turner EH, Robertson PD, et al. Targeted capture and massively parallel sequencing of 12 human exomes. *Nature.* 2009;461:272-276.
136. Cooper DN, Krawczak M, Antonorakis SE. The nature and mechanisms of human gene mutation. In: Scriver C, Beaudet AL, Sly WS, Valle D, eds. *The Metabolic and Molecular Bases of Inherited Disease.* 7th ed. New York, NY: McGraw-Hill; 1995:259-291.

CHAPTER 20

Molecular Imaging and Cancer Management: PET and MR Agents for Molecular Imaging of Cancer Metabolism

Yunkou Wu, Xiankai Sun, and A. Dean Sherry

INTRODUCTION

Clinical imaging plays an important role in cancer detection but often only after a tumor has reached a sufficient size to be easily detected. For this reason and others, most of our standard clinical imaging modalities are not suitable for early cancer detection and have limited capacity for extracting specific biological information about a tumor. Fortunately, new imaging approaches collectively referred to as molecular imaging have undergone an explosive growth over the past two decades. The power of molecular imaging over traditional cancer diagnoses such as tissue biopsies and histopathology lies in its noninvasive properties. Thus, molecular imaging can be used to interrogate cancer staging and to follow treatment response serially in the same tumor. Molecular imaging tools can be classified by energy (X-rays, positrons, photons, or sound), spatial resolution (macroscopic, mesoscopic, or microscopic), or the type of information obtained (anatomical, physiological, cellular, or molecular).[1] Magnetic resonance imaging and spectroscopy (MRI and MRS), positron emission tomography (PET), computed tomography (CT), single photon emission computed tomography (SPECT), and ultrasound are all examples of macroscopic imaging technologies. Each technology has specific strengths and limitations in terms of resolution, depth penetration, imaging time, and cost.[2] PET is considered by many as the only true molecular imaging technique because it provides indices of metabolic flux and offers superior sensitivity compared to other imaging modalities but offers little information about tissue morphology. MRI and MRS offer a wide range of information from anatomical to metabolic but have limited sensitivity compared to nuclear imaging techniques at the molecular level. With advances in combining or fusing imaging technologies, multimodality imaging systems such as PET/CT and PET/MRI are rapidly becoming the norm. These allow for the combination of the advantages of superior anatomical resolution with molecular sensitivity for a more comprehensive diagnosis.

Molecular imaging has been defined as "the visualization, characterization, and measurement of biological processes at the molecular and cellular levels in humans and other living systems using noninvasive imaging techniques such as PET, SPECT, MRI, MRS, optical imaging, ultrasound, and others."[3] Molecular imaging commonly invokes the use of either an endogenous molecule or an exogenous imaging agent to monitor various biological molecular targets that correlate with a disease progress.[3] Molecular imaging is most often associated with oncology partly because of the rapid growth of the use of ^{18}F-fluorodeoxyglucose (^{18}F-FDG) as a marker of high glycolytic activity. Tumor cells exhibit various abnormalities in metabolism, proliferation, apoptosis, signal transduction, and gene expression while the tumor microenvironment also undergoes alterations in oxygenation, pH, and extracellular matrix organization. Many of these biological processes have been targeted for direct imaging of cancer with specific agents. In contrast to receptor-targeted imaging for monitoring the expression levels of a particular receptor, imaging of metabolism interrogates the effect of metabolic milieu on cancer initiation, progression, and dissemination, thus providing unique information about the functional state of tumor tissues. In this chapter, we will focus our attention on molecular imaging agents that report on cancer metabolism using either PET or MRI/MRS for detection.

METABOLIC ALTERNATIONS AND ADAPTATIONS IN CANCER CELLS

Tumor cells display a different metabolic profile from the normal cells in a microenvironment where the concentrations of crucial nutrients are dynamic and often stressed. These metabolic alternations provide the rapid energy generation required for an increased biosynthesis of macromolecules while maintaining an appropriate cellular redox balance. Specifically, cancer cells undergo metabolic alterations of four major classes of macromolecules: carbohydrates, proteins, lipids, and nucleic acids (Fig. 20.1).[4-6]

It has been known for years that cancer cells experience a shift in ATP generation from oxidative phosphorylation to glycolysis (the Warburg effect) even when oxygen is readily available.[7] This shift in energy generation is paradoxical because ATP production from glycolysis is much less efficient than from oxidative phosphorylation. This suggests that glycolytic ATP generation represents an adaptive advantage for tumor growth and proliferation.[6] Tumor cells can live via glycolysis under conditions of fluctuating oxygen tension that would otherwise be lethal to the cells if oxidative phosphorylation was an absolute requirement.

Mutations in tumor suppression genes, such as PTEN in phosphatidylinositol 3-kinase (PI3K) signaling pathways, can activate the key mediators, serine/threonine protein kinase (AKT1) and hypoxia-inducible factor 1 (HIF1), which in turn stimulate the expression of genes that promote glycolysis.[6] Specifically, AKT1 can stimulate glycolysis by upregulating the expression of glucose transporters (GLUTs) and by phosphorylating key glycolytic enzymes. Activated HIF1 in combination with c-MYC proto-oncogene (MYC) also amplifies the transcription of genes encoding GLUTs and most glycolytic enzymes. In addition, the HIF1/MYC combination can activate pyruvate dehydrogenase kinase (PDK), an enzyme that inactivates mitochondrial pyruvate dehydrogenase complex (PDH) and thereby blocks the flow of glycolytically produced pyruvate into the tricarboxylic acid (TCA) cycle. The net consequence is that pyruvate derived from glucose is subsequently converted largely into lactate in tumor cells. Tumor cells then export excess lactate and acid produced by glycolysis to maintain normal intracellular pH (pHi) for cell survival by virtue of multiple transporters and enzymes that are upregulated by HIF1.[4] At least three factors contribute to the accumulation of excess acid in the extracellular matrix. First, the

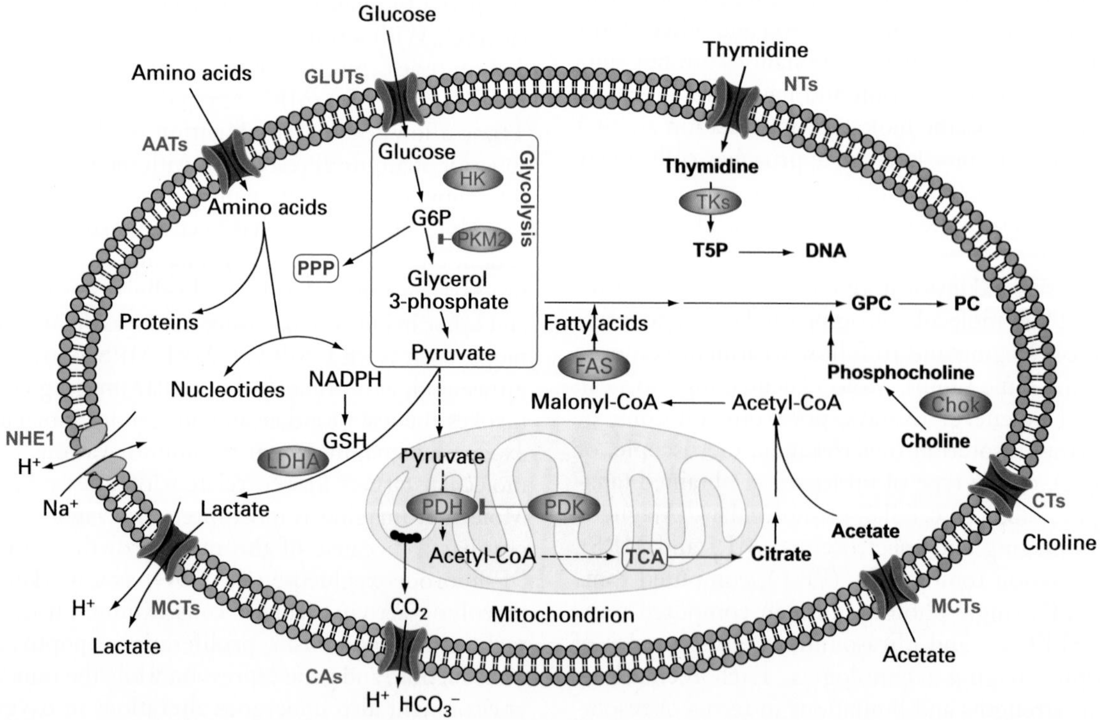

FIGURE 20–1 Metabolic reprogramming in cancer cells. The upregulated alterations are indicated in red color. GLUTs, glucose transporters; HK, hexokinase; LDHA, lactate dehydrogenase isoform; MCTs, monocarboxylate transporters; PKM2, pyruvate kinase isoform M2; CAs, carbonic anhydrases; NHE1, Na^+–H^+ exchanger; PDH, pyruvate dehydrogenase; PDK, pyruvate dehydrogenase kinase; AATs, amino acid transporters 1; GSH, glutathione; CTs, choline transporters; FAS, fatty acid synthase; ChoK, choline kinase; NTs, nucleoside transporters; TKs, thymidine kinases; PPP, pentose phosphate pathway. (The figure is reproduced from Kroemer G, Pouyssegur J, *Cancer Cell.* 2008;13:472-482 and Plathow C, Weber WA, *J Nucl Med.* 2008;49(suppl 2):43S-63S.)

monocarboxylate transporters (MCTs) that export excess lactate are known to co-transport protons along with lactate. Second, overexpressed Na^+–H^+ exchanger (NHE1) also removed protons. And last, overexpressed carbonic anhydrase (CA) isoforms 9 and 12, two transmembrane enzymes, efficiently hydrate intracellular CO_2 to generate membrane-impermeable H^+ and HCO_3^- in the extracellular space. These combined events result in an increase in extracellular acidity that in turn promotes invasion and metastasis of tumor cells (see Fig. 20.1).

In addition to enhanced glycolysis to supply the ATP needed for cellular proliferation, tumor cells must also adopt other metabolic pathways to acquire other building blocks for rapid syntheses of macromolecules either by transporting more nutrients such as amino acids into the cells or by promoting biosynthesis. mTOR, a 289-kDa serine/threonine protein kinase and a member of the PIKK (PI3K-related kinase) family, is one of the key enzymes that regulates nutrient uptake and biosynthesis. mTOR exerts its effects in two ways. First, mTOR signaling promotes uptake of amino acids by increasing the expression of specific amino acid transporters (AATs).[8] Second, activated mTOR stimulates the expression of a series of genes for promoting protein, lipid biosynthesis, mRNA translation, and ribosome biogenesis.[6] For example, two key enzymes related with lipid syntheses, fatty acid synthase (FAS) and choline kinase (ChoK), are activated by mTOR and HIF1, respectively, during the cancer cell proliferation. Activated FAS catalyzes syntheses of long-chain fatty acids from malonyl-CoA, while ChoK catalyzes the conversion of choline to phosphorylcholine (PC). In addition, MYC can also increase the mitochondrial biogenesis and function by activating the transcription of related enzymes.

The levels of reactive oxygen species (ROS), produced as a by-product of increased metabolism, must be tightly regulated in tumor cells because a high level of ROS results in damage to macromolecules and promotes apoptosis. Tumor cells require higher levels of two primary antioxidants, nicotinamide adenine dinucleotide phosphate (NADPH) and glutathione (GHS), to control ROS levels. Increased NADPH production in tumor cells is thought to occur by diverting glucose 6-phosphate (G6P) away from glycolysis into the pentose phosphate pathway (PPP), the major pathway for production of NADPH and sugar building blocks required for biosynthesis (see Fig. 20.1). This diversion is promoted by upregulation of the less active, dimeric form of pyruvate kinase isoform M2 (PKM2) in cancer cells. Slower conversion of phosphoenolpyruvate (PEP) to pyruvate results in buildup of glycolytic intermediates and this is thought to promote increased flux of G6P toward PPP. In addition, MYC drives the syntheses of GSH through glutaminolysis (see Fig. 20.1).

In summary, many metabolic pathways in cancer cells are reprogrammed. These metabolic alterations represent biological adaptations for cellular survival and a biosynthetic advantage for tumor proliferation. Some of these metabolic alterations are so significant that they become likely targets for developing molecular imaging reporters, either through the use of endogenous metabolites or by the use of exogenous agents that participate in or interact with these metabolic processes.

AGENTS FOR MOLECULAR IMAGING OF CANCER METABOLISM

Agents for Glucose Metabolism

As summarized above, tumor cells exhibit a distinct metabolic phenotype characterized by increased consumption of glucose through glycolysis. Specifically, glucose uptake is increased by 20- to 30-fold in tumor cells compared with normal cells.[9] This dramatic change in metabolism can be easily monitored by using a variety of molecular imaging agents and imaging techniques (Table 20.1).

PET Agents

^{18}F-Fluorodeoxyglucose

PET imaging with ^{18}F-FDG has dominated this field since its invention in 1977.[10,11] As the first FDA-approved PET tracer, ^{18}F-FDG has become indispensable for routine clinical imaging for staging, restaging, and monitoring therapeutic responses in many types of cancer.[11] Metabolically, ^{18}F-FDG is taken into cells by means of GLUTs and phosphorylated by hexokinase (HK) to ^{18}F-FDG-6-phosphate, but this phosphorylated intermediate cannot be metabolized further either through glycolysis or through the PPP pathway due to the presence of ^{18}F at the C2 position of glucose. Hence, after intravenous injection, ^{18}F-FDG accumulates in all healthy cells to some extent but shows greatest accumulation in tumor cells that have the most active glucose transporters. Image contrast is further enhanced by rapid renal excretion of ^{18}F-FDG because, unlike glucose, ^{18}F-FDG is not a substrate of glucose transporters in kidneys that are involved in readsorption of glucose during glomerular filtration. Thus, a whole-body PET image collected 1 to 2 hours after administration of ^{18}F-FDG allows one to distinguish those tissues that collect excess ^{18}F-FDG (Fig. 20.2). A wide range of PET analysis methods from semiquantitative techniques to full dynamic studies with kinetic analysis can be performed clinically.[12] In general, ^{18}F-FDG accumulation in tumors reflects GLUT activity and tumor aggressiveness. A decline in ^{18}F-FDG uptake after therapy correlates well with cancer survival rate.[11] It should be noted that, despite its high diagnostic accuracy (>80%) for most types of tumors,[13] ^{18}F-FDG PET often fails to distinguish tumors from benign tissues where the glycolysis is also upregulated due to infection and inflammation. In addition, many differentiated cancer cells like those in prostate cancer are not glucose avid, while tissues like the brain always show intense ^{18}F-FDG uptake. These

TABLE 20–1 Chemical Structures of Molecular Imaging Agents

Agent Name	Chemical Structure	Dectection Method	References
^{18}F-Fluorodeoxyglucose (^{18}F-FDG)	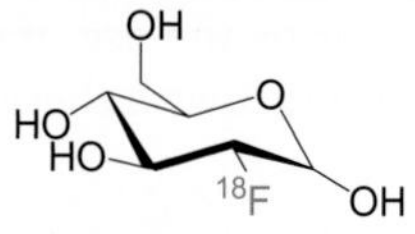	PET	10–13
[1-^{13}C]Glucose	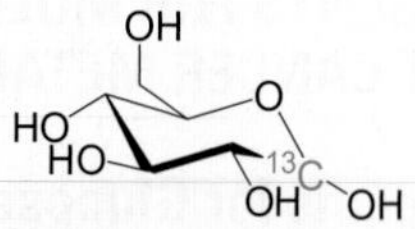	^{13}C MRS	14,15
[2-^{13}C]Fructose	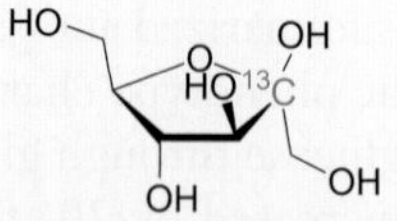	^{13}C MRS	16
[1-^{13}C]Pyruvate	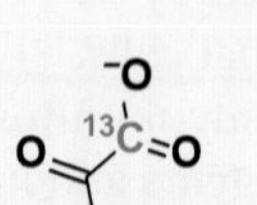	^{13}C MRS	17
Lactate	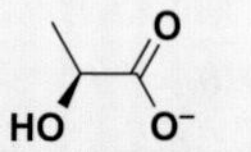	^{1}H MRS	18–20
Glucose	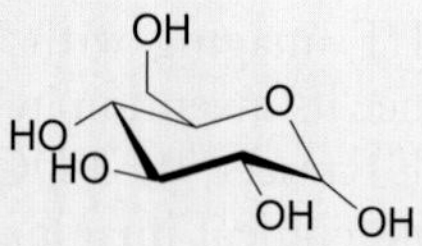	CEST	21,22
^{11}C-Acetate	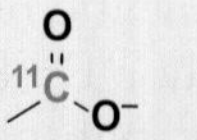	PET	23,24
^{18}F-Acetate	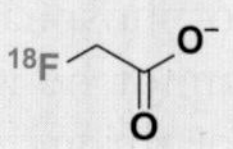	PET	25
^{11}C-Choline	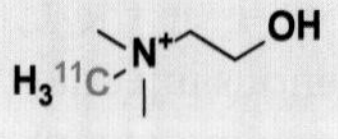	PET	26
^{18}F-Choline	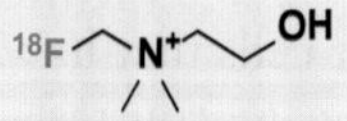	PET	27
^{18}F-Fluoroethylcholine	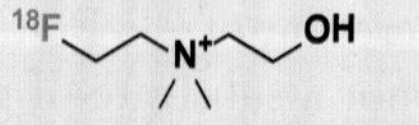	PET	28
Choline	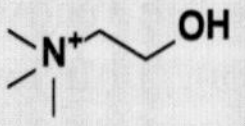	^{1}H MRS	29-33
Phosphocholine (PC)	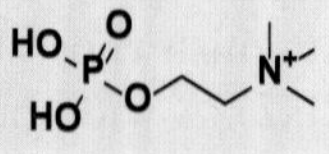	^{1}H MRS ^{31}P MRS	32,34,35
Glycerophosphocholine (GPC)	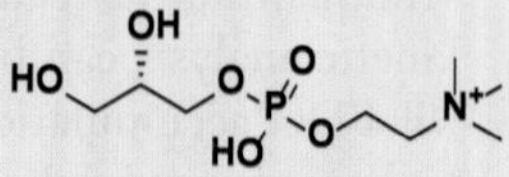	^{1}H MRS ^{31}P MRS	32,34,35
^{11}C-Methionine (^{11}C-MET)	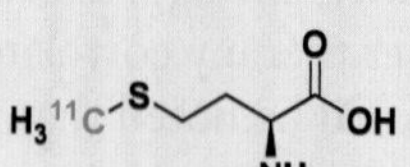	PET	36,37

^{18}F-Fluoromethyl-tyrosine (^{18}F-FMT)	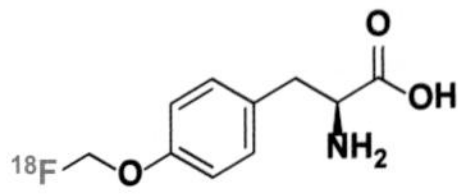	PET	38
^{18}F-Fluoroethyl-tyrosine (^{18}F-FET)	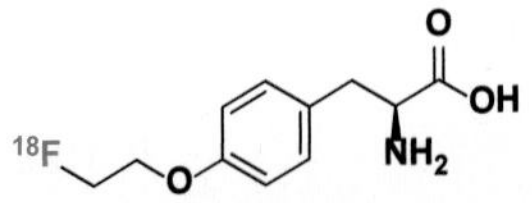	PET	38
^{18}F-Dihydroxyphenylalanine (^{18}F-DOPA)	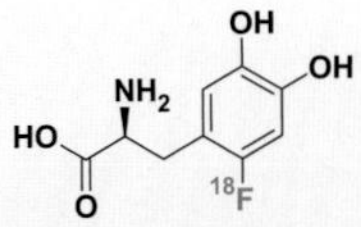	PET	39,40
[1-^{13}C]-α-Ketoisocaproate	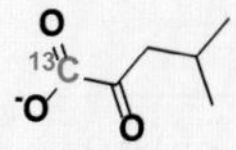	^{13}C MRS	41
GdDOTAMA-C6-Gln	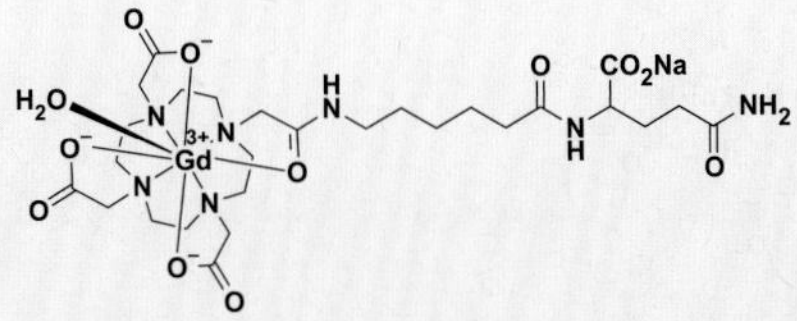	T_1 MRI	42
3′-Deoxy-3′-[^{18}F]fluorothymidine (^{18}F-FLT)	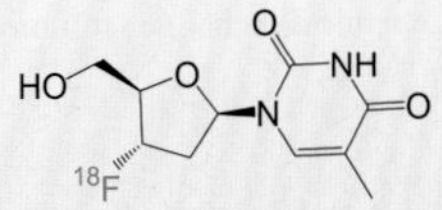	PET	43
1-(2′-Deoxy-2′fluoro-β-D-arabinofuranosyl)thymidine (^{18}F-FMAU)	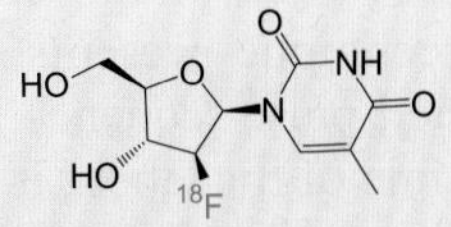	PET	43
^{11}C-Dimethyloxazolidinedione (^{11}C-DMO)	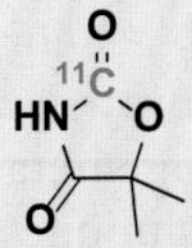	PET	44
^{64}Cu-DOTA-pHLIP	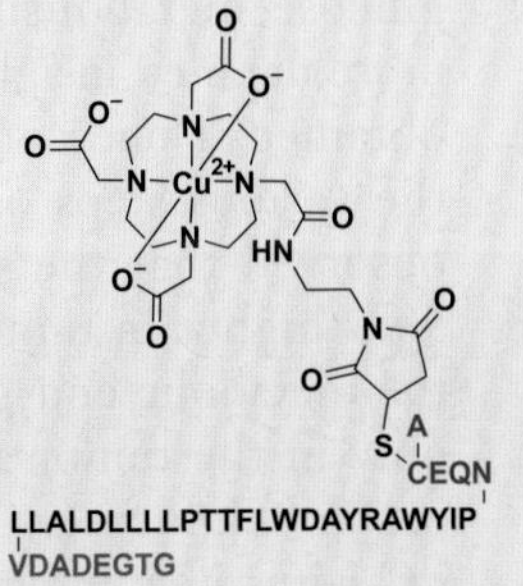 LLALDLLLLPTTFLWDAYRAWYIP VDADEGTG	PET	45
3-Aminopropylphosphonate (3-APP)	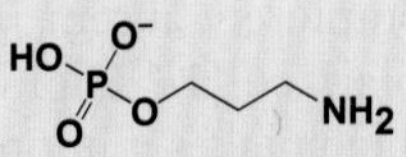	^{31}P MRS	46
(±)2-Imidazole-1-yl-3-ethoxycarbonylpropionic acid (IEPA)	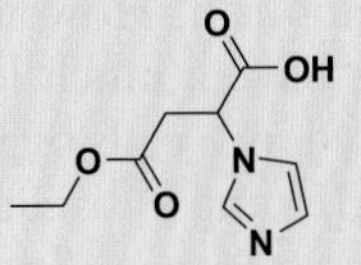	^{1}H MRS	47,48

(Continued)

TABLE 20-1 Chemical Structures of Molecular Imaging Agents (Continued)

Agent Name	Chemical Structure	Dectection Method	References
[1-^{13}C]Bicarbonate		^{13}C MRS	49
Gadolinium-1,4,7,10-tetraazacyclododecane-1,4,7,10-tetraacetic acid-tetraamide methylene phosphonate (GdDOTA-4AmP^{5-})		T_1 MRI	50,51
Ytterbium-1,4,7,10-tetraazacyclododecane-1,4,7-triacetic acid,10-o-aminoanilide (Yb-DO3A-oAA)		CEST	52

PET, positron emission tomography; MRS, magnetic resonance spectroscopy; CEST, chemical exchange saturation transfer; MRI, magnetic resonance imaging.

are major aspects that impair the diagnostic accuracy and limit the applications of ^{18}F-FDG.

MR Agents

^{13}C and ^{1}H MRS Agents

MRS can provide much more specific information about metabolic pathways beyond glucose transport that is simply not possible with ^{18}F-FDG PET. MRS has been intensively used to study many metabolic processes in cells and in tissues ex vivo and in vivo for many years. The unique strength of MRS is that it can distinguish between molecules of many types simply on the basis of differences in chemical shifts. MRS has been recognized as a global tool for the analysis of metabolic phenotypes and profiles of cancer cells, tissues, or organisms.[54] The sensitivity of MRS depends on the particular nucleus chosen for study and the abundance of that isotope. Protons, for example, are almost 100% abundant so metabolites present in tissues in the micromolar concentration range can potentially be detected by ^{1}H MRS. The MRS spin-active isotope of carbon, ^{13}C, however, is much less abundant in nature (~1.1%) and is about 1.6×10^{-2} less sensitive than ^{1}H, so applications of ^{13}C MRS are normally limited to experiments where a ^{13}C-enriched substrate has been given to tissue. The power of ^{13}C MRS compared with ^{1}H MRS is that the chemical shift of ^{13}C in molecules spans a much wider range, so it is much easier to distinguish most common metabolites by ^{13}C MRS, even phosphorylated versus non-phosphorylated substrates like G6P and glucose. Recently, an exciting technique—dynamic nuclear polarization (DNP)—was introduced to increase the detection sensitivity of ^{13}C and other nuclei by a factor of 10,000 or more.[55] Although the hyperpolarization technique presents special demands on the MR scanner, pulse sequence, data acquisition, and T_1 relaxation time of the labels, it has exciting potential for following metabolism in real time in tumors.

Various ^{13}C-enriched substrates related to the glycolytic pathway have been used as imaging agents for interrogating metabolite conversions. As a complementary technique to ^{18}F-FDG PET, imaging [1-^{13}C] glucose metabolism with MRS is attractive because more detailed insights into tumor metabolism could be obtained if one could measure or image flux through the various steps of glycolysis. As an example, it was observed that the signal of [1-^{13}C]glucose was about 50% higher in tumors than that in normal tissues and the metabolic end-product [1-^{13}C]lactate was observed only in the tumor area after 15 to 20 min of infusion of [1-^{13}C]glucose. Glutamate also became enriched in ^{13}C with time, indicating that TCA cycle activity is not completely absent in tumors.[14,15] Unfortunately, hyperpolarized [1-^{13}C]glucose has a very short ^{13}C T_1 (<2 s), which makes it impractical for in vivo imaging of glucose metabolism. However, hyperpolarized [2-^{13}C]-fructose does have a much longer T_1 (~16 s, 37°C); it is transported into cells by various GLUTs and phosphorylated by HK and subsequently enter downstream of glycolysis, so it may ultimately prove feasible to use hyperpolarized fructose as an alternative to investigate the glycolytic pathway in tumors. Early results show that [2-^{13}C]-fructose and its phosphorylation products are significantly higher in regions of prostate tumors compared with benign prostate tissues.[16] Pyruvate, another downstream metabolite of glucose, is widely used as a substrate for DNP hyperpolarization and subsequent

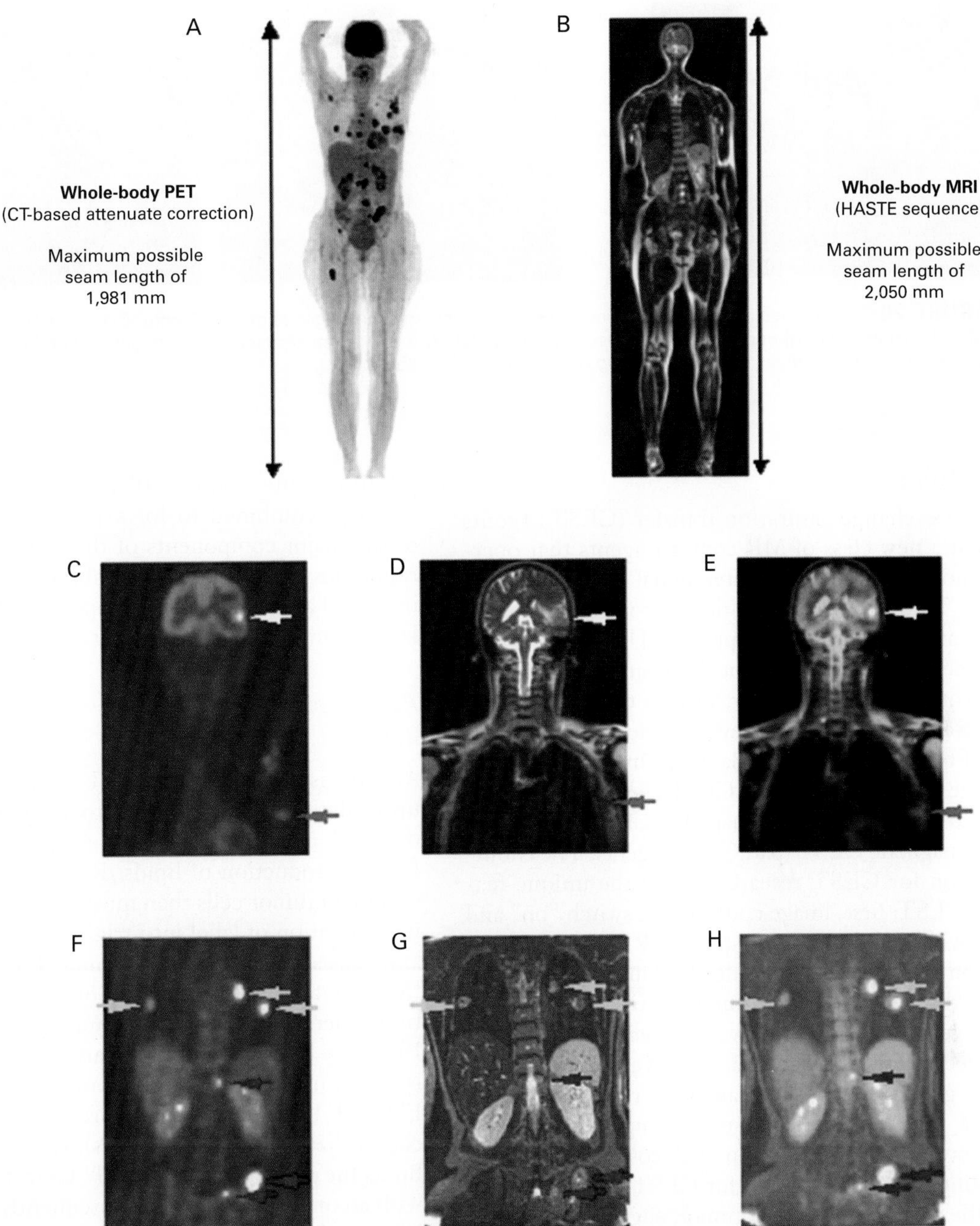

FIGURE 20–2 A patient with cerebral (arrow, white), pulmonary (arrows, yellow), lymphogen, osseous (arrows, blue), and soft-tissue metastases (arrow, red) of a malignant melanoma was examined with whole-body ^{18}F-FDG PET and T_2-weighted HASTE MRI (**A** and **B**). The coronal centered view of PET (**C** and **F**) and MRI (**D** and **G**) images, and the corresponding fused images (**G** and **H**). (Reproduced with permission from Seemann MD, *Technol Cancer Res Treat.* 2005;4:577-582.)

metabolic imaging. The metabolic products produced directly after hyperpolarized [1-^{13}C]pyruvate administration include [1-^{13}C]lactate, [1-^{13}C]alanine, $^{13}CO_2$, and $H^{13}CO_3^-$. Early observations suggest that the amount of hyperpolarized [1-^{13}C]lactate derived from hyperpolarized [1-^{13}C]pyruvate in tumors may provide a simple assay to distinguish a tumor from normal tissue in a metabolic imaging experiment. Moreover, response to therapy by imaging the ratio of hyperpolarized [1-^{13}C]lactate/[1-^{13}C]pyruvate in tumors could possibly one day become a widely used clinical tool just as ^{18}F-FDG PET is today.[17] One could argue that detection of lactate by ^{1}H MRS in tumors[18] might be just as diagnostic and certainly simpler in principle than using hyperpolarized materials. Even though high levels of lactate have been confirmed in the intermediate-grade gliomas[19] and high-grade brain tumors,[20] lactate detection by ^{1}H MRS is not that straightforward because the chemical shift of the lactate methyl group is often overwhelmed by intense ^{1}H lipid signals.

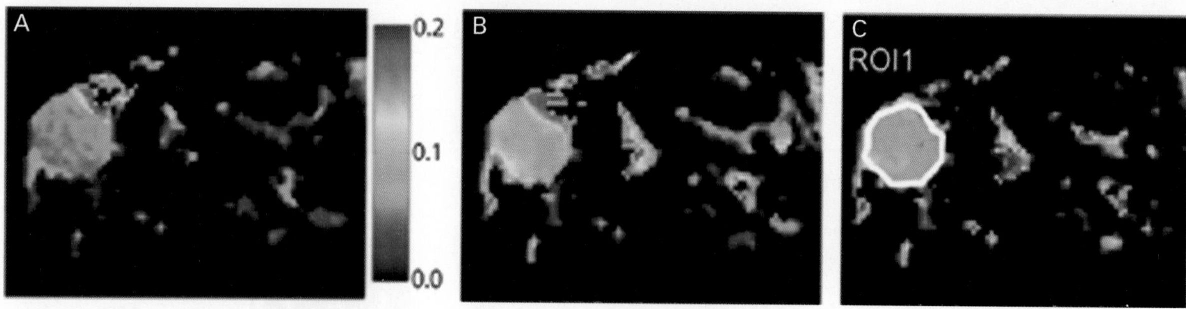

FIGURE 20–3 Summation of magnetization transfer ratio asymmetry images at offset 1.2 ppm **(C)** derived from pre-infusion **(A)** and post-infusion **(B)** of D-glucose for a mouse bearing MDA-MB-231 tumor. (Reproduced with permission from Chan KW, McMahon MC, Liu G, et al., *Proc Intl Soc Mag Reson Med.* 2011;19:551.)

CEST Agents

Chemical exchange saturation transfer (CEST) agents represent a new class of MR contrast agents that operate by modifying the total water signal intensity rather than the T_1 or T_2 relaxation times of water protons.[56] Given that the image contrast produced by CEST agents is extremely sensitive to chemical exchange rates (k_{ex}) of labile protons with bulk water, various types of responsive CEST agents have been developed for sensing a wide range of biological species.[57] Based on magnetic properties of the molecules involved, CEST agents can be separated into two categories: diamagnetic CEST (diaCEST) and paramagnetic CEST (paraCEST) agents. The enduring passion for CEST research lies in the unique features of CEST: first, image contrast can switch "on" and "off" at will by gating radiofrequency (RF) presaturation pulses on or off; second, multiplex imaging becomes possible by simultaneous administration of multiple CEST agents that can be activated selectively by an RF pulse specific for a particular agent.[56] Very recently, two research groups nearly simultaneously reported the use of CEST technique to detect glucose uptake in tumors after intravenous administration of glucose (Fig. 20.3).[21,22] Interestingly, the kinetic data for CEST contrast varied with different regions of the tumor, suggesting heterogeneous uptake of glucose by tumors.[22] The major drawback of using CEST to detect glucose is that the chemical shifts of labile glucose –OH protons are quite close to those of bulk water protons ($\Delta\omega < 2$ ppm). This makes it difficult to selectively saturate the glucose –OH protons only without indirect partial saturation of bulk water protons themselves.

Agents for Lipid Metabolism

Acetate and choline are essential nutrients for the production of lipids and phospholipids (see Fig. 20.1). Overexpressed FAS in tumors catalyzes the conversion of malonyl-CoA to fatty acids and diacyl- and triacylglycerol. At the same time, upregulated ChoK promotes phosphorylation of choline to form cytidine-diphosphocholine (CDP-choline), and CDP-choline and diacyglycerol are then combined to form phosphatidylcholine, one of the major components of the cell membrane. Thus, rapid biosynthesis of cell membranes is associated with increased acetate and choline uptake and upregulation of key enzymes in tumors.

PET Agents

^{11}C and ^{18}F-Acetate

Acetate is rapidly taken up by tumor cells through upregulated MCTs, activated to acetyl-CoA, and either oxidized in the TCA cycle or used as a starting material for the production of lipids. Retention of radiolabeled acetate in tumor cells then must reflect biosynthesis and incorporation of label into triglycerides, phospholipids, and subsequently cell membranes. For this reason, the ^{11}C-acetate PET may be a more reliable indicator of tumor activity even under conditions where ^{18}F-FDG PET may be limited.[23,24,58] In particular, ^{11}C-acetate PET is widely used as a diagnostic tool complementary to ^{18}F-FDG PET in tumors such as prostate that have low glucose utilization. However, the short half-life time of ^{11}C limits the general availability of ^{11}C-acetate to those sites with an on-site cyclotron. Consequently, ^{18}F-acetate has been used as an analogue of ^{11}C-acetate for prostate cancer diagnoses. Compared with ^{11}C-acetate, ^{18}F-acetate shows a much higher tumor/organ uptake for most tissues, but the practical applications of ^{18}F-acetate are impeded by potential safety concerns.[25]

^{18}F and ^{11}C-Choline

Choline uptake by tumor cells is facilitated by elevated levels of the choline transporter, and entry of choline into phospholipids is further stimulated by the upregulated ChoK. The combination of these two effects results in the elevated downstream choline metabolites, glycerophosphocholine (GPC) and phosphocholine (PC), a consequence of cancer progression (see Fig. 20.1).[59] Based on this observation, ^{11}C-choline has been used as a ^{11}C-acetate analogue for the detection of tumors (Fig. 20.4). It has

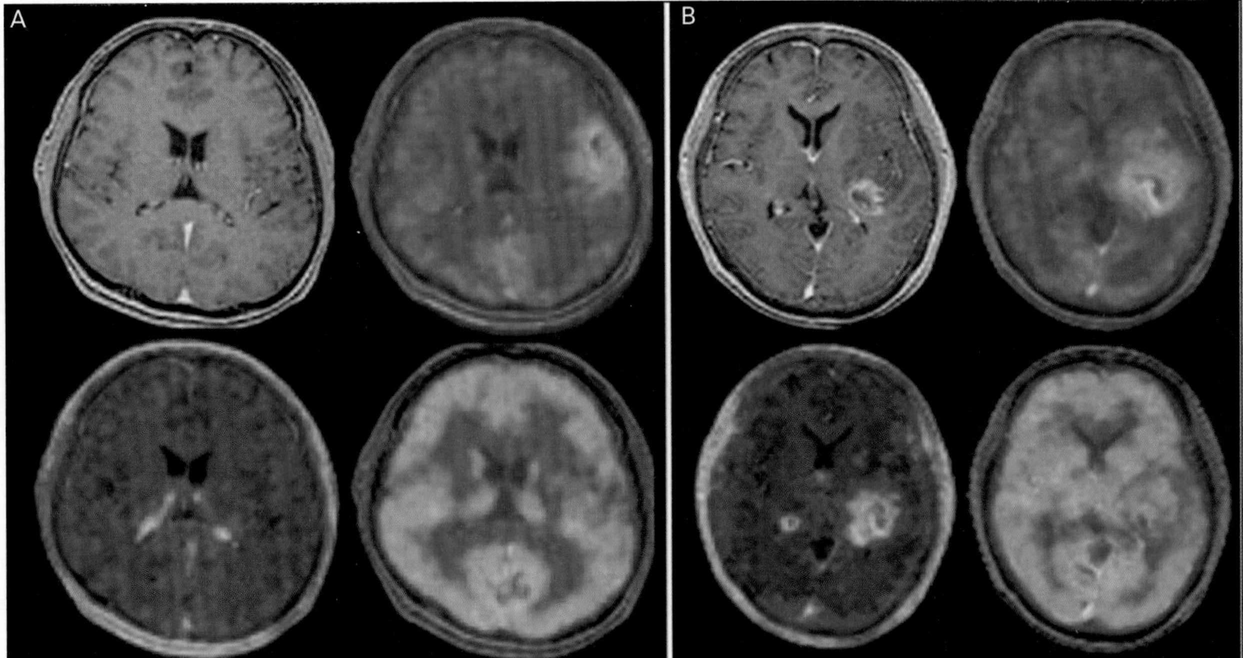

FIGURE 20–4 Representative case studies for metabolic assessment of **(A)** oligodendroglioma and **(B)** anaplastic astrocytoma using ^{11}C-methionine (MET), ^{11}C-choline (CHO), and ^{18}F-FDG PET. MET (right top), CHO (left bottom), and FDG (right bottom) PET imaging are superimposed on T_1-weighted MR imaging (left top). (Reproduced with permission from Kato T, Shinoda J, Nakayama N, et al., *AJNR Am J Neuroradiol.* 2008;29:1176-1182.)

been found that ^{11}C-choline and ^{11}C-acetate show similar sensitivities, specificities, and accuracies for the detection of prostate cancers.[26] ^{18}F-choline[27] and ^{18}F-fluoroethylcholine[28] have been made available still mainly due to the short half-life time of ^{11}C-choline. The applications of the ^{18}F-labeled tracers are exactly the same as those of ^{11}C-choline but rapid renal excretion is considered a clinical disadvantage for the ^{18}F analogues.[60]

MR Agents

^{1}H and ^{31}P MRS Agents

One consequence of enhanced lipid metabolism in tumors is that total choline (tCho), the sum of choline, PC, and GPC, becomes elevated with cancer progression. In vivo detection of endogenous tCho with ^{1}H MRS has been recognized as a convenient way to distinguish benign and malignant tissues by monitoring the signal intensity of $-N(CH_3)_3$ protons of tCho (~3.2 to 3.3 ppm) as an index of tumor grade. This method has been reported to have high sensitivity and specificity (~80%) in breast tumors,[29] and this makes it possible to exploit the decline in tCho levels after therapy as a criterion to evaluate the treatment.[29,30] Moreover, the diagnostic accuracy of measuring tCho by ^{1}H MRS can be significantly improved by careful optimization of acquisition conditions.[31]

Phospholipids can in principle also be detected by ^{31}P MRS even though spectra of tissues in vivo can be complicated by extra ^{31}P signals from metabolites in cell membranes.[32] Two phosphorus resonances are normally detected, a phosphomonoester (PME) peak around 3.9 ppm, reflecting the sum of unresolved phosphatidylcholine and phosphoethanolamine, and a phosphodiester (PDE) peak around 0.5 ppm, which reflects unresolved GPC and glycerophosphoethanolamine. As the PME peak contains largely the choline component, it is always elevated in tumors relative to normal tissues.[34] Since protons in these same molecules contribute to ^{31}P MRS linewidths, proton decoupling sharpens the ^{31}P linewidths and improves the detection accuracy.[35] It has also been shown that a switch from high GPC/low PC to low GPC/high PC reflects a malignant phenotype associated with tumor progression and this can be followed by ^{31}P MRS.[32]

Agents for Detecting Protein Metabolism

To date, more than 20 distinct AATs classified by either transport mechanism or substrate specificity have been identified in mammalian cells. A detailed review of the structure and function of AATs is beyond the scope of this chapter, so the reader is referred to Kilberg and Häussinger for details.[61] Briefly, AATs can be grouped as A, ASC, L, and cationic AATs. Type A and ASC are sodium-dependent and preferentially transport small amino acids like L-alanine, L-serine, L-glutamine, and L-serine. Type L AATs are sodium-independent and transport amino acids with large neutral side chains like L-leucine, L-phenylalanine, and L-tyrosine while cationic amino acids like L-arginine, L-lysine, and L-histidine use system cationic AATs. As mentioned earlier, mTOR signaling is found to be one of the pathways that stimulates the amino acid uptake and protein synthesis. However, more and more evidence suggests that the overexpressed AATs dominate cancer phenotype other than protein synthesis.[62]

PET Agents

Natural amino acids and synthetic analogues have been widely investigated as PET agents for molecular imaging of cancer. Natural amino acid–based agents are normally labeled with ^{11}C, while most of their analogues are labeled with ^{18}F. Here, we will focus the discussion on the agents most widely studied to date such as ^{11}C-methionine (^{11}C-MET), ^{18}F-methyl-tyrosine (^{18}F-FMT), ^{18}F-ethyl-tyrosine (^{18}F-FET), and ^{18}F-dihydroxyphenylalanine (^{18}F-DOPA). Further details about precursor synthesis, radiolabeling, and preclinical evaluation are found elsewhere.[63-65] As noted above, ^{18}F-FDG PET is of limited use in detecting central nervous system (CNS)–related tumors because CNS tissues like brain display a strong uptake of ^{18}F-FDG. PET tracers like ^{11}C-MET have been developed to overcome this limitation. Uptake of ^{11}C-MET is not significant in normal brain tissue, but does accumulate in malignant brain lesions due to the high demand for amino acids in tumors (see Fig. 20.4). This has made ^{11}C-MET quite popular for the diagnosis of CNS tumors.[36] In addition, the degree of ^{11}C-MET uptake correlates with tumor grade.[37] ^{18}F-FMT and ^{18}F-FET are examples of two unnatural amino acid tracers developed for the diagnosis of CNS tumors. These agents show similar diagnostic specificity and accuracy as ^{11}C-MET.[36] Two reasons have made ^{18}F-FMT and ^{18}F-FET potentially superior to ^{11}C-MET. First, most unnatural amino acid tracers are not metabolized further after transport into cells, so accumulation of such agents results in higher sensitivity and avoids more complicated kinetic analyses of the data. Second, unlike ^{11}C-MET and ^{18}F-FDG, these agents do not accumulate in inflammatory tissues, so tumor specificity is improved.[38] As an ^{18}F-labeled amino acid precursor, ^{18}F-DOPA is taken up by normal brain by means of type L AATs. In addition to the above mentioned application in detecting the brain neoplasms, ^{18}F-DOPA has shown great potential for diagnosis of well-differentiated tumors like neural crest tissues, where ^{18}F-FDG is limited as a consequence of low uptake.[39,40]

MR Agents

^{13}C MRS Tracers

^{13}C MRS studies of amino acid metabolism have been largely limited to ex vivo studies of tumor cells until only recently when in vivo imaging of branched chain amino acid metabolism was demonstrated using hyperpolarized [1-^{13}C]ketoisocaproate.[41] α-Ketoisocaproate is converted to leucine by branched chain amino acid transferase (BCAT), a catabolic enzyme known to be upregulated in some tumors.[66] Following injection of hyperpolarized [1-^{13}C]ketoisocaproate, the large increase in hyperpolarized [1-^{13}C]leucine was observed in murine lymphoma tumor relative to the surrounding healthy tissues, but no hyperpolarized [1-^{13}C]leucine was detected in rat mammary adenocarcinoma tumor. It is interesting that these differences paralleled the different activities of BCAT and the amount of glutamate (the amine donor for leucine) present in these two tumors, so the differentiation between tumor types by hyperpolarized ^{13}C MRS or MRI is an exciting prospect.[41]

MRI Relaxometry Agents

As indicated previously, tumor cells use glutamine as a carbon and nitrogen source for biosynthetic reactions at a faster rate than normal cells. Given that MRI is now widely available in most clinics and does not require handling of radioactive materials, there is considerable interest in developing MRI agents that highlight in tumors on the basis of differences in metabolism compared with normal cells. Monitoring enhanced glutamine metabolism is one possible target. Toward this end, two different DOTA-glutamine conjugates, GdDOTAMA-Gln (glutamine directly conjugated to one carboxyl group of DOTA) and GdDOTAMA-C6-Gln (glutamine separated by a six-bond spacer from DOTA), have been prepared and evaluated in vitro and in vivo.[42] It was found that GdDOTAMA-C6-Gln, the molecule with the extended glutamine, accumulated in tumors much more readily than did GdDOTAMA-Gln and GdHPDO3A (used as a control). Less tumor uptake of GdDOTAMA-Gln likely reflects steric hindrance between the rather large macrocyclic chelate, GdDO3A, and the directly appended glutamine molecule, which could reduce the affinity between the glutamine moiety and the active site of the transporter. In vivo MRI results showed that, after agent administration, tumor contrast was maintained at 24 and 72 hours, long after excess chelate should have been excreted. Although the contrast enhancement in tumors was lower than expected based upon the amount of GdDOTAMA-C6-Gln found in tumor cells, this study provided the first evidence that contrast-enhanced MRI may indeed be sensitive enough to detect tumors that are actively taking up glutamine for biosynthesis.

Agents as Markers of Nucleic Acid Metabolism

Rapid tumor cell proliferation features elevated DNA replication, so interest in measuring the proliferation status of tumors by either MRI or PET is high. Given that highly proliferating tumors are usually more responsive to cell cycle–specific anti-cancer agents and radiotherapy, it is important to be able to identify proliferating tumors so that one could monitor changes in proliferation rate in response to therapy.[63]

PET Agents

By analogy to ^{18}F-FDG, ^{11}C-labeled thymidine can be trapped in tumors undergoing high rates of proliferation by phosphorylation, a reaction catalyzed by thymidine kinase. However, this probe has not proven fruitful because the short half-life of ^{11}C does not provide enough time to eliminate excess unreacted probe from tissues or to allow sufficient incorporation of ^{11}C-thymidine into DNA. For this reason, ^{18}F-labeled thymidine analogues, 3′-deoxy-3′-[^{18}F]fluorothymidine (^{18}F-FLT) and 1-(2′-deoxy-2′-fluoro-β-D-arabinofuranosyl) thymidine (^{18}F-FMAU), have gained in popularity for clinical assessment of tumor proliferation.[43] The activities of cytosolic thymidine kinase (TK1) and mitochondrial thymidine kinase (TK2) are regulated in cancer cells. TK1 is upregulated in proliferating cells especially during the S phase of DNA synthesis while TK2 expression is not cell cycle dependent. Studies have shown that ^{18}F-FLT is almost exclusively phosphorylated by TK1 even though the substrate specificity of TK1 for ^{18}F-FLT is around 12% relative to thymidine (100%). On the other hand, ^{18}F-FMAU is phosphorylated by both TK1 and TK2 with a substrate specificity of 15% and 30%, respectively.[67] Phosphorylated ^{18}F-FMAU can be rapidly incorporated into DNA, while phosphorylated ^{18}F-FLT is not because it lacks the 3′-hydroxy group required for elongation of DNA. Nevertheless, ^{18}F-FLT is still useful because it accumulates more in cancer cells than in normal cells, similar to ^{18}F-FDG. Both nucleic acid tracers are capable of imaging tumor proliferation state in various kinds of cancers. In particular, ^{18}F-FLT PET is currently in clinical use for evaluating therapeutic response early in the course of treatment.[67] However, it should be noted that they show differences in detection sensitivity and specificity. Some studies have found that ^{18}F-FMAU PET is more sensitive than ^{18}F-FLT PET.[68] In addition, ^{18}F-FLT tends to accumulate in proliferating bone marrow while ^{18}F-FMAU does not.[69,70] However, Alauddin et al. suggested that the high uptake of ^{18}F-FLT in bone may be due to the existence of free ^{18}F-fluoride in ^{18}F-FLT, which exists as an impurity not detected by high-performance liquid chromatography (HPLC) during the quality assays.[67]

Agents for Measuring Extracellular pH

The extracellular pH (pHe) of many tumors can become quite acidic due to the cellular adaptations (see Fig. 20.1) associated with abnormally high glucose utilization. Studies have shown that tumor cells proliferate at a maximal rate when they are in a slightly acidic environment, typically at a pHe ~6.8 compared with normal cells at a pHe ~7.3.[71] Thus, imaging this pHe difference has become an important diagnostic goal.

PET Agents

To date, only two agents have been reported to evaluate pHe with PET. The first, ^{11}C-labeled dimethyloxazolidinedione (^{11}C-DMO), fails to measure pHe accurately because the pHe measurement is built on a questionable assumption that the distribution of ^{11}C-DMO across the semipermeable membranes varies with the pH gradient.[44] pHLIP is a pH-sensitive peptide that can insert into a cell membrane at acidic pHe but not at normal pHi. This unique property of pHLIP was recently utilized in the design of a PET probe, ^{64}Cu-DOTA-pHLIP, to detect low pHe environments.[45] However, it is challenging to apply this method in the clinical setting because ^{64}Cu-DOTA-pHLIP fails to measure absolute pH and exhibits only modest specificity.

MR Agents

^{31}P, ^{1}H, and ^{13}C MRS Agents

MRS is an excellent tool for measuring absolute pHe because many molecules show changes in chemical shift ($\Delta\omega$) with pH. ^{31}P MRS was first applied when it was shown that the chemical shift of endogenous inorganic phosphate, P_i, provides a direct measure of intracellular pH (pHi). Subsequently, exogenous, negatively charged probes like 3-aminopropylphosphonate (3-APP) also show a nice change in chemical shift with changes in pH, so these can be used to measure the absolute values of pHe.[46] The sensitivity of detection of such exogenous probes can be improved by switching to proton observation (^{1}H MRS) and molecules like 2-imidazole-1-yl-3-ethoxycarbonylpropionic acid (IEPA), where the chemical shift of the imidazole H2 resonance provides a direct readout of pHe.[47,48] However, the accuracy of the pH measurement is limited in ^{1}H MRS because of the relatively small proton chemical shift window compared with other nuclei.

One recent exciting observation was the use of hyperpolarized ^{13}C bicarbonate for measuring pHe. In biological tissue, an equilibrium is established rapidly between $H^{13}CO_3^-$ and $^{13}CO_2$ after intravenous injection of hyperpolarized $H^{13}CO_3^-$, and both species can be imaged separately (Fig. 20.5). Given the well-known pK_a of this carbonic anhydrase–catalyzed reaction, the ratio of image intensity of these two hyperpolarized species provides a direct readout of tissue pH.[49] One uncertainty involved with this method is the exact cellular location of $H^{13}CO_3^-$ and $^{13}CO_2$. Nevertheless, a pHe of 6.7 was found for a highly proliferating tumor in mice, a value very close to that anticipated for pHe in this tumor model. Given that $H^{13}CO_3^-$ is a common endogenous anion and considered nontoxic at the levels required for hyperpolarized imaging, this technique shows great potential for translation to human clinical studies if obstacles related to the relatively short T_1 of $H^{13}CO_3^-$ (~10 s) can be resolved.[72]

MRI Relaxation Agents

Several gadolinium-based pH-sensitive contrast agents have been reported but only a few have been demonstrated in vivo. One of the first of these was gadolinium-1,4,7,10-tetraazacyclododecane-1,4,7,10-tetraacetic acid-tetraamide methylene phosphonate (GdDOTA-4AmP^{5-}), a complex having a single, slowly exchanging bound water molecule. This complex has a relatively low T_1 water proton relaxivity when the solution pH is in the range 8 to 9, but upon protonation of the four appended phosphonate groups

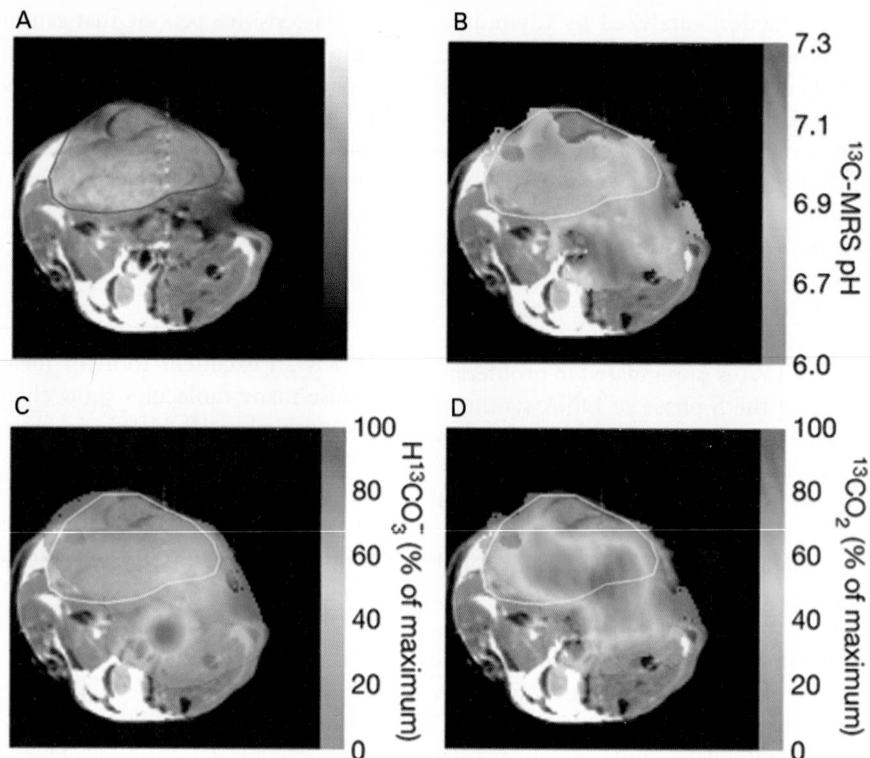

FIGURE 20–5 pH map of a mouse with a subcutaneously implanted EL4 tumor after injection of hyperpolarized $H^{13}CO_3^-$. **A:** Transverse proton MR image showing the tumor profile in red. **B:** pH map of the mouse calculated from the ratio of the $H^{13}CO_3^-$ **(C)** and $^{13}CO_2$ **(D)** voxel intensities in ^{13}C chemical shift images. (Reproduced with permission from Gallagher FA, Kettunen MI, Day SE, et al. *Nature.* 2008;453:940-943.)

beginning at pH ~8.5 and ending near pH 6, the monoprotonated phosphonate groups catalyzed proton exchange between the gadolinium-bound water molecule and solvent water.[73] This results in an increase in water proton T_1 relaxivity of about 25% over this pH range, enough to initiate a significant increase in water intensity in a proton MR image. However, the use of this agent to measure absolute pH requires knowledge of the agent concentration in each image pixel, obviously a problem in vivo. Initially, this problem was solved by sequential injection of GdDOTA-4AmP^{5-} followed by a dynamic contrast enhancement (DCE) measurement of the kinetics of agent washout. This is then followed by injection of the pH-insensitive agent, gadolinium-1,4,7,10-tetraazacyclododecane-1,4,7,10-tetrakis(methylene phosphonic acid) (GdDOTP^{5-}) and a second DCE study.[50] If one assumes an identical tissue distribution and kinetic washout curves for the two agents, then any difference in water intensity in each voxel must reflect differences in pH. This "dual agent" protocol was used to obtain pHe maps of functioning mouse kidney[74] and of gliomas grown in the brain of rats.[50] Nevertheless, this agent and dual agent imaging protocol will likely not be used in humans to image pHe for a couple of reasons: (1) highly charged phosphonate complexes such as these bind to bone, so they would remain in the body much too long and (2) the dual agent protocol is too lengthy for a typical clinical MRI exam. More recently, the experimental procedure was simplified by co-injecting a mixture of two agents, GdDOTA-4AmP^{5-} (the pH sensor) and DyDOTP^{5-} (a concentration marker as obtained from a map of T_2*), to obtain a pHe map in an acceptable time frame.[51] Thus, even though progress has been made in measuring absolute pHe by MRI, the proper compounds for translation of this technology to humans have yet to be discovered.

CEST Agents

The requirement of two agents, one for measuring pH and another as a tissue concentration marker, assumes that the molecules have identical tissue distributions and pharmacokinetics, an assumption that may not be valid under many conditions. It would clearly be preferable to administer a single agent for reporting tissue pHe. Single agent–based pH measurements are more easily envisioned using newer types of MR imaging agents, those based on CEST methods. This idea was first demonstrated by Ward and Balaban with a diamagnetic CEST agent having two types of proton exchange groups with different chemical shifts.[75] Activation at each exchange frequency sequentially then produces two different water CEST images and the ratio of these two CEST intensities can be shown to parallel pH. Thus, a standard curve of CEST ratio versus pH for any given molecule having two or more proton exchange groups allows a direct measure of pHe without knowing the agent concentration. This ratiometric method was later extended to paramagnetic CEST (paraCEST) agents and these have the advantage of having protons exchange sites much further away from the water resonance (larger $\Delta\omega$).[76-78] The use of a single paraCEST agent for measuring pHe was first demonstrated in vivo using the complex Yb^{3+}-1,4,7,10-tetraazacyclododecane-1,4,7-triacetic acid-10-o-aminoanilide (Yb-DO3A-oAA). In this molecule, two chemically distinct –NH protons can be activated selectively for ratiometric imaging of pHe.[52] Even though the Yb-DO3A-oAA is heterogeneously distributed throughout the tumor, pH mapping is still possible using ratiometric imaging. The pHe map shows that the pHe of the tumor was at or below 6.5 across the entire tumor.

CONCLUSIONS

Molecular imaging of tumor metabolism will one day serve a very important role in cancer diagnosis and therapy. Despite the remarkable advances made in the past decade, quantitative molecular imaging of tumors to characterize tumor type and morphology at early stages remains challenging. Imaging methods are now available to probe specific, select pathways in tumors without removal of tissue and these methods will become key in the design of new therapeutics. Advances in this field will require further convergence of interdisciplinary collaborators among experts in biology, chemistry, physics, and engineering. For example, the motivation for moving metabolic imaging of hyperpolarized nuclei into the clinical setting requires development of new agents with longer T_1 values and new imaging techniques to conserve the hyperpolarized signal as long as possible. Given the remarkable progress achieved to date, we envision that molecular imaging of cancer metabolism will gain even more momentum and play an ever-increasing role in the care of cancer patients in future.

REFERENCES

1. Weissleder R, Pittet MJ. Imaging in the era of molecular oncology. *Nature.* 2008;452:580-589.
2. Condeelis J, Weissleder R. In vivo imaging in cancer. *Cold Spring Harb Perspect Biol.* 2010;2:a003848.
3. Mankoff DA. A definition of molecular imaging. *J Nucl Med.* 2007;48:18N, 21N.
4. Kroemer G, Pouyssegur J. Tumor cell metabolism: cancer's Achilles' heel. *Cancer Cell.* 2008;13:472-482.
5. Plathow C, Weber WA. Tumor cell metabolism imaging. *J Nucl Med.* 2008;49(suppl 2):43S-63S.
6. Cairns RA, Harris IS, Mak TW. Regulation of cancer cell metabolism. *Nat Rev Cancer.* 2011;11:85-95.
7. Koppenol WH, Bounds PL, Dang CV. Otto Warburg's contributions to current concepts of cancer metabolism. *Nat Rev Cancer.* 2011;11:325-337.
8. Feron O. Pyruvate into lactate and back: from the Warburg effect to symbiotic energy fuel exchange in cancer cells. *Radiother Oncol.* 2009;92:329-333.
9. Ganapathy V, Thangaraju M, Prasad PD. Nutrient transporters in cancer: relevance to Warburg hypothesis and beyond. *Pharmacol Ther.* 2009;121:29-40.
10. Reivich M, Kuhl D, Wolf A, et al. Measurement of local cerebral glucose metabolism in man with 18F-2-fluoro-2-deoxy-d-glucose. *Acta Neurol Scand Suppl.* 1977;64:190-191.
11. Rohren EM, Turkington TG, Coleman RE. Clinical applications of PET in oncology. *Radiology.* 2004;231:305-332.
12. Castell F, Cook GJ. Quantitative techniques in 18FDG PET scanning in oncology. *Br J Cancer.* 2008;98:1597-1601.
13. Almuhaideb A, Papathanasiou N, Bomanji J. 18F-FDG PET/CT imaging in oncology. *Ann Saudi Med.* 2011;31:3-13.
14. Wijnen JP, Van der Graaf M, Scheenen TW, et al. In vivo 13C magnetic resonance spectroscopy of a human brain tumor after application of 13C-1-enriched glucose. *Magn Reson Imaging.* 2010;28:690-697.
15. Constantinidis I, Chatham JC, Wehrle JP, et al. In vivo 13C NMR spectroscopy of glucose metabolism of RIF-1 tumors. *Magn Reson Med.* 1991;20:17-26.
16. Keshari KR, Wilson DM, Chen AP, et al. Hyperpolarized [2-13C]-fructose: a hemiketal DNP substrate for in vivo metabolic imaging. *J Am Chem Soc.* 2009;131:17591-17596.
17. Day SE, Kettunen MI, Cherukuri MK, et al. Detecting response of rat C6 glioma tumors to radiotherapy using hyperpolarized [1- 13C]pyruvate and 13C magnetic resonance spectroscopic imaging. *Magn Reson Med.* 2011;65:557-563.
18. Thakur SB, Yaligar J, Koutcher JA. In vivo lactate signal enhancement using binomial spectral-selective pulses in selective MQ coherence (SS-SelMQC) spectroscopy. *Magn Reson Med.* 2009;62:591-598.
19. Li X, Vigneron DB, Cha S, et al. Relationship of MR-derived lactate, mobile lipids, and relative blood volume for gliomas in vivo. *AJNR Am J Neuroradiol.* 2005;26:760-769.
20. Sijens PE, Levendag PC, Vecht CJ, et al. 1H MR spectroscopy detection of lipids and lactate in metastatic brain tumors. *NMR Biomed.* 1996;9:65-71.
21. Chan KW, McMahon MC, Liu G, et al. Imaging of glucose uptake in breast tumors using non-labeled D-glucose. *Proc Intl Soc Mag Reson Med.* 2011;19:551.
22. Walker-Samuel S, Johnson P, Pedley B, et al. Assessment of tumour glucose uptake using gluco-CEST. *Proc Intl Soc Mag Reson Med.* 2011;19:962.
23. Yu EY, Muzi M, Hackenbracht JA, et al. C11-acetate and F-18 FDG PET for men with prostate cancer bone metastases: relative findings and response to therapy. *Clin Nucl Med.* 2011;36:192-198.
24. Fricke E, Machtens S, Hofmann M, et al. Positron emission tomography with 11C-acetate and 18F-FDG in prostate cancer patients. *Eur J Nucl Med Mol Imaging.* 2003;30:607-611.
25. Ponde DE, Dence CS, Oyama N, et al. 18F-fluoroacetate: a potential acetate analog for prostate tumor imaging—in vivo evaluation of 18F-fluoroacetate versus 11C-acetate. *J Nucl Med.* 2007;48:420-428.
26. Kotzerke J, Volkmer BG, Glatting G, et al. Intraindividual comparison of [11C]acetate and [11C]choline PET for detection of metastases of prostate cancer. *Nuklearmedizin.* 2003;42:25-30.
27. DeGrado TR, Coleman RE, Wang S, et al. Synthesis and evaluation of 18F-labeled choline as an oncologic tracer for positron emission tomography: initial findings in prostate cancer. *Cancer Res.* 2001;61:110-117.
28. Hara T, Kosaka N, Kishi H. Development of (18) F-fluoroethylcholine for cancer imaging with PET: synthesis, biochemistry, and prostate cancer imaging. *J Nucl Med.* 2002;43:187-199.
29. Jagannathan NR, Kumar M, Seenu V, et al. Evaluation of total choline from in-vivo volume localized proton MR spectroscopy and its response to neoadjuvant chemotherapy in locally advanced breast cancer. *Br J Cancer.* 2001;84:1016-1022.
30. Sharma U, Baek HM, Su MY, et al. In vivo (1) H MRS in the assessment of the therapeutic response of breast cancer patients. *NMR Biomed.* 2011;24:700-711.
31. Stanwell P, Gluch L, Clark D, et al. Specificity of choline metabolites for in vivo diagnosis of breast cancer using 1H MRS at 1.5 T. *Eur Radiol.* 2005;15:1037-1043.
32. Podo F. Tumour phospholipid metabolism. *NMR Biomed.* 1999;12:413-439.
33. Bolan PJ, Meisamy S, Baker EH, et al. In vivo quantification of choline compounds in the breast with 1H MR spectroscopy. *Magn Reson Med.* 2003;50:1134-1143.

34. Negendank W. Studies of human tumors by MRS: a review. *NMR Biomed.* 1992;5:303-324.
35. Bluml S, Seymour KJ, Ross BD. Developmental changes in choline- and ethanolamine-containing compounds measured with proton-decoupled (31)P MRS in in vivo human brain. *Magn Reson Med.* 1999;42:643-654.
36. Wong TZ, van der Westhuizen GJ, Coleman RE. Positron emission tomography imaging of brain tumors. *Neuroimaging Clin N Am.* 2002;12:615-626.
37. De Witte O, Goldberg I, Wikler D, et al. Positron emission tomography with injection of methionine as a prognostic factor in glioma. *J Neurosurg.* 2001;95:746-750.
38. Haubner R. PET radiopharmaceuticals in radiation treatment planning—synthesis and biological characteristics. *Radiother Oncol.* 2010;96:280-287.
39. Hoegerle S, Altehoefer C, Ghanem N, et al. Whole-body 18F dopa PET for detection of gastrointestinal carcinoid tumors. *Radiology.* 2001;220:373-380.
40. Brink I, Hoegerle S, Klisch J, et al. Imaging of pheochromocytoma and paraganglioma. *Fam Cancer.* 2005;4:61-68.
41. Karlsson M, Jensen PR, in't Zandt R, et al. Imaging of branched chain amino acid metabolism in tumors with hyperpolarized (13) C ketoisocaproate. *Int J Cancer.* 2010;127:729-736.
42. Geninatti Crich S, Cabella C, Barge A, et al. In vitro and in vivo magnetic resonance detection of tumor cells by targeting glutamine transporters with Gd-based probes. *J Med Chem.* 2006;49:4926-4936.
43. Mach RH, Dehdashti F, Wheeler KT. PET radiotracers for imaging the proliferative status of solid tumors. *PET Clin.* 2009;4:1-15.
44. Rottenberg DA, Ginos JZ, Kearfott KJ, et al. In vivo measurement of brain tumor pH using [11C]DMO and positron emission tomography. *Ann Neurol.* 1985;17:70-79.
45. Vavere AL, Biddlecombe GB, Spees WM, et al. A novel technology for the imaging of acidic prostate tumors by positron emission tomography. *Cancer Res.* 2009;69:4510-4516.
46. Gillies RJ, Liu Z, Bhujwalla Z. 31P-MRS measurements of extracellular pH of tumors using 3-aminopropylphosphonate. *Am J Physiol.* 1994;267:C195-C203.
47. Gil S, Zaderenzo P, Cruz F, et al. Imidazol-1-ylalkanoic acids as extrinsic 1H NMR probes for the determination of intracellular pH, extracellular pH and cell volume. *Bioorg Med Chem.* 1994;2:305-314.
48. Gillies RJ, Raghunand N, Garcia-Martin ML, et al. pH imaging. A review of pH measurement methods and applications in cancers. *IEEE Eng Med Biol Mag.* 2004;23:57-64.
49. Gallagher FA, Kettunen MI, Day SE, et al. Magnetic resonance imaging of pH in vivo using hyperpolarized 13C-labelled bicarbonate. *Nature.* 2008;453:940-943.
50. Garcia-Martin ML, Martinez GV, Raghunand N, et al. High resolution pH(e) imaging of rat glioma using pH-dependent relaxivity. *Magn Reson Med.* 2006;55:309-315.
51. Martinez GV, Zhang X, Garcia-Martin ML, et al. Imaging the extracellular pH of tumors by MRI after injection of a single cocktail of T(1) and T(2) contrast agents. *NMR Biomed.* 2011;24:1380-1391.
52. Liu G, Li Y, Sheth VR, et al. Imaging in vivo extracellular pH with a single paramagnetic chemical exchange saturation transfer magnetic resonance imaging contrast agent. *Mol Imaging.* 2012;11:47-57.
53. Seemann MD. Whole-body PET/MRI: the future in oncological imaging. *Technol Cancer Res Treat.* 2005;4:577-582.
54. Griffin JL, Shockcor JP. Metabolic profiles of cancer cells. *Nat Rev Cancer.* 2004;4:551-561.
55. Ardenkjaer-Larsen JH, Fridlund B, Gram A, et al. Increase in signal-to-noise ratio of >10,000 times in liquid-state NMR. *Proc Natl Acad Sci U S A.* 2003;100:10158-10163.
56. Sherry AD, Woods M. Chemical exchange saturation transfer contrast agents for magnetic resonance imaging. *Annu Rev Biomed Eng.* 2008;10:391-411.
57. Viswanathan S, Kovacs Z, Green KN, et al. Alternatives to gadolinium-based metal chelates for magnetic resonance imaging. *Chem Rev.* 2010;110:2960-3018.
58. Jadvar H. Prostate cancer: PET with 18F-FDG, 18F- or 11C-acetate, and 18F- or 11C-choline. *J Nucl Med.* 2011;52:81-89.
59. Gillies RJ, Morse DL. In vivo magnetic resonance spectroscopy in cancer. *Annu Rev Biomed Eng.* 2005;7:287-326.
60. Kato T, Shinoda J, Nakayama N, et al. Metabolic assessment of gliomas using 11C-methionine, [18F] fluorodeoxyglucose, and 11C-choline positron-emission tomography. *AJNR Am J Neuroradiol.* 2008;29:1176-1182.
61. Kilberg MS, Häussinger D. *Mammalian Amino Acid Transport: Mechanisms and Control.* New York, NY: Plenum Press; 1992.
62. Fuchs BC, Bode BP. Amino acid transporters ASCT2 and LAT1 in cancer: partners in crime? *Semin Cancer Biol.* 2005;15:254-266.
63. McConathy J, Yu W, Jarkas N, et al. Radiohalogenated nonnatural amino acids as PET and SPECT tumor imaging agents. *Med Res Rev.* 2012;32:868-905.
64. Tu Z, Mach RH. C-11 radiochemistry in cancer imaging applications. *Curr Top Med Chem.* 2010;10:1060-1095.
65. McConathy J, Goodman MM. Non-natural amino acids for tumor imaging using positron emission tomography and single photon emission computed tomography. *Cancer Metastasis Rev.* 2008;27:555-573.
66. Weggen S, Preuss U, Pietsch T, et al. Identification of amplified genes from SV40 large T antigen-induced rat PNET cell lines by subtractive cDNA analysis and radiation hybrid mapping. *Oncogene.* 2001;20:2023-2031.
67. Alauddin MM, Gelovani JG. Pyrimidine nucleosides in molecular PET imaging of tumor proliferation. *Curr Med Chem.* 2010;17:1010-1029.
68. Sun H, Sloan A, Mangner TJ, et al. Imaging DNA synthesis with [18F]FMAU and positron emission tomography in patients with cancer. *Eur J Nucl Med Mol Imaging.* 2005;32:15-22.
69. Sun H, Mangner TJ, Collins JM, et al. Imaging DNA synthesis in vivo with 18F-FMAU and PET. *J Nucl Med.* 2005;46:292-296.
70. Buck AK, Herrmann K, Shen C, et al. Molecular imaging of proliferation in vivo: positron emission tomography with [18F] fluorothymidine. *Methods.* 2009;48:205-215.
71. Zhang X, Lin Y, Gillies RJ. Tumor pH and its measurement. *J Nucl Med.* 2010;51:1167-1170.
72. Gallagher FA, Kettunen MI, Brindle KM. Imaging pH with hyperpolarized (13) C. *NMR Biomed.* 2011;24:1006-1015.
73. Zhang S, Wu K, Sherry AD. A Novel pH-sensitive MRI contrast agent. *Angew Chem Int Ed Engl.* 1999;38:3192-3194.
74. Raghunand N, Howison C, Sherry AD, et al. Renal and systemic pH imaging by contrast-enhanced MRI. *Magn Reson Med.* 2003;49:249-257.
75. Ward KM, Balaban RS. Determination of pH using water protons and chemical exchange dependent saturation transfer (CEST). *Magn Reson Med.* 2000;44:799-802.
76. Aime S, Barge A, Delli Castelli D, et al. Paramagnetic lanthanide(III) complexes as pH-sensitive chemical exchange saturation transfer (CEST) contrast agents for MRI applications. *Magn Reson Med.* 2002;47:639-648.
77. Wu YK, Soesbe TC, Kiefer GE, et al. A responsive europium(III) chelate that provides a direct readout of pH by MRI. *J Am Chem Soc.* 2010;132:14002-14003.
78. Delli Castelli D, Terreno E, Aime S. Yb(III)-HPDO3A: a dual pH- and temperature-responsive CEST agent. *Angew Chem Int Ed Engl.* 2011;50:1798-1800.

CHAPTER 21

Detection and Molecular Monitoring of Minimal Residual Diseases in Myeloid Neoplasms

C. Cameron Yin

INTRODUCTION

The term "minimal residual disease" (MRD) usually refers to the persistence of residual neoplastic cells below the threshold of conventional morphologic detection. During the last decade, the rapidly emerging molecular markers that play a role in the pathogenesis of neoplasms and the advancement in molecular technologies have revolutionized the clinical management of common neoplasms in the context of diagnosis, risk stratification, targeted therapy, and monitoring MRD. Monitoring MRD has become an important component of clinical management of many neoplasms, particularly hematological malignancies. It has been demonstrated that MRD analysis allows for early detection of impending hematologic relapse and timely therapeutic intervention and, therefore, has significantly improved clinical outcome in many hematopoietic malignancies. In this chapter, we summarize some of the important molecular markers that are currently used for the detection of MRD in several myeloid malignancies including acute myeloid leukemias (AML), *BCR/ABL1*-positive chronic myelogenous leukemia (CML), *JAK2*-mutated myeloproliferative neoplasms (MPN), and *KIT*-mutated mastocytosis (Table 21.1).

ACUTE MYELOID LEUKEMIAS

Acute myeloid leukemias are a group of genetically heterogeneous diseases characterized by abnormal proliferation of immature hematopoietic cells and disruption of normal hematopoiesis. Leukemogenesis is a complex multistep process involving mutations of two broadly defined complementary classes of molecules.[1] Class I mutations involve genes encoding receptor tyrosine kinases (RTK) (e.g., *FLT3*, *KIT*) or downstream effectors (e.g., *RAS*) that activate signal transduction pathways, providing proliferative and/or survival advantage to the leukemic cells. Class II mutations involve genes that affect transcription factors or components of the transcriptional co-activation complex (e.g., *CBF*, *CEBPA*), resulting in impaired myeloid differentiation (Fig. 21.1). Mutations within each of these complementary groups occur infrequently in the same tumor, whereas mutations between the two complementary groups often occur synergistically in the same AML patient. Screening for abnormalities of some of these molecular markers has become a routine practice in newly diagnosed AML patients. Information about the mutational status of some of these genes is useful for diagnosis, risk stratification, MRD monitoring, and targeted therapy. The monitoring of MRD in AML can be based on three major classes of molecular genetic aberrations—chromosomal translocations or inversions, gene mutations, and gene overexpression (Table 21.2).

AML with Recurrent Chromosomal Translocations or Inversions

The third and fourth editions of the World Health Organization (WHO) classification incorporated genetic abnormalities in the diagnosis and classification of AML. Most cases included in the category of AML with recurrent genetic abnormalities involve balanced chromosomal

TABLE 21–1 Molecular Genetic Aberrations and Detection Methods Used for Monitoring of Minimal Residual Diseases in Myeloid Neoplasms

Disease	Molecular Aberrations	MRD Method	Sensitivity	Comment
AML	Translocations/inversions	qRT-PCR	1×10^{-5}	Karyotyping and FISH lack sensitivity for MRD
	Gene mutations	PCR-CE	1–5%	Suitable for *FLT3* and *NPM1* with limited sensitivity
		RQ-PCR	1×10^{-5}	Sensitive but may miss certain rare mutations
		Pyrosequencing	1–5%	Good for genes with known "hot-spot" point mutations
				Sanger sequencing lacks sensitivity for MRD
	Gene overexpressions	qRT-PCR	1×10^{-5}	
CML	*BCR-ABL1*	Karyotyping	5%	Limited sensitivity but can detect clonal evolution
		Dual-fusion FISH	0.5%	Detect cryptic translocation, use interphase cells
		qRT-PCR	1×10^{-5}	
MPN	*JAK2/MPL*	RQ-PCR	1×10^{-5}	Sanger sequencing lacks sensitivity for MRD
		Pyrosequencing	1–5%	
Mastocytosis	*KIT*	RQ-PCR	1×10^{-5}	Sanger sequencing lacks sensitivity for MRD
		Pyrosequencing	1–5%	

AML, acute myeloid leukemia; CML, chronic myelogenous leukemia; MPN, myeloproliferative neoplasm; MRD, minimal residual disease; qRT-PCR, quantitative real-time reverse transcription–polymerase chain reaction; PCR-CE, PCR-capillary electrophoresis; RQ-PCR, quantitative real-time PCR; FISH, fluorescence in situ hybridization.

translocations or inversions activating transcription factors. Examples include t(8;21)(q22;q22)/*RUNX1-RUNX1T1*, inv(16)(p13.1q22) or t(16;16)(p13.1;q22)/*CBFB-MYH11*, t(15;17)(q22;q21)/*PML-RARA*, t(9;11)(p22;q23)/*MLLT3-MLL*, t(6;9)(p23;q34)/*DEK-NUP214*, inv(3)(q21q26.2) or t(3;3)(q21;q26.2)/*RPN1-EVI1*, and t(1;22)(p13;q13)/*RBM15-MKL1*. Among these entities, cases with t(8;21), inv(16)/t(16;16), or t(15;17) each constitute approximately 5% to 10% of AML and are considered acute leukemia without regard to the blast count. They have been associated with favorable prognosis.

Each of these chromosome rearrangements leads to the formation of a fusion gene. The resultant chimeric protein plays a role in leukemogenesis. At initial diagnosis, many

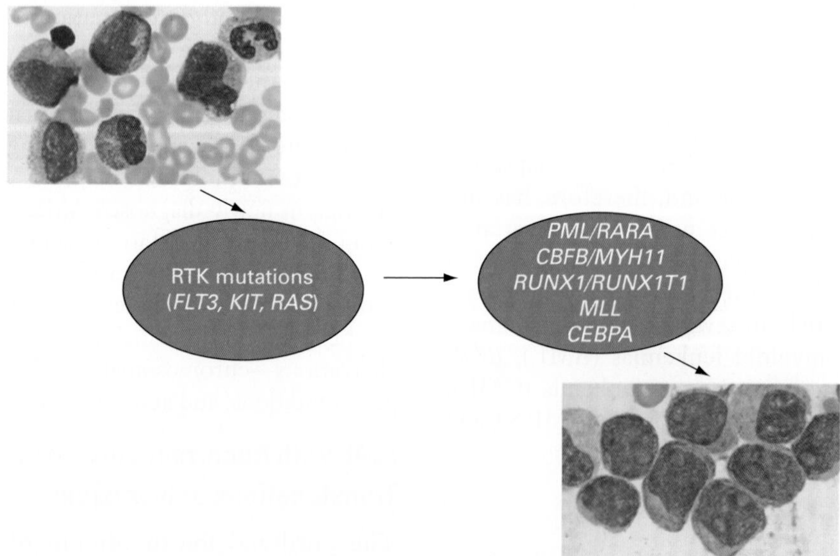

FIGURE 21–1 Leukemogenesis is a complex multistep process involving mutations of two complementary classes of molecules. Class I mutations involve genes encoding receptor tyrosine kinases (RTK) (e.g., *FLT3*, *KIT*) or downstream effectors (e.g., *RAS*) that activate signal transduction pathways, providing proliferative and/or survival advantage to the leukemic cells. Class II mutations involve genes that affect transcription factors or components of the transcriptional co-activation complex (e.g., *CBF*, *CEBPA*), resulting in impaired myeloid differentiation.

TABLE 21–2 Molecular Monitoring of Minimal Residual Disease in Acute Myeloid Leukemia

Type	Fusion/Gene	MRD Method	Sensitivity	Comment
AML with chromosomal translocations or inversions[a]	t(8;21)(q22;q22)/*RUNX1-RUNX1T1*	qRT-PCR	1×10^{-5}	Single common fusion
				Transcript persists during long-term remission
	inv(16)(p13.1q22)/t(16;16)(p13.1;q22)/*CBFB-MYH11*	qRT-PCR	1×10^{-5}	Isoform A most common
				Rare fusion types require different primer sets
	t(15;17)(q22;q21)/*PML-RARA*	qRT-PCR	1×10^{-5}	Long and short forms
				Rare fusion types require different primer sets
AML with gene mutations[b]	*NPM1*	PCR-CE	1–5%	Detects most mutations with limited sensitivity
		RQ-PCR	1×10^{-5}	Only detects the most common mutations
				Stable at relapse
	FLT3-ITD	PCR-CE	1–5%	Limited sensitivity
				Relatively unstable, lost at relapse in small subsets
AML with gene overexpressions	*WT1*	qRT-PCR	1×10^{-5}	

AML, acute myeloid leukemia; MRD, minimal residual disease; qRT-PCR, quantitative real-time reverse transcription–polymerase chain reaction; PCR-CE, PCR-capillary electrophoresis; RQ-PCR, quantitative real-time PCR.

[a]Karyotyping and FISH lack sensitivity for MRD detection. Karyotyping has high false-negative rate for inv(16)/t(16;16).

[b]Sanger sequencing is of limited value for MRD monitoring due to lack of sensitivity.

of these chromosomal translocations and inversions can be detected by conventional cytogenetic analysis, fluorescence in situ hybridization (FISH), Southern blot, or reverse transcription–polymerase chain reaction (RT-PCR). However, conventional karyotyping (with a sensitivity of about 5%) and FISH (with a sensitivity of about 0.5%) lack the sensitivity and ease of automation of PCR, especially when used to monitor responses to therapy. Quantitative real-time (RQ) PCR detects and quantifies amplicons during the exponential expansion phase rather than at the end of cycling (plateau phase) when logarithmic doubling has ceased, and offers a much higher sensitivity (1×10^{-5}) than cytogenetic analysis. It is important to design the primers/probes so that the PCR can amplify all the common types of fusion transcripts. Nested PCR is performed with two consecutive PCR reactions and two different sets of primers, both covering the region of interest, thus resulting in an even higher sensitivity (1×10^{-6}) (Table 21.3).

Quantitative real-time RT-PCR (qRT-PCR) to serially assess the transcript level of the fusion gene is now the most frequently used method for MRD detection. Association of molecular remission and long-term clinical remission has been well established in AML with inv(16)/t(16;16) and AML with t(15;17),[2-5] but the results are controversial for AML with t(8;21). Some studies have reported that the RUNX1-RUNX1T1 fusion transcript persisted in bone marrow (BM) samples from AML patients with t(8;21) who were in long-term clinical remission (up to 210 months),[6-9] which made it of limited value in MRD detection. Others showed that complete molecular remission could be achieved following intensive therapy and was associated with complete clinical remission.[10] Nevertheless, it seems that quantitative molecular monitoring of RUNX1-RUNX1T1 fusion transcript may be useful in MRD testing in patients with t(8;21), especially when using a "cutoff" (or threshold) value that could predict clinical outcome.[11,12]

Although the method for MRD detection in AML with chromosomal translocations or inversions has been

TABLE 21–3 Methodologies Used for Detection of Chromosomal Translocations and Inversions

Method	Sensitivity	Comment
Karyotyping	5%	Good for initial diagnosis, lacks sensitivity and ease of automation for MRD
FISH	0.5%	Good for initial diagnosis, lacks sensitivity and ease of automation for MRD
qRT-PCR	1×10^{-5}	Good for initial diagnosis and best for MRD monitoring
		Need to design primers/probes to cover all the common types of fusion transcripts

FISH, fluorescence in situ hybridization; qRT-PCR, quantitative real-time reverse transcription–polymerase chain reaction; MRD, minimal residual disease.

standardized, the type of specimens used for detection, optimal sampling interval, relapse kinetics, and results interpretation differs with the underlying molecular lesion and has not been well defined. Ommen et al. reported that the median doubling time of the *CBFB-MYH11* leukemic clone was significantly longer than that of clones harboring *RUNX1-RUNX1T1* and *PML-RARA* and suggested that, to obtain a relapse detection fraction of 90% and a median time of 60 days from MRD detection to hematologic relapse, a blood sampling should be performed once every 6, 4, and 2 months for AML with *CBFB-MYH11*, *RUNX1-RUNX1T1*, and *PML-RARA*, respectively.[13] In addition, by comparing peripheral blood (PB) and BM, they found that BM was superior to PB for MRD assessment in patients carrying *PML-RARA*, whereas PB and BM were comparable for MRD detection in core binding factor (CBF) leukemias.[13] Moreover, dynamic change of the transcript level is more predictive,[14] and any result of molecular relapse should be confirmed by a repeat PCR.

AML with Specific Gene Mutations

Cytogenetic abnormalities can be detected in only 55% of all AML patients. In AML patients with normal cytogenetics (CN-AML), molecular screening identifies genetic alterations in over 85% of cases. Examples include frequent mutations of *FLT3* (fms-related tyrosine kinase 3) and *NPM1* (nucleophosmin) and, less commonly, *CEBPA* (CCAAT/enhancer binding protein α) gene. Mutations of these genes have been used in risk stratification and development of targeted therapy, and detection of these mutations is very helpful for the assessment of MRD, especially in patients with CN-AML.

Sanger sequencing is the most common method of DNA sequencing and can accurately sequence up to 500 to 1,000 base pairs (bp) of DNA. However, it has a limited sensitivity of 20% and therefore has a limited value in MRD monitoring. Pyrosequencing can detect mutations that are present at 1% to 5% of the template and also allows for assessment of the ratio of mutated to unmutated clones. However, it can only sequence less than 50 bp of DNA and works best for mutational analysis of genes with known "hot-spot" point mutations. Some gene mutations, such as internal tandem duplication (ITD) of *FLT3* gene and the 4 bp insertion of *NPM1* gene, can be detected by PCR followed by capillary electrophoresis (PCR-CE, sensitivity 1% to 5%). For genes with known single base pair mutations, quantitative allele-specific PCR, using PCR primers or probes that differentially recognize the mutated and unmutated sequences, can detect the presence of a mutation as low as 0.01-0.001% of the template DNA. However, for each individual point mutation, two pairs of primers and/or probes need to be designed (Table 21.4).

NPM1 Mutation

NPM1 gene, located at chromosome 5q35, encodes a nucleolar phosphoprotein that has multiple cellular functions. A major role of NPM1 is to act as a molecular chaperone for preribosomal proteins to be transported between the nucleus and the cytoplasm. It also interacts with tumor suppressors such as p53 and ARF and is involved in cell proliferation and apoptosis.[15] *NPM1* mutations are now recognized as the most common genetic lesion in AML, seen in about 25% to 35% of adult AML overall and 45% to 65% of CN-AML.[16,17] More than 50 different mutant variants have been reported, most of which consist of 4 bp insertions in exon 12 of the *NPM1* gene. The most common is mutant A, a TCTG tetranucleotide duplication at codons 956 to 959.[16,17] The mutations create a nuclear export signal that mediates aberrant localization of NPM1 protein from the nucleus to the cytoplasm.[17] This aberrant cytoplasmic localization can be shown by immunohistochemical analysis.[18] In the absence of *FLT3*-ITD, *NPM1* mutations have been associated with a favorable clinical outcome.[17]

NPM1 mutation is found to be very stable at relapse. It has been reported that the same *NPM1* mutation is detectable in 90% to 100% of patients with *NPM1*-mutated AML 3 to 6 months prior to a hematologic relapse.[19-22] On the other hand, a hematologic relapse has been reported to be preceded by a molecular relapse in 80% of patients with *NPM1*-mutated AML.[13,22] Therefore, *NPM1* has become one of the best molecular markers for MRD monitoring in AML patients.

TABLE 21-4 Methodologies Used for Detection of Point Mutations

Method	Sensitivity	Comment
Sanger sequencing	20%	Most common method, limited value in MRD
Pyrosequencing	1–5%	Semiquantitative, suitable for genes with known "hot-spot" point mutations
PCR-CE	1–5%	Semiquantitative, suitable for some gene mutations, e.g., *FLT3*-ITD, *NPM1*
RQ-PCR	1×10^{-5}	Quantitative and most sensitive for MRD
		Suitable for genes with known "hot-spot" point mutations, needs two pairs of primers/probes for each mutation

PCR-CE, polymerase chain reaction-capillary electrophoresis; RQ-PCR, quantitative real-time PCR; MRD, minimal residual disease; ITD, internal tandem duplication.

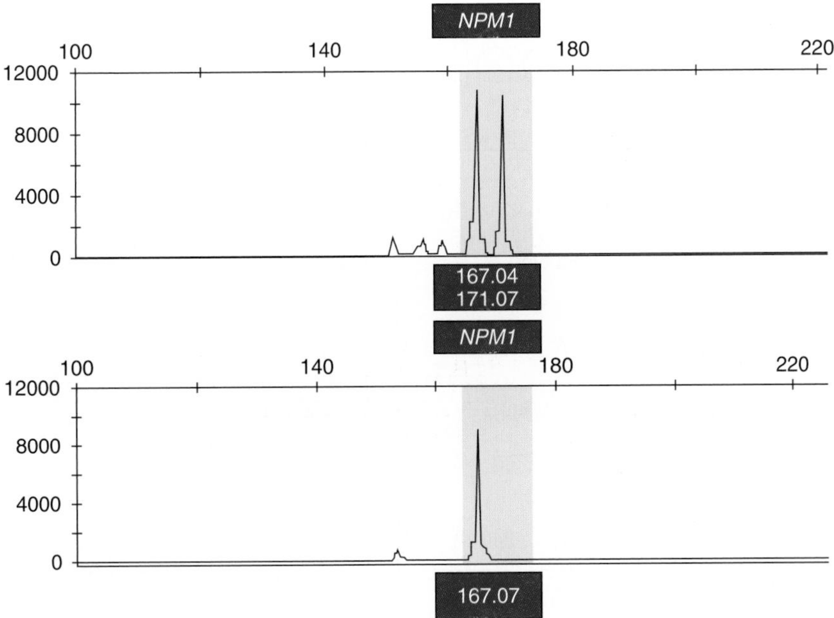

FIGURE 21–2 Detection of *NPM1* mutation by polymerase chain reaction-capillary electrophoresis. The upper panel shows a case of acute myeloid leukemia with *NPM1* mutation (4 bp insertion). The lower panel shows a negative control.

A number of methods can be used for the detection of *NPM1* mutations using genomic DNA and/or mRNA. Sanger sequencing is of limited value for MRD monitoring due to its limited analytical sensitivity. Since the majority of *NPM1* mutations are 4 bp insertions, PCR-CE has become a widely adopted screening method (Fig. 21.2). This approach provides semiquantitative results and it can detect most of the known mutations. However, it also has a limited sensitivity of 1% to 5%. RQ-PCR yields quantitative results and offers a much higher sensitivity (0.01-0.001%) and is regarded as the best method for MRD monitoring in *NPM1*-mutated cases.[22,23] Although RQ-PCR is often designed to detect only the most common *NPM1* mutations that can, therefore, miss rare mutations, this is usually not a problem since the same type of *NPM1* mutation is usually seen at initial diagnosis and at relapse.[22] In addition, Dvorakova et al. found a strong correlation between BM and PB and suggested that PB could be used as an alternative source for MRD monitoring.[22]

FLT3 Mutation

FLT3 gene, located at chromosome 13q12, encodes the class III RTK FLT3 that is essential in the differentiation and proliferation of hematopoietic stem cells. *FLT3* mutations result in cell proliferation and inhibition of apoptosis through activation of multiple signaling pathways.[24] There are two major types of *FLT3* mutations. Internal tandem duplications (ITD) within the juxtamembrane domain occur in 20% to 25% of AML overall and 35% to 40% of CN-AML.[24] Mutations at codons 835 or 836 of the second tyrosine kinase domain (TKD) are seen in 5% to 10% AML.[25] Prognosis of CN-AML with *FLT3*-ITD is significantly inferior compared with those without when treated with current standard chemotherapy, and the outcome is proportional to the ratio of mutated versus unmutated allele.[26,27] The prognostic significance of *FLT3*-TKD mutations remains controversial, although it is suggested by some groups that patients with *FLT3*-TKD mutation also have an inferior disease-free survival.[25]

The role of *FLT3*-ITD in MRD monitoring has been debated. It is generally regarded as a relatively unstable marker as compared with *NPM1* and has been reported lost at relapse in a small subset of AML patients carrying *FLT3*-ITD at initial diagnosis.[28-30] However, in a large cohort of 97 patients, Schnittger et al. found that *FLT3*-ITD was lost in only 4 patients at relapse.[29] Nevertheless, when used with caution, *FLT3*-ITD may serve as a useful marker in AML patients with no other specific MRD marker and in patients undergoing therapy with *FLT3* inhibitors.

Similar to *NPM1* mutations, Sanger sequencing is of limited value in the assessment of *FLT3* mutations in MRD monitoring. *FLT3*-ITD can be detected by fluorescent-based PCR-CE. An *Eco*RV restriction site that spans codon 835/836 can be used to detect these mutations using PCR-CE. This approach provides semiquantitative results and a sensitivity of 1% to 5% (Fig. 21.3). RQ-PCR yields quantitative results and is the most sensitive method for MRD monitoring in *FLT3*-mutated cases (sensitivity 0.01-0.001%). However, it is labor intensive in the design of primers/probes as the *FLT3*-ITDs are

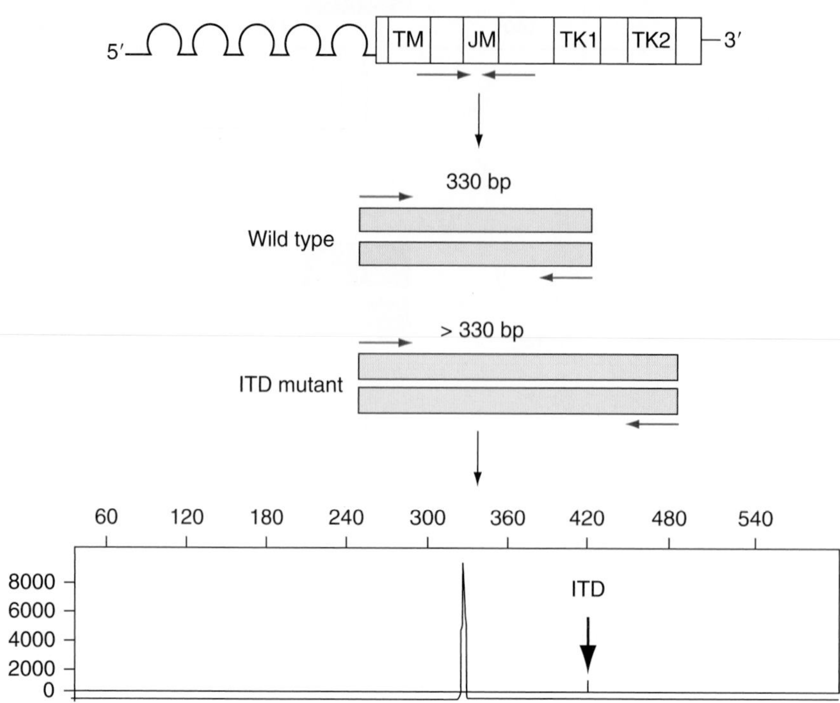

FIGURE 21–3 Detection of *FLT3* internal tandem duplication (ITD) by polymerase chain reaction-capillary electrophoresis (PCR-CE). The wild-type *FLT3* gives rise to a PCR product of 330 bp, and the *FLT3*-ITD results in a PCR product of greater than 330 bp.

highly variable in location and size. A good concordance has been reported between BM and PB in the detection of *FLT3*-ITD, though it seems that it is slightly more sensitive when measured using BM than using PB samples (1 log difference).[30]

CEBPA Mutation

CEBPA gene, located at chromosome 19q13.1, encodes a leucine zipper transcription factor that is involved in the regulation of proliferation and differentiation of granulopoiesis. *CEBPA* mutations have been reported in 5% to 15% of de novo AML, are more common in CN-AML, and are usually biallelic.[31] There are two types of *CEBPA* mutations: out-of-frame nonsense mutations in the N-terminal region that result in a truncated CEBPA protein with complete loss of CEBPA function and dominant-negative inhibition of wild-type CEBPA DNA binding and in-frame mutations in the C-terminal region that give rise to a CEBPA protein with decreased DNA binding or dimerization activity.[32] In the absence of *FLT3*-ITD, *CEBPA* mutations confer a favorable prognosis in patients with CN-AML.[31] It is noted that only biallelic (but not single) *CEBPA* mutations predict for this favorable outcome.[31] *CEBPA* mutations are usually detected by Sanger sequencing. Multiplex PCR-CE is technically challenging and often misses a significant portion of *CEBPA*-positive cases due to the marked heterogeneity of *CEBPA* mutations. The role of *CEBPA* mutation in MRD monitoring is limited and not well established.

KRAS and *NRAS* Mutations

KRAS and *NRAS* are a family of oncogenes encoding small 21 kD GTP-binding proteins that play a central role in intracellular signaling pathways involved in the regulation of proliferation, differentiation, and apoptosis. Mutations in *NRAS* and *KRAS* occur in 5% to 15% of AML cases overall and 30% to 40% of AML with monolytic differentiation lead to constitutive activation of the RAS signaling pathway.[33] It is suggested that patients with *RAS* mutations may benefit from high-dose cytarabine consolidation.[34] However, no significant prognostic impact of *KRAS/NRAS* mutation on the survival of AML patients has been identified.[34] *NRAS/KRAS* point mutations almost always occur at codons 12, 13, or 61, and can be detected by Sanger sequencing, pyrosequencing, or allele-specific PCR (Fig. 21.4).[33] Detection of *NRAS/KRAS* mutations may have a role in monitoring MRD. However, this is not well studied, and a study by Casey et al. on four cases of AML revealed no consistent pattern of association between the presence of *NRAS* mutation and disease state.[35]

KIT Mutation

KIT, located at chromosome 4q11-12, encodes the type III RTK KIT. Gain-of-function mutations of *KIT* have been identified in a variety of diseases, including gastrointestinal stromal tumors, germ cell tumors, mastocytosis, and AML. Although they occur in only 1% to 2% of AML overall, they are more frequently found in

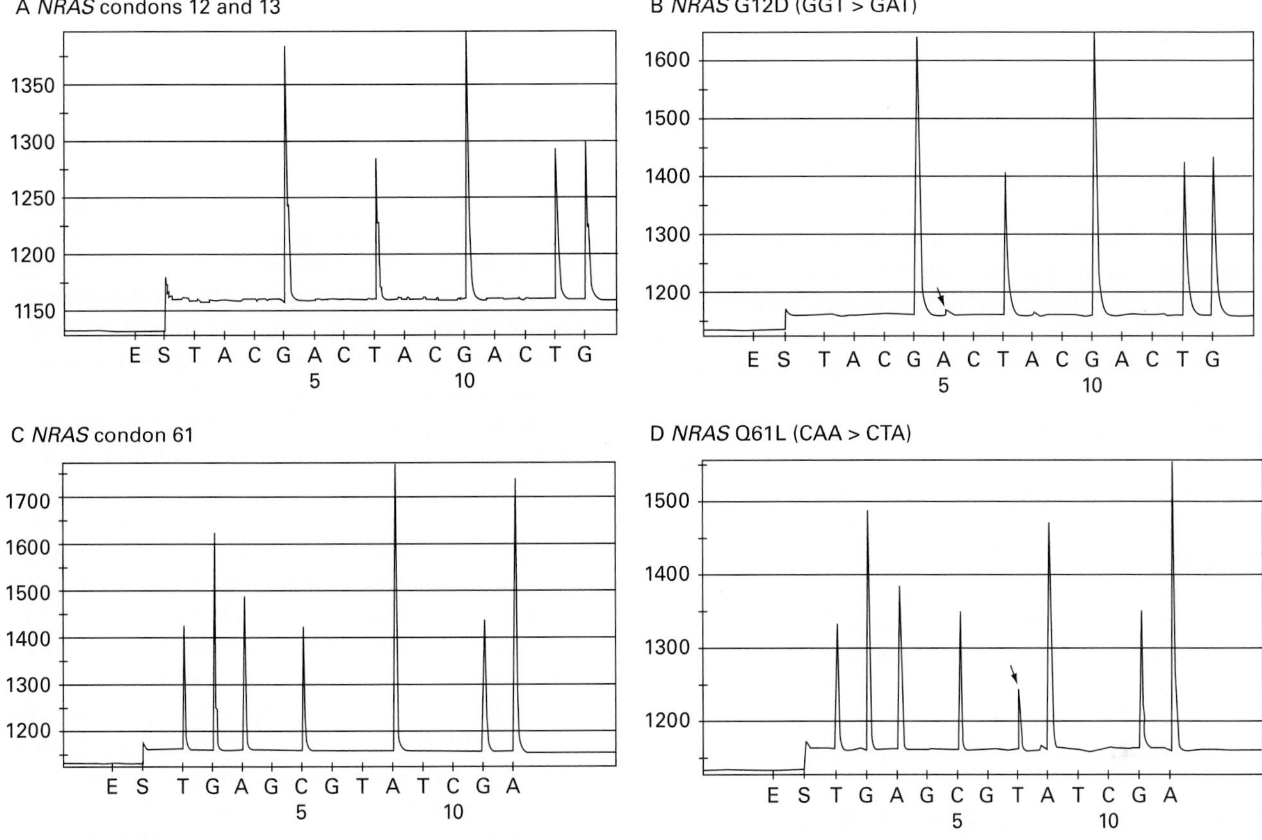

FIGURE 21–4 Detection of *NRAS* mutation by pyrosequencing. **A:** A case with wild-type *NRAS* gene at codons 12 and 13. **B:** A case with mutated *NRAS* gene at codon 12 (GGT>GAT, G12D). **C:** A case with wild-type *NRAS* gene at codon 61. **D:** A case with mutated *NRAS* gene at codon 61 (CAA>CTA, Q61L).

CBF-AML (25% to 30%).[36] In AML, *KIT* mutations mainly consist of missense amino acid substitution in exon 17 of the activation loop.[36] In most studies, *KIT* mutations have been associated with inferior clinical outcome.[37] *KIT* mutations can be detected by Sanger sequencing or allele-specific PCR. It has limited role in MRD monitoring in CBF-AML because the disease-specific fusion gene is a much more reliable marker and is amenable to detection by qRT-PCR.

MLL Abnormalities

MLL (mixed lineage leukemia, or myeloid lymphoid leukemia) gene, located at chromosome 11q23, encodes a DNA binding protein that regulates gene expression in hematopoiesis. Rearrangements of *MLL* gene through recurrent translocations involve over 80 partner genes, many of which are transcription factors. The fusion leads to a gain of function of the *MLL* gene that affects differentiation of hematopoietic stem cells by deregulating homeobox (*HOX*) gene expression.[38] It occurs in 5% to 10% of AML and is more commonly seen in AML in infants or therapy-related AML.[38] The prognosis of AML with 11q23/*MLL* rearrangement varies depending on the partner gene, the lineage of the blasts, the age of the patient, and the treatment regimen.[38] It is best detected by break-apart FISH probe. The presence of numerous fusion partners makes RT-PCR very difficult for the detection of *MLL* translocation.

Genetic alterations of *MLL* through partial tandem duplication (*MLL*-PTD) occur in 5% to 10% of AML and are more frequently seen in AML with trisomy 11.[39] It plays a role in leukemogenesis through DNA hypermethylation and epigenetic silencing of tumor suppressor genes.[39] It has been identified as a negative prognostic factor in initial studies, but more recent multivariate analysis does not confirm its role as an independent prognostic factor.[39] It is detectable by Sanger sequencing or RQ-PCR. By using RQ-PCR, Weisser et al. demonstrated that *MLL*-PTD was a stable marker and preceded hematologic relapse, and thus could be used as a marker of MRD.[40]

AML with Altered Level of Gene Expression

In addition to structural genetic aberrations, changes in the level of expression of certain genes have also been shown to have prognostic impact in AML. Examples include *WT1* (Wilms' tumor 1), *EVI1* (ecotropic viral integration site 1), *BAALC* (brain and acute leukemia, cytoplasmic), *ERG* (ETS-related genes), and *MN1* (meningioma 1). Overexpression of most of these genes has been associated with inferior clinical outcome in patients with AML.[41-45] However, with the exception of *WT1*, their role in MRD monitoring has not been well characterized.

WT1 Overexpression

WT1 (Wilms' tumor 1) gene, located at chromosome 11p13, encodes a zinc finger DNA binding protein that plays a role in the regulation of proliferation, differentiation, and apoptosis of hematopoietic stem cells. *WT1* mutations are found in approximately 10% of CN-AML and have been associated with conflict prognostic significance.[46] In most studies, *WT1* mutations have been associated with inferior clinical outcome,[46,47] but this negative impact on survival has not been confirmed by other studies.[48,49] In addition to mutation, *WT1* has been reported to be overexpressed in over 90% of AML cases, and its overexpression has been associated with poor clinical outcome.[45,50-52] It was shown that high level of *WT1* expression in both BM and PB as assessed by qRT-PCR correlated with disease burden in AML patients, and a rise in WT1 expression preceded the hematological relapse by approximately 4 months.[50-52] Failure to reduce *WT1* transcript level below the threshold limit defined in healthy controls by the end of consolidation predicted increased relapse risk, suggesting a role of *WT1* in MRD monitoring after therapy.[50]

BCR/ABL1-POSITIVE CHRONIC MYELOGENOUS LEUKEMIA

Chronic myelogenous leukemia (CML) is a myeloproliferative neoplasm that originates in an abnormal pluripotent hematopoietic stem cell and is characterized by the presence of t(9;22)(q34;q11.2)/*BCR-ABL1* fusion resulting in the Philadelphia chromosome (Ph). The t(9;22)(q34;q11.2) can be detected by conventional cytogenetic analysis in approximately 95% of the cases at initial diagnosis. The remaining cases either have variant translocations that involve a third or fourth chromosome or have a cryptic translocation of 9q34 and 22q11.2 that cannot be detected by karyotypic analysis, but can be identified by FISH, RT-PCR, or Southern blot analysis. The chimeric BCR-ABL1 fusion protein has constitutive tyrosine kinase activity that plays an essential role in CML pathogenesis by increasing proliferation, reducing apoptosis, decreasing adhesion to extracellular matrix, and causing genomic instability. The clinical course of CML usually consists of an initial chronic phase, an ill-defined accelerated phase, and a terminal blast phase. During this evolution, the neoplastic cells usually acquire additional cytogenetic abnormalities, most often trisomy 8, a second copy of Ph, isochromosome 17q, and trisomy 19.[53]

Tyrosine kinase inhibitors (TKIs) that target the BCR-ABL1, including imatinib, nilotinib and dasatinib, are very effective in treating CML patients, but their effectiveness is limited in some patients by either primary resistance or the development of secondary resistance usually due to acquisition of point mutations in the *ABL1* kinase domain (KD) as a result of selective pressure.[54] The occurrence of *ABL1* KD mutation is often associated with progression to an advanced phase and inferior clinical outcome. Early detection of TKI resistance is critical to allow timely implementation of other effective therapies. Thus, cytogenetic and molecular analyses to quantify the disease burden and identify *ABL1* mutation are critical in the monitoring of CML patients on TKI therapy.

Detection of the Level of *BCR-ABL1* Fusion Transcript

Responses to TKI can be evaluated at several levels, i.e., hematologic response (HR), cytogenetic response (CyR), and molecular response (MR) (Table 21.5). Most patients will achieve complete HR (CHR) at 3 months after initiation of imatinib. Patient compliance to imatinib should be checked if no CHR occurs at 3 months,

TABLE 21-5 Criteria for Hematologic, Cytogenetic, and Molecular Remissions in Chronic Myelogenous Leukemia

HR	CHR	Complete normalization of CBC and spleen size
		WBC < 10 × 10^9/L, platelets < 450 × 10^9/L, basophils < 5%
		Absent immature cells (blasts, promyelocytes, myelocytes) in peripheral blood
	PHR	Partial normalization of CBC and spleen size
		CBC not normalized, but <50% of pretreatment count
		Presence of splenomegaly, but <50% of pretreatment size
		Presence of immature cells in peripheral blood
CyR[a]	CCyR	0% Ph+ metaphases
	PCyR	1–35%
	MCyR	36–95%
MR	CMR	Undetectable *BCR-ABL1* fusion transcripts
	MMR	≥3 log reduction in *BCR-ABL1* fusion transcripts

HR, hematologic remission; CHR, complete HR; PHR, partial HR; CyR, cytogenetic remission; CCyR, complete CyR; PCyR, partial CyR; MCyR, minor CyR; MR, molecular remission; CMR, complete MR; MMR, major MR; CBC, complete blood cell count; WBC, white blood cell.

[a]CyR response is defined as the percentage of Ph+ metaphases measured by karyotypic analysis (not FISH), and a minimum of 20 metaphases should be examined.

and BM cytogenetic and qRT-PCR analyses should be repeated.[55] Cytogenetic response has been shown as the major prognostic factor for overall and progression-free survival.[56] Early achievement of complete CyR (CCyR, within 12 months) decreases the chances of progression.[55] Cytogenetic response is defined as the percentage of Ph+ metaphases measured by karyotypic analysis, and a minimum of 20 metaphases should be examined. It has a sensitivity of 5% and can detect additional cytogenetic aberrations. The role of interphase FISH in CML monitoring after achievement of CCyR has been controversial. The main objection to the routine use of FISH for CML monitoring is that it has not been correlated with other results in large clinical trials. However, some studies have shown that FISH analysis of PB to detect *BCR-ABL1* fusion gene is correlated with cytogenetic responsiveness.[57] It is more sensitive (sensitivity 0.5%), can detect cryptic translocation, and is particularly useful when BM metaphase is not available. The drawback of FISH is that it cannot detect cytogenetic abnormalities other than t(9;22). Therefore, periodic karyotypic analysis is still needed for assessment of clonal evolution.

Although cytogenetic response is commonly used to trigger decision points in CML patients on TKI therapy, molecular testing using qRT-PCR is still regarded as the "gold standard" for the detection and quantification of low-level disease and is the most important factor to monitor after achievement of CCyR and after allogeneic stem cell transplantation (Fig. 21.5). It was reported that major (MMR) and complete (CMR) molecular remissions were associated with more durable cytogenetic responses.[58] Molecular response is defined as the ratio of the level of *BCR-ABL1* fusion transcript to the level of a reference gene transcript (usually *ABL1*, *BCR*, *GUSB*).

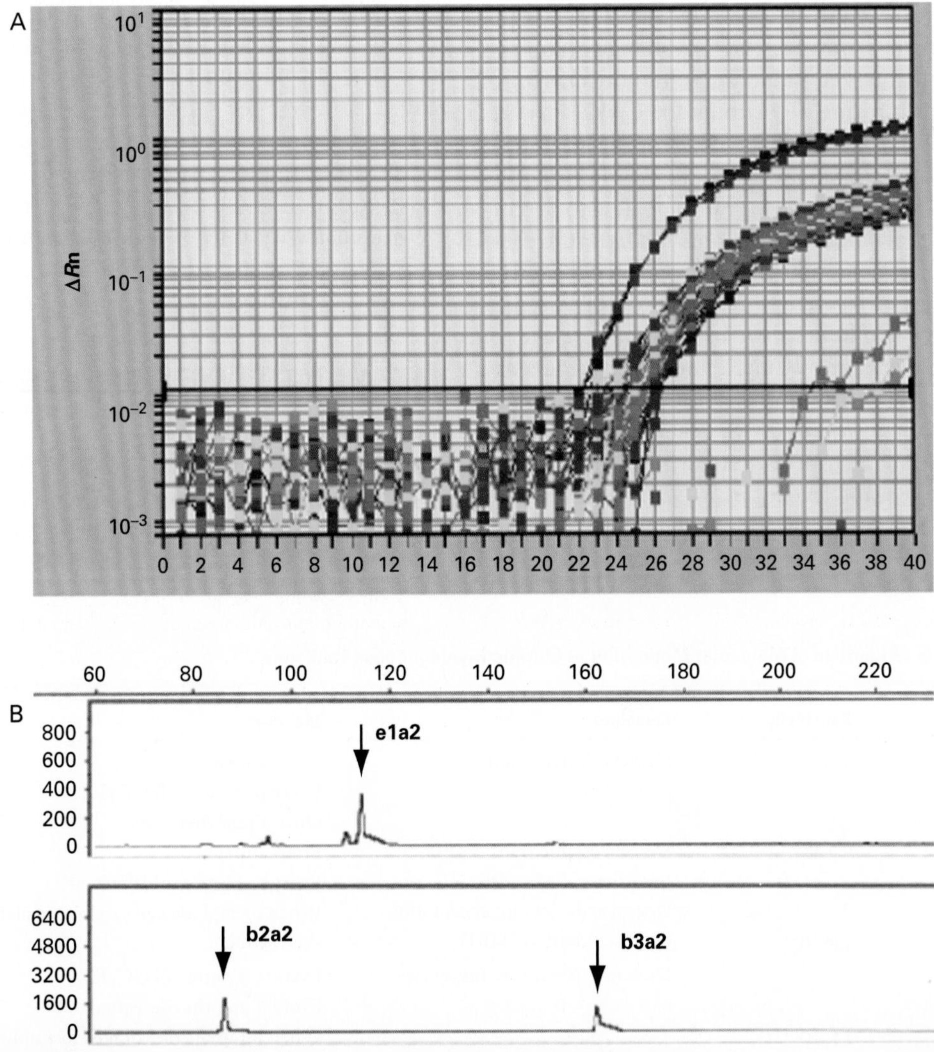

FIGURE 21–5 Detection and quantitation of *BCR-ABL1* fusion transcript in chronic myelogenous leukemia. **A:** Detection and quantitation of *BCR-ABL1* fusion transcript by quantitative real-time reverse transcription–polymerase chain reaction (qRT-PCR). RNA is extracted from bone marrow aspirate or peripheral blood specimen, reverse transcribed into cDNA, and then subject to a multiplex PCR amplifying b2a2, b3a2, and e1a2 fusion genes. The result is normalized to a control gene, e.g., *ABL1*. **B:** The PCR product is subject to capillary electrophoresis to identify the type of the *BCR-ABL1* fusion transcript.

It has a sensitivity of 1/100,000 and can be performed with either TaqMan or fluorescence resonance energy transfer (FRET) technology. Significant inter- and intra-laboratory variations exist, depending on the type of specimen, the quality of RNA, the efficiency of RT and PCR, and the reference gene. Although both BM and PB can be used, the same type of specimen should be used consistently throughout the course of monitoring. Efforts have been made to develop a universal international standard to allow for inter-laboratory comparisons, and the first WHO international genetic reference panel for quantification of *BCR-ABL1* fusion transcript has been established that comprises four different dilutions of lyophilized K562 cells diluted into HL60 cells, each assigned a fixed ratio of *BCR-ABL1* and the control gene according to the International Scale that sets the baseline defined by the IRIS trial as 100% and a 3 log reduction (i.e., MMR) as 0.1%.[59] There is also concern regarding the use of *ABL1* as internal reference since some of the primers used to amplify this transcript will also amplify *ABL1*, and thus this may underestimate the levels of the fusion transcript at diagnosis. However, this is less problematic during monitoring given a marked reduction of tumor burden.

Molecular monitoring algorithms for CML vary in different centers, but most include conventional cytogenetic analysis before treatment, then every 6 months till achievement of CCyR, and once a year thereafter to detect evidence of clonal evolution; FISH analysis before treatment and every 6 to 12 months till achievement of CCyR, or when metaphase cells are not available for karyotypic analysis; and qRT-PCR before treatment, then every 3 months till achievement of CCyR, and every 6 months thereafter. Nested RT-PCR (sensitivity 1/1,000,000) can be used when internal control (e.g., *ABL1*) fails to amplify or an alternate transcript is suspected. At any time during the course of therapy, a rising level of *BCR-ABL1* fusion transcripts mandates more frequent monitoring (Table 21.6).

Identification of *ABL1* Mutation

ABL1 KD mutation is the most common mechanism of secondary resistance to TKIs and has been described in 40% to 90% of cases with TKI resistance. The wide reported range may be due to differences in study populations, detection methodologies, definitions of resistance, and disease phases. In our experience, *ABL1* KD mutation can be detected in approximately 50% of cases that are resistant to imatinib. Over 50 different *ABL1* KD point mutations have been reported. Mutations vary in their ability to inhibit TKIs, e.g., T315I confers resistance to imatinib, nilotinib, and dasatinib. Therefore, not only the presence but also the type of mutation may guide treatment decision. *ABL1* mutation analysis is indicated when there is no CHR at 3 months, partial CyR (pCyR) not achieved by 6 months, CCyR not reached by 12 months, loss of CHR or CCyR at any point during therapy, ≥10-fold rise in *BCR-ABL1* transcript levels, patient presentation with TKI-resistant disease, and patients in accelerated phase (AP) or blast phase (BP) (Table 21.7). Several methods can be used for *ABL1* KD mutation analysis (Fig. 21.6). Sanger sequencing, despite its low sensitivity (20%), is still the most commonly used method in the initial detection of an *ABL1* KD mutation. Pyrosequencing (sensitivity 5%) and allele-specific PCR (sensitivity 0.01-0.001%) are much more sensitive and may be used for monitoring once a mutation has been identified by Sanger sequencing.[60]

JAK2-MUTATED MYELOPROLIFERATIVE NEOPLASMS

Myeloproliferative neoplasms (MPNs) comprise a variety of chronic clonal hematopoietic stem cell disorders that are characterized by proliferation of at least one of the

TABLE 21–6 Algorithm of Molecular Monitoring of Chronic Myelogeneous Leukemia

Method	Sensitivity	Comment	Monitor[a]
Karyotyping	5%	Detects clonal evolution	Pretreatment Every 6 months till CCyR Once a year thereafter
FISH	0.5%	Detects cryptic translocation Interphase, BM or PB Does not detect clonal evolution	Pretreatment Every 6–12 months till CCyR When metaphase cells are not available
qRT-PCR	1×10^{-5}	Gold standard for MRD Does not detect rare fusion types	Pretreatment Every 3 months till CCyR Every 6 months thereafter
Nested RT-PCR	1×10^{-6}		When internal control fails to amplify When an alternate transcript is suspected

[a]At any time during the course of therapy, a rising level of *BCR-ABL1* fusion transcripts mandates more frequent monitoring.
FISH, fluorescence in situ hybridization; qRT-PCR, quantitative real-time reverse transcription–polymerase chain reaction; BM, bone marrow; PB, peripheral blood; MRD, minimal residual disease; CCyR, complete cytogenetic remission.

TABLE 21–7 Methods and Indications for ABL1 Mutational Analysis

Method	Sensitivity	Comment
Sanger sequencing	20%	Most commonly used method in the initial detection of *ABL1* mutation
Pyrosequencing	1–5%	More sensitive and semiquantitative, used to follow up a previously identified mutation
Allele-specific PCR	1×10^{-5}	Most sensitive and quantitative, used to follow up a previously identified mutation
Indication	CHR not achieved by 3 months PCyR not achieved by 6 months CCyR not reached by 12 months Loss of CHR or CCyR at any point during therapy ≥10-fold rise in *BCR-ABL1* transcript levels Patients presentation with TKI-resistant disease Patients in AP or BP	

PCR, polymerase chain reaction; CHR, complete hematologic remission; CCyR, complete cytogenetic remission; PCyR, partial cytogenetic remission; TKI, tyrosine kinase inhibitor; AP, accelerated phase; BP, blast phase.

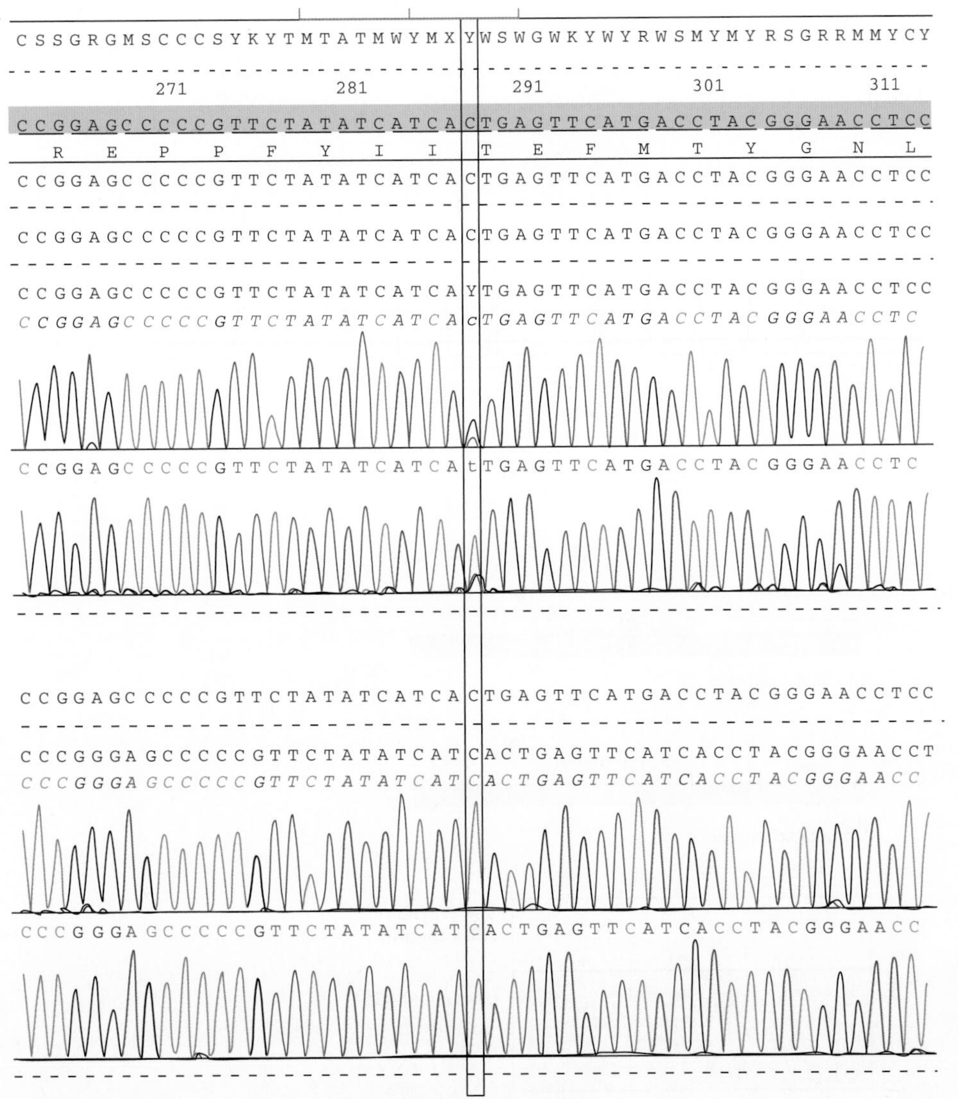

FIGURE 21–6 *ABL1* mutational analysis. **A:** Sanger sequencing identifies a point mutation at codon 315 of the *ABL1* gene (ACT>ATT, T315I). **B:** A case from a CML patient who had an *ABL1* mutation at codon 351 (ATG>ACG, M351T) detected upon development of resistance to imatinib (upper panel). Ten weeks after switching to nilotinib, the patient showed a mixed mutated and unmated *ABL1* kinase (middle panel). Twelve weeks after switching to nilotinib, the M351T is fully reverted to wild type (lower panel). **C:** An example of *ABL1* T315I (ACT>ATT) detected by quantitative allele-specific polymerase chain reaction.

B

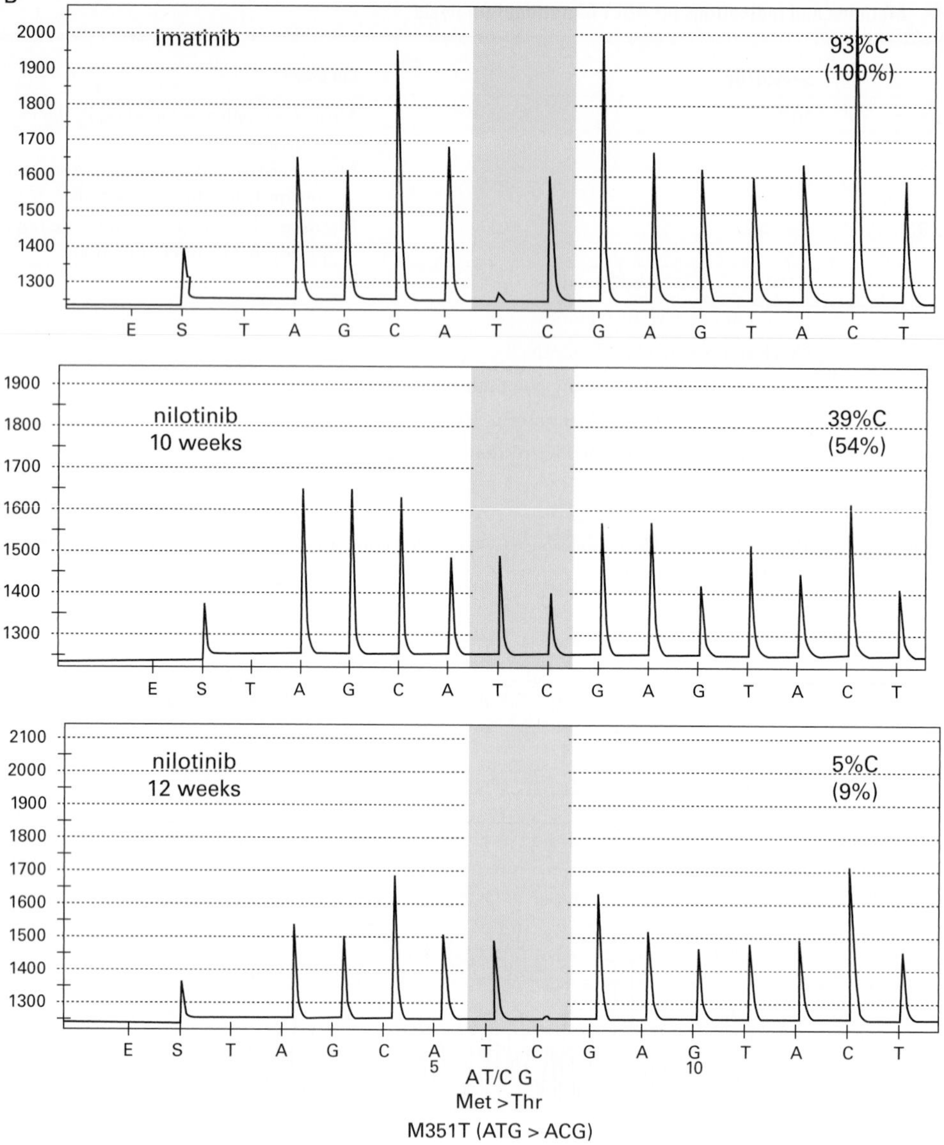

imatinib
93%C
(100%)
2000 1900 1800 1700 1600 1500 1400 1300
E S T A G C A T C G A G T A C T

nilotinib
10 weeks
39%C
(54%)
1900 1800 1700 1600 1500 1400 1300
E S T A G C A T C G A G T A C T

nilotinib
12 weeks
5%C
(9%)
2100 2000 1900 1800 1700 1600 1500 1400 1300
E S T A G C A T C G A G T A C T
5 10
AT/C G
Met > Thr
M351T (ATG > ACG)

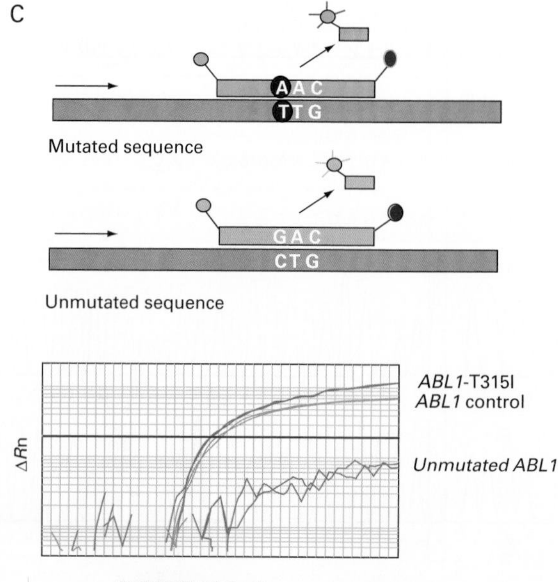

FIGURE 21–6 *(Continued)*

myeloid lineages (i.e., granulocytic, erythroid, or megakaryocytic), with minimal defects in maturation. Most MPNs are associated with abnormalities involving genes that encode protein tyrosine kinases that constitutively activate signal transduction pathways leading to abnormal cell proliferation.

JAK2 gene, located at chromosome 9p24, encodes the Janus kinase 2 that binds to cytokine receptors of granulocyte-macrophage colony-stimulating factor (GM-CSF), granulocyte colony-stimulating factor (G-CSF), erythropoietin (EPO), and thrombopoietin (TPO) and is involved in hematopoiesis, inflammation, and immune responses. Somatic missense mutation at codon 617 (c.1849 G>T, V617F) of exon 14 leads to JAK2 kinase autophosphorylation and constitutive activation that further activates STAT, MAPK, and PI3K signaling pathways and results in hypersensitivity of JAK2-linked cytokine receptors.[61-65] *JAK2* V617F has been reported in approximately 95% polycythemia vera (PV) and 40% to 50% of essential thrombocythemia (ET) and primary myelofibrosis (PMF).[61-65] It has also been detected in other hematologic malignancies such as refractory anemia with ring sideroblasts and thrombocytosis (RARS-t), chronic myelomonocytic leukemia, myelodysplastic syndrome, and AML.[66,67] Subsequent studies have identified *JAK2* exon 12 mutation in the rare PV without V617F[68,69] and W515K/L in exon 10 of thrombopoietin receptor *MPL* in approximately 5% of ET and PMF.[70,71] *MPL* mutation also leads to constitutive JAK-STAT signaling and confers hypersensitivity to TPO.[70,71] In addition, deletion of the entire exon 14 of *JAK2* due to alternative splicing has also been described, which gives rise to a truncated protein and can be detected by RNA-based (rather than DNA-based) method.[72]

JAK2-mutated PV, ET, and PMF may be better regarded as a spectrum of disorder with overlapping clinical and biologic features and the same molecular origin. The different phenotypes of these three diseases may be due to the different stem cell stage at which the *JAK2* mutation arises, dosage effect, complementary genetic events, and different host genetic background. *JAK2* and *MPL* mutational status do not appear to be strong independent predictors of inferior survival.[72] However, mutational analysis aids in diagnosis, understanding of the molecular pathogenesis, treatment strategies, as well as MRD detection.

The algorithm for the diagnosis of PV, ET, and PMF includes initial assessment of *JAK2* V617F followed by analysis of either *JAK2* exon 12 mutation for patients with suspected PV or *MPL* W515L/K for patients with suspected ET or PMF (Fig. 21.7). The choice for follow-up tests should be based on initial screening results.[73] Several methods can be used to detect *JAK2* V617F including the relatively insensitive and non-quantitative restriction fragment length polymorphism or Sanger sequencing (sensitivity 20%), as well as the more sensitive and quantitative pyrosequencing (sensitivity 1%) or allele-specific RQ-PCR (sensitivity 0.01-0.001%). Both DNA and RNA

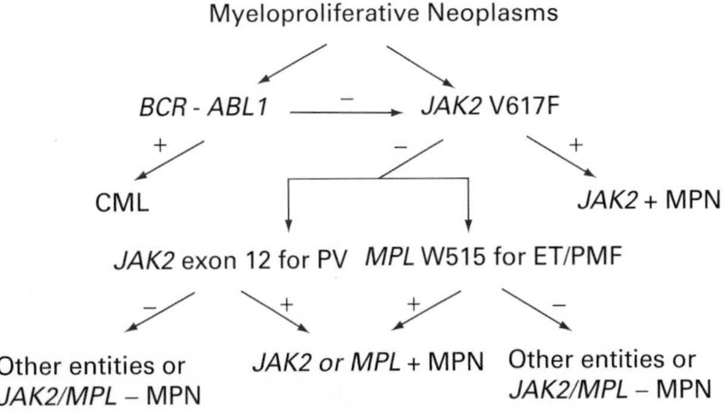

FIGURE 21–7 Algorithm of *JAK2/MPL* detection in myeloproliferative neoplasms. A reasonable approach includes initial assessment of *JAK2* V617F followed by analysis of either *JAK2* exon 12 mutation for patients with suspected polycythemia vera or *MPL* W515L/K for patients with suspected essential thrombocytosis or primary myelofibrosis. The choice for follow-up tests should be based on initial screening results.

have been used to determine the gene copy number and *JAK2*-mutated transcript level, respectively, and both BM and PB are acceptable. Cell sorting of granulocytes or megakaryocytes may improve detection sensitivity, especially for MRD monitoring when very low level of mutation is present, but this is technically challenging in the clinical setting. RQ-PCR of unsorted BM or PB is currently the most widely used method for monitoring *JAK2* V617F-mutated MPN, and it was shown that the mutation disappeared after allogeneic stem cell transplantation, and that its re-appearance preceded hemotologic relapse.[74,75] Extremely low level of *JAK2* V617F can be detected in a small subset of otherwise healthy individuals by PCR.[76] Therefore, caution needs to be practiced while interpreting the results, especially upon initial diagnosis. *MPL* W515L/K can be detected using an approach similar to that used for *JAK2* V617F. However, *JAK2* exon 12 mutations are still better detected using Sanger sequencing due to the diverse nature of the mutations, though high-resolution melting curve analysis has shown some promise recently.

KIT-MUTATED MASTOCYTOSIS

Mastocytosis is characterized by a clonal proliferation of neoplastic mast cells and is frequently associated with activating point mutations of *KIT*. *KIT* gene, located at chromosome 4q12, encodes an RTK that, upon binding of stem cell factor, plays a role in the development of myeloid cells, mast cells, neural crest (melanocytes), and gametes. *KIT* activating mutations have been described in AML (especially CBF-ABL), mastocytosis, gastrointestinal stromal tumor, and germ cell tumors. The activating mutations result in *KIT* phosphorylation and ligand-independent activation of downstream effectors including JAK-STAT, RAS-MAPK, and PI3K-AKT.[77] In mastocytosis, the majority of *KIT* mutations occur at codon 816 in exon 17 (most often D816V), with a

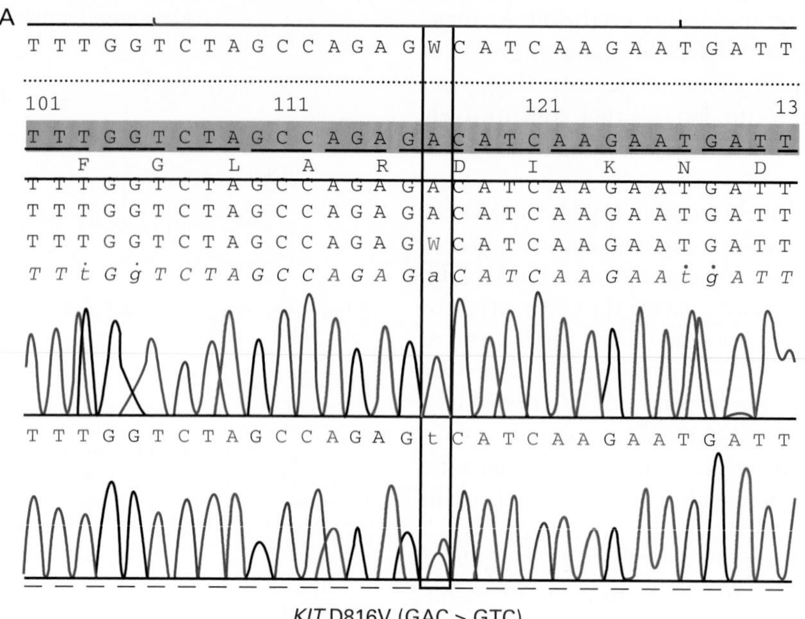

FIGURE 21–8 Detection of *KIT* D816V mutation. **A:** Sanger sequencing shows a mutation at codon 816 of the KIT gene (GAC>GTC, D816V). **B:** Allele-specific polymerase chain reaction shows amplification of the KIT D816V-mutated sequence (upper panel). The lower panel shows the amplification of the control gene, cyclophilin.

frequency of 50% to 95% in adults with systemic mastocytosis and 30% to 50% in children with cutaneous mastocytosis.[78,79] This wide reported range may reflect the difference in diagnostic criteria and the sensitivity of mutation detection methods, and our experience shows an incidence of approximately 75%. Other rare *KIT* mutations include D820G, E839K, F522C, and V560G.[77] The presence of D816V confers resistance to imatinib, but it still responds to other inhibitors such as dasatinib or PKC412.[80] *KIT* mutational analysis can therefore aid in the diagnosis, understanding of molecular pathogenesis, treatment strategies, and MRD monitoring of mastocytosis.

KIT mutation can be detected by a number of methods including allele-specific PCR, pyrosequencing, and Sanger sequencing (Fig. 21.8). Given the focal nature of mast cell aggregates and the poor sampling in BM aspirates due to fibrosis, we recommend pyrosequencing (sensitivity 1%) or allele-specific PCR (sensitivity 0.01-0.001%) on DNA extracted from grossly microdissected BM or skin. Sanger (sensitivity 20%) or non-quantitative PCR is not recommended. Cell sorting of BM aspirate specimens may further increase detection sensitivity, but is technically challenging in the clinical setting.

MRD TESTING IN POST-TRANSPLANTATION PATIENTS

Monitoring of MRD in the post-transplantation setting can be achieved by the detection of chimerism, i.e., the ratio of donor and recipient cells, using one of several methods, including PCR-based microsatellite polymorphism analysis, RQ-PCR, and interphase FISH in sex-mismatched cases. It has been shown that increasing mixed chimerism is associated with a higher risk of relapse.[81] However, an increase in recipient cells does not always predict impending relapse of the underlying disease.[82] This may be explained by the sensitivity of the detection method, the type of transplantation, the source of specimen used for analysis, the age of the patient, and the timing of the detection. Transient mixed chimerism, detected with very sensitive molecular method particularly in the first 6 to 9 months post–nonmyeloablative transplantation, has been well documented.[83] Therefore, identification of dynamic changes is more useful than a single test result.

PCR-based microsatellite analysis of short tandem repeat (STR) using primers that flank the repeating sequence, followed by fluorescence-based CE to size the PCR products and therefore calculate the number of repeats, has become the most frequently used technology for assessment of chimerism after allogeneic transplantation. It is very informative since one can almost always find at least one STR locus for each donor–recipient pair by assessing multiple STR loci with multiplex PCR. By comparing the peak area on the electropherogram, STR-PCR can be used to quantitatively discriminate the ratio of donor to recipient alleles, with a sensitivity of 1% to 5%.[84]

RQ-PCR using single nucleotide polymorphism (SNP) provides a higher sensitivity (lower limit of sensitivity 0.01% to 1%). However, SNP analysis is less informative in that it is usually necessary to evaluate many SNPs

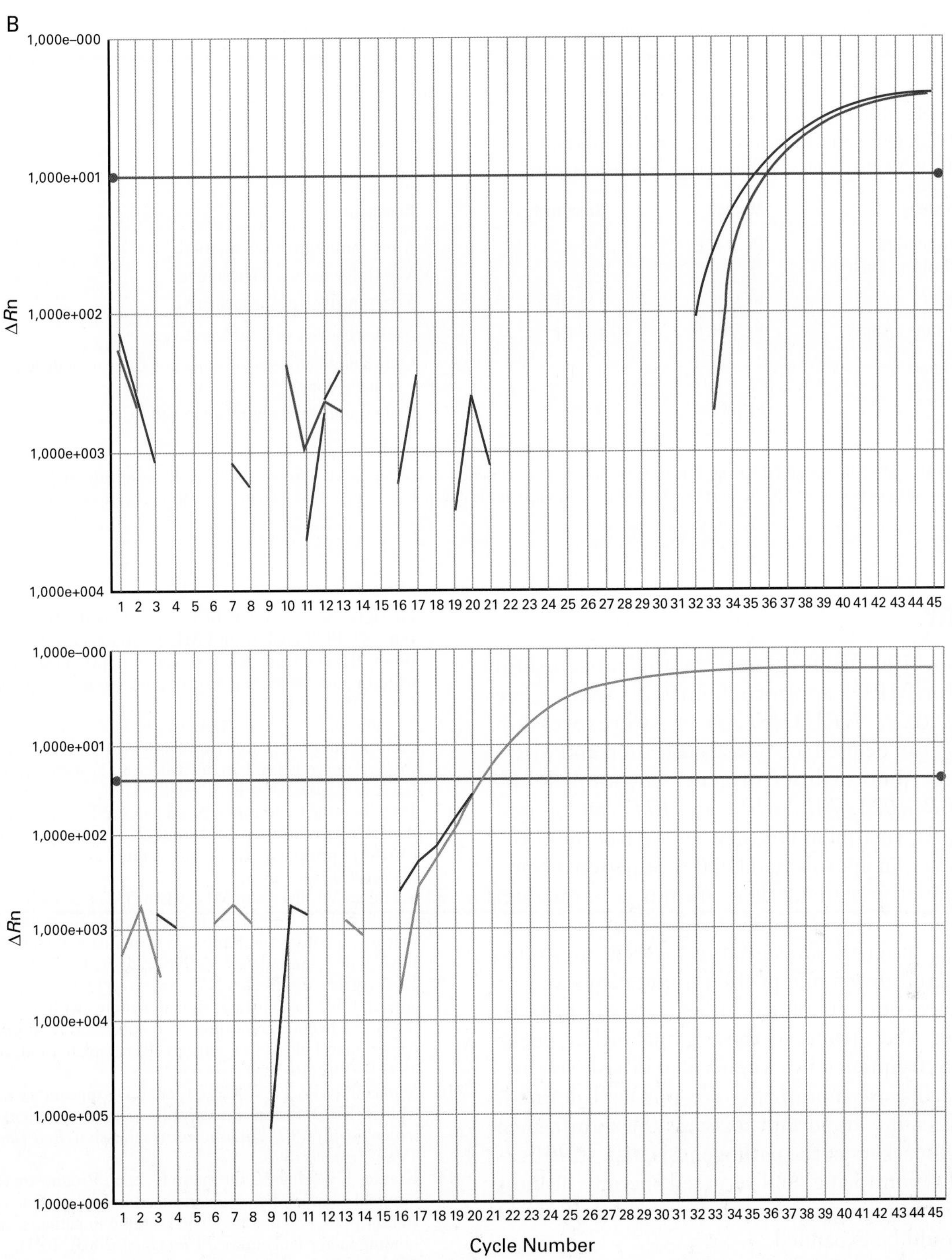

FIGURE 21–8 *(Continued)*

in order to find an informative SNP. RQ-PCR using Y-chromosome markers is very informative and provides further sensitivity (0.001% to 0.1%), but it can only be applied to sex-mismatched cases with male recipient and female donor.[85] FISH analysis has a sensitivity of 0.1% to 0.5%, but its application is also limited to sex-mismatched transplants.[86] Chimerism analysis of a subset cell population, e.g., T and B cells or $CD34^+$ cells, can further increase the sensitivity and specificity of the above assays, but it requires additional cell sorting and larger volume of samples. It is noteworthy that for patients who have a disease-specific molecular genetic abnormality, such as recurrent translocation/inversion or specific gene mutation, detection of the molecular genetic abnormality is still the preferred method for MRD monitoring due to the short interval between the increase of recipient cells and the clinical manifestation of relapse and the fact that a relapse is not always preceded by an increase in recipient cells, which limit the application of chimerism analysis in early detection of relapse (Table 21.8).

TABLE 21-8 Monitoring of Minimal Residual Diseases in Post-transplantation Patients

Disease-specific genetic markers (e.g., translocation, inversion, gene mutation, gene overexpression)
Better marker than chimerism for MRD monitoring
qRT-PCR for translocation, inversion, gene overexpression
RQ-PCR, PCR-CE, or pyrosequencing for gene mutation

Chimerism study	Method	Sensitivity	Comment
STR microsatellite polymorphism analysis	PCR-CE	1–5%	Most commonly used method Very informative, quantitative
SNP analysis	RQ-PCR	1×10^{-5}	Very sensitive, less informative
Y-chromosome analysis	RQ-PCR	1×10^{-6}	Most sensitive, very informative Only suitable for sex-mismatched cases with male recipient/female donor
	FISH	0.5%	Only suitable for sex-mismatched cases

MRD, minimal residual disease; qRT-PCR, quantitative real-time reverse transcription–polymerase chain reaction; RQ-PCR, quantitative real-time PCR; PCR-CE, PCR-capillary electrophoresis; STR, short tandem repeat; SNP, single nucleotide polymorphism; FISH, fluorescence in situ hybridization.

SUMMARY

Disease-specific fusion genes are the most useful markers for MRD monitoring. In CN-AML, gene mutations (e.g., *NPM1*, *FLT3*) or overexpression (e.g., *WT1*) can be used for risk stratification and MRD assessment. Abnormalities of genes encoding RTK, such as *BCR-ABL1*, *JAK2/MPL*, and *KIT*, can be used for diagnosis, treatment strategy, and MRD monitoring. However, in approximately 20% of patients, suitable molecular genetic markers are not yet available. With the advancement of gene expression profiling, SNP array, microRNA signature, DNA methylation array, and proteomic profiling, mutations and/or altered expressions of a lot of other genes have been discovered. Aberrations of these genes either occur at very low frequencies or their roles in risk stratification and disease monitoring are not well defined. Nevertheless, it is important to assess the significance of these biomarkers in the pathogenesis, risk stratification, MRD monitoring, and targeted therapy in light of new treatment regimens so that the panel of MRD markers could be expanded.

REFERENCES

1. Kelly LM, Gilliland DG. Genetics of myeloid leukemias. *Annu Rev Genomics Hum Genet*. 2002;3:179-198.
2. Evens PA, Short MA, Jack AS, et al. Detection and quantitation of the CBFbeta/MYH11 transcripts associated with the inv(16) in presentation and follow-up samples from patients with AML. *Leukemia*. 1997;11(3):364-369.
3. Diverio D, Rossi V, Avvisati G, et al. Early detection of relapse by prospective reverse transcriptase-polymerase chain reaction analysis of the PML/RARalpha fusion gene in patients with acute promyelocytic leukemia enrolled in the GIMEMA-AIEOP multicenter "AIDA" trial. GIM-EMA-AIEOP Multicenter "AIDA" Trial. *Blood*. 1998;92(3): 784-789.
4. Marcucci G, Caligiuri MA, Dohner H, et al. Quantification of CBFbeta/MYH11 fusion transcript by real-time RT-PCR in patients with inv(16) acute myeloid leukemia. *Leukemia*. 2001;15(7):1072-1080.
5. Gallagher RE, Yeap BY, Bi W, et al. Quantitative real-time RT-PCR analysis of PML-RARalpha mRNA in acute promyelocytic leukemia: assessment of prognostic significance in adult patients from intergroup protocol 0129. *Blood*. 2003;101(7):2521-2528.
6. Miyamoto T, Nagafuji K, Akashi K, et al. Persistence of multipotent progenitors expressing AML1/ETO transcripts in long-term remission patients with t(8;21) acute myelogenous leukemia. *Blood*. 1996;87(11):4789-4796.
7. Preudhomme C, Philippe N, Macintyre E, et al. Persistence of AML1/ETO fusion mRNA in t(8;21) acute myeloid leukemia (AML) in prolonged remission: is there a consensus? *Leukemia*. 1996;10(1):186-188.
8. Saunders MJ, Brereton ML, Adams JA, et al. Expression of AML1/MTG8 transcripts in clonogenic cells grown from bone marrow of patients in remission of acute myeloid leukaemia with t(8;21). *Br J Haematol*. 1997;99(4):921-924.
9. Elmmagacli AH, Beelen DW, Stockova J, et al. Detection of AML1/ETO fusion transcripts in patients with t(8;21) acute myeloid leukemia after allogeneic bone marrow transplantation or peripheral blood progenitor cell transplantation. *Blood*. 1997;90(8):3230-3231.
10. Statake N, Maseki N, Kozy T, et al. Disappearance of AML1-MTG8(ETO) fusion transcript in acute myeloid leukaemia patients with t(8;21) in long-term remission. *Br J Haematol*. 1995;91(4):892-898.
11. Krauter J, Gorlich K, Ottmann O, et al. Prognostic value of minimal residual disease quantification by real-time reverse transcriptase polymerase chain reaction in patients with core binding factor leukemias. *J Clin Oncol*. 2003;21(23): 4413-4422.
12. Perea G, Lasa A, Aventín A, et al. Prognostic value of minimal residual disease (MRD) in acute myeloid leukemia (AML) with favorable cytogenetics [t(8;21) and inv(16)]. *Leukemia*. 2006;20(1):87-94.
13. Ommen HB, Schnittger S, Jovanovic JV, et al. Strikingly different molecular relapse kinetics in NPM1c, PML-RARA, RUNX1-RUNX1T1, and CBFB-MYH11 acute myeloid leukemias. *Blood*. 2010;115(2):198-205.
14. Lane S, Saal R, Mollee P, et al. A >or=1 log rise in RQ-PCR transcript levels defines molecular relapse in core binding factor acute myeloid leukemia and predicts subsequent morphologic relapse. *Leuk Lymphoma*. 2008;49(3):517-523.
15. Borer RA, Lehner CF, Eppenberger HM, et al. Major nucleolar proteins shuttle between nucleus and cytoplasm. *Cell*. 1989;56(3):379-390.
16. Falini B, Mecucci C, Tiacci E, et al. Cytoplasmic nucleophosmin in acute myelogenous leukemia with a normal karyotype. *N Engl J Med*. 2005;352(3):254-266.

17. Falini B, Nicoletti I, Martelli MF, et al. Acute myeloid leukemia carrying cytoplasmic/mutated nucleophosmin (NPMc+ AML): biologic and clinical features. *Blood*. 2007;109(3):874-885.
18. Falini B, Martelli MP, Bolli N, et al. Immunohistochemistry predicts nucleophosmin (NPM) mutations in acute myeloid leukemia. *Blood*. 2006;108(6):1999-2005.
19. Palmisano M, Grafone T, Ottaviani E, et al. NPM1 mutations are more stable than FLT3 mutations during the course of disease in patients with acute myeloid leukemia. *Haematologica*. 2007;92(9):1268-1269.
20. Chou WC, Tang IL, Wu SJ, et al. Clinical implications of minimal residual disease monitoring by quantitative polymerase chain reaction in acute myeloid leukemia patients bearing nucleophosmin (NPM1) mutations. *Leukemia*. 2007;21(5):998-1004.
21. Bacher U, Badbaran A, Fehse B, et al. Quantitative monitoring of *NPM1* mutations provides a valid minimal residual disease parameter following allogeneic stem cell transplantation. *Exp Hematol*. 2009;37(1):135-142.
22. Dvorakova D, Racil Z, Jezikova I, et al. Monitoring of minimal residual disease in acute myeloid leukemia with frequent and rare patient-specific NPM1 mutations. *Am J Hematol*. 2010;85(12):926-929.
23. Barakat FH, Luthra R, Yin CC, et al. Detection of nucleophosmin 1 mutations by quantitative real-time polymerase chain reaction versus capillary electrophoresis. *Arch Pathol Lab Med*. 2011;135(8):949-1000.
24. Gilliland DG, Griffin JD. The roles of FLT3 in hematopoiesis and leukemia. *Blood*. 2002;100(5):1532-1542.
25. Mead AJ, Gale RE, Hills RK, et al. Conflicting data on the prognostic significance of FLT3/TKD mutations in acute myeloid leukemia might be related to the incidence of biallelic disease. *Blood*. 2008;112(2):444-445.
26. Schnittger S, Schoch C, Dugas M, et al. Analysis of FLT3 length mutations in 1003 patients with acute myeloid leukemia: correlation to cytogenetics, FAB subtype, and prognosis in the AMLCG study and usefulness as a marker for the detection of minimal residual disease. *Blood*. 2002;100(1):1532-1542.
27. Gale RE, Green C, Allen C, et al. The impact of FLT3 internal tandem duplication mutant level, number, size, and interaction with NPM1 mutations in a large cohort of young adult patients with acute myeloid leukemia. *Blood*. 2008;111(5):2772-2784.
28. Nakano Y, Kiyoi H, Miyawaki S, et al. Molecular evolution of acute myeloid leukaemia in relapse: unstable N-ras and FLT3 genes compared with p53 gene. *Br J Haematol*. 1999;104(4):659-664.
29. Schnittger S, Schoch C, Kern W, et al. FLT3 length mutations as marker for follow-up studies in acute myeloid leukaemia. *Acta Haematol*. 2004;112(1-2):68-78.
30. Abdelhamid E, Preudhomme C, Helevaut N, et al. Minimal residual disease monitoring based on *FLT3* internal tandem duplication in adult acute myeloid leukemia. *Leukemia Res*. 2012;36(3):316-323.
31. Dufour A, Schneider F, Metzeler KH, et al. Acute myeloid leukemia with biallelic CEBPA gene mutations and normal karyotype represents a distinct genetic entity associated with a favorable clinical outcome. *J Clin Oncol*. 2010;28(4):570-577.
32. Kato N, Kitaura J, Doki N, et al. Two types of C/EBPα mutations play distinct but collaborative roles in leukemogenesis: lessons from clinical data and BMT models. *Blood*. 2011;117(1):221-233.
33. Tyner JW, Erickson H, Deininger MW, et al. High-throughput sequencing screen reveals novel, transforming RAS mutations in myeloid leukemia patients. *Blood*. 2009;113(8):1749-1755.
34. Neubauer A, Maharry K, Mrozek K, et al. Patients with acute myeloid leukemia and RAS mutations benefit most from post remission high-dose cytarabine: a Cancer and Leukemia Group B study. *J Clin Oncol*. 2008;26(28):4603-4609.
35. Casey G, Rudzki Z, Roberts M, et al. N-ras mutation in acute myeloid leukemia: incidence, prognostic significance and value as a marker of minimal residual disease. *Pathology*. 1993;25(1):57-62.
36. Care RS, Valk PJ, Goodeve AC, et al. Incidence and prognosis of c-KIT and FLT3 mutations in core binding factor (CBF) acute myeloid leukaemias. *Br J Haematol*. 2003;121(5):775-777.
37. Paschka P, Marcucci G, Ruppert AS, et al. Adverse prognostic significance of KIT mutations in adult acute myeloid leukemia with inv(16) and t(8;21): a Cancer and Leukemia Group B study. *J Clin Oncol*. 2006;24(24):3904-3911.
38. Tamai H, Inokuchi K. 11q23/MLL acute leukemia: update of clinical aspects. *J Clin Exp Hematol*. 2010;50(2):91-98.
39. Mrózek K, Marcucci G, Paschka P, et al. Clinical relevance of mutations and gene-expression changes in adult acute myeloid leukemia with normal cytogenetics: are we ready for a prognostically prioritized molecular classification? *Blood*. 2007;109(2):431-448.
40. Weisser M, Kern W, Schoch C, et al. Risk assessment by monitoring expression levels of partial tandem duplications in the MLL gene in acute myeloid leukemia during therapy. *Haematologica*. 2005;90(7):881-889.
41. Baldus CD, Tanner SM, Ruppert AS, et al. *BAALC* expression predicts clinical outcome of de novo acute myeloid leukemia patients with normal cytogenetics: a Cancer and Leukemia Group B study. *Blood*. 2003;102(5):1613-1618.
42. Marcucci G, Maharry K, Whitman SP, et al. High expression levels of the ETS-related gene, ERG, predict adverse outcome and improve molecular risk-based classification of cytogenetically normal acute myeloid leukemia: a Cancer and Leukemia Group B study. *J Clin Oncol*. 2007;25(22):3337-3343.
43. Langer C, Marcucci G, Holland KB, et al. Prognostic importance of MN1 transcript levels, and biologic insights from MN1-associated gene and microRNA expression signatures in cytogenetically normal acute myeloid leukemia. A Cancer and Leukemia Group B study. *J Clin Oncol*. 2009;27(19):3198-3204.
44. Groschel S, Lugthart S, Schlenk RF, et al. High EVI1 expression predicts outcome in younger adult patients with acute myeloid leukemia and is associated with distinct cytogenetic abnormalities. *J Clin Oncol*. 2010;28(12):2101-2117.
45. Gray JX, McMillen L, Mollee P, et al. WT1 expression as a marker of minimal residual disease predicts outcome in acute myeloid leukemia when measured post-consolidation. *Leuk Res*. 2011. [Epub ahead of print].
46. Paschka P, Marcucci G, Ruppert AS, et al. Wilms' tumor 1 gene mutations independently predict poor outcome in adults with cytogenetically normal acute myeloid leukemia: a Cancer and Leukemia Group B study. *J Clin Oncol*. 2008;26(28): 4595-4602.
47. Virappane P, Gale R, Hills R, et al. Mutation of the Wilms' tumor 1 gene is a poor prognostic factor associated with chemotherapy resistance in normal karyotype acute myeloid leukemia: the United Kingdom Medical Research Council Adult Leukaemia Working Party. *J Clin Oncol*. 2008;26(33):5429-5435.
48. Gaidzik VI, Schlenk RF, Moschny S, et al. Prognostic impact of WT1 mutations in cytogenetically normal acute myeloid leukemia: a study of the German-Austrian AML Study Group. *Blood*. 2009;113(19):4505-4511.
49. Damm F, Heuser M, Morgan M, et al. Single nucleotide polymorphism in the mutational hotspot of WT1 predicts a favorable outcome in patients with cytogenetically normal acute myeloid leukemia. *J Clin Oncol*. 2010;28(4):578-585.
50. Cilloni D, Renneville A, Hermitte F, et al. Real-time quantitative polymerase chain reaction detection of minimal residual disease by standardized WT1 assay to enhance risk stratification in acute myeloid leukemia: a European Leukemia Net study. *J Clin Oncol*. 2009;27(31):5195-5201.
51. Nowakowska-Kopera A, Sacha T, Florek I, et al. Wilms' tumor gene 1 expression analysis by real-time quantitative polymerase chain reaction for monitoring of minimal residual disease in acute leukemia. *Leuk Lymphoma*. 2009;50(8):1326-1332.
52. Kwon M, Martínez-Laperche C, Infante M, et al. Evaluation of minimal residual disease by real-time quantitative PCR of Wilms' tumor 1 (WT1) expression in patients with acute myeloid leukemia after allogeneic stem cell transplantation. Correlation with flow cytometry and chimerism. *Biol Blood Marrow Transplant*. 2012. [Epub ahead of print].
53. Vardiman JW, Melo JV, Baccarani M, et al. Chronic myelogenous leukaemia, *BCR-ABL1* positive. In: Swerdlow SH, Campo E, Harris NL, et al., eds. *WHO Classification of Tumours of Haematopoietic and Lymphoid Tissues*. Lyon: IARC; 2008:32-37.
54. Branford S, Rudzki Z, Walsh S, et al. High frequency of point mutations clustered within the adenosine triphosphate-binding region of BCR/ABL in patients with chronic myeloid leukemia or Ph-positive acute lymphoblastic leukemia who develop imatinib (STI571) resistance. *Blood*. 2002;99(9):3472-3475.
55. Radich JP, Zelenetz AD, Chan WC, et al. NCCN Task Force Report: molecular markers in leukemias and lymphomas. *J Natl Compr Canc Netw*. 2009;(suppl 4):S1-S34.

56. De Lavallade H, Apperley JF, Khorashad JS, et al. Imatinib for newly diagnosed patients with chronic myeloid leukemia: incidence of sustained responses in an intention-to-treat analysis. *J Clin Oncol.* 2008;26(20):3658-3663.
57. Lima L, Bernal-Mizrachi L, Saxe D, et al. Peripheral blood monitoring of chronic myeloid leukemia during treatment with imatinib, second-line agents, and beyond. *Cancer.* 2011;117(6):1245-1252.
58. Cortes J, Talpaz M, O'Brien S, et al. Molecular responses in patients with chronic myelogenous leukemia in chronic phase treated with imatinib mesylate. *Clin Cancer Res.* 2005;11(9):3425-3432.
59. White HE, Matejtschuk P, Rigsby P, et al. Establishment of the first World Health Organization International Genetic Reference Panel for quantitation of BCR-ABL mRNA. *Blood.* 2010;116(22):111-117.
60. Yin CC, Cortes J, Galbincea J, et al. Rapid clonal shifts in response to kinase inhibitor therapy in chronic myelogenous leukemia are identified by quantitation mutation assays. *Cancer Sci.* 2010;101(9):2005-2010.
61. Baxter EJ, Scott LM, Campbell PJ, et al. Acquired mutation of the tyrosine kinase JAK2 in human myeloproliferative disorders. *Lancet.* 2005;365(9464):1054-1061.
62. James C, Ugo V, Le Couedic JP, et al. A unique clonal JAK2 mutation leading to constitutive signaling causes polycythaemia vera. *Nature.* 2005;434(7037):1144-1148.
63. Jones AV, Kreil S, Zoi K, et al. Widespread occurrence of the JAK2 V617F mutation in chronic myeloproliferative disorders. *Blood.* 2005;106(6):2162-2168.
64. Kralovics R, Passamonti F, Buser AS, et al. A gain-of-function mutation of JAK2 in myeloproliferative disorders. *N Engl J Med.* 2005;352(17):1779-1790.
65. Levine RL, Wadleigh M, Cools J, et al. Activating mutation in the tyrosine kinase JAK2 in polycythemia vera, essential thrombocythemia, and myeloid metaplasia with myelofibrosis. *Cancer Cell.* 2005;7(4):387-397.
66. Steensma DP, Dewald GW, Lasho TL, et al. The JAK2 V617F activating tyrosine kinase mutation is an infrequent event in both "atypical" myeloproliferative disorders and myelodysplastic syndromes. *Blood.* 2005;106(4):1207-1209.
67. Atallah E, Nussenzveig R, Yin CC, et al. Prognostic interaction between thrombocytosis and *JAK2* V617F mutation in the WHO subcategories of myelodysplastic/myeloproliferative disease—unclassifiable and refractory anemia with ringed sideroblasts and marked thrombocytosis. *Leukemia.* 2008;22(6):1295-1298.
68. Pardanani A, Lasho TL, Finke C, et al. Prevalence and clinicopathologic correlates of JAK2 exon 12 mutations in JAK2V617F-negative polycythemia vera. *Leukemia.* 2007;21(9):1960-1963.
69. Scott LM, Tong W, Levine RL, et al. JAK2 exon 12 mutations in polycythemia vera and idiopathic erythrocytosis. *N Engl J Med.* 2007;356(5):459-468.
70. Pardanani AD, Levine RL, Lasho T, et al. MPL515 mutations in myeloproliferative and other myeloid disorders: a study of 1182 patients. *Blood.* 2006;108(10):3472-3476.
71. Pikman Y, Lee BH, Mercher T, et al. MPLW515L is a novel somatic activating mutation in myelofibrosis with myeloid metaplasia. *PLoS Med.* 2006;3(7):e270.
72. Ma W, Kantarjian H, Zhang X, et al. JAK2 exon 14 deletion in patients with chronic myeloproliferative neoplasms. *PLoS One.* 2010;5(8):e12165.
73. Yin CC, Jones D. Myeloproliferative neoplasms. In: Jones D, ed. *Neoplastic Hematopathology: Experimental and Clinical Approaches.* New York, NY: Humana Press; 2010:177-192.
74. Kröger N, Badbaran A, Holler E, et al. Monitoring of the JAK2-V617F mutation by highly sensitive quantitative real-time PCR after allogeneic stem cell transplantation in patients with myelofibrosis. *Blood.* 2007;109(3):1316-1321.
75. Steckel NK, Koldehoff M, Ditschkowski M, et al. Use of the activating gene mutation of the tyrosine kinase (VAL617Phe) JAK2 as a minimal residual disease marker in patients with myelofibrosis and myeloid metaplasia after allogeneic stem cell transplantation. *Transplantation.* 2007;83(11): 1518-1520.
76. Xu X, Zhang Q, Luo J, et al. JAK2(V617F): prevalence in a large Chinese hospital population. *Blood.* 2007;109(1):339-342.
77. Lim KH, Pardanani A, Tefferi A. KIT and mastocytosis. *Acta Haematol.* 2008;119(4):194-198.
78. Furitsu T, Tsujimura T, Tono T, et al. Identification of mutations in the coding sequence of the proto-oncogene c-kit in a human mast cell leukemia cell line causing ligand-independent activation of c-kit product. *J Clin Invest.* 1993;92(4):1736-1744.
79. Nagata H, Worobec AS, Oh CK, et al. Identification of a point mutation in the catalytic domain of the protooncogene c-kit in peripheral blood mononuclear cells of patients who have mastocytosis with an associated hematologic disorder. *Proc Natl Acad Sci U S A.* 1995;92(23):10560-10564.
80. Gleixner KV, Mayerhofer M, Sonneck K, et al. Synergistic growth-inhibitory effects of two tyrosine kinase inhibitors, dasatinib and PKC412, on neoplastic mast cells expressing the D816V-mutated oncogenic variant of KIT. *Haematologica.* 2007;92(11):1451-1459.
81. Bader P, Kreyenberg H, Hoelle W, et al. Increasing mixed chimerism defines a high-risk group of childhood acute myelogenous leukemia patients after allogeneic stem cell transplantation where pre-emptive immunotherapy may be effective. *Bone Marrow Transplant.* 2004;33(8):815-821.
82. Baron F, Sandmaier BM. Chimerism and outcomes after allogeneic hematopoietic cell transplantation following nonmyeloablative conditioning. *Leukemia.* 2006;20(10):1690-1700.
83. McCann SR, Carmpe M, Molloy K, et al. Hemopoietic chimerism following stem cell transplantation. *Transfus Apher Sci.* 2005;32(1):55-61.
84. Thiede C, Bornhäuser M, Oelschlägel U, et al. Sequential monitoring of chimerism and detection of minimal residual disease after allogeneic blood stem cell transplantation (ASCT) using multiplex PCR amplification of short tandem repeat markers. *Leukemia.* 2001;15(2):293-302.
85. Fehse B, Chukhlovin A, Kühlcke K, et al. Real-time quantitative Y chromosome-specific PCR (QYCS-PCR) for monitoring hematopoietic chimerism after sex-mismatched allogeneic stem cell transplantation. *J Hematother Stem Cell Res.* 2001;10(3):419-425.
86. Najfeld V, Burnett W, Vlachos A, et al. Interphase FISH analysis of sex-mismatched BMT utilizing dual color XY probes. *Bone Marrow Transplant.* 1997;19(8):829-834.

CHAPTER 22

Molecular Assessment of Cancer Prognosis

Qing Zhao and Dongfeng Tan

INTRODUCTION

Cancer is a complex disease that requires a long-term progression. Accurately predicting prognosis for effective cancer therapy needs advanced pathologic diagnosis and molecular assessment. Pathologic assessment of the molecular features of tumors with advanced ancillary tools plays essential roles in guiding clinical decision-making for treatment and monitoring recurrence. For most solid tumors, a broad generalization regarding treatment approaches is based on the TNM staging system, which is the principal guideline in clinical management. However, considerable heterogeneity in the nature of individual tumors, the variety of subtypes and differentiation of tissues and organ-specific tumors, individual differences in patients' genetic backgrounds, and differences in cancers' clinical presentation all have been known to play important roles in patients' different responses to surgery or surgery with combined chemoradiation or neoadjuvant therapy. The introduction of targeted cancer therapies into clinical practice, in which patients are selected for certain treatments based on the results of molecular analysis of their tumor samples, has brought surgical pathology as well as clinical oncology to a new level, with new challenges and opportunities. Increasingly, demand for molecular biomarkers (e.g., cancer prognostic or predictive markers) for cancer care has been applied in clinical practice, especially in large cancer institutions. Researchers have demonstrated the role of molecular biomarkers, including those currently still under investigation or in clinical trials, in early cancer detection[1-4] and cancer prognosis[4,5] and in predicting patients' response to neoadjuvant or chemoradiation therapy.[6]

Biomarkers are physical, functional, or biochemical indicators of physiologic or disease processes. Biomarker is objectively measured and evaluated as an indicator of normal biologic processes, pathogenic processes, or pharmacologic responses to a therapeutic intervention.[7] These key indicators can provide vital information in determining disease prognosis, in predicting of response to therapies, adverse events, and drug interactions, and in establishing baseline risk. Many biomarkers and molecular pathways have been studied extensively over the last several decades. While some biomarkers appear promising, many others have failed the rigorous test of reproducibility, and many biomarker candidates are still under investigation. For example, serum cancer antigen 125 and carbohydrate antigen 19.9 are serum biomarkers for monitoring ovarian and pancreatic cancers. Cancer biomarkers have recently heightened interest in the relevance to cancer biology and clinical oncology; for example, the role of KRAS in colorectal cancer (CRC) and other cancers in which epidermal growth factor receptor (EGFR) pathways are involved.[8,9] In patients whose tumors express the mutated *KRAS* gene, the encoded KRAS protein, which is part of the EGFR signaling pathway, is constitutively activated. This constitutively overactive EGFR signaling continues downstream from EGFR; even when upstream signaling is blocked by an EGFR inhibitor, such as cetuximab (Erbitux) or panitumumab (Vectibix); cancer cell growth and proliferation are not blocked. Therefore, testing certain tumors for wild-type versus mutant *KRAS* status helps identify those patients who will benefit most from treatment with cetuximab.[10] Molecular biomarkers can be classified as diagnostic, prognostic, and predictive. Diagnostic markers are lineage-specific proteins; their preserved expression or loss of expression in certain cancer cells is useful in confirming tissue diagnoses. For instance, cytokeratin 20 is commonly expressed in colorectal and appendiceal epithelia, but renal cell antigen is unique to renal cell carcinoma and glial fibrillary acidic protein is mostly used in the diagnosis of glioma in the central nervous system. However, prognostic and predictive biomarkers are used interchangeably because of their overlapping features. By definition, prognostic markers separate a population of patients in terms of their clinical outcome in the absence of treatment, thereby defining the natural history of the disease. Therefore, validation of prognostic markers is straightforward inasmuch as it can be performed using data from a retrospective series of patients treated with standard drugs. On the other hand, predictive markers stratify patients based on clinical outcome in response to a particular treatment. Molecular biomarkers will commonly have both predictive and prognostic characteristics. Therefore, validation of predictive markers requires analysis of quality randomized clinical trials to exclude prognostic effects.

The incorporation of ancillary techniques in the field of molecular biology has had a great effect on the surgical pathology field; many of these techniques have become routine tests in surgical pathology and molecular biology laboratories. These include immunohistochemical (IHC) analysis, cytogenetic analysis, RNA in situ hybridization, fluorescence in situ hybridization (FISH), and more recently, polymerase chain reaction (PCR) and other PCR-based molecular tests (e.g., reverse transcription–polymerase chain reaction [RT-PCR], nested PCR, multiplex PCR, and methylation-specific PCR), as well as DNA sequencing and DNA microarrays. Other methods, including comparative genomic hybridization, micro-RNA analysis, and mass spectrometry, are still being used predominantly in basic and clinical translational research fields, although they have demonstrated promise in molecular biomarker discovery and in cancer prognosis and outcome prediction. Many of the molecular assays used in clinical practice are based on variations of the PCR amplification method and hybridization of complementary nucleic acids and on direct sequencing techniques. Technical applications and descriptions of methods have been discussed elsewhere in great detail.[11] In this chapter, we review the most commonly used methods in the anatomic surgical pathology laboratory and their importance in cancer prognosis. We also discuss general sampling and technical issues that are relevant to molecular methods used in surgical pathology. Finally, we discuss the advantages and disadvantages of each method. We believe that cancer prognostic biomarkers will continue to alter therapeutic regimens and that targeted personalized cancer therapies will represent the next generation of cancer management.

TISSUE COLLECTION

Specimen Sampling

Surgical tumor specimens are received directly from the operating room after being resected. Most patients will have received chemoradiation therapy before surgery, so the specimens usually represent treated tumors. Patients often had a pre-surgery diagnosis by either surgical or fine-needle aspiration biopsy, but for patients who had no definite diagnosis before surgery, resected surgical specimens become important in making the final pathologic diagnosis. Most tumor resection is for treatment, tumor staging, and evaluation of the treatment effect. Fresh tissue specimens are still needed for cytogenetic analysis and hematopoietic flow cytometry (and are kept in special medium, e.g., RPMI 1640). Tissue collected for potential electron microscopy is freshly collected and treated with a special fixative (3% glutaraldehyde in 0.1 M phosphate-buffered saline).[12] All other tests can be performed on paraffin-fixed tissues. Some solid tumors tend to have large necrotic areas; for example, untreated renal cell carcinomas and after treatment soft tissue tumors (for instance, liposarcoma and gastrointestinal stromal tumor). Therefore, sampling of the non-necrotic region becomes more relevant. Molecular testing also requires an enriched tumor tissue with minimal contamination by normal tissue for specificity. The majority of the tumor can be fixed in 10% formalin for several hours to overnight.

Tissue Fixation

Although nucleic acid preservation is best on fresh or snap-frozen tissue, this is not routinely performed and is rarely available because it requires extra effort by the pathologist. Many molecular assays are being optimized for formalin-fixed, paraffin-embedded (FFPE) tissue specimens. Formalin creates crosslinks between nucleic acids and proteins and between different proteins.[13] This crosslinking interferes with the recovery of RNA and protein from FFPE tissue and is not appropriate for RNA or protein-based assays (for example, in DNA microarrays and micro-RNA tests). Unfortunately, the protective effects of formalin are neither absolute nor everlasting, and the DNA recovered from FFPE blocks tends to be degraded into fragments <500 bp in length, becoming further degraded over time. The length or even shorter fragments, however, can be used as DNA templates in most molecular tests.[14] The use of other fixatives containing either acids (Bouin's and decalcifying solutions), which damage nucleic strands, or heavy metals (Zenker's and B5 solution), which contain mercuric chloride that inhibits enzymes used in amplification, render these specimens unsuitable for most molecular testing. Therefore, routine surgical FFPE tissues can be used in initial PCR-based amplification for further molecular tests.

Tissue Dissection and DNA or Protein Extraction

Eight or 10 sections that are 1-μm thick are cut from FFPE normal tissue and tumor samples and placed onto positive-charged glass slides. Sections containing abundant amounts of tumor are carefully scraped under microscopy and collected. If the tumor tissue is <20% or 30% of the total volume, it needs to be dissected under laser capture microdissection (LCM). DNA extraction can be performed by a standard phenol/chloroform procedure[13,15] after incubation for a minimum of 16 hours with proteinase K at 37°C. Matched control and tumor DNA can then be used for PCR amplification by approved consensus primers or markers (for example, microsatellite instability [MSI] testing of BAT25, BAT26, D2S124, D5S346, and D17S250),[16] or DNA sequencing from tumor tissue can be obtained usually after PCR amplification of/using sufficient templates. Although proteins are not extractable from FFPE samples, RNA can be isolated from FFPE tissue for downstream applications such as RT-PCR[17] and complementary DNA (cDNA) microarray.[18,19] A previous report showed that 70% ethanol is one candidate fixative that is optimal for histology and recovery of RNA,[19] although this technique has not been widely accepted in the clinical laboratory.

IHC ANALYSIS

IHC analysis is one of the most powerful and widely used ancillary methods in the surgical pathology laboratory. We include IHC analysis as a molecular ancillary test in this chapter because of its routine use in assessing tumor prognostic and predictive biomarkers. This technique is favored by surgical pathologists because it enables them to simultaneously visualize tissue histology and the expression patterns of the protein of interest. An antibody cocktail can be applied to a single slide or multiple antibodies can be tested on the same tissue section at the same time. The antibody is tagged with a colorimetric stain that differentially binds to the protein of interest, providing a visual stain showing the presence or absence of the protein. Antigens were first detected by exposing fluorescence-tagged antibodies to frozen tissue sections.[20] This technique has a long history; it has been used since 1897. Paul Ehrlich, who proposed the antigen–antibody interaction in a "lock-and-key-interaction," shared the 1908 Nobel Prize in medicine with Elie Metchnikoff.[21] In the molecular technology era, the IHC method is still used because it is simple, fast, and effective in evaluating cancer biomarkers. Here, we discuss typical examples of IHC analysis used in the diagnosis of breast carcinoma and colon adenocarcinoma and in the assessment of the proliferative index (by Ki-67) in various tumors. Another advantage of IHC analysis is that it can be performed on FFPE tissue sections that can then be stored for long periods. New amplification methods,[22] such as tyramide- and polymer-based labeling, allow for much greater sensitivity in antigen detection than conventional IHC. These new IHC methods also require less tissue. This technique is relatively inexpensive compared with other molecular techniques, such as DNA microarray and gene sequencing, and it is widely available in institutions and commercial laboratories. The disadvantage is that the results are only qualitative or semi-quantitative: positive, negative, and sometimes indeterminate. Inconsistency in interpretation can occur because of the quality of staining, as well as inter- and intra-interpreter variabilities. In addition, immunostains only identify the presence or absence of certain proteins; they do not indicate whether the proteins are functioning or not. IHC analysis is most frequently used to classify tumors (carcinoma, sarcoma, or lymphoma); identify in situ lesions versus invasive carcinomas (myoepithelial markers in breast carcinomas and basal cell markers in prostate adenocarcinoma); determine prognostic information (e.g., the proliferative index of Ki-67 in neuroendocrine tumors and glioblastomas); determine predictive factors to guide specific therapy (e.g., c-Kit, estrogen receptor [ER], progesterone receptor [PR], and human epidermal growth factor receptor 2 [HER2]/neu status); identify extracellular material (beta-2 microglobulin amyloid); and identify infectious agents (e.g., cytomegalovirus and herpes simplex virus). More detailed technical information can be found in *Modern Immunohistochemistry* by Chu and Weiss.

This chapter focuses only on those tumor biomarkers that can be detected with simple IHC analysis and discusses the markers' implications in predicting and guiding treatment.

Assessing The Expression of ER, PR, And Her2/Neu In Breast Carcinoma

IHC analysis is a well-accepted routine initial assessment for stratifying subgroups of breast cancer patients and guiding clinical therapy. There is a relatively high concordance (75% to 90%) between molecular subtypes as defined by genomic methods and IHC phenotype.[23] ER and PR expressions are weak prognostic factors but excellent predictive factors that are seen in 70% to 80% of breast cancers. Weak expression in only 1% to 10% of tumor cells can still predict response to hormonal therapy. The response to hormonal therapy is highest in patients with tumors that are ER positive/PR positive; response rates in patients with ER negative/PR positive, ER positive/PR negative, and ER negative/PR negative cancers are sequentially lower. *HER2/neu* oncogene overexpression is present in approximately 20% of all breast carcinomas and is associated with a worse clinical outcome,[24] but carcinomas that overexpress HER2/neu will respond to trastuzumab (Herceptin), a humanized monoclonal antibody directed against cells overexpressing HER2/neu.[25,26] Given the prognostic and predictive nature of HER2/neu status, there are established guidelines for standardized testing and reporting.[27] IHC analysis results for ER, PR, HER2/neu, and Ki-67 can also define triple-negative breast carcinomas as a reasonable surrogate for basal-like molecular class and can directly identify HER2/neu positive cancers. Recently, an international panel of experts proposed that patients with breast cancer be further subgrouped based on IHC analysis results correlating to four therapeutic and prognostic risk factors: (a) triple-negative breast cancer, defined as the lack of immunoreactivities to antibodies of ER and HER2/neu and/or detection of HER2/neu by FISH[22]; (b) HER2/neu positive breast cancer (either ER positive or ER negative), as determined by HER2/neu IHC analysis or FISH; and (c) ER positive/HER2/neu-negative breast cancer. The panel suggested that the last subgroup be further divided into low risk/low proliferation and high risk/high proliferation groups on the basis of semi-quantified immunoreactivity to Ki-67. The most suggested thresholds for percentages of immunoreactive cells ranged between 13% and 17%.[28] IHC testing for HER2/neu should not be done when assay requirements, such as fixative type, are not met. Studies also indicate that negative IHC analysis results on archived material should be interpreted with caution because the negative result may be associated with prolonged fixation or storage considerations. The current approved fixation time is 6 to 48 hours.[29] Several reports have verified that false-positive results are a problem in testing for HER2 status by IHC analysis.[30] The gold standard method for identifying these false-positive results is testing for *HER2/neu* gene amplification by FISH, which is covered later in the chapter.

IHC Staining For MSI Status In CRC

About 15% of CRCs arise through the (microsatellite DNA sequence instability) MSI pathway, and most of these tumors (12%) are sporadic.[31,32] The other ~3% of CRCs that arise via the MSI pathway are inherited as the result of a germline mutation in one mismatch repair (MMR) gene (e.g., *hMLH1*, *hMSH2*, or *MSH6*); these genes are responsible for Lynch syndrome (also known as hereditary nonpolyposis colorectal cancer [HNPCC]).[33-35] MMR deficiency, identified as either the loss of MMR protein expression (e.g., absence of either hMLH1 or hMSH2 by IHC analysis) or the presence of a high degree of MSI as assessed by PCR, has been associated with better outcome in resected colon cancer.[33,36] MSI screening tests by either PCR or IHC analysis are useful in determining the association between sporadic CRCs (15% of which are MSI positive) and hereditary HNPCCs (95% of which are MSI positive). The current suggested algorithm[37] is to detect MSI status by PCR testing with a panel of two mononucleotide repeats (BAT25 and BAT26) and three dinucleotide repeats (D5S346, D2S123, and D17S250). Nineteen "alternative loci" are also available. When analyzing the five-focus panel, microsatellite instability–high (MSI-H) (at least two foci are positive), microsatellite instability–low (MSI-L) (one focus is positive), or microsatellite instability–stable (MSI-S) (all foci are negative) is defined on the basis of the numbers of mutations detected relative to the number of foci. A patient found to have MSI-H by PCR testing will be tested further for *BRAF* mutation status by sequencing and/or IHC analysis to determine the expression of individual MSI repair enzymes. A panel of four individual antibodies (hMLH1, hMSH2, MSH6, and PMS2) is currently used in the IHC test. Since hMLH1 recruits its binding partner PMS2 to the site of DNA repair, when normal expression of hMLH1 is lost, PMS2 will be subsequently lost, whereas hMSH2 and MSH6 may still be preserved. The same interaction is true for hMSH2 and its binding partner MSH6. However, there are rare cases (1% to 2%) of germline mutation of either PMS2 or MSH6 in which only the affected protein is lost. In recent studies[38] based on the heterodimer pairing properties of MMR proteins, a two-antibody panel of PMS2 and MSH6 has been shown to be as effective as the four-antibody panel in detecting DNA MMR protein abnormalities. Suggested interpretations are as follows: (a) when proteins are lost in the hMLH1/PMS2 pair, further molecular testing should be performed to determine whether the hMLH1 loss is due to DNA hypermethylation (in sporadic cases) or *BRAF* mutation by sequencing (in 40% to 50% of cases), with further testing done by sequencing, which can occur simultaneously or individually in sporadic cases and (b) if proteins are lost in pairs of hMSH2/MSH6 or if individual protein loss of PMS2 or MSH6 occurs, the result will be highly suggestive of germline mutation, which requires further confirmation by genetic counseling and testing. However, IHC analysis has its limitations. IHC analysis can be used to determine the presence of MSI proteins, but it cannot determine whether the protein is functional or not. IHC analysis needs to be combined with other molecular tests (e.g., sequencing of the *BRAF* gene and PCR testing of *hMLH1* promoter methylation status), as is the current practice in determining if a CRC is derived from a genetic mutation of the chromosomal instability pathway or is sporadic due to loss of hMLH1 protein by CpG island methylator phenotype pathways or *BRAF* mutation. Small-scale studies have suggested that the expression of many other molecular biomarker candidates may predict a high likelihood of long-term favorable survival; therefore, their application as molecular biomarkers in the clinical setting needs to be verified. For example, phosphatase and tensin homolog (PTEN)[39] may be active/present in one-third of CRCs bearing activating somatic mutations in PIK3CA, which encodes the catalytic subunit of phosphatidylinositol 3-kinase (PI3K). This catalytic subunit is activated by being recruited to the cytoplasmic aspect of moieties such as EGFR and insulin-like growth factor receptor, leading to downstream activation of the protein kinase AKT via phosphorylation by adenosine-5′-triphosphate and the accompanying loss of PTEN (an inhibitor of PIK3 signaling).[39] Detection of PTEN expression in both endometrial carcinomas and CRCs indicates a favorable survival and better prognosis.[40,41] This correlation will guarantee a postoperative chemotherapy if being verified, since patients with PTEN-positive advanced endometrial cancer had a longer survival than those with PTEN-negative cancer.[42] Another example that can be tested by IHC analysis is thymidylate synthase (TS). TS is an essential enzyme needed for DNA synthesis in the S phase of the cell cycle and is the target enzyme of 5-fluorouracil, an important chemotherapeutic agent used in the treatment of CRC.[43] The clinical importance of the TS protein has been suggested by studies demonstrating that intrinsic levels of TS correlate with resistance markers of chemosensitivity,[44-49] although more studies are needed to confirm its efficacy in clinical applications.

FLUORESCENCE IN SITU HYBRIDIZATION

When initially described in 1969, FISH was performed on intact cytologic material using radiolabeled probes.[50] The development of fluorescent labeling of nucleic acid probes allows investigators now to avoid using radioactive materials; rather, they can directly analyze the hybridization results by fluorescent microscopy. Simultaneous analysis of multiple chromosomal regions was also made possible by using different probes. For many years, FISH has been a powerful research tool for investigating chromosomal aberrations in intact cells, valued especially for its application to cells in any phase of the cell cycle, unlike traditional metaphase cytogenetic techniques. In the last several years, FISH analysis has been increasingly used in diagnostic pathology and is important in determining tumor prognostic and predictive markers. FISH can be used to detect a wide variety of genomic alterations that are important in diagnostic and prognostic pathology, including locus amplification, gains and losses of either entire chromosomes or specific chromosomal regions, and chromosomal translocations. FISH can also be used in a variety of tissues, including fresh/frozen tissue, FFPE samples, and cytologic specimens. The fluorescence-tagged probes bind to chromosome-specific DNA sequences of interest, allowing for the identification of both structural and numeric aberrations that specify malignancy.

Assays for gene amplification employ a probe specific for the targeted gene of interest, often together with a differentially labeled probe of the corresponding centromere. Multiple target gene signals are observed in the setting of amplification and by calculating the ratio of the target gene signals to centromere signals, even low-level amplification can be distinguished from polysomy for the entire chromosome. High levels of gene amplification typically occur in one of two patterns: if the amplified gene is present on small extra-chromosomal segments known as double minutes, FISH will show numerous individual signals; if the gene amplification consists of contiguously arranged gene copies within a single chromosomal region, manifested as a homogeneously stained region on chromosomal banding, FISH will show regions of hybridization so close together that they coalesce into abnormally large linear or globular signals. Rough estimates are made regarding how many signals are contained within the coalescent signals on the basis of their overall size. In both settings, chromosome enumeration probes (CEPs) are often used as references of chromosome numbers, so that polysomies (i.e., gains of the entire chromosome) can be distinguished from true gene amplification. Determining the ratio of HER2/neu to CEP17 is appropriate for identifying the amplifications (ratio of 2.2 [HER2/CEP17] for breast cancer; ratio of 2.0 [HER2/CEP17] for gastroesophageal junction (GEJ) tumors or esophageal carcinomas; and ratio of 4.0 [MYCN/D2Z1] in chromosome 2 for neuroblastoma).

In breast cancer, amplification of the HER2/neu oncogene and overexpression of the protein product is associated with poor prognosis, predicts response to some chemotherapeutic regimens, such as cyclophosphamide–methotrexate–5-fluorouracil hormonal therapy and paclitaxel (Taxol),[51-53] and is the target for trastuzumab (Herceptin) treatment.[25,26] HER2 positivity predicts a response to the anti-HER2 monoclonal antibody Herceptin. Patients with strong HER2 overexpression (IHC 3+) or *HER2* gene amplification benefit most from this therapy.[30,54-56] Additionally, because of the significant risk of cardiotoxicity due to combined doxorubicin (Adriamycin) and Herceptin therapy, testing is adjusted to identify patients with a low probability of response.[57,58] Therefore, a combination of IHC analysis and FISH and/or PCR is critical in determining HER2/neu amplification status. Many studies have shown concordance between IHC and FISH results and there were very few cases (3% to 5%) that showed protein expression without gene amplification by FISH or PCR, indicating that FISH or PCR has a false-negative rate of 5% or less.[59] FISH was found to be highly sensitive (96.5% to 98.0%) and specific (100%)[60,61] unlike IHC methods. It can be used as a confirmatory test in the currently suggested algorithm.[29] The current suggested regimens in HER2/neu FISH tests in breast carcinoma use tumor samples that were initially tested by IHC. Samples with strong HER2/neu overexpression (IHC 3+) indicate eligibility for Herceptin therapy. IHC samples with 2+ staining should be retested with another method, preferably FISH, to confirm the results. Amplification of HER2 detected by FISH indicates eligibility for trastuzumab therapy. The number of cells needed to determine the level of *HER2/neu* gene amplification is between 20 and 100. Sixty nuclei should be counted and an average score taken.

Other techniques to determine HER2 amplification include Southern blotting and chromogenic in situ hybridization (CISH)[62]; PCR can also be used to measure the level of *HER2/neu* gene amplification. However, many of these assays are currently limited to research settings. In Finland, CISH has superseded FISH as the recommended method for determining *HER2* gene amplification; it is performed only in two national reference laboratories by highly trained personnel. Outside Finland, CISH is not recommended for routine diagnostic use.

About 20% of GEJ tumors overexpress HER2/neu.[63] The current role of HER2/neu inhibition as a new treatment option and the testing of HER2/neu by FISH are still in phase III clinical trials. So far, the phase III trials have shown that the addition of Herceptin (trastuzumab) to chemotherapy significantly improves the overall survival without compromising safety in patients with HER2/neu-positive metastatic gastric or GEJ adenocarcinoma. This improvement is mainly the result of the survival advantage conferred to patients with high expression of the HER2/neu protein on IHC or FISH.[64] Their study suggested that HER2/neu status be included in the diagnostic workup of patients presenting with advanced gastric and GEJ cancer.[49] The addition of Herceptin (trastuzumab) to chemotherapy is a new standard treatment for patients with locally advanced and non-resectable, recurrent, or metastatic HER2/neu-positive disease. Confirmatory results from large, multi-institutional studies are needed before definite clinical use can be recommended.

Approximately, 25% of all neuroblastomas have amplification of the *MYCN* oncogene,[65] which is located on chromosome 2 at p24.1.[66] Amplification of the *MYCN* oncogene correlates with an unfavorable prognosis and aggressive disease. In pediatric patients, neuroblastomas are routinely tested for *MYCN* amplification.[67] A similar amplification pattern is encountered in a subset of medulloblastoma, which is the central nervous system counterpart of neuroblastoma. *MYCN* and c-myc amplifications are particularly common in the highly aggressive anaplastic large cell variants. EGFR amplification is often found in combination with monosomy of chromosome 10 or chromosome 10q deletion,[68,69] which helps to distinguish the clinically aggressive and therapeutically refractory small cell variant of glioblastoma from the more biologically favorable and chemotherapeutically responsive look-alike anaplastic oligodendroglioma.

Other genetic tests by FISH include testing for *ALK1* gene rearrangement in non-small-cell lung cancer and testing for specific gene translocations in many soft tissue sarcomas (e.g., EWS-FLI1 in Ewing sarcoma/primitive neuroectodermal tumor, SYT-SSX in synovial sarcoma, and PAX3-FKHR and PAX7-FKHR in alveolar rhabdoid sarcoma). Therefore, FISH plays an important role as an ancillary molecular test in tumor diagnosis, as well as in prediction of tumor prognosis, and helps physicians determine appropriate treatments. In summary, the advantages of FISH in surgical pathology are as follows: (a) FISH can be performed in a wide range of tissue preparations, including fresh/frozen tissue, cytologic preparations, and FFPE samples; (b) there are no requirements related to tumor cell proliferative rate and FISH can be performed on non-dividing (interphase) cells; (c) FISH analysis is quantitative, reproducible, and similar to IHC analysis and the results are archivable; and (d) FISH is very sensitive.

However, the limitations of FISH in surgical pathology are that (a) FISH is unable to determine whether the tested genes are active or silent; (b) FISH is usually performed in a specialty laboratory, such as a cytogenetic laboratory, making it less accessible and more costly; (c) FISH cannot detect small intragenic mutations, deletions, or insertions; (d) signal fading and short half-life commonly occur; (e) artifacts due to aneuploidy or polyploidy may be confused with deletions or amplifications if the results are subtle; and (f) autofluorescence on FFPE tissue may require repeated analysis or render interpretation difficult.

PCR-BASED METHODS FOR MOLECULAR TESTING

Most molecular tests performed in oncologic pathology focus on testing somatic or acquired DNA variations in tumor cells; the results aid in tissue diagnosis and help determine prognostic indicators, identify patients who have increased risks of developing cancer, divide patients into groups likely to respond to different treatment options, and monitor treatment response. PCR has become an important test in molecular biology laboratories. While it has its advantages, such as being quick, reliable, and sensitive, it also has its disadvantages. The basic principles of PCR methodology have been described in molecular biology textbooks.[11] In this chapter, we summarize some of the major PCR-based molecular tests and emphasize their usefulness in determining tumor prognosis.

Example of PCR-Based Tests in Identifying MSI Status in CRC

PCR testing relies on the evaluation of certain foci in the human genome that are known to harbor microsatellites. Given the variability in size of many of the microsatellites from one individual to another, it is necessary to identify the normal (germ line) size of a particular microsatellite in the patient tested. DNA is extracted from both normal and tumor tissue and from FFPE tissue blocks, as discussed earlier. After PCR amplification of the selected microsatellite, the size of the PCR products obtained with normal DNA is compared with the PCR products amplified from tumor tissue. MSI is defined as changes of any length due to either insertion or deletion of repeated units in a microsatellite within a tumor when compared with normal tissue. A panel of microsatellites validated by a National Cancer Institute workshop, commonly referred to as the Bethesda Panel, is considered the reference panel for clinical and research testing.[16] It consists of two mononucleotide repeats (BAT25 and BAT26) and three dinucleotide repeats (D5S346, D2S123, and D17S250). Nineteen "alternative loci" are also provided. This workshop also defined diagnostic criteria for MSH-H (two or more foci), MSI-L (one focus), and MSI-S (normal foci) phenotypes. In 2002, another National Cancer Institute workshop added to these guidelines, recommending the testing of additional mononucleotide markers in tumors with instability at only dinucleotide loci, since mononucleotide markers are more reliable in the identification of MSI-H tumors.[35] The clinical significance of MSI-L and its distinction from MSI-S cancer is not clear. Testing of all tumors, regardless of patient age or family history, is indicated in current practice. To exclude sporadic MSI cases and detect potential cases of Lynch syndrome, tumors may be tested for either MSI by PCR methods or MMR protein deficiency by the IHC method. If MSI-H is suggested by PCR or there is MMR protein loss by IHC analysis, it is then recommended that *BRAF* mutational analysis be conducted. If wild-type *BRAF* is present, *hMLH1* methylation testing should then be conducted to further confirm whether the MMR protein loss is due to hypermethylation at the *hMLH1* promoter region, which is highly suggestive of a sporadic hMLH1 loss. On the other hand, if MMR protein loss detected by IHC analysis is shown as loss in MSH2, MSH6, and/or PMS2, it is probably due to a germline mutation; in that case, genetic counseling is needed.[37] In a rare Lynch syndrome phenotype, although there was MSI and absence of MSH2 expression by immunohistochemistry, no MMR mutation is present.[70] Lynch et al. found a deletion at the 3′-end of the epithelial cell adhesion molecule (*EPCAM*) gene, causing transcription read-through resulting in silencing of MSH2 through hypermethylation of its promoter. The EPCAM deletion is predominantly present in CRC but not in Lynch syndrome–associated endometrial cancer. Therefore, CRC surveillance should be performed in EPCAM mutation carriers.

Deleted in Colorectal Cancer/18q Loss of Heterozygosity in CRC

The deleted in colorectal cancer (*DCC*) gene is a putative tumor suppressor gene that has been suggested to become activated late in colorectal carcinogenesis. The tumor suppressor gene *SMAD4* is also in this region. Loss of heterozygosity (LOH) of *DCC* and *SMAD4* was found in 70% of colorectal adenocarcinomas.[71] The *SMAD4* gene encodes a protein involved in transforming growth factor-β (TGF-β) signaling. TGF-β normally has inhibitory effects on colonic epithelial cells; therefore, the loss of TGF-β function, resulting from the loss of *SMAD4* function, could be important in CRC development.[72,73] Most clinical studies of DCC have examined 18q LOH by PCR amplification of polymorphic microsatellite markers at or near 18q21 and the resulting multiplex PCR amplification of various informative polymorphic microsatellite markers at or near 18q21 by comparing tumor and nontumor tissue. LOH of the *DCC* gene region was determined by the amplification of the cancer repeat markers within the D18S58 and D18S61 loci. Additional markers used included D18S45, D18S838, D18S1099, D18S1407, and D18S70. LOH of the *SMAD4* gene region was initially determined by PCR amplification of the microsatellite cancer repeats D18S474 and D18S1110. In retrospective studies, 18q LOH was found to be predictive of shortened survival after adjustment for all other evaluated factors, including tumor differentiation, vascular invasion, and yTNM stage. These studies remain controversial because in stage II disease, 18q LOH has been found to predict shortened disease-free survival and overall survival in some studies[6,74] but not in others.[75-77] MSI occurs prior to the histologic change from adenoma to carcinoma, whereas LOH of this region is frequently a late event in the neoplastic process. Large-scale and/or multi-institutional studies are needed to validate whether DCC or other tumor suppressors can serve as predictors of adverse outcome in stage II disease. If so, detection of DCC loss by PCR may be used in the future to identify patients for whom adjuvant chemotherapy is indicated.

Advantages of using PCR-based tests include (a) the variety of specimens, including fresh/frozen tissue, FFPE tissue, and cytologic specimens that can be used; (b) the relatively small amount of tissue, e.g., 20 to 200 μg of DNA (from 10^3 to 10^4 cells) required; (c) the tests' simplicity, rapidity, and low cost; (d) the tests' high sensitivity and specificity; (e) the fact that PCR products can be easily labeled with chemical fluorophore in order for detection; and (f) the fact that phenotype–genotype correlations are possible by using microdissection of individual tumor cells or single-cell-based PCR. More precise phenotypic–genotypic analysis is achieved by collecting individual cells by LCM, flow cytometry, or immunomagnetic methods. In situ PCR performed on histologic tissue sections is perhaps the best method for morphologically localizing genotypic expression.

A disadvantage of using PCR-based tests is that testing only provides information on the targeted gene or messenger RNA (mRNA) segment amplified by specific primers. Moreover, some DNA templates are preferentially amplified versus other templates within the same reaction, a phenomenon known as PCR bias. PCR bias can be caused by changes/errors in template length, template number, or the template sequence itself as small as a single-base substitution and random variations in PCR efficiency with each cycle. PCR bias can cause 10-fold to 30-fold differences in amplification efficiency in some settings, differences that can influence quantitative PCR test results and LOH analysis. PCR bias can be particularly troublesome in multiplex PCR. Another disadvantage is that non-specific PCR inhibitors of PCR, including heparin, and uncharacterized components, are sometimes present in a patient's sample of cerebrospinal fluid, urine, or sputum. When FFPE tissues are used, degradation of DNA and mRNA that occurred prior to or during fixation may cause further nucleic acid degradation that compromises the sensitivity and specificity of the PCR, making it necessary to amplify a shorter sequence or use nested PCR, which may in turn increase the risk of contamination.

LOCUS-SPECIFIC DNA SEQUENCING VERSUS HIGH-THROUGHPUT DNA SEQUENCING

Site- and locus-specific DNA sequencing are PCR-based methods that are routinely used in most molecular diagnostic laboratories for detecting many of the known gene mutations; for example, frequent or hot spot mutations in the oncogenes *KRAS*, *BRAF*, or *EGFR* in CRC,[78,79] lung cancer,[80,81] melanoma,[81] and glioblastoma.[82] DNA extraction from FFPE primary and metastatic cancer tissue was described in the beginning of this chapter. Gene- or locus-specific exon fragments are/can be amplified by PCR and then DNA sequencing methods are performed. Dideoxynucleotide chain termination DNA sequencing (also known as Sanger sequencing)[63] is the traditional and, until recently, the most commonly used sequencing method; however, it may not detect a minority of mutant sequences present in a background of abundant wild-type DNA sequences. Solid tumors are heterogeneous tissues that contain tumor cells admixed with non-neoplastic cells, including inflammatory cells, vascular endothelial cells, and mesenchymal cells. Detection of gain-of-function mutations in oncogenes such as *KRAS* poses a particular challenge. Not only does each non-neoplastic cell in the tumor tissue contribute two wild-type alleles, but each tumor cell may also carry one copy of its own wild-type allele. A massively parallel sequencing-by-synthesis approach known as "pyrosequencing" provides a new alternative to Sanger sequencing. This approach relies on emulsion PCR–based clonal amplification of a DNA library adapted onto micron-sized beads and subsequent pyrosequencing-by-synthesis[83] of each clonally amplified template in a picotiter plate; this pyrosequencing enables the detection of low-abundance oncogene mutations in complex samples with low tumor content that conventional Sanger sequencing is not able to detect. Highly parallel sequencing approaches could make it feasible to monitor the molecular composition and evolution of tumor subtypes even in cases of low or impure tumor content without the need for laborious tumor cell enrichment methods.

Pyrosequencing is the leading technique in overcoming the limitations of traditional sequencing. It is real-time, non-electrophoretic, nucleotide extension sequencing for various applications.[84,85] In pyrosequencing, pyrophosphate is generated only when a dispensed nucleotide anneals to the template and a primer is extended by DNA polymerase. Subsequently, pyrophosphate is converted to fluorescence emission, the intensity of which is proportional to the amounts of annealed and extended nucleotide molecules. The pyrosequencing assay for single-nucleotide polymorphisms can quantify the relative amount of each allele very accurately. The assay can also be applied to quantitative CpG island methylation analysis.[86,87]

The advantages of pyrosequencing are as follows: (a) it works effectively on paraffin-embedded archival tumor tissue and DNA samples after whole genome amplification (genomic DNA is amplified by PCR using primers consisting of random sequences of 15 nucleotides); (b) it has high analytical sensitivity, even in tumors with abundant inflammatory cells, as seen in CRCs with MSI, desmoplastic pancreatic cancers with cellular and abundant stroma, or previously treated tumors with only scant remaining neoplastic cells; (c) it is a simple, robust, and high-throughput mutation detection assay that can be applied to large epidemiologic studies and clinical trials; (d) it accurately quantifies the amount of each allele; and (e) it can read a nucleotide sequence starting from the first nucleotide next to a pyrosequencing primer, so one can design relatively small PCR products. Designing smaller PCR products is especially useful for degraded DNA samples, particularly DNA derived from paraffin-embedded tissue, in which the DNA is typically fragmented into short pieces. Also, dideoxy sequencing requires purification of PCR products. There is no need for a separate purification step with pyrosequencing after PCR products are obtained. Finally, pyrosequencing is more cost effective than dideoxy sequencing in terms of both reagents and labor time.

EXAMPLES OF USING PYROSEQUENCING IN CRC

Detection of KRAS Mutation by Pyrosequencing of CRC

The Ras family (HRAS, KRAS, and NRAS) are guanosine triphosphate (GTP)–binding proteins involved in activating signal transduction. The *KRAS* homolog is one of the most prevalent human oncogenes; 17% to 25% of all tumors harbor activating *KRAS* mutations.[88] Most of these are point missense mutations of codons 12, 13, and 61 of exon 2 (rarely, mutations at codons 59, 63, and 146). These mutations result in a persistently activated GTP-bound state due to impaired intrinsic GTPase activity.[88] Activating mutations of *KRAS* are found in 30% to 40% of CRCs and lead to increased cell proliferation via the mitogen-activated protein kinase pathway. These mutations are rarely found in very early adenomas and are thought to be acquired during the intermediate phase of oncogenesis. EGFR acts via the same downstream pathways with similar downstream mitogenic effects. Molecular profiling studies indicate that activating mutations of *EGFR, KRAS, PI3CA, and BRAF* possess activating KRAS mutations that can bypass EGFR control. It is apparent that patients with KRAS-mutated tumors will not benefit from anti-EGFR therapies. The American Society of Clinical Oncology guidelines published in 2009 do not recommend anti-EGFR therapy for patients with KRAS-mutated metastatic CRC.[8] In addition, not all patients with wild-type *KRAS* will respond to EGFR inhibitors. More biomarkers are needed to better distinguish responders from non-responders based on targeted therapy information. Since most *KRAS* mutations are located in discrete regions of the gene, pyrosequencing is commonly used in clinical testing. A commercially available KRAS PCR kit (DxS/Qiagen) enables the detection of seven major mutations in *KRAS* codons 12 and 13. Some modified amplification methods for detecting *KRAS* mutations (e.g., the amplification refractory mutation system Scorpion assay[89] reportedly have increased sensitivity) result in higher quality KRAS testing and provide improved power to determine the efficacy of anti-EGFR antibodies.[89]

BRAF Mutation Testing in CRC and Melanoma

The mutation frequency of the *BRAF* oncogene has varied widely between tumor types; for example, mutations in the *BRAF* oncogene have been documented at a high frequency in cutaneous melanomas, occurring in up to 60% of cell lines and tumor samples[90,91] and in about 10% of CRCs. The most common mutation is the thymine-to-adenosine switch at nucleotide position 1799 in exon 15,[91] causing a V600E mutation[92] in both cancers. This is therapeutically relevant in patients with melanoma whose tumors harbor *BRAF* mutations and who might be more likely than others who do not carry *BRAF* mutation to respond to targeted therapies such as MEK inhibitors. This is not true, however, in the CRC mutation of *BRAF*. The resulting structural change mimics phosphorylated *BRAF* and has an elevated basal kinase activity substantially higher than that for wild-type *BRAF*, causing constitutive activation of downstream signaling in the Ras-Raf-MEK-extracellular ligand-regulated kinase pathway, which can lead to malignant transformation.[93]

In CRC, *KRAS* mutations occur in 30% to 51% of cases[94-96] and are inversely associated with *BRAF* mutations, suggesting that their involvement in cancer progression can independently induce similar cellular effects via the same pathway. BRAF is a cytosolic protein kinase and is activated by membrane-bound RAS. Mutated BRAF activates a signaling cascade involving proteins in the mitogen-activated protein kinase system, resulting in cell proliferation[97] and predisposition to inhibition of apoptosis, thus increasing invasiveness[98] and occurs earlier than wild-type patients during colorectal carcinogenesis.[99] The *BRAF* V600E mutation is mutually exclusive with *KRAS* mutations and is significantly associated with MSI, resulting from aberrant methylation of the MLH1 promoter,[100] but it also rarely occurs in patients with HNPCC.[101,102] Therefore, BRAF mutational analysis can be used to categorize MSI-H tumors of patients as germ line or sporadic in origin. Mutations are also located in exon 11 (codon 468) in addition to exon 15 (primarily in codon 600, but also rarely in codon 596). As most mutations are located in specific regions, pyrosequencing is an ideal technique for analysis.

PIK3CA Constitutive Activation in CRC

The PI3K/AKT pathway has been hypothesized to play an important role in the development of a number of human cancers, including CRC.[103] The *PIK3CA* gene encodes the p110 alpha catalytic subunit of PI3K.[104] The most activating somatic mutation of the *PIK3CA* gene in CRC [105] was frequently located in exons 9 and 20.[105] Mutation in *PIK3CA* led to constitutive activation of the AKT pathway, driving cell proliferation.[106] *PIK3CA* mutations have been found in association with 10% to 30% of CRC cases.[105,107-110]

The prognostic value of *PIK3CA* mutations was analyzed by Ogino et al.[109] using archived FFPE samples curatively resected from 450 patients with CRC. *PIK3CA* mutations were identified in 18% of specimens. In a multivariate analysis adjusting for standard risk factors, patients with PIK3CA-mutated tumors had an increased colon cancer–specific mortality compared with patients with PIK3CA wild-type tumors. When stratified by KRAS status, the higher CRC-specific mortality rate associated with the *PIK3CA* mutation was found to be confined to patients with *KRAS* wild-type tumors, but it is not evident among patients with mutated KRAS. *PIK3CA* mutations have also been reported to be an independent risk factor for local recurrence in patients with early- and late-stage colon cancer who undergo curative resection and who do not receive neoadjuvant therapy. Studies also suggest that *PIK3CA* exon 20 mutation was associated with a lack of response to cetuximab in patients with KRAS wild-type tumors.[111]

PTEN in CRC

PTEN is a key component of the PI3K/AKT pathway, and loss of PTEN is thought to constitutively activate the AKT pathway, leading to tumorigenesis.[39] PTEN activity can be lost by several mechanisms, including mutations, deletions, and promoter methylation in various cancers.[112,113] The significance of loss/inactivation of PTEN in CRC is still under investigation. In a retrospective analysis of archived FFPE tissues from 173 patients with metastatic CRC, loss of PTEN expression as detected by IHC analysis was associated with worse overall survival in a multivariate analysis.[114] In a separate report by Loupakis et al.,[115] archived tissues from 103 patients were retrospectively analyzed for a number of biomarkers, including PTEN. PTEN was detected in 58% of primary tumor samples and 60% of metastatic tumor samples. With a concordance of about 60%, PTEN expression/loss was not found to be an independent predictor of patient by IHC study survival during the follow-up period. Interestingly, retained PTEN expression in metatastatic samples was predictive of response to cetuximab, whereas this was not found for retained PTEN expression in primary tumor tissue. Large confirmatory studies are needed to further characterize the significant tumor predictive value of PTEN in CRC.

DNA MICROARRAY

DNA microarray analysis has been applied mainly in basic research settings, but it is developing so rapidly that it will probably soon be applied in molecular diagnostic pathology laboratories and surgical pathology. A DNA microarray is a cDNA array that consists of tens of thousands of oligonucleotides of known sequences aligned in rows on a solid surface (usually a glass slide). A typical cDNA array is printed onto a 30 mm by 15 mm glass microscope slide; each spot is about 50 to 150 μm in diameter. Arrays of short oligonucleotides (about 25 bp) made by photolithography in situ are also available commercially and are the basis of GeneChip technology (Affymetrix). Arrays of longer oligonucleotides (50 to 70 bp) can also be made. These longer oligonucleotide arrays have the advantage of not requiring PCR amplification and clone-insert purification before arraying. RNA is extracted from both sample and reference tissues, reverse transcribed into cDNA, and labeled with two fluorescent dyes. Samples of DNA and RNA derived from cells or tissue are hybridized to microarrays to identify targeted molecules by quantifying the levels of expressions. Computerized techniques have made it possible to reveal the complete gene expression profile in any clinical specimen.

In clinical settings, DNA microarray analysis has been used to examine histologically indistinguishable tumors. Molecular subclassification based on their significantly different molecular profiles may account for such tumors' underlying biologic differences, which may explain their different responses to treatment and which may help determine patients' long-term prognoses (e.g., in cases of B-cell lymphoma, thyroid carcinoma, leukemia, breast carcinoma, CRC, urinary bladder carcinoma, osteosarcoma, and lung carcinoma).[116-124] Gene microarray analyses of morphologically similar large B-cell lymphomas showed that there are two subtypes, which have different molecular profiles of gene expression.[122] Other studies demonstrated new gene targets that may be responsible for the amplification of tumor DNA.[124] Recently, Wang et al.[120] identified a promising predictor of outcome in patients with stage II CRC using a 23-gene signature derived from microarray gene expression data and classification methods. Anticancer drug resistance is thought to arise through numerous mechanisms, and microarrays offer a new approach to studying the cellular pathways implicated in these mechanisms and in predicting drug sensitivity and side effects.[125,126] DNA microarray analyses may also help when confronted with a metastatic tumor from an unknown primary: on the basis of typical multigene expression profile of each solid tumor, a definitive diagnosis may be possible.[127,128] Although cancers of unknown primary origin can be classified by their expression signature, they may harbor genetic traits distinct from tumors of known primaries. Such distinctive/distinguishing traits should be sought. Nevertheless, molecularly classified primary site–directed therapy may not yield a response to therapy or improve outcome, as noted by Pentheroudakis et al.[128]

Despite the enormous potential of DNA microarray technology, there are several possible barriers to applying it in the clinical pathology setting: (1) DNA microarray relies on the preservation of mRNA from the tissue of interest. However, standard FFPE tissue samples from surgical resections and biopsies are not ideal for microarray experiments. Formalin fixation leads to degradation of RNA. In addition, RNA hydrolysis and fragmentation occur at the high temperature required for paraffin embedding. In contrast, freshly frozen specimens are required for DNA microarray experiments; (2) DNA microarray requires a large quantity of RNA from tumor and normal controls. At least 5 to 15 μg of RNA is needed from tissue for oligonucleotide arrays; up to 100 μg of RNA may be needed for cDNA arrays. Therefore, amplification of RNAs obtained from fine-needle biopsies and from samples obtained after LCM is often needed. Additional verification steps are required prior to or after each amplification step using primers specific for proximal and distal exons of, for example, ubiquitous elongation factors. This makes the procedure very tedious and labor intensive; (3) As in basic research, in clinical settings some genes may be regulated at the translational rather than transcriptional level, which would preclude their detection by a DNA microarray. Moreover, proteins rather than DNA carry out most cellular functions, and the mRNA level has been known not to correlate well with the level of its protein products. A direct measurement of protein levels and activity within the tissue would be the best determinant of overall cell function (except perhaps for some transcription regulatory factors). Other choices include the use of cDNA microarrays and proteomic analysis; (4) Post-DNA microarray validation is a critical step because of patient variability and genetic heterogeneity. The validation analysis includes Northern blot analysis, semi-quantitative RT-PCR, and RNA in situ hybridization. RT-PCR is commonly used initially and can be applied in many samples simultaneously. The drawback is that RT-PCR is only a semi-quantitative method. Modified RT-PCR tests with increased quantitative abilities provide accurate and reproducible information on RNA copy number. RNA in situ hybridization and Northern blot analysis are often used together with RT-PCR for validation; (5) Finally, one of the current limiting factors for the routine use of DNA microarray analysis in the clinical setting is its high cost compared with other immunohistologic techniques. (6) Moreover, microarray technology and a microarray platform are not yet readily available to all pathologists. In addition, the complexity of the large data set that results from microarray analysis requires collaboration with bioinformatics specialists who can perform appropriate statistical analyses.

REFERENCES

1. Lilja H, Ulmert D, Björk T, et al. Long-term prediction of prostate cancer up to 25 years before diagnosis of prostate cancer using prostate kallikreins measured at age 44 to 50 years. *J Clin Oncol.* 2007;25(4):431-436.
2. Wang X, Yu J, Sreekumar A, et al. Autoantibody signatures in prostate cancer. *N Engl J Med.* 2005;353(12):1224-1235.
3. Sanchini MA, Gunelli R, Nanni O, et al. Relevance of urine telomerase in the diagnosis of bladder cancer. *JAMA.* 2005;294(16):2052-2056.
4. Cristofanilli M, Budd GT, Ellis MJ, et al. Circulating tumor cells, disease progression, and survival in metastatic breast cancer. *N Engl J Med.* 2004;351(8):781-791.
5. Paik S, Shak S, Tang G, et al. A multigene assay to predict recurrence of tamoxifen-treated, node-negative breast cancer. *N Engl J Med.* 2004;351(27):2817-2826.
6. Watanabe T, Wu TT, Catalano PJ, et al. Molecular predictors of survival after adjuvant chemotherapy for colon cancer. *N Engl J Med.* 2001;344(16):1196-1206.

7. Biomarkers Definitions Working Group. Biomarkers and surrogate endpoints: preferred definitions and conceptual framework. *Clin Pharmacol Ther*. 2001;69(3):89-95.
8. Allegra CJ, Jessup JM, Somerfield MR, et al. American Society of Clinical Oncology provisional clinical opinion: testing for *KRAS* gene mutations in patients with metastatic colorectal carcinoma to predict response to anti-epidermal growth factor receptor monoclonal antibody therapy. *J Clin Oncol*. 2009;27(12):2091-2096.
9. Wheeler DL, Dunn EF, Harari PM. Understanding resistance to EGFR inhibitors—impact on future treatment strategies. *Nat Rev Clin Oncol*. 2010;7(9):493-507.
10. Loupakis F, Ruzzo A, Cremolini C, et al. KRAS codon 61, 146 and BRAF mutations predict resistance to cetuximab plus irinotecan in KRAS codon 12 and 13 wild-type metastatic colorectal cancer. *Br J Cancer*. 2009;101(4):715-721.
11. Lodish HF. *Molecular Cell Biology*. 6th ed. New York, NY: W.H. Freeman; 2008.
12. Sabatini DD, Miller F, Barrnett RJ. Aldehyde fixation for morphological and enzyme histochemical studies with the electron microscope. *J Histochem Cytochem*. 1964;12:57-71.
13. Huang WY, Sheehy TM, Moore LE, Hsing AW, Purdue MP. Simultaneous recovery of DNA and RNA from formalin-fixed paraffin-embedded tissue and application in epidemiologic studies. *Cancer Epidemiol Biomarkers Prev*. 2010;19(4):973-977.
14. Berg D, Hipp S, Malinowsky K, Böllner C, Becker KF. Molecular profiling of signalling pathways in formalin-fixed and paraffin-embedded cancer tissues. *Eur J Cancer*. 2010;46(1):47-55.
15. Lewis F, Maughan NJ, Smith V, Hillan K, Quirke P. Unlocking the archive—gene expression in paraffin-embedded tissue. *J Pathol*. 2001;195(1):66-71.
16. Boland CR, Thibodeau SN, Hamilton SR, et al. A National Cancer Institute Workshop on MSI for cancer detection and familial predisposition: development of international criteria for the determination of microsatellite instability in colorectal cancer. *Cancer Res*. 1998;58(22):5248-5257.
17. Vilardell F, Iacobuzio-Donahue, CA. Cancer gene profiling in pancreatic cancer. *Methods Mol Biol*. 2010;576:279-292.
18. Turashvili G, Yang W, McKinney S, et al. Nucleic acid quantity and quality from paraffin blocks: defining optimal fixation, processing and DNA/RNA extraction techniques. *Exp Mol Pathol*. 2011;92(1):33-43.
19. Su JM, Perlaky L, Li XN, et al. Comparison of ethanol versus formalin fixation on preservation of histology and RNA in laser capture microdissected brain tissues. *Brain Pathol*. 2004;14(2):175-182.
20. Carlsson A, Falck B, Hillarp NA, Torp A. Histochemical localization at the cellular level of hypothalamic noradrenaline. *Acta Physiol Scand*. 1962;54:385-386.
21. Buchwalow IB. *Immunohistochemistry: Basics and Methods*. New York, NY: Springer; 2010.
22. Taylor CR, Shi SR, Chaiwun B, Young L, Imam SA, Cote RJ. Strategies for improving the immunohistochemical staining of various intranuclear prognostic markers in formalin–paraffin sections: androgen receptor, estrogen receptor, progesterone receptor, p53 protein, proliferating cell nuclear antigen, and Ki-67 antigen revealed by antigen retrieval techniques. *Hum Pathol*. 1994;25(3):263-270.
23. Kaufmann M, Pusztai L. Use of standard markers and incorporation of molecular markers into breast cancer therapy: consensus recommendations from an International Expert Panel. *Cancer*. 2011;117(8):1575-1582.
24. Wolff AC, Hammond ME, Schwartz JN, et al. American Society of Clinical Oncology/College of American Pathologists guideline recommendations for human epidermal growth factor receptor 2 testing in breast cancer. *J Clin Oncol*. 2007;25(1):118-145.
25. Di Fiore PP, Pierce JH, Kraus MH, Segatto O, King CR, Aaronson SA. erbB-2 is a potent oncogene when overexpressed in NIH/3T3 cells. *Science*. 1987;237(4811):178-182.
26. Slamon DJ, Clark GM, Wong SG, Levin WJ, Ullrich A, McGuire WL. Human breast cancer: correlation of relapse and survival with amplification of the HER-2/neu oncogene. *Science*. 1987;235(4785):177-182.
27. Mrozkowiak A, Olszewski WP, Piaścik A, Olszewski WT. HER2 status in breast cancer determined by IHC and FISH: comparison of the results. *Pol J Pathol*. 2004;55(4):165-171.
28. Feitosa AC, Ayub B, Caramelli B, et al. [I Guideline of the perioperative evaluation]. *Arq Bras Cardiol*. 2007;88(5):e139-e178.
29. Bilous M, Dowsett M, Hanna W, et al. Current perspectives on HER2 testing: a review of national testing guidelines. *Mod Pathol*. 2003;16(2):173-182.
30. Ridolfi RL, Jamehdor MR, Arber JM. HER-2/neu testing in breast carcinoma: a combined immunohistochemical and fluorescence in situ hybridization approach. *Mod Pathol*. 2000;13(8):866-873.
31. Jenkins MA, Hayashi S, O'Shea AM, et al. Pathology features in Bethesda guidelines predict colorectal cancer microsatellite instability: a population-based study. *Gastroenterology*. 2007;133(1):48-56.
32. Kim H, Jen J, Vogelstein B, Hamilton SR. Clinical and pathological characteristics of sporadic colorectal carcinomas with DNA replication errors in microsatellite sequences. *Am J Pathol*. 1994;145(1):148-156.
33. Marcus VA, Madlensky L, Gryfe R, et al. Immunohistochemistry for hMLH1 and hMSH2: a practical test for DNA mismatch repair-deficient tumors. *Am J Surg Pathol*. 1999;23(10):1248-1255.
34. Abdel-Rahman WM, Mecklin JP, Peltomaki P. The genetics of HNPCC: application to diagnosis and screening. *Crit Rev Oncol Hematol*. 2006;58(3):208-220.
35. Umar A, Boland CR, Terdiman JP, et al. Revised Bethesda guidelines for hereditary nonpolyposis colorectal cancer (Lynch syndrome) and microsatellite instability. *J Natl Cancer Inst*. 2004;96(4):261-268.
36. Lindor NM, Burgart LJ, Leontovich O, et al. Immunohistochemistry versus microsatellite instability testing in phenotyping colorectal tumors. *J Clin Oncol*. 2002;20(4):1043-1048.
37. Bedeir A, Krasinskas AM. Molecular diagnostics of colorectal cancer. *Arch Pathol Lab Med*. 2011;135(5):578-587.
38. Hall G, Clarkson A, Shi A, et al. Immunohistochemistry for PMS2 and MSH6 alone can replace a four antibody panel for mismatch repair deficiency screening in colorectal adenocarcinoma. *Pathology*. 2010;42(5):409-413.
39. Stokoe D. PTEN. *Curr Biol*. 2001;11(13):R502.
40. Risinger JI, Hayes K, Maxwell GL, et al. PTEN mutation in endometrial cancers is associated with favorable clinical and pathologic characteristics. *Clin Cancer Res*. 1998;4(12): 3005-3010.
41. Saal LH, Gruvberger-Saal SK, Persson C, et al. Recurrent gross mutations of the *PTEN* tumor suppressor gene in breast cancers with deficient DSB repair. *Nat Genet*. 2008;40(1):102-107.
42. Terakawa N, Kanamori Y, Yoshida S. Loss of PTEN expression followed by Akt phosphorylation is a poor prognostic factor for patients with endometrial cancer. *Endocr Relat Cancer*. 2003;10(2):203-208.
43. Pinedo HM, Peters GF. Fluorouracil: biochemistry and pharmacology. *J Clin Oncol*. 1988;6(10):1653-1664.
44. Lenz HJ, Danenberg KD, Leichman CG, et al. p53 and thymidylate synthase expression in untreated stage II colon cancer: associations with recurrence, survival, and site. *Clin Cancer Res*. 1998;4(5):1227-1234.
45. Allegra CJ, Paik S, Colangelo LH, et al. Prognostic value of thymidylate synthase, Ki-67, and p53 in patients with Dukes' B and C colon cancer: a National Cancer Institute–National Surgical Adjuvant Breast and Bowel Project collaborative study. *J Clin Oncol*. 2003;21(2):241-250.
46. Edler D, Glimelius B, Hallström M, et al. Thymidylate synthase expression in colorectal cancer: a prognostic and predictive marker of benefit from adjuvant fluorouracil-based chemotherapy. *J Clin Oncol*. 2002;20(7):1721-1728.
47. Johnston PG, Fisher ER, Rockette HE, et al. The role of thymidylate synthase expression in prognosis and outcome of adjuvant chemotherapy in patients with rectal cancer. *J Clin Oncol*. 1994;12(12):2640-2647.
48. Popat S, Matakidou A, Houlston RS. Thymidylate synthase expression and prognosis in colorectal cancer: a systematic review and meta-analysis. *J Clin Oncol*. 2004;22(3):529-536.
49. Sakamoto J, Hamashima H, Suzuki H, et al. Thymidylate synthase expression as a predictor of the prognosis of curatively resected colon carcinoma in patients registered in an adjuvant immunochemotherapy clinical trial. *Oncol Rep*. 2003;10(5):1081-1090.

50. Gall JG, Pardue ML. Formation and detection of RNA–DNA hybrid molecules in cytological preparations. *Proc Natl Acad Sci U S A*. 1969;63(2):378-383.
51. Piccart-Gebhart MJ, Procter M, Leyland-Jones B, et al. Trastuzumab after adjuvant chemotherapy in HER2-positive breast cancer. *N Engl J Med*. 2005;353(16):1659-1672.
52. Smith I, Procter M, Gelber RD, et al. 2-year follow-up of trastuzumab after adjuvant chemotherapy in HER2-positive breast cancer: a randomised controlled trial. *Lancet*. 2007;369(9555):29-36.
53. Bartlett JM, Going JJ, Mallon EA, et al. Evaluating HER2 amplification and overexpression in breast cancer. *J Pathol*. 2001;195(4):422-428.
54. Graziano C. HER-2 breast assay, linked to Herceptin, wins FDA's okay. *CAP Today*. 1998;12(10):1, 14-16.
55. Tubbs RR, Pettay JD, Roche PC, Stoler MH, Jenkins RB, Grogan TM. Discrepancies in clinical laboratory testing of eligibility for trastuzumab therapy: apparent immunohistochemical false-positives do not get the message. *J Clin Oncol*. 2001;19(10):2714-2721.
56. Hoang MP, Sahin AA, Ordòñez NG, Sneige N. HER-2/neu gene amplification compared with HER-2/neu protein overexpression and interobserver reproducibility in invasive breast carcinoma. *Am J Clin Pathol*. 2000;113(6):852-859.
57. Ross JS. Update on HER2 testing for breast and upper gastrointestinal tract cancers. *Biomark Med*. 2011;5(3):307-318.
58. Brien TP, Odze RD, Sheehan CE, McKenna BJ, Ross JS. HER-2/neu gene amplification by FISH predicts poor survival in Barrett's esophagus-associated adenocarcinoma. *Hum Pathol*. 2000;31(1):35-39.
59. Jacobs TW, Gown AM, Yaziji H, Barnes MJ, Schnitt SJ. Specificity of HercepTest in determining HER-2/neu status of breast cancers using the United States Food and Drug Administration-approved scoring system. *J Clin Oncol*. 1999;17(7):1983-1987.
60. Pauletti G, Dandekar S, Rong H, et al. Assessment of methods for tissue-based detection of the HER-2/neu alteration in human breast cancer: a direct comparison of fluorescence in situ hybridization and immunohistochemistry. *J Clin Oncol*. 2000;18(21):3651-3664.
61. Press MF, Bernstein L, Thomas PA, et al. HER-2/neu gene amplification characterized by fluorescence in situ hybridization: poor prognosis in node-negative breast carcinomas. *J Clin Oncol*. 1997;15(8):2894-2904.
62. Tanner M, Gancberg D, Di Leo A, et al. Chromogenic in situ hybridization: a practical alternative for fluorescence in situ hybridization to detect HER-2/neu oncogene amplification in archival breast cancer samples. *Am J Pathol*. 2000;157(5):1467-1472.
63. Jorgensen JT. Targeted HER2 treatment in advanced gastric cancer. *Oncology*. 2010;78(1):26-33.
64. Lorenzen S, Lordick F. How will human epidermal growth factor receptor 2-neu data impact clinical management of gastric cancer? *Curr Opin Oncol*. 2011;23(4):396-402.
65. Brodeur GM, Seeger RC, Schwab M, Varmus HE, Bishop JM. Amplification of N-myc in untreated human neuroblastomas correlates with advanced disease stage. *Science*. 1984;224(4653):1121-1124.
66. Hunt JD, Valentine M, Tereba A. Excision of N-myc from chromosome 2 in human neuroblastoma cells containing amplified N-myc sequences. *Mol Cell Biol*. 1990;10(2):823-829.
67. Tonini GP, Boni L, Pession A, et al. MYCN oncogene amplification in neuroblastoma is associated with worse prognosis, except in stage 4s: the Italian experience with 295 children. *J Clin Oncol*. 1997;15(1):85-93.
68. Yadav AK, Renfrow JJ, Scholtens DM, et al. Monosomy of chromosome 10 associated with dysregulation of epidermal growth factor signaling in glioblastomas. *JAMA*. 2009;302(3):276-289.
69. von Deimling A, Louis DN, von Ammon K, et al. Association of epidermal growth factor receptor gene amplification with loss of chromosome 10 in human glioblastoma multiforme. *J Neurosurg*. 1992;77(2):295-301.
70. Lynch HT, Riegert-Johnson DL, Snyder C, et al. Lynch syndrome-associated extracolonic tumors are rare in two extended families with the same EPCAM deletion. *Am J Gastroenterol*. 2011;106(10):1829-1836.
71. Thiagalingam S, Lengauer C, Leach FS, et al. Evaluation of candidate tumour suppressor genes on chromosome 18 in colorectal cancers. *Nat Genet*. 1996;13(3):343-346.
72. Downing JR. TGF-beta signaling, tumor suppression, and acute lymphoblastic leukemia. *N Engl J Med*. 2004;351(6):528-530.
73. Attisano L, Wrana JL. Signal transduction by the TGF-beta superfamily. *Science*. 2002;296(5573):1646-1647.
74. Ogino S, Nosho K, Kirkner GJ, et al. CpG island methylator phenotype, microsatellite instability, BRAF mutation and clinical outcome in colon cancer. *Gut*. 2009;58(1):90-96.
75. Carethers JM, Smith EJ, Behling CA, et al. Use of 5-fluorouracil and survival in patients with microsatellite-unstable colorectal cancer. *Gastroenterology*. 2004;126(2):394-401.
76. Ribic CM, Sargent DJ, Moore MJ, et al. Tumor microsatellite-instability status as a predictor of benefit from fluorouracil-based adjuvant chemotherapy for colon cancer. *N Engl J Med*. 2003;349(3):247-257.
77. Vasen HF, Mecklin JP, Khan PM, Lynch HT. The International Collaborative Group on Hereditary Non-Polyposis Colorectal Cancer (ICG-HNPCC). *Dis Colon Rectum*. 1991;34(5):424-425.
78. Andreyev HJ, Norman AR, Cunningham D, Oates JR, Clarke PA. Kirsten ras mutations in patients with colorectal cancer: the multicenter "RASCAL" study. *J Natl Cancer Inst*. 1998;90(9):675-684.
79. Samowitz WS, Sweeney C, Herrick J, et al. Poor survival associated with the BRAF V600E mutation in microsatellite-stable colon cancers. *Cancer Res*. 2005;65(14):6063-6069.
80. Lynch TJ, Bell DW, Sordella R, et al. Activating mutations in the epidermal growth factor receptor underlying responsiveness of non-small-cell lung cancer to gefitinib. *N Engl J Med*. 2004;350(21):2129-2139.
81. Gray-Schopfer V, Wellbrock C, Marais R. Melanoma biology and new targeted therapy. *Nature*. 2007;445(7130):851-857.
82. Ang C, Guiot MC, Ramanakumar AV, Roberge D, Kavan P. Clinical significance of molecular biomarkers in glioblastoma. *Can J Neurol Sci*. 2010;37(5):625-630.
83. Ronaghi M, Uhlen M, Nyren P. A sequencing method based on real-time pyrophosphate. *Science*. 1998;281(5375):363-365.
84. Fakhrai-Rad H, Pourmand N, Ronaghi M. Pyrosequencing: an accurate detection platform for single nucleotide polymorphisms. *Hum Mutat*. 2002;19(5):479-485.
85. Jordan JA, Butchko AR, Durso MB. Use of pyrosequencing of 16S rRNA fragments to differentiate between bacteria responsible for neonatal sepsis. *J Mol Diagn*. 2005;7(1):105-110.
86. Colella S, Shen L, Baggerly KA, Issa JP, Krahe R. Sensitive and quantitative universal Pyrosequencing methylation analysis of CpG sites. *Biotechniques*. 2003;35(1):146-150.
87. Tost J, Dunker J, Gut IG. Analysis and quantification of multiple methylation variable positions in CpG islands by Pyrosequencing. *Biotechniques*. 2003;35(1):152-156.
88. Plesec TP, Hunt JL. KRAS mutation testing in colorectal cancer. *Adv Anat Pathol*. 2009;16(4):196-203.
89. Bando H, Yoshino T, Tsuchihara K, et al. KRAS mutations detected by the amplification refractory mutation system—Scorpion assays strongly correlate with therapeutic effect of cetuximab. *Br J Cancer*. 2011;105(3):403-406.
90. Brose MS, Volpe P, Feldman M, et al. BRAF and RAS mutations in human lung cancer and melanoma. *Cancer Res*. 2002;62(23):6997-7000.
91. Davies H, Bignell GR, Cox C, et al. Mutations of the *BRAF* gene in human cancer. *Nature*. 2002;417(6892):949-954.
92. Smalley KS, Herlyn M. Loitering with intent: new evidence for the role of BRAF mutations in the proliferation of melanocytic lesions. *J Invest Dermatol*. 2004;123(4):xvi-xvii.
93. Mansour SJ, Matten WT, Hermann AS, et al. Transformation of mammalian cells by constitutively active MAP kinase kinase. *Science*. 1994;265(5174):966-970.
94. Oliveira C, Velho S, Moutinho C, et al. KRAS and BRAF oncogenic mutations in MSS colorectal carcinoma progression. *Oncogene*. 2007;26(1):158-163.
95. Rajagopalan H, Bardelli A, Lengauer C, Kinzler KW, Vogelstein B, Velculescu VE. Tumorigenesis: RAF/RAS oncogenes and mismatch-repair status. *Nature*. 2002;418(6901):934.

96. Schubbert S, Bollag G, Lyubynska N, et al. Biochemical and functional characterization of germ line KRAS mutations. *Mol Cell Biol*. 2007;27(22):7765-7770.
97. Kolch W. Meaningful relationships: the regulation of the Ras/Raf/MEK/ERK pathway by protein interactions. *Biochem J*. 2000;351(Pt 2):289-305.
98. Minoo P, Moyer MP, Jass JR. Role of BRAF-V600E in the serrated pathway of colorectal tumourigenesis. *J Pathol*. 2007;212(2):124-133.
99. Rosenberg DW, Yang S, Pleau DC, et al. Mutations in BRAF and KRAS differentially distinguish serrated versus non-serrated hyperplastic aberrant crypt foci in humans. *Cancer Res*. 2007;67(8):3551-3554.
100. Li WQ, Kawakami K, Ruszkiewicz A, Bennett G, Moore J, Iacopetta B. BRAF mutations are associated with distinctive clinical, pathological and molecular features of colorectal cancer independently of microsatellite instability status. *Mol Cancer*. 2006;5:2.
101. Ogino S, Goel A. Molecular classification and correlates in colorectal cancer. *J Mol Diagn*. 2008;10(1):13-27.
102. Vasen HF, Möslein G, Alonso A, et al. Guidelines for the clinical management of Lynch syndrome (hereditary non-polyposis cancer). *J Med Genet*. 2007;44(6):353-362.
103. Manning BD, Cantley LC. AKT/PKB signaling: navigating downstream. *Cell*. 2007;129(7):1261-1274.
104. Engelman JA, Luo J, Cantley LC. The evolution of phosphatidylinositol 3-kinases as regulators of growth and metabolism. *Nat Rev Genet*. 2006;7(8):606-619.
105. Samuels Y, Wang Z, Bardelli A, et al. High frequency of mutations of the PIK3CA gene in human cancers. *Science*. 2004;304(5670):554.
106. Samuels Y, Velculescu VE. Oncogenic mutations of PIK3CA in human cancers. *Cell Cycle*. 2004;3(10):1221-1224.
107. Kato S, Iida S, Higuchi T, et al. PIK3CA mutation is predictive of poor survival in patients with colorectal cancer. *Int J Cancer*. 2007;121(8):1771-1778.
108. Nosho K, Kawasaki T, Ohnishi M, et al. PIK3CA mutation in colorectal cancer: relationship with genetic and epigenetic alterations. *Neoplasia*. 2008;10(6):534-541.
109. Ogino S, Nosho K, Kirkner GJ, et al. PIK3CA mutation is associated with poor prognosis among patients with curatively resected colon cancer. *J Clin Oncol*. 2009;27(9):1477-1484.
110. Velho S, Oliveira C, Ferreira A, et al. The prevalence of PIK3CA mutations in gastric and colon cancer. *Eur J Cancer*. 2005;41(11):1649-1654.
111. De Roock W, Claes B, Bernasconi D, et al. Effects of KRAS, BRAF, NRAS, and PIK3CA mutations on the efficacy of cetuximab plus chemotherapy in chemotherapy-refractory metastatic colorectal cancer: a retrospective consortium analysis. *Lancet Oncol*. 2010;11(8):753-762.
112. Parsons DW, Wang TL, Samuels Y, et al. Colorectal cancer: mutations in a signalling pathway. *Nature*. 2005;436(7052):792.
113. Vivanco I, Sawyers CL. The phosphatidylinositol 3-kinase AKT pathway in human cancer. *Nat Rev Cancer*. 2002;2(7):489-501.
114. Laurent-Puig P, Cayre A, Manceau G, et al. Analysis of PTEN, BRAF, and EGFR status in determining benefit from cetuximab therapy in wild-type KRAS metastatic colon cancer. *J Clin Oncol*. 2009;27(35):5924-5930.
115. Loupakis F, Pollina L, Stasi I, et al. PTEN expression and KRAS mutations on primary tumors and metastases in the prediction of benefit from cetuximab plus irinotecan for patients with metastatic colorectal cancer. *J Clin Oncol*. 2009;27(16):2622-2629.
116. Dyrskjot L, Kruhøffer M, Thykjaer T, et al. Gene expression in the urinary bladder: a common carcinoma in situ gene expression signature exists disregarding histopathological classification. *Cancer* Res. 2004;64(11):4040-4048.
117. Harris NL, Stein H, Coupland SE, et al. New approaches to lymphoma diagnosis. *Hematol Am Soc Hematol Educ Program*, 2001;2001(1):194-220.
118. Jeffrey SS, Pollack JR. The diagnosis and management of pre-invasive breast disease: promise of new technologies in understanding pre-invasive breast lesions. *Breast Cancer Res*. 2003;5(6):320-328.
119. Leonard P, Sharp T, Henderson S, et al. Gene expression array profile of human osteosarcoma. *Br J Cancer*. 2003;89(12):2284-2288.
120. Wang Y, Jatkoe T, Zhang Y, et al. Gene expression profiles and molecular markers to predict recurrence of Dukes' B colon cancer. *J Clin Oncol*. 2004;22(9):1564-1571.
121. Rice SC, Vacek P, Homans AH, et al. Genotoxicity of therapeutic intervention in children with acute lymphocytic leukemia. *Cancer Res*. 2004;64(13):4464-4471.
122. Alizadeh AA, Eisen MB, Davis RE, et al. Distinct types of diffuse large B-cell lymphoma identified by gene expression profiling. *Nature*. 2000;403(6769):503-511.
123. Parmigiani G, Garrett-Mayer ES, Anbazhagan R, Gabrielson E. A cross-study comparison of gene expression studies for the molecular classification of lung cancer. *Clin Cancer Res*. 2004;10(9):2922-2927.
124. Wreesmann VB, Sieczka EM, Socci ND, et al. Genome-wide profiling of papillary thyroid cancer identifies MUC1 as an independent prognostic marker. *Cancer Res*. 2004;64(11):3780-3789.
125. de Bono JS, Tolcher AW, Rowinsky EK. The future of cytotoxic therapy: selective cytotoxicity based on biology is the key. *Breast Cancer Res*. 2003;5(3):154-159.
126. Shioda T. Application of DNA microarray to toxicological research. *J Environ Pathol Toxicol Oncol*. 2004;23(1):13-31.
127. Wen S, Felley CP, Bouzourene H, Reimers M, Michetti P, Pan-Hammarström Q. Inflammatory gene profiles in gastric mucosa during *Helicobacter pylori* infection in humans. *J Immunol*. 2004;172(4):2595-2606.
128. Pentheroudakis G, Golfinopoulos V, Pavlidis N. Switching benchmarks in cancer of unknown primary: from autopsy to microarray. *Eur J Cancer*. 2007;43(14):2026-2036.

CHAPTER 23

Quality Control, Assurance, and Standardization of Molecular Diagnostics

Matthew J. McGinniss, Ryan P. Bender, and Anatole Ghazalpour

INTRODUCTION

Quality control (QC) and quality assurance (QA) measures are the collective actions taken to ensure that results of clinical testing are accurate and meet all quality requirements. QC can be defined as the specific activities or techniques that are intended to ensure that certain quality requirements are being met.[1] For example, QC results may be used to show that a given clinical instrument is operating within certain predefined limits or standards. QA can be defined as the set of processes that verify or determine if a final product or service meets or exceeds all quality requirements.[1] For example, review of blinded proficiency sample results by an independent agency (e.g., College of American Pathologists [CAP]) is a QA process to ensure that a clinical laboratory is producing accurate and reliable results. In other words, QA can be thought of simply as "QC of the QC." QA monitoring can also be used to help identify errors and adverse trends that could eventually result in errors of analytic testing and that could adversely affect patient safety.

In this chapter, we summarize the current best practices for QC measures and QA practices relevant to molecular oncology laboratories (both solid tumor profiling and hematopathology). QC measures are critical within various levels of analysis including pre-analytic (such as sample collection, shipment, and storage), analytic (measures specific to certain molecular testing platforms or methods), and post-analytic processes (such as interpreting and reporting results).

BACKGROUND

Both anatomic and molecular diagnostic laboratories are at the very heart of diagnosing cancer patients and performing tests that help clinicians decide what may be the best therapeutic choice(s) for a particular cancer patient. These clinical laboratory test results are then used by health-care providers to make diagnostic and therapeutic decisions. As such, we depend on the quality of these results used to make actionable decisions on diagnosis and treatment. For example, the mislabeling rate for specimen, blocks, and slides reported in a recent CAP Q-probe survey of 136 pathology laboratories was on the order of 0.1% to 0.17%.[2] These errors in labeling occurred nearly equally throughout the entire process of accessioning, gross pathology processing, and tissue cutting. Raab and Grzybicki[3] point out that clinical practitioners play a key role in laboratory error reduction by effective test orders, providing accurate clinical histories, providing high-quality specimens, communicating effectively with the laboratory on potentially discrepant diagnoses, and advocating second opinions in certain situations.

Molecular diagnostic testing has increased significantly in the last decade and new molecular tests have been developed in molecular genetics, infectious disease, as well as oncology. New tests are constantly being developed and validated in molecular oncology. The CAP Molecular Pathology Resource Committee has recommended a set of guidelines for validating new clinical molecular tests.[4] However, some have argued that this proliferation of molecular testing has not kept pace with the availability of suitable reference materials, proficiency testing programs, and the establishment of reference methods and standards.[5]

QUALITY CONTROL

Outlined in the following sections are some of the main QC elements central to any molecular diagnostic laboratory. Molecular oncology deals with a vast array of sample types that may have challenges with regard to producing quality results, so it is pertinent to detail the challenges and pitfalls known for the various sample types. Some key QC features for the various testing methodologies (polymerase chain reaction [PCR], fragment analysis, sequencing, and microarray) encountered in a molecular oncology laboratory are also outlined.

Individual Sample

In molecular oncology, the list of various sample types that are presented for molecular testing spans a broad range including blood, bone marrow aspirates, malignant fluids, and solid tumors. In addition, each sample could be presented as they are collected (such as blood samples collected in ethylenediaminetetraacetic acid [EDTA] or heparin tubes or malignant fluids collected in a flask from the pleura or peritoneal cavity), frozen at very low temperatures, or further processed after collection to preserve the integrity of the tumor cells. The latter, which is generally applied to the solid tumors, is often achieved by treating the specimen with formalin, which then could be shipped either by embedding the treated sample in paraffin (also known as formalin-fixed paraffin-embedded or FFPE) or mounting the sample on a glass slide (typically applied to biopsies taken by fine needle aspiration). The wide range of the sample collection methods along with the various methodologies applied to process, preserve, and ship the samples, however, introduces a challenge for molecular biology laboratories to obtain high-integrity nucleic acid from the specimen. In addition, the origin of the tumor can also adversely affect the integrity of the nucleic acids in tumor cells, making it difficult and a less-than-ideal product to use for molecular testing. For example, fibrotic tissue, high calcium content (tumors of bone origin), high melanin content (typical of melanoma samples), and high albumin (typical of blood samples) are known factors that can potentially influence the quality of the nucleic acids at the time of extraction and/or downstream application of commonly used molecular methods such as PCR, restriction digestion, and hybridization-based assays. The dependence of DNA and RNA integrity on various sample collection methods, sample processing methods, and tumor types emphasizes the importance of establishing a vigorous QC system to assess the integrity of the nucleic acids isolated from such a wide range of samples types. Such a QC system must assure and set a series of well-defined parameters that can be measured in the pre-analytic phase and after the extraction of nucleic acids from the specimen to assure the reliability of the results obtained in subsequent molecular testing (Fig. 23.1).

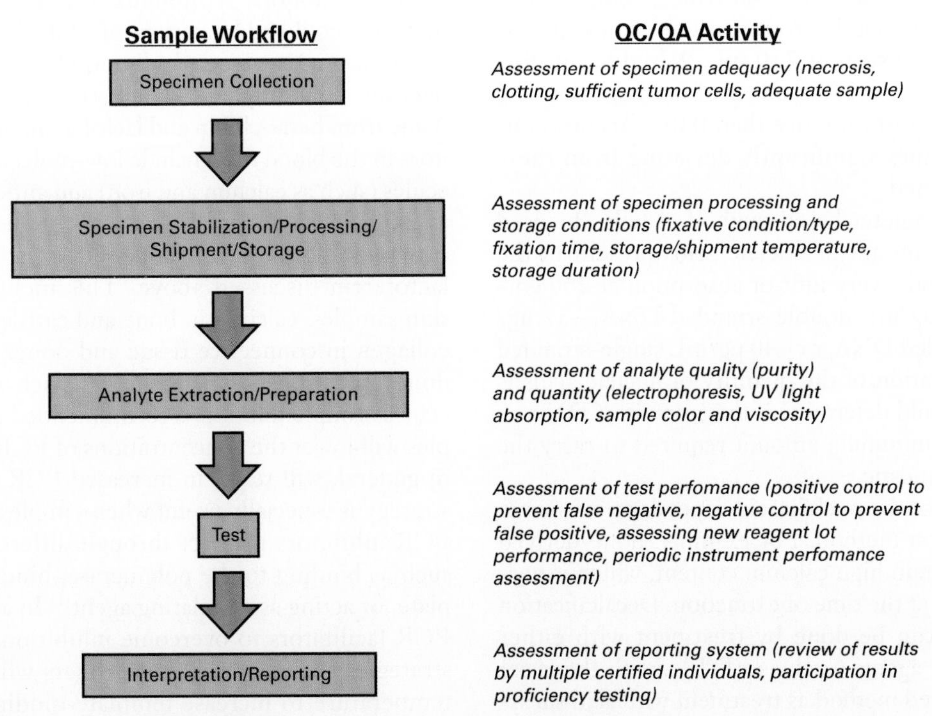

FIGURE 23–1 A molecular oncology workflow for sample processing (left) and the corresponding quality control (QC) activity (right).

Two important QC measures commonly used in molecular oncology are the yield and purity of nucleic acids. This can be done by assessing the amount of nucleic acid degradation as samples that are highly degraded may give false-negative results. A sign of DNA degradation is the presence of abundant low-molecular-weight nucleic acids among the extracted DNA. This can be observed by fractionating the nucleic acids on agarose gels and visualizing the DNA content with ethidium bromide. RNA degradation can be assessed by separating isolated product on the gel, staining the gel, and semiquantitatively measuring the ratio of 18S and 28S ribosomal RNA from the intensity of the bands on the gel. Samples with pure RNA display a 2 to 1 ratio of 28S to 18S ribosomal RNA.

Another QC measure is the purity of nucleic acids after extraction. In general, extraction methods for nucleic acids can cause carryover of other molecules, such as proteins and low-molecular-weight compounds, that can inhibit downstream diagnostic applications especially when they are present at high concentrations. The purity of nucleic acids can be determined by measuring the ratio of UV light absorption. DNA and RNA absorb UV light at the 260-nm peak and the UV light absorption for proteins is at the 280-nm peak. Ratios of 1.8 to 1.9 and 1.9 to 2.0 indicate highly purified preparations of DNA and RNA, respectively. Contaminants that absorb at 280 nm (e.g., protein) will lower this ratio.[6] A ratio below 1.6 indicates the presence of contaminating proteins and as such it may be necessary to repeat the extraction procedure to purify the sample further. UV absorption can also be used to assess the presence of organic solvents and impurity. Absorbance at 325 nm indicates particulates in the solution or dirty cuvettes used to measure the absorbance; contaminants containing peptide bonds or aromatic moieties such as urea and phenol absorb at 230 nm. A highly purified product should have a 230 reading of no more than 0.3 and a 325 reading of no more than 0.01.[6] Accordingly, samples with values significantly deviating from these should be repurified.

Spectrophotometer-based method can also be used to quantify the amount of nucleic acids present in the sample. In general, every unit of absorption at 260 corresponds to 50 µg/mL double-stranded DNA, ~37 µg/mL single-stranded DNA, or ~40 µg/mL single-stranded RNA. Determination of the quantity of nucleic acids is essential as it would determine if the amount of DNA or RNA meets the minimum amount required to carry the downstream diagnostic assay.

The quality of the nucleic acid depends on its source and the extraction method. For example, bone-derived tissues often contain high calcium content, which is necessary to remove at the time of extraction. Decalcification of such tissues can be done by treatment with either acid or chelating agents (such as EDTA), with the latter being the preferred method as treatment with acid shears nucleic acids.[7]

Blood samples offer a noninvasive method of sample collection in patients and are routinely used for diagnostic purposes in hematological malignancies. The two major factors that can adversely affect the quantity and quality of the nucleic acid extracted from blood for downstream molecular diagnostic techniques are (1) the shipment and storage condition; (2) the presence of inhibitory components and external agents that are used to stabilize the sample. For the shipment and storage condition, the best quality nucleic acid is obtained when the sample is shipped immediately and nucleic acid is extracted shortly after. In general, the storage temperature should be kept low enough to prevent the potential enzymatic degradation of nucleic acids by nucleases (DNase and RNase). It has been shown that the nucleic acid quality is preserved at room temperature if the sample is used within 24 hours and at 4°C if the sample is used within a week.[8,9] For longer storage time, nucleic acids must first be extracted from the blood prior to storage and then stored at temperatures below freezing (–20°C or –80°C). It is also recommended to create aliquots of the extracted nucleic acids for future use as repeated freezing and thawing of the sample can cause degradation of the nucleic acids.[8,9] Since storage and shipment conditions are essential in determining the quality of the nucleic acid, laboratories should maintain a log of temperature and length of storage for each sample.

Certain blood samples may contain inhibitors that can interfere with the downstream molecular techniques. For example, the two major inhibitors found in blood samples are hemoglobin and lactoferrin present in erythrocyte- and leukocyte-derived samples, respectively.[10] A sample with a reddish color, coupled with a 260/280 ratio of less than 1.6, is generally an indication of the presence of these inhibitors. To minimize the effect of these inhibitors, one could add a variety of PCR facilitators such as albumin, gp32, glycerol, dimethyl sulfoxide (DMSO), betaine, poly(ethylene glycol) (PEG), and dextran.[10,11] Aside from hemoglobin and lactoferrin, other PCR inhibitors in the blood may include low-molecular-weight molecules (such as calcium and iron) and anticoagulants (such as EDTA and heparin). Other types of specimens may also contain molecules with similar effect as hemoglobin and lactoferrin discussed above. This includes melanin in skin samples, calcium in bone and cartilage samples, and collagen in connective tissue and bone. When tests are done on samples that may carry such inhibitory molecules, sample dilution is recommended as diluting samples will lower the concentrations of PCR inhibitors and, in general, will result in increased PCR efficiency. This strategy is especially useful when samples appear viscous. PCR inhibitors may act through different mechanisms such as binding to the polymerase, binding to the template, or acting as a chelating agent.[12] In addition to using PCR facilitators to overcome inhibition, implementing strategies such as designing primers with high melting temperature to increase template-binding efficiency or production of smaller amplicons to reduce the likelihood of inhibitor–template interaction should be considered. In addition, because the type of sample determines the type of inhibitory molecules it carries and different DNA polymerases can be affected by a wide variety of compounds, the choice of the appropriate polymerase must be carefully considered in relation to the type of samples utilized in the diagnostic assay.

Other common sample types used in molecular oncology applications are frozen tissues and formalin-fixed tissues. Formalin-fixed tissues may be kept in formalin vials or embedded into paraffin blocks for storage. Comparison of DNA quality and quantity from these three sample types has shown that frozen tissues, even after prolonged storage (20 years), give the best quantity and quality of nucleic acids. The DNA obtained from FFPE samples can give acceptable quality and yield if the samples are embedded in paraffin no longer than 6 weeks after formalin fixation. Long-term storage of tissues in formalin gives the poorest quality and yield of DNA.[13] Formalin fixation is a preferred method of specimen collection for pathologists as formalin treatment of the sample preserves the cellular structure for microscopic examinations by cross-linking macromolecules. Formalin, however, is known to denature the DNA and damage both the DNA and RNA via various mechanisms including cross-linking proteins with nucleic acids, which can lead to DNA and RNA fragmentation, chemical modification of nucleotides (addition of hydroxymethyl group to the base), depurination, and production of nonreversible changes, commonly in the form of a transition (C→T or G→A), in the nucleotide sequence.[14-16] The quality and quantity of the nucleic acids extracted from FFPE samples are highly compromised, and fixation process often leads to low concentration of highly sheared DNA and RNA (typically 200-base-long fragments[17,18]) that may contain incorrect information about the true DNA sequence of the patient from whom the tumor DNA was extracted.

To overcome the limitations associated with formalin treatment, modifications to formalin fixation protocols are recommended. For example, the low yield post-extraction is mainly attributed to the cross-linking of proteins to nucleic acids and subsequent trapping of the nucleic acid during the extraction process. This can be overcome by extending the proteinase K digestion time to more than 16 hours during the extraction process[19,20] without compromising the quality of the nucleic acid.[21] Degradation of DNA can also be reduced by using neutral pH fixative buffers, as acidic pH is another source of DNA degradation during formalin fixation. It has been shown that phosphate-buffered formalin results in optimal fixation and better RNA quality.[22] Prolonged storage of tissues in paraffin will also have adverse effects on the quality of nucleic acids as it will increase damage due to oxidation, so storage time should also be kept to a minimum.

Quantification of RNA to measure single gene expression level or analyze the entire transcriptome profile of the tumor is becoming increasingly popular in molecular oncology laboratories. However, most of the deleterious properties of formalin with regard to damaging DNA, as discussed above, also apply to RNA species and consequently have raised skepticism about the utility of FFPE samples for RNA-based applications. The major obstacle is the chemical modification of nucleotides in RNA (especially adenine nucleotides in the poly-A tail of the messenger RNA) that can interfere with downstream PCR-based methods as the modified adenines will reduce the efficiency of both RNA extraction by chaotropic agents[23] and the reverse transcription process when oligo-dT is used as the primer. Several modifications that may increase the efficiency of extraction and reverse transcription process include the use of random-priming instead of oligo-dT, substituting extraction of RNA by a chaotropic agent with extended proteinase K treatment to reverse cross-linking between proteins and RNA, and incubating RNA in formalin-free buffers at 70°C.[24] Understanding the limitations of formalin fixations and implementing appropriate modifications to the fixation and extraction protocols should result in RNA with acceptable quality suitable for both real-time PCR and microarray gene expression analysis. Some recent microarray studies have in fact compared the results for RNA extracted from frozen tissues versus FFPE and demonstrated that current FFPE methods can produce RNA samples that give comparable transcript measurements as those obtained from frozen tissues.[24,25]

Quantitative PCR

Real-time or quantitative PCR (qPCR) can be used for the rapid detection of specific RNA transcripts or DNA mutations in a given biological specimen. qPCR relies on progressive amplification of a template in which the efficiency of amplification is monitored typically using a fluorescent marker. The two major detection methods utilized in performing qPCR are probes labeled with both fluorescent and quenching dyes such as TaqMan and amplification refractory mutation system or dyes that bind to double-stranded DNA such as SYBR Green. Depending on the design of a qPCR assay, the read-out can be qualitative or quantitative.

Qualitative

Qualitative qPCR is a sensitive method for detecting the presence or absence of a particular transcript or DNA variant. By its nature, this assay is unable to determine the relative or absolute abundance of a DNA variant or transcript in the sample tested. In developing, validating, and performing a qualitative PCR assay, several performance parameters need to be addressed prior to use in a clinical laboratory.

Using qPCR for detection of DNA mutations in clinical samples is not considered a gold standard method. The typical design of a qPCR-based mutation detection assay is to create one probe for every individual mutation to be detected. Each probe that is designed should be verified to be able to accurately detect each mutation or transcript that the probe was designed to identify. A sample should be identified, for each probe used, that contains the mutation or transcript targeted by the probe. The sample should be independently verified by a secondary method as a positive sample. Using clinical samples for this portion of the validation would most accurately test the ability of each probe to detect the mutation or transcript it was designed to detect. If positive control clinical samples are not available, cell lines known to harbor a mutation or express a transcript can be used. However, it is recommended that the cell line sample be prepared in a similar fashion to clinical samples. For example, if the typical sample to be analyzed is an FFPE specimen, a cell pellet should also be formalin fixed and paraffin embedded prior to analysis to simulate the conditions of a standard clinical sample tested.

As qPCR is an extremely sensitive assay, it is important to run several known negative samples to determine the appropriate number of PCR cycles the assay should be run before detecting false-positive samples. Since qPCR is much more sensitive than the other mutation methods such as Sanger sequencing, it is possible to detect DNA mutations using qualitative qPCR that are not observed when using less sensitive techniques. This is illustrated by the increased level of sensitivity for qPCR assays as compared with conventional Sanger sequencing or fragment analysis (Table 23.1). Therefore, it is recommended that samples that are confirmed as negative using secondary methods as well as samples in which a mutation or transcript is not present should be used as a negative control. For example, in designing an assay to detect somatic mutations in cancer, an appropriate negative control would be an apparently normal tissue sample from an individual that has not been diagnosed with cancer (and these tissues possibly verified as noncancerous by an experienced oncologic pathologist) and has been confirmed as a negative sample using a secondary molecular testing method. In some cases, it may be prudent to run several negative samples to ensure that the assay is performing properly. There are also several pitfalls in using tissue samples from other cancers or tumor-adjacent normal tissues. These pitfalls include the presence of mutations undetected using less sensitive methods, the limited presence of mutation-positive tumor infiltration in the surrounding normal tissue, tumor mutation heterogeneity, and other genetic anomalies that may affect the performance of the assay such as gross chromosomal rearrangements. All of these issues can cause the Ct cutoff to call a sample negative to be artificially high, increasing the risk of reporting false-negative samples. The testing of known negative samples is also essential to verify the specificity of the assay. Small amounts of nonspecific amplification during the course of performing a qPCR assay can also result in an increased risk of reporting a false-positive result.

The overall sensitivity of the assay should be determined empirically with real-world clinical samples for which the assay was validated for, such as FFPE or frozen tissues. Probe sets for the detection of DNA variants or specific transcripts are commercially available and may provide a level of sensitivity; however, this may only be a theoretical level of sensitivity and may not have been determined using material similar to what is being tested in a routine clinical diagnostic laboratory. Therefore, it is essential to determine the sensitivity using standard samples received in the laboratory.

It is important to include several controls when performing a qPCR assay to verify the performance of the assay. Using an internal amplification control is essential in assuring that the sample is of sufficient quality to be analyzed by qPCR. When performing a mutation detection assay, a good surrogate would be the detection of the wild-type (WT) allele of that gene and also

TABLE 23-1 Comparison of Common Platforms Used for Mutational Analysis

	Allele-Specific Real-Time PCR	Sanger Sequencing	Fragment Analysis by Capillary Electrophoresis	Next-Generation Sequencing
Advantages	Rapid turnaround time Closed system minimizes the risk of PCR contamination Available for certain genes as commercial kits	Considered the “gold standard” by many Detects all possible mutations	Efficient and relatively inexpensive Higher resolution than gel-based methods	Efficient way to generate multiplex sequencing results Can be used to generate whole-genome data, including copy number, expression data, and chromosomal rearrangements
Disadvantages	Commercially available More expensive than Sanger sequencing	Labor intensive and expensive	Only detects mutations that alter fragment size and/or restriction site	Emerging technology, few experienced users Relatively expensive
Sensitivity, % of mutant alleles	5–10%	20%	10%	Depends upon sequence read depth

PCR, polymerase chain reaction.

a housekeeping gene known to be expressed in all tissues for assays designed to detect transcripts. The positive surrogate should also have established performance characteristics to ensure that the negative results are not due to poor quality of the sample or reduced sample input due to quantification, normalization, or human errors. Due to the sensitive nature of qPCR assays, a WT control should be included on every batched run to verify that there is no cross-contamination of samples leading to false-positive results. A non-template control that lacks nucleic acids should also be included to verify that there is no contamination that may preclude the detection of a mutation or transcript increasing the risk of a false-negative result.

Quantitative

Quantitative qPCR is the "gold standard" method for determining the level of expression of a particular RNA transcript or the mutation load of a clinical sample. Due to the reproducibility and sensitivity of quantitative qPCR, this methodology can be used to detect low mutation loads or for minimal residual disease monitoring. In order to ensure accuracy and reproducibility of the assay, several assay and quality metrics should be addressed.

In designing a quantitative qPCR assay, the efficiency of the probes in use should be determined.[26] This can be performed by serially diluting a sample with a known copy number and determining the Ct of each dilution. This can be achieved by using cell lines or engineered controls. It is also important to use these controls to determine the upper and lower limits of detection of the probes selected for the assay.[26]

In addition to determining the efficiency of the probes in the PCR, a serial dilution should be performed to establish a standard curve. Establishing a standard curve for every batch of experiments is essential when performing serial monitoring of residual disease. Since there is the potential for variation to occur when making new formulations of reagents and between users, establishing the performance of each run is necessary. To account for variability in the quality of nucleic acids obtained from clinical samples, a standard curve should also be established for a control probe. When assessing the level of a particular transcript, a housekeeping gene could be used to assess sample variability and a probe specific to the WT allele could be used for quantitative mutation analysis. Serial dilutions of both the control and the test probes should be run with every batch of samples analyzed. Spearman correlations (R^2) should be determined on an assay to assay basis to ensure the reproducibility of the assay as well as to allow inter-experiment correlations.

Fragment Analysis

Fragment analysis is an elegant methodology to detect known point mutations, translocations, or genetic rearrangements in clinical samples. These assays typically employ fluorescently labeled primers or gel electrophoresis and detect the presence or size alterations in PCR products. Restriction enzymes to selectively digest PCR products can be used to detect variants in DNA that alter restriction enzyme cleavage sites known as restriction fragment length polymorphism analysis. One limitation of this technology is that the mutation or chromosomal rearrangement to be assayed must be known.

When validating a fragment analysis assay, a positive control should be obtained to address each individual mutation or chromosomal rearrangement to be tested. Positive controls are necessary to verify that the probes selected will accurately detect the aberration of interest. It is also essential to include known negative samples to verify the specificity of the assay. In addition, inclusion of positive and negative controls in every batch analyzed will ensure that the assay has reproducible sensitivity and specificity.

The fragment size patterns of normal and abnormal samples should be determined and verified by running a fragment size standard with every assay. The fragments produced for analysis should be of a predictable size for both negative and positive samples.

In all fragment analysis assays, an amplification control should be included for all samples assessed. An amplification control is essential in assays designed to detect a translocation or the presence of a particular genetic rearrangement, such as B- and T-cell clonality assays. Without an amplification control, it is not possible to determine whether the inability to detect a translocation or rearrangement is due to the absence of the alteration or if the sample was not of high enough quality to be assessed by this method. Furthermore, signal thresholds should be established to prevent false-negative calls due to an abnormal signal being present below the limit of detection.

Dideoxy or Sanger Sequencing

Sanger sequencing is a "gold standard" method for the detection of sequence variants. This direct sequencing methodology is more technically demanding than qPCR or fragment analysis and has the ability to identify novel variants that other methods of mutation detection are unable to do. Sanger sequencing is a multistep process that involves the selective PCR amplification of a region of interest followed by a subsequent PCR containing labeled dideoxy nucleotides producing DNA fragments of various lengths and uniquely labeled depending on the terminating nucleotide. One inherent drawback of Sanger sequencing is the reduced sensitivity of the assay. The typical expectation of this technology is the detection of mutations that comprise at least 20% of all alleles. However, it is important to determine the particular sensitivity of each assay prior to use in clinical diagnostics. It is also important to appropriately screen samples prior to analysis, such as using % tumor nuclei, to avoid processing samples with mutations below the sensitivity of the assay.

To verify the performance of a Sanger sequencing assay, positive and negative amplification controls should be included in each assay. A positive amplification control should be utilized to verify that a failure to amplify a region of interest is sample dependent. A negative or no template control should also be included in each run, for each master mix used, to ensure that contamination with exogenous DNA has not occurred.

Prior to the analysis of Sanger sequencing data, the quality of the sequence traces must be first assessed. Stringent quality metrics should be determined for both the amplitude of the peaks of the trace and the background of each peak in the trace. Peak amplitude should be of sufficient height as to not preclude the identification of low-level mutations within the limits of sensitivity as illustrated for an epidermal growth factor receptor (EGFR) deletion mutation (Fig. 23.2). Background within a trace should be $<5\%$ of the intensity of the dominant peak for each nucleotide call across the region of interest. Furthermore, the signal-to-noise ratio across the entire trace should be $<2.5\%$. There are software programs available to assess the strength of the signal-to-noise ratios and these can be quite useful for assessing the overall quality of sequence traces.[27]

Even though steps can be taken to ensure the quality of sequence traces, there is still an inherent low level of background typically present; therefore, it is highly recommended that bidirectional sequencing be employed. The use of bidirectional sequencing will greatly reduce the risk of producing false-positive results due to either background noise in sequence traces or polymerase infidelity. A negative control should also be included on each run to further distinguish background from a true mutation. Due to the subjective nature, more than one individual should also inspect each sequencing trace to reach a consensus call.[28] If a consensus cannot be reached as to the mutation status of a sample, a repeat analysis should be performed if there is sufficient material left to do so. Re-extraction from the same biological specimen to produce more material for analysis can be performed to repeat mutation analysis. However, it should be noted that re-extraction of nucleic acids from tumor samples for mutation confirmation may produce discordant results due to tumor heterogeneity. This issue of tumor heterogeneity is well illustrated in a recent KRAS proficiency challenge sponsored by the CAP. The results of this survey (CAP 2010 KRAS-B) revealed that two-thirds of participating laboratories reported detecting a KRAS mutation in the proficiency sample, while one-third of laboratories did not detect a KRAS mutation. These apparently discrepant proficiency test results were attributed to tumor heterogeneity.

Microarray

Microarray is an oligonucleotide array–based technology that can be used to detect a vast number of RNA transcripts in a single reaction or identify gene copy number losses and gains. Microarrays are typically composed of thousands to millions of DNA probes that are fixed either to a surface in a predictable pattern or to beads and randomly distributed on the array. Expression arrays are able to detect cDNA fragments that have been fluorescently labeled, while comparative genomic hybridization arrays (aCGH) detect genomic DNA fragments that have been fluorescently labeled. Due to the complexity of microarray platforms and the propensity for variation, it is essential to verify the performance of these assays prior to and during use in a clinical laboratory.

Wild-Type EGFR

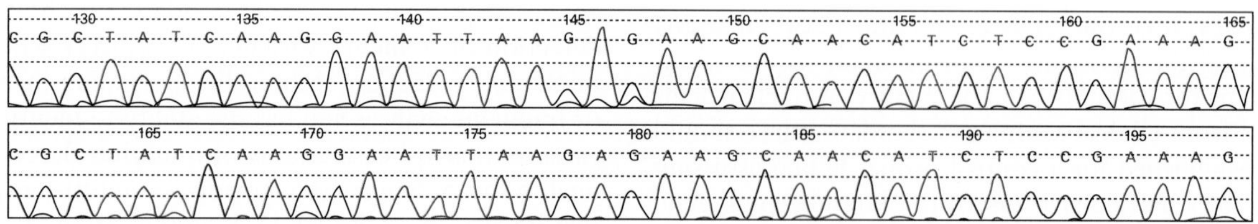

Mutated EGFR

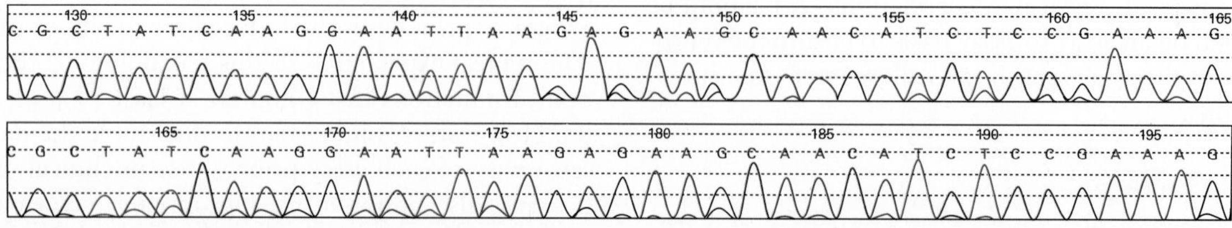

FIGURE 23–2 (Top) Portions of a forward and reverse sequence trace of exon 19 of epidermal growth factor receptor (EGFR), with mild background, from a non-mutated patient sample. (Bottom) Portions of a forward and reverse sequence trace of exon 19 of EGFR from a patient sample with a p.L747_A750delinsP mutation.

The reproducibility of any microarray platform should be verified prior to clinical use. This is typically achieved by performing the assay on separate days by different technicians, and metrics should be determined to validate the reproducibility of the array. For example, if an RNA expression signature is used to stratify patients into prognostic groups, the same samples should be segregated to the same groups when assayed on different days. When using a microarray to determine the expression level of many genes or identify gene copy number alterations, the same levels of expression or copy number changes should be obtained among runs.

There are several caveats to performing accuracy assays when validating a microarray platform. Using other expression arrays or qPCR may yield discordant results based on differences in probe design, housekeeping genes selected for normalization, and normalization techniques.[28] Performing accuracy studies using the gold standard of fluorescence in situ hybridization (FISH) for aCGH platforms can also lead to discordant results when validating very small deletions or if a well-validated FISH probe is not available for confirmatory analysis. When designing accuracy studies for microarray platforms, one must also verify that the means of normalization or detection sensitivities are equivalent between the two technologies or platforms used.

Prior to performing expression arrays, the quality of the RNA being examined should be determined. For expression arrays, a typical method for evaluating the quality of RNA is by determining the RNA integrity number (RIN) of the sample. Samples with a higher RIN tend to have more intact RNA than samples with a lower RIN. When performing microarray experiments that rely on the transcript being attached to the poly-A tail for cDNA synthesis, the RIN of the sample is incredibly important to the success of the assay. However, some microarray platforms are designed to accurately quantify degraded transcripts; therefore, the RIN may have very little correlation to the performance of the sample. Another method of determining the quality of RNA prior to microarray analysis is using qPCR directed at a housekeeping gene known to be expressed in all tissues such as β-tubulin or certain ribosomal proteins. A Ct cutoff value should be established for qPCR assays designed to evaluate the quality of RNA to avoid processing patient samples of inferior quality and possibly report inaccurate results.

When performing microarray analysis, the quality of each run should be evaluated prior to the reporting of results. Most commercially available microarray platforms have built-in controls designed to verify the performance of the entire array. Control probes should include those designed to evaluate background (negative control probes), binding specificity (mismatch probes), oligo annealing (probes with different melting temperatures), and overall performance (positive or housekeeping control probes).[29] In addition, it is vital that if normal reference materials are used for relative gene expression measurement, then the reference sample should be verified as normal by an experienced oncologic/pathologist prior to dissemination of patient data.

After identifying gene copy number gains and losses using aCGH, confirmation using FISH would be ideal. However, a FISH probe designed to interrogate a specific region of the genome may not be available or the deletion/insertion/duplication may not be of sufficient size to be detected by FISH analysis. As a minimum, a dye swap should be performed in which the patient and reference materials are labeled with the opposite dyes when compared with the initial analysis.

Next-Generation Sequencing

Next-generation sequencing (NGS) is a powerful tool that allows a user to generate a large amount of sequence data in a short period of time. NGS relies upon selective amplification of a DNA target that is then immobilized to a bead or glass chip using universal primers to generate sequence data. The sequence data produced are then aligned to a reference sequence to identify any mutations, translocations, or transcripts that may be present in a patient sample. By its nature, NGS is extremely prone to contamination and laboratories should be extremely vigilant in preventing contamination of patient samples undergoing NGS analysis. To this point, up to 20% of all non-primate sequences in public databases contain human sequences likely due to contamination.[30]

NGS platforms have the capability of being incredibly sensitive platforms. The sensitivity of any NGS platform is based on the depth of coverage of the assay or how many times a particular nucleotide is sequenced. Increasing the depth of coverage of an NGS platform will increase the sensitivity of the assay but has the ability to also decrease specificity. Therefore, the read depth should be tailored to the sensitivity desired for the use of the NGS assay. For example, when looking for inherited mutations, a read depth of 10 may be sufficient as mutations are expected to comprise 50% of the alleles. However, when using NGS to detect somatic mutations that may be present in only 5% of alleles, a much higher read depth would be required. It is imperative that the laboratory empirically determine what the appropriate coverage depth would be using positive and negative controls as outlined in the qPCR section above. When running NGS-based assays, positive and negative controls should also be used, as outlined in the Sanger sequencing section, to verify the performance of the platform.

Reporting and Laboratory Information Management Systems

Accuracy of results and continuous monitoring of clinical diagnostic test results are important features of molecular diagnostic laboratories. Reports of molecular diagnostic analyses can be complex and it is essential that the content of molecular diagnostic reports be complete, clear, and concise. Reports of test results must clearly convey the test result and test method(s), and furthermore, the analytic limitations of the particular test result must be clearly stated so that the clinical significance of the result(s) is obvious to the ordering physician.[31]

QC of laboratory information management systems (LIMS) is of particular importance for laboratories that rely upon automated systems that assist with sample tracking, workflow management, analysis, and clinical reporting. LIMS support several goals of the clinical diagnostic laboratory. First, the security of the information system and patient data must be controlled to ensure that confidentiality of medical information is maintained, and that the laboratory analytic data are secured from alterations and unauthorized access and periodically backed up. Second, LIMS usually enable result reporting including hard copy, fax, or electronic reports. Validation of LIMS is an important step to ensure that the software is performing and producing results as it was designed.[32] The CAP molecular pathology checklist item (MOL.20550) calls for the periodic review of molecular genetic statistics including the percentages of normal and abnormal findings and allele frequencies. Reviewing rates of positive or negative results can be helpful in ascertaining if test performance is changing or if there is a shift in the populations or sample types being tested. Finally, LIMS are usually employed to help with routine monitoring of certain key post-analytic quality metrics such as turnaround time, test repeat rate, first pass yield, number of PCR contaminations, and corrected analytic results.

Laboratory Design

As a variety of molecular diagnostic techniques utilize PCR amplification nucleic acids, a laboratory should be designed to reduce the risk of contaminating patient samples with nucleases or exogenous DNA. Ideally, the workflow in a molecular diagnostic laboratory is unidirectional from specimen receipt to nucleic acid extraction to analytic detection to ensure that amplified DNA products will not contaminate sample processing, DNA extraction, or PCR amplification areas.[33] Laboratories that perform DNA and RNA extractions should use distinct areas for each type of nucleic acid extraction to avoid cross-contamination of nucleases. In open laboratories where both RNA and DNA extractions are performed, it is good practice to use RNase-decontaminating wipes or solutions as a precaution against RNase contamination.[29]

Pre-PCR setup should take place preferably in a negatively pressured enclosed area that is distinct from the rest of the laboratory.[33] Air locks can also be used when passing between the open laboratory and pre-PCR area to further reduce the risk of contamination. Personal protective equipment (PPE) to be worn during pre-PCR setup should be donned after entering the pre-PCR area and should be discarded or removed prior to leaving the area. Dead air hoods or boxes should be used during PCR setup and decontaminated before and after use using both UV light and bleach. Tools such as pipettes and tube racks should also be stored in dead air hoods and regularly decontaminated as well.

One of the most common sources of contamination in a molecular laboratory is PCR amplicons. Laboratories utilizing universal PCR primers for next-generation or Sanger sequencing are especially vulnerable to amplicon contamination. PCR amplification and any processing step following PCR amplification should take place in a segregated area of the laboratory. A positively pressured room separated from the general laboratory space would be the most effective means of reducing potential contamination of patient samples.[33] Following any PCR, all reactions and materials should be considered dirty and segregated to the post-PCR area. If possible, all post-PCR materials should be removed from this area using a means of egress that does not use the main laboratory space. PPE should be donned after entering the post-PCR area and then removed or discarded prior to exiting the area.

QUALITY ASSURANCE

All laboratories should have a quality management system, and certain elements for QA are routinely applied such as audits of proficiency testing results, training, and competency. As described earlier, QA activities encompass those measures or processes that promote quality of the final end product—in our case the accuracy and timeliness of patient laboratory results. An important attribute of QA activities is the idea of independence of review—such as audits of equipment calibrations to ensure these are being completed or independent inspection of a laboratory for accreditation. One of the main goals of QA is to build quality improvements into processes through the use of performance standards, identification of outliers, and problem solving. An important concept or framework to help coordinate quality improvement activities in the laboratory is the well-known Plan-Do-Check-Act (PDCA) circle.[1] Similarly, lean techniques developed in manufacturing (also known as the Toyota Production System) can be applied to clinical diagnostic laboratories to help sustain continuous improvement activities. Lean is a system-wide culture that focuses on continuous incremental quality improvements through problem solving, visual controls, standard work, and standard accountability.[34] For example, one laboratory institution used lean techniques and laboratory process redesign to help significantly reduce diagnostic errors in patients undergoing thyroid gland fine needle aspiration biopsies.[35] A variety of methods/techniques are available for problem solving/quality improvement in the laboratory, including 5s (workplace organization and standardization), value stream mapping to assist with process redesign, standard work, Kaizen event (structured quality improvement events involving all work team members of 2 to 5 d duration), Kanban (system of pulling reagents/supplies that automatically triggers re-orders), and root cause analysis.[34] Outlined below are some key QA best practices currently used in many laboratories regarding reference materials, proficiency testing, personnel training, peer review, and laboratory accreditation.

Reference Samples and Positive Control Samples

The use of well-characterized positive and negative control samples (i.e., reference materials) is an integral element of new test validations, routine clinical diagnostic testing, and proficiency testing. In fact, the Clinical Laboratory Improvement Amendments of 1988 (CLIA '88) mandates that a positive control sample be available and run for each analyte being tested. Positive controls for mutation detection in genotyping tests are required to assure that the detection method is sensitive and all steps of the analytical testing process are performing properly. Reference materials that are certified can also provide the foundation for standardization of specific molecular tests.

The availability of standard reference materials and positive control samples is an important need of the molecular diagnostic testing community.[5,36] The rapid growth in molecular diagnostic testing methods and the availability of tests for new genetic disorders have been limited in part due to the availability of suitable positive control materials. Furthermore, the increasingly widespread practice of filing patents on disease mutations and specific test methodologies has also contributed to the shortage of freely available reference materials. In response to this apparent shortage of suitable reference materials, a process for producing and validating positive control samples from Epstein-Barr virus–transformed blood lymphocytes was developed using a network of 32 genetic testing laboratories.[37] During this 3-year study, 33 cell lines representing mutations across 11 genetic disorders were established, validated, and made available to others from the Coriell Cell Repositories. More recently, the Centers for Disease Control has established the Genetic Testing Reference Material Coordination Program (GeT-RM), and this program has made available genomic DNA reference materials for several genes including BRCA1 and BRCA2.[38] The GeT-RM program is also considering approaches to developing a characterized genomic DNA for next-generation/whole-genome sequencing.

The analytic performance of control samples and reference materials in the clinical laboratory is also very important. Performance of synthetic controls such as oligonucleotide or PCR amplicons may not be as good as the performance of genomic DNA controls derived from "real-world" samples such as FFPE. For example, in our experience, if a vendor claims 1% sensitivity of a test method, our results with real-world clinical samples may only demonstrate a 10% sensitivity.

Proficiency Testing

Proficiency testing programs are external, unbiased audit systems that help ensure the accuracy of analytical testing results through periodic inter-laboratory comparisons of testing results on the same sample. These programs are a very important measure of a laboratory's ability to produce reliable analytical test reports. Participation in an approved external proficiency program is mandated by CLIA '88 and failure to comply with these requirements can lead to severe sanctions.[39]

Both formal and informal proficiency testing or external quality assessment programs are available for molecular oncology/molecular diagnostic laboratories. For example, formal programs in molecular oncology have been offered by CAP for many years. CAP also offers proficiency programs for engraftment, microsatellite instability, DNA extraction, and amplification. Despite the potential limitations of tumor heterogeneity and shipping samples to geographically distant sites, the performance of laboratories participating in a CAP-sponsored proficiency challenge for BCL2 major breakpoint region analysis by PCR was good as 90% of the participating laboratories obtained the correct result over a 4-year period (1997 to 2000).[40] Currently, over 80 laboratories participated in the most recent CAP molecular oncology test challenge for KRAS mutational analysis (KRAS-A, 2011, CAP 2011). In this recent CAP challenge, 83 out of 88 laboratories correctly identified a specific codon 12 KRAS mutation (c.34G>A). Four laboratories reported a mutation positive in KRAS but did not indicate the specific nucleotide. However, one laboratory reported the wrong codon 12 KRAS mutation. Overall, these results suggest that virtually all participating laboratories reported the consensus result for this particular proficiency challenge. The New York State Department of Health, Clinical Laboratory Evaluation Program (NYSDOH CLEP) also provides for proficiency testing for molecular and cellular tumor markers (3 different specimens for approximately 30 distinct molecular oncology assays), and they routinely publish the results of their program online (see Internet resources below). Finally, the National External Quality Assessment Service in the United Kingdom has been offering a hemato-oncology program since 1983.

Informal programs also exist for proficiency testing of molecular diagnostic laboratories. For example, interlaboratory sample exchanges can be set up on an ad hoc basis within and between interested laboratories for analytes not currently offered by external agencies. Other professional societies (e.g., Association for Molecular Pathology [AMP]; American College of Medical Genetics [ACMG]) have been involved in some laboratory sample exchange programs.

Personnel Qualifications and Competency

In general, a PhD degree in the relevant sciences or an MD degree, with additional training as necessary, is required to run most molecular diagnostic laboratories. Other nationally recognized credentialing authorities include the American Society of Histocompatibility and Immunogenetics (ASHI) and the American Board of

Bioanalysis (ABB). The ABB is recognized by CLIA '88 as a certifying agency for the credential of high-complexity clinical laboratory director (HCLD). Applicants for HCLD certification must demonstrate at least 2 years of experience directing or supervising high-complexity clinical laboratory testing. There may also be state-specific requirements. For example, when samples are tested from patients originating in New York State, the laboratory director must hold a certificate of qualification in various specialties such as molecular genetic testing and molecular oncology. The NYSDOH CLEP currently certifies, on a biennial basis, over 3,000 certificates of qualification to individuals who serve as directors/assistant directors of these clinical laboratories across the United States. The state of California also requires that director-level personnel for molecular genetic laboratories within that state are licensed as a clinical genetic molecular biologist.

Requirements for molecular technologists typically include a bachelor's degree in the biological sciences along with a few years of experience in molecular testing in a clinical setting. National credentialing is available through several avenues including the American Society of Clinical Pathology (ASCP) that sponsors a molecular biology technologist (MB (ASCP)) certificate program. Some states such as California, New York, and Florida require licensure for laboratory technologists.

Random Peer Review

We follow a standard operating procedure in our laboratory that stipulates independent peer review of approximately 5% of the weekly case volume for molecular diagnostic results. We currently employ three board-certified clinical molecular geneticists and a random 5% selection of each person's case work is peer-reviewed by another molecular geneticist. This is a best practice adopted from pathology,[41] and we feel that this independent random review is another QA practice to help ensure quality, foster consensus, and maintain standardization of reporting nomenclature.[42]

Laboratory Accreditation

Laboratory accreditation by an authorized body is increasingly recognized as an important attribute of medical testing laboratories. In the United States, this is required by CLIA '88 and inspections can be done by the Centers for Medicare and Medicaid Services or by "deemed authorities" such as the College of American Pathologists (CAP) and the Joint Commission on Accreditation of Healthcare Organizations (JCAHO).[43] In addition, certain individual states in the United States also require laboratory licensure. The International Organization for Standardization (ISO) 15189 standard for medical laboratories is increasingly becoming a requirement throughout Europe.[1]

INTERNET RESOURCES

- Catalogue of Somatic Mutations in Cancer (Cosmic) (http://www.sanger.ac.uk/genetics/CGP/cosmic). This site offers a wealth of curated data on somatic mutations in cancer and is searchable by gene and tissue. For any given gene of interest, one can view a histogram page that graphically summarizes the spectrum of somatic mutations found within the coding sequences.
- The Human Genome Variation Society (HGVS) (http://www.hgvs.org). This site contains guidelines and recommendations for mutation nomenclature and links to mutation databases.
- College of American Pathologists (CAP) (http://www.cap.org). This site contains information on laboratory accreditation, proficiency testing surveys, QA programs, and continuing education programs.
- Association for Molecular Pathology (AMP) (http://www.amp.org). AMP is an international medical professional association dedicated to the advancement, practice, and science of clinical molecular laboratory medicine and translational research based on the applications of molecular biology, genetics, and genomics.
- The New York State Department of Health, Clinical Laboratory Evaluation Program (NYSDOH CLEP) (http://www.wadsworth.org/labcert/clep/clep.html). This program coordinates the onsite inspections of NYS-accredited laboratories in New York and throughout the United States, the certificate of qualifications of laboratory directors, and proficiency testing programs for molecular oncology among other specialties.

REFERENCES

1. Berwouts S, Morris MA, Dequeker E. Approaches to quality management and accreditation in a genetic testing laboratory. *Eur J Hum Genet.* Sep 2010;18(suppl 1):S1-S19.
2. Nakhleh RE, Idowu MO, Souers RJ, et al. Mislabeling of cases, specimens, blocks, and slides: a College of American Pathologists study of 136 institutions. *Arch Pathol Lab Med.* 2011;8:969-974.
3. Raab SS, Grzybicki DM. Quality in cancer diagnosis. *CA Cancer J Clin.* 2010;3:139-165.
4. Jennings L, Van Deerlin VM, Gulley ML. Recommended principles and practices for validating clinical molecular pathology tests. *Arch Pathol Lab Med.* 2009;5:743-755.
5. Holden MJ, Madej RM, Minor P, et al. Molecular diagnostics: harmonization through reference materials, documentary standards and proficiency testing. *Expert Rev Mol Diagn.* 2011;7:741-755.
6. Gallagher SR, Desjardins PR. Quantitation of DNA and RNA with absorption and fluorescence spectroscopy. *Curr Prot Hum Genet.* 2007;Appendix 3: Appendix 3D A.3D.1-A.3D.21.
7. Alers JC, Krijtenburg PJ, Vissers KJ, et al. Effect of bone decalcification procedures on DNA in situ hybridization and comparative genomic hybridization. EDTA is highly preferable to a routinely used acid decalcifier. *J Histochem Cytochem.* 1999;5:703-710.
8. Visvikis S, Schlenck A, Maurice M. DNA extraction and stability for epidemiological studies. *Clin Chem Lab Med.* 1998;8:551-555.
9. Farkas DH, Kaul KL, Wiedbrauk DL, et al. Specimen collection and storage for diagnostic molecular pathology investigation. *Arch Pathol Lab Med.* 1996;6:591-596.

10. Al-Soud WA, Radstrom P. Purification and characterization of PCR-inhibitory components in blood cells. *J Clin Microbiol.* 2001;2:485-493.
11. Radstrom P, Knutsson R, Wolffs P, et al. Pre-PCR processing: strategies to generate PCR-compatible samples. *Mol Biotechnol.* 2004;2:133-146.
12. Opel KL, Chung D, McCord BR. A study of PCR inhibition mechanisms using real time PCR. *J Forensic Sci.* 2010;1:25-33.
13. Ferrer I, Armstrong J, Capellari S, et al. Effects of formalin fixation, paraffin embedding, and time of storage on DNA preservation in brain tissue: a BrainNet Europe study. *Brain Pathol.* 2007;3:297-303.
14. Srinivasan M, Sedmak D, Jewell S. Effect of fixatives and tissue processing on the content and integrity of nucleic acids. *Am J Pathol.* 2002;6:1961-1971.
15. Williams C, Ponten F, Moberg C, et al. A high frequency of sequence alterations is due to formalin fixation of archival specimens. *Am J Pathol.* 1999;5:1467-1471.
16. Klopfleisch R, Weiss AT, Gruber AD. Excavation of a buried treasure—DNA, mRNA, miRNA and protein analysis in formalin fixed, paraffin embedded tissues. *Histol Histopathol.* 2011;6:797-810.
17. Lehmann U, Kreipe H. Real-time PCR analysis of DNA and RNA extracted from formalin-fixed and paraffin-embedded biopsies. *Methods.* 2001;4:409-418.
18. Gilbert MT, Haselkorn T, Bunce M, et al. The isolation of nucleic acids from fixed, paraffin-embedded tissues—which methods are useful when? *PLoS One.* 2007;6:e537.
19. McKinney MD, Moon SJ, Kulesh DA, et al. Detection of viral RNA from paraffin-embedded tissues after prolonged formalin fixation. *J Clin Virol.* 2009;1:39-42.
20. Weiss AT, Delcour NM, Meyer A, et al. Efficient and cost-effective extraction of genomic DNA from formalin-fixed and paraffin-embedded tissues. *Vet Pathol.* 2011;4:834-838.
21. Bonin S, Hlubek F, Benhattar J, et al. Multicentre validation study of nucleic acids extraction from FFPE tissues. *Virchows Arch.* 2010;3:309-317.
22. Chung JY, Braunschweig T, Williams R, et al. Factors in tissue handling and processing that impact RNA obtained from formalin-fixed, paraffin-embedded tissue. *J Histochem Cytochem.* 2008;11:1033-1042.
23. Doleshal M, Magotra AA, Choudhury B, et al. Evaluation and validation of total RNA extraction methods for microRNA expression analyses in formalin-fixed, paraffin-embedded tissues. *J Mol Diagn.* 2008;3:203-211.
24. Farragher SM, Tanney A, Kennedy RD, et al. RNA expression analysis from formalin fixed paraffin embedded tissues. *Histochem Cell Biol.* 2008;3:435-445.
25. April C, Klotzle B, Royce T, et al. Whole-genome gene expression profiling of formalin-fixed, paraffin-embedded tissue samples. *PLoS One.* 2009;12:e8162.
26. Bustin SA, Benes V, Garson JA, et al. The MIQE guidelines: minimum information for publication of quantitative real-time PCR experiments. *Clin Chem.* 2009;4:611-622.
27. Ellard S, Charlton R, Yau M, et al. Practice guidelines for Sanger sequencing analysis and interpretation. http://www.cmgs.org; 2009.
28. Shi L, Campbell G, Jones WD, et al. The MicroArray Quality Control (MAQC)-II study of common practices for the development and validation of microarray-based predictive models. *Nat Biotechnol.* 2010;8:827-838.
29. Tang W, Hu Z, Muallem H, et al. Quality assurance of RNA expression profiling in clinical laboratories. *J Mol Diagn.* 2012;14:1-11.
30. Tuma R. Genome sequencing in patient care: preventing contamination is crucial. *J Natl Cancer Inst.* 2011;11:847-848.
31. Gulley ML, Braziel RM, Halling KC, et al. Clinical laboratory reports in molecular pathology. *Arch Pathol Lab Med.* 2007;6:852-863.
32. Turner E, Bolton J. Required steps for the validation of a laboratory information management system. *Qual Assur.* 2001;3-4:217-224.
33. Mifflin TE. Setting up a PCR laboratory. *Cold Spring Harb Protoc.* 2007: pdb top14.
34. Mann DW. *Creating a Lean Culture: Tools to Sustain Lean Conversions.* Boca Raton, FL: Productivity Press; 2005.
35. Raab SS, Grzybicki DM, Sudilovsky D, et al. Effectiveness of Toyota process redesign in reducing thyroid gland fine-needle aspiration error. *Am J Clin Pathol.* 2006;4:585-592.
36. Chen B, O'Connell CD, Boone DJ, et al. Developing a sustainable process to provide quality control materials for genetic testing. *Genet Med.* 2005;8:534-549.
37. Bernacki SH, Beck JC, Muralidharan K, et al. Characterization of publicly available lymphoblastoid cell lines for disease-associated mutations in 11 genes. *Clin Chem.* 2005;11:2156-2159.
38. Barker SD, Bale S, Booker J, et al. Development and characterization of reference materials for MTHFR, SERPINA1, RET, BRCA1, and BRCA2 genetic testing. *J Mol Diagn.* 2009;6:553-561.
39. Killeen AA. Laboratory sanctions for proficiency testing sample referral and result communication: a review of actions from 1993-2006. *Arch Pathol Lab Med.* 2009;6:979-982.
40. Hsi ED, Tubbs RR, Lovell MA, et al. Detection of bcl-2/J(H) translocation by polymerase chain reaction: a summary of the experience of the Molecular Oncology Survey of the College of American Pathologist. *Arch Pathol Lab Med.* 2002;8:902-908.
41. Morton D, Sellers RS, Barale-Thomas E, et al. Recommendations for pathology peer review. *Toxicol Pathol.* 2010;7:1118-1127.
42. den Dunnen JT, Antonarakis SE. Nomenclature for the description of human sequence variations. *Hum Genet.* 2001;1:121-124.
43. Burnett D. *Practical Guide to Accreditation in Laboratory Medicine.* London: ACB Venture Publications; 2002.

CHAPTER 24

BIOSTATISTICS AND BIOINFORMATICS

Qian Shi and Daniel J. Sargent

INTRODUCTION

The inherent variability in treatment response and adverse reactions among individual cancer patients has a significant impact on therapeutic development and is the basis of personalized cancer medicine. Successful disease gene and molecular pathways identification can lead to major breakthroughs in our understanding of cancer prognosis, developing the targeted therapies, and achieving optimal clinical benefit by selecting a particular treatment that is tailored to an individual patient's disease. The scope of the research in this area covers disease-related gene identification or gene mapping, the development of risk classifications based on genetic or molecular discoveries, and the rapid screening and development of innovative molecular targeted therapies.

Regardless of the development stage of the research, a scientifically sound study design is fundamental and essential to the success of the research. The study design includes many aspects, such as focused and clear aims, a correctly targeted study population, specific study hypothesis directed at observable outcome measures, determination of effective and feasible sample size and sampling schema, careful control of confounding and bias rigorous data collection and quality control, prospectively planned statistical analysis plan, efficient presentations of the data, and interpreting results with objectiveness and cautiousness. Successful design and conduct of a study is never an easy task and always involves multidisciplinary specialists. Biostatistics and bioinformatics is one area of expertise that no evidence-based medicine research can live without.

In this chapter, we aim to present the principles of statistical study design, data analysis, and results interpretation that are tailored to research in molecular diagnosis and personalized medicine. The core intended audience of this chapter is laboratory and clinical professionals, policy makers, and applied biostatisticians who collaborate with investigators in this area. We will not discuss the mathematical theories behind the statistical methods, but rather, we will provide a high-level overview of concepts and statistical methods, provide guidance of appropriate application of the methods, and (hopefully) facilitate informative communications between biostatisticians and medical scientists.

In this chapter, we start with the review of the genetic statistics methods that are substantially utilized in the initial discoveries of genetic and molecular markers, followed by the techniques of establishing and validating diagnostic/prognostic markers and associated prediction models, which can assist decision making in individual patient care. We will then focus on the study designs for marker-driven development of targeted and personalized therapies in oncology.

GENETIC AND MOLECULAR DISCOVERIES

Due to rapid evolution of gene mapping techniques, the pace of genetic and molecular research is increasing exponentially. In this section, we present a review of the major considerations pertaining to the statistical aspects of a mapping study, either searching for one or few rare mutations in a single gene that cause a (likely rare) disease or identifying alternations in more than one gene, such as common polymorphisms, that either increase or decrease the risk of a trait. Additional details on statistical aspects of gene mapping and statistical genetics are available in Haines and Pericak-Vance[1] and Thomas.[2]

In the context of genetic analyses, traits (also called phenotype) are the observable outcomes. Indentifying the unobserved genotype that has a causal relationship with a trait is the primary aim of the genetic study. The unobserved genotype can be the disease gene, pathway marker, already cloned gene, or polymorphisms in a number of genes. It is essential to define the trait under the study. Traits (or phenotypes) can be grouped into three types based on their statistical properties—qualitative (discontinuous) traits, quantitative (continuous) traits, and censoring survival (time-to-event) traits. The presence or absence of a disease is an example of a qualitative trait, whereas blood glucose level is a quantitative trait. A censoring survival trait can be the time from surgery to the first documented recurrence for a patient. The choice of a trait should be based on etiologic and pathogenetic causal implications, with the requirement that the outcome of the trait is able to be defined in a rigorously consistent fashion. This principle is essentially the same for different stages of gene mapping or association discoveries. However, as the question at hand (i.e., the hypothesis to be tested) evolves at the different stages of research, the appropriate experimental design and statistical analysis method should be determined accordingly. We discuss the specifics of this key point in the following sections representing three critical phases of the genetic research: initial separation of the gene effect from the environmental factors, identification of the approximate chromosome of a suspicious gene, and population genetics including fine mapping and cloning, testing candidate gene associations, and characterization of the gene that has been established as causally related to disease.

Identification of Gene Causal Effect

Summarizing and examining the descriptive epidemiologic characteristics is a starting point for generating hypotheses related to genetic traits. These characteristics include geographical origin and migrations, individual's demographics (especially race/ethnicity, gender, and age), and/or social class. For example, the migrant study[3] summarizes disease incidence rates in migrants by comparing them with those in their country of origin. A significant difference between migrants and those in their country of origin in such a study may indicate that international variation is potentially explained by genetic variation beyond environmental factors.

To formally separate the genetic effects of a disease trait from environmental influences, familial aggregation studies followed by segregation analyses are commonly carried out. For the former, the hypothesis involves testing whether the disease clusters in families more than would be expected by chance, but without any assumptions of a specific genetic model. If this hypothesis is proven to be true, then segregation analysis will be performed to further test whether one or more major genes and/or polygenes can be considered to be related to the observed familial aggregation or the model of inheritance. Hence, formal genetic models are fit to the observed data on phenotypes. For both types of studies, family, rather than an individual, is the sampling unit and samples are obtained based on ascertainment of *probands* (i.e., individuals who caused a family to be identified).

Depending on the type of trait, appropriate sampling designs can be standard case–control or cohort studies (dichotomous traits) or large population-based series design (continuous traits). Based on the sampling schema, several specific study designs are commonly seen. Twin studies were done (e.g., breast cancer study conducted by Linchtenstein et al.[4]) on sample pairs of twins, where one exhibits the disease traits by including both identical and fraternal twins. The concordance rates of identical and fraternal twins are compared to examine whether the genetic effects can be separated from the environmental factors based on the assumption that the environmental factors are similar between identical and fraternal twins, but not genetic factors. Other designs include adoption studies[5] and inbreeding studies,[6] based on the assumption that the offspring of consanguineous mating are more likely to carry two copies of mutant alleles and hence be at increased risk of certain diseases. For segregation analysis, in order to maintain balance between avoiding ascertainment bias (by restricting to first-degree relatives) and maintaining sufficient power (by assembling large pedigrees), the sequential sampling of pedigrees method[7] can be considered.

Due to the complex dependences existing in genotype and phenotype data among subjects within families, and the fact that the degree of dependency varies according to familial ascertainment methods, the statistical analyses and hypothesis testing for familial aggregation and segregation analysis often involve advanced computational procedures, such as peeling algorithm,[8] Gibbs sampling (for a general background, see the textbook by Gilks et al.),[9] or generalized estimating equations[10] for an application to segregation analysis.

Linkage Analysis

Once the genetic effect on a certain disease is identified to be important, the next step is to determine the approximate chromosomal location of the disease-related gene by linkage analysis. The biological process of meiosis and recombination and their mathematical implications are the foundation of linkage analysis. Linkage happens during meiosis when two loci are situated on the same chromosome, and the degree of linkage is a function of how close the loci are to each other. Therefore, linkage analysis makes it possible to estimate the location of an unknown gene relative to one or more known markers (single gene, a set of genes, polymorphisms, etc.). In other words, the general location of a gene responsible for a trait can be estimated by linkage analysis on gene transmission within families. The parametric lod score method and the nonparametric relative pair method are two commonly used methods in linkage analysis. The relative pair methods are mainly useful for rapid screening of a large number of marker loci to look for promising linkage, but not the fine mapping of genes, as they provide simple significance hypothesis testing without the capability to estimate the recombination fraction. However, these methods are considered more robust than the lod score approach since no underlying genetic models are assumed. When the genetic models (similarity in phenotypes, similarity in marker alleles, a specific type of relationship is considered) are correctly specified based on previous knowledge of the disease, the lod score methods are more powerful than nonparametric methods.

The most widely used relative pair methods for dichotomous traits are based on affected pairs of siblings (sibs) since if a disease is rare, then an affected individual is much more likely to carry the disease gene. The hypothesis tested in such an analysis is whether the pairs of affected sibs are more likely to share marker alleles than random pairs of sibs. For an additive or rare dominant gene with two alleles, the number of alleles shared by the pairs of sibs can take values of 0, 1, and 2. The standard chi-square test with degrees of freedom (df) of 2, or the chi-square test for trend in proportion (df = 1) can be used to test the null hypothesis. In linkage analysis literature, the means test[11]—a *t*-test of comparing the mean proportion of alleles shared—is also commonly used.

Lod score methods are maximum likelihood–based methods. For the simplest situation, when all meioses can be classified as recombinants or non-recombinants in a two-point linkage problem, a standard likelihood ratio (LR) test can be used to test the null hypothesis that the recombination fraction is equal to one-half. Many times, this likelihood approach is generalized due to unknown parameters related to penetrance (probability of a phenotype given the genotype), Hardy-Weinberg population genotype probabilities, and transition probabilities. The number of unknown parameters increases substantially due to these generations; accordingly, the computational challenges increased exponentially.[8,12]

The statistical power of linkage analysis depends on many factors including the number of pairs, type of relationships, the genetic model, the magnitude of relative risk, the true recombination fraction, and the degree of polymorphism in the marker locus. Bias in selection of pedigrees and misspecifications of the genetic model and/or its parameters can further reduce the statistical power. Therefore, linkage analysis is most efficient for localizing relatively rare genes with very high penetrance. For complex traits that involve common polymorphisms with modest penetrance, multiple genes, confounding effects, and interactions, linkage analysis has very limited power and usage. For these genetic analyses, the association studies described in the next section should be considered.

Population Genetics

Although the chromosomal location of a hypothesized causal gene may be narrowed to a small region, further localization with a finer resolution is generally needed. This can be achieved by analyses of association with polymorphisms, known as linkage disequilibrium (LD) mapping, which then allows studies for casual relationship of the candidate gene with the trait of interest through gene association studies. The last step in the research of the etiology of disease is the gene characterization for the established causal gene and other factors affecting its penetrance. The key goal in such studies is to test the association between a trait (a measure representing the disease) and a candidate gene (multiple genes). Therefore, the study designs and statistical analysis methods for testing associations are essentially the same for the population genetics studies.

Generally speaking, standard statistical analysis methods are appropriate to be used in association studies when the individuals are uncorrelated (opposed to family-based sampling schema). For dichotomous traits, odds ratios (ORs) are the common estimates of the disease risks for the candidate genes. When cases and controls are not matched, chi-square test (or Fisher's exact test when sample size is not sufficient) and logistic regression are used for single categorical genetic variables and continuous or multiple genetic variables, respectively. For matched cases and controls, the analogies of the two are McNemar's test and conditional logistic regression. When the quantitative traits are under study, the gene association tests include standard *t*-test, F-test for multiple genes, and the corresponding regression analog.

A causal disease gene must present strong association between its genotype and the trait under study. However, a significant association is not sufficient to prove the causal relationship. For example, the apparent associations between genes and disease can be noncausal because they are in LD with another truly causal gene or are purely spurious, due to chance, drift, or population stratification. Although by itself alone when the true causal relationship cannot be determined, a well-designed association study is very efficient to eliminate noncausal genes whose associations are simply due to population stratification. On the other hand, by appropriately controlling confounding effects and reducing biases due to population heterogeneity (race, ethnicity, gender, etc.), other genes, and/or environmental risk factors, association studies can provide sufficient evidence to support further biological studies on an established disease gene.

The standard cohort or case–control designs are common designs for association studies. The primary characteristic to distinguish between when to use these two designs is the direction of inference. Cohort studies look forward in time from an exposure (candidate gene, for example) to disease, whereas case–control studies look backward from disease status to possible risk factors. The cohort design is preferred but generally requires large cohorts that are already established, probably for a different purpose, and the specimens can then be used to genotype the candidate gene that can be collected and stored. Since the genotypes do not change over time, it is possible to retrospectively (in a sense of data collection, not direction of inference) assess the disease risks of candidate genes with existing cohorts.[13]

In case–control studies, individuals are sampled based on their known disease status. In order to deliver valid inference regarding disease risks of genes under study, it is very important to insure that both cases and controls are representative of the target populations with respect to the expected allele frequencies. A major challenge is to obtain an appropriate control group. Different approaches will lead to different statistical analysis methods. We discuss two main approaches—population and family controls—with corresponding analysis procedures in the following paragraphs.

Population controls are sampled from the source population of cases, either with or without matching on appropriate confounders. Within this approach, the confounding bias due to a wide range of allele frequencies across subgroups is a major problem. It has been shown frequently that the noncausal associations found by case–control genetic studies are due to inadequately matched population control groups.[14] Recently, genomic control methods have been proposed to address the issue of population stratification. In this approach, a panel of polymorphic markers that are not linked to the candidate gene under study are incorporated in the analyses to detect and estimate subgroup differences.[15-19] The alternative to the challenges of population controls is to use family member controls to adjust for possible confounding impacts on gene association testing. The family members that can serve as controls in genetic case–control studies can be siblings, cousins, parents, and even extended pedigree family members. Careful consideration must be taken in the design to choose appropriate control members and corresponding statistical analysis methods.[20]

INDIVIDUALIZED RISK CLASSIFICATIONS AND OUTCOME PREDICTIONS

As more and more markers discovered through genetic association studies or biologic/pathologic research are validated to have clinical impact, it becomes feasible to explicitly and judiciously use the current best evidence to make decisions in diagnostic testing and treatment for cancer patients. In the current era of evidence-based medicine, clinical prediction models, designed to predict a diagnostic or prognostic outcome for an individual patient, increasingly play a critical role in bringing newly discovered markers into clinical practice. Prediction not only is an estimation problem but also generates a hypothesis testing problem. For example, validating a prognostic marker that has been newly developed requires one to test the hypothesis that determines whether the marker is an independent predictor of disease prognosis and provides additional value over classical, well-established predictors.[21] On the other hand, estimating the expected survival rate for a cancer patient based on the combined information that is related to the patient, the disease, and/or the treatment can provide meaningful decision-making aids for patient care. For both, appropriate study designs and sophisticated statistical modeling strategies based on available data are essential.

In this section, we discuss general concepts regarding developing, validating, updating, and presenting clinical prediction models. Suggested further reading on this topic includes textbooks by Steyerberg (2009)[22] and Harrell (2001).[23]

Study Designs for Generating and Validating Prediction Models

In general, the intended purpose of a prediction model defines the choice of study design including the specific patient population with one or more particular characteristics, the choices of outcome, and potential predictors, also including when and how the outcome and potential predicting factors should be measured and collected. Frequently, validation studies for a diagnosis are designed as a cross-sectional study, where the presence or absence of a particular symptom or sign (predictor) and the disease status (outcome) are examined on patients at one time point or over a short time span. In contrast, the cohort design is often used for prognostic studies, where the potential prognostic factors (demographics, disease characteristics, or markers of interest) are collected with the goal of predicting a clinical outcome, which usually requires following up patients over time. Data collection can be either retrospective or prospective. The case–control design may also apply to either diagnostic or prognostic studies, especially when the disease or the outcome event is relatively rare.

Single Cohort Studies

For building prognostic prediction models, there are several types of cohort studies often used including single-center retrospective studies, multicenter prospective studies, and registry studies. Table 24.1[22] tabulates the key characteristics, strengths, and limitations for each type of cohort study. In single-center studies, patients may be identified based on hospital records within a defined time period. This type of study is simple, with relatively low cost, and does not require integrated infrastructures. However, the retrospective nature of patient selection, likely inconsistent recording of predictors, and non-protocolized outcome data abstraction limit the usefulness of the prediction models based on single-center retrospective studies, due to potential selection biases, small sample size, inconsistent outcome and/or predictor assessment, frequent missing predictors, and/or poor follow-up for outcome. In general, registry studies are more attractive than single-center studies since the large databases, such as cancer registries or insurance databases, can provide a more representative study population with a larger sample size. However, registry studies still suffer from some of the same disadvantages as the single-center retrospective studies in

TABLE 24–1 Comparisons among Study Designs for Prognostic Studies[22]

Design	Characteristics	Strengths	Limitations
Retrospective cohort study	Often single-center studies	Simple, low costs	Selection of patients Definitions and completeness of predictors Outcome assessment not by protocol
Prospective cohort study	Often multicenter RCT	Well-defined selection of patients Prospective recording of predictors Prospective assessment of outcome According to protocol	Pool generalizability because of stringent inclusions and exclusion criteria
Registry cohort study	Complete coverage of an area/ participants covered by insurance	Simple, low costs Prospective recording of predictors	Outcome assessment not by protocol
Case–control	Efficient when outcome relatively rare	Simple, low costs	Selection of controls critical Definitions and completeness of predictors Outcome assessment not by protocols

RCT, randomized clinical trial.

terms of outcome assessment (i.e., not prespecified by protocol) and limited data collected on factors of interest.

It is well recognized that prospective cohort studies, especially the data collected in randomized clinical trials (RCTs), are always preferable to retrospective series. In these studies, not only is the selection of patient population well-defined but also the contents and procedures for data collection on predictors and outcomes can be predetermined in a unified fashion for patients from multiple centers. For RCTs, integrated infrastructures for trial conduct and data collection in general facilitate high-quality data, particularly regarding primary outcome measures. One may consider whether the stringent inclusion and exclusion criteria for patient selection will limit the generalizability of a prediction model based on the RCT data. However, since large RCTs usually accrue patients from multiple centers, or even multiple countries, the uniform protocol for patient selection and data collection in most cases actually strengthens the generalizability of the prediction model.

Multiple Cohort Studies

The increased awareness of collaborations among different research groups from academia, government, and industry makes it feasible to assemble large databases in a particular disease or subtype of disease. Pooled or meta-analyses data from multiple studies has emerged as a new trend in prognostic factors and patient risk/outcome prediction research. For example, the Adjuvant Colon Cancer Endpoints (ACCENT) collaborative group assembled a large database that included more than 33,000 individual patients' data from 24 large randomized phase III clinical trials worldwide. With a large sample size in a well-defined study population, proper control of unknown confounding factors, and high-quality data, this kind of collaborative large database has high potential to provide definitive inference regarding patient prognostic prediction.

It is acknowledged, however, that conducting RCTs is not always feasible in some settings, for example, in rare diseases. In this case, the series of retrospective studies will be a valuable data source for building a prediction model, if the following critical principals are closely followed: (1) the study design is prospectively defined. This includes clear and focused study objectives, the inclusion criteria of studies, and the prospectively specified statistical analysis plan; (2) individual patient data are available to consistently code important predictor variables and define relevant outcomes; (3) internal and external validation is feasible.

Outcomes and Predictors

In oncology, the outcomes of interest for diagnostic studies naturally are the disease status determined by radiological, pathological, or clinical assessments following standard guidelines. Therefore, the diagnostic outcomes are mostly binary outcomes. For prognostic research, overall survival has been used historically and will likely continue to be the primary outcome for cancer research since it is simple to measure, unambiguous, less subjective, and of unquestionable clinical relevance. Other outcomes, including tumor-related measures (for example, response rate, time to disease progression or recurrence, and recurrence-free or progression-free survival), are also of interest. The specific type of the outcomes of interest dedicates the type of statistical regression model that will be used to develop the prediction models. For example, the logistic regression and Cox proportion hazard model are very commonly used in oncology prognostic studies for binary and time-to-event outcomes, respectively.

To develop a well-performing prediction model, candidate predictors should be selected before initiating the study based on the considerations of clinical relevance, statistical strength, and practical usefulness. The selection of the potential predictors usually starts with newly discovered factors or markers with preliminary strong data, suggesting an impact on disease prognosis that is specific to the study purposes. Critically, previously established risk factors or prognostic markers should also be considered for inclusion since they could be confounders or effect modifiers. From the perspective of statistical strength, in addition to measurement accuracy (reliability and reproducibility of the predictors), the distribution or the prevalence of the predictors is also important. The strength of the predictors in the prediction model is a function of the association of the predictor with the outcome and its distribution. For example, a genetic marker with an OR of 2.0 and a prevalence of 50% is more relevant for a prediction model than a marker with an OR of 3.0 and a prevalence of 1%. Furthermore, predictors that can be obtained easily, non-invasively to the patient, at low cost, and that can be easily interpreted will make the prediction model more useful in practice.

Building a Prediction Model

Steyerberg[22] classified prediction model building strategies into seven steps: data inspection, coding of predictors, model specification, model estimation, model performance, model validation, and model presentation. Hence we provide brief descriptions of these seven modeling steps.

Data Inspection and Coding of Predictors

In prediction research, missing values of predictors in the dataset is a common problem, especially for those retrospective studies. The complete case analysis, where only patients with all predictors observed are included in the analysis, is easy to be implemented but generally statistically inefficient,[24] and the regression coefficient estimates may be biased.[25] Various imputation methods ranging from simple imputation to multiple imputation can be used to properly account for missing values in the regression analysis.[26-28] Conducting sensitivity analysis to assess the robustness of the prediction models and objectively reporting the nature of missingness and approaches to dealing with missing predictors are always recommended.

For building a prediction model, raw data from a study are usually not optimal for model selection and need to be carefully coded. For categorical predictors, combing small categories or applying penalized estimation or shrinkage provides stable estimates.[29,30] When a natural order is present among the categories for a predictor, functional forms that require less parameter estimations yet still provide sufficient fit to the data can be tested through model comparison tests, such as LR test for nested models. For continuous predictors, although categorization is thought to be suboptimal due to the loss of information, it can be very useful in prognostic prediction due to the ease of the interpretation. Continuous predictors can alternatively be modeled as smooth nonlinear functions, such as polynomials, fractional polynomials,[31] or restricted cubic spline functions.[32]

Model Specification and Estimation

Model specification is the core of the prediction model development and is also the most challenging step. There is no single best routine of model selection that can fit every prediction problem. For a particular prediction question, it is important to carefully prespecify the model selection strategies based on data availability and pay attention to critical issues including instability of selection, biased estimation of coefficients, and exaggerated *P* values.

Model specification involves reducing the number of predictors. In this step, the question of which predictor(s) is(are) of greatest importance to predict the outcome is examined through hypothesis testing procedures that are often automatic algorithms, such as stepwise selection. The common selection criterion for a predictor to stay in the model or to be removed is using a *P* value of 0.05. However, using a higher *P* value can provide better predictions in small datasets with a set of established candidate predictors.[33] Another aspect of model specification is testing interaction terms in multivariate regression models, i.e., testing whether the main effects are additive. The standard hypothesis testing in regression analysis (Score or LR tests) can be used to determine whether the interaction term is significant or not. The interpretation of a two-way interaction is that the effect of one predictor on outcome depends on the value of another predictor. Testing interaction terms usually requires large sample sizes.

Model Performance

In the development of prediction models, model performance refers to how good the predictions from the model are. In the simplest case of linear regression analysis, the coefficient of determination, R^2, is a useful overall performance measure. The interpretation of R^2 is the amount of variability seen in a continuous outcome explained by the predictors included in the linear regression model. R^2 takes values from 0 to 1, with values close to 1 indicating better overall model performance. For logistic and Cox regression models for binary and time-to-event outcomes, respectively, Nagelkerke's R^2 can be used for overall performance assessment.[34] The overall R^2 measures have two components—discrimination and calibration. These two concepts relate to each other, but have different relevance in relation to the aim of the prediction model.

In oncology, an important application of a prediction model is to classify patients into high- versus low-risk groups. In this case, the discrimination is the primary requirement for model performance assessment. The concordance (c) statistic is the most commonly used performance measure to indicate the discrimination ability of a prediction model. Harrell's overall c statistic is an extension used in Cox model for time-to-event outcome.[35] In other situations, it is more informative to provide a specific risk prediction probability for clinicians to make patient care decisions or discuss their decisions with patients. In this case, the calibration is an essential requirement. Calibration-in-the-large and calibration slope are two common measures for assessment of model calibration.[22]

Model Validation and Presentation

It is well recognized that validation of the finding from a prediction model built on the development dataset is a critical step to achieving clinical and practical usefulness. Internal validity refers to reproducibility of the model; this is often studied by assessing the validity on dataset coming from the same source as the development data. More critical is external validity that should be tested on an independent dataset, which is different but still a plausibly related population. Cross-validation[36] appears to be the most common technique used in medical research for internal validation. One extension of this method is bootstrap validation,[36] where the model is developed on bootstrapped samples and evaluated on original samples.

The simplest presentation of a prediction model is to present tables with ORs or hazard ratios (HRs) with confidence intervals. It is easy to see which predictors are more important; however, such tables are less useful to actually classify patients as being high versus low risk or calculating the absolute risk for individual patients. Depending on the purpose of the prediction model, better presentations are available. For example, a nomogram,[37] a graphical presentation of a prediction model (Fig. 24.1), is a common method to convey the inputs of patients' risk factor status or measures to a risk probability. Decision tree type of presentations based on a score chart rule[38] or a meta-model[39] can also provide an intuitive communication tool for a risk classification model.

DEVELOPING TARGETED AND PERSONALIZED THERAPIES

With increased understanding of the mechanism of the cancer at a genetic, molecular, or cellular level, cancer treatment development is continuously shifting toward targeted therapies that require the identification of a smaller subgroup of patients than standard RCTs. There are two key questions in testing targeted therapies that are essential to personalized patient care in oncology. First, one must validate that the marker predicts the differential efficacy of a targeted therapy, as assessed by a defined clinical endpoint, based on marker status.[40-42] The second is to formally verify the efficacy of a targeted therapy in the corresponding subpopulation, which can be identified by the predictive marker. Both questions need to be answered at the trial level rather than at the individual patient level. Fortunately, there are several clinical trial designs that can be applied to validate a predictive marker and establish the efficacy of a targeted therapy within a single study.

Retrospective Designs

When a prospective RCT may not be feasible due to ethical reasons or require unrealistically large sample size or a long time to complete,[42] retrospective validation using previously conducted prospective RCTs can provide the most important source of evidence and bring forward effective treatments to marker-defined subgroup of patients in a timely manner.[41-43] One example of applying this "retrospective–prospective" approach was the demonstration of the predictive value of KRAS gene status in advanced colorectal cancer. Several analyses based on the data from previously conducted RCTs in advanced

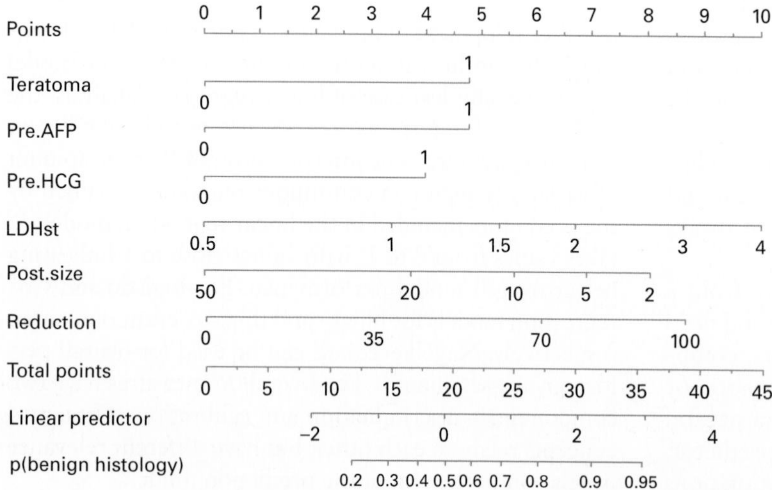

FIGURE 24–1 Example of a nomogram from a textbook written by Steyerberg.[22] Nomogram for benign histology based on six predictors in a penalized logistic regression model. Teratoma, teratoma elements in the primary tumor; Pre. AFP, pre-chemotherapy AFP normal/elevated; Pre. HCG, pre-chemotherapy HCG normal/elevated; LDHst, standardized pre-chemotherapy LDH (LDH divided by upper limit of normal values; 1 means values equal to upper normal); Post.size, post-chemotherapy mass size in mm; Reduction, % reduction in size during chemotherapy, e.g., 50–10 mm = 80%.

colorectal cancer have demonstrated that cetuximab[44-46] and panitumumab[47,48] are only effective in patients with KRAS wild-type status.

There are several essential elements that are required to provide convincing evidence for a biomarker to be validated as predictive based on retrospective data. First, in order to avoid selection bias, the samples on a large majority of patients should be available. Second, the analyses should be prospectively planned, specifically, (1) predefine the scoring system used for the biomarker measures to classify risk groups, (2) state focused hypotheses, (3) define the statistical methods, and (4) clarify the interpretational guidelines, e.g., level of statistical significance, magnitude of effect, etc. In addition, if several independent RCTs are available, concordant results across trials will provide strong evidence for a robust predictive effect.[41,42]

Enrichment or Targeted Designs

Enrichment or targeted designs have been proposed to evaluate a targeted therapy that is thought to have different activities in subgroups defined by a biomarker. In this design, only patients with biomarker-positive status (assuming this is the group where the new agent will have favorable efficacy) are enrolled and treated with the new agent. This is especially appealing when the proportion of truly benefiting patients is expected to be low.[49] In such a situation, an enrichment design can improve the efficiency of testing a drug in a targeted subpopulation (larger effect size, hence smaller sample size) and, possibly, clearly and quickly define an effective treatment for a subset of patients.[42,49] This design was utilized to evaluate the efficacy of trastuzumab in HER2-positive patients with early-stage breast cancer. Simon and Maitournam demonstrated that the enrichment design has higher relative efficiency in terms of required sample size and number of patients to be screened compared with a traditional RCT design without incorporating biomarkers. The magnitude of the efficiency gained depends on the accuracy of the assay and the prevalence of the markers in the population.[50,51] Other factors dictating an enrichment design include a well-established, reproducible assay and the infeasibility of an unselected design based on previous knowledge.[52]

Treatment-by-Marker Interaction Design

The treatment-by-marker interaction design (Fig. 24.2) uses the marker status as a stratification factor and randomizes patients in the marker-defined subgroups between experimental and control arms. The fundamental difference between this design and the common RCT is that only patients with a valid marker result are eligible and randomized. Therefore, the trial utilizing this design is truly a prospective marker validation trial that delivers the highest level of evidence.[40,41,52,53] This approach was used in the Marker Validation of Erlotinib in Lung Cancer (MARVEL) trial, in which patients were tested for epidermal growth factor receptor (EGFR) status and then randomized between erlotinib and pemetrexed as second-line treatment of non–small cell lung cancer.[54]

The sample size planning for treatment-by-marker interaction design is based on the prespecified analysis plan. A separate evaluation of the treatment effect can be tested in the two marker-defined subgroups or a preliminary test of interaction can be carried out first. Different sequential analysis plans can also be implemented. For example, when a preliminary test of interaction is not significant at a prespecified significance level, the treatment arms can be compared in the overall population (ignoring the biomarker status). If the interaction is significant, then the experimental treatment can be compared with the control arm within the strata determined by the marker.

Marker-Based Strategy Design

In this design, patients are randomized to two arms—a biomarker-directed arm and a biomarker-independent arm (Fig. 24.3). Patients in the biomarker-directed arm receive the experimental therapy if their biomarker status is positive or control treatment if their biomarker status is negative. Patients in the biomarker-independent arm receive the control treatment (or are randomized between

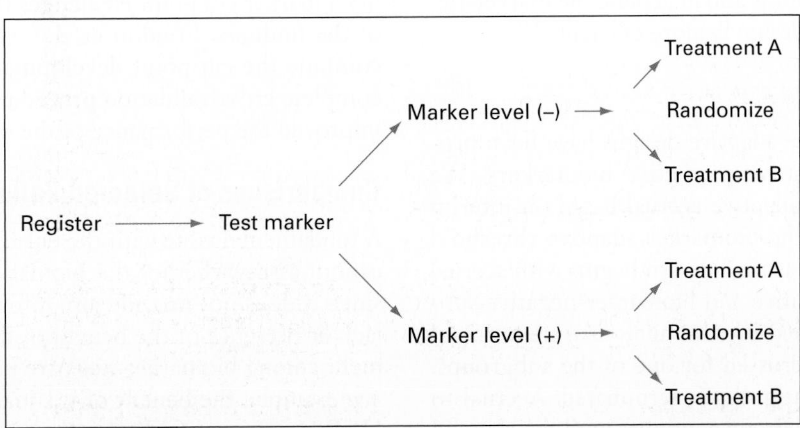

FIGURE 24–2 Treatment-by-marker interaction design as in Sargent et al.[40]

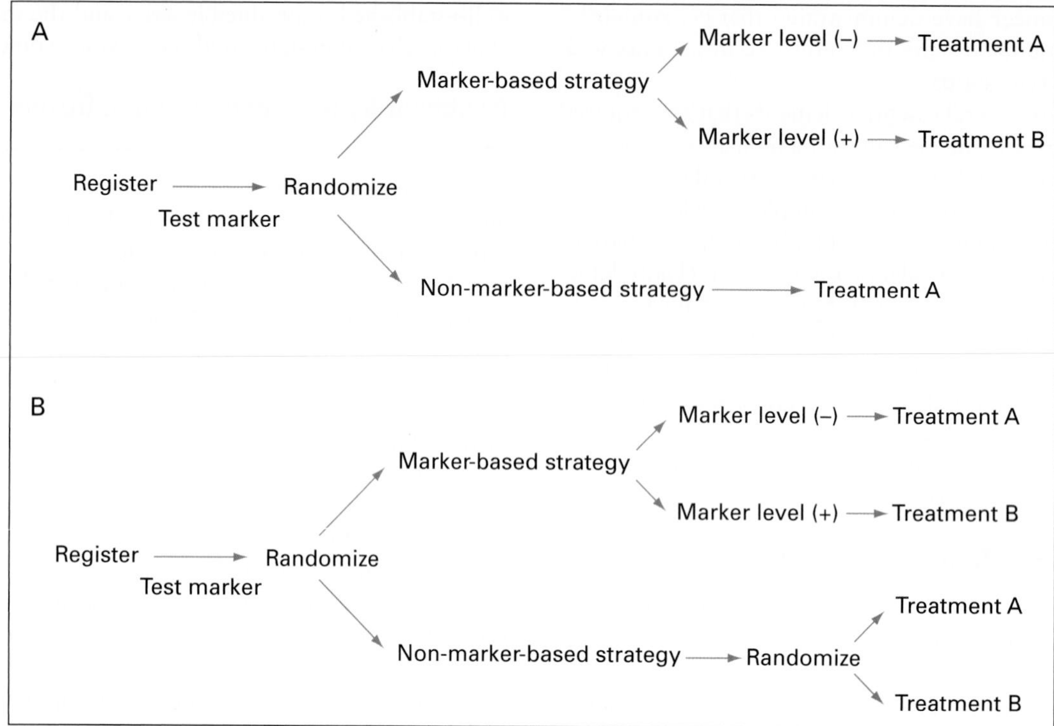

FIGURE 24–3 Marker-based strategy design as in Sargent et al.[40] **A:** Marker-based strategy design to test predictive factor question; no randomization in non–marker-based arm. **B:** Marker-based strategy design to test predictive factor question; no randomization in both arms.

experimental and control treatment) regardless of their biomarker status.[40,55,56] This design fits the paradigm of evaluating treatment effectiveness, i.e., the effect achieved when the marker is used in broad clinical practice, since it naturally estimates the "averaged" treatment effect when a biomarker-directed therapy will be used in a certain population of patients compared with control treatments.[57]

A limitation of this design is that in the absence of a very large treatment effect, it results in a very large sample size due to the significant overlap between the treatment arms. That is, in this design, there are patients in both the marker-directed and non–marker-directed arms receiving the same therapy. As such, the HR for comparing the two arms is forced toward unity, and in general the marker-by-treatment interaction design is more efficient.[52,58]

Adaptive Designs

A number of innovative adaptive designs have been proposed to validate putative predictive biomarkers. We briefly describe two—adaptive accrual based on interim analysis design[59] and the biomarker adaptive threshold design.[60] The adaptive accrual design begins with accrual to both biomarker-positive and biomarker-negative subgroups. At a prespecified interim analysis time point, if a futility boundary is crossed for one of the subgroups, then the accrual to that group is terminated. Accrual to the other biomarker subgroup continues until the planned sample size is reached, plus the unaccrued patients from the other subgroup that was terminated due to the futility analysis.[59]

The biomarker adaptive threshold design allows for the identification and validation of a cut point for a prespecified biomarker measured in an RCT. The advantages of this design are twofold. This design preserves the ability to evaluate the overall treatment effect in the unselected population. Second, it allows for the prospective validation of a biomarker without a predefined cutoff for risk group classification. This design involves testing the overall treatment effect and indentifying the optimal cut point for the biomarker.[60] However, the fact that the data from the same trial are used for both defining and validating a marker cut point challenges the external robustness of the findings. Freidlin et al.[57] extended this design to combine the cut point development and validation in a complete cross-validation procedure, which considerably improved the performance of the original design.

Comparisons of Selected Validation Designs

A fundamental issue with the enrichment design is that it cannot assess whether the biomarker is truly predictive, since it does not provide any information regarding the lack or presence of the benefit of the experimental treatment among biomarker-negative patients. In the HER2/*neu* example, the benefit of trastuzumab in patients with HER2/*neu* amplified tumors has been established by several large randomized trials.[61] However, it has been suggested that trastuzumab is perhaps beneficial in patients beyond the specific HER2/*neu* status used in the adjuvant trials when the biomarker was retested in central laboratories.[62,63] This suggests that an unselected design (treatment-by-marker interaction or marker-based strategy design) may be indicated even when the prior assumption is that the regimen will only work in marker-positive patients. In addition, in case of the therapy truly benefiting some subset of patients, if the biomarker targets the wrong subpopulation, then a promising regimen could mistakenly be abandoned.[57]

The primary goal of the treatment-by-marker interaction design is to maximize the advantage of randomization and allow the relevant questions to be addressed at both the subpopulation and overall population levels. Furthermore, this design provides rigorous evidence to determine the best treatment in both the biomarker-positive and the biomarker-negative subgroups.[31] If, however, there are a large number of regimens to be tested, or a treatment decision is to be based on a panel of biomarkers, the treatment-by-marker interaction design is not feasible but the marker-based strategy design could remain useful.

CONCLUDING REMARKS

In the current era, advances in laboratory technologies are rapidly increasing the discovery of potential medically or clinically useful markers. These markers can be the measures that reflect biological, pathogenic, or pharmacologic processes. In oncology, as genetic research advances toward whole-genome sequencing, the discovery of a large number of genetic loci has provided great insights into the molecular basis of inherited disease and the role of structural variation in disease.[64] However, at this point very few genomic or molecular markers have been successfully adapted in routine clinical practice, for example, as predictors of drug toxicities, assisting for dose adjustment, or aiding the decision of a particular targeted treatment for patients.[65] Transferring the discoveries in laboratory and genetics into clinical practice is a huge undertaking. This is a continuous and iterative process involving the following steps:

- Initial discoveries from laboratory biology research, genetic mapping studies, etc.
- Establishment of the diagnostic or prognostic value of individual molecular or genetic markers through genetic association studies or clinical retrospective studies.
- Establishment of personalized clinical usefulness of these markers at the patient level by developing the validated diagnostic or prognostic prediction models that integrate multiple markers to provide comprehensive insights into a patient's disease course.
- Development of effective targeted therapies with corresponding validated predictive markers to deliver personalized patient care.

Bioinformatics and biostatistics play critical roles in each of these steps. In this chapter, we have reviewed the study designs and statistical methods that are tailored to each area. We hope that through increased awareness of available design options, variations of statistical methods due to the nature of different research stage, and alternative powerful statistical methods that are not routinely used in medical research, progress toward timely personalized medicine can be accelerated.

REFERENCES

1. Haines JL, Pericak-Vance MA, eds. *Approaches to Gene Mapping in Complex Human Diseases*. 1st ed. New York, NY: Wiley-Liss, a John Wiley & Sons, Publication; 1998.
2. Thomas DC. *Statistical Methods in Genetic Epidemiology*. 1st ed. New York, NY: Oxford University Press; 2004.
3. Thomas DC, Karagas MR. Migrant studies. In: Schottenfeld D, Fraumeni JFJ, eds. *Cancer Epidemiology and Prevention*. 2nd ed. Oxford: Oxford University Press; 1996:63-76.
4. Linchtenstein P, Holm NV, Verkasalo PK, et al. Environmental and heritable factors in the causation of cancer—analyses of cohorts of twins from Sweden, Denmark, and Finland. *N Engl J Med*. 2000;343:78-85.
5. Ingraham LJ, Katy SS. Adoption studies of schizophrenia. *Am J Med Genet*. 2000;256:804-808.
6. Wright S. Coefficients of inbreeding and relationship. *Am Nat*. 1922;56:330-338.
7. Cannings C, Thompson EA. Ascertainment in the sequential sampling of pedigrees. *Clin Genet*. 1977;12:208-212.
8. Elston RC, Stewart J. A general model for the genetic analysis of pedigrees. *Hum Hered*. 1971;21:523-542.
9. Gilks W, Richardson S, Spiegelhalter D, eds. *Markov Chain Monte Carlo in Practice*. London: Chapman and Hall; 1996.
10. Lee H, Stram DO, Thomas D. A generalized estimating equation approach to fitting major gene models in segregation analysis of continuous phenotypes. *Genet Epidemiol*. 1993;10:61-74.
11. Blackwelder WC, Elston RC. A comparison of sib-pair linkage tests for disease susceptibility loci. *Genet Epidemiol*. 1985;2: 85-97.
12. Lander ES, Green P. Construction of multilocus genetic linkage maps in humans. *Proc Natl Acad Sci U S A*. 1987;84:2363-2367.
13. Langholz B, Rothman N, Wacholder S, et al. Cohort studies for characterizing measured genes. *Monogr Natl Cancer Inst*. 1999;26:39-42.
14. London S, Daly A, Thomas D, et al. Methodological issues in the interpretation of studies of the CYP 2D6 genotype in relation to lung cancer risk. *Pharmacogenetics*. 1994;4:107-108.
15. Devlin B, Roeder K. Genomic control for association studies. *Biometrics*. 1999;55:997-1004.
16. Pritchard JK, Stephens M, Donnelly P. Inference of population structure using multilocus genotype data. *Genetics*. 2000;155: 945-959.
17. Schork NJ, Fallin D, Thiel B, et al. The future of genetic case-control studies. In: Rao DC, Province M, eds. *Genetic Dissection of Complex Traits*. San Diego, CA: Academic Press; 2001:191-212.
18. Pritchard JK, Stephens M, Rosenberg NA, et al. Association mapping in structured populations. *Am J Hum Genet*. 2000;67:170-181.
19. Satten GA, Flanders WD, Yang Q. Accounting for unmeasured population substructure in case-control studies of genetic association using a novel latent-class model. *Am J Hum Genet*. 2001;68:466-477.
20. Schaid DJ, Rowland C. Use of parents, sibs and unrelated controls for detection of association between genetic markers and disease. *Am J Hum Genet*. 1998;63:1492-1506.
21. Kattan MW. Judging new markers by their ability to improve predictive accuracy. *J Natl Cancer Inst*. 2003;95:634-635.
22. Steyerberg EW. *Clinical Prediction Models: A Practical Approach to Development, Validation and Updating*. New York, NY: Springer; 2009.

23. Harrell FE. *Regression Modeling Strategies: With Applications to Linear Models, Logistic Regression, and Survival Analysis*. New York, NY: Springer; 2001.
24. Greenland S, Finkle WD. A critical look at methods for handling missing covariates in epidemiologic regression analyses. *Am J Epidemiol.* 1995;142:1255-1264.
25. Vach W, Blettner M. *Missing Data in Epidemiologic Studies. Encyclopedia of Biostatistics*. New York, NY: Wiley; 1998:2641-2654.
26. Enders CK. A primer on the use of modern missing-data methods in psychosomatic medicine research. *Psychosom Med.* 2006;68:427-436.
27. Little RJA, Rubin DB. *Statistical Analysis with Missing Data*. 2nd ed. Hoboken, NJ: Wiley; 2002.
28. Rubin DB. Inference and missing data. *Biometrika.* 1976;63:581-592.
29. Smits M, Dippel DW, Steyerberg EW, et al. Predicting intracranial traumatic findings on computed tomography in patients with minor head injury: the CHIP prediction rule. *Ann Intern Med.* 2007;146:397-405.
30. Verveij PJ, van Houwelingen HC. Penalized likelihood in Cox regression. *Stat Med.* 1994;13:2427-2436.
31. Royston P, Sauerbrei W. Improving the robustness of fractional polynomial models by preliminary covariate transformation: a pragmatic approach. *Comput Stat Data Anal.* 2007;51:4240-4253.
32. Harrell FE Jr, Lee KL, Pollock BG. Regression models in clinical studies: determining relationships between predictors and response. *J Natl Cancer Inst.* 1988;80:1198-1202.
33. Steyerberg EW, Eijkemans MJ, Harrell FE Jr, Habbema JD. Prognostic modeling with logistic regression analysis: a comparison of selection and estimation methods in small data sets. *Stat Med.* 2000;19:1059-1079.
34. Nagelkerke NJ. A note on a general definition of the coefficient of determination. *Biometrika.*1991:78:691-692.
35. Harrell FE Jr, Lee KL, Califf RM, Pryor DB, Rosati RA. Regression modeling strategies for improved prognostic prediction. *Stat Med.* 1984;3:143-152.
36. Efron B, Tibshirani R. *An Introduction to the Bootstrap*. New York, NY: Chapman & Hall; 1993.
37. Lubsen J, Pool J, van der Does E. A practical device for the application of a diagnostic or prognostic function. *Methods Inf Med.* 1978;17:127-129.
38. Michel P, Roques F, Nashef SA. Logistic or additive EuroSCORE for high-risk patients? *Eur J Cardiothorac Surg.* 2003;23:684-687.
39. Steyerberg EW, Keizer HJ, Habbema JD. Prediction models for the histology of residual masses after chemotherapy for metastatic testicular cancer. ReHiT study group. *Int J Cancer.* 1999;83:856-859.
40. Sargent DJ, Conley BA, Allegra C, Collette L. Clinical trial designs for predictive marker validation in cancer treatment trials. *J Clin Oncol.* 2005;23:2020-2027.
41. Buyse M, Sargent DJ, Grothey A, et al. Biomarkers and surrogate end points—the challenge of statistical validation. *Nat Rev Clin Oncol.* 2010;7:309-317.
42. Buyse M, Michiels S, Sargent DJ, et al. Integrating biomarkers in clinical trial. *Expert Rev Mol Diagn.* 2011;11:171-182.
43. Simon RM, Paik S, Hayes DF. Use of archived specimens in evaluation of prognostic and predictive biomarkers. *J Natl Cancer Inst.* 2009;101:1446-1452.
44. Karapetis CS, Khambata-Ford S, Jonker DJ, et al. K-ras mutations and benefit from cetuximab in advanced colorectal cancer. *N Engl J Med.* 2008;359:1757-1765.
45. Van Cutsem E, Lang I, D'haens G, et al. KRAS status and efficacy in the first-line treatment of patients with metastatic colorectal cancer (mCRC) treated with FOLFIRI with or without cetuximab: the CRYSTAL experience. *J Clin Oncol.* 2008;(suppl):5s.
46. Bokemeyer G, Bondarenko I, Makhson A, et al. Fluorouracil, leucovorin, and oxaliplatin with and without cetuximab in the first-line treatment of metastatic colorectal cancer. *J Clin Oncol.* 2009;27:663-671.
47. Amado RG, Wolf M, Peeters M, et al. Wild-type KRAS is required for panitumumab efficacy in patients with metastatic colorectal cancer. *J Clin Oncol.* 2008;26:1626-1634.
48. Freeman D, Juan T, Meropol NJ, et al. Association of KRAS gene mutations and clinical outcome in patients with metastatic colorectal cancer receiving panitumumab monotherapy. In 14th European Cancer Conference; September 23-27, Barcelona, Spain.
49. McShane LM, Hunsberger S, Adjei AA. Effective incorporation of biomarkers into phase II trials. *Clin Cancer Res.* 2009;15:1898-1905.
50. Simon R, Maitournam A. Evaluating the efficiency of targeted designs for randomized clinical trials. *Clin Cancer Res.* 2004;10:6759-6763.
51. Maitournam A, Simon R. On the efficiency of targeted clinical trials. *Stat Med.*2005;24:329-339.
52. Mandrekar SJ, Sargent DJ. Clinical trial designs for predictive biomarker validation: one size does not fit all. *J Biopharm Stat.* 2009;19:530-542.
53. Mandrekar SJ, Sargent DJ. Clinical trial designs for predictive biomarker validation: theoretical considerations and practical challenges. *J Clin Oncol.* 2009;27:4027-4034.
54. Pemetrexed or erlotinib as second-line therapy in treating patients with advanced non-small cell lung cancer. http://www.clinicaltrials.gov/ct2/show/NCT00738881?term=NCT00738881&rank=1, 2009.
55. Sargent D, Allegra C. Issues in clinical trial design for tumor marker studies. *Semin Oncol.* 2002;29:222-230.
56. Mandrekar SJ, Grothey A, Goetz MP, Sargent DJ. Clinical trial designs for prospective validation of biomarkers. *Am J Pharmacogenomics.* 2005;5:317-325.
57. Freidlin B, McShane LM, Korn EL. Randomized clinical trials with biomarkers: design issues. *J Natl Cancer Inst.* 2010;102:152-160.
58. Hoering A, Leblanc M, Crowley JJ. Randomized phase III clinical trial designs for targeted agents. *Clin Cancer Res.* 2008;14:4358-4367.
59. Wang SJ, O'Neill RT, Hung HM. Approaches to evaluation of treatment effect in randomized clinical trials with genomic subset. *Pharm Stat.* 2007;6:227-244.
60. Jiang W, Freidlin B, Simon R. Biomarker-adaptive threshold design: a procedure for evaluating treatment with possible biomarker-defined subset effect. *J Natl Cancer Inst.* 2007;99:1036-1043.
61. Romond EH, Perez EA, Bryant J, et al. Trastuzumab plus adjuvant chemotherapy for operable HER2-positive breast cancer. *N Engl J Med.* 2005;353:1673-1684.
62. Paik S, Kim C, Jeong J, et al. Benefit from adjuvant trastuzumab may not be confined to patient with IHC 3+ and/or FISH-positive tumors: central testing results from NSABP B-31. *J Clin Oncol.* 2007;25:511.
63. Perez EA, Romond EH, Suman VJ, et al. Updated results of the combined analysis of NCCTG N9831 and NSABP B-31 adjuvant chemotherapy with/without trastuzumab in patients with HER2-positive breast cancer. *J Clin Oncol.* 2007;25:512.
64. Green ED, Guyer MS. Charting a course for genomic medicine from base pairs to bedside. *Nature.* 2011;470:204-213.
65. Tajik P, Bossuyt PM. Genomic markers to tailor treatments: waiting or initiating? *Hum Genet.* 2011;130:15-18.

CHAPTER 25

In Vitro Companion Diagnostic and Anti-cancer Drug Co-development: Regulatory Perspectives

Reena Philip, Elizabeth Mansfield, Lea Carrington, Yun-Fu Hu, and Maria Chan

INTRODUCTION

Recently, cancer researchers and pharmaceutical and biotechnology companies have devoted greater attention to an integral part of the therapeutic equation: the so-called companion diagnostic tests that are needed to determine not only whether a patient's tumor expresses the molecule being targeted but also whether that expression correlates with the patient's response to the treatment. The importance of companion diagnostics has recently gained momentum particularly in oncology, with the realization that good biomarkers can potentially help pharmaceutical companies to find targets in discovery much faster and to design clinical trials in a more effective and efficient way. Moving away from "nonselective therapeutics" to personalized medicine has made the companion diagnostic essential to individualizing patient care. The success of personalized medicine depends in part on safe and effective in vitro diagnostics. This chapter addresses companion diagnostic tests, also considered in vitro diagnostic (IVD) devices reviewed by FDA within the Office of In Vitro Diagnostic Device Evaluation and Safety (OIVD).[1]

Co-development is the development of a diagnostic device (test) and a therapeutic (drug/biologic) that are intended to be used together. Co-development is a term used to describe the process of developing a companion diagnostic[2] to meet the need for supporting a therapeutic claim. There are several scenarios in which a drug company might choose to develop a diagnostic device to identify a population of patients, including a diagnostic that will identify patients: (1) for whom the drug is expected to be effective; (2) for whom the drug is expected to have minimal or no effect; (3) who would likely have serious adverse events; or (4) who would likely receive greater benefit or have lower probability for adverse events from one drug than another. The most common type of companion diagnostic claim to date is to select patients who match the population studies in the pivotal therapeutic trial (selection claim). A companion diagnostic device can also be intended to monitor response to drug therapy or to select doses of the drug most likely to be effective and/or safe to the patient. Co-development can be initiated at any stage of therapeutic development—whenever it is identified that the drug and the diagnostic test should be used together. Co-development as a concept does not require actual development of a *new* test or a *new* drug, but rather it requires the development of evidence that a diagnostic test adequately informed therapeutic use. Therefore, co-development may also include development of a *new use* for an already cleared or approved test or of a drug such that it requires a companion diagnostic in order to be found safe and effective for the new use.

If performance of the companion diagnostic test is poor or variable, because of poor measurement quality, poor choice of the marker of interest, or lack of sufficient

This chapter includes scientific opinions of the authors and should not be interpreted as establishing new FDA policies, procedures, or positions.

validation in the specific therapeutic context of use, the performance of the therapeutic that depends on the diagnostic result likely will be unpredictable. For example, with an incorrect diagnostic result, an unsuitable drug may be given to a patient who may as a result be harmed, or will not benefit, because the drug will cause an otherwise avoidable adverse event, or will be ineffective for that patient, or both. Therefore, appropriate design and validation of the diagnostic test is crucial in order to gain the best risk–benefit profile for the accompanying therapeutic.

IN VITRO DIAGNOSTIC DEVICES

An IVD is a type of medical device. The definition of a medical device[2] as defined in the Federal Food, Drug, & Cosmetic Act (FD&C Act) includes "an instrument, apparatus, implement, machine, contrivance, implant, in vitro reagent, or other similar or related article, including any component, part, or accessory, which is intended for use in the diagnosis of disease or other conditions, or in the cure, mitigation, treatment, or prevention of disease, in man or other animals, or intended to affect the structure or any function of the body of man ... , and which does not achieve its primary intended purposes through chemical action within or on the body of man or other animals and which is not dependent upon being metabolized for the achievement of its primary intended purposes." By regulation, FDA has further defined "in vitro diagnostic products,"[3] or IVDs, as a specific subset of medical devices that include "...those reagents, instruments, and systems intended for use in the diagnosis of disease or other conditions, including a determination of the state of health, in order to cure, mitigate, treat, or prevent disease or its sequelae." Currently, most companion diagnostics belong to the IVD category of medical devices.

CLASSIFICATION OF IVDs

Devices regulated by FDA are assigned one of three classes related to the level of FDA oversight needed in order to assure that the product is safe and effective when it is commercially marketed.[4] Classification is risk based, that is, the risk the device poses to the patient and/or the user is a major factor in the class it is assigned. Class I includes devices with the lowest risk and Class III includes those with the greatest risk.

Class I devices are those where a more general type of regulatory oversight is considered sufficient to provide reasonable assurance of safety and effectiveness. In general, Class I devices are those that are well understood and present minimal risk of harm to patients, and many of these types of devices are exempt from premarket notification to FDA.

Class II devices generally carry more risk of harm to a patient than those in Class I, and premarket submissions (termed 510(k)s) for these devices are reviewed by FDA to determine whether they are similar (substantially equivalent in terms of safety and effectiveness) to another legally marketed device that is intended for the same type of use.

Class III devices have the highest risk, or potential to present significant harm to patients, and these devices usually require a premarket application (which involves a more in-depth review of the safety and effectiveness of the device).

Some of the major risks typically considered for IVDs are the consequences of incorrect results. For example, if a consequence of a false-positive test result is an invasive medical procedure or an unnecessary therapy with toxic side effects, this type of test would generally be considered higher risk, since a falsely positive test result will likely lead to substantial harm to the patient. Similarly, a falsely negative test result might adversely alter medical management and the appropriate intervention for the patient may be unnecessarily delayed, or not pursued at all, again with the potential to result in substantial harm to the patient.

PATHWAYS TO BRING AN IVD TO MARKET

As alluded to above, there are different pathways to get an in vitro diagnostic product to market. Depending on the nature of the test and its classification, the product could be reviewed as a premarket notification (510(k))[5] submission with a 90-day review timeline or as a premarket approval (PMA)[6] submission with a 180-day review timeline.

The PMA is the most comprehensive type of premarket submission for devices within Center for Devices and Radiological Health (CDRH) and is the premarket submission type for Class III devices. In determining the safety and effectiveness of a Class III device, FDA considers the following, among other relevant factors[4]: the persons for whose use the device is represented or intended; the conditions of use for the device, including conditions of use prescribed, recommended, or suggested in the labeling or advertising of the device and other intended conditions of use; the probable benefit to health from the use of the device weighed against any probable injury or illness from such use; and the reliability of the device. FDA relies on valid scientific evidence to determine whether there is reasonable assurance that the device is safe and effective. In studies supporting PMAs (see reference[8] for examples), device results have been compared with some measure of truth, such as diagnosis or treatment outcome, determined prior to the beginning of the study. Studies have been carefully designed to show statistical and clinical significance of the results, which included clinical sensitivity and specificity as well as (where relevant) positive and negative predictive values. FDA may also require other conditions of approval for Class III devices, for example, inspection of manufacturing facilities prior to approval. In addition, required periodic reports[7] are typically submitted annually.

Thus far, several IVD companion diagnostic devices have been classified as Class III devices.[8] These determinations include consideration of a likelihood of harm to the patient if the diagnostic result is incorrect and the regulatory oversight determined to be needed to provide reasonable assurance of safety and effectiveness of the devices. Changes in diagnostic performance of these devices, for example, due to unmonitored product modifications or inconsistent manufacture have potential to severely harm patients if the therapeutic performance will depend on diagnostic results.

In addition to the 510(k) and PMA pathways, the humanitarian device exemption (HDE)[9] and investigational device exemption (IDE)[10,11] are the two other pathways that allow an IVD to be used legally for clinical diagnostic use.

Currently, where the investigational setting is a therapeutic clinical trial, investigational device requirements found in 21 Code of Federal Regulations (CFR) Part 812 can be addressed either as a part of the therapeutic investigational new drug (IND) application submitted (usually as an amendment to the IND) for review by Center for Drug Evaluation and Research (CDER) or Center for Biologics Evaluation and Research (CBER) and/or as an IDE submitted for review by CBER or CDRH. In either case, all relevant review Centers will interact to assure that both the therapeutic and the diagnostic are addressed with the appropriate investigational controls in the trial.

IN VITRO DIAGNOSTIC PRODUCTS: EVIDENCE FOR SAFETY AND EFFECTIVENESS

Review and clearance or approval of in vitro diagnostic products requires evidence of device safety and effectiveness. The concepts of safety and effectiveness can be phrased in two questions as follows:

- ***Evidence for safety:*** Are there reasonable assurances based on valid scientific evidence that the probable benefits to health from use of the device outweigh any probable risks? [US FDA: Code of Federal Regulations Title 21 §860.7(d)[1]]
- ***Evidence for effectiveness:*** Is there reasonable assurance based on valid scientific evidence that the use of the device in the target population will provide clinically significant results? [US FDA: Code of Federal Regulations Title 21 §860.7(e)[1]]

The evidence to provide a reasonable assurance of safety and effectiveness will differ somewhat from device to device, according to the way in which the device is intended to be used.

BIOMARKER VERSUS IVD

There is a misperception that a biomarker and an IVD are the same. A biomarker[12] has been defined as an analyte (or group of analytes or features) that is measurable and informative as an indicator of normal biologic processes, pathogenic processes, or pharmacologic responses to a therapeutic intervention. The validity of a biomarker is demonstrated through evidence of accurate and reproducible measurement of the biomarker in an analytical test system with well-established performance characteristics. FDA generally reviews the analytical and clinical validity of diagnostic devices (tests) for biomarkers to help determine the safety and effectiveness (or substantial equivalence in terms of safety and effectiveness) of the IVD. There may be multiple valid tests for the same biomarker. As opposed to a biomarker, which simply has an established relationship to a physiologic process, an IVD has a specific intended use, has specific performance parameters, and is shown to be safe and effective (or substantial equivalence in terms of safety and effectiveness) for its intended use. In addition, there are other controls applicable to medical devices which are not applicable to a biomarker alone. For instance, IVDs for clinical use are designed and manufactured under the Quality System Regulations.[13] IVD adverse events have to be reported[14] and procedures must be established and maintained for implementing corrective and preventive actions.[15]

BIOMARKER EFFECTS

Some biomarkers can discriminate normal from diseased states (i.e., diagnostic biomarkers), while others predict the likely course of disease progression (i.e., prognostic biomarkers), response to therapy (i.e., predictive biomarkers), or drug effect (i.e., pharmacodynamic biomarkers). It is important to understand the distinction between prognostic and predictive markers, their uses, and the information they provide. In addition, FDA review generally includes different types of supporting information depending on the use of the biomarker that a test is intended to measure.

Some biomarkers can predict which patients will benefit from a drug. For example, patients who express the particular biomarker will benefit and patients who do not express the biomarker will not benefit. This is the essence of a predictive biomarker. For an IVD intended for testing such a biomarker, comparison of the drug effect in the biomarker-positive group with the drug effect in the biomarker-negative group to support the predictive claim is generally most relevant.

If the expression of a biomarker simply denotes the aggressiveness of the disease without regard to how the disease is treated, it is in essence a prognostic biomarker. For an IVD with a prognostic claim, the future state (e.g., more aggressive disease vs. stable disease) among a group of patients who are otherwise considered to be similar is most relevant. Prognostic claims are generally not related to drug effect since only the base state, and not the different treatments applied, is part of the outcome comparisons.

COMPANION DIAGNOSTIC TEST DEVELOPMENT: ISSUES TO CONSIDER

Through the critical path initiative, several guidances, and stakeholder meetings,[16-20] FDA is collaboratively working with manufacturers to bring qualified biomarkers into the clinical setting. The following are some important points to consider during the test development.

The "Intended Use"

The device "Intended Use"[21] is key in the FDA evaluation of a submission. Manufacturers provide valid scientific evidence to FDA to provide reasonable assurance that the device is safe and effective for its intended use and conditions for use. Typically, this includes the performance characteristics based on well-designed analytical and clinical studies.

Pre-analytical Factors

One important component in understanding the performance characteristics of a new test is the impact of pre-analytical[22-28] factors on the test result. It is generally useful to determine optimal materials and methods for sample collection and processing prior to test validation. A reasonable goal is for collection procedures to minimize non-biologic variability of the analyte(s) to be measured and thus of the test results. Some steps that may impact performance are sample collection procedures and materials; storage and handling conditions for collected specimens; stability controls to assure analyte stability over time; and specimen rejection criteria, including assessment of sample quality and quantity (e.g., minimum amount of tumor tissue or peripheral blood required to yield a valid test result). Numerous other pre-analytical factors could affect the quality of test results, so careful consideration, and measures to control these factors, can be important. In addition, it is useful to build quality control steps into the assay and to provide information such as criteria for (1) sample/biopsy quality, (2) input sample quality, and (3) process quality.

Analytical Validation

Another key step in test development is the validation of the test's analytical performance parameters. Analytical performance parameters relevant for testing may vary with the intended use, the technology, quantitative versus qualitative, use setting (e.g., single laboratory vs. multiple laboratories), how results are reported (e.g., signature vs. individual markers), and the end user (e.g., laboratories vs. physicians). Analytical validation measures may include accuracy, precision/reproducibility, limit of detection, limit of quantification, analytical specificity, interfering substances, cut-off value, stability, instrumentation variability, and other appropriate parameters. For example, precision includes identifying factors that may impact the performance of the test under altered conditions, e.g., day-to-day variation, lot-to-lot variation, lab-to-lab variation, operator-to-operator variation, and variation among instruments, among operators, and/or labs. Well-designed precision studies capture the total potential test variability from specimen preparation to the final result. For tests with a cut-off value, it is typically important for precision studies to demonstrate performance estimates of the assay at or near medical decision points, e.g., around the cut-off(s). For an assay claiming a quantitative score, evaluating precision at numerous analyte levels may be relevant to estimate performance over the measurement range of the device. With a multivariate assay in which multiple analytes are measured and all results are combined in to the score, this can be a complex task. See, for example, the FDA Guidance Document: Ovarian Adnexal Mass Assessment Score Test System, http://www.fda.gov/MedicalDevices/DeviceRegulationandGuidance/GuidanceDocuments/ucm237299.htm.

If the device is used with a specific instrument and software, FDA recommends that the manufacturers refer to the following FDA Guidance documents[29]:

- Instrumentation for Clinical Multiplex Test Systems
- Content of Premarket Submissions for Software Contained in Medical Devices
- General Principles of Software Validation
- Off-the-Shelf Software Use in Medical Devices
- Cybersecurity for Networked Medical Devices Containing Off-the-Shelf (OTS) Software.

Clinical Validation

The design of clinical validation studies for companion diagnostics calls for careful consideration. For companion diagnostic devices, data regarding the therapeutic–test interaction from the drug trial are fundamental. It is ideal to have an analytically validated device prior to testing samples for the pivotal clinical trial. Generally in well-designed trials, the test, including the cut-off, is fully developed prior to the independent clinical validation or pivotal trial, which is typically one or more Phase III clinical trials or in some rare cases, a Phase II trial submitted for accelerated approval. Subject inclusion and exclusion criteria consistent with the intended use of the device are an important consideration in clinical validation. An appropriate therapeutic study design generally includes taking into account how the performance of the test in the trial will be demonstrated, using statistical principles and objective end points, prior to the start of the study. Although most companion diagnostic validation studies to date have been prospectively enrolled Phase III drug trial studies, there may be scenarios, such as for drug safety claims, where the use of prospectively collected, retrospectively analyzed samples would be appropriate. However, there are several key factors to consider regarding the suitability of retrospectively analyzed samples, including (1) whether the storage conditions for the specimens impact the assay, (2) whether available specimens are representative of the intended use of the device (and often, whether an unbiased sample set can be obtained) based on well-annotated records, (3) whether specimens meet a prespecified set of inclusion/exclusion criteria, such as consecutive collection, and (4) whether the performance assessed is comparable to that expected with a prospective study.

In some studies, investigators have opted to use more than one version of a test to select patients for a pivotal therapeutic trial. A disadvantage of this approach is that using more than one version of the test in the studies may make it difficult to understand the potential impact of test design on drug performance, i.e., differences in performance between different versions of a test may introduce variables that result in the selection of a different spectrum of subjects, without the ability to identify who the "correct" population will be when the therapy is reviewed. In some cases, there is only a subset of the therapeutic trial samples available for analysis after a change is made to the diagnostic test. In certain situations, a subset of samples from the studies may be available to bridge between the different test versions; however, the potential to introduce bias is greatly increased when subsets are used, and it is often impossible to assure that no biases are generated. Any of these situations may make it difficult to characterize which patients are appropriate (or inappropriate, if applicable) for treatment. It is important to consider the impact of using different versions of a test, and of introduction of bias by sample subsetting in bridging studies, so that questions of test performance with the approved therapy are minimized. If a test other than the one intended to be marketed is used to select subjects for a clinical trial (often referred to as a "clinical trial assay" or "CTA"), a bridging study may be able to help demonstrate performance of the device to be marketed. A bridging study is a clinical study used to demonstrate that the to-be-marketed assay has equivalent performance to that of the CTA, including factors such as selecting the same patient population and having the same predictive power. FDA typically recommends that a sponsor contemplating a bridging strategy to demonstrate performance of a new assay contact OIVD/CDRH through the pre-IDE process in the design and analysis plan of the bridging study.

In general, a trial that includes both marker-positive and marker-negative patients is considered quite valuable because it allows determination of the device sensitivity and specificity, as well as positive and negative predictive values. In the absence of both markers, there may be no information about how well the marker is correlated to the metric(s) in question (response, selection, dose, etc.) or whether the cut-offs are as optimized as possible. In some cases, adequate trials can be constructed with only one stratum of patients with a particular test result (e.g., marker-positive only), and if the therapeutic meets approval criteria, then the test is considered to be informative. However, it is important to note that single-stratum designs may not always provide sufficient information, so early consultation with the FDA may be helpful. It is also helpful to keep in mind that the effectiveness of the assay as a predictive biomarker is generally shown by demonstrating a differential in treatment effect between marker-positive and marker-negative patients. If only marker-positive patients are enrolled in the pivotal clinical study, the ability of the device to predict clinical efficacy of the therapy cannot be evaluated, and the device may be appropriate for a "selection" claim (i.e., as opposed to including a "predictive" claim).

COMPANION DIAGNOSTICS: REGULATORY CHALLENGES AT FDA

FDA is developing mechanisms for effective oversight of medical devices used for personalized medicine. FDA's oversight activities for personalized medicine products primarily include the three medical product review centers: the CDRH, the CDER, and the CBER.

Each of these centers applies specific sets of regulations, most of which have been in place for many years. Thus, not surprisingly, existing regulations for drugs, biologics, and medical devices do not directly address the current situations in personalized medicine in which different types of medical products are dependent upon one another to achieve safety and effectiveness.

FDA is now identifying these areas, establishing regulatory processes, and implementing policies that will clearly delineate the activities and responsibilities of the different centers in the oversight of personalized medicine products within each center's existing regulatory framework. These activities are intended to help coordinate premarket reviews for the different products (therapeutic and diagnostic) to provide consistency and timeliness in regulatory decision-making for these products. In an effort to begin a process for providing further clarity on its policy requiring premarket review for companion diagnostics, FDA released a draft guidance for comment (Draft Guidance for Industry and Food and Drug Administration Staff—In Vitro Companion Diagnostic Devices) on July 14, 2011, available at http://www.fda.gov/MedicalDevices/DeviceRegulationandGuidance/GuidanceDocuments/ucm262292.htm.

COMPANION DIAGNOSTICS: EXAMPLES

Companion diagnostics, such as those cited in drug indication statements, define the context in which the drug is expected to work. OIVD/CDRH has a growing history of completing review of companion diagnostics as follows. The term "companion diagnostic" applies regardless of where in the drug development/marketing cycle the diagnostic test is introduced. For example:

- Diagnostic test developed with a new drug (e.g., HER-2/*neu* for Herceptin)
- New diagnostic test for an old drug (e.g., UGT1A1 for Irinotecan)
- Existing diagnostic test for a new drug (e.g., EGFR IHC testing for Panitumumab)

There are some examples of FDA-approved tests indicated in the therapeutic label, such as HER2 and Herceptin for breast cancer, *BRAF* and Vemurafenib for melanoma, and ALK and Xalkori for non–small cell lung cancer.[8]

LABELING AND FDA REVIEW

FDA reviews labeling for (companion) diagnostic devices as well as related therapeutic products. Having the companion diagnostic sponsor identify the regulatory submissions for both the device and the therapeutic so that these can be coordinated with regard to timing and content between CDER/CBER and CDRH (OIVD) helps to increase efficiency of this process.

CONCLUSIONS

Companion diagnostics can be critical to safe and effective use of certain therapeutic products, and the performance of the drug in the intended use population may depend on the performance of the test. Recent experience is helping FDA in characterizing when a companion diagnostic test is appropriate, as well as what types of information are generally relevant for the determination of safety and effectiveness of the companion diagnostic test. In many ways, validation of companion diagnostic tests is similar to validation for any in vitro diagnostic test, yet certain therapeutic trial design issues, particulars related to bridging between assays, and ties of the companion diagnostic performance to the therapeutic performance may differ significantly enough to merit close attention by sponsors. To date, FDA's experience with development of companion diagnostics and therapeutics has been characterized by a steep learning curve, but we are highly optimistic that the model is workable and will yield a new generation of safe and effective personalized medicines.

REFERENCES

1. For further information on the Office of In Vitro Diagnostic Device Evaluation and Safety, see the OIVD website: http://www.fda.gov/AboutFDA/CentersOffices/OfficeofMedicalProductsandTobacco/CDRH/CDRHOffices/ucm115904.htm.
2. US FDA: Federal Food, Drug and Cosmetic Act. Section §201(h); 21 U.S.C. §321(h).
3. US FDA: Code of Federal Regulations Title 21 §809.3.—IVD Products for Human Use, Definitions.
4. US FDA: Code of Federal Regulations Title 21 Part 860—Medical Device Classification Procedures. For further explanation also see FDA's "Device Advice" webpage: http://www.fda.gov/MedicalDevices/DeviceRegulationandGuidance/Overview/ClassifyYourDevice/default.htm.
5. US FDA: Code of Federal Regulations Title 21 Part 807, Subpart E.—Premarket Notification Procedures.
6. US FDA: Code of Federal Regulations Title 21 Part 814, Subpart B.—Premarket Approval Application (PMA)
7. US FDA: Code of Federal Regulations Title 21 § CFR 814.84—[PMA] Reports
8. U.S. Food and Drug Administration. http://www.accessdata.fda.gov/scripts/cdrh/cfdocs/cfPMA/pma.cfm; http://www.accessdata.fda.gov/scripts/cdrh/cfdocs/cfPMA/pma.cfm?id=7806; http://www.accessdata.fda.gov/scripts/cdrh/cfdocs/cfPMA/pma.cfm?id=8239; http://www.accessdata.fda.gov/scripts/cdrh/cfdocs/cfPMA/pma.cfm?id=1430; http://www.accessdata.fda.gov/scripts/cdrh/cfdocs/cfPMA/pma.cfm?id=19977.
9. US FDA: Code of Federal Regulations Title 21 Part 814, Subpart H—Humanitarian Use Devices.
10. US FDA: Code of Federal Regulations Title 21 Part 812—Investigational Device Exemptions.
11. In Vitro Diagnostic (IVD) Device Studies—Frequently Asked Questions. http://www.fda.gov/downloads/MedicalDevices/DeviceRegulationandGuidance/GuidanceDocuments/ucm071230.pdf.
12. Biomarkers Definitions Working Group. Biomarkers and surrogate endpoints: preferred definitions and conceptual framework. *Clin Pharmacol Ther*. 2001;69:89-95.
13. US FDA: Code of Federal Regulations Title 21 §820—Quality System Regulation.
14. US FDA: Code of Federal Regulations Title 21 Part 803—Medical Device Reporting.
15. US FDA: Code of Federal Regulations Title 21 §820.100(a).
16. Workshop on Pharmacogenetics/Pharmacogenomics in Drug Development and Regulatory Decision-Making; 16-17 May, 2002; Rockville, MD.
17. Pharmacogenomics in Drug Development and Regulatory Decision-Making: The Genomic Data Submission (GDS) Proposal; 13-14 November, 2003; Washington, DC.
18. FDA/DIA Pharmacogenomics Workshop: Co-development of Drug, Biological, and Device Products; 29 July, 2004; Arlington, VA.
19. Pharmacogenomics in Drug Development and Regulatory Decision-Making: Workshop III; 11-13 April, 2005; Rockville, MD.
20. 4th Workshop in a Series on Pharmacogenomics: Biomarkers and Pharmacogenomics in Drug Development and Regulatory Decision Making; 2007; Bethesda, MD.
21. US FDA: Code of Federal Regulations Title 21 §801.4—Meaning of Intended Uses.
22. Gene Expression Profiling Test System for Breast Cancer Prognosis. http://www.fda.gov/MedicalDevices/DeviceRegulationandGuidance/GuidanceDocuments/ucm079163.htm. 2007.
23. Cardiac Allograft Gene Expression Profiling Test Systems. http://www.fda.gov/MedicalDevices/DeviceRegulationandGuidance/GuidanceDocuments/ucm187084.htm. 2009.
24. CFTR Gene Mutation detection Systems. http://www.fda.gov/downloads/MedicalDevices/DeviceRegulationandGuidance/GuidanceDocuments/UCM071104.pdf. 2005.
25. Ovarian Adnexal Mass Assessment Score test System. http://www.fda.gov/MedicalDevices/DeviceRegulationandGuidance/GuidanceDocuments/ucm237299.htm. 2011.
26. Content of Premarket Submissions for Software Contained in Medical Devices. http://www.fda.gov/MedicalDevices/DeviceRegulationandGuidance/GuidanceDocuments/ucm089543.htm. 2005.
27. General Principles of Software Validation. http://www.fda.gov/downloads/MedicalDevices/DeviceRegulationandGuidance/GuidanceDocuments/UCM085371.pdf. 2002.
28. Off-The-Shelf Software Use in Medical Devices. http://www.fda.gov/downloads/MedicalDevices/DeviceRegulationandGuidance/GuidanceDocuments/UCM073779.pdf. 1999.
29. Cybersecurity for Networked Medical Devices Containing Off-the-Shelf (OTS) Software. http://www.fda.gov/MedicalDevices/DeviceRegulationandGuidance/GuidanceDocuments/ucm077812.htm. 2005.

SECTION IV

Molecular Diagnostics of Common Malignancies

CHAPTER 26

Molecular Biology and Pathology of Lung Cancer: Genotype–Morphology Correlation

Yuichi Ishikawa and Osamu Matsubara

INTRODUCTION

Lung cancer has four major histologies: adenocarcinoma, squamous cell carcinoma (SqCC), large cell carcinoma, and small cell lung carcinoma (SCLC). Adenocarcinoma is currently a hot topic for research in a variety of areas, including epidemiology, molecular studies, and clinical medicine, because the prevalence of adenocarcinoma is rapidly increasing in many industrialized countries despite decreases in the number of smokers[1] and because it is now classified by oncogene changes. In addition, molecularly targeted therapies have been crowned with epoch-making success.

Recent evidence has shown that most cancer cells harbor only a single oncogene change, and tumor cells proliferate depending upon its altered simple pathway, a phenomenon that is called oncogene addiction. This fact explains why a molecularly targeted drug may work extremely effectively even in an advanced cancer. Because oncogene changes are usually mutually exclusive, tumors can be classified by such oncogene changes. This is particularly true for lung cancer, as adenocarcinomas of the lung are classified by mutually exclusive changes in receptor tyrosine kinases (RTKs) or signal transduction factors, such as in cancers with epidermal growth factor receptor (*EGFR*) mutations, *KRAS* mutations, anaplastic lymphoma kinase (*ALK*) rearrangements, *MET* amplifications, and other changes.

However, worldwide, most lung cancers are currently diagnosed by pathologists on the basis of their histologies. The main reasons for the prevalence of histology-based diagnosis includes the fact that lung cancers, particularly adenocarcinomas, are very heterogeneous in terms of genomic changes, gene expression, gene regulation, signal transduction pathways, and protein expression signatures. Because state-of-the-art technologies tend to focus on one or a few cellular features, they are not useful for delineating the true clinical character of a tumor. On the other hand, histologic diagnosis by pathologists is currently the most useful and convenient tool for understanding the general nature of tumor cells. Considering the comprehensive nature of histologic diagnosis, we believe that histology-based diagnosis will continue to be useful for at least decades despite the wide range of molecular tools becoming available.

Many pathologists and scientists have proved that there are associations among histologic findings, etiology, prognosis, and molecular changes. In this review article, we discuss correlations between histology and several aspects of lung adenocarcinoma, i.e., etiology, prognosis, oncogene-based classification, and other molecular characteristics.

ONCOGENE CHANGES RELATED TO THE ETIOLOGY AND HISTOLOGY OF LUNG ADENOCARCINOMA

Lung adenocarcinoma has distinct characteristics that are not seen in other common cancers, namely, it can be subclassified by mutually exclusive oncogene changes, such as *KRAS* mutation, *EGFR* mutation, *MET* amplification,

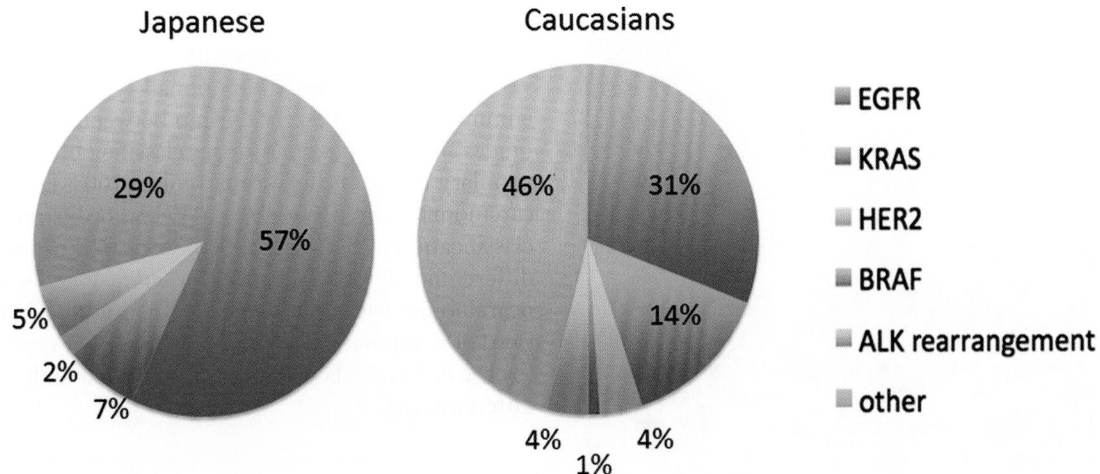

FIGURE 26–1 Comparisons between patterns of oncogene changes in lung adenocarcinomas in Japanese and Caucasian patients. Datasets are based on the JFCR Cancer Institute, Japan, and literatures.

and *ALK* fusion. The classification of lung adenocarcinoma based on oncogene changes has tremendous advantages over histology-based classification, because the molecular subtype indicates a therapeutic target. For example, *EGFR*-mutated cancers are treated with *EGFR* inhibitors and tumors with *ALK* rearrangements are highly sensitive to *ALK* inhibitors. In addition, the patterns of oncogene changes are different between Caucasians and Asians (Fig. 26.1).

Another remarkable characteristic of adenocarcinomas is the existence of correlations between genetic changes and etiology and histology. For example, *EGFR*-mutated tumors predominantly occur in non-smokers, women, and Asian populations. In addition, the tumors are characterized by bronchioloalveolar (or adenocarcinoma in situ [AIS]) histology and hobnail cell morphology. In this section, we outline the evidence that lung adenocarcinoma can be divided by the predominant cell type (hobnail cell type, columnar cell type, polygonal cell type, etc.). We also discuss *TP53* mutation patterns and etiology as well as genotype–histology correlation in *RTK*-mutated adenocarcinomas.

Adenocarcinoma: Cell Type, Etiology, and Mutation

Adenocarcinoma is now the most common type of lung cancer; thus, new approaches for its prevention, early detection, and treatment are needed. To achieve this goal, causative factors for adenocarcinoma and carcinogenic mechanisms need to be elucidated. Tobacco smoking is a well-known cause of squamous cell and small cell carcinomas, but other, as yet unknown, endogenous factors may be more important for the development of adenocarcinomas. One reason why little is known about the nature of adenocarcinomas may be that they have generally been analyzed as a single group. However, the histopathology of lung adenocarcinoma is very heterogeneous, and the several subtypes may each have their own etiology.

Subclassification by Cell Morphology

To investigate whether or not cell morphology of lung adenocarcinoma, rather than structural morphology, has clinicopathologic and etiologic relevance, we examined surgically resected 151 non–small cell lung carcinomas (NSCLCs) (113 adenocarcinomas and 38 SqCCs).[2] The study population ranged in age from 26 to 84 (median 62) years and comprised 98 men and 53 women. The location of a tumor in the lung was classified as central when it was considered to have arisen in a main or segmental bronchus and peripheral when in a subsegmental or more distal bronchus. The patient's smoking history (number of cigarettes per day, starting age, and duration of smoking) was obtained from preoperative personal interviews and patients were classified as either non-smokers or smokers, the latter including both patients with a past history of smoking and current smokers. The adenocarcinomas were subclassified by the predominant cell types, which were modified from the original description by Hashimoto et al.[2] as follows: (1) hobnail, (2) columnar, (3) polygonal, and (4) other (Fig. 26.2). The hobnail type consists of cells with cytoplasmic protrusions or a dome formation at their apices, resulting in hobnail- or tadpole-shaped cells. The columnar type is composed of columnar/cuboidal cells with flat apices. Cytoplasmic mucus is usually absent, and if it is present it is scant and is located near the free cell surface. Polygonal cells, with or without mucus in their cytoplasm, proliferating in sheets are sometimes observed in tumors with hobnail and columnar cells, but when such cells made up >95% of the tumor, it was diagnosed as the polygonal cell type.

Using the 2004 World Health Organization (WHO) classification,[3] more than half of the adenocarcinomas were classified as adenocarcinomas with mixed subtypes. Only two bronchioloalveolar carcinomas (BACs, currently known as AIS) were observed and no papillary adenocarcinomas consisting entirely of tall columnar or cuboidal cells were observed. Almost half of the tumor cells were the hobnail type, followed by columnar, polygonal,

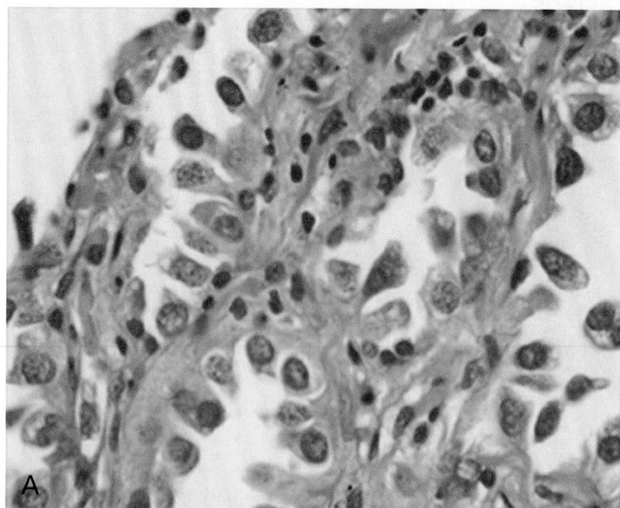

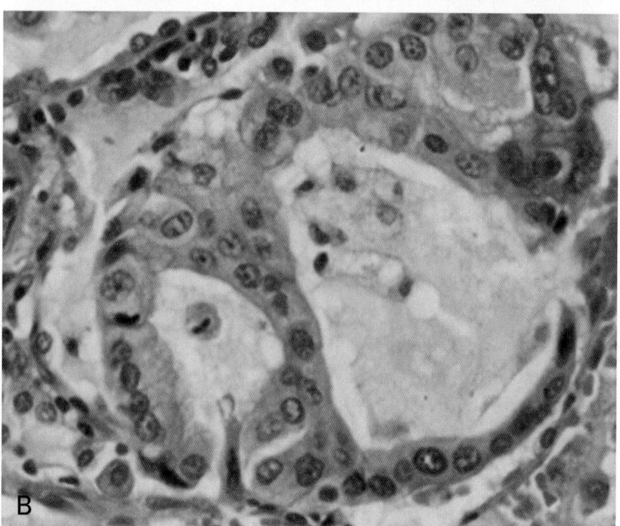

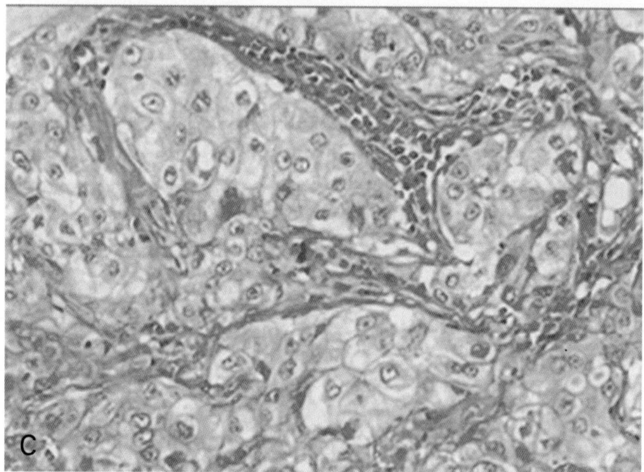

FIGURE 26–2 Major cell morphologies of lung adenocarcinomas. **A:** Hobnail cell type; **B:** columnar cell type; **C:** polygonal cell type.

and others. As compared with the WHO classifications, when tumors were classified by cell type, more than half of the acinar and papillary adenocarcinomas were classified as columnar and hobnail cell types. All of the solid adenocarcinomas with mucin were of the polygonal cell type. The adenocarcinomas with mixed subtypes included various cell types, with the hobnail type being the most common. As for the relationship between differentiation grades and subtypes, many cases classified by the WHO as papillary (94%), bronchioloalveolar (100%), and adenocarcinoma with mixed subtypes (94%) or by our cell-type classification as hobnail (100%) were well or moderately differentiated, whereas most acinar (95%) and solid adenocarcinomas with mucin (100%) (by the WHO classification) or columnar (91%) and polygonal cell types (100%) (by the cell-type classification) were moderately or poorly differentiated.

Correlations of TP53 Mutations with Adenocarcinoma Morphology and Etiology

Mutations in the *TP53* tumor suppressor gene are important for the development of many kinds of tumors, including lung cancers. The frequency and type of *TP53* mutations can reflect carcinogenesis caused by exogenous or endogenous factors and thus may be helpful for identifying the causative agents. With lung cancers, tobacco smoking has been shown to frequently cause *TP53* mutations, especially G to T transversions. On the other hand, transitions, especially C to T transitions at CpG sites, are thought to be caused by endogenous mechanisms involved in spontaneous mutations. Therefore, the frequency and types of mutations may provide information on the etiology of lung cancer. Working on the hypothesis that different subtypes of adenocarcinoma may be caused by different etiologic factors, we subclassified a large series of lung tumor samples based on our cell-type classification as well as their histologic subtype and examined *TP53* gene mutations in exons 4 to 8 and 10. We then assessed the relationships among histologic subtypes, *TP53* mutational status, and smoking history.[2]

Screening the tumor samples for *TP53* mutations in exons 4 to 8 and 10 revealed mutations in 68 of 151 NSCLCs (45%). No mutations were found in normal lung tissue samples except polymorphisms. We saw a trend toward more frequent mutations in SqCCs (58%) than in adenocarcinomas (41%). By the WHO classification, papillary adenocarcinomas and adenocarcinomas with mixed subtypes showed the lowest frequency of mutations, although statistically significant differences from other individual subtypes were not found. Using our cell-type classification, the columnar cell type (16/23 = 70%) had the most *TP53* mutations, which is similar to the finding for squamous cell lesions, followed by polygonal (6/13 = 46%), hobnail (20/54 = 37%), and other (4/23 = 17%) cell types (Table 26.1).

Most *TP53* mutations were transitions (43%) or transversions (41%), and only 16% were deletions/insertions. In adenocarcinomas, the frequencies of transitions and transversions were 46% and 35%, respectively, and in SqCCs, the frequencies were 36% and 55%,

TABLE 26–1 TP53 Mutations in Adenocarcinoma of the Lung, Sorted by the WHO Classification and Cell-Type Classification

Smoking status	Examined	Mutated	%
Non-smoker	50	17	34
Smoker	63	29	46
Adenocarcinoma subtypes			
WHO classification			
Acinar	22	12	55
Papillary	16	5	31
Bronchioloalveolar carcinoma	2	1	50
Solid adenocarcinoma with mucin	5	4	80
Adenocarcinoma with mixed subtypes	68	24	35
Cell-type classification			
Hobnail cell type	54	20	37
Columnar cell type	23	16	70
Polygonal cell type	13	6	46
Other	23	4	17

respectively. No significant differences were observed between adenocarcinoma and SqCC, in agreement with a previous Japanese report.[4] Comparison of the subtypes revealed a significant difference between the hobnail and columnar cell groups: transitions were higher in the former (65%) than in the latter (25%); transversions also tended to be less frequent in the former (20%) than in the latter (50%). With the WHO classification, we did not observe any significant differences in the frequencies of transitions or transversions between subtypes of adenocarcinomas. We next examined base substitutions by adenocarcinoma subtype. With CpG-site transitions, the hobnail cell type was more frequent (45%) than the columnar cell type and SqCCs (13% and 23%, respectively). On the other hand, G:C to T:A transversions tended to be rarer in hobnail cell-type lesions (15%) than in the columnar and SqCC types (44% and 27%, respectively; $P = 0.062$ between 15% and 44%). When adenocarcinomas were classified by the WHO criteria, no such variation was noted.

It has been hypothesized that mutations induced by exogenous or environmental carcinogens preferentially occur in nontranscribed gene alleles.[5] Therefore, evaluating the *TP53* base substitutions for strand bias may also provide clues to suspected carcinogens. In our study, we observed a marked strand bias for G:C to T:A transversions: 17 of the 18 mutations were found on the nontranscribed strand, whereas the 18 G:C to A:T transitions observed in CpG sites were equally distributed on the two strands (9 vs. 9).

The percentage of smokers with columnar cell lesions (83%) was almost the same as the percentage of smokers with SqCCs and significantly higher than the percentages of smokers with hobnail cell lesions (44%). Mutations were more frequent in lesions from smokers (46%) than in those from non-smokers (34%), consistent with previous reports.[6] As for the types of mutations, transitions were significantly less frequent among smokers (33%) than among non-smokers (65%; $P = 0.016$). By contrast, transversions were more common among smokers (48%) than among non-smokers (25%), but the significance was marginal ($P = 0.068$). Furthermore, G:C to A:T transitions at CpG sites were preferentially found in non-smokers (35%), and G:C to T:A transversions were more frequent in smokers (29%), although the differences were not significant.

EGFR Mutation and Histology of Lung Adenocarcinoma

EGFR, a member of the RTK family, dimerizes and phosphorylates several tyrosine residues after binding to specific ligands (Fig. 26.3).[7] The phosphorylated tyrosines play important roles in cell physiology, and activation of pathways downstream of EGFR can lead to abnormal cell growth and cellular transformation. Gefitinib, an orally administered agent that prevents binding of adenosine triphosphate to EGFR, inhibits tyrosine phosphorylation and signaling. Blockade of EGFR-mediated effects induces apoptosis and reduces tumor growth. EGFR is highly expressed in solid carcinomas, including NSCLCs, but despite high expectations based on biologic findings and data suggesting wide applicability, neither the expression nor phosphorylation level of EGFR in NSCLCs has been shown to predict sensitivity to gefitinib in either preclinical or clinical studies.[8]

A number of reports have referred to clinicopathologic factors of lung tumors associated with *EGFR* mutations. In two early notable studies, Lynch et al.[9] and Paez et al.[10] reported that clinical responsiveness to gefitinib was associated with somatic mutations in the TK domain of EGFR. Paez et al. indicated that such mutations are prevalent in women of Asian origin with adenocarcinoma. In terms of pathologic subtypes, Miller et al.[11] reported that of 139 cases of NSCLCs, BACs (i.e., AISs) responded best to gefitinib. This subtype appears to be prevalent among female non-smokers and is genetically relatively simple. Yatabe et al. also described a terminal respiratory unit-type adenocarcinoma, corresponding to the majority of non-mucinous BACs (AISs), which represent a distinct subset of significantly related *EGFR* mutations.[12] As these studies proved, *EGFR*-mutated adenocarcinomas are separate biologic entities depending on particular molecular pathways for their maintenance and survival and these entities exhibit a characteristic microscopic appearance presumably on that basis. In the next section, we describe a study of clinicopathologic characteristics of primary lung adenocarcinomas arising in a Japanese population, focusing on associations between *EGFR* mutations and specific pathologic features, especially cytologic subtypes and micropapillary morphology.

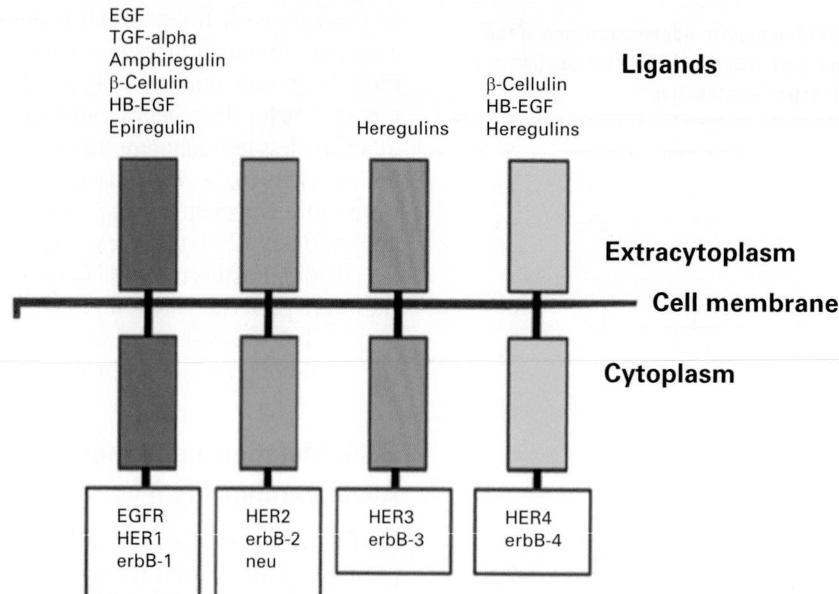

FIGURE 26–3 Epidermal growth factor receptor (EGFR) and its family proteins. Reprinted from Inamura K et al. Is the epidermal growth factor receptor status in lung cancers reflected in clinicopathologic features? Arch Pathol Lab Med. 2010;134(1):66-72.

Adenocarcinomas Harboring EGFR Mutations Show Typical Histology

To analyze the association between *EGFR* mutations and tumor histology, samples of primary lung tumors were obtained from 107 consecutive cases who underwent surgery between January 1998 and June 2002 at the Cancer Institute Hospital in Tokyo. All cases were adenocarcinomas and all but one underwent complete surgical resection. Cases with multiple and metachronous tumors at the time of surgery were excluded. We also reviewed the medical records and pathology slides to compare the characteristics of patients with or without *EGFR* mutations. The following patient characteristics were analyzed: gender, age, pathologic disease stage, smoking status, and histologic findings, including dominant cell types. Smoking status was recorded as a smoking index (SI), which was calculated as the number of cigarettes smoked per day times the number of years the patient had smoked. Fifty-two males and 55 females were included in the study. The median age was 63 years (range 43 to 83). There were 54 ever smokers (current or former smokers) and 53 never smokers.

We evaluated tumors based on either histologic structure or cell type. Classification by histologic structure included adenocarcinoma subtypes defined by the 2004 WHO criteria, such as papillary and acinar adenocarcinomas, and differentiation grades. Classification by cell type was based on our previous study as detailed above. In addition, an expert pathologist (Y.I.) described the nature of each tumor by estimating the proportion of the tumor areas occupied by each differentiation grade on the largest cut surface. Differentiation grades were defined according to Japanese Lung Cancer Society criteria.[13] Briefly, well-differentiated tumors are composed chiefly of glands lined by, or of papilla covered by, one-layered tumor cells. Also, BACs (or AISs), strictly defined to be noninvasive in this study, are included in this category. Moderately differentiated lesions comprise glands showing a cribriform pattern, fused with one another, or glands lined by, or papillae covered by, tumor cells demonstrating obvious piling-up. Poorly differentiated carcinomas show mainly solid growth and only occasionally glandular/papillary patterns and/or mucus production. In cases where two or more patterns were observed, the predominant pattern was considered. In addition, we focused on the presence of a micropapillary pattern (MPP), defined as papillary structures with tufts lacking a fibrovascular core (Fig. 26.4).[14] The micropapillary component belongs to the moderately differentiated structure because it lacks stroma and has invasive potential. When a tumor had >5% MPP, it was regarded as having MPP, since adenocarcinomas with >5% MPP exhibited poorer prognosis than those with <5% MPP, even in stage I disease. For BAC (AIS) components, the same condition was applied. As a result, each tumor was found to be a composite of some constituents.

Adenocarcinomas with EGFR Mutations Are Related to Hobnail Cells

We also classified tumors by cell types. We applied the cell-type classification to the tumor samples after slight modification. We divided tumors into hobnail, columnar, and polygonal cell types, categorizing the tumors based on the most frequent cell type rather than using the mixed cell type.

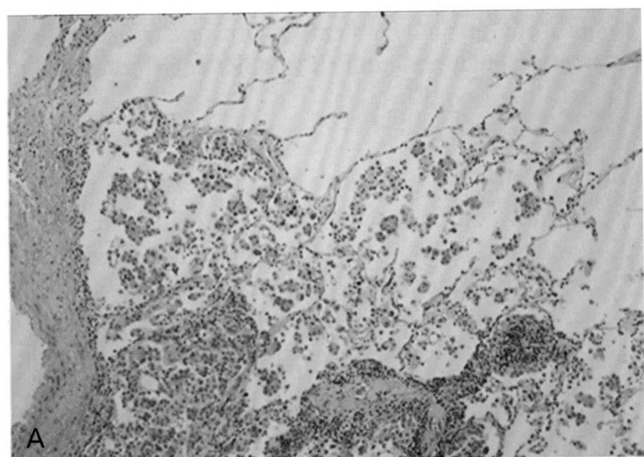

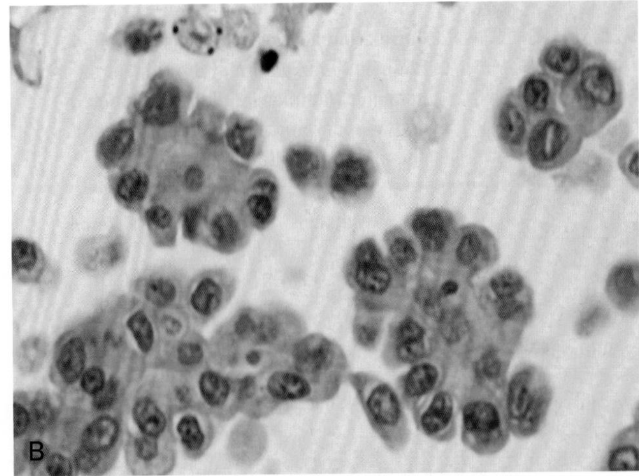

FIGURE 26–4 Micropapillary pattern of lung adenocarcinoma. It is defined as papillary structures with tufts lacking a fibrovascular core. **A:** A low power view. **B:** A high power view. Note that the pattern is characterized by protrusions of the cytoplasm and nucleus and that cellular polarity as glandular epithelia is preserved.

The overall frequency of *EGFR* mutations was 59% (63/107) and the relative frequencies of exons 18, 19, 20, 21 were 3%, 48%, 6%, and 43%, respectively. The most common mutation was an inframe deletion involving three to eight codons in exon 19. Missense mutations in exon 21 (L858R) were the second most common, while mutations were seen in exon 18 as well. Insertions of one to four codons in exon 20 were also detected. *EGFR* mutations were significantly associated with female gender ($P = 0.003$) and never smoker status ($P = 0.008$). The amount of cumulative tobacco consumption was significantly higher in patients with wild-type *EGFR* and in males ($P = 0.003$) than in those with *EGFR* mutations ($P = 0.0002$). Among smokers, there was no significant difference in *EGFR* mutation status between former and current smokers (data not shown).

We subclassified tumors into adenocarcinoma subtypes according to the 2004 WHO guidelines, and >90% (97/107) fell into the mixed subtype. This again suggested the limited usefulness of adenocarcinoma subclassification. Therefore, we attempted to characterize each tumor histologically as follows. Percentages of areas with each histologic component, such as well differentiated and MPP components, were evaluated in each case and averaged in cases with EGFR mutations ($n = 63$) and the wild-type population ($n = 44$). Among the three cell types, hobnail cells ($n = 76$) were more associated with EGFR mutations than were columnar and polygonal cells ($n = 31$; $P < 0.00001$) (Table 26.2).

In this study, we used the cytologic classification determined in our previous study to demonstrate differences in *TP53* mutation frequency and patterns.[2] The hobnail cell type, characterized by cytoplasmic protrusions and a tadpole or hobnail shape, exhibits a low frequency of *TP53* mutations, with mainly spontaneous transition type mutations at CpG nucleotides. In contrast, for the columnar cell type, we observed a high *TP53* mutational frequency, with G:C to T:A transversions thought to be caused by exogenous carcinogenic agents such as tobacco. We noted a significant difference in *EGFR* mutation rates between the hobnail cell type and the other two types examined, providing further evidence of differences in the genetic backgrounds of these tumors (see Table 26.2).

The Micropapillary Feature Is Related to EGFR Mutation

MPP is a distinct pathologic feature of lung adenocarcinoma that was first reported by Amin et al.[15] Among early-stage pulmonary adenocarcinomas, MPP-positive tumors show a significantly poorer prognosis than MPP-negative tumors.[14] We speculated that the distinct

TABLE 26–2 Clinicopathologic Features of Lung Adenocarcinoma and Epidermal Growth Factor Receptor Mutation

	N	Mutated	%	*P*-Value
Gender				
Male	52	23	44	0.003
Female	55	40	73	
Differentiation				
Well	52	36	69	
Moderately	42	22	52	
Poorly	13	5	38	
Cell type				
Hobnail	76	55	72	
Columnar	18	4	22	<0.00001
Polygonal	13	4	31	
Smoking status				
Never	53	38	72	0.008
Ever	54	25	46	

Note: The cell types are strongly related to epidermal growth factor receptor mutations.

TABLE 26-3 Correlation between the Number of Patients with Epidermal Growth Factor Receptor Mutations and the Presence of an Adenocarcinoma In Situ Component and a Micropapillary Pattern

	Mutated	Wild Type	*P*-Value
With AIS component	50	25	0.012
Without AIS component	13	19	
With MPP	41	20	0.043
Without MPP	22	24	

AIS, adenocarcinoma in situ; MPP, microcapillary pattern.

micropapillary feature reflects a step during the progression from well-differentiated papillary adenocarcinoma of the hobnail cell type to a less-differentiated state unrelated to smoking. Judging from its pathologic presentation and relatively unfavorable outcome, it is appropriate that tumors with MPP are classified as moderately differentiated rather than as well differentiated. This pattern is often found in non-smokers and correlates with a high degree of aggressiveness. Miyoshi et al. also have demonstrated that metastasis to lymph nodes, pleural invasion, intrapulmonary metastases, and non-smoking status are significantly more frequent in MPP-positive cases, with significantly poorer 5-year survival.[14]

The presence of micropapillary components is significantly related to *EGFR* mutations as given in Table 26.3, shown by Ninomiya et al.[16] using 214 Japanese adenocarcinoma cases.[17] A notable feature of MPP is that it is frequently present at the periphery of tumors and is predominant in metastatic foci. These clinicopathologic observations, accompanied by our findings that *EGFR* is frequently mutated, may explain the dramatic responses of lung adenocarcinomas with diffuse micronodular intrapulmonary metastasis to gefitinib. This is a good example of a clinically useful histology (MPP)–genotype (mutated *EGFR*) correlation.

ALK Rearrangement and Histology of Lung Adenocarcinoma

Recently, a novel transforming fusion gene joining the echinoderm microtubule associated protein-like 4 gene (*EML4*) and the *ALK* gene was found in five NSCLCs.[18] The *EML4–ALK* fusion gene is formed by a small inversion within chromosome 2p. The encoded protein contains the N-terminal part of *EML4* and the intracellular catalytic domain of *ALK*. Replacement of the extracellular and transmembrane domain of *ALK* with a region of *EML4* results in constitutive dimerization of the kinase domain and a consequent increase in its catalytic activity. In this section, we discuss the characteristic histologic features of the 11 lung tumors as well as the clinicopathologic and genetic findings from immunohistochemical analysis and confirmed by reverse transcription–polymerase chain reaction (RT-PCR) and fluorescent in situ hybridization (FISH).[19]

Immunohistochemistry or ALK Screening

Eleven lung tumors were analyzed using multiplex RT-PCR and FISH.[20] Briefly, the tumors were found from 363 individuals who underwent surgery at the Cancer Institute Hospital, Tokyo, between May 1997 and February 2004. The 363 lung cancers comprised 253 adenocarcinomas, 7 adenosquamous carcinomas, 72 SqCCs, 7 large cell carcinomas (including 4 large cell neuroendocrine carcinomas [LCNECs]), 2 pleomorphic carcinomas, and 22 SCLCs. Histologic diagnoses were made primarily based on the 2004 WHO classification, with the addition of a predominance classification of invasive components, which is mostly based on the WHO classification except for the mixed subtype, such as papillary predominant and acinar predominant. In the predominance classification of invasive components, we made a diagnosis by the component that makes up the predominant portion of the invasive lesion even if it is <50%. In addition, we used differentiation grading as mentioned above.

For screening by immunostaining, we used the intercalated antibody-enhanced polymer method, an enhancing method appropriately adjusted for *ALK*-rearranged cancers.[21] When we found positive cases by immunostaining, the rearrangements were confirmed by RT-PCR and FISH. To characterize the nature of the tumor cell, we examined the expression of TTF-1 and mutations in *KRAS*, *EGFR*, and *TP53* as described earlier.

Acinar Configuration with Mucin Is Characteristic of ALK Tumors

Histologically, the 253 adenocarcinomas comprised 246 invasive and 7 noninvasive tumors. Subtypes of the 246 invasive tumors were 206 papillary predominant, 34 acinar predominant, 5 solid predominant, and 1 other. According to the predominance subtypes in adenocarcinomas, 6 of 11 *EML4–ALK*-positive lung cancers (54.5%) were subclassified as acinar adenocarcinomas ($P < 0.0001$) (Fig. 26.4). In other words, 6 of 34 (18%) acinar-predominant adenocarcinomas had an *EML4–ALK* fusion. In adenocarcinomas not subclassified as acinar-predominant adenocarcinomas based on the above criteria, acinar structures were also frequently observed as a minor component. In differentiation grading, *EML4–ALK* lung cancers were less differentiated. In addition, they often featured mucin production with acinar structures (Fig. 26.5). As for the cell types, the columnar cell type was characteristic of *EML4–ALK* lung cancers (see Figs. 26.2 and 26.5), although tall columnar cells were not evident.

Lung adenocarcinomas with *EML4–ALK* were also found to be significantly smaller than those without, which is generally in line with the lack of in situ

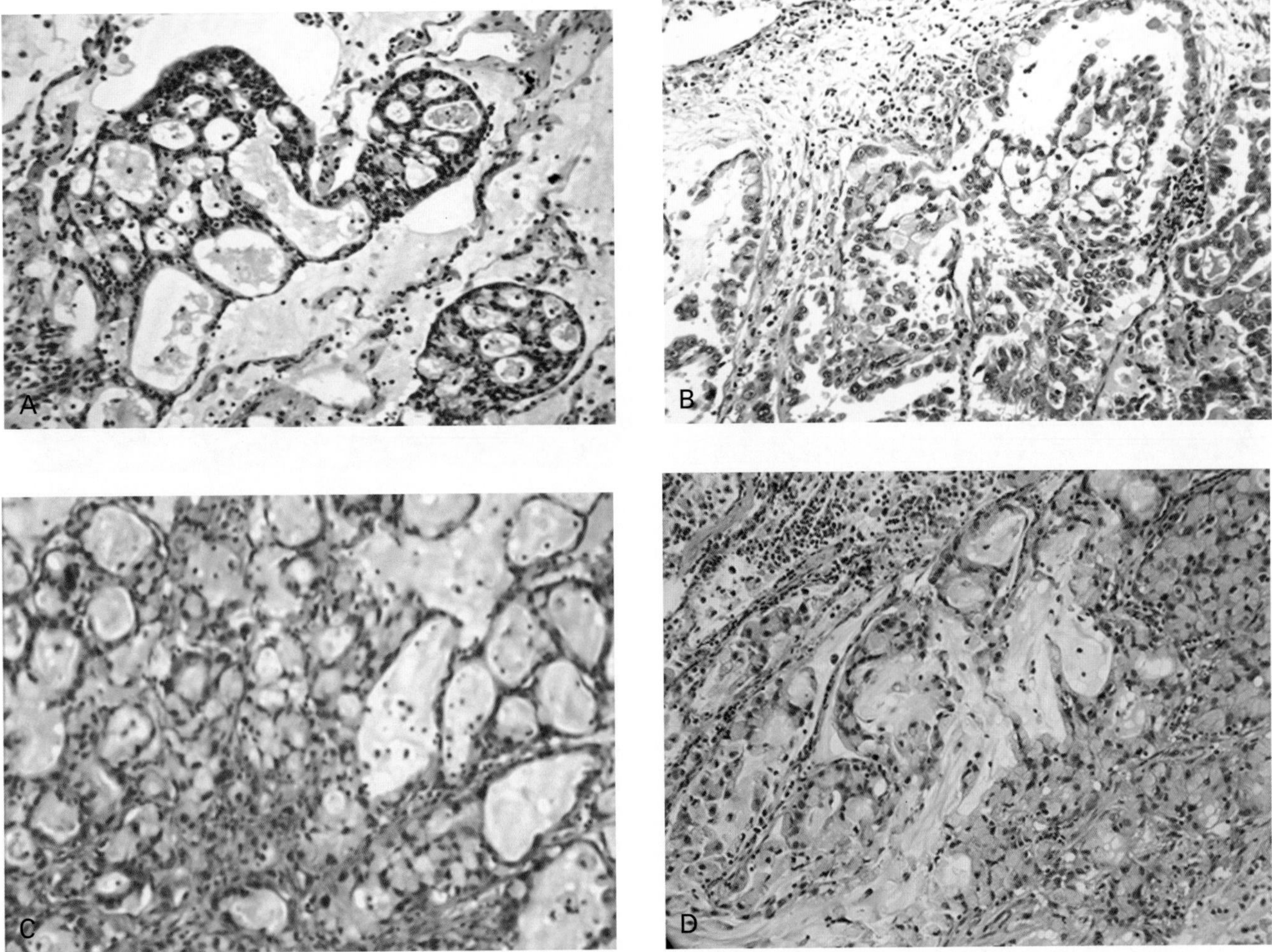

FIGURE 26–5 Typical histology of pulmonary adenocarcinoma with an EML4–ALK fusion. **A:** An acinar structure or a mucinous cribriform pattern (O-40940). **B:** A tubulopapillary structure with thin cords and occasional signet ring cells (10-3323). **C:** A tubulopapillary structure with an occasional mucinous cribriform pattern (O-39673). **D:** Combined moderately differentiated and poorly differentiated components with mucin (H1022276).

components. Patients with *EML4–ALK* lung cancers tended to be young (56 vs. 64 years for other tumor types). We defined early-onset lung cancers by classifying patients as younger or older than 50. In 253 patients with lung adenocarcinomas, 16 were diagnosed at younger than 50. Four of 11 patients (36%) with *EML4–ALK*-positive lung cancers were younger than 50 as compared with 12 of 242 patients (5.0%) with *EML4–ALK*-negative lung cancers.

It is true that the *EML4–ALK* rearrangement was first found in a smoker's lung cancer, but overall there was no significant difference between the smokers' and non-smokers' tumors with regard to *EML4–ALK* fusion. Rather, we finally have evidence that these tumors were unrelated to smoking. Actually, smoking habits can be classified into the following two grades of cumulative smoking based on the SI: non-smokers and light smokers (SI < 400) and heavy smokers (SI = 400 or more). Ten of the 11 (91%) *EML4–ALK*-positive lung cancer patients had SI < 400 as compared with 109 of 241 (45%) *EML4–ALK*-negative lung cancer patients ($P = 0.040$). In our examination of the 11 cases, *EML4–ALK* fusion was detected in only 1 heavy smoker's lung cancer (1/11 = 9.1%).

ALK, EGFR, and KRAS Changes Are Mutually Exclusive

EGFR and *KRAS* mutations are two major oncogenic drivers of lung adenocarcinoma development and they are mutually exclusive in usual cases. In our study, *EML4–ALK*-positive lung cancers lacked both *EGFR* and *KRAS* mutations ($P = 0.00018$), and only 1 of 11 (9.1%) harbored a *TP53* mutation. It is noteworthy that the single mutation was a G/A transition (GTG–ATG) (V-M) in codon 273, exon 8. This is known to be a spontaneous mutation, usually seen in non-smokers' lung cancers, rather than in the tobacco-carcinogen-induced mutation. In the 11 *EML4–ALK*-positive cases, immunohistochemical assays with an anti-ALK antibody consistently showed definite staining. As illustrated in Fig. 26.5, the cytoplasm of tumor cells was stained strongly with fine

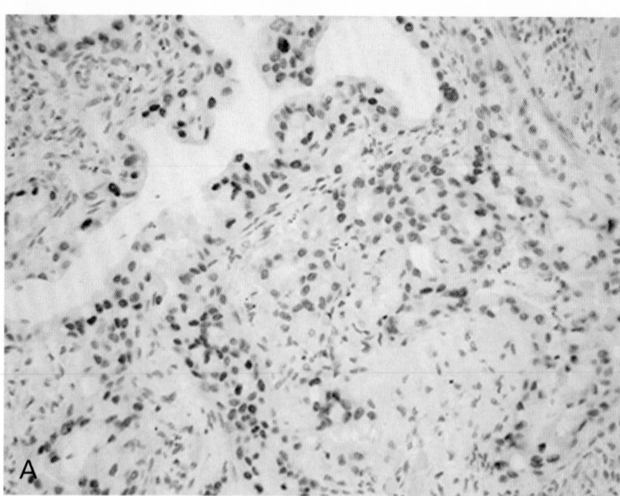

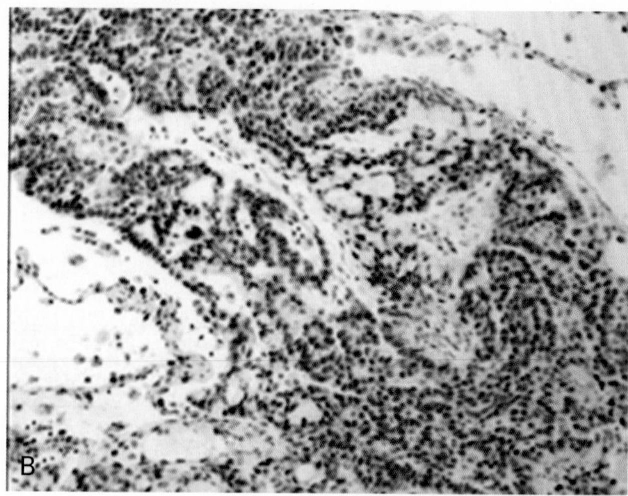

FIGURE 26–6 Tumor cells of adenocarcinomas with EML4–ALK fusion show immunoreactivity to TTF-1, an immunohistochemical marker for alveolar type II cell differentiation. **A:** Moderately to poorly differentiated adenocarcinoma with signet-ring cells are partly positive for TTF-1 (H1022276). **B:** Moderately differentiated acinar adenocarcinoma showing a mucinous cribriform pattern, entirely positive for TTF-1 (H1109043).

granular accentuation. Although we immunostained 88 *EML4–ALK*-negative lung adenocarcinoma specimens, we could discriminate all the fusion-negative specimens from fusion-positive ones by our refined immunohistochemical conditions. As expected from the fact that most *EML4–ALK* tumors arise in non- or light smokers, the tumor cells were of alveolar type II, as evidenced by TTF-1 immunoreactivity. In fact, all 11 cases were either positive (6 cases) or partially positive (5 cases) for TTF-1 immunostaining (Fig. 26.6).

Histologically, less-differentiated acinar structures composed of low columnar cells appear characteristic of *EML4–ALK* lung adenocarcinomas. It is noted that smoker's lung adenocarcinomas are often composed of columnar cells, usually taller columnar cells, whereas the hobnail cell type, characterized by cytoplasmic protrusions and with a tadpole shape, is often observed in non-smoker's lung adenocarcinomas.[2] Although *EML4–ALK* lung cancers are TTF-1 positive, their histology is somewhat similar to lung cancers developing in smokers, which is interesting in the view of histology–etiology relationships.

RTK Signal Pathway Activation and Its Association with EGFR and KRAS Mutations, Progression, and Adenocarcinoma Histology

RTK pathways are one of the major cell growth and differentiation routes of signal transduction and have emerged as therapeutic targets. There are three signal transduction pathways under RTKs: the phosphatidylinositol-3-kinase (PI3K)–Akt pathway, the RAS–extracellular signal regulated kinases 1 and 2 (ERK) pathway, and the STAT pathway. Here, we demonstrate how RTK pathway activation is associated with *EGFR* and *KRAS* oncogene mutations, tumor progression, and histology by focusing on the two major routes: the PI3K–Akt and RAS–ERK pathways[21] (Fig. 26.7). Since *KRAS* mutations in lung cancer are found most frequently in adenocarcinomas, we focus here on adenocarcinoma histology.

Akt, a serine/threonine kinase, and ERK are major target proteins downstream of EGFR and work with various other oncoproteins, such as Ras and Raf. They are known to be activated in a wide spectrum of human cancers together with various downstream substrates, such as glycogen synthase kinase 3-beta (GSK3B), mammalian target of rapamycin (mTOR), p70 ribosomal protein S6 kinase (S6K), and forkhead proteins FKHR/FKHRL1 (FKHR), and to play central roles in tumorigenesis, cell growth, or cell proliferation. By analyzing tumor tissue samples by immunohistochemistry, we examined whether there may be selective activation of pathways downstream of RTKs in lung adenocarcinomas that depend on the presence of *EGFR* and *KRAS* mutations.

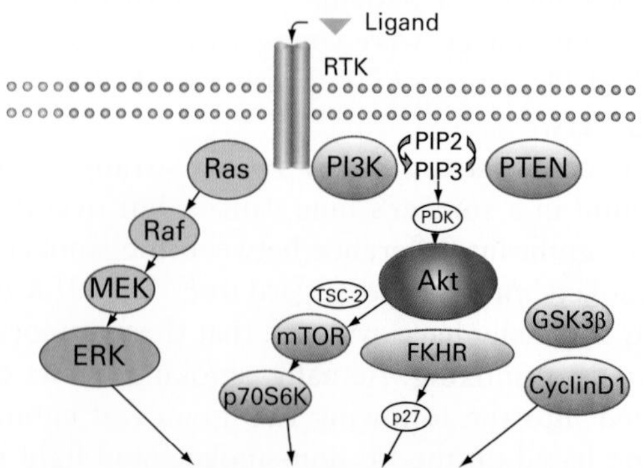

FIGURE 26–7 Cell growth and differentiation pathway under a receptor tyrosine kinase (RTK) such as epidermal growth factor receptor. For abbreviations of substrates, see text.

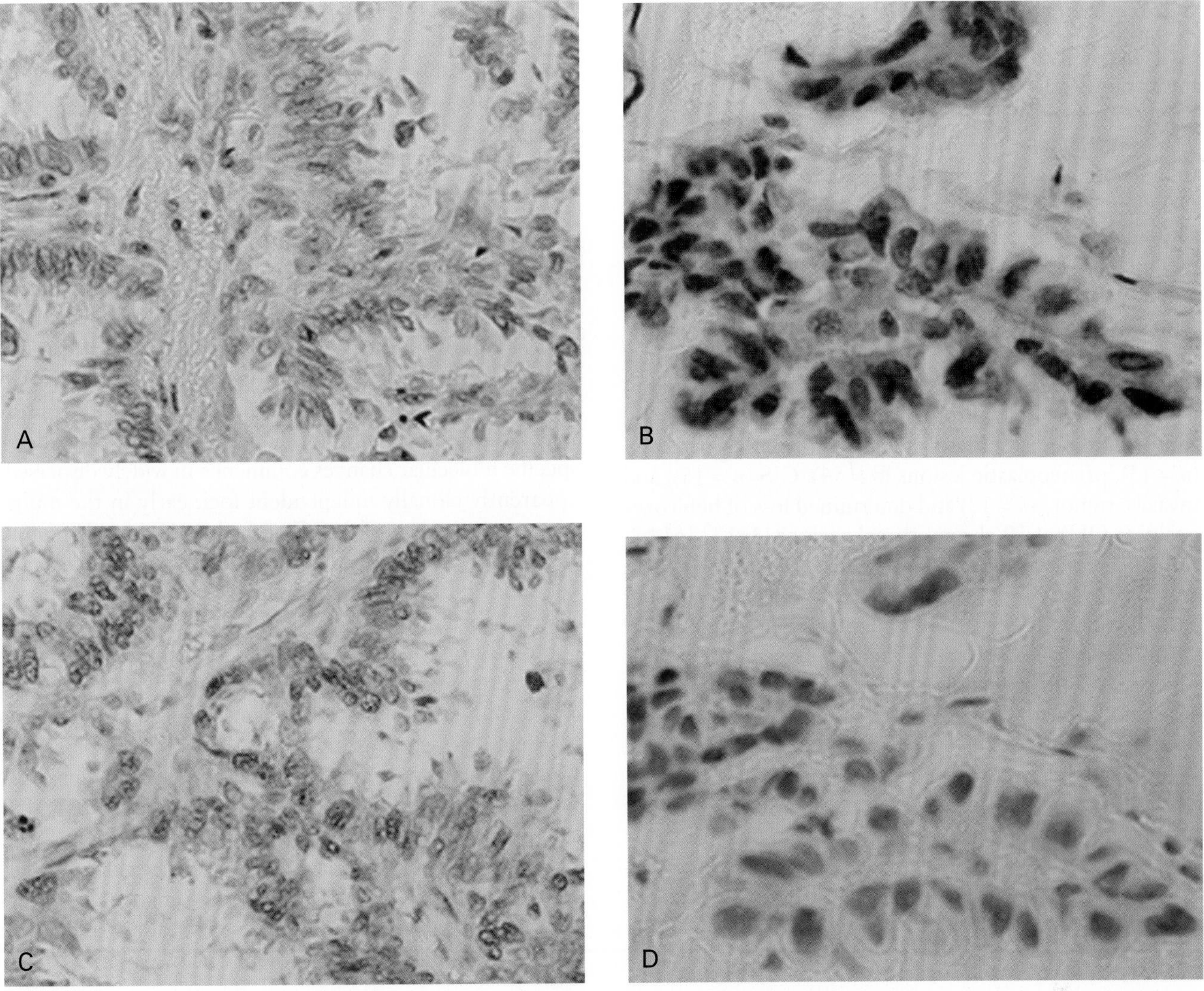

FIGURE 26–8 A–D: Proliferation signal pathways of RTKs downstream are changed from the RAS–ERK pathway to the PI3K–Akt pathway when tumors progress from preinvasive or minimally invasive to overt invasive. For abbreviations, see text.

We further evaluated the clinicopathologic and prognostic significance of such activation in various adenocarcinoma subtypes. Since we had found by expression profiling that adenocarcinoma cell lines may have different gene expression profiles than clinical adenocarcinomas,[23] we used tissue samples from 193 adenocarcinomas surgically resected at the JFCR Cancer Institute Hospital rather than cell lines. In addition, we examined TTF-1 expression as a cell lineage marker and *EGFR* and *KRAS* mutation status. As a result, we found that Akt activation, or phosphorylated Akt (pAkt) expression ($P = 0.015$), and negative TTF-1 staining ($P < 0.001$) were independent and significant markers for poor prognosis. We then analyzed the relationships between the expression of pAkt or TTF-1 and other factors, including clinicopathologic factors and oncogene mutation status.

pAkt expression was significantly associated with advanced disease stage (stages II–IV, $P = 0.021$) and lymph node metastasis ($P = 0.002$) but not with expression of any other signal proteins or TTF-1. On the contrary, TTF-1 expression was significantly associated with never-smoker status ($P = 0.013$) and a preinvasive or minimally invasive nature ($P < 0.001$), as well as with the expression of pERK ($P = 0.039$) and pmTOR ($P = 0.014$). In addition, TTF-1 expression was related to *EGFR* mutation ($P = 0.017$).

Regarding the invasiveness of the tumor, the pAkt activation frequency was lower in the preinvasive and minimally invasive adenocarcinomas (18.2%; 8/44) than in the invasive types (43.6%; 65/149), and this tendency was highly and statistically significant ($P = 0.004$). In contrast, TTF-1 staining was more frequently seen among the preinvasive and minimally invasive adenocarcinomas ($P < 0.001$). These results imply that lung adenocarcinoma cells use the RAS–ERK pathway for proliferation in their early stages, but the proliferation route switches to the PI3K–Akt pathway in advanced stages regardless of TTF-1 status (Fig. 26.8).

SQCC AND ITS PRECURSORS

SqCC is defined as "a malignant epithelial tumor showing keratinization and/or intercellular bridges that arises from bronchial epithelium," according to the WHO classification scheme. The basal cells in the bronchial epithelium are thought to be the progenitor cells for SqCC. Development of pulmonary SqCC is believed to progress sequentially from basal cell hyperplasia to squamous metaplasia, squamous dysplasia, carcinoma in situ (CIS), and invasive SqCC.[24-27]

Wistuba and Gazdar's groups examined sequential molecular abnormalities in the multistage development of pulmonary SqCC (Fig. 26.9). They obtained DNA from 94 microdissected foci from 12 archival surgically resected tumors, including histologically normal epithelium (n = 13), preneoplastic lesions (n = 54), CIS (n = 15), and invasive tumors (n = 12) and determined loss of heterozygosity (LOH) at 10 chromosomal regions (3p12, 3p14.2, 3p14.1-21.3, 3p21, 3p22-24, 3p25, 5q22, 9p21, 13q14 RB, and 17p13 *TP53*) frequently deleted in lung cancer using 31 polymorphic microsatellite markers, including 24 that spanned the entire 3p arm.[26] Their major findings were as follows: (i) 31% of histologically normal epithelium and 42% of mildly abnormal (hyperplasia/metaplasia) specimens had clones of cells with allelic loss at one or more regions; (ii) there was a progressive increase of the overall LOH frequency within clones with increasing severity of histopathologic changes; (iii) the earliest and most frequent regions of allelic loss occurred at 3p21, 3p22-24, 3p25, and 9p21; (iv) the size of the 3p deletions increased with progressive histologic changes; (v) *TP53* allelic loss was present in many histologically advanced lesions (dysplasia and CIS); (vi) analyses of 58 normal and noninvasive foci having any molecular abnormality indicated that 30 probably arose as independent clonal events, while 28 were potentially of the same clonal origin as the corresponding tumor; (vii) nevertheless, when the allelic losses in the 30 clonally independent lesions and their clonally unrelated tumors were compared, the same parental allele was lost in 113 of 125 (90%) of comparisons. The mechanism by which this phenomenon (known as allele-specific mutations) occurs is unknown; (viii) four patterns of allelic loss in clones were found. Histologically, normal or mildly abnormal foci had a negative pattern (no allelic loss) or early pattern of loss while all foci of CIS and invasive tumors had an advanced pattern. These findings indicate that multiple, sequentially occurring allele-specific molecular changes commence in widely dispersed, apparently clonally independent foci, early in the multistage pathogenesis of SqCC of the lung. They also found that allelic losses of 3p were detected in 96% of lung cancers and in 78% of preneoplastic/preinvasive lesions.[25] They reported that the allelic losses were often multiple and discontinuous, with areas of LOH interspersed with areas of retention of heterozygosity, and that most SCLCs (91%) and SqCC (95%) demonstrated larger 3p segments of allele loss, whereas most of the adenocarcinomas and preneoplastic/preinvasive lesions (71%) had smaller chromosome areas of 3p allele loss. These findings imply that there is a progressive increase in the frequency and size of 3p allele loss regions with increasing severity of histopathologic preneoplastic/preinvasive changes. An overview of the sequential molecular events leading to invasive SqCC is demonstrated in a recent review paper.[24]

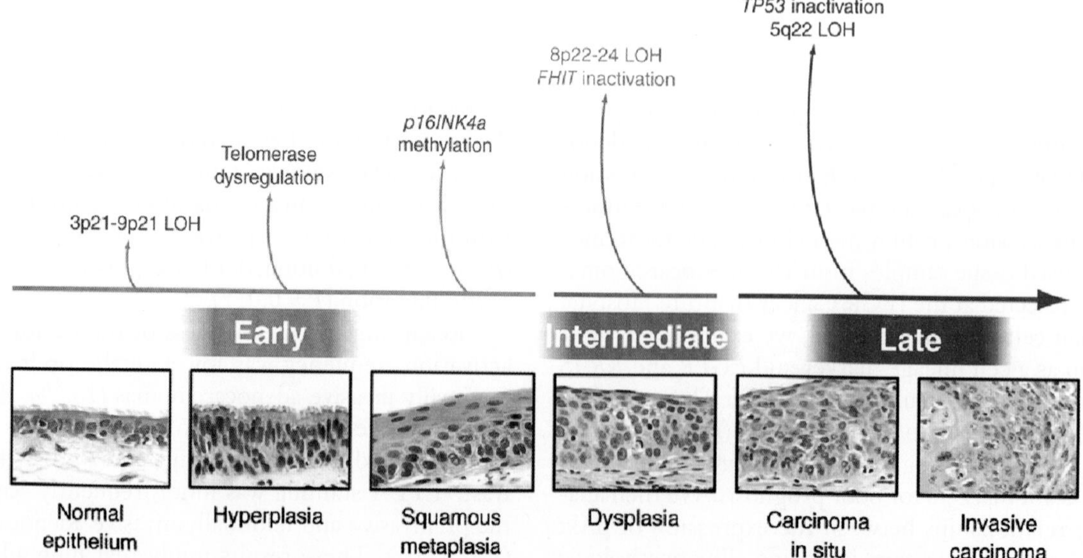

FIGURE 26–9 Sequential development of lung squamous cell carcinoma by Wistuba and Gazdar. Histologic and molecular changes in the development of pulmonary squamous cell carcinoma. These changes occur in a stepwise fashion, beginning in histologically normal epithelium. LOH, loss of heterozygosity. From Wistuba II, Gadar AF. Lung cancer preneoplasia. *Annu Rev Pathol.* 2006;1,331–348.

LARGE CELL CARCINOMA

Large cell carcinoma is an undifferentiated NSCLC without microscopic evidence of squamous, glandular, or neuroendocrine differentiation, although those characteristics can be detected by ultrastructural or immunohistochemical examinations or by molecular methods.

These tumors often demonstrate losses of 1p, lq, 3p, 6q, 7q, and 17p and gains of 5q and 7p, more closely resembling adenocarcinomas than other histologic types.[28] Although both large cell carcinomas and LCNECs show 3p LOH, it is found more frequently in LCNECs and SCLCs than in large cell carcinomas.[29] LOH at 5q33 is more often a feature of large cell carcinoma than LCNEC. LCNECs and SCLCs were more similar to each other than to large cell carcinoma, with 3pl4.2 (*FHIT*), 3p21, and 5q21 losses seen more frequently in LCNECs and SCLCs than in classic large cell carcinomas. *TP53* and 13ql4 LOHs were seen in all tumor types. Common molecular abnormalities include *C-MYC* amplification,[30] *TP53* mutation,[31] and inactivation of *p16*,[32] while *KRAS* mutation is less common.[33]

NEUROENDOCRINE NEOPLASMS, INCLUDING SMALL CELL CARCINOMA

Pulmonary neuroendocrine tumors consist of typical carcinoids, atypical carcinoids, SCLCs, and LCNECs. Molecular markers of these tumors include chromogranin A, synaptophysin, and N-CAM (CD56), which are frequently expressed by neuroendocrine tumors. Typical carcinoids and atypical carcinoids show higher frequencies of immunohistochemical staining of these molecules than SCLCs and LCNECs. Neuroendocrine neoplasms develop in many organs, and although they share some pathologic and clinical features, significant differences do exist among different tumor types and locations.[34] For easy diagnostic categorization, well-differentiated neuroendocrine neoplasms are called neuroendocrine tumors and poorly differentiated neuroendocrine neoplasms are called neuroendocrine carcinomas.

Gastrin-releasing peptide, calcitonin, and other peptide hormones have also been reported to be overexpressed by these tumors. Pedersen et al.[35] reported that the insulinoma-associated 1 (*INSM1*) promoter region was highly expressed in most SCLC cell lines, and expression was absent in cell lines of non-neuroendocrine origin. Jiang et al.[36] reported that the expression of the human homolog 1 of the Drosophila neurogenic achaete-scute genes (*hASH1*) is closely correlated with the endocrine phenotype and differentiation extent in pulmonary neuroendocrine tumors. *hASH1* is specifically expressed in fetal pulmonary neuroendocrine cells and in some neuroendocrine tumor cell lines.

Sturm et al.[37] studied the expression of TTF-1 in 270 neuroendocrine proliferations and tumors and reported that positive immunostaining for TTF-1 was detected in 47 of 55 (85.5%) pure SCLCs, in 31 of 64 (49%) pure LCNECs, but in none of 15 neuroendocrine cell hyperplasias, 23 tumorlets, or 50 carcinoid tumors (27 typical carcinoids and 23 atypical carcinoids). In 19 of 20 (95%) combined SCLCs and LCNECs, TTF-1 expression was identical both in neuroendocrine and non-neuroendocrine components. They concluded that TTF-1 is not expressed in normal and hyperplastic neuroendocrine cells or in carcinoids, but it is expressed in high-grade neuroendocrine proliferations and in lung adenocarcinomas. This report suggests the concept of a spectrum of neuroendocrine proliferations and tumors and lends credence to the alternative hypothesis of a common derivation for SCLC and NSCLC including LCNEC, with carcinoids deriving from a different stem cell. On the other hand, Du et al.[38] reported that TTF-1 expression is specific for lung primary tumors of typical and atypical carcinoids and that TTF-1 positivity is seen exclusively in pulmonary neuroendocrine tumors while all extrapulmonary neuroendocrine tumors were uniformly negative for TTF-1 staining. They also found that TTF-1 positivity was significantly higher in neuroendocrine cell hyperplasia or tumorlets than in typical carcinoids, atypical carcinoids, and LCNECs. They concluded that prevalent TTF-1 positivity in tumorlets and peripheral carcinoids suggests that they may be histogenetically distinct from the central carcinoids, which are typically composed of TTF-1-negative cells. TTF-1 expression of SCLCs and LCNECs is definitely accepted, but that of carcinoid tumors is controversial among the reporters. From our experience, we have not seen any case of typical or atypical carcinoids that show TTF-1 expression and suspect that the remnant type II pneumocytes might be stained positively for TTF-1 antibody.

SCLC showed high frequencies of deletions on chromosome 3p. The region encompasses *ROBO1/DUTT1* [3p12.13], *FHIT* [3p14.2], *RASSF1* [3p21.3], beta-catenin [3p21.3], *Fus1* [3p21.3], *SEMA3B* [3p21.3], *SEMA3F* [3p21.3], *VHL* [3p24.6], and *RAR* beta [3p24.6]). Petersen et al. reported that SCLCs are characterized by a high incidence of deletions on chromosomes 3p, 4q, 5q, 10q, 13q, and 17p.[39] SCLCs have gains on 3q, 5p, 6p, 8q, 17q, 19q, and 20q.[40-42] More than 90% of SCLCs demonstrate large often discontinuous segments of allelic loss on chromosome 3p in areas encompassing multiple candidate tumor suppressor genes, including some of those listed previously.[25] Atypical carcinoids show a higher frequency of LOH at 3p, 13q, 9p21, and 17p than typical carcinoids, but not as high as the high-grade neuroendocrine tumors.[43]

Some typical and atypical carcinoids possess mutations of the multiple endocrine neoplasia 1 (*MEN1*) gene on chromosome 11ql3 or LOH at this locus, while these abnormalities occur with lower frequencies in SCLCs and LCNECs. Debelenko et al. suggested that SCLCs and pulmonary carcinoids develop by distinct molecular pathways.[44]

Oncogenes that are frequently amplified in SCLCs are *MYC* (8q24), *MYCN* (2p24), and *MYCL1* (1p34), and additional amplified genes that represent candidate oncogenes are thought to be the antiapoptotic genes *TNFRSF4* (1p36), *DAD1* (14qll), *BCL2L1* (20qll), and *BCL2L2* (14q11).[42] Tumor suppressor genes are inactivated in the majority of SCLCs. Eighty percent to 90% of SCLCs demonstrate *TP53* mutations as compared with >50% of NSCLCs, fewer atypical carcinoids, and virtually no typical carcinoids.[40,45]

Alterations compromising the p16INK4a/cyclin D1/Rb pathway that induces G_1 arrest are consistent in high-grade pulmonary neuroendocrine carcinomas (92%), primarily through loss of the Rb protein. However, these alterations are less frequent in atypical carcinoids (59%) and uncommon in typical carcinoids.[35,36] Beasley et al.[46] reported that the Rb pathway of G_1 arrest is consistently compromised in high-grade neuroendocrine lung tumors (92%) and is intact in low-grade typical carcinoids. In atypical carcinoids, an intermediate level of alterations (59%) is seen, consistent with their less-aggressive behavior compared with high-grade tumors. The specific expression profile of the Rb pathway proteins may provide specific therapeutic targets in pulmonary neuroendocrine tumors.

Righi et al.[41] examined somatostatin receptor tissue distribution in lung neuroendocrine tumors and reported that somatostatin receptors were heterogeneously distributed with a significant progressive decrease from low- to high-grade forms. They also stressed that somatostatin receptor type 2A was strikingly overexpressed in metastatic typical carcinoids as compared with atypical carcinoids and clinically benign typical carcinoids.

CONCLUDING REMARKS

Lung adenocarcinoma is generally a very heterogeneous tumor showing complicated morphology and arising in both smokers and non-smokers. Recent advances in molecular biology techniques, however, have revealed that lung adenocarcinoma is classified by mutually exclusive oncogene changes: typically, *EGFR* mutations, *KRAS* mutations, and *ALK* rearrangements. Whereas the histology and patterns of oncogene changes are relevant to the choice of chemotherapeutic agents (Fig. 26.10), these changes are also related to etiologic factors and cell morphology. We have proposed the usefulness of classifying lung adenocarcinomas by cell type. The cell-type classification has implications for tumor etiology. We have shown that adenocarcinomas arising in non-smokers are morphologically characterized by hobnail cells, the presence of BAC (AIS) components, and MPPs, as well as by neutral TP53 mutations.

Tumors with *ALK* rearrangements have recently been discovered. They have characteristic histologic features, namely moderately differentiated acinar structures with mucin and sometimes signet-ring cell configurations. Immunohistochemical analysis is useful for screening of tumors with *ALK* translocations.

We also found that RTK signal pathways are selectively activated in adenocarcinomas depending on the tumor's stage or invasiveness. Preinvasive or minimally invasive adenocarcinomas tend to use the RAS–ERK pathway, whereas overt invasive tumors proliferate using the PI3K–Akt pathway. These results are different from those obtained from cell line studies.

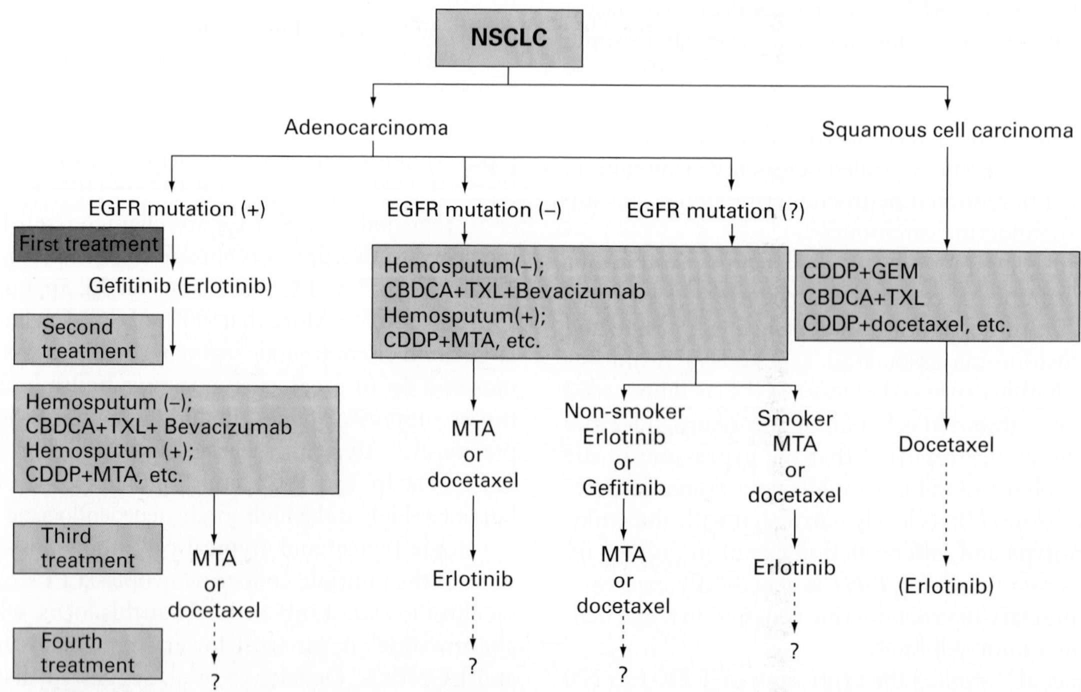

FIGURE 26–10 Choice of therapeutic agents in lung cancer based on histology and oncogene changes. NSCLC, non–small cell lung cancer; EGFR, epidermal growth factor receptor; CBDCA, carboplatin; TXL, paclitaxel; CDDP, cisplatin; MTA, pemetrexed; GEM, gemcitabine.

In the field of pulmonary adenocarcinomas, fantastic scientific progress is ongoing. The research is translational and integrates clinical medicine, histopathology and cytopathology, molecular biology, and etiologic studies. For SqCC, the multistep nature of the tumor development is based on both histology and molecular changes.

SqCC, large cell carcinomas, and neuroendocrine tumors (carcinoids, SCLCs, and LCNECs) have characteristic genetic changes, and their molecular markers and activation of signature pathways are emerging,[47] but correlations between phenotypes and genotypes remain unclear.

REFERENCES

1. Gabrielson E. Worldwide trends in lung cancer pathology. *Respirology*. September 2006;11(5):533-538.
2. Hashimoto T, Tokuchi Y, Hayashi M, et al. Different subtypes of human lung adenocarcinoma caused by different etiological factors—evidence from p53 mutational spectra. *Am J Pathol.* 2000;157:2133-2141.
3. Travis WD, Brambilla E, Muller-Hermelink H, Harris C. *WHO Classification of Tumors. Pathology and Genetics Tumors of the Lung, Pleura, Thymus and Heart.* Lyon: IARC Press; 2004:1-344.
4. Kishimoto Y, Murakami Y, Shiraishi M, Hayashi K, Sekiya T. Aberrations of the *p53* tumor suppressor gene in human non-small cell carcinomas of the lung. *Cancer Res.* 1992;52:4799-4804.
5. Greenblatt MS, Bennett WP, Hollstein M, Harris CC. Mutations in the *p53* tumor suppressor gene: clues to cancer etiology and molecular pathogenesis. *Cancer Res.* 1994;54:4855-4878.
6. Suzuki H, Takahashi T, Kuroishi T, et al. p53 mutations in non-small cell lung cancer in Japan: association between mutations and smoking. *Cancer Res.* 1992;52:734-736.
7. Inamura K, Ninomiya H, Ishikawa Y, Matsubara O. Is the epidermal growth factor receptor status in lung cancers reflected in clinicopathologic features? *Arch Pathol Lab Med.* 2010; 134(1):66-72.
8. Barbara AH, David R, Marileila VG, et al. Antitumor activity of the epidermal growth factor receptor (EGFR) tyrosine kinase inhibitor gefitinib (ZD1839, Iressa) in non-small cell lung cancer cell lines correlates with gene copy number and EGFR mutations but not EGFR protein levels. *Clin Cancer Res.* 2006;12:7117-7125.
9. Lynch TJ, Bell DW, Sordella R, et al. Activating mutations in the epidermal growth factor receptor underlying responsiveness of non-small cell lung cancer to gefitinib. *N Engl J Med.* 2004;350:2129-2139.
10. Paez JG, Janne PA, Lee JC, et al. EGFR mutations in lung cancer: correlation with clinical response to gefitinib therapy. *Science.* 2004;304:1497-1500.
11. Miller VA, Kris MG, Shah N, et al. Bronchioloalveolar pathologic subtype and smoking history predict sensitivity to gefitinib in advanced non-small-cell lung cancer. *J Clin Oncol.* 2004;22:1103-1109.
12. Yatabe Y, Kosaka T, Takahashi T, Mitsudomi T. EGFR mutation is specific for terminal respiratory unit type adenocarcinoma. *Am J Surg Pathol.* 2005;29:633-639.
13. Japan Lung Cancer Society. *General Rules for Clinical and Pathological Records of Lung Cancer.* 5th ed. Tokyo: Kanehara; 1999 [in Japanese].
14. Miyoshi T, Satoh Y, Okumura S, et al. Early-stage lung adenocarcinomas with a micropapillary pattern, a distinct pathologic marker for a significantly poor prognosis. *Am J Surg Pathol.* 2003;27:101-109.
15. Amin MB, Tamboli P, Merchant SH, et al. Micropapillary component in lung adenocarcinoma. A distinctive histological feature with possible prognostic significance. *Am J Surg Pathol.* 2002;26:358-364.
16. Ninomiya H, Hiramatsu M, Inamura K, et al. Correlation between morphology and EGFR mutations in lung adenocarcinomas. Significance of the micropapillary pattern and the hobnail cell type. *Lung Cancer.* 2009;63(2):235-240.
17. Kim YH, Ishii G, Goto K, et al. Dominant papillary subtype is a significant predictor of the response to gefitinib in adenocarcinoma of the lung. *Clin Cancer Res.* 2004;10:7311-7317.
18. Soda M, Choi Y-L, Enomoto M, et al. A novel transforming fusion gene, *EML4–ALK*, identified in non-small cell lung cancer. *Nature.* 2007;448(7153):561-566.
19. Inamura K, Takeuchi K, Togashi Y, et al. *EML4–ALK* lung cancers are characterized by rare other mutations, a TTF-1 cell lineage, an acinar histology, and young onset. *Mod Pathol.* 2009;22:508-515.
20. Takeuchi K, Choi YL, Soda M, et al. Multiplex reverse transcription-PCR screening for *EML4–ALK* fusion transcripts. *Clin Cancer Res.* 2008;14:6618-6624.
21. Takeuchi K, Choi YL, Togashi Y, et al. KIF5B–ALK, a novel fusion oncokinase identified by an immunohistochemistry-based diagnostic system for ALK-positive lung cancer. *Clin Cancer Res.* 2009;15(9):3143-3149.
22. Hiramatsu M, Ninomiya H, Inamura K, et al. Activation status of receptor tyrosine kinase downstream pathways in primary lung adenocarcinoma with reference of KRAS and EGFR mutations. *Lung Cancer.* 2010;70:94-102.
23. Virtanen C, Ishikawa Y, Honjoh D, et al. Integrated classification of lung tumors and cell lines by expression profiling. *Proc Natl Acad Sci U S A.* 2002;99:12357-12362.
24. Wistuba II, Gazdar AF. Lung cancer preneoplasia. *Annu Rev Pathol.* 2006;1:331-348.
25. Wistuba II, Behrens C, Virmani AK, et al. High resolution chromosome 3p allelotyping of human lung cancer and preneoplastic/preinvasive bronchial epithelium reveals multiple, discontinuous sites of 3p allele loss and three regions of frequent breakpoints. *Cancer Res.* April 2000;60(7):1949-1960.
26. Wistuba II, Behrens C, Milchgrub S, et al. Sequential molecular abnormalities are involved in the multistage development of squamous cell lung carcinoma. *Oncogene.* January 1999;18(3): 643-650.
27. Franklin WA, Wistuba II, Geisinger K, et al. Squamous dysplasia and carcinoma in situ. In: Travis WD, Brambilla E, Muller-Hermelink HK, Harris CC, eds. *Pathology and Genetics of Tumours of the Lung, Pleura, Thymus and Heart.* Lyon: IARC Press; 2004:68-72.
28. Johansson M, Karauzum S, Dietrich C, et al. Karyotypic abnormalities in adenocarcinomas of the lung. *Int J Oncol.* July 1994;5(1):17-26.
29. Peng WX, Sano T, Oyama T, Kawashima O, Nakajima T. Large cell neuroendocrine carcinoma of the lung: a comparison with large cell carcinoma with neuroendocrine morphology and small cell carcinoma. *Lung Cancer.* February 2005;47(2):225-233.
30. Lorenz J, Friedberg T, Paulus R, Oesch F, Ferlinz R. Oncogene overexpression in non-small-cell lung cancer tissue: prevalence and clinicopathological significance. *Clin Investig.* January 1994;72(2):156-163.
31. Liu D, Huang CL, Kameyama K, et al. Topoisomerase II alpha gene expression is regulated by the p53 tumor suppressor gene in nonsmall cell lung carcinoma patients. *Cancer.* April 2002;94(8):2239-2247.
32. Jarmalaite S, Kannio A, Anttila S, Lazutka JR, Husgafvel-Pursiainen K. Aberrant p16 promoter methylation in smokers and former smokers with nonsmall cell lung cancer. *Int J Cancer.* October 2003;106(6):913-918.
33. Eleazar JA, Borczuk AC. Molecular pathology of large cell carcinoma and its precursors. In: Zander DS, Popper HH, Jagirdar J, Haque AK, Cagle PT, Barrios R, eds. *Molecular Pathology of Lung Diseases.* New York, NY: Springer; 2008:279-292.
34. Volante M, Righi L, Berruti A, Rindi G, Papotti M. The pathological diagnosis of neuroendocrine tumors: common questions and tentative answers. *Virchows Arch.* 2011;458(4):393-402.
35. Pedersen N, Pedersen MW, Lan MS, Breslin MB, Poulsen HS. The insulinoma-associated 1: a novel promoter for targeted cancer gene therapy for small-cell lung cancer. *Cancer Gene Ther.* 2006;13(4):375-384.
36. Jiang SX, Kameya T, Asamura H, et al. hASH1 expression is closely correlated with endocrine phenotype and differentiation extent in pulmonary neuroendocrine tumors. *Mod Pathol.* 2004;17(2):222-229.

37. Du EZ, Goldstraw P, Zacharias J, et al. TTF-1 expression is specific for lung primary in typical and atypical carcinoids: TTF-1-positive carcinoids are predominantly in peripheral location. *Hum Pathol.* 2004;35(7):825-831.
38. Sturm N, Rossi G, Lantuejoul S, et al. Expression of thyroid transcription factor-1 in the spectrum of neuroendocrine cell lung proliferations with special interest in carcinoids. *Hum Pathol.* February 2002;33(2):175-182.
39. Petersen I, Langreck H, Wolf G, et al. Small-cell lung cancer is characterized by a high incidence of deletions on chromosomes 3p, 4q, 5q, 10q, 13q and 17p. *Br J Cancer.* 1997;75(1):79-86.
40. Righi L, Volante M, Rapa I, Scagliotti GV, Papotti M. Neuroendocrine tumours of the lung. A review of relevant pathological and molecular data. *Virchows Arch.* 2007;451(suppl 1):S51-S59.
41. Righi L, Volante M, Tavaglione V, et al. Somatostatin receptor tissue distribution in lung neuroendocrine tumours: a clinicopathologic and immunohistochemical study of 218 "clinically aggressive" cases. *Ann Oncol.* 2010;21(3):548-555.
42. Kim YH, Girard L, Giacomini CP, et al. Combined microarray analysis of small cell lung cancer reveals altered apoptotic balance and distinct expression signatures of MYC family gene amplification. *Oncogene.* 2006;25(1):130-138.
43. Onuki N, Wistuba II, Travis WD, et al. Genetic changes in the spectrum of neuroendocrine lung tumors. *Cancer.* 1999;85(3):600-607.
44. Debelenko LV, Swalwell JI, Kelley MJ, et al. *MEN1* gene mutation analysis of high-grade neuroendocrine lung carcinoma. *Genes Chromosomes Cancer.* 2000;28(1):58-65.
45. Wistuba II, Gazdar AF, Minna JD. Molecular genetics of small cell lung carcinoma. *Semin Oncol.* 2001;28(2 suppl 4):3-13.
46. Beasley MB, Lantuejoul S, Abbondanzo S, et al. The P16/cyclin D1/Rb pathway in neuroendocrine tumors of the lung. *Hum Pathol.* 2003;34(2):136-142.
47. Shigematsu H, Gazdar AF. Somatic mutations of epidermal growth factor receptor signaling pathway in lung cancers. *Int J Cancer.* 2006;118:257-262.

CHAPTER 27

Molecular Diagnostics of Breast Cancer

Ping Tang and David G. Hicks

INTRODUCTION

Breast cancer is a group of heterogeneous tumors with a wide spectrum of morphologic subtypes and biologic behaviors.[1] A major challenge in the treatment of breast cancer is to identify subgroups of breast cancer patients who will benefit from a particular adjuvant therapy regimen, with the goal of minimizing overtreatment or undertreatment.[2,3] Currently, the treatment strategy for clinical decision-making involves careful consideration of a group of key clinicopathologic factors that include patient age, menopausal status, tumor size, histologic type, tumor grade, lymphovascular invasion, lymph node staging, and evidence of distant metastasis along with the estrogen receptor (ER), progesterone receptor (PR), and human epidermal growth factor receptor 2 (HER2) status of the tumor. These factors have been validated in numerous clinical studies and through years of clinical experience as being helpful in determining the probability of local or distant recurrence and, along with the development of effective adjuvant therapies, has contributed to a steady decline in breast cancer mortality.

TRADITIONAL PATHOLOGIC PROGNOSTIC FACTORS

Treating physicians take into account a number of clinically validated patient factors and tumor-related factors in making important decisions regarding the most appropriate adjuvant therapy. The two major systems with robust prognostic value are the TNM staging system and the histologic grading system.[4]

TNM Staging

The TNM staging system from the American Joint Committee on Cancer (AJCC) provides useful information for determining the risk of recurrence and is used clinically to help make treatment decisions.

T = Tumor Size

The size of the primary tumor (measured in centimeters) is useful in assessing the patient's tumor burden, and the T stages are based on size (pT1 through pT4) and provide useful prognostic information. The size of the primary tumor has been shown to be an independent prognostic factor; it correlates with the number of involved lymph nodes and is associated with increasing risk of recurrence. For node-negative patients, tumor size is the second most significant prognostic factor and is routinely used to make adjuvant treatment decisions.[5,6]

N = Nodal Status

Numerous clinical studies have shown that one of the strongest and most consistent prognostic factors in breast cancer is the presence or absence of axillary lymph node involvement. In addition, there seems to be a direct linear relationship between the number of involved lymph nodes and the risk of distance recurrence. Traditionally, the status of the axilla has been assessed by a standard axillary dissection in which level I and level II lymph nodes were removed. Recently, the use of sentinel node biopsy has become more readily accepted for axillary staging, with the goal of sparing patients the potential morbidity associated with axillary dissection, while still providing staging information to guide adjuvant treatment decisions.[7,8]

M = Distant Metastasis

The extent of metastasis is often determined by clinical and/or radiologic methods (cM) or by confirmation with a biopsy of the metastatic site (pM). A newly created M0i+

category is defined by the presence of either disseminated tumor cells (DTCs) detectable in bone marrow or circulating blood or found incidentally in other tissue if the metastatic site does not exceed 0.2 mm.

Histologic Grade

The histologic or pathologic grade in primary breast cancer provides important independent prognostic information. Pathological grade is routinely used to stratify breast cancer patients into favorable (well-differentiated tumor) and less favorable (poorly differentiated tumor) outcome groups. One of the more widely used systems for grading breast tumors is the Elston and Ellis modification of the Scarff-Bloom-Richardson score, based on mitotic index, architectural differentiation, and nuclear pleomorphism.[9] Although many clinical studies have validated and confirmed the prognostic significance of tumor grade, adherence to strict morphologic criteria is needed to help ensure reproducibility between different observers, so that grade is reliably usable as a strong prognostic factor.[10,11] Rakha et al.[12] recently showed that even in this new molecular era, the Nottingham grading system still provides important clinical information regarding the tumor. Tumor grade can discriminate between different subsets of breast cancer with different risks of recurrence. Interestingly, recent molecular studies have begun to define potential mechanisms and genomic changes that may underlie breast cancer grade and may help to explain its relationship to prognosis (Fig. 27.1). High-grade breast cancers are at increased risk for early recurrence and metastasis, whereas low-grade tumors tend to follow a more indolent clinical course with fewer and later recurrences. Rakha et al.[12] also showed that accurate breast cancer grading provides prognostic information that is equivalent to that provided by the nodal status of tumors (Table 27.1).

Addition of Molecular Diagnosis

With careful documentation of all the pathologic features of each breast cancer, pathologists attempt to provide clinicians with the most accurate prognostic and predictive information possible to help guide therapeutic decision-making. However, clearly there are limitations to what can be provided by morphologic assessment alone. As an adjunct to traditional diagnosis, significant advancements in molecular biology have been translated into new tools that place breast cancers into clinically relevant classifications, with therapeutic implications. Our better understanding of the molecular alterations that underlie breast cancer has fundamentally changed our approach to classifying and treating breast cancer patients. For example, immunohistochemical (IHC) testing for ER and PR and IHC and/or fluorescence in situ hybridization (FISH) testing for HER2 have been firmly established as the standard of care for all primary and recurrent breast cancers on the basis of prospective randomized clinical trials. ER-positive tumors represent a more favorable

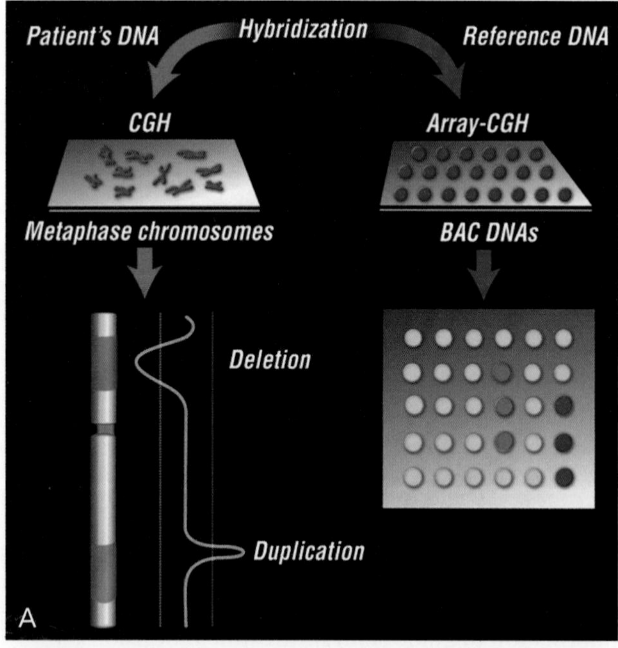

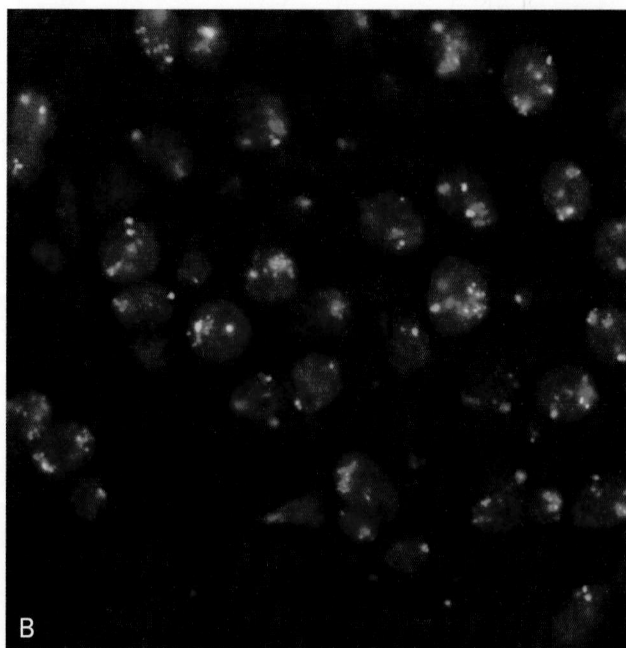

FIGURE 27–1 Breast cancers are characterized by complex genomic changes and copy number alterations (CNA). Many of these changes occur in regions that harbor known proto-oncogenes and tumor suppressor genes and these alterations can lead to gene overexpression or loss of function. Fluorescent-labeled DNA from breast cancer can be hybridized to either metaphase chromosomes (comparative genomic hybridization, CGH) or a DNA microarray (array-CGH) to evaluate CNA. Deletions or amplification of DNA is detected by comparison with reference normal DNA (**A**, **left** image). DNA CNAs discovered by CGH can be validated by fluorescence in situ hybridization. Amplification of the HER2 gene (**B**, red signal, **right** image) is the prototype for genomic changes that can be seen in high-grade breast cancers. (This figure was used with permission from Amirsys, Inc., Hicks DG, **Lester SC.** DNA analysis. In: *Diagnostic Pathology: Breast.* 1st ed. Salt Lake City, UT: Amirsys Publishing; 2012:210-211.)

TABLE 27-1 Nottingham Grade and Breast Cancer Characteristics

Tumor Features	Low Nottingham Grade	High Nottingham Grade
ER, PR, HER2	Typically ER/PR+ and HER2 non-amplified	Typically low or negative ER expression, more likely HER2 amplified
Proliferation	Low proliferative index	High proliferative index
P53	Normal function (p53 IHC negative)	Loss of p53 function (p53 IHC positive)
DNA copy number changes	Fewer copy number changes; most common changes are losses on 16q and gains on 1q.	More frequent, extensive, and complex chromosomal alterations.
	Other reported changes: gains on 8q, 11q, 16p, and 17q and losses on 1p, 8p, 11q, 13q, and 22q	Gains are often on 8q, 17q, and 20q and losses are on 17p, 1p, 19p, and 19q
		Genomic losses are rarely seen on 16q
Gene expression profiling	Most likely to show luminal A profile, some luminal B	Luminal B, HER, and basal profiles

ER, estrogen receptor; PR, progesterone receptor; HER2, human epidermal growth factor receptor 2; IHC, immunohistochemical.

subtype, with better prognosis and response to hormonal therapy. HER2-positive tumors are next in line in terms of prognosis, because of the development of effective HER2-targeted therapy. Patients with triple-negative (ER, PR, and HER2 negative) cancers continue to have a poor prognosis, with no targeted therapy currently available. The newer poly-ADP-ribose polymerase (PARP) inhibitors have shown promise for the treatment of this latter disease subtype.

The recent addition of Ki-67 IHC analysis by some centers also seems to provide additional information regarding prognosis and prediction for benefit from chemotherapy. In addition to IHC analysis, other types of molecular analysis are now being used clinically, such as testing for BRCA mutations (BRCA1 [Breast Cancer gene one] and BRCA2 [Breast Cancer gene two]) in high-risk subgroups and using multigene assays such as the 21-gene assay (OncotypeDx)[13] and MammaPrint.[14] Furthermore, what has emerged from recent molecular studies of breast cancer that have examined DNA copy number changes and gene expression profiles is the concept that there are two different pathways to the development of invasive tumors. These have been referred to as the low-grade breast neoplasia pathway and the high-grade breast neoplasia pathway. Each of these pathways is associated with unique DNA changes and gene expression profiles that appear to arise early and are shared between precursor lesions, in situ lesions, and the subsequent invasive carcinomas.

The goal of these new approaches to the study of breast cancer is to identify new molecules that can be utilized for targeted therapy and to better stratify patients into clinically relevant subsets of disease that have therapeutic implications. Here, we summarize recent developments in the molecular diagnosis of breast cancer, with a focus on those that have a significant effect on therapeutic decisions. In considering any new approach to profiling breast cancers, it is vitally important that the results be interpreted within the morphologic and clinical context for each patient and not be discordant with the traditional pathologic features of the tumor.

MANDATED MOLECULAR TESTS FOR ALL BREAST CARCINOMA RECOMMENDED BY THE AMERICAN SOCIETY OF CLINICAL ONCOLOGY (ASCO)/THE COLLEGE OF AMERICAN PATHOLOGISTS (CAP)

Despite extensive studies on many possible biomarkers for breast cancer, only three prognostic and predictive markers (ER, PR, and HER2) are recommended by the ASCO and CAP and routinely tested in breast cancer patients[15,16] (Table 27.2).

TABLE 27-2 Criterion for Selecting Targeted Therapy

Tumor Targets	Targeted Agents	Clinically Validated Testing Methodology	Treatment Thresholds per ASCO/CAP Guidelines
Endocrine blockade	Tamoxifen, aromatase inhibitors	ER positive based on validated IHC test	≥1% of invasive tumor cells showing nuclear staining
HER2 blockade	Trastuzumab Lapatinib	HER2 positive based on validated IHC or FISH test	IHC ≥ 30% intense complete membrane staining FISH = HER2/CEP17 > 2.2 or HER2 > 6

ASCO/CAP, American Society of Clinical Oncology (ASCO)/The College Of American Pathologists; IHC, immunohistochemical; HER2, human epidermal growth factor receptor 2; FISH, fluorescence in situ hybridization; CEP17, chromosome enumeration probe 17.
Accurate, reliable, and reproducible estrogen receptor, progesterone receptor, and HER2 analyses are an important prerequisite for the best possible adjuvant therapy decision-making.

ER and PR

ER is a member of an intracellular steroid hormone receptor family that is activated by interaction with the ligand estrogen. Two different forms exist, ER alpha and ER beta, each encoded by a separate gene (ESR1 and ESR2, respectively). ER alpha is the most important ER in breast cancer. After binding to its ligand, estrogen, ER is transported to the nucleus, where it functions as a transcription factor and regulates the expression of a number of genes that are important in breast cancer biology, including genes associated with proliferation.[17-19]

PR, also known as NR3C3, is another steroid hormone receptor and is activated by the ligand progesterone. PR also functions as a nuclear transcription factor and is regulated by ER. Thus, PR expression can serve as an indicator of a functionally intact nuclear ER pathway and can help in predicting the response to hormonal therapy. There are two isoforms of PR, PR-A and PR-B, and abundant PR-A has been associated with an elevated risk of breast cancer.[20] The two forms of PR induce the expression of different sets of genes that are related to both proliferation and inhibitory effects on cell growth. A breast cancer is considered positive for hormone receptors if either ER or PR is positive by IHC. Almost all well-differentiated, low-grade tumors (classic infiltrating lobular, pure mucinous, or tubular carcinomas) are expected to be ER positive. If tumors with these morphologic features test negative for ER, this suggests that the result may be a false negative and that the assay should be repeated.

The analysis of ER in breast tumors is one of the oldest and most successful examples of how a biomarker can guide therapy in breast cancer patients. The expression of hormone receptors by breast cancer has been shown to be highly predictive for a clinical benefit from a variety of endocrine therapies, and this benefit is seen only in tumors that are ER and/or PR positive. Endocrine therapy with tamoxifen or aromatase inhibitors has been shown to be the most effective and available targeted therapy for ER-positive breast cancer, being used in neoadjuvant, adjuvant, palliative, and preventive settings.[21] A 5-year course of tamoxifen adjuvant therapy after surgery almost halves the annual recurrence rate and reduces the breast cancer mortality rate by 1/3 in both pre- and postmenopausal women with ER-positive tumors.[22] Given the clinical importance of an accurate assessment of these receptors, the ASCO/CAP Task Force in 2010 provided new guidelines for standardized testing and reporting for ER and PR.[16]

Although ER and PR are good positive predictors for hormonal therapy, they are not good negative predictors, because not all ER- and PR-positive tumors will respond to hormonal therapy. A better understanding of the pathways involved in endocrine therapy resistance will help us to develop novel strategies to overcome this problem and improve breast cancer management. One of the well-studied resistance pathways comes from the metabolism of tamoxifen and the generation of active metabolites. Plasma concentration of tamoxifen metabolites can be affected by genetic polymorphism of its metabolizing enzyme cytochrome p4502D6 (CYP2D6). Indeed, recent studies have shown allelic variants in CYP2D6 to be an important determinant of tamoxifen activity.[23] Although ASCO,[24] NCCN,[25] and St. Gallen's expert consensus[26] do not endorse routine CYP2D6 genotyping, some experts have suggested such testing for selective patients who are not able to tolerate aromatase inhibitors or who have a contraindication to aromatase inhibitors.[27,28]

The epidermal growth factor receptor (EGFR)/HER2-activated signaling pathway has also been implicated in endocrine resistance. The transcriptional activities of ER have been shown to be repressed by heregulin, the ligand for both EGFR and HER2, resulting in the development of estrogen independence and in turn causing endocrine resistance.[29-31] EGFR/HER2 signaling has been reported to be involved in acquired tamoxifen resistance in a cellular model,[32] and its inhibition by gefitinib or trastuzumab resulted in growth suppression of these cells.[33] A phase II clinical trial involving patients with tamoxifen-resistant advanced breast cancer treated with gefitinib showed beneficial effects of this anti-EGFR agent.[34] Other pathways implicated in endocrine resistance include co-activators and co-repressors, kinase-activated growth pathways, the PI3K cell survival pathway, and the stress-activated protein kinase-JUNNH2 terminal kinase pathway.[35]

One important subtype of breast cancer is the ER-positive/PR-negative (ER+/PR–) tumors, which constitute about 11% of all breast cancers and 13% of ER-positive breast cancers.[36] Interestingly, recent data have suggested that the PR status of breast cancer may be independently associated with clinical outcome and that the loss of PR expression in ER-positive tumors is associated with a more aggressive clinical course.[37] These distinctive clinical features may be related to differences in tumor biology for the ER+/PR– subset of breast cancers. It now appears that ER+/PR– tumors represent a distinct subset of breast cancer characterized by aggressive behavior and tamoxifen resistance in spite of being ER positive. Clinically these tumors are larger, more likely to be lymph node positive, with higher proliferation rates,[38] greater genomic instability,[39,40] and higher levels of expression of EGFR and HER2.[20] We have shown, using a 21-gene assay, that ER+/PR– tumors are more likely to develop bone metastasis[41] and have higher recurrence scores (RSs).[42] ER-positive tumors defined by gene signature as luminal B subtypes may show loss of PR,[43] and ER-positive, high-grade tumors defined by the genomic grade index of Loi et al.[11] typically fall into the high recurrence risk category.

There are various theories to explain the downregulation of PR in the presence of ER, leading to this subset of ER+/PR– tumors. In some cases, the ER pathway is nonfunctional so that it is unable to simulate PR production or there may be low serum concentrations of estrogen.[20] Other mechanisms include hypermethylation of the PR promoter found in 20% to 40% of ER+/PR– tumors, downregulation of PR expression by molecular cross-talk between growth factor and membrane ER,[20,44] and expression of mutated epidermal growth factor receptor (EGFRvIII).[45] The data from clinical trials are unclear as to whether, in terms of endocrine therapy, the ER+/PR− and ER+/PR+ groups of patients should receive different treatment. Currently, the preferred treatment includes aromatase inhibitors, fulvestrant, and chemotherapy for ER+/PR− tumors. Overcoming tamoxifen resistance with targeted therapies such as gefitinib is being evaluated.

Human Epidermal Growth Factor Receptor 2

HER2 is a 185-kDa transmembrane glycoprotein with tyrosine kinase activity and is a member of the HER family of growth factor receptors involved in the complex regulation of cell proliferation and angiogenesis and in enhancing cell survival pathway. The HER2 gene is located on chromosome 17 and is amplified as an early event in breast cancer carcinogenesis for a subset of tumors, occurring in about 15% to 20% of breast cancers.[46,47] Gene amplification is the primary mechanism that drives HER2 overexpression in this important subset of breast cancers. HER2 overexpression resulting from gene amplification dramatically increases the likelihood of receptor activation and signaling, contributing to a more aggressive tumor biology, and is associated with worse clinical outcome and higher rates of recurrence and mortality.

Clinical assays to assess the HER2 status include IHC, which detects protein overexpression, and FISH, which detects gene amplification.[48] Both assays have been clinically validated to help predict response to agents that target overexpressed HER2. In addition, HER2 status is also predictive for the response to several systematic therapies. HER2 overexpression is associated with relative resistance to endocrine therapy, which may be selectively to tamoxifen but not to aromatase inhibitors.[49,50] HER2 status also appears to be predictive for either resistance or sensitivity to different types of chemotherapeutic agents.[51-53] Most importantly, targeted therapies against HER2-positive tumors have been developed and shown to be remarkably effective in both metastatic and adjuvant settings for patients with HER2-positive tumors as determined by clinical assays (FISH or IHC) for gene amplification or protein overexpression. Trastuzumab is a humanized monoclonal antibody that combines the mouse recognition sequence of a monoclonal antibody (clone 4D5) against an extracellular epitope of the receptors with a human IgG1. Trastuzumab demonstrates a high affinity and specificity for the HER2 receptor and has been shown to improve response rates, time to progression, and even survival when used alone[54] or added to chemotherapy in metastatic settings.[55] Several international, prospective randomized trials have demonstrated that adjuvant trastuzumab reduces the relative risk of recurrence by half and mortality by one-third in early-stage breast cancer.[56-59] Furthermore, lapatinib, a small tyrosine kinase inhibitor of HER2 kinase activity, improves clinical outcome in patients with advanced disease.[60] The findings from these clinical trials highlight the importance of accurate HER2 testing for every patient with newly diagnosed breast cancer in order to help select those patients who will be the most suitable candidates for HER2-targeted therapy.

The ASCO/CAP Task Force has provided comprehensive HER2 testing guidelines and recommends that HER2[15] be tested in patients with a new diagnosis of invasive breast cancer. The guidelines did not recommend one test over another (IHC or FISH) and on the basis of clinical trial data concluded that both IHC and FISH could be used to assess the HER2 status of breast cancer if the test had been appropriately validated and the laboratory had a rigorous quality assurance program. Those patients with evidence either of gene amplification by FISH or protein overexpression by IHC are considered suitable for HER2-targeted therapy. The guidelines also recognized that there is an equivocal category that is occasionally encountered when interpreting the results from both IHC and FISH for HER2. These equivocal categories recognize that the HER2 test results represent a continuous rather than a categorical variable and can no longer be reported simply as binary. Equivocal results for IHC assays must be confirmed by reflex FISH analysis of the sample, whereas equivocal FISH results can be confirmed by counting additional cells, repeating the FISH assay, or confirmatory IHC testing. The intention of creating these equivocal categories was to trigger additional testing so that clinicians and patients had additional information for clinical decision-making. However, the panel did not recommend withholding HER2-targeted therapy in those patients with equivocal results on the HER2 test (or tests) whose results fell within ranges that would have allowed them to be treated in the first generation of adjuvant HER2-targeted trials.[61]

Despite the remarkable clinical efficacy of HER2-targeted therapy, not all patients respond, and de novo and acquired resistance remain an important clinical issue. Currently, there are no clinically validated factors that can be used to predict trastuzumab resistance in breast cancer. Preclinical data have suggested a number of potential mechanisms of resistance—including reduction of antibody affinity and binding due to MUC4 overexpression, constitutively active downstream signaling involving p27 Kip1, PTEN, PI3K, mTOR, and Akt, as well as cross talk with other signaling pathways including IGFR-1—that can bypass the HER2 blockade.[62]

BRCA TEST FOR PATIENTS SUSPECTED TO HAVE HEREDITARY BREAST CANCER

It has long been recognized that as many as 10% to 20% women with breast cancer also have an affected first-degree relative (parent, sister, or daughter). However, only 5% to 6% of breast cancers have been linked to a specific inherited high penetrance germline mutation in a breast cancer susceptibility gene. Two well-recognized major susceptibility genes for breast cancer are BRCA1 and BRCA2. Approximately 0.1% of the population carries any of the 200+ described different mutations for the BRCA genes.[63,64] Recent meta-analysis has reported that the rate of lifetime risk of breast cancer is in the range of 47% to 66% for BRCA1 mutation carriers and 40% to 57% for BRCA2.[65,66] Interestingly, the majority of reported germline mutations that have been associated with breast cancer risk are involved in DNA repair pathways, including BRCA1 and BRCA2. Cells lacking BRCA1 and BRCA2 functional activity are prone to replication errors and genomic instability, leading to DNA abnormalities and the accumulation of mutations that would drive tumor formation. Also, BRCA1 function is required for transactivation of the ER gene promoter, which may partially explain why 90% of BRCA1-associated carcinomas are ER negative. In addition to being triple negative (TN) (negative for ER, PR, and HER2), the majority of BRCA1-associated cancers will show characteristic morphologic features (circumscribed growth pattern, high nuclear grade, geographic necrosis, and high mitotic rate) and fall into the basal phenotype subset by gene expression profiling. The reason for this relative tissue specificity for breast cancers is not well understood; however, mutation carriers are also at risk for other solid tumors, including ovarian, fallopian tube, and pancreatic adenocarcinomas. Because of the significant breast cancer risk, BRCA mutation carriers often choose to undergo interventions aimed at cancer prevention or cancer risk reduction for additional cancers once an index cancer occurs. These interventions can include frequent screenings with mammograms, screenings with magnetic resonance imaging,[67] chemoprevention with tamoxifen,[68] and prophylactic oophorectomy or mastectomy.[69]

Rapid germline testing has made it possible to identify a BRCA mutation carrier contemporaneously with a diagnosis of breast cancer. More than 200 different mutations have been reported in each gene, distributed throughout their length, requiring full direct sequencing of both genes to exclude a mutation. The majority of mutations are small deletions or insertions, resulting in frameshift mutations, or non-sense mutations, resulting in a truncated or absent protein. Often high-risk patients will need a highly specialized genetic consultation to determine whether the test is appropriate for them. Indications for BRCA germline testing include two first-degree relatives under the age of 50 years with a diagnosis of breast cancer, three or more first- or second-degree relatives with breast cancer regardless of age at diagnosis, a combination of first- or second-degree relatives with breast or ovarian cancer, a first-degree relative with bilateral breast cancer, a combination of two or more first- or second-degree relatives with ovarian cancer regardless of age, first- or second-degree relatives with both breast and ovary cancer regardless of age, and a relative with male breast cancer. On occasion, mutations not associated with a known breast cancer risk may be detected and the significance of these findings is uncertain. Once a mutation has been identified in an individual, other family members may be tested for that specific mutation at considerably less expense.

In addition to a young age at diagnosis and a strong family history, a number of pathological features have been identified that are associated with BRCA1- and BRCA2-related breast tumors and which can also suggest the need for germline testing. Breast cancers associated with BRCA1 are often invasive ductal carcinomas (IDCs), medullary-like, high-grade, ER positive in only about 10% of cases, often HER2 negative and p53 positive (Table 27.3). Tumors associated with

TABLE 27-3 Molecular Subtypes of Invasive Ductal Carcinoma: Clinical and Biologic Features

Feature	Luminal A	Luminal B	HER2 Positive	Basal/Triple Negative
% of breast cancer	55%	15%	12–18%	10–15%
Patient age	Older age	Younger age	Younger age	Younger age
Nottingham grade	1 or 2	2 or 3	2 or 3	Typically 3
ER status	Positive (high)	Positive (may be low)	60% negative (classic HER2) and 40% positive (luminal HER2)	Mostly negative
PR status	Usually positive	May be low or negative	May be low or negative	Mostly negative
HER2 status	Negative	Positive in ~40% (luminal HER2)	Positive (HER2 classic)	Negative
Ki-67 proliferative index	Low (<10%)	Typically high (>14%)	Typically high (>20%)	Typically very high (>50%)
CK5/6 or EGFR	Absent	Absent	Occasionally positive	50–85% positive
Natural history	Indolent, possible late recurrence	More aggressive	Worse natural history, sensitive to HER2-targeted therapy	Worse natural history, early recurrence more likely
Hormonal therapy	Most likely to benefit	May benefit	May benefit for ER+/HER+	No benefit
Chemotherapy	Unlikely to benefit	May benefit when added to hormonal therapy	Benefit from chemotherapy + HER2 targeted therapy	Most likely to benefit from neoadjuvant

HER2, human epidermal growth factor receptor 2; ER, estrogen receptor; PR, progesterone receptor; CK, cytokeratin; EGFR, epidermal growth factor receptor.

BRCA2 may be lobular or with minimal tubal formation, lower nuclear grade, 70% positive for ER, mostly HER2 negative and p53 negative. The histologic features that are significant in predicting BRCA1-related breast cancers include high mitotic count, prominent lymphocytic infiltrate, and pushing borders; for BRCA2-related tumors, pushing borders and minimal tubule formation are the most significant pathologic features.

OTHER IHC-BASED TESTS

Ki-67

Ki-67 was first described in 1983 by Gerdes et al.,[70] who used a mouse monoclonal antibody that reacts with a human nuclear protein associated with cell proliferation. A year later, the same group reported[71] a detailed cell cycle study showing that this nuclear antigen Ki-67 was expressed in G1, S, G2 and in mitosis but not in G0. In 1990, Gerdes et al.[72] described Ki-67 as a non-histone protein present as double bands upon immunoblot, with molecular weights of 395 and 345 kDa.

Ki-67 is now routinely used as a pathological measurement of cellular proliferation index in formalin-fixed, paraffin-embedded tissues. High levels of Ki-67 expression are associated with breast carcinomas of higher grade and positive lymph node involvement.[73] Ki-67 has been shown to have both prognostic and predictive values for breast cancer. Molino et al.[74] showed that Ki-67 is associated with tumor size, lymph node status, ER/PR expression, disease-free survival, and overall survival, and this was also confirmed by later larger studies[75,76]; Ki-67 is also predictive of axillary node metastasis.[77] Many studies have also demonstrated that the expression level of Ki-67 is predictive for benefit from chemotherapy[78,79] and hormonal therapy.[80]

In 2009, Cheang et al.[81] reported that expression of Ki-67 can be used to separate the original ER- and PR-positive luminal A subtype of breast cancer into luminal A with low Ki-67 (<14%) and luminal B with high Ki-67 (>14%). (Table 27.3) Luminal B group has a prognosis that is similar to luminal HER2 (triple positive tumor). Another study has confirmed the clinical significance of this subclassification.[82] There is increasing evidence showing that proliferation rate is perhaps the strongest determinant of outcome in patients with ER-positive tumors.[13,83,84] Ki-67 was added in 2007 to the St. Gallen consensus meeting and Adjuvant! Online because it does provide additional prognostic information.[69] Although many major cancer centers have been testing and reporting the expression of Ki-67 at the request of clinicians, currently there are no guidelines, recommendations, or international or national standards regarding how to test and report it.

MOLECULAR CLASSIFICATION OF BREAST CANCER: GENE EXPRESSION PROFILING AND IHC SURROGATES

The application of molecular gene expression analysis in clinical breast tumor samples by utilizing new array technologies has been a major advance in our understanding of the biological diversity of breast cancer. Initial evidence for molecular subtypes of breast carcinomas came from a cDNA microarray study of gene expression among a small number of tumor samples and several benign controls.[43] Two major subgroups of expression patterns were identified among the tumor samples that were reminiscent of two normal mammary cellular components: ER-positive luminal cells and ER-negative basal cells. Two other groups were also identified: one with strong HER2 expression and low expression of ER-related genes, and the other, a very small group with an expression pattern very similar to that for normal breast. Further studies with additional tumor samples from the same laboratory[85,86] added one more group by separating the luminal tumors into luminal A and B subtypes. These five molecular subtypes not only have distinct gene expression profiles but also have unique clinical outcomes. These molecular subtypes have been confirmed as reproducible and statistically robust in independent data[87-90] (Fig. 27.2).

These studies have contributed to an evolving understanding of the clinical course of disease for breast cancer patients. Each of these molecular subtypes is characterized by different clinical features, such as statistically robust differences in relapse-free survival, overall survival, and patterns of recurrence, independent of traditional pathologic factors. Although the gold standard for molecular classification remains gene expression microarray analysis, its use in clinical practice has been limited by its strict tissue requirements (fresh/frozen tissue), as well as by issues of cost, complexity, and technical feasibility. In an effort to develop a molecular classification that is clinically significant, technically simple, reproducible, and readily available, investigators have been studying molecular classifications that are IHC based, derived from the data of gene expression profiling, correlated with clinical outcome, and able to provide corroborative prognostic and predictive information (Fig. 27.3).

Currently, there are still no internationally accepted criteria for IHC-based classification. Several IHC-based systems have been used by researchers, all of which have shown a relationship to gene expression profiling and have correlated with clinical outcome. Cytokeratin (CK) classification divides breast carcinomas into a basal-like subtype (CK5/6, CK14, and CK17 positive) and a luminal subtype (CK8, CK18 positive, and basal negative).[91,92] The basal-like subtype is associated with poor prognosis,[93] BRCA1-associated tumors,[94] and more frequent metastasis to lung and brain.[95,96]

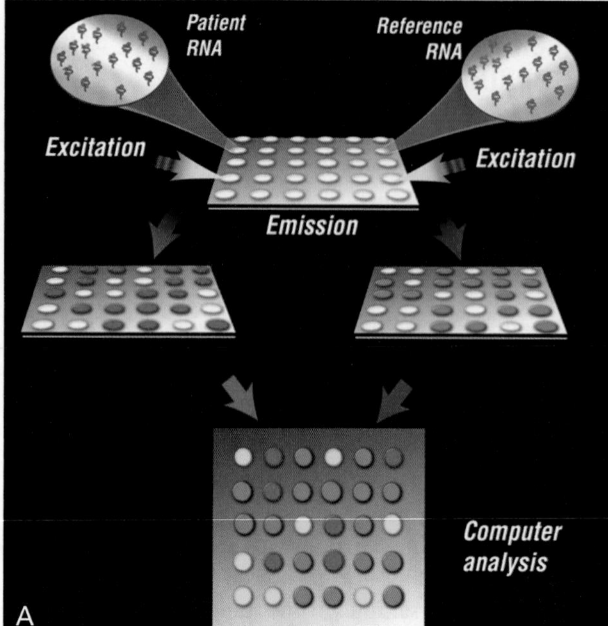

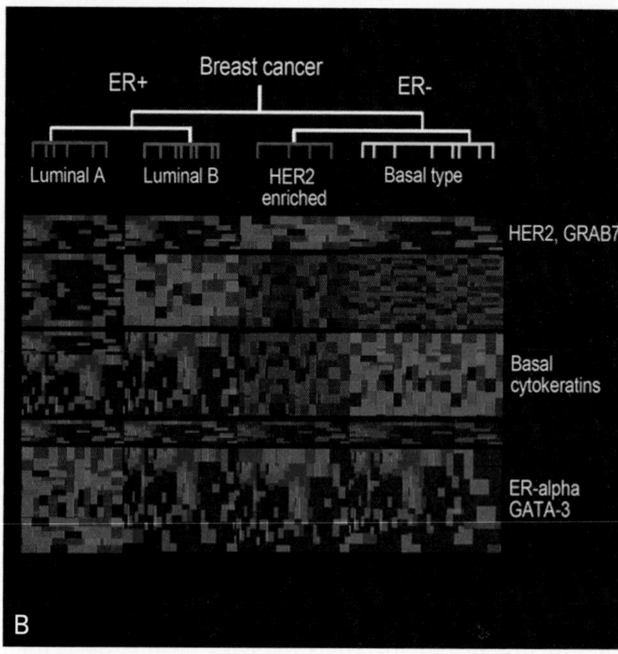

FIGURE 27–2 Gene expression profiling (GEP) using cDNA microarrays can be utilized to study global changes in the patterns of gene expression in breast cancer tissue. GEP is performed by mixing fluorescent-labeled tumor RNA (red) with labeled reference RNA (green) followed by hybridization on a cDNA microarray which contains complementary transcript sequences. The relative level of tumor RNA expression can be measured by fluorescent intensity and can be increased (red), decreased (green), or unchanged (**A**, yellow, left image) in comparison to the reference RNA. GEP data are analyzed to find biologically meaningful patterns based on similar patterns of gene expression. Using unsupervised cluster analysis, tumor can be sorted into related groups (class discovery) based on similarities in their gene expression profiles. This approach was used to develop the intrinsic molecular classification of breast cancer (**B**, right image). (This figure was used with permission from Amirsys, Inc., Hicks DG, **Lester SC.** Expression profiling, mRNA. In: *Diagnostic Pathology: Breast.* 1st ed. Salt Lake City, UT: Amirsys Publishing; 2012:212-215.)

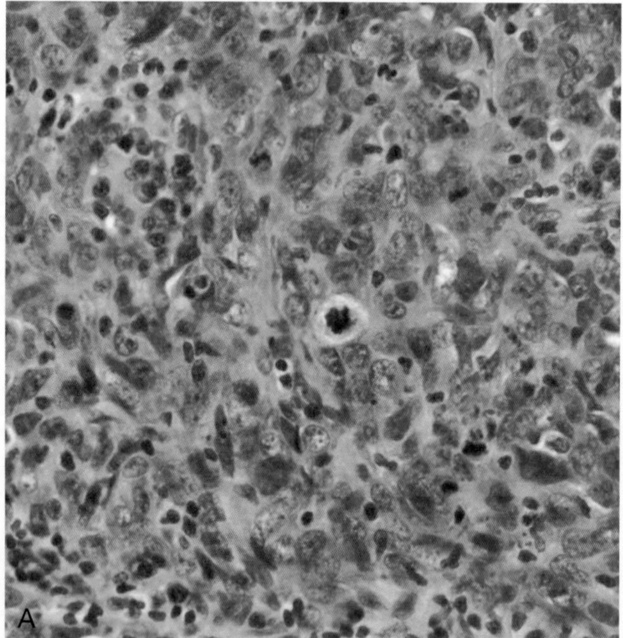

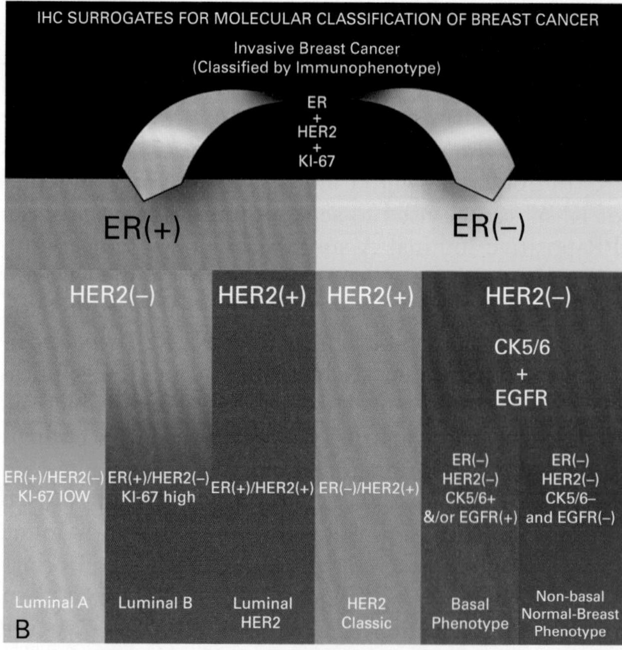

FIGURE 27–3 This high-grade invasive breast cancer (**A**, **left** image) has a high mitotic rate and will likely follow an aggressive clinical course. Additional clinically valuable information can be obtained through the use of immunohistochemical (IHC) markers to determine prognosis and guide the selection of the most appropriate adjuvant therapy. Using IHC markers in panels (**B**, right image), breast tumors can be classified into distinct cancer subsets that demonstrate differences on patient characteristics, prognosis, patterns of recurrence, and response to different adjuvant treatment regimens and targeted therapies. (This figure was used with permission from Amirsys, Inc., Hicks DG, **Lester SC.** Expression profiling, protein. In: *Diagnostic Pathology: Breast.* 1st ed. Salt Lake City, UT: Amirsys Publishing; 2012:216-223.)

TN classification defines the basal-like subtype as an absence of expression of ER, PR, and HER2. These tumors constitute 11.2% to 16.3% of IDCs.[97-99] The TN phenotype is commonly used as a clinical surrogate for basal-like tumors as it roughly correlates with the basal-like subgroup defined by gene expression profiling[43,85,86] and is resistant to currently available targeted therapies.[100] Tumors of this subtype are frequently larger, grade 3 tumors, with pushing margins, a poor Nottingham prognostic index, and higher rates for regional recurrence and distant metastasis.[97] They tend to occur in patients under the age of 40 years and portend poor survival regardless of the stage at diagnosis.[98] Furthermore, TN tumors appear to be more sensitive to anthracycline-based neoadjuvant chemotherapy than is the hormone receptor–positive luminal subtype.[101,102]

The combined CK/TN classification proposed by Nielsen et al.[103] is the classification most closely related to the intrinsic subtypes as defined by gene expression profiling. Using four antibodies, they showed that they can define the basal subtype as ER and HER2 negative, and CK5/6 and/or EGFR positive, with 76% sensitivity and 100% specificity, respectively, compared with the basal subtype defined by gene expression profiling. Livasy et al.[104] also showed that the basal subtype defined by gene expression profiling was consistently ER and HER2 negative, with varying degrees of positivity for CK8/18, EGFR, and CK5/6. Clinically, the basal-like subtypes are not only associated with poor clinical outcome[103,105] and hereditary breast cancer (BRCA1 mutant)[106] but also have different metastatic patterns[96] and could potentially benefit from EGFR-targeted therapy.[107] More recently, Cheang et al.[81] reported that the expression of Ki-67 can be used to separate the original ER- and PR-positive luminal A subtype of breast cancer into luminal A with low Ki-67 (<14%) and luminal B with high Ki-67 (>14%). The latter group has a prognosis similar to that for luminal HER2 (triple positive) (Fig. 27.4).

Morphologically, Livasy et al.[104] demonstrated that the most consistent pathologic features of basal subtypes include high grade, high mitotic count, geographic necrosis, pushing borders, prominent lymphocytic infiltrates, solid growth pattern, central fibrotic/acellular area, and less association with ductal carcinoma in situ (DCIS). Clinically, luminal cancers are generally hormone receptor positive and appropriate for endocrine therapy. The HER2 subtype is suitable for targeted therapy such as trastuzumab. Basal subtypes are resistant to current targeted therapies but seem to be more responsive to chemotherapies.[22,108,109] Some of the possible molecular targets for basal tumors that have been proposed include EGFR and VEGF. More recently, PARP inhibitors have shown great promise against this group of tumors.[110,111]

Although these classifications divide breast carcinoma into basal and non-basal and show similar clinical and pathological features in each subtype, the precise relationship between these classifications is not clear. By comparing these three molecular classifications (CK, TN, and CK/TN) as well as the ER/HER2 classification,[112] we demonstrated that these classifications are not identical. They vary greatly depending on tumor type (DCIS vs. IDCs) and tumor grade (high and non-high nuclear grade), with basal subtypes ranging from 5% to 36% for DCIS and from 14% to 40% for IDCs. Furthermore, other limitations for IHC-based molecular classifications include differences in patient cohorts, tumor grades, antibody methodology, and definitions of positive staining for each molecular marker. All of these factors can contribute to the variable results seen for different subtypes and across different studies. For example, the definition for

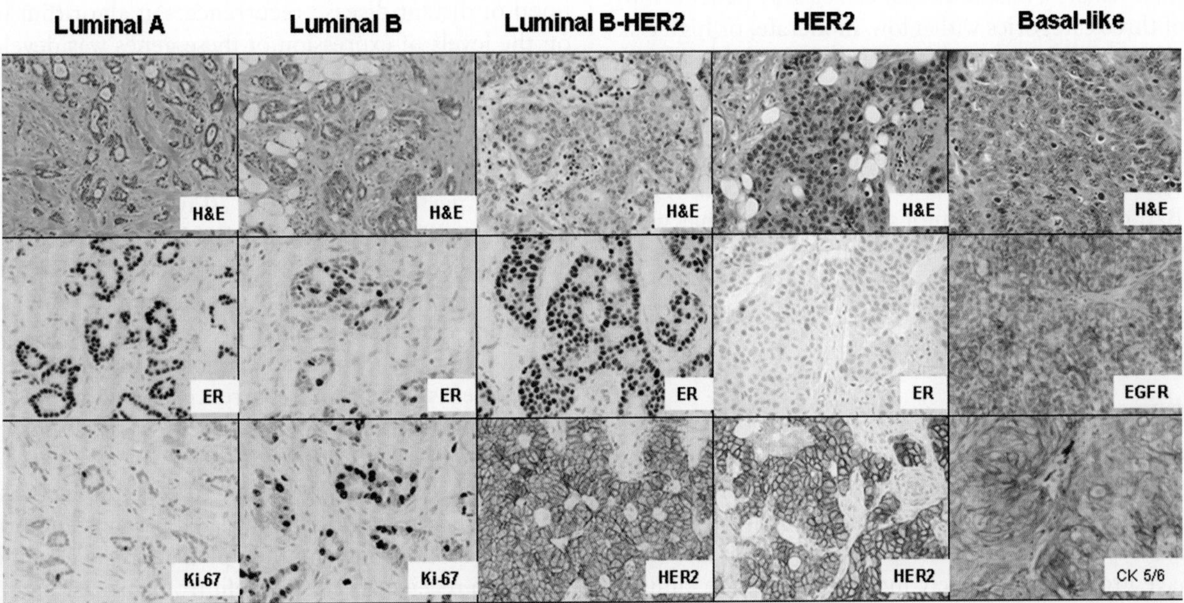

FIGURE 27–4 Typical staining patterns for hematoxylin and eosin (H&E) and immunohistochemical (IHC) surrogates for five major molecular subtypes of breast carcinomas. ER, estrogen receptor; EGFR, epidermal growth factor receptor; HER2, human epidermal growth factor receptor 2.

positive CK expression varies from any positivity[113,114] to positive in all tumor cells,[115] and the definition for positive ER and PR varies from >0%[97] to >10%.[113] Clearly, a consensus on the definitions for each subtype, as well as for the standardization of tissue fixation conditions and antibody clones, incubation conditions, and scoring criteria for each molecule, must be reached before studies with large numbers of patients and long-term follow-up can be conducted to verify the clinical significance and potential clinical utility of molecular classifications for breast carcinoma.

Mammostrat, an IHC-Based Multigene Assay

An alternative approach to profiling breast cancer patients in terms of prognosis has been an attempt to directly translate gene expression data into IHC-based markers for clinical testing. Applied Genomics, Inc. (Clarient Laboratories) in collaboration with researchers at Stanford University has undertaken the task of translating the rich biologic diversity revealed by gene expression studies into new IHC tests with potential clinical utility. These investigators have used gene expression data sets to select hundreds of novel targets for production of new antibodies. These antibodies have been screened across several thousand tumor samples to identify quality IHC reagents that could be used in the identification of clinically significant subsets of solid tumors. This approach was used to develop a five-antibody IHC panel for determining the prognosis of early-stage, ER-positive breast cancer (Mammostrat, Clarient Laboratory). The five monoclonal antibodies measure diverse tumor physiology independent of proliferation, HER2, and hormone receptors and include markers related to nutrient transport, cell cycle progression, hypoxia, and embryonic differentiation.[116] The staining results from these five antibodies are used to calculate a risk index that can classify patients into one of three categories with a low, moderate, or high risk of recurrence. This approach to classifying breast cancer into different prognostic categories has been validated in three independent institutional cohorts of patients as well as on archival tissue samples from the National Surgical Adjuvant Breast and Bowel Project (NSABP) B14 and B20 clinical trials, demonstrating results that were remarkably similar to those seen with the 21-gene reverse transcriptase polymerase chain reaction (RT-PCR) test (Onco*type* DX; Genomic Health Inc., Redwood City, CA, USA) on the same patient samples.[117]

Multigene Assays

Although clinically validated, the traditional assessment of breast cancer does not provide sufficient information to allow accurate individual risk assessment on a case-by-case basis. As the treatment options for breast cancer have grown progressively more complex, the clinical decisions regarding the suitability of adjuvant systemic therapy for individual patients require some assessment of the underlying biology of each tumor, necessitating the development of new ways to characterize, profile, and classify breast cancer. To address this need, the application of molecular approaches and multigene assays for predicting prognosis and treatment response in breast cancer has begun to move into the clinical arena with the introduction of clinically available assays such as the Onco*type* DX diagnostic test (Genomic Health Inc., Redwood City, CA, USA). This test is a validated 21-gene quantitative RT-PCR assay developed for use in formalin-fixed, paraffin-embedded breast cancer samples that are ER positive and node negative. An alternative approach that is also clinically available is the 70-gene MammaPrint assay (Agendia, Amsterdam, The Netherlands), which utilizes cDNA microarray gene expression analysis to stratify patients according to their risk of disease recurrence.

Oncotype DX

Using quantitative reverse transcriptase (QRT)-PCR adapted for formalin-fixed, paraffin-embedded clinical samples and a multi-step developmental method, a validated 21-gene assay (Oncotype DX) (Table 27.4) has been developed for breast cancer through collaborations between Genomic Health Incorporated and the NSABP. The assay quantifies the expression of 21 tumor-related genes using TaqMan quantitative PCR.[13] The assay development utilized a candidate gene approach, in which 250 genes were selected for RT-PCR assays based on the published literature, genomic databases, and cDNA microarray analysis, and these RT-PCR assays were used to study some 447 patients across 3 independent training cohorts. The data from all three studies were used to select a panel of 21 genes (16 cancer-related genes and 5 reference genes used for normalization of gene expression) that consistently showed a strong correlation with the likelihood of distant disease recurrence. An algorithm based on the levels of expression of these genes was developed and used to calculate an RS for each breast cancer sample. The calculated RS ranges from 0 to 100 and divides cases into three risk groups: low (0 to 18), intermediate (19 to 31), and high (32 to 100).

The performance of the assay was then validated using material from NSABP B-14, a clinical trial that had established the value of tamoxifen in the treatment of hormone receptor–positive breast cancer. The validation study demonstrated that the RS was an independent and highly significant predictor of recurrence-free survival. The risk of distant recurrence at 10 years was 6.8% for patients with a low RS (<18), 14.3% for those with an intermediate RS (18 to 30), and 30.5% for patients with a high RS (>31). In further studies, the RS was also shown to be prognostic in untreated patients and predictive of response to chemotherapy (patients with high RS appear to receive greatest benefit from chemotherapy).[118] Approximately 50% of patients fall within the low RS category in published cohorts, and the data suggest that these

TABLE 27-4 Multigene Assay: Oncotype Dx, 21-Gene Recurrence Score

Proliferation Gene Set	HER2 Gene Set	ER Gene Set	Invasion Gene Set	Other Gene Set	Reference Gene Set
Ki-67	GRB7	ER	Stromelysin 3	GSTM1	Beta-actin
STK15	HER2	PR	Cathepsin L2	BAG1	GAPDH
Survivin		Bcl2		CD68	RPLPO
Cyclin B1		SCUBE2			GUS
MYBL2					TFRC

The recurrence score defined as quantitative level of gene expression × coefficient

RS = + 0.47 × HER2 Group Score
– 0.34 × ER Group Score
+ 1.04 × Proliferation Group Score
+ 0.10 × Invasion Group Score
+ 0.05 × CD68
– 0.08 × GSTM1
– 0.07 × BAG1
Results scaled 0 to 100

Risk Category	RS (0–100)	10-Y Recurrence Risk (%)
Low risk	<18	6.8
Intermediate risk	≥18 and <31	14.3
High risk	>31	30.5

Results of Clinical Validation Studies of the RS

- RS is prognostic in ER+/node negative, tamoxifen-treated patients
- RS is prognostic in ER+/node negative, untreated patients
- RS is predictive for response to chemotherapy

HER2, human epidermal growth factor receptor 2; RS, recurrence score; ER, estrogen receptor.

patients are likely to be adequately treated with hormonal therapy alone and unlikely to receive any additional benefit from the addition of chemotherapy to their adjuvant treatment regimen.

The Oncotype test measures the level of expression in four groups of genes, including the ER pathway, proliferation, the HER2 amplicon, and inflammation in early-stage, ER-positive patients. However, clinical validation was not shown in two studies.[119,120] Furthermore, some have argued that the test only recapitulates the information provided by most pathologists, namely grade and ER, PR, HER2, and Ki-67 status.[84,121]

MammaPrint

The 70-gene MammaPrint assay is now available for clinical use and has recently received the Food and Drug Administration (FDA) clearance. Two large studies have utilized this supervised gene expression profiling approach to address broad prognostic questions involving recurrence and survival in node-negative breast cancer patients treated only with surgery. Investigators from the Netherlands Cancer Institute identified a cohort of 98 patients who were node negative and younger than 55 years of age. The patients from this cohort were separated into those who experienced relapse of their disease within 5 years (34 patients) and those who were disease free at 5 years or more (44 patients). From the initial study, which examined 25,000 genes, a system of supervised classification identified 70 genes that were independently correlated with poor prognosis. Subsequently, the prognostic power of the 70-gene classifier was tested in a validation study in 295 patients, some of whom were lymph node positive. The patients with a good prognostic gene signature had a <15% risk of recurrence at 10 years, whereas those who had tumor genes associated with a poor prognosis had a 50% risk of distant metastases.[87,122]

GENOMIC GRADING

Tumor grade can distinguish different subsets of breast cancer patients who fall into different risk groups for recurrence. Interestingly, recent molecular studies have begun to define potential mechanisms and genomic changes that may underlie breast cancer grade and may help to explain its relationship to prognosis. Gene expression studies have been used to define a 97-gene expression grade index that can consistently and reproducibly discriminate between two ER-positive molecular subgroups that are correlated with tumor grade and significantly different patient outcomes (low and high recurrence risk).[123] The genomic-grade signature, which is driven by proliferation and cell cycle–related genes, has challenged the clinical relevance of an intermediate grade 2 category, as these tumors could also be divided, placing them into either the low or high genomic grade category with outcomes similar to those for low- and high-grade tumors.[11,124] More recently, Ma et al.[125] reported a five-gene molecular grade index that could recognize grade I and grade III tumors with 89% accuracy; grade II tumors were stratified into the two aforementioned clinically significant groups. The results were validated in a QRT-PCR assay suitable for formalin-fixed, paraffin-embedded tissue. Thus, such indexing may help remove the subjectivity and intra/inter-observer variability associated with conventional grading. Although there is great enthusiasm about genomic grading, additional independent validation is still required.

DISSEMINATED TUMOR CELLS AND CIRCULATING TUMOR CELLS

Despite the demonstrated clinical utility of breast cancer staging, a significant number of early-stage breast cancer patients with negative margins and axillary nodes will still have disease recurrence following surgical excision. This fact suggests that the current methods used for clinical staging may be inadequate for some patients and that more sensitive methods for determining tumor cell dissemination are needed. Over the past few decades, a number of investigators have examined the value of circulating tumor cells (CTCs) as a novel marker for understanding disease progression, prognosis, and therapeutic responsiveness.[126] Interest in the potential clinical importance of CTCs arose from earlier studies that showed that DTCs in bone marrow at the time of diagnosis correlated with larger tumors, higher histologic grade, and a higher rate of cancer-related deaths.[127,128]

CTCs are rare events within the bloodstream, requiring the development of sensitive and specific methodologies for their detection. Detection strategies rely on a combination of cell enrichment techniques, using immunomagnetic selection followed by a detection step using epithelial markers to help enumerate CTCs. An FDA-cleared commercial assay for CTCs (Cell Search Assay; Veridex, Raritan, NJ, USA) is now available for use as a prognostic test in patients with metastatic cancers of the breast, prostate, and colon. Newer methods under development seek to capture viable tumor cells in the blood stream for further biological and molecular analysis.[129] Accumulating clinical data have shown that the presence of DTC and CTC is associated with a worse clinical outcome and may provide an early indication of chemotherapy resistance for patients whose circulation is not cleared of CTCs while on treatment.[130,131] The ability to capture and profile CTCs has the potential to provide additional clinically useful information on tumor biology. The seventh edition of the AJCC manual includes the addition of the M0i+ category for patients who have CTCs detected in their peripheral blood.

STANDARDIZED SPECIMEN HANDLING IS CRITICAL FOR MOLECULAR TESTING

Specimen preparation, including proper tissue handling and fixation, is critically important for the assessment of both traditional and newer prognostic and predictive factors in breast cancer. Proper tissue handling, fixation, and preparation will help ensure high-quality tissue sections for morphologic assessment and histologic grading, as well as accurate and reliable assessment of important tumor target molecules in breast tissue samples, such as ER, PR, HER2, and other potentially useful biomarkers. Studies have shown that delays between resection of the tumor to the start of fixation as well as inadequate fixation can have detrimental effects on the ability to accurately assess ER, PR, and HER2 expression in breast tissue.[132,133] The important elements involved in specimen preparation that require rigorous standardization include both tissue handling and tissue fixation.

Standardizing Breast Tissue Handling

An important variable in the analysis of macromolecules from clinical breast tissue samples is the cold ischemic time, defined as the time from tumor tissue removal by the surgeon to the initiation of tissue fixation. Numerous studies have documented the progressive loss of important tumor target molecules following the surgical interruption of blood flow, which then leads to metabolic stress, tissue ischemia, acidosis, and enzymatic degradation. Thus, excessive delay before the start of tissue fixation following surgical removal can reduce the efficacy of the subsequent analysis of clinically important target molecules, as well as compromise the quality of tissue histology for morphologic and molecular analyses. Every effort should be made to transport breast excision samples having a documented or suspected cancer from the operating room to the pathology laboratory as soon as they are available for an immediate gross assessment and placement into fixative.[134]

Standardizing Breast Tissue Fixation

For the fixative for breast tissue samples, 10% phosphate-buffered formalin should be used. This is based on the collective body of knowledge in the published literature on the expected immunoreactivity for predictive markers in breast cancer, which has been accrued over many years and which has been clinically validated with patient outcomes in numerous clinical trials. In addition, the FDA approval for assay kits analyzing ER, PR, and HER2 explicitly states that formalin fixation should be used, and the FDA approval for the kits is invalid if an alternative fixation is used. Breast tissue samples need to be fixed in 10% neutral buffered formalin for no less than 6 to 8 hours and not more than 48 to 72 hours before processing. Formalin penetrates tissue at a rate of approximately 1 mm/h, which is the reason breast excision samples need to be incised and placed into formalin in a timely fashion in order to initiate formalin fixation throughout the tissue.

TABLE 27-5 Chemotherapy Sensitivity and Indications for Adjuvant Chemotherapy

Tumor Factors	Indications Favoring Chemotherapy	Indications Against Chemotherapy
Tumor grade	Grade 3	Grade 1
Histologic type	Ductal (NST)	Classic lobular, tubular, mucinous
Nodal status	Positive (≥4)	Negative
Tumor size	>5 cm	<1 cm
ER status	ER- (high expression)	ER+
HER2 status	HER2+ (chemotherapy + HER2-targeted therapy)	+/- (depending on other factors)
Ki-67 index	High (Ki-67 > 20%)	Low (Ki-67 < 10%)
LVI	Extensive	absent
Molecular classification	Basal, HER2, and luminal B subtypes	Luminal A subtype
Oncotype Dx	High RS (>30)	Low RS(<18)
MammaPrint	High risk MammaPrint	Low risk MammaPrint
GGI	High risk GGI	Low risk GGI
Mammostrat	High risk index	Low risk index

LVI, lymphovascular invasion; NST, no special type; ER, estrogen receptor; HER2, epidermal growth factor receptor 2; RS, recurrence score; GGI, genomic grade index.

Chemical fixation takes time, with the rate-limiting step being the equilibrium between formaldehyde and methylene glycol in solution.[109] This chemical reaction, which involves protein cross-linking, is time dependent and can be measured in hours ("clock reaction"). Studies have documented that a minimum of 6 to 8 hours of formalin fixation for breast samples is needed to obtain consistent IHC assay results for ER.[132] Under- or over-fixed tissue can lead to technical problems in performing IHC assays and has the real potential for yielding false-negative or even false-positive spurious results.

CONCLUSIONS

The most clinically relevant, practical, affordable, and broadly available ancillary testing to help determine the prognosis for breast cancer patients, as well as testing to help guide the selection of the most beneficial treatment regimens, will continue to be an area of active research. Gene expression profiling has begun to provide a molecular basis for the clinical and biologic heterogeneity of breast cancer. The molecular classification of breast tumors has shown great promise and has the potential to provide important prognostic information that can be used to guide clinical decision-making. However, the clinical necessity for increasing information about the biology of a patient's breast cancer means that the tissue sample is no longer used only for microscopic interpretation and should also be considered an analyte, with greater attention paid to the quality of the sample for further molecular analysis.

Moving forward, it will also be necessary to evaluate new, potentially useful prognostic assays in a prospective fashion, in uniformly treated patient populations using standardized assay procedures and state-of-the-art statistical methods. By combining morphologic, immunohistochemical, and molecular techniques, the pathology community is rapidly moving toward providing clinicians with a more biological and clinically meaningful diagnosis for breast cancer patients (Table 27.5).

REFERENCES

1. Simpson PT, Reis-Filho JS, Gale T, Lakhani SR. Molecular evolution of breast cancer. *J Pathol.* 2005;205:248-254.
2. Eifel P, Axelson JA, Costa J, et al. National Institutes of Health Consensus Development Conference statement: adjuvant therapy for breast cancer, November 1-3, 2000. *J Natl Cancer Inst.* 2001;93:979-989.
3. Ravdin PM, Siminoff LA, Davis GJ, et al. Computer program to assist in making decisions about adjuvant therapy for women with early breast cancer. *J Clin Oncol.* 2001;19:980-991.
4. *Cancer Staging Handbook from the AJCC Cancer Staging Manual.* 7th ed. New York, NY: Springer; 2010:419-460.
5. Carter CL, Allen C, Henson DE. Relation of tumor size, lymph node status, and survival in 24,740 breast cancer cases. *Cancer.* 1989;63:181-187.
6. Koscielny S, Tubiana M, Le MG, et al. Breast cancer: relationship between the size of the primary tumour and the probability if metastatic dissemination. *Br J Cancer.* 1984;49:709-715.
7. Fisher B, Bauer M, Wickerham DL, et al. Relation of number of positive axillary nodes to the prognosis of patients with primary breast cancer. An NSABP update. *Cancer.* 1983;52:1551-1557.
8. Albertini JJ, Lyman GH, Cox C, et al. Lymphatic mapping and sentinel node biopsy in the patient with breast cancer. *JAMA.* 1996;276:1818-1822.
9. Elston CW, Ellis IO. Pathological prognostic factors in breast cancer. I. The value of histological grade in breast cancer: experience from a large study with long-term follow-up. *Histopathology.* 1991;19:403-410.
10. Frkovic-Grazio S, Bracko M. Long term prognostic value of Nottingham histological grade and its components in early (pT1N0M0) breast carcinoma. *J Clin Pathol.* 2002;55:88-92.
11. Loi S, Haibe-Kains B, Desmedt C, et al. Definition of clinically distinct molecular subtypes in estrogen receptor-positive breast carcinomas through genomic grade. *J Clin Oncol.* 2007;25:1239-1246.
12. Rakha EA, Reis-Filho JS, Baehner F, et al. Breast cancer prognostic classification in the molecular era: the role of histological grade. *Breast Cancer Res.* 2010;12:207.
13. Paik S, Shak S, Tang G, et al. A multigene assay to predict recurrence of tamoxifen-treated, node-negative breast cancer. *N Engl J Med.* 2004;351:2817-2826.

14. van de Rijn M, Perou CM, Tibshirani R, et al. Expression of cytokeratins 17 and 5 identifies a group of breast carcinomas with poor clinical outcome. *Am J Pathol.* 2002;161:1991-1996.
15. Wolff AC, Hammond ME, Schwartz JN, et al. American Society of Clinical Oncology/College of American Pathologists guideline recommendations for human epidermal growth factor receptor 2 testing in breast cancer. *Arch Pathol Lab Med.* 2007;131:18-43.
16. Hammond ME, Hayes DF, Dowsett M, et al. American Society of Clinical Oncology/College of American Pathologists guideline recommendations for immunohistochemical testing of estrogen and progesterone receptors in breast cancer. *Arch Pathol Lab Med.* 2010;134:E1-E16.
17. Gronemeyer H. Transcription activation by estrogen and progesterone receptors. *Annu Rev Genet.* 1991;25:89-123.
18. Osborne CK, Schiff R, Fuqua SA, Shou J. Estrogen receptor: current understanding of its activation and modulation. *Clin Cancer Res.* 2001;7:S4338-S4342.
19. Dunbier AK, Anderson H, Folkerd EJ, et al. Expression of estrogen responsive genes in breast cancers correlates with plasma estradiol levels in postmenopausal women. In: Presented at the 31st Annual San Antonio Breast Cancer Symposium; December 13, 2008; San Antonio, TX.
20. Cui X, Schiff R, Arpino G, et al. Biology of progesterone receptor loss in breast cancer and its implications for endocrine therapy. *J Clin Oncol.* 2005;23:7721-7735.
21. Jordan VC, Brodie AM. Development and evolution of therapies targeted to the estrogen receptor for the treatment and prevention of breast cancer. *Steroids.* 2007;72:7-25.
22. Early Breast Cancer Trialists' Collaborative Group (EBCTCG). Effects of chemotherapy and hormonal therapy for early breast cancer on recurrence and 15-year survival: an overview of the randomised trials. *Lancet.* 2005;365:1687-1717.
23. De Souza JA, Olopade OI. CYP2D6 Genotyping and tamoxifen: an unfinished story in the quest for personalized medicine. *Semin Oncol.* 2011;38:263-273.
24. Burstein HJ, Prestrud AA, Seidenfeld J, et al. American Society of Clinical Oncology clinical practice guideline: update on adjuvant endocrine therapy for women with hormone receptor-positive breast cancer. *J Clin Oncol.* 2010;28:3784-3796.
25. National Comprehensive Cancer Network Practice Guidelines in Oncology: Breast Cancer-v 1-2011. http://www.nccn.org/professionals/physician-gls/PDF/Breast.pdf
26. Goldhirsch A, Ingle JN, Gelber RD, et al. Thresholds for therapies: highlights of the St. Gallen International Expert Consensus on the primary therapy of early breast cancer 2009. *Ann Oncol.* 2009;20:1319-1329.
27. Goetz MP. Tamoxifen, endoxifen, and CYP2D6: the rules for evaluating a predictive factors. *Oncology (Williston Park).* 2009;23:1233-1234.
28. Higgins MJ, Stearns V. CYP2D6 polymorphisms and tamoxifen metabolism: clinical relevance. *Curr Oncol Rep.* 2010;12:7-15.
29. Mueller H, Kueng W, Schoumacher F, et al. Selective regulation of steroid receptor expression in MCF-7 breast cancer cells by a novel member of the heregulin family. *Biochem Biophys Res Commun.* 1995;217;1271-1278.
30. Tang CK, Perez C, Grunt T, et al. Involvement of heregulin-beta2 in the acquisition of the hormone-independent phenotype of breast cancer cells. *Cancer Res.* 1996;56:3350-3358.
31. Pietras RJ, Arboleda J, Reese DM, et al. HER2 tyrosine kinase pathway targets estrogen receptor and promotes hormone-independent growth in human breast cancer cells. *Oncogene.* 1995;10:2435-2446.
32. Nicholson RI, Staka C, Boyns F, et al. Growth factor-driven mechanisms associated with resistance to estrogen deprivation in breast cancer: new opportunities for therapy. *Endocr Relat Cancer.* 2004;11:623-641.
33. Gee JM, Harper ME, Hutcheson IR, et al. The antiepidermal growth factor receptor agent gefitinib (ZD1839/Iressa) improves antihormone response and prevents development of resistance in breast cancer in vitro. *Endocrinology.* 2003;144:5105-5117.
34. Robertson JFR, Gutterridge E, Chenung KL, et al. Gefitinib (ZD1839) is active in acquired tamoxifen(TAM)-resistant estrogen receptor (ER)-positive and ER-negative breast cancer: results from a phase II study. *Proc Am Soc Clin Oncol.* 2003;22(abstract 7).
35. Al Saleh S, Sharaf LH, Luqmani YA. Signalling pathways involved in endocrine resistance in breast cancer and associations with epithelial to mesenchymal transition. *Int J Oncol.* 2011;38:1197-1217.
36. Tai P, Wang J, Ding P, Tang P. ER+PR-breast carcinomas are more frequently associated with older patients, larger tumors and HER2 positive tumors. *Mod Pathol.* 23S:74A. Abstract 325.
37. Thakkar JP, Mehta DG. A review of an unfavorable subset of breast cancer: estrogen receptor positive progesterone receptor negative. *Oncologist.* 2011;16:276-285.
38. Arpino G, Weiss H, Lee AV, et al. Estrogen receptor-positive, progesterone receptor-negative breast cancer: association with growth factor receptor expression and tamoxifen resistance. *J Natl Cancer Inst.* 2005;97:1254-1261.
39. Viale G, Regan MM, Maiorano E, et al. Prognostic and predictive value of centrally reviewed expression of estrogen and progesterone receptors in a randomized trial comparing letrozole and tamoxifen adjuvant therapy for postmenopausal early breast cancer: BIG-1-98. *J Clin Oncol.* 2007;25:3846-3852.
40. Creighton CJ, Kent Osborne C, van de Vijver MJ, et al. Molecular profiles of progesterone receptor loss in human breast tumors. *Breast Cancer Res Treat.* 2009;114:287-299.
41. Wei B, Wang J, Bourne P, et al. Bone metastasis is strongly associated with estrogen receptor positive/progesterone receptor negative breast carcinomas. *Hum Pathol.* 2008;39:1809-1815.
42. Tang P, Wang J, Hicks DG, et al. A lower Allred score for progesterone receptor is strongly associated with a higher recurrence score of 21-gene assay in breast cancer. *Cancer Invest.* 2010;28:978-982.
43. Perou CM, Sorlie T, Eisen MB, et al. Molecular portraits of human breast tumours. *Nature.* 2000;406:747-752.
44. Osborne CK, Shou J, Massarweh S, et al. Crosstalk between estrogen receptor and growth factor receptor pathways as a cause for endocrine therapy resistance in breast cancer. *Clin Cancer Res.* 2005;11:865s-870s.
45. Zhang Y, Su H, Rahimi M, et al. EGFRvIII-induced estrogen-independence, tamoxifen-resistance phenotype correlates with PgR expression and modulation of apoptotic molecules in breast cancer. *Int J Cancer.* 2009;125:2021-2028.
46. Yaziji H, Goldstein LC, Barry TS, et al. HER-2 testing in breast cancer using parallel tissue-based methods. *JAMA.* 2004;291;1972-1977.
47. Owens MA, Horten BC, Da Silva MM. HER2 amplification ratios by fluorescence in situ hybridization and correlation with immunohistochemistry in cohort of 6556 breast cancer tissues. *Clin Breast Cancer.* 2004;5:63-69.
48. Hicks DG, Kulkarni D, Hammond ME. The role of the indispensable surgical pathologist in treatment planning for breast cancer. *Arch Pathol Lab Med.* 2008;132:1226-1227.
49. Konecny G, Pauletti G, Pegram M, et al. Quantitative association between HER-2/neu and steroid hormone receptors in hormone receptor-positive primary breast cancer. *J Natl Cancer Inst.* 2003;95:142-153.
50. Ellis MJ, Coop A, Singh B, et al. Letrozole is more effective neoadjuvant endocrine therapy than tamoxifen for ErbB-1 and/or ErbB-2 positive, estrogen receptor-positive primary breast cancer. Evidence from a phase III randomized trial. *J Clin Oncol.* 2001;19:3808-3816.
51. Menard S, Valagussa P, Pilotti S, et al. Response to cyclophosphamide, methotrexate, and fluorouracil in lymph node-positive breast cancer according to HER2 overexpression and other tumor biologic variables. *J Clin Oncol.* 2001;19:329-335.
52. Pritchard KI, Shepherd LE, O'Malley FP, et al. HER2 and responsiveness of breast cancer to adjuvant chemotherapy. *N Engl J Med.* 2006;354:2103-2111.
53. Hayes DF, Thor A, Dressler L, et al. HER2 predicts benefit from adjuvant paclitaxel after AC in node-positive breast cancer: CALGB 9344. *J Clin Oncol.* 2006;24:5S:2000. Abstract 510.
54. Cobleigh MA, Vogel CL, Tripathy D, et al. Multinational study of the efficacy and safety of humanized anti-HER2 monoclonal antibody in women who have HER2-overexpressing metastatic breast cancer that has progressed after chemotherapy for metastatic disease. *J Clin Oncol.* 1999;17:2639-2648.
55. Slamon DJ, Leyland-Jones B, Shak S, et al. Use of chemotherapy plus a monoclonal antibody against HER2 for metastatic breast cancer that overexpresses HER2. *N Engl J Med.* 2001;344:783-792.

56. Slamon D, Eiermann W, Robert N, et al. Phase III randomized trial comparing doxorubicin and cyclophosphamide followed by docetaxel (ACT) with doxonubicin and cyclophosphamide followed by docetaxel and trastuzumab (ACTH) with docetaxel, carboplatin and trastuzumab (TCH) in HER2 positive early breast cancer patients: BCIRG 006 study. *Breast Cancer Res Treat.* 2005;94(suppl, abstract 1):S4.
57. Joensuu H, Kellokumpu-Lehtinen PL, Bono P, et al. Adjuvant docetaxel or vinorelbine with or without trastuzumab for breast cancer. *N Engl J Med.* 2006;354:809-820.
58. Romond EH, Perez EA, Bryant J, et al. Trastuzumab plus adjuvant chemotherapy for operable HER2-positive breast cancer. *N Engl J Med.* 2005;353:1673-1684.
59. Piccart-Gebhart MJ, Procter M, Leyland-Jones B, et al. Trastuzumab after adjuvant chemotherapy in HER2 positive breast cancer. *N Engl J Med.* 2005;353:1659-1672.
60. Geyer CE, Forster J, Lindquist D, et al. Lapatinib plus capecitabine for HER2-positive advanced breast cancer. *N Engl J Med.* 2006;355:2733-2743.
61. Hammond ME, Hayes DF, Wolff AC. Clinical notice for American Society of Clinical Oncology–College of American Pathologists Guideline Recommendations on ER/PgR and HER2 testing in breast cancer. *J Clin Oncol.* 2011;29:e458.
62. Khoury T, Mojica W, Hicks D, et al. ERBB2 juxtamembrane domain (transtuzumab binding site) gene mutation is a rare event in invasive breast cancers overexpressing the ERBB2 gene. *Mod Pathol.* 2011;24:1055-1059.
63. Newman B, Mu H, Butler LM, et al. Frequency of breast cancer attributable to BRCA1 in a population-based series of American women. *JAMA.* 1998;279:915-921.
64. Ford D, Easton DF, Stratton M, et al. Genetic heterogeneity and penetrance analysis of the BRCA1 and BRCA2 genes in breast cancer families. The Breast Cancer Linkage Consortium. *Am J Hum Genet.* 1998;62:676-689.
65. Antoniou A, Pharoah P, Narod S, et al. Average risks of breast and ovarian cancer associated with BRCA1 or BRCA2 mutations detected in cases series unselected for family history: a combined analysis of 22 studies. *Am J Hum Genet.* 2003;72:1117-1130.
66. Chen S, Iversen ES, Friebel T, et al. Characterization of BRCA1 and BRCA2 mutations in a large United States sample. *J Clin Oncol.* 2006;24:863-871.
67. Warner E, Plewes DB, Hill KA, et al. Surveillance of BRCA1 and BRCA2 mutation carriers with magnetic resonance imaging, ultrasound, mammography, and clinical breast examination. *JAMA.* 2004;292:1317-1325.
68. Metcalfe K, Lynch HT, Ghadirian P, et al. Contralateral breast cancer in BRCA1 and BRCA2 mutation carriers. *J Clin Oncol.* 2004;22:2328-2335.
69. Kauff ND, Domchek SM, Friebel TM, et al. Risk-reducing salpingo-oophorectomy for the prevention of BRCA1 and BRCA2-associated breast and gynecologic cancer: a multicenter, prospective study. *J Clin Oncol.* 2008;26:1331-1337.
70. Gerdes J, Schwab U, Lemke H, Stein H. Production of a mouse monoclonal antibody reactive with a human nuclear antigen associated with cell proliferation. *Int J Cancer.* 1983;31:3-20.
71. Gerdes J, Lemke H, Baisch H, et al. Cell cycle analysis of a cell proliferation-associated human nuclear antigen defined by the monoclonal antibody Ki-67. *J Immunol.* 1984;133:1710-1715.
72. Gerdes J, Li L, Schlueter C, et al. Immunobiochemical and molecular biologic characterization of the cell proliferation-associated nuclear antigen that is defined by monoclonal antibody Ki-67. *Am J Pathol.* 1991;138:867-873.
73. Lelle R, Heidenreich W, Stauch G, Gerdes J. The correlation of growth fractions with histologic grading and lymph node status in human mammary carcinoma. *Cancer.* 1987;59:83-88.
74. Molino A, Micciolo R, Turazza M, et al. Ki-67 immunostaining in 322 primary breast cancers: associations with clinical and pathological variables and prognosis. *Int J Cancer.* 1997;74:433-437.
75. Wiesner FG, Magener A, Fasching PA, et al. Ki-67 as a prognostic molecular marker in routine clinical use in breast cancer patients. *Breast.* 2009;8:135-141.
76. Jung SY, Han W, Lee JW, et al. Ki-67 expression gives additional prognostic information on St. Gallen 2007 and Adjuvant! Online risk categories in early breast cancer. *Ann Surg Oncol.* 2009;16:1112-1121.
77. Susini T, Nori J, Olivieri S, et al. Predicting the status of axillary lymph nodes in breast cancer: a multiparameter approach including axillary ultrasound scanning. *Breast.* 2009;18:103-108.
78. Lee J, Im YH, Lee SH, et al. Evaluation of ER and Ki-67 proliferation index as prognostic factors for survival following neoadjuvant chemotherapy with doxorubicin/docetaxel for locally advanced breast cancer. *Cancer Chemother Pharmacol.* 2008;61:569-577.
79. Penault-Llorca F, Andre F, Sagan C, et al. Ki67 expression and docetaxel efficacy in patients with estrogen receptor-positive breast cancer. *J Clin Oncol.* 2009;27:2809-2815.
80. Dowsett M, Smith IE, Ebbs SR, et al. Prognostic value of KI67 expression after short term presurgical endocrine therapy for primary breast cancer. *J Natl Cancer Inst.* 2007;99:167-170.
81. Cheang MC, Chia SK, Voduc D, et al. KI67 index, HER2 status, and prognosis of patients with luminal B breast cancer. *J Natl Cancer Inst.* 2009;101:736-750.
82. Hugh J, Hanson J, Cheang MC, et al. Breast cancer subtypes and response to docetaxel in node-positive breast cancer: use of an immunohistochemical definition in the BCIRG 001 trial. *J Clin Oncol.* 2009;27:1168-1176.
83. Reyal F, van Vliet MH, Armstrong NJ, et al. A comprehensive analysis of prognostic signatures reveals the high predictive capacity of the proliferation, immune response and RNA spicing modules in breast cancer. *Breast Cancer Res.* 2008;10:R93.
84. Cuzick J, Dowsett M, Wale C, et al. Prognostic value of a combined ER, PgR, Ki67, HER2 immunohistochemical (IHC4) score and comparison with the GHI recurrence score—results from transATAC. *Cancer Res.* 2009;69(abstr):503s.
85. Sorlie T, Perou CM, Tibshirani R, et al. Gene expression patterns of breast carcinomas distinguish tumor subclasses with clinical implications. *Proc Natl Acad Sci U S A.* 2001;98:10869-10874.
86. Sorlie T, Tibshirani R, Parker J, et al. Repeated observation of breast tumor subtypes in independent gene expression data sets. *Proc Natl Acad Sci U S A.* 2003;100:8418-8423.
87. Van't Veer LJ, Dai H, van de Vijver MJ, et al. Gene expression profiling predicts clinical outcome of breast cancer. *Nature.* 2002;415:530-536.
88. Yu L, Lee CH, Tan PH, Tan P. Conservation of breast cancer molecular subtypes and transcriptional patterns of tumor progression across distinct ethnic populations. *Clin Cancer Res.* 2004;10:5508-5517.
89. Van Laere SJ, van den Eynden GG, van der Auwera I, et al. Identification of cell-of-origin breast tumor subtypes in inflammatory breast cancer by gene expression profiling. *Breast Cancer Res Treat.* 2006;95:243-255.
90. Weigelt B, Hu Z, He X, et al. Molecular portraits and 70-gene prognosis signature are preserved throughout the metastatic progress of breast cancer. *Cancer Res.* 2005;65:9155-9158.
91. Boecker W, Moll R, Dervan P, et al. Usual ductal hyperplasia of the breast is a committed stem (progenitor) cell lesion distinct from atypical ductal hyperplasia and ductal carcinoma in situ. *J Pathol.* 2002;198:458-467.
92. Korsching E, Packeisen J, Agelopoulos K, et al. Cytogenetic alterations and cytokeratin expression patterns in breast cancer: integrating a new model of breast differentiation into cytogenetic pathways of breast carcinogenesis. *Lab Invest.* 2002;82:1525-1533.
93. Jones C, Ford E, Gillett C, et al. Molecular cytogenetic identification of subgroups of grade III invasive ductal breast carcinomas with different clinical outcomes. *Clin Cancer Res.* 2004:10:5988-5997.
94. Laakso M, Loman N, Borg A, Isola J. Cytokeratin 5/14-positive breast cancer: true basal phenotype confined to BRCA1 tumors. *Mod Pathol.* 2005;18:1321-1328.
95. Fulford LG, Reis-Filho JS, Ryder K, et al. Basal-like grade III invasive ductal carcinoma of the breast: patterns of metastasis and long-term survival. *Breast Cancer Res.* 2007;9:R4.
96. Hicks DG, Short SM, Prescott NL, et al. Breast cancers with brain metastases are more likely to be estrogen receptor negative, expression the basal cytokeratin CK5/6, and overexpression HER2 or EGFR. *Am J Surg Pathol.* 2006;30:1097-1104.
97. Rakha EA, El-Sayed ME, Green AR, et al. Prognostic markers in triple negative breast cancer. *Cancer.* 2007;109:25-32.
98. Bauer KR, Brown M, Cress RD, et al. Descriptive analysis of estrogen receptor (ER)-negative, progesterone receptor (PR)-negative, and HER2-negative invasive breast cancer, the so-called triple-negative phenotype: a population-based study from the California Cancer Registry. *Cancer.* 2007;109:1721-1728.

99. Dent R, Trudeau M, Pritchard KI, et al. Triple-negative breast cancer: clinical features and patterns of recurrence. *Clin Cancer Res*. 2007;13:4429-4434.
100. Cleator S, Heller W, Coombes RC. Triple-negative breast cancer: therapeutic options. *Lancet Oncol*. 2007;8:235-244.
101. Carey LA, Dees EC, Sawyer L, et al. The triple negative paradox: primary tumor chemosensitivity of breast cancer subtypes. *Clin Cancer Res*. 2007:13:2329-2334.
102. Tan DS, Marchio C, Jones RL, et al. Triple negative breast cancer: molecular profiling and prognostic impact in adjuvant anthracycline-treated patients. *Breast Cancer Res Treat*. 2008;111:27-44.
103. Nielsen TO, Hsu FD, Jensen K, et al. Immunohistochemical and clinical characterization of the basal-like subtype of invasive breast carcinoma. *Clin Cancer Res*. 2004;10:5367-5374.
104. Livasy CA, Karaca G, Nanda R, et al. Phenotypic evaluation of the basal-like subtype of invasive breast carcinoma. *Mod Pathol*. 2006;19:264-271.
105. Abd El-Rehim DM, Ball G, Pinder SE, et al. High-throughput protein expression analysis using tissue microarray technology of a large well-characterized series identifies biologically distinct classes of breast cancer confirming recent cDNA expression analyses. *Int J Cancer*. 2005;116:340-350.
106. Lakhani SR, Reis-Filho JS, Fulford L, et al. Prediction of BRCA1 status in patients with breast cancer using estrogen receptor and basal phenotype. *Clin Cancer Res*. 2005;11:5175-5180.
107. Siziopikou KP, Cobleigh M. The basal subtype of breast carcinomas may represent the group of breast tumors that could benefit from EGFR-targeted therapies. *Breast*. 2007;16:104-107.
108. Colleoni M, Minchella I, Mazzarol G, et al. Response to primary chemotherapy in breast cancer patients with tumors not expressing estrogen and progesterone receptors. *Ann Oncol*. 2000;11:1057-1059.
109. Goldstein NS, Decker D, Severson D, et al. Molecular classification system identifies invasive breast carcinoma patients who are most likely and those who are least likely to achieve a complete pathologic response after neoadjuvant chemotherapy. *Cancer*. 2007;110:1687-1696.
110. Anders CK, Winer EP, Ford JM, et al. Poly(ADP-ribose) polymerase inhibition: "targeted" therapy for triple-negative breast cancer. *Clin Cancer Res*. 2010;16:4702-4710.
111. O'Shaughnessy J, Osborne C, Pippen JE, et al. Iniparib plus chemotherapy in metastatic triple-negative breast cancer. *N Engl J Med*. 2011;364:205-214.
112. Tang P, Wang J, Bourne P. Molecular classifications of breast carcinoma with similar terminology and different definitions: are they the same? *Hum Pathol*. 2008;39:506-513.
113. Banerjee S, Reis-Filho JS, Ashley S, et al. Basal-like breast carcinomas: clinical outcome and response to chemotherapy. *J Clin Pathol*. 2006;59:729-735.
114. Abd El-Rehim DM, Pinder SE, Paish CE, et al. Expression of luminal and basal cytokeratins in human breast carcinoma. *J Pathol*. 2004:203:661-671.
115. Megha T, Ferrari F, Benvenuto A, et al. p53 mutation in breast cancer. Correlation with cell kinetics and cell of origin. *J Clin Pathol*. 2003;55:461-466.
116. Ring BZ, Seitz RS, Beck R, et al. Novel prognostic immunohistochemical biomarker panel for estrogen receptor-positive breast cancer. *J Clin Oncol*. 2006;24:3039-3047.
117. Ross DT, Kim CY, Tang G, et al. Chemosensitivity and stratification by a five monoclonal antibody immunohistochemistry test in the NSABP B14 and B20 trials. *Clin Cancer Res*. 2008;14:6602-6609.
118. Paik S, Tang G, Shak S, et al. Gene expression and benefit of chemotherapy in women with node-negative, estrogen receptor-positive breast cancer. *J Clin Oncol*. 2006;24:3726-3734.
119. Esteva FJ, Sahin AA, Cristofanilli M, et al. Prognostic role of a multigene reverse transcriptase-PCR assay in patients with node-negative breast cancer not receiving adjuvant systemic therapy. *Clin Cancer Res*. 2005;11:3315-3319.
120. Mina L, Soule SE, Badve S, et al. Predicting response to primary chemotherapy: gene expression profiling of paraffin-embedded core biopsy tissue. *Breast Cancer Res Treat*. 2007;103:197-208.
121. Flanagan MB, Dabbs DJ, Brufsky AM, et al. Histopathologic variables predict Oncotype DX recurrence score. *Mod Pathol*. 2008;21:1255-1261.
122. van de Vijver MJ, He YD, van'tVeer LJ, et al. A gene-expression signature as a predictor of survival in breast cancer. *N Engl J Med*. 2002;347:1999-2009.
123. Sotiriou C, Wirapati P, Loi S, et al. Gene expression profiling in breast cancer: understanding the molecular basis of histologic grade in improve prognosis. *J Natl Cancer Inst*. 2006;98:262-272.
124. Desmedt S, Sotiriou C. Proliferation: the most prominent predictor of clinical outcome in breast cancer. *Cell Cycle*. 2006;5:2298-2302.
125. Ma XJ, Salunga R, Dahiya S, et al. A five-gene molecular grade index and HOXB13:IL17BR are complementary prognostic factors in early breast cancer. *Clin Cancer Res*. 2008;14:2601-2608.
126. Graves H, Czerniecki BJ. Circulating tumor cells in breast cancer patients: an evolving role in patient prognosis and disease progression. *Pathol Res Int*. 2011;2011:621090.
127. Braun S, Pantel K, Müller P, et al. Cytokeratin-positive cells in the bone marrow and survival of patients with stage I, II, or III breast cancer. *N Engl J Med*. 2000;342:525-533.
128. Braun S, Vogl FD, Naume B, et al. A pooled analysis of bone marrow micrometastasis in breast cancer. *N Engl J Med*. 2005;353:793-802.
129. Hayes DF, Smerage J. Is there a role for circulating tumor cells in the management of breast cancer? *Clin Cancer Res*. 2008;14:3646-3650.
130. Cristofanilli M, Budd GT, Ellis MJ, et al. Circulating tumor cells, disease progression, and survival in metastatic breast cancer. *N Engl J Med*. 2004;351:781-791.
131. Pierga JY, Bidard FC, Mathiot C, et al. Circulating tumor cell detection predicts early metastatic relapse after neoadjuvant chemotherapy in large operable and locally advanced breast cancer in a phase II randomized trial. *Clin Cancer Res*. 2008;14:7004-7010.
132. Goldstein NS, Ferkowicz M, Odish E, et al. Minimum formalin fixation time for consistent estrogen receptor immunohistochemical staining of invasive breast carcinoma. *Am J Clin Pathol*. 2003;120:86-92.
133. Khoury T, Sait S, Hwang H, et al. Delay to formalin fixation effect on breast biomarkers. *Mod Pathol*. 2009;22:1457-1467.
134. Hicks DG, Kushner L, McCarthy K. Breast cancer predictive factor testing: the challenges and importance of standardizing tissue handling. *J Natl Cancer Inst Monogr*. 2011;2011:43-45.

CHAPTER 28

Molecular Diagnostics of Colorectal Cancer

Dongfeng Tan

INTRODUCTION

Colorectal cancer (CRC) is a complex collection of genetic diseases. Based on the distinct patterns of genetic instability,[1-3] CRC can be classified, for the most part, into three groups. Approximately 70% of CRCs are associated with chromosomal instability (CIN) due to allelic imbalance of chromosomal foci, chromosome amplification, or translocation. About 15% of CRCs have microsatellite instability (MSI), i.e., frameshift mutations and base pair substitutions that commonly arise in short, tandemly repeated nucleotide sequences. The remaining 15% of CRCs do not show CIN or MSI. CIN CRCs are aneuploid and are associated with intrinsic drug resistance and poor prognosis, whereas most MSI CRCs are near-diploid, with better overall survival. Based on epigenetic characteristics, about one-third of CRCs have the CpG island methylator phenotype (CIMP). Overlap exists between MSI and CIMP tumors, because about 60% of CIMP-high tumors have methylation of the *MLH1* promoter, which leads to MSI. Molecular classification of genetically heterogenetic CRC will potentially have significant impact on clinical practice of personalized medicine of CRC. Molecular tests for CRC are being increasingly used in clinical practice where they have significant implications for risk assessment, diagnosis, prognosis, and treatment of this common malignancy.

RISK ASSESSMENT

Approximately 20% of CRC cases are associated with familial colorectal neoplasms, i.e., two or more first-degree relatives with colorectal adenomas and carcinomas.[4,5] First-degree relatives of patients with newly diagnosed familial colorectal neoplasms are at increased risk for CRC.[6,7] Genetic susceptibility to CRC mainly occurs in inherited colorectal syndromes such as Lynch syndrome and familial adenomatous polyposis.[8-10] The common hereditary syndromes and incidences of CRC are listed in Table 28.1. It is recommended that all CRC patients be queried about their family history and considered for risk assessment as detailed in the National Comprehensive Cancer Network (NCCN) Colorectal Cancer Screening Clinical Practice Guidelines.

Lynch Syndrome

Individuals with Lynch syndrome—including those with existing cancer and those who have not yet developed cancer—have a predisposition to CRC and certain other tumors. Lynch syndrome is the most common form of genetically determined colon cancer predisposition, accounting for 2% to 6% of all CRC cases,[8,9,11,12] and usually displays distinctive clinical features (Table 28.2).

Patients with Lynch syndrome are at risk for synchronous or metachronous CRC and for extracolonic neoplasms.[13] In women with Lynch syndrome, the most common extraintestinal tumor is endometrial carcinoma, with a lifetime risk of 60%. Other sites of extracolonic tumors in Lynch syndrome include the stomach, ovaries, urinary tract, small intestine, sebaceous glands, and brain; there is no increase in the frequency of lung, breast, or prostate cancers, although cancers in these sites have been reported in patients with Lynch syndrome.

Lynch syndrome is caused by germline mutations in the DNA mismatch repair (MMR) genes.[6] The presence of defective MMR genes leads to MSI of tumoral DNA. Major DNA MMR genes include *MLH1*, *MSH2*, *MSH6*, *PMS2*, and *PMS1*.[14] The frequency of MMR gene involvement in Lynch syndrome is listed in Table 28.3.

MSI, one of the hallmarks of this disease, is a clonal change in the number of repeated DNA nucleotides

TABLE 28-1 Incidence of Familial Colorectal Cancer

Type	Percentage	Absolute Number of Cases[a]
Lynch syndrome	2–6% of all CRC	4,277–7,129
FAP	<1% of all CRC	<1,426
Familial[b]	20% of all CRC	28,514

CRC, colorectal cancer; FAP, familial adenomatous polyposis.
[a]Based on the annual incidence of CRC in the United States of 142,570. *CA Cancer J Clin*. 2010;60:277-300.
[b]Family members are characterized by a microsatellite instability–stable genotype, a lower relative risk of CRC, the absence of excess extracolonic tumors, and later onset of CRC. The genetic basis of this group is currently unknown.

TABLE 28-3 Frequency of Major Mismatch Repair Genes in Lynch Syndrome

MMR Gene	Frequency (%)[a]
MLH1	35–45
MSH2	35–45
MSH6	5–10
PMS2	<5

MMR, mismatch repair.
[a]Note: In about 5% of Lynch syndrome cases, a germline mutation in a known DNA MMR gene cannot be identified.

TABLE 28-2 Cardinal Features of Lynch Syndrome

- Autosomal dominant inheritance
- Proximal colon predilection: 70–85% in colon proximal to the splenic flexure
- Earlier age at onset: average age of 45 vs. 63 y in the general population
- Accelerated progression: 2–3 y from adenomas to carcinomas vs. 8–10 y in the general population
- Extra colonic cancers
- Favorable survival

or nucleotide units (more than a single nucleotide). Examples of microsatellites are listed in Table 28.4. Although identifying a germline mutation in an MMR gene by sequencing is definitive for diagnosing Lynch syndrome, patients usually undergo two other methods of identifying this disease before sequencing: information based on family history and initial screening tests on the tumor sample. A detailed family history can give hints of possible Lynch syndrome, and national and international guidelines for clinical screening for Lynch syndrome have been proposed. The well-adopted guidelines are the Bethesda Guidelines and the Amsterdam Guidelines.[15,16] However, the screening performance of the Amsterdam (sensitivity, 30% to 45%; specificity, 95%) and Bethesda (sensitivity, 70% to 90%; specificity, 80%) criteria to identify individuals with Lynch syndrome has been heterogeneous and neither offers an adequately reliable sensitivity and specificity.[17,18] For instance, one study of 500 CRCs showed that only 72% of patients with Lynch syndrome met the criteria of the revised Bethesda guidelines.[19] In other words, restriction of molecular screening to the patients meeting the revised Bethesda guidelines would not identify 28% of Lynch syndrome cases. After a thorough evidence-based review of the current literature, the Evaluation of Genomic Applications in Practice and Prevention (EGAPP) Working Group recommended that MSI tests, regardless of the patient's family history and age, should be done in all patients with newly diagnosed CRC to reduce morbidity and mortality from Lynch syndrome,[14] although family history and age may still be important components of CRC risk assessment in the general population.

Histologically, many morphological and immunohistochemical (IHC) features indicate high-level MSI in CRC. Mucinous adenocarcinoma, signet ring cell carcinoma, medullary adenocarcinoma, and poorly differentiated carcinoma with heterogeneous morphology are reported to have higher frequency of high-level MSI (MSI-H) (Fig. 28.1). Other morphological characteristics of MSI-H CRC include increased tumor-infiltrating lymphocytes and Crohn's-like lymphocyte reaction to tumor. In addition, aberrant IHC phenotype is noted in MSI-H cancer, including unreactive for CK20, CDX2, or epithelial cell adhesion molecule (EPCAM). Table 28.5 summarizes the pathological characteristics of MSI-H CRC.

TABLE 28-4 Types of Microsatellites

Name/Type	Sequence	Repeat Location	Gene	Chromosome
BAT25/mononucleotide	AGGTAAAAAAAAAAAAA AAAAAAAAAAAAGGT (A_{25} repeat)	Intron 16	*c-kit*	4q12
D2S123/dinucleotide units	TGTACACACACACACAT CGA (CA_6 repeat)	Intron 5	*MSH2*	2p16

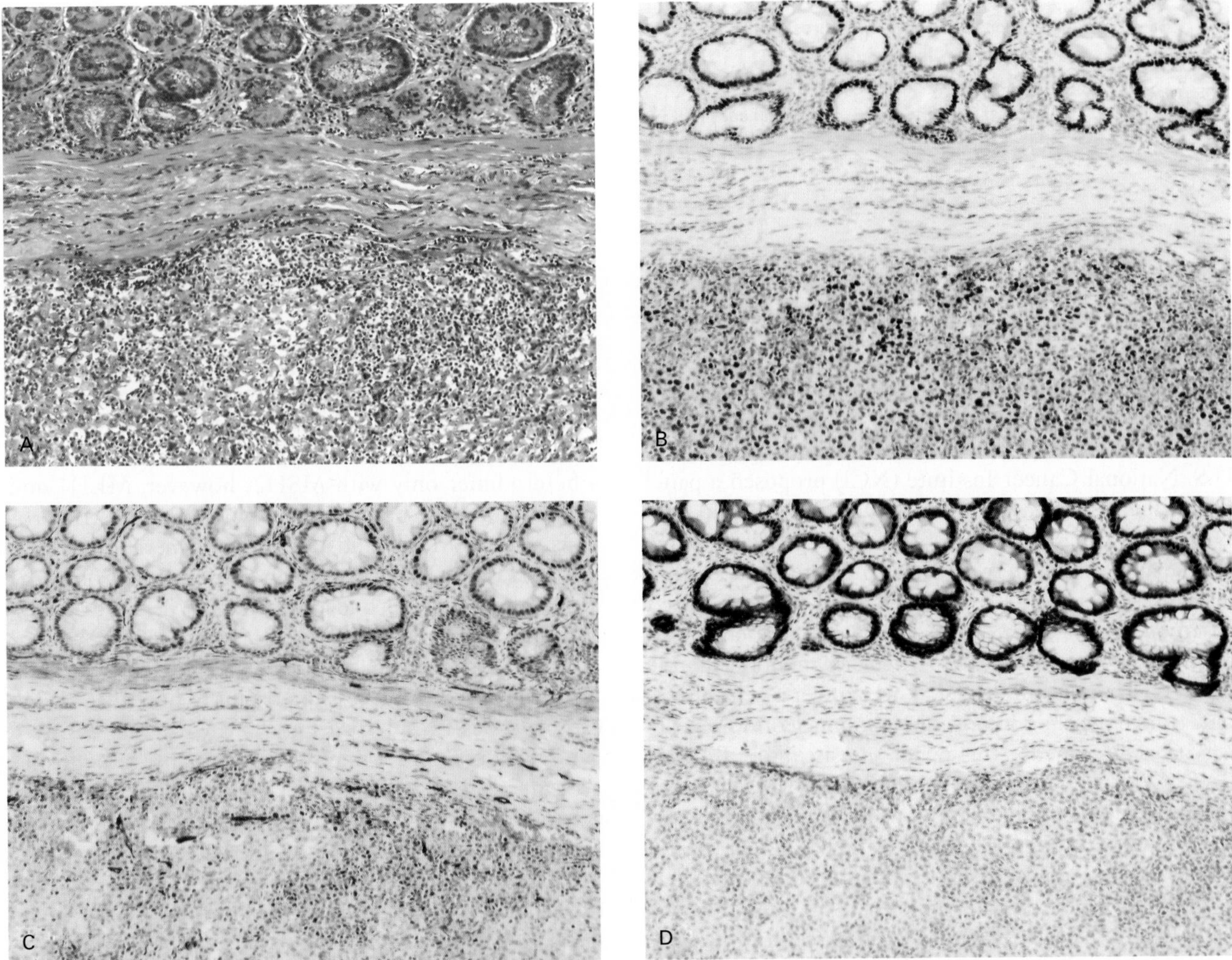

FIGURE 28–1 Immunohistochemistry of mismatch repair protein panel in colorectal cancer. MLH1, PMS2, MSH2, and MSH6 were performed in an ascending colon cancer. **A:** Invasive medullary adenocarcinoma with increased intratumoral lymphocytes and overlying colonic mucosa. **B:** MLH1 expressed in tumor cells and non-neoplastic cells. PMS2 was also positive (not shown). **C:** Loss of MSH2 expression was noted in tumor cells, while non-neoplastic cells have normal expression. **D:** Initial MSH6 staining showed primarily cytoplasmic staining of normal mucosa, while tumor cells were negative, stromal cells and lymphocytes were weakly stained. It was a false negative. Repeat staining revealed MSH6 loss with adequate internal control (not shown).

Screening Tests for Lynch Syndrome

Two tests are initially performed on CRC specimens to identify individuals who might have Lynch syndrome: IHC analysis for MMR protein expression, which is often diminished due to mutation, and analysis for MSI, which results from MMR gene deficiency and is detected as an altered amount of short, repeated DNA sequences in tumor tissue caused by the insertion or deletion of repeated units.[20-26]

TABLE 28–5 Pathological Characteristics of High-Level Microsatellite Instability in Colorectal Cancer

Increased Tumor-infiltrating lymphocytes
Crohn's-like lymphocytic reaction
Mucinous adenocarcinoma
Signet ring cell differentiation
Medullary adenocarcinoma
Poorly differentiated carcinoma with heterogeneous morphology
Aberrant CK7/CK20 expression: unreactive
Aberrant CDX2 expression: unreactive
BEREP4 (EPCAM) expression: unreactive

MSI Assay

In the clinical MSI assay, DNA is usually extracted from microdissected paraffin-embedded tumor and non-neoplastic tissue. The extracted DNA is subsequently analyzed by a polymerase chain reaction (PCR)–based method. Revelation of PCR amplification products is usually carried out by either capillary electrophoresis or polyacrylamide gel electrophoresis–silver staining. Because defective MMR genes do not affect all microsatellites in a given neoplasm, multiple microsatellites that are frequently affected by instability are needed in order to study MSI. Repeats with units ranging from two to hundreds

TABLE 28-6 Proposed Criteria for Microsatellite Instability Classification

Type	Abnormal Markers	Frequency (%)
MSI-H	≥40%	15
MSI-L	One marker or <40% of markers	5
MSS	0	80

MSI-H, high-level MSI; MSI-L, low-level MSI; MSS, MSI-stable.

TABLE 28-7 Loss of the MMR Proteins and Associated MMR Genes

Loss of MMR Proteins	Affected Genes			
	MLH1	*MSH2*	*MSH6*	*PMS2*
MLH1 and PMS2	+			Occasional
PMS2				+
MSH2 and MSH6		+	Occasional	
MSH6			+	

MMR, mismatch repair.

have been used to classify microsatellites. Although there is no consensus on the minimum number of repeated nucleotide units required to define a microsatellite, the U.S. National Cancer Institute (NCI) proposed a panel of five markers (BAT25, BAT26, D2S123, D5S346, and D17S250) as a standard test panel for MSI.[2,20,26] This "NCI panel" has been recently expanded to include other markers, such as BAT40, BAT34c4, MycL, and TGFBR2, based on evidence that MSI sensitivity can be enhanced by including more markers, particularly mononucleotide markers, in the testing panel. Therefore, a recent pentaplex of five quasimonomorphic mononucleotide repeats has been described[25]; this panel, consisting of BAT25, BAT26, NR21, NR24, and NR22 or NR27, has two potential advantages: it does not need for the corresponding normal control germline DNA and has higher (nearly 100%) specificity and sensitivity. It has been reported that analysis of MSI of the same tumor samples using the pentaplex panel in several different testing facilities had the same results with no discrepancies.[6]

Regardless of whether five, seven, or more markers are used, if 40% or more of the markers tested are abnormal (for example, when at least three of seven markers are abnormal), the CRC specimen is categorized as MSI-H. When no abnormality is detected in the tested microsatellite markers, the specimen is called MSI-stable (MSS). If one marker or less than 40% of the markers tested show abnormalities, the specimen is categorized as low-level MSI (MSI-L). The biologic significance of MSI-L is not entirely clear, and MSI-L tumors have clinical features of MSS tumors. The proposed criteria for MSI classification are listed in Table 28.6.

For external quality assessment and evaluation of inter-laboratory reproducibility, proficiency testing for MSI was introduced by the College of American Pathologists (http:www.cap.org/apps/cap.portal).

Assessment of MMR Proteins

Compared with the PCR-based MSI assay, IHC analysis is more convenient and inexpensive. More importantly, IHC analysis directly detects the MMR gene that is likely to be mutated.[24] The relationships between the loss of MMR proteins and their associated MMR genes are shown in Table 28.7.

MMR proteins function in heterodimer pairs. MLH1 and MSH2 are the obligatory dimers. PMS2 can form a heterodimer only with MLH1, and MSH6 can form a heterodimer only with MSH2; however, MLH1 and MSH2 can form heterodimers with other MMR proteins, such as MSH3 and PMS1.[21] In general, mutations in MLH1 and MSH2 result in subsequent proteolytic degradation of the secondary partners, PMS2 and MSH6, respectively. On the other hand, mutations in PMS2 or MSH6 may not result in proteolytic degradation of its primary partner. Also, it is important to note that MSH6 can be lost as a result of defective MMR because MSH6 gene itself contains a microsatellite, or it can be lost as a result of germline mutation. Accordingly, the use of a two-antibody panel consisting of PMS2 and MSH6 for screening for Lynch syndrome has been proposed.[23] Studies of two-antibody panels for examining colonic and extracolonic Lynch syndrome–related tumors have shown fairly consistent results compared with results for four-antibody panels, indicating the potential value in reducing the cost of MMR protein IHC analysis.[23]

In general, IHC analysis to interpret MMR protein is straightforward since all MMR proteins are readily recognizable on nuclear staining (Fig. 28.1A–C). It is always helpful to carefully assess the expression of MMR proteins, first in non-neoplastic cells and then in tumor cells. Cases are classified with loss of expression when there is a lack of expression in tumor cells in the presence of internal positive controls (lymphocytes and stromal cells). However, it should be noted that immunostaining of MMR proteins can be heterogeneous throughout the tumor, and difficult cases with patchy, weak immunoreactivity, particularly with MLH1 and MSH6, are encountered. Any equivocal staining should be repeated or even redone with a different antibody clone (Fig. 28.1D). It has also been reported that a subset of cases with loss of MMR protein were initially misinterpreted as tumors exhibiting intact MMR protein by individuals without knowledge of the potential pitfall of frequently present intratumoral lymphocytes, underscoring the important role of experienced pathologists in assessing MMR proteins. Furthermore, partial expression of MSH6 has been reported in colorectal carcinoma after neoadjuvant treatment; in general, a low percentage of tumors with intact expression of the mismatch enzymes can have MSI

TABLE 28-8 Comparison of Microsatellite Instability Screening Test Methodologie

	IHC Analysis	MSI Assay
Assessment level	Proteins	DNA
Sensitivity	90–93%	Up to 95%
Cost	Less expensive	More expensive
Availability	Most pathology laboratories	Molecular laboratories
Implicates genes	Yes	No
Sample	Tumor cells	Tumor and normal cells
Turnaround time	Same day	A couple of days
Variability in results	Capricious staining	Depending on tumor cellularity
Interpretation	Experienced pathologist	Relatively straightforward

MSI, microsatellite instability; IHC, immunohistochemistry.

genotype.[24] Therefore, concurrent testing for both mismatch enzymes and PCR testing for microsatellite markers are advocated.

In summary, IHC staining for MMR proteins and the MSI PCR assay are unique and complementary[26]: IHC analysis can identify tumors with low levels of MSI that may be missed by PCR studies, particularly those tumors with mutations in *MSH6*. A subset of *MSH2*-deficient patients with germline deletions in the *EpCAM* gene, also known as TACSTD1, cannot be identified by the loss of MSH2 protein expression with the use of IHC analysis, and no *MSH2* gene mutations can be identified. On the other hand, the MSI PCR assay may identify patients with abnormal DNA MMR genes, but IHC analysis cannot detect nontruncating missense alterations or defects in genes other than the four MMR proteins. For example, in a recent study ($n = 500$), both MSI (five-marker panel) and IHC analysis (all four MMR proteins) were used to identify 64 patients with MSI and 71 patients with abnormal IHC findings, and one major discrepancy was found: one Lynch syndrome case was detected by MSI, whereas IHC results were normal.[19] In short, each test platform has advantages and disadvantages. Comparisons of commonly used IHC- and PCR-based MSI tests are listed in Table 28.8.

Colorectal Adenoma and MSI

Although testing of MSI status is widely used in invasive CRC samples, such testing of colorectal adenoma samples has also been reported. Provided that the MMR gene repair deficiency is an early event in CRC tumorigenesis, testing colorectal adenomas for MSI should be a useful strategy for the early detection of Lynch syndrome (Fig. 28.2). Studies have demonstrated that coexisting adenomas and carcinomas displayed similar immunostaining patterns for MMR proteins, indicating that the MMR gene defect is indeed an early event in the carcinogenesis

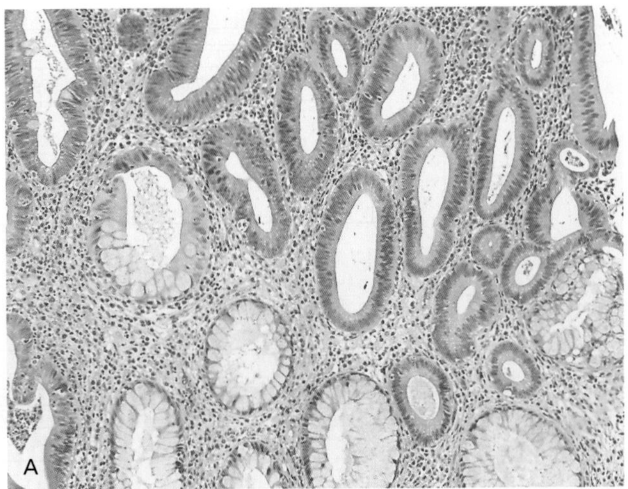

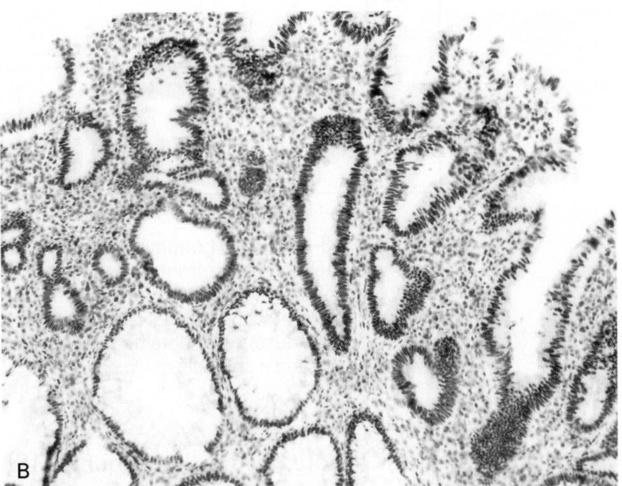

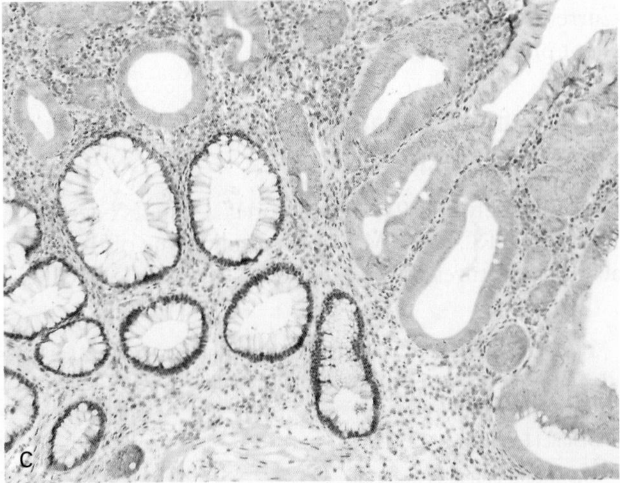

FIGURE 28–2 Immunohistochemistry of mismatch repair protein panel in colonic adenoma. MLH1, PMS2, MSH2, and *MSH6* were performed in a tubular adenoma. **A:** Tubular adenoma (surface portion of the specimen) and normal colonic mucosa (deep portion of the specimen). **B:** MSH2 expressed in both adenoma and non-neoplastic cells. MSH6 was also positive (not shown). **C:** Loss of MLH1 expression was noted in the adenoma, while non-neoplastic cells have normal expression. PMS2 is also lost in adenoma (not shown). Further workup of *hMLH1* methylation revealed that *hMLH1* was not hypermethylated, suggesting that it is likely a Lynch syndrome.

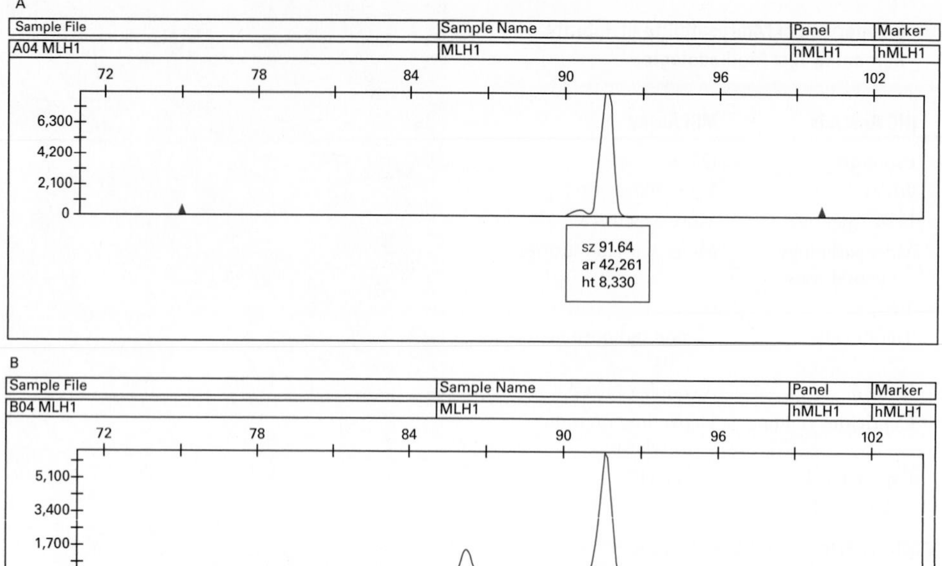

FIGURE 28–3 *hMLH1* methylation testing. DNA was extracted from microdissected paraffin-embedded tissue from a transverse colon cancer biopsy specimen. The tissue was treated with bisulfite to convert unmethylated cytosine to uracil. Polymerase chain reaction amplification of both unmethylated and methylated *hMLH1* promoter sequences was done with fluorescently labeled primers and products were detected using capillary electrophoresis. **A:** Normal control. **B:** Methylated *hMLH1*, indicating a sporadic colon cancer.

of Lynch syndrome. Of note, studies have found MSI testing to be more accurate in larger adenomas, particularly the tubulovillous type with high-grade dysplasia. Currently, testing for MSI status in all biopsied adenomas is not practical or cost-effective.

MLH1 Hypermethylation and *BRAF* Mutation in Sporadic MSI CRC

Approximately 15-19% of all colorectal tumors have MSI, and most CRCs with MSI are sporadic. One of the characteristic features of sporadic CRCs with MSI is biallelic methylation of the *MLH1* promoter (Fig. 28.3).[27] In addition, sporadic CRCs with MSI display frequent mutation of the *BRAF* gene. The common and differential features of Lynch syndrome and sporadic CRC with MSI are listed in Table 28.9.

Because of the significant clinical implications between the two subsets of MSI-associated CRCs, it is essential to distinguish them. Several workup algorithms have been proposed, although currently there is no consensus on the approach or workflow to distinguish Lynch syndrome from sporadic CRCs with MSI. One cost-effective way is to perform a *BRAF* gene mutation test when MLH1

TABLE 28–9 Common and Differential Features of Lynch Syndrome and Sporadic Colorectal Cancer with Microsatellite Instability

Distinct Features	Lynch Syndrome	Sporadic CRC with MSI
Significant familial clustering	Yes	No
Patient age	Younger	Older
Absence of MLH1 and PMS2 proteins	Yes	Yes
Mutation in *BRAF*	None	Yes (50% of cases)
Mutation in *KRAS*[a]	Often (40%)	Less frequent (20%)
Associated with CIMP	No	Yes
Better prognosis than those with non-MSI CRC	Yes	Yes

CRC, colorectal cancer; MSI, microsatellite instability; CIMP, CpG island methylator phenotype.
[a]In contrast to the *BRAF* V600E mutation, the status of the *KRAS* mutation is unlikely to benefit Lynch syndrome screening protocols because *KRAS* mutations occur in both forms of MSI CRCs (sporadic and hereditary) and in about 40% of MSI-stable CRCs.

immunoexpression is absent in the tumor.[22] The presence of *BRAF* mutation indicates that *MLH1* expression is downregulated by somatic methylation of the promoter region of the gene and not by a germline mutation,[13] ruling out Lynch syndrome. If no *BRAF* mutation is detected, the sample should further undergo a hypermethylation test of *MLH1*. If no *MLH1* hypermethylation is detected, the case is most likely a Lynch syndrome, requiring an *MLH1* mutation test for confirmation and subsequent genetic counseling.

MMR Gene Mutations

MMR gene mutation testing is required to confirm Lynch syndrome. To detect point mutations and small insertion–deletion mutations that involve DNA sequences between the primers, MMR genes are preferably analyzed by using exon-by-exon sequencing with PCR primers that include portions of the intron–exon boundaries. When DNA sequencing is performed, the tracing is examined for a double signal: the simultaneous presence of a wild-type and mutant nucleotide in the same sequence position. To detect large deletions or rearrangements, such as DNA sequences that are rejoined after a break, frequently occurring in *MSH2*- and *MSH6*-associated Lynch syndrome, multiplex ligation-dependent probe amplification is used to quantify the number of alleles at each exon.[2]

Although beyond the scope of this chapter, it should be stressed that when a sequence variation is found after analysis of mutations in DNA MMR genes, appropriate interpretation is important. Most deletions and nonsense mutations have pathologic consequences. Missense mutations are not always readily interpretable; thus, the mutant allele might need to be cloned and its product analyzed in a functional assay.

GENETIC COUNSELING

Some physicians might not be cognizant of the molecular genetic and phenotypic features of Lynch syndrome or of the clinical implications of these features for the patient and the patient's immediate family members.[28] In such cases, referral should be made to ensure appropriate genetic counseling, and appropriate clinical surveillance and management can be offered. An example of a genetic counseling report is shown below.

Genetic Counseling Initial Assessment Note

Note: Genetic consultation notes should be released only with special authorization from the patient.

Time spent: 45 minutes.

REASON FOR CONSULTATION

The patient was referred for genetic counseling after high-level microsatellite instability (MSI-H) colorectal cancer (CRC) was identified.

RELEVANT HISTORY

The patient is a 41-year-old gentleman who was diagnosed as having descending colon cancer earlier this year in a regional hospital. Fine needle aspiration also confirmed a solitary liver metastasis of the left lobe. Of note, pathological examination of the CRC revealed the presence of tumor-infiltrating lymphocytes. Immunohistochemical analysis of MLH1, PMS2, MSH2, and MSH6, performed at the outside institute, showed MSI-stable results. Four weeks after CRC was diagnosed, the patient started receiving six cycles of neoadjuvant FOLFOX. Two months after completing this chemotherapy, the patient came to our medical center and underwent an exploratory laparotomy and low anterior resection of the colon tumor. MSI assay and *KRAS* and *BRAF* mutations were performed on the resected tumor sample, which showed that seven of seven markers had shifted (BAT25, BAT26, BAT40, D2S123, D5S346, D17S250, and TGFBR2), characteristic of an MSI-H phenotype. No mutations were detected in codons 595 to 600 in exon 15 of the *BRAF* gene or in codons 12, 13, or 61 of the *KRAS* gene. Immunostaining was then performed again and showed loss of MLH1 and PMS2. Subsequently, *hMLH1* was performed and showed that the tumor did not have hypermethylation of the *MLH1* promoter. After the patient completed nine cycles of adjuvant treatment consisting of 5-fluorouracil, leucovorin, and Avastin, he underwent a wedge resection of the metastatic disease of the left lobe. Pathological examination revealed a 1.5-cm well-defined mass with necrosis, marked with foamy histiocytes, foreign body giant cell reaction, and fibrosis, consistent with treatment effect, with no tumor cells identified, indicating a pathological complete response.

FAMILY HISTORY

The patient is married and lives in ABC city, DEF state. He has one son, age 8 years, who is healthy. He has two brothers, ages 23 and 33 years, and one sister, age 27 years. None of his siblings have had a colonoscopy. The patient reports no history of cancer in his nieces and nephews. The patient's mother is living at the age of 57 years with no history of cancer. She has not had a colonoscopy or a total abdominal hysterectomy. The patient's mother has a sister in her forties with CRC and another sister in her forties with breast cancer. The patient denies cancer in his maternal first cousins. Both of the patient's maternal grandparents died in their seventies of heart disease.

The patient's father died of a heart attack at age 68 years with no history of cancer. The patient has a deceased paternal aunt and paternal uncle who both died in their fifties of myocardial infarctions. The patient has three living paternal aunts and two living paternal uncles in their sixties and seventies with no history of cancer. The patient denies a history of cancer in his paternal first cousins. The patient has no information about his paternal grandparents.

The patient denies Ashkenazi Jewish ancestry. Complete pedigree is available for the Clinical Cancer Genetics Program upon request.

(*Continued*)

Genetic Counseling Initial Assessment Note (*Continued*)

DISCUSSION

We discussed Lynch syndrome with the patient at length. He was informed that Lynch syndrome is the most commonly inherited predisposition for CRC, accounting for approximately 5% of CRC cases. The patient's tumor was tested for MSI to determine whether he has an inherited predisposition to colon cancer and was found to be MSI-H, the hallmark of tumors associated with Lynch syndrome. In addition, the tumor was tested for protein products of the four mismatch DNA repair genes and found to lack staining for the MLH1 and PMS2 proteins. Further testing of *MLH1* promoter methylation and *BRAF* studies showed that the tumor has no methylation of the *MLH1* promoter and no *BRAF* V600E mutation. Therefore, all sporadic causes of MSI have been ruled out. The patient was informed that studies of his tumor provide a presumptive diagnosis of Lynch syndrome.

We discussed the fact that the most significant risks are for CRC (up to 80%) and uterine cancer (up to 60%). Individuals with Lynch syndrome are also at increased risk (as high as 50% within 15 years of diagnosis) for a second primary CRC. Patients are therefore advised to agree to relatively strict surveillance, even after receiving a diagnosis of a primary colon cancer. In addition, individuals with Lynch syndrome have increased risk (almost 10%) of other types of cancer, such as gastric, small bowel, upper urinary tract, hepatobiliary tract, ovarian, skin, and brain tumors.

Lynch syndrome is an autosomal dominant condition, meaning that it is passed from parent to child. Individuals with Lynch syndrome have an approximate 50% chance of passing Lynch syndrome on to their children. Patients should undergo germline genetic testing of the *MLH1* gene, which is performed on a blood draw. If a mutation is identified, the patient's mother would be advised to be tested since she might have Lynch syndrome and therefore be at risk for colon, endometrial, and other cancers. If the mutation is identified in the patient's *MLH1* gene, his brothers, sister, and son (at age 18 years) should eventually undergo a blood test for *MLH1* mutation to determine whether they inherited Lynch syndrome.

All individuals with Lynch syndrome should follow the recommendations outlined by the National Comprehensive Cancer Network (NCCN) for clinical surveillance and management, including the following:

1. Colonoscopy every 1 to 2 years, beginning at age 20 to 25 years.
2. Upper endoscopy every 2 to 3 years, beginning at age 30 to 35 years.
3. Consideration of annual urinalysis with cytology.
4. For women: Yearly screening for endometrial cancer beginning at age 30 to 35 years. Consideration of prophylactic oophorectomy and hysterectomy for women who have completed childbearing.

In a small percentage of families with Lynch syndrome, current genetic testing is unable to identify a causative mutation. In the event that the patient test results are negative for an *MLH1* mutation, all individuals in his immediate family will be advised to undergo surveillance, since they are at risk for Lynch syndrome. At that point, genetic testing would not be helpful in other family members.

The patient was provided comprehensive counseling about the results of his tumor studies, the genetics and natural history of Lynch syndrome, and the next steps to take. The patient was also advised to undergo *MLH1* genetic testing to attempt to identify the causative mutations so that other individuals in his family may be tested for this mutation to determine whether they have Lynch syndrome. The patient expressed understanding that Lynch syndrome is the most likely cause for his colon cancer and puts him at risk for other cancers in the future. He was advised to undergo screening as recommended by the NCCN, as outlined above, and elected to undergo *MLH1* genetic testing. This blood draw will be scheduled when he returns to the institution the following Monday. Results will be available approximately 2 weeks after that date. The patient will be informed of the results of the genetic testing, and further recommendations for family members will be made at that time. The patient was given ample opportunity to ask questions, and all of his questions were addressed. The patient was given a patient education document about Lynch syndrome, as well as a copy of his genetic counselor's business card, and was encouraged to contact the genetic counselor with any changes to his personal or family history or with any questions.

The risk assessment here is based on history and reports provided.

RECOMMENDATIONS AND DECISIONS

1. The patient has been found to have presumptive Lynch syndrome based on an MSI-H tumor, with loss of MLH1 and PMS2; *MLH1* hypermethylation of the promoter and *BRAF* V600E mutations have been excluded.
2. The patient is advised to undergo *MLH1* genetic testing to determine the causative mutation and has elected to proceed with this testing, which is scheduled for the following Monday. The patient will be called with the results approximately 2 weeks after the test.
3. If a mutation is identified in the patient, family members will be advised to undergo predictive testing to determine whether they have inherited Lynch syndrome. If a mutation is not identified, all individuals in the patient's immediate family will be advised to undergo risk screening, since they are at risk for Lynch syndrome.
4. The patient was encouraged to contact the genetic counselor with any changes to his personal or family history, since these may alter the above risk assessment. In addition, cancer genetics is a rapidly evolving field, and new information that could benefit the patient may become available in the future.
5. The patient's pertinent medical and family histories will be reviewed at the weekly CRC genetics case conference; this report reflects a consensus of opinion.

PREDICTIVE AND PROGNOSTIC MARKERS

Predictive biomarkers indicate the likelihood of treatment benefit, allowing the identification of patients who will or will not benefit from the use of a particular therapy; *prognostic biomarkers*, independent of the treatment effect, provide information about the natural history of the disease and are associated with patient survival. We have little knowledge of why some CRC patients respond to therapy, yet others do not, or why some experience disease relapse, whereas others do not. However, progress has been made by using various techniques to refine prognostic and predictive information.

MSI and Chemotherapy—Predictive Power

MSI status is important to consider during the decision-making process for the use of adjuvant chemotherapy in CRC patients. On a molecular level, evidence has shown that patients would need intact MMR gene function to induce apoptosis of 5-fluorouracil (5-FU)–modified DNA. There is evidence that MSI has decreased benefit or even a detrimental effect from adjuvant therapy with a fluoropyrimidine alone in patients with stage II disease.[29-31]

A retrospective study involving long-term follow-up of patients with stage II or stage III disease that was evaluated according to MSI tumor status demonstrated that those with MSI-L or MSS tumors had improved outcome with 5-FU adjuvant therapy. However, patients with MSI-H tumors did not show statistically significant benefit from 5-FU after surgery and instead exhibited a lower 5-year survival rate than did those undergoing surgery alone.[29] Similarly, results from another retrospective study of pooled data from adjuvant trials by Sargent et al. showed that in tumors characterized as having a defective MMR gene, adjuvant 5-FU chemotherapy appeared to be detrimental in patients with stage II but not stage III disease.

The molecular mechanism behind the lack of 5-FU–based treatment benefit in MSI-H cancers is unclear, but it was probably related to a higher thymidylate synthase (TS) level in MMR gene–deficient cancer. Regarding molecular mechanisms, it may be reasonable to withhold 5-FU–based adjuvant therapy in patients with stage II MSI-H disease on the basis of possible detrimental treatment effect.

Moreover, studies have demonstrated that inclusion of *irinotecan* in the chemotherapeutic regimen was associated with increased survival time in patients with MSI-associated CRC, indicating that a combination of drugs without excessive immunotoxicity is best for this subset of patients.

MSI and Clinical Outcomes—Prognostic Power

MSI status is closely associated with patient prognosis. Data from the Pan-European Trial in Adjuvant Colon Cancer 3 (PETACC-3) showed that specimens characterized as MSI-H were more common in stage II disease than in stage III disease (22% vs. 12%, respectively; $P < 0.0001$).[32] In another large study, the percentage of stage IV tumors characterized as MSI-H was only 3.5%.[33] These results suggest that MSI-H tumors have decreased likelihood to metastasize. In fact, there is substantial evidence that in patients with stage II disease, a deficiency in MMR protein expression or MSI-H tumor status is a prognostic marker of more favorable outcome.[29,31]

A pooled meta-analysis of 32 studies (n = 7,642 CRCs) found that MSI was associated with better survival, demonstrating an overall hazard ratio of 0.65 for patients with MSI-associated CRC. Moreover, patients with MSI tumors had lower mortality rates when they were stratified by tumor stage, confirming the independent prognostic value of MSI. A recent study of 1,913 patients with stage II CRC from the QUASAR study, half of whom received adjuvant chemotherapy, showed that defective MMR genes were prognostic. The recurrence rate of MMR gene–defective and MMR gene–proficient tumors was 11% and 26%, respectively.[34] Overall, although the prognostic power of MMR gene status in stage II disease seems clear, there is considerable controversy surrounding the predictive power of MMR gene status.[35]

Furthermore, a recent prospective evaluation of 1,852 colon cancers demonstrated that MMR deficiency has prognostic value for stages II and III colon cancer. The NCCN CRC panel recommends that MMR gene testing,[30] as well as planned adjuvant therapy with a fluoropyrimidine alone, be considered for patients with stage II disease.

Due to the significant impact of MSI on the treatment and prognosis of CRC, both on the patient and possibly on the patient's family members, it has been recommended that all patients with newly diagnosed CRC be screened for MSI by MSI testing or IHC analysis. In fact, some centers now perform both IHC and MSI testing on all colorectal tumors to determine which patients should have genetic testing for Lynch syndrome. The cost-effectiveness of this so-called reflex testing approach has been confirmed for CRC, and this approach was endorsed by the EGAPP Working Group at the Centers for Disease Control and Prevention.[14]

KRAS Test

One of the most important developments in molecular markers for CRC has been the validation of the KRAS mutation as predictive of targeted epidermal growth factor receptor (EGFR) treatment response. *KRAS*, a member of the RAS family (*HRAS*, *KRAS*, *NRAS*), encodes small proteins with enzymatic guanosine triphosphatase activity that couple external growth signals to intracellular signaling cascades that govern cell proliferation and survival. *KRAS* mutations are an early event in the adenoma–carcinoma sequence. Approximately 40% to 45% of patients with metastatic CRC are characterized by

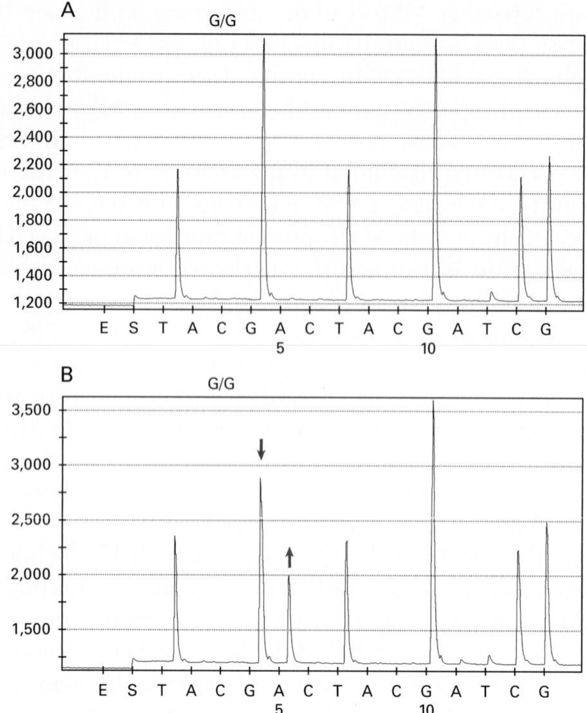

FIGURE 28–4 *KRAS* mutation analysis. Polymerase chain reaction–based DNA sequencing analysis was performed (Sanger method) in a rectal cancer. **A:** Normal control. **B:** A mutation was detected in codon 12 of *KRAS* (GGT to GAT) (*arrow*) that changes the encoded amino acid from Gly to Asp.

mutations in codons 12 and 13 in exon 2 of the coding region of the *KRAS* gene (Fig. 28.4).[32,36] Cetuximab and panitumumab are monoclonal antibodies directed against EGFR that inhibit its downstream signaling pathways. Cetuximab is a chimeric monoclonal antibody, whereas panitumumab is a fully human monoclonal antibody. These targeted drugs can be used alone or in combination with other anticancer drugs. The RAS/RAF/MAPK pathway is downstream of EGFR, and mutations in components of this pathway are being studied in search of predictive markers for efficacy of these therapies.

Studies of anti-EGFR antibody treatment showed that patients with *KRAS* mutant-type CRC had significantly less benefit than did those with *KRAS* wild-type CRC. Use of cetuximab as initial therapy for metastatic disease was investigated in a large clinical trial, in which patients were randomly assigned to receive FOLFIRI with or without cetuximab.[37] Retrospective analyses of the subset of patients with known *KRAS* tumor status showed statistically significant improvement in median progression-free survival (PFS) with the addition of cetuximab in groups with disease characterized by the *KRAS* wild-type gene. The statistically significant favorable clinical outcome for patients with *KRAS* wild-type tumors receiving cetuximab was verified in a recent publication of an updated analysis of the CRYSTAL data.[38] This recent study included a retrospective analysis of overall survival in the *KRAS* wild-type population and found improvement with the addition of cetuximab (23.5 vs. 20.0 months, $P < 0.01$). The negative predictive value of the *KRAS* mutation for anti-EGFR treatment response is high: up to 95% of patients with mutated *KRAS* do not respond to the anti-EGFR regimen.

Panitumumab in combination with either FOLFOX[39] or FOLFIRI has also been studied as a first-line treatment for patients with metastatic CRC. Results from the large, open-label, randomized PRIME trial comparing panitumumab plus FOLFOX versus FOLFOX alone in patients with *KRAS* wild-type advanced CRC showed statistically significant benefit in PFS with the addition of panitumumab.[39] It is also important to note that the addition of panitumumab had a detrimental effect on PFS for patients with tumors characterized by mutated *KRAS*.

In short, a sizable body of recent literature has revealed that CRCs with a mutation in codon 12 or 13 of the *KRAS* gene are essentially insensitive to EGFR inhibitors such as cetuximab or panitumumab[36,37,40-46] and may have a detrimental effect on survival. The NCCN panel therefore recommends that *KRAS* genotyping of tumor tissue be performed in all patients with metastatic CRC. Patients with known codon 12 or 13 *KRAS* mutations should not be treated with either cetuximab or panitumumab, either alone or in combination with other anticancer agents, because there is virtually no chance of benefit and the exposure to toxicity and the cost cannot be justified.[47,48] However, *KRAS* mutation at c.38G > A(G13D), one of *KRAS* mutations in codon 13, was reported to have no influence on anti-EGFR-regimen.[38]

It is strongly recommended that genotyping of tumor tissue be performed in all patients with metastatic CRC *at the time of diagnosis of stage IV disease*. The recommendation for *KRAS* testing at this point is not meant to indicate a preference in first-line regimen; instead, this early establishment of *KRAS* status is appropriate in order to plan the treatment continuum, to obtain information in a non–time-sensitive manner, and to allow the patient and provider to discuss the implications of a *KRAS* mutation, if present, while other treatment options exist. Since anti-EGFR agents have no role in the management of stage I, II, or III disease, *KRAS* genotyping of CRCs at these earlier stages is not recommended.

Technically, *KRAS* genotyping can be performed on archived specimens of either the primary tumor or a metastasis because *KRAS* mutations are early events in CRC formation; therefore, the mutation status between the primary tumor and metastases is very tightly correlated.[49-51] Although no specific methodologies for *KRAS* gene testing are recommended,[52] these tests should be performed only in laboratories that have been certified by the clinical laboratory improvement amendments of 1988 (CLIA-88) as qualified to perform highly complex molecular pathology testing.[52]

It should be pointed out that although *KRAS* mutations at residues G12 and G13 predominate in CRCs, broader testing is revealing other relatively uncommon mutations, such as A146 mutations in about 2% to 3% of CRCs and codon 61 mutations in about 6% of CRCs, and these mutations confer similar pathway dependence and resistance to targeted agents. Therefore, testing *KRAS* mutations beyond G12 and G13 would provide more accurate information of the status of this critical oncogene, maximizing the benefit of EGFR-targeted therapy.

Of note, in contrast to the predictive value of *KRAS* mutations, results have been mixed in attempts to determine the prognostic value of these mutations. An international study combining data from various groups showed that *KRAS* mutations generally confer a worse prognosis. However, subsequent analysis found that only the glycine to valine substitution at codon 12 was associated with poorer progress. One recent study demonstrated an association between *KRAS* mutation and poor overall survival, whereas another large trial failed to show significant association between *KRAS* status and patient outcome. Nevertheless, it is generally believed that a subset of patients with KRAS-mutated CRCs may have a poor prognosis, regardless of the treatments given.[53]

NRAS Test

NRAS and *KRAS*, mutually exclusive, are highly homologous to each other. *NRAS* mutations occur predominately in codon 61 rather than in codon 12 or 13, and the frequency of *NRAS* mutations is low (about 3% to 5% of all metastatic CRCs). A large cohort of metastatic CRCs showed that *NRAS* mutations are significantly associated with refractory cetuximab-based therapy and shorter overall survival and show a trend toward shorter PFS.[54]

BRAF Test

Although certain *KRAS* mutations indicate a lack of response to EGFR inhibitors, many tumors (40% to 60%) with wild-type *KRAS* do not respond to these drugs. In other words, the presence of wild-type *KRAS* does not dictate that anti-EGFR therapies will be effective. Additional factors such as *BRAF* mutations, or loss of phosphatase and tensin homologue (*PTEN*) or *PIK3CA* activation, might contribute to resistance to EGFR-targeted monoclonal antibody treatment. Therefore, studies have investigated factors downstream of *KRAS* as possible additional biomarkers predictive of response to cetuximab or panitumumab. *BRAF*, a cytoplasmic serine–threonine kinase, is a key component in the RAS–MAPK pathway.[54,55] Activating mutations in the *BRAF* gene exist in exon 15 and result in constitutive activation of the MAPK pathway.[55] A relatively specific mutation (V600E) that activates the *BRAF* gene occurs in about 12% of metastatic CRCs (Fig. 28.5). Activation of the protein product of the non-mutated *BRAF* gene occurs downstream of the activated *KRAS* protein in the EGFR pathway; the mutated *BRAF* protein product is believed to be constitutively active, thus putatively bypassing inhibition of EGFR by cetuximab or panitumumab.[56-58] Therefore, *BRAF* is likely a locus for a second hit affecting the same RAS–MAPK pathway.

There is evidence that mutated *BRAF* is another marker of resistance to anti-EGFR therapy in the non–first-line setting of metastatic disease.[59,60] A retrospective study of 773 CRCs from chemotherapy-refractory patients showed that *BRAF*-mutated type conferred a significantly lower response rate to cetuximab (2/24; 8.3%) compared with *BRAF* wild type (124/326; 38.0%; $P < 0.01$) (55). Overall, the data strongly suggest that *BRAF* V600E mutations confer resistance to anti-EGFR therapy in the non–first-line setting,[59,60] whereas there may be some benefit to the addition of anti-EGFR agents to

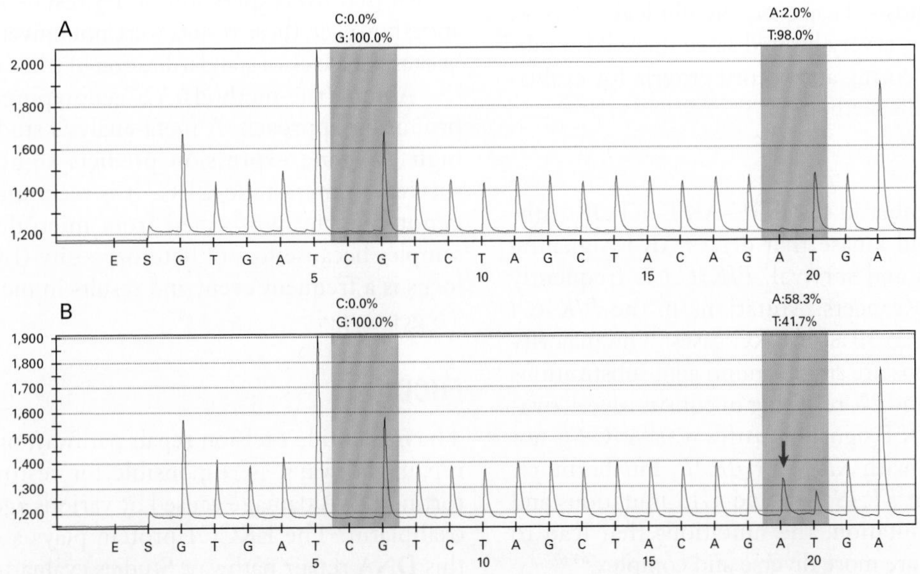

FIGURE 28–5 *BRAF* mutation analysis. Polymerase chain reaction–based DNA sequencing analysis was performed (Sanger method) in a sigmoid cancer. **A:** Normal control. **B:** Mutation was detected in codon 600 (GTG to GAG) in exon 15 (*arrow*) of the *BRAF* gene that would change the encoding amino acid from Val to Glu (V600E).

FOLFOX or FOLFIRI when given to patients with *BRAF* V600E mutations in the first-line metastatic setting.[38]

BRAF and *KRAS* mutations are mutually exclusive; for example, *RAF* mutations are, for all practical purposes, limited to those tumors that do not have *KRAS* exon 2 mutations.[55] It showed that the *BRAF* mutation may also be associated with CRC prognosis[61]; an updated analysis of the CRYSTAL trial demonstrated that patients with metastatic colorectal tumors carrying a *BRAF* V600E mutation have a worse prognosis than do those with the wild-type gene.[38] Moreover, a confirmed *prospective* analysis of tissues from stage II and III colon cancer patients enrolled in the PETACC-3 trial demonstrated that the *BRAF* mutation is a negative prognostic factor of overall survival in patients with MSI-L or MSS tumors (hazard ratio, 2.2; 95% confidence interval, 1.4-3.4; $P < 0.001$).[32] On the basis of fairly consistent clinical studies, the NCCN panel includes the option of *BRAF* genotyping of tumor tissue at the time of diagnosis of *KRAS* wild-type stage IV disease.[30]

In short, although the use of *BRAF* genotyping is currently optional for patients with tumors characterized by the wild-type *KRAS* gene, such testing is recommended, but not mandatory, when making decisions about whether to use anti-EGFR agents. With respect to the technical aspects of *BRAF* gene testing, no specific testing methodology is recommended, and the specific recommendations regarding tumor tissue sampling described for *KRAS* gene testing apply.

PTEN

The *PTEN* gene is a negative regulator of the PI3K/AKT signaling pathway. The loss of PTEN leads to persistent activation of PIK3CA and its downstream oncogenic signaling. Loss of PTEN protein expression measured by IHC analysis occurs in 30% to 45% of CRCs. Studies have shown that loss of PTEN protein by IHC analysis is associated with a lack of response to anti-EGFR antibodies and poor prognosis. However, the clinical utility of PTEN IHC analysis is very limited since there is no validated antibody or scoring and record criteria for evaluation of PTEN by this method.[62,63]

PIK3CA

PIK3CA, a key member in the PI3K-AKT-mTOR pathway, encodes a lipid kinase that drives AKT signaling to support growth and survival. *PIK3CA* is frequently mutated in human cancers. Mutations in the *PIK3CA* gene occur in 15% to 30% of CRC cases. The majority of *PIK3CA* mutations are single amino acid substitutions located in exons 9 and 20, resulting in constitutive activation of the PI3K/AKT signaling pathway. *PIK3CA* is not mutually exclusive with *KRAS* or *BRAF*. Furthermore, unlike the prevalent *KRAS* G12 and G13 mutations and the *BRAF* V600 mutation, the mutations that lead to *PIK3CA* activation are more diverse and complex.[64-67]

An initial study demonstrated that *PIK3CA* mutations were significantly associated with lack of response to anti–EGFR-targeted therapy,[66] whereas another study failed to demonstrate the predictive value of *PIK3CA* in *KRAS* wild-type patients treated with cetuximab.[67] A different proportion of exons 9 and 20 mutations in the studies may represent one of the major explanations. A recent study revealed that only *PIK3CA* exon 20 mutations were associated with a significantly lower response rate and shorter overall survival in a cohort of 370 CRC patients who were *KRAS* wild type and treated with cetuximab.

In addition to the assessment of *KRAS/BRAF/PTEN/PIK3CA* mutational status, gene copy number of EGFR through fluorescence in situ hybridization (FISH) assay has been performed to evaluate clinical response to anti-EGFR treatment in CRCs.[68,69] A positive correlation between the *EGFR* gene copy number and response to cetuximab therapy has been reported.[69] However, implementation of FISH assay, due to the lack of a clear cutoff point for interpretation, in clinical practice may be difficult. Although EGFR testing of colorectal tumor cells by IHC analysis was initially considered useful for making decisions about the use of anti-EGFR agents, many recent studies have demonstrated no predictive value of EGFR testing for colon cancer in determining the likelihood of response to either cetuximab or panitumumab.[70] Therefore, EGFR testing is no longer recommended for guiding EGFR therapy in CRC.

Thymidylate Synthase

The anti-metabolites 5-FU and 5-FU–based chemotherapy remain the central agents in the treatment of advanced CRCs. TS is an important therapeutic target for 5-FU. The metabolite of 5-FU binds to TS, blocking thymidine generation, which inhibits DNA synthesis and repair, leading to cell apoptosis. TSs have been studied by using various methods, such as IHC analysis of TS protein, TS mRNA expression, and *TS* gene amplification.[71] Studies have shown that overexpression of TS results in 5-FU resistance; however, these results were not universally consistent because of a lack of standardization of these methodologies.

Among the methods, *TS* genotyping seems to be a promising approach. A meta-analysis study showed that high *TS* gene expression predicts significantly worse survival in metastatic CRC. It is recommended that *TS* genotyping be performed from microdissected tumor samples because loss of heterozygosity (LOH) at the *TS* locus is a frequent event and results in medication of the *TS* genotype.[72]

ERCC1

The nucleotide excision repair pathway, one of the DNA repair pathways, is responsible for restoring helix-distorting DNA damage caused by various agents, including oxaliplatin. The ERCC1 protein plays a critical role in this DNA repair pathway. Studies evaluating this protein showed that high ERCC1 expression was significantly associated with lower response rate in oxaliplatin-based chemotherapy and shorter overall survival duration.[73,74]

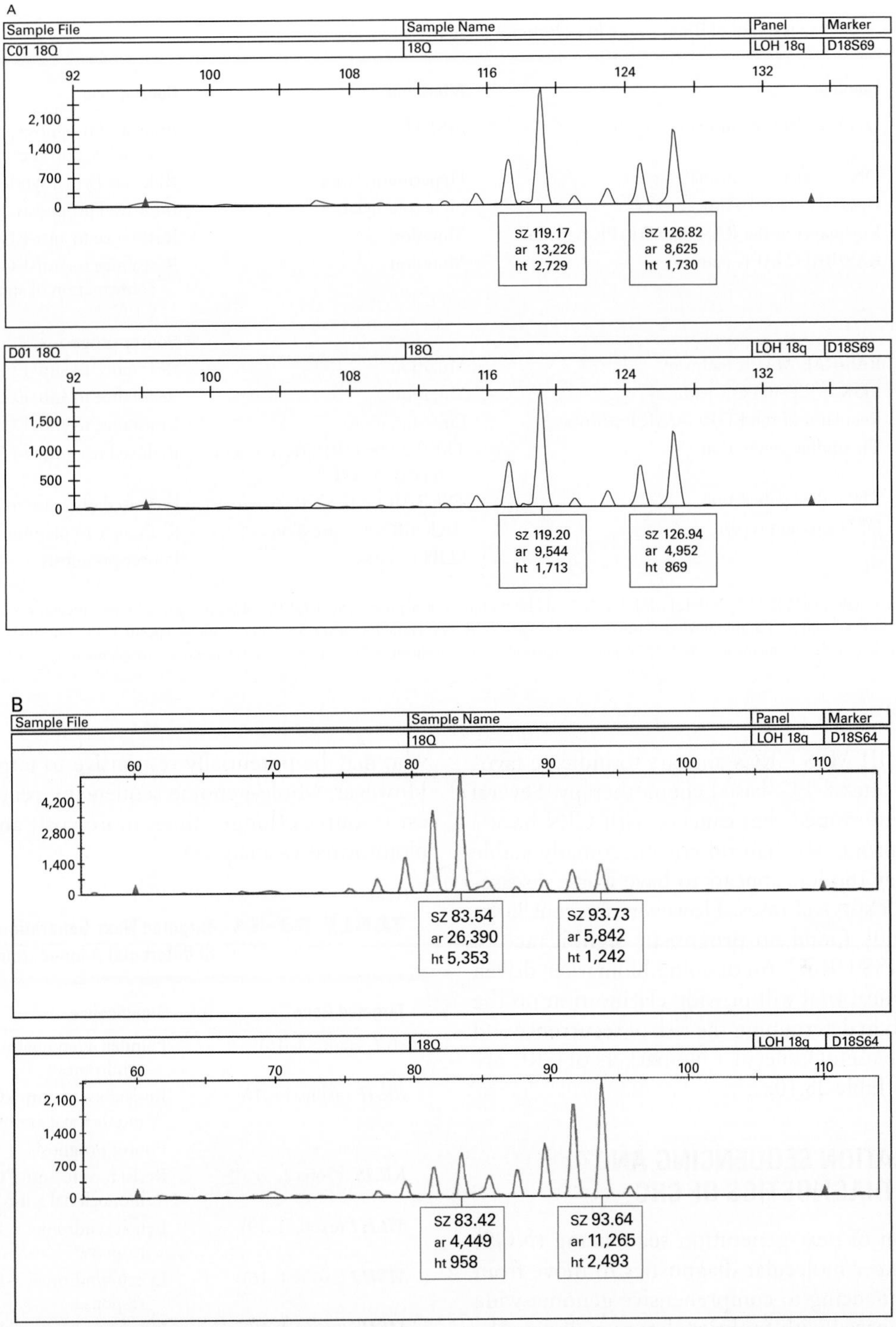

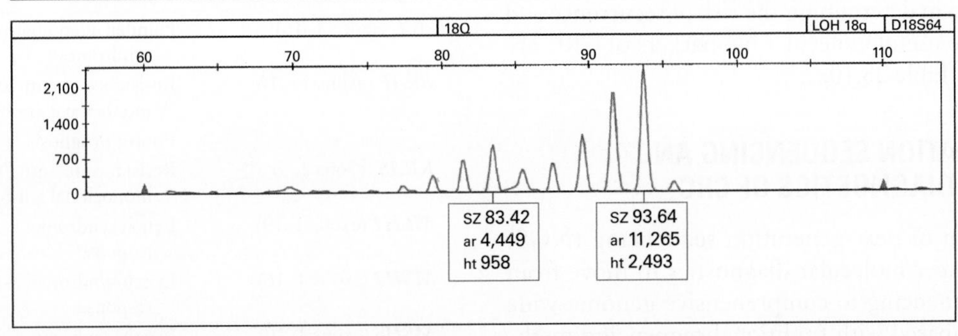

FIGURE 28–6 Chromosome 18q loss of heterozygosity (LOH) testing. Polymerase chain reaction (PCR) and capillary electrophoresis for genomic copy of the long arm(q) of chromosome 18 were performed in an ascending colon cancer. A panel of six fluorescent-labeled markers, D18S55, D18S58, D18S61, D18S64, D18S69, and D18S1147, was used in assessing the LOH of 18q by comparison of the peak areas of PCR products from the tumor to the normal tissue (T/N ratio). **A:** D18S69 was normal: tumor and normal samples were identical. **B:** The other five markers were abnormal. D18S64, one of the five informative foci, was shown.

LOH Test

Allelic imbalance of chromosomal foci (e.g., 5q, 8p, 17p, and 18q) is very common, and an association between LOH and prognosis in patients with CRC has been suggested. LOH of chromosome 18q has been studied most frequently (Fig. 28.6). The 18q region contains several important candidate genes, including *DCC*, *SMAD2*, *SMAD4*, and *SMAD7*. Reduced *SMAD4* expression has been associated with poor prognosis. Retention of 18q

TABLE 28-10 Assessment of Biomarkers in Colorectal Cancer

Biomarker	Function	Alteration	Consequence
MSI	DNA nucleotide mismatch repair	MSI-H	Improved prognosis; need to rule out Lynch syndrome
MLH1	DNA nucleotide mismatch gene	Hypermethylation	Rule out Lynch syndrome
CIMP	CpG island methylator	Hypermethylation	Improved prognosis
KRAS	Key player in the RAS/RAF/MAPK pathway	Mutation	Resistance to anti-EGFR mAB
BRAF	RAS/RAF/MAPK pathway	Mutation	Resistance to anti-EGFR mAB; confirmation of sporadic MSI-H CRC
			Poorer prognosis
NRAS	RAS/RAF/MAPK pathway	Mutation	Resistance to anti-EGFR mAB
PIK3CA	PI3K–AKT–mTOR pathway	Mutation	Resistance to anti-EGFR mAB
PTEN	Regulator of the PI3KCA/AKT pathway	Loss/mutation	Resistance to anti-EGFR mAB
TS	Thymidine generation	TSER 28 bp (2R)/(3R) tandem repeats 5′-UTR	Reduced response to 5-FU
	Thymidine generation	TSER 3R G>C SNP	Increased response to 5-FU
ERCC-1	DNA excision repair	High mRNA expression	Resistance to platinum-based therapy
18q		LOH or loss	Poorer prognosis

MSI, microsatellite instability; MSI-H, high-level MSI; CIMP, CpG island methylator phenotype; EGFR, epidermal growth factor receptor; mAB, monoclonal antibody; CRC, colorectal cancer; TS, thymidylate synthase; bp, base pairs; 2R, two tandem repeats; 3R, three tandem repeats; UTR, untranslated region; 5-FU, 5-fluorouracil; TSER, TS enhancer region; SNP, single-nucleotide polymorphism; ERCC-1, excision repair cross-complementing-1; LOH, loss of heterozygosity.

alleles in stage III MSS CRCs appears to indicate favorable outcome after 5-FU–based chemotherapy. Several studies have determined that cancers with CIN have a worse overall prognosis than do chromosomally stable tumors, and that 18q loss appears to have worse disease-free and overall survival rates. However, a recent large prospective study found no prognostic significance of 18q LOH in MSS CRC.[75] An ongoing biomarker-driven prospective clinical trial will provide clarification on the influence of 18q in determining the risk of recurrence and survival.[76] Some useful molecular biomarkers of CRC are summarized in Table 28.10.

NEXT-GENERATION SEQUENCING AND MOLECULAR DIAGNOSTICS OF CRC

The application of next-generation sequencing (NGS) has allowed cancer molecular diagnostics to move from single-gene sequencing to comprehensive genome-wide analysis.[77] Compared with traditional sequencing methods, which are analogue, NGS is digital, allowing alleles to be counted at any nucleotide in the genome.[78,79] NGS overcomes the challenges of low tumor cell percentage in the specimen, non-neoplastic tissue admixture in the tumor, heterogeneity of cancer genomes, and variable ploidy. Thus, NGS methods can provide the most comprehensive characterization of the cancer genome by detecting an array of genetic alterations in cancer cells (e.g., point and deletion mutations, nucleotide substitutions, small insertions, copy number variation, and chromosomal rearrangement). A recent study has identified *C2orf44-ALK*, a new gene fusion, in patients with CRC who may be potentially responsive to targeted therapy.[80] However, whole-genome sequencing requires the greatest resources (longer time, more cost, and complicated bioinformatics analyses).

TABLE 28-11 Targeted Next-Generation Sequencing of Colorectal Adenocarcinoma

Targeted Gene	Significance
APC (exons 1–16)	Familial adenomatous polyposis syndrome
BRAF (exons 15, 16)	Resistance to anti-EGFR monoclonal antibody treatment
	Poorer prognosis
KRAS (exons 2, 3)	Resistance to anti-EGFR monoclonal antibody treatment
MLH1 (exons 1–19)	Lynch syndrome; 5-FU therapy response
MSH2 (exons 1–16)	Lynch syndrome; 5-FU therapy response
MSH6 (exons 1–10)	Lynch syndrome; 5-FU therapy response
MUTYH (exons 1–16)	Familial adenomatous polyposis syndrome
NRAS (exons 2, 3)	Resistance to anti-EGFR monoclonal antibody treatment
PIK3CA (exons 9, 20)	Resistance to anti-EGFR monoclonal antibody treatment
PMS2 (exons 1–15)	Lynch syndrome; 5-FU therapy response
PTEN (exons 7, 8)	Resistance to anti-EGFR monoclonal antibody treatment
STK11 (exons 1–10)	Peutz-Jeghers syndrome

EGFR, epidermal growth factor receptor; 5-FU, 5-fluorouracil.

In contrast, low-cost approaches, such as targeted exome sequencing and transcriptome sequencing, have the general advantage of increased sequence coverage of regions of interest, and the mutations targeted by the panel are readily interpretable. They are also cost-efficient. For example, targeted sequencing allowed the analysis of all known coding genes, such as *KRAS*, *NRAS*, *BRAF*, *PTEN*, and *P1K3CA*, as well as *MLH1*, *MSH2*, *MSH6*, *PMS2*, *APC*, *STK11*, and *MUTHY* in CRC (Table 28.11). A dozen medical centers, including the MD Anderson Cancer Center, have launched targeted NGS in a clinical setting for cancer patient treatment. Nevertheless, the major challenges of applying NGS to cancer diagnostics will be making biological sense of the mountains of genomic data and making the test results clinically actionable. This requires integration of computational, biological, and clinical analyses of the genomic data, namely computational analyses, to assess accuracy, reproducibility, and statistical significance; biological analyses to evaluate links to cancer pathways and the functional relevance of molecular alterations to cancer; and clinical analyses to focus on the relationships of those alterations with cancer histology, prognosis, response to therapy, and cancer risk.[79]

REFERENCES

1. Cunningham D, Atkin W, Lenz HJ, et al. Colorectal cancer. *Lancet*. March 2010;375(9719):1030-1047.
2. Boland CR, Goel A. Microsatellite instability in colorectal cancer. *Gastroenterology*. June 2010;138(6):2073-2087.
3. Jass JR. Classification of colorectal cancer based on correlation of clinical, morphological and molecular features. *Histopathology*. 2001;50:113-130.
4. Hemminki K, Eng C. Clinical genetic counselling for familial cancers requires reliable data on familial cancer risks and general action plans. *J Med Genet*. November 2004;41(11):801-807.
5. Hemminki K, Chen B. Familial risk for colorectal cancers are mainly due to heritable causes. *Cancer Epidemiol Biomarkers Prev*. 2004;13(7):1253-1256.
6. Colas C, Coulet F, Svrcek M, et al. Lynch or not lynch? Is that always a question? *Adv Cancer Res*. 2012;113:121-166.
7. Ahsan H, Neugut AI, Garbowski GC, et al. Family history of colorectal adenomatous polyps and increased risk for colorectal cancer. *Ann Intern Med*. June 1998;128(11):900-905.
8. Hampel H, Frankel WL, Martin E, et al. Feasibility of screening for Lynch syndrome among patients with colorectal cancer. *J Clin Oncol*. December 2008;26(35):5783-5788. [Epub September 22, 2008].
9. Lynch HT, de la Chapelle A. Hereditary colorectal cancer. *N Engl J Med*. March 2003;348(10):919-932.
10. Walsh MD, Buchanan DD, Pearson SA, et al. Immunohistochemical testing of conventional adenomas for loss of expression of mismatch repair proteins in Lynch syndrome mutation carriers: a case series from the Australasian site of the colon cancer family registry. *Mod Pathol*. 2012;25(5):722-730.
11. Galiatsatos P, Foulkes WD. Familial adenomatous polyposis. *Am J Gastroenterol*. 2006;101:385-398.
12. Aaltonen LA, Salovaara R, Kristo P, et al. Incidence of hereditary nonpolyposis colorectal cancer and the feasibility of molecular screening for the disease. *N Engl J Med*. May 1998;338(21):1481-1487.
13. Hendriks YM, de Jong AE, Morreau H, et al. Diagnostic approach and management of Lynch syndrome (hereditary nonpolyposis colorectal carcinoma): a guide for clinicians. *CA Cancer J Clin*. July-August 2006;56(4):213-225.
14. Evaluation of Genomic Applications in Practice and Prevention (EGAPP) Working Group. Recommendations from the EGAPP Working Group: genetic testing strategies in newly diagnosed individuals with colorectal cancer aimed at reducing morbidity and mortality from Lynch syndrome in relatives. *Genet Med*. January 2009;11(1):35-41.
15. Kastrinos F, Mukherjee B, Tayob N, et al. Risk of pancreatic cancer in families with Lynch syndrome. *JAMA*. 2009;302(16):1790–1795.
16. Jenkins MA, Hayashi S, O'Shea AM, et al. Pathology features in Bethesda guidelines predict colorectal cancer microsatellite instability: a population-based study. *Gastroenterology*. 2007;133(1):48-56.
17. Rodriguez-Bigas MA, Boland CR, Hamilton SR, et al. A National Cancer Institute Workshop on hereditary nonpolyposis colorectal cancer syndrome: meeting highlights and Bethesda guidelines. *J Natl Cancer Inst*. 1997;89(23):1758-1762.
18. Umar A, Boland CR, Terdiman JP, et al. Revised Bethesda guidelines for hereditary nonpolyposis colorectal cancer (Lynch syndrome) and microsatellite instability. *J Natl Cancer Inst*. 2004;96(4):261-268.
19. Pinol V, Castells A, Andreu M, et al. Accuracy of revised Bethesda guidelines, microsatellite instability, and immunohistochemistry for the identification of patients with hereditary nonpolyposis colorectal cancer. *JAMA*. 2005;293(16):1986-1994.
20. Hampel H, Frankel WL, Martin E, et al. Screening for the Lynch syndrome (hereditary nonpolyposis colorectal cancer). *N Engl J Med*. 2005;352(18):1851-1860.
21. Wu Y, Berends MJ, Sijmons RH, et al. A role for *MLH3* in hereditary nonpolyposis colorectal cancer. *Nat Genet*. 2001;29(2):137-138.
22. Domingo E, Laiho P, Ollikainen M, et al. *BRAF* screening as a low-cost effective strategy for simplifying HNPCC genetic testing. *J Med Genet*. 2004;41(9):664-668.
23. Shia J, Tang LH, Vakiani E, et al. Immunohistochemistry as first-line screening for detecting colorectal cancer patients at risk for hereditary nonpolyposis colorectal cancer syndrome: a 2-antibody panel may be as predictive as a 4-antibody panel. *Am J Surg Pathol*. 2009;33(11):1639-1645.
24. Shia J. Immunohistochemistry versus microsatellite instability testing for screening colorectal cancer patients at risk for hereditary nonpolyposis colorectal cancer syndrome, part I: the utility of immunohistochemistry. *J Mol Diagn*. 2008;10(4):293-300.
25. Suraweera N, Duval A, Reperant M, et al. Evaluation of tumor microsatellite instability using five quasimonomorphic mononucleotide repeats and pentaplex PCR. *Gastroenterology*. 2002;123(6):1804-1811.
26. Zhang L. Immunohistochemistry versus microsatellite instability testing for screening colorectal cancer patients at risk for hereditary nonpolyposis colorectal cancer syndrome, part II: the utility of microsatellite instability testing. *J Mol Diagn*. 2008;10(4):301-307.
27. Capel E, Flejou JF, Hamelin R. Assessment of *MLH1* promoter methylation in relation to gene expression requires specific analysis. *Oncogene*. 2007;26(54):7596-7600.
28. Chubak B, Heald B, Sharp RR. Informed consent to microsatellite instability and immunohistochemistry screening for Lynch syndrome. *Genet Med*. 2011;13(4):356-360.
29. Ribic CM, Sargent DJ, Moore MJ, et al. Tumor microsatellite-instability status as a predictor of benefit from fluorouracil-based adjuvant chemotherapy for colon cancer. *N Engl J Med*. 2003;349(3):247-257.
30. NCCN Colon Cancer Panel Members. *Colorectal Cancer Screening*. Fort Washington, PA: National Comprehensive Care Network Inc; 2010. *NCCN Clinical Practice Guidelines in Oncology*; version 2.2011.
31. Sargent DJ, Marsoni S, Monges G, et al. Defective mismatch repair as a predictive marker for lack of efficacy of fluorouracil-based adjuvant therapy in colon cancer. *J Clin Oncol*. July 2010;28(20):3219-3226.
32. Roth AD, Tejpar S, Delorenzi M, et al. Prognostic role of KRAS and BRAF in stage II and III resected colon cancer: results of the translational study on the PETACC-3, EORTC 40993, SAKK 60-00 trial. *J Clin Oncol*. January 2010;28(3):466-474.
33. Koopman M, Kortman GA, Mekenkamp L, et al. Deficient mismatch repair system in patients with sporadic advanced colorectal cancer. *Br J Cancer*. January 2009;100(2):266-273.
34. Hutchins G, Southward K, Handley K, et al. Value of mismatch repair, KRAS, and BRAF mutations in predicting recurrence and

benefits from chemotherapy in colorectal cancer. *J Clin Oncol.* April 2011;29(10):1261-1270.
35. Ng K, Schrag D. Microsatellite instability and adjuvant fluorouracil chemotherapy: a mismatch? *J Clin Oncol.* July 2010;28(20):3207-3210.
36. Amado RG, Wolf M, Peeters M, et al. Wild-type KRAS is required for panitumumab efficacy in patients with metastatic colorectal cancer. *J Clin Oncol.* April 2008;26(10):1626-1634.
37. Van Cutsem E, Köhne CH, Hitre E, et al. Cetuximab and chemotherapy as initial treatment for metastatic colorectal cancer. *N Engl J Med.* April 2009;360(14):1408-1417.
38. Van Cutsem E, Köhne CH, Láng I, et al. Cetuximab plus irinotecan, fluorouracil, and leucovorin as first-line treatment for metastatic colorectal cancer: updated analysis of overall survival according to tumor KRAS and BRAF mutation status. *J Clin Oncol.* May 2011;29(15):2011-2019.
39. Douillard JY, Siena S, Cassidy J, et al. Randomized, phase III trial of panitumumab with infusional fluorouracil, leucovorin, and oxaliplatin (FOLFOX4) versus FOLFOX4 alone as first-line treatment in patients with previously untreated metastatic colorectal cancer: the PRIME study. *J Clin Oncol.* November 2010;28(31):4697-4705.
40. Bokemeyer C, Bondarenko I, Makhson A, et al. Fluorouracil, leucovorin, and oxaliplatin with and without cetuximab in the first-line treatment of metastatic colorectal cancer. *J Clin Oncol.* February 2009;27(5):663-671.
41. Baselga J, Rosen N. Determinants of RASistance to anti-epidermal growth factor receptor agents. *J Clin Oncol.* April 2008;26(10):1582-1584.
42. De Roock W, Piessevaux H, De Schutter J, et al. KRAS wild-type state predicts survival and is associated to early radiological response in metastatic colorectal cancer treated with cetuximab. *Ann Oncol.* March 2008;19(3):508-515.
43. Karapetis CS, Khambata-Ford S, Jonker DJ, et al. K-ras mutations and benefit from cetuximab in advanced colorectal cancer. *N Engl J Med.* October 2008;359(17):1757-1765.
44. Khambata-Ford S, Garrett CR, Meropol NJ, et al. Expression of epiregulin and amphiregulin and K-ras mutation status predict disease control in metastatic colorectal cancer patients treated with cetuximab. *J Clin Oncol.* August 2007;25(22):3230-3237.
45. Lièvre A, Bachet JB, Boige V, et al. KRAS mutations as an independent prognostic factor in patients with advanced colorectal cancer treated with cetuximab. *J Clin Oncol.* January 2008;26(3):374-379.
46. Dahabreh IJ, Terasawa T, Castaldi PJ, Trikalinos TA. Systematic review: anti-epidermal growth factor receptor treatment effect modification by KRAS mutations in advanced colorectal cancer. *Ann Intern Med.* January 2011;154(1):37-49.
47. Package Insert. *Cetuximab (Erbitux).* Branchburg, NJ: IMClone Systems Incorporated; 2009.
48. Package Insert. *Vectibix (Panitumumab).* Thousand Oaks, CA: Amgen Inc.; 2009.
49. Artale S, Sartore-Bianchi A, Veronese SM, et al. Mutations of KRAS and BRAF in primary and matched metastatic sites of colorectal cancer. *J Clin Oncol.* September 2008;26(25):4217-4219.
50. Etienne-Grimaldi MC, Formento JL, Francoual M, et al. K-Ras mutations and treatment outcome in colorectal cancer patients receiving exclusive fluoropyrimidine therapy. *Clin Cancer Res.* August 2008;14(15):4830-4835.
51. Knijn N, Mekenkamp LJ, Klomp M, et al. KRAS mutation analysis: a comparison between primary tumours and matched liver metastases in 305 colorectal cancer patients. *Br J Cancer.* March 2011;104(6):1020-1026.
52. Wang HL, Lopategui J, Amin MB, Patterson SD. KRAS mutation testing in human cancers: the pathologist's role in the era of personalized medicine. *Adv Anat Pathol.* January 2010;17(1):23-32.
53. Monzon FA, Ogino S, Hammond ME, Halling KC, Bloom KJ, Nikiforova MN. The role of KRAS mutation testing in the management of patients with metastatic colorectal cancer. *Arch Pathol Lab Med.* October 2009;133(10):1600-1606.
54. De Roock W, Claes B, Bernasconi D, et al. Effects of KRAS, BRAF, NRAS, and PIK3CA mutations on the efficacy of cetuximab plus chemotherapy in chemotherapy-refractory metastatic colorectal cancer: a retrospective consortium analysis. *Lancet Oncol.* August 2010;11(8):753-762.
55. Tol J, Nagtegaal ID, Punt CJ. BRAF mutation in metastatic colorectal cancer. *N Engl J Med.* July 2009;361(1):98-99.
56. Davies H, Bignell GR, Cox C, et al. Mutations of the BRAF gene in human cancer. *Nature.* June 2002;417(6892):949-954.
57. Wan PT, Garnett MJ, Roe SM, et al. Cancer Genome Project. Mechanism of activation of the RAF-ERK signaling pathway by oncogenic mutations of B-RAF. *Cell.* March 2004;116(6):855-867.
58. Tian S, Simon I, Moreno V, et al. A combined oncogenic pathway signature of BRAF, KRAS and PI3KCA mutation improves colorectal cancer classification and cetuximab treatment prediction. *Gut.* 2012 Jul 14. [Epub ahead of print]
59. Di Nicolantonio F, Martini M, Molinari F, et al. Wild-type BRAF is required for response to panitumumab or cetuximab in metastatic colorectal cancer. *J Clin Oncol.* December 2008;26(35):5705-5712.
60. Laurent-Puig P, Cayre A, Manceau G, et al. Analysis of PTEN, BRAF, and EGFR status in determining benefit from cetuximab therapy in wild-type KRAS metastatic colon cancer. *J Clin Oncol.* December 2009;27(35):5924-5930.
61. Santini D, Spoto C, Loupakis F, et al. High concordance of BRAF status between primary colorectal tumours and related metastatic sites: implications for clinical practice. *Ann Oncol.* July 2010;21(7):1565.
62. Qing H, Gong W, Che Y, et al. PAK1-dependent MAPK pathway activation is required for colorectal cancer cell proliferation. *Tumour Biol.* January 2012. [Epub ahead of print].
63. Sood A, McClain D, Maitra R, et al. PTEN gene expression and mutations in the PIK3CA gene as predictors of clinical benefit to anti-epidermal growth factor receptor antibody therapy in patients with KRAS wild-type metastatic colorectal cancer. *Clin Colorectal Cancer.* January 2012. [Epub ahead of print].
64. Ogino S, Katsuhiko N, Gregory J, et al. *PIK3CA* mutation is associated with poor prognosis among patients with curatively resected colon cancer. *J Clin Oncol.* 2009;27:1477-1484.
65. Barault L, Veyrie N, Jooste V, et al. Mutations in the RAS-MAPK, PI3K (phosphatidylinositol-3-OH kinase) signaling network correlate with poor survival in a population-based series of colon cancers. *Int J Cancer.* 2008;122:2255-2259.
66. Sartore-Bianchi A, Martini M, Molinari F, et al. PIK3CA mutations in colorectal cancer are associated with clinical resistance to EGFR-targeted monoclonal antibodies. *Cancer Res.* 2009;69:1851-1857.
67. Prenen H, De Schutter J, Jacobs B, et al. *PIK3CA* mutations are not a major determinant of resistance to the epidermal growth factor receptor inhibitor cetuximab in metastatic colorectal cancer. *Clin Cancer Res.* 2009;15:3184-3188.
68. Moroni M, Veronese S, Benvenuti S, et al. Gene copy number for epidermal growth factor receptor (EGFR) and clinical response to anti-EGFR treatment in colorectal cancer: a cohort study. *Lancet Oncol.* 2005;6:279-286.
69. Personeni N, Fieuws S, Piessevaux H, et al. Clinical usefulness of *EGFR* gene copy number as a predictive marker in colorectal cancer patients treated with cetuximab: a fluorescent in situ hybridization study. *Clin Cancer Res.* 2008;14:5869-5876.
70. Hecht JR, Mitchell E, Neubauer MA, et al. Lack of correlation between epidermal growth factor receptor status and response to panitumumab monotherapy in metastatic colorectal cancer. *Clin Cancer Res.* April 2010;16(7):2205-2213.
71. Ghosh S, Hossain MZ, Borges M, et al. Analysis of polymorphisms and haplotype structure of the human thymidylate synthase genetic region: a tool for pharmacogenetic studies. *PLoS One.* 2012;7(3):e34426.
72. Hwang HY. A practical approach for assessing chemosensitivity in colorectal cancer cell lines by comparative analysis of cell viability and thymidylate synthase mRNA expression. *J Korean Surg Soc.* January 2012;82(1):28-34.
73. Fariña Sarasqueta A, van Lijnschoten G, Lemmens VE, et al. Pharmacogenetics of oxaliplatin as adjuvant treatment in colon carcinoma: are single nucleotide polymorphisms in GSTP1, ERCC1, and ERCC2 good predictive markers? *Mol Diagn Ther.* October 2011;15(5):277-283.
74. Yin M, Yan J, Martinez-Balibrea E, et al. ERCC1 and ERCC2 polymorphisms predict clinical outcomes of oxaliplatin-based chemotherapies in gastric and colorectal cancer: a systemic review and meta-analysis. *Clin Cancer Res.* March 2011;17(6):1632-1640.

75. Melcher R, Hartmann E, Zopf W, et al. LOH and copy neutral LOH (cnLOH) act as alternative mechanism in sporadic colorectal cancers with chromosomal and microsatellite instability. *Carcinogenesis*. April 2011;32(4):636-642.
76. Watanabe T, Kobunai T, Yamamoto Y, et al. Chromosomal instability (CIN) phenotype, CIN high or CIN low, predicts survival for colorectal cancer. *J Clin Oncol*. April 2012. [Epub ahead of print].
77. Metzker ML. Sequencing technologies—the next generation. *Nat Rev Genet*. 2010;1:31-46.
78. Gerlinger M, Rowan AJ, Horswell S, et al. Intratumor heterogeneity and branched evolution revealed by multiregion sequencing. *N Engl J Med*. 2012;366(10):883-892.
79. Meyerson M, Gabriel S, Getz G. Advances in understanding cancer genomes through second-generation sequencing. *Nat Rev Genet*. 2010;11:685-696.
80. Lipson D, Capelletti M, Yelensky R, et al. Identification of new ALK and RET gene fusions from colorectal and lung cancer biopsies. *Nat Med*. 2012;18(3):382-384.

CHAPTER 29

Molecular Diagnostics of Esophageal and Gastric Cancers

Wataru Yasui, Naohide Oue, Kazuhiro Sentani, and Dongfeng Tan

INTRODUCTION

Gastric cancer is the fourth most common cancer worldwide, and mortality from gastric cancer is second only to that of lung cancer.[1] The areas with the highest rates of gastric cancer are in Eastern Asia, South America, and Eastern Europe. Of note, approximately 60% of all gastric cancers occur in Japan, China, and Korea. The incidence of gastric cancer is declining worldwide, mainly due to changes in eating habits such as decreased consumption of high-salt diets and availability of fresh fruits and vegetables throughout the year. One of the most important etiologic factors is *Helicobacter pylori* (HP) infection. Infection with HP causes chronic atrophic gastritis and intestinal metaplasia, conditions that are considered as predisposing to cancer development. In Japan and to some degree in Korea, screening for early disease by double-contrast barium X-ray followed by endoscopy has been widely performed. Advances in endoscopic diagnosis and treatment have enabled us to offer excellent long-term survival for patients with early cancer. However, in other parts of the world, the majority of gastric cancers are diagnosed as advanced disease after symptoms appear, and prognosis of advanced cancer remains poor.

Esophageal cancer is the sixth most common human malignant disease worldwide, with more than 400,000 new cases per year.[2] Two major types, squamous cell carcinoma (SCC) and adenocarcinoma, account for over 95% of esophageal cancers. SCC commonly occurs in developing countries and is typically associated with consumption of tobacco and alcohol. Adenocarcinoma typically occurs in white men in developed countries, and the important etiologic factors are obesity, chronic gastro-esophageal reflux, and Barrett esophagus. Although endoscopic screening is useful for early cancer detection, 50% of superficial esophageal cancers (those confined to the submucosa) have nodal metastasis. Most esophageal cancers are diagnosed at an advanced stage, and prognosis after surgical resection with neoadjuvant chemoradiotherapy remains unsatisfactory; the 5-year survival rate is <50% after curative surgery.

Cancer is a chronic proliferative disease that develops and progresses by accumulation of multiple genetic and epigenetic alterations. Great efforts have been made to clarify the precise molecular mechanisms of esophageal and gastric carcinogeneses. Multiple alterations include abnormalities in tumor suppressor genes, oncogenes, growth factors and receptors, DNA mismatch repair genes, cell adhesion molecules, and matrix metalloproteinases.[3-6] In recent years, the role of microRNA (miRNA) in epigenetic regulation and biologic function in cancers has been extensively studied.[7] Better knowledge of molecular carcinogenesis will lead to new methods of diagnosis and treatment. At present, although molecular-targeted therapy has been introduced widely against a variety of cancers, for esophago-gastric and gastric cancers only trastuzumab against HER2 has been approved for clinical use in advanced cases. Molecular diagnosis still remains challenging in the practical setting. This chapter describes molecular diagnosis of gastric and esophageal cancers and possible clinical implications (Table 29.1).

TABLE 29–1 Molecular Diagnosis of Esophageal and Gastric Cancers and Its Clinical Implication

Diagnosis	Method	Implication
DNA methylation–targeted diagnosis	Methylation-specific PCR and bisulfite sequencing	Detection, aggressiveness, prognosis, and serum marker
Molecular target	IHC and FISH/DISH	Target detection and patient selection
Micrometastasis	RT-PCR and OSNA	Detection of cancer cells and CTC
miRNA-based diagnosis	RT-PCR and microarray	Detection, aggressiveness, prognosis, and serum marker
Genetic polymorphism	Sequencing and RFLP	Cancer risk, efficacy, and toxicity of chemotherapy

IHC, immunohistochemistry, FISH, fluorescence in situ hybridization; DISH, dual-color silver-enhanced in situ hybridization; CTC, circulating tumor cell; OSNA, one-step nucleic acid amplification; RFLP, restriction fragment length polymorphism; PCR, polymerase chain reaction; RT-PCR, reverse transcription–polymerase chain reaction.

MOLECULAR DIAGNOSIS OF GASTRIC CANCER

Molecular Pathologic Diagnosis Routinely Implemented

From 1993 to 2000, a project was implemented to perform molecular diagnosis using histopathologic samples from the gastrointestinal tract as a routine service.[8,9] This system of molecular diagnosis was designed mainly for the differential diagnosis of benign and malignant tumors, diagnosis of the degree of malignancy, and identification of susceptibility to multiple primary cancers (Fig. 29.1). Molecular examination was performed on about 5,000 gastric lesions, and much useful information in addition to histopathologic findings was obtained. During routine microscopic observation, pathologists observed cancer, adenoma/dysplasia, borderline lesions, and suspicious lesions of neoplasia. The sections were immunostained for molecular markers (including p53, TGF-α, EGF, EGFR, c-met, c-erbB2/HER2, cyclin E, p27, and CD44) for differential diagnosis and/or evaluation of degree of malignancy. With polymerase chain reaction (PCR)–single-strand conformation polymorphism and PCR–restriction fragment length polymorphism, deletion and mutation of *APC* and *p53* genes were examined by the pathologist using portions of formalin-fixed, paraffin-embedded, hematoxylin and eosin–stained sections. For detection of genetic instability, human mutL homolog 1 (hMLH1) staining was used for screening, and genetic instability was assessed by microsatellite assay using four loci of CA repeats and two poly(A) tracts. Ten percent of histologically diagnosed adenomas were diagnosed as adenoma with malignant potential and 2% were considered suspicious for adenocarcinoma. Adenocarcinoma was identified in more than 20% of histologically diagnosed borderline lesions. Twelve percent of adenocarcinomas were regarded as showing high-grade malignancy, and their prognosis

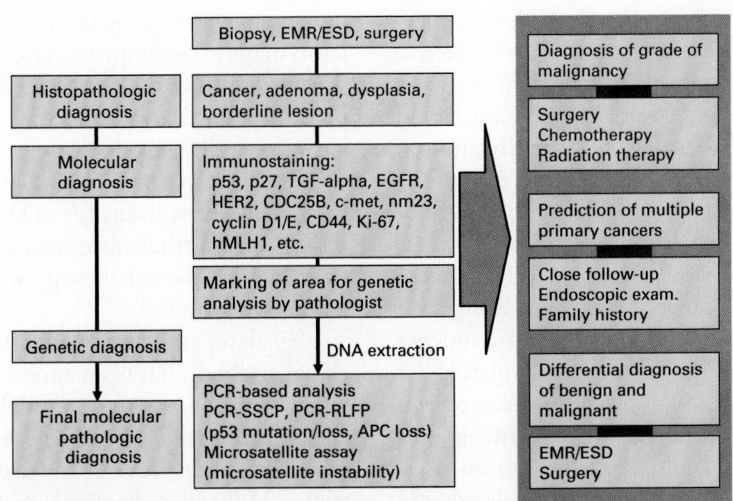

FIGURE 29–1 Proposed workflow of molecular evaluation of esophageal and gastric cancers. EMR (endoscopic mucosal resection), ESD (endoscopic submucosal dissection), PCR (polymerase chain reaction), SSCP (single strand conformation polymorphism), RFLP (restriction fragment length polymorphism), APC (adenomatous polyposis coli)

tended to be poor on follow-up observation. About 4% of gastric cancers were judged to have high-frequency microsatellite instability (MSI-H) by microsatellite assay, and half of the patients showing MSI-H were confirmed to have clinically synchronous or asynchronous multiple primary cancers. Detailed methods and results were described elsewhere.[8,9] This system may be applicable to molecular diagnosis in the future if appropriate molecular and genetic markers are selected.

DNA Methylation–Targeted Molecular Diagnosis

DNA methylation is the most important event among various epigenetic alterations in cancers. To regulate gene expression at the transcriptional level, DNA methylation, histone modification, and chromatin remodeling function as an on–off switch, while transcription factors act as a volume switch.[10] Hypermethylation of CpG islands is associated with gene silencing of many tumor suppressors, including hMLH1, p16, CDH1 (E-cadherin), RAR-β, RUNX3, and O^6-methylguanine-DNA methyltransferase (MGMT) in gastric cancer. Aberrant DNA methylation is readily detected in cancer-derived DNA in the serum of patients with gastric cancer. Many reports have indicated that aberrant DNA methylation is a useful diagnostic marker and a prognostic indicator.[11-14] DNA methylation of p16 and of CDH1 was detected in the serum of 20% to 50% of gastric cancer patients, whereas none of the controls without cancer showed aberrant methylation.[11-14] Some of the DNA methylation is associated with tumor stage and prognosis. For instance, gastric cancer patients with CDH1 methylation showed significantly poorer prognosis than those without aberrant methylation[15] RUNX3 methylation was detected in the peripheral circulation of 30% of gastric cancer patients and was concordant with tumor stage and lymphatic and vascular invasion.[16] After surgical removal of gastric cancer, RUNX3 methylation in serum decreases significantly. Detection of aberrant DNA methylation in serum is a useful and effective tool in cancer screening, monitoring, and prognosis.

Infection with HP, a potent gastric carcinogenic factor, has been shown to induce aberrant DNA methylation in gastric mucosa and produce a predisposed field of cancerization.[17] Methylation levels of p16, LOX, FLNc, HRASLS, HAND1, THBD, and p41ARC in gastric mucosa are higher in HP-positive individuals than in HP-negative persons among healthy volunteers.[18] Among HP-negative individuals, methylation levels in non-neoplastic mucosa are higher in gastric cancer cases than in controls.[19,20] Furthermore, significant increasing levels of methylation are present in the following order: healthy volunteers, single gastric cancer cases, and multiple gastric cancer cases. Among HP-positive individuals, methylation levels are highly variable. The evidence indicates that the measurement of methylation levels among individuals without current HP infection is a promising risk marker for gastric cancer and can be used in molecular diagnosis to predict future risk of gastric cancer.

Endoscopy followed by pathologic examination has been proven to be useful for the detection and diagnosis of gastric cancer; however, the diagnostic power depends on the technical skill of the endoscopist, although the sensitivity and specificity are generally high. Detection of molecular markers in stomach juice or gastric washes is a possible non-invasive approach to screen for gastric cancer. There is evidence that methylation analysis of DNA recovered from gastric washes can be used to detect gastric cancer.[21] The methylation status of six genes (*MINT25*, *RORA*, *GDNF*, *ADAM23*, *PRDM5*, and *MLF1*) in gastric washes differs significantly between patients with gastric cancer and those without. *GDNF* and *MINT25* are the most sensitive molecular markers of early cancer, while *PRDM5* and *MLF1* are potential markers of epigenetic field defects. There is a close association between the methylation levels in tissue samples and gastric washes. *MINT25* methylation in gastric washes shows the best sensitivity (90%) and specificity (96%) and may have value as a powerful molecular tool for screening of gastric cancer. Genomic variations of HP can be analyzed in samples recovered from gastric washes.[22] Antibiotic-resistant HP is correlated with 23S rRNA single-nucleotide polymorphisms (SNPs). Gastric wash–based PCR and pyrosequencing are useful for detecting SNPs and diagnosing drug resistance.

Molecular Diagnosis for Molecular-Targeted Therapy

Molecular-targeted therapy refers to drugs (inhibitor or monoclonal antibody) that selectively inhibit specific molecular pathways that are involved in the development, progression, and metastasis of cancers. A number of biologic agents modulating different signaling pathways are currently in clinical development, such as agents targeting angiogenesis, growth factor receptor, cell cycle regulator, matrix metalloproteinase, and mammalian target of rapamycin (mTOR).[23-25] Several randomized multicenter phase III studies are underway in molecularly unselected patients with gastric cancer, considering cetuximab for EGFR, lapatinib for EGFR/HER2, panitumumab for EGFR, everolimus for mTOR, and ramucirumab for VEGFR-2. Furthermore, a stromal cell–targeted strategy, such as anti-stromal therapy with imatinib for PDGFR, has been advocated.[26]

To date, only trastuzumab, an anti-HER2 monoclonal antibody, has been approved for use in combination with chemotherapy to treat HER2-positive advanced gastric and esophago-gastric junction cancers, on the basis of the results of the ToGA (Trastuzumab for Gastric Cancer) trial.[27] Molecular diagnosis of HER2 status is made by immunohistochemistry (IHC) and fluorescence in situ hybridization (FISH) or dual-color silver-enhanced in situ hybridization (DISH). DISH is an alternative to FISH

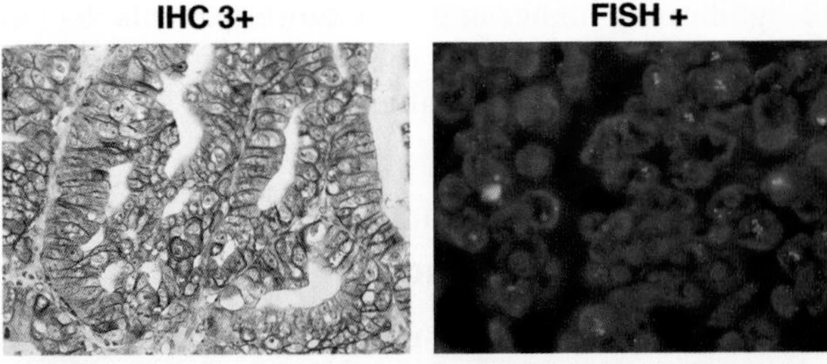

FIGURE 29–2 Evaluation of HER2 in gastro-esophageal junctional and gastric adenocarcinoma. **A:** Immunohistochemistry reveals diffuse and strong membranous expression of HER2 protein in a gastric cancer. **B:** Fluorescence in situ hybridization confirms amplification of the *HER2* gene (*red signal*), indicating this patient may benefit from targeted therapy of Herceptin.

with the same accuracy (concordance rate is 97%), and signals can be observed under conventional light microscopy.[28] Tumors showing as IHC 3+ (strong membrane staining in over 10% of cancer cells) and FISH/DISH positive (HER2:CEP17 ratio>2) are regarded as HER2 positive (Fig. 29.2) and subjected to trastuzumab therapy. Because HER2 status in gastric cancer shows marked heterogeneity, it is recommended that the order of testing for HER2 is IHC followed by FISH/DISH. IHC 2+ (moderate membrane staining in >10% of cancer cells) is judged as borderline or equivocal, and subsequent HER2 amplification should be confirmed by FISH/DISH. Total HER2-positive rate is 12% to 18%, with 20% to 30% as the differentiated type and 3% to 6% as the undifferentiated type. However, evaluation of HER2 status by this method may not be definitive for patient selection, because not all HER2-positive patients respond to trastuzumab treatment.

Molecular Diagnosis of Micrometastasis and Circulating Tumor Cells

Lymph node metastasis is an important determinant of patient outcome. Routine pathologic examination of representative sections of the cut surface may overlook micrometastasis. Molecular detection of mRNAs for cytokeratin (CK) 19 and CEA by RT-PCR is useful for detecting micrometastasis. In recent years, the sentinel lymph node concept has been validated for gastrointestinal cancer in addition to breast cancer.[29] The sentinel node is defined as the first node to receive lymphatic drainage from the primary tumor. According to this concept, lymph node dissection can be avoided if no metastases are detected in the sentinel node. Therefore, examination for micrometastasis in the sentinel node must be made intraoperatively during sentinel node navigation surgery. The real-time multiplex RT-PCR assay for the expression of CK19, CK20, and CEA is more sensitive and accurate than histopathologic diagnosis and generates results within 80 minutes intraoperatively.[30] A more rapid molecular diagnosis system has been developed using one-step nucleic acid amplification (OSNA).[31,32] The OSNA system consists of homogenization of lymph node tissue followed by a reverse transcription loop–mediated isothermal amplification (RT-LAMP) and the quantification of a target mRNA, CK19, directly from the lysate. RT-LAMP measurement of CK19 mRNA is performed using an RD-100i gene amplification detector (Sysmex, Kobe, Japan). The whole procedure takes approximately 30 minutes to obtain a final result. The OSNA system is effective and efficient for intraoperative molecular diagnosis during sentinel node navigation surgery in gastric cancer.

Circulating tumor cells (CTCs) are considered a reflection of tumor aggressiveness because hematogenous spreading of CTCs from a primary tumor is a crucial step in the metastatic cascade leading to the formation of metastatic tumor.[33] Molecular methods can detect CTCs in blood with high sensitivity and specificity and can be a useful tool for judging tumor stage, predicting distant metastasis and patient survival, and monitoring the response to cancer therapy.[34] Although clinical relevance remains to be verified in large-scale clinical trials, many detection methods have been established including the above-mentioned RT-PCR–based method.[33] The detection of free cancer cells in the peritoneal cavity has important therapeutic and prognostic implications. The RT-PCR–based technique with the same markers as CTCs, such as CK19 and CEA, is useful for detecting free cancer cells in peritoneal lavage fluid.[35] The clinical significance of establishing the presence of peritoneal metastasis has been assessed by several studies and most have confirmed the predictive value of molecular detection of peritoneal metastasis and recurrence using peritoneal washes.[35]

miRNA-based Molecular Diagnosis

The role of miRNA in cancer development and progression through epigenetic gene regulation has become a recent focus in cancer research.[6,7] Mature RNAs are composed of 19–25 nucleotides that are cleaved from 60- to 110-nucleotide pre-miRNA precursors by RNase III Dicer.[36] Single-stranded miRNAs bind through partial sequence homology to the 3′-untranslated region of potentially hundreds of target genes and cause degradation of mRNAs and inhibition of translation. miRNAs possess either anti-tumorigenic or oncogenic properties depending on the target genes.[37] In gastric cancer, many miRNAs are expressed differentially, and unique miRNAs are associated with the development, progression, and prognosis of gastric cancer by modulating several biologic pathways.[38] By miRNA microarray analysis, 22 miRNAs were upregulated and 13 were downregulated in gastric cancer in comparison with corresponding non-neoplastic gastric tissue.[39] miR-125b, miR-199a, and miR-433 are important miRNAs involved in cancer progression, while low expressions of let-7g and miR-433 and high expression of miR-214 are independent unfavorable prognostic markers. miR-146a targeting EGFR and interleukin-1 receptor–associated kinase (IRAK1) is an independent prognostic factor in gastric cancer.[40] miR-148a functions as a tumor metastasis suppressor in gastric cancer, and downregulation of miR-148a contributes to lymph node metastasis and progression.[41] Furthermore, miR-335 also acts as a metastasis suppressor in gastric cancer by targeting Bcl-w and specificity protein 1 (SP-1).[42] The metastasis-associated miR-516a-3p appears to be a potential therapeutic target for inhibiting peritoneal dissemination of scirrhous-type gastric cancer.[43] miR-486 targets olfactomedin 4 (OLFM4), and genomic loss and downregulation of miR-486 are associated with gastric cancer progression.[44] Downregulation of miR-125a-5p targeting HER2 is associated with invasion, metastasis, and poor prognosis of gastric cancer, and its growth inhibitory effect is enhanced in combination with trastuzumab.[45] Therefore, these miRNAs as tumor biomarkers are potential targets for molecular diagnosis in gastric cancer.

As in protein-coding genes, miRNA genes are also transcriptionally regulated by DNA methylation and chromatin remodeling. DNA methylation of *miR-34b* and *miR-129* genes causes downregulation in gastric cancer and is associated with poor clinicopathologic features.[46] In stomach carcinogenesis, a mucosal field with HP infection is a condition predisposing to cancer development. Methylation levels of three miRNA genes (*miR-124a-1*, *miR-124a-2*, and *miR-124a-3*) are higher in gastric mucosa with HP infection than in gastric mucosa without HP infection, and the methylation levels are higher in non-cancerous gastric mucosa taken from gastric cancer patients than in those from healthy individuals.[47] Methylation-associated silencing of miR-34b and miR-34c is detected in a majority of gastric cancers, and the methylation levels are higher in gastric mucosa from patients with multiple gastric cancers than in mucosa from patients with single gastric cancer or mucosa from HP-positive healthy individuals.[48] Thus, methylation-associated silencing of miRNAs contributes to the formation of field defects and may serve as a predictive marker of gastric cancer risk.

miRNAs are stable in human circulation in a cell-free form and may be a powerful new class of blood-based biomarkers for gastric cancer.[49] Stability of extracellular miRNAs is believed to be due to vesicular encapsulation in exosomes and/or binding with argonaute 2 (Ago2) to make Ago2–miRNA complexes.[49] By genome-wide serum miRNA expression profiling, five miRNA signatures (miR-1, miR-20a, miR-27a, miR-34a, and miR-423-5p) for gastric cancer diagnosis have been identified.[50] The levels of the five miRNAs in serum assessed by quantitative RT-PCR are correlated with tumor stage, and the sensitivity and specificity of gastric cancer detection by the five miRNAs as biomarkers are 80% and 81%, respectively. The plasma concentrations of miRNAs (miR-17-5p, miR-21, miR-106a, and miR-106b) are significantly higher in gastric cancer patients than in non-cancerous controls, and the plasma concentrations of these miRNAs are reduced after surgery.[51]

Diagnosis of Gastric Cancer Risk and Chemotherapeutic Efficacy

Stomach carcinogenesis is modulated by such genetic polymorphisms as mucosal protection by HP infection inflammatory response, carcinogen detoxification and antioxidant protection, DNA damage repair, and cell proliferation. Therefore, genetic polymorphisms are increasingly used for molecular assessment of gastric cancer risk.[6,52,53] Variations of IL-1β (*IL1B*) and IL-1 receptor antagonist (*IL1RN*) genes affect IL-1β production and gastric acid secretion, causing an increased risk of chronic hypochlorhydric response to HP infection and gastric cancer risk.[54] Upon HP infection, CagA in gastric epithelial cells interacts with src homology 2 domain–containing protein tyrosine phosphatase (SHP-2) and transduces signal to downstream molecules participating in atrophic gastritis and stomach carcinogenesis.[55] Frequent G/A SNP in the intron 3 of the *PTPN11* gene encoding SHP-2 is associated with gastric atrophy in the Asian population.[53] Genetic polymorphisms significantly associated with gastric cancer risk include cyclin D1, CDH1, EGFR, $p16^{INK4A}$, $p21^{WAF1/CIP1}$, and HER2.[53] A genome-wide study using Japanese and Korean cohorts found that genetic variation in prostate stem cell antigen (PSCA) is associated with susceptibility to diffuse-type gastric cancer.[56] Furthermore, the same group recently found that *MUC1* is the second major susceptibility gene for diffuse-type gastric cancer, and the SNPs (rs2070803 and rs4072037) in the *MUC1* gene might be used to identify individuals at risk for this type of gastric cancer.[57]

Genetic polymorphisms are also associated with therapeutic efficacy and toxicity of anti-cancer drugs. Pharmacogenomics in gastric cancer has provided a number of putative biomarkers and genetic polymorphisms for the prediction of tumor response to chemotherapies and for prediction of toxicity, and these are summarized in the review by Nishiyama and Eguchi.[58] Polymorphisms of thymidylate synthetase (TYMS) and variation of glutathione-*S*-transferase pi 1 (GSTP1) are associated with responses to the 5-FU–based regimen and platinum-containing therapy, respectively, in gastric cancer. Nucleotide excision repair modulates platinum-based chemotherapeutic efficacy by removing drug-produced DNA damage. Polymorphisms of excision repair cross-complementing 1 (ERCC1) (rs11615C > T) and ERCC2 (rs13181T > G) predict clinical outcomes of oxaliplatin-based chemotherapy in gastric cancer and are useful prognostic factors.[59] In regard to chemotherapeutic toxicity, among the various polymorphisms in the dihydropyrimidine dehydrogenase (*DPYD*) gene, exon 14-skipping mutation (DPYD*2A) is a prominent genotype marker related to deficiency of enzyme activity resulting in severe toxicity caused by 5-FU–based therapy. Another important consideration regarding drug toxicity is the polymorphism of UDP-glucuronosyltransferase 1A1 (*UGT1A1*) gene (UGT1A1*28), which reduces enzyme activity and results in irinotecan toxicity, especially neutropenia. Molecular examination of such genetic polymorphisms is directly connected to personalized cancer prevention and treatment.

Novel Molecular Markers Identified through Transcriptome Dissection

Many molecules and genes have been identified as novel diagnostic and therapeutic targets in patients with gastric cancer through transcriptome dissection by using microarray and other techniques. Serial analysis of gene expression (SAGE) is a powerful tool for the global analysis of gene expression in a quantitative manner.[60,61] A comparison of SAGE data between gastric cancers and systemic normal tissues in combination with quantitative RT-PCR, IHC, and biologic studies has identified many genes, including regenerating islet–derived family, member 4 (*Reg IV*) and *OLFM4*, as candidate diagnostic markers and therapeutic targets.[62,63] *Reg IV* is expressed in about 30% of gastric cancers, and Reg IV protein is detectable in sera of about 30% of gastric cancer patients.[64] Reg IV, induced by CDX2, participates in 5-FU resistance in gastric cancer. CDX2 also induces multidrug resistance 1 (*MDR1*) gene, resulting in resistance to chemotherapy.[65] There is an intestinal phenotype of gastric cancer defined by the expression of MUC2, CDX2, and/or CD10. Molecular detection of intestinal phenotype predicts chemoresistance in gastric cancer. OLFM4 is detected in 60% of gastric cancers, with a significant association with the gastric phenotype defined by the expression of gastric-type mucins such as MUC5AC and MUC6.[66] Combined measurement of Reg IV and OLFM4 protein levels in sera shows a sensitivity of 57% and specificity of 95% for detecting gastric cancer. *MMP-10* is one of the cancer-specific genes identified by SAGE data analysis, with serum *MMP-10* diagnostic sensitivity and specificity of 94% and 85%, respectively, indicating that *MMP-10* is suitable for gastric cancer screening.[67] CLDN18 (encoding claudin-18, a major component of tight junction in the stomach) is reduced in HP-positive atrophic gastritis, intestinal metaplasia, gastric adenoma, and the intestinal phenotype of gastric cancer.[68] CLDN18 knockout mice show atrophic gastritis and spasmolytic polypeptide–expressing metaplasia (SPEM) through paracellular H^+ leakage, upregulation of proinflammatory cytokines, and loss of parietal cells.[69] Therefore, the detection of loss of CLDN expression is a predictive marker of a precancerous condition. Cell surface and secreted proteins are potential drug targets and tumor markers when they are overexpressed in cancer. The CAST (*Escherichia coli* ampicillin trap) method systemically and efficiently detects gene expression profiles encoding transmembrane and secreted proteins. By this method, several genes that are upregulated in gastric cancer have been identified, including desmocollin 2 (*DSC2*).[70] Because *DSC2* expression is induced by CDX2 and is significantly associated with the MUC2-positive intestinal phenotype, *DSC2* is also a novel diagnostic marker for chemoresistant gastric cancer of the intestinal phenotype. In short, information obtained from transcriptome dissection greatly contributes to our understanding of the molecular characteristics of gastric cancer and will be connected to new developments in diagnosis and treatment.

Molecular Testing to Assess Hereditary Gastric Cancer Syndrome

It is estimated that about 10% to 15% of gastric cancers are familial, though the majority of gastric cancers are classified as sporadic. Among the familial gastric malignancies, hereditary diffuse gastric cancer (HDGC) syndrome is the most important condition that leads to familial gastric cancer. Other hereditary cancer syndromes, such as hereditary non-polyposis colorectal cancer, familial adenomatous polyposis, Peutz-Jeghers syndrome, Li-Fraumeni syndrome, and hereditary breast and ovarian cancer, are also associated with a significantly higher risk compared with the general population for developing gastric cancer.[71-73] HDGC patients typically present with diffuse-type signet-ring cell gastric cancer. In addition to a high susceptibility of developing gastric cancer, HDGC patients also have an increased risk of lobular breast carcinoma.

It is now known that germline mutations of *CDH1* gene, encoding E-cadherin, plays an essential role in HDGC.[71-75] Specifically, *CDH1* germline mutations occur in approximately 30% to 40 % of HDGC and missense mutations, such as c.1748T>G(p.Leu583Arg), are frequent. *CDH1* mutation has also been found to have synergistic effect along with other genetic alterations. To examine the synergistic effect of the loss of E-cadherin and p53 on gastric cancer development, a mouse line was established in which E-cadherin and p53 were specifically inactivated in the gastric parietal cell lineage.[71] Mouse diffuse gastric cancer developed at 100% penetrance within a year, frequently associated with lymph node metastasis. Gene expression profiling study of diffuse gastric cancer in DCKO mice resembled those of human HDGC. In addition, the mesenchymal markers and epithelial-mesenchymal transition-related genes were highly expressed in mouse diffuse gastric cancer as in human HDGC. Thus, genetically engineered mouse model of diffuse gastric cancer is very useful for clarifying the mechanism underlying gastric carcinogenesis and provides potentially a novel approach to management of HDGC.

The penetrance of *CDH1* is 70% to 80%, and the average age for the diagnosis of gastric cancer is 37 years.

Currently, there is no consensus regarding who should be tested for *CDH1* mutation.[75] Though age is an important factor, it has been reported that the age at onset and aggressiveness of gastric carcinoma is highly variable, which has to be included in counseling on mutation testing and potentially planning prophylactic gastrectomies.[72] Since early gastric cancer of HDGC is not readily identified by endoscopic examination, prophylactic gastrectomy is the sole preventive treatment for *CDH1* mutation carriers. Because of the occult nature of this special type of specimen, examination of the entire mucosa of prophylactic gastrectomy specimens is essential. Analysis of prophylactic gastric resection specimens has led to the detection of in situ signet-ring cell carcinomas. Usually multiple (20 to >100) foci of in situ signet-ring cell carcinoma (SRCC) and invasion in the superficial lamina propria can be detected by careful examination (Fig. 29.3). Frequently, the foci of carcinoma are very small (Fig. 29.4), and cytokeratin and PAS staining may highlight the signet-ring cells and facilitate the diagnosis.[76]

It is reported that SRCC arises from the upper isthmus of the neck region of the gastric mucosa.[72] In addition, de novo germline *CDH1* mutation is reported in an HDGC kindred presenting with early-onset diffuse gastric cancer.[74] The incident case was a woman with a personal history of Hodgkin lymphoma and diffuse gastric cancer, who was then confirmed to have a germline mutation in *CDH1* (c.1792 C > T (R598X)). The patient's mother had the same *CDH1* germline mutation, while neither maternal grandparent was found to carry this mutation, indicating that the proband's mother's mutation is of de novo origin. This report highlights the importance of recognition of the HDGC syndrome and of testing for *CDH1* germline mutations in young individuals with diffuse gastric cancer without a family history of the disease.

Does *CDH1* represent a target for treatment of HDGC? This is another area with several studies.[71,73] Using cells stably expressing WT E-cadherin and two HDGC-associated missense mutations, a recent study

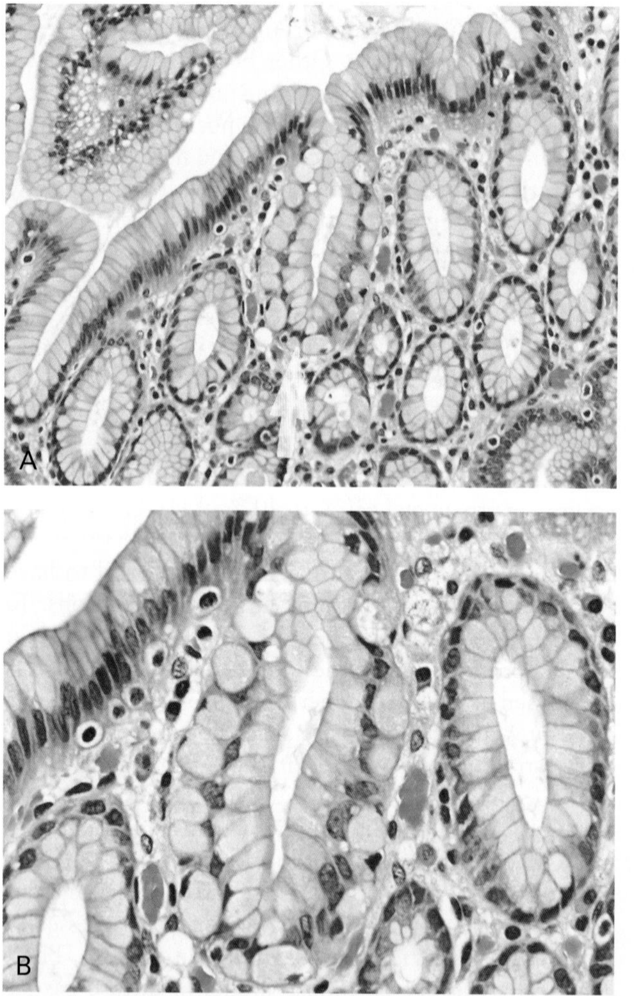

FIGURE 29–3 In situ signet-ring cell carcinoma in the superficial epithelium of a gastrectomy specimen from a CDH1 mutation carrier. **A:** Serial sections of a representative SRCC (*arrowed*) at intermediate power magnification (×200). **B:** Higher magnification of Figure 29.3A (×400).

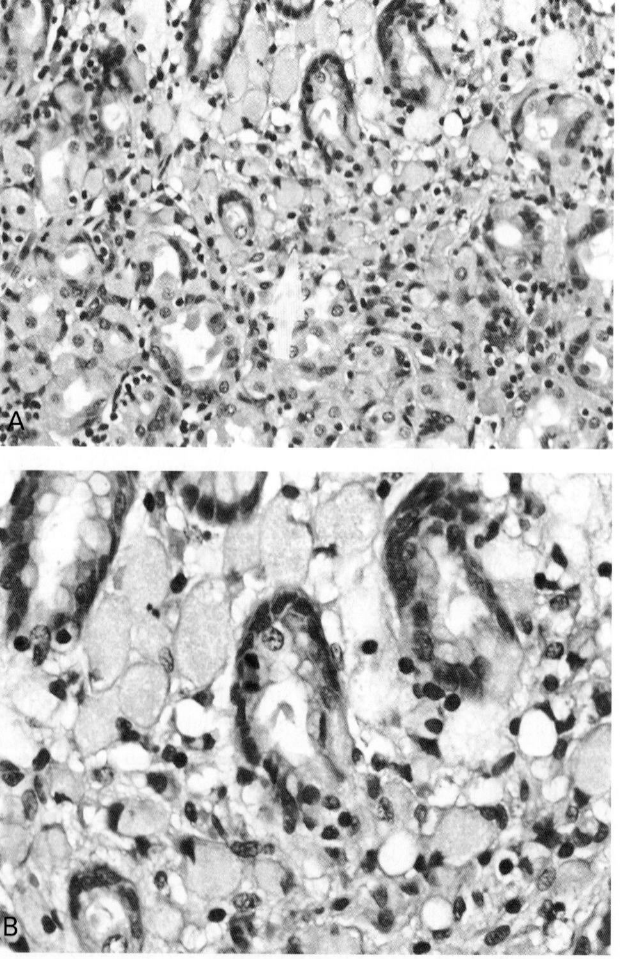

FIGURE 29–4 Invasive diffuse gastric carcinoma with signet-ring cell morphology from a gastrectomy specimen from a CDH1 mutation carrier. **A:** Notice that the size of the invasive focus is small (*arrowed*), frequently <0.5 mm in size, and located in the superficial lamina propria, intermediate magnification (×200). **B:** Higher magnification of Figure 29.4A (×400).

shows that upon DMSO treatment, mutant E-cadherin can be restored and stabilized at the cell membrane, which is associated with altered expression of Arf6 and PIPKIr.[73] Modulation of Arf6 expression partially mimics the effect of chemical chaperones (CCs), indicating that the cellular effects observed upon CCs treatment are mediated by Arf6. The investigators concluded that direct influence of CCs in cellular trafficking machinery and its effects are of crucial importance in the context of juxtamembrane E-cadherin missense mutations associated with HDGC, and they proposed that this influence should be considered when exploring the therapeutic potential of this type of chemicals in genetic diseases associated with protein misfolding.[73]

MOLECULAR DIAGNOSIS OF ESOPHAGEAL CANCER

General Concept of the Molecular Basis of Esophageal Cancer

The principle of molecular diagnosis of esophageal cancer is the same as that of gastric cancer. There are differences and similarities in the genes and molecules involved in the development and progression between gastric cancer and esophageal cancer. Furthermore, among esophageal cancers, SCC and adenocarcinomas preceded by Barrett esophagus also show distinct and similar molecular characteristics that are important in molecular diagnosis for the selection of biomarkers suitable for each histologic type of esophageal cancer.[1,77,80] Esophageal SCC develops in sequential steps through normal squamous epithelium, basal cell hyperplasia, dysplasia, and SCC, whereas esophageal adenocarcinoma is believed to develop through the dysplasia–carcinoma sequence in Barrett esophagus, by serial accumulation of genetic and epigenetic alterations.[79]

Genetic and Epigenetic Alterations in Esophageal Cancer and Diagnostic Implications

In esophageal SCC, mutation of the *p53* gene occurs at an early stage of carcinogenesis and is found in 40% to 60% of SCC and less commonly in non-cancerous mucosa adjacent to the cancer.[77,78] EGFR overexpression, partly due to gene amplification, is correlated with tumor progression, minimal response to chemotherapy, and poor prognosis. Gene amplification and overexpression of cyclin D1 are detected in 25% to 50% of esophageal SCC and cyclin D1 is an independent prognostic marker confirmed by multivariate analysis.[77,78] Homozygous deletion and hypermethylation of the *p16*^{INK4a} gene are found in 50% to 60% of esophageal SCC and cause dysregulation of the G_1/S checkpoint and abnormal proliferation, resulting in metastasis and poor prognosis.[79] Loss of FHIT expression occurs even in normal-appearing squamous epithelium that has been heavily exposed to environmental carcinogens such as tobacco and alcohol.

In esophageal adenocarcinoma, p53 mutation is also an early event in carcinogenesis, as it is detected in Barrett esophagus and dysplasia.[77,80] Alterations in transcription of FHIT and p16^{INK4a} also occur in adenocarcinoma at an early stage. HER2 amplification and overexpression are found in 20% to 30% of esophago-gastric and Barrett esophagus–related adenocarcinomas. In Barrett esophagus and esophageal adenocarcinoma, lack of p27 expression is associated with malignant transformation and poor prognosis.[80]

In regard to epigenetic alterations in esophageal SCC, genes including *APC*, *CDH1*, *p16*^{INK4a}, *RAR*β, and Ras association domain family protein 1 (*RASSF1A*) are highly methylated.[79] CDH1 methylation is observed in 70% of esophageal SCC and is associated with invasion, metastasis, and poor prognosis. Hypermethylation of *RAR*β and *RASSF1A* that causes cell cycle deregulation is found in 50% to 60% of esophageal SCC. As in SCC, esophageal adenocarcinoma is also characterized by frequent methylation of *APC*, *CDH1*, and *p16*^{INK4a}.[79] CDH1 methylation and reduced expression are associated with metastatic ability. Hypermethylation of p14^{ARF} and p15^{INK4b} is uncommon in Barrett esophagus–associated carcinogenesis. The lower frequency (10%) of hMLH1 methylation is consistent with the lower prevalence of MSI in esophageal adenocarcinoma compared with gastric and colorectal adenocarcinomas. MGMT inactivation by DNA methylation is frequently found in Barrett esophagus (40%) and esophageal adenocarcinoma (60%), whereas 20% of normal squamous epithelia show MGMT methylation.

The aberrant methylations mentioned above can be used as biomarkers for the molecular diagnosis of esophageal cancer. Methylation profiles of multiple genes including *APC*, *CDH1*, *MGMT*, *p16*, and *RUNX3* serve as indicators of the neoplastic progression of Barrett esophagus and are independent prognostic factors for esophageal adenocarcinoma.[81,82] DNA methylation detected in serum is useful for screening and monitoring of esophageal cancers. P16 methylation is found in the sera of 10% to 20% of esophageal SCC patients and correlates with poor prognosis.[83-85] APC methylation is observed in the sera of 25% of esophageal adenocarcinoma patients and in the sera of <10% of esophageal SCC patients, and high serum levels of APC methylation are significantly associated with reduced patient survival.[86]

Molecular Diagnosis of Micrometastasis and CTCs

Sentinel node mapping for esophageal cancer is relatively complicated compared with that for gastric cancer, but it provides useful information on individualized selective lymphadenectomy, which reduces morbidity and maintains the quality of life for esophageal cancer patients.[87] Detection rates of sentinel nodes by the ^{99m}Tc–tin colloid method or fluorescent dye imaging have been reported to be satisfactory; the sensitivity is 90% to 100% for clinical stage T1 to T3 patients and 45% for patients who received neoadjuvant chemoradiation therapy, respectively.[88,89] A sensitive real-time RT-PCR system, using CK19, CK20, SCC antigen, and CEA as marker mRNAs, efficiently detects micrometastasis in sentinel nodes. CTCs in the blood can also be detected in esophageal cancer patients by the RT-PCR–based molecular method. CEA mRNA is detected in the sera of 60% of esophageal SCC patients and is correlated with tumor invasion, vessel involvement, nodal metastasis, and advanced stage.[90,91] The presence of CTCs detected by CEA expression is an independent factor for a shortened hematogenous disease-free interval. CTC positivity is correlated with reduced E-cadherin expression in the primary tumor. Detection of CTC by the RT-PCR–based method is useful for predicting recurrence in patients with esophageal SCC.

miRNA-Based Molecular Diagnosis

Altered expression pattern of miRNAs has potential clinical applications toward developing biomarkers to identify the presence and progression of esophageal cancer and to assess tumor chemosensitivity and radiosensitivity.[92,93] In esophageal SCC, expressions of miR-10b, miR-92a, miR-93, miR-192, miR-194, and miR-205 are increased in tumor tissues compared with normal esophageal mucosa, while expressions of miR-100, miR-125b, miR-133a, miR-133b, miR-143, miR-145, miR-203, miR-205, and miR-375 are reduced. Overexpression of miR-21, miR-23a, miR-26a, miR-96, miR-103, miR-107, miR-128b, and miR-129 detected in esophageal SCC is correlated with prognosis. Increased expression of miR-200c correlates not only with poor prognosis but also with diminished sensitivity to chemotherapy in patients with esophageal SCC. Increased expression of miR-296 is also associated with chemoresistance. Detection of circulating miRNAs provides a new complementary tumor marker for esophageal SCC. The plasma level of miR-21 is higher and that of miR-375 is lower in SCC patients than in controls.[94] High plasma concentrations of miR-21 show significant correlation with recurrence.

On the other hand, increased expression of miR-21, miR-192, miR-195, and miR-223 and reduced expression of miR-203 are found in esophageal adenocarcinoma.[93] The levels of miR-30e and miR-200a correlate with survival of esophageal adenocarcinoma patients, whereas reduced miR-375 expression is associated with shorter survival.[95] Overexpression of miR-148 enhances the effect of cisplatin and 5-FU, providing a basis for the potential use of miRNAs to predict or improve the response to chemotherapy.[96] During the progression from normal mucosa to adenocarcinoma via Barrett esophagus, sequential upregulation of miR-21, miR-93, miR-192, and miR-194 is observed.[97] Upregulation of miR-192 and miR-215 and downregulation of miR-203, miR-205, and let7c are a "progression signature" for the progression from Barrett esophagus to adenocarcinoma and may serve as molecular markers for neoplastic progression.[98]

Genetic Polymorphism and Esophageal Cancer Risk

Many studies have evaluated genetic polymorphism and esophageal cancer risk, with a majority of these studies conducted in Asian countries.[99-101] Meta-analyses of ALDH2, MTHFR, CYP1A1, CYP2E1, GSTP1, GSTM1, and GSTT1 have found significant correlations between ALDH2*1*2 and CYP1A1 Val allele and increased risk of esophageal cancer. *ALDH2* is a polymorphic gene, and individual genotypes determine blood concentrations of acetaldehyde after drinking, whereas *CYP1A1* is involved in the activation of major classes of tobacco procarcinogens such as polyaromatic hydrocarbons and aromatic amines. Increased risk of esophageal SCC is associated with ADH2*1*2 and p53 codon 72 Pro/Pro genotypes. GSTP1 (Ile105Val) is a risk factor for Barrett esophagus and adenocarcinoma in Caucasian males.[100] GSTP1 is the major isoform expressed in the esophagus and eliminates DNA oxidative products. In addition to protein-coding genes, pre-miRNAs also possess polymorphisms that affect esophageal cancer risk.[92] For instance, C–T SNP in pre-miR-196a (rs11614913) and G > C variant in pre-miR-146a increase esophageal SCC in the Chinese population.[92] These findings are applicable to molecular diagnosis in identifying individuals at high risk for developing esophageal cancer.

Novel Molecular Markers Identified through SAGE Data Analysis

Although conventional serum tumor markers such as SCC antigen and CYFRA21-1 (fragment of CK19) have been used clinically as biomarkers, they have low sensitivity and low specificity. To search for novel biomarkers for esophageal cancer, a SAGE library was generated from esophageal SCC and compared with the library from normal esophageal mucosa.[102] Many upregulated and downregulated genes were identified that might be candidate diagnostic markers and therapeutic targets (Table 29.2). ADAM metalloproteinase with thrombospondin type 1 motif 16 (ADAMTS16) was the most upregulated gene in esophageal SCC. ADAMTS16 is expressed in 40% of esophageal SCC at high levels, as shown by quantitative RT-PCR, whereas SCCA1-encoding SCC antigen is expressed in only 20% of esophageal SCC. ADAMTS protein is secreted from cancer cells, and knockdown of ADAMTS16 inhibits cell growth and invasion ability. Thus, ADAMTS16 could be a novel diagnostic and therapeutic target in patients with esophageal SCC. SAGE data provide a list of genes associated with the development and progression of esophageal cancer.

TABLE 29-2 The 10 Most Upregulated and Downregulated Tags/Genes in Esophageal Squamous Cell Carcinoma in Comparison with Normal Esophagus by Sage Data Analysis

Upregulated Tag Sequence	Tags per Million: SCC	Tags per Million: Normal Esophagus	Symbol	Description
TCCCCTACAT	2564[a] (37)[b]	0 (0)	*ADAMTS16*	ADAM metallopeptidase with thrombospondin type 1 motif, 16
GAAATAAAGC	2495 (36)	0 (0)	*IGHG1*	Immunoglobulin heavy constant gamma 1 (G1m marker)
TTCGGTTGGT	2148 (31)	0 (0)	*OGFOD1*	2-Oxoglutarate and iron-dependent oxygenase domain containing 1
AGGCATTGAA	5336 (77)	20 (1)	*NUTF2*	Nuclear transport factor 2
CAGTTACAAA	5544 (80)	40 (2)	*RYBP*	RING1 and YY1 binding protein
TGGAAATGAC	1317 (19)	0 (0)	*COL1A1*	Collagen, type I, alpha 1
ACCAAAAACC	1663 (24)	20 (1)	*COL1A1*	Collagen, type I, alpha 1
GGCAGCACAA	1455 (21)	20 (1)	*NBEAL2*	Neurobeachin-like 2
TTTATTAGAA	1455 (21)	20 (1)	*CCDC75*	Coiled-coil domain containing 75
AGCCAAAAAA	2980 (43)	40 (2)	*MAP3K12*	Nuclear casein kinase and cyclin-dependent kinase substrate 1
GTGGCCACGG	0 (0)	25283 (1277)	*S100A9*	S100 calcium binding protein A9 (calgranulin B)
GGCAGAGAAG	0 (0)	8454 (427)	*KRT4*	Keratin 4
ATGAGCTGAC	0 (0)	3762 (190)	*CSTB*	Cystatin B (stefin B)
			XPO7	Exportin 7
GAAGCACAAG	0 (0)	2475 (125)	*KRT6C*	Keratin 6C
TAATTTGCAT	0 (0)	2455 (124)	*EMP1*	Epithelial membrane protein 1
			GNA13	Guanine nucleotide binding protein (G protein), alpha 13
AAAGCGGGGC	0 (0)	2356 (119)	*KRT13*	Keratin 13
TGTGTTGAGA	0 (0)	2257 (114)	*EEF1A1*	Eukaryotic translation elongation factor 1 alpha 1
CACAAACGGT	0 (0)	2079 (105)	*TSPAN9*	Tetraspanin 9
			RPS27	Ribosomal protein S27
TGGTGTTGAG	0 (0)	1841 (93)	*RPS18*	Ribosomal protein S18
GCCAATCCAG	0 (0)	1802 (91)	*CRNN*	Cornulin

[a]The absolute tag counts are normalized to 1,000,000 total tags/sample.

[b]Number in parentheses indicates the absolute tag counts.

REFERENCES

1. Ohgaki H, Matsukura N. Stomach cancer. In: Stewart BW, Kleihues P, ed. *World Cancer Report*. Lyon: IARC Press; 2003:194-197.
2. Boffetta P, Hainaut P. Oesophageal cancer. In: Stewart BW, Kleihues P, ed. *World Cancer Report*. Lyon: IARC Press; 2003:223-231.
3. Ushijima T, Sasako M. Focus on gastric cancer. *Cancer Cell*. 2004;5:121-125.
4. Yasui W, Oue N, Aung PP, et al. Molecular-pathological prognostic factors of gastric cancer: a review. *Gastric Cancer*. 2005;8:86-94.
5. Yasui W, Sentani K, Motoshita J, et al. Molecular pathobiology of gastric cancer (review). *Scand J Surg*. 2006;95:225-231.
6. Yasui W, Sentani K, Sakamoto N, et al. Molecular pathology of gastric cancer: research and practice. *Pathol Res Pract*. 2011;207:608-612
7. Calin GA, Croce CM. MicroRNA–cancer connection: the beginning of a new tale. *Cancer Res*. 2006;66:7390-7394.
8. Yasui W, Yokozaki H, Shimamoto F, et al. Molecular-pathological diagnosis of gastrointestinal tissues and its contribution to cancer histopathology. *Pathol Int*. 1999;49:763-774.
9. Yasui W, Oue N, Kuniyasu H, et al. Molecular diagnosis of gastric cancer: present and future. *Gastric Cancer*. 2001;4:113-121.
10. Yasui W, Oue N, Ono S, et al. Histone acetylation and gastrointestinal carcinogenesis. *Ann NY Acad Sci*. 2003;983:220-231.
11. Lee TL, Leung WK, Chan MW, et al. Detection of gene promoter hypermethylation in the tumor and serum of patients with gastric carcinoma. *Clin Cancer Res*. 2002;8:1761-1766.
12. Kanyama Y, Hibi K, Nakayama H, et al. Detection of p16 promoter hypermethylation in serum of gastric cancer patients. *Cancer Sci*. 2003;94:418-420.
13. Leung WK, To KF, Chu ES, et al. Potential diagnostic and prognostic values of detecting promoter hypermethylation in the serum of patients with gastric cancer. *Br J Cancer*. 2005;92:2190-2194.
14. Ikoma H, Ichikawa D, Daito I, et al. Clinical application of methylation specific-polymerase chain reaction in serum of patients with gastric cancer. *Hepatogastroenterology*. 2007;54:946-950.

15. Ikoma H, Ichikawa D, Koike H, et al. Correlation between serum DNA methylation and prognosis of gastric cancer patients. *Anticancer Res.* 2006;26:2313-2316.
16. Sakakura C, Hamada T, Miyagawa K, et al. Quantitative analysis of tumor-derived methylated RUNX3 sequences in the serum of gastric cancer patients. *Anticancer Res.* 2009;29:2619-2625.
17. Nakajima T, Yamashita S, Maekita T, et al. The presence of a methylation fingerprint of *Helicobacter pylori* infection in human gastric mucosa. *Int J Cancer.* 2009;124:905-910.
18. Maekita T, Nakazawa K, Mihara M, et al. High levels of aberrant DNA methylation in *Helicobacter pylori*-infected gastric mucosae and its possible association with gastric cancer risk. *Clin Cancer Res.* 2006;12:989-995.
19. Nakajima T, Maekita T, Oda I, et al. High methylation levels in gastric mucosae significantly correlate with higher rink of gastric cancers. *Cancer Epidemiol Biomarkers Prev.* 2006;15:2317-2321.
20. Ushijima T. Epigenetic field for cancerization. *J Biochem Mol Biol.* 2007;40:142-150.
21. Watanabe Y, Kim HS, Castoro RJ, et al. Sensitive and specific detection of early gastric cancer with DNA methylation analysis of gastric washes. *Gastroenterology.* 2009;136:2149-2159.
22. Baba S, Oishi Y, Watanabe Y, et al. Gastric wash-based molecular testing for antibiotic resistance in *Helicobacter pylori. Digestion.* 2011;84:299-305.
23. Ohtsu A. Chemotherapy for metastatic gastric cancer: past, present, and future. *J Gastroenterol.* 2008;43:256-564.
24. Zagouri F, Papadimitriou CA, Dimopoulos MA, et al. Molecular targeted therapies in unresectable-metastatic gastric cancer. *Cancer Treat Rev.* 2011;37:599-610.
25. Fornaro L, Lucchesi M, Caparello, et al. Anti-HER2 agents in gastric cancer: from bench to bedside. *Nat Rev Gastroenterol Hepatol.* 2011;8:369-383.
26. Sumida T, Kitadai Y, Shinagawa K, et al. Anti-stromal therapy with imatinib inhibits growth and metastasis of gastric carcinoma in an orthotopic mouse model. *Int J Cancer.* 2011;128: 2050-2062.
27. Bang YJ, Custem EV, Feyereislova A, et al. Trastuzumab in combination with chemotherapy versus chemotherapy alone for treatment of HER2-positive advanced gastric and gastro-oesophageal junction cancer (ToGA): a phase 3, open-label, randomized controlled trial. *Lancet.* 2010;376:687-697.
28. Koh YW, Lee HJ, Lee JW, et al. Dual-color silver-enhanced in situ hybridization for assessing *HER2* gene amplification in breast cancer. *Modern Pathol.* 2011;24:794-800.
29. Takeuchi H, Ueda M, Oyama T, et al. Molecular diagnosis and translymphatic chemotherapy targeting sentinel lymph nodes of patients with early gastrointestinal cancers. *Digestion.* 2010;82:187-191.
30. Shimizu Y, Takeuchi H, Sakakura Y, et al. Molecular detection of sentinel node micrometastases in patients with clinical N0 gastric carcinoma with real-time multiplex reverse transcription-polymerase chain reaction assay. *Ann Surg Oncol.* 2012;19:469-477.
31. Yaguchi Y, Sugasawa H, Tsujimoto H, et al. One-step nucleic acid amplification (OSNA) for the application of sentinel node concept in gastric cancer. *Ann Surg Oncol.* 2011;18:2289-2296.
32. Muto Y, Matsubara H, Tanizawa T, et al. Rapid diagnosis of micrometastasis of gastric cancer using reverse transcription loop-mediated isothermal amplification. *Oncol Rep.* 2011;26:789-794.
33. Sun YF, Yang XR, Zhou J, et al. Circulating tumor cells: advances in detection methods, biological issues, and clinical relevance. *J Cancer Res Clin Oncol.* 2011;137:1151-1173.
34. Takeuchi H, Kitagawa Y. Circulating tumor cells in gastrointestinal cancer. *J Hepatobiliary Pancreat Sci.* 2010;17:577-582.
35. Fujiwara Y, Doki Y, Taniguchi H, et al. Genetic detection of free cancer cells in the peritoneal cavity of the patient with gastric cancer: present status and further perspectives. *Gastric Cancer.* 2007;10:197-204.
36. Bartel DP. MicroRNAs: genomics, biogenesis, mechanism, and function. *Cell.* 2004;116:281-297.
37. Spizzo R, Nicoloso MS, Croce CM, et al. SnapShot: microRNAs in cancer. *Cell.* 2009;137:586.
38. Wu WK, Lee CW, Cho CH, et al. MicroRNA dysregulation in gastric cancer: a new player enters the game. *Oncogene.* 2010;29:5761-5771.
39. Ueda T, Volinia S, Okumura H, et al. Relation between microRNA expression and progression and prognosis of gastric cancer: a microRNA expression analysis. *Lancet Oncol.* 2010;11: 136-146.
40. Kogo R, Mimori K, Tanaka F, et al. Clinical significance of miR-146a in gastric cancer cases. *Clin Cancer Res.* 2011;17: 4277-4284.
41. Zheng B, Liang L, Wang C, et al. MicroRNA-148a suppress tumor cell invasion and metastasis by downregulating ROCK1 in gastric cancer. *Clin Cancer Res.* 2011;17:7574-7583.
42. Xu Y, Zhao F, Wang Z, et al. Micro-RNA-335 acts as a metastasis suppressor in gastric cancer by targeting Bcl-w and specificity protein 1. *Oncogene.* 2012;31:1398-1407.
43. Takei T, Takigahira M, Mihara K, et al. The metastasis-associated microRNA miR-516a-3p is a novel therapeutic target for inhibiting peritoneal dissemination of human scirrhous gastric cancer. *Cancer Res.* 2011;71:1442-1453.
44. Oh HK, Das K, Ooi CH, et al. Genomic loss of miR-486 regulated tumor progression of the OLFM4 antiapoptotic factor in gastric cancer. *Clin Cancer Res.* 2011;17:2657-2667.
45. Nishida N, Mimori K, Fabbri M, et al. MicroRNA-125a-5p is an independent prognostic factor in gastric cancer and inhibits the proliferation of human gastric carcinoma cells in combination with trastuzumab. *Clin Cancer Res.* 2011;17:2725-2733.
46. Tsai KW, Wu CW, Hu LY, et al. Epigenetic regulation of miR-34b and miR-129 expression in gastric cancer. *Int J Cancer.* 2011;129: 2600-2610.
47. Ando T, Yoshida T, Enomoto S, et al. DNA methylation of microRNA genes in gastric mucosa of gastric cancer patients: its possible involvement in the formation of epigenetic field defect. *Int J Cancer.* 2009;124:2367-2374.
48. Suzuki H, Yamamoto E, Nojima M, et al. Methylation-associated silencing of microRNA-34b/c in gastric cancer and its involvement in an epigenetic field defect. *Carcinogenesis.* 2010;31:2066-2073.
49. Arroyo JD, Chevillet JR, Kroh EM, et al. Argonaute2 complexes carry a population of circulating microRNAs independent of vesicles in human plasma. *Proc Natl Acad Sci U S A.* 2011;108:5003-5008.
50. Liu R, Zhang C, Hu Z, et al. A five-microRNA signature identified from genome-wide serum microRNA expression profiling serves as a fingerprint for gastric cancer diagnosis. *Eur J Cancer.* 2011;47:784-791.
51. Tsujiura M, Ichikawa D, Komatsu S, et al. Circulating microRNAs in plasma of patients with gastric cancers. *Br J Cancer.* 2010;102:1174-1179.
52. Gonzalez CA, Sala N, Capella G. Genetic susceptibility and gastric cancer risk. *Int J Cancer.* 2002;100:249-260.
53. Hamajima N, Naito M, Kondo T, et al. Genetic factors involved in the development of *Helicobacter pylori*-related gastric cancer. *Cancer Sci.* 2006;97:1129-1138.
54. El-Omar EM, Carrington M, Chow WH, et al. Interleukin-1 polymorphisms associated with increased risk of gastric cancer. *Nature.* 2000;404:398-402.
55. Hatakeyama M. Anthropological and clinical implications for the structural diversity of the *Helicobacter pylori* CagA oncoprotein. *Cancer Sci.* 2011;102:36-43.
56. The Study Group of Millennium Genome Project for Cancer. Genetic variation in PSCA is associated with susceptibility to diffuse-type gastric cancer. *Nat Genet.* 2008;40:730-740.
57. Saeki N, Saito A, Choi IJ, et al. A functional single nucleotide polymorphism in mucin 1, at chromosome 1q22 determines susceptibility to diffuse-type gastric cancer. *Gastroenterology.* 2011;140:892-902.
58. Nishiyama M, Eguchi H. Pharmacokinetics and pharmacogenomics in gastric cancer chemotherapy. *Adv Drug Deliv Rev.* 2009;61:402-407.
59. Yin M, Yan J, Martinez-Balibrea E, et al. ERCC1 and ERCC2 polymorphisms predict clinical outcomes of oxaliplatin-based chemotherapies in gastric and colorectal cancer: a systemic review and meta-analysis. *Clin Cancer Res.* 2011;17:1632-1640.
60. Yasui W, Oue N, Ito R, et al. Search for new biomarkers of gastric cancer through serial analysis of gene expression and its clinical implications. *Cancer Sci.* 2004;95:385-392.
61. Oue N, Hamai Y, Mitani Y, et al. Gene expression profile of gastric carcinoma: identification of genes and tags potentially involved in invasion, metastasis, and carcinogenesis by serial analysis of gene expression. *Cancer Res.* 2004;64:2397-2405.
62. Yasui W, Oue N, Sentani K, et al. Transcriptome dissection of gastric cancer: identification of novel diagnostic and therapeutic targets from pathology specimens. *Pathol Int.* 2009;59:121-136.

63. Yasui W, Sentani K, Sakamoto N, et al. Histological and serological tumor markers of gastric cancer. In: Hellberg D, ed. *Histological and Serological Tumor Markers and Gene Expression and Their Clinical Usefulness in Cancers*. New York, NY: Nova Biomedical Books; 2009:93-111.
64. Mitani Y, Oue N, Matsumura S, et al. Reg IV is a serum biomarker for gastric cancer patients and predicts response to 5-fluorouracil-based chemotherapy. *Oncogene*. 2007;26:4383-4393.
65. Takakura Y, Hinoi T, Oue N, et al. CDX2 regulates multidrug resistance 1 gene expression in malignant intestinal epithelium. *Cancer Res*. 2010;70:6767-6778.
66. Oue N, Sentani K, Noguchi T, et al. Serum olfactomedin 4 (GW112, hGC-1) in combination with Reg IV is a highly sensitive biomarker for gastric cancer patients. *Int J Cancer.* 2009;125:2383-2392.
67. Aung PP, Oue N, Mitani Y, et al. Systematic search for gastric cancer-specific genes based on SAGE data: melanoma inhibitory activity and matrix metalloproteinase-10 are novel prognostic factors in patients with gastric cancer. *Oncogene*. 2006;25:2546-2557.
68. Sanada Y, Oue N, Mitani Y, et al. Down-regulation of the claudin-18 gene, identified through serial analysis of gene expression data analysis, in gastric cancer with an intestinal phenotype. *J Pathol*. 2006;208:633-642.
69. Hayashi D, Tamura A, Tanaka H, et al. Deficiency of claudin-18 causes paracellular H^+ leakage, up-regulation of interleukin-1beta, and atrophic gastritis in mice. *Gastroenterology*. 2012;29: 1649-1659.
70. Anami K, Oue N, Noguchi T, et al. Search for transmembrane protein in gastric cancer by the *Escherichia coli* ampicillin secretion trap: expression of DSC2 in gastric cancer with intestinal phenotype. *J Pathol*. 2010;221:275-284.
71. Shimada S, Mimata A, Sekine M, et al. Synergistic tumour suppressor activity of E-cadherin and p53 in a conditional mouse model for metastatic diffuse-type gastric cancer. Gut. 2012;64:344-353.
72. Sereno M, Aguayo C, Guillén Ponce C, et al. Gastric tumours in hereditary cancer syndromes: clinical features, molecular biology and strategies for prevention. *Clin Transl Oncol*. 2011;13:599-610.
73. Figueiredo J, Simões-Correia J, Söderberg O, et al. ADP-ribosylation factor 6 mediates E-cadherin recovery by chemical chaperones. *PLoS One*. 2011;6(8):e23188.
74. Shah M, Salo-Mullen E, Stadler Z, et al. De novo CDH1 mutation in a family presenting with early-onset diffuse gastric cancer. *Clin Genet* 2011. In press.
75. Kluijt I, Siemerink EJ, Ausems MG, et al.; on behalf of the Dutch Working Group on Hereditary Gastric Cancer. CDH1-related hereditary diffuse gastric cancer syndrome: clinical variations and implications for counseling. *Int J Cancer* 2011. In press.
76. Lee A, Rees H, Owen DA, et al. Periodic acid–Schiff is superior to hematoxylin and eosin for screening prophylactic gastrectomies from CDH1 mutation carriers. *Am J Surg Pathol* 2010 34(7): 1007-1013
77. Kuwano H, Kato H, Miyazaki T, et al. Genetic alterations in esophageal cancer. *Surg Today*. 2005;35:7/18.
78. Lin DC, Du XL, Wang MR. Protein alterations in ESCC and clinical implications: a review. *Dis Esophagus*. 2009;22:9-20.
79. Sato F, Meltzer SJ. CpG island hypermethylation in progression of esophageal and gastric cancer. *Cancer*. 2006;106:483-493.
80. Moyes LH, Going JJ. Still waiting for predictive biomarkers in Barrett's oesophagus. *J Clin Pathol*. 2011;64:742-750.
81. Schulmann K, Sterian A, Berki A, et al. Inactivation of p16, RUNX3, and HPP1 occurs early in Barrett's-associated neoplastic progression and predicts progression risk. *Oncogene*. 2005;24:4138-4148.
82. Brock MV, Gou M, Akiyama Y, et al. Prognostic importance of promoter hypermethylation of multiple gene in esophageal adenocarcinoma. *Clin Cancer Res*. 2003;9:2912-2919.
83. Hibi K, Taguchi M, Nakayama H, et al. Molecular detection of p16 promoter methylation in the serum of patients with esophageal squamous cell carcinoma. *Clin Cancer Res*. 2001;7:3135-3138.
84. Ikoma D, Ichikawa D, Ueda Y, et al. Circulating tumor cells and aberrant methylation as tumor markers in patients with esophageal cancer. *Anticancer Res*. 2007;27:535-539.
85. Fujiwara S, Noguchi T, Takeno S, et al. Hypermethylation of p16 gene promoter correlates with loss of p16 expression that results in poorer prognosis in esophageal squamous cell carcinoma. *Dis Esophagus*. 2008;21:125-131.
86. Kawakami K, Brebender J, Lord RV, et al. Hypermethylated APC DNA in plasma and prognosis of patients with esophageal adenocarcinoma. *J Natl Cancer Inst*. 2000;92:1805-1811.
87. Takeuchi H, Kitagawa Y. Sentinel node navigation surgery for esophageal cancer. *Gen Thorac Cardiovasc Surg*. 2008;56: 393-396.
88. Uenosono Y, Arigami T, Yanagida S, et al. Sentinel node navigation surgery is acceptable for clinical T1 and N0 esophageal cancer. *Ann Surg Oncol*. 2011;18:2003-2009.
89. Yuasa Y, Seike J, Yoshida T, et al. Sentinel lymph node biopsy using intraoperative indocyanine green fluorescence imaging navigated with preoperative CT lymphography for superficial esophageal cancer. *Ann Surg Oncol*. 2012;19:486-493.
90. Nakashima D, Natsugoe S, Matsumoto M, et al. Clinical significance of circulating tumor cells in blood by molecular detection and tumor markers in esophageal cancer. *Surgery*. 2003;133:162-169.
91. Setoyama T, Natsugoe S, Okumura H, et al. Isolated tumor cells in blood and E-cadherin expression in oesophageal squamous cell cancer. *Br J Cancer*. 2007;94:984-991.
92. David S, Meltzer SJ. MicroRNA involvement in esophageal carcinogenesis. *Curr Opin Pharmacol*. 2011;11:612-616.
93. Mathe EA, Nguyen GH, Bowman ED, et al. MicroRNA expression in squamous cell carcinoma and adenocarcinoma of the esophagus: association with survival. *Clin Cancer Res*. 2009;15:6193-6200.
94. Komatsu S, Ichikawa D, Takeshita H, et al. Circulating microRNAs in plasma of patients with oesophageal squamous cell carcinoma. *Br J Cancer*. 2011;105:104-111.
95. Hu Y, Correa AM, Hoque A, et al. Prognostic significance of differentially expressed miRNAs in esophageal cancer. *Int J Cancer*. 2011;128:132-143.
96. Hummel R, Watson DI, Smith C, et al. Mir-148 improves response to chemotherapy in sensitive and resistant oesophageal adenocarcinoma and squamous cell carcinoma cells. *J Gastrointest Surg*. 2011;15:429-438.
97. Feber A, Xi L, Luketich JD, et al. MicroRNA expression profiles of esophageal cancer. *J Thorac Cardiovasc Surg*. 2008;135:255-260.
98. Fassan M, Volinia D, Palatini J, et al. MicroRNA expression profiling in human Barrett's carcinogenesis. *Int J Cancer*. 2011;129:1661-1670.
99. Hiyama T, Yoshihara M, Tanaka S, et al. Genetic polymorphisms and esophageal cancer risk. *Int J Cancer*. 2007;121:1643-1658.
100. Bull LM, White DL, Bray M, et al. Phase I and II enzyme polymorphisms as risk factors for Barrett's esophagus and esophageal adenocarcinoma: a systematic review and meta-analysis. *Dis Esophagus*. 2009;22:571-587.
101. Li T, Suo Q, He D, et al. Esophageal cancer risk is associated with polymorphisms of DNA repair genes *MSH2* and *WRN* in Chinese population. *J Thorac Oncol*. 2012 7(2):448-52.
102. Sakamoto N, Oue N, Noguchi T, et al. Serial analysis of gene expression of esophageal squamous cell carcinoma: ADAMTS16 is upregulated in esophageal squamous cell carcinoma. *Cancer Sci*. 2010;101:1038-1044.

CHAPTER 30

Molecular Biology of Prostate Cancer: Practical Considerations for Diagnosis and Prognosis

David G. Bostwick

INTRODUCTION

In recent years, advances in our understanding of the molecular biology of prostate cancer have spawned optimism that these new markers will allow greater sensitivity and specificity in diagnosis as well as more accurate prediction of outcome after treatment for the individual patient. This chapter summarizes the current state of prostate cancer biomarkers, with emphasis on tissue expression and genetic abnormalities. We begin with a brief discussion of the pathogenesis of prostate cancer.

PATHOGENESIS OF PROSTATE CANCER

The pathogenesis of prostate cancer is uncertain but may be classified as genotoxic or non-genotoxic.[1] The genotoxic theory hypothesizes that genetic mutations may be inherited owing to familial or racial predilection or may be induced by a wide variety of agents. One possible genotoxic trigger may be continuous cell division, driven by hormones such as testosterone, resulting in the accumulation of spontaneous mutations, and thereby activating select oncogenes and inactivating tumor suppressor genes. Another possible trigger could be small amounts of dietary carcinogens, such as PhiP in cooked fish and meat, that may cause mutations in prostate tissue. If this finding is confirmed in humans, it would suggest that consumption of foods containing PhiP over a lifetime may result in the consumption of a substantial prostate carcinogen. Since PhiP is mutagenic, forms DNA adducts, and is carcinogenic in the rat prostate, this could provide evidence for a genotoxic mechanism of human prostate carcinogenesis. However, there is currently no strong evidence that chemical carcinogens or endocrine-disrupting chemicals play a role in the induction or evolution of human prostate cancer.

The non-genotoxic theory hypothesizes that testosterone plays a significant role in the evolution of human prostatic cancer by acting as a stimulus for prostate cell growth. It may function as a mitogen or a tumor promoter. Testosterone induces cell division, and, over a lifetime, the large number of cell divisions may result in the accumulation of spontaneous mutations in prostate cells. Testosterone is at least a necessary factor (necessary but not sufficient?) for prostatic carcinogenesis, but may serve as a cofactor rather than the ultimate trigger. Another trigger could be oxidative stress induced by smouldering longstanding chronic inflammation and the unique biochemical milieu of the prostate (e.g., high citrate and zinc levels), ultimately resulting in mitogenesis. This latter mechanism is currently favored by us and most investigators.

GENETIC BASIS OF FAMILIAL PROSTATE CANCER

Genome-wide association studies to date have revealed about 35 single-nucleotide polymorphisms (SNPs) that are consistently associated with familial prostate cancer, although none have been linked to cancer stage or outcome.[2] Cancer risk is minimal (<1.3) for individual SNPs, accounting in total for only about 25% of inherited risk.[3] Conversely, linkage analysis of families with hereditary prostate cancer has usually yielded inconsistent findings. However, a recent report found by linkage analysis in combination with targeted massively parallel sequencing that a recurrent mutation in HOXB13 G84E variant on chromosome 17 was associated with early-onset and hereditary prostate cancer, but accounted for only a small fraction of cases (3.1%).[4]

The best model to predict genetic susceptibility to prostate cancer may be a mixed model of inheritance that included both a recessive major gene component and a polygenic component composed of all SNPs known to be associated with prostate cancer and a residual polygenic component due to the postulated but as yet unknown genetic variants.[5] Such a model may be able to predict the probability of developing prostate cancer in the future based on the combination of SNP profiles and family history.

Genetic Confirmation of Patient Identity

Genotypic analysis to verify patient identity in cases of "vanishing cancer" is becoming increasingly popular and appears prudent to reassure patients that their diagnosis is accurate.[6,7] The inability to identify residual cancer in radical prostatectomy specimens—referred to as vanishing cancer—raises the question of accuracy of the original diagnosis of cancer. In one report, biopsies were overdiagnosed as cancer in two of four cases with no residual cancer after radical prostatectomy.[7]

In a series of 38 patients with pT0 cancer, we found that none developed clinical evidence of cancer recurrence with a mean follow-up of almost 10 years.[8] Those that died of other causes had no evidence of prostate cancer at the time of death. These cumulative data strongly suggest that these patients are cured of cancer and no residual therapy is indicated.

IMMUNOHISTOCHEMICAL MARKERS IN PROSTATIC INTRAEPITHELIAL NEOPLASIA (PIN) AND PROSTATE CANCER

Tissue (Immunohistochemical) Determination of Prostatic Origin

Determination of tissue of origin (prostatic vs. nonprostatic) relies chiefly on prostate-specific antigen (PSA), prostatic acid phosphatase (PAP), and prostate-specific membrane antigen (PSMA).

Prostate-Specific Antigen

PSA is a 34-kDa, single-chain glycoprotein of 237-amino acids produced almost exclusively by prostatic epithelial cells. PSA, a serine protease, is a member of the kallikrein gene family and has a high sequence homology with human glandular kallikrein 2. It exhibits chymotrypsin-like, trypsin-like, and esterase-like activity. In serum, PSA is present mainly as a complex with alpha-1-antichymotrypsin. It is secreted in seminal plasma and is responsible for gel dissolution in freshly ejaculated semen by proteolysis of the major gel-forming proteins, semenogelin I and II, and fibronectin. A small amount of PSA in semen is complexed. The free, non-complexed form of PSA constitutes a minor fraction of serum PSA, and derivatives of PSA such as free/total ratio of PSA may be superior to PSA alone. Production of PSA appears to be under the control of circulating androgens acting through the androgen receptors (ARs).[9]

In the normal and hyperplastic prostate, PSA was uniformly present at the apical portion of the glandular epithelium of secretory cells (Fig. 30.1A). The intensity of the staining decreased in poorly differentiated adenocarcinoma.[10] PSA immunoreactivity has been described in extraprostatic tissues and tumors but is usually patchy and weak when present. PSA is also a sensitive and specific

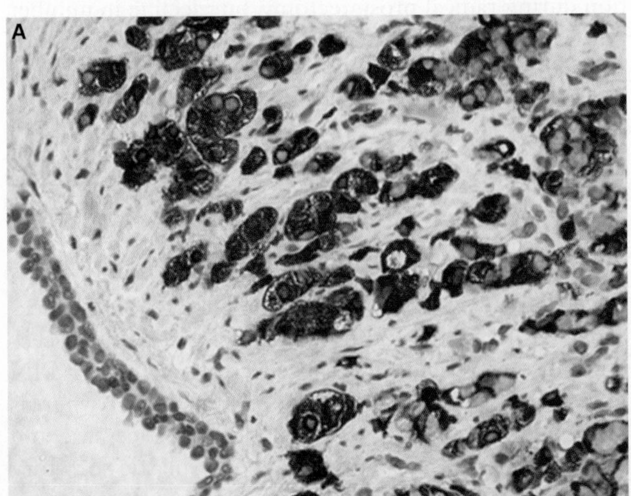

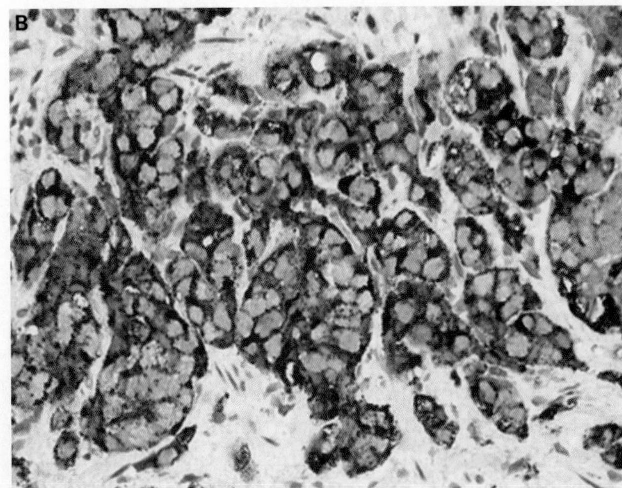

FIGURE 30–1 Intense cytoplasmic immunoreactivity in high-grade prostatic adenocarcinoma (brown reaction product) for **A (left):** prostate-specific antigen and **B (right):** prostatic acid phosphatase.

immunohistochemical marker for tumors of prostatic origin. This is very useful for the differential diagnosis of poorly differentiated or undifferentiated carcinomas.[10]

Serum PSA may become elevated by conditions other than benign prostatic hyperplasia and cancer, including prostatitis, PIN, acute urinary retention, renal failure, and sialadenitis. Earlier detection through screening for elevated levels of PSA has been shown to decrease prostate cancer mortality.[11] PSA accurately predicts cancer status and can detect recurrence several months before detection by any other method. However, this test is hampered by its low specificity (47% with a cut point of 4.0 ng/ml). In two of three men with a serum PSA level of 4 ng/ml or greater, biopsies will be negative. Furthermore, the rate of cancer in men with a PSA level of 2.5 to 4 ng/ml undergoing systematic biopsies reaches 20% to 23%.[12] It has been suggested to use PSA level of 2.5 as cut point for prostate cancer screening.

PSA is particularly sensitive and accurate in the detection of residual cancer, recurrence, and cancer progression following treatment, irrespective of the treatment modality. Serum PSA concentration exceeding 0.2 ng/ml following radical prostatectomy is often considered as evidence of biochemical tumor recurrence.[13] However, in 26% to 29% of radical prostatectomy specimens, the surgical margin contains benign prostatic glands with or without tumor. In 45% of whole mounted prostatectomies, only benign glands were present at the margins.[14] In one-third of these patients, postoperative serum PSA was measurable, and, in half of these, the PSA concentration indicated recurrence.

Prostatic Acid Phosphatase

The immunohistochemical localization and distribution of prostatic-specific acid phosphatase (PAP) in normal, hyperplastic, and cancerous human prostate has been used as a prostate-specific marker for many years.[15-17] In the normal and hyperplastic prostate, PAP was uniformly present at the apical portion of the glandular epithelium of secretory cells. There was more intense and uniform staining of cancer cells and the glandular epithelium of well-differentiated adenocarcinoma, whereas less intense and more variable staining was seen in moderately and poorly differentiated adenocarcinoma (Fig. 30.1B).[18,19] We consider PAP to be a more reliable marker than PSA in difficult cases and routinely employ both when needed to confirm prostatic identity.

Prostate-Specific Membrane Antigen

PSMA is a membrane-bound antigen that is highly specific for benign and malignant prostatic epithelial cells. It is present in the serum of normal men, according to studies with monoclonal antibody 7E11.C5, and an elevated concentration is associated with the presence of prostatic adenocarcinoma, clinical progression of carcinoma, and hormone-refractory carcinoma.[20,21]

PSMA has partial homology with the transferrin receptor, and its extracellular domain also possesses properties of the NAALADase enzyme activity.[22] The 7E11.C5 antibody has been successfully used with SPECT (single photon emission computed tomography) scanning to detect soft tissue and bone metastatic prostate cancer, as well as cancer in the preoperative and postoperative prostate and prostate bed.[23,24] There is intense cytoplasmic epithelial immunoreactivity for PSMA in every prostate.[21,25] The number of immunoreactive cells increased from benign epithelium to high-grade PIN and prostatic adenocarcinoma.[26] The most extensive and intense staining for PSMA was observed in high-grade carcinoma, with immunoreactivity in virtually every cell in Gleason primary patterns of 4 or 5.[27] PSMA expression is upregulated in prostate cancer, and the ratio of the mRNA encoding PSMA is nearly 100-fold greater than its splice variant, PSMA′, in cancer.[27,28]

Extraprostatic expression of PSMA is highly restricted and has been reported in the duodenal mucosa, a subset of proximal renal tubules, a subset of colonic crypt neuroendocrine cells, lactating breast, and salivary and submaxillary glands.[20,21,25]

PSMA immunoreactivity in cancer cells was not predictive of PSA biochemical failure or recurrence in a cohort of organ-confined margin-negative cancers treated by surgery[26]; these findings differ from serum studies in which elevated concentration of PSMA indicated surgical treatment failure.[20,29,30]

PSMA is clinically useful for diagnostic and therapeutic applications. PSMA is expressed in lymph node[21,25] and bone marrow metastases[25] of prostate cancer, underscoring its utility in identifying cancer of unknown primary site. Serum PSMA was of prognostic significance, especially in the presence of metastases, and correlated well with cancer stage in a screened population. It is also useful in reverse transcriptase-polymerase chain reaction (RT-PCR) assays that detect circulating PSMA-containing cells (presumptive tumor cells), providing positive results in 42% and 75%[31] of patients with localized prostate cancer.[32] Such PSMA-containing cells apparently spill into the circulation during radical prostatectomy, but decline in number following androgen deprivation therapy (ADT).[25] In suicide gene therapy, anti-PSMA–liposome complex exerted a significant inhibitory effect on the growth of LNCaP xenograft, in contrast to normal IgG–liposome complex.[33]

Tissue (Immunohistochemical) Diagnosis of PIN and Cancer (versus Benign Mimicks)

Select antibodies such as anti-keratin 34βE12 (high molecular weight keratin) and p63 are used to stain tissue sections for the presence of basal cells, recognizing that PIN retains an intact or fragmented basal cell layer whereas cancer does not (Fig. 30.2). In addition, racemase and c-myc are useful for staining of the dysplastic secretory cells of PIN (see below). We routinely generate unstained intervening sections of all prostate biopsies for possible future immunohistochemical staining, recognizing that

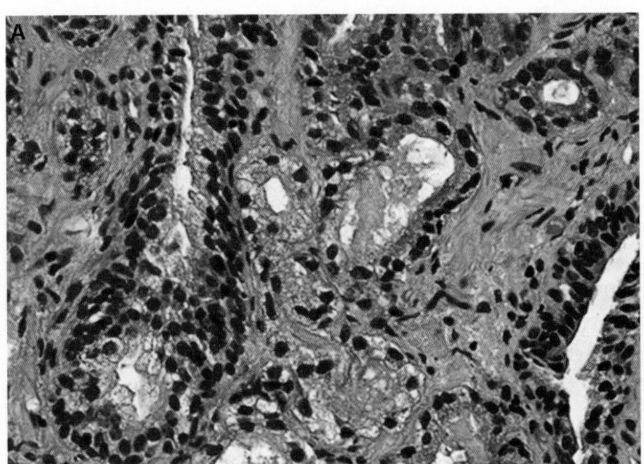

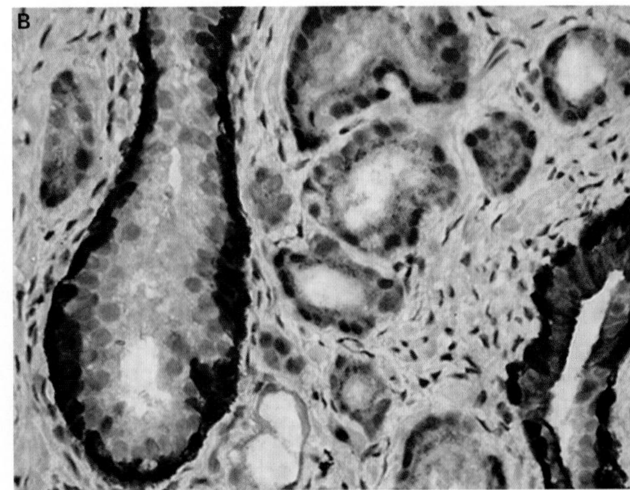

FIGURE 30–2 **A (left):** Routine hematoxylin and eosin–stained section of small adenocarcinoma adjacent to benign large acini. Compare with **B (right):** Triple multiplex immunostain, including brown cytoplasmic staining for keratin 34βE12 and brown nuclear staining for p63, completely staining virtually every basal cell at the periphery of the benign large acini on the left and right sides of the image. Compare with the smaller centrally located malignant acini that are decorated by the red reaction product for racemase.

small foci of concern are often lost when the tissue block is recut; one study reported loss of the suspicious focus in 31 of 52 cases when deeper sectioning was attempted.[34]

Multiple stain combinations (multiplex immunohistochemistry) such as triple staining with racemase, high molecular weight cytokeratin, and p63 are commonly used to confirm the diagnosis of prostate cancer, especially in diagnostically challenging cases (see Fig. 30.2). Routine dual-color immunostaining of all prostate biopsies for keratin 34βE12 and racemase in combination with routine H&E staining reportedly produced better diagnostic sensitivity with a smaller microscopy workload for the pathologist.[35,36] The recent addition of c-myc to create a quadruple stain provides additional invaluable diagnostic support for cancer, recognizing that there may be heterogeneity or complete lack of staining for some of the other markers.[37] These stain combinations must, of necessity, be used together on one slide owing to common loss of the focus of concern on deeper sections. Other antibodies directed against neuroendocrine markers may be useful in the diagnosis of small cell carcinoma of the prostate.

Cytokeratin 34βE12

Monoclonal basal cell–specific anti-keratin 34βE12 stains the cytoplasm of most normal basal cells of the prostate, with continuous intact circumferential staining in many instances. There is no staining in secretory and stromal cells. This marker was the first and remains the most commonly used immunostain for prostatic basal cells,[38,39] and methods of use with paraffin-embedded sections have been optimized.[40,41] Keratin 34βE12 is sensitive to formalin fixation and requires pretreatment by enzymes or heat if formalin-based fixatives are used. After pepsin predigestion or microwaving, there is progressive loss of immunoreactivity from 1 week or longer of formalin fixation. Heat-induced epitope retrieval with a hot plate yielded consistent results with no decrease in immunoreactivity with as long as 1 month of formalin fixation.[40] Staining intensity was consistently stronger at all periods of formalin fixation when the hot plate method was used, compared with pepsin predigestion or microwaving. Weak immunoreactivity was rarely observed in cancer cells after hot plate treatment, but not with pepsin predigestion or microwave antigen retrieval. Steam-EDTA (ethylenediaminetetraacetic) in combination with protease significantly enhanced basal cell immunoreactivity compared with protease treatment alone in benign prostatic epithelium.[42] Nonreactive benign acini were always the most peripheral acini in a lobule, a small cluster of outpouched acini furthest from a large duct, at the terminal end of a large duct, or showing simple atrophy.[43] More proximal acini had a discontinuous pattern of immunoreactivity.

Increasing grades of PIN have progressive disruption of the basal cell layer, according to studies utilizing anti-keratin 34βE12. Basal cell layer disruption is present in 56% of cases of high-grade PIN and is more frequent in acini adjacent to invasive carcinoma than in distant acini. Early invasive carcinoma occurs at sites of glandular out-pouching and basal cell discontinuity in association with PIN.[44] The cribriform pattern of PIN may be mistaken for the cribriform pattern of ductal adenocarcinoma, referred to as non-invasive ductal carcinoma, and the use of anti-keratin staining may be useful in making this distinction in combination with histologic features.[45] Cancer cells consistently fail to react with this antibody, although admixed benign acini may be misinterpreted as cancerous staining. Thus, immunohistochemical stains for anti-keratin 34βE12 may show the presence or absence of basal cells in a small focus of atypical glands, helping to establish a benign or malignant diagnosis, respectively. We believe that this antibody can be employed successfully if one judiciously interprets the results in combination with the light microscopic findings; relying solely on the absence of immunoreactivity (absence of basal cell staining) to render the diagnosis of cancer is without precedent in diagnostic immunohistochemistry and is discouraged. Nonetheless, some studies have noted that the rate of equivocal cases can be reduced considerably,[46] by 68%,[38] or from 5.1% to 1.0%[47] by addition of this immunohistochemical marker. Evaluation of prostate biopsies following therapy such as radiation therapy may be one of the most useful roles for anti-keratin 34βE12 (see below).

In addition to PIN and cancer, basal cell layer disruption or loss also occurs in inflamed acini, atypical adenomatous hyperplasia, and atrophy and postatrophic hyperplasia and may be misinterpreted as cancer if one relies exclusively on the immunohistochemical profile of a suspicious focus. Furthermore, basal cells of Cowper's glands may not express keratin 34βE12,[48] although this has been disputed.[49] Rare (0.2%) cases of adenocarcinoma have been reported that focally or weakly express keratin 34βE12, including foci of metastatic high-grade adenocarcinoma.[50] Basal cell hyperplasia is a histologic mimic of cancer, and use of anti-keratin 34βE12 is recommended in any equivocal cases that include this lesion in the differential considerations as it is invariably positive in that lesion.[51]

p63

p63 is a nuclear protein that is at least as sensitive and specific for the identification of basal cells in diagnostic prostate specimens as high molecular weight cytokeratin staining.[41,52-55] Shah et al.[56] found that p63 was more sensitive than keratin 34βE12 in staining benign basal cells, particularly in transurethral resection of the prostate specimens, offering slight advantage over keratins in diagnostically challenging cases. Zhou et al. demonstrated that the basal cell cocktail (34βE12 and p63) increased the sensitivity of the basal cell detection and reduced staining variability, thus rendering basal cell immunostaining more consistent.[41,57]

Racemase

The molecular marker, racemase (α-methylacyl-CoA racemase [AMACR], P504S) assists in discrimination of benign and neoplastic acini. This well-characterized enzyme catalyzes the conversion of several (2*R*)-methyl-branched-chain fatty acyl-CoAs to their (*S*)-stereoisomers. Analysis of mRNA levels of racemase revealed an average upregulation of ninefold in prostate cancer. The gene for AMACR is greatly overexpressed in prostate cancer cells. Its advantage over anti-keratin 34βE12 is its positive granular cytoplasmic staining in cancer cells, with little or no staining in benign acini.[41] In PIN, monoclonal and polyclonal antibodies to AMACR (P504S) were positive in 77% and 91% of foci, respectively, consistent with other studies. Since racemase is not specific for prostate cancer and is present in high-grade PIN (>90%), this staining must be interpreted with caution and the diagnosis of PIN or prostate cancer should be rendered only with convincing histologic evidence. Moderate to strong racemase expression in PIN is strongly suggestive of nearby coexistent adenocarcinoma.

c-myc

Most studies suggest that c-myc plays a role in the regulation of prostate growth and carcinogenesis. C-myc is a well-known oncogene that is activated in many human cancers and is amplified with increasing grade of prostate cancer, particularly in metastases. C-myc expression correlates with the growth of androgen-responsive prostate epithelium.[58]

Other Cytokeratins

CK5 and CK14 mRNA and protein are expressed in the basal cells of benign acini and PIN, and CK14 mRNA is present in low levels in the luminal cells of the most of some foci of PIN; thus, if PIN is derived from basal cells, as is currently believed, CK14 translation is depressed and a low level of CK14 mRNA may persist.[59] CK8 mRNA and protein are constitutively expressed in all epithelia of the normal and neoplastic prostate. CK19 mRNA and protein were expressed in both basal and luminal cells of benign acini. CK16 mRNA was expressed in a similar pattern as CK19, but CK16 protein was not detected.[59]

Basal cells display immunoreactivity at least focally for keratins 5, 10, 11, 13, 14, 16, and 19; of these, only keratin 19 is also found in secretory cells. Keratins found exclusively in the secretory cells include 7, 8, and 18.

Other Basal Cell Markers

Other markers of basal cells include proliferation markers, differentiation markers, and genetic markers. The preferential localization of many of these markers in basal cells but not in secretory cells suggests that they play a role in growth regulation. Basal cells usually do not display immunoreactivity for PSA, PAP, and S-100 protein, and only rare single cells stain with chromogranin and neuron-specific enolase. Conversely, the normal secretory luminal cells invariably stain with PSA and PAP. Prostatic basal cells do not usually display myoepithelial differentiation, in contrast with basal cells in the breast, salivary glands, pancreas, and other sites.

Proliferation Markers' PCNA and KI67/MIB-1

Proliferating cell nuclear antigen (PCNA) is an auxiliary protein for DNA polymerase that reaches maximal expression during the S-phase of the cell cycle. Hence, PCNA has been widely used as an index of the proliferative activity of cancers. The PCNA labeling index is reported to be lowest in benign normal prostatic epithelium and organ-confined cancer but to increase progressively from PIN to well-differentiated and poorly differentiated invasive prostate cancer, although there is wide variance (Table 30.1).[60] The correlation of PCNA index is strong with cancer stage. Hence, high PCNA

TABLE 30–1 Select Markers with Progressively Decreased or Increased Expression in Prostatic Intraepithelial Neoplasia and Cancer Compared with Benign Epithelium

Decreased Expression
Activated caspase-3
Androgen receptor expression
Annexin I
Annexin II
Blood group antigens
CD-10
Fibroblast growth factor-2
Hepatocyte growth factor activator inhibitor-1
Inhibin
Insulin-like growth factor binding protein-3
Interstitial collagenase (MMP-1)
Neuroendocrine cells
NKX3.1 homeobox gene-encoded protein
Ornithine decarboxylase
Prostate-specific antigen
Prostatic acid phosphatase
p-Cadherin
Prostate-specific transglutaminase
Telomerase
p27KIP1
5α-Reductase type 2
15-Lipoxygenase 1 and 2

Increased Expression
Amphiregulin
Aneuploidy
Apoptotic bodies
Aurora-A (Aurora 2 kinase, STK-15), a protein found in centrosomes
bcl-2 oncoprotein
Cell growth regulatory protein LIM domain only 2
Cell proliferation–associated protein Cdc46
Centrosome-associated protein Aurora-A (Aurora 2 kinase, STK-15)
c-erbB-2 (Her-2/neu) and c-erbB-3 oncoproteins
c-met proto-oncogene
Cyclooxygenase-2
Cysteine-rich secretory protein 3
Dentin sialophosphoprotein
Ep-Cam transmembrane glycoprotein
Epidermal growth factor and epidermal growth factor receptor
Estrogen receptor-α
FAS-related apoptosis signaling pathway markers "FAS associating protein with death domain, pro-caspase-8, and caspase-8"
Gelatinase B (MMP-9), matrilysin-1 (MMP-7), and the membrane-type 1-MMP
G-protein coupled receptor PSGR2
G1 cell cycle arrest regulator p16(INK4a)
Heat shock protein-90
Human glandular kallikrein 2
Hypoxia-inducible factor 1α
IL-6 and IL-10
Insulin-like growth factor binding protein rP1
Ki-67 expression
Lewis Y antigen
Macrophage inhibitory cytokine-1
Matriptase, a type II transmembrane serine protease
MMP-26
Metallothionein isoform II
MIB-1 expression
Microvessel density
Minichromosome maintenance protein-2
Mitochondrial protein MAGMAS
Mitotic figures
mTOR signaling pathway markers 4E-BP1 and p-4E-BP1
Mutator (RER (+)) phenotype
Neuropeptide Y
NOS-1 and NOS-2
Osteopontin
PCNA
Polo-like kinase-1
Prolactin receptor
Promoter methylation of GSTP1 gene
Prostate-specific membrane antigen
Prothymosin-α
Rac-specific guanine nucleotide exchange factor Tiam1
RNase III endonuclease Dicer
Serine/threonine kinase Pim-1
Tenascin-C
Transforming growth factor-α
Tissue inhibitor of metalloproteinases-4
TXA(2) synthase and TXA(2) receptors
Type IV collagenase
Vascular endothelial growth factor
p21
p53
p62 sequestosome 1 (SQSTM1) gene product
5α-Reductase type 1

MMP, matrix metalloproteinase; PCNA, proliferating cell nuclear antigen.

labeling indices may indicate progression of prostate cancer[61,62] and may be an independent prognostic indicator.

A high proliferation index for Ki-67 or MIB-1 appears to add little predictive information for patient outcome above the traditional indicators of Gleason score, pathologic stage, and DNA ploidy.[63] However, the Ki-67 labeling index may discriminate between organ-confined and metastatic cancer. Hence, elevation in the proliferation indices of Ki-67/MIB-1 appears to reflect progression.[64] This is further reflected in an association between expression of Ki-67 and epidermal growth factor receptor,[65] mutant p53,[65,66] particular chromosomal aberrations,[67] and perineural invasion.[68] In combination, these findings suggest that Ki-67 expression may be a weak predictor of recurrence, progression, and survival.[69]

Neuroendocrine Markers

Neuroendocrine cells are part of the widely dispersed diffuse neuroendocrine regulatory system, also known as endocrine–paracrine cells. In the human prostate, subpopulations of neuroendocrine cells have been identified based upon morphology and secretory products.[70-72] In LNCaP cell lines, the paracrine–endocrine phenotype can be induced by agents that increase intracellular dbcAMP levels (such as dbcAMP, forskolin, isoproterenol, and epinephrine). Tissue-specific expression of FoxA2 combined with Siah2-dependent hypoxia-inducible factor 1α availability enables a transcriptional program required for neuroendocrine tumor development and phenotype.[73]

Most neuroendocrine cells of the prostate contain serotonin, chromogranin A,[74,75] manserin,[76] and other neuroendocrine markers that are not consistently expressed. Neuroendocrine cells in the prostate are probably involved in regulation of growth, differentiation, and secretory functions.

There are three patterns of neuroendocrine differentiation in prostatic carcinoma: (1) as infrequent small cell neuroendocrine carcinoma; (2) rare carcinoid-like cancer; and (3) conventional prostatic cancer with focal neuroendocrine differentiation. Virtually all prostatic adenocarcinomas contain at least a small number of neuroendocrine cells, but special studies such as histochemistry and immunohistochemistry are usually necessary to identify these cells.[77] Neuroendocrine differentiation typically consists of scattered cells that are inapparent by light microscopy but revealed by immunoreactivity for one or more markers. Neuroendocrine cells in prostate cancer are malignant and lack AR expression. About 10% of adenocarcinomas contain cells with large eosinophilic granules (formerly referred to as adenocarcinoma with Paneth cell–like change), usually consisting of only rare foci of scattered cells and small clusters that may be overlooked.[78,79] Cells with large eosinophilic granules in the normal epithelium and adenocarcinoma resemble Paneth cells of the intestine and other sites by light microscopy, but they differ from Paneth cells by neuroendocrine differentiation (producing chromogranin, neuron-specific enolase, and serotonin) and lack of lysozyme expression.[78] The number of neuroendocrine cells in benign prostatic epithelium and adenocarcinoma is substantially greater than the number of cells with large eosinophilic granules, indicating that most neuroendocrine cells are not apparent on hematoxylin and eosin–stained sections.

Most cases of neuroendocrine carcinoma have typical local signs and symptoms of prostatic adenocarcinoma, although paraneoplastic syndromes are frequent in these patients. Cushing's syndrome is most common, invariably in association with adrenocorticotrophin (ACTH) immunoreactivity in tumor cells[80]; other clinical conditions include malignant hypercalcemia, syndrome of inappropriate antidiuretic hormone (SIADH) secretion, and myasthenic (Eaton-Lambert) syndrome. Small cell carcinoma is aggressive and rapidly fatal. Neuroendocrine carcinoma of the prostate varies histopathologically from carcinoid-like pattern (low-grade neuroendocrine carcinoma) to small cell undifferentiated (oat cell) carcinoma (high-grade neuroendocrine carcinoma). These tumors are morphologically identical to their counterparts in the lung and other sites. Typical acinar adenocarcinoma is present, at least focally, in most cases, and transition patterns may be seen. In cases with solid Gleason 5 pattern suggestive of neuroendocrine carcinoma, immunohistochemical stains are recommended. Mixed patterns may be observed, including one case with small cell carcinoma, adenocarcinoma, typical carcinoid, and spindle cell carcinoma.[79] A wide variety of secretory products may be detected within the malignant cells, including serotonin, calcitonin, ACTH, human chorionic gonadotropin, thyroid-stimulating hormone, bombesin, calcitonin gene-related peptide, amphiregulin, survivin, and inhibin. The same cells may express peptide hormones and PSA and PAP, but pure small cell carcinoma does not usually display immunoreactivity for PSA. Serotonin, chromogranin, and synaptophysin are the most useful markers of neuroendocrine cells in formalin-fixed sections of prostate.[81] Ultrastructurally, small cell carcinoma and carcinoid tumor of the prostate contain a variable number of round regular membrane-bound neurosecretory granules. Well-defined cytoplasmic processes are usually present which contain neurosecretory granules. The cells are small, with dispersed chromatin and small inconspicuous nucleoli.

Neuroendocrine cells have no apparent clinical or prognostic significance in benign epithelium, primary prostatic adenocarcinoma, and lymph node metastases, according to most but not all reports. Aprikian and colleagues[82] found no correlation between neuroendocrine differentiation and pathologic stage or metastases. We previously found no apparent relationship between the number of immunoreactive neuroendocrine cells in high-grade PIN and cancer and a variety of clinical and pathologic factors, including stage. Allen et al.[83] studied 120 patients and found no significant association between neuroendocrine differentiation and patient prognosis. Conversely, Weinstein and colleagues[84] studied 104 patients with clinically localized prostate cancer and found that neuroendocrine differentiation was associated with patient survival, although they restricted their study to cancers with Gleason scores of

5 and 6, so their findings may be influenced by selection bias. Frierson et al.[85] showed that neuroendocrine differentiation predicted patient survival, but this was only true for the analysis with one variable model. Krijnen et al.[86] reported that neuroendocrine differentiation was associated with early hormone therapy failure, indicating that these cells are androgen independent. Their findings suggested that the presence of large numbers of neuroendocrine cells in cancer may indicate a poor prognosis, perhaps due to insensitivity to hormonal growth regulation, but this has been refuted by most studies.[81,87] A recent study found that tissue chromogranin A expression, evaluated in prostate cancer needle biopsies at diagnosis, was an independent prognostic factor of survival in prostate cancer patients.[88] After radiation therapy, chromogranin A staining concentration independently predicted biochemical and clinical failure, distant metastases, and cause-specific survival.[89] We reported that lymph node metastases contain fewer chromogranin and serotonin-immunoreactive cells than benign prostatic epithelium and primary prostate cancer, suggesting that decreased expression of neuroendocrine markers is involved in cancer progression.[77] Neuroendocrine expression was not clinically useful for predicting outcome in patients with node-positive prostate cancer treated by radical prostatectomy.

Immunohistochemical Findings after Therapy

Immunohistochemical Findings after ADT

PSA, PAP, and racemase expression are retained in tumor cells after 3 months of therapy, but decline with longer duration of therapy[90]; keratin 34βE12 and p63 remain negative, regardless of duration, indicating an absent basal cell layer.[90] No differences were found in expression of neuroendocrine differentiation markers such as chromogranin, neuron-specific enolase, β-HCG, and serotonin following ADT, although some claim a significant increase. PCNA immunoreactivity declines after ADT, indicating that androgens regulate cyclically expressed proteins involved in cell proliferation. Some investigators reported that, after ADT, there was residual cancerous proliferative activity in lymph nodes, assessed by PCNA staining, and this was greater than that in primary tumors (4.5% and 1.3%, respectively).[91] This could be attributed to a metastatic phenotype that is less responsive to hormonal therapy than the primary tumor. In another study, PCNA was the same for tumors with lower and higher Gleason scores, suggesting that cellular dedifferentiation after neoadjuvant androgen deprivation represents a mere morphologic phenomenon and not a real increase in tumor aggressiveness.

Quantitative comparative genomic hybridization studies of untreated and treated prostate cancer revealed similar level of genetic alterations, suggesting that untreated cancer contains most of the chromosomal changes necessary for recurrence.[92]

The value of immunohistochemistry in predicting outcome after androgen deprivation has not been sufficiently validated to warrant routine clinical use (Table 30.2). However, one report found that shorter time to hormonal relapse was associated with high expression of aromatase and BCAR1 on diagnostic biopsy, together

TABLE 30–2 Prognostic Value of Immunohistochemical Findings in Prostate Cancer Treated with Androgen Deprivation Therapy

Biomarker	Prognostic Value
Androgen receptors	Not related to cancer-specific death
	Predictive of survival in advanced stage
	Decreased staining is predictive of failure of hormonal therapy
PSA	Increased expression predicted earlier relapse
Neuroendocrine cells	Not predictive of clinical outcome
HER2/neu	Competing data on cancer-specific survival
	Predicts time to biochemical failure
Bcl-2	Not predictive of cancer-specific survival
Ki-67	Higher values predictive of cancer recurrence
Fibroblast growth factor 8	Predicts worse survival in patients with androgen-independent cancer
Protein kinase C	Predicts decreased survival after relapse
BAG-1	Predicts earlier relapse
p53 immunoreactivity	Predicts androgen receptor gene amplification and cancer progression in patients with androgen-independent cancer
P21/WAF1/CIP1	Predictive of worse clinical outcome

PSA, prostate-specific antigen; HER2, human epidermal growth factor receptor 2.

with low staining for estrogen receptor-α in stromal cells. Overall survival was significantly shorter when tissues collected after relapse showed a high proliferation index and low estrogen receptor-α expression.[93] Another biomarker, N-cadherin, was more frequently found in tumors from patients treated with ADT than in those from patients with no prior hormonal treatment, and expression was associated with metastasis and Gleason score.[94]

ADT induced oxidative stress in in vitro and human prostate cancer according to immunohistochemical and Western blot studies.[95] Short-term administration of ADT interferes with BCL-2 expression, suggesting that androgen-mediated mechanisms may act through BCL-2-mediated apoptotic pathways, probably at the posttranscriptional level.[96]

Immunohistochemical Findings after Radiation Therapy

PSA, PAP, keratin 34βE12, p63, racemase, and c-myc expressions in the prostatic epithelium are not altered by radiation therapy and are often of value in separating treated adenocarcinoma and its mimics. Prostate cancer after radiation therapy has increased p53 nuclear accumulation and Ki-67 labeling index associated with a greater risk of distant metastasis and disease-specific survival.[97] Also, overexpression of survivin, Ki67, MDM2, and protein kinase A type I (PKA (RIα)) was associated with improved overall and prostate cancer survival on multivariate analysis.[98-100]

GENETIC MARKERS AND MOLECULAR CHANGES

Genetics of High-Grade PIN

High-grade PIN and prostate cancer share similar genetic alterations (see Table 30.1).[101-103] For example, 8p12-21 allelic loss is commonly found in cancer and microdissected PIN.[103] Other genetic changes found in carcinoma that already exist in PIN include loss of heterozygosity (LOH) at 8p22, 12pter-p12, and 10q11.2[103] and gain of chromosomes 7, 8, 10, and 12,[104] and the 8p24 and PTEN genes. LOH frequencies at 13q (one of the most common chromosomal alterations in high-stage cancer) is 0% vs. 49% in PIN and clinical prostate cancer, respectively. Alterations in oncogene bcl-2 expression and RER+ phenotype are similar for PIN and prostate cancer. Up to 64% of patients with PIN have LOH for the mannose 6-phosphate/insulin-like growth factor 2 receptor gene.

PIN is epigenetically similar to carcinoma according to the percentage of methylated alleles for the APC, glutathione S-transferase class π gene (GSTP1), and RARβ2 genes.[105] Methylation of the apoptosis-associated ASC promoter region was increased in PIN and cancer. TMPRSS2 exon 1 was fused in-frame with ERG exon 4 in 50% of prostate carcinomas and in 19% to 21% of cases of PIN, but not in benign prostatic controls, suggesting that the TMPRSS2–ERG fusion molecular rearrangement is an early event that may precede chromosome-level alterations in prostate carcinogenesis.

PIN is associated with progressive abnormalities of phenotype and genotype, which are intermediate between normal prostatic epithelium and cancer, indicating impairment of cell differentiation and regulatory control with advancing stages of prostatic carcinogenesis. There is progressive loss of some markers of secretory differentiation, cytoskeletal proteins, and multiple gene products. Other markers show progressive increase in expression from benign epithelium through PIN to cancer.[1] A model of prostatic carcinogenesis has been proposed based on the morphologic continuum of PIN and the multistep theory of carcinogenesis.[101]

Genetics of Adenocarcinoma

Prostate carcinogenesis involves multiple genetic changes, including loss of specific genomic sequences that may be associated with inactivation of tumor suppressor genes and gain of specific chromosome regions that may be associated with activation of oncogenes. The most common chromosomal aberrations in PIN and carcinoma are TMPRSS2–ETS translocations, gain of chromosome 7 (particular 7q31), loss of 8p and gain of 8q, and loss of 10q, 16q, and 18q.[106]

Despite decades of gene expression and sequencing studies, including next-generation sequencing, we have not succeeded in defining a unified molecular classification of prostate cancer.[107] Our efforts are hampered by the enormous complexity of this cancer—even when the earliest or smallest cancer is detected, it already contains hundreds of deregulated, aberrantly expressed, or mutated genes. This creates great difficulty in identifying gene-signaling pathways that are potential drivers of pathogenesis suitable for therapeutic intervention. Further, there is marked heterogeneity of prostate cancer at both the cellular level and the level of multifocality (e.g., "men don't get prostate cancer, they get prostate cancers.").

DNA Ploidy

DNA ploidy analysis of prostate cancer provides important predictive information that supplements histopathologic examination. Patients with diploid tumors have a more favorable outcome than those with aneuploid tumors. Among patients with lymph node metastases treated with radical prostatectomy and ADT, those with diploid tumors may survive 20 years or more, whereas those with aneuploid tumors die within 5 years.[108] However, the ploidy pattern of prostate cancer is often heterogeneous, creating potential problems with sampling error.[109] Analysis of multiple biopsies is important for correct preoperative ploidy estimation.[109] A good correlation exists between DNA ploidy and histologic grade,[110] and DNA ploidy adds clinically useful predictive information for some patients.[110] The incidence of aneuploidy in high-grade PIN varies from 32% to 68% and is somewhat lower than carcinoma (55% to 62%). There is a high level of concordance of DNA content of PIN and cancer. About 70% of aneuploid cases of PIN are associated with aneuploid carcinoma; conversely, only 29% of cases of aneuploid cancer are associated with aneuploid PIN. DNA ploidy pattern by flow cytometry correlates with cancer grade, volume, and stage. Most low-stage tumors are diploid and high-stage tumors are non-diploid, but numerous exceptions occur.

The 5-year cancer-specific survival is about 95% for diploid tumors, 70% for tetraploid tumors, and 25% for aneuploid tumors.[111] Biopsy ploidy status independently predicted cancer recurrence in patients treated by prostatectomy. Patients with diploid lymph node metastases treated by ADT alone had longer progression-free survival and overall survival than those with aneuploid metastases.[112] Digital image analysis appears to have a high level of concordance (about 85%) with radical prostatectomy specimens evaluated by flow cytometry.[113] For T1a prostate cancer, DNA ploidy was not predictive of progression or survival, but these patients have a very favorable prognosis.[114]

The popularity of DNA ploidy testing in the 1990s has waned this decade, replaced by more specific contemporary tests. (DG Bostwick, personal observations and communications, January 2012.)

Chromosome 7

Fluorescence in situ hybridization[115] studies showed that aneusomy of chromosome 7 is frequent in prostate cancer and associated with higher cancer grade, higher pathologic stage, and early patient death from prostate cancer.[116] PCR analysis of microsatellite markers identified frequent imbalance of alleles mapped to 7q31 in prostate cancer.[115,117] Allelic imbalance of 7q31 was strongly correlated with cancer aggressiveness, progression, and cancer-specific death.[118] These findings suggest that genetic alterations of the 7q-arm play an important role in the development of prostate cancer.

Chromosome 8

Chromosome 8p is one of the most frequently deleted regions in prostate cancer. The rate of 8p22 loss ranged from 29% to 50% in PIN, 32% to 69% in primary cancer, and 65% to 100% in metastatic cancer.[119] Other frequently deleted 8p regions include 8p21 and 8p12.[103,119] Emmert-Buck et al.[103] found the loss of 8p12–21 in 63% of PIN foci and 91% of cancer foci using microdissected frozen tissue. Bostwick et al.[120] detected the loss of 8p21–12 in 37% of PIN foci and 46% of cancer foci. These findings suggest that more than one tumor suppressor gene may be located on 8p, and inactivation of these tumor suppressor genes may be important for the initiation of prostate cancer. In addition to loss of the 8 p-arm, gain of the 8 q-arm has been reported in prostate cancer.[119,121] Bova et al.[122] found the gain of 8q in 11% of primary cancers and 40% of lymph node metastases. Van Den Berg et al.[123] found amplification of 8q DNA sequences in 75% of cancers metastatic to lymph nodes. Similarly, Visakorpi et al.[124] found gain of 8q far more frequently in locally recurrent cancer than in primary cancer. Cher et al.[125] also detected frequent gain of 8q in metastatic and androgen-independent prostate cancer. Four putative target genes for 8q gain have been identified and they are Elongin C at 8q21, as well as EIF3S3, KIAA0196, and RAD21 at 8q23–q24 regions. They seem to be overexpressed and amplified in about 20% to 30% of the hormone-refractory prostate carcinomas.[126,127] Gain of the chromosome 8 centromere or the 8 q-arm occurs simultaneously with loss of portions of the 8 p-arm in PIN and carcinoma.[121,124] One simple genetic mechanism that could explain these prior observations is the presence of multiple copies of isochromosome 8q in cancer cells.

Chromosome 10

There is also a high frequency of allelic imbalance at 10p and 10q in prostate cancer.[128] The most commonly deleted region on the 10 q-arm includes bands 10q23–24, and allelic loss of this region may inactivate the MXI-1 gene. Loss of PTEN, a tumor suppressor gene on chromosome 10q23, has been reported in 25% to 33% of advanced prostate cancer (Fig. 30.3). It has been associated with increased Gleason score and risk of clinical recurrence.[129]

Chromosome 16

Chromosome 16 had frequent allelic imbalance in prostate cancer. Allelic imbalance at 16q was present in about 30% of cases of clinically localized prostate cancer,[130] and there was a high frequency of allelic imbalance at 16q23–q24.[131] The most commonly deleted region was located at 16q24.1–q24.2, and this deletion was significantly associated with cancer progression.[131]

Other Chromosomes

The frequency of loss of 18q22.1 varied from 20% to 40%.[132] Other regions demonstrating frequent allelic imbalance include 3p25–26, 5q12–23, 6q, 13q, 17p31.1, and 21q22.2–22.3.[133] Loss of 10q, 16q, and 18q has also been reported in PIN.[120]

TMPRSS2 and ETS Family Gene Fusions

Gene fusions between the androgen-responsive gene TMPRSS2 and members of the ETS family of DNA-binding transcription factor genes were found in up to 70% of prostate cancers and a lower percentage of cases of high-grade PIN. Recurrent fusions were identified between the 5′-noncoding region of TMPRSS2 and ERG. These gene fusions are the driving mechanism for overexpression of the three members of the ETS transcription factor family, including ERG (21q22.3), ETV1 (7p21.2), and ETV4 (17q21). Considering the high incidence of prostate cancer and the high frequency of this

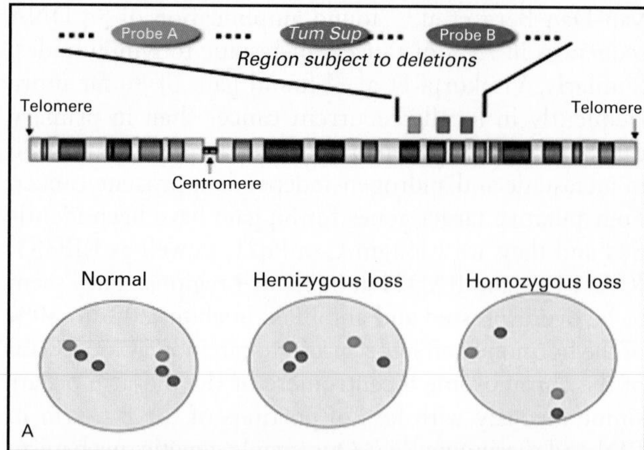

FIGURE 30–3 **A (left):** Changes to PTEN proteins are caused by deletion of the gene in cells. **B (left):** This deletion can be detected reliably by fluorescence in situ hybridization (FISH), which shows homozygous deletion detected by red FISH probe.

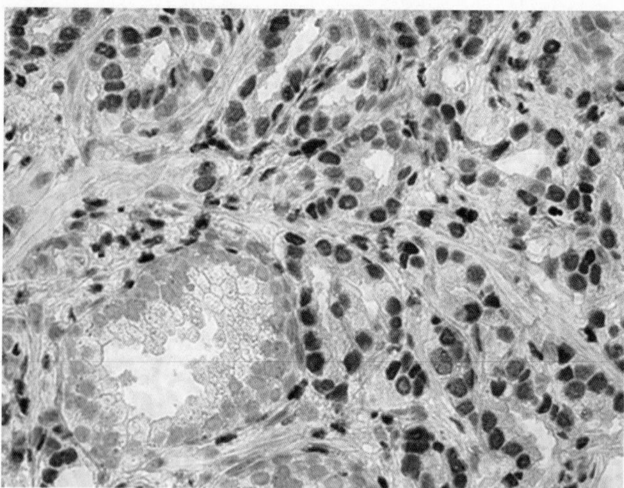

FIGURE 30–4 Adenocarcinoma displays intense nuclear reactivity (brown reaction product) for ERG, which stands in contrast with the absence of staining in large benign acinus in lower left of image.

gene fusion, the TMPRSS2–ETS gene fusion is the most common genetic aberration described to date in human malignancies (Fig. 30.4).

Fusion-positive tumors were associated with higher Gleason grade, higher stage, and poorer survival than fusion-negative tumors. Five morphological features were associated with TMPRSS2–ERG fusion prostate cancer, including blue-tinged mucin, cribriform growth pattern, macronucleoli, cancer spread with preexisting ducts and ductules, and signet-ring cell features. Distinct hybrid transcript patterns were found in samples taken from multifocal cancer, suggesting that TMPRSS2–ERG gene fusions arise independently in different foci. TMPRSS2:ERG gene fusions were also detected clinically in the urine of patients with prostate cancer.

Prostate Cancer Antigen 3 (PCA3)

The PCA3 gene, located on chromosome 9q21–22, is overexpressed more than 60-fold in more than 90% of prostate cancers but is not present in the benign prostate. Moreover, no PCA3 transcripts are detectable in a wide range of human extraprostatic benign and cancerous tissues, indicating that PCA3 is the most specific prostate cancer gene identified to date. The PCA3 mRNA includes a high density of stop codons; thus, it does not have an open reading frame, resulting in a noncoding RNA.

Independent studies showed that this test is a very promising adjunct tool for the early diagnosis of prostate cancer from urine samples. Radical prostatectomy specimens removed for carcinoma indicate that PCA3 is a significant and independent biomarker of prostate cancer that shows no correlation with serum PSA or prostate volume. However, it is predictive of cancer volume, stage, Gleason score, and positive surgical margins[134,135] and is not influenced by inflammation.[136] PCA3 gene testing holds valuable potential in PSA quandary situations: (1) men with elevated PSA levels but no cancer on initial biopsy; (2) men found to have cancer despite normal levels of PSA; (3) men with PSA elevations associated with varying degrees of prostatitis; and (4) men undergoing active surveillance for presumed microfocal disease.[137] In a large prospective multicenter study of biopsies, we found that PCA3 had a specificity of 78% and sensitivity of 49% for prostate cancer detection, and both parameters for serum PSA test were 21% and 87%, respectively.[138] We found that the PCA3 score is associated with Gleason score and cancer volume (Fig. 30.5). A higher PCA3 score was also correlated with an increased probability of detecting prostate cancer by histopathologic evaluation. The PCA3 urine test can be utilized after negative biopsy results are obtained to help determine which patients may be a candidate to undergo active surveillance and, possibly, a second biopsy.

Apoptosis-Suppressing Oncoprotein bcl-2

bcl-2 is considered to be an apoptosis suppressor gene. Overexpression of the protein in cancer cells may block

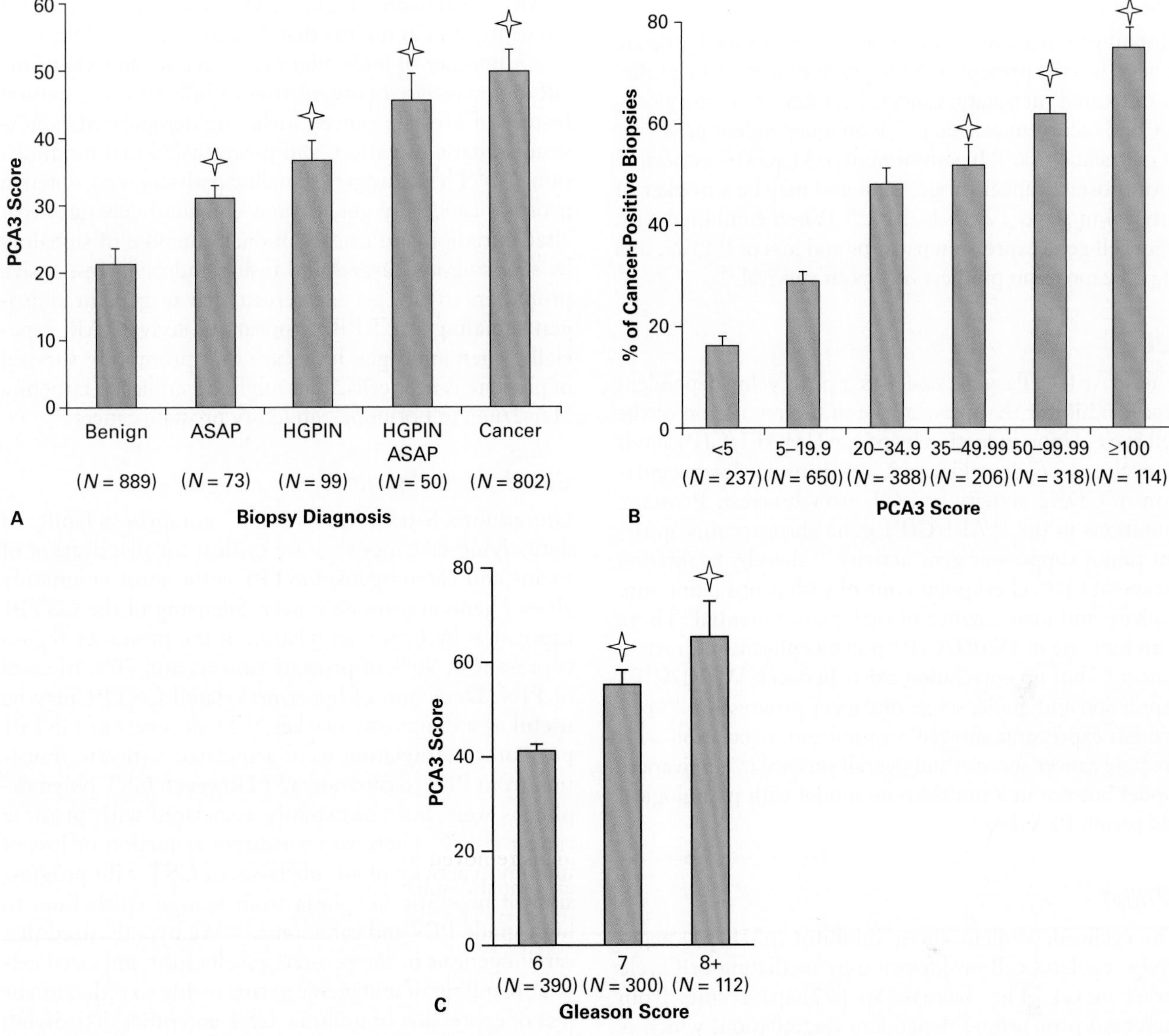

FIGURE 30–5 **A:** Relationship between PCA3 score and diagnosis of biopsy. **B:** Relationship between PCA3 score and detection rate (%) of prostate cancer–positive biopsies. **C:** Relationship between PCA3 score and Gleason score. *N* = number of evaluated biopsy cases. (A) and (C) * $P < 0.05$; (B) * $P < 0.0001$ to $P < 0.001$ (reprinted with permission from Crawford et al. 2012).

or delay onset of apoptosis by selecting and maintaining long-living cells and arresting cells in the G0 phase of the cell cycle.

Expression of bcl-2 is usually restricted to the basal cell layer of the normal and hyperplastic prostatic epithelium.[139] However, overexpression of bcl-2 is present in PIN. In cancer, the prevalence and expression pattern of bcl-2 are controversial. Over 70% of prostate carcinomas are bcl-2 negative, 18% have weak expression, and 11% exhibit strong expression.[140] One study found moderate heterogeneous bcl-2 overexpression in localized cancer[141] that was inversely correlated with Gleason grade.

Expression of bcl-2 correlated with high stage, high grade, metastases, response to therapy, biochemical recurrence-free survival, and cancer-specific survival.[142] Bcl-2 was positive in 46% cases, and Bax expression altered in 54% of cases after radiation therapy[143]; abnormal Bcl-2 was not related to any of the failure end points tested. Altered Bax expression was significantly associated with any failure and marginally with biochemical failure. The combination of negative Bcl-2/normal Bax expression seemed more robust after radiation and ADT, being significantly related to reduced biochemical failure and any failure.[143] ADT decreased bcl-2 expression in cancer, suggesting that these cells develop resistance to apoptotic signals.[141] Targeted suppression of bcl-2 anti-apoptotic family members using multi-target inhibition strategies through the effective induction of apoptosis is considered a research modality for the treatment of prostate cancer.[144]

p53

Mutant p53 expression is a late event in localized prostate cancer, usually present in high-grade cancer and elevated in untreated metastatic cancer, hormone-refractory cancer, and recurrent cancer. p53 is an independent predictor of metastatic risk.[145] Inactivation of p53 (-p53) is associated with prostate cancer progression and may be a marker of survival in stage T2-3N1-3M0.[146] When combined with stem cell gene expression patterns and loss of PTEN, loss of p53 expression predicts very poor survival.[147]

p21

The WAF1/CIP1 gene encodes a p21 cyclin-dependent kinase inhibitor that plays a role in the regulation of the cell cycle. Upon induction by p53, p21WAF1/CIP1 binds to cyclin-dependent kinase 2, resulting in downregulation of CDK2 activity and G1 growth arrest. Prostatic mutations in the WAF1/CIP1 gene abrogate this apparent tumor suppressor gene activity,[148] thereby facilitating escape of G1/S checkpoint control with propagation into S-phase and maintenance of malignant potential. There is an increase in WAF1/CIP1 polymorphisms in prostate cancer,[149] but no correlation exists between WAF1/CIP1 expression and grade, stage, or cancer progression.[150] p21 protein expression showed a significant association with prostate cancer survival and overall survival in a univariate model but not in a multivariate model with pathological and serum PSA data.[151]

p27Kip1

The cyclin-dependent kinase inhibitor (p27Kip1) negatively regulates cell proliferation by mediating cell cycle arrest in G1. The decrease in p27Kip1 results from increased proteasome-dependent degradation, which is mediated by its specific ubiquitin ligase subunits S-phase kinase protein 2 and cyclin-dependent kinase subunit 1. Cyclin-dependent kinase subunit 1 is involved in p27Kip1 downregulation and it may have an important causative role in the development of aggressive tumor behavior in prostate cancer.[152] p27Kip1 expression decreases with higher Gleason score and seminal vesicle involvement by cancer.[153] Further, p27Kip1 expression is an independent predictor of treatment failure of node-negative cancer following radical prostatectomy.[153,154]

Androgen Receptors

Androgen action in target cells is mediated by ARs. Mutations of AR are rare in untreated prostate cancer and are present in up to 25% of cancers from patients treated with anti-androgens.[155,156] No amplifications are found in untreated cancer, suggesting that androgen withdrawal selected the gene amplification. AR gene amplification leads to overexpression of the gene, and almost all hormone-refractory prostate carcinomas express high levels of AR.[157] It remains enigmatic what mechanisms exist for AR expression in tumors that do have gene amplification.

A number of molecular events act at the level of the AR and associated coregulators to influence the natural history of prostate cancer, including deregulated expression, somatic mutation, and posttranslational modification.[158,159] The androgen-signaling pathway is co-opted in prostate cancer by genetic and epigenetic changes that alter initiation and transcriptional outcome of signaling by silencing key targets and fusing androgen-responsive promoters to new genes to create new targets for androgen signaling.[160] ERBB[161] appears to activate AR, especially when androgen levels are low, promoting survival of prostate cancer cells. This might be similar to targeting Her-2/neu in hormone-refractory prostate cancer.[161]

GST Hypermethylation

Glutathione S-transferases (GST) comprise a family of detoxifying enzymes that are critical for inactivation of toxins and carcinogens. GSTP1 is the most commonly altered gene in prostate cancer. Silencing of the GSTP1 expression by hypermethylation of the promoter region is present in 90% of prostate cancers and 70% of cases of PIN. Detection of hypermethylated GSTP1 may be useful as a diagnostic marker.[162] High levels of GSTP1 promoter methylation were associated with the transition from PIN to carcinoma.[105] However, GST polymorphisms were not consistently associated with prostate cancer risk.[163] There was consistent reduction or loss of immunoreactivity of all subclasses of GST with progression of prostatic neoplasia from benign epithelium to high-grade PIN and carcinoma.[164] We hypothesized that carcinogenesis in the prostate results from impaired cellular handling of mutagenic agents owing to reduction or loss of expression of multiple GST and other detoxifying and anti-mutagenesis agents.

Mitochondrial DNA Testing

Mitochondrial DNA deletion was measured by quantitative PCR assay in negative biopsies from 101 patients who had repeat biopsy within a year.[165] Using an empirically established cycle threshold cutoff of 31, sensitivity and specificity were 84% and 54%, respectively, with the area under the receiver-operating characteristic curve of 0.75. The assay was predictive of missed cancer in 17 out of 20 men a year before diagnosis. This test appears to identify men who do not require a repeat biopsy with a high degree of accuracy. They also found that the majority of men with atypical small acinar proliferation have a concurrent missed tumor and therefore require close monitoring for early detection.

Integrins

Integrins participate in multiple cellular processes, including cell adhesion, migration, proliferation, survival, and activation of growth factor receptors. Several integrin α-subunits are downregulated, while β-subunits are upregulated.[166] The expression of several cadherins and catenins has specific prognostic value. There is an association between the expression of the E-cadherin/catenin complex and high-grade prostate cancer. Several integrin α-subunits are downregulated, while β-subunits are upregulated. The expression of several cadherins and catenins has specific prognostic value. There is an association between the expression of the E-cadherin/catenin complex and high-grade prostate cancer. Several integrin α-subunits are downregulated, while β-subunits are upregulated. The expression of several cadherins and catenins has specific prognostic value. There was an association between the expression of the E-cadherin/catenin complex and high-grade prostate cancer.

Multivariate analysis showed that immunohistochemical expression of α3 and α3β1 was related to worse outcome after radical prostatectomy.[167] When α3 expression was strong and α3β1 expression was positive, the odds of recurrence were 3.0- and 2.5-fold higher, respectively. Only 19% and 28% of patients were recurrence free in a mean period of 123 months of follow-up when their tumors showed strong α3 or positive α3β1 immunoreactivity, respectively.

Investigators from MD Anderson Cancer Center in Houston undertook a meta-analysis of gene expression data from 18 gene array data sets targeting the transition from normal to localized prostate cancer and from localized to metastatic prostate cancer.[168] They functionally annotated the top 500 differentially expressed genes and found the top differentially expressed genes to be clustered in pathways involving integrin-based cell adhesion: integrin signaling, the actin cytoskeleton, cell death, and cell motility pathways. Integrins were downregulated in the transition from benign tissue to primary localized cancer. Based on the results of their study, they developed the collagen hypothesis of prostate carcinogenesis in which the initiating event is the age-related decrease in the expression of collagen genes and other genes encoding integrin ligands. Concomitant depletion of integrin ligands leads to the accumulation of ligandless integrin and activation of integrin-associated cell death. To escape integrin-associated death, cells suppress the expression of integrins, which in turn alters the actin cytoskeleton, elevates cell motility and proliferation, and disorganizes prostate histology, contributing to the histologic progression of prostate cancer and its increased metastasizing potential.

Heat Shock Protein 90 (hsp90)

Cell surface Hsp90 is involved in prostate cancer cell invasion through the integrin β1/FAK/c-Src signaling pathway, and molecular targeting of cell surface Hsp90 may be a novel target for the effective treatment of metastatic prostate cancer. The hsp90 chaperone, tumor necrosis factor receptor-associated protein-1 (TRAP-1), is abundantly expressed in PIN and cancer but not in the benign prostate.[169]

Pro-PSA

Pro-PSA, the precursor of PSA, is an inactive 244-amino acid protein secreted by prostatic cells. It is found in serum as a distinct molecular form of free PSA in serum, including native and truncated forms. Truncated (−2) pro-PSA accounts for up to 19% of free PSA in the serum of patients without prostate cancer but represents up to 95% of free PSA.

Percent pro-PSA was superior to percent free and calculated complexed PSA for early detection in the PSA range of 2 to 10 ng/ml and it had selectivity for detecting more aggressive cancers, as indicated by Gleason score 7 or greater and/or extraprostatic extension of cancer.[170] However, this claim was recently challenged.[171]

In tissue samples, we found that 100% and 99% of cases of PIN and cancer were immunoreactive for [−5/−7] pro-PSA and [−2] pro-PSA, respectively.[172] A total of 31% of high-grade PIN and 11% of cancer cases with negative racemase staining showed strong staining for [−5/−7] pro-PSA. Both forms were sensitive markers for prostatic epithelium, making them possible candidates for investigating carcinoma with an unknown primary, particularly in cases in which PSA staining is negative and the level of suspicion is high.

Engrailed Nuclear Protein-2 (EN2)

EN2 gene is a homeobox-containing transcription factor overexpressed in prostate cancer cells when compared with benign epithelial cells. Downregulation of EN2 expression by siRNA resulted in decreased PAX2 expression and cancer cell proliferation. Recently, investigators from the University of Surrey (UK) demonstrated that EN2 in urine was highly predictive of prostate cancer, with a sensitivity of 66% and a specificity of 88.2%, with no relation to PSA concentration.[173]

Sarcosine and Other Metabolites

Sreekumar and colleagues[174] profiled more than 1,126 metabolites across 262 clinical samples related to prostate cancer (42 tissues and 110 each of urine and plasma) and identified sarcosine, an N-methyl derivative of the amino acid glycine, as a differential metabolite that was highly increased during prostate cancer progression to metastasis and that was detectable non-invasively in urine. Sarcosine levels were also increased in invasive prostate cancer cell lines relative to benign epithelial cells. Knockdown of glycine-*N*-methyl transferase, the enzyme that generates sarcosine from glycine, attenuated cancer invasion. Addition of exogenous sarcosine or knockdown of the enzyme that leads to sarcosine degradation, sarcosine dehydrogenase, induced an invasive phenotype in benign epithelial cells. AR and the ERG gene fusion product coordinately regulate components of the sarcosine pathway. However, Jentzmik and colleagues[175] noted that sarcosine had no clinical value as a marker for prostate cancer detection and identification of aggressive cancer.

Other Factors

A wide variety of other predictive factors have been evaluated in prostate cancer, but none are recommended at this time for routine use by the College of American Pathologists or the World Health Organization.[176-178]

Combining Multiple Predictive Factors

The combination of predictive factors provides the greatest accuracy of predicting stage and outcome. The American Joint Committee on Cancer recommends the use of neural network analysis or nomograms to improve prostate cancer survival prediction.[179]

CONCLUSION

This is arguably the most exciting time ever for the study of the molecular biology of prostate cancer. There is an urgent need for more sensitive and specific diagnostic and prognostic tests—despite the abundance of knowledge already known as described above—and the emergence of new technologies such as next-generation sequencing holds great promise for significant breakthroughs that will contribute to patient care. Further, the combination of diagnostics linked to therapy (e.g., Her2 in breast cancer) has not yet found a role in prostate cancer treatment but is likely to in the near future owing to the considerable effort being expended.

REFERENCES

1. Bostwick DG, Burke HB, Djakiew D, et al. Human prostate cancer risk factors. *Cancer*. 2004;101:2371-2490.
2. Aly M, Wiklund F, Gronberg H. Early detection of prostate cancer with emphasis on genetic markers. *Acta Oncol*. 2011;50(suppl 1): 18-23.
3. Kote-Jarai Z, Olama AA, Giles GG, et al. Seven prostate cancer susceptibility loci identified by a multi-stage genome-wide association study. *Nat Genet*. 2011;43:785-791.
4. Ewing CM, Ray AM, Lange EM, et al. Germline mutations in HOXB13 and prostate-cancer risk. *N Engl J Med*. 2012;366:141-149.
5. Macinnis RJ, Antoniou AC, Eeles RA, et al. A risk prediction algorithm based on family history and common genetic variants: application to prostate cancer with potential clinical impact. *Genet Epidemiol*. 2011;35:549-556.
6. Cao D, Hafez M, Berg K, Murphy K, Epstein JI. Little or no residual prostate cancer at radical prostatectomy: vanishing cancer or switched specimen?: a microsatellite analysis of specimen identity. *Am J Surg Pathol*. 2005;29:467-473.
7. DiGiuseppe JA, Sauvageot J, Epstein JI. Increasing incidence of minimal residual cancer in radical prostatectomy specimens. *Am J Surg Pathol*. 1997;21:174-178.
8. Bostwick DG, Bostwick KC. "Vanishing" prostate cancer in radical prostatectomy specimens: incidence and long-term follow-up in 38 cases. *BJU Int*. 2004;94:57-58.
9. Rocchi P, Muracciole X, Fina F, et al. Molecular analysis integrating different pathways associated with androgen-independent progression in LuCaP 23.1 xenograft. *Oncogene*. 2004;23:9111-9119.
10. Bostwick DG. Prostate-specific antigen. Current role in diagnostic pathology of prostate cancer. *Am J Clin Pathol*. 1994;102:S31-S37.
11. Schroder FH, Hugosson J, Roobol MJ, et al. Screening and prostate-cancer mortality in a randomized European study. *N Engl J Med*. 2009;360:1320-1328.
12. Andriole GL, Bostwick DG, Brawley OW, et al. Effect of dutasteride on the risk of prostate cancer. *N Engl J Med*. 2011;362:1192-1202.
13. Ishibashi M. Progress in standardization of total PSA immunoassays. *Rinsho Byori*. 2004;52:618-624.
14. Cheng L, Darson MF, Bergstralh EJ, Slezak J, Myers RP, Bostwick DG. Correlation of margin status and extraprostatic extension with progression of prostate carcinoma. *Cancer*. 1999;86:1775-1782.
15. De Marzo AM, Bradshaw C, Sauvageot J, Epstein JI, Miller GJ. CD44 and CD44v6 downregulation in clinical prostatic carcinoma: relation to Gleason grade and cytoarchitecture. *Prostate*. 1998;34:162-168.
16. Bettencourt MC, Bauer JJ, Sesterhenn IA, Connelly RR, Moul JW. CD34 immunohistochemical assessment of angiogenesis as a prognostic marker for prostate cancer recurrence after radical prostatectomy. *J Urol*. 1998;160:459-465.
17. Sinha AA, Quast BJ, Wilson MJ, et al. Immunocytochemical localization of an immunoconjugate (antibody IgG against prostatic acid phosphatase conjugated to 5-fluoro-2′-deoxyuridine) in human prostate tumors. *Anticancer Res*. 1998;18:1385-1392.
18. Goldstein NS. Immunophenotypic characterization of 225 prostate adenocarcinomas with intermediate or high Gleason scores. *Am J Clin Pathol*. 2002;117:471-477.
19. Varma M, Berney DM, Jasani B, Rhodes A. Technical variations in prostatic immunohistochemistry: need for standardisation and stringent quality assurance in PSA and PSAP immunostaining. *J Clin Pathol*. 2004;57:687-690.
20. Murphy GP, Elgamal AA, Su SL, Bostwick DG, Holmes EH. Current evaluation of the tissue localization and diagnostic utility of prostate specific membrane antigen. *Cancer*. 1998;83:2259-2269.
21. Troyer JK, Beckett ML, Wright GL Jr. Detection and characterization of the prostate-specific membrane antigen (PSMA) in tissue extracts and body fluids. *Int J Cancer*. 1995;62:552-558.
22. Brooks JD, Bova GS, Ewing CM, et al. An uncertain role for p53 gene alterations in human prostate cancers. *Cancer Res*. 1996;56:3814-3822.
23. Hessels D, Verhaegh GW, Schalken JA, Witjes JA. Applicability of biomarkers in the early diagnosis of prostate cancer. *Expert Rev Mol Diagn*. 2004;4:513-526.
24. Ghosh A, Heston WD. Tumor target prostate specific membrane antigen (PSMA) and its regulation in prostate cancer. *J Cell Biochem*. 2004;91:528-539.
25. Zaviacic M, Danihel L, Ruzickova M, et al. Immunohistochemical localization of human protein 1 in the female prostate (Skene's gland) and the male prostate. *Histochem J*. 1997;29:219-227.
26. Sweat SD, Pacelli A, Murphy GP, Bostwick DG. Prostate-specific membrane antigen expression is greatest in prostate adenocarcinoma and lymph node metastases. *Urology*. 1998;52:637-640.
27. Marchal C, Redondo M, Padilla M, et al. Expression of prostate specific membrane antigen (PSMA) in prostatic adenocarcinoma and prostatic intraepithelial neoplasia. *Histol Histopathol*. 2004;19:715-718.
28. Chang SS. Monoclonal antibodies and prostate-specific membrane antigen. *Curr Opin Investig Drugs*. 2004;5:611-615.
29. Ross JS, Sheehan CE, Fisher HA, et al. Correlation of primary tumor prostate-specific membrane antigen expression with disease recurrence in prostate cancer. *Clin Cancer Res*. 2003;9:6357-6362.
30. Schmidt B, Anastasiadis AG, Seifert HH, Franke KH, Oya M, Ackermann R. Detection of circulating prostate cells during radical prostatectomy by standardized PSMA RT-PCR: association with positive lymph nodes and high malignant grade. *Anticancer Res*. 2003;23:3991-3999.
31. Israeli RS, Powell CT, Corr JG, Fair WR, Heston WD. Expression of the prostate-specific membrane antigen. *Cancer Res*. 1994;54:1807-1811.

32. Yates DR, Roupret M, Drouin SJ, et al. Quantitative RT-PCR analysis of PSA and prostate-specific membrane antigen mRNA to detect circulating tumor cells improves recurrence-free survival nomogram prediction after radical prostatectomy. *Prostate*. 2012; 72:1382-1388.
33. Ikegami S, Yamakami K, Ono T, et al. Targeting gene therapy for prostate cancer cells by liposomes complexed with anti-prostate-specific membrane antigen monoclonal antibody. *Hum Gene Ther*. 2006;17:997-1005.
34. Green R, Epstein JI. Use of intervening unstained slides for immunohistochemical stains for high molecular weight cytokeratin on prostate needle biopsies. *Am J Surg Pathol*. 1999;23:567-570.
35. Tolonen TT, Kujala PM, Laurila M, et al. Routine dual-color immunostaining with a 3-antibody cocktail improves the detection of small cancers in prostate needle biopsies. *Hum Pathol*. 2011;42:1635-1642.
36. Kumaresan K, Kakkar N, Verma A, Mandal AK, Singh SK, Joshi K. Diagnostic utility of alpha-methylacyl CoA racemase (P504S) & HMWCK in morphologically difficult prostate cancer. *Diagn Pathol*. 2010;5:83.
37. Koh CM, Bieberich CJ, Dang CV, Nelson WG, Yegnasubramanian S, De Marzo AM. MYC and Prostate Cancer. *Genes Cancer*. 2010;1:617-628.
38. Novis DA, Zarbo RJ, Valenstein PA. Diagnostic uncertainty expressed in prostate needle biopsies. A College of American Pathologists Q-probes Study of 15,753 prostate needle biopsies in 332 institutions. *Arch Pathol Lab Med*. 1999;123:687-692.
39. Kahane H, Sharp JW, Shuman GB, Dasilva G, Epstein JI. Utilization of high molecular weight cytokeratin on prostate needle biopsies in an independent laboratory. *Urology*. 1995;45:981-986.
40. Varma M, Linden MD, Amin MB. Effect of formalin fixation and epitope retrieval techniques on antibody 34betaE12 immunostaining of prostatic tissues [see comments]. *Mod Pathol*. 1999;12:472-478.
41. Boran C, Kandirali E, Yilmaz F, Serin E, Akyol M. Reliability of the 34betaE12, keratin 5/6, p63, bcl-2, and AMACR in the diagnosis of prostate carcinoma. *Urol Oncol*. 2011;29:614-623.
42. Iczkowski KA, Cheng L, Crawford BG, Bostwick DG. Steam heat with an EDTA buffer and protease digestion optimizes immunohistochemical expression of basal cell-specific antikeratin 34betaE12 to discriminate cancer in prostatic epithelium. *Mod Pathol*. 1999;12:1-4.
43. Goldstein NS, Underhill J, Roszka J, Neill JS. Cytokeratin 34 beta E-12 immunoreactivity in benign prostatic acini. Quantitation, pattern assessment, and electron microscopic study. *Am J Clin Pathol*. 1999;112:69-74.
44. Bostwick DG, Brawer MK. Prostatic intra-epithelial neoplasia and early invasion in prostate cancer. *Cancer*. 1987;59:788-794.
45. Amin MB, Schultz DS, Zarbo RJ. Analysis of cribriform morphology in prostatic neoplasia using antibody to high-molecular-weight cytokeratins. *Arch Pathol Lab Med*. 1994;118:260-264.
46. Shin M, Fujita MQ, Yasunaga Y, Miki T, Okuyama A, Aozasa K. Utility of immunohistochemical detection of high molecular weight cytokeratin for differential diagnosis of proliferative conditions of the prostate. *Int J Urol*. 1998;5:237-242.
47. Freibauer C. Diagnosis of prostate carcinoma on biopsy specimens improved by basal-cell-specific anti-cytokeratin antibody (34 beta E12). *Wien Klin Wochenschr*. 1998;110:608-611.
48. Saboorian MH, Huffman H, Ashfaq R, Ayala AG, Ro JY. Distinguishing Cowper's glands from neoplastic and pseudoneoplastic lesions of prostate: immunohistochemical and ultrastructural studies. *Am J Surg Pathol*. 1997;21:1069-1074.
49. Cina SJ, Silberman MA, Kahane H, Epstein JI. Diagnosis of Cowper's glands on prostate needle biopsy. *Am J Surg Pathol*. 1997;21:550-555.
50. Yang XJ, Lecksell K, Gaudin P, Epstein JI. Rare expression of high-molecular-weight cytokeratin in adenocarcinoma of the prostate gland: a study of 100 cases of metastatic and locally advanced prostate cancer. *Am J Surg Pathol*. 1999;23:147-152.
51. Devaraj LT, Bostwick DG. Atypical basal cell hyperplasia of the prostate. Immunophenotypic profile and proposed classification of basal cell proliferations. *Am J Surg Pathol*. 1993;17:645-659.
52. Zhou M, Shah R, Shen R, Rubin MA. Basal cell cocktail (34betaE12 + p63) improves the detection of prostate basal cells. *Am J Surg Pathol*. 2003;27:365-371.
53. Tacha DE, Miller RT. Use of p63/P504S monoclonal antibody cocktail in immunohistochemical staining of prostate tissue. *Appl Immunohistochem Mol Morphol*. 2004;12:75-78.
54. Humphrey PA. Diagnosis of adenocarcinoma in prostate needle biopsy tissue. *J Clin Pathol*. 2007;60:35-42.
55. Hameed O, Sublett J, Humphrey PA. Immunohistochemical stains for p63 and alpha-methylacyl-CoA racemase, versus a cocktail comprising both, in the diagnosis of prostatic carcinoma: a comparison of the immunohistochemical staining of 430 foci in radical prostatectomy and needle biopsy tissues. *Am J Surg Pathol*. 2005;29:579-587.
56. Shah RB, Kunju LP, Shen R, LeBlanc M, Zhou M, Rubin MA. Usefulness of basal cell cocktail (34betaE12 + p63) in the diagnosis of atypical prostate glandular proliferations. *Am J Clin Pathol*. 2004;122:517-523.
57. Zhou M, Epstein JI. The reporting of prostate cancer on needle biopsy: prognostic and therapeutic implications and the utility of diagnostic markers. *Pathology*. 2003;35:472-479.
58. Kokontis J, Takakura K, Hay N, Liao S. Increased androgen receptor activity and altered c-myc expression in prostate cancer cells after long-term androgen deprivation. *Cancer Res*. 1994;54:1566-1573.
59. Yang Y, Hao J, Liu X, Dalkin B, Nagle RB. Differential expression of cytokeratin mRNA and protein in normal prostate, prostatic intraepithelial neoplasia, and invasive carcinoma. *Am J Pathol*. 1997;150:693-704.
60. Wang X, Hickey RJ, Malkas LH, et al. Elevated expression of cancer-associated proliferating cell nuclear antigen in high-grade prostatic intraepithelial neoplasia and prostate cancer. *Prostate*. 2011;71:748-754.
61. Idikio HA. Expression of proliferating cell nuclear antigen in node-negative human prostate cancer. *Anticancer Res*. 1996;16:2607-2611.
62. Taftachi R, Ayhan A, Ekici S, Ergen A, Ozen H. Proliferating-cell nuclear antigen (PCNA) as an independent prognostic marker in patients after prostatectomy: a comparison of PCNA and Ki-67. *BJU Int*. March 2005;95(4):650-654.
63. Coetzee LJ, Layfield LJ, Hars V, Paulson DF. Proliferative index determination in prostatic carcinoma tissue: is there any additional prognostic value greater than that of Gleason score, ploidy and pathological stage? [see comments]. *J Urol*. 1997;157:214-218.
64. Casella R, Bubendorf L, Sauter G, Moch H, Mihatsch MJ, Gasser TC. Focal neuroendocrine differentiation lacks prognostic significance in prostate core needle biopsies. *J Urol*. 1998;160:406-410.
65. Glynne-Jones E, Goddard L, Harper ME. Comparative analysis of mRNA and protein expression for epidermal growth factor receptor and ligands relative to the proliferative index in human prostate tissue. *Hum Pathol*. 1996;27:688-694.
66. Moul JW. Angiogenesis, p53, bcl-2 and Ki-67 in the progression of prostate cancer after radical prostatectomy. *Eur Urol*. 1999;35:399-407.
67. Henke RP, Kruger E, Ayhan N, Hubner D, Hammerer P. Numerical chromosomal aberrations in prostate cancer: correlation with morphology and cell kinetics. *Virchows Arch A Pathol Anat Histopathol*. 1993;422:61-66.
68. Aaltomaa S, Lipponen P, Vesalainen S, Ala-Opas M, Eskelinen M, Syrjanen K. Value of Ki-67 immunolabelling as a prognostic factor in prostate cancer. *Eur Urol*. 1997;32:410-415.
69. Li R, Wheeler T, Dai H, Frolov A, Thompson T, Ayala G. High level of androgen receptor is associated with aggressive clinicopathologic features and decreased biochemical recurrence-free survival in prostate: cancer patients treated with radical prostatectomy. *Am J Surg Pathol*. 2004;28:928-934.
70. Mahapokai W, Xue Y, van Garderen E, van Sluijs FJ, Mol JA, Schalken JA. Cell kinetics and differentiation after hormonal-induced prostatic hyperplasia in the dog. *Prostate*. 2000;44:40-48.
71. Mucci NR, Akdas G, Manely S, Rubin MA. Neuroendocrine expression in metastatic prostate cancer: evaluation of high throughput tissue microarrays to detect heterogeneous protein expression. *Hum Pathol*. 2000;31:406-414.
72. Kamiya N, Akakura K, Suzuki H, et al. Pretreatment serum level of neuron specific enolase (NSE) as a prognostic factor in metastatic prostate cancer patients treated with endocrine therapy. *Eur Urol*. 2003;44:309-314; discussion 314.
73. Qi J, Nakayama K, Cardiff RD, et al. Siah2-dependent concerted activity of HIF and FoxA2 regulates formation of neuroendocrine

phenotype and neuroendocrine prostate tumors. *Cancer Cell.* 2010;18:23-38.
74. McCormick DL, Rao KV. Chemoprevention of hormone-dependent prostate cancer in the Wistar-Unilever rat. *Eur Urol.* 1999;35:464-467.
75. Pruneri G, Galli S, Rossi RS, et al. Chromogranin A and B and secretogranin II in prostatic adenocarcinomas: neuroendocrine expression in patients untreated and treated with androgen deprivation therapy. *Prostate.* 1998;34:113-120.
76. Nishikawa K, Soga N, Ishii K, et al. Manserin as a novel histochemical neuroendocrine marker in prostate cancer. *Urol Oncol.* 2012. In press.
77. Bostwick DG, Qian J, Pacelli A, et al. Neuroendocrine expression in node positive prostate cancer: correlation with systemic progression and patient survival. *J Urol.* 2002;168:1204-1211.
78. Adlakha H, Bostwick DG. Paneth cell-like change in prostatic adenocarcinoma represents neuroendocrine differentiation: report of 30 cases. *Hum Pathol.* 1994;25:135-139.
79. Weaver MG, Abdul-Karim FW, Srigley JR. Paneth cell-like change and small cell carcinoma of the prostate. Two divergent forms of prostatic neuroendocrine differentiation. *Am J Surg Pathol.* 1992;16:1013-1016.
80. Watanabe K, Hoshi N, Hiraki H, Yamaki T, Tsu-Ura Y, Suzuki T. Neoplastic endocrine cells in prostatic carcinoma: a case report with immunocytochemical and electron microscopic findings. *Fukushima J Med Sci.* 1995;41:51-60.
81. Dizeyi N, Bjartell A, Nilsson E, et al. Expression of serotonin receptors and role of serotonin in human prostate cancer tissue and cell lines. *Prostate.* 2004;59:328-336.
82. Aprikian AG, Cordon-Cardo C, Fair WR, Reuter VE. Characterization of neuroendocrine differentiation in human benign prostate and prostatic adenocarcinoma. *Cancer.* 1993;71:3952-3965.
83. Allen FJ, Van Velden DJ, Heyns CF. Are neuroendocrine cells of practical value as an independent prognostic parameter in prostate cancer? *Br J Urol.* 1995;75:751-754.
84. Weinstein MH, Partin AW, Veltri RW, Epstein JI. Neuroendocrine differentiation in prostate cancer: enhanced prediction of progression after radical prostatectomy. *Hum Pathol.* 1996;27:683-687.
85. Theodorescu D, Broder SR, Boyd JC, Mills SE, Frierson HF Jr. Cathepsin D and chromogranin A as predictors of long term disease specific survival after radical prostatectomy for localized carcinoma of the prostate. *Cancer.* 1997;80:2109-2119.
86. Krijnen JL, Janssen PJ, Ruizeveld de Winter JA, van Krimpen H, Schroder FH, van der Kwast TH. Do neuroendocrine cells in human prostate cancer express androgen receptor? *Histochemistry.* 1993;100:393-398.
87. Yu DS, Hsieh DS, Chen HI, Chang SY. The expression of neuropeptides in hyperplastic and malignant prostate tissue and its possible clinical implications. *J Urol.* 2001;166:871-875.
88. Berruti A, Bollito E, Cracco CM, et al. The prognostic role of immunohistochemical chromogranin a expression in prostate cancer patients is significantly modified by androgen-deprivation therapy. *Prostate.* 2010;70:718-726.
89. Krauss DJ, Hayek S, Amin M, et al. Prognostic significance of neuroendocrine differentiation in patients with Gleason score 8-10 prostate cancer treated with primary radiotherapy. *Int J Radiat Oncol Biol Phys.* 2011;81:e119-e125.
90. Patterson RF GM, Jones EC, Zubovits JT, Goldenberg SL, Sullivan LD. Immunohistochemical analysis of radical prostatectomy specimens after 8 months of neoadjuvant hormonal therapy. *Mol Urol.* 1999;3: 277-286.
91. Minardi D, Galosi AB, Giannulis I, Montironi R, Polito M, Muzzonigro G. Comparison of proliferating cell nuclear antigen immunostaining in lymph node metastases and primary prostate adenocarcinoma after neoadjuvant androgen deprivation therapy. *Scand J Urol Nephrol.* 2004;38:19-25.
92. Cher ML, Bova GS, Moore DH, et al. Genetic alterations in untreated metastases and androgen-independent prostate cancer detected by comparative genomic hybridization and allelotyping. *Cancer Res.* 1996;56:3091-3102.
93. Celhay O, Yacoub M, Irani J, Dore B, Cussenot O, Fromont G. Expression of estrogen related proteins in hormone refractory prostate cancer: association with tumor progression. *J Urol.* 2010;184:2172-2178.
94. Jennbacken K, Tesan T, Wang W, Gustavsson H, Damber JE, Welen K. N-cadherin increases after androgen deprivation and is associated with metastasis in prostate cancer. *Endocr Relat Cancer.* 2010;17:469-479.
95. Shiota M, Song Y, Takeuchi A, et al. Antioxidant therapy alleviates oxidative stress by androgen deprivation and prevents conversion from androgen dependent to castration resistant prostate cancer. *J Urol.* 2012;187:707-714.
96. Fuzio P, Ditonno P, Lucarelli G, et al. Androgen deprivation therapy affects BCL-2 expression in human prostate cancer. *Int J Oncol.* 2011;39:1233-1242.
97. Li R, Heydon K, Hammond ME, et al. Ki-67 staining index predicts distant metastasis and survival in locally advanced prostate cancer treated with radiotherapy: an analysis of patients in radiation therapy oncology group protocol 86-10. *Clin Cancer Res.* 2004;10:4118-4124.
98. Zhang M, Ho A, Hammond EH, et al. Prognostic value of survivin in locally advanced prostate cancer: study based on RTOG 8610. *Int J Radiat Oncol Biol Phys.* 2009;73:1033-1042.
99. Khor LY, Bae K, Paulus R, et al. MDM2 and Ki-67 predict for distant metastasis and mortality in men treated with radiotherapy and androgen deprivation for prostate cancer: RTOG 92-02. *J Clin Oncol.* 2009;27:3177-3184.
100. Pollack A, Bae K, Khor LY, et al. The importance of protein kinase A in prostate cancer: relationship to patient outcome in Radiation Therapy Oncology Group trial 92-02. *Clin Cancer Res.* 2009;15:5478-5484.
101. Bostwick DG, Pacelli A, Lopez-Beltran A. Molecular biology of prostatic intraepithelial neoplasia. *Prostate.* 1996;29:117-134.
102. Bostwick DG. Progression of prostatic intraepithelial neoplasia to early invasive adenocarcinoma. *Eur Urol.* 1996;30:145-152.
103. Emmert-Buck MR, Vocke CD, Pozzatti RO, et al. Allelic loss on chromosome 8p12-21 in microdissected prostatic intraepithelial neoplasia. *Cancer Res.* 1995;55:2959-2962.
104. Qian J, Jenkins RB, Bostwick DG. Chromosomal anomalies in atypical adenomatous hyperplasia and carcinoma of the prostate using fluorescence in situ hybridization. *Urology.* 1995;46:837-842.
105. Henrique R, Jeronimo C, Teixeira MR, et al. Epigenetic heterogeneity of high-grade prostatic intraepithelial neoplasia: clues for clonal progression in prostate carcinogenesis. *Mol Cancer Res.* 2006;4:1-8.
106. Qian J, Jenkins RB, Bostwick DG. Determination of gene and chromosome dosage in prostatic intraepithelial neoplasia and carcinoma. *Anal Quant Cytol Histol.* 1998;20:373-380.
107. Farooqi AA, Bhatti S, Nawaz A, Khalid AM. One size fits all in prostate cancer: a story tale whose time has come and gone. *Int J Biol Markers.* 2011;26:75-81.
108. Zincke H, Bergstralh EJ, Larson-Keller JJ, et al. Stage D1 prostate cancer treated by radical prostatectomy and adjuvant hormonal treatment. Evidence for favorable survival in patients with DNA diploid tumors. *Cancer.* 1992;70:311-323.
109. Haggarth L, Auer G, Busch C, Norberg M, Haggman M, Egevad L. The significance of tumor heterogeneity for prediction of DNA ploidy of prostate cancer. *Scand J Urol Nephrol.* 2005;39:387-392.
110. Bantis A, Gonidi M, Athanassiades P, et al. Prognostic value of DNA analysis of prostate adenocarcinoma: correlation to clinicopathologic predictors. *J Exp Clin Cancer Res.* 2005;24:273-278.
111. Deitch AD, deVere-White RW. Flow cytometry as a predictive modality in prostate cancer. *Hum Pathol.* 1992;23:352-359.
112. Pollack A, Zagars GK. External beam radiotherapy dose response of prostate cancer. *Int J Radiat Oncol Biol Phys.* 1997;39:1011-1018.
113. Takai K, Goellner JR, Katzmann JA, Myers RP, Lieber MM. Static image and flow DNA cytometry of prostatic adenocarcinoma: studies of needle biopsy and radical prostatectomy specimens. *J Urol Pathol.* 1994;2:39-48.
114. Abaza R Diaz LK Jr, Laskin WB, Pins MR. Prognostic value of DNA ploidy, bcl-2 and p53 in localized prostate adenocarcinoma incidentally discovered at transurethral prostatectomy. *J Urol.* December 2006;176(6 pt 1):2701-2705.
115. Jenkins RB, Qian J, Lee HK, et al. A molecular cytogenetic analysis of 7q31 in prostate cancer. *Cancer Res.* 1998;58:759-766.
116. Das K, Lau W, Sivaswaren C, et al. Chromosomal changes in prostate cancer: a fluorescence in situ hybridization study. *Clin Genet.* July 2005;68(1):40-47.

117. Takahashi S, Shan AL, Ritland SR, et al. Frequent loss of heterozygosity at 7q31.1 in primary prostate cancer is associated with tumor aggressiveness and progression. *Cancer Res.* 1995;55:4114-4119.
118. Takahashi S, Qian J, Brown JA, et al. Potential markers of prostate cancer aggressiveness detected by fluorescence in situ hybridization in needle biopsies. *Cancer Res.* 1994;54:3574-3579.
119. Macoska JA, Trybus TM, Benson PD, et al. Evidence for three tumor suppressor gene loci on chromosome 8p in human prostate cancer. *Cancer Res.* 1995;55:5390-5395.
120. Bostwick DG, Shan A, Qian J, et al. Independent origin of multiple foci of prostatic intraepithelial neoplasia: comparison with matched foci of prostate carcinoma. *Cancer.* 1998;83:1995-2002.
121. Jenkins RB, Qian J, Lieber MM, Bostwick DG. Detection of c-myc oncogene amplification and chromosomal anomalies in metastatic prostatic carcinoma by fluorescence in situ hybridization. *Cancer Res.* 1997;57:524-531.
122. Bova GS, Fox WM, Epstein JI. Methods of radical prostatectomy specimen processing: a novel technique for harvesting fresh prostate cancer tissue and review of processing techniques. *Mod Pathol.* 1993;6:201-207.
123. Van Den Berg C, Guan XY, Von Hoff D, et al. DNA sequence amplification in human prostate cancer identified by chromosome microdissection: potential prognostic implications. *Clin Cancer Res.* 1995;1:11-18.
124. Visakorpi T, Kallioniemi AH, Syvanen AC, et al. Genetic changes in primary and recurrent prostate cancer by comparative genomic hybridization. *Cancer Res.* 1995;55:342-347.
125. Cher ML, MacGrogan D, Bookstein R, Brown JA, Jenkins RB, Jensen RH. Comparative genomic hybridization, allelic imbalance, and fluorescence in situ hybridization on chromosome 8 in prostate cancer. *Genes Chromosomes Cancer.* 1994;11:153-162.
126. Porkka K, Saramaki O, Tanner M, Visakorpi T. Amplification and overexpression of Elongin C gene discovered in prostate cancer by cDNA microarrays. *Lab Invest.* 2002;82:629-637.
127. Porkka KP, Tammela TL, Vessella RL, Visakorpi T. RAD21 and KIAA0196 at 8q24 are amplified and overexpressed in prostate cancer. *Genes Chromosomes Cancer.* January 2004;39(1):1-10.
128. Ittman M, Mansukhani A. Expression of fibroblast growth factors (FGFs) and FGF receptors in human prostate. *J Urol.* 1997;157:351-356.
129. Halvorsen OJ, Haukaas SA, Akslen LA. Combined loss of PTEN and p27 expression is associated with tumor cell proliferation by Ki-67 and increased risk of recurrent disease in localized prostate cancer. *Clin Cancer Res.* April 2003;9(4):1474-1479.
130. Carter BS, Epstein JI, Isaacs WB. ras gene mutations in human prostate cancer. *Cancer Res.* 1990;50:6830-6832.
131. Latil A, Cussenot O, Fournier G, Driouch K, Lidereau R. Loss of heterozygosity at chromosome 16q in prostate adenocarcinoma: identification of three independent regions. *Cancer Res.* 1997;57:1058-1062.
132. Gray IC, Phillips SM, Lee SJ, Neoptolemos JP, Weissenbach J, Spurr NK. Loss of the chromosomal region 10q23-25 in prostate cancer. *Cancer Res.* 1995;55:4800-4803.
133. Bergheim USR, Kunimi K, Collins VP, Ekman P. Deletion of chromosome 8, 10 and 16 in human prostatic carcinoma. *Genes Chromosomes Cancer.* 1991;3:215-220.
134. Durand X, Xylinas E, Radulescu C, et al. The value of urinary prostate cancer gene 3 (PCA3) scores in predicting pathological features at radical prostatectomy. *BJU Int.* 2012;110:43-49.
135. de la Taille A, Irani J, Graefen M, et al. Clinical evaluation of the PCA3 assay in guiding initial biopsy decisions. *J Urol.* 2011;185:2119-2125.
136. Vlaeminck-Guillem V, Bandel M, Cottancin M, Rodriguez-Lafrasse C, Bohbot JM, Sednaoui P. Chronic prostatitis does not influence urinary PCA3 score. *Prostate.* 2011;72:549-554.
137. Marks LS, Bostwick DG. Prostate cancer specificity of PCA3 gene testing: examples from clinical practice. *Rev Urol.* 2008;10:175-181.
138. Crawford ED, Rove KO, Trabulsi EJ, et al. Diagnostic performance of PCA3 to detect prostate cancer in men with elevated PSA: a prospective study of 1,952 cases. *J Urol.* 2012. In press.
139. Foster CS, Ke Y. Stem cells in prostatic epithelia. *Int J Exp Pathol.* 1997;78:311-329.
140. Lipponen P, Vesalainen S. Expression of the apoptosis suppressing protein bcl-2 in prostatic adenocarcinoma is related to tumor malignancy. *Prostate.* 1997;32:9-15.
141. Hockenbery DM, Zutter M, Hickey W, Nahm M, Korsmeyer SJ. BCL2 protein is topographically restricted in tissues characterized by apoptotic cell death. *Proc Natl Acad Sci U S A.* 1991;88:6961-6965.
142. Concato J, Jain D, Uchio E, Risch H, Li WW, Wells CK. Molecular markers and death from prostate cancer. *Ann Intern Med.* 2009;150:595-603.
143. Khor LY, Moughan J, Al-Saleem T, et al. Bcl-2 and Bax expression predict prostate cancer outcome in men treated with androgen deprivation and radiotherapy on radiation therapy oncology group protocol 92-02. *Clin Cancer Res.* 2007;13:3585-3590.
144. Yamanaka K, Rocchi P, Miyake H, et al. Induction of apoptosis and enhancement of chemosensitivity in human prostate cancer LNCaP cells using bispecific antisense oligonucleotide targeting Bcl-2 and Bcl-xL genes. *BJU Int.* June 2006;97(6):1300-1308.
145. Petrescu A, M Cerzan L, Codreanu O, Niculescu L. Immunohistochemical detection of p53 protein as a prognostic indicator in prostate carcinoma. *Rom J Morphol Embryol.* 2006;47(2):143-146.
146. Moul JW, Bettencourt MC, Sesterhenn IA, et al. Protein expression of p53, bcl-2, and KI-67 (MIB-1) as prognostic biomarkers in patients with surgically treated, clinically localized prostate cancer. *Surgery.* 1996;120:159-166; discussion 166-167.
147. Markert EK, Mizuno H, Vazquez A, Levine AJ. Molecular classification of prostate cancer using curated expression signatures. *Proc Natl Acad Sci U S A.* 2011;108:21276-21281.
148. Gao X, Chen YQ, Wu N, et al. Somatic mutations of the WAF1/CIP1 gene in primary prostate cancer. *Oncogene.* 1997;11:1395-1398.
149. Facher EA, Becich MJ, Deka A, Law JC. Association between human cancer and two polymorphisms occurring in the p21WAF1/CIP1 cyclin-dependent kinase inhibitor gene. *Cancer.* 1997;79:2424-2429.
150. Byrne RL, Horne CH, Robinson MC, et al. The expression of waf-1, p53 and bcl-2 in prostatic adenocarcinoma. *Br J Urol.* 1997;79:190-195.
151. Kudahetti SC, Fisher G, Ambroisine L, et al. Immunohistochemistry for p16, but not Rb or p21, is an independent predictor of prognosis in conservatively treated, clinically localised prostate cancer. *Pathology.* 2010;42: 519-523.
152. Shapira M, Ben-Izhak O, Slotky M, Goldin O, Lahav-Baratz S, Hershko DD. Expression of the ubiquitin ligase subunit cyclin kinase subunit 1 and its relationship to S-phase kinase protein 2 and p27Kip1 in prostate cancer. *J Urol.* 2006;176:2285-2289.
153. Tsihlias J, Kapusta LR, DeBoer G, et al. Loss of cyclin-dependent kinase inhibitor p27Kip1 is a novel prognostic factor in localized human prostate adenocarcinoma. *Cancer Res.* 1998;58:542-548.
154. Ananthanarayanan V, Deaton RJ, Amatya A, et al. Subcellular localization of p27 and prostate cancer recurrence: automated digital microscopy analysis of tissue microarrays. *Hum Pathol.* 2011;42:873-881.
155. Taplin ME, Bubley GJ, Shuster TD, et al. Mutation of the androgen-receptor gene in metastatic androgen-independent prostate cancer. *N Engl J Med.* 1995;332:1393-1398.
156. Haapala K, Hyytinen ER, Roiha M, et al. Androgen receptor alterations in prostate cancer relapsed during a combined androgen blockade by orchiectomy and bicalutamide. *Lab Invest.* 2001;81:1647-1651.
157. Linja MJ, Savinainen K, Saramaki OR, Tammela TL, Vessella RL, Visakorpi T. Amplification and overexpression of androgen receptor gene in hormone-refractory prostate cancer. *Cancer Res.* May 2001;61(9):3550-3555.
158. Chmelar R, Buchanan G, Need EF, Tilley W, Greenberg NM. Androgen receptor coregulators and their involvement in the development and progression of prostate cancer. *Int J Cancer.* February 2007;120(4):719-733.
159. Burd CJ, Morey LM, Knudsen KE. Androgen receptor corepressors and prostate cancer. *Endocr Relat Cancer.* 2006;13:979-994.
160. Marker PC. Does prostate cancer co-opt the developmental program? *Differentiation.* 2008;76:736-744.
161. Berger R, Lin DI, Nieto M, et al. Androgen-dependent regulation of Her-2/neu in prostate cancer cells. *Cancer Res.* 2006;66:5723-5728.
162. Reibenwein J, Pils D, Horak P, et al. Promoter hypermethylation of GSTP1, AR, and 14-3-3sigma in serum of prostate cancer patients and its clinical relevance. *Prostate.* 2006;67:427-432.

163. Sivonova M, Waczulikova I, Dobrota D, et al. Polymorphisms of glutathione-S-transferase M1, T1, P1 and the risk of prostate cancer: a case-control study. *J Exp Clin Cancer Res*. 2009;28:32.
164. Bostwick DG, Meiers I, Shanks JH. Glutathione S-transferase: differential expression of alpha, mu, and pi isoenzymes in benign prostate, prostatic intraepithelial neoplasia, and prostatic adenocarcinoma. *Hum Pathol*. 2007;38:1394-1401.
165. Robinson K, Creed J, Reguly B, et al. Accurate prediction of repeat prostate biopsy outcomes by a mitochondrial DNA deletion assay. *Prostate Cancer Prostatic Dis*. 2010;13:126-131.
166. Karlou M, Tzelepi V, Efstathiou E. Therapeutic targeting of the prostate cancer microenvironment. *Nat Rev Urol*. 2010;7:494-509.
167. Pontes-Junior J, Reis ST, de Oliveira LC, et al. Association between integrin expression and prognosis in localized prostate cancer. *Prostate*. 2010;70:1189-1195.
168. Gorlov IP, Byun J, Gorlova OY, Aparicio AM, Efstathiou E, Logothetis CJ. Candidate pathways and genes for prostate cancer: a meta-analysis of gene expression data. *BMC Med Genomics*. 2009;2:48.
169. Leav I, Plescia J, Goel HL, et al. Cytoprotective mitochondrial chaperone TRAP-1 as a novel molecular target in localized and metastatic prostate cancer. *Am J Pathol*. 2010;176:393-401.
170. Catalona WJ, Bartsch G, Rittenhouse HG, et al. Serum pro-prostate specific antigen preferentially detects aggressive prostate cancers in men with 2 to 4 ng/ml prostate specific antigen. *J Urol*. 2004;171:2239-2244.
171. Liang Y, Ankerst DP, Ketchum NS, et al. Prospective evaluation of operating characteristics of prostate cancer detection biomarkers. *J Urol*. 2011;185:104-110.
172. Hull D, Ma J, Singh H, Hossain D, Qian J, Bostwick DG. Precursor of prostate-specific antigen expression in prostatic intraepithelial neoplasia and adenocarcinoma: a study of 90 cases. *BJU Int*. 2009;104:915-918.
173. Morgan R, Boxall A, Bhatt A, et al. Engrailed-2 (EN2): a tumor specific urinary biomarker for the early diagnosis of prostate cancer. *Clin Cancer Res*. 2011;17:1090-1098.
174. Sreekumar A, Poisson LM, Rajendiran TM, et al. Metabolomic profiles delineate potential role for sarcosine in prostate cancer progression. *Nature*. 2009;457:910-914.
175. Jentzmik F, Stephan C, Miller K, et al. Sarcosine in urine after digital rectal examination fails as a marker in prostate cancer detection and identification of aggressive tumours. *Eur Urol*. 2011;58:12-18; discussion 20-21.
176. Brawer MK, Benson MC, Bostwick DG, et al. Prostate-specific antigen and other serum markers: current concepts from the World Health Organization Second International Consultation on Prostate Cancer. *Semin Urol Oncol*. 1999;17:206-221.
177. Bostwick DG, Montironi R, Sesterhenn IA. Diagnosis of prostatic intraepithelial neoplasia: Prostate Working Group/consensus report. *Scand J Urol Nephrol Suppl*. 2000;205:3-10.
178. Srigley JR. Key issues in handling and reporting radical prostatectomy specimens. *Arch Pathol Lab Med*. 2006;130:303-317.
179. Burke HB, Goodman PH, Rosen DB, et al. Artificial neural networks improve the accuracy of cancer survival prediction. *Cancer*. 1997;79:857-862.

CHAPTER 31

Molecular Diagnostics of Hepatocellular Carcinoma

Seung Kew Yoon, Hyun Goo Woo, Dongfeng Tan, and Yoon Jun Kim

INTRODUCTION

Hepatocellular carcinoma (HCC) is the sixth most common cancer worldwide and the third leading cause of cancer-related death.[1] Liver cirrhosis, irrespective of etiology, caused by hepatitis C virus (HCV) infection, heavy alcohol consumption, nonalcoholic steatohepatitis, hemochromatosis, autoimmune diseases, and hepatitis B virus (HBV)–related liver diseases even in the absence of cirrhosis, are major risk factors for developing HCC. Although the overall prevalence of HBV infection has decreased globally with the development of an effective vaccine, the incidence of HCV infection has been increasing in the United States and Europe, resulting in an increase in the incidence of HCC.[2,3]

Geographically, China alone accounts for more than 55% of the world's cases of HCC.[4] This may be due to the prevalence of HBV infection and endemic exposure to aflatoxin B_1 (AFB_1), a well-known carcinogenic mycotoxin. Other geographic areas of endemic HBV infection, including sub-Saharan Africa and Asia, also account for the high incidence of HCC. Indeed, a handful of evidence has demonstrated that HBV causes HCC development. Chronic HBV infection and its replication are associated with an increased risk of HCC. Consequently, the World Health Organization includes HBV in a list of "group 1" human carcinogens classifying it among the most important oncogenic agents after tobacco smoking. Noticeably, the coexistence of HBV infection with other risk factors, such as HCV infection, AFB_1 exposure, alcohol abuse, obesity, and diabetes, synergistically increases the risk of HCC development. For example, molecular and epidemiological studies have shown the cooperative interaction of HBV infection with AFB_1, indicating the epidemiological and clinical importance of HBV infection in HCC development.[5,6]

PATHOGENESIS OF HBV-RELATED HEPATOCARCINOGENESIS

Hepatocarcinogenesis has been proposed as a slow, progressive multistep process evolving from hepatitis, cirrhosis, and dysplasia to HCC. The molecular mechanisms by which HBV infection promotes the development and progression of HCC have been studied extensively and form the basis of our understanding of HCC carcinogenesis. The mechanisms can be summarized into four categories (Fig. 31.1): (1) chronic inflammation accompanied by repetitive hepatocyte destruction and regeneration, resulting in fibrosis and cirrhosis; (2) integration of the HBV genome into the host–cell genome, resulting in the cis-activation of target genes, genome instability, and mutagenesis; (3) trans-activation of cellular genes by viral proteins, which alters cancer-associated signaling cascades; and (4) epigenetic regulation, including altered DNA methylation, histone modification, and deregulation of microRNAs (miRNAs), which may induce oncogenic potential in HBV-infected livers.

Inflammation in HBV-Related Hepatocarcinogenesis

The great majority of HBV-related HCCs (70% to 90%) occurs in patients with liver cirrhosis. Although HBV is not directly cytopathic, immune-mediated destruction of HBV-infected hepatocytes results in liver regeneration.[6] During liver regeneration, wound healing–related signals are activated, causing fibrosis. The continual destruction of hepatocytes and consequent liver regeneration persist repeatedly during chronic HBV infection. Activation and production of inflammatory cytokines, such as nuclear factor-kappa B (NF-κB), tumor necrosis factor-alpha (TNFα), and interleukin-6, may also contribute to the

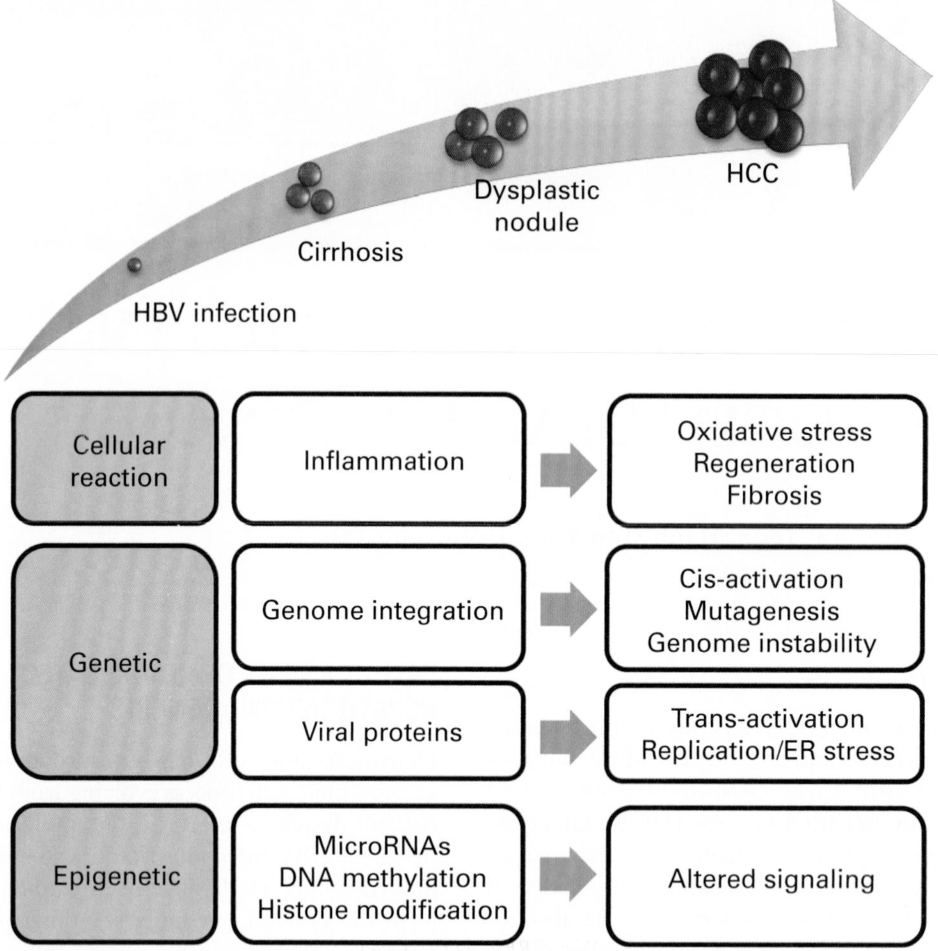

FIGURE 31–1 Schematic illustration of the molecular mechanism of HBV-induced hepatocarcinogenesis.

altered cellular signaling cascades. In addition, viral genes and proteins decrease the mitochondrial membrane potential, resulting in the generation of reactive oxygen intermediates, which can activate various transcription factors, such as NF-κB and STAT3, and provoke chromosomal alterations. The activation of those inflammatory signals perpetuates the progression of liver disease to fibrosis, cirrhosis, and eventually HCC.

HBV DNA Integration and Alteration of Cancer-Associated Signaling Cascades

In the initial step of HBV-related hepatocarcinogenesis, HBV DNA integrates into the host genome. The integration of HBV into the host genome is one of the most important mechanisms, which plays a direct pro-oncogenic role by inducing genomic alterations and producing oncoproteins such as HBx. For many years, HBV DNA integration was thought to occur randomly across the human genome. However, more recent reports have shown that the integration events appear to occur frequently in actively transcribed chromosomal regions.[7] In particular, chromosomal fragile sites and cancer-associated regions are often targets for HBV integration, resulting in altered expression of cellular genes and signaling pathways that are known to contribute importantly to the pathogenesis of cancer cell growth.[8]

Once the HBV DNA has integrated into the human genome, it can exert its effects through cis- and trans-activation mechanisms (Table 31.1). HBV integrates into cis-acting promoters often targeting genes encoding cyclin A, cyclin E1, hTERT, MLL, PDGFR, EGFR, BIRC3, and ErbB, which induce various cellular signaling cascades associated with cell survival, proliferation, and immortalization.[11,13] Several tumor suppressors, including retinoic acid receptor-β (RAR-β), p53, KLF4, and PTEN, are also targets for HBV integration.

HBV integration also promotes genomic aberrations, such as DNA copy number alteration, mutations, genome instability, and rearrangement. Indeed, higher rates of chromosomal alterations and instability have been observed in HBV-related HCC than in HCCs related to other risk factors.[18,19] This is because HBV integrates into host DNA, while HCV does not. Fusion proteins such as HBV-cyclin A, which has strong tumorigenic properties, are also produced by HBV integration.[12] Gene mutations have been shown to play important roles in the development and progression of various types of cancers.

TABLE 31–1 HBV Integration and Its Action in Hepatitis B Virus–Related Hepatocellular Carcinomas

Site	Action	Targets	Functions	References
		Cis-activation and genomic alteration by HBV integration		
1p36	Instability	miRNA-200a, RAB30	RAS activation	8,9
1q	Amplification	CHML	Cell survival	8
3p24	Mutation	RAR-β	Cell growth, differentiation	10
3q25	Amplification	IRAK2	Inflammation	11
4q	Fusion	Cyclin A	Cell cycle	12
5p14	Amplification	hTERT	Immortalization	11,13
5q31	Transcription	PDGFRβ, miRNA-224	Cell growth	7
7q11	Amplification	NCF1	Oxidative stress	7
9q	LOH	CASPR3	Differentiation	7
		KLF4	Tumor suppression	8
		miR-32, miR-123	Tumorigenesis	8
10q	LOH	PTEN	Cell growth, metastasis	8
11q	Amplification	EMS1, cyclin D1, FGF4	Metastasis	8
12q	Amplification	ErbB3, MLL2	Cell survival	8
13q32	Amplification	miRNA-17–92 cluster	Tumor growth	8
14q	LOH	SMOC1	Ca^{2+} signaling	8
16p	LOH	SERCA1	Ca^{2+} signaling	7
17p	LOH	TP53	Genome instability	8
18q	LOH	DCC, ODC4	Tumor suppression	8
19p	Deletion	miRNA-199a-1	Activate JUNB	14
19q	Amplification	Cyclin E	Cell cycle	8
		Trans-activation by HBV proteins		
Surface proteins	Protein interaction, accumulation in ER	c-Myc, c-Jun, TNF-α, TGF-β, NF-κB, src, ras, AP-1, PI3K/Akt, Jak/STAT, Smad, Wnt, CREB, ATF-2, Oct-1, TBP, P53, hTERT	Tumorigenesis Activate ER stress pathways	2,8,10
HBx	Protein interaction	p53, TNF, Fas, TGF-β, SERCA1 (TF)IIB, TFIIH, TBP, CREB,NF-κB, AP-1, NFAT, STAT3	Inhibit apoptosis Transcription	15,8
	DNA methylation DNMT activation	p16, p21, E-cadherin, and GSTP1	Hypermethylation of tumor suppressors	16,17
	Histone modification	Histone acetyltransferase CBP/P300 Histone deacetylase	Epigenetic regulation of viral genome	16

HBV, hepatitis B virus; HCC, hepatocellular carcinoma; LOH, loss of heterozygosity; ER, endoplasmic reticulum; DNMT, DNA methyltransferase.

According to the COSMIC database (http://www.sanger.ac.uk/cosmic), more than 100 genes with somatic mutations have been reported in HCC. Of these, p53 and CTNNB1 are the most frequently mutated. However, the types of mutations in these genes are quite different depending on the geographic and etiological background of HCC. For example, p53 is mutated most frequently in HBV-associated HCC but less frequently in HCV-related HCC. By contrast, CTNNB1 mutation, which results in aberrant β-catenin activation, is less frequently mutated in HBV-related HCC than in HCV-related HCC. It is of interest to note that the p53 mutation rate in HBV-related HCC has increased by up to 40% in China.[20] This may be associated with dietary exposure to AFB1 in China, which is known to accelerate p53 mutation, especially at codon 249, in the presence of HBV infection.[21]

p53 mutations can induce gain-of-function as well as loss-of-function of wild-type genes. For example, some p53 mutants such as R273 can bind to target DNAs perturbing transcription activation which may promote aggressive cancer phenotypes.[22] By contrast, some p53 mutations cause transcriptional repression of wild-type tumor suppressors. Those functional gains or losses of the mutated p53 protein may be derived from structural conformational changes that alter its physico-chemical properties. However, a recent study has revealed that mutations at hotspot sites (codons 157 and 249), and not mutations altering structural or functional properties, are associated with poor prognosis in Chinese patients with HBV-associated HCC.[20] The expression of stem cell–like traits in p53-mutated tumors has also been observed, suggesting that the acquisition of stem-like features may contribute to the aggressive behaviors of p53 mutated tumors. Undoubtedly, these results emphasize that p53 mutations play pivotal roles in HCC progression; however, its functional effects on cellular signaling are likely complicated, requiring further investigation.

On the other hand, integrated viral sequences also contribute "in trans" to tumorigenesis. For example, HBx has been reported to play several roles during hepatocarcinogenesis, including effects on apoptosis, anti-apoptosis, cell-cycle regulation, and angiogenesis and/or oncogenic potential.[15] The target genes trans-activated by HBV include oncogenes (c-Myc and c-Jun), cytokines (TNF-α and TGF-β [transforming growth factor]), and signal transduction pathway genes (e.g., NF-κB, src, ras, AP-1, AP-2, PI3K/Akt, Jak/STAT, Smad, Wnt, CREB, ATF-2, Oct-1, and TBP). In addition, the production of truncated and mutated viral proteins, such as truncated pre-S2/S, HBx, and hepatitis B spliced protein, has been shown to have effects on cellular growth and apoptosis by trans-activating cellular target genes.[23] Accumulation of the truncated viral proteins may also activate endoplasmic reticulum stress pathways[15] (see Table 31.1). Together, HBV integration events and the consequent cis- and trans-activation of target genes and genomic alteration play pivotal roles in HCC development and progression.

Epigenetic Regulation in HBV-Related HCC

Besides genomic alterations, epigenetic factors such as DNA methylation, histone modification, and non-coding RNAs, including miRNAs, have been shown to be frequently involved in the deregulation of cellular functions in HCC.[16] For example, DNA methylation is frequently found in HBV- and HCV-related HCC, while virus-negative tumors have fewer epigenetic and genetic alterations.[18] Indeed, HBx can increase total DNA methyltransferase (DNMT) activities (e.g., DNMT1, DNMT3A, and DNMT3B), promoting methylation of CpG groups, an effect which is often increased in livers affected with chronic hepatitis and cirrhosis, as well as in HCC.[17] Hypermethylation of the Ras pathway and angiogenesis-related genes has also been reported to be associated with poor prognosis in HBV-related HCC.[24] Silencing of tumor suppressors, including p16, p21, E-cadherin, and GSTP1, results in the deregulation of the RB1, p53, and Wnt pathways in HBV-related HCC. Together, these findings suggest that HBV may be, at least in part, responsible for the methylator phenotype seen in HBV-related HCC.

Histone modification is also affected by HBV infection. For example, HBx directly interacts with the histone deacetylase complex CBP/P300, promoting its trans-activation activity. HBx also influences the histone modification of the viral genome, which regulates the replication and transcription of intracellular viral genome.

miRNAs have recently been found to play critical roles in HCC development and progression by regulating gene expression, mostly at the post-transcriptional level. For example, the miRNAs Let-7a, miR-602, miR-143, and miR-152 have been reported to be deregulated in HBV-related HCC.[25] In addition, because miRNAs are frequently located at fragile sites or genomic regions involved in cancers,[14] altered expression of miRNAs within those viral insertion sites, such as miR-200a, (1p36), miR-224 (5q31-32), Let-7a-2(11q22), the miR-17–92 cluster (13q32), miR-195 (17p12), and miR-199a-1 (19p13.2), could act as oncogenes or tumor suppressors depending on their target genes (see Table 31.1). Moreover, some cellular miRNAs were found to inhibit or stimulate viral replication by directly targeting viral RNAs.[26] Overall, it is clear that HBV proteins can alter the levels of various cellular miRNAs, suggesting their important roles in HCC development.

MOLECULAR PROFILING OF HBV-RELATED HCC

Recent advances in microarray and sequencing technologies have provided genome-wide profiles of genomes and transcriptomes as well as epigenomes. During the past 10 years, microarrays have been successfully used to stratify heterogeneous HCC into homogeneous subgroups revealing distinct biological determinants. Some of these distinct characteristics of HBV-related HCC include increased genetic instability, poor differentiation, p53 mutations, poor prognosis, activation of the mitotic cell cycle, and deregulated activation of IGF2 and AKT pathways.[27,28] Differential expression of mRNAs and miRNAs in HBV- and HCV-related HCCs has also been observed, revealing an etiology of these biological differences.[29,30] In addition, gene-expression signatures used to predict patient outcomes, such as survival, tumor recurrence, and metastasis, have been identified. For example, a gene-expression signature that is predictive of early recurrence has been identified in HBV-related HCC (Fig. 31.2A and B).[31] Noticeably, CD24 was identified as a putative biomarker for the prediction of early recurrence, a finding that needs to be validated by an independent study (Fig. 31.2C).[32] Indeed, a recent study has demonstrated that the CD24-positive tumor cells have tumor-initiating properties caused by Nanog regulation, indicating an aggressive phenotype of CD24-positive tumors.[33] Together, these subsequent studies consistently support the biological and clinical significance of CD24 expression in HCC.

Metastasis signatures are also found in non-tumoral surrounding tissues, as well as tumors from HBV-related HCC patients.[34,35] Interestingly, the expression of inflammation-related gene signatures was identified in non-tumoral tissues from metastatic HCC, suggesting

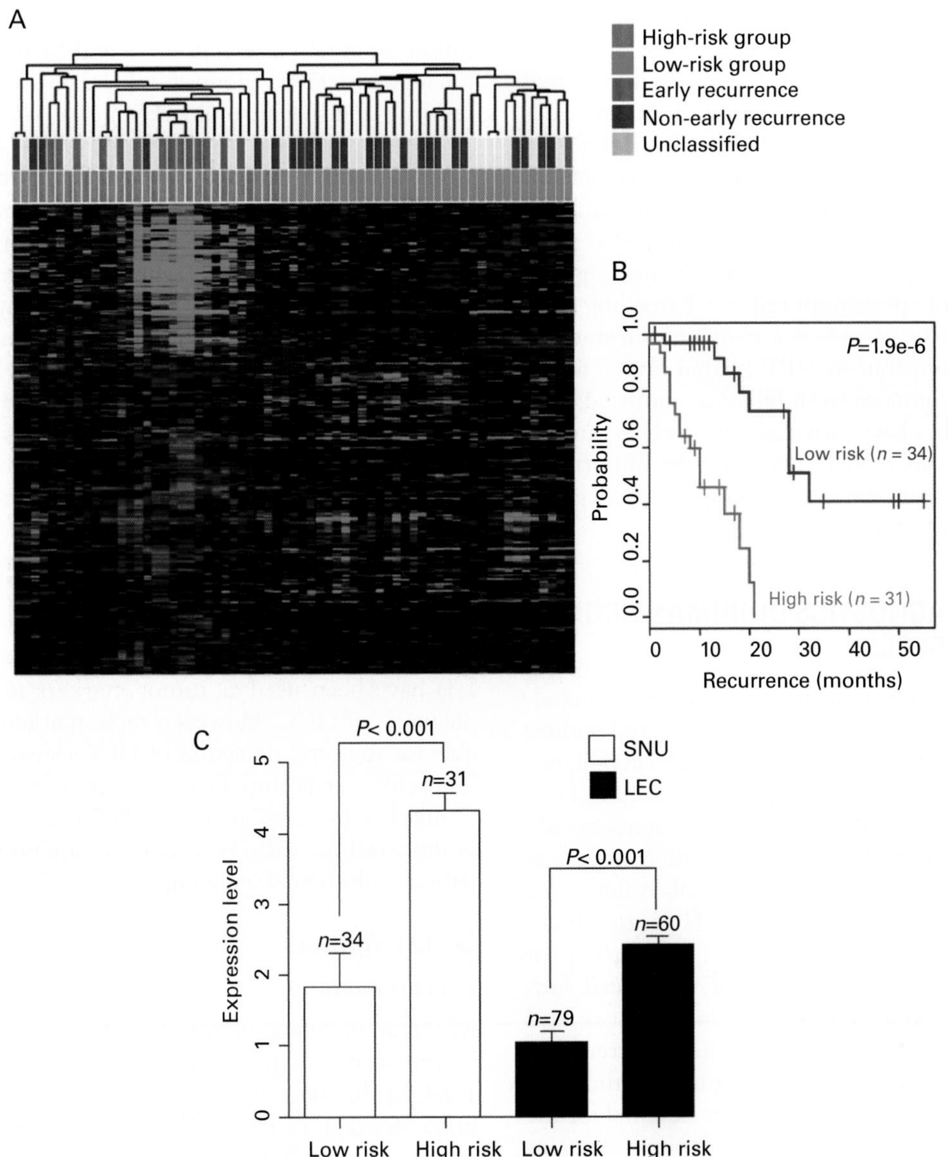

FIGURE 31–2 Identification of a gene-expression signature for predicting early recurrence in HBV-related hepatocellular carcinomas (HCCs). **(A)** Hierarchical clustering was done on the expression profile of genes identified by Cox proportional hazards analysis ($P < 0.005$, log-rank test). Patients with early recurrence (recurrence within 1 y after curative resection) and late recurrence are indicated. **(B)** Kaplan-Meier plot of recurrence-free survival of HCCs stratified by hierarchical clustering of the expression profile of genes associated with recurrence. **(C)** Expression levels of CD24 in group with high and low risks of early recurrence. The average expression levels of CD24 between high-risk and low-risk groups were compared in independent data sets from Seoul National University ($n = 65$) and the Laboratory of Experimental Carcinogenesis at the National Cancer Institute ($n = 139$), respectively. Reprinted from a previous study.[29]

the importance of the expression of inflammatory traits in the acquisition of the metastatic phenotype, particularly in HBV-related HCC.

In addition to these, several genomic profiling studies of mRNAs, DNA copy number, and miRNAs have been performed on tissue samples from HCC cohorts with a predominance of HBV infections. The largest miRNA profiling was performed on 455 HCC patients, a majority of whom had HBV infection.[36] This analysis revealed that miR-26 is overexpressed in non-tumoral liver tissues from HBV-positive HCC patients. In addition, alterations in DNA copy number are also common events in cancers, including HCC. Genome-wide profiling of DNA copy number has revealed chromosomal amplification and deletions in HCC.[37] Frequent chromosomal gains were observed at 1q, 3q, 6p, 7q, 8q, 17q, 20q, and 22q and frequent losses were observed at 1p, 6q, 8p, 9p, 14q, 16q, and 17p. However, additional studies, requiring further large-scale evaluation in a cohort of HBV-infected HCC patients, are needed to determine whether the findings are specific for HBV-related HCC.

The delineation of tumor heterogeneity is one of the challenges in studying cancer, because proper classification of cancers and linking the classes with functional and clinical outcomes, such as chemical or drug responses, would be a promising strategy to develop personalized cancer treatments. In this context, recent identification of the expression profiles of the origins of progenitor cells has provided novel biological and clinical insights into classifying cancer on the basis of the cancer development model. The expression of stem cell–like traits or stemness-related markers (e.g., EpCam) has been proposed to be associated with poor prognosis of HCC patients, suggesting it originates from progenitor cells.[38,39] Extending these studies, we recently proposed a cholangiocarcinoma-like gene-expression trait in HBV-related HCC, which suggests that it originates from biliary-committed stem cells.[40] These studies have provided new insights into the hepatocarcinogenesis model, indicating the importance of cellular origins from different developmental stages in heterogeneous HCC progression.

MOLECULAR DIAGNOSTICS OF HUMAN HCC TUMOR BIOMARKERS

Despite recent advances in the treatment of HCC, including molecularly targeted agents, there are limited options for curing this disease. Moreover, although surveillance programs for HCC in high-risk populations have been established in different countries, many patients cannot be cured owing to the advanced stage of their disease at the time of diagnosis. Thus, it is essential to develop a tumor marker for the early detection of HCC to achieve the highest likelihood of survival. A tumor marker (or biomarker) is defined as an abnormally produced substance in the body of a patient with cancer that is used to help diagnose cancer or predict tumor recurrence or the therapeutic response following treatment. Although a histological examination of liver tissue is essential for the diagnosis of HCC, the routine use of liver biopsy remains controversial because of bleeding and local tumor spread along the needle track.[41] Moreover, a liver biopsy is often difficult or dangerous for patients with advanced liver disease with accompanying ascites or coagulopathy. Consequently, the clinical diagnosis of HCC based on radiological imaging and tumor markers has been widely accepted in clinical practice for decades. However, currently, the diagnosis of HCC is greatly dependent on radiological techniques because of the inadequate sensitivity and specificity of serum α-fetoprotein (AFP), which is the most widely used tumor marker for HCC.[9,10] Radiologically, HCC is characterized by the presence of arterial enhancement followed by contrast washout on dynamic computed tomography or magnetic resonance imaging. Thus, the most recent guidelines of the American Association for the Study of Liver Disease state that surveillance has to be based on an ultrasound examination, and the diagnosis of HCC should be based on imaging techniques and/or a biopsy.[42] Nevertheless, tumor markers play a critical role in the management of HCC, because HCC recurs in over 70% of patients following curative resection,[43,44] and earlier detection in the high-risk HCC group should be possible with a more sensitive and specific biomarker.

Tumor markers can be found in the blood, urine, stool, and other tissues. An ideal biomarker should be reliable, reproducible, easy to detect, and obtained in a minimally invasive manner. With recent advances in high-throughput "omics" technologies, a large number of potential candidate biomarkers for the early detection or prediction of the prognosis of HCC have been reported, although further validation as suggested by the Early Detection Research Network[45] is required to develop a tumor-specific biomarker for HCC. These biomarkers can be divided into two groups according to their clinical role: (1) diagnostic and (2) prognostic markers.

BIOMARKERS FOR DIAGNOSING HCC

Until recently, serum AFP, des-γ-carboxy prothrombin (DCP), and *Lens culinaris* agglutinin-reactive AFP (AFP-L3) have been used as tumor markers for the clinical diagnosis of HCC. However, these markers are not reliable for the early detection of HCCs smaller than 2 cm. Therefore, it is imperative to identify a confirmative biomarker for early diagnosis because late-stage HCC is devastating, with very few therapeutic options for patients, ultimately reducing survival.

Serum Markers

α-Fetoprotein

AFP is an oncofetal glycoprotein that was first described in the serum of patients with HCC by Tatarinov in 1964.[46] It has been used widely as a diagnostic and prognostic marker in HCC. When using a cutoff value of 20 ng/mL for HCC diagnosis, the reported sensitivity and specificity of AFP range from 41% to 65% and 80% to 94%, respectively.[10,47] This low sensitivity has been an impediment to detecting early HCC, and false-positive results can occur in benign liver diseases, resulting in reduced specificity. Nevertheless, serum AFP has been used widely as a tumor marker for screening and surveillance of HCC in high-endemic areas of HBV and HCV infection.

Des-γ-Carboxyprothrombin

Des-γ-carboxyprothrombin, also known as protein induced by vitamin K absence or antagonist-II (PIVKA-II), has been used as a tumor marker for HCC since it was first reported by Liebman et al. in 1984.[48] The reported sensitivity and specificity of DCP for HCC diagnosis ranges from 28% to 89% and 87% to 96%, respectively.[49] Although it is difficult to compare the diagnostic accuracy of serum AFP and DCP because of variable results in different studies, a recent study demonstrated that the diagnostic utility of DCP was poorer than that of AFP for small HCC, but better for large HCC.

Lens culinaris Agglutinin-Reactive AFP

Lens culinaris agglutinin-reactive AFP is a fucosylated variant of AFP with a high affinity for the sugar chain of *Lens culinaris*. Since AFP-L3 was first reported by Taketa et al. in 1990,[50] subsequent studies of AFL-3 have shown sensitivities of 36% to 96% and specificities of 89% to 94% for the detection of HCC.[20] In recent years, however, the AFP-L3 test has limited use for screening or diagnosing HCC because of its low sensitivity and high cost.

Glypican-3

Glypican-3 (GPC3), also known as an oncofetal protein composed of cell surface heparin sulfate proteoglycan, plays a key role in the development of cellular process.[51] Recent studies have demonstrated the diagnostic value of GPC3 as a tissue and serological marker for the early detection of HCC.[52,53] Hippo et al.[54] reported a sensitivity of 51% and specificity of 90% for serum GPC3 for HCC diagnosis. GPC3 has been validated in a number of studies and is considered a strong candidate as a molecular signature of early HCC.

Other Markers

Other serological markers are under investigation as candidates for the diagnosis of HCC. They include proteins, growth factors, cytokines, enzymes or isoenzymes, autoantibodies, DNA, RNA, and miRNA. The characteristics of these serological candidate biomarkers for HCC are shown in Table 31.2.[55-64] Moreover, a recent genome-wide association study identified several serum biomarkers for the early detection of HCC, including heat shock protein 70,[65,66] midkine,[67] serine/threonine kinase 15, glutamate carboxypeptidase phospholipases A2, complement C3A, and cystatin B.[68-70]

Immunohistochemistry (IHC) plays a role in assessment and differential diagnosis of hepatocellular neoplasms and secondary (metastatic) tumor. A summary of IHC used in the diagnosis of hepatocellular neoplasms is presented in Table 31.3

GENE-EXPRESSION SIGNATURES FOR HCC DIAGNOSIS

HCC can be discriminated from premalignant lesions or the disease-free state by its molecular signature. With recent advances in high-throughput technologies, including cDNA/oligonucleotides, non-coding RNA microarrays, protein arrays, tissue microarrays, and array comparative genomic hybridization, tumor-specific gene-expression profiles have been defined. The development of these technologies has contributed tremendously to the differential diagnosis of chronic liver disease by addressing complex molecular pathogenesis and identifying target molecules for HCC. Nevertheless, the routine clinical application of microarray-based tests remains impractical owing to difficulty interpreting the differences between HCC and controls and their high cost.

Recent microarray studies have compared the gene-expression profile of HCC with that of surrounding non-tumor tissues or normal liver tissues. Nam et al.[71] identified 240 genes that can discriminate precancerous nodules, including low- and high-grade dysplastic nodules, from overt HCC. HBV and HCV are the major causative viruses of HCC. However, it is unclear whether the two viruses have different mechanisms of

TABLE 31-2 Sensitivity and Specificity of Candidate Biomarkers for Hepatocellular Carcinoma Diagnosis

Marker	No. of Cases	Sensitivity (%)	Specificity (%)	Authors
γ-Glutamyl transferase	210	74.0	82.2	Cui et al.[55]
α-L-Fucosidase	168	77.6	78.7	Takahashi et al.[56]
Golgi protein 73	4217	74.6	97.4	Mao et al.[57]
miR-16	283	72.1	88.8	Qu et al.[58]
Transforming growth factor-β1	92	68	95	Song et al.[59]
Insulin-like growth factor (IGF-II)+	150	42	95.1	Tsai et al.[60]
Interleukin-6	128	46	95	Hsia et al.[61]
Interleukin-10	128	50	96	Hsia et al.[61]
Hepatocyte growth factor	128	58	53	Hsia et al.[61]
Human cervical cancer oncogene	570	78.2	95.5	Yoon et al.[62]
Hypermethylation biomarkers (P16, P15, RASSF1A)	100	84	94	Zhang et al.[63]
Squamous cell carcinoma antigen	210	84.2	48.9	Giannelli et al.[64]

TABLE 31-3 Immunohistochemistry Commonly Used in Diagnosis and Differential Diagnosis of Tumors in the Liver[a]

Immunohistochemistry	Comments on Results
	Cancer viral antigens
HBV surface antigen	Detection of HBV infection and evaluation of the status of HBV replication
HBV core antigen	Assessment of levels of viral replication (staining intensity usually corresponds to disease activity)
Hepatitis C virus	No reliable antibody commercially available
	Diagnosis and classification of epithelial tumors in the liver
α-Fetoprotein	Positive in 30% HCC Cirrhotic hepatocytes may reveal focal staining
CD 10	Positive in HCC (canalicular pattern)
CD31	Sinusoidal endothelial cells are negative in normal liver, but positive in HCC and some chronic liver diseases
CD56, chromogranin, synaptophysin	Neuroendocrine tumors, metastatic or primary
CK7, CK8, CK18, CK19, and CK20	CK7/CK20 are both negative in HCC Hepatocytes are positive for CK8 and CK18. CK7 and CK19 are positive in the presence of cholangiocellular differentiation
Epithelial membrane antigen	Negative in HCC Positive in cholangiocarcinoma and metastatic adenocarcinoma
Glypican 3	Positive in HCC Negative in benign hepatocellular neoplasms
Hepatocyte (HepPar1)	Hepatocyte differentiation
MOC-31	Negative in HCC Positive in cholangiocarcinoma and metastatic adenocarcinoma
Polyclonal CEA	Positive in HCC (canalicular pattern) Positive in cholangiocarcinoma and adenocarcinoma (cytoplasmic and membranous)

HBV, hepatitis B virus; HCC, hepatocellular carcinoma.

[a]The immunostain should consist of a panel of antibodies to work out a tumor in the liver, because no single immunohistochemistry (IHC) stain is specific. In addition, IHC results should correlate with morphology and clinical presentations to arrive at a meaningful conclusion.

hepatocarcinogenesis. To examine this question, a recent cDNA microarray study revealed that the gene-expression profiles of HBV- and HCV-related HCC were different.[72] HBV-related HCC involved different cellular pathways that control apoptosis, p53 signaling, and G1/S transition, whereas HCV-related HCC showed a more heterogeneous pattern, with overexpression of TGF-β. In another study, Paradis et al.[73] suggested that a molecular index consisting of a 13-gene set (TERT, IGF2, Connexin 26/GJB2, Tie2/TEK, TIAM1, CXCL12, TOP2A, A2M, PLG, p14ARF/CDKN2A, PDGFRA, MKI67, and THBS1) was an efficient tool for discriminating early HCC from premalignant lesions and for classifying HCC. More recently, a cDNA array study showed that the integrin and Akt/NFκB signaling pathways linked to osteopontin, GPC3, annexin 2 (ANXA2), S100A10, and vimentin (VIM) were upregulated in HCC, making them potential novel targets.

Serum proteomics has also been used to search for new biomarkers for the early detection of HCC. In particular, a recently developed surface-enhanced laser desorption/ionization-time of flight mass spectrometry protein chip system has been used in studies of cancer biomarkers. Recent proteomic studies for the diagnosis of HCC have demonstrated sensitivities of 83% to 94% and specificities of 76% to 100%, suggesting that the tumor-specific proteomic features used in the diagnosis of HCC are useful for the detection and classification of HCC.[74-77]

Numerous recent studies have provided evidence that miRNA plays an important role in tumorigenesis and may be useful for diagnosing cancer.[78] Wang et al.[79] revealed that miR-224 is upregulated in HCC and sensitizes cells to apoptosis by reducing apoptosis inhibitor-5 mRNA levels and increasing cell proliferation. In another study, circulating miR-16 was used to diagnose HCC with higher sensitivity than that of conventional markers, such as AFP, DCP, and AFP-L3. Furthermore, the combined use of miR-16 with conventional markers improved the sensitivity (92.4%) and specificity (78.5%) for the diagnosis of HCC.[58]

PROGNOSTIC MARKERS IN HCC

The long-term outcome for patients with HCC is still very poor owing to the high recurrence rate, even after curative resection or local ablation therapy. In addition, because the prognosis is related to liver function status in addition to tumor factors, identifying the predictors of patient survival is even harder. Numerous studies have described serum markers or gene-expression signatures that predict prognosis. However, no definitive biomarkers have yet emerged. Therefore, it is critical for patient survival to identify a predictor of recurrence or metastasis after curative treatment.

Serum Markers

The markers AFP, DCP, and AFP-L3, currently used for HCC diagnosis, have also been used to predict recurrence and monitor the response of the tumor to treatment.[80-83] Other serum biomarkers have also been proposed as prognostic markers, including human carbonyl reductase, chromogranin A, vascular endothelial growth factors, and HGF.[84-90] A recent study by Li et al.[91] suggested that serum miR-221, which is upregulated in HCC, can be used to predict the prognosis of HCC patients.

GENE-EXPRESSION SIGNATURES OF RECURRENCE, METASTASIS, AND SURVIVAL

The long-term survival of HCC patients is still unsatisfactory, with no more than 30% of patients surviving more than 5 years after surgical resection.[44] In addition to the clinicopathological features of HCC, specific molecular signatures to predict prognosis, including recurrence, metastasis, and survival, have been reported.

Several studies have reported using gene-expression profiling to predict HCC recurrence after surgical resection.[92-99] For example, Iizuka et al.[92] established a predictive system consisting of 12 genes that could be used to predict early intrahepatic recurrence, with a positive predictive value of 88%. In another study, Kurokawa et al.[93] demonstrated that a 20-gene-expression signature identified by a polymerase chain reaction–based array predicted early intrahepatic recurrence with approximately 70% accuracy. More recently, Wang et al.[94] identified a 57-gene signature identified by oligonucleotide probe arrays that could predict recurrent disease at diagnosis, with 84% accuracy (sensitivity 86% and specificity 82%). In addition, the recurrence of HCC after treatment has been reported to be associated with the host's human leukocyte antigen type.[95]

Recent studies have searched for molecular markers linked to HCC metastasis following curative treatment.[35,100] Ye et al. identified osteopontin as a lead gene from the 153 HCC metastasis gene signatures identified by a cDNA microarray. Osteopontin may be a diagnostic marker for discriminating metastatic HCC accurately and a potential therapeutic target for metastatic HCC.[101] In another study, Hu et al. established a metastatic HCC cell line and identified eight genes upregulated in response to the primary HCC cell line using a cDNA microarray. Among the metastasis-associated genes, VIM and clusterin were significantly overexpressed in metastatic HCC,[102,103] suggesting that these genes play key roles in the metastasis of HCC. More recently, Budhu et al.[103] investigated the expression profiles of metastasis-associated miRNA in paired tumor/non-tumor tissues from HCC patients. They found a 20-miRNA metastasis signature that could predict vascular metastasis from primary HCC. In addition, this molecular signature was significantly associated with both survival and relapse. Another study analyzed the association between the genetic variant of phosphatidic acid phosphatase (HTPAP), known as a metastatic suppressor of HCC, and HCC recurrence.[104] Patients with the +357G/C genotype had earlier recurrence and shorter overall survival than patients with the +357CC genotype. To evaluate the potential mechanism of the HTPAP +357G/C genotype in HCC metastasis, the gene-expression profiles were analyzed using an oligonucleotide array. Of 38,500 genes, 41 were significantly overexpressed in HCC patients with the +357G/C genotype.

In recent years, numerous studies have addressed HCC survival.[20,105,106] However, it is difficult to specify the cause of death of these patients, because most HCC patients have accompanying decompensated liver disease and, eventually, liver failure. Lee et al.[105] initially reported that the expression of 406 unique genes was significantly correlated with the survival time. Most recently, Woo et al.[20] investigated the prognostic significance of a TP53 mutation and found that patients with the mutation had a shorter overall survival time than patients with wild-type TP53. A gene-expression analysis that explored the underlying mechanism by which TP53 mutations exert these effects demonstrated the existence of stem cell–like traits, reflecting the aggressive behavior of tumors with TP53 mutations. The gene-expression signatures associated with the prognosis of HCC after surgery are shown in Table 31.4.

Although recent studies have attempted to find a role for cancer stem cells in the prognosis of HCC, Lee et al.[107] demonstrated through comparative genomic investigations in both human and animal models that individuals with HCC who expressed markers for fetal progenitor cells (hepatoblast-like) had a poor prognosis. In another study, HCCs expressing cytokeratin 7 and 19, which are markers for early hepatoblasts and mature hepatic stem/progenitor cells, were associated with HCC recurrence owing to its aggressive tumor characteristics after surgery.[108] More recently, clinical studies revealed that patients with HCC expressing CD133 and EpCAM, which are cancer stem cell markers, showed early tumor recurrence and shorter survival time after treatment.[38,109,110]

Overall, with advances in high-throughput "omics" technologies, the comprehensive prediction of prognosis following treatment may be feasible but remains to be resolved. Therefore, it is crucial to develop new biomarkers and to validate new surrogate end points in HCC.

TABLE 31-4 Gene-Expression Signatures Associated with Prognosis in HCC after Surgery

Prediction	No. of Cases	No. of Genes in Signature	Method	Authors
Recurrence	60	12	Oligonucleotide microarray	Iizuka et al.[92]
	100	92	PCR-based array	Kurokawa et al.[93]
	80	57	Oligo-Affymetrix	Wang et al.[94]
	1000	100	DNA microarray	Uchimura et al.[95]
Metastasis	67	153	cDNA microarray	Ye et al.[35]
	200 primary + 60 pairs	Vimentin	Tissue microarray	Hu et al.[101]
	104 pairs	Clusterin	Tissue microarray	Lau et al.[102]
	482	20 miRNAs	miRNA microarray	Budhu et al.[103]
	665	41	Oligonucleotide array	Ren et al.[104]
Survival	592	20 miRNAs	miRNA microarray	Budhu et al.[103]
	91	406	DNA microarray	Lee et al.[105]
	409	366	Oligonucleotide array	Woo et al.[20]

REFERENCES

1. El-Serag HB, Rudolph KL. Hepatocellular carcinoma: epidemiology and molecular carcinogenesis. *Gastroenterology.* 2007;132:2557-2576.
2. Pollicino T, Saitta C, Raimondo G. Hepatocellular carcinoma: the point of view of the hepatitis B virus. *Carcinogenesis.* 2011;32(8): 1122-1132.
3. Kew MC. Synergistic interaction between aflatoxin B1 and hepatitis B virus in hepatocarcinogenesis. *Liver International.* 2003;23:405-409.
4. Hassan MM, Hwang L-Y, Hatten CJ, et al. Risk factors for hepatocellular carcinoma: synergism of alcohol with viral hepatitis and diabetes mellitus. *Hepatology.* 2002;36:1206-1213.
5. Hussain SP, Schwank J, Staib F, et al. TP53 mutations and hepatocellular carcinoma: insights into the etiology and pathogenesis of liver cancer. *Oncogene.* 2007;26:2166-2176.
6. Ganem D, Prince AM. Hepatitis B virus infection—natural history and clinical consequences. *N Engl J Med.* 2004;350:1118-1129.
7. Murakami Y, Saigo K, Takashima H, et al. Large scaled analysis of hepatitis B virus (HBV) DNA integration in HBV related hepatocellular carcinomas. *Gut.* 2005;54:1162-1168.
8. Feitelson MA, Lee J. Hepatitis B virus integration, fragile sites, and hepatocarcinogenesis. *Cancer Lett.* 2007;252:157-170.
9. Singal A, Volk ML, Waljee A, et al. Meta-analysis: surveillance with ultrasound for early-stage hepatocellular carcinoma in patients with cirrhosis. *Aliment Pharmacol Ther.* 2009;30:37-47.
10. Lok AS, Sterling RK, Everhart JE, et al. Des-gamma-carboxy prothrombin and alpha-fetoprotein as biomarkers for the early detection of hepatocellular carcinoma. *Gastroenterology.* 2010;138:493-502.
11. Paterlini-Brechot P, Saigo K, Murakami Y, et al. Hepatitis B virus-related insertional mutagenesis occurs frequently in human liver cancers and recurrently targets human telomerase gene. *Oncogene.* 2003;22:3911-3916.
12. Wang J, Chenivesse X, Henglein B, et al. Hepatitis B virus integration in a cyclin A gene in a hepatocellular carcinoma. *Nature.* 1990;343:555-557.
13. Horikawa I, Barrett JC. cis-Activation of the human telomerase gene (hTERT) by the hepatitis B virus genome. *J Natl Cancer Inst.* 2001;93:1171-1173.
14. Calin GA, Sevignani C, Dumitru CD, et al. Human microRNA genes are frequently located at fragile sites and genomic regions involved in cancers. *Proc Natl Acad Sci U S A.* 2004;101:2999-3004.
15. Bouchard MJ, Navas-Martin S. Hepatitis B and C virus hepatocarcinogenesis: lessons learned and future challenges. *Cancer Lett.* 2011;305:123-143.
16. Herceg Z, Paliwal A. Epigenetic mechanisms in hepatocellular carcinoma: how environmental factors influence the epigenome. *Mutat Res.* 2011;727:55-61.
17. Park IY, Sohn BH, Yu E, et al. Aberrant epigenetic modifications in hepatocarcinogenesis induced by hepatitis B virus X protein. *Gastroenterology.* 2007;132:1476-1494.
18. Katoh H, Shibata T, Kokubu A, et al. Epigenetic instability and chromosomal instability in hepatocellular carcinoma. *Am J Pathol.* 2006;168:1375-1384.
19. Marchio A, Pineau P, Meddeb M, et al. Distinct chromosomal abnormality pattern in primary liver cancer of non-B, non-C patients. *Oncogene.* 2000;19:3733-3738.
20. Woo HG, Wang XW, Budhu A, et al. Association of TP53 mutations with stem cell-like gene expression and survival of patients with hepatocellular carcinoma. *Gastroenterology.* 2011;140:1063-1070.
21. Aguilar F, Harris CC, Sun T, et al. Geographic variation of p53 mutational profile in nonmalignant human liver. *Science.* 1994;264:1317-1319.
22. Bullock AN, Fersht AR. Rescuing the function of mutant p53. *Nat Rev Cancer.* 2001;1:68-76.
23. Fernandez PC, Frank SR, Wang L, et al. Genomic targets of the human c-Myc protein. *Genes Dev.* 2003;17:1115-1129.
24. Calvisi DF, Ladu S, Gorden A, et al. Mechanistic and prognostic significance of aberrant methylation in the molecular pathogenesis of human hepatocellular carcinoma. *J Clin Invest.* 2007;117:2713-2722.
25. Liu WH, Yeh SH, Chen PJ. Role of microRNAs in hepatitis B virus replication and pathogenesis. *Biochim Biophys Acta.* 2011; 1809:678-685.
26. Lin Z, Flemington EK. MiRNAs in the pathogenesis of oncogenic human viruses. *Cancer Lett.* 2011;305:186-199.
27. Laurent-Puig P, Legoix P, Bluteau O, et al. Genetic alterations associated with hepatocellular carcinomas define distinct pathways of hepatocarcinogenesis. *Gastroenterology.* 2001;120:1763-1773.
28. Boyault S, Rickman DS, de Reynies A, et al. Transcriptome classification of HCC is related to gene alterations and to new therapeutic targets. *Hepatology.* 2007;45:42-52.
29. Iizuka N, Oka M, Yamada-Okabe H, et al. Comparison of gene expression profiles between hepatitis B virus- and hepatitis C virus-infected hepatocellular carcinoma by oligonucleotide microarray data on the basis of a supervised learning method. *Cancer Res.* 2002;62:3939-3944.
30. Ura S, Honda M, Yamashita T, et al. Differential microRNA expression between hepatitis B and hepatitis C leading disease progression to hepatocellular carcinoma. *Hepatology.* 2009;49:1098-1112.

31. Woo HG, Park ES, Cheon JH, et al. Gene expression-based recurrence prediction of hepatitis B virus-related human hepatocellular carcinoma. *Clin Cancer Res.* 2008;14:2056-2064.
32. Yang X-R, Xu Y, Yu B, et al. CD24 is a novel predictor for poor prognosis of hepatocellular carcinoma after surgery. *Clin Cancer Res.* 2009;15:5518-5527.
33. Lee Terence Kin W, Castilho A, Cheung Vincent Chi H, et al. CD24+ liver tumor-initiating cells drive self-renewal and tumor initiation through STAT3-mediated NANOG regulation. *Cell Stem Cell.* 2011;9:50-63.
34. Budhu A, Forgues M, Ye QH, et al. Prediction of venous metastases, recurrence, and prognosis in hepatocellular carcinoma based on a unique immune response signature of the liver microenvironment. *Cancer Cell.* 2006;10:99-111.
35. Ye QH, Qin LX, Forgues M, et al. Predicting hepatitis B virus-positive metastatic hepatocellular carcinomas using gene expression profiling and supervised machine learning. *Nat Med.* 2003;9:416-423.
36. Ji J, Shi J, Budhu A, et al. MicroRNA expression, survival, and response to interferon in liver cancer. *N Engl J Med.* 2009;361:1437-1447.
37. Woo HG, Park ES, Lee JS, et al. Identification of potential driver genes in human liver carcinoma by genomewide screening. *Cancer Res.* 2009;69:4059-4066.
38. Lee JS, Heo J, Libbrecht L, et al. A novel prognostic subtype of human hepatocellular carcinoma derived from hepatic progenitor cells. *Nat Med.* 2006;12:410-416.
39. Yamashita T, Forgues M, Wang W, et al. EpCAM and alpha-fetoprotein expression defines novel prognostic subtypes of hepatocellular carcinoma. *Cancer Res.* 2008;68:1451-1461.
40. Woo HG, Lee JH, Yoon JH, et al. Identification of a cholangiocarcinoma-like gene expression trait in hepatocellular carcinoma. *Cancer Res.* 2010;70:3034-3041.
41. Durand F, Regimbeau JM, Belghiti J, et al. Assessment of the benefits and risks of percutaneous biopsy before surgical resection of hepatocellular carcinoma. *J Hepatol.* 2001;35:254-258.
42. Bruix J, Sherman M. Management of hepatocellular carcinoma: an update. *Hepatology.* 2011;53:1020-1022.
43. Poon RT, Fan ST, Lo CM, et al. Improving survival results after resection of hepatocellular carcinoma: a prospective study of 377 patients over 10 years. *Ann Surg.* 2001;234:63-70.
44. Yeh CN, Chen MF, Lee WC, et al. Prognostic factors of hepatic resection for hepatocellular carcinoma with cirrhosis: univariate and multivariate analysis. *J Surg Oncol.* 2002;81:195-202.
45. Pepe MS, Etzioni R, Feng Z, et al. Phases of biomarker development for early detection of cancer. *J Natl Cancer Inst.* 2001;93:1054-1061.
46. IuS T. Detection of embryo-specific alpha-globulin in the serum of a patient with primary liver cancer. *Vopr Med Khim.* 1964; 10:90-91.
47. Gupta S, Bent S, Kohlwes J. Test characteristics of alpha-fetoprotein for detecting hepatocellular carcinoma in patients with hepatitis C. A systematic review and critical analysis. *Ann Intern Med.* 2003;139:46-50.
48. Liebman HA, Furie BC, Tong MJ, et al. Des-gamma-carboxy (abnormal) prothrombin as a serum marker of primary hepatocellular carcinoma. *N Engl J Med.* 1984;310:1427-1431.
49. Marrero JA, Lok AS. Newer markers for hepatocellular carcinoma. *Gastroenterology.* 2004;127:S113-S119.
50. Taketa K, Sekiya C, Namiki M, et al. Lectin-reactive profiles of alpha-fetoprotein characterizing hepatocellular carcinoma and related conditions. *Gastroenterology.* 1990;99:508-518.
51. Grozdanov PN, Yovchev MI, Dabeva MD. The oncofetal protein glypican-3 is a novel marker of hepatic progenitor/oval cells. *Lab Invest.* 2006;86:1272-1284.
52. Capurro M, Wanless IR, Sherman M, et al. Glypican-3: a novel serum and histochemical marker for hepatocellular carcinoma. *Gastroenterology.* 2003;125:89-97.
53. Di Tommaso L, Franchi G, Park YN, et al. Diagnostic value of HSP70, glypican 3, and glutamine synthetase in hepatocellular nodules in cirrhosis. *Hepatology.* 2007;45:725-734.
54. Hippo Y, Watanabe K, Watanabe A, et al. Identification of soluble NH2-terminal fragment of glypican-3 as a serological marker for early-stage hepatocellular carcinoma. *Cancer Res.* 2004;64:2418-2423.
55. Cui R, He J, Zhang F, et al. Diagnostic value of protein induced by vitamin K absence (PIVKAII) and hepatoma-specific band of serum gamma-glutamyl transferase (GGTII) as hepatocellular carcinoma markers complementary to alpha-fetoprotein. *Br J Cancer.* 2003;88:1878-1882.
56. Takahashi H, Saibara T, Iwamura S, et al. Serum alpha-l-fucosidase activity and tumor size in hepatocellular carcinoma. *Hepatology.* 1994;19:1414-1417.
57. Mao Y, Yang H, Xu H, et al. Golgi protein 73 (GOLPH2) is a valuable serum marker for hepatocellular carcinoma. *Gut.* 2010;59:1687-1693.
58. Qu KZ, Zhang K, Li H, et al. Circulating microRNAs as biomarkers for hepatocellular carcinoma. *J Clin Gastroenterol.* 2011;45:355-360.
59. Song BC, Chung YH, Kim JA, et al. Transforming growth factor-beta1 as a useful serologic marker of small hepatocellular carcinoma. *Cancer.* 2002;94:175-180.
60. Tsai JF, Jeng JE, Chuang LY, et al. Serum insulin-like growth factor-II and alpha-fetoprotein as tumor markers of hepatocellular carcinoma. *Tumour Biol.* 2003;24:291-298.
61. Hsia CY, Huo TI, Chiang SY, et al. Evaluation of interleukin-6, interleukin-10 and human hepatocyte growth factor as tumor markers for hepatocellular carcinoma. *Eur J Surg Oncol.* 2007;33:208-212.
62. Yoon SK, Lim NK, Ha SA, et al. The human cervical cancer oncogene protein is a biomarker for human hepatocellular carcinoma. *Cancer Res.* 2004;64:5434-5441.
63. Zhang YJ, Wu HC, Shen J, et al. Predicting hepatocellular carcinoma by detection of aberrant promoter methylation in serum DNA. *Clin Cancer Res.* 2007;13:2378-2384.
64. Giannelli G, Marinosci F, Trerotoli P, et al. SCCA antigen combined with alpha-fetoprotein as serologic markers of HCC. *Int J Cancer.* 2005;117:506-509.
65. Chuma M, Sakamoto M, Yamazaki K, et al. Expression profiling in multistage hepatocarcinogenesis: identification of HSP70 as a molecular marker of early hepatocellular carcinoma. *Hepatology.* 2003;37:198-207.
66. Sakamoto M, Mori T, Masugi Y, et al. Candidate molecular markers for histological diagnosis of early hepatocellular carcinoma. *Intervirology.* 2008;51(suppl 1):42-45.
67. Kato M, Shinozawa T, Kato S, et al. Increased midkine expression in hepatocellular carcinoma. *Arch Pathol Lab Med.* 2000;124:848-852.
68. Smith MW, Yue ZN, Geiss GK, et al. Identification of novel tumor markers in hepatitis C virus-associated hepatocellular carcinoma. *Cancer Res.* 2003;63:859-864.
69. Lee IN, Chen CH, Sheu JC, et al. Identification of complement C3a as a candidate biomarker in human chronic hepatitis C and HCV-related hepatocellular carcinoma using a proteomics approach. *Proteomics.* 2006;6:2865-2873.
70. Lee MJ, Yu GR, Park SH, et al. Identification of cystatin B as a potential serum marker in hepatocellular carcinoma. *Clin Cancer Res.* 2008;14:1080-1089.
71. Nam SW, Park JY, Ramasamy A, et al. Molecular changes from dysplastic nodule to hepatocellular carcinoma through gene expression profiling. *Hepatology.* 2005;42:809-818.
72. Delpuech O, Trabut JB, Carnot F, et al. Identification, using cDNA macroarray analysis, of distinct gene expression profiles associated with pathological and virological features of hepatocellular carcinoma. *Oncogene.* 2002;21:2926-2937.
73. Paradis V, Bieche I, Dargere D, et al. Molecular profiling of hepatocellular carcinomas (HCC) using a large-scale real-time RT-PCR approach: determination of a molecular diagnostic index. *Am J Pathol.* 2003;163:733-741.
74. Poon TC, Yip TT, Chan AT, et al. Comprehensive proteomic profiling identifies serum proteomic signatures for detection of hepatocellular carcinoma and its subtypes. *Clin Chem.* 2003;49:752-760.
75. Paradis V, Degos F, Dargere D, et al. Identification of a new marker of hepatocellular carcinoma by serum protein profiling of patients with chronic liver diseases. *Hepatology.* 2005;41:40-47.
76. Ward DG, Cheng Y, N'Kontchou G, et al. Changes in the serum proteome associated with the development of hepatocellular carcinoma in hepatitis C-related cirrhosis. *Br J Cancer.* 2006;94:287-292.

77. Kanmura S, Uto H, Kusumoto K, et al. Early diagnostic potential for hepatocellular carcinoma using the SELDI ProteinChip system. *Hepatology.* 2007;45:948-956.
78. Vandenboom Ii TG, Li Y, Philip PA, et al. MicroRNA and cancer: tiny molecules with major implications. *Curr Genomics.* 2008;9:97-109.
79. Wang Y, Lee AT, Ma JZ, et al. Profiling microRNA expression in hepatocellular carcinoma reveals microRNA-224 up-regulation and apoptosis inhibitor-5 as a microRNA-224-specific target. *J Biol Chem.* 2008;283:13205-13215.
80. Han SJ, Yoo S, Choi SH, et al. Actual half-life of alpha-fetoprotein as a prognostic tool in pediatric malignant tumors. *Pediatr Surg Int.* 1997;12:599-602.
81. Yamashita F, Tanaka M, Satomura S, et al. Prognostic significance of *Lens culinaris* agglutinin A-reactive alpha-fetoprotein in small hepatocellular carcinomas. *Gastroenterology.* 1996;111:996-1001.
82. Hayashi K, Kumada T, Nakano S, et al. Usefulness of measurement of *Lens culinaris* agglutinin-reactive fraction of alpha-fetoprotein as a marker of prognosis and recurrence of small hepatocellular carcinoma. *Am J Gastroenterol.* 1999;94:3028-3033.
83. Yamashiki N, Seki T, Wakabayashi M, et al. Usefulness of *Lens culinaris* agglutinin A-reactive fraction of alpha-fetoprotein (AFP-L3) as a marker of distant metastasis from hepatocellular carcinoma. *Oncol Rep.* 1999;6:1229-1232.
84. Hsu IC, Metcalf RA, Sun T, et al. Mutational hotspot in the p53 gene in human hepatocellular carcinomas. *Nature.* 1991;350:427-428.
85. Liu S, Ma L, Huang W, et al. Decreased expression of the human carbonyl reductase 2 gene HCR2 in hepatocellular carcinoma. *Cell Mol Biol Lett.* 2006;11:230-241.
86. Leone N, Pellicano R, Brunello F, et al. Elevated serum chromogranin A in patients with hepatocellular carcinoma. *Clin Exp Med.* 2002;2:119-123.
87. Malaguarnera M, Cristaldi E, Cammalleri L, et al. Elevated chromogranin A (CgA) serum levels in the patients with advanced pancreatic cancer. *Arch Gerontol Geriatr.* 2009;48:213-217.
88. Spadaro A, Ajello A, Morace C, et al. Serum chromogranin-A in hepatocellular carcinoma: diagnostic utility and limits. *World J Gastroenterol.* 2005;11:1987-1990.
89. Li XM, Tang ZY, Qin LX, et al. Serum vascular endothelial growth factor is a predictor of invasion and metastasis in hepatocellular carcinoma. *J Exp Clin Cancer Res.* 1999;18:511-517.
90. Yamagamim H, Moriyama M, Matsumura H, et al. Serum concentrations of human hepatocyte growth factor is a useful indicator for predicting the occurrence of hepatocellular carcinomas in C-viral chronic liver diseases. *Cancer.* 2002;95:824-834.
91. Li J, Wang Y, Yu W, et al. Expression of serum miR-221 in human hepatocellular carcinoma and its prognostic significance. *Biochem Biophys Res Commun.* 2011;406:70-73.
92. Iizuka N, Oka M, Yamada-Okabe H, et al. Oligonucleotide microarray for prediction of early intrahepatic recurrence of hepatocellular carcinoma after curative resection. *Lancet.* 2003;361:923-929.
93. Kurokawa Y, Matoba R, Takemasa I, et al. Molecular-based prediction of early recurrence in hepatocellular carcinoma. *J Hepatol.* 2004;41:284-291.
94. Wang SM, Ooi LL, Hui KM. Identification and validation of a novel gene signature associated with the recurrence of human hepatocellular carcinoma. *Clin Cancer Res.* 2007;13:6275-6283.
95. Uchimura S, Iizuka N, Tamesa T, et al. Resampling based on geographic patterns of hepatitis virus infection reveals a common gene signature for early intrahepatic recurrence of hepatocellular carcinoma. *Anticancer Res.* 2007;27:3323-3330.
96. Cheung ST, Leung KL, Ip YC, et al. Claudin-10 expression level is associated with recurrence of primary hepatocellular carcinoma. *Clin Cancer Res.* 2005;11:551-556.
97. Iizuka N, Tamesa T, Sakamoto K, et al. Different molecular pathways determining extrahepatic and intrahepatic recurrences of hepatocellular carcinoma. *Oncol Rep.* 2006;16:1137-1142.
98. Sato F, Hatano E, Kitamura K, et al. MicroRNA profile predicts recurrence after resection in patients with hepatocellular carcinoma within the Milan Criteria. *PLoS One.* 2011;6:e16435.
99. Chuma M, Sakamoto M, Yasuda J, et al. Overexpression of cortactin is involved in motility and metastasis of hepatocellular carcinoma. *J Hepatol.* 2004;41:629-636.
100. Fidler IJ. Critical determinants of metastasis. *Semin Cancer Biol.* 2002;12:89-96.
101. Hu L, Lau SH, Tzang CH, et al. Association of vimentin overexpression and hepatocellular carcinoma metastasis. *Oncogene.* 2004;23:298-302.
102. Lau SH, Sham JS, Xie D, et al. Clusterin plays an important role in hepatocellular carcinoma metastasis. *Oncogene.* 2006;25:1242-1250.
103. Budhu A, Jia HL, Forgues M, et al. Identification of metastasis-related microRNAs in hepatocellular carcinoma. *Hepatology.* 2008;47:897-907.
104. Ren N, Wu JC, Dong QZ, et al. Association of specific genotypes in metastatic suppressor HTPAP with tumor metastasis and clinical prognosis in hepatocellular carcinoma. *Cancer Res.* 2011;71:3278-3286.
105. Lee JS, Chu IS, Heo J, et al. Classification and prediction of survival in hepatocellular carcinoma by gene expression profiling. *Hepatology.* 2004;40:667-676.
106. Chen R, Cui J, Xu C, et al. The significance of MMP-9 over MMP-2 in HCC invasiveness and recurrence of hepatocellular carcinoma after curative resection. *Ann Surg Oncol.* 2012;19 (Suppl 3):375-384.
107. Lee JS, Chu IS, Mikaelyan A, et al. Application of comparative functional genomics to identify best-fit mouse models to study human cancer. *Nat Genet.* 2004;36:1306-1311.
108. Durnez A, Verslype C, Nevens F, et al. The clinicopathological and prognostic relevance of cytokeratin 7 and 19 expression in hepatocellular carcinoma. A possible progenitor cell origin. *Histopathology.* 2006;49:138-151.
109. Song W, Li H, Tao K, et al. Expression and clinical significance of the stem cell marker CD133 in hepatocellular carcinoma. *Int J Clin Pract.* 2008;62:1212-1218.
110. Yamashita T, Ji J, Budhu A, et al. EpCAM-positive hepatocellular carcinoma cells are tumor-initiating cells with stem/progenitor cell features. *Gastroenterology.* 2009;136:1012-1024.

CHAPTER 32

Molecular Diagnostics of Pancreatic Cancer

Marco Dal Molin and Anirban Maitra

CURRENT DIAGNOSTIC APPROACH TO PANCREATIC CANCER

The vast majority of pancreatic ductal adenocarcinomas (aka pancreatic cancer) are diagnosed at a late stage. It is estimated that only 15% to 20% of all diagnoses are achieved in an ideal time frame in which the disease is still amenable to cure.[1–3] More frequently, clinicians are able to formulate the correct diagnosis when the tumor has already metastasized to other organs or is locally advanced, and therefore not surgically resectable. There are several reasons for such a delay: first, because of its anatomic location, the pancreas is not easily accessible with conventional diagnostic tools, rendering screening tests that have been extremely successful for the early diagnosis of other tumor types (e.g., breast, colorectal, and cervical) difficult to apply. Second, since initial signs and symptoms of pancreatic cancer are usually aspecific, the clinical workup is often procrastinated until the onset of more suspicious signs, such as obstructive jaundice, new-onset diabetes, and weight loss, that are more often associated with advanced disease. Third, cystic precursor lesions of pancreatic cancer (intraductal papillary mucinous neoplasms [IPMNs] and mucinous cystic neoplasms [MCNs]) are not easily distinguishable from benign cysts and may represent a diagnostic dilemma that eventually delays the correct diagnosis.

The capability to diagnose pancreatic cancer at an early stage would represent an invaluable resource for improving cure rates of this devastating disease. In fact, a clear benefit in overall survival from early-stage surgical resection has been shown by several studies in literature. Sohn and colleagues[4] prospectively evaluated 616 resected pancreatic cancer patients and observed that patients with tumors less than 3 cm in diameter without nodal involvement and negative resection margins had significantly higher 5-year survival rates (31%) compared with the study's overall survival rate (17%).

Currently, the diagnosis of pancreatic cancer relies almost exclusively on imaging tests, including computed tomography (CT) scan, magnetic resonance imaging (MRI)/magnetic resonance cholangio-pancreatography, endoscopic ultrasonography (EUS), and endoscopic retrograde cholangio-pancreatography (ERCP). In recent years, the sensitivity of CT scan and EUS has significantly improved, and both these techniques are now considered the diagnostic gold-standard for pancreatic cancer.[5,6] However, several limitations hamper the accuracy of such tests: the detection of small pancreatic lesions (<5 mm) is still difficult to achieve, leading to potentially curable tumors being missed. Furthermore, macroscopic precursor lesions of pancreatic cancer (either IPMNs or MCNs) may be difficult to differentiate from other benign cystic lesions, based upon imaging. In this context, the availability of new diagnostic tools that help discriminate potentially malignant lesions from "innocent" benign cysts would be extremely beneficial. Finally, tests such as EUS and ERCP represent invasive procedures, and although rarely, they can lead to iatrogenic complications, such as acute pancreatitis and intra-abdominal hemorrhage.

Ideally, the introduction of accurate diagnostic biomarkers, harboring high sensitivity and specificity, would greatly enhance the armamentarium available to clinicians in the diagnostic setting. Currently, the serum marker, sialylated Lewis-A blood group antigen CA 19-9, is widely employed in clinical practice, but because of lack of sensitivity and specificity as a diagnostic marker, its use is limited to monitoring responses to therapy.[7–12] Elevated levels of CA 19-9 are commonly seen in patients with benign pancreatic and biliary disorders. Furthermore, up to 30% of patients with pancreatic cancer do not present elevated serum levels of CA 19-9, and it is estimated that 5% to 10% of the population do not express Lewis antigens and do not have detectable CA 19-9 levels. CA 19-9 is also unable to reliably differentiate patients with pancreatic cancer from those with chronic pancreatitis, since up to 40% of patients with chronic pancreatitis display an elevated CA 19-9 level.[8,13,14]

New diagnostic biomarkers that overcome such limitations would complement current imaging techniques and allow a more rapid definition of the disease in patients with symptoms suspicious for pancreatic cancer. They would also represent a fundamental tool for the surveillance of individuals at high risk for pancreatic cancer. Ideally, a correct diagnosis could be achieved in those individuals, when microscopic lesions are present, even before the onset of symptoms.[15]

MOLECULAR ALTERATIONS AS TOOLS FOR EARLY DIAGNOSIS

A wealth of studies over the last two decades have unquestionably proved that cancer is a genetic disease, in which tumorigenesis is driven by both somatic and inherited alterations in the DNA. The recently uncovered genomic sequence of pancreatic cancer has offered an unprecedent opportunity to better characterize the genetic landscape of this disease and identify potential candidates for biomarker discovery.[16] Genomic DNA abnormalities are frequently observed in pancreatic cancer, including copy number changes, activating mutations of oncogenes, and silencing mutations or inactivation of tumor-suppressor and caretaker genes. In addition, epigenetic modifications, alterations in telomeres, and mutations in mitochondrial DNA (mt-DNA) are also features of pancreatic cancer as well as other cancer types. Based on these observations, the unique molecular features displayed by cancer cells as opposed to their normal counterparts indeed constitute an invaluable resource that can be exploited for diagnostic purposes.

Circulating tumor cells (CTCs) could represent an ideal diagnostic biomarker, as they display the molecular characteristics of the bulk tumor, with the advantage of being isolated directly from blood of patients. Not only do they indicate the presence of a tumor, but they may also be used to test tumor sensitivity to specific anticancer agents. Although extremely appealing as biomarkers, CTCs are rare and their isolation represents a tremendous challenge from a technical standpoint. Recently, researchers have developed and optimized a microfluidic device (CTC-chip) consisting of an array of microposts coated with antiepithelial cell-adhesion molecule (EpCAM) antibodies.[17] The presence of antibodies specific for epithelial cells ensures adequate power for discriminating CTCs from the much more abundant hematologic cells, directly in unfractioned blood samples. Such a technique, tested in blood samples from metastatic pancreatic cancer patients, as well as patients with other tumor types, demonstrated a sensitivity of 99.1% and a specificity of 100%. Although mainly tested in metastatic patients, in whom CTCs may differ in concentration and characteristics when compared with CTCs from patients at earlier stages, this novel approach may represent a promising tool for early detection, if validated by additional studies.

GENETIC ALTERATIONS AS BIOMARKERS OF PANCREATIC CANCER

DNA-based biomarkers may represent advantageous diagnostic tools, as they aim to identify cancer-specific alterations. The accuracy of DNA markers has been greatly improved in recent years by novel technologies such as chip-based arrays and quantitative polymerase chain reaction (PCR). Despite the tremendous accuracy of most of the new available technologies, only a few DNA mutations have been discovered that display ideal diagnostic features. In fact, a perfect DNA marker would be widespread among the cancer cell population and would be limited to a small portion of DNA, in order to be easily detectable. *KRAS2* gene is an example of such appealing molecular markers. It has been shown that missense mutations in the *KRAS2* gene are present in over 90% of pancreatic adenocarcinomas and can be readily detected using molecular assays since they are generally limited to one codon (codon 12 > 13 > 61).[18-20] Furthermore, *KRAS2* mutations are among the earliest genetic abnormalities observed in pancreatic intraepithelial neoplasia (PanINs), before cancer develops, and may therefore represent ideal candidates for the early diagnosis of pancreatic cancer.[21] However, several obstacles have mitigated the initial enthusiasm toward *KRAS2* mutations as diagnostic markers. The presence of abundant wild-type DNA, as opposed to a limited number of mutant molecules, makes *KRAS2* mutations difficult to detect in biologic samples, such as serum, pancreatic juice, and stool. Furthermore, *KRAS2* mutations are not only present in pancreatic cancer, but they can also occur in patients with chronic pancreatitis, in individuals who smoke, and in low-grade PanINs of patients without pancreatic cancer.[22-25]

In recent years, several more sensitive assays for the detection of mutant *KRAS2* have been developed that could help identify low-concentration mutant molecules and allow the quantification of differences in the concentration of mutant *KRAS2* between pancreatic cancer and benign conditions. Recently, a technique termed LigAmp, which involves DNA ligation and PCR amplification, has been successfully used to detect *KRAS2* mutations in pancreatic juice samples.[26] This method has shown exquisite sensitivity, as it was able to identify 1 mutant molecule in 10,000 wild-type molecules. Moreover, LigAmp quantification of mutant *KRAS2* has demonstrated significantly higher levels of mutant molecules among patients with pancreatic cancer, compared with patients affected by chronic pancreatitis. Another robust technology termed BEAMing (based on its four main components: beads, emulsion, amplification, and magnetics) has been recently shown to represent an ultrasensitive method for detection of mutant alleles.[27] This technology converts single DNA molecules to single magnetic beads so that, after PCR amplification, each bead contains thousands of copies of the sequence of the original DNA molecule. Fluorescent-labeled oligonucleotides are used to assess mutant molecule specificity, and the number of mutant DNA molecules in a population is determined by quantifying fluorescence using flow cytometry. Given the frequency of mutant *KRAS2* in pancreatic cancer, these new quantitative assays could greatly improve its role as a diagnostic biomarker.

TP53 gene mutations have been widely investigated as diagnostic markers in a variety of cancers, including pancreatic cancer. It has been estimated that *TP53* mutations are found in ~50% to 75% of invasive pancreatic cancers[28] and tend to occur late in the progression from low-grade PanINs toward cancer. This feature renders *TP53* particularly appealing as a biomarker, since it could help discriminate precursor lesions with low malignant potential from lesions that are more likely to progress toward cancer. In addition, *TP53* mutations might be helpful for differentiating cancer from chronic pancreatitis, as it has been shown that *TP53* mutations rarely occur in chronic pancreatitis.[29] However, mutant *TP53* has been found in individuals who smoke or have been exposed to environmental toxins (e.g., aflatoxins), limiting its specificity as a diagnostic marker.[30] In addition, unlike mutant *KRAS2*, *TP53* mutations can occur throughout the entire gene,[30] although hotspot regions of a few nucleotides have been described. The widespread susceptibility to mutations that characterizes the *TP53* gene has minimized the application of specific nucleotide detection strategies to diagnosis. To overcome this limitation, researchers have focused on new detection strategies that harbor the potential to identify the entire mutational spectrum of *TP53*. In a recent study, PCR single-strand conformational polymorphism followed by direct sequencing was used for analyses of p53 mutations in exons 5–8 in pancreatic juice from patients with pancreatic cancer.[31] By a combined assay with supernatant and sediment, *TP53* mutations were detected in 52.4% of patients with cancer, approximately the mutation rate that would be expected in primary cancers from these patients. Immunohistochemistry represents another useful assay to detect *TP53* mutations in pancreatic cancer. This technique relies on highly specific antibodies against mutant p53 protein, which accumulates in the nucleus of neoplastic cells. Recently, investigators have used a panel consisting of combined markers to improve the molecular diagnosis of pancreatic cancer.[32] Markers included in the panel included mutant K-ras, aberrantly methylated p16, and a functional yeast assay for the detection of mutant p53. Of all markers analyzed, the presence of p53 mutations was the most specific. These results suggest that improvements in technology may allow for a more sensitive and specific detection of p53 mutations in pancreatic juice, even at very low concentration.

The expansion of high-throughput technologies over the last decade, and the increasing knowledge of the genomic alterations that characterize pancreatic cancer, will more easily allow the detection of multiple mutated genes in a single sample using a single assay. Assays that use "capture" technology to enrich for specific exomic regions or genes, followed by library preparation and next-generation sequencing, will allow the assessment of somatic mutations in multiple genetic regions in one experiment. In addition, because of the high sensitivity (at least 1% of mutant DNA), such techniques are particularly suitable for the analysis of heterogeneous biologic samples, in which the amount of mutant molecules can be very low. Therefore, the analysis of mutant *KRAS2* or *TP53* can be implemented by adding other mutated genes, for example, *p16/CDKN2A* or *DPC4/SMAD4*, to gain sensitivity and specificity.

The *p16/CDKN2A* gene on chromosome 9p is inactivated in more than 95% of pancreatic cancers, representing the most frequently inactivated tumor-suppressor gene in this tumor type. In 40% of the cancers, this is caused by a homozygous deletion of both alleles of the gene, in another 40% by an intragenic mutation in one allele coupled with loss of the other allele, and in 15% by hypermethylation of the *p16/CDKN2A* gene promoter.[24,33,34] The *p16/CDKN2A* gene is also inactivated in PanINs, suggesting its potential use as a biomarker for early detection.[34,35] *DPC4/SMAD4* is involved in the transforming growth factor beta transduction signaling pathway and functions as a key tumor suppressor; homozygous deletion or intragenic mutation of somatic *DPC4/SMAD4* gene frequently occurs in pancreatic cancer.[36] Loss of heterozygosity (LOH) at 18q, where *DPC4/SMAD4* gene is located, also occurs in 90% of pancreatic cancer.[37] Homozygous deletion or intragenic inactivating mutations of *DPC4/SMAD4* gene, as well as the complete loss of Smad4 protein expression, are observed in 50% ductal adenocarcinomas.[36] The loss of Smad4 appears to be rather a late event in the pathogenesis of pancreatic cancer and it is uncommon in nonductal pancreatic cancer or other malignancies.[36,38,39] Remarkably, inactivation of the *DPC4/SMAD4* gene has been shown to correlate with high histopathologic grade and poorer prognosis. Furthermore, it has been found that pancreatic cancers with an increased propensity to metastasize rapidly display a significantly higher proportion of mutant *DPC4*/SMAD4, compared with tumors in which *DPC4*/SMAD4 is intact.[40] An immunohistochemical labeling for Smad4 protein expression has been developed that correlates with *DPC4/SMAD4* gene status and is widely used in clinical biopsies or aspiration cytology samples where an occult pancreatic primary is suspected[41] (Fig. 32.1).

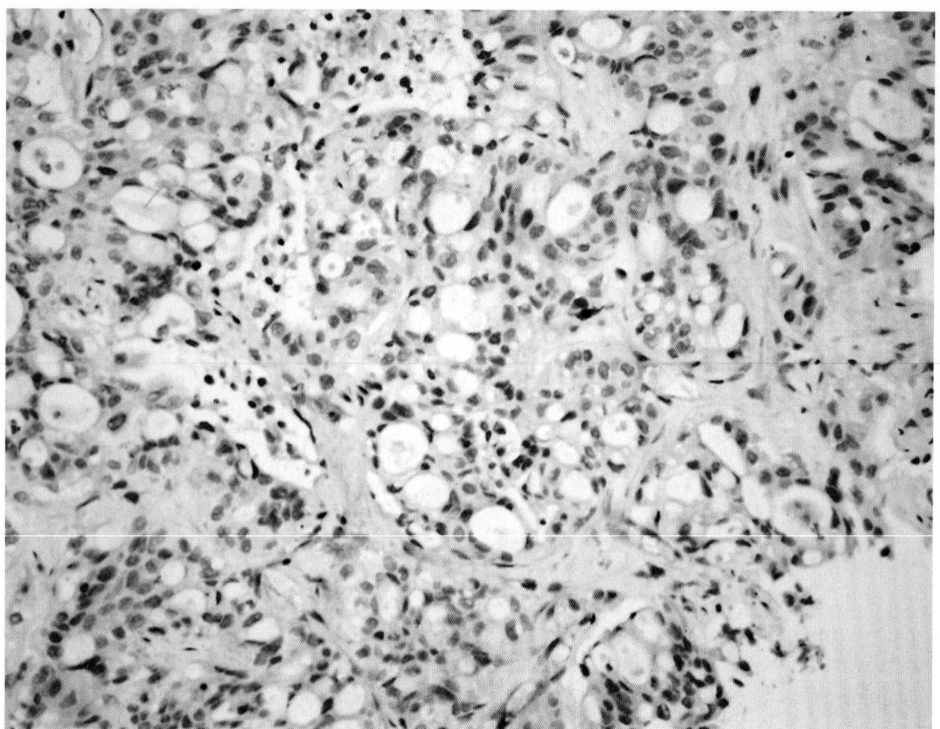

FIGURE 32–1 Loss of Dpc4 immunostain in a liver metastasis from a pancreatic ductal adenocarcinoma. The neoplastic cells lack any discernible expression of Dpc4, while entrapped non-neoplastic cells retain expression.

The expansion of sequencing analysis to entire cancer genomes or exomes, including pancreatic cancer, has allowed for the identification of rare genetic alterations in an unprecedented detail. Remarkably, such rare mutations have acquired considerable attention over the last few years, as they may identify specific subsets of patients who benefit from tailored anticancer therapies. An example of such a therapeutic advantage has been shown in tumors harboring mutations in the *BRCA2* gene. It is reported that 7% to 10% of infiltrating ductal adenocarcinomas of the pancreas present an inactivating inherited mutation of one copy of the second breast cancer gene (*BRCA2*) accompanied by LOH.[42,43] Pancreatic cancers harboring *BRCA2* gene mutations are clinically relevant for two reasons: first, the *BRCA2* gene in these cancers is usually inactivated by a germline mutation in one allele, coupled with somatic loss of the remaining allele in the cancer. Therefore, patients with germline *BRCA2* mutations can be identified and followed even before the onset of cancer. Second, *BRCA2*-mutant cancers may benefit from targeted therapeutic options. In fact, the protein product of the *BRCA2* gene interacts with the protein products of the Fanconi anemia complementation genes (the *FANC* genes) to promote homologous recombination, preventing dangerous gene rearrangements that can occur as a consequence of DNA double-strand breaks.[44] It has been shown that pancreatic cancer cells harboring mutations in the FANC/BRCA2 pathway are hypersensitive to DNA-interstrand cross-linking agents, such as mitomycin C, cisplatin, and poly (ADP-ribose) polymerase inhibitors (PARP-i).[45] The clinical use of such specific anticancer therapies is currently under investigation for other tumor types that harbor BRCA2 mutations, such as breast and ovarian cancer.[46] Preliminary data in pancreatic cancer, although on a small cohort of patients, have suggested a potential benefit from PARP-i and platinum-based therapies in a selected subset of patients, in which early detection of BRCA1-2 mutations had been demonstrated.[47]

Along with high-resolution mutational analyses of nuclear coding genes, a substantial area of cancer genetic research has focused on mt-DNA mutations. mt-DNA mutations are commonly observed in a variety of human cancers, including pancreatic cancer. Although they are more likely to represent a bystander effect rather than being directly involved in the pathogenesis of cancer, mutations of mt-DNA have been proposed as candidates for the early diagnosis of pancreatic cancer.[48] In fact, mt-DNA offers several advantages as a biomarker, since hundreds to thousands of copies of the mitochondrial genome are present inside a single human cell, and cancer cells present significantly higher levels of mt-DNA, compared with normal tissue. The MitoChip (Custom Reseq), an array-based sequencing platform for high-throughput analysis of mt-DNA, has demonstrated its usefulness to detect mitochondrial mutation in pancreatic juice of patients with pancreatic cancer.[48] Interestingly, mt-DNA mutations are also found in precursor lesions of pancreatic cancer, suggesting that mutations occur in early stages of tumor development and rendering their analysis for early detection particularly attractive.

EPIGENETIC ALTERATIONS

Epigenetic changes such as DNA methylation, post-translational modifications of histones, and changes in micro-RNAs expression have gained considerable importance in the context of cancer research. Aberrant methylation of gene promoters is commonly observed in a broad spectrum of tumors and it is thought to represent a contributing factor for inactivation of tumor-suppressor genes.[49] In human cells, methylation of DNA involves the cytosines of CG dinucleotides (CpGs). Often CpGs are located at a high concentration in specific regions of the DNA (CpG islands) that are usually found in the 5′ regulatory regions of genes in an unmethylated status. Aberrant methylation of genes represents a particularly attractive feature, since it can be readily identified using a sensitive methylation-specific PCR (MSP). This technique relies on the fact that unmethylated cytosines can be effectively converted into uracils by bisulfite treatment, whereas methylated cytosines are insensitive to bisulfite treatment. After bisulfite treatment, methylated and unmethylated regions can be easily differentiated by MSP. Recently, the analysis of a large panel of pancreatic cancers, using this technique, has identified several specific hypermethylated genes.[50]

An increasing number of genes that play a role in the pathogenesis of pancreatic cancer, such as *APC*,[51] *TSLC/IGSF4*,[52] *SOCS-1*,[53] *RASSF1A*,[54] *CCDN2*,[55] *WWOX*,[56] *RUNX3*,[57] *CDH13*,[58] *DUSP6*,[59] *SLC5A8*,[60] and *HHIP*,[61] have been shown to undergo aberrant methylation, resulting in reduced or lost expression. Aberrant methylation status represents an attractive feature that can be investigated for diagnostic purposes, as multiple studies indicate that the detection of aberrantly methylated genes in the pancreatic juice and other biologic fluids of patients with pancreatic cancer is feasible.[62-66] In addition to the assessment of hypermethylated genes, recent studies have shown that aberrant *hypo*methylation of genes is also involved in cancer development and progression. The reduction or loss of DNA methylation determines the induction of gene expression which, in turn, drives tumorigenesis. Several hypomethylated genes, such as S100A4,[67] have been identified in pancreatic cancer that could have important biologic implications. In fact, some of those genes may represent candidates for early diagnosis tests, as well as molecular targets for novel therapies directed to suppress gene function.

Although encouraging, DNA methylation analysis studies present several caveats that need to be taken into account. First, the evaluation of hyper- or hypomethylation is based on the comparison between cancer and normal tissues. It has been shown that some of the genes aberrantly methylated in pancreatic cancer when compared with normal pancreas are also methylated in normal duodenum[62]; furthermore, genes are more likely to become aberrantly methylated as patient's age increases limiting the specificity of this technique.[68,69] It is expected that more sophisticated and specific methods will overcome soon these limitations, providing a deeper understanding of the mechanisms that regulate methylation, as well as the effects of methylation on cancer cell metabolism.

MicroRNAs (miRNAs) are recently described small RNA molecules 18 to 24 nucleotide long that regulate the stability and translational efficiency of their complementary target mRNAs. Approximately 1,000 miRNAs have been identified so far, and widespread alterations in these miRNAs have been reported in various types of cancer.[70-74] While the expression of most miRNAs appears to be reduced in cancer, several are overexpressed and could be potential targets for early detection of pancreatic cancer. A recent study performed by Bloomston and colleagues[75] compared miRNAs expression in 65 microdissected pancreatic cancers, in their adjacent non-neoplastic pancreatic tissues and in a set of chronic pancreatitis specimens, demonstrating that miRNA expression profile associated with chronic pancreatitis samples was closer to normal pancreas profiles than to pancreatic cancer profiles.[75] Furthermore, aberrant expression of certain miRNAs has been shown to correlate with precursor lesions of pancreatic cancer, engendering the hope that these can serve as biomarkers for early detection. For example, a recent study showed that aberrant expression of miR-155 appears to be an early event in the progression model of pancreatic cancer.[76] The expression of miR-155 was assessed using quantitative reverse transcription PCR in 31 microdissected PanINs and then was tested using locked nucleic acid in situ hybridization (LNA-ISH) in PanIN tissue microarrays. Overexpression of miR-155 was confirmed in both PanIN-2 and PanIN-3 when compared with normal ductal epithelium (Fig. 32.2), suggesting a role for this miRNA in the progression of pancreatic cancer. miRNAs can be feasibly detected in biologic fluids, such as blood, pancreatic juice, and cyst fluid, as they have been shown to accurately discriminate between cancer and non-invasive conditions. For example, significant overexpression of miR-200a and miR-200b in the sera of patients with pancreatic cancer or chronic pancreatitis has been found compared with healthy controls.[77] Furthermore, miRNAs profiling in pancreatic cyst fluid samples has been shown to be an efficient method for discriminating between benign and potentially malignant cysts of the pancreas. Among five miRNAs known to be overexpressed in pancreatic cancer (miR-155, miR-21, miR-221, miR-17-3, and miR-191), miR-155, miR-21, and miR-17-3 were found to be overexpressed in mucinous *versus* non-mucinous pancreatic cystic neoplasms. Of these three miRNAs, miR-21 resulted in the most specific marker associated with mucinous cysts, with a sensitivity of 80% and a specificity of 76%.[78]

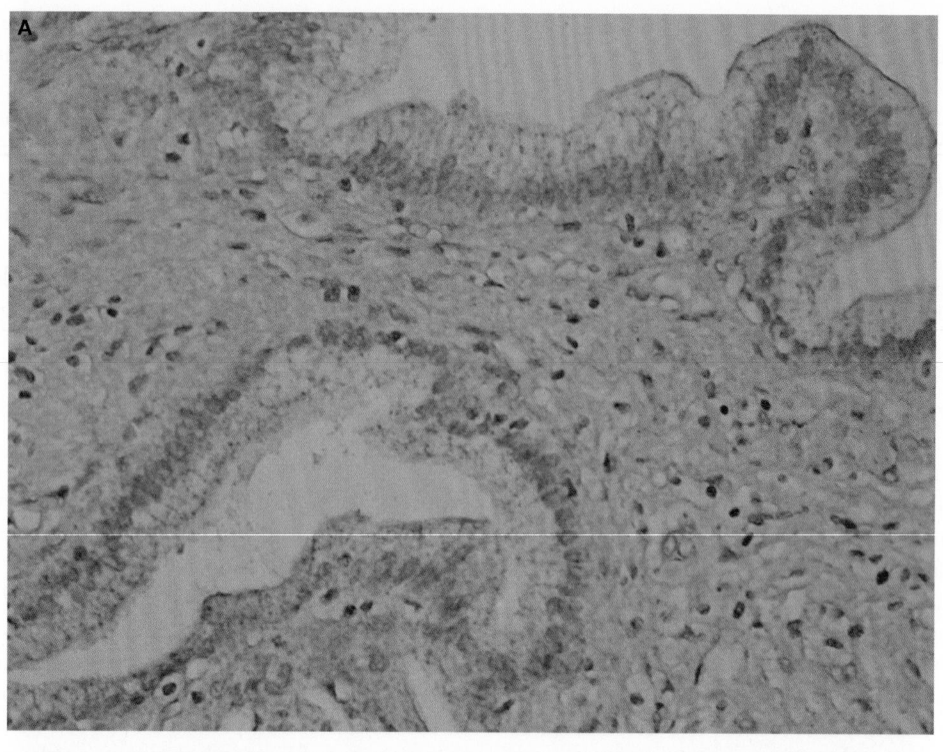

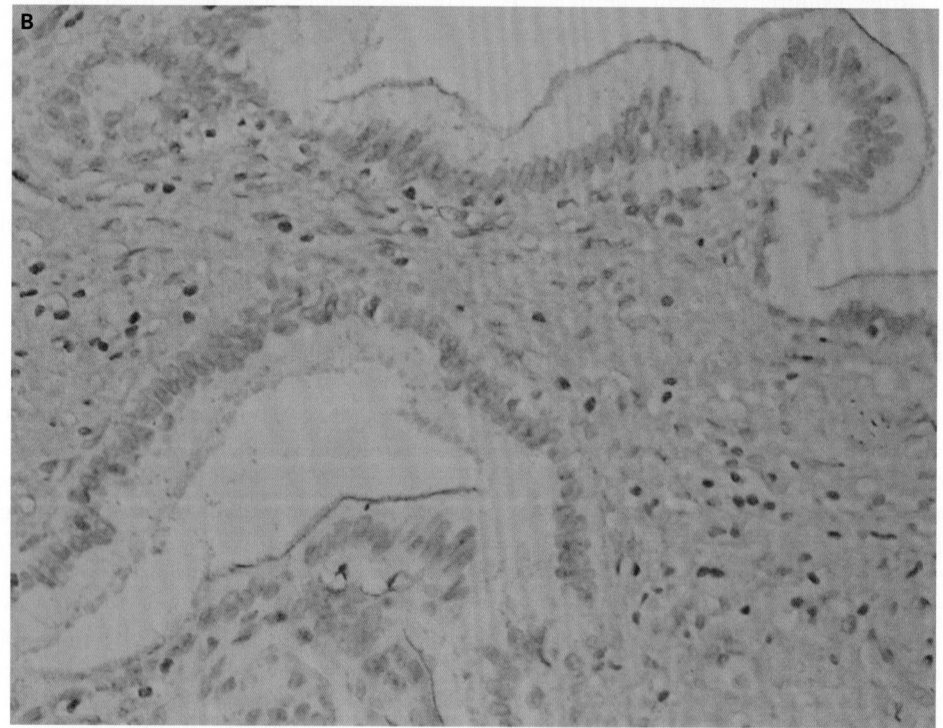

FIGURE 32–2 Overexpression of microRNA miR-155 in non-invasive precursor lesion of pancreatic adenocarcinoma (pancreatic intraepithelial neoplasia). In situ hybridization for miR-155 was performed **(A)**, with scrambled sequence used as control **(B)**.

TRANSCRIPTOMIC AND PROTEOMIC ALTERATIONS

The development of sophisticated gene expression analysis methods in recent years has enormously increased the detection of abnormalities at the transcriptional (RNA) level in most human cancers. Several transcriptome profiling studies have identified differentially expressed genes in pancreatic cancer[79-88] compared with non-neoplastic tissues. These data can be used to evaluate the expression profiling of cancer genomes and identify altered proteins that may represent candidates for either diagnosis and targeted therapy. One of the better studied RNA-based marker of cancer to date has been the human telomerase reverse transcriptase gene (*hTERT*). *hTERT*, which represents one of the subunits of telomerase, has been extensively investigated as a diagnostic marker of pancreatic cancer.[89,90] One study has demonstrated *hTERT* expression to be highly specific, as it has been detected in 88% of the pancreatic cancer samples examined, and only in 17% of chronic pancreatitis samples but not in normal controls.[89] Furthermore, quantitative analysis of *hTERT* mRNA in pancreatic juice has been shown to be advantageous over cytologic analysis for differentiation between pancreatic cancer and IPMNs.[90]

Gene expression profiling studies have identified numerous genes overexpressed at the transcriptional level in pancreatic cancer, and these alterations can be confirmed by the analysis of expression changes at the tissue level using immunohistochemistry or in situ hybridization. The importance of determining protein expression lies in the fact that it can elucidate the specific compartment (epithelial, stromal, angiolymphatic, etc.) where the aberrant expression is occurring. For example, the actin-associated protein palladin has been recently identified as overexpressed in many sporadic pancreatic tumors and in precursor lesions of pancreatic cancer.[91] There are two major palladin isoforms expressed in pancreas: 65 and 85 to 90 kDa. Immunohistochemical studies have shown that the 85 to 90 kDa palladin isoform is highly expressed in tumor-associated fibroblasts in both primary and metastatic tumors, compared with normal pancreas. Thus, palladin abnormalities are a reflection of stroma, rather than epithelial, misexpression, in pancreatic cancer. In contrast, mesothelin mRNA transcripts and proteins are consistently overexpressed in virtually all primary pancreatic adenocarcinomas, and here the expression is entirely epithelial.[92] Furthermore, mesothelin-specific T cells can be induced in patients with pancreatic cancer. This observation suggests that mesothelin may not only be a diagnostic marker of pancreatic cancer but also a potential target for immune-based therapies.[93-95] Deregulation of several other transcripts and their correspondent proteins has been demonstrated in pancreatic cancer. For example, the gene expression profiles of primary infiltrating ductal adenocarcinomas of the pancreas from surgical specimens and non-neoplastic samples demonstrated that Claudin 18 and Annexin A8 are frequently highly overexpressed in infiltrating ductal adenocarcinomas but not in normal ducts.[96]

Pyruvate kinase (PK) is a key enzyme of glucose metabolism, with various isoforms of PK expressed in different cell types (L-PK, R-PK, and M1-PK).[97] The pyruvate kinase isoenzyme type M2 (M2-PK) is expressed in proliferating cells and tumor cells.[97] A recent study has shown that elevated blood levels of M2-PK had a sensitivity of 85% and specificity of 41% for the diagnosis of pancreatic cancer.[98] Interestingly, the presence of chronic pancreatitis or jaundice, that can limit the reliability of the only available biomarker CA 19-9, does not influence M2-PK levels, rendering it attractive for clinical use.[99] However, M2-PK is reported to have less sensitivity in detecting pancreatic cancer compared with CA 19-9 and the combination of the two markers did not improve the diagnostic sensitivity compared with CA 19-9 alone.

In a recent immunohistochemical study, fatty acid synthase (FAS) labeling was assessed in primary pancreatic adenocarcinomas, IPMNs, and in chronic pancreatitis tissues.[100] FAS catalyzes the synthesis of long-chain fatty acids, and its overexpression has been demonstrated in a variety of solid tumors.[101-106] Elevated levels of FAS were also found in serum of patients with pancreatic cancer and IPMNs suggesting a potential use, in combination with other markers, to quantify the risk of developing cancer in patients affected by premalignant lesions, such as IPMNs.[100]

Remarkable improvements in technology over the last two decades have allowed researchers to explore the proteomes of cancer cells in unprecedented detail. Mass spectrometry (MS) is a widely used unbiased technology for proteomic profiling studies in human cancer. It has been shown that such a sensitive technique is able to accurately identify and quantify rare protein products, such as mutant cancer-specific proteins. Ideally, these proteins provide unique opportunities for biomarker development. Unlike other protein-based biomarkers, such as CA 19-9, carcinoembryonic antigen (CEA), and prostate-specific antigen, mutant proteins are exclusively produced by tumor cells. Furthermore, they not only stand as indirect signals of tumor presence but are also involved in tumor generation and maintenance, in the case they represent the product of a mutated driver gene. As elegantly shown by Wang and colleagues,[107] a new MS approach was able to identify and directly quantify mutant proteins in both cancer cell lines and biologic specimens. When dealing with extremely low quantities of proteins in the context of complex samples, such as tissue lysates and biologic fluids, the sensitivity of conventional proteomic analysis methods can be greatly compromised. To overcome these limitations, the authors enriched a specific fraction of heterogeneous samples by immunoprecipitation, and selectively detected products of normal and mutant alleles by selected reaction monitoring (SRM). The SRM method presents considerable advantages, compared with classic MS, to focus upon a limited number of preselected ions of interest, that are characteristics of certain peptides only, providing therefore a much greater sensitivity. With this approach, the authors demonstrated that it is possible to quantify the number and fraction of normal and mutant Kras protein present in cancer cell lines. Moreover, they also found that mutant Ras proteins can be detected and quantified in complex tissue specimens such as pancreatic and colorectal tumors and in fluid samples from premalignant pancreatic cysts. This new method not only accurately estimated the relative levels of genetically abnormal proteins in the tumors analyzed but also effectively proved to be useful in the diagnostic setting.

PRECURSOR LESIONS OF PANCREATIC CANCER: KEY MOLECULAR TARGETS FOR EARLY DETECTION

Over the last two decades, substantial efforts have been made to elucidate the pathogenesis of pancreatic cancer, and a progression model from non-invasive intraductal precursor lesions toward cancer has been proposed.[108] Precursor lesions of pancreatic cancer include PanIN, IPMNs, and MCNs.

PanINs are microscopic lesions in the smaller (<5 mm) pancreatic ducts[109,110] and are subclassified into PanIN-1, PanIN-2, and PanIN-3 lesions, depending upon the degree of cytologic and architectural atypia. PanINs are often present in the pancreatic parenchyma adjacent to infiltrating adenocarcinomas, and several case reports have documented patients with PanINs who later developed pancreatic cancer. In addition, the high frequency of *KRAS2* gene mutations in human PanINs supports its role as an initiating event for pancreatic cancer formation. Mutations of the *KRAS2* gene are one of the earliest genetic abnormalities observed in the progression model of pancreatic cancer.[111] Interestingly, PanIN lesions and associated cancer within the same pancreas may harbor different *KRAS2* gene mutations, suggesting that some precursors evolve as independent clones from the one that eventually progress to the invasive cancer.[112] Three tumor-suppressor genes, *p16INK4A/CDKN2A*, *TP53*, and *DPC4/SMAD4*, are inactivated in a significant proportion of PanINs, similarly to what is found in invasive adenocarcinomas. Loss of function of *p16INK4A/CDKN2A* is seen in all progression steps toward invasive carcinoma,[34] whereas *TP53* and *DPC4/SMAD4* are believed to be late genetic events in pancreatic carcinoma progression[28,36] (Fig. 32.3).

The recognition of the biologic connection that links PanINs to cancer has led to a plethora of studies on PanINs, including morphologic studies that may harbor clinically relevant implications. For example, Brune et al.[113] and Detlefsen et al.[114] have shown that PanINs are often associated with a distinctive lobulocentric atrophy and fibrosis. These inflammatory lesions are often larger than the PanINs themselves, suggesting their potential use for diagnostic purposes. In fact, although PanINs are too small to be detected by currently available imaging technologies, focal areas of pancreatic fibrosis may represent an indirect marker for their presence.[113]

IPMNs are grossly visible non-invasive mucin-producing epithelial neoplasms that usually form long finger-like papillae and, by definition, involve the main pancreatic duct or one of its branches.[115] IPMNs represent the most frequent macroscopic precursor lesion of pancreatic cancer and, since the progression toward carcinoma is usually slow in these neoplasms, they represent a particularly appealing target for the development of diagnostic biomarkers. From a molecular perspective, IPMNs share certain genetic features with PanINs and ductal adenocarcinoma, such as a relatively high frequency of *KRAS2* gene mutations and inactivation of *TP53* and *p16/CDKN2A*[116,117]; in contrast, other common mutational events in pancreatic cancer such as *SMAD4* gene mutations are relatively infrequent.[118] The serine/threonine kinase encoded by the *LKB1/STK11* gene (which is mutated in the germline in patients with Peutz-Jeghers syndrome [PJS]) is silenced in ~25% of IMPNs (likely through non-mutational events like epigenetic inactivation), and the *PIK3CA* gene has been shown to be mutated in approximately 10% of IPMNs.[119,120] Neither of these genes is frequently altered in usual ductal adenocarcinoma, suggesting underlying genetic differences between IPMNs and "garden variety" adenocarcinomas.[121,122]

In addition to the aforementioned genetic features, a recent study has provided a deeper insight into the pathogenesis of IPMNs,[123] underscoring the unique molecular genetics of this disease. Researchers studied a panel of cyst fluid samples obtained from non-invasive IPMNs, and DNA isolated from these cyst fluid samples was assessed by next-generation sequencing following capture of 169 genes (including oncogenes and tumor-suppressor genes)

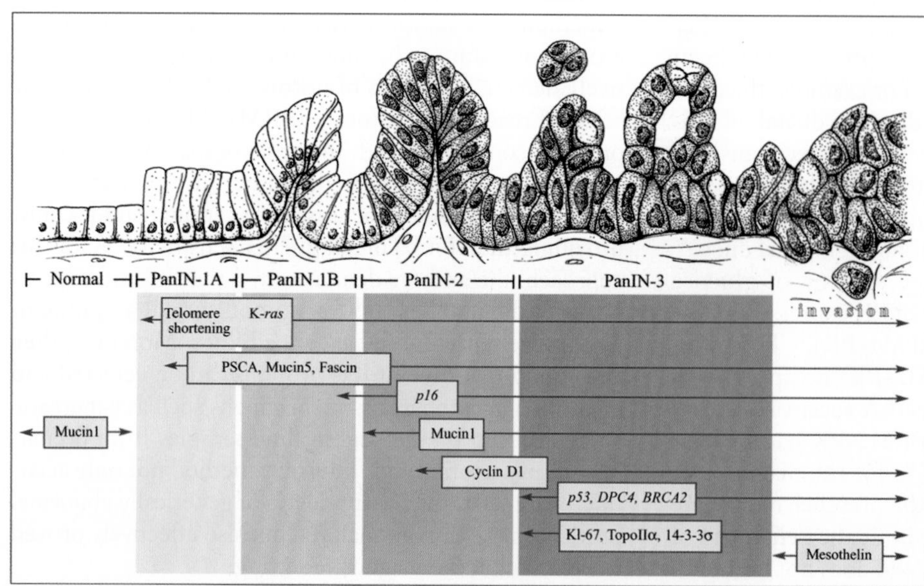

FIGURE 32–3 "PanINgram" model of genetic progression of pancreatic intraepithelial neoplasia to invasive carcinoma. Genetic alterations listed include those that are "early," "intermediate," and "late." Many additional alterations described in the chapter are not illustrated due to space. (Adapted from Maitra et al., *Mod Pathol.* 2003;16:902.)

previously associated with cancer. Somewhat unexpectedly, besides mutant *KRAS2*, which was confirmed to be the most frequently mutated gene in IPMNs, the authors found *GNAS* to be a recurrent abnormal gene in IPMNs. *GNAS* mutations were found in 6 out of 19 cyst fluid specimens analyzed, and this finding was confirmed combining a much more substantial number of samples (cyst fluid and cyst wall from FFPE [formalin-fixed paraffin-embedded] tissues) analyzed in the validation set. In total, 66% of 132 specimens analyzed harbored a somatic *GNAS* mutation, which were always located at a "hot spot" on codon 201 (Fig. 32.4). This newly discovered molecular alteration in IPMNs represents a promising target for both diagnostic and therapeutic options in the most common cystic neoplasm of the pancreas. In fact, more than 96% of the IPMN cyst fluids studied harbored either a *KRAS2* or a *GNAS* mutation, rendering the identification of both mutations particularly attractive for discriminating IPMN from other pancreatic cysts.

MCNs represent the other cystic precursor lesion of pancreatic cancer. MCNs are defined as mucin-producing cyst-forming epithelial neoplasms of the pancreas with a distinctive ovarian-type stroma.[124] It is estimated that one-third of MCNs present with an associated cancer,[125] that is usually of the tubular or ductal type.[126] Mutations of *KRAS* gene are considered early events in the development of MCNs, whereas *TP53* and *SMAD4* gene mutations represent late changes.[127,128] Aberrant methylation of the *p16/CDKN2A* gene occurs infrequently, manifesting in approximately 14% of cases.[127] A recent whole exome

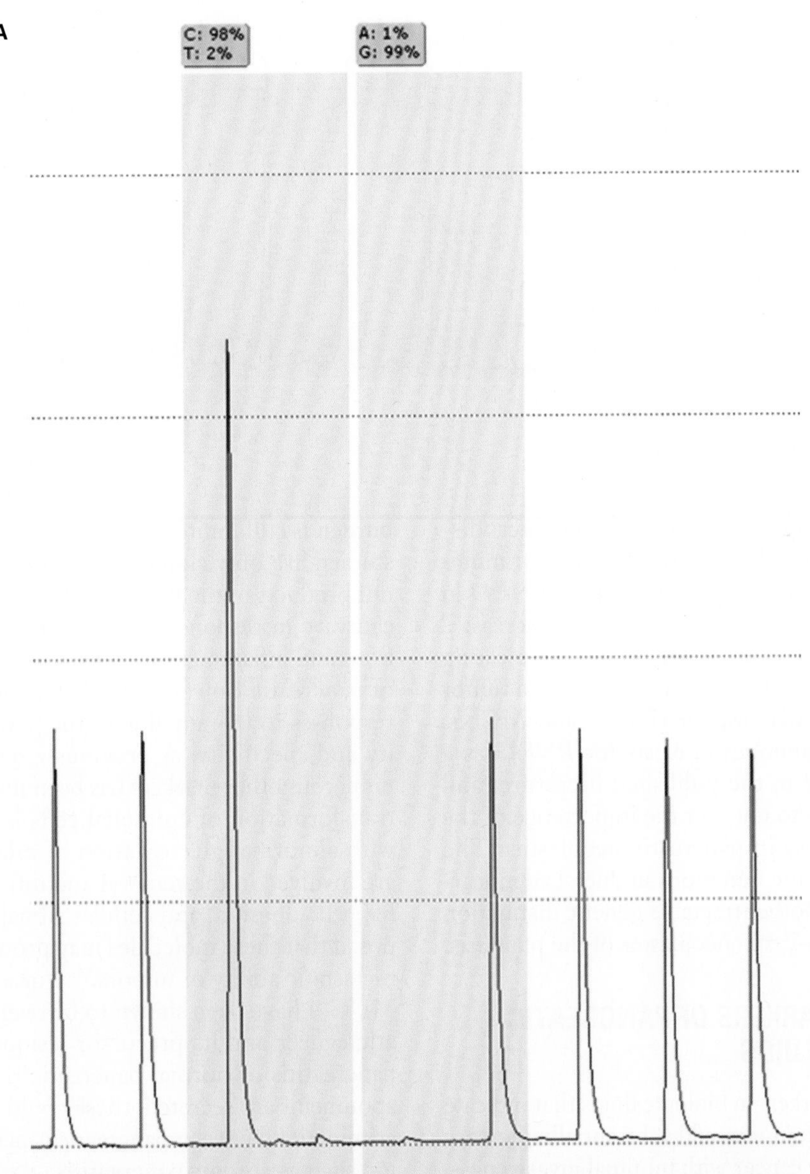

FIGURE 32–4 Mutations of *GNAS* oncogene at codon 201 in a non-invasive intraductal papillary mucinous neoplasm (IPMN) identified by pyrosequencing. Non-neoplastic germline DNA is used as control **(A)**. The pyrogram demonstrates the presence of a heterozygous CGT–TGT mutation **(B)**.

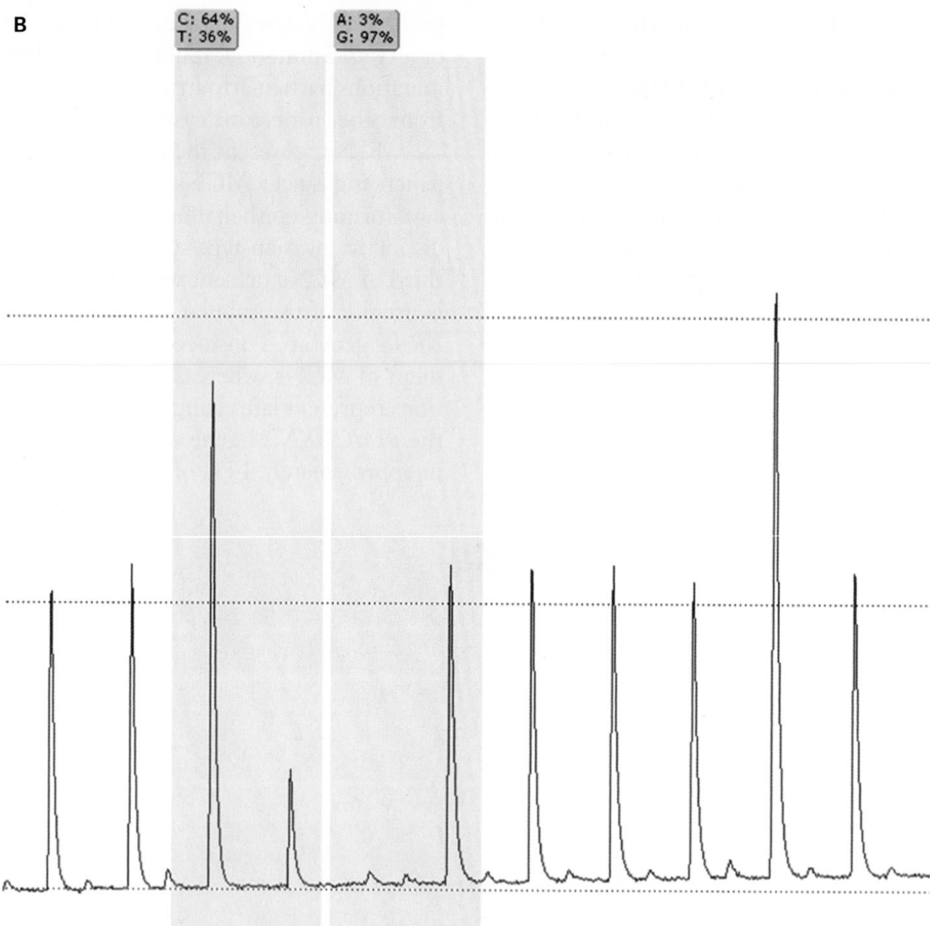

FIGURE 32–4 (*Continued*)

study using next-generation sequencing on microdissected MCNs and IPMNs has identified recurrent mutations of the E3 ubiquitin ligase encoding gene *RNF43* in at least 50% of mucinous cystic lesions of the pancreas.[129] The vast majority of somatic mutations were truncating in nature, suggesting that the gene is behaving as a tumor suppressor in the pathogenesis of IPMNs and MCNs. Very little functional annotation exists for *RNF43* as a cancer-associated gene in the published literature, and future studies are likely to uncover the importance of the encoded ubiquitin ligase in pancreatic neoplasms. The absence of *RNF43* somatic mutations in ductal adenocarcinomas suggests yet another tractable genetic distinction between cystic and non-cystic neoplasms of the pancreas.

DIAGNOSTIC BIOMARKERS OF PANCREATIC CANCER IN BODY FLUIDS

The detection of biomarkers in biologic fluids that indicate the presence of a solid tumor would substantially increase the chances to diagnose cancer with minimal invasiveness, before it becomes unresectable. Unfortunately, several drawbacks have hampered this scenario from becoming a reality in the clinical setting. First, serum markers are usually present at a very low concentration when the tumor burden is still limited. Furthermore, most of the markers studied are only signals of the presence of a tumor, but not products of the tumor itself, and therefore their levels can vary in response to other conditions, such as infections and inflammation. The only available serum marker of pancreatic cancer, CA 19-9, is limited to monitoring responses to therapy due to the poor diagnostic sensitivity and specificity, as previously discussed. The role of numerous other markers has been investigated. Malignant transformation of epithelial cells is generally associated with abnormal glycosylation of mucins (MUCs), which are involved in the renewal and differentiation of epithelia, cell adhesion, and cellular signaling. It has been proposed that these molecules may promote invasiveness and metastatic ability of tumors.[130] For example, MUC-1 and MUC-4 have been shown to be overexpressed in pancreatic cancer and its precursor lesions but not in chronic pancreatitis or normal pancreatic tissue.[131,132] Since both apomucins are secreted, these could be useful for the discrimination between pancreatic cancer from benign mimics, such as chronic pancreatitis.

Using in situ hybridization, *macrophage inhibitory cytokine-1* (MIC-1) RNA levels have been found to be highly expressed in pancreatic cancer, IPMNs, and pancreatic cancer cell lines, as opposed to non-neoplastic pancreatic ductal epithelium.[133] In clinical samples, elevated MIC-1 serum levels were found in 80% of patients with pancreatic cancer, 50% of patients with ampullary adenocarcinoma, 70% of patients with cholangiocarcinoma, but also in 42% of patients with chronic pancreatitis, 67% patients with pancreatic neuroendocrine tumors, and only 4% of healthy controls.[134] Although MIC-1 was significantly better than CA 19-9 in differentiating patients with pancreatic cancer from healthy controls, it was not useful in distinguishing pancreatic cancer from chronic pancreatitis. Nevertheless, elevated serum MIC-1 performed as well as CA 19-9, and the combination of MIC-1 and CA 19-9 significantly improved the diagnosis of pancreatic cancer, rendering this combination particularly attractive.

Pancreatic juice also represents a relevant proximate source for a variety of different molecules that could be used as candidate biomarkers. A distinct advantage of using pancreatic juice is that it can be collected during upper gastrointestinal endoscopy, following secretin infusion. Recent studies have shown that the quantification of altered DNA methylation across a panel of genes in pancreatic juice samples can help in distinguishing between patients with pancreatic cancer and those with chronic pancreatitis, as well as healthy controls. Thus, detection and quantification of aberrantly methylated DNA in pancreatic juice can be regarded as a promising approach to the diagnosis of pancreatic cancer.[65]

Gene expression alterations indicative of pancreatic cancer can also be detected by profiling the RNA of pancreatic juice. A recent study has shown that pancreatic juice samples from patients with pancreatic cancer contain increased levels of *IL8*, *IFITM1*, *fibrinogen*, *osteopontin*, *CXCR4*, and *DAF* transcripts, genes that have been previously reported as overexpressed in primary pancreatic cancers or pancreatic cancer cell lines compared with control tissues.[135] According to these results, RNA analysis of pancreatic juice may represent a potential diagnostic tool, similar to epigenetic or genomic alterations analysis.

The recognition that most pancreatic cysts have a benign behavior, whereas only MCNs and IPMNs harbor a malignant potential, has led researchers to pursue tests that are able to predict whether or not a certain pancreatic cyst will give rise to cancer. Current imaging technologies are not always sufficient to accurately discriminate between different pancreatic cysts; however, in recent years, a molecular approach for the analysis of pancreatic cyst fluid has emerged as a promising tool for complementing the available diagnostic methods. There are several advantages to studying cyst fluid: first, being in direct contact with tumor cells, cyst fluid is more likely to contain tumor cells and tumor-specific molecules, such as DNA, RNA, miRNAs, and proteins, at a higher concentration compared with serum or other biologic fluids. Second, cyst fluid can be visualized by CT scan or EUS and collected using EUS–fine needle aspiration, with limited invasiveness.[136-140] Currently, the most important distinction among pancreatic cysts is the differentiation between serous (and usually benign) cysts and mucinous (potentially malignant) cysts. Overall, the sensitivity and specificity of the cytologic diagnosis are highly variable, depending on the technical expertise.[136-139] Analysis of cyst fluid for CEA is currently considered the most accurate predictor of mucinous cysts.[141] The presence of CA 19-9 in cyst fluid has also been investigated, as a potential test for diagnosis of mucinous cystic tumors. One recent study showed that the detection of CA 19-9 in cyst fluid, in combination with a glycan variant on MUC5AC, was helpful in discriminating mucin-producing cystic neoplasms from benign pancreatic cystic lesions.[142] A team of researchers recently performed the analysis of cyst fluid specimens using a multiplexed Luminex (bead-based) protein assay specifically customized for pancreatic cancer.[143] Differential protein expression between serous cystadenomas (SCAs) and IPMNs was observed in 92% of patients, showing accurate discrimination power. In this study, CEA and CA72.4 were the only proteins that proved to be overexpressed in the cyst fluid of patients with mucinous neoplasms, whereas the majority of other included proteins were downregulated in IPMNs and MCNs compared with SCA.

An increasing number of studies have shown that the molecular analysis of cyst fluid may have a fundamental role as an ancillary test to the current multimodal approach. Given its frequency in pancreatic cancer and mucinous cystic tumors, mutant *KRAS2* represents a very attractive alteration that can be investigated in cyst fluid. In several recent studies, the presence of *KRAS2* gene mutations in cyst fluid specimens was correlated with the presence of an underlying mucinous cyst.[144-146] As previously discussed, however, the low sensitivity of current methods limits the reliability of those techniques in the everyday clinical practice. It is expected that the validation of more sensitive next-generation assays will permit the identification of mutant genes, such as *KRAS2*, with higher sensitivity and specificity. In addition, the recent discovery of the high prevalence of activating *GNAS* mutations in IPMNs[123] will likely be responsible for increasing our ability to accurately discriminate among different pancreatic cysts. Mutant *GNAS* has been shown to act as an oncogene in pituitary and other uncommon tumor types, but has been rarely associated with epithelial neoplasms. Remarkably, all previous studies have shown that *GNAS* mutations tend to cluster in two codons, codon 201 and codon 227. In IPMNs, all *GNAS* mutations were limited to a single "hot spot" on codon 201 (either R201C or R201H), providing an unprecedented opportunity to design a readily applicable ultrasensitive assay for early detection. The presence of either *GNAS* or *KRAS2* mutations was able to reliably exclude the presence of SCAs. Furthermore, although not as sensitive, the presence of *GNAS* mutations can effectively help to discriminate IPMNs from MCNs, since this mutation has not been identified in the latter cysts.

Stool has also been considered an attractive source of biomarkers for the early detection of gastrointestinal cancers. The retrieval of neoplastic pancreatic cells in stool appears feasible, given the excretion of ~1.5 L of pancreatic juice per day and because the majority of pancreatic adenocarcinomas are anatomically connected to the ductal system. Regarding the range of potential marker candidates, the use of non-DNA markers, for instance, proteins or mRNA produced by tumor cells, which have been intensely investigated in blood or pancreatic juice, may be limited in fecal analysis, due to the rapid degradation operated by digestive enzymes or other components inside stool. A few studies have investigated the potential use of genetic markers such as *KRAS2* and *TP53* in stool.[147-151] However, *KRAS2* and *TP53* alterations were not sensitive and specific enough to be considered as reliable fecal biomarkers in pancreatic cancer, as opposed to the large number of stool markers that have been investigated in connection with the early detection of colorectal cancer.[151-157] The introduction of novel technologies that allow for a more sensitive detection will likely improve our ability to identify mutant molecules at a very low concentration. In addition, the emerging field of epigenetics has recently become a focus of current research in the field of stool testing. This has been shown to be a promising method for the early detection of colorectal cancer.[157] Given the fact that aberrant DNA methylation has been extensively studied in pancreatic cancer cells, the identification of epigenetic alterations may represent a valuable resource for improving stool analysis in pancreatic cancer.

Saliva is a readily accessible and informative biofluid, rendering it ideal for the early detection of a wide range of diseases. Saliva is a filtration of blood, reflecting the physiologic conditions of the body; thus, it could be potentially used to monitor clinical status and predict systemic diseases. Compared with blood or other body fluids, its collection is cost-effective, safe, easy, and non-invasive. High-throughput analysis indicates that the mRNA in saliva supernatant is relatively stable and informative and is a suitable source of disease discriminatory biomarkers.[158,159] Of interest, a recent study by Zhang et al.[160] demonstrated that the combination of four messenger RNA biomarkers (*KRAS2*, *MBD3L2*, *ACRV1*, and *DPM1*) could differentiate pancreatic cancer patients from subjects with chronic pancreatitis or healthy controls, with 90.0% sensitivity and 95.0% specificity. However, because of circadian variations, some concerns exist about the use of saliva as a biomarker. Furthermore, the possible fluctuation of its components in response to systemic conditions such as stress and local alterations limits its diagnostic power.[161,162]

SCREENING MODALITIES IN HIGH-RISK INDIVIDUALS

Recent studies suggest that about 10% of all patients diagnosed with pancreatic cancer harbor a genetic predisposition. The mechanisms underlying the genetic predisposition to all pancreatic cancers are not yet fully understood; however, individuals with a strong family history of pancreatic cancer involving at least two close relatives and individuals with certain cancer predisposition syndromes have been shown to harbor a significantly increased risk of developing pancreatic cancer. Although multiple cases of pancreatic cancer within the same family may be due to chance, or exposure to environmental factors (e.g., cigarette smoking), a common genetic basis has been shown to play an important role in the development of this disease.[163] In fact, over the last several years, several germline mutations responsible for an inherited susceptibility to pancreatic cancer in families have been identified.

The *BRCA2* gene, also known to be involved in the pathogenesis of familial breast/ovarian cancer, represents one of the more common susceptibility genes identified so far. It has been estimated that individuals with germline *BRCA2* mutations present an approximately 3.5-fold increased risk of developing pancreatic cancer, compared with the normal population.[164-168] The *p16/CDKN2A* gene, whose germline mutations are responsible for the familial atypical multiple mole melanoma syndrome, is also involved in the pathogenesis of familial pancreatic cancer. Individuals that harbor this mutation have a 13- to 37-fold increased risk of developing pancreatic cancer.[169-173] Inherited mutations in the *LKB1/STK11* gene cause PJS, characterized by intestinal hamartomatous polyps in association with a distinct pattern of skin and mucosal macular melanin deposition. Patients with PJS not only harbor a 15-fold increased risk of developing intestinal cancer compared with that of the general population but also harbor a 130-fold increased risk of pancreatic cancer.[119,174-178] More recently, exome sequencing of germline DNA in patients with familial pancreatic cancer has led to the identification of *PALB2* gene as a new pancreatic cancer susceptibility gene.[179] This discovery is particularly relevant for two reasons: first, germline mutant *PALB2* represents an important genetic marker that can be tested in first-degree relatives of patients affected by hereditary pancreatic cancer. Second, the *PALB2* encoded protein functions in the same pathway of DNA homologous recombination repair as Brca2, and thus, the resultant tumors are also susceptible to agents like Mitomycin C and PARP-i discussed previously. The discovery of familial pancreatic cancer genes has certainly provided new insights into the cellular pathways important for the development of pancreatic cancer. Furthermore, members of families with high incidence of pancreatic cancer can be screened for mutations in those genes and clinically followed in the hope for detecting early, pre-invasive disease.

Although the identification of individuals at risk for pancreatic cancer represents a remarkable opportunity for early diagnosis and effective cure for those patients, the timing and frequency for such screenings remain an unsolved question. Serum CA 19-9 levels have been suggested as a possible screening test, but the sensitivity and specificity of the assay are too low to be applied in the clinical setting. There are, however, a number of screening tests that are being currently evaluated in clinical trials. Thus, EUS has been tested as a screening method for asymptomatic members of families considered at risk for pancreatic cancer.[38,180] The Cancer of the Pancreas Screening trial (CAPS trial) has used EUS for the screening of asymptomatic patients with a strong family history of pancreatic cancer, as well as asymptomatic patients with genetic syndromes associated with pancreatic cancer.[38,180] About 10% of the asymptomatic individuals screened were found to have a lesion in their pancreas that was subsequently treated with surgery. The most frequent final pathologic diagnosis of the lesions included was IPMNs, displaying high-grade dysplasia in one-fourth of cases. Other studies using either EUS-based or abdominal MRI to screen high-risk individuals, with a strong family history of pancreatic cancer, have also demonstrated the presence of IPMNs, PanIN, and invasive pancreatic ductal adenocarcinomas.[181] More recently, the CAPS-3 trial was developed to test which of the three most commonly used imaging modalities (CT scan, EUS, and MRI with secretin infusion) was more accurate in detecting preneoplastic pancreatic lesions in individuals at high risk for hereditary pancreatic cancer.[182] The study demonstrated that EUS was the technique of choice, being able to detect pancreatic cystic lesions with higher sensitivity, compared with MRI and CT scan.

The screening and surgical resection of early detected pancreatic lesions in at-risk individuals has also allowed researchers to formulate important observations. While pancreatic cystic lesions are large enough to be effectively detected by EUS at an early stage, PanINs are too small to be identified. However, PanINs are often associated with larger areas of lobulocentric atrophy and fibrosis lobulocentric atrophy, as discussed above. Furthermore, PanINs in the specimens of patients with a strong family history of pancreatic cancer are often multifocal, and it was estimated that as many as 20% of the smaller ducts in some patients contain PanIN lesions. Therefore, macroscopic changes in the pancreas determined by the combination of lobulocentric atrophy and multifocal PanINs can be used as indicators of an underlying lesion and detected by EUS.[113]

Thus, EUS-based studies might help identify "curable" pancreatic neoplasms in asymptomatic high-risk patients. The results so far suggest that the identification of pre-invasive lesions of the pancreas is possible, although the risk of overtreating patients in whom atypical lesions are found represents a concern. The discovery of new biomarkers, or the application of new technologies that increase the accuracy of EUS-based screening approaches, will hopefully improve our ability to predict the natural history of pancreatic lesions in patients at risk. As an expected consequence, such specific markers might help the creation of a decisional algorithm to apply into the clinical practice, once a pancreatic lesion has been detected by imaging.

FUTURE DIRECTIONS IN MOLECULAR DIAGNOSTICS OF PANCREATIC CANCER

Until recently, the discovery of specific molecular alterations in human cancers was based on candidate gene approaches, such as studies of familial cancer, in vitro transformation assays, and positional cloning. These methods are effective tools in finding the frequently mutated genes, but they are unable to find infrequently mutated genes or novel candidate genes, not previously associated with cancer. The completion of the Human Genome Project and the availability of new high-throughput sequencing technologies have led to a much greater insight into the complexity of cancer genomes, including pancreatic cancer. Recently, in-depth mutational analysis of individual pancreatic cancers and correspondent metastases has shed light on the genomic instability of this disease, as well as on its development and progression timeline.[183] Sequencing of tumor DNA from patients with pancreatic cancer clarified the clonal relationships among primary and metastatic cancers. While the majority of mutations were present both in the primary tumor and in all metastases from the same patient, a minority of mutations were found in one or more metastases but not in the parental clone. Systematic analysis of mutations from several areas of primary tumors and metastases from different anatomical regions allowed for the identification of subclones in the primary tumor that had given rise to distinct metastases. Based upon these data, the timing of events that lead to pancreatic cancer development and progression was estimated. It was proposed that an average of 11.7 years was required, from tumor initiation to the development of the parental clone, and 6.8 additional years to the development of metastatic subclones that were responsible for patients' death after an average of 2 years. This proposed timeline has important implications: first, pancreatic cancer is probably not as a rapidly growing tumor as it was thought to be. The time span between the onset of suspicious symptoms of pancreatic cancer and diagnosis represents just the "tip of the iceberg," but a far longer period of time, required for cancer to develop, remains asymptomatic and undiagnosed. Second, and even more important, the time frame needed for tumor formation represents a huge window of opportunity for early detection and intervention. The next decades of research toward the discovery of new diagnostic modalities will indeed represent a very exciting time. New sophisticated technologies have been developed that, if approved for clinical use, may allow for detection of pancreatic cancer at an early, even preinvasive stage. For example, researchers recently used a cathepsin-activatable near-infrared probe combined with flexible confocal fluorescence laser microscopy in a genetically engineered mouse model of pancreatic cancer, to investigate in vivo the presence of pancreatic cancer and microscopic precursor lesions.[184] This new endoscopic approach was able to detect and grade murine pancreatic cancer and all grades of PanIN lesions with high sensitivity and specificity. Ideally, translation of such a sensitive technique into the clinic, associated with newer high-resolution imaging methods and more accurate molecular biomarkers, could have the potential to greatly improve early detection of pancreatic cancer.

In conclusion, the last decade has been characterized by an explosion of data about the molecular features of pancreatic cancer and other pancreatic neoplasms, along with increasingly more accurate imaging technologies. This new breadth of knowledge harbors tremendous expectations that our ability to diagnose pancreatic cancer will soon improve. In addition to early diagnosis, the molecular profiling of individual pancreatic cancers will also help us predict their biologic behavior and their responsiveness to targeted therapies that are more likely to benefit each individual patient affected by this devastating disease.

REFERENCES

1. Jemal A, Siegel R, Ward E, et al. Cancer statistics, 2009. *CA Cancer J Clin.* 2009;59:225-249.
2. Yeo TP, Hruban RH, Leach SD, et al. Pancreatic cancer. *Curr Probl Cancer.* 2002;26:176-275.
3. Simianu V, Zyromski N, Nakeeb A, Lillemoe KD. Pancreatic cancer: progress made. *Acta Oncol.* 2010;49:407-417.
4. Sohn TA, Yeo CJ, Cameron JL, et al. Resected adenocarcinoma of the pancreas-616 patients: results, outcomes, and prognostic indicators. *J Gastrointest Surg.* November-December 2000;4(6):567-579.
5. Fishman EK, Horton KM. Imaging pancreatic cancer: the role of multidetector CT with three-dimensional CT angiography. *Pancreatology.* 2001;1(6):610-624.
6. Legmann P, Vignaux O, Dousset B, et al. Pancreatic tumors: comparison of dual-phase helical CT and endoscopic sonography. *AJR Am J Roentgenol.* May 1998;170(5):1315-1322.
7. Goonetilleke KS, Siriwardena AK. Systematic review of carbohydrate antigen (CA 19-9) as a biochemical marker in the diagnosis of pancreatic cancer. *Eur J Surg Oncol.* April 2007;33(3):266-270.
8. Steinberg W. The clinical utility of the CA 19-9 tumor-associated antigen. *Am J Gastroenterol.* 1990;85:350-355.
9. Lamerz R. Role of tumour markers, cytogenetics. *Ann Oncol.* 1999;10(suppl 4):145-149.
10. Tumour markers in gastrointestinal cancers—EGTM recommendations. European Group on Tumour Markers. *Anticancer Res.* 1999;19:2811-2815.
11. Takahashi H, Ohigashi H, Ishikawa O, et al. Serum CA19-9 alterations during preoperative gemcitabine-based chemoradiation therapy for resectable invasive ductal carcinoma of the pancreas as an indicator for therapeutic selection and survival. *Ann Surg.* March 2010;251(3):461-469.
12. Katz MH, Varadhachary GR, Fleming JB, et al. Serum CA 19-9 as a marker of resectability and survival in patients with potentially resectable pancreatic cancer treated with neoadjuvant chemoradiation. *Ann Surg Oncol.* 2010 Jul;17(7):1794-801.
13. Boeck S, Stieber P, Holdenrieder S, Wilkowski R, Heinemann V. Prognostic and therapeutic significance of carbohydrate antigen 19-9 as tumor marker in patients with pancreatic cancer. *Oncology.* 2006;70:255-264.
14. Safi F, Schlosser W, Kolb G, Beger HG. Diagnostic value of CA 19-9 in patients with pancreatic cancer and nonspecific gastrointestinal symptoms. *J Gastrointest Surg.* 1997;1:106-112.
15. Rosty C, Goggins M. The early detection of pancreatic cancer. *Hematol Oncol Clin North Am.* 2002;16:37-52.
16. Jones S, Zhang X, Parsons DW, et al. Core signaling pathways in human pancreatic cancers revealed by global genomic analyses. *Science.* 2008;321:1801-1806.
17. Nagrath S, Sequist LV, Maheswaran S, et al. Isolation of rare circulating tumour cells in cancer patients by microchip technology. *Nature.* December 2007;450(7173):1235-1239.
18. Caldas C, Kern SE. K-ras mutation and pancreatic adenocarcinoma. *Int J Pancreatol.* 1995;18:1-6.
19. Yamada T, Nakamori S, Ohzato H, et al. Detection of K-ras gene mutations in plasma DNA of patients with pancreatic adenocarcinoma: correlation with clinicopathological features. *Clin Cancer Res.* June 1998;4(6):1527-1532.
20. Wilentz RE, Chung CH, Sturm PD, et al. K-ras mutations in the duodenal fluid of patients with pancreatic carcinoma. *Cancer.* January 1998;82(1):96-103.
21. Feldmann G, Beaty R, Hruban RH, Maitra A. Molecular genetics of pancreatic intraepithelial neoplasia. *J Hepatobiliary Pancreat Surg.* 2007;14(3):224-232.
22. Berger DH, Chang H, Wood M, et al. Mutational activation of K-ras in nonneoplastic exocrine pancreatic lesions in relation to cigarette smoking status. *Cancer.* 1999 Jan 15;85(2):326-32.
23. Kalthoff H, Schmiegel W, Roeder C. p53 and K-RAS alterations in pancreatic epithelial cell lesions. *Oncogene.* 1993;8:289-298.
24. Schutte M, Hruban RH, Geradts J, et al. Abrogation of the Rb/p16 tumor-suppressive pathway in virtually all pancreatic carcinomas. *Cancer Res.* 1997;57:3126-3130.
25. Tada M, Komatsu Y, Kawabe T, et al. Quantitative analysis of K-ras gene mutation in pancreatic tissue obtained by endoscopic ultrasonography-guided fine needle aspiration: clinical utility for diagnosis of pancreatic tumor. *Am J Gastroenterol.* 2002;97:2263-2270.
26. Shi C, Eshleman SH, Jones D. LigAmp for sensitive detection of single-nucleotide differences. *Nat Methods.* 2004;1:141-147.
27. Dressman D, Yan H, Traverso G. Transforming single DNA molecules into fluorescent magnetic particles for detection and enumeration of genetic variations. *Proc Natl Acad Sci U S A.* 2003;100:8817-8822.
28. Redston MS, Caldas C, Seymour AB, et al. p53 mutations in pancreatic carcinoma and evidence of common involvement of homocopolymer tracts in DNA microdeletions. *Cancer Res.* 1994;54:3025-3033.
29. Löhr M, Müller P, Mora J, et al. p53 and K-ras mutations in pancreatic juice samples from patients with chronic pancreatitis. *Gastrointest Endosc.* June 2001;53(7):734-743.
30. Hollstein M, Sidransky D, Vogelstein B, Harris CC. p53 mutations in human cancers. *Science.* July 1991;253(5015):49-53.
31. Sturm PD, Hruban RH, Ramsoekh TB. The potential diagnostic use of K-ras codon 12 and p53 alterations in brush cytology from the pancreatic head region. *J Pathol.* 1998;186:247-253.
32. Yan L, McFaul C, Howes N, et al. Molecular analysis to detect pancreatic ductal adenocarcinoma in high-risk groups. *Gastroenterology.* June 2005;128(7):2124-2130.
33. Hruban RH, Goggins M, Parsons J, Kern SE (2000) Progression model for pancreatic cancer. *Clin Cancer Res.* 2000;6:2969-2972.
34. Wilentz RE, Geradts J, Maynard R, et al. Inactivation of the p16 (INK4A) tumor-suppressor gene in pancreatic duct lesions: loss of intranuclear expression. *Cancer Res.* 1998;58:4740-4744.
35. Heinmöller E, Dietmaier W, Zirngibl H, et al. Molecular analysis of microdissected tumors and preneoplastic intraductal lesions in pancreatic carcinoma. *Am J Pathol.* 2000;157:83-92.
36. Wilentz RE, Iacobuzio-Donahue CA, Argani P, et al. Loss of expression of Dpc4 in pancreatic intraepithelial neoplasia: evidence that DPC4 inactivation occurs late in neoplastic progression. *Cancer Res.* 2000;60:2002-2006.
37. Massague J, Blain SW, Lo RS. TGFbeta signaling in growth control, cancer, and heritable disorders. *Cell.* 2000;103:295-309.
38. Canto MI, Goggins M, Hruban RH, et al. Screening for early pancreatic neoplasia in high-risk individuals: a prospective controlled study. *Clin Gastroenterol Hepatol.* June 2006;4(6):766-781; quiz 665.
39. Schutte M, Hruban RH, Hedrick L, et al. DPC4 gene in various tumor types. *Cancer Res.* 1996;56:2527-2530.
40. Blackford A, Serrano OK, Wolfgang CL, et al. SMAD4 gene mutations are associated with poor prognosis in pancreatic cancer. *Clin Cancer Res.* July 2009;15(14):4674-4679.
41. Wilentz RE, Su GH, Dai JL, et al. Immunohistochemical labeling for dpc4 mirrors genetic status in pancreatic adenocarcinomas: a new marker of DPC4 inactivation. *Am J Pathol.* January 2000;156(1):37-43.
42. Goggins M, Schutte M, Lu J, et al. Germline BRCA2 gene mutations in patients with apparently sporadic pancreatic carcinomas. *Cancer Res.* 1996;56:5360-5364.

43. Schutte M, da Costa LT, Hahn SA, et al. Identification by representational difference analysis of a homozygous deletion in pancreatic carcinoma that lies within the BRCA2 region. *Proc Natl Acad Sci U S A*. 1995;92:5950-5954.
44. van der Heijden MS, Brody JR, Dezentje DA, et al. In vivo therapeutic responses contingent on Fanconi anemia/BRCA2 status of the tumor. *Clin Cancer Res*. 2005;11:7508-7515.
45. McCabe N, Lord CJ, Tutt AN, Martin NM, Smith GC, Ashworth A. BRCA2- deficient CAPAN-1 cells are extremely sensitive to the inhibition of Poly (ADP- Ribose) polymerase: an issue of potency. *Cancer Biol Ther*. 2005;4:934-936.
46. Gelmon KA, Tischkowitz M, Mackay H, et al. Olaparib in patients with recurrent high-grade serous or poorly differentiated ovarian carcinoma or triple-negative breast cancer: a phase 2, multicentre, open-label, non-randomised study. *Lancet Oncol*. September 2011;12(9):852-861.
47. Lowery MA, Kelsen DP, Stadler ZK, et al. An emerging entity: pancreatic adenocarcinoma associated with a known BRCA mutation: clinical descriptors, treatment implications, and future directions. *Oncologist*. 2011;16(10):1397-1402.
48. Maitra A, Cohen Y, Gillespie SE, et al. The human MitoChip: a high-throughput sequencing microarray for mitochondrial mutation detection. *Genome Res*. 2004;14:812-819.
49. Weber M, Davies JJ, Wittig D, et al. Chromosome-wide and promoter- specific analyses identify sites of differential DNA methylation in normal and transformed human cells. *Nat Genet*. 2005;37:853-862.
50. Ueki T, Toyota M, Sohn T, et al. Hypermethylation of multiple genes in pancreatic adenocarcinoma. *Cancer Res*. 2000; 60:1835-1839.
51. Esteller M, Sparks A, Toyota M, et al. Analysis of adenomatous polyposis coli promoter hypermethylation in human cancer. *Cancer Res*. 2000;60:4366-4371.
52. Jansen M, Fukushima N, Rosty C, et al. Aberrant methylation of the 5′ CpG island of TSLC1 is common in pancreatic ductal adenocarcinoma and is first manifest in high-grade PanINs. *Cancer Biol Ther*. 2002;1:293-296.
53. Fukushima N, Sato N, Sahin F, Su GH, Hruban RH, Goggins M. Aberrant methylation of suppressor of cytokine signalling-1 (SOCS-1) gene in pancreatic ductal neoplasms. *Br J Cancer*. 2003;89:338-343.
54. Dammann R, Schagdarsurengin U, Liu L, et al. Frequent RASSF1A promoter hypermethylation and K-ras mutations in pancreatic carcinoma. *Oncogene*. 2003;22:3806-3812.
55. Matsubayashi H, Sato N, Fukushima N, et al. Methylation of cyclin D2 is observed frequently in pancreatic cancer but is also an age-related phenomenon in gastrointestinal tissues. *Clin Cancer Res*. 2003;9:1446-1452.
56. Kuroki T, Yendamuri S, Trapasso F, et al. The tumor suppressor gene WWOX at FRA16D is involved in pancreatic carcinogenesis. *Clin Cancer Res*. 2004;10:2459-2465.
57. Wada M, Yazumi S, Takaishi S, et al. Frequent loss of RUNX3 gene expression in human bile duct and pancreatic cancer cell lines. *Oncogene*. 2004;23:2401-2407.
58. Sakai M, Hibi K, Koshikawa K, et al. Frequent promoter methylation and gene silencing of CDH13 in pancreatic cancer. *Cancer Sci*. 2004;95:588-591.
59. Xu S, Furukawa T, Kanai N, Sunamura M, Horii A. Abrogation of DUSP6 by hypermethylation in human pancreatic cancer. *J Hum Genet*. 2005;50:159-167.
60. Park JY, Helm JF, Zheng W, et al. Silencing of the candidate tumor suppressor gene solute carrier family 5 member 8 (SLC5A8) in human pancreatic cancer. *Pancreas*. 2008;36:e32-e39.
61. Martin ST, Sato N, Dhara S, et al. Aberrant methylation of the Human Hedgehog interacting protein (HHIP) gene in pancreatic neoplasms. *Cancer Biol Ther*. 2005;4:728-733.
62. Fukushima N, Walter KM, Ueki T, et al. Diagnosing pancreatic cancer using methylation specific PCR analysis of pancreatic juice. *Cancer Biol Ther*. January-February 2003;2(1):78-83.
63. Sato N, Fukushima N, Maitra A. Discovery of novel targets for aberrant methylation in pancreatic carcinoma using high-throughput microarrays. *Cancer Res*. 2003;63:3735-3742.
64. Sato N, Parker AR, Fukushima N. Epigenetic inactivation of TFPI-2 as a common mechanism associated with growth and invasion of pancreatic ductal adenocarcinoma. *Oncogene*. 2005;24:850.
65. Matsubayashi H, Canto M, Sato N, et al. DNA methylation alterations in the pancreatic juice of patients with suspected pancreatic disease. *Cancer Res*. January 2006;66(2):1208-1217.
66. Schumacher A, Kapranov P, Kaminsky Z. Microarray-based DNA methylation profiling: technology and applications. *Nucleic Acids Res*. 2006;34:528-542.
67. Rosty C, Ueki T, Argani P, et al. Overexpression of S100A4 in pancreatic ductal adenocarcinomas is associated with poor differentiation and DNA hypomethylation. *Am J Pathol*. January 2002;160(1):45-50.
68. Issa JP, Ahuja N, Toyota M, Bronner MP, Brentnall TA. Accelerated age-related CpG island methylation in ulcerative colitis. *Cancer Res*. May 2001;61(9):3573-3577.
69. Issa JP, Ottaviano YL, Celano P, Hamilton SR, Davidson NE, Baylin SB. Methylation of the oestrogen receptor CpG island links ageing and neoplasia in human colon. *Nat Genet*. August 1994;7(4):536-540.
70. Di Leva G, Gasparini P, Piovan C, et al. MicroRNA cluster 221-222 and estrogen receptor alpha interactions in breast cancer. *J Natl Cancer Inst*. May 2010;102(10):706-721. [Epub 2010 Apr 13].
71. Yanaihara N, Caplen N, Bowman E. Unique microRNA molecular profiles in lung cancer diagnosis and prognosis. *Cancer Cell*. 2006;9:189-198.
72. Lee HC, Kim JG, Chae YS, et al. Prognostic impact of microRNA-related gene polymorphisms on survival of patients with colorectal cancer. *J Cancer Res Clin Oncol*. July 2010;136(7):1073-1078.
73. Incoronato M, Garofalo M, Urso L, et al. miR-212 increases tumor necrosis factor-related apoptosis-inducing ligand sensitivity in non-small cell lung cancer by targeting the antiapoptotic protein PED. *Cancer Res*. May 2010;70(9):3638-3646.
74. Volinia S, Galasso M, Costinean S, et al. Reprogramming of miRNA networks in cancer and leukemia. *Genome Res*. May 2010;20(5):589-599.
75. Bloomston M, Frankel WL, Petrocca F, et al. MicroRNA expression patterns to differentiate pancreatic adenocarcinoma from normal pancreas and chronic pancreatitis. *JAMA*. 2007;297:1901-1908.
76. Ryu JK, Hong SM, Karikari CA, Hruban RH, Goggins MG, Maitra A. Aberrant microRNA-155 expression is an early event in the multistep progression of pancreatic adenocarcinoma. *Pancreatology*. 2010;10:66-73.
77. Li A, Omura N, Hong SM, et al. Pancreatic cancers epigenetically silence SIP1 and hypomethylate and overexpress miR-200a/200b in association with elevated circulating miR-200a and miR-200b levels. *Cancer Res*. July 2010;70(13):5226-5237.
78. Ryu JK, Matthaei H, Dal Molin M, et al. Elevated microRNA miR-21 levels in pancreatic cyst fluid are predictive of mucinous precursor lesions of ductal adenocarcinoma. *Pancreatology*. 2011;11(3):343-350.
79. Peng DF, Kanai Y, Sawada M, et al. DNA methylation of multiple tumor-related genes in association with overexpression of DNA methyltransferase 1 (DNMT1) during multistage carcinogenesis of the pancreas. *Carcinogenesis*. 2006;27:1160-1168.
80. Buchholz M, Braun M, Heidenblut A, et al. Transcriptome analysis of microdissected pancreatic intraepithelial neoplastic lesions. *Oncogene*. 2005;24:6626-6636.
81. Iacobuzio-Donahue CA, Ashfaq R, Maitra A, et al. Highly expressed genes in pancreatic ductal adenocarcinomas: a comprehensive characterization and comparison of the transcription profiles obtained from three major technologies. *Cancer Res*. 2003; 63:8614-8622.
82. Iacobuzio-Donahue CA, Maitra A, Olsen M, et al. Exploration of global gene expression patterns in pancreatic adenocarcinoma using cDNA microarrays. *Am J Pathol*. 2003;162:1151-1162.
83. Van Heek NT, Maitra A, Koopmann J, et al. Gene expression profiling identifies markers of ampullary adenocarcinoma. *Cancer Biol Ther*. 2004;3:651-656.
84. Crnogorac-Jurcevic T, Efthimiou E, Capelli P, et al. Gene expression profiles of pancreatic cancer and stromal desmoplasia. *Oncogene*. 2001;20:7437-7446.
85. Crnogorac-Jurcevic T, Efthimiou E, Nielsen T, et al. Expression profiling of microdissected pancreatic adenocarcinomas. *Oncogene*. 2002;21:4587-4594.
86. Crnogorac-Jurcevic T, Gangeswaran R, Bhakta V, et al. Proteomic analysis of chronic pancreatitis and pancreatic adenocarcinoma. *Gastroenterology*. 2005;129:1454-1463.

87. Crnogorac-Jurcevic T, Missiaglia E, Blaveri E, et al. Molecular alterations in pancreatic carcinoma: expression profiling shows that dysregulated expression of S100 genes is highly prevalent. *J Pathol.* 2003;201:63-74.
88. Friess H, Ding J, Kleeff J, et al. Microarray-based identification of differentially expressed growth- and metastasis-associated genes in pancreatic cancer. *Cell Mol Life Sci.* 2003;60:1180-1199.
89. Seki K, Suda T, Aoyagi Y, et al. Diagnosis of pancreatic adenocarcinoma by detection of human telomerase reverse transcriptase messenger RNA in pancreatic juice with sample qualification. *Clin Cancer Res.* 2001;7:1976-1981.
90. Ohuchida K, Mizumoto K, Yamada D, et al. Quantitative analysis of human telomerase reverse transcriptase in pancreatic cancer. *Clin Cancer Res.* 2006;12:2066-2069.
91. Goicoechea SM, Bednarski B, Stack C, et al. Isoform-specific upregulation of palladin in human and murine pancreas. *Tumors PLoS One.* April 2010;5(4):e10347.
92. Argani P, Iacobuzio-Donahue C, Ryu B, et al. Mesothelin is overexpressed in the vast majority of ductal adenocarcinomas of the pancreas: identification of a new pancreatic cancer marker by serial analysis of gene expression (SAGE). *Clin Cancer Res.* 2001;7:3862-3868.
93. Circulating mesothelin protein and cellular antimesothelin immunity in patients with pancreatic cancer. *Clin Transl Sci.* December 2008;1(3):228-239.
94. Leao IC, Ganesan P, Armstrong TD, Jaffee EM. Effective depletion of regulatory T cells allows the recruitment of mesothelin-specific CD8 T cells to the antitumor immune response against a mesothelin-expressing mouse pancreatic adenocarcinoma. *Clin Transl Sci.* December 2008;1(3):228-239.
95. Johnston FM, Tan MC, Tan BR Jr, et al. Circulating mesothelin protein and cellular antimesothelin immunity in patients with pancreatic cancer. *Clin Cancer Res.* November 2009; 15(21):6511-6518.
96. Karanjawala ZE, Illei PB, Ashfaq R, et al. New markers of pancreatic cancer identified through differential gene expression analyses: claudin 18 and annexin A8. *Am J Surg Pathol.* February 2008;32(2):188-196.
97. Mazurek S, Boschek CB, Hugo F, Eigenbrodt E. Pyruvate kinase type M2 and its role in tumor growth and spreading. *Semin Cancer Biol.* 2005;15:300-308.
98. Ventrucci M, Cipolla A, Racchini C, Casadei R, Simoni P, Gullo L. Tumor M2-pyruvate kinase, a new metabolic marker for pancreatic cancer. *Dig Dis Sci.* August 2004;49(7-8):1149-1155.
99. Joergensen MT, Heegaard NH, Schaffalitzky de Muckadell OB. Comparison of plasma Tu-M2-PK and CA19-9 in pancreatic cancer. *Pancreas.* March 2010;39(2):243-247.
100. Walter K, Hong SM, Nyhan S, et al. Serum fatty acid synthase as a marker of pancreatic neoplasia. *Cancer Epidemiol Biomarkers Prev.* September 2009;18(9):2380-2385.
101. Swinnen JV, Roskams T, Joniau S, et al. Overexpression of fatty acid synthase is an early and common event in the development of prostate cancer. *Int J Cancer.* 2002;98:19-22.
102. Pizer ES, Lax SF, Kuhajda FP, Pasternack GR, Kurman RJ. Fatty acid synthase expression in endometrial carcinoma: correlation with cell proliferation and hormone receptors. *Cancer.* 1998;83:528-537.
103. Gansler TS, Hardman W III, Hunt DA, Schaffel S, Hennigar RA. Increased expression of fatty acid synthase (OA-519) in ovarian neoplasms predicts shorter survival. *Hum Pathol.* 1997;28:686-692.
104. Rashid A, Pizer ES, Moga M, et al. Elevated expression of fatty acid synthase and fatty acid synthetic activity in colorectal neoplasia. *Am J Pathol.* 1997;150:201-208.
105. Visca P, Sebastiani V, Botti C, et al. Fatty acid synthase (FAS) is a marker of increased risk of recurrence in lung carcinoma. *Anticancer Res.* 2004;24:4169-4173.
106. Milgraum LZ, Witters LA, Pasternack GR, Kuhajda FP. Enzymes of the fatty acid synthesis pathway are highly expressed in in situ breast carcinoma. *Clin Cancer Res.* 1997;3:2115-2120.
107. Wang Q, Chaerkady R, Wu J, et al. Mutant proteins as cancer-specific biomarkers *Proc Natl Acad Sci U S A.* February 2011;108(6):2444-2449.
108. Brat DJ, Lillemoe KD, Yeo CJ, Warfield PB, Hruban RH. Progression of pancreatic intraductal neoplasias to infiltrating adenocarcinoma of the pancreas. *Am J Surg Pathol.* 1998;22:163-169.
109. Hruban RH, Adsay NV, Albores-Saavedra J, et al. Pancreatic intraepithelial neoplasia: a new nomenclature and classification system for pancreatic duct lesions. *Am J Surg Pathol.* 2001;25:579-586.
110. Hruban RH, Takaori K, Klimstra DS, et al. An illustrated consensus on the classification of pancreatic intraepithelial neoplasia and intraductal papillary mucinous neoplasms. *Am J Surg Pathol.* 2004;28:977-987.
111. Lohr M, Kloppel G, Maisonneuve P, Lowenfels AB, Luttges J. Frequency of K-ras mutations in pancreatic intraductal neoplasias associated with pancreatic ductal adenocarcinoma and chronic pancreatitis: a meta-analysis. *Neoplasia.* 2005;7:17-23.
112. Laghi L, Orbetegli O, Bianchi P, et al. Common occurrence of multiple K-RAS mutations in pancreatic cancers with associated precursor lesions and in biliary cancers. *Oncogene.* 2002;21:4301-4306.
113. Brune K, Abe T, Canto M, et al. Multifocal neoplastic precursor lesions associated with lobular atrophy of the pancreas in patients having a strong family history of pancreatic cancer. *Am J Surg Pathol.* September 2006;30(9):1067-1076.
114. Detlefsen S, Sipos B, Feyerabend B, Klöppel G. Pancreatic fibrosis associated with age and ductal papillary hyperplasia. *Virchows Arch.* November 2005;447(5):800-805.
115. Matthaei H, Schulick RD, Hruban RH, Maitra A. Cystic precursors to invasive pancreatic cancer. *Nat Rev Gastroenterol Hepatol.* March 2011;8(3):141-150.
116. Yoshizawa K, Nagai H, Sakurai S, et al. Clonality and K-ras mutation analyses of epithelia in intraductal papillary mucinous tumor and mucinous cystic tumor of the pancreas. *Virchows Arch.* 2002;441(5):437-443.
117. Shi C, Daniels JA, Hruban RH. Molecular characterization of pancreatic neoplasms. *Adv Anat Pathol.* 2008;15:185-195.
118. Sasaki S, Yamamoto H, Kaneto H, et al. Differential roles of alterations of p53, p16, and SMAD4 expression in the progression of intraductal papillary-mucinous tumors of the pancreas. *Oncol Rep.* 2003;10:21-25.
119. Su GH, Hruban RH, Bova GS, et al. Germline and somatic mutations of the STK11/LKB1 Peutz-Jeghers gene in pancreatic and biliary cancers. *Am J Pathol.* 1999;154(6):1835-1840.
120. Schonleben F, Qiu W, Ciau NT, et al. PIK3CA mutations in intraductal papillary mucinous neoplasm/carcinoma of the pancreas. *Clin Cancer Res.* 2006;12(12):3851-3855.
121. Adsay NV, Pierson C, Sarkar F, et al. Colloid (mucinous noncystic) carcinoma of the pancreas. *Am J Surg Pathol.* 2001; 25(1):26-42.
122. D'Angelica M, Brennan MF, Suriawinata AA, Klimstra DS, Conlon KC. Intraductal papillary mucinous neoplasms of the pancreas: an analysis of clinicopathologic features and outcome. *Ann Surg.* 2004;239(3):400-408.
123. Wu J, Matthaei H, Maitra A, et al. Recurrent GNAS mutations define an unexpected pathway for pancreatic cyst development. *Sci Transl Med.* July 2011;3(92):92ra66.
124. Klöppel G, Kosmahl M. Cystic lesions and neoplasms of the pancreas. The features are becoming clearer. *Pancreatology.* 2001;1(6):648-655.
125. Le Borgne J, de Calan L, Partensky C. Cystadenomas and cystadenocarcinomas of the pancreas: a multiinstitutional retrospective study of 398 cases. French Surgical Association. *Ann Surg.* 1999 Aug;230(2):152-61.
126. Zamboni G, Scarpa A, Bogina G, et al. Mucinous cystic tumors of the pancreas: clinicopathological features, prognosis, and relationship to other mucinous cystic tumors. *Am J Surg Pathol.* 1999;23(4):410-422.
127. Kim SG, Wu TT, Lee JH, et al. Comparison of epigenetic and genetic alterations in mucinous cystic neoplasm and serous microcystic adenoma of pancreas. *Mod Pathol.* 2003;16(11): 1086-1094.
128. Iacobuzio-Donahue CA, Wilentz RE, Argani P, et al. Dpc4 protein in mucinous cystic neoplasms of the pancreas: frequent loss of expression in invasive carcinomas suggests a role in genetic progression. *Am J Surg Pathol.* 2000;24(11):1544-1548.
129. Wu J, Jiao Y, Dal Molin M, et al. Whole-exome sequencing of neoplastic cysts of the pancreas reveals recurrent mutations in components of ubiquitin-dependent pathways. *Proc Natl Acad Sci U S A.* 2011 Dec 27;108(52):21188-93.

130. Strous GJ, Dekker J. Mucin-type glycoproteins. *Crit Rev Biochem Mol Biol.* 1992;27:57-92.
131. Balague C, Gambus G, Carrato C, et al. Altered expression of MUC2, MUC4, and MUC5 mucin genes in pancreas tissues and cancer cell lines. *Gastroenterology.* 1994;106:1054-1061.
132. Andrianifahanana M, Moniaux N, Schmied BM, et al. Mucin (MUC) gene expression in human pancreatic adenocarcinoma and chronic pancreatitis: a potential role of MUC4 as a tumor marker of diagnostic significance. *Clin Cancer Res.* 2001;7:4033-4040.
133. Koopmann J, Buckhaults P, Brown DA, et al. Serum macrophage inhibitory cytokine 1 as a marker of pancreatic and other periampullary cancers. *Clin Cancer Res.* 2004;10:2386-2392.
134. Koopmann J, Rosenzweig CN, Zhang Z, et al. Serum markers in patients with resectable pancreatic adenocarcinoma: macrophage inhibitory cytokine 1 versus CA19-9. *Clin Cancer Res.* 2006;12:442-446.
135. Rogers CD, Fukushima N, Sato N, et al. Differentiating pancreatic lesions by microarray and QPCR analysis of pancreatic juice RNAs. *Cancer Biol Ther.* October 2006;5(10):1383-1389.
136. Tseng JF, Warshaw AL, Sahani DV, et al. Serous cystadenoma of the pancreas: tumor growth rates and recommendations for treatment. *Ann Surg.* 2005;242:413-419.
137. Matthes K, Mino-Kenudson M, Sahani DV, Holalkere N, Brugge WR. Concentration-dependent ablation of pancreatic tissue by EUS-guided ethanol injection. *Gastrointest Endosc.* 2007; 65:272-277.
138. Lahav M, Maor Y, Avidan B, Novis B, Bar-Meir S. Nonsurgical management of asymptomatic incidental pancreatic cysts. *Clin Gastroenterol Hepatol.* 2007;5:813-817.
139. Tanaka M, Chari S, Adsay V, et al. International consensus guidelines for management of intraductal papillary mucinous neoplasms and mucinous cystic neoplasms of the pancreas. *Pancreatology.* 2006;6:17-32.
140. Crippa S, Salvia R, Warshaw AL, et al. Mucinous cystic neoplasm of the pancreas is not an aggressive entity: lessons from 163 resected patients. *Ann Surg.* April 2008;247(4):571-579.
141. Brugge WR, Lewandrowski K, Lee-Lewandrowski E, et al. Diagnosis of pancreatic cystic neoplasms: a report of the Cooperative Pancreatic Cyst Study. *Gastroenterology.* 2004;126: 1330-1336.
142. Haab BB, Porter A, Yue T, et al. Glycosylation variants of mucins and CEACAMs as candidate biomarkers for the diagnosis of pancreatic cystic neoplasms. *Ann Surg.* May 2010; 251(5):937-945.
143. Allen PJ, Qin LX, Tang L, Klimstra D, Brennan MF, Lokshin A. Pancreatic cyst fluid protein expression profiling for discriminating between serous cystadenoma and intraductal papillary mucinous neoplasm. *Ann Surg.* November 2009;250(5):754-760.
144. Khalid A, McGrath KM, Zahid M, et al. The role of pancreatic cyst fluid molecular analysis in predicting cyst pathology. *Clin Gastroenterol Hepatol.* 2005;3:967-973.
145. Khalid A, Finkelstein S, McGrath K. Molecular diagnosis of solid and cystic lesions of the pancreas. *Gastroenterol Clin North Am.* 2004;33:891-906.
146. Schoedel KE, Finkelstein SD, Ohori NP. K-Ras and microsatellite marker analysis of fine-needle aspirates from intraductal papillary mucinous neoplasms of the pancreas. *Diagn Cytopathol.* 2006;34:605-608.
147. Caldas C, Hahn SA, Hruban RH, Redston MS, Yeo CJ, Kern SE. Detection of K-ras mutations in the stool of patients with pancreatic adenocarcinoma and pancreatic ductal hyperplasia. *Cancer Res.* July 1994;54(13):3568-3573.
148. Berndt C, Haubold K, Wenger F, et al. K-ras mutations in stools and tissue samples from patients with malignant and nonmalignant pancreatic diseases. *Clin Chem.* October 1998;44(10): 2103-2107.
149. Wenger FA, Zieren J, Peter FJ, Jacobi CA, Müller JM. K-ras mutations in tissue and stool samples from patients with pancreatic cancer and chronic pancreatitis. *Langenbecks Arch Surg.* April 1999;384(2):181-186.
150. Lu X, Xu T, Qian J, Wen X, Wu D. Detecting K-ras and p53 gene mutation from stool and pancreatic juice for diagnosis of early pancreatic cancer. *Chin Med J.* November 2002;115(11):1632-1636.
151. Pezzilli R, Barassi A, Melzi d'Eril G, et al. The search of the stool and blood K-ras mutations in patients with pancreatic mass. *Pancreas.* August 2006;33(2):199-200.
152. Müller HM, Oberwalder M, Fiegl H, et al. Methylation changes in faecal DNA: a marker for colorectal cancer screening? *Lancet.* April 2004;363(9417):1283-1285.
153. Belshaw NJ, Elliott GO, Williams EA, et al. Use of DNA from human stools to detect aberrant CpG island methylation of genes implicated in colorectal cancer. *Cancer Epidemiol Biomarkers Prev.* September 2004;13(9):1495-501.
154. Leung WK, To KF, Man EP, et al. Detection of epigenetic changes in fecal DNA as a molecular screening test for colorectal cancer: a feasibility study. *Clin Chem.* November 2004;50(11): 2179-2182.
155. Petko Z, Ghiassi M, Shuber A, et al. Aberrantly methylated CDKN2A, MGMT, and MLH1 in colon polyps and in fecal DNA from patients with colorectal polyps. *Clin Cancer Res.* February 2005;11(3):1203-1209.
156. Itzkowitz S, Brand R, Jandorf L, et al. A simplified, noninvasive stool DNA test for colorectal cancer detection. *Am J Gastroenterol.* November 2008;103(11):2862-2870.
157. Huang ZH, Li LH, Yang F, Wang JF. Detection of aberrant methylation in fecal DNA as a molecular screening tool for colorectal cancer and precancerous lesions. *World J Gastroenterol.* February 2007;13(6):950-954.
158. Li Y, Zhou X, St. John MA, et al. RNA profiling of cell-free saliva using microarray technology. *J Dent Res.* 2004;83:199-203.
159. Park NJ, Li Y, Yu T, et al. Characterization of RNA in saliva. *Clin Chem.* 2006;52:988-994.
160. Zhang L, Farrell JJ, Zhou H, et al. Salivary transcriptomic biomarkers for detection of resectable pancreatic cancer. *Gastroenterology.* March 2010;138(3):949-957.e1-7.
161. Dawes C. Circadian rhythms in human salivary flow rate and composition. *J Physiol.* 1972;220:529-545.
162. Fabian TK, Fejerdy P, Csermely P. Salivary genomics, transcriptomics and proteomics: the emerging concept of the oral ecosystem and their use in the early diagnosis of cancer and other diseases. *Curr Genomics.* 2008;9:11-21.
163. Klein AP, Beaty TH, Bailey-Wilson JE, Brune KA, Hruban RH, Petersen GM. Evidence for a major gene influencing risk of pancreatic cancer. *Genet Epidemiol.* August 2002;23(2):133-149.
164. Couch FJ, Johnson MR, Rabe KG, et al. The prevalence of BRCA2 mutations in familial pancreatic cancer. *Cancer Epidemiol Biomarkers Prev.* February 2007;16(2):342-346.
165. Cancer risks in BRCA2 mutation carriers. The Breast Cancer Linkage Consortium. *J Natl Cancer Inst.* August 1999;91(15): 1310-1316 .
166. Hahn SA, Greenhalf B, Ellis I, et al. BRCA2 germline mutations in familial pancreatic carcinoma. *J Natl Cancer Inst.* February 2003;95(3):214-221.
167. Lal G, Liu G, Schmocker B, et al. Inherited predisposition to pancreatic adenocarcinoma: role of family history and germline p16, BRCA1, and BRCA2 mutations. *Cancer Res.* January 2000;60:409-416.
168. Murphy KM, Brune KA, Griffin CA, et al. Evaluation of candidate genes MAP2K4, MADH4, ACVR1B, and BRCA2 in familial pancreatic cancer: deleterious BRCA2 mutations in 17%. *Cancer Res.* July 2002;62(13):3789-3793.
169. Lynch HT, Fusaro RM. Pancreatic cancer and the familial atypical multiple mole melanoma (FAMMM) syndrome. *Pancreas.* 1991;6:127-131.
170. Bartsch DK, Sina-Frey M, Lang S, et al. CDKN2A germline mutations in familial pancreatic cancer. *Ann Surg.* December 2002;236(6):730-737.
171. Borg A, Sandberg T, Nilsson K, et al. High frequency of multiple melanomas and breast and pancreas carcinomas in CDKN2A mutation-positive melanoma families. *J Natl Cancer Inst.* August 2000;92(15):1260-1266.
172. De Snoo FA, Bishop DT, Bergman W, et al. Increased risk of cancer other than melanoma in CDKN2A founder mutation (p16-Leiden)-positive melanoma families. *Clin Cancer Res.* November 2008;14(21):7151-7157.
173. de vos tot Nederveen Cappel WH, Offerhaus GJ, van Puijenbroek M, et al. Pancreatic carcinoma in carriers of a specific 19 base pair deletion of CDKN2A/p16 (p16-leiden). *Clin Cancer Res.* September 2003;9(10 pt 1):3598-3605.
174. Bowlby LS. Pancreatic adenocarcinoma in an adolescent male with Peutz-Jeghers syndrome. *Hum Pathol.* 1986;17:97-99.

175. Giardiello FM, Welsh SB, Hamilton SR, et al. Increased risk of cancer in the Peutz-Jeghers syndrome. *N Engl J Med.* 1987;316(24):1511-1514.
176. Giardiello FM, Brensinger JD, Tersmette AC, et al. Very high risk of cancer in familial Peutz-Jeghers Syndrome. *Gastroenterology.* 2000;119:1447-1453.
177. Hearle N, Schumacher V, Menko FH, et al. Frequency and spectrum of cancers in the Peutz-Jeghers syndrome. *Clin Cancer Res.* May 2006;12(10):3209-3215.
178. Latchford A, Greenhalf W, Vitone LJ, Neoptolemos JP, Lancaster GA, Phillips RK. Peutz-Jeghers syndrome and screening for pancreatic cancer. *Br J Surg.* December 2006;93(12): 1446-1455.
179. Jones S, Hruban RH, Kamiyama M, et al. Exomic sequencing identifies PALB2 as a pancreatic cancer susceptibility gene. *Science.* 2009 Apr 10;324(5924):217.
180. Canto MI, Goggins M, Yeo CJ, et al. Screening for pancreatic neoplasia in high-risk individuals: an EUS-based approach. *Clin Gastroenterol Hepatol.* July 2004;2(7):606-621.
181. Poley JW, Kluijt I, Gouma DJ, et al. The yield of first-time endoscopic ultrasonography in screening individuals at a high risk of developing pancreatic cancer. *Am J Gastroenterol.* 2009 Sep;104(9):2175-81.
182. Canto MI, Schulick RD, Kamel IR, et al. Screening for familial pancreatic neoplasia: a prospective, multicenter, blinded study of EUS, CT and secretin-MRCP. Presented at Digestive Disease Week DDW 2010; New Orleans, LA, USA; May 1-5, 2010. Abstract 415g.
183. Yachida S, Jones S, Bozic I, et al. Distant metastasis occurs late during the genetic evolution of pancreatic cancer. *Nature.* October 2010;467(7319):1114-1117.
184. Eser S, Messer M, Eser P, et al. In vivo diagnosis of murine pancreatic intraepithelial neoplasia and early-stage pancreatic cancer by molecular imaging. *Proc Natl Acad Sci U S A.* June 2011;108(24):9945-9950. [Epub 2011 May 31].

CHAPTER 33

Molecular Diagnostics of Head and Neck Cancer

Adel K. El-Naggar

INTRODUCTION

Head and neck regions comprise anatomically complex sites and organs that give rise to diverse and heterogeneous tumor types. Traditional pathologic classification and diagnosis of neoplasms at these sites are based on light microscopic evaluation and in a few instances by the selective use of immunohistochemical cell lineage marker evaluation. Recent efforts to define the molecular events of different head and neck tumors have led to valuable information that will soon be integrated in the pathologic evaluation to guide patients strategically and for targeted therapy. This chapter provides a contemporary view of the pathologic and molecular characterization of the spectrum of head and neck tumors for clinical management.[1,2]

SQUAMOUS MUCOSAL TUMORIGENESIS

Squamous carcinoma is the most common malignancy of all head and neck sites and the fifth ranking cancer type worldwide with an annual rate of 500,000 new cases per year.[3] The mortality of this disease is 45% to 50% and has remained largely constant in the last three decades despite improvement in diagnostic and multidisciplinary management.[2] Head and neck squamous carcinoma (HNSC) arises from the stratified non-keratinizing squamous epithelial lining of the mucosal sites as a result of progressive cellular alterations caused by prolonged exposure to risk factors in susceptible individuals. Patients are traditionally males in their late fifties and sixties with tumors mainly at the oral cavity, tongue, larynx, and sino-nasal mucosa.[3] Other rare sites include the nasopharynx and the oropharynx, and these carcinomas are etiologically and demographically distinct from conventional squamous carcinoma.[3] The majority of conventional squamous tumorigenesis is based on the concept of field carcinogenesis, which assumes that the entire mucosal lining is genetically altered and susceptible to tumorigenesis.[1-4]

Conventional Squamous Neoplasia

The pathologic assessment of mucosal lesions at the head and neck mucosal sites is based on the evaluation of biopsy specimens from premalignant and malignant lesions.[3]

Premalignant Lesions

Early head and neck mucosal pre-cancerous lesions are clinically identified as a white leukoplakia and red (erythroplakia) appearing mucosa and pathologically as hyperplasia, dysplasia, and severe dysplasia/carcinoma in situ.[1]

Leukoplakia/Hyperplasia and Dysplasia with Hyperkeratosis

These lesions are morphologically recognized by an increase in the thickness of the squamous epithelium without (hyperplasia) and with cellular alterations (dysplasia). Several genetic, phenotypic, and epigenetic alterations associated with these phenotypic stages have been identified. Although the majority of these lesions occur in patients with high risk factors, they may also be encountered in individuals without risk factors.[2]

The potential progression of dysplastic oral premalignant lesions to invasive squamous carcinoma ranges from 17% to 39%, respectively. Concerted efforts to identify the genetic and phenotypic alterations that predict the biological progression of these lesions have led to the characterization of several markers associated with the process of epithelial–mesenchymal transitions (EMTs).[5]

The characterization of these premalignant lesions is critical to morphologic and biological understanding of the molecular events associated with their progression. Although major obstacles such as the lack of genetic inheritance, the multitude of risk factors, and paucity of biological models hinder progress in this field, recent progress in molecular and informative technologies provides new opportunities for advances in this field.

Verrucous Hyperplasia

Grossly, verrucous hyperplasia appears as a warty white and exophytic lesion most commonly in oral or laryngeal sites. Histologically, it is characterized by mature squamous proliferation with broad-based exophytic growth.

Proliferative Verrucous Leukoplakia

This is a clinically aggressive form of leukoplakia that mostly affects elderly females with no risk factors. In this condition, early lesions cannot be differentiated from conventional leukoplakia and only with the subsequent progressive clinical expansion and the acquisition of the verrucoid appearance this condition is recognized. Currently, no known etiologic factor or genetic marker has been linked to this condition.

Squamous Carcinoma Variants

Conventional Squamous Carcinoma

This is the most common form of HNSC[6-8]. These tumors are graded into well- (grade 1), moderately (grade 2), and poorly (grade 3)[1] differentiated carcinoma based on the degree and the extent of keratinization and squamous maturation features manifested.

Verrucous Carcinoma

This is a locally aggressive form of HNSC characterized by downward broad pushing borders of mature warty looking squamous lesions. The most common sites for this type are the oral cavity and larynx. In their pure form, these lesions never metastasize.

Papillary Squamous Carcinoma

Not uncommonly, a hybrid of verrucous and conventional squamous carcinoma is encountered. This form is characterized by finger-like projections with fibrovascular core lined by malignant squamous epithelial cells. They may be invasive or non-invasive and commonly present in the naso- and hypopharynx. An association with certain types of human papillomavirus (HPV) infection has been documented.

Basaloid Squamous Carcinoma

This is a unique form of poorly differentiated squamous carcinoma comprised of basal-like cell proliferation with thick eosinophilic deposition, homogenized necrosis, and occasional abrupt and localized keratinization. On small biopsy evaluation, this phenotype may mimic the solid form of adenoid cystic carcinoma (ACC), neuroendocrine carcinoma, or melanoma. Basaloid squamous carcinoma is the most common form of HPV associated with oropharyngeal carcinoma.

Sarcomatoid Squamous Carcinoma

Sarcomatoid squamous carcinoma is a rare form of squamous carcinoma with sarcoma-like morphology in the presence or absence of conventional squamous components and may be mistaken for sarcoma or a reactive process.[8] Immunostaining and close consultation with the surgeon prior to reporting is critical. Grossly, they may present as exophytic or ulcerative endophytic forms. The exophytic form is believed to behave better than the ulcerative form. Their main differential diagnoses are sarcoma, pseudo-sarcoma, myofibroblastic proliferative lesion, and spindle cell melanoma.

Pathologic features of clinical relevance include (1) tumor size; (2) distance of closest margin; (3) pattern of invasion (broad pushing vs. finger-like single file); (4) perineural permeation; and (5) the presence or absence of high-grade dysplasia at margins.

Features related to the lymph node status include the level and number of positive to total lymph nodes identified, size of the largest lymph node with metastasis, and presence or absence of extranodal extension in involved nodes.

VIRAL-ASSOCIATED SQUAMOUS CARCINOMAS

Carcinomas arising at certain head and neck anatomic locations characterized by lymphoid-rich stroma are phenotypically, etiologically, and epidemiologically distinct entities.

Nasopharyngeal Carcinoma

This entity is characterized by dominant geographic and ethnic distribution. Although Epstein-Barr virus (EBV) infection is strongly linked to this tumor especially in endemic location, it is believed that other contributing factors such as genetic susceptibility and dietary and/or environmental factors play a major role.[9] Histopathologically, nasopharyngeal carcinoma is graded according to the World Health Organization classification into grade I, differentiated squamous carcinoma and grades II and III, undifferentiated carcinoma. Keratin and EBV in situ testing is one important diagnostic marker. These tumors are radiosensitive and are rarely excised in the Western countries.

Oropharyngeal Carcinoma

Recently, a progressive rise in the incidence of poorly differentiated carcinoma of the Waldeyer's ring has been reported.[10] Similar to their northern neighbor at the nasopharynx, the mucosa is lymphoid-based and the tumors are poorly differentiated or undifferentiated (basaloid) and typically positive for the papilloma virus-type 16. The detection of HPV-16 by in situ hybridization and/or polymerase chain reaction (PCR) techniques and/or the elevation of p16 expression in tumor cells is important in the diagnosis. The majority of the patients are

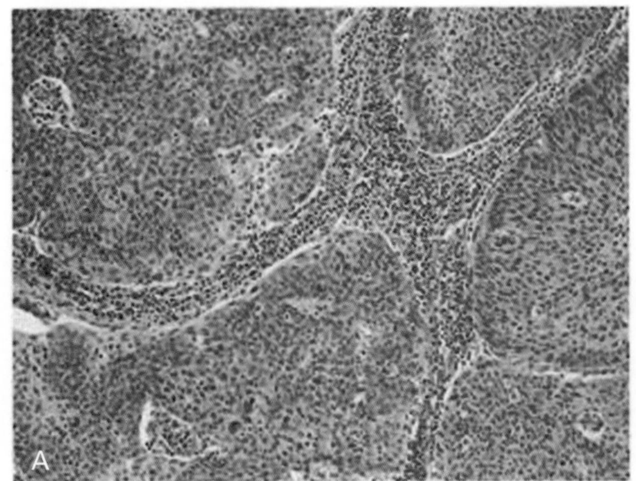

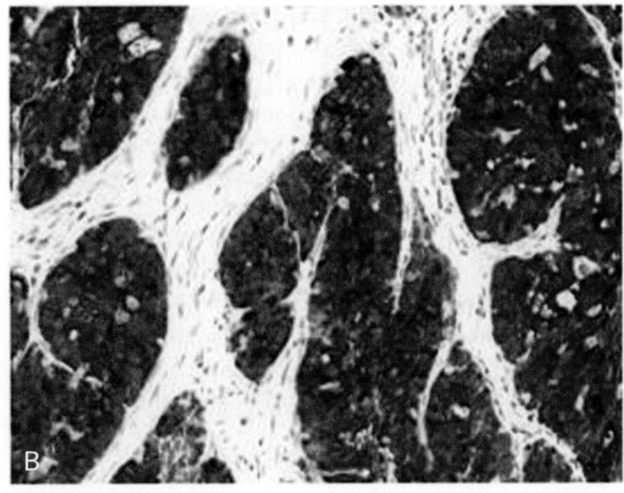

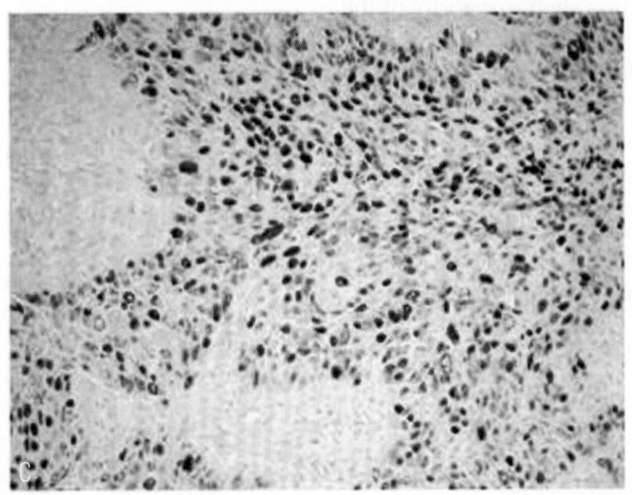

FIGURE 33–1 **A:** Poorly differentiated oropharyngeal squamous carcinoma, with basaloid features. **B:** Typical p16 immunostaining of an oropharyngeal tumor with strong homogeneous staining in cytoplasm and nuclei. **C:** An in situ hybridization for high-risk HPV subtypes depicting positive viral particles with variable intranuclear patterns.

young adults, well educated, and do not have the typical risk factors of patients with HNSC. Moreover, a strong putative association with the disease in this population is attributed to sexual practice.

Central to the pathogenesis of the HPV-16 is the integration of the circular double-stranded viral DNA, in the host DNA genome. Such integration results in the loss of the regulatory exon 2 of the virus genome leading to unregulated E6 and E7 viral oncogenes.[11]

The E6 and E7 bind and degrade the p53 and retinoblastoma (Rb) tumor suppressor proteins, respectively. It is believed that the loss of the cell regulatory functions of these genes underlies the pathogenesis of this subtype. Interestingly, a near universal upregulation of the p16 protein is presumably due to the degradation of the Rb protein and the release of the E-F transcription factor.

The upregulation of the p16 proteins is currently considered a reliable surrogate marker for HPV-positive oropharyngeal cancer. Molecular and immunohistochemical methods are critical to the diagnosis of viral-associated oropharyngeal carcinoma. These include DNA and RNA viral detection by quantitative or qualitative PCRs, fluorescent in situ hybridization, and p16 protein expression (Fig. 33.1A-C).

MOLECULAR AND BIOLOGICAL EVENTS IN CONVENTIONAL (NON–VIRAL) SQUAMOUS CARCINOMA

Squamous tumorigenesis is a multistage process as a result of the accumulation of successive genomic alterations that precede and coincide with the phenotypic epithelial alterations (dysplastic).[1] The type, order, and composition of these events are currently unknown, but current data indicate that the cumulative occurrence of genetic and epigenetic events is associated with the progressive dysplastic lesions and that subsequent epithelial/mesenchymal (subepithelial) modification determines invasion and progression. Although this model may conform to the majority of HNSCs at common mucosal sites, it does not relate to carcinoma associated with viral etiology at the nasopharyngeal and oropharyngeal sites. Although no definitive molecular events and/or pathways have been firmly established for head and neck squamous tumorigenesis, significant progress in identifying critical chromosomal genomic alterations has been achieved. Among these are loss of heterozygosity (LOH) at chromosomes 3p and 9p, mutation of the p53, methylation of the p16, ΔNp63, high podoplanin expression, and increase in copy number and overexpression of the epidermal growth factor receptor (EGFR). Although none of these factors are being used clinically, LOH and EGFR are being performed on biopsies from patients enrolled in prospective clinical trials.[1-4]

Cellular-Related Molecular Markers

Loss of Heterozygosity

Numerous studies using the unique heterozygosity of the microsatellite repeats in the human genome were used to identify loci of LOH in HNSC. Comparative analysis of constitutional DNA extracted from either histologically normal mucosa or lymphocytes to tumor specimens identified LOH at chromosomes 3p, 9p, and 17p in more than 30% of the tumors.[2] Interestingly, these chromosomal regions house the F-hit (fragile histidine triad), p16, and the p53 tumor suppressor genes. The frequency of these alterations in both early and advanced cancer led to the belief that they are involved in early development of these tumors. This is also supported by similar studies of premalignant lesions. LOH at 4p, 8p, 11q, 13q, and 18q loci was predominantly found in a subset of advanced cancer along with those loci found at 3p, 9p, and 17p suggesting their acquisition with tumor progression.[1,4]

More recently, chromosomal aberration, including 3q24, 8p23.1, 8q12.2k, and gain of chromosome 20, distinguishes two major subgroups with different biological progression and metastasis.[12]

Tumor Suppressor Genes

P53 Gene Family

Mutations at certain hotspot exons of the p53 gene, located on chromosome 17p13, are the most frequent finding in HNSC. These hotspots are located at exons 5 to 9. Recently, certain high-risk deleterious mutations have been found to be associated with poor response to therapy and aggressive outcome.

P16 Gene[13,14]

The p16 gene is located at 9p21 region and plays a central role in the regulation of the cell cycle. Loss of this gene, most commonly, is due to methylation of its promoter and the first exons were frequently found in HNSC.

F-HIT Gene

F-HIT gene is a suppressor gene located on the short arm of chromosome 3 region 14.2. Studies of this gene in HNSC, albeit few, have shown similar alterations to those reported in pulmonary carcinoma. However, the role of this as a driver in HNSC remains unclear.

Oncogenes

Cyclin D1 is located on chromosome 11p and is a critical cycle gene. Amplification and overexpression have been amply reported in approximately 30% of HNSCs and were found to be associated with advanced and more aggressive tumors. Recently, a polymorphism of this gene has been linked to increased risk of developing squamous carcinoma.[15]

P63 is a putative oncogene located at chromosome 3q27 region. Two main isotopes by alternative promoters and six isotopes by alternative splicing at the carboxyl domain are identified. P36ΔN isotype is found to be highly expressed in progressive premalignant and aggressive HNSC.[12]

Epigenetic Alterations

Epigenetic modifications, including methylation of 5′-cytosine at CpG islands active gene, chromatin modeling, and histone acetylation, play a major role in tumorigenesis. Several genes have been found to be hypermethylated in studies of head and neck squamous cell carcinoma (HNSCC). These include CDKN1, p16, DAP-K, E-cadherin, cyclin A1, and MGMT. Alterations of these genes lead to disruption of key cancer pathways such as proliferation, differentiation, apoptosis, invasion, and migration.[16,17] Recently, a profile of these genes has been tested on DNA extracted from saliva and mouthwash, and methylation was found to diagnose an increased risk of squamous carcinoma and is predictive of recurrence. Epigenetics refers to heritable changes in gene expression without DNA alterations. These modifications occur in carcinogenesis and may play an important early or later role in tumor development and/or progression.[18-20]

Genomics and Transcriptomics

Recent advances in molecular genetics, epigenetics, proteomics, and array comparative genomic hybridization (CGH) along with sophisticated bioinformatics tools permit the integration of complex data that may allow for characterizing pathways and critical central driving events in these tumors. The results of these studies have allowed better appreciation of the complexity and the heterogeneity of these tumors. Although some of these studies have correlated differential genomic patterns with aggressive behavior, response, and/or resistance to therapy, the practical application of these findings is unclear. Further efforts to limit the analysis to critically important events are needed for reliable testing and potential clinical application.

Genetic Analysis

Although genetic studies have shown a correlation between certain molecular alterations and traditional clinicopathologic factors which may allow the segregation of patients for treatment response and toxicity, they are generally unvalidated and of no practical clinical use. There is an increasing need for molecular and biologic predictors of response and targets for novel therapy.[20]

Expression Analysis

Several gene expression array studies have been conducted on HNSC. In these studies correlation between, gene expression and tumor sites and clinicopathologic and biologic features were reported. Moreover, gene expression profiling were found to predict lymph node metastasis better than current clinicopathologic predictors.[20] However, clinical application of these techniques is currently impractical and requires further validity. In addition, none of these profiles have been validated in a prospective analysis. Recently, a set of differentially expressed genes representing proteasome, MYC gene, and ribosomal elements were identified in patients with squamous carcinoma. Further validation and technical and interpretive guidelines are needed.[20]

MicroRNA

MicroRNAs are short non–coding RNA sequences that have been found to regulate post-transcription RNA transcript by pairing with their 3′-untranslated region. The degree of complementarity between these microRNAs and their RNA transcript targets determines the degree of repression. The majority of these molecules share sequences with multiple targets. Studies of these markers in HNSC indicate either loss or overproduction of certain microRNAs. Some of the microRNAs are critical to the regulation of cell proliferation, differentiation, and apoptosis (MiR-375, MiR-221, and MiR-184). These molecules are attractive targets for novel therapeutic applications in HNSC patients.[21]

Growth Factors

Several growth factors have been investigated in HNSCC. EGFR has been consistently reported to play an important role in these tumors.[22] EGFR is a transmembrane glycoprotein receptor that upon stimulation and through its ligand plays a central role in vital cell pathways. They comprise four closely related receptors that include EGFR (human epidermal growth factor receptor [HER]-1), EGFR-2 (HER-2), HER-3, and HER-4. These are transmembrane receptors with an extracellular ligand binding and intracellular receptor tyrosine kinase domain. The alterations in these pathways by overexpression and/or constitutive activation can lead to tumorigenesis. These receptors show considerable homology in the intracellular tyrosine kinase domain. They, however, differ in their extracellular and terminal COOH domain composition.

Two members of this family are independent in regard to their ligand binding and activation of downstream signaling, while HER-2 and HER-3 lack the ligand-binding autonomy. They activate similar signaling pathways through heterodimerization with other members. EGFR gene, a member of the HER-1 family, is located on chromosome 7p. Binding of the ligand growth factors, epidermal growth factors, transforming growth factor (TGF-x), heparin-binding epidermal growth factor (EGF), or betacellulin to the extracellular domain induces receptor internalization and activation of the intracellular protein tyrosine kinase and the induction of downstream signaling pathways, including the Ras/Raf/MAPK (mitogen-activated protein kinase), the phosphoinositide 3 (PI3)L/AKT/mTOR (mammalian target of rapamycin), and the STAT and the Src kinase pathways. The most common manifestation of dysregulated EGFR is overexpression and gene amplification but mutations of this gene in HNSCC are very rare.

Overexpression of EGFR has been associated with invasion and metastasis by inducing upregulation of the metalloproteinases (Fig. 33.2A and B). Similarly, overexpression has been positively correlated with nodal metastasis, high stage, and poor outcome. The EGFR involvement in HNSC has attracted considerable attention because of the availability of reagents that can be used to target this factor. Dysregulation of EGFR pathway by either overexpression or constitutive activation can induce angiogenesis, invasion, and metastasis. Therefore, inhibition or blockade of the EGFR by monoclonal antibodies (MoAbs) or small molecule tyrosine kinase inhibitors (TKIs) can inhibit these processes and lead to the treatment of certain patients with head and neck carcinoma.

EGFR Signaling and Therapy[2]

Several growth factors bind to those receptors, including EGF, TGF-α, amphiregulin, epiregulin, neuroregulin, heparin-binding EGF, and betacellulin.

This signaling pathway is complex and multilayered with cross-linkage to multiple vital cellular pathways, including the Ras/RAf/MAPK, PI3k/AKT, STAT, and the Src kinase pathways.

Monoclonal Antibodies

Antibodies (cetuximab and panitumumab) bind to the extracellular domain and block ligand binding and internalization. Antibody-based therapy has been effective in the treatment of patients with HNSC.[2]

Tyrosine Kinase Inhibitors

Tyrosine Kinase Inhibitors, TKIs (gefitinib and erlotinib) disrupting exert their effect by the binding of adenosine phosphate to the tyrosine kinase domain of the EGFR and block the activation of downstream signaling. Treatment success has been achieved in a subset of patients using TKIs such as gefitinib and erlotinib. However, resistance to therapy may develop over time in patients who have shown response initially. This resistance may develop

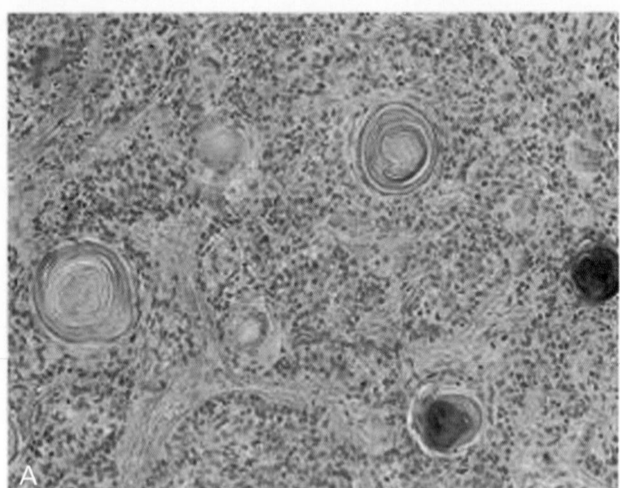

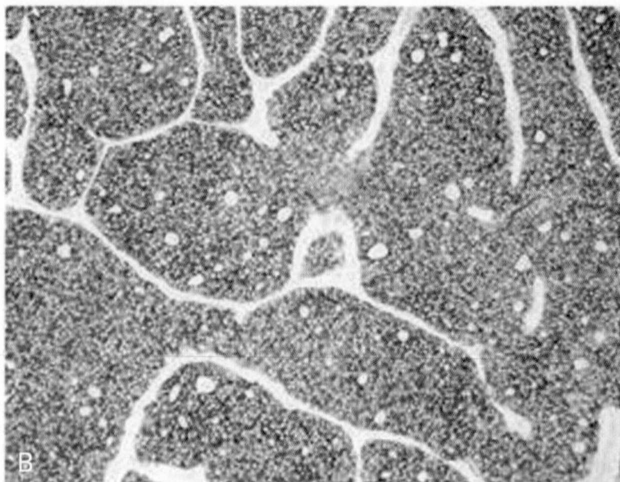

FIGURE 33–2 **A:** A moderately differentiated squamous carcinoma of the oral tongue. **B:** Tumor cells express high EGFR membranous and cytoplasmic staining in tumor.

through activation of alternative mechanism, EGFR amplification/mutation, or constitutive activation of downstream targets.[22] Potential markers for EGFR resistance include BRAF mutations, PTEN loss and k-ras alterations, and EGFR amplification.

Future strategy should focus on biomarker-based stratification of patients for efficient treatment and reduction of morbidity. Moreover, a multifaceted treatment approach using combined agents targeting diverse pathways to overcome the complexity and the escape routes of the EGFR network should be considered.

VEGF and FGF

Elevated expression of vascular endothelial growth factor (VEGF) and FGF (fibroblast growth factor) and their receptors has been reported to be associated with angiogenesis and aggressive behavior in HNSC.[23,24] The regulation of this growth factor is primarily through the hypoxia-inducible factor-1α (HIF-1α)–dependent and HIF-1α–independent processes and involves both PI3L and AkT pathways.[42-47]

A humanized VEGF MoAb (bevacizumab) has recently been tested and shown to inhibit angiogenesis.[48,49]

P13K/AKT/mTOR Pathways

This is a complex pathway that has been shown to be activated in the majority of HNSC (>70%). The PTEN gene on chromosome 10q is a negative regulator of the PI3k. Loss of this gene results in the upregulation of AKT and mTOR and is associated with poor behavior of these tumors.[25] Activation of these pathways plays an important role in the development and progression of HNSC. Mutation of the PI3K gene leads to cellular transformation of HNSC. Restoration of this pathway may lead to inhibition of PI3K phosphorylation and expression, which is responsible for radioresistance to targeted treatment. The mTOR has been shown to regulate critical cellular processes, including motility, proliferation, survival, and transcription. mTOR inhibition, however, may lead to negative feedback of the insulin-like growth factor, which may lead to activation of PI3k and AkT and potentially counteracting the mTOR inhibitor. Multiple agents or single agents targeting multiple pathways may be an ideal strategy. Given the complexity of HNSC development, it is difficult to conceive that a single marker or target would result in the characterization of these tumors or in therapeutic success. The development of TKI that targets multiple components of diverse pathways and/or the combination of different agents is a likely strategy for the successful management of patients with these tumors.

Mesenchymal–Epithelial Transformation

In the last two decades, minimal attention has been paid to the role of epithelial/stromal interactions of invasion, progression, and metastasis in HNSC.[5] Recent investigations in several solid tumor models have shown that invasion and metastasis are associated with disruption of cell–cell and cell–matrix adhesion, altered epithelial cell polarity, and increased motility. Several studies have shown that this process is initiated in response to extracellular stimuli and factors. Growth factors and their receptors play a central role in the transduction of key events associated with this process. Among the most important of these are the RAS, SRC, PI3K, and the MAPK pathways. The activation of these pathways has been shown to lead to the downregulation of adhesion molecules (e.g., E-cadherin) and elevation of surrogate mesenchymal markers (e.g., vimentin).[3,5,26] Metalloproteinase enzymes (MMPs) play a critical role in the digestion of the extracellular matrix components. Studies have linked the overexpression of MMP-2 in squamous carcinoma with invasion and metastasis. E-cadherin is another important adhesion factor in cell to cell and cell basement adhesion through Ca-dependent homotypic interactions.

Several growth factors, including TGF, lead to the downregulation of E-cadherin and other cellular features associated with EMT. However, the manifestation of EMT in HNSC may vary considerably from tumor to tumor and within a given tumor. Not infrequently, minimal EMT changes are observed in well-differentiated broad invasive fronts while complete mesenchymal transformations are found in the sarcomatoid form of these tumors. In addition to the semiquantitative changes in these molecules, qualitative changes may also occur. This is clearly manifested in the phenotypic distribution of E-cadherin from membranous to cytoplasmic localization. EMT, therefore, is a dynamic and heterogeneous process that underlies the biology of a squamous carcinoma and the degree and extent of these changes reflect their aggressive nature.

BIOMARKER APPLICATIONS IN HEAD AND NECK TUMORIGENESIS

Early diagnosis in individuals at high risk for HNSC is key to improving treatment and prognosis of this disease. Similarly, predicting the biological behavior response to nonsurgical therapy, and toxicity is important in stratifying patients for treatment and targeted therapy. Therefore, the identification of sensitive and reproducible markers is critical to the success of these efforts. The application of tissue-based assay requires that they accurately and reproducibly reflect the underlying pathological and biological processes. These processes are dynamically varied in and between individuals. Quantitation of lesional variabilities and confounding non-neoplastic processes is necessary for accurate interpretation and the exclusion of false-positive and false-negative results. Integrating tissue assessment and biomarker results might ultimately be the best model of risk assessment for head and neck cancer patients.[2,24]

Current molecular findings support the fact that defined genetic events precede the morphologic alterations of the squamous epithelium and lead to the clonal development, tumor formation, and progression. These changes occur throughout the mucosal field as evidenced by the findings of similar molecular alterations in metachronous and synchronous lesions in the same patients. However, this may run counter to the known heterogeneity of these tumors considering the wide range of genetic and epigenetic alterations identified within and between tumors. This impacts not only on our understanding of this entity but also on the conceptual approach for the identification of diagnostic and biological markers.

Because of the inherent variability of the risk factors and the events leading to the development of individual tumors, the goal of identifying specific marker for the molecular classification must be considered. Molecular findings of future clinical potential include specific genes (p16, p53, and cyclin D1), localized genetic alterations (LOH at 3p, 9p, and 17p), methylation (MGMT and p16), growth factors (EGFR and VEGF), and localized novel microRNA. Concurrently, efforts to standardize specimen, techniques, scoring, and interpretive criteria should equally be addressed. Moreover, investigations of surrogate materials, including saliva, mouthwash, scrapping, and serum, should be encouraged. All these efforts will advance and expedite the availability of defined markers profiling for biological, prognostic stratification and targeted management of HNSC patients.[27,28]

Similar efforts to establish risk assessment and early detection and screening of high-risk patients are critical to combating this cancer.

SALIVARY GLAND TUMORS

Salivary gland tumors comprise only 2% to 3% of all head and neck neoplasms, with an overall incidence of approximately 2.5 to 3 per 100,000 persons per year.[57,58] The three major salivary glands are the most commonly afflicted sites, with 80% of tumors occurring in the parotid, 10% to 15% in the submandibular gland, and 5% to 10% in the sublingual and minor glands.[30] The majority of tumors (80%) arising in the parotid gland are benign, whereas those of the submandibular, sublingual, and minor gland origins are more often malignant (50% to 60%). Generally, salivary neoplasms are present in middle and older age (mean age, 56 years), patients with slight male predominance. Only 2% to 3% of salivary gland tumors afflict children under 10 years of age.[31]

Fine needle aspiration (FNA) is conventionally used in the initial evaluation of a salivary mass. The main indication of this procedure is to exclude lymphoreticular disorder, inflammatory and granulocytic reactive lesions, and metastasis. FNA may not be recommended in the diagnosis of primary salivary gland tumors and cystic lesions. Not uncommonly, FNA may induce neurosis, reactive inflammatory, and reparative manifestations that may obscure the underlying neoplastic conditions. Occasionally, however, especially in the planning of the extent of the operation, surgeons may utilize this technique to obtain a malignant diagnosis. Pathologic features of clinical importance are as follows:

1. Tumor size
2. Histologic diagnosis
3. Malignancy grade (when applicable)
4. Margin status
5. Perineural involvement

Benign Tumors

Pleomorphic Adenoma

Pleomorphic adenomas (PAs) are the most common benign salivary tumors that primarily occur in the parotid gland. Clinically, these tumors pursue a benign clinical course with a tendency for local recurrence mainly due to nodular extension. Rarely, some PAs may metastasize while retaining their benign phenotypic features.

Histologically, they manifest varied cellular components, comprising epithelial and myoepithelial cells in a variable background of myxoid and/or chondroid stroma.

Karyotypic analysis has identified recurrent and specific cytogenetic abnormalities, with t(3;8) (p21;q12) reported in more than 40%, and a small subset manifesting rearrangements of the 12q14-15 region.[33] The latter include translocation involving 12q14-15 with chromosome 9p12 or different partners and/or inversion of both chromosomes at the same breakpoint. Random clonal abnormalities have also been detected in more than 20% of PAs. Molecular studies using microsatellite repeat markers reported frequent LOH at the long arm of chromosomes 8 and 12p loci. Two specific genetic markers have been consistently identified in PAs; the PLAG1 on chromosome 3p21 is the most frequently upregulated gene, but its biological significance in the development of PA remains uncertain.

The second recurrent and specific chromosomal alteration involving 12q14-15 leads to overexpression of the high mobility group A2 gene (HMGA2). The gene is an architectural factor that regulates transcription through binding to AT-rich DNA. Microarray analysis of PA and PLAG1-transduced cells has identified most of the unregulated genes to be growth factors, such as IGF, BDGF1, CRABP2, SMARCD1, and EFNB1. Together these findings indicate that the PLAG1 gene contributes to oncogenesis through the induction of growth factors.[34]

Warthin's and Oncocytic Tumors

Warthin's tumor (WT) is the second most common benign salivary gland tumor. It arises almost exclusively in intraparotid or periparotid lymphoid stroma. Histopathologically, the tumor manifests oncotypic epithelial cell proliferation within lymphoid stroma with and without cystic formation. A spectrum of oncocytic tumors ranging from nodular oncocytic hyperplasia, adenoma, and carcinoma have been described and are most likely related to WTs. Current molecular and cytogenetic studies indicate that the majority of these lesions manifest a normal karyotype, while approximately 10% have cytogenetic abnormalities; the most common cytogenetic alteration identified is the t(11;19) (q21-22;p13). The same translocation and its fusion gene product CRTC1/MAML2 were also found in mucoepidermoid carcinoma (MEC). The finding of this abnormality in both tumors, along with their reported simultaneous occurrence, indicated a genetic link between these lesions. Collectively, the data supports a clonal origin in a subset of these tumors with a propensity to transform to MEC or oncocytic carcinoma.

Basal Cell Adenoma

Basal cell salivary neoplasms are rare and constitute approximately 2% to 3% of all salivary gland tumors. These tumors may not infrequently pose diagnostic difficulties due to their cytomorphologic similarities. They are typically formed of bland basal cell proliferation in nests and/or cords with intercellular eosinophilic homogeneous material deposition. These are classified into benign and malignant subtypes based on the invasive nature of a given tumor. Because of the infrequency of these tumors, only small numbers have been genetically analyzed; a common cytogenetic alteration in a few tumors was trisomy 8, but other sporadic cytogenetic alterations, including t(7;13) translocation, have also been reported. CGH analysis of samples of these tumors showed loss of chromosomes 2, 6, and 7, gain of chromosomes 1 and 8, and amplification of 12q region. Molecular analysis of these tumors has reported frequent LOH at chromosome 16q12-13, a region that houses the cylindromatosis gene.[35]

Canalicular Adenoma

Canalicular adenoma is characterized by columnar epithelial cells forming anastomosing bilayered cellular formations including nests and is trabecular in vascular stroma. The lesions are typically well circumscribed and encapsulated.[30] Differential diagnosis of canalicular adenoma from basal cell adenoma and ACC may occasionally be difficult, especially on biopsy specimens. Because of their rarity and benign nature, molecular studies of this entity are very rare.

Myoepithelioma

Myoepithelial tumors are formed almost exclusively of myoepithelial cells, which are rare and are less than 1% of all salivary gland neoplasms.[30] Some tumors may show focal areas of PA. They may manifest a variety of phenotypic forms, including plasmacytoid, spindle, clear, and/or epithelial features. Current molecular genetic data on these lesions are sparse and preclude any definitive findings that contribute to either their development or biology. Cytogenetic analyses of a few samples have reported nonspecific chromosomal abnormalities and were insufficient for commenting on their contribution to these tumors. Upregulation of the WT1 mRNA has been detected in some benign and malignant myoepithelial tumors, but the oncogenic role of this event in their development is unknown.

Malignant Neoplasms

Mucoepidermoid Carcinoma

MECs compose approximately 30% of malignant salivary neoplasms and are more common in children and adolescents. MEC manifests three distinctive phenotypic grades based on the cellularity and architectural features of the tumors. Of all salivary neoplasms, MEC is the only entity in which both cytogenetic and molecular analyses have led to the identification of consistent unique alterations that may constitute an initiating event in the development of a subset of these tumors. Several cytogenetic analyses of MEC have shown translocation t(11;19)(q21;p13) either alone or with other nonspecific alterations.[30] Cloning of this translocation has identified a fusion oncogene composed of exon 1 of the MECT1 (CRTC1/WAMTP) gene on chromosome 19p13 and exons 2 to 5 of the MAML2 gene on chromosome 11q21 regions. MAML2, a member of the mastermind gene family, encodes a nuclear protein that binds to the CSL transcriptional factor and the intracellular domain of the Notch receptor to activate the Notch target gene. The fusion partner is the CRTC1 (MECT1), a member of the highly conserved CREβ/cAMP coactivator gene family.[35,36] Studies of this fusion transcript in a series of MEC have reported a correlation between fusion-positive tumors and low tumor grade and better behavior. Fusion-negative MEC may evolve from a different evolutionary pathway and may represent a biologically distinctive category. The results also suggest that tumors lacking the fusion transcript behave more aggressively. In addition, fusion transcript–positive tumors have been shown to behave less aggressively than those with fusion-negative counterparts. The finding of the fusion transcript in both sporadic WT and MEC and concomitant tumors supports an early or etiologic linking of a subset of these tumors. Epithelial ductal cells in heterotypic salivary tissue in intraparotid or paraparotid lymphoid stroma acquiring the t(11;19)[37-39] fusion gene give rise to WT, while the same alteration in the salivary tissue gives rise to MEC in sporadic presentations. The development of MEC in a WT may therefore result from metaplastic changes in ductal cells with the fusion transcript. Although an attractive therapeutic target, obstacles remained in its application in clinical settings. Until this goal is achieved, the detection of CRTC1-MAML2 fusion transcript can serve in the differential diagnosis of poorly differentiated carcinoma and intraosseous MEC using fine needle aspirations.[40]

Salivary Duct Carcinoma and Adenocarcinoma Ex-pleomorphic Adenoma

Salivary duct carcinoma (SDC) and adenocarcinomas present either de novo or in the setting of PA and manifest remarkable similarity to mammary duct carcinoma.[41] Cytogenetic studies of some of these tumors have shown that rearrangements of chromosome 8q12, alteration of chromosome 12q13-15 regions, and amplification of both the HMG1C and MDM2 genes may be potentially associated with these tumors. Other studies have shown that translocations of chromosome 5(q22-23, q32-33) and t(10;12)(p15;q14-14) resulted in transportations of the entire HMG1C gene to chromosome 10 marker.

Using microsatellite markers on microdissected benign and matching malignant components of salivary gland carcinoma, ex-pleomorphic adenoma has shown alterations at 8q and/or 12q in both components and restricted alterations at chromosome 17p loci in the malignant component.[42] These findings suggest that alterations at 8q and 12q regions represent early events, whereas alteration at 17p is associated or coincident with the malignant transformation. Studies of specific genes and loci have also reported homozygous deletion of the p16 gene on chromosome, and p53 alterations and LOH at different loci on chromosome. A subset of SDC, as in mammary ductal carcinoma, express hormonal and growth factor overexpression that may be used in their biological and therapeutic stratification. Overexpression of HER-2, EGFR, and androgen receptors is found in more than one-third of these tumors (Fig. 33.3A-C). Since targeting individual receptors has limited therapeutic potential, dual anti-EGFR and HER-2 target therapy may overcome some of the resistance to new single agents such as lapatinib. High EGFR and/or HER-2 expression are reported in approximately 25% to 35% of salivary gland adenocarcinomas and have been associated with aggressive behaviors. These findings provide strong rationale for patients' stratification and targeted therapy.[43,44]

Adenoid Cystic Carcinoma

ACC is the second most common malignant salivary gland tumor and the most clinically relentless malignancy. ACC is known for its indolent and persistent clinical behavior and propensity for perineural invasion. ACC manifests three phenotypic subtypes, which nearly always present in the majority of tumors but in variable proportions. These include tubular, cribriform, and the solid morphologic variants. In both the tubular and the cribriform phenotypes, the tumor units consist of myoepithelial and ductal epithelial cells. Cytogenetic studies of these tumors have reported frequent alterations at chromosomes 6q, 9p, and 17p, with the most consistent alteration at the 6q regions.[46] Studies of ACC have reported frequent LOH at 6q23-25, 12q, 6q23-qter, 13q21-33, and 19q regions in these tumors.

A recent CGH of ACCs identified a novel gain at chromosome 22q13 region in 30% of the tumors in addition to the loss of chromosome 6q and gains of chromosome 16p and 17q regions.[47-49] Microarray analysis of a few samples of these tumors has shown amplification of MDM2, HMG1C, MYC, and other genes located on chromosomes 8q and 12q14. A frequent finding in these tumors is the overexpression of the C-Kit protein. C-Kit (CD117) is a transmembrane tyrosine kinase receptor encoded by the C-Kit gene on chromosome 4. The C-Kit ligand, a stem cell factor (also known as steel factor and mast cell growth factor), induces signal transduction pathways affecting development, cell growth, and migration of different cell functions (Fig. 33.4 A-C). The role and the cellular distribution of this gene product in the biology and as a target in these tumors remain to be determined. Recently, a fusion gene resulting from the t(6;9) translocation was identified in ACC. This fusion gene comprised the MYB gene on 6q13 and the NFIB on chromosome 9p13. This translocation resulted in high expression of the MYB gene. Although complex and variable alterations have been identified as a consequence of the translocation, the MYB expression remained elevated. Targeting the MYB gene is being considered in the treatment.

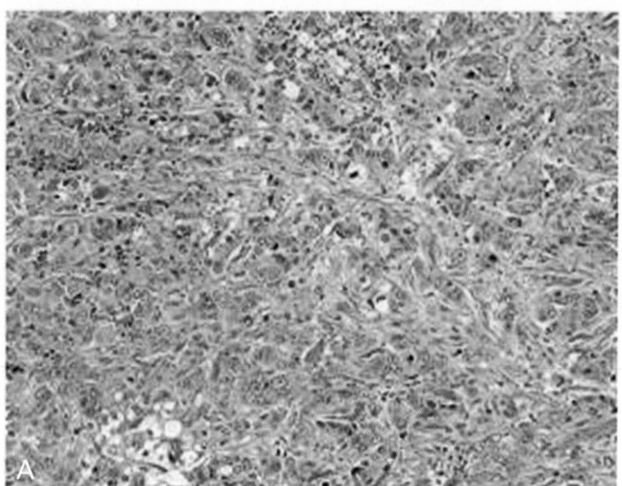

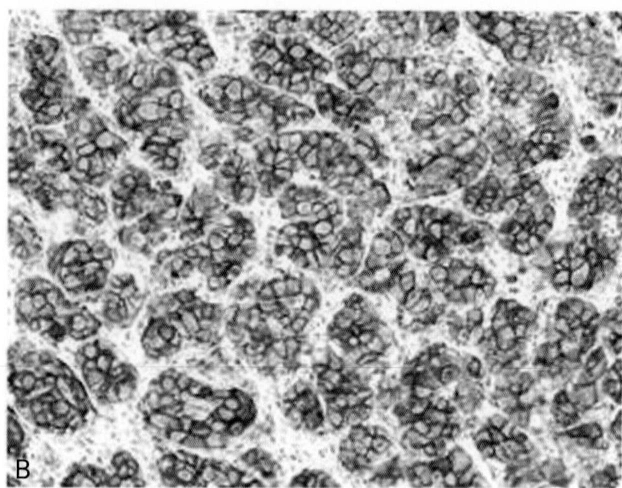

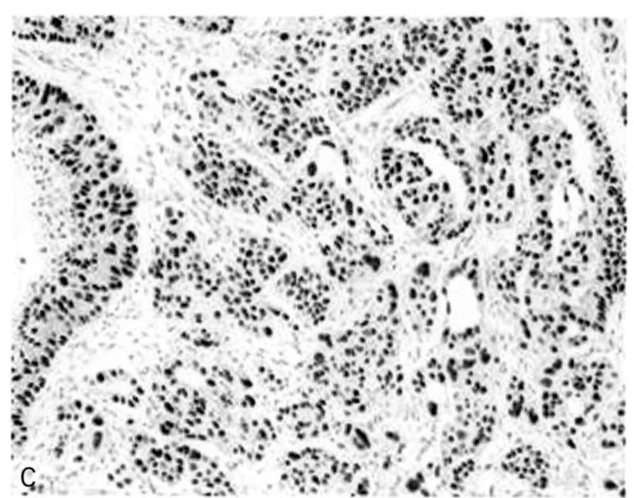

FIGURE 33–3 **A:** A light-optic micrograph of a salivary duct carcinoma. Note the resemblance to mammary duct carcinoma. **B:** Similar to breast ductal carcinoma, 25% of salivary duct carcinomas highly express HER-2 as in this example. **C:** Homogeneous nuclear staining of androgen receptor in a salivary duct carcinoma.

Acinic Cell Carcinomas

Acinic cell carcinoma is a distinctive salivary malignancy that develops almost exclusively in the parotid gland. These tumors arise from acinar cells and manifest granular serous cellular features with variable and overlapping morphologic subtypes.[50] They are generally low-grade indolent carcinomas, occasionally presenting as high-grade carcinomas with high mitotic figures, necrosis, and lymph node metastasis. In addition, several examples of transformation into dedifferentiation or anaplastic carcinomas have been reported. Cytogenetic and molecular studies of these tumors are few and inconclusive. One study cites evidence for a frequent LOH at limited chromosomal regions,[51] including 4p15-16, 6p25-qter, and 17p11, suggesting that these regions may contain critical genes related to their development. In another study of multiple samples of an ACC, variable clonal alterations were obtained, suggesting multiclonal origin. Studies of dedifferentiated acinic cell carcinoma have shown an association of such transformation with cyclin D upregulation. The lack of confirmatory and validated follow-up studies precludes any speculation on the role of these findings in this entity.

Recently, the conditional inactivation of both the APC and the PTEN suppressor genes in a mouse model led to the development of acinic cell carcinoma after short latency implicating the canonical Wnt and the mammalian target of rapamycin (mTOR) pathways in the pathogenesis of this phenotype.[51] Interestingly, treatment with mTOR inhibitors leads to the eradication of these tumors. Human studies are needed to explore the validity of these findings.

Polymorphous Salivary Adenocarcinoma (Terminal Duct Carcinoma)

This entity is characterized by intratumoral growth pattern variabilities and uniform monotonous cellular composition. The hard palate is the most frequent site but they may rarely occur in major salivary glands.[30] The tumor constitutes 19.6% of malignant minor gland tumors. Because of the lack of encapsulations, these tumors typically infiltrate adjacent tissue and are prone to perineural

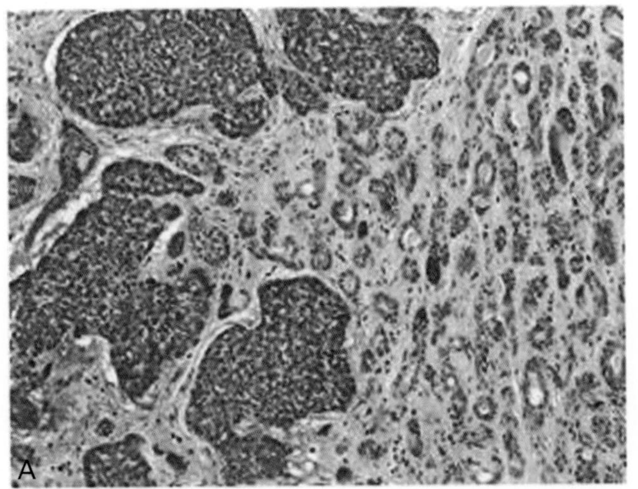

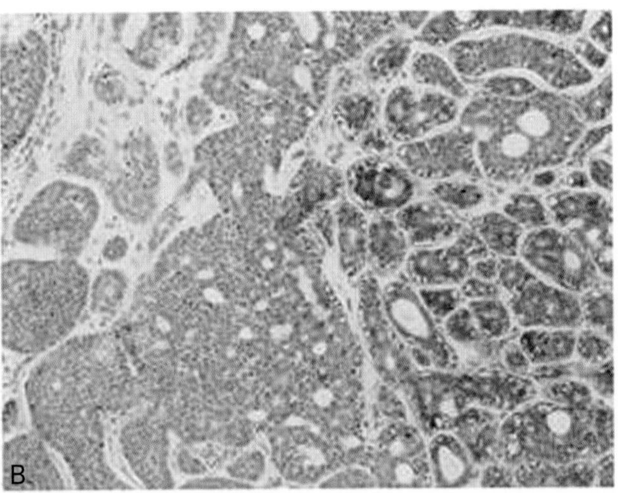

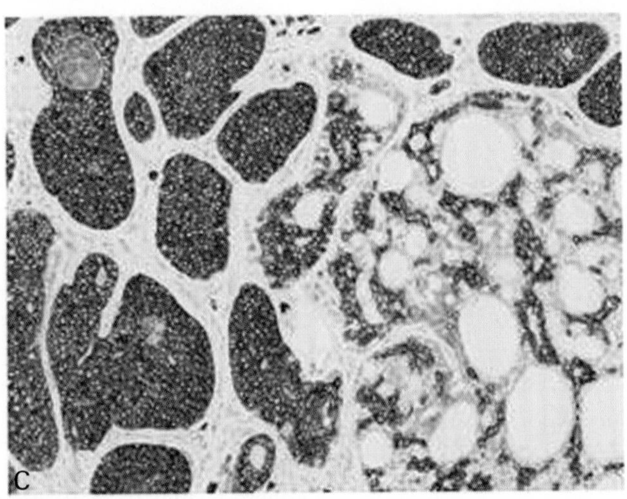

FIGURE 33–4 **A:** Adenoid cystic carcinoma with ductal, cribriform, and solid components. **B:** An EGFR staining of the same tumor showing paradoxical positivity in myoepithelial cells. **C:** A c-kit immunostaining highlighting the differential cellular localization of this marker in this entity. Note that only epithelial not myoepithelial cells are positive.

invasions. The recurrence rate for these tumors is approximately 17% and regional metastasis occurs in approximately 9%.

Epi-myoepithelial Carcinoma

This rare entity represents a malignancy of low grade and indolent course and is composed of dual myoepithelial and ductal tumor cells.[30] Histopathologically, the tumor forms duct and tubular formations of relatively prominent clear myoepithelial cells and inner cuboidal and uniform duct cells.

Salivary Tumors in Children

The majority of salivary neoplasms in children are nonepithelial and mainly of vascular origin. The most common malignant neoplasm in this age group is mucoepidermoid followed by acinic cell carcinomas, forming approximately 60% of malignant neoplasms.[30] The most common benign epithelial neoplasm in this age group is PA. Rarely, tumors including embryoma or sialoblastoma are present at birth and occur prenatally. Histologically, these tumors represent a neoplastic growth of embryonic, primitive, and basaloid epithelial cells of salivary gland. These lesions are considered low-grade malignancy.[31] The differential diagnosis includes basal cell adenocarcinoma and adenoid cystic carcinoma.

Genomic Studies

Several genomic studies have been conducted to characterize these tumors. The results, however, are contradictory and remain to be validated.

Rare Salivary Gland Neoplasms

Squamous Carcinoma

Rarely, squamous carcinoma may arise de novo in major salivary glands and if presented, are not underlined. The exclusion of metastasis from other sites must be proved.[30] Rare carcinomas reported to be of primary origin include small cell carcinoma and lymphoepithelial carcinoma (LEC).

Small Cell Carcinoma

This is very rare in salivary gland, and metastasis from distant sites should be excluded before considering a primary origin.[52]

Lymphoepithelial Carcinoma

Primary LEC may not be uncommonly encountered in the parotid gland. These tumors are histologically identical to those of nasopharyngeal origin. Epstein-Barr virus may or may not be present in these tumors.[53]

Mesenchymal Neoplasms

Nonepithelial neoplasms form less than 5% of all salivary gland tumors. They represent lesions arising from salivary gland supporting connective tissue. The most common lesions are angioma, lipoma, neurofibroma, and hemangiopericytoma. The growth and microscopic features of these lesions are identical to those encountered in other sites.

Primary Lymphoma

Lymphomas are very rare and are mainly found in the parotid gland. The majority of primary lymphomas are of the MALT type. They may arise in either intraparotid lymph nodes or parenchyma. The vast majority of them are of the follicular B-cell derivation with rare instances of T-cell origin.[53]

Metastasis to Salivary Glands

The most common metastasis to major salivary glands, especially the parotid, is squamous carcinoma followed by melanoma of the skin. This is largely due to the lymphatic drainage of the skin of the face. Hematogenous spread to the parotid originates primarily from kidney, breast, and lung carcinomas. Metastasis to the submandibular gland is very rare due to the lack of intraglandular lymph nodes. Epithelial neoplasms are rare and disproportionately malignant.[30]

THYROID TUMORS

Thyroid nodules are one of the most common clinical conditions. The vast majority of these are reactive lesions or benign tumors and only 10% are malignant.[55] Thyroid neoplasms represent a wide spectrum of histogenetically and biologically variable entities. Approximately 14,000 new cases of thyroid carcinomas are diagnosed per year in the USA. The histologic subtypes of thyroid malignancies include papillary, follicular, poorly differentiated, anaplastic, and medullary carcinomas. Broadly, these tumors can be categorized into differentiated (papillary, follicular, and medullary) and undifferentiated (poorly differentiated and anaplastic) carcinomas. The papillary, follicular, poorly differentiated (insular), and the majority of anaplastic carcinomas arise from the follicular epithelial cells while the medullary thyroid carcinoma (MTC) is derived from parafollicular calcitonin-producing C cells.

Etiology

The etiology of thyroid malignancies is largely unknown. However, exposure to radiation during childhood (papillary) and iodine deficiency (follicular) have been linked to the development of certain carcinoma subtypes. Papillary thyroid carcinoma (PTC) may affect people of any age, including children and young adults with no prior radiation history, and typically present as an enlarged mass with or without ipsilateral nodal involvement.[56]

Radiology

Initial radioscintigraphy is helpful in distinguishing between hot (benign) and cold (malignant) nodules. Computer-guided tomography is routinely used in the initial FNA cytology.

Pathology

FNA is the first line of diagnostic technique for thyroid tumor diagnosis. In general, an accurate diagnosis of PTC and MTC can be readily made on FNA. The sensitivity and the specificity of FNA in diagnosing follicular lesions, including follicular variant of papillary carcinoma, however, are low. It is estimated that up to 30% of FNA-based diagnosis of follicular neoplasms are indeterminate.

Histology

Thyroid neoplasms are generally classified based on their histogenesis from epithelial (follicular cell) and neuroectodermal (C-cell) neoplasms. Epithelial neoplasms are broadly benign follicular adenomas and differentiated neoplasms and poorly differentiated and anaplastic carcinomas.

Follicular forming tumors are pathologically divided into adenoma and carcinoma based on whether capsular and/or vascular invasion is found. The papillary form is typically malignant but may present with follicular component. The latter may dominate a given tumor and lead to differential diagnostic difficulties. Both the follicular and the papillary subtypes may progress to poorly differentiated and/or anaplastic carcinoma.[55,56]

Follicular Adenoma

Adenomas are characterized by a well-circumscribed nodular growth with thin encapsulation. They may present as solitary or multiple nodules at any age and in any gender. Microscopically, they may manifest microfollicular, trabecular, and macrofollicular forms. The main differential diagnosis for adenomas is follicular hyperplasia (Goiter) and follicular carcinoma. Oncocytic changes due to the high content of mitochondria are most likely secondary to respiratory cellular demands. The biological behavior of these neoplasms is similar to those of corresponding follicular tumors.[55]

Differentiated Carcinomas

Follicular Thyroid Carcinoma

Follicular carcinomas comprise approximately 5% to 10% of all thyroid malignances. They generally afflict females in their middle age than males. A high incidence of these tumors is reported in iodine deficient regions, suggesting a role for continuous TSH stimulation in the genesis of this entity. The diagnosis of this entity is based on the findings of a thick fibrous capsule and the presence of capsular and/or vascular penetration. These tumors can be further classified as minimally invasive or encapsulated, if invasion did not extend beyond the capsule. Follicular carcinoma is typically solitary and may present or be preceded by metastasis typically to bone, lung, and brain.

Patients present with a singly palpable cold mass with a high propensity for radioactive iodine uptake.[56,57]

Papillary Thyroid Carcinoma

Papillary carcinoma is the most common of all thyroid carcinomas, accounting for more than 70% of these tumors. They may present at any age with peak incidence between 30 and 40 years of age. Females are far more affected than males, and young patients typically have a better and long protracted course than older patients, especially men. There is strong evidence for increased incidence of PTC in patients with Hashimoto's thyroiditis. PTC may not uncommonly present as multifocal disease and total thyroidectomy is generally the treatment of choice. Presentation with concurrent lymph node metastasis occurs in approximately 20% of patients. The hallmark of papillary carcinoma is the formation of finger-like structures lined by cuboidal or columnar cells with clear and/or cleaved nuclei. The nuclear features are especially helpful in the diagnosis of the follicular variant of this entity. Not uncommonly present (40%) is the concentric calcification (psammoma bodies). This is a common feature in this tumor and may aid in the diagnosis.[55] Several histopathologic variants of this entity have been described with some being associated with a more aggressive clinical course. However, the lack of prospective studies with long-term follow-up renders the significance of these subtypes tenuous. The clinical aggressiveness of PTC varies depending on the gender, age, and size of the tumors with older males having a more aggressive course, as well as patients with large invasive tumors.

Medullary Thyroid Carcinoma

MTC arises from the C cell, a neuroectodermally derived cell, and accounts for 3% to 10% of thyroid cancer. The tumors present in two forms: sporadic, the most common, which accounts for 70% to 80%; and the familial form, which represents the remaining 20% to 30%. The tumors affect both genders equally and also patients in their middle age.

The familial and the sporadic forms have mutations in the RET gene, and the frequency and the type of these mutations vary. Tumors in the sporadic form present with a solitary mass with or without neck enlargement and paraneoplastic syndrome. Tumors in the familial form are generally multifocal and affect the younger adults and children.[57]

The most common location of these tumors is the lateral aspect of the upper two-thirds of the thyroid lobes, where a high aggregation of C cells can be found. Histopathologically, tumors consist of nests and cords and organized structures composed of small- to medium-sized cells with uniform nuclei. Tumor clusters are encircled by delicate vessels and fibrous tissue. Not uncommonly, deposition of dense homogeneous eosinophotic materials representing amyloid deposition is noted. The amyloid nature of these materials can be verified by either Congo red staining or light microscopic birefringence.

Immunostaining for calcitonin and other neuroendocrine markers may be used for confirmation. The most common sites of metastasis for MTC are regional lymph nodes, lung, liver, and bone. The prognosis of MTC depends on several factors, including age, gender, size, and stage. Generally, the young and females have better outcomes. Patients with multiple endocrine neoplasia (MEN)-2B have a worse outcome. The differential diagnosis of these tumors includes metastasis from neuroendocrine carcinoma, renal cell carcinoma, and microfollicular thyroid neoplasm.

Sclerosing MEC

This is a rare malignancy of the thyroid gland, typically in association with Hashimoto's thyroiditis. It is characterized by infiltrating sclerotic stroma with infiltrating nests of squamoid cells with occasional mucinous cells. The stroma is characteristically infiltrated by numerous eosinophils.

Undifferentiated Thyroid Carcinomas

Poorly Differentiated

This histologic variant represents a tumor that lacks follicular or papillary differentiation and the cellular anaplasia of anaplastic carcinoma. Tumors typically manifest cell nests or cords with monotonous cellular features. The differential diagnosis is mostly with MTC. Tumor cells react positively to antithyroglobulin antibodies and they are negative for calcitonin. Their behavior is considered more aggressive than the fully differentiated tumors.[57]

Anaplastic Thyroid Carcinomas

Anaplastic thyroid carcinoma (ATC) is the most clinically aggressive neoplasm and accounts for 4% to 10% of all thyroid malignancies. This entity afflicts elderly individuals and is more common in females than in males (3:1). Clinically, patients present with rapidly progressive local disease.[58] The majority of these tumors arise from preexisting differentiated thyroid carcinoma, most commonly the papillary phenotype. In resected specimens of these tumors, evidence for a differentiated carcinoma can be found. The etiology of ATC is unknown, but previous radiation of thyroid lesions has been linked to the development of these tumors. Histopathologically, these tumors manifest highly malignant tumor cell composition with heterogeneous features and tumor necrosis.[32] The most common pathologic phenotypes are sarcomatous, giant cell, and squamous variants. The differential diagnoses of these tumors include sarcomatoid carcinoma of the upper aerodigestive tract, sarcoma, and melanoma.[29] Immunostaining assists in excluding sarcoma and melanoma. The prognosis of these patients is very poor.

MOLECULAR ANALYSIS OF THYROID NEOPLASMS

Papillary Thyroid Carcinoma

Frequent alterations at the BRAF and the RAS genes and RET/PTC rearrangement are found in PTC. These alterations are in large part mutually exclusive and lead to the activation of the MAPK. Less frequent alterations in PTC include rearrangements of the tyrosine receptor kinase pathway (5%).

BRAF

The frequency of BRAF mutations in PTC is 35% to 75%. The majority of these mutations involve the 1799 (T1799A) nucleotide resulting in thymine to adenine transversion at codon 600 (V600E). Other mutations include K601E point mutation, deletion, or insertion at codon 600. Interestingly, RET-PTC rearrangement has been found in PTC associated with radiation exposure. Although unconfirmed, an association between BRAF mutations and aggressive features has been reported.[61]

RET/PTC

The RET/PTC rearrangement is formed by binding of the 3′-segment of the RET gene to the 5′-segment of either the PTC1 or PTC3 by intrachromosomal inversion of chromosome 10.[62] These rearrangements contain the RET tyrosine kinase receptor domain. This alteration has been reported in approximately 15% to 20% of PTC. It is highly associated with radiation exposure and found in children and young adults with PTC.[62,63]

RAS Gene

All RAS genes (H-, N-, and K-RAS) are G-protein with considerable homology-associated transmitting cell membrane signals to their intracellular targets. All types of the RAS genes have been reported in different thyroid neoplasms, including follicular adenoma.[65]

Mutations in these genes lead to constitutional activation and persistent stimulation of the MAPK and PI3K/AKT pathways. Future studies linking these alterations to either biological progression and response to iodine therapy are needed to define the use of these markers in clinical practice.

Follicular Thyroid Neoplasms

In contrast to PTC, follicular thyroid neoplasms are characterized by frequent mutations of the RAS gene and PAX8/PPAR-γ gene rearrangements and constitute up to 75% of these tumors.[66]

RAS mutations are reported in 40% of follicular carcinomas and less frequently in histologically diagnosed follicular adenomas (20%). The finding of RAS mutations in hyperplastic nodules and benign follicular lesions renders the diagnostic potential of this event unlikely.[67]

PAX8/PPARγ

The translocation involving chromosomes 2q and 3p results in the fusion of the PAX8/PPARγ genes. The PAX8 gene encodes for paired domain transcription factor specific to the thyroid gland. The final outcome of this translocation is the overexpression of the PPARγ protein. This molecular event is so far restricted to follicular carcinoma, in which it occurs in approximately 30% to 45% of cases. The biological effect of this event in follicular carcinoma is largely uncertain since a small percentage occurs in follicular adenomas (5%) and follicular variant of PTC. It may be that follicular adenomas with this alteration constitute a premalignant stage. Studies of benign adenomas with temporal malignant behaviors should shed more light on this issue.

These molecular alterations may have a potential diagnostic and biological significance. This is especially the case in follicular thyroid nodules prior to surgery. The use of fresh high-quality cellular materials of FNA lends this as an excellent source in future diagnostic applications.

However, only the detection of these alterations may be useful. Negative results are not a ground for exclusion of malignancy. Approximately, 25% of PTC harbors RAS mutations and this has been predominantly found in the follicular variant.[68,69]

Evidence for molecular progression of thyroid differentiated carcinoma to the poorly differentiated and the anaplastic carcinoma provides important new information on the events associated with such transformations. Validating these events allow for the characterization and validation of predictor and prognostic markers in the assessment of these tumors.[70]

Genomics

Gene expression analyses of several thyroid neoplasms have been performed. Upregulation of MET, SGRPINA, FNI, CD44, and DPP4 and downregulation of TFF3 gene have been reported in some of these studies. Although genomic analysis is allowed for the identification of thyroid neoplasm and the biological categorization within carcinomas, the utilization of these assays in the clinical diagnosis is limited and impractical.[70]

Parathyroid Tumors

Parathyroid glands are derived from the third and fourth pharyngeal pouches and are recognized by the fifth to the sixth weeks of gestation. The majority of humans have two pairs of parathyroid glands but multiple glands (13%) may occur, and as few as one has been reported in humans.

Normal glands are encapsulated, small, soft, and tan to red-brown in color. Parathyroid cells are organized in lobules with fat cells and vascular stroma. The percentage of fat in normal parathyroid varies but in general is approximately 60%. Although literally a non-neoplastic process, evidence of clonality and evolution to adenoma and carcinoma based on clonality analysis has been documented.

Parathyroid Hyperplasia

Parathyroid hyperplasia is pathologically characterized by increased parathyroid cells with reduction of fat cells in parathyroid lobules. This may occur in all four glands with a variable degree. Generally, this may signify a systemic etiology such as calcium deficiency, vitamin D alterations, and kidney diseases. Hyperplasia of the parathyroid can also be a manifestation of MEN type I syndrome. Histopathologically, they manifest diffuse or nodular cellular proliferation. The cellular feature varies and may include clear and oncocytic cytoplasm.[71-73]

Parathyroid Adenoma

Parathyroid adenoma is a benign parathyroid gland neoplasm and is the most common cause of hyperparathyroidism accounting for more than 80% of cases. Parathyroid adenoma affects more females than males in the middle age. These lesions are considered clonal in origin and present as a single well-circumscribed nodule with a peripheral rim of parathyroid tissue. Adenoma is typically homogeneous and contains no adipose tissue cells. Although they may arise in any gland, they are more frequently reported in the lower glands.

Locally Infiltrative Parathyroid Neoplasm (Atypical Parathyroid Adenoma)

Occasionally, parathyroid neoplasms with cytomorphologic features identical to those of hyperplasia or adenoma and infiltrative growth into surrounding soft tissue with intersecting fibrous bands may be encountered. The lack of high and abnormal mitotic figures, necrosis, and marked cellular pleomorphism preclude a definitive malignant diagnosis. These lesions are typically prone to local recurrence because of the difficulties in completely excising them. These lesions may also be called atypical parathyroid adenoma.

Parathyroid Carcinoma

Parathyroid carcinoma is a rare, highly malignant neoplasm which accounts for less than 5% of patients with hyperparathyroidism. This entity may be hormonally active or inactive. The inactive carcinoma has reportedly been more aggressive. These tumors present as a solid mass that is difficult to excise due to its infiltrative nature. Histopathologically, these tumors are characterized by a proliferation of markedly pleomorphic cells, high and abnormally mitotic figures, broad intersecting fibrous bands, vascular and soft tissue invasion, and necrosis. This is a surgically treated disease but more than a third of these patients experience metastasis.[74]

Molecular Analysis of Parathyroid Neoplasms

Alterations in overexpression of cyclin D and chromosome 11q13 regions have been shown to characterize parathyroid nodular hyperplasia and adenoma. Other clonal and molecular findings support a clonal basis for the development of at least a subset of these lesions. The cyclin D and Rb glue have frequently been found in parathyroid carcinoma alterations. Mutation at the MEN1 gene on chromosome 11q13 region has been reported in up to 50% of cases. Genome-wide studies have also shown the loss of 11q region in addition to other chromosomes.[75-77]

Molecular alterations of parathyroid carcinoma are rare and inconclusive, but alterations of the Rb and the MEN1 genes have been reported. Proteins have been reported to be limited to these tumors. LOH and mutation of the HPRT2 gene, which encodes for the parafibromin, have also been documented in parathyroid carcinoma and are believed to be restricted to malignancy. If validated, this may have a diagnostic and therapeutic implication. Somatic mutations as well as germline mutations of the HPRT2 have been implicated to underlie primary hyperparathyroidism.

REFERENCES

1. El-Naggar AK. Pathobiology of head and neck squamous tumorigenesis. *Curr Cancer Drug Targets*. 2007;7:606-612.
2. Forastiere A, Koch W, Trotti A, et al. Head and neck cancer. *N Engl J Med*. 2001;345:1890-1900.
3. Barnes L, Eveson JW, Reichart P, et al. *World Health Organization Classification of Tumours. Pathology & Genetics. Head and Neck Tumours*. Lyon: IARC;2005.
4. Braakhuis BJ, Tabor MP, Kimmer JA, et al. A genetic explanation of Slaughter's concept of field cancerization: evidence and clinical implications. *Cancer Res*. 2003;63:1727-1730.
5. Mandal M, Myers JN, Lippman SM, et al. Epithelial to mesenchymal transition in head and neck squamous carcinoma: association of Src activation with E-cadherin down-regulation, vimentin expression, and aggressive tumor features. *Cancer*. 2008;112:2088-2100.
6. Mete O, Keskin Y, Hafiz G, Kayhan KB, Unur M. Oral proliferative verrucous leukoplakia: underdiagnosed oral precursor lesion that requires retrospective clinicopathological correlation. *Dermatol Online J*. 2010;16:6.
7. Choi HR, Roberts DB, Johnigan RH, et al. Molecular and clinicopathologic comparisons of head and neck squamous carcinoma variants: common and distinctive features of biological significance. *Am J Surg Pathol*. 2004;28:1299-1310.
8. Choi HR, Stugis EM, Rosenthal DI, et al. Sarcomatoid carcinoma of the head and neck: molecular evidence for evolution and progression from conventional squamous cell carcinomas. *Am J Surg Pathol*. 2003;27:1216-1220.
9. Dahlstrand H, Nasman A, Romanitan M, et al. Human papillomavirus accounts both for increased incidence and better prognosis in tonsillar cancer. *Anticancer Res*. 2008;28:1133-1138.

10. Begum S, Westra WH. Basaloid squamous cell carcinoma of the head and neck is a mixed variant that can be further resolved by HPV status. *Am J Surg Pathol.* 2008;32:1044-1050.
11. Kumar B, Cordell KG, Lee JS, et al. Response to therapy and outcomes in oropharyngeal cancer are associated with biomarkers including human papilloma, epidermal growth factor receptor, gender and smoking. *Int J Radiat Oncol Biol Phys.* 2007;69:S109-S111.
12. Weber A, Bellmann U, Bootz F, et al. Expression of p53 and its homologues in primary and recurrent squamous cell carcinomas of the head and neck. *Int J Cancer.* 2002;99:22-28.
13. Wang D, Grecula JC, Gahbauer RA, et al. p16 gene alterations in locally advanced squamous cell carcinoma of the head and neck. *Oncol Rep.* 2006;15:661-665.
14. Coombes MM, Briggs KL, Bone JR, et al. Resetting the histone code at CDKN2A in HNSCC by inhibition of DNA methylation. *Oncogene.* 2003;22:8902-8911.
15. Papadimitrakopoulou VA, Izzo J, Mao L, et al. Cyclin D1 and p16 alterations in advanced premalignant lesions of the upper aerodigestive tract: role in response to chemoprevention and cancer development. *Clin Cancer Res.* 2001;7:3127-3134.
16. Maruya S, Issa JP, Weber RS, et al. Differential methylation status of tumor-associated genes in head and neck squamous carcinoma: incidence and potential implications. *Clin Cancer Res.* 2004;10:3825-3830.
17. Poage GM, Houseman EA, Christensen BC, et al. Global hypomethylation identifies loci targeted for hypermethylation in head and neck cancer. *Clin Cancer Res.* 2011;17:3579-3589.
18. Chen YJ, Lin SC, Kao T, et al. Genome-wide profiling of oral squamous cell carcinoma. *J Pathol.* 2004;204:326-332.
19. Roepman P, Wessels LF, Kettelarij N, et al. An expression profile for diagnosis of lymph node metastases from primary head and neck squamous cell carcinomas. *Nat Genet.* 2005;37:182-186.
20. Saintigny P, Zhang L, Fan YH, et al. Gene expression profiling predicts the development of oral cancer. *Cancer Prev Res (Phila).* 2011;4:218-229.
21. Li J, Huang H, Sun L, et al. MiR-21 indicates poor prognosis in tongue squamous cell carcinomas as an apoptosis inhibitor. *Clin Cancer Res.* 2009;15:3998-4008.
22. Temem S, Kawaguchi H, El-Naggar AK, et al. Epidermal growth factor receptor copy number alterations correlate with poor clinical outcome in patients with head and neck squamous cancer. *J Clin Oncol.* 2007;25:2164-2170.
23. Joo YH, Jung CK, Kim MS, et al. Relationship between vascular endothelial growth factor and Notch1 expression and lymphative metastasis in tongue cancer. *Otolaryngol Head Neck Surg.* 2009;140:512-518.
24. Montag M, Dyckhoff G, Lohr J, et al. Angiogenic growth factors in tissue homogenates of HNSCC: expression pattern, prognostic relevance, and interrelationships. *Cancer Sci.* 2009;100:1210-1218.
25. Qiu W, Schonleben F, Li X, et al. PIK3CA mutations in head and neck squamous cell carcinoma. *Clin Cancer Res.* 2006;12:1441-1446.
26. Bockmühl U, Ishwad CS, Ferrell RE, Gollin SM. sociation of 8p23 deletions with poor survival in head and neck cancer. *Otolaryngol Head Neck Surg.* 2001;124(4):451-455.
27. Shah SI, Yip L, Greenberg B, Califano JA, Chow J, Eisenberger CF, Lee DJ, Sewell DA, Reed AL, Lango M, Jen J, Koch WM, Sidransky D. Two distinct regions of loss on chromosome arm 4q in primary head and neck squamous cell carcinoma. *Arch Otolaryngol Head Neck Surg.* 2000;126(9):1073-1076.
28. Matsuura K, Shiga K, Yokoyama J, Saijo S, Miyagi T, Takasaka T. Loss of heterozygosity of chromosome 9p21 and 7q31 is correlated with high incidence of recurrent tumor in head and neck squamous cell carcinoma. *Anticancer Res.* 1998;18(1A):453-458.
29. Li X, Lee NK, Ye YW, Waber PG, Schweitzer C, Cheng QC, Nisen PD. Allelic loss at chromosomes 3p, 8p, 13q, and 17p associated with poor prognosis in head and neck cancer. *J Natl Cancer Inst.* 1994;86(20):1524-1529.
30. Day TA, Deveikis j, Gillespie MB, et al. Salivary gland neoplasms. *Curr Treat Options Oncol.* 2004;5:11-26.
31. Shapiro NL, Bhattacharyya N. Clinical characteristics and survival for major salivary gland malignancies in children. *Otolaryngol Head Neck Surg.* 2006;134:631-634.
32. Bradley PJ. Recurrent salivary gland pleomorphic adenoma: etiology, management, and results. *Curr Opin Otolaryngol Head Neck Surg.* 2001;9:100-108.
33. Gillenwater A, Hurr K, Wolf P, et al. Microsatellite alterations as chromosome 8q loci pleomorphic adenoma. *Otolaryngol Head Neck Surg.* 1997;117:448-452.
34. Martins C, Fonseca I, Roque L, et al. PLAG1 gene alterations in salivary gland pleomorphic adenoma and carcinoma ex-pleomorphic adenoma: a combined study using chromosome banding in situ hybridization and immunocytochemistry. *Mod Pathol.* 2005;18:1048-1055.
35. Choi HR, Batsakis JG, Callendar DL, et al. Molecular analysis of chromosome 16q regions in dermal analogue tumors of salivary glands: a genetic link to dermal cylindroma? *Am J Surg Pathol.* 2002;26:778-783.
36. Enlund F, Behboudi A, Andren Y, et al. Altered notch signaling resulting from expression of a WAMTP1-MAML2 gene fusion in mucoepidermoid carcinomas and benign Warthin's tumors. *Exp Cell Res.* 2004;292:21-28.
37. El-Naggar AK, Lovell M, Killary AM, et al. A mucoepidermoid carcinoma of minor salivary gland with t(11;19)(q21;913.1) as the only karyotypic abnormality. *Cancer Genet Cytogenet.* 1996;87:29-33.
38. Komiya T, Park Y, Modi S, et al. Sustained expression of Mect1-Maml2 is essential for tumor cell growth in salivary gland cancers carrying the t(11;19) translocation. *Oncogene.* 2006;25:6128-6132.
39. Kyakumoto S, Kito N, Sato N. Expression of cAMP response element binding protein (CREB)-binding protein (CBP) and the implication in retinoic acid-inducible transcription activation in human salivary gland adenocarcinoma cell line HSG. *Endocr Res.* 2003;29:277-289.
40. Tonon G, Modi S, Wu L, et al. t(11;19)(q21;p13) translocation in mucoepidermoid carcinoma creates a novel fusion product that disrupts a Notch signaling pathway. *Nat Genet.* 2003;33:208-213.
41. Lewis JE, Olsen KD, Sebo TJ. Carcinoma ex pleomorphic adenoma: pathologic analysis of 73 cases. *Hum Pathol.* 2001;32:596-604.
42. El-Naggar AK, Callendar D, Coombes MM, et al. Molecular genetic alterations in carcinoma ex-pleomorphic adenoma: a putative progression model? *Genes Chromosomes Cancer.* 2000;27:162-168.
43. Williams MD, Chakravarti N, Kies MS, et al. Implications of methylation patterns of cancer genes in salivary gland tumors. *Clin Cancer Res.* 2006;12:7353-7358.
44. Williams MD, Roberts D, Blumenschein GR Jr, et al. Differential expression of hormonal and growth factor receptors in salivary duct carcinomas: biologic significance and potential role in therapeutic stratification of patients. *Am J Surg Pathol.* 2007;31:1645-1652.
45. Fordice J, Kershaw C, El-Naggar AK, et al. Adenoid cystic carcinoma of the head and neck: predictors of morbidity and mortality. *Arch Otolaryngol Head Neck Surg.* 1999;125:149-152.
46. Rutherford S, Yu Y, Rumpel CA, et al. Chromosome 6 deletion and candidate tumor suppressor genes in adenoid cystic carcinoma. *Cancer Lett.* 2006;236:309-317.
47. Presson M, Andrén Y, Mark J, Horlings HM, Persson F, Stenman G. Recurrent fusion of MYB and NFIB transcription factor genes in carcinomas of the breast and head and neck. *Proc Natl Acad Sci.* 2009;106:18740-18744.
48. Mitani Y, Li J, Rao PH, et al. Comprehensive analysis of the MYB-NFIB gene fusion in salivary adenoid cystic carcinoma: incidence, variability, and clinicopathologic significance. *Clin Cancer Res.* 2010;16(19):4722-31.
49. Mitani Y, Rao PH, Futreal PA, et al. Novel chromosomal rearrangements and break points at the t(6;9) in salivary adenoid cystic carcinoma: association with MYB-NFIB chimeric fusion, MYB expression, and clinical outcome. *Clin Cancer Res.* 2011;17(22):7003-7014.
50. Lewis JE, Olsen KD, Weiland LH. Acinic cell carcinoma. Clinicopathologic review. *Cancer.* 1991;67:172-179.
51. Diegel CR, Cho KR, El-Naggar AK, Williams BO, Lindvall C. Mammalian target of rapamycin-dependent acinar cell neoplasia after inactivation of Apc and Pten in the mouse salivary gland: implications for human acinic cell carcinoma. *Cancer Res.* 2010;70(22):9143-9152.

52. Zhang Q, Qing J, Wei WW, Guo ZM. Clinical analysis of sixteen cases of lymphoepithelial carcinoma of salivary gland. *Ai Zheng*. 2005;24:1384-1387.
53. Dispenza F, Cicero G, Mortellaro G, Marchese D, Kulamarva G, Dispenza C. Primary non-Hodgkins lymphoma of the parotid gland. *Braz J Otorhinolaryngol*. 2011;77:639-644.
54. Kondo T, Ezzat S, Asa SL. Pathogenetic mechanisms in thyroid follicular-cell neoplasia. *Nat Rev Cancer*. 2006;6:292-306.
55. Lloyd RV, Erickson LA, Casey MB, et al. Observer variation in the diagnosis of follicular variant of papillary thyroid carcinoma. *Am J Surg Pathol*. 2004;28:1336-1340.
56. Kebebew E, Ituarte PH, Siperstein AE, et al. Medullary thyroid carcinoma: clinical characteristics, treatment, prognostic factors, and a comparison of staging systems. *Cancer*. 2000;88:1139-1148.
57. Pulcrano M, Boukheris H, Talbot M, et al. Poorly differentiated follicular thyroid carcinoma: prognostic factors and relevance of histological classification. *Thyroid*. 2007;17:639-646.
58. Giuffrida D, Gharib H. Anaplastic thyroid carcinoma: current diagnosis and treatment. *Ann Oncol*. 2000;11:1083-1089.
59. Lima J, Trovisco V, Soares P, et al. BRAF mutations are not a major event in post-Chernobyl childhood thyroid carcinomas. *J Clin Endocrinol Metab*. 2004;89:4267-4271.
60. Mitsiades CS, Negri J, McMullan C, et al. Targeting BRAFV600E in thyroid carcinomas: therapeutic implications. *Mol Cancer Ther*. 2007;6:1070-1078.
61. Gujral TS, van Veelen W, Richardson DS, et al. A novel RET kinase-beta-catenin signaling pathway contributes to tumorigenesis in thyroid carcinoma. *Cancer Res*. 2008;68:1338-1346.
62. Bongarzone I, Vigneri P, Mariani L, et al. RET/NTRK1 rearrangement in thyroid gland tumors of the papillary carcinoma family: correlation with clinicopathological features. *Clin Cancer Res*. 1998;4:223-228.
63. Garcia-Rostan G, Zhao H, Camp RL, et al. ras mutations are associated with aggressive tumor phenotypes and poor prognosis in thyroid cancer. *J Clin Oncol*. 2003;21:3226-3235.
64. Di CristoJ, Marcy M, Vasko V, et al. Molecular genetic study comparing follicular variant versus classic papillary thyroid carcinomas: association of N-ras mutation in codon 61 with follicular variant. *Hum Pathol*. 2006;37:824-830.
65. Castro P, Rebocho AP, Soares RJ, et al. PAX8-PPARgamma rearrangement is frequently detected in the follicular variant of papillary thyroid carcinomas. *J Clin Endocrinol Metab*. 2006;91:213-220.
66. Barden CD, Shister KW, Zhu B, et al. Classification of follicular thyroid tumors by molecular signature: results of gene profiling. *Clin Cancer Res*. 2003;9:1792-1800.
67. Nikiforov YE. Molecular analysis of thyroid tumors. *Mod Pathol*. 2011;24(suppl 2):S34-S43.
68. Nikiforov YE, Nikiforova MN. Molecular genetics and diagnosis of thyroid cancer. *Nat Rev Endocrinol*. 2011;7:569-580.
69. Fagin JA, Matsuo K, Karmakar A, et al. High prevalence of mutations of the p53 gene in poorly differentiated human thyroid carcinomas. *J Clin Invest*. 1993;91:179-184.
70. Vasko V, Espinosa AV, Scouten W, et al. Gene expression and functional evidence of epithelial-to-mesenchymal transition in papillary thyroid carcinomas invasion. *Proc Natl Acad Sci U S A*. 2007;104:2803-2808.
71. DeLellis RA, Mazzaglia P, Mangray S. Primary hyperparathyroidism: a current perspective. *Arch Pathol Lab Med*. 2008;132:1251-1262.
72. Scarpelli D, D'Aloiso L, Arturi F, et al. Novel somatic MEN1 gene alterations in sporadic primary hyperparathyroidism and correlations with clinical characteristics. *J Endocrinol Invest*. 2004;27:1015-1021.
73. Cetani F, Pardi E, Ambrogini E, et al. Difference somatic alterations of the HRPT2 gene in a patient with recurrent sporadic primary hyperparathyroidism carrying an HRPT2 germline mutation. *Endocr Relat Cancer*. 2007;14:493-499.
74. Lumachi F, Basso SM, Basso U. Parathyroid cancer: etiology, clinical presentation and treatment. *Anticancer Res*. 2006;26:4803-4807.
75. Morrison C, Farrar W, Kneile J, et al. Molecular classification of parathyroid neoplasia by gene expression profiling. *Am J Pathol*. 2004;165:565-576.
76. Juhlin CC, Villablanca A, Sandelin K, et al. Parafibromin immunoreactivity: its use as an additional diagnostic marker for parathyroid tumor classification. *Endocr Relat Cancer*. 2007;14:501-512.
77. Cetani F, Pardi E, Viacava P, et al. A reappraisal of the Rb1 gene abnormalities in the diagnosis of parathyroid cancer. *Clin Endocrinol (Oxf)*. 2004;60:99-106.

CHAPTER 34

IMMUNOHISTOCHEMICAL AND MOLECULAR DIAGNOSIS OF MELANOMA

Andrea Suárez and Whitney A. High

INTRODUCTION

The availability of immunohistochemical (IHC) and genotypic testing modalities has impacted directly our ability to diagnose melanoma and to differentiate it from mimics and related conditions. While interpretation of hematoxylin and eosin (H&E)–stained tissue sections remains the cornerstone of histopathologic assessment, IHC and genotypic analysis improves our diagnostic capabilities; it may even provide a means to assess disease severity, guide prognosis, or select appropriate management.

In this chapter, we review the means for IHC-based assessment of melanocytic processes and review known mutations that impact biomolecular pathways in melanoma development and progression. Because many melanomas acquire measurable chromosomal abnormalities that distinguish them from benign nevi, comparative genomic hybridization (CGH) and fluorescence in situ hybridization (FISH) represent additional diagnostic technologies, and these techniques will also be reviewed and summarized. Lastly, polymerase chain reaction (PCR)–based diagnostic modalities, particularly as such techniques apply to the selection of therapy, will be reviewed.

IHC ASSESSMENT OF MELANOCTYIC PROCESSES

IHC assessment in histopathology refers to a process of detecting proteins in tissue sections via specific interactions between applied antibodies and targeted antigens. Modern IHC is a highly automated endeavor, readily performed at dermatopathology laboratories of all sizes. Clearly, a complete review of the specific techniques involved in IHC is beyond the scope of this chapter. Instead, we will focus our attention upon specific, commercially available antibodies that are routinely employed in the assessment of pigmented lesions and the diagnosis of melanoma.

Chromogens

Before a discussion of specific antibodies, a brief segue regarding chromogen use is appropriate. In IHC, chromogens are reagents that react with enzymes, notably horseradish peroxidase (HRP) or alkaline phosphatase (AP), to form insoluble colored precipitates detected by light microscopy. One of the most widely used chromogens in histology is 3,3-diaminobenzidine (DAB), which forms an alcohol-insoluble, brown-colored precipitant in the presence of HRP.

However, when studying melanocytic lesions, which often appear pigmented due to melanin production, a brown-colored IHC chromogen may be suboptimal. To this end, some laboratories utilize aminoethyl carbazole (AEC), an alcohol-soluble chromogen that generates a red-colored precipitant upon reaction with peroxidase, or Fast red/AP red, two additional alcohol-soluble reagents that generate a red-colored precipitate with AP. In fact, at our own large academic dermatopathology referral practice, where we perform over 30,000 IHC-stained sections each year upon skin sections, including a majority of pigmented lesions, we use red chromogen detection kits for all our melanocytic markers.

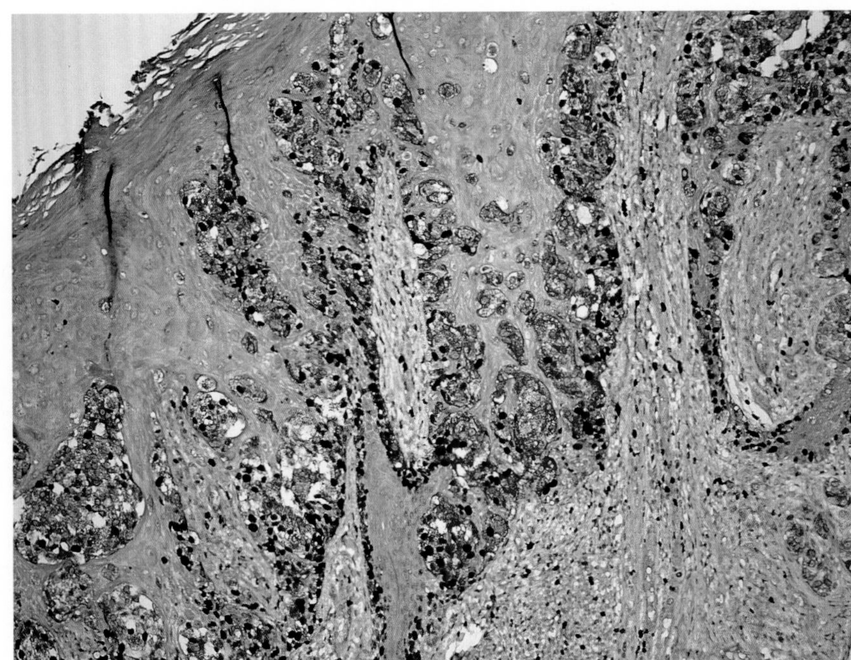

FIGURE 34–1 Immunohistochemical "double stain" of melanoma using Ki67 (brown chromogen) and Mart-1 (red chromogen) facilitates the assessment of an elevated proliferative index of melanocytes in particular, including an elevated proliferative index in the pagetoid nests.

Additionally, the availability of multiple detection systems with different colors yields another opportunity in dermatopathology—use of the "double stain." In "double stain," one antigen is marked brown via DAB system, while another is marked red with either an AEC or Fast red/AP red system, using either simultaneous or sequential staining (depending upon the speciation of the antibodies, the enzyme system employed, and the desired result).[1] In some situations, it may be necessary to elute the first antibody, or allow the reaction to adequately or fully develop, before employing the second reaction.[2] For example, a stain utilizing HRP/DAB for Ki67, a proliferation marker, and AP/Fast red for Mart-1, a melanocyte marker, performed consecutively at our laboratory, allows for inspection of a proliferative index among highlighted melanocytes. We refer to this stain as a "KiMart" stain (Fig. 34.1). Other double stains of utility in melanoma include a CD34(brown)/Mart-1 ("CDMart") stain to study vascular invasion or a D2-40/Mart ("DuMart") stain to study lymphatic invasion (Fig. 34.2).

No Single "Melanoma Marker" Exists

Before discussing commercially available IHC markers employed in pigmented lesions, it is important to address bluntly an important caveat in our understanding—*no*

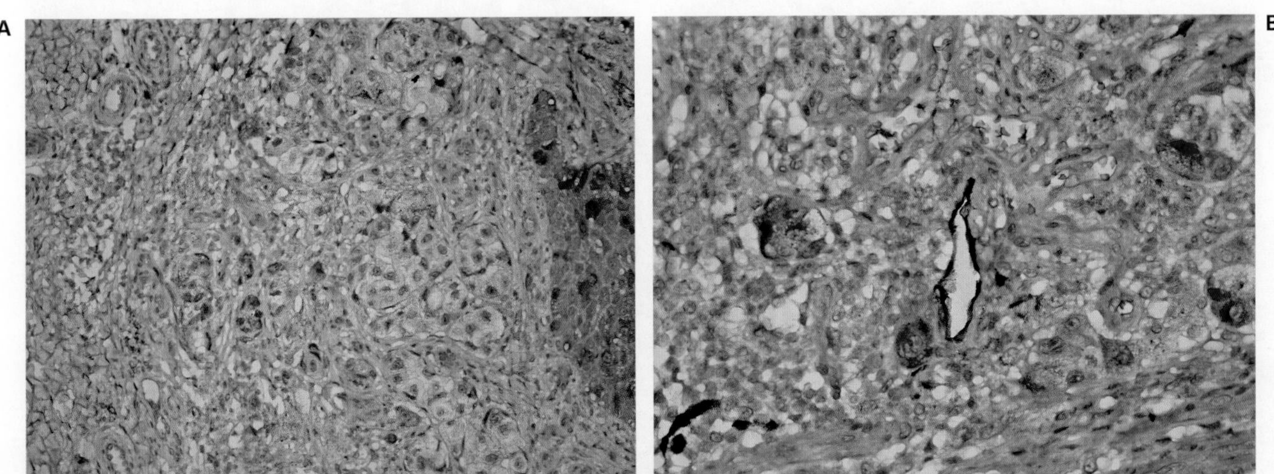

FIGURE 34–2 **A:** Immunohistochemical "double stain" of melanoma using CD34 (brown chromogen) and Mart-1 (red chromogen) facilitates the inclusion or exclusion of vascular invasion, as the endothelium of vessels marks brown and the melanocytes mark red. **B:** Immunohistochemical "double stain" of melanoma using D2-40 (brown chromogen), and Mart-1 (red chromogen) facilitates the inclusion or exclusion of lymphatic invasion, as the endothelium of lymphatics marks brown and the melanocytes mark red.

single "MELANOMA MARKER" exists. In other words, while some IHC markers are useful in suggesting melanoma, the result must be interpreted in the context of all available data, specifically including a morphological assessment by H&E staining alone.

For example, aberrant retention of HMB-45 positivity in the dermal nests of a melanocytic process, while abnormal in many situations, does not indicate unequivocally that a proliferation is melanoma. On the contrary, if other morphologic features of the lesion suggest benignity, and aberrant retention of HMB-45 in the dermal component is discovered, it is incumbent upon the dermatopathologist to recognize this marking; while anomalous, it is most likely spurious and inconsequential. "Overcall," based solely upon any single piece of data, including that of IHC markers interpreted in isolation, without corroborating features by morphologic analysis, must be avoided.

In sum, the IHC markers discussed specifically in the passages to follow are only single "tools," existing in a larger "tool kit," carried by an expert dermatopathologist. Results from IHC studies must be in context and do not supplant traditional morphologic clues provided by traditional light microscopy (such as asymmetry, pagetoid extent, nuclear pleomorphism, hyperchromasia, irregular nuclear contour, irregular nesting of melanocytes, lack of maturation with decent into the dermis, and dermal mitotic activity) or clinical data (such as asymmetry, irregular borders, color variegation, large size, unusual/rapid growth, and other evolving and atypical clinical behavior).

Melanocytic Markers in Common Use

The following IHC markers are often utilized in the evaluation of pigmented lesions and the characteristics of each are discussed below.

S100

S100 is a family of 24 calcium-binding proteins that regulate a variety of cellular processes. These proteins are often involved in tumorigenesis and metastasis. S100 proteins exist as combinations of two polypeptide chains, S100a and S100b.[3] Most commercially available S100 antibodies react mainly with S100b polypeptide-containing cells, unless otherwise specified (see S100A6 discussed below). S100 antibodies of all forms are both nuclear and cytoplasmic markers.

S100 is widely considered the most sensitive marker of dermal melanoma, particularly desmoplastic melanoma (DM) and spindle cell melanoma (SCM) (Fig. 34.3), with about 95% of primary cutaneous melanomas expressing reactivity with this antibody.[4-7] However, and importantly, S100 is not specific for melanoma, and reactivity with this antibody is also exhibited by normal melanocytes, nerve sheath cells, myoepithelial cells, adipocytes, chondrocytes, and Langerhans' cells, as well as tumors derived from these cell types.[4] In fact, the myoepithelial spindled cells of scars may express S100, a point of concern when evaluating a re-excision specimen, as this may generate undue concern for a desmoplastic component to the melanoma.[8]

Lastly, while S100 is a sensitive but non-specific marker for melanocytic proliferations, S100-negative

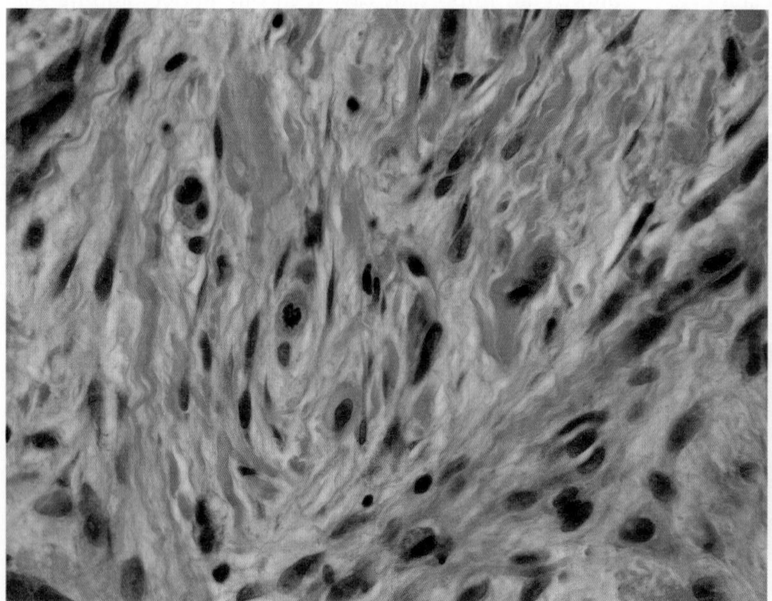

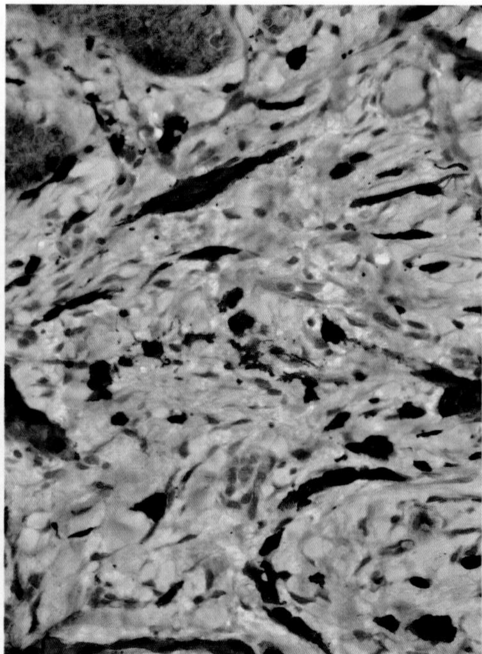

FIGURE 34–3 S100 protein is the most sensitive marker of melanoma that possesses a spindled/desmoplastic morphology. **A:** Staining with hematoxylin and eosin reveals a desmoplastic atypical spindled population in the dermis, and dermal mitotic figures are noted. **B:** Staining with S100 protein reveals a spindled component that did not mark with Mart-1.

melanoma has been described in the literature.[9] In general, S100 negative melanoma occurs more often in metastatic disease, especially metastatic disease from an ocular primary melanoma, and most often if the diagnosis of melanoma can still be established via exclusion of other malignancies (carcinoma, lymphoproliferative, or sarcomatous disease), affirmative marking with HMB45 or Melan A/MART-1, and/or correlation with a history of primary melanoma.[10] S100 reactivity may also be lost due to poor tissue fixation in formaldehyde, accidental extraction of low-molecular weight and soluble S100 protein during processing, or by destruction with protease during pre-treatment of tissue.[3]

S100A6

Antibodies that bind specifically and exclusively with S100a subtypes of S100 are commercially available. This allows for the detection of different variants of the S100 chains.[3] S-100A6 is a specific S100 subtype expressed in some melanocytic lesions, as well as fibrohistiocytic lesions, and neurothekeomas.[11] S100A6 is a nuclear and cytoplasmic marker.

Ribe and McNutt[12] studied the expression of S100A6 protein in melanoma and Spitz nevi, as well as other melanocytic nevi, and found that S100A6 protein was strongly expressed in all Spitz nevi cases, but expression in melanoma was generally weak and spotty. Therefore, strong and diffuse expression of this marker often favors interpretation of a Spitz nevus over that of melanoma, assuming of course that other clinical and morphologic features are compatible with that diagnosis.

However, within pigmented spindle cell nevus (of Reed), considered by some authorities to be a superficial and pigmented variant of a Spitz nevus, melanocytes often show patchy marking, or fail to mark entirely, with S100A6. Therefore, this pattern of expression within this entity should not be interpreted as evidence of supporting a diagnosis of melanoma.[13]

HMB-45

HMB-45 is an antibody directed at a particular protein contained within melanocytes, known as gp100. HMB-45 is a cytoplasmic marker. HMB-45 expression is seen predominantly in intraepidermal melanocytes,[14] activated melanocytes,[15] and immature melanocytes.[16] Therefore, in common acquired nevi, HMB-45 positivity is often limited to melanocytes in the junctional component, of nests of cells in the papillary dermis or adventitial dermis of adnexa, with lesser marking in melanocytes of the deeper dermis. This pattern reinforces that of normal maturation of nevomelanocytic processes by light microscopy and is often referred to as "zonation" (Fig. 34.4).

In contrast, primary cutaneous melanoma typically demonstrates an altered pattern of HMB-45 expression, with either rather homogenous aberrant retention in the deeper dermal component or at least retention within clusters of melanocytes at all levels of the dermis. Therefore, lack of normal "zonation" with HMB-45 in a pigmented lesion is a concerning finding in some situations, but it should be specifically noted that melanocytes with dusty cytoplasm, such as those of clonal nevi or deep penetrating nevi, represent important exceptions to this pattern of "zonation," with HMB-45 often labeling the deeper extents or even the entirety of the population of dusty melanocytes, seemingly without any malignant connotation.[17]

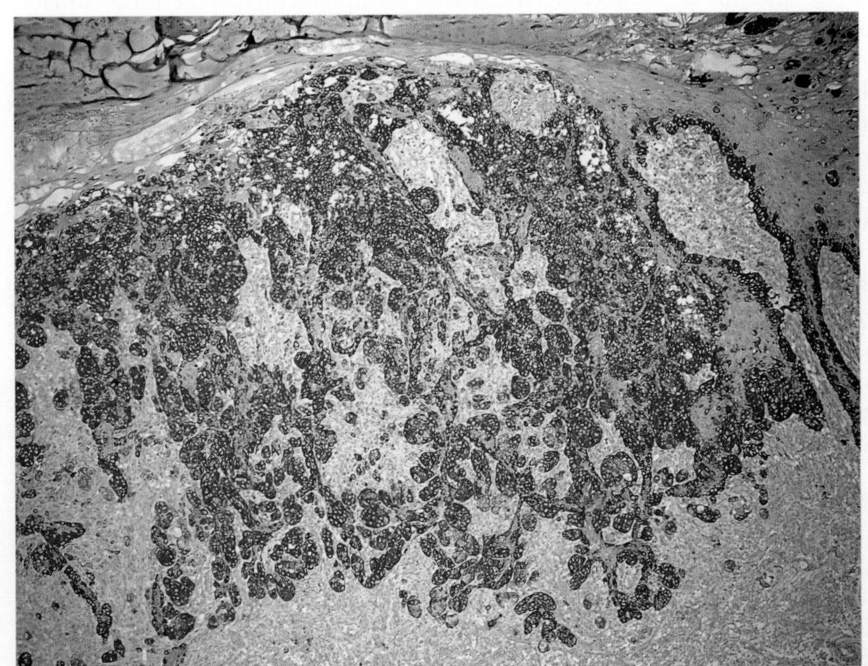

FIGURE 34–4 In most benign nevi the degree of marking with HMB-45 normally diminishes with descent into the dermis ("zonation"), and this parallels normal maturation of nevomelanocytic processes, but in melanoma (such as that here) there is often aberrant retention of HMB-45 expression at all levels of the melanocytic process.

HMB-45 does not reliably stain DM/SCM,[17] and use in this setting should be avoided. Other lesions, including angiomyolipoma, sugar cell tumor of the lung, lymphangioleiomyomatosis, and PEComa, also express gp100 and possess HMB45 positivity[18]; however, these tumors are not common concerns in the skin.

Melan-A/MART-1

Most benign and malignant melanocytes express the Melan A/MART-1 antigen, which is detected by the A103 clone and the M2-7C10 clonal antibodies, respectively, making them useful markers for melanocytic processes in general.[19-21] The names for this antigen (MART-1 and Melan-A) were derived from two groups of researchers who independently sequenced the gene for this antigen; however, in truth, in practical parlance the terms such as "Melan A" or "MART-1" are used in rather equivalent fashion, and distinction at the clinical level is of no clinical importance. Melan A/MART-1 is a cytoplasmic marker.

While a sensitive and specific marker for melanocytes in general, from the outset, it is important to recognize that DM/SCM is consistently negative for Melan A/MART-1 antibodies, as well as for HMB-45. In this setting, S100 is the most widely recommended marker, along with p75 and possibly KBA.62.

Steroid-producing tumors may demonstrate Melan A/MART-1 positivity, and metastatic melanoma should be included in the differential of Melan A/MART-1–positive tumors of the pelvis and retroperitoneum. Also, like HMB-45, angiomyolipoma, sugar cell tumor of lung, lymphangioleiomyomatosis, and pecoma also express Melan A/MART-1 positivity.[18]

Furthermore, sun-exposed skin that contains large, dendritic melanocytes ("sun-damaged" melanocytes) may mark excessively with Melan A/MART-1. This may raise genuine concern for melanoma in situ,[22] and this is particularly problematic as excessive solar exposure, with resultant dermatoheliosis (histologic manifestations of sun damage), is associated with melanoma; however, in general, a true diagnosis of melanoma in situ can usually be distinguished on other histopathologic grounds.[23]

Lastly, beginning in 2003, there are reports of Melan A/MART-1–positive "pseudonesting," where the immunostain marks a disputed mixture of inflammatory cells, melanocytes, and keratinocytes, along the dermoepidermal junction, and this may lead to an erroneous impression of melanoma in situ.[24,25] This phenomenon must be kept in mind during evaluation with this immunostain, and it is justification to employ more than one immunomarker when studying melanocytic processes along the dermoepidermal junction.[26]

Ki67/MIB-1

Ki67 is a proliferation marker, and antibody directed against a Ki67, also referred to as MIB-1, is an IHC marker known to show significant differences in the proliferative index among melanocytic proliferations, namely, melanoma and its mimics.[27] Ki67/MIB-1 is a nuclear marker.

In one study, common and dysplastic nevi showed about 1% of melanocyte nuclei to mark (most often near the dermoepidermal junction or in the superficial dermis), while in melanoma, about 16.4% of melanocyte nuclei marked (particularly in the deeper extents). This study, as well as other similar investigations, led to postulated "rule of thumb" that for difficult pigmented processes, such as spitzoid neoplasms, benignity is favored by a Ki67/MIB-1 proliferative index of <2%, while malignancy favored by a Ki67/MIB-1 proliferative index of >10%, with indeterminate lesions occupying a middle ground of 2% to 10%.[28,29]

Of course, these, or any other numerical schema, are perhaps valid only for the study population examined. Certainly, all matrices are subject to the caution that a diagnosis of melanoma depends upon the totality of data, but it is entirely logical that in a general sense a high proliferative index is an unfavorable quality in a pigmented process, while a low proliferative index is a favorable quality.

Additionally, Ki67/MIB-1 may be of utility in distinguishing DM from benign melanocytic proliferations, as DM often has a significantly higher proliferative index.[30]

Microphthalmia-Associated Transcription Factor

Microphthalmia-associated transcription factor (MiTF) is a nuclear protein involved in the development, differentiation, and survival of melanocytes.[31] Tissue microarray studies show MiTF amplification in 10% to 20% of primary melanomas, and this finding was associated with a decreased 5-year survival.[32] Being a strong and relatively specific nuclear marker, the expression of MiTF is often useful in quantifying the number of intraepidermal melanocytes in areas of a pigmented epidermis.[33] In fact, recent investigation found MiTF immunostaining to be as informative and technically less demanding for making the diagnosis of melanoma in situ (lentigo maligna–type) when compared with combined immunostaining and special staining with Melan A and azure blue.[34]

However, while the nuclear staining of MiTF is appealing for some applications in dermatopathology, it is not a particularly specific marker for melanocytes. Histiocytes, mast cells, lymphocytes, fibroblasts, Schwann cells, and smooth muscle cells have all, on occasion, been described to label with MiTF.[20] Also, MiTF, like Melan A, has been described to yield false-positive results with inflammatory pseudonesting within inflammatory conditions.[26]

p75 (Nerve Growth Factor Receptor)

p75 (nerve growth factor receptor, NGFR) is a membrane-associated, tyrosine kinase receptor that is expressed in cells derived from both the neural crest and mesenchyma.[35] This protein is expressed in a variety of cells with spindle or dendritic morphology, such as follicular dendritic cells, macrophages, myoepithelial cells, and vascular adventitia.[35,36] While normal melanocytes do not express p75 (NGFR), it is expressed in benign neurotized nevi, as well as invasive desmoplastic and/or spindled melanomas.[36,37]

For example, DM/SCM are entities that pose a diagnostic dilemma given a cryptic histologic appearance and limited immunoreactivity with melanocytic markers, such as HMB45, melan A, and MiTF.[38,39] Reports of immunostaining with p75 NGF-R suggest that it may be useful as a confirmatory antibody within a panel of melanoma markers, especially with regard to SCM and DM.[40-44] In one study, all 13 cases of SCM and DM marked strongly for p75 NGF-R, whereas only 12 cases were positive for S100.[45] While the number of cases included is small, the authors of the study believed the data to show that p75 NGF-R was superior to S100 for identifying SCM and DM.

However, in a second study, p75 (NGFR) antibody was ineffective in detecting residual disease within re-excision specimens of melanoma, marking myofibroblasts, nerve twigs, and Schwann cells, leading to diagnostic confusion.[46] Therefore, at least at present, it would seem that while p75 (NGFR) antibody may be of utility as an ancillary stain for the diagnosis of primary DM/SCM, it may not be a suitable marker in the evaluation of re-excision scars, given its limited specificity.

Sry-Related HMG-BOX Gene 10

Sry-related HMG-BOX gene 10 (Sox10) is a neural crest transcription factor that plays a role in the differentiation of Schwann cells and melanocytes.[47] Like MiTF, Sox10 is a nuclear protein and, as mentioned, nuclear immunostains may afford certain advantages, such as improvement in signal to noise, preservation of cellular architecture, and improved distinction of the chromogen from cytoplasmic melanin in pigmented lesions.

Sox10 activates the transcription of MiTF and can be detected at various stages of melanoma progression in established melanoma cell lines.[48] Nonaka et al.[49] demonstrated Sox10 immunopositivity in ≥75% tumor cells in 76/78 (97.4%) cases of melanoma examined. In this same study, among the six cases of S100-negative metastatic melanoma, four showed Sox10 expression, and there were no cases of Sox10-negative/S100-positive melanoma, or Sox10-negative/MiTF-positive melanoma. Despite the high sensitivity of S100 protein for melanoma, there are reported cases of S100-negative melanoma, and these results, at least in the opinion of the authors, suggested that Sox10 may be more sensitive than S100 or MiTF for melanoma detection.

In a comparison study examining 26 cases of melanoma and 18 excision scars alone, Sox10 strongly highlighted all in situ, invasive, and DM/SCM but was less likely than S100 or MiTF to have results that were confounded by background expression of fibrocytes and histiocytes within the scar.[50] The results of this study confirmed the utility of Sox10 in detecting in situ and DM/SCM melanoma and suggested that Sox10 is superior to MiTF in the evaluation of melanoma in situ, given its increased expression in subtle underlying DM that might otherwise be missed. Furthermore, these findings underscore a useful role for Sox10 in discriminating residual DM/SCM from scar.

Tyrosinase

Tyrosinase is an enzyme involved in the synthesis of melanin within melanocytes. T311 (anti-tyrosinase or simply tyrosinase) is a monoclonal IgG antibody that detects tyrosinase expression in paraffin wax–embedded tissue sections, and it has been shown to have a sensitivity that is less than S100, but greater than HMB-45 and is more equivalent to that of Melan A/MART-1.[51] In this same study, tyrosinase stained most benign and malignant lesions strongly, but in some common nevi there was lesser staining of more mature melanocytes. In our own experience, studying thousands of melanocytic lesions with tyrosinase, we have found it to often demonstrate the pattern of "zonation," similar to, but probably less dramatic than, HMB-45. In fact, in a study of melanoma, tyrosinase demonstrated 94% sensitive for melanomas overall, but the sensitivity was inversely correlated with stage.[52] Also, and similar to Melan A/MART-1 and HMB-45, tyrosinase does not suitably or reliably detect DM/SCM.

KBA.62

KBA.62 is a monoclonal antibody directed at a novel melanocyte antigen that survives tissue processing and appears to be distinct from gp100 (HMB-45). Pagés (2008) demonstrated this antibody to mark around 93% of all melanomas tested, including three cases of DM. Overall, in the study, the sensitivity of KBA.62 was similar to that of HMB-45, but KBA.62 had a lesser sensitivity than did S100. KBA.62 is a cytoplasmic marker.

Recently, Bernaba et al.[53] examined a small series of 12 DM and found that 9 of 12 cases marked affirmatively with KBA.62 (>5% of cells marking), with an average of 49% of cells with the melanoma marking. While less than the number of DM marking with S100, marking with KBA.62 was significantly higher than the aggregate of reports using other melanoma markers such as Melan A/MART-1, HMB-45, and MiTF, and, in the author's opinion, it marked melanoma cells more specifically than S100.

Anecdotally, we, at the University of Colorado, were one of the first labs to utilize KBA.62, having maintained this antibody in our repertoire since 2004, and we keep it on hand, specifically, as an adjunct to S100 in the detection of DM/SCM, where we find it to be of great utility.

TABLE 34–1 Common Melanocyte Markers Useful in the Diagnosis of Melanoma

Antigen	Sensitivity	Specificity	Staining	Also Expressed in
S100	97–100%[20]	75–87%[20]	Nuclear and cytoplasmic	Tumors of nerve sheath, myoepithelial, adipocyte, chondrocyte, and Langherhans cells
HMB5	69–93%[20]	95%[54]	Cytoplasmic	PEComas (angiomyolipomas, lymphangiomyomatosis, pulmonary "sugar" tumors), meningeal melanocytomas, clear cell sarcoma of the tendons and aponeurosis, some ovarian steroid cell tumors, sweat gland tumors, some breast cancers, t(6,11)(p21;q12) translocation harboring renal cell carcinomas
MART-1	75–92%[20]	95–100%[20]	Cytoplasmic	PEComas (angiomyolipomas, lymphangiomyomatosis, pulmonary "sugar" tumors), some clear cell sarcomas
MITF	81–100%[20]	88–100%[20]	Nuclear	Spindle cell tumors, lymphoid neoplasms, angiomyolipomas, rare breast carcinomas and renal carcinomas, histiocytes, lymphocytes, fibroblasts, Schwann cells, smooth muscle cells, and mast cells

Detecting Melanocyte and Melanogenesis Markers in Combination

From our primer on antibodies used in studying melanocytic lesions, it should be readily apparent that many IHC-based "tools" exist to study melanocytic processes. As outlined in Table 34.1,[54] the most common of these markers have variable sensitivities and specificities and often stain other tumors or cell types, beyond melanoma or melanocytes, respectively. As mentioned prior, while no single antibody is specific for the melanocytes of melanoma, when used in combination, these markers enhance the diagnostic accuracy of malignant melanoma in complicated cases.

Tumor infiltrating cells can complicate the IHC analysis of melanomas when certain stains are assessed in isolation. When a prominent proliferative lymphatic infiltrate is present in melanomas and nevi, interpreting the Ki67 index becomes more challenging, and a double stain allows for assessment of the proliferative index of just melanocytes, to the exclusion of lymphocytes, stromal cells, histiocytes, and epithelial cells.[33] In one study, misclassification rates for melanomas and nevi were significantly lower using MART-1/Ki67 and HMB45/MiTF combined stains compared with each stain in isolation.[55] This study also reported consistently lower estimates of proliferative indices by MART-1/Ki67 versus Ki67 alone. These findings demonstrate the value of combination staining in improving the evaluation of melanocyte-specific proliferation and in the diagnosis of melanocytic lesions.

Sentinel lymph node involvement portends important prognostic information, but because lymphovascular invasion (LVI) is rarely seen in primary melanomas by routine histology, evaluation with IHC lymphatic markers is often necessary. D2-40 is an IHC stain specific for lymphatic endothelium that is widely used in the analysis of LVI.[56] This reagent increases the sensitivity of detection of LVI in melanoma.[57] When D2-40 is applied simultaneously with S-100, there is enhanced detection of LVI by melanoma tumor cells,[58,59] and when LVI was evaluated with D2-40 and the panvascular marker CD34 the rate of detection of LVI positivity was increased compared with routine H&E-stained sections alone.[60] Cases of LVI missed by H&E-stained sections may create false prognostic impressions, and such studies suggest that combination IHC staining improves LVI detection.

Other antibodies/antigens that are promising future reagents to include in combinatorial stains for the diagnosis and evaluation of melanocytic lesions are NKI-C3, p16, galectin-3, COX-2, TRP, survivin, and claudin-1.[33]

Assessment of Cell Cycle Checkpoint Alterations by IHC and Involvement in Melanoma Development and Progression

The cell cycle is a highly regulated series of molecular interactions governing cellular division (Fig. 34.5). One critical function of checkpoints in the cell cycle is to allow for the assessment of DNA damage, as cells with damaged DNA have the potential to become immortalized (as tumor cells) and, ideally, should instead be shunted toward senescence or apoptosis. Such damage control is exerted at the G1-S checkpoint, prior to the cell's entrance into the phase of DNA synthesis. The retinoblastoma protein (Rb) inhibits G1-S transition, and inactivation of Rb by cyclin-dependent kinases (CDKs), such as CDK4, must occur before entry into the DNA synthesis phase of the cell cycle. Mutations in these and other regulators of the cell cycle result in uncontrolled cellular proliferation, with propagation of cells with DNA damage conveying the properties of transformed growth and immortalization characteristic of cancer cells.

p16

The INK4A protein, also referred to as p16^{INK4A}, functions to inactivate CDK4, effectively arresting cells at the G1-S checkpoint.[61] Encoded by the CDKN2A gene locus, this critical gatekeeper of the G1-S checkpoint is often

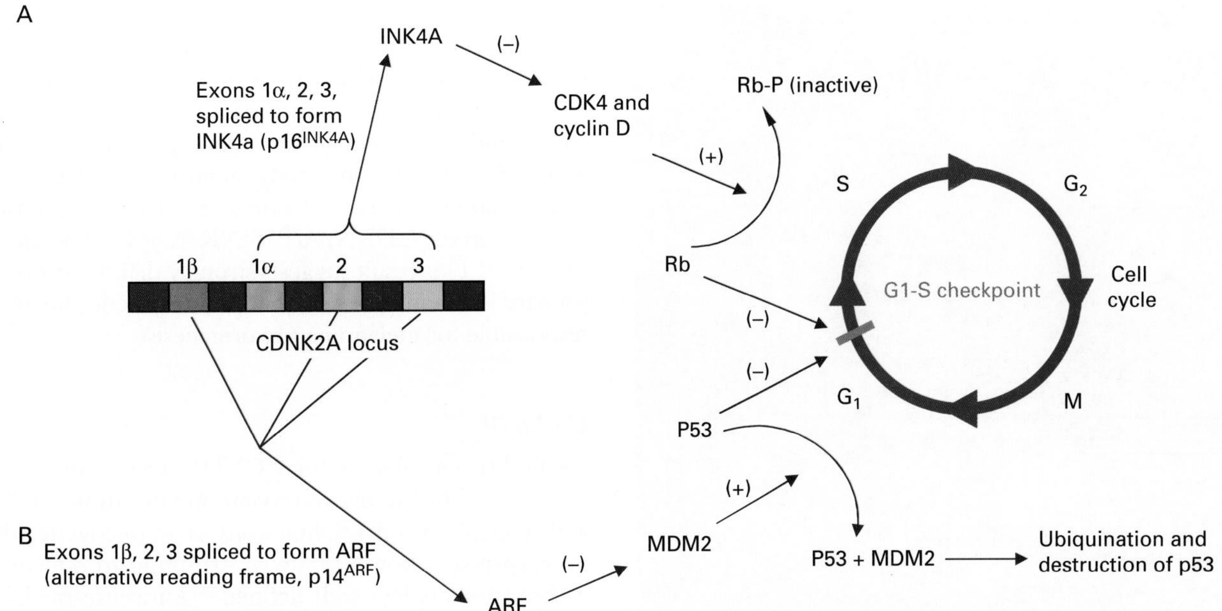

FIGURE 34–5 Cell cycle checkpoints ensure fidelity of DNA replication and cell division. **A:** In normal cells, INK4A acts as an inhibitor of cyclin-dependent kinases, including CDK4 and cyclin D1. These proteins function to phosphorylate and inactivate Rb, a protein inhibitor of cell cycle progression. When Rb is phosphorylated by unchecked/mutant cyclin-dependent kinases, it no longer can function to halt G1-S progression. **B:** Alternative exon splicing within the CDKN2A gene gives rise to ARF, a protein that inhibits MDM2 to p53 binding. Upon binding together, MDM2 and p53 result in MDM2-mediated ubiquitination and destruction of p53. Thus, mutations in ARF result in faulty protection of p53 from destruction, with subsequent diminished levels of p53 and a defect in G1-S interruption. +, activation/disinhibition; –, inhibition. (Adapted from High WA, Robinson WA, *Adv Dermatol.* 2007;23:61-79.)

inactivated in human tumors, with inherited p16^{INK4A} mutations identified in up to 40% of familial melanomas.[62] Furthermore, there is a higher incidence of other types of tumors (such as pancreatic cancer, meningioma, non–small cell lung cancer, and other cancers of the head and neck) in some p16^{INK4A}-deficient relatives of probands.[63,64] Low expression of p16 is a marker of adverse prognosis in many human cancers, especially pancreas, esophagus, and head and neck cancer.[65]

While the vast majority of hereditary INK4A mutations occur in individuals heterozygous for the defect, it is unclear whether loss or mutation of the second functional allele is required to acquire an increased risk of melanoma, or if INK4A haploinsufficiency alone impairs cell cycle regulation to affect tumorigenesis.[66] Inactivation of the wild-type, functional INK4A allele might occur by homozygous deletion,[67] loss of heterozygosity,[68,69] promoter methylation,[70] or other mutations resulting in a nonfunctional protein. Overall, sporadic melanomas outnumber familial cases. CDKN2A mutations comprise approximately 20% to 40% of familial cases, whereas other mutations (CDK4, CCND1, and ARF) are more rare (~1%). Importantly, in 60% of cases a known mutation is not identified, underscoring our limited knowledge of the genetics of familial melanoma.

While INK4A mutations in sporadic melanomas are considered rare,[71,72] Kumar et al.[73] noted a 26% mutation frequency in microdissected cases. Rb pathway inactivation in sporadic melanomas mostly occurs by non-mutational silencing of INK4A expression or CKD4/CCND1 activation.[74] In general, the progressive and gradual loss of p16INK4A correlates with advanced stages of melanoma progression. Nevi do not tend to exhibit altered INK4A expression,[75,76] nor does melanoma in situ.[77,78] However, more recent studies demonstrate that the percentage of p16INK4A-positive nevus cells and the intensity of staining are heterogeneous.[79-81] It has been suggested that the clinical presentation of larger, more numerous, and dysplastic nevi in patients heterozygous for p16INK4A mutations[82] is perhaps related to reduced p16INK4A expression in nevi and a clonal expansion of nevus cells.

Straume and Akslen[83] showed a loss of P16/INK4A expression, by IHC analysis, in cutaneous melanomas located on the trunk and extremities when compared with lesions on the head and neck. While 85% of melanomas arising de novo showed a loss of INK4A immunoreactivity, only 24% of melanomas associated with a nevus showed loss of INK4A by IHC staining.[84] Atypical (dysplastic) melanocytic nevi are considered by many experts to be an intermediate step in a continuous process from acquired melanocytic nevi to melanoma, which, in turn, proceeds through radial and linear growth phases.[85] Mean values of CDKN2A expression in low-grade atypical melanocytic nevi and high-grade atypical melanocytic nevi were significantly higher than those recorded in radial- and vertical-growth phase melanomas.[86] In one study of p16 immunostaining of 15 desmoplastic Spitz nevi and

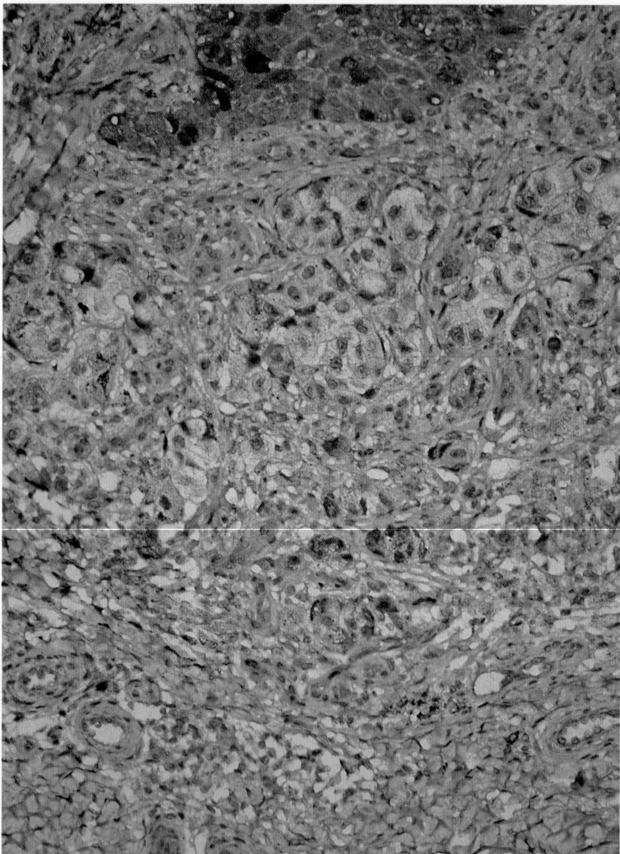

FIGURE 34–6 Loss of P16 expression, assessed by immunohistochemical means, is a relatively common finding in melanoma, and it is correlated with other negative prognostic indicators such as ulceration, vascular invasion, mitotic index, advanced tumor stage, presence of lymph node metastases, and decreased recurrence-free and 5-y survival.

11 DMs, all cases of Spitz nevi showed affirmative p16 immunoreactivity, whereas 81.2% of DMs were negative and 18.8% of melanomas were only weakly positive.[87] Furthermore, detailed IHC analyses of p16 expression reveal the loss of p16 in melanoma to correlate significantly with ulceration, vascular invasion, mitotic index, advanced tumor stage, presence of lymph node metastases, and decreased recurrence-free and 5-year survival (Fig. 34.6).[88]

Cyclin-Dependent Kinase 4 (CDK4)

CDK4 binds with CCND1 and phosphorylates Rb to its inactivated state, thus allowing for progression to DNA synthesis.[89] INK4A binds to and inhibits CDK4, abrogating cell cycle progression. Therefore, mutations in the INK4A gene result in loss of tumor suppression and loss of inhibition of cyclin-dependent kinases, including CDK4.

Activating germline mutations and amplification of CDK4 can yield uncontrolled cellular proliferation, and such mutations have been described in familial melanoma,[90,91] as well as in sporadic melanoma.[92] Whereas INK4A mutations represent defects in tumor suppression, altered CDK4 functions as an oncogene. CDK4 amplification is more common in acral and mucosal melanoma.[93] Uveal melanoma, arising from melanocytes in the uveal tract, is the most common intraocular malignancy in adults, and like its cutaneous counterpart, it can present within families. In one study, genotypic analysis of 25 cases of familial uveal melanoma revealed no deleterious mutation in the CDKN2A/P16INK4A or CDK4 genes in any case.[94] This result suggests strongly that the site of the primary lesion may govern the specific genetic alterations responsible for melanoma tumorigenesis.

Cyclin D1

Cyclin D1, encoded by the CCND1 gene, forms a complex with CDK4 to phosphorylate and inactivate Rb.[89] As with CDK4, cyclin D1 functions as an oncogene when overexpressed; however, its contribution to melanoma pathogenesis is less well defined.[95] Antisense-mediated knockdown of CCDN1 caused apoptosis in vitro and led to significant tumor shrinkage of melanoma xenografts in mice, enforcing a role for cyclin D1 in melanoma oncogenesis.[96] Up to 44% of acral lentiginous melanomas studied revealed CCND1 amplification, while this observation was less common with other melanoma subtypes.[96,97] A normal copy number was demonstrated in 25% of cases where increased cyclin D1 expression was demonstrated by IHC, a finding that suggests other mechanisms, besides copy number, may influence cyclin D1 expression.[96]

In fact, the expression of ROC1, a protein involved in cyclin D1 degradation, was deficient in cutaneous melanomas and correlated negatively with cyclin D1.[98] Furthermore, compared with other nevi and melanomas, melanomas with decreased ROC1 expression had increased cyclin D1 expression,[98] suggesting that impairment in cyclin D1 degradation may account for cyclin D1 overexpression in cases of melanoma without CCND1 amplification.

In studies using IHC markers and examining cyclin D1 expression in benign nevi, primary melanoma, and metastatic melanomas, there were significant differences in the expression between nevi and primary melanomas, and between thin and thick melanomas, suggesting the utility of cyclin D1 in diagnosis of malignant melanoma and as a marker for tumor progression.[99]

Additionally, as cyclin D1 functions downstream from p-ERK in the mitogen-activated protein kinase (MAPK) pathway, and induction of cyclin D1 requires sustained ERK activation,[100] a correlation between p-ERK and cyclin D1 expression in primary melanoma has been noted.[99] There were no such associations noted in metastatic melanoma, however, which instead demonstrated high expression of p-ERK and decreased expression of cyclin D1, suggesting that the regulation of cyclin D1 expression might differ in metastatic melanoma, when compared with primary melanoma.

p27

p27, like p16, is a cyclin-dependent kinase inhibitor (CDKI), which functions to halt G1-S progression by blocking phosphorylation and activation of cyclins by CDKs. Reduction of CDKIs leads to uncontrolled cell cycling. Low expression of p27 is a marker of adverse prognosis in many human cancers, especially bowel, breast, and prostate cancer.[101,102] p27 knockout mice display gigantism, organ hyperplasia, retinal dysplasia, pituitary tumors, and increased tumorigenesis when subjected to γ-irradiation or chemical carcinogens, phenotypic characteristics that lend support to the tumor suppressor function of p27.[103,104] Despite this phenotype in murine models, there are few reports of specific p27 gene mutations in human tumors,[104] and instead p27 expression appears to predominately be affected at the post-translational level.[105]

Reports of p27 expression in melanoma range from unchanged,[106] to elevated,[107] or even reduced.[108] Sanki et al.[109] demonstrated positive p27 expression in all of 19 compound and dysplastic nevi analyzed, but only in 43.6% of primary melanomas, with greater expression in lymph node and in-transit metastases (63.6%) than in soft tissue metastases (36.4%). Normally, p27 expression decreases as cells pass from G1 to S phase by ubiquitin-proteasome–mediated degradation involving the protein Skp2. Skp2 is inversely related to p27 levels in benign and malignant melanocytic lesions, suggesting increasing malignant potential with acquired defects in p27 degradation.[105] Additionally others have shown p27 silencing in melanoma cells by DNA methylation.[110]

CGH IN THE ASSESSMENT OF MELANOCYTIC LESIONS

CGH is a technique for the genome-wide detection of changes in DNA copy number, and it compares a tumor genome with a selected (presumably) normal genome, allowing detection and mapping of chromosomal alterations that result in DNA copy number differences.[111] The use of chromosomal analysis in the diagnosis of melanocytic lesions is attractive, as genomic aberrations observed in melanoma are relatively absent in benign nevi, with most melanomas possessing an average of greater than five aberrations.[112]

Common abnormalities in melanoma include loss of chromosome 9, namely 9p21-22 (81%), loss of chromosome 10 (63%), and gain of chromosome 7 (50%).[113] Furthermore, even among the most skilled dermatopathology experts, there exist a subset of melanocytic lesions for which morphologic analysis and IHC analysis are insufficient for unequivocal distinction between benign and malignant processes.[114,115] Atypical Spitz nevi, persistent or recurrent melanocytic nevi, mechanically irritated or recently sun-exposed nevi, proliferative nodules in congenital nevi, and melanocytic nevi occurring on "special sites" (acral, genital, or mammary line regions) are examples of lesions with a greater incidence of diagnostic ambiguity.

Spitz nevi are an ongoing source of diagnostic difficulty, as these lesions have morphologic overlap with melanoma.[116-119] While the majority of Spitz nevi are without chromosomal abnormalities, 10% to 20% have a gain of chromosome 11p, associated with a mutation in HRAS that results in constitutive MAPK pathway activation.[120,121] Additionally, Spitz nevi can possess gains of chromosome 7q.[120] These chromosomal abnormalities, while not present in all Spitz nevi, are different from those found in melanomas, suggesting that cytogenic tests may help distinguish these two entities.

Additionally, cytogenic abnormalities vary with the subtype of melanoma studied. Acral melanomas possess amplifications of 11q13 (47%), 22q11-13 (40%), and 5p15 (20%). Less than 10% of superficial spreading melanomas, however, possess chromosomal amplifications. Distinct DNA copy number changes were identified by CGH in four melanoma groups, classified by body site and level of sun damage: acral, mucosal, non-acral skin with chronic sun damage, and non-acral skin without chronic sun damage.[93] This heterogeneity of chromosomal aberration in different melanomas may explain their distinct clinical and morphological characteristics.

CGH thus offers the opportunity to assess the entire genome and has the capacity of discovering novel abnormalities.[122] Nevertheless, there are several limitations to the routine use of CGH in the diagnosis and analysis of melanocytic lesions, particularly in the clinical environment. For example, CGH requires a significant amount of tissue in order to extract sufficient DNA. This requirement may hinder the analysis of smaller specimens. Tissue specimens with only a few atypical melanocytes or with abundant inflammatory infiltrates also pose a challenge, as the DNA from nonmalignant cells can dilute and mask the chromosomal abnormalities of the malignant population. CGH requires DNA copy number changes present in 30% to 50% of cells for detections.[122] Lastly, CGH requires special equipment and expertise not widely available, and at present, it is most often employed in research settings, rather than in routine clinical care.

FISH AND THE ASSESSMENT OF MELANOCYTIC LESIONS

FISH is a technique that has garnered much attention for the diagnosis of melanoma,[123] as it allows visualization of cytogenic abnormalities, such as chromosomal deletions, amplifications, and translocations, frequently present in many cancers. Loss of heterozygosity analyses at polymorphic microsatellites demonstrate DNA copy number abnormalities at specific loci,[124-126] and centromere-specific probes can identify gains and losses of chromosomes in melanomas.[127-129] Such probes offer the advantage that they can be applied directly to formalin-fixed, paraffin-embedded tissue sections, allowing assessment of interphase cells. Early cytogenic studies identified a number of nonrandom and recurrent chromosomal aberrations in melanomas, including losses on chromosomes 6, 8, 9, and 10, and gains on chromosome 1.[112,117,130-132]

FISH has many desirable qualities over CGH, as FISH probes are sensitive, can demonstrate balanced translocations, and are lower cost. FISH-based detection of chromosomal abnormalities is governed by the specificity of the probes utilized. Multiple probes are required for sufficient sensitivity in the diagnostic evaluation of melanocytic lesions. Specificity is less of a concern, as benign nevi do not harbor any detectable chromosomal aberrations, and even the rare cytogenic abnormalities found in Spitz nevi do not significantly overlap with those of melanoma, with only one Spitz nevus reported, to date, to carry a gain of 7q also seen in melanoma.[112]

Selection of FISH probes is vital to enhancing diagnostic value, and the number of probes is important as too few probes may impair sensitivity, whereas too many may increase technical difficulty, with the potential for lower specificity. From a technical standpoint, one option is to combine several probes, each with a distinct fluorophore, into a single multicolor FISH analysis.

A set of four probes targeting 6p25 (RREB1), 6q23 (MYB), 11q13 (CCND1), and centromere 6 (CEP6) seem to offer the best combination of sensitivity and specificity.[133] Positive results for a diagnosis of melanoma is defined by the presence of one or more of the following four criteria: >55% nuclei with more 6p25 than CEP6 signals, >29% nuclei with >2 6p25 signals, >40% nuclei with fewer 6q23 than CEP6 signals, or >38% nuclei with >2 11q13 signals. These four probes are commercially available and have subsequently undergone evaluation in other studies, with overall sensitivities and specificities ranging from 83% to 100% and 94% to 100%, respectively.[133-139]

Intranodal nevi, while a benign entity, can be located in the parenchyma of lymph nodes, making them difficult to distinguish from metastatic melanoma.[140] In this setting, four-probe FISH showed 83% sensitivity and 94% specificity.[137] Four-probe FISH can also be helpful when pagetoid melanocytosis is present, as lesions under this differential include melanomas, Spitz nevi, and de novo melanocytic dysplasia and are subject to discordance in interpretation. In a recent study, a four-probe FISH analysis correctly identified five of seven pagetoid melanomas, as identified and agreed upon by an expert panel, but this same probe set was negative in six of six cases of pagetoid lesions with a benign consensus diagnosis.[141]

FISH also has utility in the staging and subtyping of melanocytic lesions. Lentiginous junctional melanomas ("lentigo maligna") of the elderly are frequently positive by FISH analysis and have the same chromosomal aberrations as common melanomas, lending credence to the classification of these lesions as a distinct melanoma subtype.[142] Measuring Breslow depth of melanomas arising within or lying in contiguity with nevi can be challenging, and in a study of 36 melanomas occurring in association with nevi, a four-probe FISH analysis revealed 78% sensitivity in the areas suspected to be melanoma, while the histologically benign appearing areas were negative.[135] In this same study, there were 16 cases with melanoma in situ and 75% of them were positive upon FISH analysis, suggesting this modality may be sensitive for melanoma in situ, as well as invasive melanoma. To this end, a case of melanoma arising within nevus of ota demonstrated positive areas by FISH analysis in areas where the morphologic features were also consistent with melanoma.[143]

Spitz nevi are a type of melanocytic process occurring most often in children, and these lesions typically follow a benign clinical course. However, a distinct subset of Spitz nevi may possess remarkably atypical and unusual features, making them difficult to distinguish from melanoma. Suggested nomenclature for these latter spitzoid neoplasms include "atypical melanocytic proliferation with spitzoid features," "atypical Spitz tumor" (AST), "malignant spindled and epithelioid cell nevus," "minimum deviation melanoma of the Spitz nevus–like type," "melanocytic tumor of unknown malignant potential," and "spitzoid tumor of uncertain malignant potential". These controversial lesions present with sufficient atypia to warrant consideration of a diagnosis of melanoma, and some authorities have advocated the use of FISH-based technologies to assist in rendering a diagnosis and selecting management.[144]

One group sought to characterize genetic abnormalities that might facilitate distinction of AST, both from frank melanoma and Spitz nevus, and found that the vast majority of chromosomal abnormalities observed in AST were uncommon to melanoma.[145] FISH probes developed to distinguish melanoma from benign melanocytic processes failed to detect one case of spitzoid melanoma, one fatal (metastatic) AST case (arguably itself a melanoma), and the other chromosomally aberrant ASTs in this series, although it did detect one spitzoid melanoma and one more conventional melanoma. However, a comprehensive, genome-wide approach to evaluating these lesions offered greater sensitivity and specificity than the current FISH probe sets used in the series.

Similarly, in another study evaluating the validity of multicolor FISH in histologically ambiguous melanocytic lesions, using locus-specific probes for RREB/MYB and CCND1 did not achieve clinically useful sensitivity and specificity.[146]

RAS/RAF/MEK/ERK ACTIVATION IN MELANOMA

The RAS and RAF families of oncogenes, which include NRAS and BRAF, respectively, are kinases that act as molecular "on/off" switches for cell growth. RAS is a small G protein that binds to the inner surface of the plasma membrane, and RAS, MEK, and ERK are protein kinases that form a three-tiered kinase cascade. In the activated state, these kinases recruit and activate proteins necessary for receptor-mediated signaling, with downstream effects upon gene expression, metabolism, and cytoskeletal functions involved in proliferation, differentiation, senescence, and death.

Dysregulation of the ERK pathway is a well-established connection to cancer pathogenesis in light of its roles in cell proliferation and position relative to several oncogenes. Activation of RAF/MEK/ERK plays a major role in the pathogenesis of one-third of all human cancers.[147]

In 2002, a pivotal large-scale resequencing of ERK pathway components revealed a high frequency of BRAF mutations in human melanoma.[148] While NRAS mutations had already been identified, resequencing efforts revealed BRAF mutations in 44% of melanomas and NRAS mutations in 21% of cases. Additionally, the receptor tyrosine kinase c-KIT and the heterotrimeric G protein α-subunit GNAQ, which both signal through ERK, are mutated in a significant number of mucosal, acral, and uveal melanomas.[149,150]

Detecting Mutations in RAS/RAF Signaling in Melanocytic Lesions

Mutations that persistently activate NRAS or BRAF lead to continuous and unregulated cell growth. NRAS mutations occur most frequently in melanocytes, occurring at rates of 56% in congenital nevi, 33% in primary melanomas, and 26% in metastatic melanoma.[151,152] Somatic missense mutations of BRAF were identified in approximately 65% of melanomas, with a single substitution of glutamic acid for valine at position 600 (V600E), accounting for 80% to 90% of mutations.[148] CGH analysis of genomic DNA extracted from 126 melanoma specimens demonstrated that melanomas without surrounding evidence of chronic sun damage had the highest incidence of BRAF mutation, while those melanomas associated with chronic sun damage instead had frequent CCND1 mutations.[93] No lesions with BRAF/N-RAS mutations had concomitant CDK4 or CCND1 mutations, suggesting that these mediators function independently in melanoma tumorigenesis.

Spitz nevi are notoriously difficult to distinguish from melanomas; however, unlike melanoma, they are associated with an overall favorable prognosis, making distinction between these two entities important. There is a paucity of BRAF mutations in Spitz nevi, suggesting the value of this marker in distinguishing it from melanoma. In one analysis of Spitz nevi, atypical Spitz nevi, suspected spitzoid melanomas, primary spitzoid melanoma, and metastases of spitzoid melanoma, neither Spitz nevi nor atypical Spitz nevi, had mutations in BRAF or NRAS, while only 35% of suspected spitzoid melanomas showed mutations in either of these genes.[153] However, 86% of spitzoid melanoma and 86% of metastases from spitzoid melanoma harbored BRAF or NRAS mutations, suggesting some utility of BRAF or NRAS mutation status in discriminating between histologically classifiable Spitz nevus and spitzoid melanoma.

Conversely, in a separate series of 68 spitzoid proliferations, 10 demonstrated BRAF mutations, including 5 Spitz tumors with atypical features.[154] While these findings would seem to diminish the support of BRAF mutational analysis as a discriminatory test, several individuals have criticized the conclusions of this study and continue to produce results that support BRAF mutation analysis as a viable diagnostic methodology.[155] Therefore, while the prevalence of BRAF mutations observed in all spitzoid neoplasms is low, at present, these data are insufficient to fully advocate for the routine use of mere presence or absence of BRAF mutations in discriminating between benign spitzoid proliferations from melanoma.

In a study with similar methodology, investigators analyzed true congenital melanocytic nevi (CMN) present since birth, proliferating nodules in CMN, and congenital pattern nevi (nevi that resemble histologically CMN but were not definitively present since birth) for BRAF and NRAS mutations.[156] Proliferative nodules are dermal proliferations that can occur in congenital nevi and can exhibit an atypical histologic appearance, making their distinction from melanoma difficult. NRAS mutations were present in 81% of congenital nevi. Of the congenital pattern nevi examined, 71% had BRAF mutations, while only 25% had mutations in NRAS. Similar to CMN, 70% of proliferating nodules harbored NRAS mutations, but none had mutations in BRAF.

Another group of investigators compared 18 benign and 25 atypical proliferative nodules, 10 congenital nevi, and 3 dermal melanomas arising in CMN.[157] BRAF mutations were detected in 40% of CMN control cases, 31% of background CMN, and 34% of proliferative nodules (31% benign and 37% atypical). NRAS mutations were detected in 14% to 81% of CMN and in 70% of proliferative nodules. Similar to the findings of Bauer et al.,[156] giant congenital nevi and associated proliferative nodules in this series possessed significantly more frequent NRAS mutations and infrequent BRAF mutations when compared with the remaining congenital nevi. Thus, it would seem that the mere presence of BRAF and/or NRAS mutations does not confer an increased risk of malignant transformation in the lesion, per se. However, the presence of NRAS mutations seems to favor a congenital melanocytic nevus.

While 66% of melanomas harbor BRAF somatic missense mutations, the same mutations pattern is seen in benign melanocytic nevi.[158] BRAF mutation status, however, may identify a distinct melanoma histologic subtype with a predictable clinical outcome. Melanomas harboring BRAF mutations showed distinct histologic features, which included increased pagetoid migration, nesting of intraepidermal melanocytes, epidermal acanthosis, and sharper circumscription of the surrounding skin.[159] Tumor cells from BRAF mutant melanomas exhibited large, round, and more pigmented cytoplasm, as opposed to NRAS mutant melanomas, which did not reveal specific histologic features.

Knowledge of BRAF as a commonly mutated target in human cancer, particularly in melanoma, warrants sensitive methods for detection and accurate quantification of the amount of mutant DNA from biopsy specimens. PCR methods are most commonly employed, particularly the recent, FDA-approved, *cobas* 4800 BRAF V600 PCR assay for detection of the canonical V600E mutation.[160] This test is designed to be the diagnostic companion used with the new FDA-approved BRAF inhibitor, vemurafenib.

However, PCR is limited in its inability to selectively amplify low percentages of variant alleles in a wild-type allele background. Co-amplification at lower denaturation temperature-PCR (COLD-PCR) is a newer approach for pre-analytical enrichment of mutant alleles from samples and shows promise for increasing the sensitivity of PCR detection of this mutation.[161]

Traditional methods of testing include Sanger dideoxy sequencing, but using this method the results may vary because of biopsy specimen contamination with normal tissue. For a mutation to be detected, it must be present in at least 20% of the sample.[162] Pyrosequencing is a method that may be more appropriate for detecting mutations when low amounts of mutant template are present in the biopsy, as it measures the fraction of mutant template present.[163,164] Amplification refractory mutation system (*ARMS*) is an allele-specific PCR-based method that can detect at least 1% mutant DNA in a normal DNA background, and unlike traditional sequencing, detects only the mutation of interest.[165] ARMS was superior to sequencing in both sensitivity and robustness on a large set of melanoma samples for the analysis of RAS, BRAF, and EGFR mutations.[166]

SUMMARY

The diagnosis of melanoma, and its distinction from other melanocytic processes, is often quite difficult. IHC markers have emerged as additional tools to supplement an impression based on classic morphologic analysis. In this regard, an elevated proliferative index among melanocytes (assessed by Ki67), abnormal preservation of HMB45 among melanocytes of the deeper dermis, or lack of expression of P16 expression among melanocytes are findings that would augment and/or reinforce an impression of melanoma, in the appropriate clinical and histological setting.

Similarly, as our understanding of the biochemical and genetic aberrations in melanoma continues to evolve, specific molecular analysis of melanocytic lesions serves as another means to supplement the classic histologic assessment, and in this regard both CGH and FISH-based analysis have been commercially offered.

In specific instances, where there is great confusion and consternation regarding the diagnosis of melanoma, such as the assessment of spitzoid neoplasms that may overlap considerably with frank melanoma, molecular approaches are beginning to offer some assistance in this diagnostic dilemma. While CGH may be more often appropriate for the research setting, as this technique's strength lies in its capacity to assess the entire genome of a tumor or lesion of interest in comparison with normal tissue, it is tedious and labor intensive. Furthermore, specific chromosomal aberrations unique to melanoma may, in many instances, be detected with a reasonable sensitivity via FISH-based analysis, a technique that is more widely available and commercially offered.

Certainly, as we develop treatment modalities targeted at specific mutations present in some melanomas, such as the recent FDA-approved release of vemurafenib (a BRAF inhibitor), there have been corresponding approvals in commercial assay techniques to detect the presence of a requisite mutation (V600E) necessary for drug efficacy. It is anticipated that this latter development is but the first of a pattern for "mated" drug and diagnostic techniques that will soon burgeon, not only in this arena, but in oncology as a whole. In fact, these targeted molecular therapies offer the potential to revolutionize the diagnosis, treatment, and outcome of melanoma in the coming years.

REFERENCES

1. Mason DY, Sammons R. Alkaline phosphatase and peroxidase for double immunoenzymatic labelling of cellular constituents. *J Clin Pathol.* May 1978;31(5):454-460.
2. Kenny-Moynihan MB, Unger ER. Immunohistochemical and in situ hybridization techniques. In: O'Leary TJ, ed. *Advanced Diagnostic Methods in Pathology*. New York, NY: Elsevier; 2003:101.
3. McNutt NS. The S100 family of multipurpose calcium-binding proteins. *J Cutan Pathol.* November 1998;25(10):521-529.
4. Cochran AJ, Wen DR. S-100 protein as a marker for melanocytic and other tumours. *Pathology*. April 1985;17(2):340-345.
5. Bishop PW, Menasce LP, Yates AJ, Win NA, Banerjee SS. An immunophenotypic survey of malignant melanomas. *Histopathology*. August 1993;23(2):159-166.
6. Fernando SS, Johnson S, Bate J. Immunohistochemical analysis of cutaneous malignant melanoma: comparison of S-100 protein, HMB-45 monoclonal antibody and NKI/C3 monoclonal antibody. *Pathology*. January 1994;26(1):16-19.
7. Kaufmann O, Koch S, Burghardt J, Audring H, Dietel M. Tyrosinase, melan-A, and KBA62 as markers for the immunohistochemical identification of metastatic amelanotic melanomas on paraffin sections. *Mod Pathol.* August 1998;11(8):740-746.
8. Chorny JA, Barr RJ. S100-positive spindle cells in scars: a diagnostic pitfall in the re-excision of desmoplastic melanoma. *Am J Dermatopathol.* August 2002;24(4):309-312.
9. Argenyi ZB, Cain C, Bromley C, et al. S-100 protein-negative malignant melanoma: fact or fiction? A light-microscopic and immunohistochemical study. *Am J Dermatopathol.* June 1994;16(3):233-240.
10. Aisner DL, Maker A, Rosenberg SA, Berman DM. Loss of S100 antigenicity in metastatic melanoma. *Hum Pathol.* September 2005;36(9):1016-1019.
11. Fullen DR, Lowe L, Su LD. Antibody to S100a6 protein is a sensitive immunohistochemical marker for neurothekeoma. *J Cutan Pathol.* February 2003;30(2):118-122.
12. Ribe A, McNutt NS. S100A6 protein expression is different in Spitz nevi and melanomas. *Mod Pathol.* May 2003;16(5):505-511.
13. Puri PK, Elston CA, Tyler WB, Ferringer TC, Elston DM. The staining pattern of pigmented spindle cell nevi with S100A6 protein. *J Cutan Pathol.* January 2011;38(1):14-17.

14. Gown AM, Vogel AM, Hoak D, Gough F, McNutt MA. Monoclonal antibodies specific for melanocytic tumors distinguish subpopulations of melanocytes. *Am J Pathol.* May 1986;123(2):195-203.
15. Smoller BR, McNutt NS, Hsu A. HMB-45 recognizes stimulated melanocytes. *J Cutan Pathol.* April 1989;16(2):49-53.
16. Cummings TJ, Shea CR, Reed JA, Burchette JL, Prieto VG. Expression of the intermediate filament peripherin in extraskeletal myxoid chondrosarcoma. *J Cutan Pathol.* March 2000;27(3):141-146.
17. Skelton HG 3rd, Smith KJ, Barrett TL, Lupton GP, Graham JH. HMB-45 staining in benign and malignant melanocytic lesions. A reflection of cellular activation. *Am J Dermatopathol.* December 1991;13(6):543-550.
18. Fetsch PA, Fetsch JF, Marincola FM, Travis W, Batts KP, Abati A. Comparison of melanoma antigen recognized by T cells (MART-1) to HMB-45: additional evidence to support a common lineage for angiomyolipoma, lymphangiomyomatosis, and clear cell sugar tumor. *Mod Pathol.* August 1998;11(8):699-703.
19. Busam KJ. The use and application of special techniques in assessing melanocytic tumours. *Pathology.* October 2004;36(5):462-469.
20. Ohsie SJ, Sarantopoulos GP, Cochran AJ, Binder SW. Immunohistochemical characteristics of melanoma. *J Cutan Pathol.* May 2008;35(5):433-444.
21. Jungbluth AA, Busam KJ, Gerald WL, et al. A103: an anti-melan-a monoclonal antibody for the detection of malignant melanoma in paraffin-embedded tissues. *Am J Surg Pathol.* May 1998;22(5):595-602.
22. El Shabrawi-Caelen L, Kerl H, Cerroni L. Melan-A: not a helpful marker in distinction between melanoma in situ on sun-damaged skin and pigmented actinic keratosis. *Am J Dermatopathol.* October 2004;26(5):364-366.
23. Prieto VG, Mourad-Zeidan AA, Melnikova V, et al. Galectin-3 expression is associated with tumor progression and pattern of sun exposure in melanoma. *Clin Cancer Res.* November 2006;12(22):6709-6715.
24. Maize JC Jr, Resneck JS Jr, Shapiro PE, McCalmont TH, LeBoit PE. Ducking stray "magic bullets": a Melan-A alert. *Am J Dermatopathol.* April 2003;25(2):162-165.
25. Nicholson KM, Gerami P. An immunohistochemical analysis of pseudomelanocytic nests mimicking melanoma in situ: report of 2 cases. *Am J Dermatopathol.* August 2010;32(6):633-637.
26. Abuzeid M, Dalton SR, Ferringer T, Bernert R, Elston DM. Microphthalmia-associated transcription factor-positive pseudonests in cutaneous lupus erythematosus. *Am J Dermatopathol.* October 2011;33(7):752-754.
27. Rudolph P, Schubert C, Schubert B, Parwaresch R. Proliferation marker Ki-S5 as a diagnostic tool in melanocytic lesions. *J Am Acad Dermatol.* August 1997;37(2 pt 1):169-178.
28. Vollmer RT. Use of Bayes rule and MIB-1 proliferation index to discriminate Spitz nevus from malignant melanoma. *Am J Clin Pathol.* October 2004;122(4):499-505.
29. Barnhill RL. The Spitzoid lesion: rethinking Spitz tumors, atypical variants, 'Spitzoid melanoma' and risk assessment. *Mod Pathol.* February 2006;19(suppl 2):S21-S33.
30. Harris GR, Shea CR, Horenstein MG, Reed JA, Burchette JL Jr, Prieto VG. Desmoplastic (sclerotic) nevus: an underrecognized entity that resembles dermatofibroma and desmoplastic melanoma. *Am J Surg Pathol.* July 1999;23(7):786-794.
31. Widlund HR, Fisher DE. Microphthalamia-associated transcription factor: a critical regulator of pigment cell development and survival. *Oncogene.* May 2003;22(20): 3035-3041.
32. Garraway LA, Widlund HR, Rubin MA, et al. Integrative genomic analyses identify MITF as a lineage survival oncogene amplified in malignant melanoma. *Nature.* July 2005;436(7047):117-122.
33. Prieto VG, Shea CR. Immunohistochemistry of melanocytic proliferations. *Arch Pathol Lab Med.* July 2011;135(7):853-859.
34. Hillesheim PB, Slone S, Kelley D, Malone J, Bahrami S. An immunohistochemical comparison between MiTF and MART-1 with Azure blue counterstaining in the setting of solar lentigo and melanoma in situ. *J Cutan Pathol.* July 2011;38(7):565-569.
35. Thompson SJ, Schatteman GC, Gown AM, Bothwell M. A monoclonal antibody against nerve growth factor receptor. Immunohistochemical analysis of normal and neoplastic human tissue. *Am J Clin Pathol.* October 1989;92(4):415-423.
36. Reed JA, Finnerty B, Albino AP. Divergent cellular differentiation pathways during the invasive stage of cutaneous malignant melanoma progression. *Am J Pathol.* August 1999;155(2): 549-555.
37. Ross AH, Grob P, Bothwell M, et al. Characterization of nerve growth factor receptor in neural crest tumors using monoclonal antibodies. *Proc Natl Acad Sci U S A.* November 1984;81(21):6681-6685.
38. Kay PA, Pinheiro AD, Lohse CM, et al. Desmoplastic melanoma of the head and neck: histopathologic and immunohistochemical study of 28 cases. *Int J Surg Pathol.* January 2004;12(1):17-24.
39. Busam KJ, Iversen K, Coplan KC, Jungbluth AA. Analysis of microphthalmia transcription factor expression in normal tissues and tumors, and comparison of its expression with S-100 protein, gp100, and tyrosinase in desmoplastic malignant melanoma. *Am J Surg Pathol.* February 2001;25(2):197-204.
40. Kanik AB, Yaar M, Bhawan J. p75 nerve growth factor receptor staining helps identify desmoplastic and neurotropic melanoma. *J Cutan Pathol.* June 1996;23(3):205-210.
41. Iwamoto S, Odland PB, Piepkorn M, Bothwell M. Evidence that the p75 neurotrophin receptor mediates perineural spread of desmoplastic melanoma. *J Am Acad Dermatol.* November 1996;35(5 pt 1):725-731.
42. Iwamoto S, Burrows RC, Agoff SN, Piepkorn M, Bothwell M, Schmidt R. The p75 neurotrophin receptor, relative to other Schwann cell and melanoma markers, is abundantly expressed in spindled melanomas. *Am J Dermatopathol.* August 2001;23(4):288-294.
43. Radfar A, Stefanato CM, Ghosn S, Bhawan J. NGFR-positive desmoplastic melanomas with focal or absent S-100 staining: Further evidence supporting the use of both NGFR and S-100 as a primary immunohistochemical panel for the diagnosis of desmoplastic melanomas. *Am J Dermatopathol.* April 2006;28(2):162-167.
44. Huttenbach Y, Prieto VG, Reed JA. Desmoplastic and spindle cell melanomas express protein markers of the neural crest but not of later committed stages of Schwann cell differentiation. *J Cutan Pathol.* October 2002;29(9):562-568.
45. Lazova R, Tantcheva-Poor I, Sigal AC. P75 nerve growth factor receptor staining is superior to S100 in identifying spindle cell and desmoplastic melanoma. *J Am Acad Dermatol.* November 2010;63(5):852-858.
46. Otaibi S, Jukic DM, Drogowski L, Bhawan J, Radfar A. NGFR (p75) expression in cutaneous scars; Further evidence for a potential pitfall in evaluation of reexcision scars of cutaneous neoplasms, in particular desmoplastic melanoma. *Am J Dermatopathol.* February 2011;33(1):65-71.
47. Kelsh RN. Sorting out Sox10 functions in neural crest development. *Bioessays.* August 2006;28(8):788-798.
48. Harris ML, Baxter LL, Loftus SK, Pavan WJ. Sox proteins in melanocyte development and melanoma. *Pigment Cell Melanoma Res.* August 2010;23(4):496-513.
49. Nonaka D, Chiriboga L, Rubin BP. Sox10: a pan-schwannian and melanocytic marker. *Am J Surg Pathol.* September 2008;32(9):1291-1298.
50. Ramos-Herberth FI, Karamchandani J, Kim J, Dadras SS. SOX10 immunostaining distinguishes desmoplastic melanoma from excision scar. *J Cutan Pathol.* September 2010;37(9):944-952.
51. Clarkson KS, Sturdgess IC, Molyneux AJ. The usefulness of tyrosinase in the immunohistochemical assessment of melanocytic lesions: a comparison of the novel T311 antibody (anti-tyrosinase) with S-100, HMB45, and A103 (anti-melan-A). *J Clin Pathol.* March 2001;54(3):196-200.
52. Hofbauer GF, Kamarashev J, Geertsen R, Boni R, Dummer R. Tyrosinase immunoreactivity in formalin-fixed, paraffin-embedded primary and metastatic melanoma: frequency and distribution. *J Cutan Pathol.* April 1998;25(4):204-209.
53. Bernaba BN, Vogiatzis PI, Binder SW, Cassarino DS. Potentially useful markers for desmoplastic melanoma: an analysis of KBA.62, p-AKT, and ezrin. *Am J Dermatopathol.* June 2011;33(4):333-337; quiz 338-340.
54. El Tal AK, Abrou AE, Stiff MA, Mehregan DA. Immunostaining in Mohs micrographic surgery: a review. *Dermatol Surg.* March;36(3):275-290.

55. Nielsen PS, Riber-Hansen R, Steiniche T. Immunohistochemical double stains against Ki67/MART1 and HMB45/MITF: promising diagnostic tools in melanocytic lesions. *Am J Dermatopathol.* June 2011;33(4):361-370.
56. Evangelou E, Kyzas PA, Trikalinos TA. Comparison of the diagnostic accuracy of lymphatic endothelium markers: Bayesian approach. *Mod Pathol.* November 2005;18(11):1490-1497.
57. Niakosari F, Kahn HJ, Marks A, From L. Detection of lymphatic invasion in primary melanoma with monoclonal antibody D2-40: a new selective immunohistochemical marker of lymphatic endothelium. *Arch Dermatol.* April 2005;141(4):440-444.
58. Petitt M, Allison A, Shimoni T, Uchida T, Raimer S, Kelly B. Lymphatic invasion detected by D2-40/S-100 dual immunohistochemistry does not predict sentinel lymph node status in melanoma. *J Am Acad Dermatol.* November 2009;61(5):819-828.
59. Xu X, Gimotty PA, Guerry D, et al. Lymphatic invasion revealed by multispectral imaging is common in primary melanomas and associates with prognosis. *Hum Pathol.* June 2008;39(6):901-909.
60. Rose AE, Christos PJ, Lackaye D, et al. Clinical relevance of detection of lymphovascular invasion in primary melanoma using endothelial markers D2-40 and CD34. *Am J Surg Pathol.* October 2011;35(10):1441-1449.
61. Serrano M, Lee H, Chin L, Cordon-Cardo C, Beach D, DePinho RA. Role of the INK4a locus in tumor suppression and cell mortality. *Cell.* April 1996;85(1):27-37.
62. Goldstein AM, Chan M, Harland M, et al. High-risk melanoma susceptibility genes and pancreatic cancer, neural system tumors, and uveal melanoma across GenoMEL. *Cancer Res.* October 2006;66(20):9818-9828.
63. Foulkes WD, Flanders TY, Pollock PM, Hayward NK. The CDKN2A (p16) gene and human cancer. *Mol Med.* January 1997;3(1):5-20.
64. Liggett WH Jr, Sidransky D. Role of the p16 tumor suppressor gene in cancer. *J Clin Oncol.* March 1998;16(3):1197-1206.
65. Rocco JW, Sidransky D. p16(MTS-1/CDKN2/INK4a) in cancer progression. *Exp Cell Res.* March 2001;264(1):42-55.
66. Fujimoto A, Morita R, Hatta N, Takehara K, Takata M. p16INK4a inactivation is not frequent in uncultured sporadic primary cutaneous melanoma. *Oncogene.* April 1999;18(15):2527-2532.
67. Peng HQ, Bailey D, Bronson D, Goss PE, Hogg D. Loss of heterozygosity of tumor suppressor genes in testis cancer. *Cancer Res.* July 1995;55(13):2871-2875.
68. Funk JO, Schiller PI, Barrett MT, Wong DJ, Kind P, Sander CA. p16INK4a expression is frequently decreased and associated with 9p21 loss of heterozygosity in sporadic melanoma. *J Cutan Pathol.* July 1998;25(6):291-296.
69. Flores JF, Walker GJ, Glendening JM, et al. Loss of the p16INK4a and p15INK4b genes, as well as neighboring 9p21 markers, in sporadic melanoma. *Cancer Res.* November 1996;56(21):5023-5032.
70. van der Velden PA, Metzelaar-Blok JA, Bergman W, et al. Promoter hypermethylation: a common cause of reduced p16(INK4a) expression in uveal melanoma. *Cancer Res.* July 2001;61(13):5303-5306.
71. Gruis NA, Weaver-Feldhaus J, Liu Q, et al. Genetic evidence in melanoma and bladder cancers that p16 and p53 function in separate pathways of tumor suppression. *Am J Pathol.* May 1995;146(5):1199-1206.
72. Aitken J, Welch J, Duffy D, et al. CDKN2A variants in a population-based sample of Queensland families with melanoma. *J Natl Cancer Inst.* March 1999;91(5):446-452.
73. Kumar R, Lundh Rozell B, Louhelainen J, Hemminki K. Mutations in the CDKN2A (p16INK4a) gene in microdissected sporadic primary melanomas. *Int J Cancer.* January 1998;75(2):193-198.
74. Fecher LA, Cummings SD, Keefe MJ, Alani RM. Toward a molecular classification of melanoma. *J Clin Oncol.* April 2007;25(12):1606-1620.
75. Reed JA, Loganzo F Jr, Shea CR, et al. Loss of expression of the p16/cyclin-dependent kinase inhibitor 2 tumor suppressor gene in melanocytic lesions correlates with invasive stage of tumor progression. *Cancer Res.* July 1995;55(13):2713-2718.
76. Sparrow LE, Eldon MJ, English DR, Heenan PJ. p16 and p21WAF1 protein expression in melanocytic tumors by immunohistochemistry. *Am J Dermatopathol.* June 1998;20(3):255-261.
77. Keller-Melchior R, Schmidt R, Piepkorn M. Expression of the tumor suppressor gene product p16INK4 in benign and malignant melanocytic lesions. *J Invest Dermatol.* June 1998;110(6):932-938.
78. Talve L, Sauroja I, Collan Y, Punnonen K, Ekfors T. Loss of expression of the p16INK4/CDKN2 gene in cutaneous malignant melanoma correlates with tumor cell proliferation and invasive stage. *Int J Cancer.* June 1997;74(3):255-259.
79. Michaloglou C, Vredeveld LC, Soengas MS, et al. BRAFE600-associated senescence-like cell cycle arrest of human naevi. *Nature.* August 2005;436(7051):720-724.
80. Gray-Schopfer VC, Cheong SC, Chong H, et al. Cellular senescence in naevi and immortalisation in melanoma: a role for p16? *Br J Cancer.* August 2006;95(4):496-505.
81. Scurr LL, McKenzie HA, Becker TM, et al. Selective loss of wild-type p16(INK4a) expression in human Nevi. *J Invest Dermatol.* July 2011;131:2329-2332.
82. Bishop JA, Wachsmuth RC, Harland M, et al. Genotype/phenotype and penetrance studies in melanoma families with germline CDKN2A mutations. *J Invest Dermatol.* January 2000;114(1):28-33.
83. Straume O, Akslen LA. Alterations and prognostic significance of p16 and p53 protein expression in subgroups of cutaneous melanoma. *Int J Cancer.* October 1997;74(5):535-539.
84. Winnepenninckx V, van den Oord JJ. p16INK4A expression in malignant melanomas with or without a contiguous naevus remnant: a clue to their divergent pathogenesis? *Melanoma Res.* August 2004;14(4):321-322.
85. Clark WH Jr, Elder DE, Guerry DT, Epstein MN, Greene MH, Van Horn M. A study of tumor progression: the precursor lesions of superficial spreading and nodular melanoma. *Hum Pathol.* December 1984;15(12):1147-1165.
86. Husain EA, Mein C, Pozo L, Blanes A, Diaz-Cano SJ. Heterogeneous topographic profiles of kinetic and cell cycle regulator microsatellites in atypical (dysplastic) melanocytic nevi. *Mod Pathol.* April 2011;24(4):471-486.
87. Hilliard NJ, Krahl D, Sellheyer K. p16 expression differentiates between desmoplastic Spitz nevus and desmoplastic melanoma. *J Cutan Pathol.* July 2009;36(7):753-759.
88. High WA, Robinson WA. Genetic mutations involved in melanoma: a summary of our current understanding. *Adv Dermatol.* 2007;23:61-79.
89. Miller AJ, Mihm MC Jr. Melanoma. *N Engl J Med.* July 2006;355(1):51-65.
90. Soufir N, Avril MF, Chompret A, et al. Prevalence of p16 and CDK4 germline mutations in 48 melanoma-prone families in France. The French Familial Melanoma Study Group. *Hum Mol Genet.* February 1998;7(2):209-216.
91. Zuo L, Weger J, Yang Q, et al. Germline mutations in the p16INK4a binding domain of CDK4 in familial melanoma. *Nat Genet.* January 1996;12(1):97-99.
92. Walker GJ, Flores JF, Glendening JM, Lin AH, Markl ID, Fountain JW. Virtually 100% of melanoma cell lines harbor alterations at the DNA level within CDKN2A, CDKN2B, or one of their downstream targets. *Genes Chromosomes Cancer.* June 1998;22(2):157-163.
93. Curtin JA, Fridlyand J, Kageshita T, et al. Distinct sets of genetic alterations in melanoma. *N Engl J Med.* November 2005;353(20):2135-2147.
94. Buecher B, Gauthier-Villars M, Desjardins L, et al. Contribution of CDKN2A/P16 (INK4A), P14 (ARF), CDK4 and BRCA1/2 germline mutations in individuals with suspected genetic predisposition to uveal melanoma. *Fam Cancer.* December 2010;9(4):663-667.
95. Li W, Sanki A, Karim RZ, et al. The role of cell cycle regulatory proteins in the pathogenesis of melanoma. *Pathology.* August 2006;38(4):287-301.
96. Sauter ER, Yeo UC, von Stemm A, et al. Cyclin D1 is a candidate oncogene in cutaneous melanoma. *Cancer Res.* June 2002;62(11):3200-3206.
97. Bastian BC, Kashani-Sabet M, Hamm H, et al. Gene amplifications characterize acral melanoma and permit the detection of occult tumor cells in the surrounding skin. *Cancer Res.* April 2000;60(7):1968-1973.

98. Nai G, Marques M. Role of ROC1 protein in the control of cyclin D1 protein expression in skin melanomas. *Pathol Res Pract.* March 2011;207(3):174-181.
99. Oba J, Nakahara T, Abe T, Hagihara A, Moroi Y, Furue M. Expression of c-Kit, p-ERK and cyclin D1 in malignant melanoma: an immunohistochemical study and analysis of prognostic value. *J Dermatol Sci.* May 2011;62(2):116-123.
100. Weber JD, Raben DM, Phillips PJ, Baldassare JJ. Sustained activation of extracellular-signal-regulated kinase 1 (ERK1) is required for the continued expression of cyclin D1 in G1 phase. *Biochem J.* August 1997;326(pt 1):61-68.
101. Lloyd RV, Erickson LA, Jin L, et al. p27kip1: a multifunctional cyclin-dependent kinase inhibitor with prognostic significance in human cancers. *Am J Pathol.* February 1999;154(2): 313-323.
102. Slingerland J, Pagano M. Regulation of the cdk inhibitor p27 and its deregulation in cancer. *J Cell Physiol.* April 2000;183(1): 10-17.
103. Nakayama K, Ishida N, Shirane M, et al. Mice lacking p27(Kip1) display increased body size, multiple organ hyperplasia, retinal dysplasia, and pituitary tumors. *Cell.* May 1996;85(5):707-720.
104. Fero ML, Randel E, Gurley KE, Roberts JM, Kemp CJ. The murine gene p27Kip1 is haplo-insufficient for tumour suppression. *Nature.* November 1998;396(6707):177-180.
105. Li Q, Murphy M, Ross J, Sheehan C, Carlson JA. Skp2 and p27kip1 expression in melanocytic nevi and melanoma: an inverse relationship. *J Cutan Pathol.* November 2004;31(10):633-642.
106. Morgan MB, Cowper SE. Expression of p-27 (kip1) in nevi and melanomas. *Am J Dermatopathol.* April 1999;21(2):121-124.
107. Bales ES, Dietrich C, Bandyopadhyay D, et al. High levels of expression of p27KIP1 and cyclin E in invasive primary malignant melanomas. *J Invest Dermatol.* December 1999;113(6):1039-1046.
108. Florenes VA, Maelandsmo GM, Kerbel RS, Slingerland JM, Nesland JM, Holm R. Protein expression of the cell-cycle inhibitor p27Kip1 in malignant melanoma: inverse correlation with disease-free survival. *Am J Pathol.* July 1998;153(1): 305-312.
109. Sanki A, Li W, Colman M, Karim RZ, Thompson JF, Scolyer RA. Reduced expression of p16 and p27 is correlated with tumour progression in cutaneous melanoma. *Pathology.* December 2007;39(6):551-557.
110. Thompson JF, Scolyer RA, Kefford RF. Cutaneous melanoma. *Lancet.* February 2005;365(9460):687-701.
111. Kallioniemi A, Kallioniemi OP, Sudar D, et al. Comparative genomic hybridization for molecular cytogenetic analysis of solid tumors. *Science.* October 1992;258(5083):818-821.
112. Bastian BC, LeBoit PE, Hamm H, Brocker EB, Pinkel D. Chromosomal gains and losses in primary cutaneous melanomas detected by comparative genomic hybridization. *Cancer Res.* May 1998;58(10):2170-2175.
113. Bastian BC, Olshen AB, LeBoit PE, Pinkel D. Classifying melanocytic tumors based on DNA copy number changes. *Am J Pathol.* November 2003;163(5):1765-1770.
114. Cook MG. Diagnostic discord with melanoma. *J Pathol.* July 1997;182(3):247-249.
115. Corona R, Mele A, Amini M, et al. Interobserver variability on the histopathologic diagnosis of cutaneous melanoma and other pigmented skin lesions. *J Clin Oncol.* April 1996;14(4):1218-1223.
116. Barnhill RL. Childhood melanoma. *Semin Diagn Pathol.* August 1998;15(3):189-194.
117. Crotty KA, Scolyer RA, Li L, Palmer AA, Wang L, McCarthy SW. Spitz naevus versus Spitzoid melanoma: when and how can they be distinguished? *Pathology.* February 2002;34(1):6-12.
118. Dahlstrom JE, Scolyer RA, Thompson JF, Jain S. Spitz naevus: diagnostic problems and their management implications. *Pathology.* October 2004;36(5):452-457.
119. Mooi WJ, Krausz T. Spitz nevus versus spitzoid melanoma: diagnostic difficulties, conceptual controversies. *Adv Anat Pathol.* July 2006;13(4):147-156.
120. Bastian BC, Wesselmann U, Pinkel D, Leboit PE. Molecular cytogenetic analysis of Spitz nevi shows clear differences to melanoma. *J Invest Dermatol.* December 1999;113(6): 1065-1069.
121. Bastian BC, LeBoit PE, Pinkel D. Mutations and copy number increase of HRAS in Spitz nevi with distinctive histopathological features. *Am J Pathol.* September 2000;157(3):967-972.
122. Bauer J, Bastian BC. Distinguishing melanocytic nevi from melanoma by DNA copy number changes: comparative genomic hybridization as a research and diagnostic tool. *Dermatol Ther.* January-February 2006;19(1):40-49.
123. McCalmont TH. Gone FISHing. *J Cutan Pathol.* February 2010;37(2):193-195.
124. Millikin D, Meese E, Vogelstein B, Witkowski C, Trent J. Loss of heterozygosity for loci on the long arm of chromosome 6 in human malignant melanoma. *Cancer Res.* October 1991;51(20):5449-5453.
125. Isshiki K, Elder DE, Guerry D, Linnenbach AJ. Chromosome 10 allelic loss in malignant melanoma. *Genes Chromosomes Cancer.* November 1993;8(3):178-184.
126. Isshiki K, Seng BA, Elder DE, Guerry D, Linnenbach AJ. Chromosome 9 deletion in sporadic and familial melanomas in vivo. *Oncogene.* June 1994;9(6):1649-1653.
127. Matsuta M, Kon S, Thompson C, LeBoit PE, Weier HU, Gray JW. Interphase cytogenetics of melanocytic neoplasms: numerical aberrations of chromosomes can be detected in interphase nuclei using centromeric DNA probes. *J Cutan Pathol.* February 1994;21(1):1-6.
128. Wolfe KQ, Southern SA, Herrington CS. Interphase cytogenetic demonstration of chromosome 9 loss in thick melanomas. *J Cutan Pathol.* August 1997;24(7):398-402.
129. D'Alessandro I, Zitzelsberger H, Hutzler P, et al. Numerical aberrations of chromosome 7 detected in 15 microns paraffin-embedded tissue sections of primary cutaneous melanomas by fluorescence in situ hybridization and confocal laser scanning microscopy. *J Cutan Pathol.* February 1997;24(2):70-75.
130. Kakati S, Song SY, Sandberg AA. Chromosomes and causation of human cancer and leukemia. XXII. Karyotypic changes in malignant melanoma. *Cancer.* September 1977;40(3): 1173-1181.
131. Balaban G, Herlyn M, Guerry DT, et al. Cytogenetics of human malignant melanoma and premalignant lesions. *Cancer Genet Cytogenet.* April 1984;11(4):429-439.
132. Thompson FH, Emerson J, Olson S, et al. Cytogenetics of 158 patients with regional or disseminated melanoma. Subset analysis of near-diploid and simple karyotypes. *Cancer Genet Cytogenet.* September 1995;83(2):93-104.
133. Gerami P, Jewell SS, Morrison LE, et al. Fluorescence in situ hybridization (FISH) as an ancillary diagnostic tool in the diagnosis of melanoma. *Am J Surg Pathol.* August 2009;33(8):1146-1156.
134. Morey AL, Murali R, McCarthy SW, Mann GJ, Scolyer RA. Diagnosis of cutaneous melanocytic tumours by four-colour fluorescence in situ hybridisation. *Pathology.* 2009;41(4):383-387.
135. Newman MD, Lertsburapa T, Mirzabeigi M, Mafee M, Guitart J, Gerami P. Fluorescence in situ hybridization as a tool for microstaging in malignant melanoma. *Mod Pathol.* August 2009;22(8):989-995.
136. Pouryazdanparast P, Newman M, Mafee M, Haghighat Z, Guitart J, Gerami P. Distinguishing epithelioid blue nevus from blue nevus-like cutaneous melanoma metastasis using fluorescence in situ hybridization. *Am J Surg Pathol.* September 2009;33(9):1396-1400.
137. Dalton SR, Gerami P, Kolaitis NA, et al. Use of fluorescence in situ hybridization (FISH) to distinguish intranodal nevus from metastatic melanoma. *Am J Surg Pathol.* February 2010;34(2):231-237.
138. Gerami P, Mafee M, Lurtsbarapa T, Guitart J, Haghighat Z, Newman M. Sensitivity of fluorescence in situ hybridization for melanoma diagnosis using RREB1, MYB, Cep6, and 11q13 probes in melanoma subtypes. *Arch Dermatol.* March 2010;146(3):273-278.
139. Busam KJ, Fang Y, Jhanwar SC, Pulitzer MP, Marr B, Abramson DH. Distinction of conjunctival melanocytic nevi from melanomas by fluorescence in situ hybridization. *J Cutan Pathol.* February 2010;37(2):196-203.
140. Biddle DA, Evans HL, Kemp BL, et al. Intraparenchymal nevus cell aggregates in lymph nodes: a possible diagnostic pitfall with malignant melanoma and carcinoma. *Am J Surg Pathol.* May 2003;27(5):673-681.

141. Gerami P, Barnhill RL, Beilfuss BA, LeBoit P, Schneider P, Guitart J. Superficial melanocytic neoplasms with pagetoid melanocytosis: a study of interobserver concordance and correlation with FISH. *Am J Surg Pathol.* June 2010;34(6):816-821.
142. Newman MD, Mirzabeigi M, Gerami P. Chromosomal copy number changes supporting the classification of lentiginous junctional melanoma of the elderly as a subtype of melanoma. *Mod Pathol.* September 2009;22(9):1258-1262.
143. Gerami P, Pouryazdanparast P, Vemula S, Bastian BC. Molecular analysis of a case of nevus of ota showing progressive evolution to melanoma with intermediate stages resembling cellular blue nevus. *Am J Dermatopathol.* May 2010;32(3):301-305.
144. Tom WL, Hsu JW, Eichenfield LF, Friedlander SF. Pediatric "STUMP" lesions: evaluation and management of difficult atypical Spitzoid lesions in children. *J Am Acad Dermatol.* March 2011;64(3):559-572.
145. Raskin L, Ludgate M, Iyer RK, et al. Copy number variations and clinical outcome in atypical spitz tumors. *Am J Surg Pathol.* February 2011;35(2):243-252.
146. Gaiser T, Kutzner H, Palmedo G, et al. Classifying ambiguous melanocytic lesions with FISH and correlation with clinical long-term follow up. *Mod Pathol.* March 2010;23(3):413-419.
147. Malumbres M, Barbacid M. RAS oncogenes: the first 30 years. *Nat Rev Cancer.* June 2003;3(6):459-465.
148. Davies H, Bignell GR, Cox C, et al. Mutations of the BRAF gene in human cancer. *Nature.* June 2002;417(6892):949-954.
149. Curtin JA, Busam K, Pinkel D, Bastian BC. Somatic activation of KIT in distinct subtypes of melanoma. *J Clin Oncol.* September 2006;24(26):4340-4346.
150. Van Raamsdonk CD, Bezrookove V, Green G, et al. Frequent somatic mutations of GNAQ in uveal melanoma and blue naevi. *Nature.* January 2009;457(7229):599-602.
151. Demunter A, Stas M, Degreef H, De Wolf-Peeters C, van den Oord JJ. Analysis of N- and K-ras mutations in the distinctive tumor progression phases of melanoma. *J Invest Dermatol.* December 2001;117(6):1483-1489.
152. Papp T, Pemsel H, Zimmermann R, Bastrop R, Weiss DG, Schiffmann D. Mutational analysis of the N-ras, p53, p16INK4a, CDK4, and MC1R genes in human congenital melanocytic naevi. *J Med Genet.* August 1999;36(8):610-614.
153. van Dijk MC, Bernsen MR, Ruiter DJ. Analysis of mutations in B-RAF, N-RAS, and H-RAS genes in the differential diagnosis of Spitz nevus and spitzoid melanoma. *Am J Surg Pathol.* September 2005;29(9):1145-1151.
154. Fullen DR, Poynter JN, Lowe L, et al. BRAF and NRAS mutations in spitzoid melanocytic lesions. *Mod Pathol.* October 2006;19(10):1324-1332.
155. Takata M, Lin J, Takayanagi S, et al. Genetic and epigenetic alterations in the differential diagnosis of malignant melanoma and spitzoid lesion. *Br J Dermatol.* June 2007;156(6):1287-1294.
156. Bauer J, Curtin JA, Pinkel D, Bastian BC. Congenital melanocytic nevi frequently harbor NRAS mutations but no BRAF mutations. *J Invest Dermatol.* January 2007;127(1):179-182.
157. Phadke PA, Rakheja D, Le LP, et al. Proliferative nodules arising within congenital melanocytic nevi: a histologic, immunohistochemical, and molecular analyses of 43 cases. *Am J Surg Pathol.* May 2011;35(5):656-669.
158. Pollock PM, Meltzer PS. A genome-based strategy uncovers frequent BRAF mutations in melanoma. *Cancer Cell.* July 2002;2(1):5-7.
159. Viros A, Fridlyand J, Bauer J, et al. Improving melanoma classification by integrating genetic and morphologic features. *PLoS Med.* June 2008;5(6):e120.
160. Chan M. Approval letter. In: Health Cfdar, ed. Silver Spring, MD: U.S. Food and Drug Administration, Center for Devices and Radiological Health. CobasÒ 4800 BRAF V600 Mutation Test approval letter, August 17, 2011. Retrieved July 28 2012, from www.accessdata.fda.gov/cdrh_docs/pdf11/p110020a.pdf. 2011.
161. Pinzani P, Santucci C, Mancini I, et al. BRAFV600E detection in melanoma is highly improved by COLD-PCR. *Clin Chim Acta.* May 2011;412(11-12):901-905.
162. Bakker E. Is the DNA sequence the gold standard in genetic testing? Quality of molecular genetic tests assessed. *Clin Chem.* April 2006;52(4):557-558.
163. Spittle C, Ward MR, Nathanson KL, et al. Application of a BRAF pyrosequencing assay for mutation detection and copy number analysis in malignant melanoma. *J Mol Diagn.* September 2007;9(4):464-471.
164. Borras E, Jurado I, Hernan I, et al. Clinical pharmacogenomic testing of KRAS, BRAF and EGFR mutations by high resolution melting analysis and ultra-deep pyrosequencing. *BMC Cancer.* 11:406.
165. Newton CR, Graham A, Heptinstall LE, et al. Analysis of any point mutation in DNA. The amplification refractory mutation system (ARMS). *Nucleic Acids Res.* April 1989;17(7):2503-2516.
166. Ellison G, Donald E, McWalter G, et al. A comparison of ARMS and DNA sequencing for mutation analysis in clinical biopsy samples. *J Exp Clin Cancer Res.* 2010;29:132.

CHAPTER 35

Molecular Diagnostics of Hematopoietic Neoplasms

Qiulu Pan and Dan Jones

The classification of lymphomas, cancers involving the lymphoid organs, and leukemias, neoplasms of the blood and bone marrow, has evolved greatly over the last 50 years through the application of molecular diagnostics. This has been a stepwise process of delineating the molecular and genetic characteristics underlying the morphologically defined lymphoma and leukemia subtypes followed by the incorporation of cytogenetic and molecular testing into routine diagnostics. Molecular subtyping has also discovered several new lymphoma and leukemia subtypes that were not well recognized by routine histopathology and immunophenotyping.

The myeloid leukemias have also been the paradigm for other tumor types in linking molecular alterations that define diagnostic entities with therapeutic agents that target these same pathways within the tumor. This connection has been most successful in the BCR-ABL1-translocated chronic myelogenous leukemia (CML), where the treating drugs are kinase inhibitors that block BCR-ABL1 kinase activity and thus inhibit CML growth.

We review here the separate classification and testing algorithms for B-cell lymphoproliferative disorders (B-LPDs), T-cell lymphoproliferative disorders (T-LPDs), and myeloid neoplasms. We also review the impact of molecular diagnostics in individualizing therapy for these tumor types.

APPROACHES TO CLASSIFICATION OF LYMPHOMAS AND LEUKEMIAS

The hematologic malignancies, including leukemias and lymphomas, were the first tumor types to develop a standardized diagnostic schema based on morphology and genetics, beginning in the 1960s. The current standard for diagnosis in hematopathology, the World Health Organization (WHO) classification of tumors of hematopoietic and lymphoid tissues (2008), represents an evolution and integration of the previous largely separate efforts in lymphomas and myeloid neoplasms in the preceding 30 years.[1,2]

The general principle of classification in the WHO schema and its predecessors is to map neoplasms to the maturation stage of the normal counterpart to which they most resemble. Although this simplistic model does not account for all the observed heterogeneity in tumors, it has been incredibly successful in placing tumor entities in a comprehensible and easy-to-remember framework for diagnosis. Therefore, we will mirror this approach here, beginning with a short discussion of the normal maturation of each hematolymphoid cell type before proceeding to discuss diagnosis, testing, and therapy selection.

B-CELL LYMPHOPROLIFERATIVE NEOPLASMS

Normal B-Cell Biology and Its Relationship to Lymphoma

B lymphocytes, abbreviated B cells throughout this chapter, represent the immune cell type responsible for antibody production through cell-bound IgD and IgM and secreted IgA, IgE, and IgG and for maintaining one aspect of immunologic memory. This latter function is due to the persistence of long-lived memory B cells whose surface antibody recognizes previously encountered foreign antigens and thus shorten the time to respond when an antigen is reencountered in later life.

Given the unique natural history of B cells, lymphomas and leukemias arising from these cells can have antigenic triggers due to persistent B-cell expansions in autoimmune and chronic infections.[3] Other causes are related to immunosuppression, when regulatory T cells that control B cell expansion are missing.[4] In these

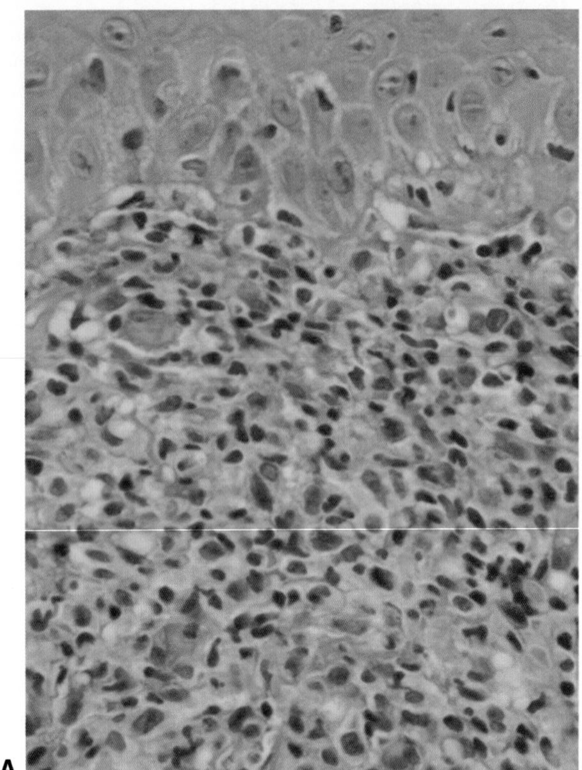

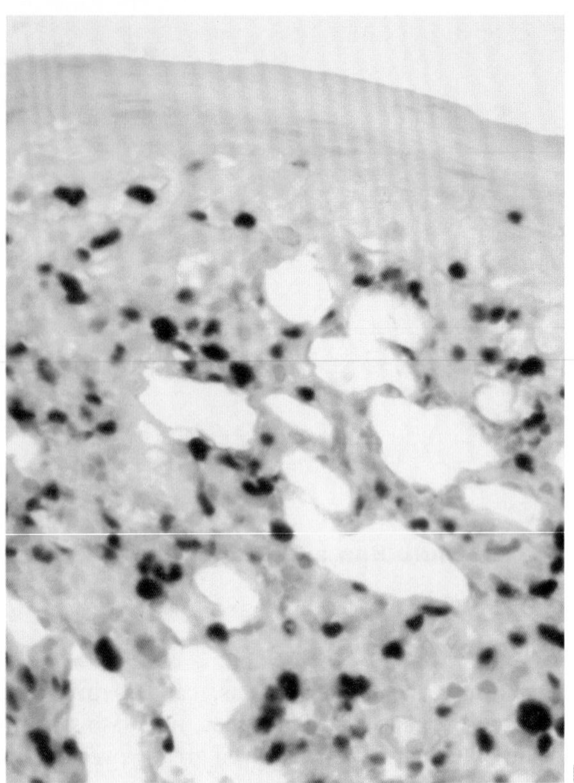

FIGURE 35–1 Epstein-Barr virus (EBV)–positive large B-cell lymphoma. **A:** Cutaneous involvement by a lymphoma in an immunosuppressed patient (hematoxylin and eosin–stained tissue section, 60×). **B:** EBV in the larger tumor cells is detected by in situ hybridization with probes for the viral EBER gene products.

instances, B-cells infected with lymphotropic transforming viruses, particularly Epstein-Barr virus, can proliferate and produce a clonal expansion (Fig. 35.1). Other etiologies of B-LPDs are iatrogenic and environmental causes due to induced mutations and chromosome breaks in this rapidly expanding cell type (Table 35.1).

Normal B cells arise as precursors in the bone marrow called lymphoblasts and then migrate into the peripheral blood as long-lived naïve forms, a process that is largely completed in childhood. Further maturation of B cells is dependent on recognition of an appropriate antigen that binds to a specific antibody molecule, also known as the B-cell receptor (BCR) comprised of immunoglobulin heavy chain (IGH) and one of two types of immunoglobulin light chain (IGK or IGL).

Triggering of the BCR by antigen, as well as costimulation by T–cell–derived soluble cytokines, leads to proliferation of that specific B cell and its progeny.[5] Further

TABLE 35–1 General Etiologic Causes of B-Cell Lymphomas

General Class	LPD Types	Initiating Condition	Treatment Approaches
Exogenous antigen	MALT lymphoma	*Helicobacter* infection (gastric) *Campylobacter* infection (bowel) *Chlamydia* infection (ocular)	Antibiotics therapy
Viral transformation	EBV+ PTLD EBV+ S-LBCL HHV8+ MCD Hodgkin lymphoma EBV+ B-LPDs	Iatrogenic immunosuppression Immune dysregulation with age Age of primary infection Germline immune defects (e.g., Wiskott-Aldrich syndrome)	Modify drug levels Early diagnosis and close monitoring
Germline DNA repair defects	Various types	Ataxia-telangiectasia, others	Early diagnosis and close monitoring
Germline defects in apoptosis	Various types	Autoimmune lymphoproliferative syndrome (ALPS), others	Early diagnosis and close monitoring

LPD, lymphoproliferative disorder; EBV, Epstein-Barr virus; HHV8, human herpesvirus 8; MCD, multicentric Castleman disease. See abbreviations in Table 35.2 for lymphoma types.

maturation occurs when the activated B cells move to the lymph nodes and other secondary lymphoid origins (e.g., intestinal Peyer patch, spleen, and tonsil). Sequential migration of B cells through the lymph node and back into the blood and other tissues is related to additional functional stages of maturation. These include movement to mantle zone of follicles (associated with phenotypic shifts in surface BCR), to the germinal center/secondary follicle (where further changes in the sequence of the BCR occur due to somatic hypermutation), to the paracortical/marginal zone areas (where shift to IgA, IgE or IgG expression often occurs), and finally either to the blood as long-lived memory B cells or to lymph node medullary areas (and the bone marrow) as plasma cells.

Diagnostic Categories of B-Cell Neoplasms

The classification of B-LPDs is largely related to mapping specific neoplasms to the above stages of B-cell maturation (Table 35.2). Thus, the principal B-cell tumors are lymphoblastic leukemias/lymphomas (LBL) and its blood counterpart acute lymphoblastic leukemia (ALL), mantle cell lymphoma (MCL), follicular lymphoma (FL), extranodal and nodal marginal zone lymphoma (MZL), and plasma cell neoplasms, including the most aggressive variant termed multiple myeloma, that each represent one stage of the B-cell life cycle.[2]

Several additional clinical subtypes, chronic lymphocytic leukemia/small lymphocytic lymphoma (CLL/SLL), Burkitt lymphoma (BL), and diffuse large B-cell lymphoma (DLBCL), do not precisely map to B-cell maturation types but generally can be associated with development stages based on their functional properties, immunophenotype, and BCR status.[2] Hodgkin disease/lymphoma, once thought to be a non-lymphoid malignancy, is now understood to represent, in nearly all cases, a B-cell malignancy in which the tumor cells have lost expression of many B-cell markers during the process of transformation.[6,7]

Molecular Diagnostic Testing for Diagnosis of B-LPDs

There are two primary challenges in the diagnosis of B-LPDs, namely the separation of small cell or low-grade neoplasms from reactive B-cell expansions and the appropriate classification of large cell or higher grade B-cell neoplasms. For diagnosis of low-grade lesions, the two most commonly used ancillary techniques are IGH PCR and clonal κ/λ-immunoglobulin restriction detected by in situ hybridization using kappa and lambda gene probes on formalin-fixed tissue sections or by flow cytometry on fresh cells. B-cell clonality by flow cytometry is determined using antibodies that detect surface or cytoplasmic

TABLE 35-2 B-Cell Lymphoproliferative Disorders (2008 WHO Classification)

B-lymphoblastic leukemia/lymphoma
Chronic lymphocytic leukemia/small lymphocytic lymphoma
B-cell prolymphocytic leukemia
Splenic marginal zone lymphoma
Hairy cell leukemia
Splenic lymphoma/leukemia, unclassifiable
  Splenic diffuse red pulp small B-cell lymphoma[a]
  Hairy cell leukemia variant[a]
Lymphoplasmacytic lymphoma
Waldenström macroglobulinemia
Heavy chain diseases
  α-Heavy chain disease
  γ-Heavy chain disease
  μ-Heavy chain disease
Plasma cell myeloma
Solitary plasmacytoma of bone
Extraosseous plasmacytoma
Extranodal marginal zone B-cell lymphoma of mucosa-associated lymphoid tissue (MALT lymphoma)
Nodal marginal zone B-cell lymphoma (MZL)
  Pediatric type nodal MZL
Follicular lymphoma
  Pediatric type follicular lymphoma
Primary cutaneous follicle center lymphoma
Mantle cell lymphoma
Diffuse large B-cell lymphoma (DLBCL), not otherwise specified
T-cell/histiocyte-rich large B-cell lymphoma
  DLBCL associated with chronic inflammation[a]
  Epstein-Barr virus (EBV)+ DLBCL of the elderly[a]
Lymphomatoid granulomatosis
Primary mediastinal (thymic) large B-cell lymphoma
Intravascular large B-cell lymphoma
Primary cutaneous DLBCL, leg type
ALK+ large B-cell lymphoma
Plasmablastic lymphoma
Primary effusion lymphoma
Large B-cell lymphoma arising in HHV8-associated multicentric Castleman disease
Burkitt lymphoma
B-cell lymphoma, unclassifiable, with features intermediate between diffuse large B-cell lymphoma and Burkitt lymphoma
B-cell lymphoma, unclassifiable, with features intermediate between diffuse large B-cell lymphoma and classical Hodgkin lymphoma

Hodgkin Lymphoma

Nodular lymphocyte-predominant Hodgkin lymphoma
Classical Hodgkin lymphoma
Nodular sclerosis classical Hodgkin lymphoma
Lymphocyte-rich classical Hodgkin lymphoma
Mixed cellularity classical Hodgkin lymphoma
Lymphocyte-depleted classical Hodgkin lymphoma

[a]Provisional entities.

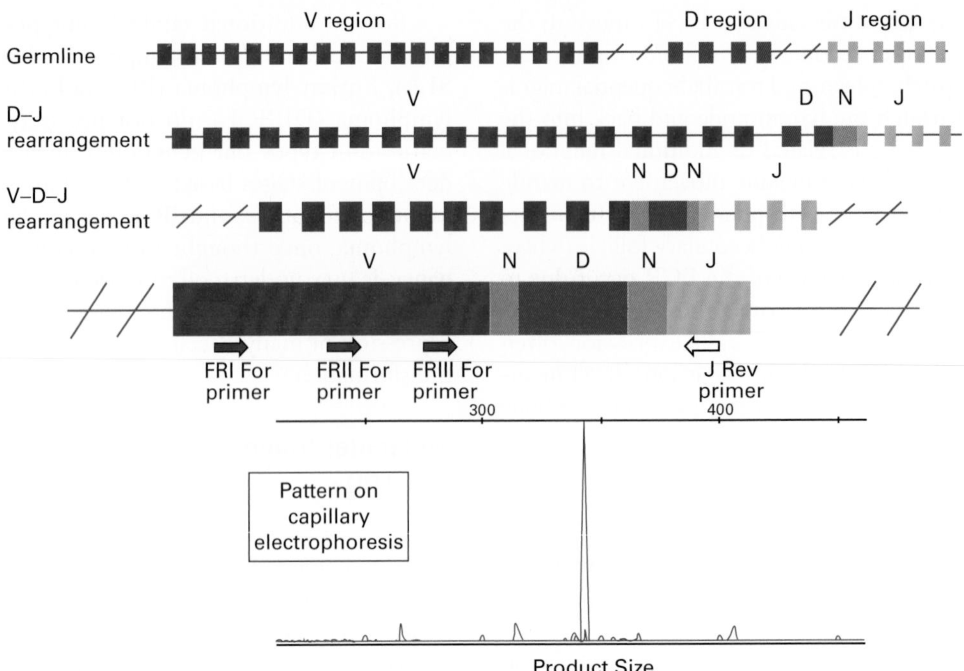

FIGURE 35–2 Principle of B-cell clonality assessment: Rearrangement of the IGH gene. (**Top**) Schematic representations of the IGH gene locus on chromosome 14. The variable region (V) segments are represented in blue, the diversity region (D) segments are represented in green, and the joining (J) region segments are shown in light blue. The sequential D–J and V–D–J rearrangements are shown with the clone-specific unique template-independent regions (N) added during each rearrangement DNA break-ligation process. (**Middle**) The location of the primers used in the IGH assay are shown including three different forward (For) primers each binding to the conserved framework regions (FRI, FRII, and FRIII) of the V regions and a reverse (Rev) primer that anneals to a conserved region of the J regions. (**Bottom**) Results of an IGH PCR assay with a clonal rearrangement shown. The distinct clonal peak is detected by fragment analysis with fluorochrome-labeled PCR products detected by capillary electrophoresis following PCR with peak height proportional to the intensity of the signal.

immunoglobulin, looking for an excess of B cells over the expected percentage of those expressing κ-chain versus λ-light chain (normal ratio of κ:λ is ~2:1).

The basis of IGH PCR is that all progeny from a founder B cell will share the same BCR which has a particular amplicon size due to the process of *VDJ recombination* that occurs in the DNA of the IGH, IGK, and IGL genes at the lymphoblast stage.[8,9] Any B-cell neoplasm derived from this founder cell thus will share the same antibody specificity/IGH sequence and thus an identically sized VDJ IGH gene amplicon that is detected as a single electrophoretic peak or band following DNA-based PCR (Fig. 35.2). In contrast, mixed/polyclonal non-neoplastic B-cell expansions will have IGH loci of varying sizes giving a normal distribution of PCR products.

For the diagnosis of specific WHO entities, immunophenotyping by flow cytometry and/or immunohistochemistry (IHC) complemented by fluorescence in situ hybridization (FISH) or PCR are the primary techniques (Table 35.3). Because individual IHC or flow cytometry markers lack absolute specificity, panels or markers are typically used.

Most of the developmental stage–specific B-cell subtypes also have specific defining chromosomal translocations that can be used for diagnosis (Table 35.3). These include the t(14;18)(q32;q21) BCL2-IGH fusion in FL, the t(11;14)(q13;q32) BCL1(cyclin D1)/IGH fusion, the 18q21/MALT1 alterations seen in extranodal MZLs (MALTomas), and the 3q27/BCL6 alterations associated with large B-cell lymphomas.[10] In general, FISH is the preferred diagnostic method since PCR assays cannot usually cover the wide range of breakpoints involved in these fusions. The minority of neoplasms in each WHO category that lack the characteristic gene alterations often have closely related mechanisms, such as overexpression of cyclin D2 and D3 homologues instead of cyclin D1 in MCL.[11] These alterations can be detected by additional testing.

Molecular Prognostic and Predictive Markers in Therapy of B-LPDs

Subtypes of B-LPD have widely differing incidences and ages at presentation as well as variable outcomes with ALL/LBL, BL, and DLBCL having the most aggressive clinical behavior and the worst outcomes.

The three primary modalities in treatment of B-LPDs are combination cytotoxic chemotherapy to target rapidly dividing cells, radiotherapy to trigger tumor cell apoptosis, and immunotherapy. The rituximab antibody directed against the pan-B–cell antigen CD20 is the most commonly used therapeutic antibody, incorporated into both frontline or salvage regimens for all B-LPDs except B-ALL/LBL which usually lacks CD20 expression.

TABLE 35–3 Protein and Molecular Markers Used to Diagnose B-Cell Lymphoproliferative Disorder Subtypes

Tumor Type	Protein Markers Used	FISH/PCR (P) Assays
Follicular lymphoma	CD10+ BCL6++ HGAL+	t(14;18) (F&P)
Mantle cell lymphoma	Cyclin D1+ CD5+ CD23–	t(11;14) (F&P)
Marginal zone lymphoma	CD5– CD10–	t(11;18) (F&P) MALT1/18q21 (BA)
Burkitt lymphoma	CD10+ Ki67(100%)+ BCL2–	t(8;14) (F), MYC/8q24 (BA)
Large cell lymphoma	BCL-6, CD10 (better prognosis) MUM1 (worse prognosis)	BCL6 3q27 (BA) BA for MYC/8q24 (dual-hit/high-grade cases)

FISH, fluorescence in situ hybridization, F, dual-color dual-fusion FISH; BA, dual-color breakapart FISH, P, PCR.

Given that standard therapies for B-LPDs produce responses in the majority of patients, there has been relatively little use of prognostic markers and therapy response predictors in routine practice. An exception is in CLL/SLL, where cytogenetic changes have been shown to have strong prognostic utility influencing the timing of therapy, These abnormalities, usually detected by multiprobe FISH assays, include deletions at the TP53 loci at chr 17p13, the ATM gene at chr 11q23, and a microRNA cluster at chr 13q14, as well as an extra copy of chromosome 12 (Fig. 35.3B and C). Loss of 17p13/TP53 and 11q22/ATM are adverse prognostic markers seen in patients likely to need earlier treatment[12,13]; del13q14 in the absence of other changes signals a favorable prognosis. Given the complexity of some gene rearrangements (Fig. 35.3D), array-based methods may be a more accurate method of identifying locus deletion/amplification in CLL and other B-LPDs.[14,15]

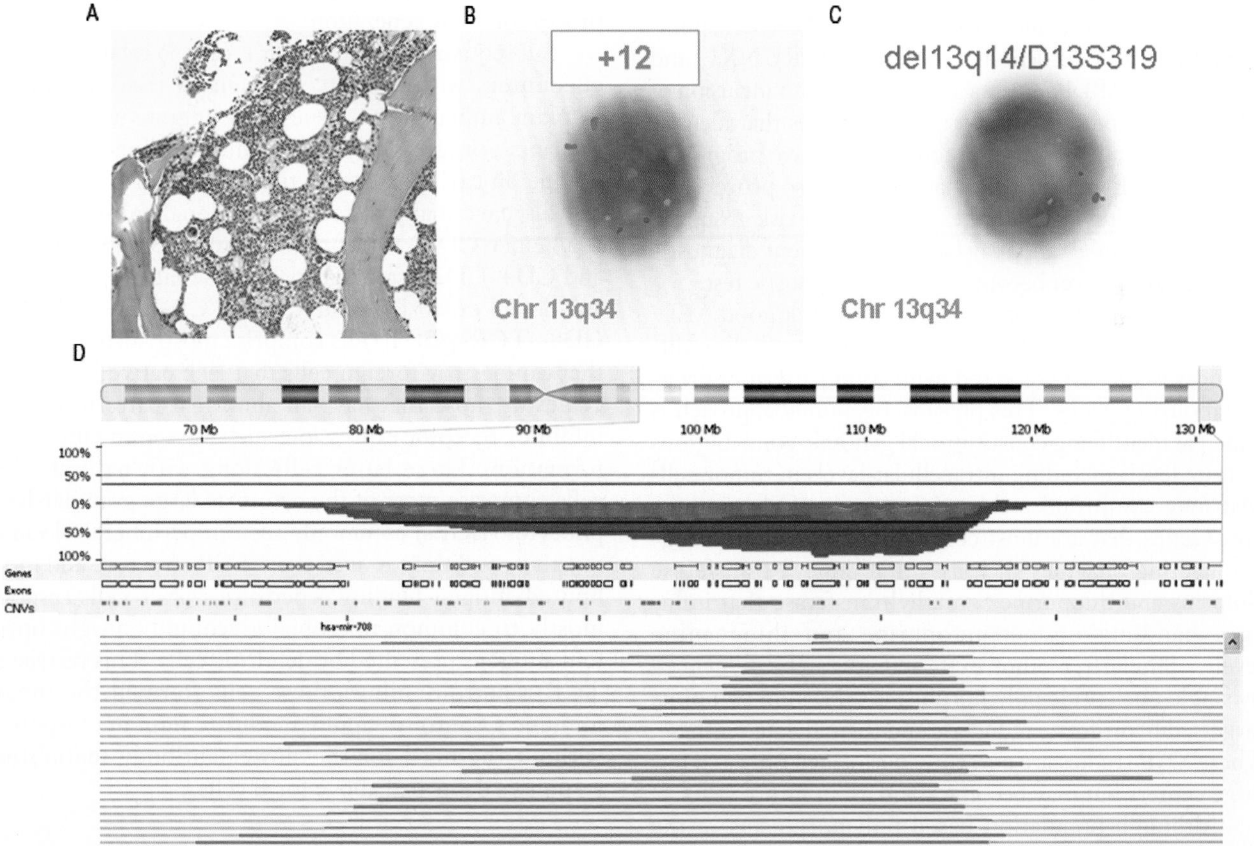

FIGURE 35–3 Outcome prediction in CLL/SLL. **A:** A typical case of CLL involving bone marrow (hematoxylin and eosin–stained tissue section, 10×). **B:** Multiprobe FISH shows trisomy of chromosome 12 (+12) in cell (three green probe signals) with the normal two copies of the 13q14 (red) and 13q34 (blue) probes. **C:** In another CLL case, multiprobe FISH showing localized deletion of chr 13q14 (loss of one red probe) with the normal two signals at 13q34 (blue). **D:** Results of array comparative genomic hybridization (CGH) in CLL show variably sized deletions spanning the ATM locus at 11q23. All cases illustrated also showed either one or two deletions detected by the 11q23/ATM probe by FISH analysis.

In the more aggressive tumor types, namely LBL/ALL in adults and DLBCL, molecular prognostic assays might be expected to have patient impact. In DLBCL, this has led to the development of microarray and PCR gene expression panels to molecular stratify subgroups that have a worse outcome with conventional combination immunotherapy–chemotherapy and may therefore benefit from dose intensification or alternate treatment strategies such as stem cell transplant.[16] However, these efforts have not yet become standard practice, but some centers utilize immunohistochemical detection of some of these prognostic markers, namely CD10, BCL6, BCL2, and IRF4. MUM1 in an analogous prognostic panel in DLBCL.

In B-LBL/ALL, the current standard therapy includes five or more drugs in complex chemotherapy regimens so a primary goal of molecular diagnostics is to identify those patients with poor prognostic subtypes who may need higher drug concentrations or longer maintenance therapy to prevent relapse. In childhood ALL/LBL, this has led to the development of two different types of assays that can be used to individualize therapy.

As discussed above, the particular type of chromosomal translocation observed in B-ALL/LBL can impart differing risks of relapse. Therefore, an efficient approach to diagnosis and risk stratification in childhood ALL/LBL is FISH panels that include detection of 11q23/MLL alteration, t(1;19)/TCF3-PBX1, t(12;21)/TEL-RUNX1, and t(9;22)/BCR-ABL1 gene rearrangements, with inclusion of additional chromosome copy number probes that identify hyperdiploid and hypodiploid groups that have prognostic significance. Expression microarrays have also proven successful in identifying all of these cytogenetic risk groups in a robust fashion[17,18] and may be a more efficient diagnostic test but have not yet become a routine diagnostic test.

The second type of testing used in childhood ALL/LBL has been the detection of inherited/germline differences in the structure and expression pattern of drug-metabolizing genes. This pharmacogenomic approach is aimed at identifying constitutional genomic contributions to drug levels including intracellular levels in tumor cells that may compromise the effectiveness of chemotherapy. Genes that are most commonly assessed are drug-conjugating enzymes such as glutathione S-transferase isoforms and thiopurine S-methyltransferase that influence handling of mercaptopurine and thioguanine levels.[19] Similarly, methotrexate activity can be influenced by single nucleotide polymorphisms (SNPs) in two of its targets, dihydrofolate reductase and thymidylate synthase. These SNP studies are currently performed only at a few large centers but may become standard in future years.

Although population-based polymorphisms in the Fc gamma receptor genes are present that can influence the efficacy and half-life of immunotherapy agents such as rituximab,[20] their detection in routine clinical settings for B-LPDs has been limited to date. Similarly, common SNPs in cytokine and immune response genes likely influence outcome in B-cell lymphomas[21] but have not been routinely identified in clinical practice.

T-CELL LYMPHOPROLIFERATIVE DISORDERS

Normal T-Cell Biology and Its Relationship to Lymphoma

Thymic-derived lymphocytes, abbreviated as T cells throughout this chapter, have many different functions in the immune system that are determined not only by the type of T-cell receptor (TCR) that they bear on their surface but also on their pattern of cytokine secretion. During maturation within the thymus, T cells undergo sequential and programmed rearrangement of their TCR genes (first the TCR-γ chain, then δ, then β, then α) in order to generate functional and properly folded TCRs with a particular antigen specificity on their surface. This clonotypic TCR is tried out for the ability to signal properly (termed "positive selection") in the thymic cortex. In the thymic medullae, autoreactive T cells are then eliminated if the expressed TCR binds to human leukocyte antigen (HLA) complexes too avidly (i.e., autoreactive T cells) or signals too strongly in the absence of any antigen (termed "negative selection"). Mature T cells emerging from the thymus thus expresses either a clonotypic TCR-α/β or a TCR-γ/δ receptor, although all mature T cells exhibit TCR-γ genomic rearrangement in their DNA reflective of the initial common process of TCR generation.

Subsequent maturation of T cells is related to their encounters with cognate antigens in tissues, and the cytokine milieu of the tissues they migrate within which imprints a progressively more committed functional phenotype on each T cell over time. Therefore, TCR-α/β+ T cells have many different functional subsets including helper CD4+ forms that stimulate B-cell expansion and CD4+CD25+ regulatory T cells that suppress B-cell and T-cell expansion. The CD8+ TCR-α/β+ and CD4– CD8– TCR-γ/δ+ T cells comprise mostly cytotoxic cells that can destroy foreign cells that lack native HLA molecules or those that have an abnormal pattern of killer inhibitor receptor expression, such as seen in viral transformation. These latter cells along with natural killer cells comprise most of the cytotoxic large granular lymphocytes (LGLs) commonly seen in peripheral blood in reactive conditions. Given their TCR structure and more limited antigen-binding repertoire, γ-δ-T cells respond mostly to common microbial glycolipid and glycoprotein antigens presented by dendritic cells. This restricted TCR repertoire allows these cells (termed the innate immune system) to rapidly modulate immune responses without the need for the slower antibody maturation responses described above for B cells.

Diagnostic Categories of T-Cell Neoplasms

For a variety of reasons, T-cell neoplasms are much less common than B-cell neoplasms and mostly arise following many years of abnormal immune dysregulation, such as can occur with chronic allergic states or autoimmune conditions. A classical example of this pathogenesis is

TABLE 35-4 T-Cell and NK-Cell Lymphoproliferative Disorders (2008 WHO Classification)

T-cell prolymphocytic leukemia
T-cell large granular lymphocytic leukemia
Chronic lymphoproliferative disorder of NK cells[a]
Aggressive NK-cell leukemia
Systemic EBV+ T-cell lymphoproliferative disease of childhood (associated with chronic active EBV infection)
Hydroa vacciniforme–like lymphoma
Adult T-cell leukemia/lymphoma
Extranodal NK/T-cell lymphoma, nasal type
Enteropathy-associated T-cell lymphoma
Hepatosplenic T-cell lymphoma
Subcutaneous panniculitis–like T-cell lymphoma
Mycosis fungoides
Sézary syndrome
Primary cutaneous CD30+ T-cell lymphoproliferative disorder
Lymphomatoid papulosis
Primary cutaneous anaplastic large cell lymphoma
Primary cutaneous aggressive epidermotropic CD8+ cytotoxic T-cell lymphoma[a]
Primary cutaneous γ–δ-T-cell lymphoma
Primary cutaneous small/medium CD4+ T-cell lymphoma[a]
Peripheral T-cell lymphoma, not otherwise specified
Angioimmunoblastic T-cell lymphoma
Anaplastic large cell lymphoma (ALCL), ALK+
Anaplastic large cell lymphoma (ALCL), ALK−[a]

[a]Provisional entities.

LGL leukemia, a low-grade T-LPD usually arising from CD8+ T-cell LGLs, some of which can be demonstrated to have specificity against cytomegalovirus (CMV) antigens.[22] Thus, the presumed mechanism of transformation is gradual expansion due to periodic or reactivated chronic CMV infection, followed by genetic transforming events.

Unlike the largely morphogenetic classification used for B-LPDs, T-LPD classification schema rely on a mixture of genetic alterations, predominant tissue site of involvement, and immunophenotype (Table 35.4). With the exception of T-LBL, which arises from thymic T-cell precursors, and some anaplastic large cell lymphomas (ALCL), most T-LPDs affect older adults. This is likely because most evolve slowly out of the preexisting reactive T-cell expansions, similarly to LGL leukemia. Most T-LPDs have a CD4+ TCR-α/β immunophenotype with TCR-γ/δ+ and CD8+ T-cell neoplasms being much rarer.

T-cell lymphomas involving the skin are the most common. Cutaneous entities include the epidermotropic mycosis fungoides (MF), which typically evolves out of chronic (atopic) dermatitis and progresses through plaque and tumor stages in skin before spreading to lymph node and blood as Sézary syndrome.[23] An unusual T-cell neoplasm is cutaneous CD30+ T-LPD which usually starts as spontaneously regressing lymphomatoid papulosis before evolving into a variant of ALCL. These tumors, despite their anaplastic appearance, remain confined to the skin except in rare circumstances and have a good outcome. Some cutaneous ALCL cases have translocations involving the IRF4 gene[24,25] but the etiology of the others remains unclear as of this date.

An epitheliotropic intestinal lymphoma, enteropathy-associated T-cell lymphoma (EATL) typically evolves from celiac disease and/or lymphocytic gastritis.[26] Although it appears to have a similar antigen-driven, slowly evolving pathogenesis as MF, EATL is usually diagnosed at late stage (often following bowel perforation) and has a poor outcome. T-cell gene rearrangement studies can be helpful in the earlier low-grade stages of EATL in dissecting evolving lymphoma from polyclonal celiac disease or other causes of enteropathy.

Among T-LPDs involving lymph node, some cases present as monomorphous high-grade lesions (such as systemic ALCL) and others show evolution from lower grade lesions, particularly angioimmunoblastic T-cell lymphoma (AITL) and its perifollicular variants.[27] Molecular heterogeneity within each group is common such as with ALCL, where a variant that shows gene fusions involving the ALK tyrosine kinase has a good outcome and occurs in younger patients. In contrast, systemic ALCL cases that lack this alteration occur in older patients and behave more aggressively.[28]

T-LPDs expressing TCR-γ/δ are rare and include hepatosplenic[29] and cutaneous variants[30] that probably reflect expansions of the different γ–δ-T-cell populations that are normally resident at those sites. For these tumors, in addition to surface TCR-γ/δ immunophenotyping (usually performed by flow cytometry), the pattern of disease involvement is critical to accurate prognostication.[31]

Molecular Diagnostic Testing for Diagnosis of T-LPDs

Like with B-LPDs, a major challenge in the diagnosis of T-LPDs is separating benign T-cell expansions from significant clonal disorders. Unlike with B-cell neoplasms, no unequivocal immunophenotyping assay is currently available to establish T-cell clonality. The most helpful immunophenotypic feature of T-LPDs by flow cytometry or IHC is their tendency to lose expression of one or more commonly expressed (pan-T) antigens, such as CD2, CD3, CD5, and CD7, but this feature is often not seen in the earliest stages of T-LPDs.

FISH analysis is highly useful in the diagnosis of ALK-translocated ALCL and TCL1+ T-cell prolymphocytic leukemia (T-PLL) that show t(14;14) or inv(14). FISH analysis can also be used for diagnosis and subtyping of T-ALL/LBL which have chromosomal translocations that juxtapose the TCR promoters with HOX transcriptional factors that are responsible for blocking the maturation of the tumor beyond the thymic stage (Table 35.5). However, most post-thymic T-LPDs lack defining chromosomal alterations. Therefore, FISH is much less helpful for diagnosis in general than in B-LPDs.

TABLE 35–5 Genetic Alterations in T-Cell Lymphoproliferative Disorders

T-LPD Type	Molecular Aberrations	Diagnostic Assays
T-LBL/ALL	NOTCH mutation	DNA sequencing
	Translocations involving TCRA/14q11 and TCRB enhancers	TCRA FISH (BA)
		Fusion gene PCR panels
T-PLL	TCL1A activation through t(14;14)(q11;q32.1) or inv14(q11;q32.1)	TCL1 FISH (BA)
AITL/PTCL	SYK translocations (~10%)	FISH or PCR
ALCL, systemic	ALK/2p23 translocations	ALK FISH (BA)
ALCL, cutaneous	IRF4 translocations (10–30% of cutaneous ALCL/MF cases)	IRF4 FISH (BA)

Abbreviations as in text and Table 35.3.

Therefore, PCR analysis of the TCR genes is a much more critical element of the diagnosis of T-LPDs (Fig. 35.4). As with IGH PCR, TCR PCR using either the TCR-γ locus or the TCR-β locus allows the separate lesions into polyclonal (multiple peaks), monoclonal (one or two peaks), or oligoclonal (three or more discrete peaks) proliferations. Given the natural history of many T-LPDs such as MF, EATL, T-LGL, and AITL that often arise from preexisting reactive T-cell expansions, oligoclonality is much more common in T-cell disorders.[32] Therefore, the correlation between clinically significant T-cell lesions and clonality identified by PCR studies is not absolute and these studies must be interpreted with caution.[23]

Molecular Prognostic and Predictive Markers in Therapy of T-LPDs

With the exception of MF, cutaneous CD30+ T-LPDs, T-cell LGL leukemia, and ALK-translocated ALCL, most T-LPDs behave very aggressively. Treatments are also not particularly efficacious and typically involved multiagent chemotherapy followed by stem cell transplantation, if adequate disease control can be obtained.

Because of this poor outcome, treatment of T-LPDs has recently become an active area of investigation to uncover new targeted and biologic therapies with personalized approaches quite common. These therapies have

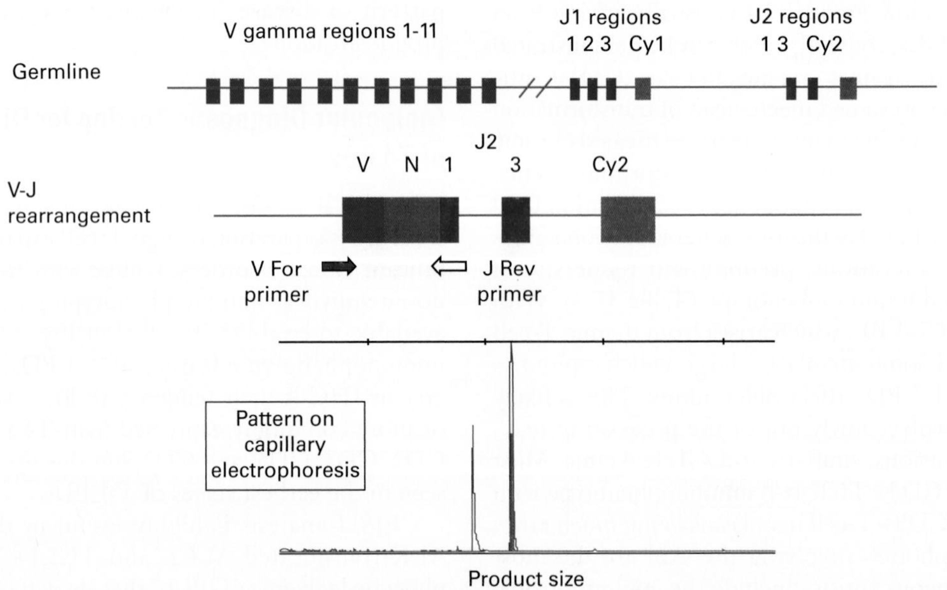

FIGURE 35–4 Principle of T-cell clonality assessment. (**Top**) Schematic representations of the TCRG locus on chromosome 7. The variable region (V) segments are shown in green with the joining region (J) segments depicted in blue. (**Middle**) A complete clonotypic V–J rearrangement shown with the clone-specific unique template-independent region in red (N) added during the DNA break-ligation process. The location of the primer used in the TCRG PCR assay, with the forward primer (for) annealing to the V region and the reverse primer (rev) annealing to the J region. The constant regions (Cγ1 and Cγ2) do not get fused to V–J sequences in the DNA but are spliced together during RNA processing to generate the functional TCR-γ chain (not shown). (**Bottom**) Results of a TCRG PCR assay with a clonal rearrangement are shown. Two distinct clonal peaks (representing the two rearranged TCRG alleles present in the neoplastic T-cell clone) are detected by fragment analysis when fluorochrome-labeled PCR products are analyzed by capillary electrophoresis following PCR with peak height proportional to the intensity of the signal.

TABLE 35-6 Targetable Pathways in T-Cell Neoplasms Under Investigation

Tumor Type	Target	Therapy Type
T-LBL/ALL	NOTCH	Secretase inhibitors
ALCL	CD30	Immunotherapy (brentuximab vedotin)
PTCL/AITL	SYK, LCK, TCR pathway	Kinase inhibitors
MF	CD25	Immunotoxins (denileukin diftitox)
ATLL/MF	CCR4	Immunotherapy

Abbreviations as in text. All of these therapies are currently investigational and not standard FDA-approved therapies with the exception of denileukin diftitox for MF.

included immunotherapy against T-cell antigens such as CD25,[33] CD30,[34] and CCR4[35] and epigenetic modulation with histone deacetylase inhibitors. Other potential targetable alterations in T-LPDs include the ALK kinase in ALCL, PTCLs with activated LYN and SYK,[36] and AKT activation in TCL1-translocated T-PLL.[37] Table 35.6 summarizes some of these approaches.

MYELOID AND OTHER BONE MARROW–DERIVED NEOPLASMS

Normal Hematopoiesis and Its Relationship to Myeloid Leukemias

The principal hematopoietic constituents in bone marrow include precursor B cells and myeloid forms that develop into granulocytes (comprising neutrophils, eosinophils, basophils, and mast cells), monocytes/macrophages, and classical and plasmacytoid dendritic cells. The erythroid lineage leads to the anucleate red blood cells (erythrocytes) and the megakaryocytes mature into platelets upon cell fragmentation.

Hematopoiesis is initiated in a pluripotent stem cell or blast that then undergoes subsequent lineage commitment with expansion of the different bone marrow compartments at different rates, related to the lifetime and condition of their mature counterparts (Fig. 35.5).

Diagnostic Categories of Bone Marrow–Derived Neoplasms

Bone marrow–derived neoplasms are distinct from most mature lymphoid tumors in that the initiating neoplastic alteration often appears to involve an early/pluripotent stem cell precursor/blast[38] that has the capability to affect maturation and proliferation in myeloid, monocytic, erythroid, and megakaryocytic lineages simultaneously (see Fig. 35.5). So although pure erythroid or megakaryocytic tumors are quite rare, pre-leukemic myelodysplastic syndromes (MDSs) affecting all of these lineages are very common. Similarly, although proliferative neoplasms involving bone marrow elements almost always lead to some degree of leukocytosis, the other lineages are also usually differentially involved. Furthermore, the same molecular genetic change is often present in tumor types that have different histomorphologic findings, clinical presentation, and therapeutic approaches.

Despite this shared pathogenesis, myeloid tumors are divided into cases of acute myeloid leukemia (AML) that show impairment in maturation beyond the blast stage and (chronic) myeloproliferative neoplasms (MPNs) that show unregulated growth but largely intact maturation (Table 35.7). These differences reflect the underlying initiating molecular alteration, with AML having a variety of different chromosomal gene fusions and inactivating and activating mutations in myeloid differentiation genes that block maturation in the tumor at a particular stage of maturation. The specific regulatory gene(s) affected drives

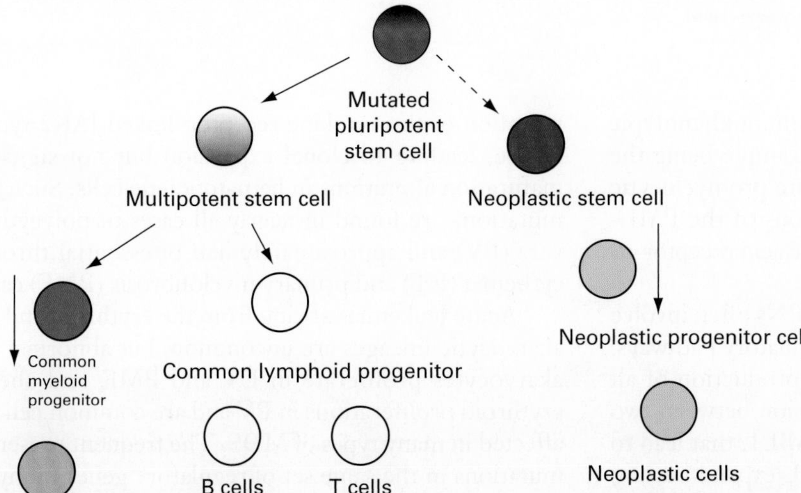

FIGURE 35–5 Stem cell properties of bone marrow neoplasms. Schematic representation of the development of "normal" and leukemic clones before and after DNA damage or mutation in a pluripotent stem cell. Depending on the particular alteration in the pluripotent stem cell, differential expansions of particular cell lineages may occur producing different bone marrow neoplasms. Further mutations may arise in expanded leukemic stem cell populations at later stages of maturation influencing the transformation to acute leukemia and the neoplasm doubling time.

TABLE 35–7 Myeloid and Related Neoplasms Involving the Blood and Bone Marrow (2008 WHO Classification)

MPN
Chronic myelogenous leukemia, *BCR-ABL1* positive
Chronic neutrophilic leukemia
Polycythemia vera
Primary myelofibrosis
Essential thrombocythemia
Chronic eosinophilic leukemia, NOS
Mastocytosis
MPNs, unclassifiable
Myeloid and lymphoid neoplasms associated with *PDGFRA* rearrangement
Myeloid neoplasms associated with *PDGFRB* rearrangement
Myeloid and lymphoid neoplasms associated with *FGFR1* abnormalities
MDS/MPN
Chronic myelomonocytic leukemia
Atypical chronic myeloid leukemia, *BCR-ABL1* negative
Juvenile myelomonocytic leukemia
MDS/MPN, unclassifiable
Provisional entity: refractory anemia with ring sideroblasts and thrombocytosis
MDS
Refractory cytopenia with unilineage dysplasia
Refractory anemia
Refractory neutropenia
Refractory thrombocytopenia
Refractory anemia with ring sideroblasts
Refractory cytopenia with multilineage dysplasia
Refractory anemia with excess blasts
MDS with isolated del(5q)
MDS, unclassifiable
Childhood MDS
Provisional entity: refractory cytopenia of childhood
AML and related neoplasms
AML with recurrent genetic abnormalities
AML with t(8;21)(q22;q22); *RUNX1-RUNX1T1*
AML with inv(16)(p13.1q22) or t((16;16)(p13.1;q22); *CBFB-MYH11*
APL with t(15;17)(q22;q12); *PML-RARA*
AML with t(9;11)(p22;q23); *MLLT3-MLL*
AML with t(6;9)(p23;q34); *DEK-NUP214*
AML with inv(3)(q21q26.2) or t(3;3)(q21;q26.2); *RPN1-EVI1*
AML (megakaryoblastic) with t(1;22)(p13;q13); *RBM15-MKL1*
Provisional entity: AML with mutated NPM1
Provisional entity: AML with mutated CEBPA
AML with myelodysplasia-related changes
Therapy-related myeloid neoplasms
AML, NOS
AML with minimal differentiation
AML without maturation
AML with maturation
Acute myelomonocytic leukemia
Acute monoblastic/monocytic leukemia
Acute erythroid leukemia
Pure erythroid leukemia
Erythroleukemia, erythroid/myeloid
Acute megakaryoblastic leukemia
Acute basophilic leukemia
Acute panmyelosis with myelofibrosis
Myeloid sarcoma
Myeloid proliferations related to Down syndrome
Transient abnormal myelopoiesis
Myeloid leukemia associated with Down syndrome
Blastic plasmacytoid dendritic cell neoplasm
Acute leukemias of ambiguous lineage
Acute undifferentiated leukemia
Mixed phenotype acute leukemia with t(9;22)(q34;q11.2); *BCR-ABL1*
Mixed phenotype acute leukemia with t(v;11q23); *MLL* rearranged
Mixed phenotype acute leukemia, B/myeloid, NOS
Mixed phenotype acute leukemia, T/myeloid, NOS
Provisional entity: NK-cell lymphoblastic leukemia/lymphoma

MPN, myeloproliferative neoplasms; MDS/MPN, myelodysplastic syndrome/myeloproliferative neoplasms; MDS, myelodysplastic syndrome; AML, acute myeloid leukemia; NK, natural killer; NOS, not otherwise specified.

the characteristic morphologic and immunophenotypic properties of each AML subtype. An example being the predominance of promyelocytes in acute promyelocytic leukemia (APL/AML-M3) due to actions of the PML-RARA (promyelocytic leukemia–retinoic acid receptor-α) gene fusion blocking RAR signaling.[39]

Genetic alterations that produce MPNs often involve cytokine and tyrosine kinase growth regulatory pathways. CML, an MPN characterized by overproduction of all types of granulocytes, shows a gene fusion between two growth regulatory proteins, BCR and ABL1, that lead to cell stimulation. Myeloid forms in CML expand beyond the available marrow space and spill out into the blood. Similarly, another common alteration in MPNs involves mutation of the cytokine receptor–linked JAK2 tyrosine kinase, leading to clonal expansion but not significant maturation alterations in hematopoietic cells. Such JAK2 mutations are found in nearly all cases of polycythemia vera (PV) and approximately half of essential thrombocythemia (ET) and primary myelofibrosis (PMF) cases.[40]

Acute leukemias arising from the erythroid and megakaryocytic lineages are uncommon, but abnormal megakaryocytes proliferate in ET and PMF, and aberrant erythroid proliferations in PV and are common cell types affected in many types of MDS. The frequent presence of mutations in the same set of regulatory genes in myeloid neoplasms[41,42] has now led to diagnostic algorithms that incorporate mutation testing (Fig. 35.6).

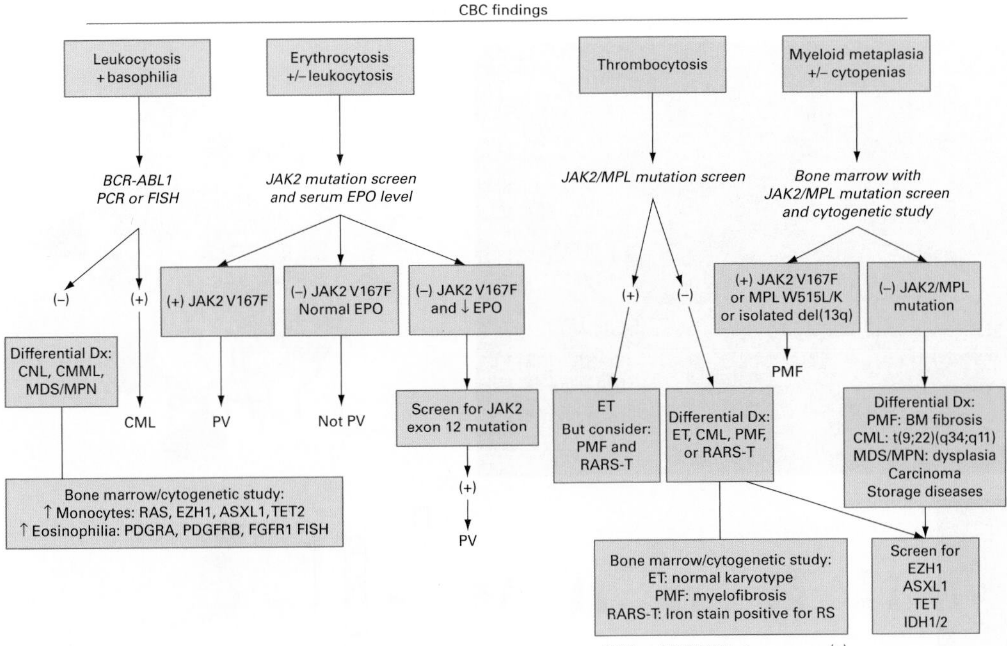

FIGURE 35–6 Algorithm for diagnosis of myeloproliferative neoplasms. Abbreviations as in text.

Testing for Diagnosis of Myeloid Malignancies

Stress conditions or peripheral consumption of blood cells lead to reactive expansions in the bone marrow that can often simulate neoplasms. Therefore, molecular and cytogenetic studies that can demonstrate a clonal alteration play a much larger role than immunophenotyping in the diagnosis of these tumor types.

Aside from ruling out a reactive condition, the primary tasks in diagnosis of myeloid neoplasms are placing a tumor in the correct WHO diagnostic category and the identification of any targetable tumor alteration that may influence initial therapy. In that regard, a number of myeloid malignancies are defined by the presence of gene fusions manifested by chromosomal translocations that can be detected by PCR or FISH.

Examples include the t(9;22)(q34;q11.2)/BCR-ABL1 fusion associated with CML (Fig. 35.7A), the t(15;17)(q22-24;q21)/PML-RARA in APL, and the t(8;21) and inv(16;16)/t(16;16) rearrangements in AMLs that involve the core-binding transcription factors. Another group of AMLs lack cytogenetically detectable gene fusions but instead have activating or inactivating mutations in transcriptional regulatory genes such as RUNX1, WT1, and CEBPA that can be detected by PCR-based DNA sequencing.[43,44]

Several common genetic alterations in AML are not associated with any particular WHO subtypes but provide a growth stimulus for many tumor types. Foremost among these is activation of the FLT3 tyrosine kinase, by point mutation or genomic duplications that lead to growth signaling. AML cases with tandem duplications in FLT3 that activate the kinase have adverse clinical outcome.[45] Other growth regulatory oncogenes include KIT, KRAS, and NRAS, each mutated in 5% to 10% of AML. More recently described mutations in TET2, DMNT3A, and ASXL1 affect the epigenetic program in myeloid cells and are commonly seen in both MDS and MPNs and the blast transformation of these neoplasms.[46]

Molecular Prognostic and Predictive Markers in Therapy of Myeloid Leukemias

In general, acute leukemias are treated with multiagent chemotherapy and chronic MPNs are treated with cytoreductive agents or biologic therapies that target rapidly dividing cells (e.g., lenalidomide) or stem cell transplantation when disease progression has occurred.

However, several myeloid leukemias have been treated successfully with targeted therapies that act on the specific molecular alteration in that tumor type. The foremost example has been the use of imatinib mesylate, a kinase inhibitor that selectively blocks the ABL1 kinase, in CML, which has led to dramatically improved outcomes. However, a small subset of patients with CML treated with imatinib become resistant to the drug through several different mechanisms (Fig. 35.7B). The most common of these resistance mechanisms is the emergence of point mutations in the BCR-ABL1 kinase that cause imatinib to fail to bind or to not inhibit the kinase effectively. Alternative kinases can be selected for therapy of such imatinib-resistant disease based on clinical experience or by matching the experimentally derived in vitro inhibitory properties of the kinase inhibitor to the specific mutation detected.[47]

Other mechanisms of imatinib resistance in CML include overexpression of BCR-ABL1 due to locus amplification, detectable by FISH, which may be overcome by dose escalation (Fig. 35.7C), and secondary genetic changes, detectable by cytogenetic or array comparative genomic hybridization analysis (Fig. 35.7D), which render the tumor resistant to imatinib. The latter changes are often related to accelerated or blast phases of CML.

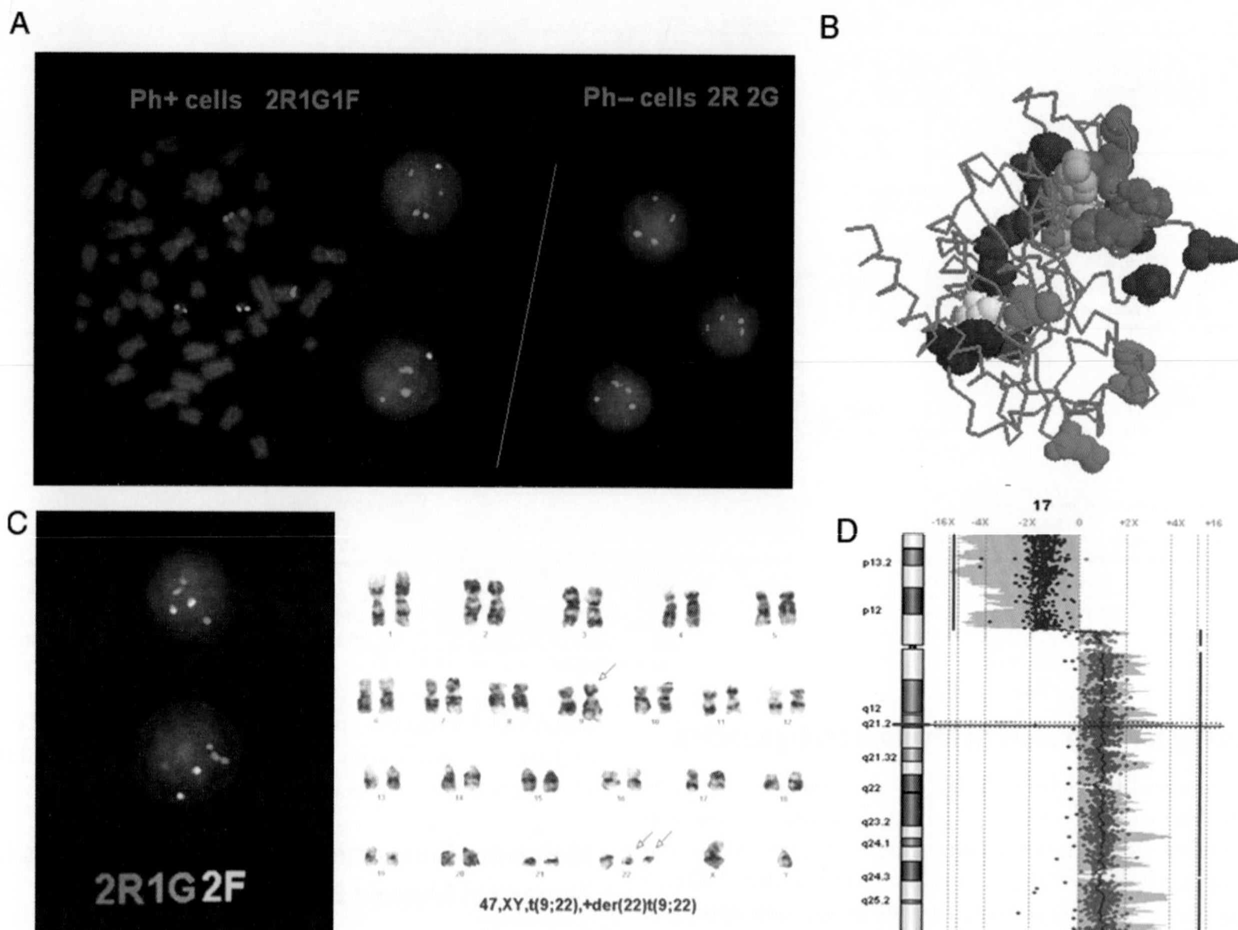

FIGURE 35–7 Diagnostic and prognostic assays in chronic myelogenous leukemia. **A:** Diagnosis of CML using fusion FISH. Left-sided figure shows chromosome spread and inset of cells with one RG fusion from red (ABL1 on 9q34) and green (BCR on 22q11) locus-specific probes associated with the presence of the t(9;22)/BCR-ABL chromosomal fusion. Right side shows 2R2G pattern in normal cells. **B:** Space-filling diagram of common ABL1 kinase domain mutations associated with imatinib-resistant chronic myeloid leukemia. Gray structure is imatinib present in the binding pocket. Green, codons mutated in the activation loop; blue, C-terminal loop mutated; magenta, P-loop mutation; brown, activation/catalytic domain mutations; white, SH2 contact area. **C:** Extra copy of the t(9;22) Philadelphia chromosome in a case of imatinib-resistant CML, as seen by fusion FISH (left, 2F2R1G pattern) and conventional karyotype. **D:** Pictogram of array CGH results in a case of imatinib-resistant CML demonstrating del17p associated with deletion of the TP53 locus.

Similar to imatinib, therapy for APL includes the RARA ligand all-*trans*-retinoic acid (ATRA) which relieves the PML-RARA–induced block in myeloid maturation and has resulted in high cure rates in this previously fatal leukemia, especially in combination with arsenic trioxide and immunotherapy.[48] Mechanisms of resistance to ATRA are not well characterized and occur only rarely. New targeted approaches to treatment for myeloid neoplasms have involved adding kinase inhibitors targeting FLT3 or other myeloid-expressed kinases to standard chemotherapy.[49]

BARRIERS TO TRULY PERSONALIZED THERAPY IN LYMPHOMAS AND LEUKEMIAS

In this chapter, we presented an overview of progress in understanding the biologic and genetic alterations underlying various types of leukemias and lymphomas. This understanding has occasionally led to dramatic improvements in therapies, such as in CML and APL. Indeed, the rapid adoption of imatinib for treatment of CML, becoming the nearly universal therapy within several years of availability, was a seminal event in the history of personalized therapy.[50] However, its success and that of ATRA in APL were exceptional due in part to the relative simplicity of the oncogenic alterations in these neoplasms and the favorable pharmacologic properties of kinase inhibitors and ATRA for treating indolent leukemias. However, treatment for more common and more aggressive leukemias and lymphomas has not progressed to individualized therapy to any substantial degree.

Such a personalized approach requires a set of readily available and affordable diagnostic assays that can localize the change(s) in the tumor genome and those in the patient's constitutional genome and epigenome that are critical in delivering an individualized treatment plan. This is a daunting task given the genomic and epigenomic complexity of many hematolymphoid neoplasms. The genomewide arrays and high-throughput sequencing approaches required for even a partial listing of targetable pathways within any leukemia or lymphoma are only now beginning to be developed for the routine clinical environment.

A desire for personalized therapy is also opposed by the trend toward more structured algorithmic approaches to treatment. Indeed, despite the large number of different tumor entities that comprise hematology, most therapeutic regimens developed for leukemias and lymphoma are currently standardized. This approach has been critical to improving outcomes since most leukemias and lymphomas are treated in the smaller regional medical centers and in private practice, and not in the highly specialized academic cancer centers that might be able to support an individualized approach.

Furthermore, since most oncologists even at very busy centers see very few of any given lymphoma and leukemia type in a year, they prefer standardized protocols where there is knowledge on how to manage the dosing and complications of complex regimens rather than customized/personalized therapies for each patient. This critical need for standardization will remain the principal barrier to the adoption of new therapeutic modalities in hematologic malignancies and slow the adoption of truly personalized therapies based on the particulars of any patient's tumor.

REFERENCES

1. Campo E, Swerdlow SH, Harris NL, Pileri S, Stein H, Jaffe ES. The 2008 WHO classification of lymphoid neoplasms and beyond: evolving concepts and practical applications. *Blood.* 2011;117(19):5019-5032.
2. Jaffe ES, Harris NL, Stein H, Isaacson PG. Classification of lymphoid neoplasms: the microscope as a tool for disease discovery. *Blood.* 2008;112(12):4384-4399.
3. Sinkovics JG. Molecular biology of oncogenic inflammatory processes. I. Non-oncogenic and oncogenic pathogens, intrinsic inflammatory reactions without pathogens, and microRNA/DNA interactions (review). *Int J Oncol.* 2012;40(2):305-349.
4. Jones D. Dismantling the germinal center: comparing the processes of transformation, regression, and fragmentation of the lymphoid follicle. *Adv Anat Pathol.* 2002;9(2):129-138.
5. Phan TG, Gray EE, Cyster JG. The microanatomy of B cell activation. *Curr Opin Immunol.* 2009;21(3):258-265.
6. Piccaluga PP, Agostinelli C, Gazzola A, et al. Pathobiology of Hodgkin lymphoma. *Adv Hematol.* 2011;2011:920898.
7. Stein H, Hummel M. Cellular origin and clonality of classic Hodgkin's lymphoma: immunophenotypic and molecular studies. *Semin Hematol.* 1999;36(3):233-241.
8. Evans PA, Pott C, Groenen PJ, et al. Significantly improved PCR-based clonality testing in B-cell malignancies by use of multiple immunoglobulin gene targets. Report of the BIOMED-2 Concerted Action BHM4-CT98-3936. *Leukemia.* 2007;21(2):207-214.
9. Langerak AW, Molina TJ, Lavender FL, et al. Polymerase chain reaction-based clonality testing in tissue samples with reactive lymphoproliferations: usefulness and pitfalls. A report of the BIOMED-2 Concerted Action BMH4-CT98-3936. *Leukemia.* 2007;21(2):222-229.
10. Willis TG, Dyer MJ. The role of immunoglobulin translocations in the pathogenesis of B-cell malignancies. *Blood.* 2000;96(3):808-822.
11. Wlodarska I, Dierickx D, Vanhentenrijk V, et al. Translocations targeting CCND2, CCND3, and MYCN do occur in t(11;14)-negative mantle cell lymphomas. *Blood.* 2008;111(12):5683-5690.
12. Stilgenbauer S, Sander S, Bullinger L, et al. Clonal evolution in chronic lymphocytic leukemia: acquisition of high-risk genomic aberrations associated with unmutated VH, resistance to therapy, and short survival. *Haematologica.* 2007;92(9):1242-1245.
13. Dohner H, Stilgenbauer S, James MR, et al. 11q deletions identify a new subset of B-cell chronic lymphocytic leukemia characterized by extensive nodal involvement and inferior prognosis. *Blood.* 1997;89(7):2516-2522.
14. Liebisch P, Viardot A, Bassermann N, et al. Value of comparative genomic hybridization and fluorescence in situ hybridization for molecular diagnostics in multiple myeloma. *Br J Haematol.* 2003;122(2):193-201.
15. Sargent R, Jones D, Abruzzo LV, et al. Customized oligonucleotide array-based comparative genomic hybridization as a clinical assay for genomic profiling of chronic lymphocytic leukemia. *J Mol Diagn.* 2009;11(1):25-34.
16. Lossos IS, Czerwinski DK, Alizadeh AA, et al. Prediction of survival in diffuse large-B-cell lymphoma based on the expression of six genes. *N Engl J Med.* 2004;350(18):1828-1837.
17. Ferrando AA, Look AT. DNA microarrays in the diagnosis and management of acute lymphoblastic leukemia. *Int J Hematol.* 2004;80(5):395-400.
18. Ferrando AA, Neuberg DS, Staunton J, et al. Gene expression signatures define novel oncogenic pathways in T cell acute lymphoblastic leukemia. *Cancer Cell.* 2002;1(1):75-87.
19. Cheok MH, Pottier N, Kager L, Evans WE. Pharmacogenetics in acute lymphoblastic leukemia. *Semin Hematol.* 2009;46(1):39-51.
20. Paiva M, Marques H, Martins A, Ferreira P, Catarino R, Medeiros R. FcgammaRIIa polymorphism and clinical response to rituximab in non-Hodgkin lymphoma patients. *Cancer Genet Cytogenet.* 2008;183(1):35-40.
21. Cerhan JR, Wang S, Maurer MJ, et al. Prognostic significance of host immune gene polymorphisms in follicular lymphoma survival. *Blood.* 2007;109(12):5439-5446.
22. Rossi D, Franceschetti S, Capello D, et al. Transient monoclonal expansion of CD8+/CD57+ T-cell large granular lymphocytes after primary cytomegalovirus infection. *Am J Hematol.* 2007;82(12):1103-1105.
23. Vega F, Luthra R, Medeiros LJ, et al. Clonal heterogeneity in mycosis fungoides and its relationship to clinical course. *Blood.* 2002;100(9):3369-3373.
24. Feldman AL, Law M, Remstein ED, et al. Recurrent translocations involving the IRF4 oncogene locus in peripheral T-cell lymphomas. *Leukemia.* 2009;23(3):574-580.
25. Pham-Ledard A, Prochazkova-Carlotti M, Laharanne E, et al. IRF4 gene rearrangements define a subgroup of CD30-positive cutaneous T-cell lymphoma: a study of 54 cases. *J Invest Dermatol.* 2010;130(3):816-825.
26. Delabie J, Holte H, Vose JM, et al. Enteropathy-associated T-cell lymphoma: clinical and histological findings from the international peripheral T-cell lymphoma project. *Blood.* 2011;118(1):148-155.
27. Warnke RA, Jones D, Hsi ED. Morphologic and immunophenotypic variants of nodal T-cell lymphomas and T-cell lymphoma mimics. *Am J Clin Pathol.* 2007;127(4):511-527.
28. Savage KJ, Harris NL, Vose JM, et al. ALK- anaplastic large-cell lymphoma is clinically and immunophenotypically different from both ALK+ ALCL and peripheral T-cell lymphoma, not otherwise specified: report from the International Peripheral T-Cell Lymphoma Project. *Blood.* 2008;111(12): 5496-5504.
29. Belhadj K, Reyes F, Farcet JP, et al. Hepatosplenic gammadelta T-cell lymphoma is a rare clinicopathologic entity with poor outcome: report on a series of 21 patients. *Blood.* 2003;102(13):4261-4269.
30. Jones D, Vega F, Sarris AH, Medeiros LJ. CD4-CD8-"Double-negative" cutaneous T-cell lymphomas share common histologic features and an aggressive clinical course. *Am J Surg Pathol.* 2002;26(2):225-231.
31. Garcia-Herrera A, Song JY, Chuang SS, et al. Nonhepatosplenic gammadelta T-cell lymphomas represent a spectrum of aggressive cytotoxic T-cell lymphomas with a mainly extranodal presentation. *Am J Surg Pathol.* 2011;35(8):1214-1225.
32. Sandberg Y, Heule F, Lam K, et al. Molecular immunoglobulin/T- cell receptor clonality analysis in cutaneous lymphoproliferations. Experience with the BIOMED-2 standardized polymerase chain reaction protocol. *Haematologica.* 2003;88(6):659-670.

33. Talpur R, Jones DM, Alencar AJ, et al. CD25 expression is correlated with histological grade and response to denileukin diftitox in cutaneous T-cell lymphoma. *J Invest Dermatol.* 2006;126(3):575-583.
34. Younes A, Bartlett NL, Leonard JP, et al. Brentuximab vedotin (SGN-35) for relapsed CD30-positive lymphomas. *N Engl J Med.* 2010;363(19):1812-1821.
35. Ishii T, Ishida T, Utsunomiya A, et al. Defucosylated humanized anti-CCR4 monoclonal antibody KW-0761 as a novel immunotherapeutic agent for adult T-cell leukemia/lymphoma. *Clin Cancer Res.* 2010;16(5):1520-1531.
36. Feldman AL, Sun DX, Law ME, et al. Overexpression of Syk tyrosine kinase in peripheral T-cell lymphomas. *Leukemia.* 2008;22(6):1139-1143.
37. Herling M, Patel KA, Teitell MA, et al. High TCL1 expression and intact T-cell receptor signaling define a hyperproliferative subset of T-cell prolymphocytic leukemia. *Blood.* 2008;111(1):328-337.
38. Jamieson CH, Barroga CF, Vainchenker WP. Miscreant myeloproliferative disorder stem cells. *Leukemia.* 2008;22(11):2011-2019.
39. Reiter A, Lengfelder E, Grimwade D. Pathogenesis, diagnosis and monitoring of residual disease in acute promyelocytic leukaemia. *Acta Haematol.* 2004;112(1-2):55-67.
40. Millecker L, Lennon PA, Verstovsek S, et al. Distinct patterns of cytogenetic and clinical progression in chronic myeloproliferative neoplasms with or without JAK2 or MPL mutations. *Cancer Genet Cytogenet.* 2010;197(1):1-7.
41. Jankowska AM, Makishima H, Tiu RV, et al. Mutational spectrum analysis of chronic myelomonocytic leukemia includes genes associated with epigenetic regulation: UTX, EZH2, and DNMT3A. *Blood.* 2011;118(14):3932-3941.
42. Tefferi A. Mutational analysis in BCR-ABL-negative classic myeloproliferative neoplasms: impact on prognosis and therapeutic choices. *Leuk Lymphoma.* 2010;51(4): 576-582.
43. Foran JM. New prognostic markers in acute myeloid leukemia: perspective from the clinic. *Hematology Am Soc Hematol Educ Program.* 2010;2010:47-55.
44. Schnittger S, Schoch C, Kern W, et al. Nucleophosmin gene mutations are predictors of favorable prognosis in acute myelogenous leukemia with a normal karyotype. *Blood.* 2005;106(12):3733-3739.
45. Santos FP, Jones D, Qiao W, et al. Prognostic value of FLT3 mutations among different cytogenetic subgroups in acute myeloid leukemia. *Cancer.* 2011;117(10):2145-2155.
46. Abdel-Wahab O, Manshouri T, Patel J, et al. Genetic analysis of transforming events that convert chronic myeloproliferative neoplasms to leukemias. *Cancer Res.* 2010;70(2): 447-452.
47. Jabbour E, Jones D, Kantarjian HM, et al. Long-term outcome of patients with chronic myeloid leukemia treated with second-generation tyrosine kinase inhibitors after imatinib failure is predicted by the in vitro sensitivity of BCR-ABL kinase domain mutations. *Blood.* 2009;114(10):2037-2043.
48. Ravandi F, Estey E, Jones D, et al. Effective treatment of acute promyelocytic leukemia with all-trans-retinoic acid, arsenic trioxide, and gemtuzumab ozogamicin. *J Clin Oncol.* 2009;27(4):504-510.
49. Prescott H, Kantarjian H, Cortes J, Ravandi F. Emerging FMS-like tyrosine kinase 3 inhibitors for the treatment of acute myelogenous leukemia. *Expert Opin Emerg Drugs.* 2011;16(3):407-423.
50. Hughes TP, Hochhaus A, Branford S, et al. Long-term prognostic significance of early molecular response to imatinib in newly diagnosed chronic myeloid leukemia: an analysis from the International Randomized Study of Interferon and STI571 (IRIS). *Blood.* 2010;116(19):3758-3765.

CHAPTER 36

MOLECULAR DIAGNOSTICS OF LYMPHOMAS

Keila Rivera-Roman and Christopher D. Gocke

INTRODUCTION

Lymphomas are the most common and most diverse group of hematopoietic malignancies, comprising 56% of all hematologic neoplasms. They represent a little over 5% of all cancers (excluding skin cancers) in the United States. Mature B-cell neoplasms are far more common than their T-cell and natural killer cell counterparts, representing more than 85% of all lymphomas. Follicular lymphoma (FL) and diffuse large B-cell lymphoma (DLBCL) taken together encompass 50% of mature lymphoid neoplasms in developed countries, while T/NK malignancies are more common in Asia than in western countries.

Molecular analysis of lymphoid neoplasms has become a fundamental portion in the workup of these diseases. Not only does molecular genetic analysis provide diagnostic information in most cases, but it also brings forth important prognostic information and is essential in the follow-up of these patients. On the other hand, molecular analysis should not be taken as the sole component of a lymphoid neoplasm workup. Other tools and modalities need to be considered in order to make a comprehensive diagnosis, including tumor cell morphology, immunophenotyping, and cytogenetics.

IMMUNOGLOBULIN AND T-CELL RECEPTOR GENE REARRANGEMENT

In order to achieve optimal reactivity when facing foreign pathogens, and simultaneously be prepared to distinguish self from non-self, the immune system and lymphocytes, specifically, undergo gene rearrangement of their antigen receptors in order to have a large number cells with a variable and diverse repertoire that could theoretically face any threat.

Immunoglobulin Gene Rearrangement

In order to be able to develop an appropriate variety of surface immunoglobulins (Ig) that will serve as antigen-binding receptors, gene rearrangement must occur from the germline (Fig. 36.1). The first step consists of recombination at the immunoglobulin heavy chain (IGH@) gene at chromosome 14q32.2 by splicing of a diversity (D) segment with a joining (J) segment as D–J arrangement occurs.[1] The end-joining process is imprecise, sometimes leading to deletion at the ends. To increase diversity further, non-templated bases are added between the D and J segments by the terminal deoxynucleotidyl transferase enzyme. The second step is the addition of a V region to the D–J segment that has already recombined. This joint also has additional bases randomly added or deleted, creating further diversity.

After heavy-chain gene recombination occurs, the next step is rearrangement at the immunoglobulin kappa light-chain locus (IGK@) on chromosome 2p12. Recombination only involves a V region and a J segment as the IGK@ does not contain a D region. It is important to note that if recombination at the first IGK@ allele fails, an attempt to form an Ig using the second allele will happen. If this fails as well, the cell will attempt to recombine one of the immunoglobulin lambda genes (IGL@) on chromosome 22q11.2, where rearrangement follows an identical process to the one occurring at IGK@.[2]

After rearrangement occurs, further diversity is introduced at and near the joints by the activation-induced deaminase protein in a process termed somatic hypermutation. Somatic hypermutation consists of point mutation and, perhaps, insertion and deletion of nucleotides in the hypervariable regions of each of the Ig genes.[3] In aggregate, these changes alter the composition and length of each individual Ig gene.

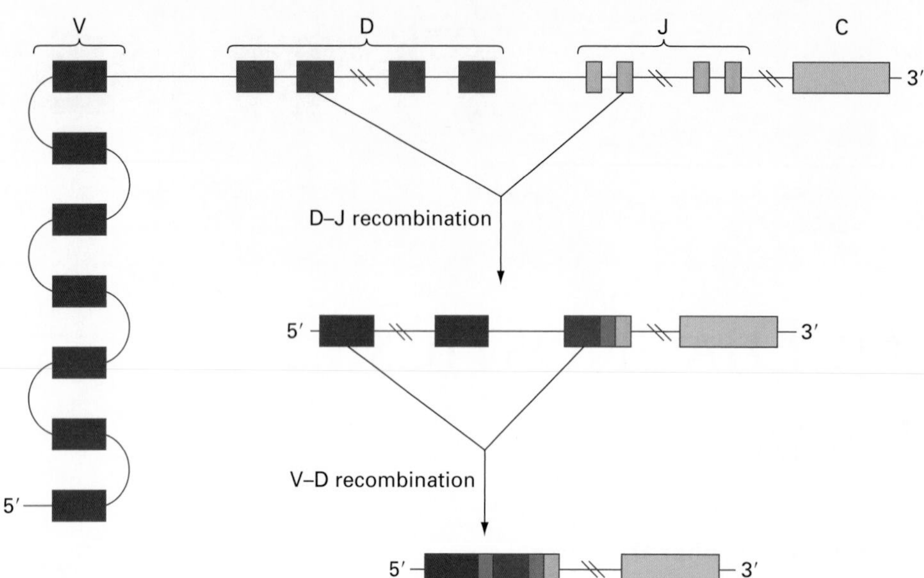

FIGURE 36–1 Schematic of a generic B-cell immunoglobulin or T-cell receptor rearrangement. The variable (V, plum), diversity (D, red), and joining (J, pink) regions are combined to create a single V–D–J segment. The constant region (C, green) is spliced in at transcription. Random nucleotides (in blue) may be inserted at the V–D and D–J junctions by the enzyme terminal deoxynucleotidyl transferase to produce further variability.

T-Cell Receptor Gene Rearrangement

The human genes for the γ- and β-subunits of the T-cell receptor (TCR) are located on the short and long arms of chromosome 7, respectively, whereas the δ- and α-chain genes are located on the centromeric half of the long arm of chromosome 14, with delta embedded within the alpha locus. Like their B-cell counterparts, TCR genes are also assembled through V(D)J segment recombination. There exist two possible TCR heterodimers: those with α- and β-polypeptides and those with γ- and δ-peptides (termed α/β or γ/δ, respectively). The vast majority of TCR proteins are of the α/β variety (roughly 95%).

The TCR V(D)J recombination process is guided by the lymphoid-specific recombinases (recombination activating genes, RAG1 and RAG2).[4] These enzymes make breaks in double-stranded DNA at recombination signal sequences that flank the V, D, and J gene segments. The order of gene rearrangement is generally as follows: δ (TRD@), γ (TRG@), β (TRB@), and α (TRA@). The α- and γ-peptides, much like their light-chain counterparts in B cells, do not contain D segments. TRD@ is the first to recombine, with V(D)J rearrangement, followed by TRG@ (with V–J joining only). In αβ-cells this is followed by TRB@ (V(D)J rearrangement as well) and TRA@ (like TRG@, only V–J joining occurs). As TRD@ is located within the TRA@ locus, if the final recombination of TRA@ happens, deletion of the TRD@ locus occurs.[5]

It is thought that following rearrangement and recombination events of the V, D, and J genes, the approximate diversity of molecules for Ig is 2×10^6, for TCRαβ is 3×10^6, and TCRγδ 5×10^3. With further random nucleotide excision and insertion that occurs following gene rearrangements, the full panoply of Ig and TCR units may be more than an astonishing 10^{125}.[6]

Historically, clonality assays were performed using Southern blot analysis (Fig. 36.2). Named after British scientist Edwin Southern, the method uses restriction endonucleases to cut high molecular weight DNA at conserved sites throughout the human genome. The DNA is electrophoresed through an agarose gel to separate according to the fragment size and then transferred ("blotted") to a nylon membrane by capillary action. The membrane is then heated or exposed to ultraviolet radiation in order to permanently bind the DNA to the membrane. This is followed by hybridization of the DNA on the membrane to target-specific probes (probes are usually radioactively or fluorescently labeled) and detection of the appropriate sequence (target-probe hybrid) with film or a fluorescence detector. If the assay is performed using carefully chosen enzymes and probes for detection, nearly all Ig and TCR gene arrangements are detectable. This approach is most useful for the detection of IGH@, IGK@, and TRB@ rearrangements due to the extensive repertoire of combinations available in these genes.[7] The same utility is not achievable using TRG@ and TRD@ rearrangements due to the limited repertoire of combinatorial possibilities in these two genes.

Important caveats to this gold standard in clonality studies are the hands-on time involved in the assay, resulting in turnaround times of days to weeks, and the need for very high quality, high molecular weight DNA, which almost always must be obtained from fresh tissue. In addition, exposure to radiation in various forms (ultraviolet light and radioactive probes) poses an occupational hazard. Fluorescent probes are used in place of radioactive ones, but there is usually a trade-off in sensitivity. False-negative results with Southern blotting analysis are a problem because of the relatively low detection limit of the assay (approximately 10% clonal molecules among all target molecules must be present to recognize a band).

Currently, polymerase chain reaction (PCR) techniques have replaced Southern blotting for the detection

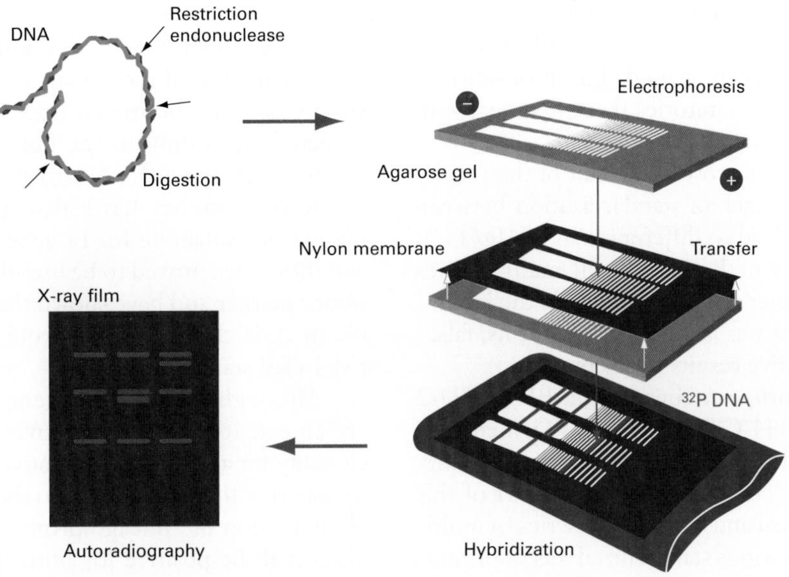

FIGURE 36–2 Southern blot analysis.

of clonal Ig and TCR gene rearrangements.[8] PCR—developed in 1983 by Kary Mullis during a moonlit inspirational drive—utilizes the concept of thermal cycling, consisting of cycles of repeated heating and cooling of a reaction mixture, in order to permit DNA melting, oligonucleotide primer annealing, and enzymatic replication by a thermostable polymerase. Primers complementary to the target sequence are included in the reaction mixture. As PCR progresses, the DNA generated is itself used as a template for replication, resulting in exponential amplification of the target sequence. In this way, billions of copies of short stretches of the target molecule are created (Fig. 36.3).

For antigen receptor clonality determination, primers straddling the Ig or TCR of interest are manufactured. These typically include an upstream (V or D region) and a downstream (J region) pair.[9] Commonly, a "consensus" oligonucleotide that is homologous or partly homologous to the targets is used. For example, there are six IGHJ regions; because they are evolutionarily related, the most homologous portion of each IGHJ is selected for primer design. The resulting PCR primer may not match any single IGHJ precisely, but will have only one or a few base mismatch with each so that hybridization during PCR is possible by appropriate adjustment of the annealing temperature. There are several advantages to PCR-based analysis with respect to Southern blotting. Turnaround time is significantly reduced (often to a few days), and this assay is more cost-effective, especially in a high-volume lab. In addition, because of the power of replicating billions of copies of the target, radioactive materials are no longer needed. Blood or fresh tissue are suitable substrates, as with Southern analysis. However, a substantial

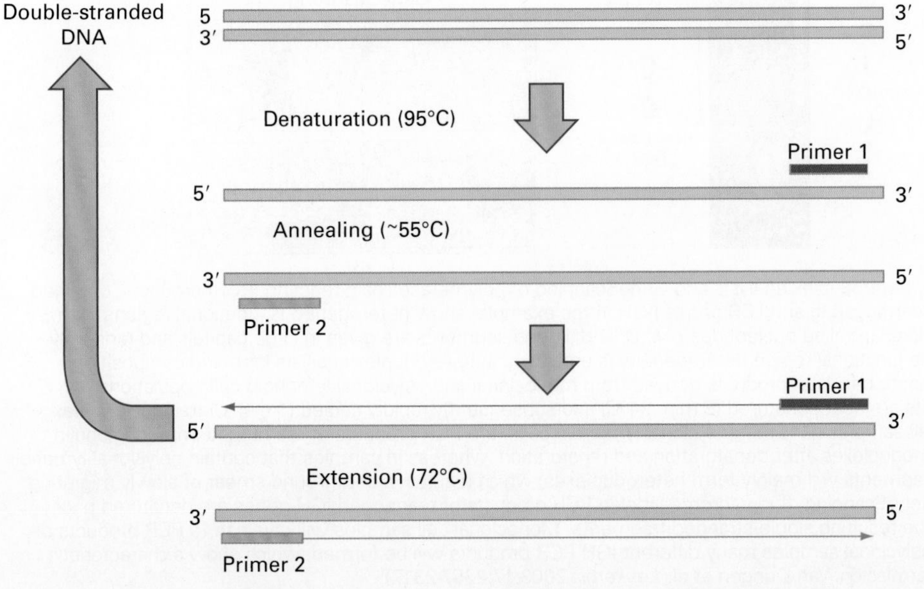

FIGURE 36–3 Polymerase chain reaction. A template molecule (double-stranded DNA) is used. The two strands are separated by a denaturing step at high temperature. The temperature is lowered and primers to a segment of interest are annealed to each single strand. By increasing the temperature once more, a DNA polymerase extends the primers in the directions indicated. This cycle is repeated 25–45 times to produce billions of copies of the segment of interest.

limitation of Southern blotting (high molecular weight DNA) no longer holds, so paraffin-embedded tissue that has been fixed in formalin can be used. This is of substantial benefit to pathology laboratories that often deal with consultation or archived samples.[10]

Historically, problems arose as a result of the variety of primers used and the lack of standardization between different labs, and this lead to differences in the Ig/TCR rearrangement profiles of B- and T-cell malignancies depending on what primer sets and conditions the laboratory performing the test was using. Because of this, false-negative and false-positive results were common.

In the 1990s, a European consortium, BIOMED-2 Concerted Action BMH4-CT98-3936, was formed with the aim of establishing standards for PCR-based clonality testing of B-cell and T-cell malignancies. As part of this effort, the group designed and developed a series of multiplex PCR assays using various standardized sets of primers for Ig and TCR gene rearrangement analysis. A total of 107 primers were developed, to be multiplexed in only 18 PCR reactions, including three VH–JH, two DH–JH, two IGK@, one IGL@, three TRB@, two TRG@, one TRD@, three BCL1-IGH@ and one BCL2-IGH@. They reported that using a combination of IGH@ and IGK@ primer tubes, nearly all clonal rearrangements in B-cell lymphoid populations can be detected (Fig. 36.4). A combination of TRB@ and TRG@ primers mirrors these results for T-cell lymphoid lesions. This is an important advance in clinical molecular diagnosis; the clinical sensitivity is much improved (nearly all clonal lesions are detected, according to the authors) as is the technical sensitivity (may reach a 5% to 10% limit of detection).[11]

Recent studies have also investigated the use of plasma as a substrate for Ig gene clonal rearrangements, and these have proved to be useful as a lymphoma-specific tumor marker and have shown that patients who are unable to clear clonal Ig DNA from plasma may be at high risk to fail standard therapy.[12]

Although Ig and TCR gene rearrangement studies are an essential part in the investigation of lineage and clonality for a lymphoproliferative process, it is important to note that there are pitfalls to their interpretation.[13] The phenomenon of "lineage promiscuity," in which a neoplasm will be positive for both Ig and TCR gene rearrangements, has long been recognized in the field. This challenges an overly simplistic conception of lymphocyte development and maturation. The standard example of this is precursor B- or T-cell leukemias, which frequently exhibit gene rearrangements of the heterologous cell type.[14] Occasional examples of non-lymphoid malignancies bearing antigen receptor gene rearrangements are also reported.[15] Of course, different lineage rearrangements

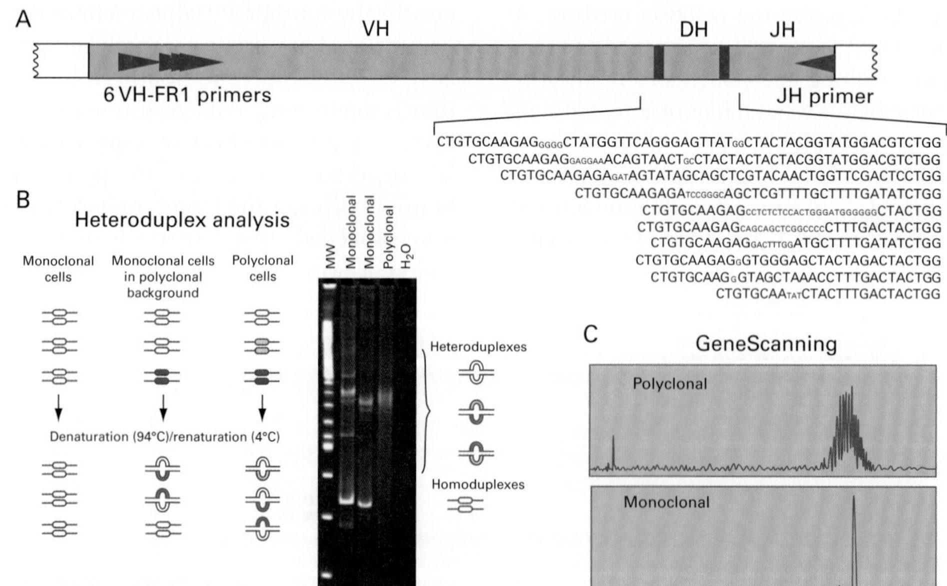

FIGURE 36–4 Schematic diagram of heteroduplex analysis and GeneScanning of polymerase chain reaction (PCR) products, obtained from rearranged Ig and TCR genes. **A:** Rearranged Ig and TCR genes (IGH in the example) show heterogeneous junctional regions with respect to size and nucleotide composition. Germline nucleotides of V, D, and J gene segments are given in large capitals and randomly inserted nucleotides in small capitals. The junctional region heterogeneity is employed in heteroduplex analysis (size and composition) and GeneScanning (size only) to discriminate between products derived from monoclonal and polyclonal lymphoid cell populations.
B: In heteroduplex analysis, PCR products are heat denatured (5 min, 94°C) and subsequently rapidly cooled (1 h, 4°C) to induce duplex (homo- or heteroduplex) formation. In cell samples consisting of clonal lymphoid cells, the PCR products of rearranged immunoglobulin heavy chain (IGH) genes give rise to homoduplexes after denaturation and renaturation, whereas in samples that contain polyclonal lymphoid cell populations the single-strand PCR fragments will mainly form heteroduplexes, which result in a background smear of slowly migrating fragments upon electrophoresis. **C:** In GeneScanning, fluorochrome-labeled PCR products of rearranged IGH genes are denatured prior to high-resolution fragment analysis of the resulting single-stranded fragments. Monoclonal cell samples will give rise to PCR products of identical size (single peak), whereas in polyclonal samples many different IGH PCR products will be formed, which show a characteristic Gaussian size distribution. (Used with permission, Van Dongen et al. *Leukemia* 2003;17:2257-2317.)

may be detected in samples with dual or mixed lineages, in which two or more populations of malignant cells with different types of clonal rearrangements (both Ig and TCR) exist. Perhaps the biggest limitation to PCR-based gene rearrangement analysis is the lack of widely accepted interpretive standards. The BIOMED-2 consortium has emphasized the need for a comprehensive evaluation of patient findings when interpreting TCR or Ig electropherograms or heteroduplex analysis gels, including correlation with morphology and immunology studies.[16] However, interpretation of the molecular lab results continues to be a somewhat subjective act.

Finally, it is imperative to recognize that although a rearrangement study result is clearly clonal, it may not be diagnostic of a malignancy. The occurrence of oligoclonality, in which (usually) three or more obvious, otherwise clonal peaks are identified, may signal an exuberant immune response that may be associated with a reactive process or an autoimmune disease, among other causes. Pseudoclonality, in which a relative paucity of lymphocytes produces a single prominent peak with a lack of a polyclonal background, may also give false-positive results. In this case, the results are usually not reproducible. Lastly, there are clearly clonal lymphoid disorders (e.g., lymphomatoid papulosis and several pediatric B-cell "lymphomas") which have benign clinical behaviors. To avoid these pitfalls, it is highly recommended to clinically correlate all cases and establish a proper diagnosis in conjunction with other ancillary tests.

B-CELL LYMPHOMAS

Chronic Lymphocytic Leukemia/Small Lymphocytic Lymphoma (CLL/SLL)

CLL is the most common leukemia in adults. The term SLL refers to the non-leukemic (i.e., nodal or splenic) presentation of this entity. This neoplasm is composed of small, round, monomorphic B cells that usually co-express CD5 and CD23.[17] The neoplastic B cells show highly selected immunoglobulin heavy-chain variable region (IGHV) genes. Bone marrow and peripheral blood are commonly involved; lymph nodes and other extranodal sites may or may not be involved.

Although molecular diagnostic techniques are not usually necessary to confirm a case as CLL/SLL, they do have prognostic significance. Poor prognostic factors that have been established include CD38 antigen expression (usually performed by flow cytometric analysis), lack of IGHV mutation ("unmutated" status), and distinct cytogenetic abnormalities. Therapeutic decisions are usually determined by the genetic diagnosis in these cases.[18]

IGHV Status

In approximately one-half of CLL/SLL cases, IGHV analysis demonstrates an unmutated gene status, suggesting origin from a naïve B cell that has not undergone the maturational process of somatic hypermutation. DNA sequencing of the rearranged IGH@ gene is performed. An IGHV differing from published germline reference sequences by less than 2% of the sequenced bases is defined as unmutated and equal to or greater than 2% is defined as mutated. There is not uniformity in the literature with regard to these cutoffs. An unmutated status has historically correlated with a poorer clinical outcome.[19] CLL/SLL with mutated status, arising from putative post-germinal center B cells, by comparison, shows a better prognosis. Some studies, however, have shown that the distinction in outcome between mutated and unmutated IGHV CLL/SLL may be trumped by associated anomalies, such as CD38 positivity and TP53 mutations, as patients with normal TP53 function and absent CD38 antigen show better prognosis regardless of IGHV mutation status.

IGHV analysis is performed following extraction of total RNA from blood or bone marrow samples. The IGH@ gene is amplified by reverse transcription-PCR (RT-PCR) and sequenced by dideoxy chain termination cycle sequencing. Comparison is made to germline IGH@ sequences in several widely available databases.

Cytogenetic Anomalies

Fluorescence in situ hybridization (FISH) is the method of choice to identify cytogenetic abnormalities in lymphomas, although traditional metaphase spread cytogenetics are also usually performed. FISH employs fluorescent probes that bind to complimentary sequences on the cognate chromosomal locations. Fluorescence microscopy is then used to visualize the bound probes.

13q Deletions

When present as an isolated anomaly, 13q deletion portends the best prognosis in CLL/SLL. These patients usually have associated IGHV hypermutated status. A recent study published by Gladstone et al. shows that patients with del(13q) usually follow an indolent course only in those patients that have an IGHV mutated status, while those with unmutated IGHV and 13q deletion have a poor overall survival rate.[20]

Trisomy 12

Once believed to be the most common cytogenetic anomaly in CLL/SLL, trisomy 12 correlates with an intermediate clinical outcome. Patients usually have unmutated IGHV genes.

11q22-23 (ATM Locus) Deletions

Approximately one-third of CLL/SLL cases show mutations in the ATM locus, which is located at 11q22-23. These mutations are associated with a poor prognosis.

17p13.3 (TP53 Locus) Deletions

A small subset of CLL/SLL patients demonstrates deletions centered on the TP53 locus, in chromosome 17. This mutation predicts poor clinical outcome.

Follicular Lymphoma

FL affects older adults, and usually involves lymph nodes, but may involve spleen, bone marrow, blood, or occasionally an extranodal site such as skin or gastrointestinal (GI) tract. In about 70% to 95% of all cases a specific translocation, t(14;18)(q32;q31), is present. These translocations involve the BCL2 gene on 18q21 with the IGH gene on 14q32 and ultimately cause overexpression of BCL2, leading to lymphoma development. This is a common theme in lymphoma biology: an oncogene (BCL2 in the case of FL, BCL1 in mantle cell lymphoma [MCL]) is translocated to an antigen receptor locus (typically, an Ig gene in B-cell lymphomas and a TCR gene in T-cell lymphomas). The antigen receptor locus, acting in cis through enhancer elements active in lymphocytes, upregulates expression of the intact oncogene, resulting in malignant transformation. In the t(14;18), the majority of breakpoints occur in the major breakpoint cluster region (M-bcr), and the remaining ones occur in the minor breakpoint cluster region (m-bcr), intermediate cluster region (icr), 3′BCL2, and 5′mcr.[21]

The characteristic BCL2 t(14;18) rearrangement can be detected in a different variety of ways, including Southern blot analysis, FISH, and PCR. The BIOMED-2-developed PCR primers include standardized oligonucleotides for BCL2-IGH@ detection, which comprise a consensus JH primer and other primers that flank the known breakpoint cluster regions. In those cases where the specific BCL2-IGH@ breakpoint of the patient is identified, minimal residual disease by PCR analysis is possible.

Mantle Cell Lymphoma

MCL is composed of monotonous small- to medium-sized cells with minimally irregular nuclei in the majority of cases. This is a disease predominantly seen in older individuals and is commonly present in males. Although it most commonly affects lymph nodes, it also involves extranodal sites, particularly the GI tract (e.g., lymphomatous polyposis of the GI tract). Molecularly, MCL is identified by t(11;14) in which the CCDN1 locus on chromosome 11 is juxtaposed to the IGH@ gene on chromosome 14, resulting in overexpression of the cyclin D1 protein.[22] It is noteworthy that a translocation may not be unique to one type of lymphoma; for example, the t(11;14) is also seen in multiple myeloma.

The breakpoints on chromosome 11 are situated far from the CCDN1 gene. Close to one-third of MCL cases have a breakpoint within an 85-bp region called MTC, but the majority of cases will have breakpoints scattered across a large genomic area upstream of CCDN1. This fact makes detection of the fusion gene by PCR methods problematic, as only those patients with breakpoints at MTC will be able to be identified using a primer specific to this region. The preferred method of detection is FISH.

Diffuse Large B-cell Lymphoma

DLBCL is a lymphoid neoplasm composed of large B cells—with sizes up to twice those of a normal lymphocyte—and a diffuse growth pattern. It is usually a lymphoma of older individuals, although it may occur in children and younger adults. It is the most common non-Hodgkin lymphoma in the Western hemisphere. This neoplasm usually arises as a primary tumor; however, it may also represent a transformation of an existing low-grade lymphoma.

In the majority of cases of this entity, the neoplastic cell has undergone Ig rearrangement and somatic hypermutation. Mutations involving the BCL6 gene (at chromosome 3q27) are the most common in DLBCL.[23] Translocations involving this gene have been reported in approximately 40% of cases, with the most common partner being the IGH@ gene at 14q32. This type of anomaly results in transcriptional activation of genes involved in proliferation although, interestingly, it does not associate with overexpression of either the BCL6 mRNA or protein.

BCL6 overexpression can be detected by multiple modalities, including molecular methods. Real-time PCR has been the method of choice for quantitative techniques. Patients with high BCL6 levels have a better prognosis in terms of longer survival time when compared with those with low levels of BCL6.

The vast majority of DLBCL will be positive for clonal Ig rearrangements and, when so, have a poorer prognosis. For this reason, it is recommended that at the time of diagnosis Ig clonality studies be performed, as this is useful when establishing patient-specific minimal residual disease detection. In addition, in the case of questionable central nervous system (CNS)–associated disease, cerebrospinal fluid can be analyzed for clones, thus establishing the diagnosis of CNS involvement.

In the earliest application of cancer classification by mRNA expression analysis, Alizadeh et al.[24] applied cDNA from DLBCL to expression microarrays. This analysis divided DLBCL into two distinct groups based on their similarity to normal lymphocyte types: germinal center B cells (GCB-like) and activated peripheral blood B cells (ABC-like). The differences in the two populations relate to many dozens of genes, although the investigators have subsequently proposed that a more limited set of genes suffices to separate the categories. In addition to different expression patterns, the two groups are associated with different chromosomal abnormalities: the GCB-like DLBCL shows BCL6 and BCL2 translocations and gains of 12q12. On the other hand, ABC-like DLBCL has gains of 3q, 18q21-22 and losses of 6q.[25] Most importantly, the classification scheme accurately stratifies patient prognosis, indicating that intrinsic biologic characteristics are being revealed.

Burkitt Lymphoma

Burkitt lymphoma (BL), a highly aggressive B-cell lymphoma, is composed of a population of monotonous, medium-sized cells. Three clinical variants are defined: endemic (occurs in equatorial Africa and common in childhood), sporadic (seen throughout the world, mainly in children and young adults), and immunodeficiency-associated (usually seen in association with HIV infection).

The classic molecular abnormality associated with BL is abnormal MYC expression due to a translocation between the MYC locus (at 8q24) and one of the Ig genes. For the most part (around 80% of cases), the partner is the IGH@ locus resulting in t(8;14)(q24;q32). The second most commonly found translocation is the one involving IGK@, thus resulting in a t(2;8)(p12;q24) rearrangement. In a subset of cases, less than 5%, the translocation involves the IGL@ locus with a resulting t(8;22)(q24;q11). All of these translocations will ultimately result in dysregulated expression of MYC.[26] In addition, the translocated MYC genes often undergo point mutation, which may influence the rate of protein turnover.

The breakpoints described for the translocation partners of IGH@ and MYC are specific in terms of what clinical variant is involved. In the endemic variant, the breakpoint is usually found approximately 100 kb upstream of MYC and the IGH@ breakpoint is found within the JH domain. On the other hand, in the sporadic and immunodeficiency variants the MYC breakpoint lies within exon or intron 1 and the IGH@ breakpoint is found in one of the Ig heavy-chain switch domains.[27]

The wide distribution of breakpoints within MYC makes translocation detection difficult using conventional PCR. Usually, multiplexing or use of multiple PCR primers is needed. Even with multiple primers, very long amplicons must be prepared to cover as many potential breakpoints as possible. In all practicality, FISH is a more efficient approach for the detection of MYC rearrangements. Two approaches are possible. A pair of adjacent, different-color probes spanning the MYC locus reveals a translocation in the locus by their separation ("break-apart" probes). Alternatively, "dual-fusion" probes, one directed to the MYC locus and another to one of the Ig loci, show which Ig gene is involved in a translocation by the merging of their signals.

Marginal Zone B-Cell Lymphoma

Extranodal marginal zone lymphoma of mucosa-associated lymphoid tissue (MALT) is usually composed predominantly of small B cells, either centrocyte-like or monocytoid, mixed with large cells. There may also be plasma cell differentiation. Lymphoepithelial lesions, in which the malignant B cells infiltrate and destroy epithelium, are usually present.

They represent 8% of all non-Hodgkin lymphoma and up to 50% of primary gastric lymphoma. The majority of cases occurs in older adults and presents in extranodal sites such as stomach, lung, salivary glands, skin, and ocular adnexae. Gastric MALT lymphomas are remarkable in that they are attributable to chronic infection with the bacterium *Helicobacter pylori*.

The most common chromosomal anomalies in cases of MALT lymphomas are t(11;18) and t(14;18), and less frequently t(3;14) and t(1;14). t(11;18) translocation joins API2 and MALT1 and is most commonly seen in gastric, intestinal, and pulmonary tumors. Detection of this translocation is prognostically important in gastric MALT lymphoma as it is a strong predictor of lymphoma progression after *H. pylori* eradication. The t(14;18)(q32;p21) arrangement puts the MALT1 gene under the control of the IGH@ enhancer, resulting in MALT1 overexpression. t(1;14)(p22;q32) and t(1;2)(p22;p12) juxtapose the oncogene BCL10 to the IGH@ or IGK@ enhancer regions, resulting in BCL10 overexpression.[28] t(3;14)(p14;q32) results in upregulation of FOXP1 by its placement near the IGH@ locus. FOXP1 is a transcriptional repressor. All of these translocations can be detected by real-time PCR assays.

Table 36.1 summarizes the genetic alterations in B-cell lymphomas and methods for their analysis.

Lymphoplasmacytic Lymphoma

Lymphoplasmacytic lymphoma (LPL) is composed of small B cells, plasmacytoid lymphocytes, and plasma cells, usually involving the bone marrow, lymph nodes, and spleen. In most instances, IgM production by the tumor cells leads to the clinical syndrome of Waldenstrom macroglobulinemia. The t(9;14) translocation that had been previously described in a large number of cases is in fact rarely observed. Deletion of chromosome 6q has been reported in approximately half of cases but is not specific. Cases with this deletion of 6q reportedly carry a poor prognosis. Trisomy 4 has been described in a subset of cases. No other B-cell lymphoma–associated translocations have been shown in LPL.

Plasma Cell Myeloma

Plasma cell myeloma is a bone marrow–based, multifocal disease, associated with a monoclonal Ig in serum and/or urine. It is more common in males, and twice as common in African-Americans as in Caucasians. The median age of affected patients is 70 years.

By definition, myeloma is a clonal plasma cell neoplasm that originates from mature, post-germinal B cells. In some cases, a premalignant form, known as monoclonal gammopathy of undetermined significance may be identified, although de novo presentations are the most common. Approximately half of myeloma cases carry an IGH@ locus translocation. The most common

TABLE 36-1 B-Cell Lymphomas

Lymphoma Subtype	Genetic Alteration	Diagnostic Tool
CLL/SLL	IGHV mutation status	Direct DNA sequencing
	CD38 antigen expression	Immunophenotyping
	TP53 mutations (del 11q22-23)	FISH
	ATM mutations (del 17p13.3)	FISH
	Del 13q	FISH, conventional cytogenetics
FL	IGH-BCL2 fusion (t(14;18))	SBA, FISH, PCR
MCL	IGH-CCDN1 (t(11;14))	FISH
DLBCL	BCL6 rearrangements	SBA, FISH, PCR
	BCL2 rearrangements	SBA, FISH, PCR
	Gain of 3q, 18p21-22	FISH, conventional cytogenetics
	Loss of 6q	FISH, conventional cytogenetics
BL	MYC-IGH (t(8;14))	SBA, FISH, PCR
	IGK-MYC (t(2;8))	SBA, FISH, PCR
	MYC-IGL (t(8;22))	SBA, FISH, PCR
MZL	AP12-MALT1 (t(11;18))	FISH, PCR
	IGH-BCL2 (t(14;18))	FISH, PCR
	FOXP1-MALT1 (t(3;14)	FISH, PCR
LPL	PAX5-IGH (t(9;14))[a]	FISH
	Trisomy 3	FISH, conventional cytogenetics

[a]Uncommon, but listed for historical purposes.

SBA, Southern blot analysis; FISH, fluorescence in situ hybridization; PCR, polymerase chain reaction; CLL/SLL, chronic lymphocytic leukemia/small lymphocytic lymphoma; FL, follicular lymphoma; MCL, mantle cell lymphoma; DLBCL, diffuse large B-cell lymphoma; BL, Burkitt lymphoma; MZL, marginal zone lymphoma; LPL, lymphoplasmacytic lymphoma.

translocations are t(11;14) (involving CCND1), t(6;14) (involving CCND3), t(4;14) (involving MMSET and FGFR3), t(14;16) (involving MAF), and t(14;20) (involving MAFB). It has been reported that essentially all myeloma cases will show expression of cyclin D proteins (one or more of CCND1, CCND2, or CCND3). CCND1 expression in myelomas, as well as the t(11;14), has been associated with a good prognosis.[29]

As with other B-cell lymphoid neoplasms, minimal residual disease can be monitored by detecting clone-specific Ig V(D)J arrangements. This can be performed using qualitative or quantitative (real-time) PCR techniques.[30] The genetic abnormalities in plasma cell myeloma and methods suitable for diagnosing them are summarized in Table 36.2.

TABLE 36-2 Plasma Cell Myeloma

Genetic Alterations	Diagnostic Tool
14q32 locus • IGH-CCND1 (t(11;14)) • IGH-CCND3 (t(6;14)) • IGH-MMSET/FGFR3 (t(4;14)) • MAF-IGH (t(14;16)) • MAFB-IGH (t(14;20))	FISH, PCR

FISH, fluorescence in situ hybridization; PCR, polymerase chain reaction.

Hodgkin Lymphoma

Hodgkin lymphoma (HL) is a distinct form of B-cell lymphoma with a characteristic clinical behavior and a unique cellular composition. HL comprises two distinct disease entities: nodular lymphocyte predominant Hodgkin lymphoma (NLPHL) and classical Hodgkin lymphoma (cHL). The two entities differ in their clinical features and behavior as well as in the composition of their cellular background. Most important to diagnosis is the difference in morphology and immunophenotype.

cHL, which accounts for approximately 95% of all Hodgkin lymphomas, is composed of small numbers of large mononuclear Hodgkin cells and multinucleated Reed-Sternberg cells in a mixed inflammatory background. Four subtypes are recognized: lymphocyte-rich cHL, nodular sclerosis cHL, mixed cellularity cHL, and lymphocyte-depleted cHL. All four subtypes share immunophenotypic and genetic characteristics. cHL shows a bimodal age curve, showing a peak in the second to third decades (15–30 years) and another in the seventh to eighth decades. Hodgkin/Reed-Sternberg (HRS) cells do not immunophenotype like any other cell in the hematopoietic cell system.

NLPHL, on the other hand, is characterized by a nodular growth of scattered large cells with folded or multilobulated nuclei known as "popcorn" or lymphocyte predominant (LP) cells. Most of the LP cells are ringed by CD3-expressing T cells within a large background of follicular dendritic cells and B cells. NLPHL frequently occurs in mid-adulthood.

For quite some time, the cell of origin of Hodgkin lymphoma remained elusive. This has been attributed to the scarcity of the cell of interest in tissue samples, making it difficult to extract and analyze molecularly. In addition, the odd immunophenotype of HRS cells created further questions regarding the lineage of this neoplasm. The origin of HL was finally ascertained when HRS cells were dissected from tumor tissue of cases of HL and analyzed individually for IGH@ gene rearrangements by PCR.[31] In each case, a single clone was identified from the HRS cells, establishing it as derived from mature B cells at a germinal center or post-germinal center stage of differentiation. Several key transcription factors that regulate the expression of many B-cell-specific genes are either not expressed in HRS cells or are expressed at reduced levels, thus explaining the lack of expression of typical B-cell markers in HRS cells.[32] There have been a few cases, though, in which cHL has been molecularly assigned to the T-cell lineage on the basis of clonal TCR rearrangements in HRS cells. These rearrangements are not possible to detect in whole tissue DNA preparations; it is crucial to isolate individual HRS cells or LP cells for demonstration of clonality in HL.

The lineage of LP cells is also GCB cells because of the presence of clonally rearranged IGH@ genes and somatic hypermutation in a subset of cases. More recently, gene profiling of mature B-cell lymphomas and normal B cells showed that LP cells are similar to GCB cells and also have features of memory B cells, indicating that they may originate from late germinal center subsets at the transition to memory B cells.[33,34] Gene expression studies also demonstrated that LP cells are more similar to HRS cells than to FL, in spite of morphologic resemblance and immunophenotypic similarities to the latter.

Epstein-Barr virus (EBV) infection has been identified in approximately 40% of cHL. EBV can immortalize B cells, suggesting that EBV may play a crucial role in the pathogenesis of cHL. By the expression of EBV nuclear antigen 1 (EBNA1) and two latent membrane proteins (LMP1 and LMP2a), EBV provides the GCB cell with two signals that are essential for survival, thus preventing apoptotic destruction of virally infected cells.[35]

MATURE T-CELL LYMPHOMAS

Cutaneous T-Cell Lymphomas (CTCL)

Mycosis fungoides is a T-cell lymphoma that is by definition limited to the skin (albeit in a widespread fashion) and may have a slow progression over many years. When there is generalized lymphadenopathy and neoplastic T cells are found in the peripheral blood, the disease is classified as Sezary syndrome. The identification of a clonal population of T cells is an extremely useful tool in the diagnosis of these lymphomas. Gene rearrangements of the TCR loci (TRG@ and/or TRB@) may be detected in close to 75% of cases of true CTCL.[36] Peripheral blood involvement may be confirmed by the gene rearrangement analysis. The caveat of this type of testing is, as discussed before, the fact that clonality does not signify malignancy, as 1 out of 12 patients with a benign diagnosis will show clonal results when tested for TCR rearrangements. This is particularly true in the peripheral blood; many healthy individuals carry apparent clonal T cells, presumably restricted populations responding to an antigenic stimulus. Diagnostic difficulties can be avoided by examining tumor tissue in parallel with blood and relying only on the presence of the same clone in both tissues.

Anaplastic Large Cell Lymphoma

Anaplastic large cell lymphoma (ALCL) is a T-cell lymphoma composed of large lymphoid cells that express the antigen CD30 and have highly pleomorphic nuclei (Fig. 36.5). Subsets of ALCL are defined by expression of the anaplastic lymphoma kinase (ALK) protein. The ALK (+) subset of cases is most prevalent in children and young adults, commonly involving lymph nodes and less commonly extranodal sites, including skin, lung, liver, bone, and soft tissue. It may also involve the mediastinum. ALK (+) ALCL carries a better prognosis than ALK (–) cases.

Abnormal ALK expression occurs when there is a gene rearrangement causing a fusion between the ALK gene at 2p33 and another partner gene. The most common fusion gene is NPM1-ALK, as a consequence of a t(2;5) which is seen in approximately 75% of ALK-positive cases. Other partner genes may be TPM3 [t(1;2)], TFG [t(2;3)], ATIC [t(2;2)], and CTCL [t(2;17)].

Since the ALK gene translocations create truncations of the partner genes, molecular analysis of ALCL can be performed on the mRNA using RT-PCR. Primers are designed to hybridize to the exons flanking the joint of the chimeric mRNA. The reported sensitivity of detecting fusion transcripts is 1 copy in 10^6, which is significantly better than morphology and flow cytometric studies in identifying minimal residual disease post treatment. As such, this is the preferred mode of follow-up studies.

In addition, ALCL-associated mutations may also be detected using immunohistochemistry via detection of aberrant expression of ALK protein, or by FISH. When dual-fusion probes are used, other partner genes with ALK on chromosome 2 can be detected.

Adult T-Cell Leukemia/Lymphoma

Adult T-cell leukemia/lymphoma (ATLL) is a rare peripheral T-cell neoplasm composed of pleomorphic T cells, which is usually widely disseminated at the time of diagnosis. It is directly caused by infection with the human T-cell leukemia virus type 1(HTLV-1). This virus is endemic to some regions of the Caribbean, Northern Australia, central Africa, and southwestern Japan. As with other retroviral diseases, this disease has a long latency period and occurs in adults ranging from the third to the eighth decade.

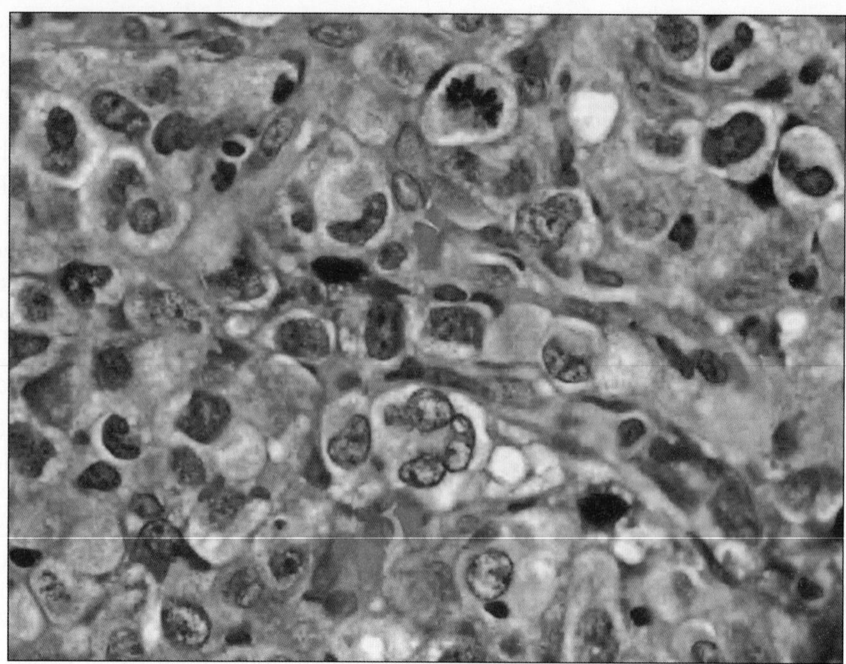

FIGURE 36–5 Morphology of anaplastic large cell lymphoma.

After integration of the HTLV-1 virus into the human genome, the p40 tax viral protein leads to transcription of many genes in lymphocytes infected with the virus. The HTLV-1 basic leucine zipper gene HBZ is thought to be involved in T-cell oncogenesis and proliferation.

Integration of the HTLV-1 virus into the human genome can be shown by Southern transfer analysis or by PCR. TCR genes are clonally rearranged. It has been shown that a clonal population of T cells in healthy carriers predicts the risk of developing ATLL. Cytogenetic abnormalities that can be identified via traditional cytogenetics or FISH are abnormalities in 14q, which could portend a poor risk, and isochromosome or trisomy of 7q, which are associated with a better outcome.

Angioimmunoblastic T-Cell Lymphoma

Angioimmunoblastic T-cell lymphoma (AITL) is a peripheral T-cell malignancy defined by systemic symptomatology and a polymorphic cellular lymph node infiltrate including a proliferation of high endothelial venules and follicular dendritic cells.

Most cases show TCR gene rearrangements, although a subset of patients also demonstrate Ig clones. The malignant cell of AITL is a T lymphocyte derived from germinal center helper T cells. EBV can be detected in most cases of this entity, although the infection is in B lymphocytes (immunoblasts) rather than the malignant T cells. In a substantial minority of cases, clonality by Ig PCR is identified, and it is hypothesized that the disruption to the immune system accompanying the T-cell malignancy permits EBV-infected B cells to proliferate in a clonal fashion. Interestingly, when there is histologic progression of AITL it is typically DLBCL that arises rather than a more aggressive-appearing T-cell malignancy.

The most common cytogenetic abnormalities are trisomy 3, trisomy 5, and an extra X chromosome.

Peripheral T-Cell Lymphoma, NOS

Peripheral T-cell lymphoma, not otherwise specified (PTCL, NOS), is a diverse group of mature T-cell lymphomas that can present in lymph nodes or extranodally and that does not meet criteria for any other defined T-cell malignancy. It is a diagnosis of exclusion, and likely contains several biologically distinct entities that are not separable with our current tools and understanding. PTCL, NOS comprises approximately 30% of all peripheral T-cell lymphomas and occurs primarily in adults.

Almost all of the PTCL, NOS carry TCR gene rearrangements, indicating their derivation from mature, post-thymic T cells. These neoplasms are characterized genetically by complex karyotypes. Comparative genomic hybridization studies have shown chromosomal gains in 7q, 8q, 17q, and 22q. Deletions have been described in 5q, 10q, and 10q and are associated with a better clinical outcome.

Hepatosplenic T-Cell Lymphoma

An aggressive neoplasm originating from cytotoxic $\gamma\delta$ T cells and presenting in an extranodal form, hepatosplenic T-cell lymphoma usually demonstrates systemic disease. This is a very rare form of lymphoma and mainly occurs in adolescents and young adults, with a male predominance. A subset of hepatosplenic T-cell lymphoma develops after a history of immunosuppression, such as after solid organ transplantation or another, unrelated malignancy.

These cells show rearranged TRG@ genes. TRB@ is not productively rearranged in the cases studied. Most cases show an isochromosome 7q.

TABLE 36-3 T-Cell Lymphomas

Lymphoma Subtype	Genetic Alteration	Diagnostic Tool
CTCL	TCR gene rearrangements in 75% of cases	SBA, FISH
ALCL	NPM-ALK (t(2;5)) seen in 75% of ALK (+) cases	SBA, FISH, PCR
	TPM3-ALK (t(1;2))	
	ALK-TFG (t(2;3))	
	ALK-ATIC (t(2;2))	
ATLL	HTLV1 virus integration	SBA, PCR
	14q abnormalities	FISH, conventional cytogenetics
	Gain of 7q	
AITL	TCR and IGH rearrangements	SBA, PCR
	Trisomy 3	FISH, conventional cytogenetics
	Trisomy 8	
	+X chromosome	
PTCL, NOS	Gains of 7q, 8q, 17q, 22q	FISH, conventional cytogenetics
	Deletions of 5q, 10q	
HSTL	Isochromosome 7q	FISH, conventional cytogenetics
T-LBL	TRA@/TRD@ at 14q11.2	SBA, PCR
	TRB@ at 7q35	FISH, conventional cytogenetics
	TRG@ at 7p14-15	
	HOX11 (10q24)	
	HOX11L2 (5q35)	
	Del 9p (loss of CDKN2A)	
	NOTCH1 gene	

CTCL, cutaneous T-cell lymphomas, ALCL, anaplastic large cell lymphoma; ATLL, adult T-cell leukemia/lymphoma; AITL, angioimmunoblastic T-cell lymphoma; PTCL, peripheral T-cell lymphoma; NOS, not otherwise specified; HSTL, hepatosplenic T-cell lymphoma; FISH, fluorescence in situ hybridization; PCR, polymerase chain reaction; SBA, Southern blot analysis.

T-Cell Lymphoblastic Lymphoma/Leukemia

T-cell lymphoblastic lymphoma/leukemia is a disease of lymphoblasts of medium size and high nuclear/cytoplasm ratio, which are indistinguishable from precursor B-cell lymphoblasts on morphologic grounds. This neoplasm presents mostly in its lymphomatous form (T-cell lymphoblastic lymphoma or T-LBL) rather than with the bone marrow and peripheral blood involvement and is commonly seen in adolescent boys and young men in the anterior mediastinum. The leukemic form is essentially identical, differing only in its site of presentation.

T-LBL will show clonal TCR rearrangements in almost all cases, but there are concomitant IGH@ rearrangements in about 20% of cases. An abnormal karyotype is also frequently found, with the most common abnormalities involving the TRA@ and TRD@ loci at 14q11.2, the TRB@ locus at 7q35, and the TRG@ locus at 7p14-15. Translocations involving these loci usually result in dysregulation of a partner oncogene. The most commonly involved genes are TLX1 (also known as HOX11, on chromosome 10q24) and TLX3 (or HOX11L2, on chromosome 5q35), occurring in 20% to 30% of all childhood T-cell lymphoblastic lymphoma/leukemia and 10% to 15% of all adult cases. The two translocations are reported to be mutually exclusive. In many cases, these translocations cannot be detected by conventional cytogenetics and must be studied by molecular genetic methods, mainly due to cryptic interstitial breaks.

Deletions may also occur in these neoplasms, the most significant one being del(9p), which results in loss of CDKN2A, leading to loss of G1 cell cycle control. Many cases have been described that show activating mutations in the NOTCH1 gene, which is critical for early T-cell development, and it has been associated with a poor outcome in adults but not childhood cases of T-cell lymphoblastic lymphoma/leukemia.

A summary of the major genetic abnormalities in T-cell lymphomas is presented in Table 36.3.

REFERENCES

1. Borghesi L, Milcarek C. From B cell to plasma cell: regulation of V(D)J recombination and antibody secretion. *Immunol Res*. 2006;36:27-32.
2. Maizels N. Immunoglobulin gene diversification. *Annu Rev Genet*. 2005;39:23-46.
3. Di Noia JM, Neuberger MS. Molecular mechanisms of antibody somatic hypermutation. *Annu Rev Biochem*. 2007;76:1-22.
4. Nikolich-Zugich J, Slifka MK, Messaoudi I. The many important facets of T cell repertoire diversity. *Nat Rev Immunol*. 2004;4:123-132.
5. Krangel MS. Mechanics of T cell receptor gene rearrangement. *Curr Opin Immunol*. 2009;21:133-139. *Nature*. 2004;4: 123-132.
6. Rajewsky K. Clonal selection and learning in the antibody system. *Nature*. 1996;381:751-758.
7. Van Dongen JJM, Langerak AW, Brüggemann M, et al. Design and standardization of PCR primers and protocols for detection of clonal immunoglobulin and T cell receptor gene recombinations in suspect lymphoproliferations: report of the BIOMED-2 Concerted Action BMH4-CT98-3936. *Leukemia*. 2003;17:2257-2317.

8. Nikiforova MN, Hsi ED, Braziel RM, et al. Detection of clonal IGH gene rearrangements: summary of molecular oncology surveys of the College of American Pathologists. *Arch Pathol Lab Med*. 2007;131:185-189.
9. Bagg A, Chu AY, Braziel RM, et al. Immunoglobulin heavy chain gene analysis in lymphomas: a multi-center study demonstrating the heterogeneity of performance of polymerase chain reaction assays. *J Mol Diagn*. 2002;4:81-89.
10. Chen YL, Huang W, Su IJ, et al. BIOMED-2 protocols to detect clonal immunoglobulin and T cell receptor gene rearrangements in B- and T cell lymphomas in southern Taiwan. *Leuk Lymphoma*. 2010;51:650-655.
11. Kuo SY, Hongxiang L, Liao YL, et al. A parallel comparison of T cell clonality assessment between an in-house PCR assay and the BIOMED-2 assay leading to an efficient and cost-effective strategy. *J Clin Pathol*. 2011;64:536-542.
12. Wagner-Johnston ND, Ambinder RF, Gocke CD, et al. Clonal immunoglobulin DNA in the plasma of patients with AIDS lymphoma. *Blood*. 2011;117:4860-4862.
13. Bagg A. Immunoglobulin and T cell receptor gene rearrangements: minding your B's and T's in assessing lineage and clonality in neoplastic lymphoproliferative disorders. *J Mol Diagn*. 2006;8:426-429.
14. Tan BT, Warnke RA, Arber DA. The frequency of B and T cell gene rearrangements and EBV in T cell lymphomas: a comparison between angioimmunoblastic T cell lymphoma and peripheral T cell lymphoma, unspecified, with and without associated B cell proliferations. *J Mol Diagn*. 2006;8:466-475.
15. Matsuda K, Nakazawa Y, Yanagisawa R, et al. Detection of T cell receptor gene rearrangement in children with Epstein–Barr virus-associated hemophagocytic lymphohistiocytosis using the BIOMED-2 multiplex polymerase chain reaction combined with GeneScan analysis. *Clin Chim Acta*. 2011;412:1554-1558.
16. Langerak AW, Molina TJ, Lavender FL. Polymerase chain reaction-based clonality testing in tissue samples with reactive lymphoproliferations: usefulness and pitfalls. A report of the BIOMED-2 Concerted Action BMH4-CT98-3936. *Leukemia*. 2007;21:222-229.
17. Swerdlow SH, Campo E, Harris NL, Jaffe ES, eds. *Pathology and Genetics of Tumours of Haematopoietic and Lymphoid Tissues*. World Health Organization Classification of Tumours. Lyon, France: IARC Press; 2008.
18. Zenz T, Mertens D, Dohner H, et al. Molecular diagnostics in chronic lymphocytic leukemia – pathogenetic and clinical implications. *Leuk Lymphoma*. 2008;49:864-873.
19. Hamblin TJ, Stevenson FK, Davis Z, et al. Unmutated Ig Vh genes are associated with a more aggressive form of chronic lymphocytic leukemia. *Blood*. 1999;94:1848-1854.
20. Gladstone DE, Jones RJ, Gocke CD, et al. Importance of immunoglobulin heavy chain variable region mutational status in del(13q) chronic lymphocytic leukemia. *Leuk Lymphoma*. 2011;52:1873-1881.
21. Wrench D, Montoto S, Fitzgibbon J. Molecular signatures in the diagnosis and management of follicular lymphoma. *Curr Opin Hematol*. 2010;17:333-340.
22. Rezuke WN, Tsongalis GJ, Abernathy EC. Molecular diagnosis of B- and T cell lymphomas: fundamental principles and clinical applications. *Clin Chem*. 1997;43:1814-1823.
23. Arber DA. Molecular diagnostic approach to non-Hodgkin's lymphoma. *J Mol Diagn*. 2000;2:178-190.
24. Alizadeh AA, Eisen MB, Davis RE, et al. Distinct types of diffuse large B-cell lymphoma identified by gene expression profiling. *Nature*. 2000;403:503-511.
25. Iqbal J, ZhongFeng L, Deffenbacher K, et al. Gene expression profiling in lymphoma diagnosis and management. *Best Pract Res Clin Haematol*. 2009;22:191-210.
26. Leich E, Hartmann EM, Burek C, et al. Diagnostic and prognostic significance of gene expression profiling in lymphomas. *APMIS*. 2007;115:1135-1146.
27. Dave SS, Fu K, Wright GW, et al. Molecular diagnosis of Burkitt's lymphoma. *N Engl J Med*. 2006;354:2431-2442.
28. Thieblemont C, Nasser V, Felman P, et al. Small lymphocytic lymphoma, marginal zone B cell lymphoma, and mantle cell lymphoma exhibit distinct gene expression profiles allowing molecular diagnosis. *Blood*. 2004;103:2727-2737.
29. Zhan F, Huang Y, Colla S, et al. The molecular classification of multiple myeloma. *Blood*. 2006;108:2020-2028.
30. Bruggeman M, Molina TJ, White H, et al. Powerful strategy for polymerase chain reaction-based clonality assessment in T-cell malignancies: report of the BIOMED-2 concerted action BHM4 CT98-3936. *Leukemia*. 2007;21:215-221.
31. Kuppers R, Hansmann ML, Rajewsky K, et al. Hodgkin disease: Hodgkin and Reed-Sternberg cells picked from histological sections show clonal immunoglobulin gene rearrangements and appear to be derived from B cells at various stages of development. *Proc Natl Acad Sci U S A*. 1994;91:10962-10966.
32. Kadin ME, Drews R, Samel A, et al. Hodgkin's lymphoma of T cell type: clonal association with a CD30+ cutaneous lymphoma. *Hum Pathol*. November 2001;32(11):1269-1272.
33. Kuppers R. Molecular biology of Hodgkin lymphoma. *Hematology Am Soc Hematol Educ Program*. 2009;491-495.
34. Re D, Kuppers R, Diehl V. Molecular pathogenesis of Hodgkin's lymphoma. *J Clin Oncol*. 2005;26:6379-6386.
35. Mueller NE, Lennette ET, Dupnik K, et al. Antibody titers against EBNA1 and EBNA2 in relation to Hodgkin lymphoma and history of infectious mononucleosis. *Int J Cancer*. 2012;130:2886-2891.
36. Bench AJ, Erber WN, Follows GA, et al. Molecular genetic analysis of haematological malignancies II: mature lymphoid neoplasms. *Int J Lab Hematol*. 2007;29:229-260.

CHAPTER 37

MOLECULAR DIAGNOSTICS OF GYNECOLOGIC NEOPLASMS

Robert J. Kurman, Christina M. Bagby, and Ie-Ming Shih

INTRODUCTION

This chapter describes the molecular genetic features of endometrial carcinomas and surface epithelial carcinomas of the ovary. In this discussion, we compare their similarities and differences as they offer important insights into the pathogenesis of these two malignancies, which in turn is important for the development of new approaches to diagnosis and treatment.

ENDOMETRIAL CARCINOMA

Endometrial carcinoma is the most common invasive gynecologic malignancy. It represents the sixth most frequently diagnosed carcinoma worldwide but is the fourth most frequently diagnosed carcinoma in the United States.[1] Based on 2011 estimates, approximately 46,470 new cases of endometrial carcinoma will be diagnosed in the United States, and 8,120 deaths are expected.[2]

Immunohistochemical and molecular analyses demonstrate that endometrial carcinoma can be divided into two major categories. Type I carcinomas represent 80% of endometrial carcinomas and generally develop in the presence of atypical endometrial hyperplasia due to unopposed estrogen exposure in pre- and post-menopausal women. Type I carcinomas are low-grade, are indolent, and are associated with microsatellite instability (MSI) and mutations in *PTEN*, *PIK3CA*, *KRAS*, and *CTNNB1*. Type II carcinomas are aggressive, are high grade, and are not related to estrogen exposure; they occur in postmenopausal women with *TP53* mutations (Table 37.1).[3]

Endometrioid Carcinoma

Endometrioid carcinoma (EMCA) is the prototypical type I endometrial carcinoma and is the most commonly diagnosed type of endometrial carcinoma. EMCA typically develops in a background of endometrial hyperplasia.

Molecular Genetic Features

The phosphatidylinositol 3-kinase (PI3K)/AKT signaling pathway plays an important role in cell cycle control, as activated AKT regulates the expression of genes involved in apoptosis and cell cycle progression.[4] The *PTEN* gene, on chromosome 10q23, functions as a tumor suppressor gene and encodes a phosphatase that normally antagonizes the PI3K/AKT pathway.[4] The PI3K/AKT pathway is frequently activated in endometrial carcinoma.

PTEN alterations are the most common molecular abnormality encountered in endometrial carcinoma. Loss of *PTEN* activity, either by mutations, loss of heterozygosity of chromosome 10q23, or promoter hypermethylation, leads to constitutive activation of the PI3K/AKT pathway and uncontrolled cell proliferation. Somatic mutations in *PTEN* are thought to occur early in the pathogenesis of, and almost exclusively in, pure EMCA.[5] *PTEN* mutations have been detected in 20% to 55% of endometrial hyperplasia[6-9] and in 50% to 86% of EMCA.[7,10-12] Loss of heterozygosity of 10q23 has been detected in up to 40% of EMCA[13] and hypermethylation of *PTEN* in 18%.[12]

PIK3CA is an oncogene on chromosome 3q26.3 that encodes a catalytic subunit of PIK3, which is responsible for downstream activation of the AKT pathway. *PIK3CA* mutations occur in 26% to 39% of EMCA[6,10,14] and are detected in both low-grade and high-grade EMCAs. *PIK3CA* mutations possibly represent a later occurrence in endometrial carcinoma, with only 7% of complex endometrial hyperplasias harboring a mutation.[6] *PIK3CA* mutations may also serve as a marker of invasion.[6] A study by

TABLE 37–1 Type I versus Type II Endometrial Carcinoma

	Type I	Type II
Risk factor	Unopposed estrogen	
Age	Pre- and post-menopausal	Post-menopausal
Precursor lesion	Atypical hyperplasia	Serous endometrial intraepithelial carcinoma
Tumor subtype	Endometrioid Mucinous	Serous Clear cell
Tumor grade	Low	High
Molecular alterations	*PTEN* mutation *PIK3CA* mutation Microsatellite instability *KRAS* mutation	*TP53* mutation
Behavior	Indolent	Aggressive

Catasus et al.[9] revealed that all EMCAs with *PIK3CA* mutations exhibited some degree of invasion, while none of the non-invasive carcinomas harbored mutations; furthermore, lymphovascular invasion was more common in the mutated tumors. *PIK3CA* mutations most frequently involve exons 9 and 20 of the gene,[10] and distinguishing which exon is mutated has some importance. Exon 20 mutations tend to display deeper myometrial invasion and are more frequently high-grade carcinomas, while mutations in exon 9 occur more often in low-grade carcinomas.[5,9]

The *KRAS* oncogene encodes a membrane-associated GTPase involved in signal transduction to the nucleus; *KRAS* also has the ability to directly bind to and activate PIK3.[13] *KRAS*-activating point mutations in codon 12 occur in both endometrial hyperplasia and EMCAs,[15] and in one study, the rate of *KRAS* mutation occurrence was similar between the two groups.[16] *KRAS*-activating mutations occur in 10% to 30% of EMCAs overall,[9,15-18] have been shown to be inversely associated with death, and may represent a good prognostic marker for EMCA.[16]

MSI occurs more frequently in EMCA compared with other subtypes of endometrial carcinoma, with incidence ranging from 18% to 34%.[9,18-20] MSI is detected equally among the three grades of EMCA.[18] MSI occurs in patients with Lynch syndrome due to germline mutations in mismatch repair (MMR) genes MSH6, MSH2, MLH1, and PMS2 (in descending order of frequency).[3,20] However, in patients with known MSH6 mutations, only a low frequency of MSI has been detected.[21] MSI is also detected in sporadic EMCA but occurs via hypermethylation of the MLH1 promoter rather than MMR gene mutation.[22,23] Hypermethylation of the MLH1 promoter has also been seen in 7% of endometrial hyperplasias, but only in cases with coexisting EMCA, which suggests MSI is an early event in EMCA pathogenesis.[19,23]

Mutations in the β-catenin gene, *CTNNB1*, on chromosome 3p21 have been detected in approximately 15% to 20% of EMCAs,[9,24,25] which results in nuclear accumulation of β-catenin[24] and activation of downstream genes including c-myc and cyclin D1. Alterations in β-catenin expression also occur in complex atypical endometrial hyperplasia, most frequently in hyperplasia with associated squamous morules.[26]

Other rarely encountered molecular alterations involve *CCND1*, *Her2/neu*, and *TP53*. Cyclin D1 overexpression due to *CCND1* gene amplification is seen in only 2% of EMCAs.[27] Both *Her2/neu* and *TP53* alterations occur more frequently in higher grade EMCAs and may be considered late events in pathogenesis. *Her2/neu* gene amplification is uncommon in EMCA, with grade 1 EMCA showing the lowest rate of amplification (1%) compared with 4% of grade 2 and 8% of grade 3 EMCA.[28] Of the approximately 17% of *TP53* mutations detected in EMCA in one study, none occurred in grade 1, 8% in grade 2, and 43% in grade 3.[18]

Multiple mutations may occur during endometrial carcinogenesis. *PIK3CA* and *PTEN* mutations coexist in 17% to 24% of endometrial carcinomas, with *PIK3CA* mutations occurring more commonly in tumors harboring *PTEN* mutations compared with those without.[9,14] The dual mutations are thought to have an additive effect on PIK3 activation.[14] *PIK3CA* and *KRAS* mutations, on the other hand, have been shown to be mutually exclusive,[10] with coexistence demonstrated in only 4% of carcinomas in another study.[9] *PIK3CA* mutations also do not correlate with MSI or *CTNNB1* mutations.[9,10] *KRAS*, *PTEN*, *CTNNB1*, and *CCND1* mutations each occur more frequently in endometrial carcinomas with MSI.[15,24,27,29]

Immunohistochemical Features

EMCAs express pan-cytokeratins, epithelial membrane antigen (EMA), CA125, BerEP4, and B72.3, while carcinoembryonic antigen (CEA) is uncommon. The majority of EMCAs are CK7 positive and CK20 negative.[3,30] Approximately 80% of FIGO grade 1 and 2 EMCA are estrogen and progesterone receptor positive (ER and PR), while only 50% of FIGO grade 3 carcinomas express ER and 42% PR (Fig. 37.1).[31,32] PAX 8, a transcription factor important for embryonic development of müllerian organs, is expressed in 95% of EMCA.[33]

Nuclear expression of β-catenin has been associated with *CTTNB1* mutations, particularly in exon 3.[25] Abnormal nuclear accumulation of β-catenin has been detected in up to 73% of EMCA with concentration in areas of squamous differentiation.[24-26,34] However, nuclear expression of β-catenin is also observed in EMCA without *CTTNB1* mutations, suggesting other alterations in the Wnt/β-catenin pathway may exist.[24,25] β-Catenin also shows strong, diffuse nuclear staining in areas of

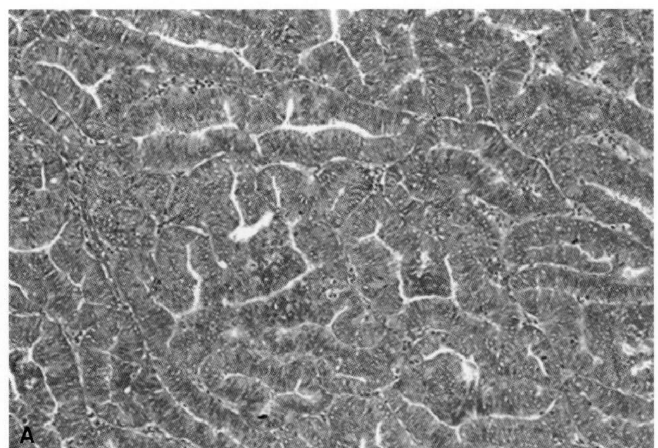

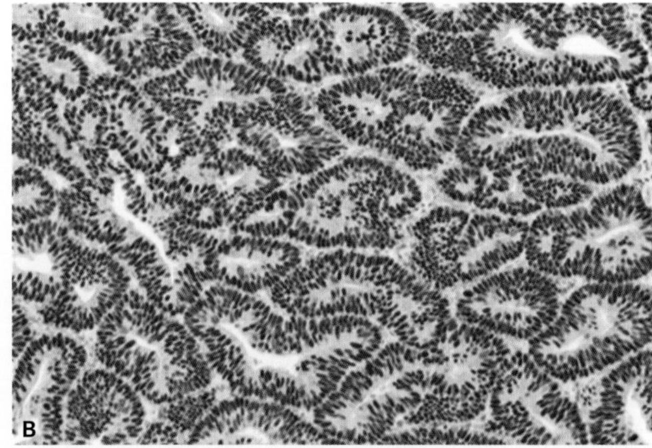

FIGURE 37–1 Endometrial endometrioid carcinoma, FIGO grade 1. **A:** EMCA, FIGO grade 1, displaying back-to-back and fused well-differentiated glands with low-grade nuclei. **B:** Low-grade EMCA typically shows strong nuclear expression of estrogen receptors.

squamous morules associated with complex atypical endometrial hyperplasia.[26]

Alterations in MLH1, whether via inherited germline mutations or sporadic hypermethylation of the MLH1 promoter, lead to the loss of MLH1 expression.[22] Therefore, DNA MMR protein immunohistochemistry has a slightly lower sensitivity of predicting MSI in EMCA compared with colon cancer.[35] In a study comparing MSI-High (MSI-H) versus non–MSI-H endometrial carcinomas, immunohistochemical staining for MLH1 and MSH2 was able to detect 69% of MSI-H tumors when the two stains were analyzed together; up to 91% were identified after the addition of PMS2 and MSH6 to the immunohistochemical panel.[35] Loss of expression of MLH1 in tumor cell nuclei occurred in 28% of all cases, with only 6% of cases showing loss of MSH2. The most common phenotype seen in MSI-H cases is concurrent loss of MLH1 and PMS2.[35]

Cyclin D1 overexpression is seen in approximately 13.8% of EMCAs; however, it does not appear to be related to *CCND1* gene amplification. Cyclin D1 expression has been significantly associated with MSI.[27]

P53 expression is extremely rare in grade 1 and occurs occasionally in grade 2 EMCA, but is present in a significant number of grade 3 EMCA.[3] In the study by Lax et al., 80% of EMCAs were immunonegative or showed a low immunoreactive score for p53 staining, with only 3% showing a high score. Of the high scoring cases, all were grade 3, with the exception of one grade 2 EMCA. Despite the high immunoreactive scores, the staining pattern is typically patchy.[18] As in the ovary, nonsense p53 mutations may occur resulting in complete absence of staining for p53 in the EMCA.[18]

Differentiating high-grade EMCA from serous carcinoma can at times be difficult, and p16 and WT1 immunomarkers may be helpful in this situation. P16 expression is patchy with weak to moderate staining in up to 7% of grade 1 and 2 carcinomas and 25% of grade 3,[32] but regardless of the grade, p16 expression is always less diffuse and intense in endometrial carcinoma compared with serous or endocervical carcinoma.[36] Nuclear WT1 immunoreactivity is rare in EMCA; however, a heterogeneous pattern of cytoplasmic staining has been detected in a significant number of cases.[37,38]

Genetics

Lynch syndrome has been detected in at least 1.8% of newly diagnosed endometrial carcinomas.[20] Endometrial carcinoma is the most common non-gastrointestinal carcinoma associated with Lynch syndrome, with the majority being of endometrioid subtype.[39] Women with Lynch syndrome have a lifetime risk of 40% to 60% for developing EMCA, which is equal to or possibly even higher than their risk of colorectal carcinoma.[40,41] In a study of women with known Lynch syndrome and metachronous colon and endometrial carcinomas, 49% presented initially with colorectal carcinoma and 46% with endometrial carcinoma.[41]

There are currently no validated guidelines for implementing Lynch syndrome screening in women with endometrial carcinoma, and importantly screening without the consent of the patient may not even be considered legal. Nonetheless, one approach is to screen all endometrial carcinomas with polymerase chain reaction genotyping for MSI.[20] Alternatively, DNA MMR protein immunohistochemistry could be used to screen for MSI since MMR gene mutations lead to the loss of expression of their related genes,[20,35] keeping in mind that IHC is less sensitive for endometrial carcinoma and the loss of expression of MLH1 is more likely due to sporadic promoter hypermethylation rather than a germline mutation. DNA sequencing for germline mutations in the MMR genes MSH6, MSH2, MLH1, and PMS2 is the confirmatory test for diagnosing Lynch syndrome. Anyone with an MSI-positive tumor should be offered genetic counseling and DNA sequencing to detect germline mutations, as these women and their children will require increased cancer surveillance.

Serous Carcinoma

Uterine serous carcinoma (USC) is the prototype for type II endometrial carcinoma. Serous endometrial intraepithelial carcinomas (EICs) are thought to represent the precursor lesions to invasive USC and demonstrate similar molecular characteristics.

Molecular Genetic Features

The overwhelming majority (>90%) of USCs are associated with *TP53* mutations.[18,42] Loss of p53 tumor suppressor function leads to inhibition of apoptosis and genetic instability. Up to 78% of serous EICs harbor *TP53* missense mutations, and identical mutations have been detected in uteri with synchronous EICs and USCs.[42] Loss of heterozygosity of chromosome 17p has been detected in 100% of USCs and 43% of EICs.[42] These findings suggest that loss of the wild-type *TP53* allele is an early event in uterine serous carcinogenesis.

ERBB2 (HER2/neu) amplification detected by fluorescent in situ hybridization (FISH) occurs in 29% to 47% of USCs.[28] Patients with HER2/neu amplification experience overall shorter survival times.[28] HER2 amplification has also been significantly correlated with a higher tumor grade and stage, non-endometrioid subtype, positive lymph node status, and greater than 50% myometrial invasion.[28] Cyclin D1 gene (*CCND1*) amplification has also been detected by FISH in up to 26% of non-EMCA.[27] Very recently, whole exome sequencing and DNA copy number analysis have revealed that molecular genetic aberrations involving cyclin E-FBXW7 and PI3K pathways also represent major mechanisms in the development of uterine serous carcinoma.[43]

Mutations in *PTEN* and *KRAS* are almost never encountered in USC.[3,18] MSI also has not been detected in USC.[18]

Immunohistochemical Features

USCs, like most gynecologic neoplasms, commonly express pan-cytokeratins, EMA, vimentin, CA125, Ber EP4, B72.3, CK7, and PAX8 and are usually negative for CK20.[3,33]

Wild-type p53 protein is rapidly degraded, whereas p53 with missense mutations resists degradation leading to nuclear accumulation and strong diffuse nuclear staining by immunohistochemistry. Strong overexpression of p53 is seen in over 60% to 80% of USCs,[5,18,42,44] with similar staining patterns in corresponding areas of serous EIC (Fig. 37.2).[42,44] Some tumors show a complete absence of p53 expression but are still associated with *TP53* mutations. This occurs with nonsense *TP53* mutations which

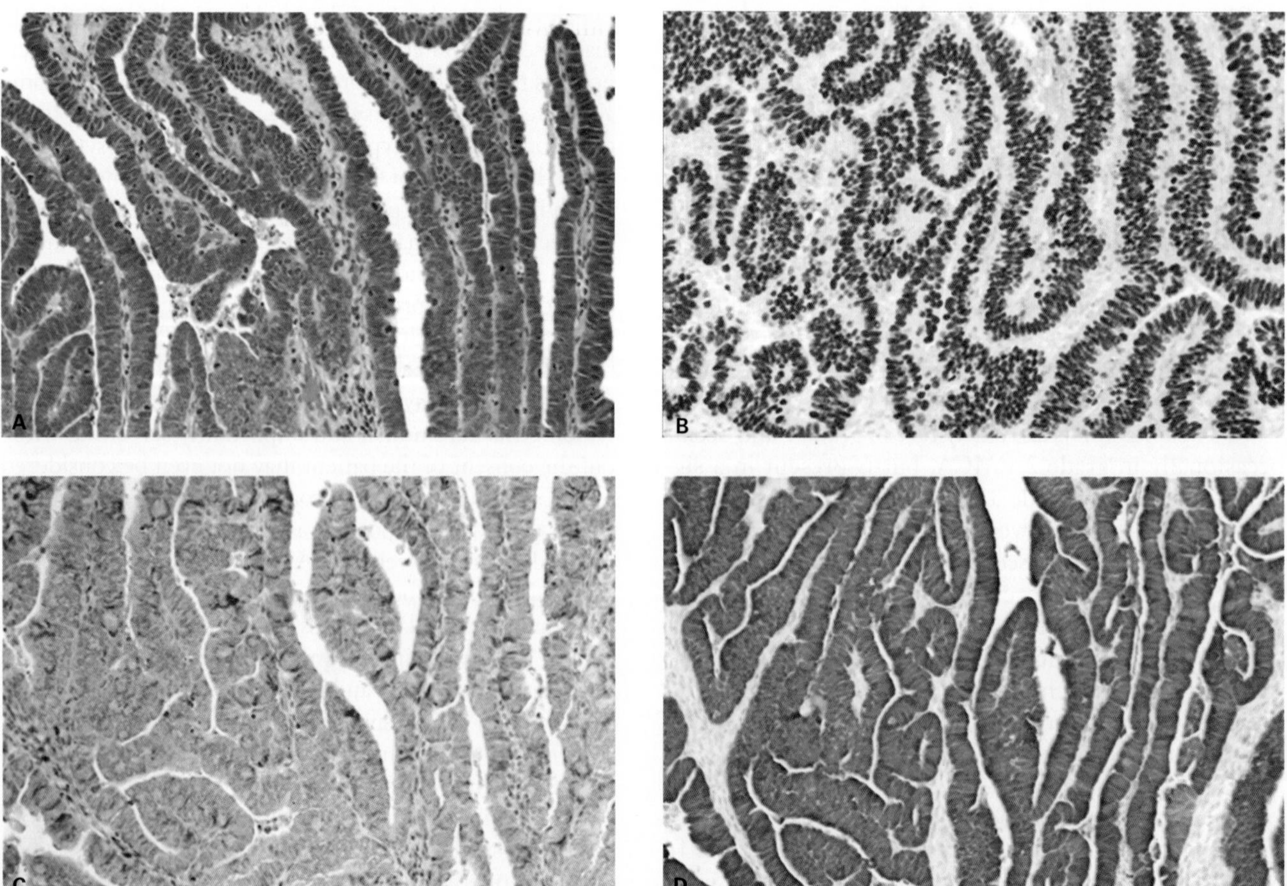

FIGURE 37–2 Uterine serous carcinoma. **A:** USC composed of papillae lined by markedly atypical epithelium. **B:** USCs typically show strong/diffuse nuclear expression of p53 due to *TP53* missense mutations. **C:** However, some USCs demonstrate complete absence of p53 staining, corresponding to *TP53* nonsense mutations. **D:** USCs typically show strong/diffuse nuclear staining for p16.

result in a truncated p53 protein that cannot be detected immunohistochemically (see Fig. 37.2).[42]

The Ki-67 proliferation index is extremely high in high-grade serous carcinoma (HGSC).[31] In comparison to EMCA, p16 shows a diffuse, strong expression pattern in 90% to 100% of tumor cells in over 90% of USC (see Fig. 37.2).[3,32,36] USC infrequently expresses WT1, in comparison to HGSC of ovarian or fallopian tube.[37,45,46] ER and PR expression is frequently negative but may show weak to moderate expression in up to approximately 50% of serous carcinomas.[32,47] PR is less frequently expressed compared with ER.[3]

Other immunohistochemical features differentiating USC from high-grade EMCA include a lack of staining for β-catenin and e-cadherin and no loss of PTEN expression in USC.[3,34] On the other hand, serous carcinomas show a higher frequency of cyclin D1 overexpression in association with *CCND1* gene amplification.[27]

Clear Cell Carcinoma

Definitive classification of uterine clear cell carcinoma (CCC) as type I or type II is difficult, as CCC shares some features of both endometrioid and serous carcinomas. Morphologically, CCCs with serous features have been associated with serous EIC but not endometrial hyperplasia, whereas pure CCCs have been associated with endometrial hyperplasia but not serous EIC.[47] CCC tends to behave more like a high-grade carcinoma with advanced stage at presentation and frequent association with high nuclear grade, deep myometrial invasion, lymphovascular invasion, and pelvic lymph node metastasis.[3]

Molecular Genetic Features

Few molecular studies are available for uterine CCC. An et al. reported that MSI and mutations in *TP53* are uncommon in pure CCCs. However, in two cases of mixed serous and CCCs, both components harbored the same *TP53* mutations, while one case with mixed endometrioid and clear cell components displayed MSI and identical mutations in both *TP53* and *PTEN*.[48] In addition to *PTEN*, a few CCCs harbor mutations of *CTNNB1* (β-catenin gene).[48,49]

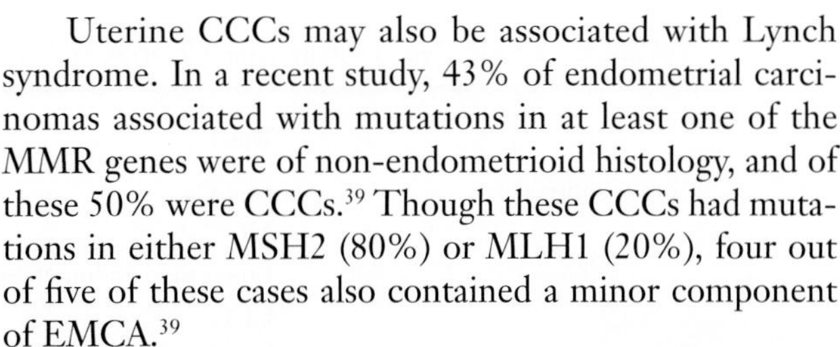

Uterine CCCs may also be associated with Lynch syndrome. In a recent study, 43% of endometrial carcinomas associated with mutations in at least one of the MMR genes were of non-endometrioid histology, and of these 50% were CCCs.[39] Though these CCCs had mutations in either MSH2 (80%) or MLH1 (20%), four out of five of these cases also contained a minor component of EMCA.[39]

Immunohistochemical Features

Uterine CCCs characteristically express CAM 5.2, 34βE12, CEA, Leu-M1, vimentin, bcl-2, CA-125, CK7, and PAX8, similar to other gynecologic tract carcinomas.[33,50] Up to 20% of uterine CCCs are immunoreactive for Her2/neu.[50] CK20 and WT1 are typically negative.[3,50]

CCCs show immunohistochemical expression patterns intermediate between those of EMCA and USC for several markers. Uterine CCCs are typically ER and PR negative, with expression patterns similar to USC and significantly lower expression compared with EMCA.[47] ER expression ranges from 0% to 9%, while PR ranges from 0% to 45%.[32,50] Variable p53 reactivity has been demonstrated,[47,48] with up to 100% of cases showing strong diffuse nuclear expression in one study.[50] Another study suggests that p53 expression occurs in only 25% of CCCs, which is significantly less expression than in serous carcinoma, but higher (though not statistically significant) compared with EMCA.[47] Ki-67 proliferation index is intermediate between endometrioid and serous carcinoma.[47] P16 staining is patchy in up to 45% of uterine CCC.[32]

Hepatocyte nuclear factor-1β (HNF-1β) is expressed in several normal organs, including liver, kidney, and pancreas, where it is involved in glucose homeostasis and glycogen accumulation. The expression of HNF-1β is significantly upregulated in CCCs of endometrium and ovary resulting in diffuse nuclear staining (Fig. 37.3). Nuclear expression of HNF-1β appears to be specific to uterine CCC, when compared with other endometrial carcinomas; however, diffuse nuclear staining can also be seen in mid-to-late secretory phase endometrium as well as in gestational endometrium with Arias-Stella reaction.[51]

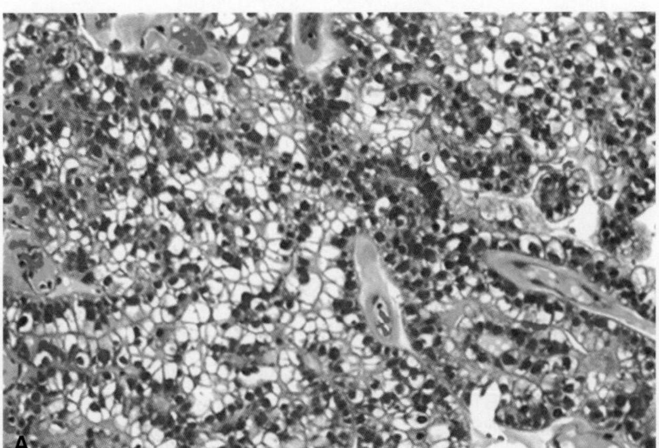

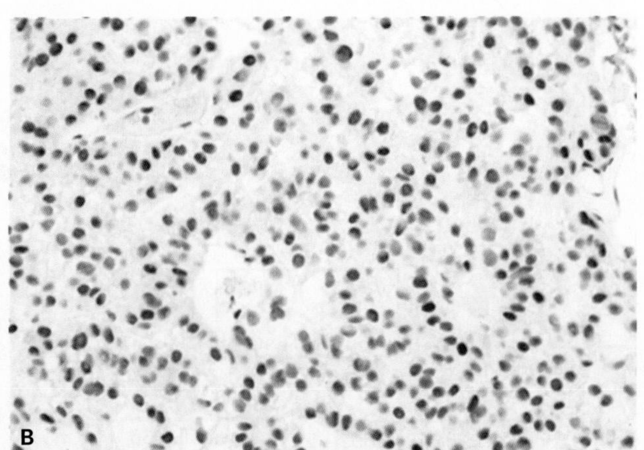

FIGURE 37–3 Uterine clear cell carcinoma (CCC). **A:** Uterine CCC composed of a solid sheet of cells with prominent clear cytoplasm. **B:** Uterine CCCs are typically diffusely positive for HNF-1β.

TABLE 37–2 Type I versus Type II Ovarian Epithelial Carcinoma

	Type I		Type II
Tumor subtype	LGSC		High-grade serous
	MOC		High-grade endometrioid
	Low-grade endometrioid (OEC)		Undifferentiated carcinoma
	CCC		Carcinosarcoma
Precursor lesions	LGSC	APST, non-invasive MPSC	STIC
	MOC	APMT and APSMT	Unknown
	OEC	Endometriosis, APET	
	CCC	Endometriosis	
Tumor grade	Low		High
Most common mutations	LGSC	*KRAS, BRAF*	TP53 mutation
	MOC	*KRAS*	
	OEC	*CTNNB1, PTEN, ARID1A*	
	CCC	*ARID1A, PIK3CA*	
Chromosome instability	Low		High
Behavior	Indolent		Aggressive

LGSC, low-grade serous carcinoma; MOC, mucinous ovarian carcinoma; OEC, ovarian endometrioid carcinoma; CCC, clear cell carcinoma; APST, atypical proliferative serous tumor; MPSC, micropapillary serous carcinoma; APMT, atypical proliferative mucinous tumor; APSMT, atypical proliferative seromucinous "endocervical" tumor; APET, atypical proliferative endometrioid tumor; STIC, serous tubal intraepithelial carcinoma.

OVARIAN CARCINOMA

Ovarian carcinoma is expected to be the ninth most frequently diagnosed carcinoma in women in the United States, with an estimated 21,990 new cases diagnosed in 2011.[2] It represents the seventh most frequent cause of cancer-related death globally and the fifth in the United States, making ovarian carcinoma the leading cause of gynecologic carcinoma–related death.[2]

As in endometrial carcinoma, a two-tier classification system exists for ovarian surface epithelial carcinomas (Table 37.2). Type I carcinomas, which include low-grade serous, low-grade endometrioid, clear cell, mucinous, and Brenner cell tumors, represent 25% of ovarian cancer diagnoses. These carcinomas usually follow an indolent course and are responsible for approximately 10% of ovarian cancer–related deaths. As a group, these tumors tend to be genetically stable and involve mutations in *KRAS/BRAF*, *PTEN*, *PIK3CA*, *CTNNB1*, *ARID1A*, and *PPP2R1A*. Seventy-five percent of ovarian carcinomas fall into the type II category, which is comprised of high-grade serous, high-grade endometrioid, malignant müllerian mixed tumors (carcinosarcoma), and undifferentiated carcinomas. These carcinomas are highly aggressive, tend to present at advanced stages, and contribute to 90% of ovarian cancer–related deaths. Type II tumors frequently show marked chromosome instability and *TP53* mutations.[52-54]

Low-Grade Serous Carcinoma

Low-grade serous carcinomas (LGSC) are the prototypical type I ovarian carcinomas. They typically progress stepwise from serous cystadenomas/adenofibromas to atypical proliferative (borderline) serous tumors (APSTs) and non-invasive micropapillary serous carcinomas (MPSC) to invasive LGSCs (also termed "invasive MPSC") (Fig. 37.4).

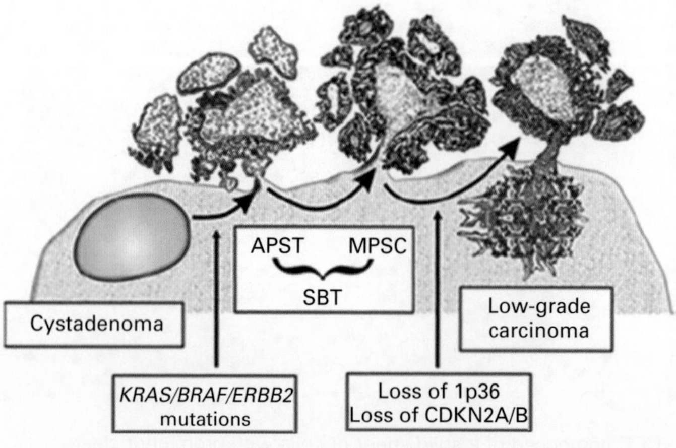

FIGURE 37–4 Pathogenesis of ovarian low-grade serous carcinoma. LGSCs follow a stepwise progression from benign serous cystadenomas to serous borderline tumors (SBTs), which include atypical proliferative serous tumors (APST) and micropapillary serous carcinoma (MPSC), and finally to invasive low-grade serous carcinoma. Figure was modified from Singer et al.[59]

Molecular Genetic Features

Alterations in the mitogen-activated protein kinase (MAPK) pathway are important in the pathogenesis of LGSC; activating *KRAS* or *BRAF* mutations lead to constitutive activation of the MAPK pathway.[3] Up to two-thirds of low-grade serous tumors have a mutation in one of *KRAS*, *BRAF*, or *ERBB2* genes. These mutations are mutually exclusive, with only one of them occurring in a single tumor.[53,55-59] *KRAS* and *BRAF* mutations appear early in the development of LGSCs, with mutations found throughout the entire spectrum of low-grade serous tumors. *KRAS* mutations have been identified in serous cystadenoma epithelium adjacent to an APST, with identical mutations in both components of the tumor.[57] *KRAS* mutations also occur in up to 50% of APSTs, 36% of non-invasive MPSC, and 54% of LGSC.[53,58,60,61] *BRAF* mutations are detected in approximately 36% of low-grade serous tumors overall,[55] with 24% to 35% of APSTs, 50% of non-invasive MPSC, and 50% of LGSC harboring mutations.[55,58] Mutations of *ERBB2* (Her2/neu) activate an upstream regulator of KRAS and are found in 6% to 9% of APSTs lacking *KRAS/BRAF* mutations.[58,62]

In comparison to HGSCs, LGSCs typically lack *TP53* mutations; these mutations have been detected in only 8% of APSTs and LGSCs.[59] LGSC also exhibits a significantly lower chromosomal instability index.[63] LGSCs display fewer hypermethylated genes as they progress from serous cystadenomas to APST and LGSC, and low-grade serous tumors have significantly more hypermethylated genes compared with HGSC.[64]

Immunohistochemical Features

APST and LGSC are positive for CK7, CA 125, EMA, and PAX8 and are typically negative for CK20.[3,33] APSTs are usually weakly positive for WT1.[3] LGSCs typically express WT1 in a strong diffuse nuclear pattern, with no significant differences in staining compared with HGSC.[65,66]

Expression of p53, p16, Her2/neu, BCL2, and Ki-67 is significantly lower in APST and LGSC, compared with HGSC (Fig. 37.5). APSTs may demonstrate patchy p53 expression, consistent with wild-type *TP53*,[59] while p53 may be focally expressed in up to 43% of LGSC, with weak to moderate staining intensity. Only up to 18% of LGSCs show high expression of p53.[65,67] APST and LGSC typically show a weak/moderate patchy staining pattern for p16.[68] Only 14% of LGSCs demonstrate a Ki-67 proliferation index of greater than 50%, with a mean proliferation index of 23% in one study.[65]

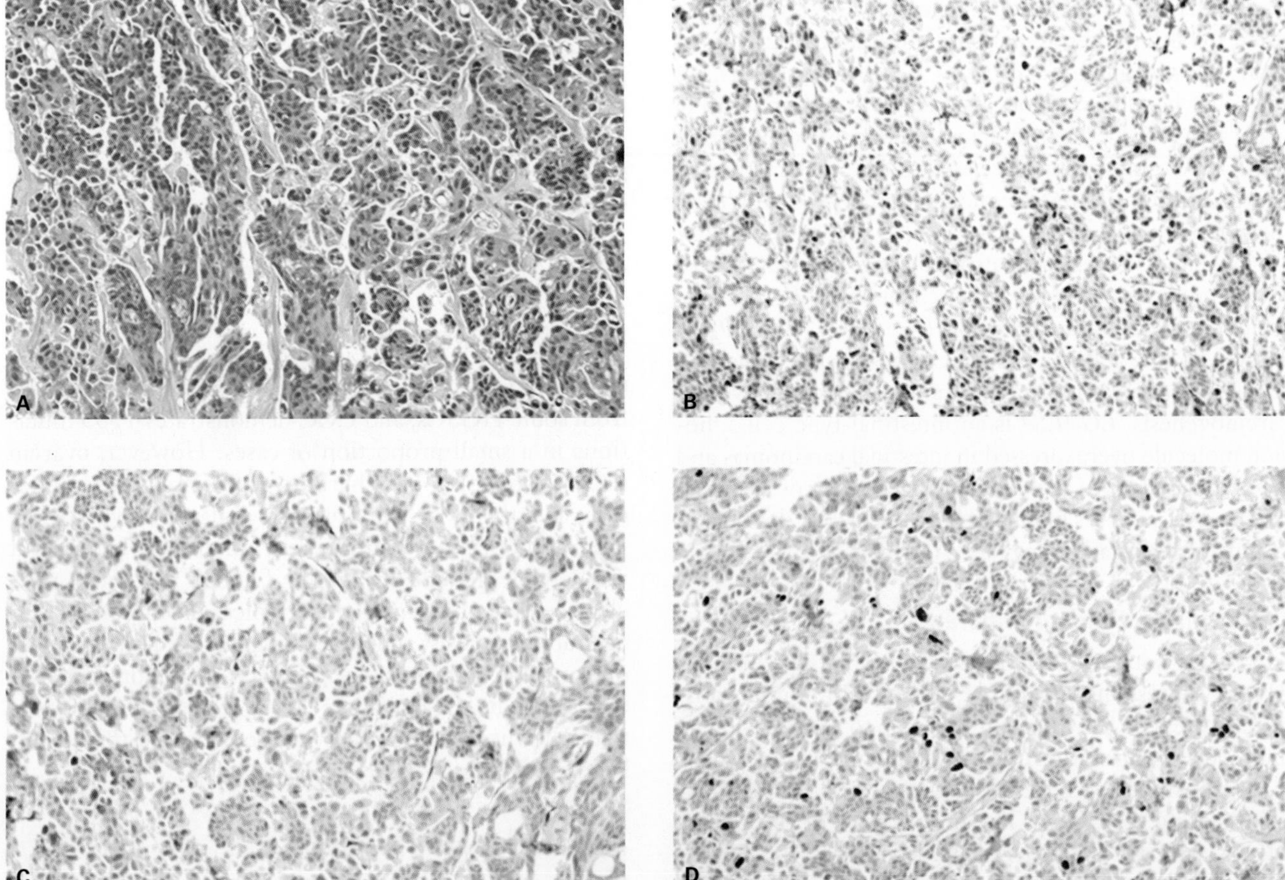

FIGURE 37–5 Ovarian low-grade serous carcinoma. LGSC displaying haphazard infiltrative growth of numerous micropapillae **(A)**. LGSCs show patchy expression of p53 **(B)** and p16 **(C)** and have a mildly increased **(D)** Ki-67 proliferation index.

Her2/neu and BCL2 have been detected in only 4.5% and 5% of LGSC, respectively.[65] Approximately 50% of LGSCs show nuclear positivity for ER and PR, which is significantly more than expressed in HGSC.[67]

Mucinous Carcinoma

Mucinous carcinomas, another type I ovarian carcinoma, follow a path similar to LGSCs with progression from mucinous cystadenomas to atypical proliferative (borderline) mucinous and seromucinous tumors (APMT and APSMT, respectively) and then to invasive mucinous ovarian carcinomas (MOCs).

Molecular Genetic Features

Gene expression analysis reveals that though MOC can be distinguished based on their own unique expression profile, they tend to cluster closer to endometrioid than serous carcinomas. Most APMTs cluster closely with MOC.[69]

Activating *KRAS* mutations, particularly those involving codon 12, are important in the pathogenesis of MOC and have been detected in up to 63% of mucinous cystadenomas, 73% of APMTs, and 85% of MOCs.[56,61,70-72] In carcinomas with adjacent cystadenoma or APMT, identical mutations have been found in each component, which suggests activating *KRAS* mutations occur early in MOC carcinogenesis.[72] *KRAS* mutations occur in both the seromucinous (endocervical) and intestinal types of mucinous tumors.[71] *BRAF* mutations, on the other hand, do not occur in APMTs and only rarely occur in MOCs.[56,71] Seromucinous (endocervical) ovarian borderline tumors may be related to endometrial tumors based on their similar frequency and type of *ARID1A* mutations.[73]

Mucinous carcinomas express genes associated with mucin production and mucinous carcinomas of other sites including the intestine, such as *MUC2*, *MUC3A*, *MUC17*, *CDX1*, *CDX2*, and *LGALS4*.[69] Of these genes, *galectin 4* (*LGALS4*) may be more important in mucinous ovarian carcinogenesis. *LGALS4* is an intestinal-type cell adhesion molecule overexpressed in intestinal carcinomas and is upregulated in MOCs compared with other ovarian carcinomas. *LGALS4* is highly expressed in MOC, but less so in mucinous cystadenomas and APMTs.[69]

Immunohistochemical Features

In comparison to other ovarian epithelial carcinomas, MOCs express more variable CK7/CK20 immunoprofiles. Expression of CK7 is diffuse in up to 98% of APMTs and 100% of primary MOCs.[74,75] The majority of MOC is also positive for CK20, but typically shows less diffuse staining than CK7. The majority (79%) of primary MOCs are CK7+/CK20+, compared with (17%) CK7+/CK20– and (5%) CK7–/CK20+, with no cases of CK7–/CK20–.[76] Up to 83% of APMTs are also CK7+/CK20+, followed by 11% showing CK7+/20–.[74]

LGALS4 is highly and specifically expressed in MOC, with a median of 72% of carcinoma cells staining positive, compared with ovarian serous and EMCAs and to normal ovarian mucosa, all with a median of zero expression.[69] Benign mucinous cysts show median expression levels of LGALS4 (approximately 30% of cells positive), while APMTs show an expression profile similar to MOCs.[69] Primary MOCs are generally negative for hormone receptors.[77] APMTs (gastrointestinal [GI] type) are also negative for ER/PR; however, all APMTs (seromucinous type) express ER to some degree and some express PR.[77] Compared with other epithelial ovarian tumors, MOCs show more limited expression of PAX8, with only approximately 20% of both benign/borderline and MOCs positive for PAX8.[33] MOCs are also typically negative for WT1.[37]

Distinguishing primary MOC from metastatic mucinous carcinomas can be difficult. The CK7+/20+ expression profile of MOC is only somewhat helpful, as this cytokeratin pattern is also the most common pattern seen in upper GI and endocervical carcinomas. In contrast, the pattern of distribution of CK7/CK20 is more helpful in distinguishing primary MOC from lower GI tract carcinomas, as colorectal and appendiceal carcinomas typically demonstrate a CK7–/CK20+ pattern.[74] CDX2 expression may be more useful because it is less frequently positive in primary ovarian carcinoma compared with metastatic GI cancer.[76] DPC4 is also useful for distinguishing metastatic pancreatic carcinoma involving the ovary from primary MOC since metastasis from pancreatic carcinomas lose expression of DPC4 in 46% of cases, while primary MOC, endocervical, colorectal, gastric, jejunal, and appendiceal carcinomas typically retain expression.[75] P16, when present in APMT and MOC, is generally patchy compared with the strong diffuse positivity seen in HPV-related endocervical carcinomas metastatic to the ovary.[78]

Clear Cell Carcinoma

Ovarian CCC can be difficult to distinguish histologically from some HGSCs, and CCC demonstrates *TP53* mutations in a small proportion of cases. However, ovarian CCC more commonly harbors type I associated mutations and, therefore, is more closely related to type I ovarian carcinomas. In addition, like other type I tumors it is relatively genetically stable. Though extremely rare, clear cell adenofibromas and atypical proliferative clear cell tumors do exist and, based on clonality, may represent one possible pathway of ovarian CCC.[79] Endometriosis is thought to be the major precursor of ovarian CCC, particularly when the CCC is cystic compared with adenofibromatous (Fig. 37.6).[80]

Molecular Genetic Features

Several common type I pathway mutations have been detected in ovarian CCC, including *ARID1A*, *PIK3CA*, *KRAS*, *PTEN*, *CTNNB1*, and *BRAF*.[81] Somatic

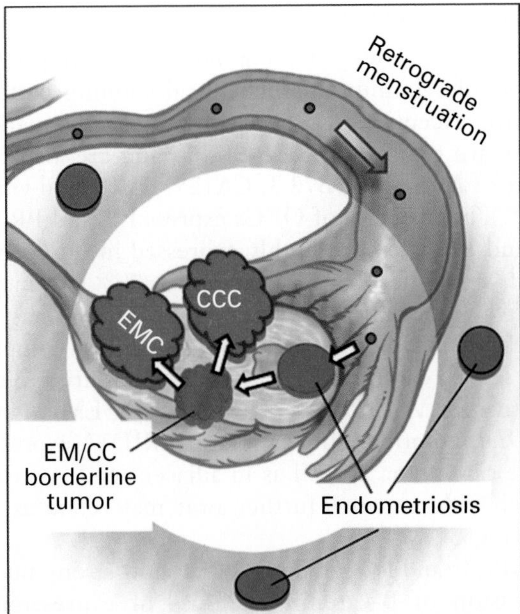

FIGURE 37–6 Pathogenesis of ovarian clear cell and low-grade endometrioid carcinoma. Ovarian CCC and OEC develop from endometriotic cysts, which likely develop from implanted endometrial tissue by retrograde menstruation. These carcinomas frequently harbor ARID1A mutations and PIK3CA mutations. Figure was modified from Kurman and Shih.[54]

inactivating mutations of *ARID1A* have recently been demonstrated to occur in 46% to 57% of CCCs.[82,83] *ARID1A* encodes BAF250a, a protein of the SWI–SNF complex that participates in chromatin remodeling, and is believed to function as a tumor suppressor gene in ovarian CCC and EMCAs.[82,83] Activating PIK3CA mutations occur in up to 46% of pure CCC.[81,83-85] Most of the *PIK3CA* mutations map to exons 9 and 20, similar to other carcinomas with *PIK3CA* mutations.[81] The other type 1 mutations are much less common, with *KRAS* mutations ranging from 0% to 7%,[56,81,83,86] *PTEN* 0% to 8%,[81,84,86] *CTNNB1* 0% to 3%,[81,84] and extremely rare *BRAF* mutations.[56,81] Though *PTEN* mutations are rare, up to 27% of CCCs show allelic loss at the *PTEN* locus on 10p23.3.[86] Jones et al.[83] have reported *PPP2R1A* mutations in 7% of ovarian CCC. *PPP2R1A* functions as an oncogene and encodes a regulatory subunit of serine/threonine phosphatase 2.

Up to 15% of ovarian CCCs harbor *TP53* mutations, which more commonly occur in advanced stage carcinomas.[81,84] However, unlike HGSCs and despite showing loss of heterozygosity for *BRCA1* in 11% of ovarian CCCs, these carcinomas are not associated with *BRCA1* null mutations.[87]

Ovarian CCCs are more commonly associated with endometriosis than any other type of ovarian carcinoma, with up to 91% of ovarian cystic CCCs and 62% of adenofibromatous CCCs showing adjacent endometriosis, compared with 21% of ovarian EMCAs, 3% of ovarian serous carcinomas, and 3% of MOCs.[80,88] Atypical endometriosis is thought to represent the transition between endometriosis and carcinoma, and up to 62% of cystic CCCs are associated with atypical endometriosis/intraepithelial carcinoma.[80] *PIK3CA* mutations are thought to be a very early event in the development of endometriosis-associated ovarian CCC.[85] Identical *PIK3CA* mutations have been detected in ovarian CCC and coexisting endometriotic epithelium in up to 90% of cases, even when there is no atypia present within the endometriosis.[85] Interestingly, all coexisting *PIK3CA* mutations identified in associated endometriosis involved exon 20, with no mutations occurring in exon 9.[85] *ARID1A* mutations also appear to be early events in endometriosis-associated CCC. Wiegand et al.[82] demonstrated similar *ARID1A* mutations in ovarian CCC and adjacent atypical endometriosis. Another study demonstrated that 43% of ovarian CCC with synchronous endometriosis display common loss of heterozygosity events in both components; they also documented loss of heterozygosity of 10q23 and *PTEN* mutations in 56.5% and 20% of solitary endometriotic cysts, respectively.[86]

Immunohistochemical Features

Ovarian CCCs show strong diffuse staining for CK7, CAM5.2, EMA, LeuM1, B72.3, and PAX8 but are negative for CK20.[3,33,50] Hormone receptor expression is usually negative; when positive, ER is expressed more frequently than PR.[50,89,90]

Ovarian CCC can be difficult to distinguish from HGSCs, but correct classification is important due to their very different responses to chemotherapy. P53 expression is generally negative in pure ovarian CCC, though there may be some patchy expression, and CCCs are typically negative for WT1.[3,37,81,89,91] The Ki-67 proliferation index is also lower compared with HGSC.[89] However, ovarian carcinomas with mixed clear cell and high-grade serous components are thought to be variants of HGSC. Immunoreactivity for p53 and WT1 in these mixed clear cell/HGSCs, even in the clear cell component, is more similar to that of pure HGSC, and Ki-67 proliferation is significantly higher compared with pure ovarian CCC.[91]

Loss of BAF250a (ARID1A) expression occurs in 73% of ovarian CCC with known *ARID1A* mutations.[82] Loss of ARID1A also occurs in ovarian endometriosis, but only in the atypical endometriotic areas harboring ARID1A mutations.[82] In a follow-up study, ARID1A expression was lost in both the endometriotic cyst and the associated carcinoma in 90% of CCCs, 90% of EMCAs, and 100% of mixed clear cell carcinomas and EMCAs. In contrast, ARID1A immunoreactivity was retained in the endometriotic cyst and lost in the carcinoma in 9% of CCCs and 10% of EMCAs. None of the cases demonstrated ARID1A loss in the endometriotic cyst with ARID1A retention in the associated carcinoma.[92]

As with uterine CCC, over 80% of ovarian CCCs display diffuse nuclear staining with HNF-1β.[51,89,93] Among ovarian tumors, HNF-1β is a marker that appears unique to CCC. In mixed ovarian carcinomas, the clear cell component shows diffuse staining, while endometrioid and serous components show sparse staining at best.[51] Not only is HNF-1β a good marker for CCC, but its gene may also be a possible target for molecular-based therapy. Tsuchiya et al.[93] demonstrated that reducing HNF-1β expression through gene silencing by an RNA interference technique induces apoptosis in ovarian CCC cells.

Endometrioid Carcinoma

Ovarian endometrioid carcinomas (OECs) may actually follow two different pathways of carcinogenesis. Low-grade EMCAs are best classified as type I ovarian carcinomas, which develop from endometriosis and atypical proliferative (borderline) endometrioid tumors (APETs). High-grade EMCAs show molecular features, specifically a high frequency of *TP53* mutations, more consistent with type II carcinomas.

Molecular Genetic Features

Low-grade EMCAs demonstrate mutations in the Wnt/β-catenin and PI3K/PTEN pathways. Defects in β-catenin signaling occur frequently in ovarian endometrioid borderline tumors and carcinomas, mostly due to activating mutations in the *CTNNB1* gene.[49,84,94,95] Loss of heterozygosity of chromosome 10q23 has been detected in up to 60% of EMCAs,[86,96] with *PTEN* mutations identified in approximately 14% to 30%.[49,84,86,96,97] *KRAS* mutations occasionally occur and when present are mutually exclusive with *PTEN* mutations.[98] When combined, *PTEN* and *KRAS* mutations occur in 80% of low-grade OEC.[96] *PIK3CA* mutations are identified with slightly lower frequency.[3,84] Co-mutations of *PTEN/PIK3CA* have been shown to occur in a subset of OECs.[98] Up to 20% of OECs are MSI high and are associated most frequently with loss of hMLH1 and hMSH2 either by mutation or MLH1 promoter hypermethylation.[49,99] Low-grade EMCAs lack *TP53* mutations.[96,98]

EMCAs are the second most common ovarian carcinoma encountered in association with endometriosis (Fig. 37.6).[88] Somatic truncating or missense *ARID1A* mutations are detected in approximately 30% of EMCAs.[82] As in ovarian CCC, similar loss of heterozygosity events of the PTEN locus on 10q23.3 occur in EMCAs and their adjacent endometriotic lesions.[86]

High-grade EMCAs are classified as type II epithelial ovarian carcinomas due to their high prevalence of *TP53* mutations and relative lack of both MSI and Wnt/β-catenin and PI3K/PTEN pathway mutations.[49,84,96,98,99] *TP53* mutations are much more common in FIGO grade 3 and advanced stage OECs.[84] In a recent study, 90% of high-grade OECs had *TP53* mutations.[96]

Immunohistochemical Features

EMCAs, regardless of their molecular pathway, display similar immunohistochemical staining patterns, with the exception of a few pathway-specific markers. OECs are typically CK7+/CK20– and are also positive for EMA, CEA, B72.3, CA125, PAX8, and vimentin.[3,33] The majority of OECs express ER and PR, and ER and PR are more highly expressed in OECs compared with other ovarian carcinomas.[90,100] P16 may be positive, especially in higher grade carcinomas, but expression is typically patchy and less diffuse compared with serous carcinoma.[78] Primary OECs are typically negative for WT1.[37,46,66,95] Up to 90% of EMCAs with *ARID1A* mutations show a loss of ARID1A expression in the carcinoma as well as in adjacent endometriosis, though endometriosis further away may retain expression (Fig. 37.7).[82,92]

APETs and low-grade EMCAs show strong nuclear expression of β-catenin and loss of expression of PTEN.[49,66,95] Loss of nuclear staining for hMLH1 and/or hMSH2 occurs in the majority of low-grade tumors that are MSI high.[49,99] High-grade OECs, on the other hand, show strong diffuse nuclear immunostaining for p53.[95,101]

High-Grade Serous Carcinoma

HGSCs are the prototypical type II ovarian carcinomas arising in association with *TP53* mutations. The origin of HGSC is a subject of much debate, with many now believing that serous tubal intraepithelial carcinomas (STICs) arising in the fallopian tube fimbria represent the precursor lesion to HGSC in a large proportion of cases. Very rarely, HGSCs may arise from an LGSC after accumulating a *TP53* mutation (Fig. 37.8).

Molecular Genetic Features

TP53 mutations represent the major event in the pathogenesis of HGSCs. *TP53* mutations have been detected in 96% of HGSCs.[59,84,102,103] STICs have been identified in association with a high proportion of ovarian HGSC and display identical *TP53* mutations when the two lesions coexist.[104,105]

The Cancer Genome Atlas Research Network identified several additional low prevalence, but statistically significant, recurrent somatic mutations occurring in HGSC including in *NF1*, *BRCA1*, *BRCA2*, *RB1*, and *CDK12*.[102] Of these genes, *BRCA* may be particularly important in HGSCs considering that nearly 25% of women with epithelial ovarian carcinomas have some form of *BRCA* dysfunction, including germline or somatic mutations, or *BRCA* promoter hypermethylation.[87] At least 10% of women with epithelial ovarian carcinoma have germline mutations in *BRCA*,[106] with more recent estimates reaching 13% to 15%.[107,108] *BRCA1* mutations are more common than *BRCA2*; however, the majority of women 60 years and older typically have *BRCA2* mutations and women less than 50 years old, *BRCA1* mutations.[107,109] Of

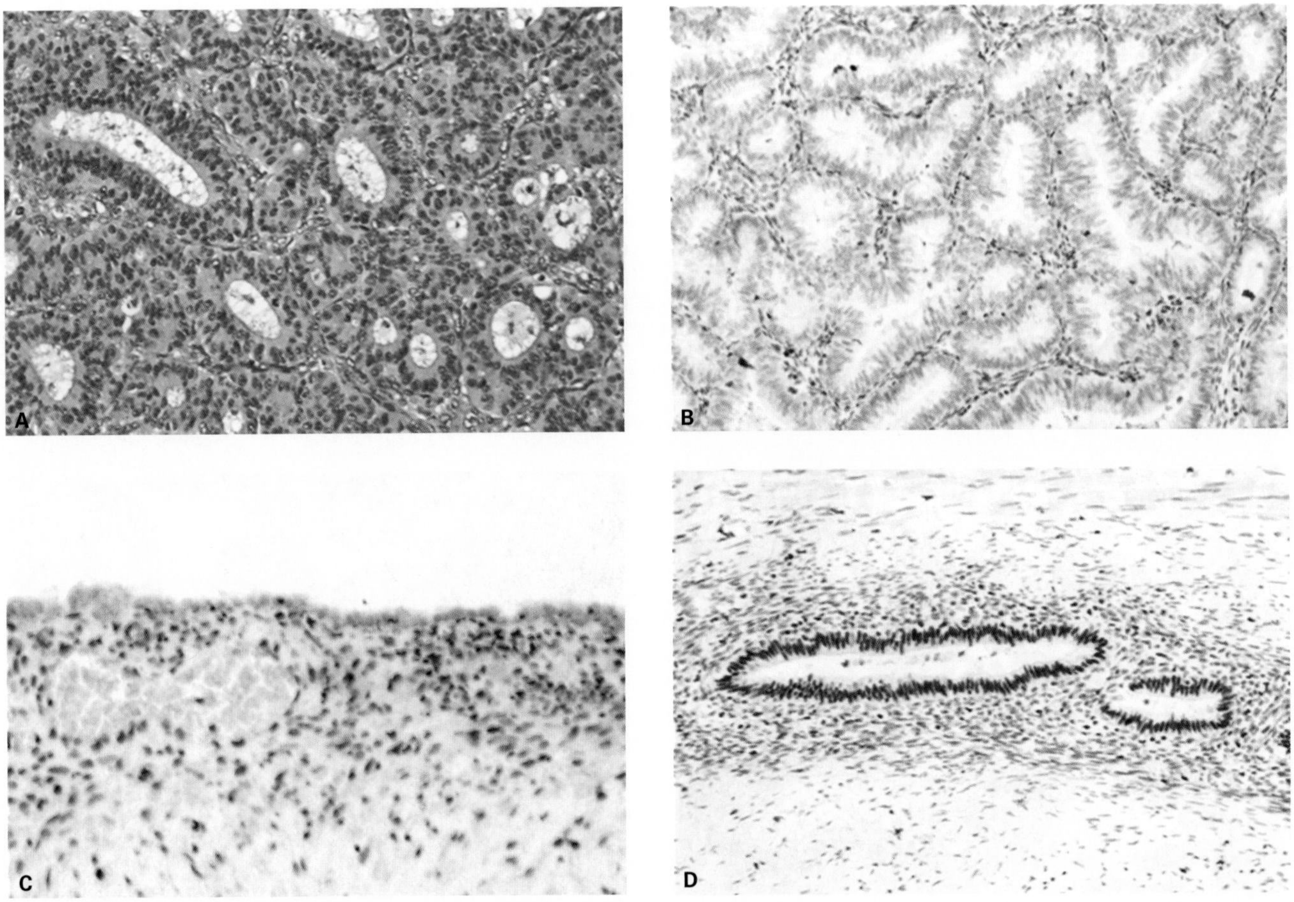

FIGURE 37–7 Ovarian endometrioid carcinoma. Well-differentiated OEC showing confluent glandular proliferation **(A)**. OEC **(B)** and adjacent endometriotic cyst epithelium **(C)** frequently show loss of ARID1A (BAF250a) expression due to *ARID1A* mutations, while the underlying stroma retains expression. Endometriosis further away **(D)** may retain ARID1A expression.

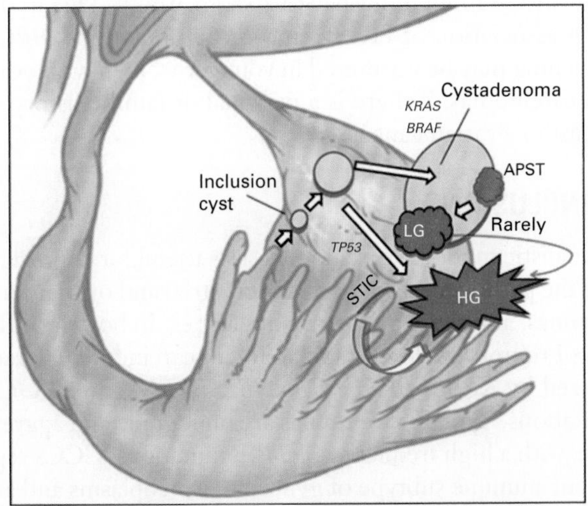

FIGURE 37–8 Pathogenesis of type I and II ovarian serous carcinomas. Type I low-grade serous carcinomas typically harbor *KRAS* and *BRAF* mutations and develop from benign serous cystadenomas and atypical proliferative tumors (APST). Type II carcinomas arise from *TP53* mutations that give rise to serous tubal intraepithelial carcinomas (STIC) which deposit cells on the ovarian surface leading to ovarian high-grade serous carcinoma (HGSC). In very rare circumstances, an HGSC may develop from an LGSC. Figure was modified from Kurman and Shih.[54]

the women with a *BRCA* mutation and ovarian carcinoma, over 75% have an HGSC, with significantly fewer displaying endometrioid histology and none with mucinous carcinomas or borderline tumors.[107,108]

Compared with LGSCs, ovarian HGSCs more frequently show chromosome instability with an increase in allelic imbalance[53] and a higher number of DNA copy number changes.[63] HGSCs lack *KRAS*,[53] *CTNNB1*,[84] and *PIK3CA*[84] mutations. However, activation of *PIK3CA* rarely occurs, but through gene amplification rather than mutations.[58,84] *PTEN* mutations are rarely detected.[84]

Immunohistochemical Features

Ovarian HGSCs express the usual markers seen in ovarian surface epithelial carcinomas, including CAM 5.2, CK7, BER-EP4, CA125, EMA, B72.3, and PAX8.[3,33] They may also show weak CEA expression and are typically negative for CK20.[3]

Similar to USC, the majority of p53 mutations in ovarian HGSC are missense mutations that produce a mutant p53 protein with a longer half-life that leads to protein accumulation in the nucleus. This mutation produces a strong/diffuse nuclear immunohistochemical

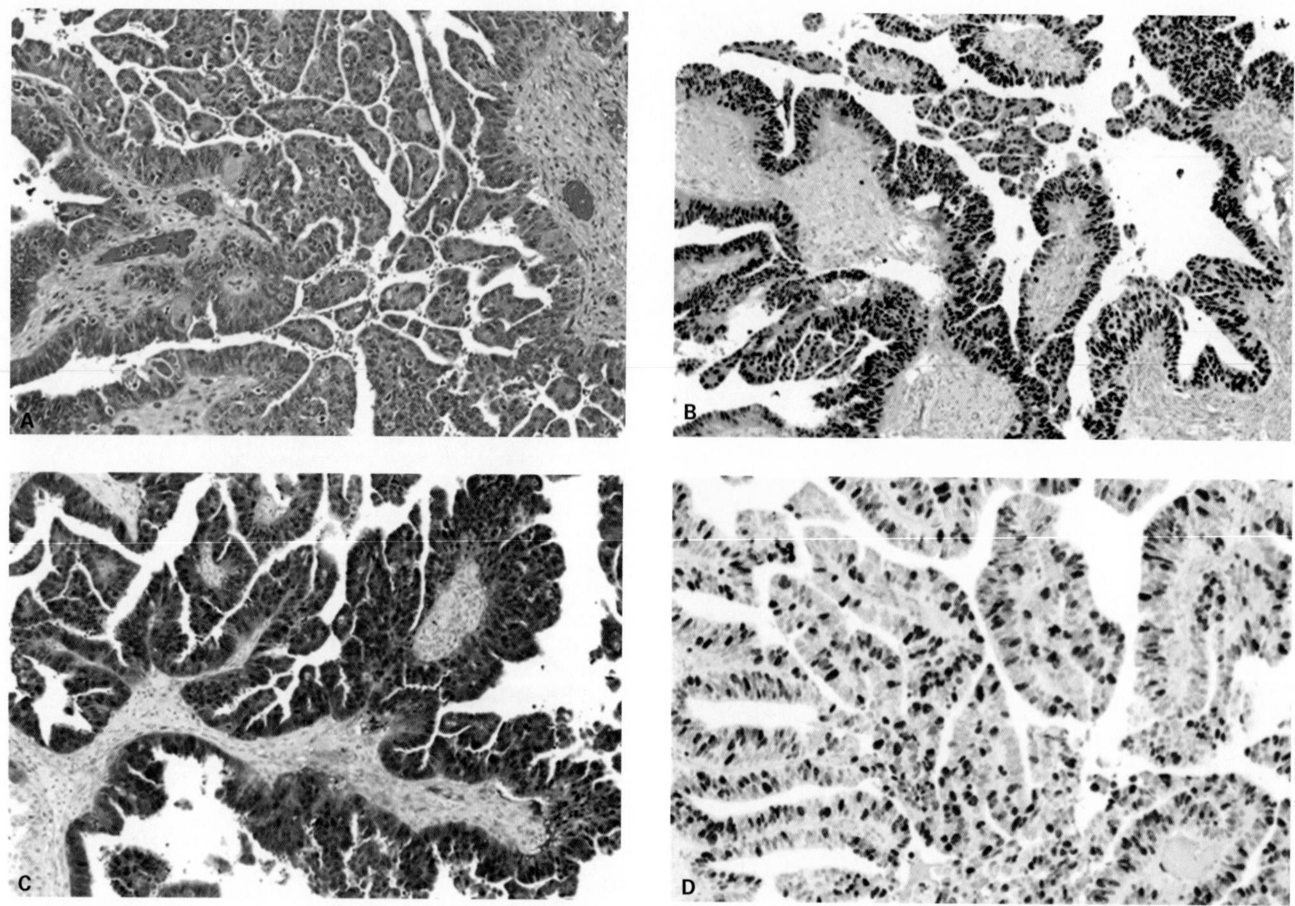

FIGURE 37–9 Ovarian high-grade serous carcinoma. HGSC with papillary architecture and markedly atypical epithelium **(A)**. HGSCs show strong/diffuse nuclear expression of p53 **(B)** and p16 **(C)** and have a markedly increased **(D)** Ki-67 proliferation index.

staining pattern in the majority of ovarian HGSC (Fig. 37.9).[65,66,89,101,103] A small percentage of HGSCs have *TP53* nonsense mutations that form a truncated, non-immunoreactive protein that results in complete absence of p53 staining.[103] STICs demonstrate a similar p53 staining pattern.[101,104,105]

In addition to p53, ovarian HGSCs and STICs express p16[68,101] and WT1[37,65,66,89,101] in a strong diffuse pattern. These carcinomas also have a markedly high Ki-67 proliferation index compared with other ovarian carcinomas (see Fig. 37.9).[65] Loss of BRCA1 expression occurs in a significant proportion of ovarian HGSC, with HGSC showing the greatest loss of BRCA1 compared with all other ovarian carcinoma subtypes.[109] Hormone receptor expression is variable with more frequent loss of PR than ER; up to 75% of HGSC may retain strong expression of ER with only approximately 25% expressing PR.[89,100]

Genetics

BRCA mutations account for approximately 90% of hereditary cases of epithelial ovarian carcinomas.[106] Women with BRCA1 mutations have a 40% to 50% lifetime risk of developing ovarian carcinoma, and women with BRCA2 mutations have a 20% to 30%.[106] Due to the high association of HGSC and *BRCA* mutations, *BRCA* screening may be warranted in younger women with ovarian carcinomas, if there is a personal or family history of breast or ovarian cancer.

CONCLUSIONS

A dualistic model of carcinogenesis is useful for appreciating the pathogenesis of both endometrial and ovarian carcinomas, and there are many similarities. In both models, type I tumors are low-grade, indolent carcinomas characterized by *KRAS*, *BRAF*, *CTNNB1*, *PTEN*, and *PIK3CA* mutations. Type II carcinomas are high grade and aggressive, with a high frequency of *TP53* mutations. CCCs represent a unique subtype of gynecologic neoplasms and are difficult to classify; they display a mixture of type I and II features.

The dualistic model of epithelial ovarian neoplasms shows some distinct differences compared with that of endometrial carcinoma. First, ovarian epithelial carcinomas follow a more complicated pathogenesis compared with endometrial carcinoma, though they share similar molecular abnormalities. Endometrial carcinomas are believed to arise solely within the uterus, while ovarian carcinomas may actually represent secondary tumors. Both low- and high-grade ovarian serous carcinomas may develop in the fallopian tube or from fallopian tube epithelium implanting on the ovary, followed by secondary involvement of the ovary. Low-grade ovarian carcinomas arising from endometriosis could also potentially be regarded as secondary ovarian involvement, if one accepts that endometriosis develops from retrograde menstruation. Second, LGSCs are unique to the ovary.

Molecular analysis is not routinely used to diagnose endometrial and ovarian carcinomas but may become more important as new targeted therapies become available. Immunohistochemical analysis can be useful in diagnosis. For example, an immunohistochemical panel of ER, PR, p53, p16, Ki-67, and WT1 is useful for differentiating many of the endometrial and ovarian neoplasms when necessary.

REFERENCES

1. Jemal A, Bray F, Center MM, et al. Global cancer statistics. *CA Cancer J Clin.* 2011;61:69-90.
2. Siegel R, Ward E, Brawley O, et al. Cancer statistics, 2011: the impact of eliminating socioeconomic and racial disparities on premature cancer deaths. *CA Cancer J Clin.* 2011;61:212-236.
3. Kurman RJ, Ellenson LH, Ronnett BM. *Blaustein's Pathology of the Female Genital Tract.* 2011;Springer. New York. 6th ed. Pages 394-452 and 680-784.
4. Vazquez F, Sellers WR. The PTEN tumor suppressor protein: an antagonist of phosphoinositide 3-kinase signaling. *Biochim Biophys Acta.* 2000;1470:M21-35.
5. Catasus L, Gallardo A, Cuatrecasas M, et al. Concomitant PI3K-AKT and p53 alterations in endometrial carcinomas are associated with poor prognosis. *Mod Pathol.* 2009;22:522-529.
6. Hayes MP, Wang H, Espinal-Witter R, et al. PIK3CA and PTEN mutations in uterine endometrioid carcinoma and complex atypical hyperplasia. *Clin Cancer Res.* 2006;12:5932-5935.
7. Mutter GL, Lin MC, Fitzgerald JT, et al. Altered PTEN expression as a diagnostic marker for the earliest endometrial precancers. *J Natl Cancer Inst.* 2000;92:924-930.
8. Maxwell GL, Risinger JI, Gumbs C, et al. Mutation of the PTEN tumor suppressor gene in endometrial hyperplasias. *Cancer Res.* 1998;58:2500-2503.
9. Catasus L, Gallardo A, Cuatrecasas M, et al. PIK3CA mutations in the kinase domain (exon 20) of uterine endometrial adenocarcinomas are associated with adverse prognostic parameters. *Mod Pathol.* 2008;21:131-139.
10. Velasco A, Bussaglia E, Pallares J, et al. PIK3CA gene mutations in endometrial carcinoma. Correlation with PTEN and K-RAS alterations. *Hum Pathol.* 2006;37:1465-1472.
11. Tashiro H, Blazes MS, Wu R, et al. Mutations in PTEN are frequent in endometrial carcinoma but rare in other common gynecological malignancies. *Cancer Res.* 1997;57:3935-3940.
12. Salvesen HB, Stefansson I, Kretzschmar EI, et al. Significance of PTEN alterations in endometrial carcinoma: a population-based study of mutations, promoter methylation and PTEN protein expression. *Int J Oncol.* 2004;25:1615-1623.
13. Catasus L, Gallardo A, Prat J. Molecular genetics of endometrial carcinoma. *Diagn Histopathol.* 2009;15:554-563.
14. Oda K, Stokoe D, Taketani Y, et al. High frequency of coexistent mutations of PIK3CA and PTEN genes in endometrial carcinoma. *Cancer Res.* 2005;65:10669-10673.
15. Lagarda H, Catasus L, Arguelles R, et al. K-ras mutations in endometrial carcinomas with microsatellite instability. *J Pathol.* 2001;193:193-199.
16. Sasaki H, Nishii H, Takahashi H, et al. Mutation of the Ki-ras protooncogene in human endometrial hyperplasia and carcinoma. *Cancer Res.* 1993;53:1906-1910.
17. Enomoto T, Inoue M, Perantoni AO, et al. K-ras activation in premalignant and malignant epithelial lesions of the human uterus. *Cancer Res.* 1991;51:5308-5314.
18. Lax SF, Kendall B, Tashiro H, et al. The frequency of p53, K-ras mutations, and microsatellite instability differs in uterine endometrioid and serous carcinoma: evidence of distinct molecular genetic pathways. *Cancer.* 2000;88:814-824.
19. Catasus L, Machin P, Matias-Guiu X, et al. Microsatellite instability in endometrial carcinomas: clinicopathologic correlations in a series of 42 cases. *Hum Pathol.* 1998;29:1160-1164.
20. Hampel H, Frankel W, Panescu J, et al. Screening for Lynch syndrome (hereditary nonpolyposis colorectal cancer) among endometrial cancer patients. *Cancer Res.* 2006;66:7810-7817.
21. Garg K, Soslow RA. Lynch syndrome (hereditary non-polyposis colorectal cancer) and endometrial carcinoma. *J Clin Pathol.* 2009;62:679-684.
22. Simpkins SB, Bocker T, Swisher EM, et al. MLH1 promoter methylation and gene silencing is the primary cause of microsatellite instability in sporadic endometrial cancers. *Hum Mol Genet.* 1999;8:661-666.
23. Esteller M, Catasus L, Matias-Guiu X, et al. hMLH1 promoter hypermethylation is an early event in human endometrial tumorigenesis. *Am J Pathol.* 1999;155:1767-1772.
24. Machin P, Catasus L, Pons C, et al. CTNNB1 mutations and [beta]-catenin expression in endometrial carcinomas. *Hum Pathol.* 2002;33:206-212.
25. Moreno-Bueno G, Hardisson D, Sanchez C, et al. Abnormalities of the APC/beta-catenin pathway in endometrial cancer. *Oncogene.* 2002;21:7981-7990.
26. Brachtel EF, Sanchez-Estevez C, Moreno-Bueno G, et al. Distinct molecular alterations in complex endometrial hyperplasia (CEH) with and without immature squamous metaplasia (squamous morules). *Am J Surg Pathol.* 2005;29:1322-1329.
27. Moreno-Bueno G, Rodriguez-Perales S, Sanchez-Estevez C, et al. Molecular alterations associated with cyclin D1 overexpression in endometrial cancer. *Int J Cancer.* 2004;110:194-200.
28. Morrison C, Zanagnolo V, Ramirez N, et al. HER-2 is an independent prognostic factor in endometrial cancer: association with outcome in a large cohort of surgically staged patients. *J Clin Oncol.* 2006;24:2376-2385.
29. Bussaglia E, del Rio E, Matias-Guiu X, et al. PTEN mutations in endometrial carcinomas: a molecular and clinicopathologic analysis of 38 cases. *Hum Pathol.* 2000;31:312-317.
30. Castrillon DH, Lee KR, Nucci MR. Distinction between endometrial and endocervical adenocarcinoma: an immunohistochemical study. *Int J Gynecol Pathol.* 2002;21:4-10.
31. Lax SF, Pizer ES, Ronnett BM, et al. Comparison of estrogen and progesterone receptor, Ki-67, and p53 immunoreactivity in uterine endometrioid carcinoma and endometrioid carcinoma with squamous, mucinous, secretory, and ciliated cell differentiation. *Hum Pathol.* 1998;29:924-931.
32. Reid-Nicholson M, Iyengar P, Hummer AJ, et al. Immunophenotypic diversity of endometrial adenocarcinomas: implications for differential diagnosis. *Mod Pathol.* 2006;19:1091-1100.
33. Ozcan A, Liles N, Coffey D, et al. PAX2 and PAX8 expression in primary and metastatic mullerian epithelial tumors: a comprehensive comparison. *Am J Surg Pathol.* 2011;35:1837-1847.
34. Schlosshauer PW, Ellenson LH, Soslow RA. Beta-catenin and E-cadherin expression patterns in high-grade endometrial carcinoma are associated with histological subtype. *Mod Pathol.* 2002;15:1032-1037.
35. Modica I, Soslow RA, Black D, et al. Utility of immunohistochemistry in predicting microsatellite instability in endometrial carcinoma. *Am J Surg Pathol.* 2007;31:744-751.
36. Yemelyanova A, Ji H, Shih I, et al. Utility of p16 expression for distinction of uterine serous carcinomas from endometrial endometrioid and endocervical adenocarcinomas: immunohistochemical analysis of 201 cases. *Am J Surg Pathol.* 2009;33:1504-1514.
37. Acs G, Pasha T, Zhang PJ. WT1 is differentially expressed in serous, endometrioid, clear cell, and mucinous carcinomas of the peritoneum, fallopian tube, ovary, and endometrium. *Int J Gynecol Pathol.* 2004;23:110-118.
38. Coosemans A, Moerman P, Verbist G, et al. Wilms' tumor gene 1 (WT1) in endometrial carcinoma. *Gynecol Oncol.* 2008;111:502-508.
39. Carcangiu ML, Radice P, Casalini P, et al. Lynch syndrome—related endometrial carcinomas show a high frequency of nonendometrioid types and of high FIGO grade endometrioid types. *Int J Surg Pathol.* 2010;18:21-26.

40. Dunlop MG, Farrington SM, Carothers AD, et al. Cancer risk associated with germline DNA mismatch repair gene mutations. *Hum Mol Genet.* 1997;6:105-110.
41. Lu KH, Dinh M, Kohlmann W, et al. Gynecologic cancer as a "sentinel cancer" for women with hereditary nonpolyposis colorectal cancer syndrome. *Obstet Gynecol.* 2005;105:569-574.
42. Tashiro H, Isacson C, Levine R, et al. P53 gene mutations are common in uterine serous carcinoma and occur early in their pathogenesis. *Am J Pathol.* 1997;150:177-185.
43. Kuhn E, Wu RC, Guan B, et al. Identification of molecular pathway aberrations in uterine serous carcinoma by genome wide analyses. *J Natl Cancer Inst.* 2012 Epub Aug 23.
44. Sherman ME, Bur ME, Kurman RJ. P53 in endometrial cancer and its putative precursors: evidence for diverse pathways of tumorigenesis. *Hum Pathol.* 1995;26:1268-1274.
45. Goldstein NS, Uzieblo A. WT1 immunoreactivity in uterine papillary serous carcinomas is different from ovarian serous carcinomas. *Am J Clin Pathol.* 2002;117:541-545.
46. Al-Hussaini M, Stockman A, Foster H, et al. WT-1 assists in distinguishing ovarian from uterine serous carcinoma and in distinguishing between serous and endometrioid ovarian carcinoma. *Histopathology.* 2004;44:109-115.
47. Lax SF, Pizer ES, Ronnett BM, et al. Clear cell carcinoma of the endometrium is characterized by a distinctive profile of p53, Ki-67, estrogen, and progesterone receptor expression. *Hum Pathol.* 1998;29:551-558.
48. An HJ, Logani S, Isacson C, et al. Molecular characterization of uterine clear cell carcinoma. *Mod Pathol.* 2004;17:530-537.
49. Catasús L, Bussaglia E, Rodríguez I, et al. Molecular genetic alterations in endometrioid carcinomas of the ovary: similar frequency of beta-catenin abnormalities but lower rate of microsatellite instability and PTEN alterations than in uterine endometrioid carcinomas. *Hum Pathol.* 2004;35:1360-1368.
50. Vang R, Whitaker BP, Farhood AI, et al. Immunohistochemical analysis of clear cell carcinoma of the gynecologic tract. *Int J Gynecol Pathol.* 2001;20:252-259.
51. Yamamoto S, Tsuda H, Aida S, et al. Immunohistochemical detection of hepatocyte nuclear factor 1beta in ovarian and endometrial clear-cell adenocarcinomas and nonneoplastic endometrium. *Hum Pathol.* 2007;38:1074-1080.
52. Kurman RJ, Shih I. Molecular pathogenesis and extraovarian origin of epithelial ovarian cancer—shifting the paradigm. *Hum Pathol.* 2011;42:918-931.
53. Singer G, Kurman RJ, Chang HW, et al. Diverse tumorigenic pathways in ovarian serous carcinoma. *Am J Pathol.* 2002;160:1223-1228.
54. Kurman RJ, Shih I. The origin and pathogenesis of epithelial ovarian cancer: a proposed unifying theory. *Am J Surg Pathol.* 2010;34:433-443.
55. Sieben NL, Macropoulos P, Roemen GM, et al. In ovarian neoplasms, BRAF, but not KRAS, mutations are restricted to low-grade serous tumours. *J Pathol.* 2004;202:336-340.
56. Mayr D, Hirschmann A, Löhrs U, et al. KRAS and BRAF mutations in ovarian tumors: a comprehensive study of invasive carcinomas, borderline tumors and extraovarian implants. *Gynecol Oncol.* 2006;103:883-887.
57. Ho C-, Kurman RJ, Dehari R, et al. Mutations of BRAF and KRAS precede the development of ovarian serous borderline tumors. *Cancer Res.* 2004;64:6915-6918.
58. Nakayama K, Nakayama N, Kurman RJ, et al. Sequence mutations and amplification of PIK3CA and AKT2 genes in purified ovarian serous neoplasms. *Cancer Biol Ther.* 2006;5:779-785.
59. Singer G, Stöhr R, Cope L, et al. Patterns of p53 mutations separate ovarian serous borderline tumors and low- and high-grade carcinomas and provide support for a new model of ovarian carcinogenesis: a mutational analysis with immunohistochemical correlation. *Am J Surg Pathol.* 2005;29:218-224.
60. Singer G, Oldt R III, Cohen Y, et al. Mutations in BRAF and KRAS characterize the development of low-grade ovarian serous carcinoma. *J Natl Cancer Inst.* 2003;95:484-486.
61. Vereczkey I, Serester O, Dobos J, et al. Molecular characterization of 103 ovarian serous and mucinous tumors. *Pathol Oncol Res.* 2011;17:551-559.
62. Anglesio MS, Arnold JM, George J, et al. Mutation of ERBB2 provides a novel alternative mechanism for the ubiquitous activation of RAS-MAPK in ovarian serous low malignant potential tumors. *Mol Cancer Res.* 2008;6:1678-1690.
63. Kuo KT, Guan B, Feng Y, et al. Analysis of DNA copy number alterations in ovarian serous tumors identifies new molecular genetic changes in low-grade and high-grade carcinomas. *Cancer Res.* 2009;69:4036-4042.
64. Shih I, Chen L, Wang CC, et al. Distinct DNA methylation profiles in ovarian serous neoplasms and their implications in ovarian carcinogenesis. *Am J Obstet Gynecol.* 2010;203:584.e1-584.22.
65. O'Neill CJ, Deavers MT, Malpica A, et al. An immunohistochemical comparison between low-grade and high-grade ovarian serous carcinomas: significantly higher expression of p53, MIB1, BCL2, HER-2/neu, and C-KIT in high-grade neoplasms. *Am J Surg Pathol.* 2005;29:1034-1041.
66. Madore J, Ren F, Filali-Mouhim A, et al. Characterization of the molecular differences between ovarian endometrioid carcinoma and ovarian serous carcinoma. *J Pathol.* 2010;220:392-400.
67. Wong KK, Lu KH, Malpica A, et al. Significantly greater expression of ER, PR, and ECAD in advanced-stage low-grade ovarian serous carcinoma as revealed by immunohistochemical analysis. *Int J Gynecol Pathol.* 2007;26:404-409.
68. O'Neill CJ, McBride HA, Connolly LE, et al. High-grade ovarian serous carcinoma exhibits significantly higher p16 expression than low-grade serous carcinoma and serous borderline tumour. *Histopathology.* 2007;50:773-779.
69. Heinzelmann-Schwarz VA, Gardiner-Garden M, Henshall SM, et al. A distinct molecular profile associated with mucinous epithelial ovarian cancer. *Br J Cancer.* 2006;94:904-913.
70. Ichikawa Y, Nishida M, Suzuki H, et al. Mutation of K-ras protooncogene is associated with histological subtypes in human mucinous ovarian tumors. *Cancer Res.* 1994;54:33-35.
71. Gemignani ML, Schlaerth AC, Bogomolniy F, et al. Role of KRAS and BRAF gene mutations in mucinous ovarian carcinoma. *Gynecol Oncol.* 2003;90:378-381.
72. Cuatrecasas M, Villanueva A, Matias-Guiu X, et al. K-ras mutations in mucinous ovarian tumors: a clinicopathologic and molecular study of 95 cases. *Cancer.* 1997;79:1581-1586.
73. Wu CH, Mao TL, Vang R, et al. Endocervical-type mucinous borderline tumors are related to endometrioid tumors based on mutation and loss of expression of ARID1A. *Int J Gynecol Pathol.* 2012;31;297-303.
74. Vang R, Gown AM, Barry TS, et al. Cytokeratins 7 and 20 in primary and secondary mucinous tumors of the ovary: analysis of coordinate immunohistochemical expression profiles and staining distribution in 179 cases. *Am J Surg Pathol.* 2006;30:1130-1139.
75. Ji H, Isacson C, Seidman JD, et al. Cytokeratins 7 and 20, Dpc4, and MUC5AC in the distinction of metastatic mucinous carcinomas in the ovary from primary ovarian mucinous tumors: Dpc4 assists in identifying metastatic pancreatic carcinomas. *Int J Gynecol Pathol.* 2002;21:391-400.
76. Vang R, Gown AM, Wu L, et al. Immunohistochemical expression of CDX2 in primary ovarian mucinous tumors and metastatic mucinous carcinomas involving the ovary: comparison with CK20 and correlation with coordinate expression of CK7. *Mod Pathol.* 2006;19:1421-1428.
77. Vang R, Gown AM, Barry TS, et al. Immunohistochemistry for estrogen and progesterone receptors in the distinction of primary and metastatic mucinous tumors in the ovary: an analysis of 124 cases. *Mod Pathol.* 2006;19:97-105.
78. Vang R, Gown AM, Farinola M, et al. p16 expression in primary ovarian mucinous and endometrioid tumors and metastatic adenocarcinomas in the ovary: utility for identification of metastatic HPV-related endocervical adenocarcinomas. *Am J Surg Pathol.* 2007;31:653-663.
79. Yamamoto S, Tsuda H, Takano M, et al. Clear-cell adenofibroma can be a clonal precursor for clear-cell adenocarcinoma of the ovary: a possible alternative ovarian clear-cell carcinogenic pathway. *J Pathol.* 2008;216:103-110.
80. Veras E, Mao TL, Ayhan A, et al. Cystic and adenofibromatous clear cell carcinomas of the ovary: distinctive tumors that differ in their pathogenesis and behavior: a clinicopathologic analysis of 122 cases. *Am J Surg Pathol.* 2009;33:844-853.
81. Kuo KT, Mao TL, Jones S, et al. Frequent activating mutations of PIK3CA in ovarian clear cell carcinoma. *Am J Pathol.* 2009;174:1597-1601.
82. Wiegand KC, Shah SP, Al-Agha OM, et al. ARID1A mutations in endometriosis-associated ovarian carcinomas. *N Engl J Med.* 2010;363:1532-1543.

83. Jones S, Wang TL, Shih I, et al. Frequent mutations of chromatin remodeling gene ARID1A in ovarian clear cell carcinoma. *Science.* 2010;330:228-231.
84. Willner J, Wurz K, Allison KH, et al. Alternate molecular genetic pathways in ovarian carcinomas of common histological types. *Hum Pathol.* 2007;38:607-613.
85. Yamamoto S, Tsuda H, Takano M, et al. PIK3CA mutation is an early event in the development of endometriosis-associated ovarian clear cell adenocarcinoma. *J Pathol.* 2011 225:189-194.
86. Sato N, Tsunoda H, Nishida M, et al. Loss of heterozygosity on 10q23.3 and mutation of the tumor suppressor gene PTEN in benign endometrial cyst of the ovary: possible sequence progression from benign endometrial cyst to endometrioid carcinoma and clear cell carcinoma of the ovary. *Cancer Res.* 2000;60:7052-7056.
87. Geisler JP, Hatterman-Zogg MA, Rathe JA, et al. Frequency of BRCA1 dysfunction in ovarian cancer. *J Natl Cancer Inst.* 2002;94:61-67.
88. Yoshikawa H, Jimbo H, Okada S, et al. Prevalence of endometriosis in ovarian cancer. *Gynecol Obstet Invest.* 2000;50(suppl 1):11-17.
89. Kobel M, Kalloger SE, Carrick J, et al. A limited panel of immunomarkers can reliably distinguish between clear cell and high-grade serous carcinoma of the ovary. *Am J Surg Pathol.* 2009;33:14-21.
90. Fujimura M, Hidaka T, Kataoka K, et al. Absence of estrogen receptor-alpha expression in human ovarian clear cell adenocarcinoma compared with ovarian serous, endometrioid, and mucinous adenocarcinoma. *Am J Surg Pathol.* 2001;25:667-672.
91. Han G, Gilks CB, Leung S, et al. Mixed ovarian epithelial carcinomas with clear cell and serous components are variants of high-grade serous carcinoma: an interobserver correlative and immunohistochemical study of 32 cases. *Am J Surg Pathol.* 2008;32:955-964.
92. Ayhan A, Mao TL, Wu CH, et al. Evidence supporting endometriosis as a precursor of ovarian clear cell and endometrioid carcinoma based on expression of ARID1A. Submitted for USCAP *Mod Pathol.* 2012; 25(S2): 259A.
93. Tsuchiya A, Sakamoto M, Yasuda J, et al. Expression profiling in ovarian clear cell carcinoma: identification of hepatocyte nuclear factor-1 beta as a molecular marker and a possible molecular target for therapy of ovarian clear cell carcinoma. *Am J Pathol.* 2003;163:2503-2512.
94. Wu R, Zhai Y, Fearon ER, et al. Diverse mechanisms of beta-catenin deregulation in ovarian endometrioid adenocarcinomas. *Cancer Res.* 2001;61:8247-8255.
95. Geyer JT, Lopez-Garcia MA, Sanchez-Estevez C, et al. Pathogenetic pathways in ovarian endometrioid adenocarcinoma: a molecular study of 29 cases. *Am J Surg Pathol.* 2009;33:1157-1163.
96. Kolasa IK, Rembiszewska A, Janiec-Jankowska A, et al. PTEN mutation, expression and LOH at its locus in ovarian carcinomas. Relation to TP53, K-RAS and BRCA1 mutations. *Gynecol Oncol.* 2006;103:692-697.
97. Obata K, Morland SJ, Watson RH, et al. Frequent PTEN/MMAC mutations in endometrioid but not serous or mucinous epithelial ovarian tumors. *Cancer Res.* 1998;58:2095-2097.
98. Wu R, Hendrix-Lucas N, Kuick R, et al. Mouse model of human ovarian endometrioid adenocarcinoma based on somatic defects in the Wnt/β-catenin and PI3K/Pten signaling pathways. *Cancer Cell.* 2007;11:321-333.
99. Liu J, Albarracin CT, Chang K, et al. Microsatellite instability and expression of hMLH1 and hMSH2 proteins in ovarian endometrioid cancer. *Mod Pathol.* 2004;17:75-80.
100. Lee P, Rosen DG, Zhu C, et al. Expression of progesterone receptor is a favorable prognostic marker in ovarian cancer. *Gynecol Oncol.* 2005;96:671-677.
101. Roh MH, Yassin Y, Miron A, et al. High-grade fimbrial-ovarian carcinomas are unified by altered p53, PTEN and PAX2 expression. *Mod Pathol.* 2010;23:1316-1324.
102. Cancer Genome Atlas Research Network. Integrated genomic analyses of ovarian carcinoma. *Nature.* 2011;474:609-615.
103. Yemelyanova A, Vang R, Kshirsagar M, et al. Immunohistochemical staining patterns of p53 can serve as a surrogate marker for TP53 mutations in ovarian carcinoma: an immunohistochemical and nucleotide sequencing analysis. *Mod Pathol.* 2011.
104. Kindelberger DW, Lee Y, Miron A, et al. Intraepithelial carcinoma of the fimbria and pelvic serous carcinoma: evidence for a causal relationship. *Am J Surg Pathol.* 2007;31:161-169.
105. Kuhn E, Kurman RJ, Vang R, et al. TP53 mutations in serous tubal intraepithelial carcinoma and concurrent pelvic high-grade serous carcinoma—evidence supporting the clonal relationship of the two lesions. *J Pathol.* 2011.
106. Prat J, Ribe A, Gallardo A. Hereditary ovarian cancer. *Hum Pathol.* 2005;36:861-870.
107. Zhang S, Royer R, Li S, et al. Frequencies of BRCA1 and BRCA2 mutations among 1,342 unselected patients with invasive ovarian cancer. *Gynecol Oncol.* 2011;121:353-357.
108. Thrall M, Gallion HH, Kryscio R, et al. BRCA1 expression in a large series of sporadic ovarian carcinomas: a GynecologicOncology Group study. *Int J Gynecol Cancer.* 2006;16:166-171.
109. Pal T, Permuth-Wey J, Betts JA, et al. BRCA1 and BRCA2 mutations account for a large proportion of ovarian carcinoma cases. *Cancer.* 2005;104:2807-2816.

CHAPTER 38

MOLECULAR DIAGNOSTICS OF BLADDER AND KIDNEY CANCERS

Hikmat A. Al-Ahmadie, Ying-Bei Chen, and Victor E. Reuter

INTRODUCTION

It is estimated that more than 128,000 new cancer cases are caused by cancers of the urinary bladder and kidney in 2010, resulting in more than 28,000 cancer-related deaths.[1] Until recently, management approaches to these tumors have not incorporated molecular biomarkers in the diagnosis, risk stratification, and treatment, which is in contrast to what has become an integral component of the clinical management in other tumors such as cancers of the lung, colon, and breast. Recent major advances in cancer genetics and genomics are changing the landscape and rapidly affecting the clinical management of solid tumors, which undoubtedly includes cancers of the urinary bladder and kidney.

TUMORS OF THE URINARY BLADDER

Bladder cancer is the second most common genitourinary malignancy, accounting for more than 70,000 new cases a year and is estimated to cause more than 14,000 yearly deaths in the United States alone.[1] The cornerstone of diagnosis remains cystoscopic evaluation with transurethral biopsy or resection. Due to the propensity for superficial lesions to recur following transurethral resection despite intravesical immunologic or chemotherapeutic agents, and the high probability of progression of carcinoma in situ (CIS) and invasive disease, frequent follow-up is required. Urinary cytology, either voided or instrumented, has long been used as an important adjunct to bladder cancer detection and surveillance.[2] Improvements to the diagnostic and prognostic abilities of both traditional histology and cytology have been always sought and are becoming more feasible with greater understanding of the molecular biology of urothelial tumors as well as the advent of new technologies that allow for better utilization and application of this knowledge.

Approximately 98% of malignant tumors arising in the urinary bladder are of epithelial origin, and of these, 90% are "usual" urothelial carcinomas (UC).[3] At initial presentation, most UCs are papillary and superficial and characterized by a prolonged clinical course manifested by multiple recurrences following local resection without tumor progression.[4] There is, however, a small but significant percentage of patients whose tumors present with an aggressive clinical course over a short period of time.

Classification of urothelial tumors has undergone many revisions in the past but the most commonly followed system is that of the World Health Organization (WHO) (Table 38.1). This classification was adopted in 2003 and was largely based on the 1998 classification of the WHO and the International Society of Urological Pathologists.[5,6] As with most classifications based on subtle cytomorphological features, it suffers from some degree of interobserver variability.

Molecular Alterations in UC

Many genetic and epigenetic alterations have been described in bladder cancer. Much of the work is pointing toward two distinct pathways that correspond to two main groups of tumors; superficial (noninvasive papillary and flat UC and UC invasive into lamina propria) and muscularis propria (MP)–invasive UC.[7-11] Molecular, genetic, and epigenetic aberrations commonly involved in UC are listed in Tables 38.2 and 38.3. Briefly, most studies of low-grade papillary UC show few molecular alterations apart from deletions involving chromosome 9 and mutations of *FGFR3* (Fig. 38.1) and *HRAS*.[12-23] These tumors are often near-diploid with loss of chromosome 9, by far the most common cytogenetic finding (refer to Tables 38.1 and 38.2 for more details).[24-26] In a recent study utilizing whole-exome sequencing, it was reported that *UTX*, one of the genes involved in chromatin remodeling, was

TABLE 38-1 The World Health Organization/International Society of Urological Pathology Consensus Classification of Urothelial (Transitional Cell) Neoplasms of the Urinary Bladder

Normal	
Flat lesions	Flat hyperplasia
	Flat lesions with atypia: reactive (inflammatory) atypia, atypia of unknown significance, dysplasia (low-grade intra-urothelial neoplasia), carcinoma in situ (high-grade intra-urothelial neoplasia)
Papillary lesions	Papillary hyperplasia
	Papillary neoplasms: papilloma, papillary urothelial neoplasm of low malignant potential, papillary carcinoma (low grade and high grade)

Adapted from Epstein JI, et al. *Am J Surg Pathol.* 1998;22(12):1435-1448.

significantly more frequently mutated in low-grade and low-stage UCs.[27] Urothelial CIS commonly has high frequency of *TP53* mutation but a relatively low frequency of chromosome 9 loss, unless it is associated with a papillary lesion, in which case loss of chromosome 9 is more frequent.[28]

In invasive UC, many genetic alterations have been reported in addition to frequent chromosome 9 deletions, involving dysregulation of several oncogenes and tumor suppressor genes.[7-9] It has been recently shown that tumors with aberrations in *p53/MDM2*, *RB1*, and *E2F3* are associated with more genomic instability compared with tumors without such aberrations.[29] In another recent publication, frequent genetic aberrations of the chromatin remodeling genes (*UTX*, *MLL-MLL3*, *CREBBP-EP300*, *NCOR1*, *ARID1A*, and *CHD6*) have been reported, suggesting a potential role for these genes in the development of bladder cancer.[27]

There seems to be two distinct signaling pathways in UC. While *FGFR3* or *HRAS* mutations in the majority of superficial tumors suggest that they share changes in pathway activation, the common inactivation of *RB1* and *TP53* pathways in invasive tumors may indicate a distinct signaling status.[7,8,10]

TABLE 38-2 Common Genetic and Epigenetic Aberrations in Urothelial Carcinoma

Gene	Location	Role	Abnormality	Clinicopathological Association	Diagnostic Role	Prognostic Role
TP53	17p13.1	Tumor suppressor	Deletion/mutation	HGUC	Y/N	Y/N
MDM2	12q14.3-q15	Oncogene	Amplification	HGUC	N	N
HRAS	11p15	Oncogene	Activating mutations	All grades and stages, up to 15%	N	N
FGFR3	4p16.3	Oncogene	Activating mutations	Predominantly low-grade/stage	N	Y/N
E2F3	6p22	Oncogene	Amplification	Invasive HGUC	N	N
CCND1	11q13	Oncogene	Amplification	All grades and stages, up to 20%	N	N
CDKN2A	9p21	Tumor suppressor	Deletion/mutation/ methylation	All stages and grades, primarily HGUC	N	N
RB1	13q14.2	Tumor suppressor	Deletion/mutation	Invasive HGUC	N	Y/N
ERBB2	17q21-q22	Oncogene	Amplification	Invasive HGUC	N	N
MYC	8q24.21	Oncogene	Amplification	Invasive HGUC	N	N
PTEN	10q23.3	Tumor suppressor	Deletion/mutation	HGUC, all stages	N	N
RASSF1A	3p21.3	Tumor suppressor	Methylation	Invasive HGUC, associated with progression	N	N
FHIT	3p14.2	Tumor suppressor	Deletion/methylation	HGUC, associated with progression	N	Y/N
PTCH	9q22.3	Tumor suppressor	Deletion/mutation	All grades and stages	N	N
DBC1	9q32-33	Tumor suppressor	Deletion/methylation	All grades and stages	N	N
TSC1	9q34	Tumor suppressor	Deletion/mutation	All grades and stages	N	N

HGUC, high-grade urothelial carcinoma.

TABLE 38–3 Common Aberrations in Urothelial Carcinoma as Detected by Loss of Heterozygosity and Comparative Genomic Hybridization Analyses

LOH		CGH		
Location	**Clinical Association**	**Location**	**Type of Aberration**	**Clinicopathological Association**
3p	High grade/high stage	9p, 9q, 10q, 11p,Y	Loss	Noninvasive UC
4p	High grade/high stage	1q, 17, 20q	Gain	Noninvasive UC
4q	High grade/high stage	11q	Amplification	Noninvasive UC
8p	High grade/high stage	2q, 4p, 4q, 5q, 6q, 8p, 9p, 9q, 10q, 11p, 11q, 13q, 15q, 17p, 18p, 18q, Y	Loss	Invasive UC
9q	All stages/grades	1q, 3p, 3q, 5p. 6p, 7p, 8q, 10p, 17q, 19p, 19q, 20p, 20q, Xq	Gain	Invasive UC
11p	High grade/high stage	1q22–24, 3p24–25, 6p22, 8p12, 8q22, 10p12–14, 10q22–23, 11q13, 12q12–21, 17q21, 20q13	Amplification	Invasive UC
11q	Recurrence			
14q	Carcinoma in situ			

UC, urothelial carcinoma.

Activation of the *PI3K/Akt* pathway in UC could occur via the known mutation of *PTEN* and *TSC1*.[30,31] A number of therapeutic applications targeting molecules in these pathways have been developed and are being tested for potential roles in treating UC.

MOLECULAR DIAGNOSTICS

Immunohistochemistry

In the majority of cases, an accurate diagnosis of UC as well as the presence and extent of invasion is achieved by regular histologic examination without the need for ancillary studies such as immunohistochemistry (IHC). However, there is still a role for IHC in certain situations.

(1) In flat urothelial lesions, IHC with CK20, CD44, p53, and Ki-67 may be utilized to aid in the distinction of reactive flat urothelial lesions from urothelial CIS.[32-34] In the normal state, CK20 and CD44 expression is limited to the umbrella cell layer and basal cell layer, respectively. Urothelial CIS is expected to express CK20 in the majority of tumor cells (full thickness) with total loss of CD44 expression. It is also expected to exhibit diffuse labeling with p53 and the proliferation marker Ki-67. On the other hand, reactive urothelial lesions are expected to express CD44 with the other markers exhibiting limited expression. It is important to note that none of these markers should be used individually to establish a malignant or benign diagnosis. Aberrant reactions of these markers are well established and their interpretation must be made in the correct context. Moreover, IHC should not be used in all cases as a screening test, but rather as an adjunctive tool to aid in the histologic classification of atypical flat urothelial lesions or in the de novo diagnosis of CIS where the morphologic features are questionable.

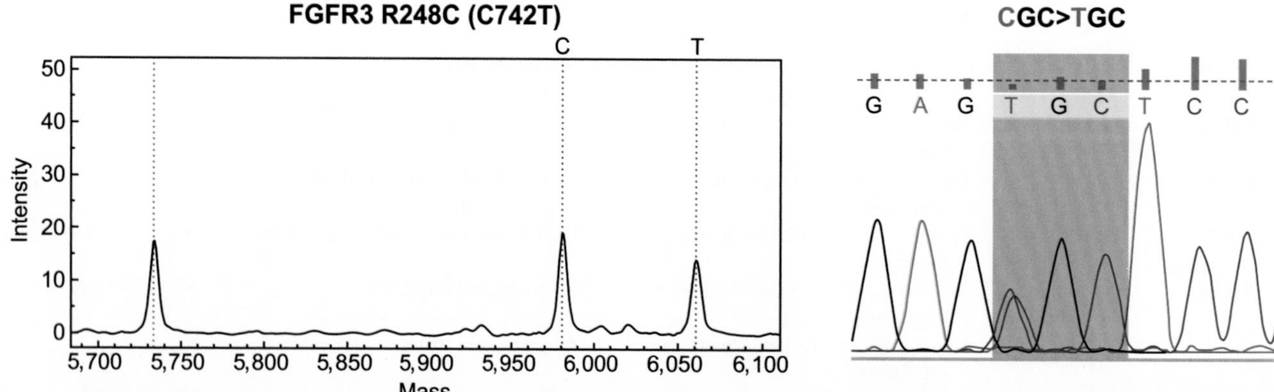

FIGURE 38–1 Somatic FGFR-3 mutation in urothelial carcinoma. Representative mass spectrometry (left) and Sanger (right) sequencing traces for a tumor harboring FGFR-3 mutation R248C, which is one of the more common (hotspot) mutations of this gene.

(2) In papillary urothelial tumors, a number of markers have shown promising results, particularly in distinguishing between low-grade and high-grade papillary UC and decreasing the interobserver variability in this category. Ki-67 and survivin were two markers that have been frequently studied and whose increased expression correlates with recurrence and progression of papillary tumors.[35,36] Similar results were reported when the mRNA levels of survivin were measured in both urine cytology and tumor tissue.[35,37-39]

(3) Lymphovascular invasion (LVI) in UC has been reported to be an independent prognostic factor for metastasis, recurrence, and survival.[40-42] Identifying LVI, however, can be complicated by the presence of peritumoral stromal retraction, which is a relatively common finding in invasive UC and mimicker of LVI. This is particularly problematic within the lamina propria. As a result, assessing LVI suffers from a considerable lack of diagnostic reproducibility, which limits its utility as a prognostic factor.[43,44] If LVI is to retain its clinical significance, it should be reported with caution and after applying rigid criteria for its identification. In this regard, a number of endothelial/vascular IHC markers can be used to confirm the presence of LVI such as CD31, CD34, and D2-40. It is not recommended, however, to use these markers as a screening tool in all cases of invasive UC and they should be used only in histologically equivocal cases for confirmation.

(4) Documenting tumor invasion of the MP is an important parameter in staging UC, upon which major management decisions depend, such as proceeding to radical cystectomy and the administration of neoadjuvant chemotherapy. The distinction between MP and muscularis mucosae (MM), although readily achieved by light microscopy in most cases, may be challenging in some situations, such as diffuse tumor infiltration of tissue fragments, post-biopsy changes that mask the normal anatomy, and marked thermal artifact of tumor-bearing tissue or hyperplastic MM. Several muscle markers have been tried in the past but were found to be of limited utility such as smooth muscle actin, desmin, and caldesmon. Recent reports have identified a new marker, smoothelin, expressed by terminally differentiated smooth muscle cells, to be differentially expressed in smooth muscle of the MP compared with that of the MM.[45-49] It should be noted, however, that other studies reported overlap of staining intensity of smoothelin between MM and MP.[50] Hence, it is still early to determine the exact role of smoothelin as a diagnostic marker to determine tumor invasion into MP and should be used with caution.

(5) Distinguishing invasive UC from carcinomas secondarily involving the bladder is of paramount significance, but can at times be difficult due to significant morphologic overlap. Examples of such scenarios include adenocarcinoma of the gastrointestinal tract, prostatic adenocarcinoma, squamous cell carcinoma of the uterine cervix, carcinomas of the uterus or ovary, and rarely from the breast, lung, stomach, and skin.[51,52] Clinical correlation is essential and remains the mainstay to establish the primary site. IHC is of limited use in these situations except perhaps in the case of prostatic adenocarcinoma, which is typically positive for prostate-specific antigen, prostate-specific acid phosphatase, and prostate-specific membrane antigen and usually negative for keratins CK7, CK20, and high-molecular weight cytokeratin (34be12) as well as p63.[53,54]

Molecular Biomarkers with Diagnostic/Prognostic Values in Urine Samples

Fluorescence In Situ hybridization (UroVysion)

UroVysion is a fluorescent in situ hybridization (FISH) probe set with Food and Drug Administration (FDA) approval for use in monitoring tumor recurrence and primary detection of UC in voided urine specimens from patients with gross or microscopic hematuria, but no previous history of UC. The UroVysion test probe set contains a mixture of four fluorescent-labeled DNA probes, a locus-specific probe to the 9p21 band on chromosome 9 and to the centromere of chromosomes 3, 7, and 17 (Fig. 38.2). The individual sensitivity of the centromeric probes for chromosomes 3, 7, and 17 is reported to be 73.7%, 76.2%, and 61.9%, respectively, while the sensitivity of homozygous 9p21 deletion for UC has been reported as 28.6%.[55] The UroVysion test is based on combination of these probes and the sensitivity and specificity have been reported to be 72% and 83%, respectively.[56] This test, however, is not free of false-positive and false-negative results.[57] Inflammation may interfere with proper interpretation of the test.

The Bladder Tumor Antigen (BTA) Tests

This test is based on the detection of the human complement factor H-related protein, which is reported to be expressed only in bladder tumor cells.[58,59] There are two types of BTA tests, one can be used in the physician's office or even in the patient's home (BTA stat), while the other has to be sent to a reference laboratory for analysis (BTA trak). The sensitivity of the BTA stat is reported to be 50% for low-grade UCs, which is higher than cytology. Conversely, the specificity of BTA stat is reportedly lower than cytology.[60,61] The BTA stat test is FDA approved for use by patients undergoing monitoring for recurrent bladder cancer.

Nuclear Matrix Protein 22 (NMP22)

This test is based on the detection of NMP22, which is a member of a family of proteins that is part of the structural framework of the nucleus and provides support for

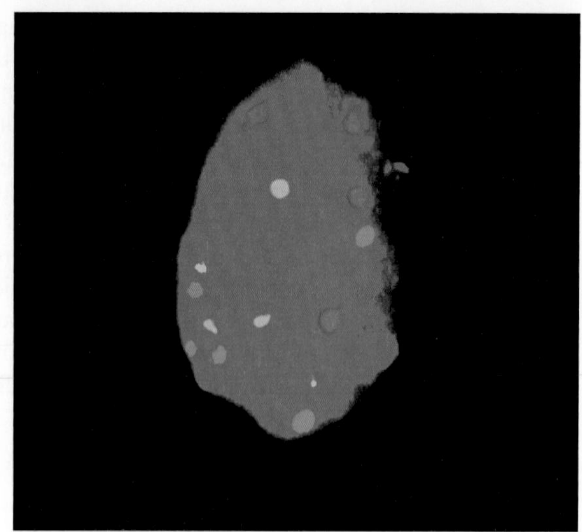

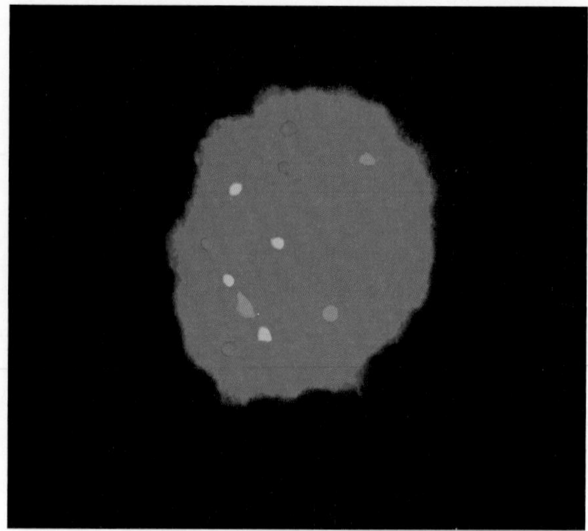

FIGURE 38–2 UroVysion in urine cytology. Abnormal cell with multiple signals (polysomy) for chromosome 3 (red), chromosome 7 (green), and chromosome 17 (aqua). Note the presence of two signals for 9p21 locus (yellow) **(A)**. Abnormal cell with multiple signals for chromosomes 3, 7, and 17 as well as the absence of locus-specific signals for 9p21 (no yellow signals) **(B)**.

the nuclear shape. It is also involved in DNA replication, RNA transcription, and regulation of gene expression.[62] This protein is reported to have a concentration as high as 25 times in UC when compared with normal urothelial cells.[62,63] This assay is FDA approved for both the detection of new cancers and the follow-up of patients with a prior history of UC. The reported sensitivity ranges are 34.6% to 100%, and 49.5% to 65.0%, but false-positive results have been reported.[64,65]

Bladder Cancer Immunofluorescence Assay (Former Immunocyt)

This is an immunofluorescence assay designed to improve the sensitivity of urine cytology. It employs a cocktail of three monoclonal antibodies: M344, LDQ10, and 19A211.[66] The first two detect a mucin-like antigen, while the third one recognizes a high molecular weight glycosylated form of carcinoembryonic antigen in exfoliated tumor cells. This assay is FDA approved only for use as a surveillance test if used in conjunction with cytology. The overall sensitivity of the combined bladder cancer immunofluorescence assay and cytology is approximately 84%, which is better than either test alone. It performs better at the detection of low-grade UC.[67,68]

Telomerase

Telomeres are repetition sequences at the end of chromosomes that protect genetic stability during DNA replication. As a result of telomeric loss during each cell division, chromosomal instability and cell senescence develop. Bladder cancer cells express telomerase, which is an enzyme that regenerates telomeres at the end of each DNA replication. The detection of the ribonucleoprotein telomerase (the telomerase subunits human telomerase RNA and human telomerase reverse transcriptase) in urine samples may offer diagnostic applications as the activity of this enzyme is generally limited to malignant cells and tissues. Detection of telomerase activity is available by the TRAP assay (telomeric repeat amplification protocol), which is a polymerase chain reaction–based method.[69,70] Most studies on telomerase activity in bladder cancer report good sensitivity of the tests but low specificity. Moreover, test results can be influenced by the patient's age and inflammatory conditions of the urinary system, making this assay a suboptimal test for the detection of bladder cancer.[69,71]

TUMORS OF THE KIDNEY

Kidney cancer is the seventh most common cancer among men and the eighth among women in United States. In 2010, there are over 58,000 new cases diagnosed and more than 13,000 patients died of the disease.[72] Accounting for about 85% of all kidney cancer, renal cell carcinoma (RCC) is a heterogeneous disease and consists of renal cell neoplasms with a broad spectrum of pathologic characteristics and clinical behaviors. Although the current 2004 WHO classification of renal cell neoplasms[6] (Table 38.4) is still mainly based on histologic features, molecular and cytogenetic characterizations have been increasingly utilized to improve histologic classification, to guide treatment decisions, and to provide prognostic information. Recent studies have shed light on the biology of renal tumorigenesis and led to the advent of targeted therapies for metastatic RCC in routine clinical practice.[73] While routine hematoxylin and eosin stains, IHC, conventional cytogenetics, and FISH remain our primary diagnostic

TABLE 38-4 Histologic Subtypes of Renal Epithelial Tumors

WHO 2004 classification of renal epithelial tumors
Malignant
Clear cell RCC
Multilocular clear cell RCC
Papillary RCC (type 1 or type 2)
Chromophobe RCC
Collecting duct carcinoma
Renal medullary carcinoma
RCC associated with Xp11.2 translocations
RCC associated with neuroblastoma
Mucinous tubular spindle cell carcinoma
Unclassified RCC
Benign
Oncocytoma
Papillary adenoma
Recently described RCC subtypes not included in the WHO classification
Tubulocystic RCC
Clear cell papillary RCC
Acquired cystic disease–associated renal cell carcinoma
RCC in hereditary leiomyomatosis and RCC

RCC, renal cell carcinoma.

tools, array-based comparative genomic hybridization (CGH) and single nucleotides polymorphism (SNP) studies have been shown to enhance our diagnostic accuracy in clinical settings.[74,75]

The majority of RCCs occur as sporadic cases, but a small percentage of cases present as part of hereditary syndromes (Table 38.5). Genetic alterations discovered in these familial/hereditary forms of RCC provide the foundation of our current understanding of the molecular basis of kidney cancer and implicate genes, including von Hippel-Lindau (*VHL*), met proto-oncogene (*MET*), fumarate hydratase (*FH*), folliculin (*FLCN*), hamartin and tuberin (*TSC1* and *TSC2*), and succinate dehydrogenase B (*SDHB*), in the pathogenesis of various subtypes of RCC.[76] Some of these genes have been shown to be also essential in sporadic tumors (i.e., *VHL*), whereas the role of others remains unclear (i.e., *FH* and *TSC1/2*). Harboring chromosomal level alterations is another important feature of RCC. Certain copy number alterations as well as translocation events have been utilized as characteristic molecular features to help define subtypes of RCC. The common copy number alterations and translocations seen in subtypes of renal epithelial neoplasms are summarized in Table 38.6. What follows is a review of the key molecular diagnostic information available for the main subtypes of RCC, as well as a discussion of the utility of molecular markers in establishing a precise diagnosis, predicting biologic behavior and response to therapy.

Clear Cell RCC

Clear cell RCC is the most common type of RCC and comprises approximately 60% of all renal cortical tumors and 90% of RCCs that metastasize. Histologically, the clear cell cytology, acinar growth pattern, and a rich vascular network are often characteristic features (Fig. 38.3A). However, in high-grade tumors, it is not uncommon to see tumor cells with granular eosinophilic cytoplasm, less conspicuous vascularity, or even predominantly sarcomatoid differentiation (Fig. 38.3B). Careful sampling of the tumor often reveals focal areas of more typical clear cell RCC morphology. In tumors without such areas identified, a diffuse membranous staining pattern of carbonic anhydrase (CA-IX) in non-necrotic area (Fig. 38.3C and D) is an adjunctive marker with high specificity in combination with membranous staining for CD10 while CK7 and α-methylacyl coenzyme A racemase (AMACR) are mostly negative.[77] Difficult differential diagnosis also includes Xp11 translocation–associated RCC, the newly described clear cell papillary carcinoma and other tumors with clear cell histology, where additional immunohistochemical studies will be helpful.[78]

Common molecular alterations identified in clear cell RCC are 3p loss and *VHL* (3p25) mutation. *VHL* inactivation via mutation or methylation has been reported as high as 91% in sporadic cases.[79] Under normoxic conditions, VHL protein (pVHL) binds to hydroxylated hypoxia-inducible factor (HIF)-α (HIF-1α and HIF-2α) and targets it for ubiquitination and proteasome degradation. In hypoxia, HIF-α is unhydroxylated and cannot bind pVHL and, therefore, accumulates and regulates the transcription of a number of genes involved in the regulation of angiogenesis, cell proliferation and survival, glucose metabolism, and extracellular matrix remodeling, etc., such as vascular endothelial growth factor (VEGF), platelet-derived growth factor (PDGF), epidermal growth factor receptor (EGFR), glucose transporter GLUT1, and CA-IX. In clear cell RCC, lacking functional pVHL caused by *VHL* inactivation also inhibits the degradation of HIF-α and the increased level of HIF-α enables the tumor cells to activate hypoxia signaling pathway in a non-hypoxic condition. The high prevalence of *VHL* inactivation in clear cell RCC suggests it is likely an early event in carcinogenesis and additional genetic aberrations are needed for tumor progression. Mutation of *PBRM1*, an SWI/SNF chromatin remodeling complex gene that is located at 3p21, was recently identified as a second major clear cell RCC gene, with truncating mutations in 41% of cases.[80] Inactivating mutations of histone-modifying genes *SETD2* and *JARID1C* (*KDM5C*) were also found in a small percentage of cases.[81] At chromosomal level, besides 3p loss (60% to 90%), 5q gain and loss of 14q are also relatively frequent (20% to 50%).[82] Other regions such as 7, 9p, and 8p are less frequently affected in sporadic tumors.

TABLE 38–5 Hereditary Renal Cell Carcinoma Syndromes and Associated Molecular Alterations

Syndrome	Clinical Manifestations	Gene (Chromosome)	Protein	Normal Protein Function
von Hippel-Lindau	Clear cell RCC, pheochromocytoma, pancreatic endocrine tumors, CNS, and retinal hemangioblastomas	*VHL* (3p25)	pVHL	Tumor suppressor; destabilizes HIF transcription factors
Hereditary papillary RCC	Type I papillary RCC	*MET* (7q31)	MET	Proto-oncogene; receptor tyrosine kinase; binds hepatocyte growth factor
Birt-Hogg-Dubé	Renal tumors (hybrid oncocytic and other types) Fibrofolliculomas Pulmonary cysts	*BHD/FLCN* (17p11.2)	Folliculin (FLCN)	Possible tumor suppressor Interacts with mTOR pathway
Hereditary Leiomyomatosis and RCC	Type II papillary RCC Leiomyomas of skin and uterus (leiomyosarcoma)	*FH* (1q42.3-q43)	Fumarate hydratase	Krebs cycle enzyme, converts fumarate to malate
Tuberous sclerosis	Multiple renal AML Cardiac rhabdomyomas Hamartomas, neurologic disorders/seizures Renal cell carcinoma	*TSC1* (9q34) *TSC2* (16p13.3)	Hamartin Tuberin	TSC1/2 complex inhibits mTOR signaling
Succinate dehydrogenase B–associated pheochromocytoma/paraganglioma syndrome type 4	Bilateral and extra-adrenal pheochromocytoma/paraganglioma, RCC, and other malignancies	*SDHB* (1p36)	Succinate dehydrogenase	Complex II of the respiratory chain, oxidation of succinate, carries electrons from FADH to CoQ

RCC, renal cell carcinoma; CNS, central nervous system; HIF, hypoxia-inducible factor; AML, angiomyolipoma; mTOR, mammalian target of rapamycin.

Understanding of the molecular pathways in clear cell RCC has led to dramatic opportunities for targeted therapies. Currently, there are six agents that have been approved by the FDA for metastatic RCC, including the VEGF and PDGF receptor tyrosine kinase inhibitors sunitinib, sorafenib, and pazopanib, and the VEGF neutralizing antibody bevacizumab, as well as two mammalian target of rapamycin (mTOR) inhibitors, temsirolimus

TABLE 38–6 Common Copy Number Variations and Translocations in Renal Epithelial Tumors

Tumor Type	Copy Number Variations/Translocations
Clear cell RCC	−3p (3p14.2, 3p21, 3p25) +5q −14q −8p, −9p
Papillary RCC	+7, +17 (trisomy or gain)
Chromophobe RCC	−1, −2, −6, −10, −13, −17, −21, −Y (monosomy or loss)
Collecting duct Carcinoma	−1, −6, −13q, −14, −15, −22 (monosomy or loss) −1q32.1-32.2
MiTF/TFE translocation-associated RCC	t(X;1)(p11.2;q21.2): *PRCC-TFE3* t(X;1)(p11.2;p34): *PSF-TFE3* t(X;17)(p11.2;q25): *ASPL-TFE3* t(X;17)(p11.2;q23): *CLTC-TFE3* t(X;3)(p11.2;q23): *?-TFE3* inv(X)(p11.2;q12): *NonO-TFE3* t(6;11)(p21;q12): *Alpha-TFEB*
Mucinous tubular and spindle cell carcinoma	−1, −4, −6, −8, −9, −11, −13, −14, −15, −18, −22
Oncocytoma	−1, −14, −11q13

RCC, renal cell carcinoma; MiTF/TFE, microphthalmia-associated transcription factor/transcription factor E.

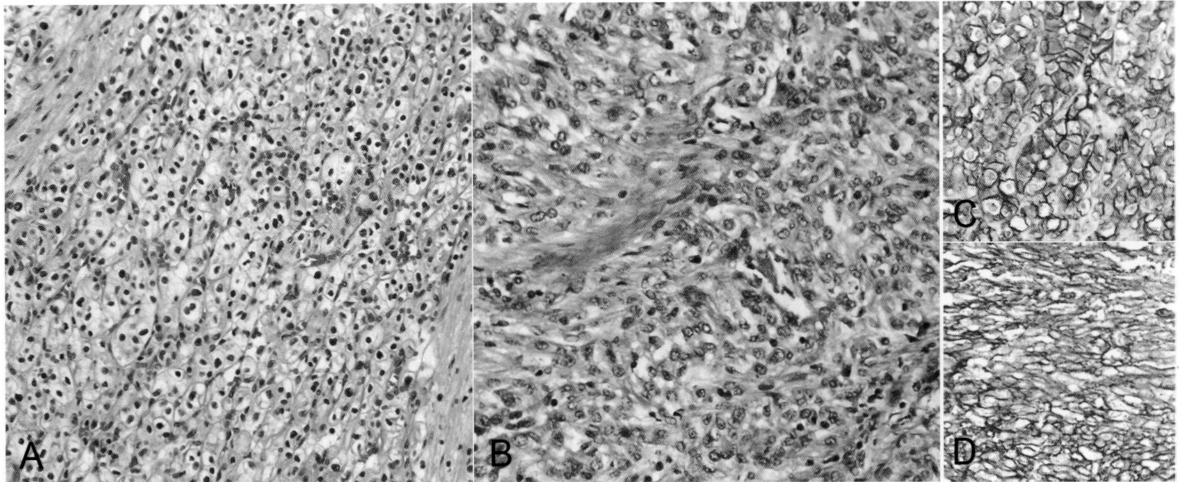

FIGURE 38–3 The histology of clear cell renal cell carcinoma has a wide spectrum. While the characteristic morphology is easy to recognize **(A)**, some tumors can have predominantly sarcomatoid differentiation **(B)**. Carbonic anhydrase (CA-IX) immunohistochemical stain often shows diffuse membranous staining pattern not only in areas with typical histology **(C)** but also in sarcomatoid areas **(D)**.

and everolimus. The effect of tyrosine kinase inhibitors on clear cell RCC could be due to a combination of anti-angiogenic activity and direct anti-tumor effect. The exact mechanism as well as how tumor develops resistance remains to be further elucidated. On the other hand, the mTOR1 pathway regulates the expression and stability of HIF1α,[83] and mTOR inhibitors have been used as second-line treatment for metastatic clear cell RCC. Other potential therapeutic targets under investigation include additional targets within the VHL–HIF signaling pathway, the PI3K/AKT/mTOR pathway, and other putative targets revealed by novel molecular alterations in RCC.[84] Noteworthy, the ongoing genomic research effort in clear cell RCC, such as the International Genomics Consortium and the NCI-sponsored Cancer Genome Atlas project, will soon generate a much more comprehensive land map for the molecular alterations in clear cell RCC.

Papillary RCC

Papillary RCC represents about 10% to 15% of all renal epithelial tumors and is the second most common renal neoplasm after clear cell RCC. The current WHO classification divides papillary RCC into two types: type 1 with papillae covered by smaller cuboidal cells with scant to moderate amphophilic cytoplasm and type 2 with large tumor cells, often higher nuclear grade, eosinophilic cytoplasm and nuclear pseudostratification (Fig. 38.4A and B). Tumors categorized as type 2 papillary RCC particularly have more variations in their histologic features and clinical behavior. Although a papillary architectural pattern is

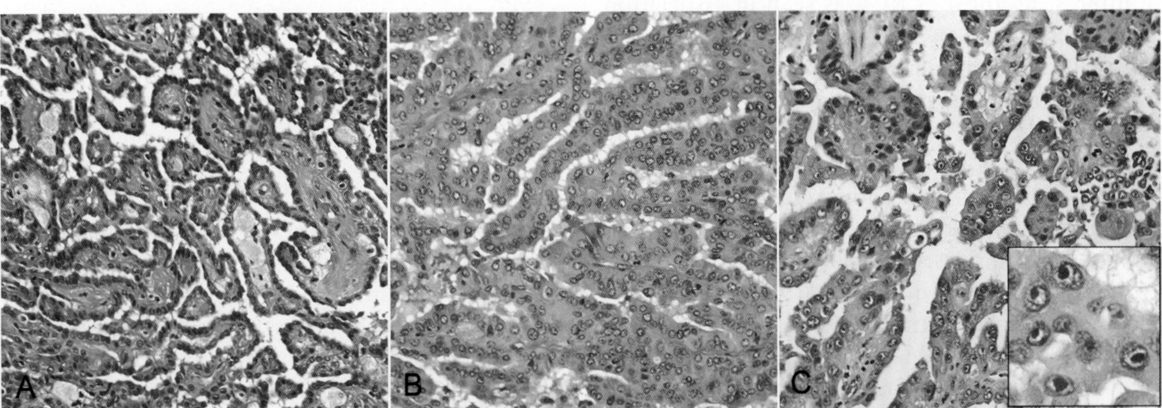

FIGURE 38–4 Papillary renal cell carcinoma (PRCC). Examples of PRCC, type 1 **(A)** and type 2 **(B)**. Renal cell carcinoma arising in a patient with hereditary leiomyomatosis and renal cell carcinoma (HLRCC) syndrome and a germline *FH* mutation **(C)**. Note the large nuclei with very prominent orangeophilic or eosinophilic nucleoli, surrounded by a clear halo (inset).

a characteristic feature, many papillary RCC exhibit other growth patterns such as tubular or solid. Meanwhile, other renal tumors can show variable or prominent papillary architecture and mimic papillary RCC, including Xp11 translocation-associated RCC, collecting duct carcinoma (CDC), and newly described entities such as acquired cystic disease-associated RCC, and clear cell papillary RCC.[85]

By IHC, most papillary RCCs show diffuse positivity for CK7, but more so in type 1 than type 2 tumors. AMACR displays diffuse cytoplasmic granular staining. In contrast to clear cell RCC, CA-IX is either negative or at the most focally positive, and the positivity is often limited to the papillary tips or perinecrotic areas. While histologic features and immunostaining are often helpful to separate most of the mimics from papillary RCC, the distinction between high-grade type 2 papillary RCC and CDC as well as some tumors in the unclassified RCC category, two groups of high-grade tumors that are often diagnosed based on exclusion from other subtypes, can be very challenging. Adjunct molecular markers are sorely needed to improve the classification in these tumors that often exhibit aggressive behavior.

The majority of sporadic papillary RCC are characterized by trisomy of chromosomes 7 and 17 as well as loss of chromosome Y. However, copy number gains in 17 and 7 are more often seen in type 1 than type 2 tumors. Absence of trisomy 17 has been associated with poorer prognosis in some studies.[86-88] Molecular characterizations by microarray expression profiling and aCGH studies suggest that it may be possible to subclassify type 2 tumors to better correlate with clinical outcome.[89] *MET* gene, identified from hereditary papillary RCC, has been reported in up to 13% of sporadic type 1 cases.[90] The overall prognosis of papillary RCC is better than clear cell RCC and either slightly worse or similar to chromophobe RCC (CRCC). However, type 2 papillary tumors have been found to have worse prognosis than type 1 papillary RCC, while there are data suggesting that metastatic papillary RCC has clinically worse outcome than metastatic clear cell RCC.[91]

An interesting form of RCC is seen in association with the hereditary leiomyomatosis and renal cell carcinoma (HLRCC) syndrome. Because of their predominant papillary growth pattern, high nuclear grade, and eosinophilic cytoplasm, this tumor has been historically classified by pathologists as type 2 papillary RCC, but recently genetic analysis has identified germline *FH* inactivating mutations in this subset of patients.[92] The most diagnostic and consistent feature observed so far is the presence of large nuclei with very prominent orangeophilic or eosinophilic nucleoli, surrounded by a clear halo (Fig. 38.4C). Meanwhile, the architectural pattern in HLRCC renal tumors is not always papillary. Some of these tumors demonstrate multifocality, solid and infiltrating growth, as well as associated desmoplasia, histologically resembling CDC.[93] Independent of the growth pattern, these HLRCC tumors are very aggressive. A high percentage (47%) of cases develop metastasis, including pT1 tumors measuring less than 3 cm.[94] Penetrance for RCC in the HLRCC syndrome is lower than for cutaneous and uterine leiomyomas, and patients often present with unilateral, solitary mass that does not necessarily raise the suspicion for a syndromic form of RCC. Somatic mutation of *FH* gene has yet to be identified in true sporadic cases of papillary RCC.[95,96] Although more data are needed to establish the relationship of these HLRCC tumors with other type 2 papillary RCC, we favor the idea that loss of functional FH is the defining molecular event of this subset of RCC, which distinguishes them from other type 2 papillary tumors not harboring this mutation.

In spite of the advances in the treatment of metastatic clear cell RCC, several agents currently available only demonstrate modest activity in metastatic non-clear cell RCC; more effective systemic therapies remain to be identified.[97] Better understanding of the molecular aberrations underlying sporadic and hereditary type 2 papillary RCC will likely be critical for the discovery of novel therapeutic targets in these tumors.

Chromophobe RCC

CRCC comprises 6% to 11% of renal epithelial neoplasms. Composed of large polygonal cells with translucent and finely reticulated cytoplasm in large nests/acini or solid sheets, CRCC mimics some histologic features of clear cell RCC. Yet CRCC, stage-by-stage, has a significantly better prognosis than clear cell RCC; thus, it is important to be able to distinguish these two subtypes of RCC. On the other hand, the "eosinophilic variant" of CRCC consists of cells with densely eosinophilic cytoplasm and may closely imitate other oncocytic renal tumors, including benign oncocytomas. Immunoreactivity to CK7 (diffuse) and CD117 (c-kit, membranous), while lacking staining for CA-IX and AMACR, often supports a diagnosis of CRCC over other subtypes of RCC. Cytogenetically, CRCC is characterized by loss of chromosomes 1 and Y, as well as combined chromosomal losses involving chromosomes 1, 2, 6, 10, 13, 17, and 21.[98-100]

CDC and Renal Medullary Carcinoma

CDC is a rare and very aggressive form of RCC that likely originates from cells of the collecting ducts of renal medulla.[101,102] Although it is a well-recognized subtype of RCC, the histologic spectrum and diagnostic features of this entity are not entirely specific. By IHC, CDC is generally, but not always, positive for high molecular weight cytokeratin (34BE12), EMA, CK7, and CD117. Based on a few cases with cytogenetic data, CDCs have been shown to harbor monosomies of chromosomes 1, 6, 14, 15, and

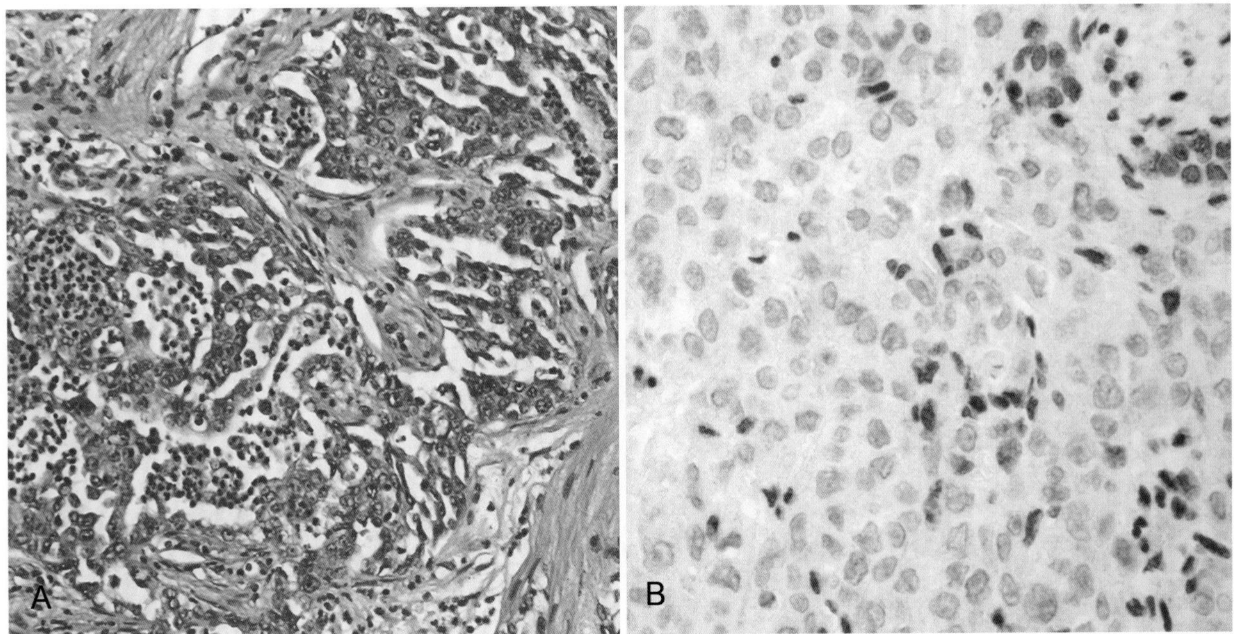

FIGURE 38–5 Renal medullary carcinoma **(A)** shows the loss of INI1 expression by immunohistochemistry **(B)**. Note the intact expression of INI1 in infiltrating inflammatory cells and stromal cells.

22. Loss of heterozygosity (LOH) of multiple chromosomal arms, including 1q, 6p, 8p, 13q, and 21q, have also been described in some cases. A minimal area of deletion located at 1q32.1-32.2 has been detected. Amplification of *HER2* is present in some cases. Trisomies of 7 and 17 (typical of papillary RCC) and 3p loss (typical of clear cell RCC) are not present in CDC.[103-107]

Renal medullary carcinoma (RMC) is a rare and distinctive entity occurring almost exclusively in young patients with sickle cell (SC) trait, and rarely in patients with other hemoglobinopathies such as hemoglobin SC disease.[108,109] Given the overlapping morphologic features with CDC, many consider it to be a particularly aggressive variant of CDC. The loss of nuclear expression of INI1 (SNF5/BAF47) protein is a consistent finding in RMC (Fig. 38.5).[110] Studies in pediatric rhabdoid tumors have shown that both mutation/deletion of *INI1* gene and epigenetic regulatory mechanism can be the reason for loss of INI1 expression,[111,112] but the exact molecular aberration in RMC remains unknown.

MiTF-TFE Translocation-Associated RCC

These translocation-associated RCC accounts for less than 5% of all renal neoplasms in children, but it is the most common type of RCC in this age group. Approximately 10% to 15% of cases in children have a history of prior exposure to chemotherapy.[113] An increasing number of cases are being recognized in adults (Fig. 38.6A).[114] These tumors are defined by translocation involving microphthalmia-associated transcription factor/transcription factor E (*MiTF/TFE*) family genes (*TFE3* or *TFEB*). The *TFE3* gene, located on Xp11.2, may fuse with one of multiple chromosomal sites (Table 38.6, i.e., *PRCC* or *ASPL* on 1q21 and 17q25, respectively) and result in overexpression of the TFE3 protein.[115,116] The *TFEB* gene located on 6p21 is fused to *alpha* gene on 11q12, resulting in overexpression of TFEB.[117] Both TFE3 and TFEB overexpression can be detected by IHC (Fig. 38.6B), a relatively specific assay, but difficult to standardize in a routine laboratory setting.[118] Cathepsin-K, a target of MiTF transcriptional factor, is another marker expressed in TFEB translocation and a subset of TFE3 translocation tumors in comparison to other renal cell neoplasms, but with less sensitivity.[119] FISH assays for TFE3 and TFEB translocations have also been developed (Fig. 38.6C).[120-123]

The diagnosis of translocation-associated RCC should always be considered in renal tumors negative for epithelial markers. Noteworthy, up to 50% of TFEB translocation RCCs express melanocytic markers such as HMB-45 and A-103, and a small percentage of TFE3 translocation tumors can also stain for these markers. Given the shared homology among TFE3, TFEB, and MiTF transcription factors in DNA-binding and activation domains, the expression of melanocytic markers (targets of MiTF) in these tumors has been hypothesized to be mediated by the overexpressed TFEB or TFE3.

The clinical behavior of translocation tumors in children is usually not aggressive, although long follow-up data

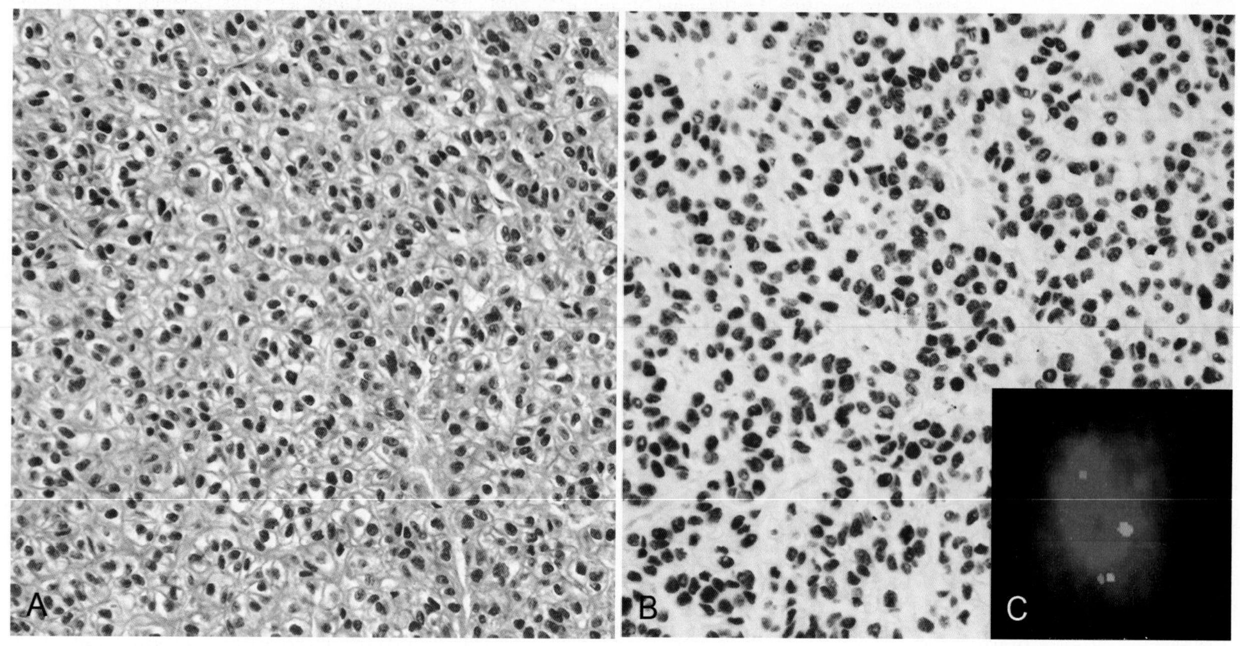

FIGURE 38–6 Xp11.2 translocation-associated renal cell carcinoma in a 60-year-old female **(A)**. The tumor shows diffuse overexpression of TFE3 **(B)**. The translocation is confirmed by a FISH assay using TFE3 breakapart probes (**C**, courtesy of Dr. Juan-Miguel Mosquera).

are lacking.[124] In contrast, the tumors in adults are reported to be more aggressive.[114] Targeted therapy with tyrosine kinase inhibitors and/or mTOR inhibitors has been suggested to have induced responses in some patients.[125]

Methodology

Immunohistochemistry

The immunohistochemical work-up for renal epithelial neoplasms may vary depending on histologic features. Markers with diagnostic utility in various contexts include CA-IX, CD10, CK7, AMACR, TFE3, TFEB, CD117, kidney-specific cadherin, parvalbumin, S100A1, PAX2 or PAX8, 34BE12, P63, HMB-45, Melan A, and synaptophysin.[78,85,126] Kidney-specific cadherin and parvalbumin are additional markers for CRCC and oncocytoma, whereas S100A1 is useful to differentiate oncocytoma from CRCC.[127] PAX2 and PAX8, when combining with tumor histologic features and other pertinent immunostains, are relatively specific markers to help establish the renal origin in a metastatic setting.

Fluorescence In Situ Hybridization

FISH assays are very useful tools in the differential diagnosis of renal epithelial tumors. Tests for trisomy 7 and 17 are commonly used clinically to help establish a diagnosis of papillary RCC. However, the specificity of this test needs to be further explored in tumors with overlapping features such as mucinous tubular spindle cell carcinoma, HLRCC-associated RCC, as well as unclassified RCC with papillary areas, in the context of other molecular alterations identified in these cases. FISH probes for detecting TFE3 and TFEB translocations have been developed and validated for clinical use.[120-123] Although FISH assays for detecting copy number loss, i.e., 3p loss, are available, given the epigenetic regulation often seen with tumor suppressor genes, they are less used clinically.

Molecular Studies

With rapid advance in technology, array-based SNP or CGH assays are being adapted to clinical use in ever increasing circumstances, providing fast and comprehensive assessment of copy number variations and LOH including formalin-fixed paraffin-embedded tissue. Mass spectrometry-based technology (Sequenom) is not only an alternative for targeted SNP genotyping but also a highly sensitive and effective method for somatic mutation detection.[128] In addition, large-scale mutation screen by next-generation sequencing, gene expression analysis, microRNA characterization, as well as methylation analysis are all becoming increasingly accessible research tools for identifying molecular alterations. The ongoing effort in the direction will serve as the groundwork for developing diagnostic, prognostic, and predication markers.

REFERENCES

1. Jemal A, Siege lR, Xu J, Ward E. Cancer statistics, 2010. *CA Cancer J Clin.* 2010;60(5):277-300.
2. Droller MJ. Bladder cancer: state-of-the-art care. *CA Cancer J Clin.* 1998;48(5):269-284.

3. Oyasu R. World Health Organization and International Society of Urological Pathology classification and two-number grading system of bladder tumors. *Cancer.* 2000;88(7):1509-1512.
4. Loening S, Narayana A, Yoder L, Slymen D, Penick G, Culp D. Analysis of bladder tumor recurrence in 178 patients. *Urology.* 1980;16(2):137-141.
5. Epstein JI, Amin MB, Reuter VR, Mostofi FK. The World Health Organization/International Society of Urological Pathology consensus classification of urothelial (transitional cell) neoplasms of the urinary bladder. Bladder Consensus Conference Committee. *Am J Surg Pathol.* 1998;22(12):1435-1448.
6. Eble JN, Sauter G, Epstein JI, Sesterhenn IA, eds. *Pathology and Genetics of Tumours of the Urinary System and Male Genital Organs.* World Health Classification of Tumours. Lyon: IARC Press; 2004.
7. Castillo-Martin M, Domingo-Domenech J, Karni-Schmidt O, Matos T, Cordon-Cardo C. Molecular pathways of urothelial development and bladder tumorigenesis. *Urol Oncol.* 2010;28(4): 401-408.
8. Knowles MA. Molecular subtypes of bladder cancer: Jekyll and Hyde or chalk and cheese? *Carcinogenesis.* 2006;27(3):361-373.
9. Mitra AP, Datar RH, Cote RJ. Molecular pathways in invasive bladder cancer: new insights into mechanisms, progression, and target identification. *J Clin Oncol.* 2006;24(35):5552-5564.
10. Pollard C, Smith SC, Theodorescu D. Molecular genesis of non-muscle-invasive urothelial carcinoma (NMIUC). *Expert Rev Mol Med.* 2010;12:e10.
11. Wu XR. Urothelial tumorigenesis: a tale of divergent pathways. *Nat Rev Cancer.* 2005;5(9):713-725.
12. Tsai YC, Nichols PW, Hiti AL, Williams Z, Skinner DG, Jones PA. Allelic losses of chromosomes 9, 11, and 17 in human bladder cancer. *Cancer Res.* 1990;50(1):44-47.
13. Cairns P, Shaw ME, Knowles MA. Initiation of bladder cancer may involve deletion of a tumour-suppressor gene on chromosome 9. *Oncogene.* 1993;8(4):1083-1085.
14. Habuchi T, Devlin J, Elder PA, Knowles MA. Detailed deletion mapping of chromosome 9q in bladder cancer: evidence for two tumour suppressor loci. *Oncogene.* 1995;11(8):1671-1674.
15. Linnenbach AJ, Pressler LB, Seng BA, Kimmel BS, Tomaszewski JE, Malkowicz SB. Characterization of chromosome 9 deletions in transitional cell carcinoma by microsatellite assay. *Hum Mol Genet.* 1993;2(9):1407-1411.
16. Cappellen D, De Oliveira C, Ricol D, et al. Frequent activating mutations of FGFR3 in human bladder and cervix carcinomas. *Nat Genet.* 1999;23(1):18-20.
17. Billerey C, Chopin D, Aubriot-Lorton MH, et al. Frequent FGFR3 mutations in papillary non-invasive bladder (pTa) tumors. *Am J Pathol.* 2001;158(6):1955-1959.
18. van Rhijn BW, Lurkin I, Radvanyi F, Kirkels WJ, van der Kwast TH, Zwarthoff EC. The fibroblast growth factor receptor 3 (FGFR3) mutation is a strong indicator of superficial bladder cancer with low recurrence rate. *Cancer Res.* 2001;61(4):1265-1268.
19. Al-Ahmadie HA, Iyer G, Janakiraman M, et al. Somatic mutation of fibroblast growth factor receptor-3 (FGFR3) defines a distinct morphological subtype of high-grade urothelial carcinoma. *J Pathol.* 2011;224(2):270-279.
20. Theodorescu D, Cornil I, Fernandez BJ, Kerbel RS. Overexpression of normal and mutated forms of HRAS induces orthotopic bladder invasion in a human transitional cell carcinoma. *Proc Natl Acad Sci U S A.* 1990;87(22):9047-9051.
21. Czerniak B, Cohen GL, Etkind P, et al. Concurrent mutations of coding and regulatory sequences of the Ha-ras gene in urinary bladder carcinomas. *Hum Pathol.* 1992;23(11):1199-1204.
22. Knowles MA, Williamson M. Mutation of H-ras is infrequent in bladder cancer: confirmation by single-strand conformation polymorphism analysis, designed restriction fragment length polymorphisms, and direct sequencing. *Cancer Res.* 1993;53(1):133-139.
23. Zhang ZT, Pak J, Huang HY, et al. Role of Ha-ras activation in superficial papillary pathway of urothelial tumor formation. *Oncogene.* 2001;20(16):1973-1980.
24. Fadl-Elmula I, Gorunova L, Mandahl N, et al. Karyotypic characterization of urinary bladder transitional cell carcinomas. *Genes Chromosomes Cancer.* 2000;29(3):256-265.
25. Aboulkassim TO, LaRue H, Lemieux P, Rousseau F, Fradet Y. Alteration of the PATCHED locus in superficial bladder cancer. *Oncogene.* 2003;22(19):2967-2971.
26. Simoneau M, Aboulkassim TO, LaRue H, Rousseau F, Fradet Y. Four tumor suppressor loci on chromosome 9q in bladder cancer: evidence for two novel candidate regions at 9q22.3 and 9q31. *Oncogene.* 1999;18(1):157-163.
27. Gui Y, Guo G, Huang Y, et al. Frequent mutations of chromatin remodeling genes in transitional cell carcinoma of the bladder. *Nat Genet.* 2011;43(9):875-878.
28. Hopman AH, Kamps MA, Speel EJ, Schapers RF, Sauter G, Ramaekers FC. Identification of chromosome 9 alterations and p53 accumulation in isolated carcinoma in situ of the urinary bladder versus carcinoma in situ associated with carcinoma. *Am J Pathol.* 2002;161(4):1119-1125.
29. Lindgren D, Frigyesi A, Gudjonsson S, et al. Combined gene expression and genomic profiling define two intrinsic molecular subtypes of urothelial carcinoma and gene signatures for molecular grading and outcome. *Cancer Res.* 2010;70(9):3463-3472.
30. Wu X, Obata T, Khan Q, Highshaw RA, De Vere White R, Sweeney C. et al. The phosphatidylinositol-3 kinase pathway regulates bladder cancer cell invasion. *BJU Int.* 2004;93(1): 143-150.
31. Chen M, Gu J, Delclos GL, et al. Genetic variations of the PI3K-AKT-mTOR pathway and clinical outcome in muscle invasive and metastatic bladder cancer patients. *Carcinogenesis.* 2010;31(8):1387-1391.
32. McKenney JK, Desai S, Cohen C, Amin MB. Discriminatory immunohistochemical staining of urothelial carcinoma in situ and non-neoplastic urothelium: an analysis of cytokeratin 20, p53, and CD44 antigens. *Am J Surg Pathol.* 2001;25(8):1074-1078.
33. Kunju LP, Lee CT, Montie J, Shah RB. Utility of cytokeratin 20 and Ki-67 as markers of urothelial dysplasia. *Pathol Int.* 2005;55(5):248-254.
34. Mallofre C, Castillo M, Morente V, Sole M. Immunohistochemical expression of CK20, p53, and Ki-67 as objective markers of urothelial dysplasia. *Mod Pathol.* 2003;16(3):187-191.
35. Chen YB, Tu JJ, Kao J, Zhou XK, Chen YT. Survivin as a useful adjunct marker for the grading of papillary urothelial carcinoma. *Arch Pathol Lab Med.* 2008;132(2):224-231.
36. Yin W, Chen N, Zhang Y, et al. Survivin nuclear labeling index: a superior biomarker in superficial urothelial carcinoma of human urinary bladder. *Mod Pathol.* 2006;19(11):1487-1497.
37. Karam JA, Lotan Y, Ashfaq R, Sagalowsky AI, Shariat SF. Survivin expression in patients with non-muscle-invasive urothelial cell carcinoma of the bladder. *Urology.* 2007;70(3):482-486.
38. Schultz IJ, Kiemeney LA, Karthaus HF, et al. Survivin mRNA copy number in bladder washings predicts tumor recurrence in patients with superficial urothelial cell carcinomas. *Clin Chem.* 2004;50(8):1425-1428.
39. Moussa O, Abol-Enein H, Bissada NK, Keane T, Ghoneim MA, Watson DK. Evaluation of survivin reverse transcriptase-polymerase chain reaction for noninvasive detection of bladder cancer. *J Urol.* 2006;175(6):2312-2316.
40. Gondo T, Nakashima J, Ozu C, et al. Risk stratification of survival by lymphovascular invasion, pathological stage, and surgical margin in patients with bladder cancer treated with radical cystectomy. *Int J Clin Oncol.* 2011 Sep 7 [Epub ahead of print]. DOI:10.1007/s10147-011-0310-7.
41. Lotan Y, Gupta A, Shariat SF, et al. Lymphovascular invasion is independently associated with overall survival, cause-specific survival, and local and distant recurrence in patients with negative lymph nodes at radical cystectomy. *J Clin Oncol.* 2005;23(27):6533-6539.
42. Bolenz C, Herrmann E, Bastian PJ, et al. Lymphovascular invasion is an independent predictor of oncological outcomes in patients with lymph node-negative urothelial bladder cancer treated by radical cystectomy: a multicentre validation trial. *BJU Int.* 2010;106(4):493-499.
43. Algaba F. Lymphovascular invasion as a prognostic tool for advanced bladder cancer. *Curr Opin Urol.* 2006;16(5):367-371.
44. Reuter VE. Lymphovascular invasion as an independent predictor of recurrence and survival in node-negative bladder cancer remains to be proven. *J Clin Oncol.* 2005;23(27):6450-6451.
45. Paner GP, Shen SS, Lapetino S, et al. Diagnostic utility of antibody to smoothelin in the distinction of muscularis propria from muscularis mucosae of the urinary bladder: a potential ancillary tool in the pathologic staging of invasive urothelial carcinoma. *Am J Surg Pathol.* 2009;33(1):91-98.

46. Council L, Hameed O. Differential expression of immunohistochemical markers in bladder smooth muscle and myofibroblasts, and the potential utility of desmin, smoothelin, and vimentin in staging of bladder carcinoma. *Mod Pathol.* 2009;22(5):639-650.
47. Paner GP, Brown JG, Lapetino S, et al. Diagnostic use of antibody to smoothelin in the recognition of muscularis propria in transurethral resection of urinary bladder tumor (TURBT) specimens. *Am J Surg Pathol.* 2010;34(6):792-799.
48. Hansel DE, Paner GP, Nese N, Amin MB. Limited smoothelin expression within the muscularis mucosae: validation in bladder diverticula. *Hum Pathol.* 2011;42(11):1770-6.
49. Khayyata S, Dudas M, Rohan SM, et al. Distribution of smoothelin expression in the musculature of the genitourinary tract. *Lab Invest.* 2009;89:175a
50. Miyamoto H, Sharma RB, Illei PB, Epstein JI. Pitfalls in the use of smoothelin to identify muscularis propria invasion by urothelial carcinoma. *Am J Surg Pathol.* 2010;34(3):418-422.
51. Coleman JF, Hansel DE. Utility of diagnostic and prognostic markers in urothelial carcinoma of the bladder. *Adv Anat Pathol.* 2009;16(2):67-78.
52. Bates AW, Baithun SI. Secondary neoplasms of the bladder are histological mimics of nontransitional cell primary tumours: clinicopathological and histological features of 282 cases. *Histopathology.* 2000;36(1):32-40.
53. Chuang AY, DeMarzo AM, Veltri RW, Sharma RB, Bieberich CJ, Epstein JI. Immunohistochemical differentiation of high-grade prostate carcinoma from urothelial carcinoma. *Am J Surg Pathol.* 2007;31(8):1246-1255.
54. Genega EM, Hutchinson B, Reuter VE, Gaudin PB. Immunophenotype of high-grade prostatic adenocarcinoma and urothelial carcinoma. *Mod Pathol.* 2000;13(11):1186-1191.
55. Sokolova IA, Halling KC, Jenkins RB, et al. The development of a multitarget, multicolor fluorescence in situ hybridization assay for the detection of urothelial carcinoma in urine. *J Mol Diagn.* 2000;2(3):116-123.
56. Hajdinjak T. UroVysion FISH test for detecting urothelial cancers: meta-analysis of diagnostic accuracy and comparison with urinary cytology testing. *Urol Oncol.* 2008;26(6):646-651.
57. Ferra S, Denley R, Herr H, Dalbagni G, Jhanwar S, Lin O. Reflex UroVysion testing in suspicious urine cytology cases. *Cancer.* 2009;117(1):7-14.
58. Burchardt M, Burchardt T, Shabsigh A, De La Taille A, Benson MC, Sawczuk I. Current concepts in biomarker technology for bladder cancers. *Clin Chem.* 2000;46(5):595-605.
59. Heicappell R, Wettig IC, Schostak M, et al. Quantitative detection of human complement factor H-related protein in transitional cell carcinoma of the urinary bladder. *Eur Urol.* 1999;35(1):81-87.
60. Murphy WM, Rivera-Ramirez I, Medina CA, Wright NJ, Wajsman Z. The bladder tumor antigen (BTA) test compared to voided urine cytology in the detection of bladder neoplasms. *J Urol.* 1997;158(6):2102-2106.
61. Sanchez-Carbayo M, Herrero E, Megias J, et al. Initial evaluation of the diagnostic performance of the new urinary bladder cancer antigen test as a tumor marker for transitional cell carcinoma of the bladder. *J Urol.* 1999;161(4):1110-1115.
62. Berezney R, Coffey DS. Identification of a nuclear protein matrix. *Biochem Biophys Res Commun.* 1974;60(4):1410-1417.
63. Fey EG, Krochmalnic G, Penman S. The nonchromatin substructures of the nucleus: the ribonucleoprotein (RNP)-containing and RNP-depleted matrices analyzed by sequential fractionation and resinless section electron microscopy. *J Cell Biol.* 1986;102(5):1654-1665.
64. Budman LI, Kassouf W, Steinberg JR. Biomarkers for detection and surveillance of bladder cancer. *Can Urol Assoc J.* 2008;2(3):212-221.
65. Chang YH, Wu CH, Lee YL, Huang PH, Kao YL, Shiau MY. Evaluation of nuclear matrix protein-22 as a clinical diagnostic marker for bladder cancer. *Urology.* 2004;64(4):687-692.
66. Fradet Y, Lockhard C. Performance characteristics of a new monoclonal antibody test for bladder cancer: ImmunoCyt trade mark. *Can J Urol.* 1997;4(3):400-405.
67. Tetu B, Tiguert R, Harel F, Fradet Y. ImmunoCyt/uCyt+ improves the sensitivity of urine cytology in patients followed for urothelial carcinoma. *Mod Pathol.* 2005;18(1):83-89.
68. Sullivan PS, Nooraie F, Sanchez H, et al. Comparison of ImmunoCyt, UroVysion, and urine cytology in detection of recurrent urothelial carcinoma: a "split-sample" study. *Cancer.* 2009;117(3):167-173.
69. Muller M. Telomerase: its clinical relevance in the diagnosis of bladder cancer. *Oncogene.* 2002;21(4):650-655.
70. Kim NW, Piatyszek MA, Prowse KR, et al. Specific association of human telomerase activity with immortal cells and cancer. *Science.* 1994;266(5193):2011-2015.
71. Weikert S, Krause H, Wolff I, et al. Quantitative evaluation of telomerase subunits in urine as biomarkers for noninvasive detection of bladder cancer. *Int J Cancer.* 2005;117(2):274-280.
72. Siegel R, Ward E, Brawley O, Jemal A. et al. Cancer statistics, 2011: the impact of eliminating socioeconomic and racial disparities on premature cancer deaths. *CA Cancer J Clin.* 2011;61(4):212-236.
73. Molina AM, Motzer RJ. Clinical practice guidelines for the treatment of metastatic renal cell carcinoma: today and tomorrow. *Oncologist.* 2011;16(suppl 2):45-50.
74. Kim HJ, Shen SS, Ayala AG, et al. Virtual-karyotyping with SNP microarrays in morphologically challenging renal cell neoplasms: a practical and useful diagnostic modality. *Am J Surg Pathol.* 2009;33(9):1276-1286.
75. Vieira J, Henrique R, Ribeiro FR, et al. Feasibility of differential diagnosis of kidney tumors by comparative genomic hybridization of fine needle aspiration biopsies. *Genes Chromosomes Cancer.* 2010;49(10):935-947.
76. Linehan WM, Srinivasan R, Schmidt LS. The genetic basis of kidney cancer: a metabolic disease. *Nat Rev Urol.* 2010;7(5):277-285.
77. Tickoo SK, Alden D, Olgac S, et al. Immunohistochemical expression of hypoxia inducible factor-1alpha and its downstream molecules in sarcomatoid renal cell carcinoma. *J Urol.* 2007;177(4):1258-1263.
78. Reuter VE, Tickoo SK. Differential diagnosis of renal tumours with clear cell histology. *Pathology.* 2010;42(4):374-383.
79. Nickerson ML, Jaeger E, Shi Y, et al. Improved identification of von Hippel-Lindau gene alterations in clear cell renal tumors. *Clin Cancer Res.* 2008;14(15):4726-4734.
80. Varela I, Tarpey P, Raine K, et al. Exome sequencing identifies frequent mutation of the SWI/SNF complex gene PBRM1 in renal carcinoma. *Nature.* 2011;469(7331):539-542.
81. Dalgliesh GL, Furge K, Greenman C, et al. Systematic sequencing of renal carcinoma reveals inactivation of histone modifying genes. *Nature.* 2010;463(7279):360-363.
82. Zhang Z, Wondergem B, Dykema K. A comprehensive study of progressive cytogenetic alterations in clear cell renal cell carcinoma and a new model for ccRCC tumorigenesis and progression. *Adv Bioinformatics.* 2010:428325.
83. Thomas GV, Tran C, Mellinghoff IK, et al. Hypoxia-inducible factor determines sensitivity to inhibitors of mTOR in kidney cancer. *Nat Med.* 2006;12(1):122-127.
84. Rasmussen N, Rathmell WK. Looking beyond inhibition of VEGF/mTOR: emerging targets for renal cell carcinoma drug development. *Curr Clin Pharmacol.* 2011;6(3):199-206.
85. Tickoo SK, Reuter VE. Differential diagnosis of renal tumors with papillary architecture. *Adv Anat Pathol.* 2011;18(2): 120-132.
86. Jiang F, Richter J, Schraml P, et al. Chromosomal imbalances in papillary renal cell carcinoma: genetic differences between histological subtypes. *Am J Pathol.* 1998;153(5):1467-1473.
87. Sanders ME, Mick R, Tomaszewski JE, Barr FG. Unique patterns of allelic imbalance distinguish type 1 from type 2 sporadic papillary renal cell carcinoma. *Am J Pathol.* 2002;161(3):997-1005.
88. Klatte T, Pantuck AJ, Said JW, et al. Cytogenetic and molecular tumor profiling for type 1 and type 2 papillary renal cell carcinoma. *Clin Cancer Res.* 2009;15(4):1162-1169.
89. Yang XJ, Tan MH, Kim HL, et al. A molecular classification of papillary renal cell carcinoma. *Cancer Res.* 2005;65(13):5628-5637.
90. Schmidt L, Junker K, Nakaigawa N, et al. Novel mutations of the MET proto-oncogene in papillary renal carcinomas. *Oncogene.* 1999;18(14):2343-2350.
91. Margulis V, Tamboli P, Matin SF, Swanson DA, Wood CG. et al. Analysis of clinicopathologic predictors of oncologic outcome provides insight into the natural history of surgically managed papillary renal cell carcinoma. *Cancer.* 2008;112(7):1480-1488.

92. Tomlinson IP, Alam NA, Rowan AJ, et al. Germline mutations in FH predispose to dominantly inherited uterine fibroids, skin leiomyomata and papillary renal cell cancer. *Nat Genet.* 2002;30(4):406-410.
93. Merino MJ, Torres-Cabala C, Pinto P, Linehan WM. The morphologic spectrum of kidney tumors in hereditary leiomyomatosis and renal cell carcinoma (HLRCC) syndrome. *Am J Surg Pathol.* 2007;31(10):1578-1585.
94. Grubb RL 3rd, Franks ME, Toro J, et al. Hereditary leiomyomatosis and renal cell cancer: a syndrome associated with an aggressive form of inherited renal cancer. *J Urol.* 2007;177(6):2074-2079; discussion 2079-2080.
95. Kiuru M, Lehtonen R, Arola J, et al. Few FH mutations in sporadic counterparts of tumor types observed in hereditary leiomyomatosis and renal cell cancer families. *Cancer Res.* 2002;62(16):4554-4557.
96. Gardie B, Remenieras A, Kattygnarath D, et al. Novel FH mutations in families with hereditary leiomyomatosis and renal cell cancer (HLRCC) and patients with isolated type 2 papillary renal cell carcinoma. *J Med Genet.* 2011;48(4):226-234.
97. Singer EA, Bratslavsky G, Linehan WM, Srinivasan R. Targeted therapies for non-clear renal cell carcinoma. *Target Oncol.* 2010;5(2):119-129.
98. Bugert P, Gaul C, Weber K, et al. Specific genetic changes of diagnostic importance in chromophobe renal cell carcinomas. *Lab Invest.* 1997;76(2):203-208.
99. Kovacs A, Kovacs G. Low chromosome number in chromophobe renal cell carcinomas. *Genes Chromosomes Cancer.* 1992;4(3):267-268.
100. Schwerdtle RF, Storkel S, Neuhaus C, et al. Allelic losses at chromosomes 1p, 2p, 6p, 10p, 13q, 17p, and 21q significantly correlate with the chromophobe subtype of renal cell carcinoma. *Cancer Res.* 1996;56(13):2927-2930.
101. Srigley JR, Eble JN. Collecting duct carcinoma of kidney. *Semin Diagn Pathol.* 1998;15(1):54-67.
102. Srigley JR, Delahunt B. Uncommon and recently described renal carcinomas. *Mod Pathol.* 2009;22(suppl 2):S2-S23.
103. Polascik TJ, Bostwick DG, Cairns P. Molecular genetics and histopathologic features of adult distal nephron tumors. *Urology.* 2002;60(6):941-946.
104. Polascik TJ, Cairns P, Epstein JI, et al. Distal nephron renal tumors: microsatellite allelotype. *Cancer Res.* 1996;56(8):1892-1895.
105. Schoenberg M, Cairns P, Brooks JD, et al. Frequent loss of chromosome arms 8p and 13q in collecting duct carcinoma (CDC) of the kidney. *Genes Chromosomes Cancer.* 1995;12(1):76-80.
106. Steiner G, Cairns P, Polascik TJ, et al. High-density mapping of chromosomal arm 1q in renal collecting duct carcinoma: region of minimal deletion at 1q32.1-32.2. *Cancer Res.* 1996;56(21):5044-5046.
107. Gregori-Romero MA, Morell-Quadreny L, Llombart-Bosch A. Cytogenetic analysis of three primary Bellini duct carcinomas. *Genes Chromosomes Cancer.* 1996;15(3):170-172.
108. Davidson AJ, Choyke PL, Hartman DS, Davis CJ, Jr. Renal medullary carcinoma associated with sickle cell trait: radiologic findings. *Radiology.* 1995;195(1):83-85.
109. Davis CJ Jr, Mostofi FK, Sesterhenn IA. Renal medullary carcinoma. The seventh sickle cell nephropathy. *Am J Surg* Pathol. 1995;19(1):1-11.
110. Cheng JX, Tretiakova M, Gong C, Mandal S, Krausz T, Taxy JB. Renal medullary carcinoma: rhabdoid features and the absence of INI1 expression as markers of aggressive behavior. *Mod Pathol.* 2008;21(6):647-652.
111. Biegel JA. Molecular genetics of atypical teratoid/rhabdoid tumor. *Neurosurg Focus.* 2006;20(1):E11.
112. Biegel JA, Zhou JY, Rorke LB, Stenstrom C, Wainwright LM, Fogelgren B. Germ-line and acquired mutations of INI1 in atypical teratoid and rhabdoid tumors. *Cancer Res.* 1999;59(1): 74-79.
113. Argani P, Lae M, Ballard ET, et al. Translocation carcinomas of the kidney after chemotherapy in childhood. *J Clin Oncol.* 2006;24(10):1529-1534.
114. Argani P, Olgac S, Tickoo SK, et al. Xp11 translocation renal cell carcinoma in adults: expanded clinical, pathologic, and genetic spectrum. *Am J Surg Pathol.* 2007;31(8):1149-1160.
115. Argani P, Hicks J, De Marzo AM, et al. Xp11 translocation renal cell carcinoma (RCC): extended immunohistochemical profile emphasizing novel RCC markers. *Am J Surg Pathol.* 2010;34(9):1295-1303.
116. Ross H, Argani P, Xp11 translocation renal cell carcinoma. *Pathology.* 2010;42(4):369-373.
117. Argani P, Lae M, Hutchinson B, et al. Renal carcinomas with the t(6;11)(p21;q12): clinicopathologic features and demonstration of the specific alpha-TFEB gene fusion by immunohistochemistry, RT-PCR, and DNA PCR. *Am J Surg Pathol.* 2005;29(2):230-240.
118. Argani P, Lal P, Hutchinson B, Lui MY, Reuter VE, Ladanyi M. et al. Aberrant nuclear immunoreactivity for TFE3 in neoplasms with TFE3 gene fusions: a sensitive and specific immunohistochemical assay. *Am J Surg Pathol.* 2003;27(6):750-761.
119. Martignoni G, Gobbo S, Camparo P, et al. Differential expression of cathepsin K in neoplasms harboring TFE3 gene fusions. *Mod Pathol.* 2011;24(10):1313-1319.
120. Zhong M, De Angelo P, Osborne L, et al. Dual-color, break-apart FISH assay on paraffin-embedded tissues as an adjunct to diagnosis of Xp11 translocation renal cell carcinoma and alveolar soft part sarcoma. *Am J Surg Pathol.* 2010;34(6):757-766.
121. Mosquera JM, Dal Cin P, Mertz KD, et al. Validation of a TFE3 break-apart FISH assay for Xp11.2 translocation renal cell carcinomas. *Diagn Mol Pathol.* 2011;20(3):129-137.
122. Kim SH, Choi Y, Jeong HY, Lee K, Chae JY, Moon KC. Usefulness of a break-apart FISH assay in the diagnosis of Xp11.2 translocation renal cell carcinoma. *Virchows Arch.* 2011;459(3):299-306.
123. Pecciarini L, Cangi MG, Lo Cunsolo C, et al. Characterization of t(6;11)(p21;q12) in a renal-cell carcinoma of an adult patient. *Genes Chromosomes Cancer.* 2007;46(5):419-426.
124. Geller JI, Argani P, Adeniran A, et al. Translocation renal cell carcinoma: lack of negative impact due to lymph node spread. *Cancer.* 2008;112(7):1607-1616.
125. Malouf GG, Camparo P, Oudard S, et al. Targeted agents in metastatic Xp11 translocation/TFE3 gene fusion renal cell carcinoma (RCC): a report from the Juvenile RCC Network. *Ann Oncol.* 2010;21(9):1834-1838.
126. Truong LD, Shen SS. Immunohistochemical diagnosis of renal neoplasms. *Arch Pathol Lab Med.* 2011;135(1):92-109.
127. Li G, Barthelemy A, Feng G, et al. S100A1: a powerful marker to differentiate chromophobe renal cell carcinoma from renal oncocytoma. *Histopathology.* 2007;50(5):642-647.
128. Thomas RK, Baker AC, Debiasi RM, et al. High-throughput oncogene mutation profiling in human cancer. *Nat Genet.* 2007;39(3):347-351.

CHAPTER 39

MOLECULAR DIAGNOSIS OF SOFT TISSUE SARCOMAS

Jorge Torres-Mora and Andre M. Oliveira

Soft tissue sarcomas can be defined as a miscellaneous group of mesenchymal and neuroectodermal tumors of varying degrees of malignancy. The sites of origin of these tumors include fibrous connective tissue, adipose tissue, skeletal muscle, blood/lymph vessels, and the peripheral nervous system. Although in a large number of cases the diagnosis of soft tissue sarcomas can be made based on histologic analysis, supportive molecular pathology is currently considered an indispensable diagnostic tool for the diagnosis, treatment, and prognostication of these tumors.

From the molecular/cytogenetics perspective, soft tissue sarcomas can be classified broadly into those neoplasms with complex and apparently non-specific cytogenetic and molecular genetic features and those harboring relatively simple cytogenetic profiles with consistent and recurrent genetic aberrations (such as reciprocal translocations or mutations) (Table 39.1). The number of recognized subtypes of sarcomas is already large and that number is rapidly increasing as a result of the refinement of molecular methods. Since it is not possible to comment on all of them, this chapter will be focused on the most important molecular features of the most commonly encountered soft tissue sarcomas, with special emphasis on molecular diagnosis.

SOFT TISSUE TUMORS WITH COMPLEX CYTOGENETIC FEATURES

Neoplasms in this category have complex karyotypes and lack known and consistent chromosomal translocations that are useful for diagnosis. It is still useful to karyotype these lesions as the presence of a complex karyotype can be useful in supporting a difficult diagnosis as more complex karyotypes usually imply greater malignant potential (e.g., it is quite unusual to see highly complex cytogenetic signatures in benign tumors). Furthermore, much has been learned about the tumors in this category as summarized below. Unless explicitly stated, molecular tests usually do not play a role in the diagnosis or prognosis of soft tissue tumors with complex cytogenetic features.

Angiosarcoma

Angiosarcoma is a malignant neoplasm of endothelial differentiation that can affect all ages with a peak incidence in the seventh decade of life. Histologically, angiosarcomas are composed of malignant, hyperchromatic, spindle to epitheliod cells lining rudimentary and complex vascular channels.[1] Soft tissue angiosarcomas are aggressive tumors with 20% local recurrence rate; up to 50% of patients are expected to succumb to their disease within the first year after the diagnosis.[2]

Cytogenetic analysis shows complex cytogenetic numeric and structural changes.[1] *KRAS2* and *TP53* mutations have been identified in both sporadic angiosarcomas and angiosarcomas induced by thorium and vinyl chloride exposure.[3] Approximately 10% of angiosarcomas show activating mutations in the vascular-specific protein tyrosine kinase KDR, which may be targeted by KDR antagonists.[4] Amplification of *MYC* and *FLT4* has been identified in many angiosarcomas secondary to radiation therapy or chronic lymphedema, but not in primary angiosarcoma.[5] Atypical vascular lesions occurring after breast radiation are difficult to differentiate from angiosarcomas but lack *MYC* amplification.[6] This molecular finding could be explored as a diagnostic tool to discriminate other vascular lesions from angiosarcoma in histologically challenging cases.

TABLE 39–1 Fusion Genes in Sarcomas

Sarcoma	Translocation	Gene fusion
Alveolar rhabdomyosarcoma	t(2;13)(q35;q14)	*PAX3–FOXO1A*
	t(1;13)(p36;q14)	*PAX7–FOXO1A*
	t(2;2)(q35;p23)	*PAX3–NCOA1*
	t(X;2)(q13; q36)	*PAX3–AFX*
Alveolar soft part sarcoma	t(X;17)(p11;q25)	*TFE3–(ASPSCRI)*
Angiomatoid fibrous histiocytoma	t(12 ;16)(q13;p11)	*FUS–ATF1*
	t(12 ;22)(q13;q12)	*EWSR1–ATF1*
	t(2;22)(q33;q12)	*EWSR1–CREB1*
Clear cell sarcoma	t(12;22)(q13;q12)	*EWSR1–ATF1*
	t(2;22)(q33;q12)	*EWSR1–CREB1*
Desmoplastic small round cell tumor	t(11;22)(p13;q12)	*EWSR1–WT1*
Dermatofibrosarcoma protuberans	Ring form of chromosomes 17 and 22	*COL1A1–PDGFB*
	t(17;22)(q21;q13)	*COL1A1–PDGFB*
Epithelioid hemangioendothelioma	t(1;3)(p36;q25)	*WWTR1/CAMTA1*
Ewing sarcoma/PNET	t(11;22)(q24;q12)	*EWSR1–FLI1*
	t(21;22)(q12;q12)	*EWSR1–ERG*
	t(2;22)(q33;q12)	*EWSR1–FEV*
	t(7;22)(p22;q12)	*EWSR1–ETV1*
	t(17;22)(q12;q12)	*EWSR1–E1AF*
	inv(22)(q12q12)	*EWSR1–ZSG*
	t(16;21(p11;q22)	*FUS–ERG*
Extraskeletal myxoid chondrosarcoma	t(9;22)(q22;q12)	*EWSR1–NR4A3*
	t(9;17)(q22;q11)	*TAF2N–NR4A3*
	t(9;15)(q22;q21)	*TCF12–NR4A3*
	t(3;9)(q11;q22)	*TFG–NR4A3*
Fibrosarcoma, infantile	t(12;15)(p13;q26)	*ETV6–NTRK3*
Inflammatory myofibroblastic tumor	t(1;2)(q22;p23)	*TPM3–ALK*
	t(2;19)(p23;p13)	*TPM4–ALK*
	t(2;17)(p23;q23)	*CLTC–ALK*
	t(2;2)(p23;q13)	*RANB2–ALK*
Low-grade fibromyxoid sarcoma	t(7;16)(q33;p11)	*FUS–CREB3L2*
	t(11;16)(p11;p11)	*FUS–CREB3L1*
Mesenchymal chondrosarcoma	del(8)(q13.3q21.1)	*HEY1–NCOA2*
Myxoid/round cell liposarcoma	t(12;16)(q13;p11)	*FUS–DDIT3*
	t(12;22)(q13;q12)	*EWSR1–DDIT3*
Synovial sarcoma		
Biphasic	t(X;18)(p11;q11)	Predominantly *SS18–SSX1*
Monophasic	t(X;18)(p11;q11)	*SS18–SSX2*, *SS18–SSX1* or *SS18–SSX4*

PNET, primitive neuroectodermal tumor.

Leiomyosarcoma

Leiomyosarcoma (LMS) is a malignant tumor of smooth muscle differentiation that usually affects middle-aged and older adults; younger patients may be occasionally affected. LMSs occur most frequently in the retroperitoneum and pelvis. Other common sites include large vessels, soft tissues of the extremities, and skin. Histologically, they are composed of intersecting fascicles of spindle cells with cigar-shaped nuclei and eosinophilic cytoplasm, with varying degrees of differentiation.[1] The prognosis of LMSs varies according to the site, with no metastasis observed in cutaneous tumors confined to the dermis, to very aggressive behavior in retroperitoneal LMSs that show 5-year survival rates of approximately 50%.[7]

Cytogenetic studies on more than 100 LMSs have shown complex structural and numeric abnormalities more commonly involving chromosomes 1, 7, 10, 13, 14, and 17p. LMS often shows loss of *RB1* and *TP53* mutations, which have been correlated with adverse prognostic factors.[8] Germline mutations in the fumarate hydratase gene have been described in occasional cases in the setting of hereditary leiomyomatosis and renal cell cancer complex.[9] Abnormalities in other cell cycle regulators, including *CDKN2A*, *CCND1*, and *CCND3*, are also seen in sporadic LMS.[10] Furthermore, three candidate genes in the 5p13–p15 region, *TRIO*, *NKD2*, and *IRX2*, seem to be involved in tumor progression.[11]

Recently, by a combination of immunohistochemical markers and gene expression profiling, it was suggested that at least 7% of undifferentiated pleomorphic sarcomas are actually LMSs.[12] In addition, myocardin (*MYOCD*), a transcriptional cofactor of serum response factor involved in smooth muscle differentiation located in chromosome 17p12, has been found to be amplified in retroperitoneal LMSs and possibly through upregulation of *LLP* (a *MYOCD* target involved in smooth muscle cell migration) contributes to the high rate of metastasis in retroperitoneal LMSs. This latter finding can have therapeutic implications in the future.[13]

Pediatric malignant smooth muscle tumors are very rare but can be found in the setting of immunosuppression such as in human immunodeficiency virus–positive or post-transplant patients with concomitant infection by Epstein-Barr virus (EBV).[14,15] In this context, immunohistochemistry or in situ hybridization for EBV mRNA may be diagnostically useful.

Malignant Peripheral Nerve Sheath Tumor

Malignant peripheral nerve sheath tumors (MPNSTs) are malignant neoplasms with Schwannian or rarely perineurial differentiation. Most are thought to arise from neurofibromas and are frequently associated with neurofibromatosis type 1 (NF-1). Histologically, MPNSTs have a variety of appearances, but most commonly they are composed of wavy cells arranged in fascicles, with alternate areas of low and high cellularity and frequent necrosis. Uncommonly, other variants such as epithelioid morphology or tumors with mesenchymal differentiation or gland formation can be seen.[1] The local recurrence and metastatic rates for these tumors range from 40% to 65% and 40% to 68%, respectively, with approximately 50% 5-year survival rate.[16]

Cytogenetic studies reveal MPNST to have very complex karyotypes.[17] There are no significant cytogenetic differences between sporadic and NF-1–associated MPNST. Biallelic loss of *NF1* is common in both sporadic and NF-1–associated MPNST but loss of *NF1* function is thought to be an initiating event that is more relevant in the development of precursor neurofibromas than in progression from neurofibroma to MPNST. Mutation of *TP53* and P53 pathway members including Ink4a (*CDKN2A*) is found in MPNST but not in neurofibromas, thus implicating loss of the P53 pathway in progression from neurofibroma to MPNST.[17,18] Recently, amplifications, deletions, and copy number changes of several genes were identified suggesting the putative role of p70S6K pathway in NF1 tumor progression.[19] *CDK4* gain/amplification and increased FOXM1 protein expression are related to poor survival in MPNST patients.[20]

MPNST is usually a diagnosis of exclusion. The histologic features of MPNST often closely mimic synovial sarcoma and thus the absence of an *SYT–SSX* translocation or its fusion gene either by fluorescence in situ hybridization (FISH) or reverse transcriptase polymerase chain reaction (RT-PCR), respectively, can be helpful in supporting the diagnosis of MPNST.

Pleomorphic Sarcomas: The So-Called Malignant Fibrous Histiocytoma, Pleomorphic Rhabdomyosarcoma, Pleomorphic Liposarcoma, and Extraskeletal Osteosarcoma

Sarcomas in this category exhibit pleomorphic histology. They range from unclassifiable sarcomas (also known as malignant fibrous histiocytoma) to those with either focal or diffuse rhabdomyoblastic differentiation (pleomorphic rhabdomyosarcoma) or focal or diffuse lipoblastic differentiation (pleomorphic liposarcoma) (Fig. 39.1). They are usually high-grade tumors with numerous atypical mitotic figures, frequent necrosis, and malignant bone formation in the case of extraskeletal osteosarcoma.[21]

Most show complex cytogenetic rearrangements with intratumoral heterogeneity in the form of clonal and non-clonal cytogenetic aberrations. More aggressive lesions tend to demonstrate highly complex cytogenetic signatures.[21]

BONE AND SOFT TISSUE TUMORS WITH SIMPLE CYTOGENETIC FEATURES

Alveolar Soft Part Sarcoma

Alveolar soft part sarcoma (ASPS) is very rare tumor of uncertain cell of origin. It can occur at any age but affects predominantly patients from 15 to 35 years. It affects more commonly the extremities, especially the deep soft tissues of the thigh. Histologically, ASPS is composed of large round or polygonal cells with prominent nucleoli. The cells are arranged in nests of varying sizes surrounded by sinusoidal vessels.[1] Periodic acid Schiff–positive intracytoplasmic inclusions are commonly identified that have a characteristic crystalline rhomboid shape on ultrastructural analysis. These inclusions were

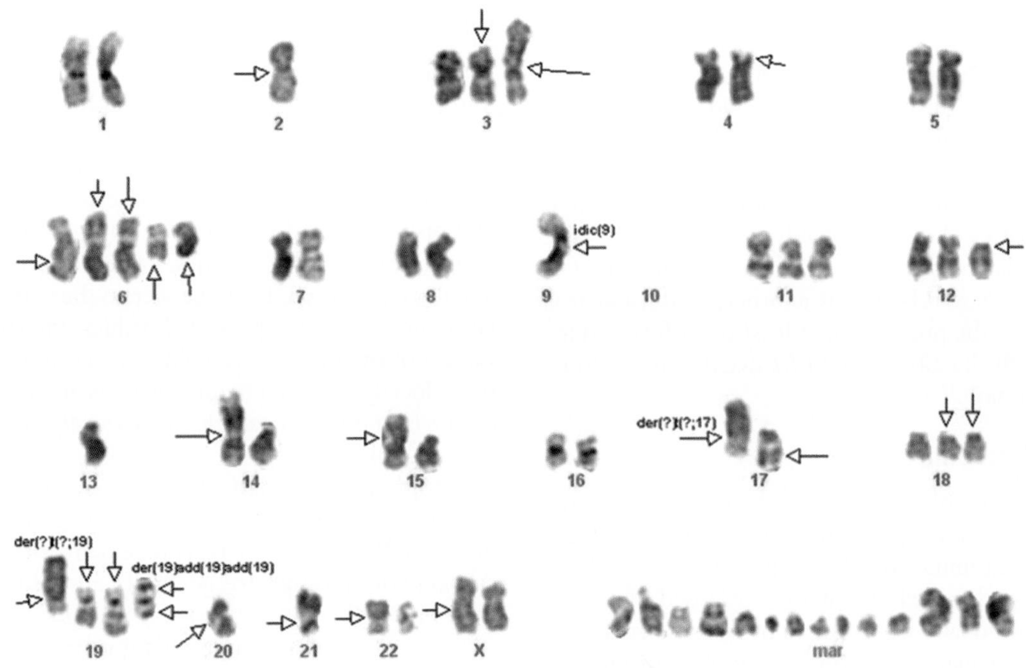

FIGURE 39–1 Pleomorphic sarcomas, including this example of pleomorphic liposarcoma. show very complex cytogenetic signatures characterized by several structural and numeric abnormalities.

recently shown to contain monocarboxylate transporter 1 (MCT1) and its partner CD147.[22] The survival rate of patients with no evidence of metastasis at the time of diagnosis was 60% at 5 years, 38% at 10 years, and 15% at 20 years.[23]

Cytogenetic and molecular studies have shown that the non-balanced translocation der(17)t(X;17)(p11;q25) is characteristic of ASPS and results in fusion of the novel gene *ASPSCR1* (formerly, *ASPL*) to the transcription factor *TFE3*. The fusion product retains the DNA-binding domains of *TFE3* and appears to work as an aberrant transcriptional factor.[24] Two types of *ASPSCR1/TFE3* fusion transcripts have been described: type I (75%) and type II (25%). Interestingly, type II is a longer transcript that also retains the activation domain of *TFE3*. *ASPSCR1/TFE3* is also seen in pediatric renal cell carcinomas with unique histologic features. However, in these cases the fusion gene results from an apparently balanced rearrangement between chromosomes X and 17 while the translocation in ASPS is unbalanced.[25] Gene expression profiling in ASPS identified elevated expression of transcripts related to angiogenesis, cell proliferation, metastasis, steroid biosynthesis, and a number of muscle-restricted transcripts.[26]

Either FISH or RT-PCR can be used for the molecular diagnosis of ASPS. The advantage of FISH for *TFE3* rearrangements is that the same probe can be used not only for the diagnosis of ASPS but also for the identification of renal cell carcinomas with *TFE3* rearrangements in the appropriate clinico-pathologic context. However, immunohistochemistry for *TFE3* is a very attractive alternative to molecular approaches because the identification of *TFE3* protein overexpression is highly specific and sensitive for tumors with *TFE3* rearrangements.[27]

Angiomatoid Fibrous Histiocytoma

Angiomatoid fibrous histiocytoma (AFH), previously known as angiomatoid malignant fibrous histiocytoma, is a rare subcutaneous tumor that arises predominantly in the extremities of young patients. Histologically, AFH is composed of a proliferation of histiocytic or myoid cells with pseudoangiomatous spaces, a thick fibrous pseudocapsule, and a dense pericapsular lymphoplasmacytic infiltrate.[28] AFH is characterized by low rates of local recurrence (2% to 11%) and limited metastatic potential (<1%). Surgical excision is considered the treatment of choice.[1]

Specific chromosomal translocations are present in practically all AFHs. The most common one, present in 75% of the cases, harbors the fusion gene *EWSR1/CREB1* due to the chromosomal t(2;22)(q33;q12). Other fusion genes are *EWSR1/ATF1* and *FUS/ATF1*.[29,30] Both ATF and related paralogue—*CREM*—belong to the cyclic adenosine monophosphate response element (CRE)-binding protein (CREB) family of transcription factors. These genes are involved in several processes, including cellular metabolism and growth factor–dependent cell survival. Interestingly, *EWSR1–CREB1* is also seen in a subset of clear cell sarcomas that occur in the gastrointestinal tract[31] (see section on Clear Cell Sarcoma). AFH is often diagnosed by its distinct morphology but unusual histologic features such as nuclear pleomorphism and myxoid changes may occasionally be seen. In these cases, molecular confirmation may be useful. Given the number of fusion partners, FISH for *EWSR1* or *FUS* may be used and in theory, the use of both probes should detect all three translocations/gene fusions reported in AFH; however, when used alone, FISH results are negative in up to 24% of the cases. This is probably due to the presence of alternate fusions or due to a cryptic rearrangement of *EWSR1* or *FUS*.[32]. RT-PCR is another option but it is complicated by the presence of at least three fusion transcripts, though the *EWSR1/CREB1* event appears to be the most common.[30]

Clear Cell Sarcoma

Clear cell sarcoma, also known as melanoma of soft parts, is a rare soft tissue neoplasm that predominantly occurs in the distal extremities of adolescents and young adults. Histologically, clear cell sarcoma is composed of nest of spindle to polygonal cells separated by fibrous septa. The nuclei have vesicular chromatin with prominent nucleoli and the cytoplasm is clear to eosinophilic. Clinically, clear cell sarcoma is characterized by the development of metastasis in 50% of patients, most commonly to lungs and lymph nodes. The mortality rate ranges from 37% to 59%.[1]

Cytogenetically, clear cell sarcoma is characterized by t(12;22)(q13;q12) in almost all cases, which results in fusion of *EWSR1* to the CREB family transcription factor *ATF1*.[33] The fusion protein *EWSR1/ATF1* was shown to bind to the promoter of the microphthalmia-associated transcription factor (MITF) and stimulate the activity of the melanocyte-stimulating hormone, an oncogene observed in melanomas and an important regulator of melanocytic differentiation.[34] At least four major *EWSR1/ATF1* splicing variants have been described. Type I is the most common and results in fusion of *EWSR1* exon 8 to *ATF1* exon 4 (85% of cases). In all splicing variants, the transcriptional activation domain of *EWSR1* and the ATF1 bZIP DNA domain are preserved.[35] The type of fusion transcript(s) does not appear to effect clinical outcome.[36]

Both RT-PCR and FISH may be used for molecular diagnosis of clear cell sarcoma. RT-PCR is specific and sensitive but can be challenging on paraffin-embedded tissues. FISH for *EWSR1* lacks specificity given the involvement of this locus in multiple neoplasms; however, in a tumor showing immunohistochemical evidence of melanocytic differentiation, clear cell sarcoma can be readily distinguished from melanoma since *EWSR1* rearrangements have not been described in melanoma.[36]

More recently, a unique type of clear cell sarcoma that occurs in the gastrointestinal tract has been described. Two fusion genes have been described for this variant: the classic *EWSR1/ATF1* and a novel *EWSR1/CREB1* that is characterized at the chromosomal level by t(2;22)(q32;q12).[31] *EWSR1/CREB1* has also been recently described in AFH.[30]

Desmoid Fibromatosis

Desmoid-type fibromatosis (DF) is a locally aggressive fibroblastic/myofibroblastic proliferation without metastatic potential. DF can present in the extremities, trunk or intra-abdominal locations, and head and neck. DFs are generally classified into two broad classes—intra-abdominal and extra-abdominal. The tumors arise in young patients, often in their thirties. Primarily intra-abdominal, but also extremity DF, can be seen in the context of familial adenomatous polyposis or Gardner syndrome where a variant of the tumor is termed Gardner fibroma. DF can recur locally when incompletely excised and occasionally can be fatal due to local effects, especially in the head and neck region.[1]

Approximately half of DF cases show evidence of clonal chromosomal aberrations, more often trisomies of 8 and 20 and loss or rearrangements of 5q21. These cytogenetic findings are generally absent in superficial fibromatosis.[37]

The most common known genetic event in DF is activating mutation of exon 3 of *CTNNB1*, the gene encoding β-catenin. This protein directly interacts with the tumor suppressor protein APC and is also a key effector in Wnt signaling.[38] β-Catenin is involved in proliferation, migration, and cell division. Mutations in exon 3 of *CTNNB1* are seen in many tumor types, both benign and malignant. Mutations in β-catenin block makes it resistant to degradation and thus it accumulates in the nucleus, resulting in constitutive signaling and transcriptional activation of target genes such as *MYC*, *JUN*, and *Cyclin D*.[38,39]

Interestingly, the mutations are present almost exclusively at codons 41 (Thr41Ala) and 45 (Ser45Phe and Ser45Pro).[38] Greater than 80% of sporadic desmoids harbor these mutations.[40] The Ser45Phe mutation correlates with poorer 5-year recurrence-free survival.[39] In DF associated with familial adenomatous polyposis or Gardner syndrome, loss of heterozygosity at the *APC* locus (5q) is present and leads to inability to form a phosphorylation complex with β-catenin, which targets the complex for destruction in the proteosome.[38]

Clinical and histologic features are usually sufficient for making the diagnosis of DF. Immunohistochemistry for nuclear β-catenin can sometimes be useful, especially in small biopsies.[41] PCR for the detection of *CTNNB1* is also diagnostically useful in small biopsies.

Desmoplastic Small Round Cell Tumor

Desmoplastic small round cell tumor (DSRCT) is a rare and highly malignant soft tissue tumor with polyphenotypic differentiation that tends to occur in adolescents and young adults and shows a striking male predominance. Histologically, DSRCT is composed of sharply outlined nest of small primitive blue cells embedded in a desmoplastic stroma. DSRCT is a tumor with poor prognosis despite multimodal therapy.[1]

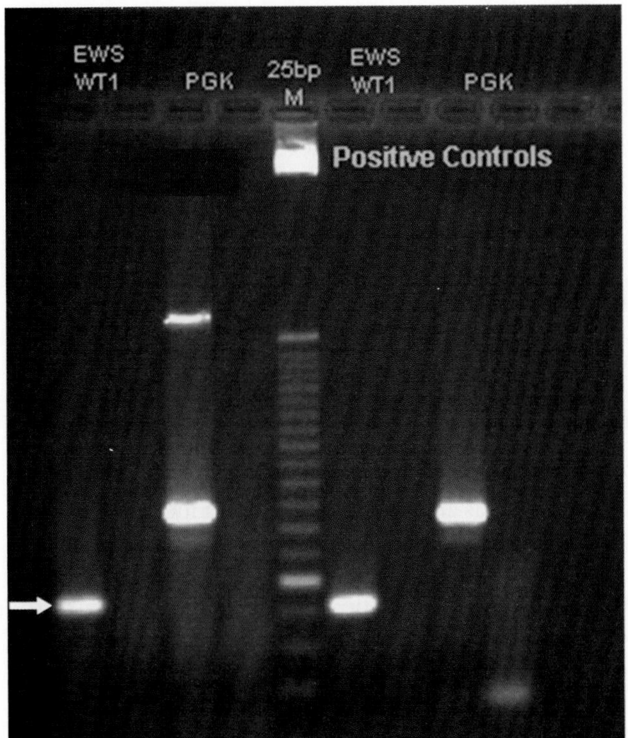

FIGURE 39–2 Agarose gel showing RT-PCR products consistent with the presence of the *EWSR1/WT1* fusion gene (arrow). Controls are displayed on the left and patient's samples on the right (PGK, phosphoglycerate kinase, used as a control for RNA integrity).

DSRCT is characterized by t(11;22)(p13;q12) in the vast majority of cases, leading to a fusion of the N-terminal domain (NTD) of Ewing sarcoma gene (*EWS*) to the C-terminal DNA-binding domain of Wilms' tumor suppressor gene, *WT1*. *EWS* encodes a putative RNA-binding protein, which together with TLS/FUS and TAFII68/TAF15 forms the TET family of proteins with presumptive roles in transcription and splicing.[42] *WT1* encodes four Cys2His2 zinc fingers in the C-terminus that mediate sequence-specific DNA binding and the NTD containing both transcriptional activation and repression domains.[43] While *WT1* is a classical tumor suppressor gene, the fusion protein behaves as an oncogene.[44]

Cytogenetic analysis can readily demonstrate t(11;22)(p13;q12) but the diagnosis of DSRCT can also be supported by RT-PCR (Fig. 39.2) or FISH for *EWSR1* locus in the context of a supportive immunohistochemical profile.

Epithelioid Hemangioendothelioma

Epithelioid hemangioendothelioma (EHE) is a rare malignant vascular neoplasm that affects all age groups, except early childhood years, with no gender predilection. The tumor occurs most commonly in bone, soft tissue, lungs, and liver. Multicentricity is often observed. Histologically, the tumor is composed of epithelioid endothelial cells with frequent intracytoplasmic lumina dispersed in a chondromyxoid matrix. Local recurrence, metastatic, and mortality rates are 10% to 15%, 20% to 30%, and 10% to 20%, respectively.[1]

Most EHE harbor the chromosomal translocation t(1;3)(p36.3;q25),[45] resulting in the fusion gene *WWTR1/CAMTA1*.[46,47] *WWTR1* is a transcriptional co-activator involved in the Hippo pathway and the *CAMTA1* encodes a transcription factor of which little is known but it is expressed almost exclusively in the brain. Interestingly, data suggest that native *CAMTA1* is a tumor suppressor, but in this gene fusion, *CAMTA1* seems to behave as an oncogene. This phenomenon is similar to the one observed in DSRCT. Cytogenetic analysis, FISH, or RT-PCR can be employed to support the diagnosis of EHE.[47]

Ewing Sarcoma/Primitive Neuroectodermal Tumor

Ewing sarcoma/primitive neuroectodermal tumor (EWS/PNET) is a neoplasm of neuroectodermal differentiation. The histological appearance represents a spectrum ranging from the prototypic "small round cell cancer" in the classic Ewing sarcoma cases to sheets of larger more atypical cells with the presence of neural rosettes or pseudorosettes in the classic PNET examples. Both subtypes represent variants of the same entity. This tumor usually involves the long bones of children and young adults but can also involve the soft tissues.[1,16] Currently, patients with localized disease have a 75% cure rate, which decreases to less than 30% in patients with metastatic disease.[48]

EWS/PNET was the first sarcoma to be associated with a recurrent chromosomal translocation.[49] The most common one, present in about 90% of cases, is t(11;22)(q24;q12) that fuses the *EWSR1* to *FLI1*. *EWSR1* is a gene containing 17 exons that encodes a multifunctional protein that is involved in various cellular processes, including gene expression, cell signaling, and RNA processing and transport. The protein includes an N-terminal transcriptional activation domain and a C-terminal RNA-binding domain. *FL1* belongs to a subset of ETS-transcription factor gene family members and is probably involved in blood and endothelial development. The *EWSR–FLI1* fusion shows multiple splice variants. The two most common are type I (*EWSR1* exon 7 fused to *FLI1* exon 6) and type II (*EWSR1* exon 7 to *FLI1* exon 5), together accounting for about 90-95% of EWSR1–FLI1 fusion. Several other fusion genes have been identified in EWS/PNET, additional members of the ETS family of genes form fusion transcripts with *EWSR1*, including *ERG* (21q22), *ETV1* (7p22), *1E1A-F* (17q21), and *FEV* (2q35–36), though *FLI1* (> 90%) and *ERG* (up to 5%) are by far the most common.[50] More recently, *EWSR1* gene fusions with genes not belonging to the ETS family have been reported in EWS/PNET tumors, including *Zinc finger gene*, *SP3*, N*FATc2*, and *SMARCA5*[51] and also rare cases with *FUS/ERG* fusion due to t(16;21).[52]

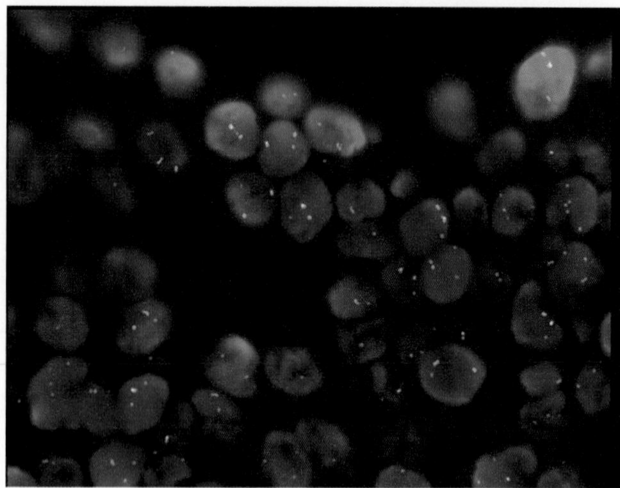

FIGURE 39–3 Molecular cytogenetic analysis of Ewing sarcoma using a break-apart FISH probe for the *EWSR1* locus. The separation of the green and orange signals consistent with the rearrangement of this locus is observed. Yellow fusion signals represent the normal allele locus (DAPI, blue counterstain).

The majority of the translocations can be detected by FISH using break-apart probes at the *EWSR1* in appropriate histologic and immunophenotypic context since *EWSR1* gene is involved in multiple other tumors (Fig. 39.3). RT-PCR is more specific and can be used to directly demonstrate the *EWSR1/FLI1* fusion transcript.

Extraskeletal Myxoid Chondrosarcoma

Extraskeletal myxoid chondrosarcoma (EMC) is a malignant tumor that was initially thought to be of cartilaginous differentiation; more recently, however, this idea has been reconsidered. Interestingly, features of neuroendocrine differentiation have been observed in this tumor.[53] EMC affects older adults with a male predominance, usually involving the deep soft tissues of the lower extremities. Most patients exhibit long survival with 5-, 10-, and 15-year survival rates of 90%, 70%, and 60%, respectively.[1]

EMC is characterized at the molecular level by the fusion of the *EWSR1* on 22q12, to the *NR4A3* on chromosome 9q22, which is detected in about 75% of cases. As often seen in chimeric transcripts involving *EWSR1*, the transactivation domain of *EWSR1* is fused to the DNA-binding domain of *NR4A3*. *NR4A3* is an orphan nuclear receptor that can activate the *FOS* promoter and plays a poorly understood role in the regulation of hematopoietic growth and differentiation. Alternate *NR4A3* gene partners include *TAF2N*, t(9;17)(q22;q11); *TCF12*, t(9;15)(q22;q21); and *TFG* gene on chromosome 3q11-q12. Interestingly, recent evidence indicates that tumors with these various translocations have similar gene expression profiles.[54] Very little is known about the molecular biology of the *EWSR1/NR4A3* fusion gene function in the development and pathogenesis of EMC. Upregulation of *PPARG* is the only direct transcriptional effect identified to date as a result of the *EWSR1/NR4A3* fusion gene in EMC.[55]

FISH with break-apart available probes for the EWSR1 locus may be used as the diagnostic option in the appropriate histological context. Even better is the use of an *NR4A3* break-apart probe, which should be more sensitive and specific for EMC. RT-PCR is a less attractive option because of the large number of fusion partners.

Infantile Fibrosarcoma

Infantile fibrosarcoma (IFS) (also known as congenital fibrosarcoma) is a rare neoplasm of infancy with a predilection for the distal extremities and a favorable prognosis. It is composed of a monomorphic cellular proliferation of spindle cells with fine chromatin and minimal cytoplasm. IFS usually has a good prognosis with a mortality ranging from 4% to 25% and up to 50% recurrence rate.[1]

IFS is characterized by the chromosomal t(12;15)(p13;q26), which can be difficult to recognize at the cytogenetic level because it involves the distal bands of chromosomes 12p and 15q. This rearrangement leads to the fusion of *ETV6* (also known as *TEL*) to *NTRK3* (also known as *TRKC*).[56] ETV6 is a nuclear transcription factor and NTRK3 is a receptor tyrosine kinase (RTK). The fusion gene encodes a chimeric constitutively activated RTK composed of the N-terminal oligomerization domain of *ETV6* and the kinase domain of *NTRK3*.[56] Trisomies of chromosomes 8, 11, 17, and 20 are also characteristic of IFS and represent secondary changes involved in tumor progression subsequent to initiation by *ETV6/NTRK3* gene fusion.[57] Trisomy 11, in particular, is a very characteristic finding and may be diagnostically useful in selected contexts. Cellular and mixed cellularity mesoblastic nephroma, a renal neoplasm of infancy with histologic features almost identical to IFS, also harbors the *ETV6/NTRK3* gene fusion and likely represents the same entity. This gene fusion has also been demonstrated in a few examples of acute myeloid leukemia, in secretory breast carcinoma[58] and recently in a rare tumor designated as mammary analogue secretory carcinoma of salivary gland.[59]

Cytogenetics is helpful in confirming the diagnosis of IFS but may be challenging due to the nature of the rearrangement (see above). Interestingly, the identification of trisomy 11 may be a warning sign for the presence of an apparently unrecognized t(12;15)[60] (Fig. 39.4). FISH and RT-PCR are useful in making the diagnosis when cytogenetics is not available or in cytogenetically ambiguous cases. By RT-PCR, the fusion gene can be identified in about 90% of cases.

ETV6/NTRK3 has a transforming activity in multiple cell lineages via association of Scr, a tyrosine kinase known to activate PI3K–AKT pathway and the MAP/extracellular signal-regulated kinase (ERK) kinase (MEK)/ERK cascades. In experimental models, the use of the Scr inhibitor SU6656 blocks the *ETV6/NTRK3* transforming activity, an interesting finding with possible therapeutic implications.[61]

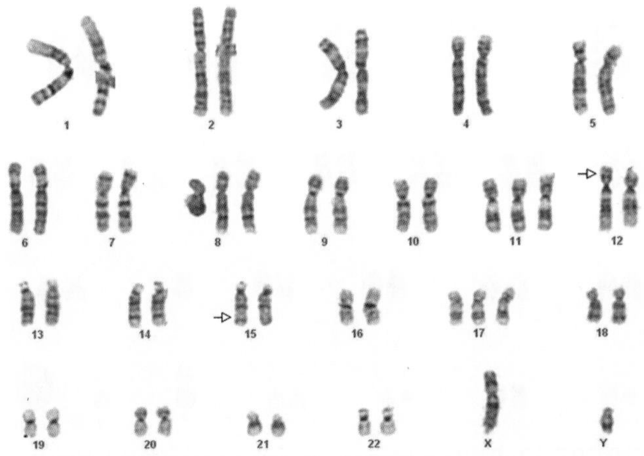

FIGURE 39–4 Infantile fibrosarcoma is characterized by t(12;15)(p13;q27), which results in the formation of the *ETV6/NTRK3* fusion gene. Note also the extra copy of chromosome 11, a common numeric abnormality seen in these tumors.

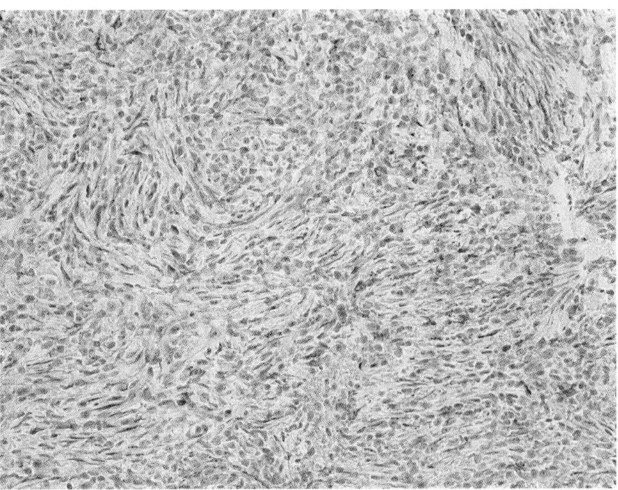

FIGURE 39–5 Inflammatory myofibroblastic tumor showing cytoplasmic anaplastic lymphoma kinase (ALK) detected by immunohistochemistry. This tumor contained the *TPM3–ALK* fusion gene.

Inflammatory Myofibroblastic Tumor

Inflammatory myofibroblastic tumor (IMT) is a mesenchymal neoplasm of myofibroblastic differentiation that was first described in the lung but is now recognized in virtually any anatomic location. IMT should not be confused with inflammatory pseudotumors encountered in a variety of locations. Histologically, IMT is composed of a mixture of myofibroblast and fibroblast intermixed with abundant lymphocytes and plasma cells. Overall, IMT can recur locally in up to 25% of cases and metastases are found in less than 5% of patients. Morbidity and mortality in IMT are due primarily to destructive local involvement.[1]

The major recurrent chromosomal aberrations are balanced translocations involving the *ALK* (anaplastic lymphoma kinase) locus at 2p23. This cytogenetic feature is more commonly encountered in younger patients and may portend a more favorable course of disease.[62] Approximately 30% to 50% cases diagnosed in patients younger than 30 are associated with translocations involving *ALK*.[63]

ALK encodes a membrane-bound TRK that is normally expressed in certain areas of the brain. Several ALK fusion genes have been described, involving tropomyosins (*TPM3* on 1q25 and *TPM4* on 19p13), clathrin heavy-chain polypeptide (*CLTC*; 17q23), *CARS* (11p15), *ATIC* (2q35), *SEC31L1* (4q21), *RANBP2* (2q13),[64] and *PPFIBP1* (12p11).[65] The most common fusions in IMT are *TPM3–ALK* and *TPM4–ALK*. In each case, the C-terminal cytoplasmic portion of *ALK* with its kinase domain is fused to the N-terminus of the partner. The fusion partner with *ALK* appears to provide an oligomerization domain that leads to constitutive activation of *ALK*. In the first four fusion partners, the chimeric protein is present in the cytosol whereas with the last, RANBP2, the fusion protein, is targeted to the nuclear membrane.[64] Similar translocations are present in anaplastic large cell lymphoma. In contrast, anaplastic large cell lymphoma employs *NPM* (5q35) in approximately 75% of cases with distinct nuclear localization.[64] By comparative genomic hybridization, IMT showed decreased expression of a few putative tumor suppression genes (*SEMA3B*, *SEMA3F*, and *SULT2A1*) and overexpression of four potential cancer-related genes (*GSTT1*, *ESR1*, *EVI1*, and *MITF*).[66]

Immunohistochemistry analysis demonstrates nuclear or cytoplasmic distribution of *ALK*, which may suggest the nature of the *ALK* fusion gene involved[64] (Fig. 39.5). Of note, the presence of *ALK* reactivity in a variety of sarcomas lacking *ALK* rearrangements has been reported,[67] and thus molecular cytogenetic confirmation is often helpful. Break-apart FISH strategies for the *ALK* locus are also commonly employed given the broad array of potential binding partners. Regarding the therapeutic implications of the molecular findings, the study of the *ALK* inhibitor crizotinib has shown encouraging results in the treatment of IMTs with *ALK* translocation.[68]

Low-Grade Fibromyxoid Sarcoma

Low-grade fibromyxoid sarcoma (LGFMS) is a neoplasm that more commonly affects the proximal extremities and trunk of young patients. Histologically, LGFMS is characterized by a bland spindle cell proliferation with a fascicular growth pattern with alternating hypo- and hypercellular areas. Although originally thought to be more aggressive tumors, more recent series reveal a local recurrence, metastatic, and death from disease rates of 9%, 6%, and 2%, respectively.[1]

The tumor is cytogenetically characterized by the chromosomal translocation t(7;16)(q33;p11), which leads to the formation of the fusion gene *FUS/CREB3L2*.[69] *FUS* gene encodes a multifunctional protein component of the heterogeneous nuclear ribonucleoprotein complex that has been implicated in cellular processes that include regulation of gene expression, maintenance of genomic integrity, and mRNA/microRNA processing.[70] *CREB3L2* encodes a member of the oasis bZIP transcription factor family that functions as a transcriptional activator.[69] More recently, a second fusion gene has been described—*FUS/CREB3L1*—due to t(11;16)(p11;p11).[71] These fusions can be detected by RT-PCR in 88% to 96% of cases.[71,72] Cytogenetically, the fusion gene may be present in supernumerary ring chromosomes containing this translocation.[73] It seems that the transcriptional upregulation of *CREBL1* is driven by the strong *FUS* promoter, which provides a transcriptional activation domain to the DNA-binding domain of *CREB3L1*. The fusion breakpoints occur within exons 6 and 7 of *FUS* and exon 5 of *CREB3L1*. The fusion genes seem to be specific for LGFMS and have not been detected in other tumors.[74] A recent study showed that the fusion gene *FUS/CREB3L1* can be successfully amplified by RT-PCR from paraffin-embedded tissues for diagnostic confirmation.[72] Another approach uses FISH to identify *FUS* in histologically suspicious cases. Despite the fact that FISH is less specific than RT-PCR (other sarcomas contain *FUS* rearrangements), the most common differential diagnoses of LGFMS—myxofibrosarcoma and perineurioma—do not harbor *FUS* rearrangements.[72]

Well-Differentiated and Dedifferentiated Liposarcoma

Well-differentiated liposarcoma (WDL) is a locally aggressive neoplasm showing adipocytic differentiation that arises most commonly in the extremities and retroperitoneum. Middle-aged adults are most commonly affected with no gender predilection. The clinical course of extremity WDL is usually excellent with only about 2% of them undergoing dedifferentiation and an overall 5-year survival rate of 100%. Because of the excellent prognosis, WDL in the extremities is referred to as atypical lipomatous tumor. A much worse prognosis is found in retroperitoneal tumors, which transform into dedifferentiated liposarcoma (DL) in up to 20% of cases. DL is defined by the transition of WDL into a non-lipogenic sarcoma of variable histologic grades. They are more aggressive tumors with rates of local recurrence of about 40% that can metastasize in up to 20% of cases with a 5-year mortality rate of 30%.[1]

Cytogenetic studies of WDL and DL frequently show ring or giant marker chromosomes (Fig. 39.6). The karyotypes can be relatively simple or may show substantial numeric and structural abnormalities with multiple subclones, especially in DL. The ring and giant marker chromosomes consistently contain amplified

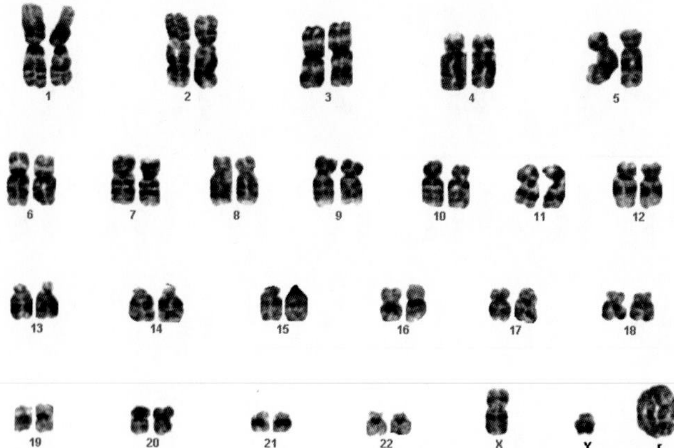

FIGURE 39–6 Well-differentiated liposarcoma is characterized by the presence of ring or giant rod chromosomes, mainly composed of amplified sequences from chromosome 12q13–q15. These sequences contain several copies of *MDM2* and other genes.

sequences derived from chromosome 12q13–q15, which includes *MDM2*, *CPM*, *FRS2*, *SAS*, *HMGA2*, and *CDK4*, among other genes.[75] Amplification of these genes is not specific for WDL or DL since they can be seen in many other sarcomas, including LMSs and non-mesenchymal tumors.[76,77] A subset of undifferentiated sarcomas may represent dedifferentiated liposarcomas since they show consistent high-level amplification of the 12q14 chromosome region accompanied with amplification of either 6q23 or 1p32, as seen in the undifferentiated relapses of liposarcomas. Based on this, the *JUN* oncogene on 1p32 has been implicated in the dedifferentiation process.[78] Assays that can detect amplification of these genes on clinical specimens are widely used because the discrimination between WDL with minimal cytologic atypia and lipoma may be histologically challenging. Amplification of at least one of these genes, especially *MDM2*, *CPM or FRS2*, is seen in almost all cases of WDL but not in lipoma.[79] Several diagnostic methodologies have been used in this regard, including immunohistochemistry for the detection of MDM2 and CDK4 protein overexpression and PCR and FISH for gene amplification. FISH seems the most specific and sensitive one because even cells devoid of cytologic atypia exhibit high levels of *MDM2* and *CPM* amplification[77,80] (Fig. 39.7).

Currently, molecular-based therapeutics is not the mainstay in the treatment of liposarcoma. However, several antagonists of some of the genes overexpressed in WDL and DL are under investigation, including *MDM2* antagonists such as Nutlin-3a, spiro-oxindoles, and *CDK4* antagonists like P1446A05.[81-83] However, to date none of them has a well-established role in the therapy of liposarcoma. More recently, in experimental settings, aberrant AKT activation seems to have a role in WDL pathogenesis and the small molecule inhibitor BEZ235 can be used as a potential therapeutic agent through inhibition of AKT activation.[84]

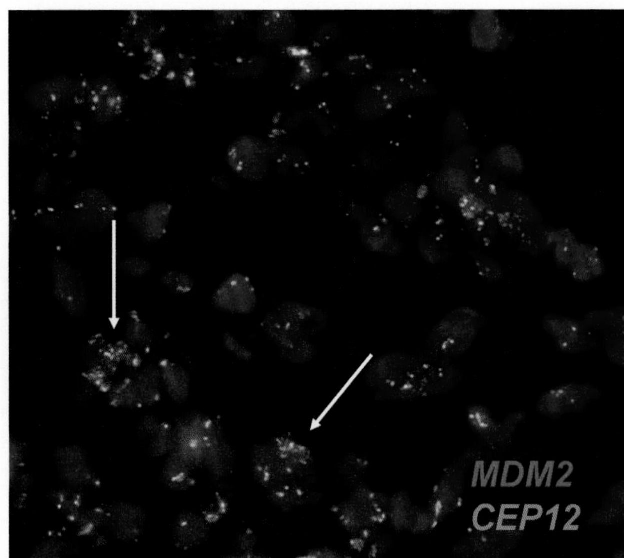

FIGURE 39–7 Fluorescent in situ hybridization (FISH) of a well-differentiated liposarcoma showing *MDM2* amplification (clusters of orange signal). Green signal represents the centromere region of chromosome 12 (CEP12).

Mesenchymal Chondrosarcoma

Mesenchymal chondrosarcoma is a rare sarcoma that occurs more commonly in bone but may also arise in the soft tissues. It affects predominantly young adults without gender predominance.[1] Histologically, mesenchymal chondrosarcoma exhibits a biphasic pattern composed of sheets of undifferentiated small to spindle cells intermixed with islands of well-differentiated cartilage. Mesenchymal chondrosarcoma behaves in an aggressive fashion and frequently metastasizes to lungs and lymph nodes. The reported 5- and 10-year survival rates are 54% and 27%, respectively.[85]

The cartilaginous nature of mesenchymal chondrosarcoma seems to be supported by the fact that both components of the tumor (cartilaginous and round cell/primitive) show immunohistochemical expression of Sox9, a transcription factor that acts as a master regulator of the differentiation of mesenchymal cells into chondrocytes.[86]

Until recently, only a few reports with cytogenetic data on mesenchymal chondrosarcoma had been published, most of them showing complex cytogenetic alterations, including identical Robertsonian translocation t(13;21)(q10;q10) in a few cases.[87] However, in a recent work based on genome-wide screen of exon-level expression data, the novel recurrent *HEY1–NCOA2* gene fusion was identified.[88] This fusion was present in all the mesenchymal chondrosarcomas tested and was negative in other subtypes of chondrosarcomas. *NCOA2* is a member of the p160 nuclear hormone receptor transcriptional co-activator family that facilitates chromatin remodeling and transcription of nuclear receptor target genes. *NCOA2* has been reported in other fusion genes such as *MYST3–NCOA2* and *ETV6–NCOA2* (both found in some subsets of acute myeloid leukemias) and is also present in the fusion *PAX3–NCOA2*, which is a rare variant fusion in alveolar rhabdomyosarcomas. *HEY1* seems to participate in the regulation of BMP9-induced osteoblastic lineage differentiation of mesenchymal stem cells.[88] Future studies are needed to decipher the molecular events driven by this gene fusion. Limited data suggest that *NCOA2* could cause a reverse effect in the *HEY1* function, that is, recruiting co-activators instead of co-repressors of the target genes of Notch signaling.[88]

The *HEY1–NCOA2* fusion or its product can be identified by FISH or RT-PCR, respectively, and may prove to be an invaluable tool for the diagnosis of mesenchymal chondrosarcoma.

Myxoid/Round Cell Liposarcoma

Myxoid liposarcoma (ML) is the second most common type of liposarcoma and occurs mainly during the fourth to fifth decades of life; most arise in the lower extremities. Histologically, ML is composed of spindle and stellate cells immersed in a myxoid matrix with a characteristic branching capillary vascular pattern ("chicken-wire"). Round cell liposarcoma is the cellular and poorly differentiated/high-grade form of ML.[1] This tumor has been associated with a relatively good prognosis. One study revealed a cumulative 5- and 10-year survival of 82% and 67% respectively, but the presence of round cell differentiation, age >45 years, and presence of necrosis were independent variables related to poor survival.[89]

Cytogenetic and molecular studies have shown that both myxoid and round cell liposarcomas share the same genetic abnormalities, and the former progress to the latter probably via activation of the PI3K/AKT pathway.[90]

Both exhibit the chromosomal translocation t(12;16)(q13;p11) in up to 90% to 95% of cases, which results in fusion of *FUS* to *DDIT3* (a.k.a. *FUS/CHOP*).[91] Several *FUS/DDIT3* splicing variants have been described in myxoid/round cell liposarcoma but their discrimination has been shown to have no prognostic relevance.[91] *FUS* (previously termed *TLS*) encodes for an RNA-binding protein similar to the EWSR1 protein. *DDIT3* encodes for a DNA-damage-inducible negative transcription regulator involved in adipocyte differentiation. The second most common chromosomal translocation—t(12;22)(q13;q12)—results in the fusion gene *EWSR1/DDIT3*.[92] Both FUS/DDIT3 and EWSR1/DDIT3 chimeric proteins can transform NIH3T3 fibroblasts and more recent work has shown that an ML-like phenotype is induced by transfecting *FUS/DDIT3* in mesenchymal progenitor cells or HT1080 sarcoma cells.[93] DNA microarray analysis of ML showed overexpression of *RET*, *CDK4*, *cyclin D2*, and *MYC* in ML.[94] By kinome profiling, kinases associated with the atypical nuclear factor-κB and Src pathways have been found to be active in ML cell lines. This finding has therapeutic implications, since the use of the casein kinase 2 inhibitor 4,5,6,7-tetrabromobenzotriazole

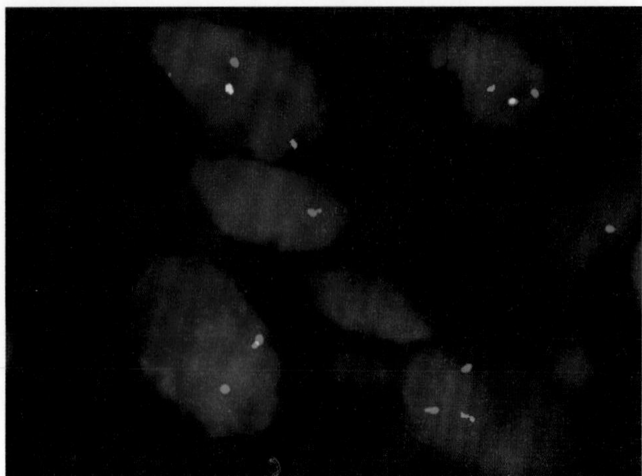

FIGURE 39–8 Molecular cytogenetic analysis of a myxoid liposarcoma using a break-apart fluorescence in situ hybridization (FISH) probe for the *DDIT3* locus. Observed the separation of the green and orange signals, consistent with the rearrangement of this locus. Yellow fusion signals represent the normal allele locus (DAPI, blue counter stain).

plus dasatinib has been shown to decrease in vitro ML tumor cell viability.[95]

Traditional cytogenetics, FISH, and RT-PCR may be helpful diagnostically. FISH for *DDIT3* rearrangements is more feasible at the clinical level, and specifically for paraffin-embedded tissues, because rearrangements of this gene have been only seen in myxoid/round cell liposarcoma (Fig. 39.8). RT-PCR–based assays can also be employed, but they have to be designed to be able to detect at least the most common fusions, since several splice variants exist.[96]

Rhabdomyosarcoma

Rhabdomyosarcomas (RMS) are sarcomas that exhibit skeletal muscle differentiation and are divided into alveolar, embryonal, and pleomorphic subtypes. Botryoid and spindle cell RMS are generally considered as subtypes of embryonal. Embryonal RMS is usually encountered in children to young adults while alveolar has a wider age distribution.[1] Pleomorphic RMS is usually encountered in elderly patients and is discussed in the pleomorphic sarcoma section. Prognostically, RMS can be divided into those with superior prognosis (botryoid and spindle cell types), intermediate prognosis (embryonal type), and poor prognosis (alveolar type). The 5-year survival rates for these groups are 95%, 67%, and 54%, respectively.[97]

Most embryonal RMS cases are sporadic but a small percentage of them are known to occur in association with NF1, Li-Fraumeni syndrome, Costello syndrome, and pleuropulmonary blastoma predisposition syndrome.[98,99] Cytogenetic analysis of embryonal RMS often shows trisomies of chromosomes 2, 8, and 20.[100] More recently, evidence shows that some congenital embryonal RMS share the recurrent t(2;8)(q35;q13).[101] Loss of heterozygosity at 11p15 is present in most instances.[102] Microcell hybridization transfer experiments have indicated at least two tumor suppressor loci in this chromosome band.[103] Experimental work in mice suggested that synergistic loss of INK4a/ARF and MET signaling disruption as well as concomitant inactivation of *TP53* and *FOS* may be important for the pathogenesis of RMS.[104,105] By comparative genomic hybridization and other methods, additional genes have been identified, including *Ras*, Hedgehog, and *FGRF4*. These findings open the possibility of treatment with small molecule inhibitors.[106]

Two major chromosomal translocations are noted in alveolar rhabdomyosarcoma: t(2;13)(q35;q14) and t(1;13)(p36;q14). Both of the translocations in alveolar rhabdomyosarcoma involve *FOXO1A* (also known as *FKHR*) at 13q14. These translocations fuse the paired box transcription factors *PAX3* and *PAX7*, respectively, to *FOXO1A*.[107] *PAX3/FOXO1A* is the most common fusion gene and occurs in approximately 55% to 75% of the cases; *PAX7/FOXO1A* occurs in 10% to 15% of the cases.[107,108] The fusion proteins stimulate transcription on PAX-binding sites with higher potency than the corresponding wild-type PAX proteins.[109] In addition, *PAX7/FOXO1A* is often amplified in the form of double minutes. *PAX3* and *PAX7* are specifically expressed during the development of the dorsal neural tube and somites, and *PAX3* plays an important role for the myoblast migration to the limbs.[110] Gene expression analyses using cDNA microarrays in alveolar rhabdomyosarcoma have shown that the *PAX3/FOXO1A* fusion transcript induces the expression of several genes involved in myogenic differentiation. In experimental models, the fusion *PAX/FOXO1A* is not sufficient to induce the tumor in mice unless other genetic modifications such as *TP53* mutations were also included.[111]

More recently, additional novel fusion genes have been identified in alveolar rhabdomyosarcoma: *PAX3/NCOA1* due to t(2;2)(q35;p23), *PAX3/AFX* due to t(2;8)(q35;q13), and a fusion involving *FOXO1* gene at 13q14 and the *FGFR1* gene at 8p12p11.2.[111-113] These findings support the notion that at least some fusion-negative alveolar rhabdomyosarcomas may in fact carry previously unknown chromosomal rearrangements.

Clinical testing is important as the alveolar subtype has a worse prognosis than does the embryonal subtype.[97] This is well established in children but is less clear in adults. Cytogenetic analysis is useful to detect the translocations. Alternatively, break-apart FISH strategies at the *FOXO1A* locus can be used. PCR-based methodologies are also practical and can readily differentiate between the *PAX3* and *PAX7* as fusion partners. Some studies have shown that *PAX7* fusion genes may have a better prognosis than *PAX3*, while others have failed to reproduce these findings.[114] Further confirmation in prospective, randomized controlled trials is needed to clarify this issue.

Synovial Sarcoma

Synovial sarcoma (SS) is a malignant tumor of uncertain line of differentiation, possibly arising from multipotent stem cells.[115] It represents approximately 10% to 15% of all soft tissue sarcomas and particularly affects the lower extremities of adolescents and young adults. Histologically, SS is classified into monophasic (most common and composed purely of spindle cells), biphasic (composed of spindle cells and glands), and poorly differentiated (composed of more primitive small round cells). Immunohistochemical analysis shows multifocal expression of EMA, cytokeratins, and TLE1 in most cases.[1,116] SS metastasizes in 40% of cases, most commonly to lungs, and 5-year overall survival rates between 36% and 76% have been reported.[1]

Cytogenetic and molecular studies demonstrated the translocation t(X;18)(p11.2;q11.2) in most cases, including the poorly differentiated variant. This chromosomal translocation results in fusion of *SYT* with members of the *SSX* family of genes on chromosome Xp11.2.[117] The most common fusion gene is *SYT/SSX1* (65%), followed by *SYT/SSX2* (35%), and very rarely *SYT–SSX4* (only a few cases reported).[118-120] While biphasic SS usually harbors the *SYT–SSX1* fusion gene, *SYT/SSX2* is predominantly associated with monophasic morphology. *SYT* encodes for a ubiquitously expressed nuclear protein that seems to function as a transcriptional coactivator. The *SSX* genes encode for transcription repressor proteins. The fusion gene encodes a chimeric protein that contains both the transcription activation domain of *SYT* and the repressor domain of the *SSX* genes.[118] The target genes of the *SYT/SSX* fusion are still largely unknown but recent experimental work suggests that *SYT/SSX2* reprograms mesenchymal/progenitor stem cells via activation of a set of neural genes and other genes involved in cell differentiation, including *FGFR2*.[115,121]

Despite initial claims that tumors harboring the *SYT/SSX1* fusion transcript had more aggressive clinical behavior, more recent and larger studies have not confirmed this association.[122,123] Therefore, the prognostic value of the different fusion genes remains uncertain at this time.

The clinical molecular diagnosis of SS is mainly done by RT-PCR (and real-time RT-PCR) or FISH for *SYT* rearrangements. Both are highly sensitive and specific. While RT-PCR has the advantage of discriminating the type of fusion gene, this is of questionable clinical value (see above). One of the major advantages of FISH is its ability to detect all three fusion genes in a single assay.

REFERENCES

1. Fletcher CDM, Umi K K, Merteus F. *Pathology and Genetics of Tumours of Soft Tissue and Bone*. World Health Organization Classification of Tumours. Lyon: IARC Press; 2002:427 p.
2. Meis-Kindblom JM, Kindblom LG. Angiosarcoma of soft tissue: a study of 80 cases. *Am J Surg Pathol*. 1998;22(6):683-697.
3. Przygodzki RM, et al. Sporadic and Thorotrast-induced angiosarcomas of the liver manifest frequent and multiple point mutations in K-ras-2. *Lab Invest*. 1997;76(1):153-159.
4. Antonescu CR, et al. KDR activating mutations in human angiosarcomas are sensitive to specific kinase inhibitors. *Cancer Res*. 2009;69(18):7175-7179.
5. Manner J, et al. MYC high level gene amplification is a distinctive feature of angiosarcomas after irradiation or chronic lymphedema. *Am J Pathol*. 2010;176(1):34-39.
6. Mentzel T, et al. Postradiation cutaneous angiosarcoma after treatment of breast carcinoma is characterized by MYC amplification in contrast to atypical vascular lesions after radiotherapy and control cases: clinicopathological, immunohistochemical and molecular analysis of 66 cases. *Mod Pathol*. 2012;25(1):75-85.
7. Stoeckle E, et al. Prognostic factors in retroperitoneal sarcoma: a multivariate analysis of a series of 165 patients of the French Cancer Center Federation Sarcoma Group. *Cancer*. 2001;92(2):359-368.
8. Sandberg AA. Updates on the cytogenetics and molecular genetics of bone and soft tissue tumors: leiomyosarcoma. *Cancer Genet Cytogenet*. 2005;161(1):1-19.
9. Lehtonen HJ. Hereditary leiomyomatosis and renal cell cancer: update on clinical and molecular characteristics. *Fam Cancer*. 2011;10(2):397-411.
10. Dei Tos AP, et al. Tumor suppressor genes and related molecules in leiomyosarcoma. *Am J Pathol*. 1996;148(4):1037-1045.
11. Adamowicz M, et al. Frequent amplifications and abundant expression of TRIO, NKD2, and IRX2 in soft tissue sarcomas. *Genes Chromosomes Cancer*. 2006;45(9):829-838.
12. Mills AM, et al. Expression of subtype-specific group 1 leiomyosarcoma markers in a wide variety of sarcomas by gene expression analysis and immunohistochemistry. *Am J Surg Pathol*. 2011;35(4):583-589.
13. Perot G, et al. Strong smooth muscle differentiation is dependent on myocardin gene amplification in most human retroperitoneal leiomyosarcomas. *Cancer Res*. 2009;69(6):2269-2278.
14. Chadwick EG, et al. Tumors of smooth-muscle origin in HIV-infected children. *JAMA*. 1990;263(23):3182-3184.
15. McClain KL, et al. Association of Epstein-Barr virus with leiomyosarcomas in children with AIDS. *N Engl J Med*. 1995;332(1):12-18.
16. Weiss SW, Goldblum JR. *Enzinger & Weiss's Soft Tissue Tumors*. 5th ed. Philadelphia, PA: Mosby Elsevier; 2008:1258.
17. Mertens F, et al. Cytogenetic characterization of peripheral nerve sheath tumours: a report of the CHAMP study group. *J Pathol*. 2000;190(1):31-38.
18. Louis DN, et al. *WHO Classification of Tumours of the Central Nervous System*. 4th ed. Lyon, France: IARC; 2007:160-162.
19. Mantripragada KK, et al. High-resolution DNA copy number profiling of malignant peripheral nerve sheath tumors using targeted microarray-based comparative genomic hybridization. *Clin Cancer Res*. 2008;14(4):1015-1024.
20. Yu J, et al. Array-based comparative genomic hybridization identifies CDK4 and FOXM1 alterations as independent predictors of survival in malignant peripheral nerve sheath tumor. *Clin Cancer Res*. 2011;17(7):1924-1934.
21. Mertens F, et al. Cytogenetic analysis of 46 pleomorphic soft tissue sarcomas and correlation with morphologic and clinical features: a report of the CHAMP Study Group. Chromosomes and MorPhology. *Genes Chromosomes Cancer*. 1998;22(1):16-25.
22. Ladanyi M, et al. The precrystalline cytoplasmic granules of alveolar soft part sarcoma contain monocarboxylate transporter 1 and CD147. *Am J Pathol*. 2002;160(4):1215-1221.
23. Lieberman PH, et al. Alveolar soft-part sarcoma. A clinico-pathologic study of half a century. *Cancer*. 1989;63(1):1-13.
24. Ladanyi M, et al. The der(17)t(X;17)(p11;q25) of human alveolar soft part sarcoma fuses the TFE3 transcription factor gene to ASPL, a novel gene at 17q25. *Oncogene*. 2001;20(1):48-57.
25. Argani P, et al. Primary renal neoplasms with the ASPL-TFE3 gene fusion of alveolar soft part sarcoma: a distinctive tumor entity previously included among renal cell carcinomas of children and adolescents. *Am J Pathol*. 2001;159(1):179-192.
26. Stockwin LH, et al. Gene expression profiling of alveolar soft-part sarcoma (ASPS). *BMC Cancer*. 2009;9:22.
27. Argani P, et al. Aberrant nuclear immunoreactivity for TFE3 in neoplasms with TFE3 gene fusions: a sensitive and specific

immunohistochemical assay. *Am J Surg Pathol*. 2003;27(6): 750-761.
28. Enzinger FM. Angiomatoid malignant fibrous histiocytoma: a distinct fibrohistiocytic tumor of children and young adults simulating a vascular neoplasm. *Cancer*. 1979;44(6):2147-2157.
29. Waters BL, Panagopoulos I, Allen EF. Genetic characterization of angiomatoid fibrous histiocytoma identifies fusion of the FUS and ATF-1 genes induced by a chromosomal translocation involving bands 12q13 and 16p11. *Cancer Genet Cytogenet*. 2000;121(2):109-116.
30. Antonescu CR, et al. EWSR1-CREB1 is the predominant gene fusion in angiomatoid fibrous histiocytoma. *Genes Chromosomes Cancer*. 2007;46(12):1051-1060.
31. Antonescu CR, et al. EWS-CREB1: a recurrent variant fusion in clear cell sarcoma—association with gastrointestinal location and absence of melanocytic differentiation. *Clin Cancer Res*. 2006;12(18):5356-5362.
32. Tanas MR, et al. Utilization of fluorescence in situ hybridization in the diagnosis of 230 mesenchymal neoplasms: an institutional experience. *Arch Pathol Lab Med*. 2010;134(12):1797-1803.
33. Zucman J, et al. EWS and ATF-1 gene fusion induced by t(12;22) translocation in malignant melanoma of soft parts. *Nat Genet*. 1993;4(4):341-345.
34. Davis IJ, et al. Oncogenic MITF dysregulation in clear cell sarcoma: defining the MiT family of human cancers. *Cancer Cell*. 2006;9(6):473-484.
35. Panagopoulos I, et al. Molecular genetic characterization of the EWS/ATF1 fusion gene in clear cell sarcoma of tendons and aponeuroses. *Int J Cancer*. 2002;99(4):560-567.
36. Coindre JM, et al. Diagnosis of clear cell sarcoma by real-time reverse transcriptase-polymerase chain reaction analysis of paraffin embedded tissues: clinicopathologic and molecular analysis of 44 patients from the French sarcoma group. *Cancer*. 2006;107(5):1055-1064.
37. De Wever I, et al. Cytogenetic, clinical, and morphologic correlations in 78 cases of fibromatosis: a report from the CHAMP Study Group. CHromosomes And Morphology. *Mod Pathol*. 2000;13(10):1080-1085.
38. Tejpar S, et al. Predominance of beta-catenin mutations and beta-catenin dysregulation in sporadic aggressive fibromatosis (desmoid tumor). *Oncogene*. 1999;18(47):6615-6620.
39. Lazar AJ, et al. Specific mutations in the beta-catenin gene (CTNNB1) correlate with local recurrence in sporadic desmoid tumors. *Am J Pathol*. 2008;173(5):1518-1527.
40. Amary MF, et al. Detection of beta-catenin mutations in paraffin-embedded sporadic desmoid-type fibromatosis by mutation-specific restriction enzyme digestion (MSRED): an ancillary diagnostic tool. *Am J Surg Pathol*. 2007;31(9):1299-1309.
41. Bhattacharya B, et al. Nuclear beta-catenin expression distinguishes deep fibromatosis from other benign and malignant fibroblastic and myofibroblastic lesions. *Am J Surg Pathol*. 2005;29(5):653-659.
42. Bertolotti A, et al. hTAF(II)68, a novel RNA/ssDNA-binding protein with homology to the pro-oncoproteins TLS/FUS and EWS is associated with both TFIID and RNA polymerase II. *EMBO J*. 1996;15(18):5022-5031.
43. Lee SB, Haber DA. Wilms tumor and the WT1 gene. *Exp Cell Res*. 2001;264(1):74-99.
44. Sandberg AA, Bridge JA. Updates on the cytogenetics and molecular genetics of bone and soft tissue tumors. desmoplastic small round-cell tumors. *Cancer Genet Cytogenet*. 2002;138(1):1-10.
45. Mendlick MR, et al. Translocation t(1;3)(p36.3;q25) is a nonrandom aberration in epithelioid hemangioendothelioma. *Am J Surg Pathol*. 2001;25(5):684-687.
46. Errani C, et al. A novel WWTR1-CAMTA1 gene fusion is a consistent abnormality in epithelioid hemangioendothelioma of different anatomic sites. *Genes Chromosomes Cancer*. 2011;50(8):644-653.
47. Tanas MR, et al. Identification of a disease-defining gene fusion in epithelioid hemangioendothelioma. *Science Transl Med*. 2011;3(98):98ra82.
48. Krasin MJ, et al. Definitive surgery and multiagent systemic therapy for patients with localized Ewing sarcoma family of tumors: local outcome and prognostic factors. *Cancer*. 2005;104(2):367-373.
49. Aurias A, et al. Translocation of chromosome 22 in Ewing's sarcoma. *C R Acad Sci Ser III*. 1983;296(23):1105-1107.
50. Sandberg AA, Bridge JA. Updates on cytogenetics and molecular genetics of bone and soft tissue tumors: Ewing sarcoma and peripheral primitive neuroectodermal tumors. *Cancer Genet Cytogenet*. 2000;123(1):1-26.
51. Sumegi J, et al. A novel t(4;22)(q31;q12) produces an EWSR1-SMARCA5 fusion in extraskeletal Ewing sarcoma/primitive neuroectodermal tumor. *Mod Pathol*. 2011;24(3):333-342.
52. Shing DC, et al. FUS/ERG gene fusions in Ewing's tumors. *Cancer Res*. 2003;63(15):4568-4576.
53. Domanski HA, et al. Extraskeletal myxoid chondrosarcoma with neuroendocrine differentiation: a case report with fine-needle aspiration biopsy, histopathology, electron microscopy, and cytogenetics. *Ultrastruct Pathol*. 2003;27(5):363-368.
54. Sjogren H, et al. Studies on the molecular pathogenesis of extraskeletal myxoid chondrosarcoma-cytogenetic, molecular genetic, and cDNA microarray analyses. *Am J Pathol*. 2003; 162(3):781-792.
55. Filion C, et al. The EWSR1/NR4A3 fusion protein of extraskeletal myxoid chondrosarcoma activates the PPARG nuclear receptor gene. *J Pathol*. 2009;217(1):83-93.
56. Knezevich SR, et al. A novel ETV6-NTRK3 gene fusion in congenital fibrosarcoma. *Nat Genet*. 1998;18(2):184-187.
57. Bourgeois JM, et al. Molecular detection of the ETV6-NTRK3 gene fusion differentiates congenital fibrosarcoma from other childhood spindle cell tumors. *Am J Surg Pathol*. 2000;24(7):937-946.
58. Lannon CL, Sorensen PH. ETV6-NTRK3: a chimeric protein tyrosine kinase with transformation activity in multiple cell lineages. *Semin Cancer Biol*. 2005;15(3):215-223.
59. Skalova A, et al. Mammary analogue secretory carcinoma of salivary glands, containing the ETV6-NTRK3 fusion gene: a hitherto undescribed salivary gland tumor entity. *Am J Surg Pathol*. 2010;34(5):599-608.
60. Rubin BP, et al. Congenital mesoblastic nephroma t(12;15) is associated with ETV6-NTRK3 gene fusion: cytogenetic and molecular relationship to congenital (infantile) fibrosarcoma. *Am J Pathol*. 1998;153(5):1451-1458.
61. Jin W, et al. Cellular transformation and activation of the phosphoinositide-3-kinase-Akt cascade by the ETV6-NTRK3 chimeric tyrosine kinase requires c-Src. *Cancer Res*. 2007;67(7):3192-3200.
62. Coffin CM, Hornick JL, Fletcher CD. Inflammatory myofibroblastic tumor: comparison of clinicopathologic, histologic, and immunohistochemical features including ALK expression in atypical and aggressive cases. *Am J Surg Pathol*. 2007;31(4):509-520.
63. Lawrence B, et al. TPM3-ALK and TPM4-ALK oncogenes in inflammatory myofibroblastic tumors. *Am J Pathol*. 2000;157(2): 377-384.
64. Ma Z, et al. Fusion of ALK to the Ran-binding protein 2 (RANBP2) gene in inflammatory myofibroblastic tumor. *Genes Chromosomes Cancer*. 2003;37(1):98-105.
65. Takeuchi K, et al. Pulmonary inflammatory myofibroblastic tumor expressing a novel fusion, PPFIBP1-ALK: reappraisal of anti-ALK immunohistochemistry as a tool for novel ALK fusion identification. *Clin Cancer Res*. 2011;17(10):3341-3348.
66. Jung SH, et al. Copy number alterations and expression profiles of candidate genes in a pulmonary inflammatory myofibroblastic tumor. *Lung Cancer*. 2010;70(2):152-157.
67. Cessna MH, et al. Expression of ALK1 and p80 in inflammatory myofibroblastic tumor and its mesenchymal mimics: a study of 135 cases. *Mod Pathol*. 2002;15(9):931-938.
68. Butrynski JE, et al. Crizotinib in ALK-rearranged inflammatory myofibroblastic tumor. *N Engl J Med*. 2010;363(18):1727-1733.
69. Storlazzi CT, et al. Fusion of the FUS and BBF2H7 genes in low grade fibromyxoid sarcoma. *Hum Mol Genet*. 2003;12(18): 2349-2358.
70. Vance C, et al. Mutations in FUS, an RNA processing protein, cause familial amyotrophic lateral sclerosis type 6. *Science*. 2009; 323(5918):1208-1211.
71. Mertens F, et al. Clinicopathologic and molecular genetic characterization of low-grade fibromyxoid sarcoma, and cloning of a novel FUS/CREB3L1 fusion gene. *Lab Invest*. 2005;85(3): 408-415.
72. Matsuyama A, et al. Molecular detection of FUS-CREB3L2 fusion transcripts in low-grade fibromyxoid sarcoma using formalin-fixed, paraffin-embedded tissue specimens. *Am J Surg Pathol*. 2006;30(9):1077-1084.

73. Bartuma H, et al. Fusion of the FUS and CREB3L2 genes in a supernumerary ring chromosome in low-grade fibromyxoid sarcoma. *Cancer Genet Cytogenet*. 2010;199(2):143-146.
74. Panagopoulos I, et al. The chimeric FUS/CREB3l2 gene is specific for low-grade fibromyxoid sarcoma. *Genes Chromosomes Cancer*. 2004;40(3):218-228.
75. Pedeutour F, et al. Structure of the supernumerary ring and giant rod chromosomes in adipose tissue tumors. *Genes Chromosomes Cancer*. 1999;24(1):30-41.
76. Momand J, et al. The MDM2 gene amplification database. *Nucleic Acids Res*. 1998;26(15):3453-3459.
77. Binh MB, et al. MDM2 and CDK4 immunostainings are useful adjuncts in diagnosing well-differentiated and dedifferentiated liposarcoma subtypes: a comparative analysis of 559 soft tissue neoplasms with genetic data. *Am J Surg Pathol*. 2005;29(10):1340-1347.
78. Mariani O, et al. JUN oncogene amplification and overexpression block adipocytic differentiation in highly aggressive sarcomas. *Cancer Cell*. 2007;11(4):361-374.
79. Erickson-Johnson MR, et al. Carboxypeptidase M: a biomarker for the discrimination of well-differentiated liposarcoma from lipoma. *Mod Pathol*. 2009;22(12):1541-1547.
80. Weaver J, et al. Fluorescence in situ hybridization for MDM2 gene amplification as a diagnostic tool in lipomatous neoplasms. *Mod Pathol*. 2008;21(8):943-949.
81. Muller CR, et al. Potential for treatment of liposarcomas with the MDM2 antagonist Nutlin-3A. *Int J Cancer*. 2007;121(1):199-205.
82. Shangary S, Wang S. Targeting the MDM2-p53 interaction for cancer therapy. *Clin Cancer Res*. 2008;14(17):5318-5324.
83. Lapenna S, Giordano A. Cell cycle kinases as therapeutic targets for cancer. *Nature Rev Drug Discov*. 2009;8(7):547-566.
84. Gutierrez A, et al. Aberrant AKT activation drives well-differentiated liposarcoma. *Proc Natl Acad Sci U S A*. 2011;108(39):16386-16391.
85. Nakashima Y, et al. Mesenchymal chondrosarcoma of bone and soft tissue. A review of 111 cases. *Cancer*. 1986;57(12):2444-2453.
86. Wehrli BM, et al. Sox9, a master regulator of chondrogenesis, distinguishes mesenchymal chondrosarcoma from other small blue round cell tumors. *Human Pathol*. 2003;34(3):263-269.
87. Naumann S, et al. Translocation der(13;21)(q10;q10) in skeletal and extraskeletal mesenchymal chondrosarcoma. *Mod Pathol*. 2002;15(5):572-576.
88. Wang L, et al. Identification of a novel, recurrent HEY1-NCOA2 fusion in mesenchymal chondrosarcoma based on a genome-wide screen of exon-level expression data. *Genes Chromosomes Cancer*. 2012;51(2):127-139.
89. Kilpatrick SE, et al. The clinicopathologic spectrum of myxoid and round cell liposarcoma. A study of 95 cases. *Cancer*. 1996;77(8):1450-1458.
90. Demicco EG, et al. Involvement of the PI3K/Akt pathway in myxoid/round cell liposarcoma. *Mod Pathol*. 2012;25(2):212-221.
91. Antonescu CR, et al. Prognostic impact of P53 status, TLS-CHOP fusion transcript structure, and histological grade in myxoid liposarcoma: a molecular and clinicopathologic study of 82 cases. *Clin Cancer Res*. 2001;7(12):3977-3987.
92. Panagopoulos I, et al. Fusion of the EWS and CHOP genes in myxoid liposarcoma. *Oncogene*. 1996;12(3):489-494.
93. Engstrom K, et al. The myxoid/round cell liposarcoma fusion oncogene FUS-DDIT3 and the normal DDIT3 induce a liposarcoma phenotype in transfected human fibrosarcoma cells. *Am J Pathol*. 2006;168(5):1642-1653.
94. Lanckohr C, et al. [Identification of genes over-expressed in myxoid/round cell liposarcoma. DNA microarray analysis and immunohistochemical correlation]. *Pathologe*. 2010;31(1):60-66.
95. Willems SM, et al. Kinome profiling of myxoid liposarcoma reveals NF-kappaB-pathway kinase activity and casein kinase II inhibition as a potential treatment option. *Mol Cancer*. 2010;9:257.
96. Powers MP, et al. Detection of myxoid liposarcoma-associated FUS-DDIT3 rearrangement variants including a newly identified breakpoint using an optimized RT-PCR assay. *Mod Pathol*. 2010;23(10):1307-1315.
97. Newton WA Jr, et al. Classification of rhabdomyosarcomas and related sarcomas. Pathologic aspects and proposal for a new classification—an Intergroup Rhabdomyosarcoma Study. *Cancer*. 1995;76(6):1073-1085.
98. Doros L, et al. DICER1 mutations in embryonal rhabdomyosarcomas from children with and without familial PPB-tumor predisposition syndrome. *Pediatr Blood Cancer.* 2012;59(3):558-560.
99. Kratz CP, et al. Uniparental disomy at chromosome 11p15.5 followed by HRAS mutations in embryonal rhabdomyosarcoma: lessons from Costello syndrome. *Hum Mol Genet*. 2007;16(4):374-379.
100. Gordon T, et al. Cytogenetic abnormalities in 42 rhabdomyosarcoma: a United Kingdom Cancer Cytogenetics Group Study. *Med Pediatr Oncol*. 2001;36(2):259-267.
101. Meloni-Ehrig A, et al. Translocation (2;8)(q35;q13): a recurrent abnormality in congenital embryonal rhabdomyosarcoma. *Cancer Genet Cytogenet*. 2009;191(1):43-45.
102. Anderson J, et al. Disruption of imprinted genes at chromosome region 11p15.5 in paediatric rhabdomyosarcoma. *Neoplasia*. 1999;1(4):340-348.
103. Loh WE Jr, et al. Human chromosome 11 contains two different growth suppressor genes for embryonal rhabdomyosarcoma. *Proc Natl Acad Sci U S A*. 1992;89(5):1755-1759.
104. Sharp R, et al. Synergism between INK4a/ARF inactivation and aberrant HGF/SF signaling in rhabdomyosarcomagenesis. *Nat Med*. 2002;8(11):1276-1280.
105. Fleischmann A, et al. Rhabdomyosarcoma development in mice lacking Trp53 and Fos: tumor suppression by the Fos protooncogene. *Cancer Cell*. 2003;4(6):477-482.
106. Paulson V, et al. High-resolution array CGH identifies common mechanisms that drive embryonal rhabdomyosarcoma pathogenesis. *Genes Chromosomes Cancer*. 2011;50(6):397-408.
107. Barr FG. Molecular genetics and pathogenesis of rhabdomyosarcoma. *J Pediatr Hematol Oncol*. 1997;19(6):483-491.
108. de Alava E, et al. Detection of chimeric transcripts in desmoplastic small round cell tumor and related developmental tumors by reverse transcriptase polymerase chain reaction. A specific diagnostic assay. *Am J Pathol*. 1995;147(6):1584-1591.
109. Bennicelli JL, Edwards RH, Barr FG. Mechanism for transcriptional gain of function resulting from chromosomal translocation in alveolar rhabdomyosarcoma. *Proc Natl Acad Sci U S A*. 1996;93(11):5455-5459.
110. Borycki AG, et al. Pax3 functions in cell survival and in pax7 regulation. *Development*. 1999;126(8):1665-1674.
111. Liu J, et al. FOXO1-FGFR1 fusion and amplification in a solid variant of alveolar rhabdomyosarcoma. *Mod Pathol*. 2011;24(10):1327-1335.
112. Wachtel M, et al. Gene expression signatures identify rhabdomyosarcoma subtypes and detect a novel t(2;2)(q35;p23) translocation fusing PAX3 to NCOA1. *Cancer Res*. 2004;64(16):5539-5545.
113. Barr FG, et al. Genetic heterogeneity in the alveolar rhabdomyosarcoma subset without typical gene fusions. *Cancer Res*. 2002;62(16):4704-4710.
114. Stegmaier S, et al. Prognostic value of PAX-FKHR fusion status in alveolar rhabdomyosarcoma: a report from the cooperative soft tissue sarcoma study group (CWS). *Pediatr Blood Cancer*. 2011;57(3):406-414.
115. Naka N, et al. Synovial sarcoma is a stem cell malignancy. *Stem Cells*. 2010;28(7):1119-1131.
116. Terry J, et al. TLE1 as a diagnostic immunohistochemical marker for synovial sarcoma emerging from gene expression profiling studies. *Am J Surg Pathol*. 2007;31(2):240-246.
117. Clark J, et al. Identification of novel genes, SYT and SSX, involved in the t(X;18)(p11.2;q11.2) translocation found in human synovial sarcoma. *Nat Genet*. 1994;7(4):502-508.
118. Sandberg AA, Bridge JA. Updates on the cytogenetics and molecular genetics of bone and soft tissue tumors. Synovial sarcoma. *Cancer Genet Cytogenet*. 2002;133(1):1-23.
119. Skytting B, et al. A novel fusion gene, SYT-SSX4, in synovial sarcoma. *J Natl Cancer Inst*. 1999;91(11):974-975.
120. Mancuso T, et al. Analysis of SYT-SSX fusion transcripts and bcl-2 expression and phosphorylation status in synovial sarcoma. *Lab Invest*. 2000;80(6):805-813.
121. Garcia CB, et al. Reprogramming of mesenchymal stem cells by the synovial sarcoma-associated oncogene SYT-SSX2. *Oncogene*. 2012;31(18):2323-2334.
122. Kawai A, et al. SYT-SSX gene fusion as a determinant of morphology and prognosis in synovial sarcoma. *N Engl J Med*. 1998;338(3):153-160.
123. Guillou L, et al. Histologic grade, but not SYT-SSX fusion type, is an important prognostic factor in patients with synovial sarcoma: a multicenter, retrospective analysis. *J Clin Oncol*. 2004;22(20):4040-4050.

CHAPTER 40

MOLECULAR DIAGNOSIS OF GLIOMA

Adriana Olar and Gregory N. Fuller

INTRODUCTION

Primary brain tumors are currently classified by the World Health Organization (WHO) based primarily upon morphologic characteristics, and molecular biomarkers have previously been viewed as confirmatory or supplementary data.[1] Many markers have been used by the pathologist as ancillary studies to confirm or further inform a hematoxylin and eosin (H&E)–based tissue diagnosis as, for example, demonstration of the lack of INI1 protein expression confirms a diagnosis of atypical teratoid/rhabdoid tumor, or the finding of epidermal growth factor receptor (*EGFR*) gene amplification supplements the characterization of a glioblastoma (GBM) that exhibits that feature.[1] However, the landscape of brain tumor diagnosis and classification, in particular that of the diffuse gliomas, has very recently undergone dramatic change as consensus builds around specific clinically relevant, objective molecular criteria, which are now supplanting traditional classification schemes based exclusively on morphologic features. This molecular paradigm is most strikingly illustrated by the speed with which two molecular signatures in particular, isocitrate dehydrogenase (*IDH*) mutation status and 1p/19q deletion status, have been incorporated as essential diagnostic elements into prospective clinical trials and, increasingly, into the daily clinical practice of oncologic neuropathologists in the classification of diffuse glioma.

In this chapter, the morphology-based WHO classification system, currently the international standard, is presented in the context of these two emerging clinically significant diagnostic, prognostic, and, as the most recent data suggest, predictive molecular markers. The last section of the chapter presents a model of the newer molecular classification system taking shape in neuro-oncology centers worldwide.

BACKGROUND: THE CURRENT MORPHOLOGIC FEATURE–BASED (WHO) CLASSIFICATION OF GLIOMAS WITH MOLECULAR CORRELATES

Astrocytic Tumors

Astrocytic tumors, whose cellular components by definition display astrocytic morphologic differentiation features, are the most common type of primary central nervous system tumor, accounting for more than 60% of all brain tumors.[2] Diffusely infiltrating astrocytomas are subdivided into three grades based on the presence or absence of three principal morphologic features: brisk mitotic activity, vascular proliferation, and tumor necrosis. Low-grade diffuse astrocytomas (WHO grade II) typically display nuclear atypia, cellular pleomorphism, and fibrillary cytoplasmic processes (astrocytic morphologic features) but do not show conspicuous mitotic activity. Anaplastic astrocytoma (WHO grade III) is characterized by the presence of brisk mitotic activity. GBM (WHO grade IV), in addition to nuclear atypia, cellular pleomorphism, and increased mitotic activity, is also characterized by the presence of microvascular proliferation and/or areas of tumor necrosis. GBMs have traditionally been subdivided into two general classes: "primary" and "secondary." Primary or "de novo" GBM is by far the more common subtype and is characterized by different molecular signatures compared with secondary GBM, which accounts for only 5% to 10% of cases.[3-7] The mean time to progression to secondary GBM is 2 years for the WHO grade II glioma and 5 years for the WHO grade III glioma.[8] Diffuse astrocytomas, including GBM, are highly infiltrative neoplasms.[9]

More than half of diffuse astrocytomas are characterized by mutations involving the *TP53* tumor suppressor gene located at 17p13.1, with concomitant loss of heterozygosity (LOH) on chromosome 17p.[6,10] Recently, IDH mutations have been identified in the WHO grade II and III astrocytic, oligodendroglial, and mixed oligoastrocytic gliomas,[11,12] as well as in secondary GBM, suggesting a common cellular precursor. It could be postulated that the subsequent acquisition of either a *TP53* mutation or of translocation-based whole arm loss of 1p and 19q would then be associated with classical astrocytic and oligodendroglial morphologic features, respectively.[3] How the traditional rubric of mixed oligoastrocytic tumors fit into this scheme is problematic.

Additional genetic abnormalities predispose to anaplastic progression, including loss of tumor suppressors *CDKN2A*, *CDKN2B*, and *p14ARF* on 9p21, deletions on chromosomes 6, 11p, 22q, and/or inactivation of *RB1*.[13]

The full catalogue of molecular alterations described in GBM is complex, with the inactivation of multiple tumor suppressor genes and activation of multiple proto-oncogenes.[14]

The *EGFR* gene, located at 7p12, is the most commonly overexpressed gene in primary GBM, present in approximately 40%.[1,15] In about half of the *EGFR* amplified GBMs, an *EGFR* rearrangement (*EGFRvIII*) gives rise to an activated truncated protein lacking the ligand-binding domain.[1] *EGFR* activation upregulates genes involved in neural stem cell proliferation, such as *ASPM* (abnormal spindle-like microcephaly associated), which promotes neuroblast proliferation and symmetric division. Inhibition of *ASPM* inhibits GBM cell growth and neural stem cell proliferation.[16] Detection of *EGFR* amplification and/or the presence of *EGFRvIII* is indicative of high-grade diffuse astrocytoma (GBM)[1,17] and predicts poor response to radiation and chemotherapy.[18,19] However, treatment with EGFR inhibitors has not shown prolonged progression-free survival, with only a small fraction of patients showing response.[13] In this regard, Verhaak et al.[20] have described four molecular subtypes of GBM: classical, mesenchymal, proneural, and neural. *EGFR* amplification is a characteristic of the classical molecular subtype.

It should be noted briefly while discussing astrocytic tumors that the other major type of astrocytoma, pilocytic astrocytoma, is a completely different neoplasm than the diffuse astrocytomas and is characterized by different molecular features. Most pilocytic astrocytomas display mitogen-activated protein kinase (MAPK)/extracellular signal-regulated kinase (ERK) pathway abnormalities, with the activation of the BRAF proto-oncogene (7q34) by duplication, fusion (*BRAF–KIAA1549* fusion gene), or, less likely, by point mutation (*BRAF*^{V600E}).[13,21-24] In pilocytic astrocytomas developing in the context of neurofibromatosis 1 (NF1), homozygous inactivation of the *NF1* gene is an alternative mechanism for MAPK/ERK activation and seems to be a mutually exclusive alternative to *BRAF* mutation.[25] An aggressive, anaplastic subtype of pilocytic astrocytoma associated with decreased survival has been described that is characterized by increased mitotic activity and alterations in the PI3K/AKT pathway.[26,27]

Oligodendroglial Tumors

As classically defined, oligodendroglial tumors account for about 2.5% of all brain tumors.[2] Oligodendroglioma (WHO grade II) is a diffusely infiltrating glioma that displays a monotonous cytologic histologic pattern, with round nuclei surrounded by cytoplasmic clearing, imparting a classical "perinuclear halo" or "fried egg" appearance. The perinuclear halo effect is a formalin fixation artifact and is not seen in frozen tissues, smears, or rapidly fixed specimens.

Anaplastic oligodendroglioma (WHO grade III) is distinguished from low-grade (WHO grade II) oligodendroglioma by increased mitotic activity, microvascular proliferation, and/or necrosis.[1] The quantitative level of mitotic activity required as the minimum criterion for upgrading to WHO grade II is not defined, and thus constitutes an area of subjectivity and potential diagnostic variability. This issue is addressed in the last section of the chapter. One study showed that 6 or more mitoses per 10 high-power fields are associated with decreased survival[28]; however, this is not a formally codified criterion.[1]

Mixed oligoastrocytoma is a WHO-codified diffuse glioma subtype in which the tumor cells display various morphological features of both oligodendroglioma and astrocytoma. This category has the most subjective diagnostic criteria, resulting in low interobserver diagnostic reproducibility.[29-31] Molecular classification has provided an alternative solution to this long-standing problematic issue, as discussed in the last section of this chapter.

MOLECULAR TESTING IN CLINICAL PRACTICE

Mutations Involving Isocitrate Dehydrogenase 1 (IDH1)

IDHs are members of a family of metabolic enzymes that catalyze the nicotinamide adenine dinucleotide phosphate (NADP+)/nicotinamide adenine dinucleotide (NAD+)–dependent oxidative decarboxylation of isocitrate to α-ketoglutarate, with subsequent NADPH/NADH release.[32,33] There are three IDH isoenzymes, subclassified into two distinct groups that utilize either $NADP^+$ or NAD^+, as an electron acceptor.[32] Two NADP+-dependent IDH homodimers have been described: a cytosolic form (IDH1)[34-37] and a mitochondrial form (IDH2).[38] IDH3 is a mitochondrial NAD+-dependent heterotetramer composed of two α-subunits, one β-subunit, and one γ-subunit.[39]

The complex functions of IDH family members have been extensively characterized. In addition to a catabolic role in the Krebs cycle, the $NADP^+$-depended IDHs (IDH1 and IDH2), as sources of NADPH, have been shown to play a key role in cellular defense against oxidative stress-induced damage.[40-42] Cytosolic IDH (IDH1) has been localized to peroxisomes, providing NADPH for the β-oxidation of unsaturated fatty acids.[35,43,44] The mitochondrial isoforms, IDH2 and IDH3, play a central role in energy production via the tricarboxylic acid cycle.[32]

In 2008, Parsons et al.,[45] as part of a genome-wide mutational analysis of GBM, identified IDH mutations. Numerous confirmatory studies followed, detailing IDH mutation in large number of diffuse gliomas of all histologic subtypes and grades. Although mutations of *IDH1* and *IDH2* have been described, *IDH1* is by far the most commonly mutated in diffuse gliomas.[11,46,47] Of major clinical significance, IDH mutation confers a favorable prognosis compared with wild type.[11,48,49]

The single most common *IDH1* mutation is a heterozygous point mutation with a change of guanine to adenine at position 395 (G395A), leading to the replacement of arginine at position 132 with histidine (*R132H*), which is located at the IDH1 active site. Other mutations involving *IDH1* and *IDH2* have been well documented, albeit at a markedly lower frequency compared with *IDH1 (R132H)*. The most commonly identified mutations and their reported frequencies are shown in Table 40.1.[11,12,45-47,50]

IDH1 is coded by the *IDH1* gene located on 2q33.3.[51] IDH2 is coded by *IDH2*, located on 15q26.1.[52] The IDH enzymes share approximately 70% of their structure. As mentioned earlier, IDH1 is a homodimer and contains two active sites, each of which has an NADP+-binding site and a metal ion–binding site. IDH1 has three biologically relevant conformational states that differ in overall structure and in the structure of the active site. The protein transitions between an inactive (open, loop conformation), a semi-open (partially unraveled α-helix), and a catalytically active (closed, α-helix) conformational state. In the inactive (open) conformation, Asp279 occupies the isocitrate-binding site and forms hydrogen bonds with Ser94. In the active form, Asp279 chelates the metal ion. The active, closed conformation of the enzyme relieves Asp279, permitting isocitrate binding. During this release process, Asp279 interacts with Arg132. Arg132, which is replaced by histidine in the mutated form, therefore plays a critical role in the transition between inactive and active IDH1 conformations.[33,53]

Numerous investigators have catalogued *IDH* mutations in cancers other than diffuse glioma[54-60]; the majority of the *IDH1/2* mutations were found in syndromic[60] and non-syndromic[56] conventional central and periosteal cartilaginous neoplasms, with a frequency as high as 92.5% in one study.[60] The most common mutation is R132C and is found in 65% of cases. *IDH1* mutations have also been identified in significantly lower incidences in acute myelogenous leukemia,[57-59] with a frequency of 23% in one study,[58] prostate carcinoma (2.7%),[55] and B-cell acute lymphoblastic leukemia (1.7%).[55] Unlike diffuse glioma, mutated *IDH1* in acute myelogenous leukemia and cartilaginous neoplasms is not associated with a favorable prognosis.[56,59]

Pathobiologic Mechanism

Intensive recent investigation has shown that *IDH1 (R132H)* has both loss-of-function and gain-of-function effects. The loss of function involves the reduction of oxidative decarboxylation of isocitrate, thus decreasing the levels of α-KG and NADPH.[11,12,61] Gain of function involves the NADPH-dependent reduction of α-KG to 2-hydroxyglutarate (2HG), principally the R(–) stereoisomer (R(–)-2HG) (Fig. 40.1).[58,62-64]

The bioavailability of α-KG is influenced by its cellular equilibrium resulting from transamination of glutamate, the major neurotransmitter in the central nervous system.[65-67] Enhanced α-KG production by residual wild-type IDH1 may also play a role.[62] The former hypothesis might explain the high frequency of *IDH1* mutations within the central nervous system and the absence or paucity of *IDH1* mutations in other cancers; however,

TABLE 40–1 IDH1 and IDH2 Mutation Frequency in Diffuse Glioma[11,12,45-47,50]

Nucleotide Substitution	Amino Acid Substitution	Frequency Range from Published Studies
IDH1		
G395A	R132H	**85–100%**
C394A	R132S	1.5–5%
C394T	R132C	1.5–4%
C394G	R132G	1–3%
G395T	R132L	0.5–3%
C394G G395T	R132V	0.5%
IDH2		
G515A	R172K	Up to 64.5%[a]
A514T	R172W	Up to 16.2%[a]
G515T	R172M	Up to 19.3%[a]

Nucleotides: A, adenine; G, guanine; C, cytosine; T, thymidine.
Amino acids: R, arginine; H, histidine; S, serine; C, cysteine; G, glycine; L, leucine; V, valine; K, lysine; W, tryptophan; M, methionine.
[a]Values obtained from a study on a very large number of gliomas.[46]

the glutamate hypothesis does not account for the high frequency of *IDH1/2* mutations in cartilaginous tumors.

Under normoxic conditions, prolyl hydroxylases act upon hypoxia-inducible factor-1α (HIF-1α) by hydroxylating proline residues, allowing further ubiquitination and proteasome degradation.[68] Under hypoxic conditions, prolyl hydroxylases are inhibited, requiring oxygen as a cofactor.[69] Prolyl hydroxylases utilize α-KG as a cofactor[70-72]; therefore, decreased levels of α-KG are associated with an increase in HIF-1α.[61] HIF-1α is a transcription factor that promotes the expression of genes involved in glycolysis, angiogenesis, and other signaling pathways involved in tumorigenesis.[61,73] Xu et al. demonstrated that prolyl hydroxylase is only one member of the α-KG–dependent dioxygenases, competitively inhibited by 2-HG, which has a similar chemical structure with α-KG. Inhibition of α-KG–dependent dioxygenases was shown to lead to a genome-wide change of histone and DNA methylation, potentially leading to tumorigenesis.[64]

Clinical Features

IDH1 (R132H) is expressed in up to 10% of pilocytic astrocytomas, 60% to 65% of WHO grades II and III astrocytoma, 75% to 80% of WHO grades II and III oligodendroglioma, 80% to 85% of WHO grades II and III mixed oligoastrocytoma, 80% of secondary GBM, and 5% of primary GBM.[3,5,11,12,46-49,74,75] *IDH1* mutations have also been reported in up to 8% of gangliogliomas.[46,47]

IDH1 mutation-positive diffuse gliomas arise in patients significantly younger than those with *IDH1* wild-type tumors,[3,5,7,45,76] have a favorable prognosis compared with wild-type tumors,[5,11,45,48,49,76] and are characteristic of secondary GBM.[5,45] In one study of gangliogliomas, however, the presence of mutant *IDH1* correlated with a greater risk of recurrence and malignant transformation and/or death compared with *IDH1* wild-type tumors. The age of patients with IDH1-mutant gangliogliomas was higher compared with those without mutation.[77]

IDH1 mutation is an early event in gliomagenesis. *IDH1* mutations do not arise after the acquisition of *TP53* mutation or 1p/19q codeletion.[3] *IDH1* mutation is highly associated with *TP53* mutation, 1p19q codeletion, and *MGMT*—promoter methylation status and is inversely correlated with loss of chromosome 10 and with *EGFR* amplification, which are signatures seen with high incidence in primary GBM.[3,4,45,48,49,74,78] Mutated *IDH1*, per se, is associated with longer progression-free survival irrespective of histology, treatment, 1p/19q status, or *MGMT* promoter methylation status.[79]

Accumulating evidence strongly suggests that *IDH* mutation status is of greater prognostic relevance than traditional WHO morphology-based grade.[74,80-82] Hartmann et al.[74] have shown that patients with *IDH1* wild-type anaplastic astrocytoma (WHO grade III) exhibit worse prognosis compared with *IDH1*-mutated GBM (WHO grade IV). Another study of gliomas of low histological grade identified the *IDH1* wild-type group as having a more highly infiltrative nature and a significantly more dismal outcome.[82] Yet another recent study described the association of absence of *IDH* mutation in non-enhancing diffuse glioma with rapid anaplastic progression and poor outcome.[83] These studies collectively highlight the importance of IDH mutation status as a critical molecular signature, impacting diffuse glioma classification, grading, treatment and prognosis, as further described in the last section of this chapter.

Laboratory Testing

The widespread availability of a mutation-specific antibody directed against the mutant IDH1 (R132H) protein,[84] permitting a simple immunohistochemical (IHC) test that can be performed at low cost on formalin-fixed paraffin-embedded (FFPE) tissue, has dramatically changed routine diffuse glioma diagnosis and classification in a very short period of time. When clinically indicated, a negative IDH1 (R132H) IHC test can be followed by sequence-based molecular assay for the rarer *IDH1* and *IDH2* mutations.

IDH1 (R132H) IHC has a number of practical applications in clinical neuropathology; for example, to help distinguish diffuse glioma from reactive astrogliosis or other conditions that mimic glioma, such as therapy changes, viral infection, and infarction.[84-88]

1p/19q Deletion Status

Early studies observed that 50% to 70% of low-grade and anaplastic oligodendrogliomas exhibit a specific molecular alteration in the form of allelic loss occurring preferentially on chromosome 1p and/or 19q.[89-92] It was noted that these alterations distinguish oligodendroglial tumors from other glial neoplasms, and a role in oligodendroglial tumorigenesis was hypothesized.[93] It had already been observed that anaplastic oligodendrogliomas showed unusual sensitivity to PCV (procarbazine, lomustine, and vincristine) chemotherapy.[94-97] In 1998, Cairncross et al.[98] linked the loss of 1p/19q to chemosensitivity. This finding was independently confirmed and extended to include patients treated with temozolomide.[99-102] Temozolomide can be administered orally and often has milder side effects compared with other alkylating agents.[103]

Oligodendrogliomas tend to occur in adults and are rare in children. Pediatric oligodendrogliomas rarely exhibit combined 1p/19q loss.[104-106] Allelic loss is seen in 80% to 90% of WHO grade II adult oligodendrogliomas and 50% to 70% of adult anaplastic oligodendrogliomas.[107] A wide range of frequencies has been reported in mixed oligoastrocytomas, likely attributable to the subjective and poorly reproducible nature of this morphology-based diagnosis.[108]

Laboratory Testing

A number of techniques, as briefly described below, can be used to determine 1p/19q deletion status. Each has relative benefits and drawbacks.

Fluorescence in situ hybridization (FISH) uses unique fluorescence-labeled probes that are hybridized directly on tissue sections, permitting evaluation of chromosomal copy number in tumor cells. FISH has relatively low cost and can be performed on FFPE tissue. However, FISH preparation and assessment can be time-consuming and the setting of multiple assays is relatively labor intensive. FISH has the singular advantage of allowing the pathologist to correlate molecular analysis with tissue morphology. FISH assessment of 1p/19q deletion status is currently the most popular technique that may likely be replaced by next-generation sequencing platforms in the near future.

Polymerase chain reaction (PCR)–based LOH assays are based on the comparison of several polymorphic alleles in tumor DNA versus a negative control (usually leukocyte DNA from peripheral blood). PCR primers are designed against unique microsatellite sequences at each chromosomal region of interest. Because not all alleles are informative, multiple loci need to be amplified for each chromosomal arm to ensure that enough loci will be available to detect loss. Selection of optimal, representative tumor tissue with minimal contamination from nonneoplastic tissue or necrosis is important. PCR-based assay is of relatively low cost, but it does require a control sample.

Array comparative genomic hybridization (CGH) is a technique that uses genome-wide differential labeling of tumor and control DNA for a comparative hybridization to arrays of DNA and provides an estimate of copy number at all chromosomal loci examined on the microarray. Array CGH is a very powerful technique but its clinical use is currently restricted by relatively high cost of specialized equipment, data processing, and analysis.

MOLECULAR CLASSIFICATION OF DIFFUSE GLIOMAS BASED ON IDH MUTATION STATUS AND 1P/19Q CODELETION STATUS

Traditional morphology-based classification of diffuse gliomas has served the neuro-oncology community and our patients well in the past. However, this system is plagued by subjectivity and lack of interobserver concordance, particularly with respect to the diagnosis of imprecisely defined category of mixed oligoastrocytoma. The recent emergence of the two robust molecular classifiers discussed above, 1p/19q codeletion status and IDH mutation status, now permit more reproducible substratification of diffuse gliomas for clinical trial purposes and also for routine clinical diagnosis. Using these two molecular signatures, diffuse gliomas can be separated into major groups based on the presence or absence of IDH mutation and combined 1p/19q codeletion (see Fig. 40.1). 1p/19q codeleted tumors (of which virtually 100% also exhibit IDH mutation) have the most favorable response to treatment and best prognosis, with noncodeleted tumors that exhibit IDH mutation occupying the prognostic middle ground, and "double-negative" noncodeleted, non-IDH mutated tumors having the poorest treatment response and prognosis. This stratification holds for both WHO grade II and grade III diffuse gliomas, and the weight of accumulated evidence to date supports the contention that this molecular model is a more objective, more reproducible, and more powerful predictor of response to therapy and of survival than the traditional partitioning of diffuse gliomas based on morphologic features. This is a very encouraging prospect in view of the fact that there are no objective consensus criteria for diagnosing "mixed oligoastrocytoma" or for the "cutoff" level of cellular proliferation (mitotic activity or proliferation marker index) required for separating grade II from grade III diffuse glioma.

Molecular diagnosis and classification of diffuse glioma begins with routine histologic assessment, which determines that the patient's lesion is a diffuse glioma and not another type of primary brain tumor or a metastasis, infection, inflammatory disease, or other type of disease. This is followed by relatively simple and increasingly rapid and cost-effective testing for IDH mutation status and 1p/19q deletion status (which will become even more efficiently obtained with the advent of next-generation sequencing platforms).

Examples of the diffuse glioma tissue diagnosis format used at MD Anderson Cancer Center are illustrated

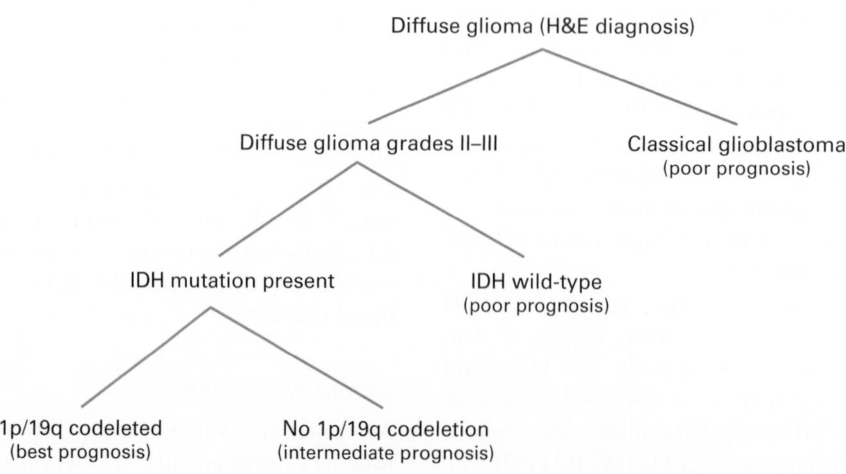

FIGURE 40–1 Diffuse glioma molecular classification.

TABLE 40-2 Illustrative Molecular Diagnosis Format for Diffuse Glioma (MD Anderson Cancer Center Format)

Diffuse Glioma

IDH status: IDH1 (R132H) mutation present
1p/19q status: codeletion present
Mitotic index (PHH3): 1/1,000
Ki-67 index (MIB1): 3%
(see comment)

Comment

Examination of H&E-stained sections shows a diffuse glioma with morphological features corresponding to oligodendroglioma, grade II, of the WHO classification system. IDH1 (R132H) mutation is determined by immunohistochemistry. 1p/19q deletion status is determined by fluorescence in situ hybridization (FISH) assay. Mitotic index of 1 mitosis per 1,000 cells is determined by automated quantitation of phosphohistone H3 (PHH3) immunostain. Ki-67 antigen index of 3% is determined by automated quantitation of MIB-1 immunostain.

in Table 40.2. This format highlights in the Diagnosis section of the pathology report the critical biomarker data needed by neuro-oncologists to formulate a treatment plan, with additional supplementary information, such as the morphological features of the tumor with correspondence to traditional WHO histologic subtype and estimation of grade and details of the technical procedures used for proliferation index and molecular marker determination, included in a Comment section.

The molecular classification scheme shown in Figure 40.1 and companion illustrative diagnosis format shown in Table 40.2 will undoubtedly undergo modification with further advance in knowledge, but both present significant advantages over morphology-based classification schemes in terms of objectivity, reproducibility, and, most importantly, clinical utility.

REFERENCES

1. Louis DN, Ohgaki H, Wiestler OD, et al. *WHO Classification of Tumors of the Central Nervous System*. 4th ed. Lyon (France): IARC; 2007.
2. Love S, Louis DN, Ellison, D, eds. *Greenfield's Neuropathology*. 8th ed. London: Edward Arnold Publishers; 2008.
3. Watanabe T, Nobusawa S, Kleihues P, et al. IDH1 mutations are early events in the development of astrocytomas and oligodendrogliomas. *Am J Pathol*. 2009;174:1149-1153.
4. Ohgaki H, Kleihues P. Genetic pathways to primary and secondary glioblastoma. *Am J Pathol*. 2007;170:1445-1453.
5. Nobusawa S, Watanabe T, Kleihues P, et al. IDH1 mutations as molecular signature and predictive factor of secondary glioblastomas. *Clin Cancer Res*. 2009;15:6002-6007.
6. Ohgaki H, Kleihues P. Genetic profile of astrocytic and oligodendroglial gliomas. *Brain Tumor Pathol*. 2011;28:177-183.
7. Ohgaki H, Dessen P, Jourde B, et al. Genetic pathways to glioblastoma: a population-based study. *Cancer Res*. 2004;64:6892-6899.
8. Ohgaki H, Kleihues P. Population-based studies on incidence, survival rates, and genetic alterations in astrocytic and oligodendroglial gliomas. *J Neuropathol Exp Neurol*. 2005;64:479-489.
9. Burger PC, Heinz ER, Shibata T, et al. Topographic anatomy and CT correlations in the untreated glioblastoma multiforme. *J Neurosurg*. 1988;68:698-704.
10. Okamoto Y, Di Patre PL, Burkhard C, et al. Population-based study on incidence, survival rates, and genetic alterations of low-grade diffuse astrocytomas and oligodendrogliomas. *Acta Neuropathol*. 2004;108:49-56.
11. Yan H, Parsons W, Jin G, et al. IDH1 and IDH2 mutations in gliomas. *N Engl J Med*. 2009:360(8):765-773.
12. Balss J, Meyer J, Mueller W, et al. Analysis of the IDH1 codon 132 mutation in brain tumors. *Acta Neuropathol*. 2008;116:597-602.
13. Riemenschneider MJ, Jeuken JW, Wesseling P, et al. Molecular diagnostics of gliomas: state of the art. *Acta Neuropathol*. 2010;120:567-584.
14. Cancer Genome Atlas Research Network. Comprehensive genomic characterization defines human glioblastoma genes and core pathways. *Nature*. 2008;455:1061-1068.
15. Yip S, Iafrate AJ, Louis DN. Molecular diagnostic testing in malignant gliomas: a practical update on predictive markers. *J Neuropathol Exp Neurol*. 2008;67:1-15.
16. Horvath S, Zhang B, Carlson M, et al. Analysis of oncogenic signaling networks in glioblastoma identifies ASPM as a molecular target. *Proc Natl Acad Sci U S A*. 2006;103(46):17402-17407.
17. Jeuken J, Sijben A, Alenda C, et al. Robust detection of EGFR copy number changes and EGFR variant III: technical aspects and relevance for glioma diagnostics. *Brain Pathol*. 2009;19:661-671.
18.Weppler SA, Li Y, Dubois L, et al. Expression of EGFR variant vIII promotes both radiation resistance and hypoxia tolerance. *Radiother Oncol*. 2007;83:333-339.
19. Chakravarti A, Chakladar A, Delaney MA, et al. The epidermal growth factor receptor pathway mediates resistance to sequential administration of radiation and chemotherapy in primary human glioblastoma cells in a RAS dependent manner. *Cancer Res*. 2002;62:4307-4315.
20. Verhaak RG, Hoadley KA, Purdom E, et al. Integrated genomic analysis identifies clinically relevant subtypes of glioblastoma characterized by abnormalities in PDGFRA, IDH1, EGFR, and NF1. *Cancer Cell*. 2010;17:98-110.
21. Pfister S, Janzarik WG, Remke M, et al. BRAF gene duplication constitutes a mechanism of MAPK pathway activation in low-grade astrocytomas. *J Clin Invest*. 2008;118:1739-1749.
22. Jones DT, Kocialkowski S, Liu L, et al. Tandem duplication producing a novel oncogenic BRAF fusion gene defines the majority of pilocytic astrocytomas. *Cancer Res*. 2008;68:8673-8677.
23. Forshew T, Tatevossian RG, Lawson AR, et al. Activation of the ERK/MAPK pathway: a signature genetic defect in posterior fossa pilocytic astrocytomas. *J Pathol*. 2009;218:172-181.
24. Lin A, Rodriguez FJ, Karajannis MA, et al. BRAF alterations in primary glial and glioneuronal neoplasms of the central nervous system with identification of 2 novel KIAA1549: BRAF fusion variants. *J Neuropathol Exp Neurol*. 2012;71:66-72.
25. Yu J, Deshmukh H, Gutmann RJ, et al. Alterations of BRAF and HIPK2 loci predominate in sporadic pilocytic astrocytoma. *Neurology*. 2009;73:1526-1531.
26. Rodriguez FJ, Scheithauer BW, Burger PC, et al. Anaplasia in pilocytic astrocytoma predicts aggressive behavior. *Am J Surg Pathol*. 2010;34:147-160.
27. Rodriguez EF, Scheithauer BW, Giannini C, et al. PI3K/AKT pathway alterations are associated with clinically aggressive and histologically anaplastic subsets of pilocytic astrocytoma. *Acta Neuropathol*. 2011;121:407-420.
28. Giannini C, Scheithauer BW, Weaver AL, et al. Oligodendrogliomas: reproducibility and prognostic value of histologic diagnosis and grading. *J Neuropathol Exp Neurol*. 2001;60:248-262.
29. Kros JM, Gorlia T, Kouwenhoven MC, et al. Panel review of anaplastic oligodendroglioma from European Organization for Research and Treatment of Cancer Trial 26951: assessment of consensus in diagnosis, influence of 1p/19q loss, and correlations with outcome. *J Neuropathol Exp Neurol*. 2007;66:545-51.
30. Aldape K, Burger PC, Perry A. Clinicopathologic aspects of 1p/19q loss and the diagnosis of oligodendroglioma. *Arch Pathol Lab Med*. 2007;131:242-251.

31. CBTRUS. CBTRUS Statistical Report: primary brain and central nervous system tumors diagnosed in the United States in 2004-2007. http://www.cbtrus.org/. Accessed December 24, 2011.
32. Haselbeck RJ, McAlister-Henn L. Function and expression of yeast mitochondrial NAD- and NADP-specific isocitrate dehydrogenases. *J Biol Chem*. 1993;268:12116-12122.
33. Reitman ZJ, Yan H. Isocitrate dehydrogenase 1 and 2 mutations in cancer: alterations at a crossroads of cellular metabolism *J Natl Cancer Inst*. 2010;102:932-941.
34. Jennings GT, Sechi S, Stevenson PM, et al. Cytosolic NADP(+)-dependent isocitrate dehydrogenase. Isolation of rat cDNA and study of tissue-specific and developmental expression of mRNA. *J Biol Chem*. 1994;269:23128-23134.
35. Henke B, Girzalsky W, Berteaux-Lecellier V, et al. IDP3 encodes a peroxisomal NADP-dependent isocitrate dehydrogenase required for the beta-oxidation of unsaturated fatty acids. *J Biol Chem*. 1998;273:3702-3711.
36. Geisbrecht BV, Gould SJ. The human PICD gene encodes a cytoplasmic and peroxisomal NADP(+)-dependent isocitrate dehydrogenase. *J Biol Chem*. 1999;274:30527-30533.
37. Yoshihara T, Hamamoto T, Munakata R, et al. Localization of cytosolic NADP-dependent isocitrate dehydrogenase in the peroxisomes of rat liver cells: biochemical and immunocytochemical studies. *J Histochem Cytochem*. 2001;49:1123-1131.
38. Plaut GW, Cook M, Aogaichi T. The subcellular location of isozymes of NADP-isocitrate dehydrogenase in tissues from pig, ox and rat. *Biochim Biophys Acta*. 1983;760:300-308.
39. Ramachandran N, Colman RF. Chemical characterization of distinct subunits of pig heart DPN-specific isocitrate dehydrogenase. *J Biol Chem*. 1980;255:8859-8864.
40. Jo SH, Son MK, Koh HJ, et al. Control of mitochondrial redox balance and cellular defense against oxidative damage by mitochondrial NADP+-dependent isocitrate dehydrogenase. *J Biol Chem*. 2001;276:16168-16176.
41. Lee SM, Koh HJ, Park DC, et al. Cytosolic NADP(+)-dependent isocitrate dehydrogenase status modulates oxidative damage to cells. *Free Radic Biol Med*. 2002;32:1185-1196.
42. Kim SY, Park JW. Cellular defense against singlet oxygen-induced oxidative damage by cytosolic NADP+-dependent isocitrate dehydrogenase. *Free Radic Res*. 2003;37:309-316.
43. van Roermund CW, Hettema EH, Kal AJ, et al. Peroxisomal beta-oxidation of polyunsaturated fatty acids in *Saccharomyces cerevisiae*: isocitrate dehydrogenase provides NADPH for reduction of double bonds at even positions. *EMBO J*. 1998;17:677-687.
44. Minard KI, McAlister-Henn L. Dependence of peroxisomal beta-oxidation on cytosolic sources of NADPH. *J Biol Chem*. 1999;274:3402-3406.
45. Parsons DW, Jones S, Zhang X, et al. An integrated genomic analysis of human glioblastoma multiforme. *Science*. 2008;321:1807-1812.
46. Hartmann C, Meyer J, Balss J, et al. Type and frequency of IDH1 and IDH2 mutations are related to astrocytic and oligodendroglial differentiation and age: a study of 1,010 diffuse gliomas. *Acta Neuropathol*. 2009;118:469-474.
47. Horbinski C, Kofler J, Kelly LM, et al. Diagnostic use of IDH1/2 mutation analysis in routine clinical testing of formalin-fixed, paraffin-embedded glioma tissues. *J Neuropathol Exp Neurol*. 2009;68:1319-1325.
48. Sonoda Y, Kumabe T, Nakamura T, et al. Analysis of IDH1 and IDH2 mutations in Japanese glioma patients. *Cancer Sci*. 2009;100:1996-1998.
49. Sanson M, Marie Y, Paris S, et al. Isocitrate dehydrogenase 1 codon 132 mutation is an important prognostic biomarker in gliomas. *J Clin Oncol*. 2009;27:4150-4154.
50. Felsberg J, Wolter M, Seul H, et al. Rapid and sensitive assessment of the IDH1 and IDH2 mutation status in cerebral gliomas based on DNA pyrosequencing. *Acta Neuropathol*. 2010;119:501-507.
51. Narahara K, Kimura S, Kikkawa K, et al. Probable assignment of soluble isocitrate dehydrogenase (IDH1) to 2q33.3. *Hum Genet*. 1985;71:37-40.
52. Grzeschik KH. Assignment of a gene for human mitochondrial isocitrate dehydrogenase (ICD-M, EC 1.1.1.41) to chromosome 15. *Hum Genet*. 1976;34:23-28.
53. Xu X, Zhao J, Xu Z, et al. Structures of human cytosolic NADP-dependent isocitrate dehydrogenase reveal a novel self-regulatory mechanism of activity. *J Biol Chem*. 2004;279:33946-33957.
54. Bleeker FE, Lamba S, Leenstra S, et al. IDH1 mutations at residue p.R132 (IDH1(R132)) occur frequently in high-grade gliomas but not in other solid tumors. *Hum Mutat*. 2009;30:7-11.
55. Kang MR, Kim MS, Oh JE, et al. Mutational analysis of IDH1 codon 132 in glioblastomas and other common cancers. *Int J Cancer*. 2009;125:353-355.
56. Amary MF, Bacsi K, Maggiani F, et al. IDH1 and IDH2 mutations are frequent events in central chondrosarcoma and central and periosteal chondromas but not in other mesenchymal tumours. *J Pathol*. 2011;224:334-343.
57. Dang L, Jin S, Su SM: IDH mutations in glioma and acute myeloid leukemia. *Trends Mol Med*. 2010;16:387-397.
58. Ward PS, Patel J, Wise DR, et al. The common feature of leukemia-associated IDH1 and IDH2 mutations is a neomorphic enzyme activity converting alpha-ketoglutarate to 2-hydroxyglutarate. *Cancer Cell*. 2010;17:225-234.
59. Boissel N, Nibourel O, Renneville A, et al. Prognostic impact of isocitrate dehydrogenase enzyme isoforms 1 and 2 mutations in acute myeloid leukemia: a study by the Acute Leukemia French Association group. *J Clin Oncol*. 2010;28:3717-3723.
60. Amary MF, Damato S, Halai D, et al. Ollier disease and Maffucci syndrome are caused by somatic mosaic mutations of IDH1 and IDH2. *Nature genetics*. 2011;43:1262-1265.
61. Zhao S, Lin Y, Xu W, et al. Glioma-derived mutations in IDH1 dominantly inhibit IDH1 catalytic activity and induce HIF-1alpha. *Science*. 2009;324:261-265.
62. Dang L, White DW, Gross S, et al. Cancer-associated IDH1 mutations produce 2-hydroxyglutarate. *Nature*. 2009;462:739-744.
63. Gross S, Cairns RA, Minden MD, et al. Cancer-associated metabolite 2-hydroxyglutarate accumulates in acute myelogenous leukemia with isocitrate dehydrogenase 1 and 2 mutations. *J Exp Med*. 2010;207:339-344.
64. Xu W, Yang H, Liu Y, et al. Oncometabolite 2-hydroxyglutarate is a competitive inhibitor of α-ketoglutarate-dependent dioxygenases. *Cancer Cell*. 2011;19:17-30.
65. Tsacopoulos M. Metabolic signaling between neurons and glial cells: a short review. *J Physiol Paris*. 2002;96:283-288.
66. Bak LK, Schousboe A, Waagepetersen HS. The glutamate/GABA-glutamine cycle: aspects of transport, neurotransmitter homeostasis and ammonia transfer. *J Neurochem*. 2006;98:641-653.
67. Seltzer MJ, Bennett BD, Joshi AD, et al. Inhibition of glutaminase preferentially slows growth of glioma cells with mutant IDH1. *Cancer Res*. 2010;70:8981-8987.
68. Maxwell PH, Wiesener MS, Chang GW, et al. The tumour suppressor protein VHL targets hypoxia-inducible factors for oxygen-dependent proteolysis. *Nature*. 1999;399:271-275.
69. Semenza GL. Hydroxylation of HIF-1: oxygen sensing at the molecular level. *Physiology (Bethesda)*. 2004;19:176-182.
70. Tuderman L, Myllylä R, Kivirikko KI. Mechanism of the prolyl hydroxylase reaction. 1. Role of co-substrates. *Eur J Biochem*. 1977;80:341-348.
71. Myllylä R, Tuderman L, Kivirikko KI. Mechanism of the prolyl hydroxylase reaction. 2. Kinetic analysis of the reaction sequence. *Eur J Biochem*. 1977;80:349-357.
72. Kaelin WG Jr, Ratcliffe PJ: Oxygen sensing by metazoans: the central role of the HIF hydroxylase pathway. *Mol Cell*. 2008;30:393-402.
73. Semenza GL. HIF-1: mediator of physiological and pathophysiological responses to hypoxia. *J Appl Physiol*. 2000;88:1474-1480.
74. Hartmann C, Hentschel B, Wick W, et al. Patients with IDH1 wild type anaplastic astrocytomas exhibit worse prognosis than IDH1-mutated glioblastomas, and IDH1 mutation status accounts for the unfavorable prognostic effect of higher age: implications for classification of gliomas. *Acta Neuropathol*. 2010;120:707-718.
75. Ichimura K, Pearson DM, Kocialkowski S, et al. IDH1 mutations are present in the majority of common adult gliomas but rare in primary glioblastomas. *Neuro Oncol*. 2009;11:341-347.
76. Bleeker FE, Atai NA, Lamba S, et al. The prognostic IDH1 (R132) mutation is associated with reduced NADP+-dependent IDH activity in glioblastoma. *Acta Neuropathol*. 2010;119: 487-494.

77. Horbinski C, Kofler J, Yeaney G, et al. Isocitrate dehydrogenase 1 analysis differentiates gangliogliomas from infiltrative gliomas. *Brain Pathol.* 2011;21:564-574.
78. van den Bent MJ, Dubbink HJ, Marie Y, et al. IDH1 and IDH2 mutations are prognostic but not predictive for outcome in anaplastic oligodendroglial tumors: a report of the European Organization for Research and Treatment of Cancer Brain Tumor Group. *Clin Cancer Res.* 2010;16:1597-1604.
79. Wick W, Hartmann C, Engel C, et al. NOA-04 randomized phase III trial of sequential radiochemotherapy of anaplastic glioma with procarbazine, lomustine, and vincristine or temozolomide. *J Clin Oncol.* 2009;27:5874-5880.
80. Gravendeel LA, Kouwenhoven MC, Gevaert O, et al. Intrinsic gene expression profiles of gliomas are a better predictor of survival than histology. *Cancer Res.* 2009;69:9065-9072.
81. Hartmann C, Hentschel B, Tatagiba M, et al. Molecular markers in low-grade gliomas: predictive or prognostic? *Clin Cancer Res.* 2011;17:4588-4599.
82. Metellus P, Coulibaly B, Colin C, et al. Absence of IDH mutation identifies a novel radiologic and molecular subtype of WHO grade II gliomas with dismal prognosis. *Acta Neuropathol.* 2010;120:719-729.
83. Olar A, Raghunathan A, Albarracin CT, et al. Absence of IDH1-R132H mutation predicts rapid progression of non-enhancing diffuse glioma in older adults. *Ann Diagn Pathol.* 2012;16(3):161-170.
84. Capper D, Zentgraf H, Balss J, et al. Monoclonal antibody specific for IDH1 R132H mutation. *Acta Neuropathol.* 2009;118:599-601.
85. Camelo-Piragua S, Jansen M, Ganguly A, et al. Mutant IDH1-specific immunohistochemistry distinguishes diffuse astrocytoma from astrocytosis. *Acta Neuropathol.* 2010;119:509-511.
86. Camelo-Piragua S, Jansen M, Ganguly A, et al. A sensitive and specific diagnostic panel to distinguish diffuse astrocytoma from astrocytosis: chromosome 7 gain with mutant isocitrate dehydrogenase 1 and p53. *J Neuropathol Exp Neurol.* 2011;70:110-115.
87. Capper D, Sahm F, Hartmann C, et al. Application of mutant IDH1 antibody to differentiate diffuse glioma from nonneoplastic central nervous system lesions and therapy-induced changes. *Am J Surg Pathol.* 2010;34:1199-1204.
88. Capper D, Weissert S, Balss J, et al. Characterization of R132H mutation-specific IDH1 antibody binding in brain tumors. *Brain Pathol.* 2010;20:245-254.
89. Reifenberger J, Reifenberger G, Liu L, et al. Molecular genetic analysis of oligodendroglial tumors shows preferential allelic deletions on 19q and 1p. *Am J Pathol.* 1994;145:1175-1190.
90. Kraus JA, Koopmann J, Kaskel P, et al. Shared allelic losses on chromosomes 1p and 19q suggest a common origin of oligodendroglioma and oligoastrocytoma. *J Neuropathol Exp Neurol.* 1995;54:91-95.
91. Bello MJ, Vaquero J, de Campos JM, et al. Molecular analysis of chromosome 1 abnormalities in human gliomas reveals frequent loss of 1p in oligodendroglial tumors. *Int J Cancer.* 1994;57:172-175.
92. von Deimling A, Louis DN, von Ammon K, et al. Evidence for a tumor suppressor gene on chromosome 19q associated with human astrocytomas, oligodendrogliomas, and mixed gliomas. *Cancer Res.* 1992;52:4277-4279.
93. Louis DN, Gusella JF. A tiger behind many doors: multiple genetic pathways to malignant glioma. *Trends Genet.* 1995;11:412-415.
94. Cairncross JG, Macdonald DR. Successful chemotherapy for recurrent malignant oligodendroglioma. *Ann Neurol.* 1988;23:360-364.
95. Cairncross JG, Macdonald D, Ludwin S, et al. Chemotherapy for anaplastic oligodendroglioma. National Cancer Institute of Canada Clinical Trials Group. *J Clin Oncol.* 1994;12:2013-2021.
96. Glass J, Hochberg FH, Gruber ML, et al. The treatment of oligodendrogliomas and mixed oligodendroglioma–astrocytomas with PCV chemotherapy. *J Neurosurg.* 1992;76:741-745.
97. Kim L, Hochberg FH, Thornton AF, et al. Procarbazine, lomustine, and vincristine (PCV) chemotherapy for grade III and grade IV oligoastrocytomas. *J Neurosurg.* 1996;85:602-607.
98. Cairncross JG, Ueki K, Zlatescu MC, et al. Specific genetic predictors of chemotherapeutic response and survival in patients with anaplastic oligodendrogliomas. *J Natl Cancer Inst.* 1998;90:1473-1479.
99. Chinot O. Chemotherapy for the treatment of oligodendroglial tumors. *Semin Oncol.* 2001;28:13-18.
100. Kaloshi G, Benouaich-Amiel A, Diakite F, et al. Temozolomide for low-grade gliomas: Predictive impact of 1p/19q loss on response and outcome. *Neurology.* 2007;68:1831-1836.
101. Hoang-Xuan K, Capelle L, Kujas M, et al. Temozolomide as initial treatment for adults with low-grade oligodendrogliomas or oligoastrocytomas and correlation with chromosome 1p deletions. *J Clin Oncol.* 2004;22:3133-3138.
102. Kouwenhoven MC, Kros JM, French PJ, et al. 1p/19q loss within oligodendroglioma is predictive for response to first line temozolomide but not to salvage treatment. *Eur J Cancer.* 2006;42: 2499-2503.
103. Wesolowski JR, Rajdev P, Mukherji SK. Temozolomide (Temodar). *AJNR Am J Neuroradiol.* 2010;31:1383-1384.
104. Kreiger PA, Okada Y, Simon S, et al. Losses of chromosomes 1p and 19q are rare in pediatric oligodendrogliomas. *Acta Neuropathol (Berl).* 2005;109:387-392.
105. Raghavan R, Balani J, Perry A, et al. Pediatric oligodendrogliomas: a study of molecular alterations on 1p and 19q using fluorescence in situ hybridization. *J Neuropathol Exp Neuro.* 2003;62:530-537.
106. Kim SH, Kim H, Kim TS. Clinical, histological, and immunohistochemical features predicting 1p/19q loss of heterozygosity in oligodendroglial tumors. *Acta Neuropathol.* 2005;110: 27-38.
107. Reifenberger G, Louis DN. Oligodendroglioma: toward molecular definitions in diagnostic neuro-oncology. *J Neuropathol Exp Neurol.* February 2003;62(2):111-126.
108. Jeuken JW, von Deimling A, Wesseling P. Molecular pathogenesis of oligodendroglial tumors. *J Neurooncol.* 2004;70:161-181.

CHAPTER 41

Molecular Diagnostics of Pediatric Neoplasms

Jennifer Picarsic, Marina Nikiforova, and Miguel Reyes-Múgica

INTRODUCTION

Pediatric tumors constitue a heterogeneous group of primitive clonal proliferations usually composed of hyperchromatic nuclei, with a small amount of cytoplasm imparting the nonspecific appearance of "small blue cell tumors" to many of these neoplasias. In classic cases with ample material, routine histology and selective immunohistochemistry help narrow the differential diagnoses and aid in arriving at a precise diagnosis. However, the current tendency of "doing more with less" is to receive little amounts of tissue for diagnosis, and pathologists only rarely encounter these classic cases. More often diagnosticians are confronted with small biopsies or cytologic specimens. Furthermore, with the advancement of neoadjuvant therapy regimens, we frequently receive small histologic remnants among necrotic and hemorrhagic debris of treated tumors. In addition, the ability to combine information derived from histological and immunohistochemical (IHC) studies (phenotype) with that obtained from molecular analyses has allowed us not only to make more accurate diagnoses but also to define families of pediatric tumors like the "Ewing sarcoma (ES)/primitive neuroectodermal tumor (PNET) family of tumors" and further refine variants of neoplasias that may feature differential therapeutic responses. For all of these reasons, molecular testing has become a vital ancillary diagnostic and often predictive tool in pediatric oncology (Table 41.1). Molecular research has led to an explosion of novel new markers not only helping to improve pathologist's diagnostic capabilities but also providing clinicians novel prognostic markers that help give insight into the biology and behavior of these tumors. Many pediatric clinical trials have now incorporated molecular markers into their risk stratification models as prognostic predictive indicators. However, diagnostic tissue is progressively scarce, and cost-effective utilization of resources is increasingly important, leaving the pathologists at the center of a complex diagnostic exercise to properly triage tissue at the time of procurement. Adequate formalin-fixed tissue for histology and immunohistochemistry is imperative, which can also be used for fluorescence in situ hybridization (FISH) studies. Imprints and smear preparations on charged slides can also be used for FISH studies, especially useful when faced with limited material or cytologic specimens. Fresh tissue for conventional cytogenetic karyotyping studies should be obtained in a sterile manner and stored in culture medium such as the popular Roswell Park Memorial Institute medium (RPMI-1640) at 4°C during transportation to ensure cell growth. Small sections of tumor should also be snap-frozen for future DNA/RNA extraction both for routine molecular testing (i.e., reverse-transcription polymerase chain reaction [RT-PCR] studies) and for research study protocols (genome-wide studies and sequencing). Additionally, tissue fixed in glutaraldehyde for ultrastructural analysis is also recommended when there is sufficient material. Furthermore, obtaining paired blood samples at the time of the procedure has become increasingly important, notably for the use of white blood cells as normal nucleic acid controls for molecular studies, such as in loss of heterozygosity (LOH) analysis. Over the past decade, we have witnessed a shift in the molecular studies of pediatric tumors from primarily adjunctive tests for diagnostics to now prognostic and predictive tools for risk stratification. Pediatric pathology and pathology as a whole now rest heavily on molecular diagnostics to better classify and predict biologic behavior. Collaboration among pathologists, surgeons, oncologists, and patient families is needed not only to obtain, triage, and process adequate tissue but also to facilitate continued understanding of the implications of this new knowledge in order to best treat and manage children with malignancy.

TABLE 41–1 Known Molecular Alterations in Pediatric Solid Tumors

Neoplasm	Gene	Locus/Translocation	Prognosis/Genetic Associations
Neuroblastoma	*MYCN*	2p23-24	Unfavorable, especially in stages 1 and 2
		1p36 LOH	Independent poor prognosis
		11q LOH	Independent poor prognosis
	DNA index	Hyperdiploidy (>1.0), near triploidy	Favorable in ages less than 1 y
	DNA index	Diploidy (1.0)	Early treatment failure in ages less than 1 y
		17q gain	Complex, related to other factors
	PHOX2B	4p12	Familial NB
	NBPF1	t(1;17)(p36.2;q11.2)	Familial NB
Ewing sarcoma/primitive neuroectodermal tumor	*EWS/FLI1*	t(11;22)(q24;q12)	Most common translocation
	EWS/ERG	t(21;22)(q22;q12)	
	EWS/ETV1	t(7;22)(p22;q12)	
	EWS/ETV4	t(17;22)(q21;q12)	
	EWS/FEV	t(2;22)(q33;q12)	
Alveolar rhabdomyosarcoma	*PAX3/FKHR*	t(2;13)(q35;q14)	Unfavorable prognosis in those presenting with metastatic disease
	PAX7/FKHR	t(1;13)(p36;q14)	
Embryonal rhabdomyosarcoma		11p15.5 LOH	Possible correlation with Beckwith-Wiedemann and WAGR syndromes
Synovial sarcoma	*SYT/SSX1* or *SYT/SSX2*	t(X;18)(p11.2;q11.2)	
Alveolar soft part sarcoma	*ASPSCR1/TFE3*	der(17)t(X;17)(p11;q25)	Unbalanced translocation
Mesenchymal hamartoma of the liver	*MHLB1* locus	19q13.3 or 19q13.4	See Table 41.3 for more details
	MALAT1	11q13	See Table 41.3 for more details
Hepatoblastoma	*β-catenin/CTNNB1*	3p22-p21.3	Nuclear accumulation of the β-catenin protein, unfavorable
	APC	5q21	Familial adenomatous polyposis coli syndrome
	GPC3	Xq26.1	Simpson-Golabi-Behmel syndrome
	WT2	11p15.5	Beckwith-Wiedemann syndrome
	TP53	17p13	Li-Fraumeni syndrome
	Copy number variants	Trisomies 8, 20	Unfavorable
Nephroblastoma (Wilms tumor)	*IRXB* gene cluster	16q LOH	Unfavorable (even in favorable histology)
		1p LOH	Unfavorable (even in favorable histology)
	WT2	11p15.5	More commonly found in association with Beckwith-Wiedemann syndrome; less common in sporadic cases
	WT1	11p13	More commonly found in association with WAGR, Frasier, and Denys-Drash syndrome; less common in sporadic cases
	GPC3	Xq26.1	Simpson-Golabi-Behmel syndrome
	NSD1	5q35	Sotos' syndrome
Renal cell carcinoma	*ASPSCR1-TFE3*	t(X;17)(p11.2;q25)	Balanced translocation
	PRCC-TFE3	t(X;1)(p11.2;q21)	
	Alpha/TFEB	t(6;11)(p21;q12)	
Clear cell sarcoma		t(10;17)	
Rhabdoid tumor	*SWI/hSNFa/INI*	22q11.2	Loss of nuclear protein staining; somatic mutations and less frequently germline mutations
Congenital infantile fibrosarcoma and congenital cellular mesoblastic nephroma	*ETV6/NTRK*	t(12;15)(p13;q25)	
PPB	*DICER1*	14q32	Familial PPB

NB, neuroblastoma; LOH, loss of heterozygosity; PPB, pleuropulmonary blastoma.

NEURAL CREST–DERIVED TUMORS

Neuroblastoma

The term "blastoma" refers to a tumor that recapitulates its embryological origin. Although the true cellular origin of many pediatric tumors is presumed and even accepted in many cases, it is important to emphasize that they are labeled with terms derived from their morphological differentiation patterns. With this caveat in mind, we will use the well-established terms that conform to the pediatric oncological nomenclature.

Neuroblastic tumors (NTs) represent a spectrum with variable degrees of cell maturation along the sympathetic nervous system embryological development and include neuroblastoma (NB), ganglioneuroblastoma, and ganglioneuroma. These are tumors arising from neural crest cells of the embryonic sympathetic nervous system and are thus most frequently found in those locations with highest density of their normal counterparts, especially the adrenal medulla and sympathetic ganglia of the retroperitoneal region, as well as the mediastinum. The histopathologic classification of NTs is based on the amount of Schwannian stroma development (positive for S-100 IHC staining) and ganglion cell differentiation. We will focus our discussion on the immature end of the spectrum (i.e., NB) where molecular findings are most relevant.

NB is the most common solid extracranial tumor throughout the world in those under 15 years of age, and among all childhood malignancies it is just behind leukemia/lymphoma and central nervous system (CNS) tumors. Most NBs are diagnosed in children under the age of 5 years. NB is classified according to the criteria that incorporate histopathologic classification based on the International Neuroblastoma Pathology Committee (INPC) terminology and criteria (e.g., undifferentiated, poorly differentiated, and differentiating NB subtypes). Favorable and unfavorable histology incorporates the mitosis and karyorrhexis cellular index (MKI) along with the age of the patient (Table 41.2). All types of NBs are stroma-poor and are composed of small- to medium-sized cells, with round to slightly oval nuclei and a "salt and pepper" chromatin with inconspicuous nucleoli. The undifferentiated subtype has no identifiable neuropil, while the poorly differentiated and differentiating subtypes have readily apparent neuropil. A poorly differentiating NB features less than 5% of neuroblasts undergoing synchronous differentiation toward ganglion cells, while a differentiating NB has between 5% and 50% of neuroblasts undergoing ganglion cell differentiation (Fig. 41.1). Table 41.2 outlines the favorable and unfavorable histology groups based on the INPC. This classification together with molecular studies, and clinical staging, based on the International Neuroblastoma Staging System, all help predict biologic behavior.[1,2] The Children's Oncology Group's (COG) NB Risk Stratification System uses clinical and biologic factors to predict biologic behavior and outcomes.

TABLE 41–2 International Neuroblastoma Pathology Classification for Neuroblastoma[a]

	Favorable Histology	Unfavorable Histology
Undifferentiated NB		
Any age	NA	Any MKI
Poorly differentiated		
<1.5 y	MKI < 200/5,000 cells	MKI > 200/5,000 cells
1.5–5 y	NA	Any MKI
>5 y	NA	Any MKI
Differentiating		
<1.5 y	MKI < 200/5,000 cells	MKI > 200/5,000 cells
1.5–5 y	MKI < 100/5,000 cells	MKI > 100/5,000 cells
>5 y	NA	Any MKI

NB, neuroblastoma; MKI, mitosis and karyorrhectic cells.

[a]Neuroblastoma defined as less than 50% Schwannian stroma development and without macroscopic nodule formation.

Molecular Diagnostics

The key morphologic diagnostic element in NBs is neural differentiation, which includes neuropil, Homer-Wright rosettes, and/or partial ganglion cell differentiation. Almost by definition, the undifferentiated subtype requires ancillary testing, including laboratory evidence of elevated urine and serum catecholamine metabolites (vanillylmandelic acid and homovanillic acid) and neural-specific IHC markers (e.g., neuron-specific enolase, protein gene product 9.5, synaptophysin, NB84, and CD56). Molecular analysis of the *MYCN* status is an essential step in classifying NBs. Up to 40% of aggressive NBs (predominantly undifferentiated and poorly differentiated

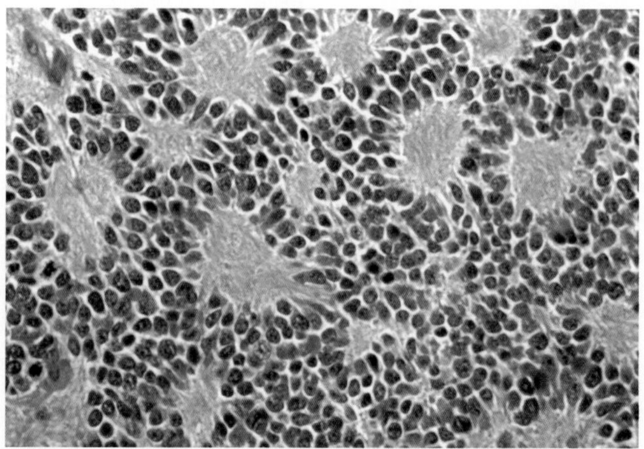

FIGURE 41–1 Neuroblastoma featuring classic Homer-Wright rosettes, with a center made of prolongations (neurites) of immature neuroblasts (H&E, ×20. Courtesy of J. Carrillo-Farga).

subtypes) demonstrate *MYCN* amplification defined by the International NB Risk Group Biology Committee as more than a fourfold increase in the 2p23-24/*MYCN* signal number compared with reference FISH centromeric probe. Conventional cytogenetic studies demonstrate extrachromosomal double-minute chromatin bodies or homogeneously staining chromosomal regions at chromosomes other than 2p in karyograms, which represent nuclear areas of amplified *MYCN* material. The nuclear fusion protein product results in an *MYCN–MAX* heterodimer thought to prevent cellular differentiation and promote proliferation. Other molecular findings of significant value in NBs include 1p deletion and TrkA expression, although the latter usually correlates inversely with the *MYCN* status and is, therefore, frequently assumed based on FISH for *MYCN* results. While hereditary NBs only account for 1% of cases, they provide further insight into the molecular basis of this tumor. Hereditary NB is associated with two congenital diseases, congenital central hypoventilation syndrome, which results in ventilation failure during sleep due to dysfunction of the autonomic control of respiration, and Hirschsprung disease, a congenital absence of ganglion cells in the distal colon with secondary constipation and megacolon. Studies have shown frameshift and missense mutations on chromosome 4p12 at the *PHOX2B* gene involved in five families of familial NB. This paired-like homeobox transcription factor is the main regulator of the autonomous nervous system by promoting the dopamine-b-hydroxylase promoter and is thought to be involved in cellular development differentiation pathways.[3] The direct involvement of this gene is not fully worked out, as some familial NB cases with mutations lead to a mutant protein with stable functional capability while mutations in *PHOX2B* are rarely found in sporadic NB cases.[3] Additional copy number variants and balanced and unbalanced translocations have been reported in the literature with the Neuroblastoma Breakpoint Family (*NBPF1*) gene at chromosome 1 involved in the constitutional translocation t(1;17)(p36.2;q11.2) and a related gene in the same family, *NBPF23*, at 1q21.1 are thought to play a role in familial NB.[3] However, further work is needed to investigate how these mutations alter pathways to make these patients susceptible to NB and what role, if any, they play in developmental pathways so as to unlock further understanding of the molecular pathogenesis of sporadic NB. One such promising gene is the *ALK* gene at chromosome 2p23-p24 in which three activating mutations were found in nine familial NB families as well as a number of sporadic cases. While the exact function of this membrane receptor is not fully characterized, mutations in this kinase receptor seem to be oncogenic with strong in vitro kinase activity. While some have shown that *ALK* mutations are associated with more aggressive tumors or advanced/metastatic tumors, this has not been validated in prospective large groups.[4,5] *ALK* as a target for small kinase inhibitors is an attractive target for therapeutic intervention used successfully in other human malignancies (i.e., *BCR/ABL* in chronic myeloid leukemia and *c-KIT* in gastrointestinal stromal tumors). The downregulation of the ALK receptor has been shown in some NB xenograft models to decrease cell proliferation; however, further work to understand the pathogenesis of *ALK* in NB is needed for successful therapeutic interventions to be fully realized.[3]

Molecular Prognostics

Investigation of molecular events that predict biologic behavior and outcome has led to an explosion of potential prognostic markers in NB and is redefining the way patients are classified in staging systems. *MYCN* amplification has been at the forefront as a prognostic molecular marker, predicting poor outcomes, most notably in those with localized (stages 1 and 2) disease, or in patients less than 1 year of age with metastatic disease of special type (stage 4S). *MYCN* amplification status has less effect on prognostic outcomes in older children with metastatic disease (stage 4). While the prognosis is generally good in children less than 1 year of age, even with metastasis to special sites (stage 4S), only half of those with *MYCN* amplification will have a 5-year survival. The COG's NB risk group schema is based on the staging, age, *MYCN* status combined with DNA ploidy index, and the INPC (Table 41.2).[2,6] Recently, however, the proposed International Neuroblastoma Risk Group Staging System has also included 11q LOH in its stratification model, because the loss of 11q is a predictor of decreased event-free and progression-free survival, independent of *MYCN* amplification.[7] COG studies for NB now include 1p loss with unbalanced 11q deletion, *MYCN* status, and DNA ploidy in their risk stratification models.

A whole chromosome copy number alteration (e.g., ploidy status) is a well-recognized prognostic marker. Triploid DNA index has better outcomes than diploid and tetraploid DNA indexes in NBs, especially in ages less than 1 year. Isolated copy number alterations, such as partial deletions, gains, and unbalanced translocations, have been reported to correlate with outcome measures in NB and may also better predict relapse.[3] Demonstration of segmental, unbalanced deletions of chromosomes 1p, 3p, and 11q and gains of 1q, 2p, and 17q have been reported as recurrent aberrations, but only recently have their prognostic implications begun to be elucidated.

Recently, microRNA (miRNAs) expression signature profile studies have distinguished favorable and unfavorable outcome groups in those NB with 11q LOH. miRNAs are small regulatory RNAs that bind to the noncoding 3′-untranslated region of mRNA. They negatively regulate the expression of protein coding genes on post-transcriptional level via several mechanisms, including translational repression of mRNA. As previously mentioned, studies have shown that unbalanced loss of 11q is an independent predictor of poor outcomes.[7] However, it was not known why some NBs with 11q deletion fare better than others. Buckley et al. have shown that miRNA expression profiling divides tumors with 11q loss into two groups, which differ by frequency of chromosomal imbalances and clinical outcome, suggesting that this miRNA expression signature can be used for patient prognostication. Several upregulated miRNAs in the prognostically unfavorable group were predicted to target a cluster of NB survival genes; however, these findings are not yet validated.[8] The unfavorable 11q LOH group also had increased segmental genomic imbalances including the concurrent loss of 3p, with additional loss identified at 4p and 14q, with gains of 7q, 2p, and 11p. Interestingly, however, gains of 17q were seen equally in both the favorable and unfavorable 11q LOH groups. Furthermore, others have noted 17q gains are not predictive of survival in those NB lacking *MYCN* amplification. These findings may suggest that while gains of 17q are one of the most prevalent chromosomal aberrations (50% to 80% of cases) in NB, it may not be a strong or an independent prognostic factor as 11q LOH.

Loss of 1p, in particular the region of band 1p36, has been demonstrated in 25% to 35% of NBs, associated with overall poor outcomes (event-free survival and overall survival), and is usually associated with *MYCN* amplification (Fig. 41.2). However, it has also been shown to be an independent prognostic marker, associated with poor outcomes even in those subgroups without *MYCN* amplification. Both 1p36 and unbalanced 11q LOH have emerged as independent predictors of poor outcomes, even in those low-risk and intermediate-risk disease groups.[7]

Others have noted that the high expression of TrkA, a high-affinity nerve growth factor receptor, from the family of nerve growth factor tyrosine kinase receptors induces terminal differentiation of sympathetic nervous system neuroblasts and is associated with good outcomes.[6] However, as mentioned above, TrkA expression is also reciprocally correlated with *MYCN* amplification. Therefore, its expression has not been adopted as a prognostic marker in clinical practice. Lastly, while the expression of the cell adhesion molecule CD44, which is lost in aggressive NB, has been associated with poor outcomes, it has also not been adopted into routine clinical practice as a marker for prognosis.

Many other markers of potential value in prognostication and staging of NBs have been studied, underscoring the extreme complexity of this group of neoplasms, which makes it very difficult to identify features for more generalized application.

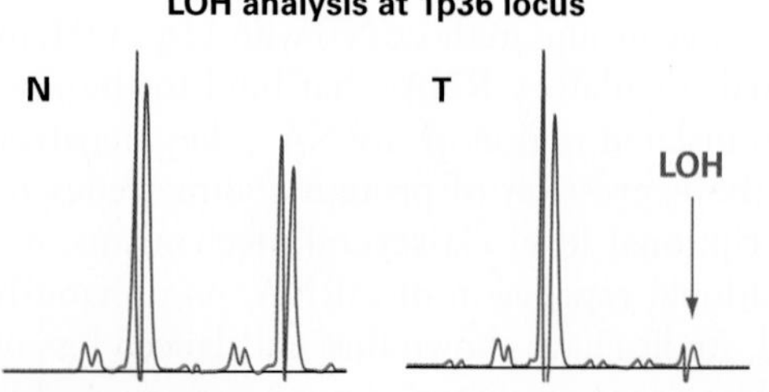

FIGURE 41–2 Loss of heterozygosity (LOH) analysis demonstrates deletion of the 1p36 chromosomal locus in tumor (T) tissue.

Ewing Sarcoma/Primitive Neuroectodermal Tumor

The Ewing family of tumors was one of the first groups of pediatric tumors to be defined by a signature translocation that includes ES, peripheral PNET, and the Askin tumor (a PNET of the chest wall). These tumors harbor a translocation that involves the fusion of the transcription factor domain of the Ewing sarcoma gene (EWS) at 22q12 to a partner belonging to the ETS family of DNA-binding domain genes, with *FLI1* at 11q24 being the most common (Fig. 41.3). This family of tumors is the second most common bone and soft tissue malignancy in adolescents and young adults, with a male predominance. Classic ES is more common in the diaphysis of long bones while PNET is seen at soft tissue sites.[9] The key histologic features of ES include a monomorphic population of densely packed sheets of cells with scant cytoplasm, alternating with lighter cells. The nuclei of light cells are round with evenly dispersed chromatin, while darker cells have slight nuclear contour irregularities with clumped chromatin (Fig. 41.4). A periodic acid–Schiff (PAS) stain often highlights the cytoplasm of tumor cells due to their glycogen content, which is best appreciated after alcohol fixation, or on cytologic preparations with a Diff-Quik stain. The histologic features of a PNET include plumper spindle cells and evidence of partial neural differentiation represented by Homer-Wright or Flexner-Wintersteiner rosettes. This family of tumors classically shows a strong and diffuse membranous expression of CD99 and is negative for CD43, CD45, and myogenin. Some examples may express low-molecular-weight keratins and neural markers, such as synaptophysin. Membranous CD99 and nuclear FLI1 IHC markers can be expressed in lymphomas; thus, a lymphoid marker is imperative in the IHC panel to rule out lymphoid origin.

While it has long been thought that this family of tumors is derived from a neural origin in which ES is at

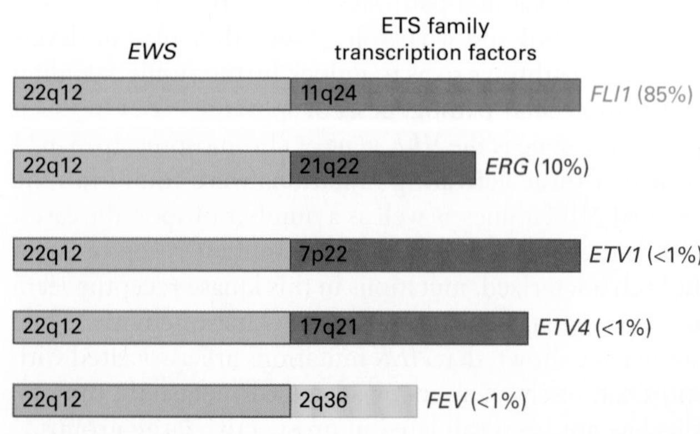

FIGURE 41–3 Schematic illustration of chromosomal alterations and aberrant gene products in Ewing sarcoma/primitive neuroectodermal tumor. *EWS*, Ewing sarcoma gene.

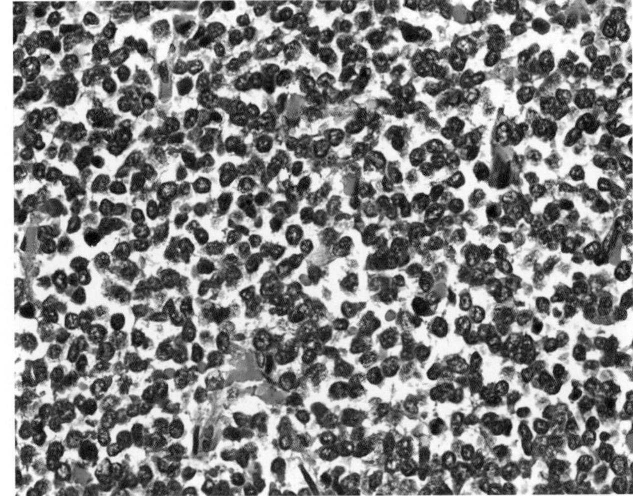

FIGURE 41–4 Ewing sarcoma composed of small, round, and poorly differentiated neoplastic elements (H&E, ×20).

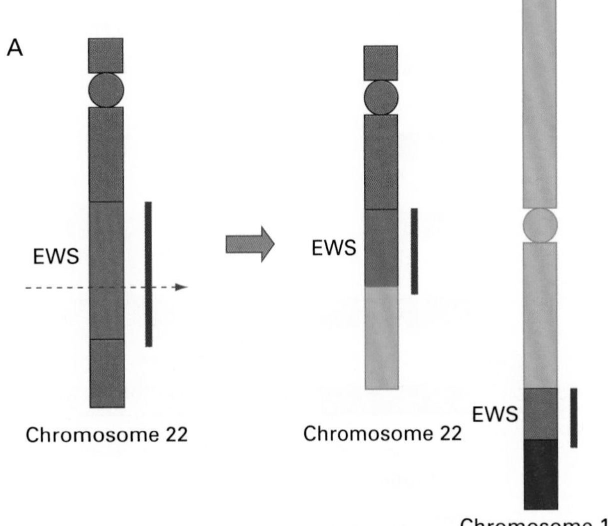

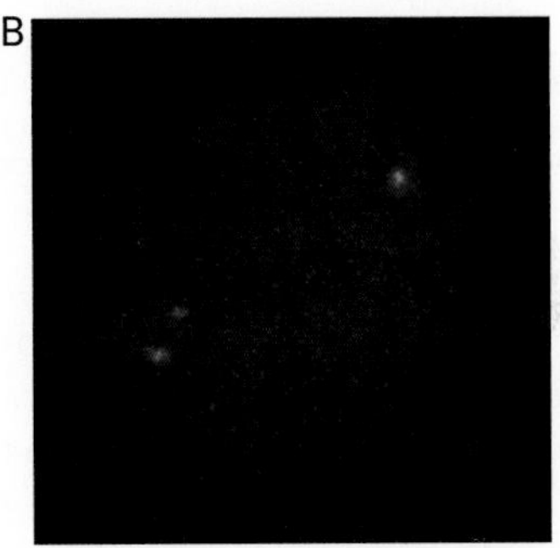

FIGURE 41–5 Fluorescence in situ hybridization for detection of chromosomal alterations in Ewing sarcoma. The break-apart design of the probe **(A)** allows to detect *EWS/FLI1* and other *EWS/PNET* translocations resulting in one green signal corresponding to the intact *EWS* gene and a pair of signals corresponding to the rearranged *EWS* gene **(B)**. In this design, the *EWS* translocation partner is unknown.

the more undifferentiated spectrum and PNET is more partially differentiated, more recent evidence has suggested that the cell of origin may arise from a subpopulation of bone marrow stromal cells, often loosely referred to in the literature as "mesenchymal stem cells."[10,11] However, the search for this cell of origin is complex and remains unfinished; it is possible that there is no "normal" counterpart of the ES cell but is rather the result of multiple molecular aberrations. In vitro studies have demonstrated that in non-transformed cells, introduction of the *EWS/FLI1* chimeric gene actually induces cell arrest without tumorigenesis, implying that other molecular alterations must occur either before or after the translocation to induce the oncogenic properties of these tumors.[11]

Molecular Diagnostics

While the ES/PNET family of tumors does share histological and immunophenotypical features with a variety of small round cell tumors, the molecular demonstration of the *EWS* gene translocation can both help provide a diagnosis in cases of scant or limited tissue and provide definite confirmation in other cases. The most prevalent partners with the *EWS* gene are *FLI1* at 11q24 which is seen in 85% of tumors and *ERG* at 21q22 in 10% of cases, while the remaining 5% of cases may have partners with *ETV1* (7p22), *ETV4* (17q21), or *FEV* (2q33).[9] Most often a single dual-color EWS break-apart probe spanning the known common breakpoints on chromosome 22 (introns 7 through 10) is used for the detection of EWS rearrangements (Fig. 41.5). Such design allows for the detection of all possible fusion transcripts with a small cost. Another method for detection of these rearrangements is real-time RT-PCR amplification (Fig. 41.6). This method is more labor intensive due to the presence of multiple splicing variants in a fusion transcript but it allows for precise identification of translocation partner. A number of other tumors harbor *EWS* rearrangements, including desmoplastic small round cell tumor with partner gene Wilms tumor 1 (*WT1*) at 11p13, clear cell sarcoma with partner gene *ATF1* at 12q13, extraskeletal myxoid chondrosarcoma with partner gene nuclear receptor subfamily 4, group A, member 3 (*NR4A3*) at 9q22, and rare variants of myxoid liposarcoma with partner gene *DDIT3* (previously *CHOP*) at 12q13; however, these tumors are often eliminated from the differential diagnosis based on adequate histology and immunophenotyping. In cases of diagnostic uncertainty, specific fusion probes or cytogenetic karyotyping is of utmost utility. ETS family of genes (*FLI1*, *ERG*, *ETV1*, *ETV4*, and *FEV*) are tissue-specific transcription factors, while the *EWS* gene belongs to the TET family of proteins, which are ubiquitously expressed in all cell types along with liposarcoma (*TLS*), Ewing sarcoma (*EWS*), and TATA-binding protein–associated factor 15 (*TAF15*) tumors. The TET proteins also control cell growth via various steps in gene transcription and/or RNA processing.

In most cases, diagnosing ES/PNET is fairly straightforward with a combination of histology, immunophenotyping, and demonstrating the *EWS* rearrangement.

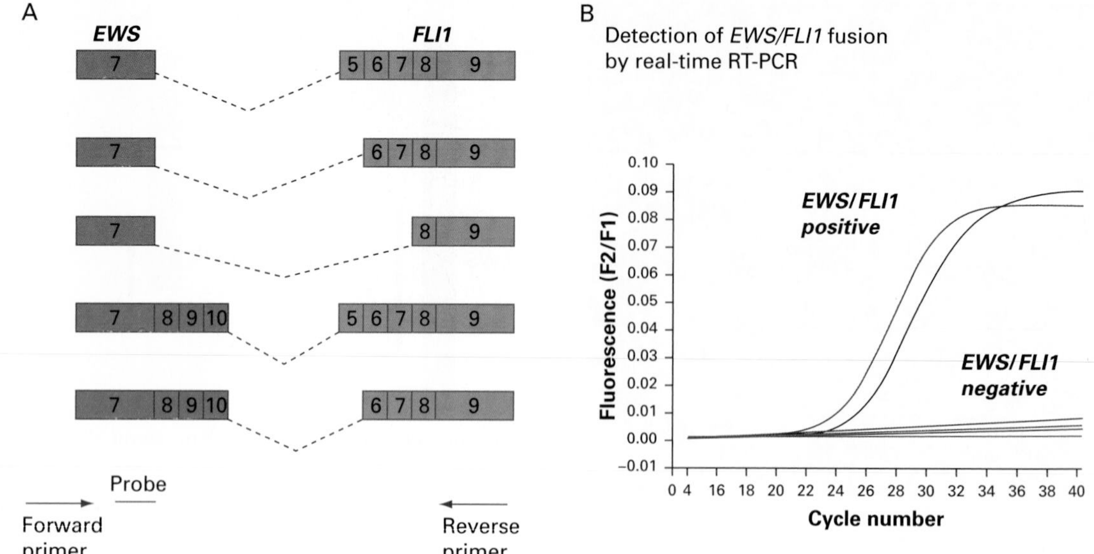

FIGURE 41–6 Detection of EWS/FLI1 translocation by real-time reverse-transcription polymerase chain reaction (RT-PCR) on ABI7500. **A:** In order to detect all splicing variants, forward primer and fluorescent probe are located in exon 7 of the *EWS* gene and reverse primer is located in exon 9 of the *FLI1* gene. **B:** Tumor samples positive for *EWS/FLI1* translocation show exponential increase in fluorescence during RT-PCR amplification and tumors negative for translocation show no amplification (flat lines on amplification plot).

Recently, new case reports identifying novel, variant genetic aberrations with and without EWS translocations have been demonstrated.[12-14] Four cases have been shown to have t(16;21)(p11;q22), *FUS/ERG* fusion transcript.[12] One case had a three-way translocation t(16;21;22)(p11;q22;p11.2), while the other cases only showed a balanced translocation t(16;21)(p11.2;q22.3).[13] Another case report demonstrated a novel t(2;16)(q35;p11) balanced translocation with the *FUS–FEV* fusion transcript.[14] Still others have demonstrated a novel t(2;22)(q31;q12), *EWS–SP3* fusion transcript. This chimeric mRNA encodes an in-frame transcript of the EWS amino-terminal domain fused to the zinc finger DNA-binding domain of SP3, which is devoid of its inhibitory domain.[13] These cases highlight the importance of a multiparameter approach for the diagnosis of non-classical cases, utilizing genome-wide studies to identify novel molecular events. In cases with molecular negative results despite appropriate clinical history, histology, and IHC findings, further investigation with *FUS* probes may be warranted. This also highlights the clinical utility of preserving fresh, sterile material for karyotypic studies, which can help orient the pathologist to these rare, novel molecular events, as was demonstrated in the above-quoted cases. Furthermore, with the advent of integrating genome-wide array comparative genomic hybridization chips to analyze copy number variants in combination with RNA expression array profiles, more robust data can be correlated with outcome survival data. Studies using these molecular tools have identified new copy number aberrations with gains of 1q, 2q, 8q, and 12 and losses at 9p and 16q in 20% of ES/PNET cases, along with identifying a novel translocation involving the *EWS* gene with a partner gene at 20q.[15]

Molecular Prognostics

Unfavorable prognosis in ES/PNET has traditionally been focused on clinical parameters, including the presence of metastasis (i.e., lung metastasis only in intermediate prognosis), location (i.e., axial vs. peripheral), ≥14 years of age, tumor size > 8 cm, viable gross tumor after chemotherapy, elevated serum lactate dehydrogenase, fever, and anemia. Recently, new molecular tools have provided additional risk stratification. The absence of a type 1 fusion (e.g., *EWS* [exon 7]/*FLI1* [exon 6]) was once thought to be an unfavorable prognostic factor; however, recent work by the COG showed similar 5-year event-free survival and overall survival rates for patients with type 1 and non–type 1 fusions diagnosed between 2001 and 2005.[16] On the other hand, Savola and colleagues have demonstrated that ES patients with >3 copy number changes had both worse cumulative event-free survival and overall survival compared with those with ≤3 copy number changes. They have also suggested that the gene of interest associated with poor prognosis in ES with del(16q) may be either *HEATR3* (16q12.1) or *ANKRD11* (16q24.3), as these genes appear to function as p53 co-activators, with deletions leading to loss of the normal regulatory feedback loop.[15] This supports previous work showing worse survival in those ES/PNETs with p53 homozygous deletions.[17]

Possible new therapeutic regimens in ES/PNET include targets of the *IGF/mTOR* signaling pathways. Recent work with miRNAs has shown that a group of miRNAs (miR-100, miR-125b, miR-22, miR-221/222, miR-27a, and miR-29a) are downregulated by *EWS/FLI1* chimeric mRNA. In a normal state, these miRNAs are thought to repress targets in the insulin-like growth factor

(IGF) signaling pathway preventing tumorigenesis.[18] Thus, these oncogenic IGF pathways in ES may serve as potential therapeutic targets with rapamycin.

SOFT TISSUE SARCOMAS

Rhabdomyosarcoma

Rhabdomyosarcoma (RMS) is the most prevalent soft tissue sarcoma of the pediatric population. There are two recognized subtypes that predominate in childhood, which include the embryonal (ERMS) and alveolar (ARMS) types (Figs. 41.7 and 41.8), while the pleomorphic type is more frequently diagnosed in the adult population. The RMS cell of origin is thought to be derived from a primitive mesenchymal cell with skeletal muscle lineage, having a variable amount of differentiating rhabdomyoblasts present in the tumor. The ERMS is more frequently seen in the head and neck, abdomen, and genitourinary sites. The botryoid and spindle cell subtypes (considered under the ERMS heading) are found with more frequency in the genitourinary tract/biliary tract and in the paratesticular/orbital sites, respectively, although they have been reported in many other locations. The ARMS is more frequently found within the soft tissues of the extremities and within parameningeal and paranasal sinuses but can occur at any site in the body. Younger age (<5 years) children usually present with ERMS (or botryoid subtypes), while those of older ages (>5 years) usually present with ARMS (and spindle cell subtypes). Recently, Jo et al have described a new morphological variant called epithelioid RMS with histologic and clinical parameters similar to poorly differentiated carcinoma or melanoma, mainly with an older median age of 70.5 years (range 14 to 78 years). It demonstrates sheets of epithelioid cells with large vesicular nuclei, prominent nucleoli, increased mitoses, and necrosis with infiltrative morphology.[19] The key histologic feature of RMS is evidence of rhabdomyoblastic differentiation, including ample eosinophilic cytoplasm and an eccentric large nucleus. ERMS typically displays a loose

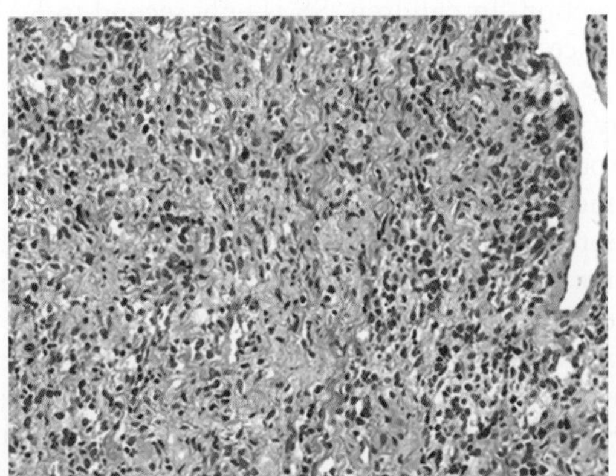

FIGURE 41–7 Embryonal rhabdomyosarcoma showing moderate cellularity of spindly elements, mild pleomorphism, and myxoid background (H&E, ×20).

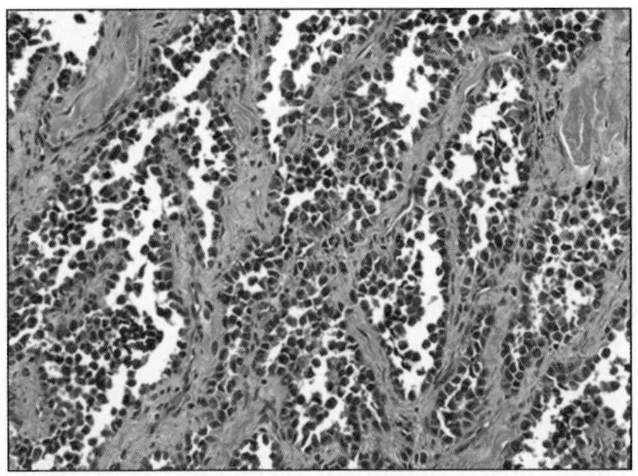

FIGURE 41–8 Alveolar rhabdomyosarcoma with characteristic septa lined by neoplastic elements with eosinophilic cytoplasm and hyperchromatic nuclei (H&E, ×20).

and cellular pattern of neoplastic elements surrounded by a myxoid background and has a more primitive mesenchymal appearance. The spindle cell subtype has interlacing bundles of elongated cells with fusiform nuclei and a cytoplasm containing PAS-positive glycogen; this subtype shares histologic overlapping features with fibrosarcoma and leiomyosarcoma. The botryoid subtype is characterized by macroscopic appearance of grape-like structures, which microscopically feature vaguely papillary clusters that have a condensed subepithelial cellular *cambium* layer. The classic ARMS subtype is highly vascular, with cellular nests or cystic spaces of small round blue cells loosely lining pseudoalveolar spaces formed by stromal septa to which the neoplastic cells are attached. A "solid alveolar" variant closely resembles lymphoma due to its compact and poorly differentiated microscopic appearance, and it requires IHC evidence of rhabdomyoblastic differentiation (myogenin, vide infra) for its precise diagnosis. The most useful set of IHC stains for RMS includes cytoplasmic desmin, muscle-specific actin, and the nuclear presence of the transcription markers myogenin and MyoD1. Furthermore, molecular analysis can differentiate between ARMS and other RMS types, especially important in cases without classic histologic patterns.

Molecular Diagnostics

Although no specific molecular alteration has been described for ERMS, some studies have found ERMS examples with LOH at the 11p15.5 locus, linked with the Beckwith-Wiedemann syndrome (BWS) and WAGR syndrome (both of which carry RMS predisposition), possibly related to abnormalities in the imprinted *IGF2* gene at this locus.[20] In contrast, ARMS is characterized by the fusion of the DNA-binding domain of the paired box *PAX* genes, *PAX3* at 2q35 or *PAX7* at 1p36, to the transcriptional activation domain of the forkhead homolog 1 RMS transcription factor (*FOX01A/FKHR)* at 13q14. The chimeric *PAX3/FKHR* mRNA transcript produces an oncogenic protein responsible for inducing a skeletal muscle genetic expression program through transcription factors such as myogenin, MyoD1, SIX1, and SLUG.[21] Recently, transgenic mice studies have shown that the oncogenic protein fusion arrests cells from completing myogenesis, since they cannot upregulate *p57/KIP2*, a cyclin cell cycle inhibitor.[22] It has been shown that about 55% of ARMS harbor the "unfavorable" t(2;13)(q35;q14), 22% harbor the t(1;13)(p36;q14), while the rest are so-called fusion-negative ARMSs. The *PAX3-FKHR* chimeric protein was shown to portend a worse outcome in patients presenting with metastatic disease but did not show a difference in those presenting with locoregional ARMS.[23] Furthermore, the significant portion of "fusion-negative" ARMS may cause a diagnostic challenge due to difficulties in confirming the typing as either fusion-negative ARMS or ERMS with ambiguous histology (i.e., solid alveolar or dense embryonal pattern). Previous work has shown that "fusion-negative" ARMS may only express the chimeric fusion in rare cells or, alternatively, these tumors may have novel chimeric fusions involving similar functional genes or have novel breakpoints in the fusion transcripts, which are not recognized by the standard RT-PCR primers or FISH probe sets. A smaller set of these fusion-negative tumors are considered truly negative without further explanation[24] and preliminary evidence has emerged to suggest that these ARMSs may have better prognosis, more similar to the outcomes for ERMS.[25] With differences in outcomes based on histologic subtype, continued improvement in accurate molecular diagnosis and confirmatory testing is needed to appropriately triage children into optimal treatment protocols to more accurately predict prognosis. Refined molecular testing to better classify these cases based on more encompassing molecular profiles, rather than a single molecular event, will be needed for the future.

Molecular Prognostics

The COG low-, intermediate-, and high-risk group stratification for RMS is based on the location of primary site (all sites are unfavorable except for orbit, head and neck, genitourinary, and biliary tract), histology (alveolar is a higher risk group than embryonal), tumor size (5 cm cutoff), lymph node involvement, distant metastasis, and clinical stage.[26] Further, risk stratification has shown that nodal disease, even regional lymph node metastasis (N1), predicts poor outcomes. Localized disease with N1 has more similar outcomes to distant metastatic disease compared with local disease without nodal disease (N0). In the Regional lymph node disease (RLND) N1 group, gene expression profiling has shown that mRNA transcripts related to immune-response genes as well as B-cell markers are overexpressed. While these findings have not yet been validated in a larger cohort, the poorer prognosis in the N1 group may be related to immune-response escape from tumor-mediated apoptosis.[27]

Previous studies on molecular prognostic markers suggested that the variant fusion protein with *PAX7* predicted better outcomes in metastatic ARMS compared with *PAX3* fusion.[23] More recently, it has been demonstrated that true fusion-negative alveolar subtypes may have better outcomes, more akin to ERMS, based both on similar clinical data and gene expression profiles in this group compared with the typical fusion-positive group[25]; however, there is no consensus agreed upon about these results and additional work is needed to confirm/validate the data.[28]

miRNAs have emerged as important molecular targets in a variety of pediatric tumors, and RMS is no exception. A group of miRNAs (miR-1, miR-133a, miR-133b, and miR-206) have been identified in modulating myogenesis by repressing translational mRNA expression of myogenin and myocyte enhancer factor-2 (MEF2) function, while also repressing non-muscle isoforms of both adenylate cyclase–associated protein (CAP1) and a non-muscle isoform of myosin (MYH9). When compared with normal skeletal muscle, ERMS and ARMS cell lines have demonstrated the downregulation of miR-1 and miR-133a and upregulation of their target genes.[29] Furthermore, transfection of the ERMS cell line with miR-1 and miR-133a showed growth suppression,[29] and introduction of miR-206 into xenografted mice promoted skeletal differentiation and blocked tumor growth.[30] The tumor suppressor action of these myogenic miRNAs appears to have selective potential in ERMS. However, further work is needed to validate these results, as miRNAs are recognized to have promiscuous mRNA binding and thus could have unrecognized mRNA targets at other organ sites with unforeseen downstream targets.[29] Careful optimism leads our progress from promising in vitro studies into clinical application in treating human tumors.

Synovial Sarcoma

Synovial sarcoma (SS) is a rare tumor, most common within the periarticular connective spaces of the distal lower extremity around the knee and less common in the upper extremity. SS is not limited to the joints and can be found in axial locations in 25% of cases (head–neck, trunk, lung-pleura, and retroperitoneum). These axial sites are often associated with worse outcomes, primarily from lower success rates in achieving complete surgical resection. In children, SS is only second to RMS in prevalence, with about 15% to 30% of SS cases occurring in those less than 20 years of age.[31] While it has a propensity to arise in the periarticular connective tissue of joint spaces, it is not derived from synovial cells, despite its name, and is rather thought to be derived from the pluripotential mesenchymal cells capable of partial or aberrant epithelial differentiation.[29] There are two major histologic subtypes of SS: a classic biphasic pattern with both glandular and uniform spindle cells whose nuclei are pale with finely granular chromatin, rare to absent mitotic figures, and inconspicuous cytoplasm; and a second, more common monophasic pattern, with a more spindled cell component and alternating light and dark areas imparted by variable cell density, often mimicking a malignant peripheral nerve sheath tumor (MPNST). Rarely, a pure poorly differentiated subtype, or calcifying/ossifying and myxoid subtypes, can be seen; however, these patterns are more commonly seen as foci within a monophasic or biphasic tumor.[32] IHC stains are diffusely positive for vimentin and epithelial membrane antigen (EMA) in the spindled component, while cytokeratins, especially CK7 and CK19, highlight the epithelioid cells and are positive in the spindle cells only in a smaller proportion of cases. Additionally, cytoplasmic CD99 and nuclear bcl2 are positive in SS. Not infrequently, SS can show S100 staining, which causes additional diagnostic confusion with MPNST. A recent nuclear marker overexpressed in SS is TLE1, a competitor with β-catenin causing repression of the Wnt signaling pathway via transcriptional repression of important downstream targets. TLE1 is expressed in both components of SS and appears to be a sensitive but not completely specific marker, as it is positive in a small fraction of solitary fibrous tumor/hemangiopericytomas (30%) and schwannomas (30%) with rare staining in MPNST (4.5%).[33] The diagnostic translocation t(X;18)(p11.2:q11.2) is seen in at least 90% of cases and has aided in the correct classification of these spindle cell sarcomas.

Molecular Diagnostics

The fusion transcript *SYT/SSX* results from a translocation of the 78 amino acids at the terminal carboxy end of the *SSX* gene at Xp11.2 to the carboxy terminal of the *SYT* (SS18) gene at 18q11.2, which replaces its last eight amino acids.[32,34] The exact pathogenesis of how the fusion transcript exerts its tumorigenic function is not completely worked out but is thought to be complexed with DNA-binding proteins to epigenetically signal downstream targets. *SS18* indirectly has a transcriptional coactivator function by forming complexes of DNA-binding proteins (i.e., AF10, SIN3A, and p300) with its N-terminal homology domain, after which it induces the SWI/hSNFa/hBRM complex to coactivate transcription via chromatin modification. The *SSX* chimera indirectly functions as a transcriptional corepressor after inducing the formation of a complex between DNA-binding LIM-homeobox protein and LHX4, to recruit chromatin modifiers and Polycomb group proteins.[35] The interesting paradox is that the chimeric transcript expresses both the activation (*SS18-QPGY*) and repression (*SSX-SSXRD*) domains. Examples of the dual translational activation–repression hypothesis include upregulation of the methylated-*IGF2* gene in SS, modification by histone methylation, and downregulation of the *CD44* gene, which is modified by the SWI/hSNFa complex and by DNA methylation.[35] The SSX family has nine genetic variants but only three are known to be involved in SS: *SSX1* is most frequent, followed by *SSX2*, with rare involvement by *SSX4*.[34] *SYT/SSX* translocation can be detected in tumor samples either by FISH or by RT-PCR (Fig. 41.9).[36] A novel translocation involving the *SS18L1* gene, a homolog of the *SS18* gene on chromosome 20, and the *SSX1* gene has been detected by classical cytogenetics and confirmed with FISH and RT-PCR.[37] While nearly all SSs demonstrate the *SS18/SSX* fusion transcript, those cases without the fusion transcript, but with distinct morphologic and IHC findings, may benefit from additional genome-wide studies to further explore variant translocations.

Molecular Prognostics

The traditional favorable prognostic factors in SS include low tumor grade, age younger than 15 years at the time of diagnosis, tumor size < 5 cm (which holds true in all pediatric sarcomas), and location in the distal extremity.[34] The significance of fusion transcript type has varying reproducibility in the literature as being an independent prognostic factor in SS. The largest multi-institutional, retrospective study with 238 fusion-positive cases, including adult and pediatric cases, demonstrated a better 5-year survival for those with localized disease at presentation that harbored the *SSX2* partner.[38] However, the significance of fusion type was lost in Cox regression modeling which only identified disease status at presentation (e.g., localized vs. metastasis) and primary tumor size as independent predictors of worse prognosis. Additional smaller studies have not been able to show the significance of fusion-type on prognosis.[39,40] Other molecular events described in the context of prognosis include evaluation of the family of cadherins, through which SS may function independently from the Wnt signaling pathway to promote tumorigenesis.[41] Saito and colleagues[41] showed that E-cadherin and α-cadherin protein expression was associated with better prognosis, whereas widespread aberrant expression of β-catenin (defined as >75% of cells with nuclear and/or cytoplasmic staining) had worse outcomes; however, only 8% of these cases showed a *CTNNB1* mutation by sequence analysis, which should not be too surprising since only nuclear β-catenin protein accumulation is associated with the *CTNNB1* mutation. However, Pretto and colleagues have shown that the *SYT/SSX2* fusion transcript protein recruits β-catenin to the nucleus and associates within it an active complex containing both *SYT/SSX2* and β-catenin, in a novel signaling pathway independent of the canonical Wnt pathway. The primary action of the 78-amino acid addition of *SSX2* to *SS18*, which results in a deletion of eight amino acids at the SS18 COOH terminus, is through SSX2 gain of function.[42] Further supporting evidence of the gain-of-function mutation was shown after depletion of *SYT/SSX2* in vitro in primary SS cells, which resulted in loss of previously demonstrated aberrant nuclear β-catenin expression and drop in the β-catenin signaling activity. Thus, in SS there may be a novel β-catenin pathway, independent of the Wnt signaling pathway that controls tumorigenesis in *SYT/SSX2* fusion-positive tumors.[43]

Alveolar Soft Part Sarcoma

Alveolar soft part sarcoma (ASPS) is a very rare tumor of uncertain lineage that is most often found in the lower

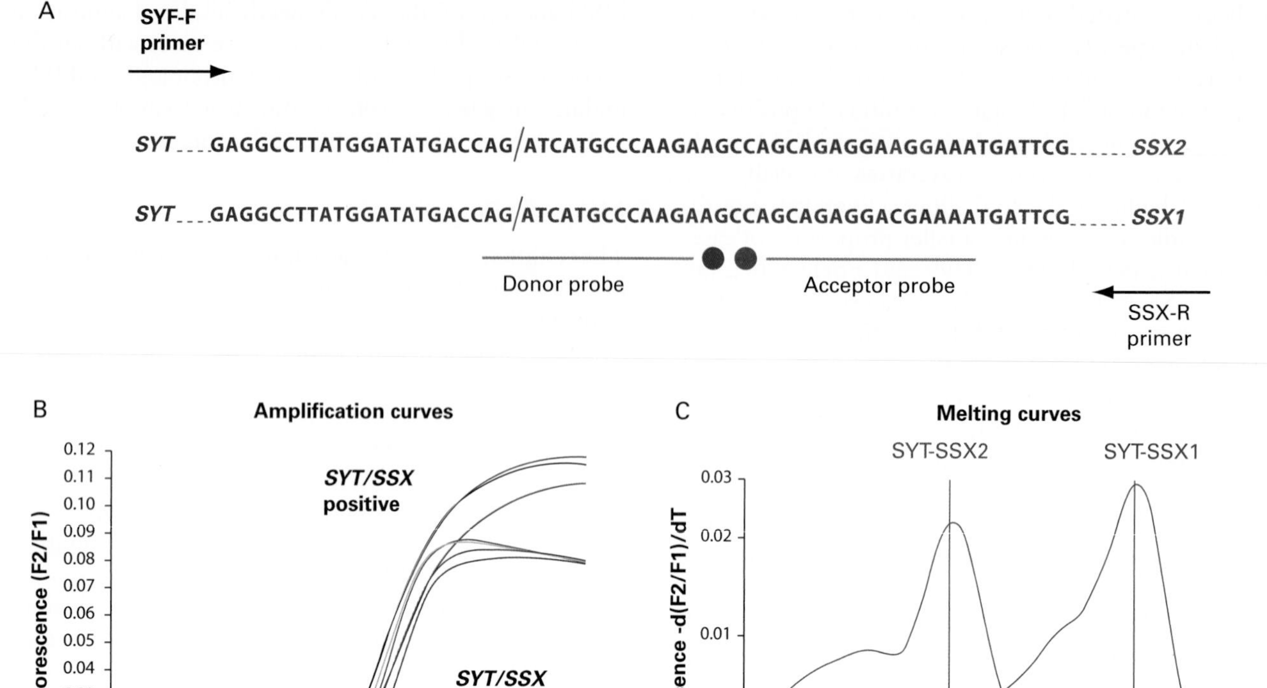

FIGURE 41–9 Detection of SYT/SSX translocation by real-time reverse-transcription polymerase chain reaction (RT-PCR). **A:** Design of real-time RT-PCR primers and probes for simultaneous detection of *SYT/SSX1* and *SYT/SSX2* rearrangements. **B:** LightCycler RT-PCR amplification of nine cases of synovial sarcoma, indicating the presence of *SYT/SSX* rearrangement. **C:** Post-PCR fluorescent melting curve analysis allows to determine the rearrangement type based on difference in melting temperatures.

extremities of adolescents and young adults, while typically more predominant in the head and neck, including the orbit and tongue, in younger children.[43] The key histological features include intermediate to large polygonal cells with a granular, eosinophilic cytoplasm, nested within surrounding fibrovascular septa that impart a pseudoalveolar pattern to the tumor. However, it has been reported that up to 40% of ASPS have variant nonalveolar patterns making histologic distinction difficult.[44] The cytoplasm is PAS and diastase resistant, and ultrastructural analysis shows cytoplasmic crystalloid rhomboid structures. In the COG non-rhabdomyosarcomatous pediatric sarcomas grading schema, ASPS is a grade 3 sarcoma. While the actuarial 5-year survival is often good (74%), most of these patients have poor long-term survival with frequent metastasis to the lung, brain, and bone.[45] The *ASPSCR1/TFE3* fusion transcript typically involves a nonreciprocal translocation der(17) t(X;17)(p11;q25), which has greatly aided the diagnostic confirmation of this tumor. In addition, immunohistochemistry for the nuclear transcription factor binding to immunoglobulin heavy constant-μ enhancer 3 (TFE) protein overexpression is a sensitive surrogate to FISH or RT-PCR (sensitivity, 97.5%; specificity, 99.6%).[46]

Molecular Diagnostics

The defining molecular fusion transcript *ASPSCR1/TFE3* is a result of the der(17)t(X;17)(p11;q25) nonreciprocal translocation. The typical ASPS type 1 chimeric fusion is a result of the duplicated ASPSCR at 17q25 in which the nitro-terminal constant portion of the gene fuses with the active site of the *TFE* gene at Xp11, which includes the basic helix-loop-helix domain and the leucine zipper domain (exons 6 through 10) (GenBank NM_006521).[45] More frequently, in pediatric translocation tumors, and less commonly in ASPS, a type 2 chimeric fusion occurs in which the break point at *TFE* includes the activation domain of exon 5 and results in a balanced translocation.[47] The *TFE3* gene, which is a member of the tripartite motif family, plays many roles in functional developmental pathways and is involved in pro-oncogenic cellular pathways. The *TFE3* has a DNA-binding site, while the *ASPSCR* domain functions as a transcription factor.[48] The chimeric transcript results in a transcriptional deregulation in the tumor and is seen in 88% to 100% of ASPS with equal diagnostic sensitivity using either FISH or RT-PCR techniques. It is thought that the few ASPS cases not reporting a translocation are likely due to poor quality RNA. The advantage of FISH techniques is that *TFE* break-apart probe can have further analytical functionality for translocation renal tumors, thus serving a dual cost-effective function in some laboratories.

Molecular Prognostics

Currently, there are no useful factors to predict which patient will have distant metastasis. Hoshino and colleagues[49] have demonstrated that a nested PCR assay was able to diagnose *ASPSCR/TFE3* fusion transcript in peripheral blood with an analytical sensitivity of 50 tumor cells/2 mL of blood in four patients with ASPS metastasis. Given the high metastatic rate in these tumors, this method may serve as an early prediction tool in monitoring patients before a metastasis is diagnostically visible; however, validation in a larger prospective cohort is needed. Lazar and colleagues have also found a unique set of angiogenesis-promoting genes (*Jag-1*, *Midkine*, and *Angiogenin*) using an RT-PCR and angiogenesis oligomicroarray in a small cohort confirmed with protein expression studies. The upregulation of these specific transcripts along with protein expression suggests that therapeutic targets targeting vasculogenesis in these tumors may play a role in modulating the metastatic potential of this tumor.[45] Recently, an in vivo mouse model of ASPS has shown that targeting vascular endothelial growth factor (VEGF) and hypoxia inducible factor-1 alpha using therapeutic modalities (i.e., bevacizumab and topotecan) showed a 70% growth delay and an effective 0.7 net log tumor cell death. This is a novel pre-clinical animal model for ASPS that has potential therapeutic value, utilizing antiangiogenic therapies in this highly vascular and metastatic tumor.[50] A few case reports have shown promise with VEGF receptor inhibitors (cediranib and bevacizumab) in metastatic ASPS; however, only one case was in a child[51,52] and no further published studies have demonstrated experience with long-term outcomes. The limiting issue in ASPS is that it is a rare tumor and thus collecting enough cases to do meaningful prospective studies is difficult, with a dependence on animal models and retrospective samples.

LIVER TUMORS

Mesenchymal Hamartoma of the Liver

Mesenchymal hamartoma of the liver (MHL), second only to hemangiomas, is the most common benign hepatic tumor occurring in children, albeit with a very low overall prevalence. More than 85% of such cases are discovered in the first 3 years of life, most commonly in the right lobe.[53] While once thought to be a developmental lesion derived from a ductal plate malformation, hence its name, increasing evidence, including demonstration of recurrent cytogenetic abnormalities, supports its neoplastic nature.[54] The cell of origin remains elusive in MHL. The key histologic features show poorly developed biliary structures and islands of normal hepatocytes within a mesenchymal stroma of loose connective tissue, dilated blood, and lymphatic vessels. IHC stains are nonspecific and highlight the various components. Secondary cystic degeneration can be seen in cases with rapid enlargement. A handful of case reports suggest the possibility of a pathogenic continuum between MHL and an undifferentiated embryonal sarcoma (UES, vide infra) with the potential link being the common chromosomal breakpoint at 19q13.4, which has been shown in an increasing number of case reports (Table 41-3).[55-59]

Molecular Diagnostics

While most cases are diagnosed by the combination of appropriate clinical presentation and histological findings, an increasing number of reports have demonstrated recurrent cytogenetic abnormalities in MHL, specifically involving aberrations to the long arm of chromosome 19, and have further supported its nature as a bona fide neoplasm. Table 41.3 lists the case reports that have described changes involving the 19q13.3 or 19q13.4 breakpoints in MHL[57,60-67] and those cases of UES arising from MHL.[55,58,59] The candidate gene at 11q13 was identified as the metastasis-associated lung adenocarcinoma transcript 1 gene (*MALAT1*) and the breakpoint at 19q13.3-13.4 was identified as the mesenchymal hamartoma of the liver breakpoint1 (*MHLB1*) by the Rajaram et al. group in 2007.[59] While the *MALAT1* gene has been implicated in other neoplasms, including renal cell carcinoma (RCC), the *MHLB1* locus has not been previously described in other human tumors. There are currently no know genes in this highly conserved region, but several human expressed sequence tags (ESTs) map to this locus. The 19q13.3-13.4 breakpoint occurs within a coding region that shares homologous sequences between several mammalian species, including regions that are highly homologous to *NFX2* or *NFX3*, members of the nuclear RNA export factor (NXF) gene family, suggesting that this novel locus contains a conserved coding region.[59]

Other genes around the chromosome 19 locus include those encoding for DNA repair enzymes, kallikrein enzymes (trypsin-like serine proteases), imprinted genes, and the immunoglobulin family of transmembrane molecules.[53] While there have been case reports linking aberrations at 19q13 to UES arising in an MHL,[56,58,59] others have not shown such a relationship.[68] However, in most cases of MHL/UES progression, complex karyotypes with hyperdiploidy were observed (Table 41.3), suggesting that there is an accumulation of cytogenetic changes that take place, in which the aberration at 19q13 may be but just one change. Further confounding most of the UES + MLH cases in the literature is that few studies state which histology type (i.e., MLH, UES, and transition between) was taken for classical cytogenetic karyotyping and thus it is difficult to explicitly conclude if there is a definite clonal progression.

Molecular Prognostics

Most outcome reports suggest that MHL is a benign tumor with excellent outcomes, with some cases even featuring spontaneous regression. There is a known risk of

TABLE 41-3 Chromosomal Translocation in Mesenchymal Hamartomas and Undifferentiated Embryonal Sarcoma of the Liver

First Author (Year)	Age (Months)	Tumor	Karyotype
Speleman (1989)	36	MHL	45,XY,t(15;19)(q15;q13.4),-21
Mascarello (1992)	6	MHL	46,XY,t(11;19)(q13;q13.4)
Bove (1998)	24	MHL	46,XX,t(11;19)(q13;q13.4)
Murthi (2003)	14	MHL	46,XY,t(11;17;19)(q12;p11;q13.3)
Rakheja (2004)	8	MHL	46,XY,t(11;19)(q13;q13.4), 22ps+c
Sharif (2006)	12	MHL	46, XX,t(11,19)(q13,q13.3)
Talmon (2006)	10	MHL	46,XX,del(19)(q13.1q13.4)
Sugito (2010)	35	MHL	46,XX,t(11;19)(q13;q13.4)
Shetty (2011)	20	MHL	46,XX,inv(19)(p13q13.4)
Sawyer (1996)	72	UES	43-53,XY,-Y[2],complex karyotype involving **del(19)(p13.1)**[6]
O'Sullivan (2001)	36	UES (<5%) arising from MHL	46,XY,t(11;19)(q11;q13.3/13.4)
Rajaram (2007)	NA	UES arising from MHL	t(11;19)(q11;q13.4) FISH and DNA sequencing; no classical cytogenetics performed
Lauwers (1997)	180	UES arising from MHL	51-55, XX, complex karyotype involving del(11)(p13)×2, add(19)(q13)

MHL, mesenchymal hamartomas; UES, undifferentiated embryonal sarcoma; FISH, fluorescence in situ hybridization.

local recurrence with incomplete excision, and a still controversial risk of concurrent or progression to an UES, with 5 of 11 cases of UES showing progression from initial MHL.[53] There is also a slightly increased risk of MHL in those with placental mesenchymal dysplasia, thought to be a result of genetic imprinting dysregulation, including androgenetic-biparental mosaicism and association with BWS.[54] The paternally expressed 3 gene (*PEG3*) maps to the 19q13 locus and could serve as a potential genetic target for future studies.[54,67] At the current time, there are no definite molecular prognostic factors.

Hepatoblastoma

Hepatoblastoma (HB) is the most recognized pediatric liver malignancy but represents only about 1% of all tumors of children. It is predominantly a tumor of early childhood, with the vast majority occurring under 5 years of age. They are classified as epithelial, mixed epithelial, and mesenchymal with or without heterologous elements. The accepted cell of origin is a primitive hepatocyte, and the identified patterns of this tumor (i.e., fetal, embryonal, and small cell) reflect stages of hepatic development/differentiation. A pure epithelial fetal type (well-differentiated cords of fetal-appearing hepatocytes and low mitotic index) is a favorable histologic pattern, while the embryonal type (resembling hepatocytes at 6 to 8 weeks of gestation) is the most common pattern. The small cell undifferentiated epithelial subtype is the most primitive pattern and can have anaplastic cytology often with rhabdoid-type cells. Often there is a mixture of epithelial and mesenchymal patterns that may contain variable amounts of osteoid, chondroid, muscle, adipose, or primitive spindle cell components, which share an IHC staining pattern similar to the HB epithelial component, thus helping to differentiate it from the chemotherapy-induced secondary mesenchyme differentiation. A final histologic type is called "teratoid," or HB with heterologous elements and contain neural-melanocytic components. A number of genetic syndromes are associated with an increased risk of HB. They include familial adenomatous polyposis coli syndrome (*APC* gene; 5q21.2), BWS (*WT2* gene; 11p15.5), Li-Fraumeni syndrome (*TP53* gene; 17p13), trisomy 18, Simpson-Golabi-Behmel syndrome (*glypican 3* gene; Xq26), along with other syndromes without defined chromosomal abnormalities (e.g., glycogen storage diseases I–IV and hemihypertrophy). Laboratory testing, especially an increased level of α-fetal protein (AFP), helps in diagnosis, except for its near absence in the small cell undifferentiated HB pattern, a histologic challenge that must be differentiated from other pediatric small round blue cell tumors. In addition, exceptional cases of MHL have been reported with significant elevations of AFP.[69]

Molecular Diagnostics

A large study of over 100 HBs with classical cytogenetics has shown that half are associated with karyotypic aberrations, most commonly demonstrating at least one copy number variant, in which trisomies 2, 8, and 20 and gains in Xp and Xq are among the most prevalent. Other common molecular events are structural chromosomal changes, including a translocation t(1;4)(q12;q33-35) in seven cases.[70,71] Further work with mRNA gene expression profiles has shown a number of signaling pathways important for cellular growth, including those upregulated in HB samples when compared with normal fetal liver (i.e., Wnt signaling pathways, cyclin D1 cell cycle control, TGF β, *PPAR* signaling, and extracellular matrix–receptor interaction pathways), while other pathways are downregulated (i.e., pathways involved in cellular apoptosis).[70] Mutations involving the canonical Wnt/β-catenin pathway have been known to play a significant role in tumorigenesis and are found in the majority of syndromic FAP and sporadic HB.[72] In sporadic HB, *CTNNB1* mutations are within the phosphorylation sites of serine/threonine residues of exon 3, which are critical for normal APC degradation. Thus, β-catenin accumulates within the cytosol as it is resistant to the APC protein complex (e.g., the complex of the adenomatous polyposis coli protein, axin, WTX, and glycogen synthase kinase-3β)–mediated degradation. The cytosolic excess results in translocation to the nucleus, which in turn leads to upregulation of the downstream genes, including cyclin D1, an antiapoptotic cell cycle gene, and *MYCC*, an oncogenic target gene leading to tumorigenesis.[73,74] In FAP-associated syndromic HB, 5q21 mutations of the *APC* gene results in functional loss of the adenomatous polyposis coli protein with a similar outcome of increased cytosolic β-catenin accumulation and subsequent increased nuclear expression with activation of downstream Wnt canonical pathway target genes. Mutations in the 5′-region of the APC gene are most common, but various rearrangements including a novel mutation at the 3′-end have also been described in an FAP kindred.[75] Glypican-3 (*GPC3*) at Xq26.1 is a membrane-bound heparan sulfate proteoglycan that can negatively regulate the Wnt and Hedgehog signaling pathways in both HB and Wilms tumors (WTs). *GPC3* can also bind to *IGF2* promoting cell growth. The *IGF2*, *p57/KIP2*, and *H19* genes, all found at 11p15.5, have been found to have aberrant mRNA expression profiles in HB, which may explain the increased risk of HB in BWS. Furthermore, gene expression analysis has revealed molecular signatures that better characterize the histological subtypes of HB (differentiated/fetal, proliferative/embryonal, and undifferentiated/small cell) that may provide future prognostic and diagnostic markers as well as therapeutic targets for these tumors. For example, in those examples with more aggressive histology (not fetal histology), the gene expression profile showed greater Wnt or *MAPK* signaling pathway deregulation and preferentially upregulated antiapoptotic signaling pathways when compared with the more differentiated/fetal HB types.[70] Significant upregulation of *MAPK* signaling pathway genes was demonstrated in epithelial tumors with small cell component when compared with those with pure-fetal histology. Others have shown that the relative expression of Wnt activation signaling (i.e., highest expression in embryonal and mixed cell types) compared with NOTCH pathway activation through expression of *DLK1*, a bipotential oval cell marker (i.e., highest in fetal cell type), may further define a molecular signature that better stratifies the different histologic subtypes.[76]

Molecular Prognostics

Unfavorable prognostic factors in HB include stage of the tumor, multilobular involvement, multifocal growth pattern, and undifferentiated small cell pattern. In addition, various genetic markers that appear to be significant for unfavorable outcomes include aneuploidy, with gains of 8q and 20, nuclear overexpression of β-catenin protein, high cyclin D1, *PLK1* oncogene and telomerase expression, along with low nuclear *p57/KIP2* expression. However, to date these molecular factors are based on numerous small retrospective series and have not yet been used in prospective clinical trials collectively to predict outcome measures on a large number of patients.[77] Newer gene expression mRNA profiles using formalin-fixed paraffin-embedded tissue on a cDNA-mediated annealing, selection, extension, and ligation (DASL) chip assay have shown a number of new potential targets that could also serve as both prognostic markers and potential therapeutic aims for future research. One such marker discovered from DASL gene expression assay is Ying-yang 1 (*YY1*), a transcription factor located at 14q32, whose normal function in tissues is to bind various cell cycle pathway factors to promote synthesis and proliferation (i.e., p53 degradation, MDM2, and cyclin D), while interacting with apoptosis-related factors to prevent cell death (i.e., *MYCN*, *BIRC5*, NF-kB, Fas, and DR5).[78] In gene expression studies, *YY1* and *IGF1* mRNA were upregulated when compared with normal liver and were associated with poor prognostic factors, including recurrence and metastasis, thus serving as an attractive target to predict behavior. Unfortunately, these results need to be validated in prospective studies, as Shin et al.[79] were only able to correlate *YY1* protein expression with poorly differentiated histologic features and not with overall prognosis, and analysis of protein expression for *IGF1* was not performed to validate the mRNA data to poor outcomes. Finally, it seems that altered miRNA expression may serve a central role in the development of HB and offer new prognostic and therapeutic markers, as seen in other pediatric malignancies, by altering the expression of genes involved in many of the above-mentioned cellular pathways along with helping to discover new pathways that may regulate these tumors.[80]

RENAL TUMORS

Nephroblastoma (Wilms Tumor)

Commonly known by the eponym WT, nephroblastoma is an embryonic malignancy thought to be derived from transformed clonal renal stem cells, which remain in their embryonic multipotent state. The exact initiating cellular event is still under investigation.[81] Nephroblastoma is the most common renal cell malignancy in children, with the vast majority (95% to 98% of cases) occurring in those under 10 years of age with a slight female predominance.[82] It rates among the top 10 of all pediatric malignancies and fourth among childhood cancers. The key histologic

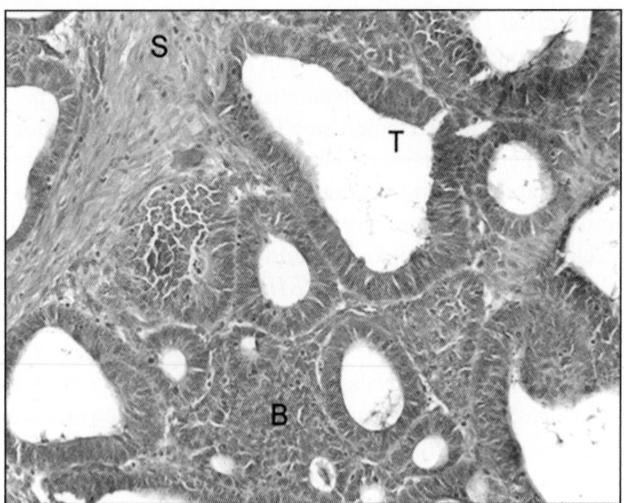

FIGURE 41–10 Triphasic (classic) Wilms tumor showing several neoplastic tubules (T); blastema, the round cell tumor component (B); and neoplastic stroma (S) composed of spindle elements (H&E, ×20).

features classically include a triphasic pattern of epithelial (immature tubular differentiation), stromal (renal interstitial/stromal counterpart with occasional heterologous elements), and undifferentiated blastema (metanephric mesenchymal counterpart) components (Fig. 41.10). The blastema cells represent the "small blue cell" component of nephroblastoma and create diagnostic confusion with other pediatric tumors when it represents the only component. The cells are round to oval with scant cytoplasm, fine chromatin, and overlapping nuclei with small to inconspicuous nuclei. There are multiple blastema-only growth patterns, including the most common and specific ones: nodular/serpentine pattern, invasive diffuse pattern, and basaloid. Most nephroblastomas are considered to have "favorable histology" with good outcomes. Conversely, poor outcomes associated with unfavorable histology are reserved for those cases with anaplastic cytologic features that include hyperchromatic/aneuploid nucleomegaly, with nuclei at least three times the size of adjacent non-anaplastic nuclei, and atypical mitoses (e.g., multipolar, clearly aneuploid mitotic figures). These cases represent about 5% of all WT cases, which are more frequent in children 5 years of age and older, as well as in patients of African American ethnicity. The utility of immunohistochemistry in nephroblastoma is limited, as the various diagnostic components are readily identifiable by hematoxylin and eosin staining. One useful nuclear stain expressed in blastema and often also in the epithelial components is the *WT1* marker, which is also expressed in desmoplastic small round cell tumor.

While the majority of sporadic and syndromic cases present as unilateral renal masses at diagnosis, bilateral nephroblastomas should prompt an investigation for a nephroblastoma predisposition syndrome. Syndromes with the highest risk of nephroblastoma include BWS (hemihypertrophy, macroglossia, omphalocele, and organomegaly) with associated mutation of the *WT2* gene at 11p15.5; WAGR (WT, aniridia, genitourinary malformation, and mental retardation) and Denys-Drash (mesangial sclerosis and 46XY ambiguous external male phenotype), both associated with chromosomal aberrations at *WT1* gene at 11p13; and familial nephroblastoma associated with mutations at either *FWT1/WT4* at 17q12-21 or *FWT2* at 19q13.3-13.4. Other syndromes with a higher nephroblastoma risk include Frasier syndrome (*WT1*, 11p13: similar spectrum to Denys-Drash, with only one abnormal *WT1* allele which cannot produce the +KTS isoform), Simpson-Golabi-Behmel syndrome (*GPC3*, Xq26: overgrowth, coarse facies, congenital heart defects, and other congenital abnormalities), and Sotos' syndrome (*NSD1*, 5q35: an overgrowth disorder with overlapping features with BWS).[82]

Molecular Diagnostics

While it has been recognized that the triphasic pattern of growth is most likely derived from an early progenitor cell, the exact WT "cell of origin" has remained elusive. Genomic array studies using unsupervised clustering of gene expression have revealed many common associations between nephroblastoma and normal fetal kidney at about 8 weeks of gestation.[83] These gene clusters include normal nephron progenitor genes (e.g., *PAX2*, *WT1*, *LIM1*, *EYA1*, *SIX1*, and *SIX2*), Wnt/β-catenin signaling pathway genes (e.g., *FZD7*, *FZD2*, and *CTNNBIP1*-β-catenin at 3p22.1), along with several imprinted genes (*IGF2*, *H19*, and *LIT1*) and genes of the Polycomb group (*EZH2* and *BMI-1*). The Wnt/β-catenin and Polycomb group genes are integral in maintaining stem cell pluripotency and plasticity during normal epithelial induction and development.[81]

Mutations in *WT1* gene at chromosome 11p13, a zinc finger transcription factor integral in genitourinary (e.g., ureteric branching and survival of the metanephric mesenchyme) and mesothelial development, are usually a nonsense mutation type, which leads to truncation and results in transcripts of different sizes. Tumors with *WT1* mutations also appear to have a stromal predominant histology.[84] The majority of syndromic cases harbor a *WT1* mutation, but only a fraction of sporadic nephroblastomas (5% to 33%) demonstrate a *WT1* mutation. The Denys-Drash syndrome shows a germline inactivating *WT1* point mutation of one allele and loss of the other normal allele in the tumor. The WAGR syndrome demonstrates a constitutional 11p13 deletion, most notably in the middle part of the band that affects several genes within this locus, thus resulting in a collection of defects. Germline aberrations of *WT2* gene in BWS are complex and involve deletions, translocations, duplications, and hypermethylation of the imprinted genes in the 11p15 locus, including p57 (*KIP2*), *CDKN1C*, *H19*, and *LIT*. Sporadic nephroblastomas with *WT2* alterations show somatic homozygosity in the tumor with either maternal allelic loss and subsequent paternal uniparental disomy or hypermethylation at the *H19* differentially methylated region (OMIM ID #19407). Mutations in the WT family of genes have been noted in sporadic cases, which include *WT3* at 16q, *WT4* at 17q12-21, and *WT5* at 7p11.2-15. The glypican-3 gene (*GPC3*) at Xq26, which negatively regulates signaling of Wnt and Hedgehog pathways as a tumor suppressor, is also associated with the Simpson-Golabi-Behmel syndrome. In one series, about a third of sporadic cases demonstrated an inactivating "single-hit" somatic mutation in the *WTX* gene at Xq11.1, which regulates the *Wnt*/β-catenin pathway as a tumor suppressor involved in the protein complex with the APC protein, axin, and glycogen synthase kinase-3β.[85] Interestingly, however, cases of germline *WTX* mutations in *osteopathia striata congenita* with hyperostosis and craniofacial malformations do not have a documented predisposition to nephroblastoma.[86]

Molecular Prognostics

Previously, prognostic factors in nephroblastoma were related to age, clinical stage, and unfavorable histology; however, LOH at 1p and 16q is now included in the risk stratification, as they are both associated with poor outcomes in favorable histology nephroblastomas, regardless of stage.[87] Stages 1 and 2 with 1p and 16q LOH are now considered standard risk while stage 3 with LOH is now high risk.[88] The area of 16q deletion in nephroblastoma appears to be preferentially lost within the blastema and/or anaplastic elements and was recently mapped to a 1.8 Mb area that contains the *IRXB* gene cluster, of which the *IRX3* gene has been identified as a target for tubular maturation during nephrogenesis.[89] Additionally, *WT1* mutation and 11p15 LOH in those children with very low risk Wilms tumor (VLRWT), defined by age less than 24 months, tumor weight less than 550 g, and stage 1, were found to have higher rates of disease relapse when treated with surgery alone. Further work has shown that this subgroup of VLRWT defined by molecular alterations benefit from more aggressive therapy. Those children with VLRWT but with constitutional *WT1* mutations who were treated with chemotherapy shared similar outcomes as compared with those VLRWT without mutations who are treated by surgery alone.[90]

Renal Cell Carcinoma

Non-WTs account for approximately 15% of childhood renal tumors and include mesoblastic nephroma, RCC, rhabdoid tumor (RT), and clear cell sarcoma. Mesoblastic nephroma, given its morphological and genetic features, is discussed under infantile fibrosarcoma (vide infra).

Pediatric RCCs are rare (2%) and mostly comprise translocation-associated tumors. These tumors are most common in older adolescents but can occur in the pediatric age group.[91] A handful of translocation RCCs in adults have been noted to have a more aggressive course compared with their pediatric counterpart.[92] These tumors have key histologic features, including voluminous clear to eosinophilic cytoplasm with prominent nucleoli (Fuhrman grade 3 typically), arranged in tubules, nests, acini, or papillae. Unlike papillary and clear cell RCC, translocation RCCs lack cytokeratin expression and almost universally express *TFE3* as a nuclear IHC stain. The transcription factor gene (*TFE*3) located at Xp11.2 is involved in the translocation with either the *ASPSCR1* gene at 17q25 or the *PRCC* gene at 1q21.

Molecular Diagnostics

The TFE family of genes in translocation-associated RCC are members of the microphthalmia-associated transcription factor (MiTF/TFE) family, which includes *MiTF*, *TFE3*, *TFEB*, and *TFEC*. *TFE3* is more frequently involved in both the *ASPSCR1–TFE3* fusion from the t(X;17)(p11.2;q25) and the *PRCC–TFE3* fusion from the t(X;1)(p11.2;q21), while fewer cases emerge involving the *Alpha/TFEB* fusion transcript from the t(6;11)(p21;q12). The t(X;17) is the same translocation involved in ASPS; however, translocation-associated RCCs feature a balanced translocation, while the ASPS translocation is unbalanced.[93] The breakpoint of the *TFE3* gene is at its amino terminal where *ASPSCR1* gene is fused, with retention of the *TFE3* transcription factor–binding domain, along with both the activation and nuclear localization domains. The resultant fusion transcript overexpresses *TFE3*, which allows binding to and autophosphorylation of the MET promoter with downstream activation of hepatocyte growth factor.[92]

The IHC stain for TFE3 is the most specific marker, with strong nuclear expression in tumors with the fusion transcript, without appreciable background staining of the normal TFE3. However, suboptimal fixation of tissue may result in high background staining of the native TFE3.[94] Additionally, expression of cathepsin-K is also another potential diagnostic marker, which is involved in overexpression of MiTF in osteoclasts. The sensitivity of cathepsin-K in translocation-associated tumors was demonstrated to be slightly lower than that of TFE3 with equal specificity.[94] The other member of the TFE family of transcription factors, *TFEB*, involved in the *Alpha-TFEB* fusion transcript induces lysosomal biogenesis with increased degradation of complex molecules, such as glycosaminoglycans, which may help these tumors in their clonal survival and proliferation.[93] The *PRCC/TFE3* fusion transcript binds the MET promoter and can also bind promoters in the MiTF pathway for melanocytic differentiation, as demonstrated by the melanocytic IHC marker expression in the TFB translocation-associated tumors.[92] The *Alpha/TFEB* fusion transcript also binds the MET promoter and can additionally bind promoters in the MiTF pathway for melanocytic differentiation, as demonstrated by the HMB-45 staining in the TFB translocation–associated tumors but not TFE3 tumors.[92] The FISH break-apart probe spanning the region of the *TFE* genes can be used for confirmation after positive IHC staining, in which two signals will be demonstrated from the TFE break-apart probe.

Molecular Prognostics

RCC in children generally has a mean 10-year survival prognosis of about 70%. While most outcome studies have documented a significant proportion of cases that present with lymph node metastasis at diagnosis (33% to 50%), some show a good prognosis despite lymph node metastasis while others report poor outcomes regardless of stage. This discrepancy may be a result of the differing follow-up times since these tumors have a propensity for long-term recurrences.[91] To date, there are no meaningful prognostic molecular marker for translocation-associated tumors; however, the MET tyrosine kinase is an attractive therapeutic target. In vitro growth restriction was demonstrated in an *ASPSCR1/TFE3* cell line subjected to selective inhibitor of the MET tyrosine kinase or miRNA-mediated knockdown of MET in vitro.[95]

Clear Cell Sarcoma

Clear cell sarcoma of the kidney (CCSK) accounts for less than 5% of primary pediatric renal tumors and is believed to be derived from a clonal undifferentiated mesenchymal cell.[96] Most patients are diagnosed between 1 and 2 years of age and with a male predominance. The key histologic features include sheaths, nests, and cords of 6 to 10 cells thick separated by a fine fibrovascular meshwork. The proliferating cells have inconspicuous cytoplasm whose vacuolization imparts to them the appearance of being separated by clear spaces; nuclei are small and feature finely dispersed chromatin.

Molecular Diagnostics

Cytogenetic studies of CCSK have reported three cases with balanced translocations involving t(10;17)(q22;p13) and t(10;17)(q11;p12). The genetic and molecular events resulting from these translocations remain elusive, as does their correlation with clinicopathologic parameters. Although the chromosome 17p13 breakpoint was thought to affect the tumor suppressor gene *TP53*, p53 abnormalities are rarely present in these tumors, and other genes are likely involved in their pathogenesis.[97] Gene expression profiling studies have helped narrow the candidate cell of origin in CCSK to a family of upregulated genes associated with neural differentiation, development, and function within both the Sonic hedgehog (Shh) and the phosphoinositide-3-kinase/Akt cell proliferation pathways.[98]

Molecular Prognostics

The overall 10-year survival for CCSK of 79% is slightly better than that of pediatric RCC of 70% and significantly better than renal malignant rhabdoid tumors of 29% (vide infra).[99] To date, there have been no specific molecular markers to predict prognosis in CCSK, but gene expression profiles have identified *EGFR*, *KIT*, and *PDGFRa* as unregulated genes that may serve as potential therapeutic targets in the future.

Rhabdoid Tumor

RTs are highly aggressive, high-stage malignancies seen as primary tumors in the preferred sites of the kidney, CNS, and soft tissues of young children, with a median age at presentation of 8 to 17 months. RTs may constitute only about 2% of pediatric renal tumors but are important to histologically distinguish from other renal neoplasms because of their universal dismal prognosis. The accepted cell of origin is an undifferentiated cell that demonstrates both neuroepithelial and mesenchymal markers. The key histologic features include a monomorphous population of discohesive cells with eosinophilic cytoplasm and a large, paranuclear, glassy, cytoplasmic pseudoinclusion of intermediate filaments and an eccentric nucleus with a prominent nucleolus. IHC stains show vimentin, cytokeratin, EMA, desmin, and neurofilament positivity in variable amounts. The majority of RTs demonstrate aberrations of the gene SWI/*hSNFa/INI* at 22q11.2, which transcribes the INI protein responsible for chromatin-histone remodeling for transcription regulation. Biallelic loss of the tumor suppressor function of this gene can occur either sporadically in the tumor or less commonly as a result of a constitutional deletion and loss of the subsequent normal allele in the tumor. Two possible *INI* targets are cyclin D1 and p16/INKa, a cyclin D1 inhibitor, both able to control cell cycle via the retinoblastoma regulator.[100]

Molecular Prognostics

RT has a universally poor prognosis with a median survival of 10.1 months. Younger patients under 3 years of age have worse outcomes compared with older children, regardless of primary tumor location.[101] Loss of nuclear INI expression helps confirm RT, but this loss is increasingly becoming less specific for RT, as it has been seen in a number of different tumors, including epithelioid sarcoma and familial schwannomas in NF2 patients (e.g., mosaic pattern of nuclear lost). Currently, there are no defined molecular prognostic markers for RT. Some have suggested that rapamycin may serve as a potential therapeutic target for RT given a probable upregulation of mTOR kinase pathway in these tumors; however, this is still under investigation.[102]

Congenital Infantile Fibrosarcoma and Congenital Mesoblastic Nephroma

We have elected to include congenital/infantile fibrosarcoma (CIFS) and cellular congenital mesoblastic nephroma (cellular CMN) under the same heading, as an increasing amount of molecular data have established that these tumors are a common entity[103] rather than two separate tumors with a similar translocation (as seen with ASPS and the Xp11 translocation-associated RCC).

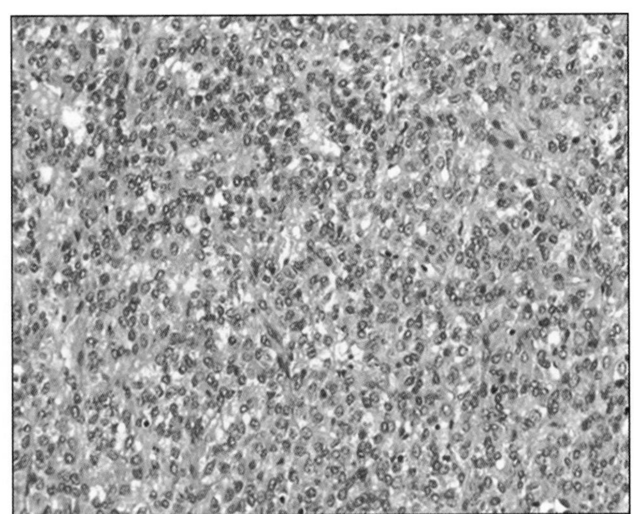

FIGURE 41–11 Congenital (infantile) fibrosarcoma (congenital mesoblastic nephroma). Compact, monomorphic neoplasm of proliferating small-sized cells with eosinophilic cytoplasm and vesicular nuclei (H&E, ×20).

CIFS/cellular CMN is a tumor of infancy with the median age of <2 months, making it the most common mesenchymal malignancy below 2 years of age.[104] Many cases are diagnosed in utero with improved ultrasound imaging. It is now recognized that cellular CMN is CIFS in a renal location. Outside the kidney, the most common location of CIFS is within the distal extremities, but cases occurring in the head, neck, and trunk are not uncommon. The key histologic findings of CIFS/cellular CMN include a circumscribed but unencapsulated mass of tightly packed round to elongate monomorphic cells with moderate eosinophilic cytoplasm and vesicular nuclei with a high proliferative rate (Fig. 41.11). In contrast, classic CMN has an irregular, interdigitating border and has longer interlacing fascicles of plump spindle cells intermixed with a variable collagenous stroma and thin, dilated blood vessels. The dual histologic pattern of classic and cellular types is seen in about 20% of renal cases.[82] All patterns of these tumors express myofibroblast IHC markers, including smooth muscle actin, vimentin, and desmin. While the so-called classic CMN of the kidney does not display the *ETV6/NTRK* fusion transcript, when compared with cellular CMN, the classic CMN, initially described by Bolande, may according to some, in fact, represent infantile fibromatosis rather than a fibrosarcoma of the kidney. Some have demonstrated that the cellular subtype is more aggressive and associated with recurrence[82]; however, others have not been able to demonstrate a difference in outcome based on histology.[104] Complete surgical excision with wide margins, usually without adjuvant chemotherapy, is the standard treatment.

Molecular Diagnostics

CIFS/cellular CMNs are confirmed by the t(12;15)(p13;q25) in which the dimerization domain of the *ETV6* transcriptional regulator gene (12p13) fuses with the tyrosine kinase domain of the neurotrophic tyrosine kinase receptor type 3 (*NTRK3*) at 15q25. The fusion protein results in autophosphorylation of the *NTRK3* and activation of downstream signaling pathways.[105] Other common but less specific molecular aberrations include trisomies of chromosomes 8, 11, 17, and 20, and their sole finding should prompt investigation for the fusion transcript by FISH or RT-PCR, if not demonstrated by classical cytogenetics. A case report of a unique three-way translocation has been described in a retroperitoneal mass of a 5-month-old boy with a novel 19p13.1 involvement (e.g., a complex karyotype: 49,XY,+8,+11, t(12;15;19)(p13.2;q25.3;p13.1),+20).[106]

Molecular Prognostics

A large British study of 47 CMN (23 classic, 14 cellular, and 10 mixed) and others[104] as well as other smaller series[107] could not demonstrate differences in outcomes based on histologic types, as CMN uniformly has good prognosis if margins are free of tumor. Thus, the *ETV6/NTRK3* fusion transcript found exclusively in the nonclassic CMN histologic subtypes would appear to be more of a diagnostic marker rather than a prognostic one.[104] Incomplete surgical excision and/or tumor spill or positive margins are the most informative risk factor for local tumor recurrence.[104,107,108] Tumors that are not amenable to surgical resection have good response to chemotherapy.[108] While there are no definite molecular prognostic markers, the diagnostic utility of identifying the fusion transcript in these tumors is helpful in distinguishing between aggressive RTs which can occasionally share some histological overlap with cellular CMN, especially when displaying foci of necrosis. The distinction between the nearly fatal RT from CMN, which has excellent outcomes, even if stage 3, is of paramount importance.

Pleuropulmonary Blastoma

Pleuropulmonary blastoma (PPB) is a rare childhood primary intrathoracic neoplasm categorized into three main pathologic subtypes (types I, II, and III, vide infra). The tumor, composed of immature pleuropulmonary mesenchyme, can arise from the lung, pleura, or mediastinum. While the cell origin is derived from the early primitive interstitial mesenchyme, the exact derivation remains a question of debate. Both boys and girls, typically 5 to 6 years old or younger, are affected. Early or type I PPB is a cystic neoplasm with a benign ciliated respiratory epithelium lining and an underlying condensed immature malignant mesenchyme of the cyst wall. These tumors share some histologic features with cystic pulmonary airway malformations (CPAMs); however, type I PPBs and CPAMs are separate entities, and PPBs are not thought to arise from these airway malformations.[109] Type II PPB has progression with sarcomatous overgrowth, having solid features intermixed with cystic areas to produce an intermediate phenotype. Type III PPB is a purely solid neoplasm with complete sarcomatous overgrowth. The solid components of both type II and III have characteristic cellular islands of blastema encircling loose immature mesenchyme, along with variable amounts of cartilage, rhabdomyoblasts, and anaplastic cells. IHC stains for desmin and myogenin help to highlight the rhabdomyosarcomatous differentiation. In familial PPB, these lung neoplasms are harbingers of other dysplasias and malignancies in the patient and/or in closely related kindred (i.e., cystic nephroma, RMSs, ovarian Sertoli-Leydig, medulloblastoma, etc.). Recently, the familial PPB locus has been mapped to a germline aberration in chromosome 14q32, the target of interest being the *DICER1* gene, which encodes a 218 kDa ribonuclease (dsRNase III endonuclease) that catalyzes the cleavage of miRNA precursor (pre-miRNA) into mature miRNA. Therefore, abnormalities in *DICER1* gene may lead to decreased production of mature miRNAs with subsequent deregulation of corresponding miRNA target genes and alteration of gene expression.[110] For the other 80% of non-familial PPB cases, gains of chromosome 8, including trisomy 8, have emerged as a recurrent cytogenetic abnormality, even in type 1 PPB, while trisomy 2 and 17p deletion have been reported less frequently.

Molecular Diagnostics

The molecular genetics of PPB has had a recent surge of activity with the discovery of the heterozygous germline mutation in the *DICER1* gene at the 14q32 locus in 11 PPB families. The RNase gene product is integral for the production of miRNAs, which have numerous functions in regulating genes in cell cycle control, oncogenesis, and organ development.[110] The loss of this gene in mouse models has led to cystic airways with disruption of pulmonary branching and mesenchymal expansion, a mouse model of type I PPB. A heterozygous germline nonsense mutation resulting in either a premature stop codon or a frameshift mutation with a resultant truncated protein product was identified in 10 familial PPB families. The 11th family had a novel germline missense mutation resulting in lysine to arginine amino acid at codon 1583 (L1583R). The non-polar to polar amino acid change has not been previously reported but is thought to result in protein dysfunction; however, there was no material for subsequent RNA analysis. The *DICER1* mutation alone is not sufficient for tumorigenesis but rather acts in a haploinsufficient manner working in combination with the germline mutation to cause tumorigenesis. Further complicating the situation, Slade et al.[111] have shown that in a subset of eight tumors (e.g., three PPBs, four Sertoli-Leydig tumors, and one cystic nephroma) from six individuals with a constitutional *DICER1* mutation, all eight tumors showed retention of the wild-type *DICER1* allele. Furthermore, many constitutional carriers and haploinsufficient mice have a normal phenotype without development of "DICER1 syndrome" tumors/dysplasia (i.e., PPB, cystic nephroma, ovarian Sertoli-Leydig, medulloepithelioma, and thyroid cysts/nodules). In support of retained wild-type expression, Hill and colleagues'[110] unexpected IHC finding at the time showed that protein expression of *DICER1* was retained in the malignant stromal mesenchyme but not expressed in the normally developed overlying respiratory epithelium in type I PPB. The cross-talk interaction between the epithelial and mesenchymal components in PPB and the pathogenesis and variable penetrance between constitutional *DICER1* mutations and phenotype remain an area of active investigation.

While gain of chromosome 8 has emerged as a predominant recurrent cytogenetic abnormality for all subtypes of PPB,[112,113] it is not found in all sporadic PPBs. A genome-wide analysis of five sporadic PPBs (e.g., type I n = 1; type II n = 2; type III n = 2) shows that gain of chromosome 8q is the most frequent abnormality, which was confirmed with FISH studies.[113] Other abnormalities include gains of 1q, 2, 7q, 20q, and 22; amplification of 5q33-34, 11q22.2–ter, 15q25–ter, and 19q11-13.2; and losses of 17p, 10 or 10q, 9p21-24, and X or Xp, and both loss and rearrangements of 11p.[112,113] Trisomies of both chromosomes 8 and 2 are not unique to PPB and have been described in other embryonal type tumors, such as HB and RMS.[112] Loss of the short arm of 17 may have association with p53 alterations while loss of 10/10q may be associated with loss of the *PTEN* tumor suppressor gene. Furthermore, rare cases of 11p rearrangements involving partial 11p deletion and/or 11p13-15 duplication could affect *WT1* and *WT2* genes, which is thought to play a role in other embryonal type tumors.

Molecular Prognostics

While there appears to be a new molecular signature for familial PPB, the prognostic significance of a constitutional *DICER1* mutation is unclear, as there is low penetrance and variable expressivity without a clear understanding of its interplay between genotype and the *DICER1* syndrome tumor phenotype. It is therefore difficult to accurately predict what screening should be done in these individuals and families. It has been suggested that patients with a *DICER1* syndrome tumor should be offered genetic testing. In sporadic PPB, certain cytogenetic abnormalities have been identified but no gene target has emerged as a clear prognostic marker. The finding of recurrent cytogenetic abnormalities in early cystic tumors and locally recurrent PPB cases may suggest evidence of an early type I PPB with a propensity to progress to type II or III and thus may help predict a worse outcome.[112]

CONCLUSION

The field of pediatric molecular diagnostics has become an important adjunct for proper classification and diagnosis over the past few decades. The new challenge for pediatric pathologists in the next decade is deciphering the endless amount of molecular data streaming through the literature in order to help guide multidisciplinary clinical trials for designing trials to study those molecular markers that could serve as meaningful prognostic markers. Many pediatric tumors have high cure rates but this comes at the expense of maximum-dose chemotherapy and often radiotherapy. It is the hope that with greater molecular understanding of biologic pathways, we may better predict prognosis and thus begin to stratify subsets of patients based on molecular markers who may be treated with less aggressive traditional chemotherapeutic regimens and help offer more targeted molecular-based therapies with this knowledge. It is important to remember that the role of the 21st century pathologist will be one that integrates and orchestrates the coordination of tissue, pathologic understanding, and interpretation of molecular pathology to best guide and educate their colleagues and patients for optimal outcomes.

REFERENCES

1. Shimada H, Ambros I, Dehner L, Hata J, Joshi V, Roald B. Terminology and morphologic criteria of neuroblastic tumors: recommendations by the International Neuroblastoma Pathology Committee. *Cancer*. 1999;86:349-363.
2. Peuchmaur M, d'Amore ES, Joshi VV, et al. Revision of the International Neuroblastoma Pathology Classification: confirmation of favorable and unfavorable prognostic subsets in ganglioneuroblastoma, nodular. *Cancer*. 2003;98(10):2274-2281.
3. Janoueix-Lerosey I, Schleiermacher G, Delattre O. Molecular pathogenesis of peripheral neuroblastic tumors. *Oncogene*. March 2010;29(11):1566-1579.
4. Wang Q, Diskin S, Rappaport E, et al. Integrative genomics identifies distinct molecular classes of neuroblastoma and shows that multiple genes are targeted by regional alterations in DNA copy number. *Cancer Res*. 2006;66:6050-6062.
5. Passoni L, Longo L, Collini P, et al. Mutation-independent anaplastic lymphoma kinase overexpression in poor prognosis neuroblastoma patients. *Cancer Res*. 2009;69:7338-7346.
6. Weinstein JL, Katzenstein HM, Cohn SL. Advances in the diagnosis and treatment of neuroblastoma. *Oncologist*. 2003;8(3):278-292.
7. Attiyeh EF, London WB, Mossé YP, et al.; Children's Oncology Group. Chromosome 1p and 11q deletions and outcome in neuroblastoma. *N Engl J Med*. November 2005;353(21):2243-2253.
8. Buckley PG, Alcock L, Bryan K, et al. Chromosomal and microRNA expression patterns reveal biologically distinct subgroups of 11q-neuroblastoma. *Clin Cancer Res*. June 2010;16(11):2971-2978.
9. Jedlicka P. Ewing sarcoma, an enigmatic malignancy of likely progenitor cell origin, driven by transcription factor oncogenic fusions. *Int J Clin Exp Pathol*. March 2010;3(4):338-347.
10. Tirode F, Laud-Duval K, Prieur A, Delorme B, Charbord P, Delattre O. Mesenchymal stem cell features of Ewing tumors. *Cancer Cell*. 2007;11:421-429.
11. Lin PP, Wang Y, Lozano G. Mesenchymal stem cells and the origin of Ewing's sarcoma. *Sarcoma*. 2011;2011:pii: 276463. [Epub October 5, 2010].
12. Shing DC, McMullan DJ, Roberts P, et al. FUS/ERG gene fusions in Ewing's tumors. *Cancer Res*. August 2003;63(15):4568-4576.
13. Wang L, Bhargava R, Zheng T, et al. Undifferentiated small round cell sarcomas with rare EWS gene fusions: identification of a novel EWS-SP3 fusion and of additional cases with the EWS-ETV1 and EWS-FEV fusions. *J Mol Diagn*. September 2007;9(4):498-509.
14. Ng TL, O'Sullivan MJ, Pallen CJ, et al. Ewing sarcoma with novel translocation t(2;16) producing an in-frame fusion of FUS and FEV. *J Mol Diagn*. September 2007;9(4):459-463.
15. Savola S, Klami A, Tripathi A, et al. Combined use of expression and CGH arrays pinpoints novel candidate genes in Ewing sarcoma family of tumors. *BMC Cancer*. 2009;9:17.
16. van Doorninck JA, Ji L, Schaub B, et al. Current treatment protocols have eliminated the prognostic advantage of type 1 fusions in Ewing sarcoma: a report from the Children's Oncology Group. *J Clin Oncol*. 2010;28(12):1989-1994.
17. Huang H-Y, Illei PB, Zhao Z, et al. Ewing sarcomas with p53 mutation or p16/p14ARF homozygous deletion: a highly lethal subset associated with poor chemoresponse. *J Clin Oncol*. 2005;23(3):548-558.
18. McKinsey EL, Parrish JK, Irwin AE, et al. A novel oncogenic mechanism in Ewing sarcoma involving IGF pathway targeting by EWS/Fli1-regulated microRNAs. *Oncogene*. 2011. [Epub ahead of print].
19. Jo VY, Mariño-Enríquez A, Fletcher CD. Epithelioid rhabdomyosarcoma: clinicopathologic analysis of 16 cases of a morphologically distinct variant of rhabdomyosarcoma. *Am J Surg Pathol*. 2011;35(10):1523-1530.
20. Pedone PV, Tirabosco R, Cavazzana AO, et al. Mono- and bi-allelic expression of insulin-like growth factor II gene in human muscle tumors. *Hum Mol Genet*. 1994;3:1117-1121.
21. Khan J, Bittner ML, Saal LH, et al. cDNA microarrays detect activation of a myogenic transcription program by the PAX3-FKHR fusion oncogene. *Proc Natl Acad Sci U S A*. 1999;96:13264-13269.
22. Roeb W, Boyer A, Cavenee WK, Arden KC. PAX3-FOXO1 controls expression of the p57Kip2 cell-cycle regulator through degradation of EGR1. *Proc Natl Acad Sci U S A*. 2007;104:18085-18090.
23. Sorensen PH, Lynch JC, Qualman SJ, et al. PAX3-FKHR and PAX7-FKHR gene fusions are prognostic indicators in alveolar rhabdomyosarcoma: a report from the Children's Oncology Group. *J Clin Oncol*. 2002;20:2672-2679.
24. Barr FG, Qualman SJ, Macris MH, et al. Genetic heterogeneity in the alveolar rhabdomyosarcoma subset without typical gene fusions. *Cancer Res*. 2002;62:4704-4710.
25. Williamson D, Missiaglia E, de Reyniès A, et al. Fusion gene-negative alveolar rhabdomyosarcoma is clinically and molecularly indistinguishable from embryonal rhabdomyosarcoma. *J Clin Oncol*. May 2010;28(13):2151-2158.
26. Rodary C, Gehan EA, Flamant F, et al. Prognostic factors in 951 nonmetastatic rhabdomyosarcoma in children: a report from the International Rhabdomyosarcoma Workshop. *Med Pediatr Oncol*. 1991;19(2):89-95.
27. Rodeberg DA, Garcia-Henriquez N, Lyden ER, et al. Prognostic significance and tumor biology of regional lymph node disease in patients with rhabdomyosarcoma: a report from the Children's Oncology Group. *J Clin Oncol*. April 2011;29(10):1304-1311.
28. Anderson JR, Barr FG, Hawkins DS, Parham DM, Skapek SX, Triche TJ. Fusion-negative alveolar rhabdomyosarcoma: modification of risk stratification is premature. *J Clin Oncol*. October 2010;28(29):e587-e588; author reply e589-e590.
29. Rao PK, Missiaglia E, Shields L, et al. Distinct roles for miR-1 and miR-133a in the proliferation and differentiation of rhabdomyosarcoma cells. *FASEB J*. September 2010;24(9):3427-3437.
30. Taulli R, Bersani F, Foglizzo V, et al. The muscle-specific microRNA miR-206 blocks human rhabdomyosarcoma growth in xenotransplanted mice by promoting myogenic differentiation. *J Clin Invest*. August 2009;119(8):2366-2378.
31. Ferrari A, Bisogno G, Alaggio R, et al. Synovial sarcoma of children and adolescents: the prognostic role of axial sites. *Eur J Cancer*. June 2008;44(9):1202-1209.
32. Fisher C. Soft tissue sarcomas with non-EWS translocations: molecular genetic features and pathologic and clinical correlations. *Virchows Arch*. February 2010;456(2):153-166.
33. Terry J, Saito T, Subramanian S, et al. TLE1 as a diagnostic immunohistochemical marker for synovial sarcoma emerging from gene expression profiling studies. *Am J Surg Pathol*. February 2007;31(2):240-246.
34. Haldar M, Randall RL, Capecchi MR. Synovial sarcoma: from genetics to genetic-based animal modeling. *Clin Orthop Relat Res*. September 2008;466(9):2156-2167.
35. de Bruijn DR, Nap JP, van Kessel AG. The (epi)genetics of human synovial sarcoma. *Genes Chromosomes Cancer*. February 2007;46(2):107-117.

36. Nikiforova MN, Groen P, Mutema G, Nikiforov YE, Witte D. Detection of SYT-SSX rearrangements in synovial sarcomas by real-time one-step RT-PCR. *Pediatr Dev Pathol.* March-April 2005;8(2):162-167.
37. Storlazzi CT, Mertens F, Mandahl N, et al. A novel fusion gene, SS18L1/SSX1, in synovial sarcoma. *Genes Chromosomes Cancer.* June 2003;37(2):195-200.
38. Ladanyi M, Antonescu CR, Leung DH, et al. Impact of SYT-SSX fusion type on the clinical behavior of synovial sarcoma: a multi-institutional retrospective study of 243 patients. *Cancer Res.* 2002;62(1):135-140.
39. Guillou L, Benhattar J, Bonichon F, et al. Histologic grade, but not SYT-SSX fusion type, is an important prognostic factor in patients with synovial sarcoma: a multicenter, retrospective analysis. *J Clin Oncol.* October 2004;22(20):4040-4050.
40. Takenaka S, Ueda T, Naka N, et al. Prognostic implication of SYT-SSX fusion type in synovial sarcoma: a multi-institutional retrospective analysis in Japan. *Oncol Rep.* February 2008;19(2):467-476.
41. Saito T, Oda Y, Sakamoto A, et al. Prognostic value of the preserved expression of the E-cadherin and catenin families of adhesion molecules and of beta-catenin mutations in synovial sarcoma. *J Pathol.* November 2000;192(3):342-350.
42. Pretto D, Barco R, Rivera J, Neel N, Gustavson MD, Eid JE. The synovial sarcoma translocation protein SYT-SSX2 recruits beta-catenin to the nucleus and associates with it in an active complex. *Oncogene.* 2006;25:3661-3669.
43. Kushner BH, LaQuaglia MP, Cheung NK, et al. Clinically critical impact of molecular genetic studies in pediatric solid tumors. *Med Pediatr Oncol.* 1999;33:530-535.
44. Williams A, Bartle G, Sumathi VP, et al. Detection of ASPL/TFE3 fusion transcripts and the TFE3 antigen in formalin-fixed, paraffin-embedded tissue in a series of 18 cases of alveolar soft part sarcoma: useful diagnostic tools in cases with unusual histological features. *Virchows Arch.* March 2011;458(3):291-300.
45. Lazar AJ, Das P, Tuvin D, et al. Angiogenesis-promoting gene patterns in alveolar soft part sarcoma. *Clin Cancer Res.* December 2007;13(24):7314-7321.
46. Argani P, Antonescu CR, Illei PB, et al. Primary renal neoplasms with the ASPLeTFE3 gene fusion of alveolar soft part sarcoma: a distinctive tumor entity previously included among renal cell carcinomas of children and adolescents. *Am J Pathol.* 2001;159:179e92.
47. Ladanyi M, Lui MY, Antonescu CR, et al. The der(17)t(X;17)(p11;q25) of human alveolar soft part sarcoma fuses the TFE3 transcription factor gene to ASPL, a novel gene at 17q25. *Oncogene.* January 2001;20(1):48-57.
48. Zarrin-Khameh N, Kaye KS. Alveolar soft part sarcoma. *Arch Pathol Lab Med.* March 2007;131(3):488-491.
49. Hoshino M, Ogose A, Kawashima H, et al. Molecular analyses of cell origin and detection of circulating tumor cells in the peripheral blood in alveolar soft part sarcoma. *Cancer Genet Cytogenet.* April 2009;190(2):75-80.
50. Vistica DT, Hollingshead M, Borgel SD, et al. Therapeutic vulnerability of an in vivo model of alveolar soft part sarcoma (ASPS) to antiangiogenic therapy. *J Pediatr Hematol Oncol.* August 2009;31(8):561-570.
51. Gardner K, Judson I, Leahy M, et al. Activity of cediranib, a highly potent and selective VEGF signaling inhibitor, in alveolar soft part sarcoma. *J Clin Oncol.* 2009;27(15S):10523.
52. Azizi AA, Haberler C, Czech T, et al. Vascular-endothelial-growth-factor (VEGF) expression and possible response to angiogenesis inhibitor bevacizumab in metastatic alveolar soft part sarcoma. *Lancet Oncol.* June 2006;7(6):521-523.
53. Stringer MD, Alizai NK. Mesenchymal hamartoma of the liver: a systematic review. *J Pediatr Surg.* November 2005;40(11):1681-1690.
54. Lin J, Cole BL, Qin X, Zhang M, Kapur RP. Occult androgenetic-biparental mosaicism and sporadic hepatic mesenchymal hamartoma. *Pediatr Dev Pathol.* May 2011. [Epub ahead of print].
55. Sawyer JR, Roloson GJ, Bell JM, Thomas JR, Teo C, Chadduck WM. Telomeric associations in the progression of chromosome aberrations in pediatric solid tumors. *Cancer Genet Cytogenet.* 1996;90:1-13.
56. Lauwers GY, Grant LD, Donnelly WH, et al. Hepatic undifferentiated (embryonal) sarcoma arising in a mesenchymal hamartoma. *Am J Surg Pathol.* 1997;21:1248-1254.
57. Bove KE, Blough RI, Soukup S. Third report of t(19q)(13.4) in mesenchymal hamartoma of liver with comments on link to embryonal sarcoma. *Pediatr Dev Pathol.* 1998;1:438-442.
58. O'Sullivan MJ, Swanson PE, Knoll J, et al. Undifferentiated embryonal sarcoma with unusual features arising within mesenchymal hamartoma of the liver: report of a case and review of the literature. *Pediatr Dev Pathol.* 2001;4:482-489.
59. Rajaram V, Knezevich S, Bove KE, Perry A, Pfeifer JD. DNA sequence of the translocation breakpoints in undifferentiated embryonal sarcoma arising in mesenchymal hamartoma of the liver harboring t(11;19)(q11;q13.4) translocation. *Genes Chromosomes Cancer.* 2007;46:508-513.
60. Speleman F, De Telder V, De Potter KR, et al. Cytogenetic analysis of a mesenchymal hamartoma of the liver. *Cancer Genet Cytogenet.* July 1989;40(1):29-32.
61. Mascarello JT, Krous HF. Second report of a translocation involving 19q13.4 in a mesenchymal hamartoma of the liver. *Cancer Genet Cytogenet.* February 1992;58(2):141-142.
62. Murthi GV, Paterson L, Azmy A. Chromosomal translocation in mesenchymal hamartoma of liver: what is its significance? *J Pediatr Surg.* October 2003;38(10):1543-1545.
63. Rakheja D, Margraf LR, Tomlinson GE, Schneider NR. Hepatic mesenchymal hamartoma with translocation involving chromosome band 19q13.4: a recurrent abnormality. *Cancer Genet Cytogenet.* August 2004;153(1):60-63.
64. Sharif K, Ramani P, Lochbühler H, Grundy R, de Ville de Goyet J. Recurrent mesenchymal hamartoma associated with 19q translocation. A call for more radical surgical resection. *Eur J Pediatr Surg.* February 2006;16(1):64-67.
65. Talmon GA, Cohen SM. Mesenchymal hamartoma of the liver with an interstitial deletion involving chromosome band 19q13.4: a theory as to pathogenesis? *Arch Pathol Lab Med.* August 2006;130(8):1216-1218.
66. Sugito K, Kawashima H, Uekusa S, Inoue M, Ikeda T, Kusafuka T. Mesenchymal hamartoma of the liver originating in the caudate lobe with t(11;19)(q13;q13.4): report of a case. *Surg Today.* 2010;40(1):83-87.
67. Shetty S, Pinto A, Roland B. Mesenchymal hamartoma of the liver with inversion of chromosome 19. *Pediatr Dev Pathol.* March 2011. [Epub ahead of print].
68. Shehata BM, Gupta NA, Katzenstein HM, et al. Undifferentiated embryonal sarcoma of the liver is associated with mesenchymal hamartoma and multiple chromosomal abnormalities: a review of eleven cases. *Pediatr Dev Pathol.* 2011;14(2):111-116.
69. Cajaiba MM, Sarita-Reyes C, Zambrano E, Reyes-Múgica M. Mesenchymal hamartoma of the liver associated with features of Beckwith-Wiedemann syndrome and high serum alpha-fetoprotein levels. *Pediatr Dev Pathol.* May-June 2007;10(3):233-238.
70. Adesina AM, Lopez-Terrada D, Wong KK, et al. Gene expression profiling reveals signatures characterizing histologic subtypes of hepatoblastoma and global deregulation in cell growth and survival pathways. *Hum Pathol.* June 2009;40(6):843-853.
71. Tomlinson GE, Douglass EC, Pollock BH, Finegold MJ, Schneider NR. Cytogenetic evaluation of a large series of hepatoblastomas: numerical abnormalities with recurring aberrations involving 1q12-q21. *Genes Chromosomes Cancer.* October 2005;44(2):177-184.
72. Koch A, Denkhaus D, Albrecht S, Leuschner I, von Schweinitz D, Pietsch T. Childhood hepatoblastomas frequently carry a mutated degradation targeting box of the beta-catenin gene. *Cancer Res.* January 1999;59(2):269-273.
73. Cairo S, Armengol C, De Reyniès A, et al. Hepatic stem-like phenotype and interplay of Wnt/beta-catenin and Myc signaling in aggressive childhood liver cancer. *Cancer Cell.* December 2008;14(6):471-484.
74. Ranganathan S, Tan X, Monga SP. beta-Catenin and met deregulation in childhood hepatoblastomas. *Pediatr Dev Pathol.* July-August 2005;8(4):435-447.
75. Hirschman BA, Pollock BH, Tomlinson GE. The spectrum of APC mutations in children with hepatoblastoma from familial adenomatous polyposis kindreds. *J Pediatr.* August 2005;147(2):263-266.
76. López-Terrada D, Gunaratne PH, Adesina AM, et al. Histologic subtypes of hepatoblastoma are characterized by differential

canonical Wnt and Notch pathway activation in DLK+ precursors. *Hum Pathol.* June 2009;40(6):783-794.
77. Weber RG, Pietsch T, von Schweinitz D, Lichter P. Characterization of genomic alterations in hepatoblastomas: a role for gains on chromosomes 8q and 20 as predictors of poor outcome. *Am J Pathol.* 2000;157:571-578.
78. Gordon S, Akopyan G, Garban H, Bonavida B. Transcription factor YY1: structure, function, and therapeutic implications in cancer biology. *Oncogene.* 2006;25:1125-1142.
79. Shin E, Lee KB, Park SY, et al. Gene expression profiling of human hepatoblastoma using archived formalin-fixed and paraffin-embedded tissues. *Virchows Arch.* April 2011;458(4):453-465.
80. Magrelli A, Azzalin G, Salvatore M, et al. Altered microRNA expression patterns in hepatoblastoma patients. *Transl Oncol.* August 2009;2(3):157-163.
81. Pode-Shakked N, Dekel B. Wilms tumor—a renal stem cell malignancy? *Pediatr Nephrol.* September 2011;26(9):1535-1543.
82. Murphy WM, Grignon DJ, Perlman EJ. Kidney tumors in children. In: Siverberg SG, Sobin LH, eds. *AFIP Atlas of Tumor Pathology: Tumors of the Kidney, Bladder, and Related Urinary Structures.* Washington, DC: Armed Forces Institute of Pathology; 2004:1-88.
83. Dekel B, Amariglio N, Kaminski N, et al. Engraftment and differentiation of human metanephroi into functional mature nephrons after transplantation into mice is accompanied by a profile of gene expression similar to normal human kidney development. *J Am Soc Nephrol.* April 2002;13(4):977-990.
84. Schumacher V, Schneider S, Figge A, et al. Correlation of germ-line mutations and two-hit inactivation of the WT1 gene with Wilms tumors of stromal-predominant histology. *Proc Natl Acad Sci U S A.* 1997;94:3972-3977.
85. Rivera MN, Kim WJ, Wells J, et al. An X chromosome gene, WTX, is commonly inactivated in Wilms tumor. *Science.* February 2007;315(5812):642-645.
86. Jenkins ZA, van Kogelenberg M, Morgan T, et al. Germline mutations in WTX cause a sclerosing skeletal dysplasia but do not predispose to tumorigenesis. *Nat Genet.* 2009;41:95-100.
87. Grundy PE, Breslow NE, Li S, et al.; National Wilms Tumor Study Group. Loss of heterozygosity for chromosomes 1p and 16q is an adverse prognostic factor in favorable-histology Wilms tumor: a report from the National Wilms Tumor Study Group. *J Clin Oncol.* October 2005;23(29):7312-7321.
88. Davidoff AM. Wilms' tumor. *Curr Opin Pediatr.* June 2009;21(3):357-364.
89. Mengelbier LH, Karlsson J, Lindgren D, et al. Deletions of 16q in Wilms tumors localize to blastemal-anaplastic cells and are associated with reduced expression of the IRXB renal tubulogenesis gene cluster. *Am J Pathol.* November 2010;177(5):2609-2621.
90. Breslow NE, Norris R, Norkool PA, et al.; National Wilms Tumor Study Group. Characteristics and outcomes of children with the Wilms tumor-Aniridia syndrome: a report from the National Wilms Tumor Study Group. *J Clin Oncol.* December 2003;21(24):4579-4585.
91. Wu A, Kunju LP, Cheng L, Shah RB. Renal cell carcinoma in children and young adults: analysis of clinicopathological, immunohistochemical and molecular characteristics with an emphasis on the spectrum of Xp11.2 translocation-associated and unusual clear cell subtypes. *Histopathology.* November 2008;53(5):533-544.
92. Armah HB, Parwani AV. Xp11.2 translocation renal cell carcinoma. *Arch Pathol Lab Med.* January 2010;134(1): 124-129.
93. Argani P, Laé M, Hutchinson B, et al. Renal carcinomas with the t(6;11)(p21;q12): clinicopathologic features and demonstration of the specific alpha-TFEB gene fusion by immunohistochemistry, RT-PCR, and DNA PCR. *Am J Surg Pathol.* February 2005;29(2):230-240.
94. Ross H, Argani P. Xp11 translocation renal cell carcinoma. *Pathology.* June 2010;42(4):369-373.
95. Tsuda M, Davis IJ, Argani P, et al. TFE3 fusions activate MET signaling by transcriptional up-regulation, defining another class of tumors as candidates for therapeutic MET inhibition. *Cancer Res.* 2007;67(3):919-929.
96. Argani P, Perlman EJ, Breslow NE, et al. Clear cell sarcoma of the kidney: a review of 351 cases from the National Wilms Tumor Study Group Pathology Center. *Am J Surg Pathol.* 2000;24:4-18.
97. Brownlee NA, Perkins LA, Stewart W, et al. Recurring translocation (10;17) and deletion (14q) in clear cell sarcoma of the kidney. *Arch Pathol Lab Med.* March 2007;131(3):446-451.
98. Cutcliffe C, Kersey D, Huang CC, Zeng Y, Walterhouse D, Perlman EJ; Renal Tumor Committee of the Children's Oncology Group. Clear cell sarcoma of the kidney: up-regulation of neural markers with activation of the sonic hedgehog and Akt pathways. *Clin Cancer Res.* November 2005;11(22):7986-7994.
99. Zhuge Y, Cheung MC, Yang R, Perez EA, Koniaris LG, Sola JE. Pediatric non-Wilms renal tumors: subtypes, survival, and prognostic indicators. *J Surg Res.* October 2010;163(2): 257-263.
100. Venneti S, Le P, Martinez D, et al. p16INK4A and p14ARF tumor suppressor pathways are deregulated in malignant rhabdoid tumors. *J Neuropathol Exp Neurol.* July 2011;70(7):596-609.
101. Morgenstern DA, Gibson S, Brown T, Sebire NJ, Anderson J. Clinical and pathological features of paediatric malignant rhabdoid tumours. *Pediatr Blood Cancer.* January 2010;54(1):29-34.
102. Lünenbürger H, Lanvers-Kaminsky C, Lechtape B, Frühwald MC. Systematic analysis of the antiproliferative effects of novel and standard anticancer agents in rhabdoid tumor cell lines. *Anticancer Drugs.* June 2010;21(5):514-522.
103. Sandberg AA, Bridge JA. Updates on the cytogenetics and molecular genetics of bone and soft tissue tumors: congenital (infantile) fibrosarcoma and mesoblastic nephroma. *Cancer Genet Cytogenet.* January 2002;132(1):1-13.
104. England RJ, Haider N, Vujanic GM, et al. Mesoblastic nephroma: a report of the United Kingdom Children's Cancer and Leukaemia Group (CCLG). *Pediatr Blood Cancer.* May 2011;56(5):744-748.
105. Rubin BP, Chen CJ, Morgan TW, et al. Congenital mesoblastic nephroma t(12;15) is associated with ETV6-NTRK3 gene fusion: cytogenetic and molecular relationship to congenital (infantile) fibrosarcoma. *Am J Pathol.* November 1998;153(5):1451-1458.
106. Mariño-Enríquez A, Li P, Samuelson J, Rossi MR, Reyes-Múgica M. Congenital fibrosarcoma with a novel complex 3-way translocation t(12;15;19) and unusual histologic features. *Hum Pathol.* December 2008;39(12):1844-1848.
107. Gormley TS, Skoog SJ, Jones RV, Maybee D. Cellular congenital mesoblastic nephroma: what are the options. *J Urol.* August 1989;142(2 pt 2):479-483.
108. McCahon E, Sorensen PH, Davis JH, Rogers PC, Schultz KR. Non-resectable congenital tumors with the ETV6-NTRK3 gene fusion are highly responsive to chemotherapy. *Med Pediatr Oncol.* May 2003;40(5):288-292.
109. Priest JR, Williams GM, Hill DA, Dehner LP, Jaffé A. Pulmonary cysts in early childhood and the risk of malignancy. *Pediatr Pulmonol.* January 2009;44(1):14-30.
110. Hill DA, Ivanovich J, Priest JR, et al. DICER1 mutations in familial pleuropulmonary blastoma. *Science.* August 2009;325(5943):965.
111. Slade I, Bacchelli C, Davies H, et al. DICER1 syndrome: clarifying the diagnosis, clinical features and management implications of a pleiotropic tumour predisposition syndrome. *J Med Genet.* 2011;48(4):273-278.
112. Taube JM, Griffin CA, Yonescu R, et al. Pleuropulmonary blastoma: cytogenetic and spectral karyotype analysis. *Pediatr Dev Pathol.* November-December 2006;9(6):453-461.
113. de Krijger RR, Claessen SM, van der Ham F, et al. Gain of chromosome 8q is a frequent finding in pleuropulmonary blastoma. *Mod Pathol.* November 2007;20(11):1191-1199.

CHAPTER 42

Molecular Diagnostics of Metastatic Malignancies

Mikhail Lisovsky, Laura J. Tafe, and Joel A. Lefferts

INTRODUCTION

A significant proportion of patients with solid tumors present initially with metastatic disease from a malignancy of uncertain origin. In many cases, thorough clinical and pathological evaluation does not reveal an anatomic primary tumor at the time of diagnosis or by the time treatment is initiated and the majority of these patients will be diagnosed with a carcinoma of unknown origin or of unknown primary site (CUP). In the vast majority of them, the primary localization of cancer will not be found during life. The reasons why some cancers present as a CUP are not well understood; however, it appears increasingly likely that CUPs represent a heterogeneous group of unrelated metastatic cancers rather than a distinct entity with specific genetic and phenotypic features.[1] It is thought that the primary site of a CUP cannot be found, because the tumor is too small or involutes after seeding a metastasis.[2]

Lymphomas and granulocytic sarcomas, metastatic melanomas, and soft tissue sarcomas can also present as malignancies of unknown origin; however, they represent a small minority of cases and can be usually separated from carcinomas during evaluation. In the United States, CUPs account for 2% to 5% of all invasive cancers.[3,4] The incidence varies depending on the definition, extent of diagnostic workup, patient base, and availability of specialized health care. For example, only 0.3% of cancer patients were diagnosed with CUP at the Mayo Clinic from 1984 to 1999.[5] The definition of CUP has been changing over time and is currently defined as a histologically proven metastatic carcinoma with a non-revealing standardized diagnostic workup consisting of thorough history and physical examination; basic blood and biochemistry screens; urinalysis; fecal occult blood testing; computed tomography (CT) scans of thorax, abdomen, and pelvis; mammography in women; serum prostate-specific antigen (PSA) levels in men; and, in certain conditions, head and neck CT/PET scan and endoscopic evaluations.[3,6] However, the consensus on the necessary diagnostic evaluation is poor, and the constant introduction of new imaging, immunohistochemical, and molecular diagnostic techniques changes the extent of examination, affects the spectrum of patients diagnosed with CUP, and confounds comparisons with older studies.[5]

CUPs can be subdivided into three major groups. The first group includes patients with more favorable prognosis. There is a strong clinicopathological suspicion of a primary site in these patients and therapy has proved effective (see below). In the second group, a primary site is suspected on the basis of largely immunohistochemical and/or gene expression profiles. These profiles are derived from the evaluation of metastatic tumors for which primary sites are known. There is an expectation, not yet proven in randomized trials, that treatment with an appropriate site-specific regimen will be superior to empirical, relatively ineffective platinum/taxane-based chemotherapy. The latter is commonly used in patients with CUP of the third group consisting of cases where the primary site remains entirely unknown.[7] In the current era of improved site-specific treatment regimens for many solid tumors, molecular analyses, such as immunohistochemistry and, possibly, gene expression profiling, have become essential in the management of patients with CUP.

CLINICOPATHOLOGICAL ASPECTS

CUP usually presents with symptoms related to the site of the metastasis (palpable mass, bowel obstruction, and ascites). It is usually a high volume disease with more than 50% of patients having at least two sites of metastasis and 30% having involvement of three and more organs. The

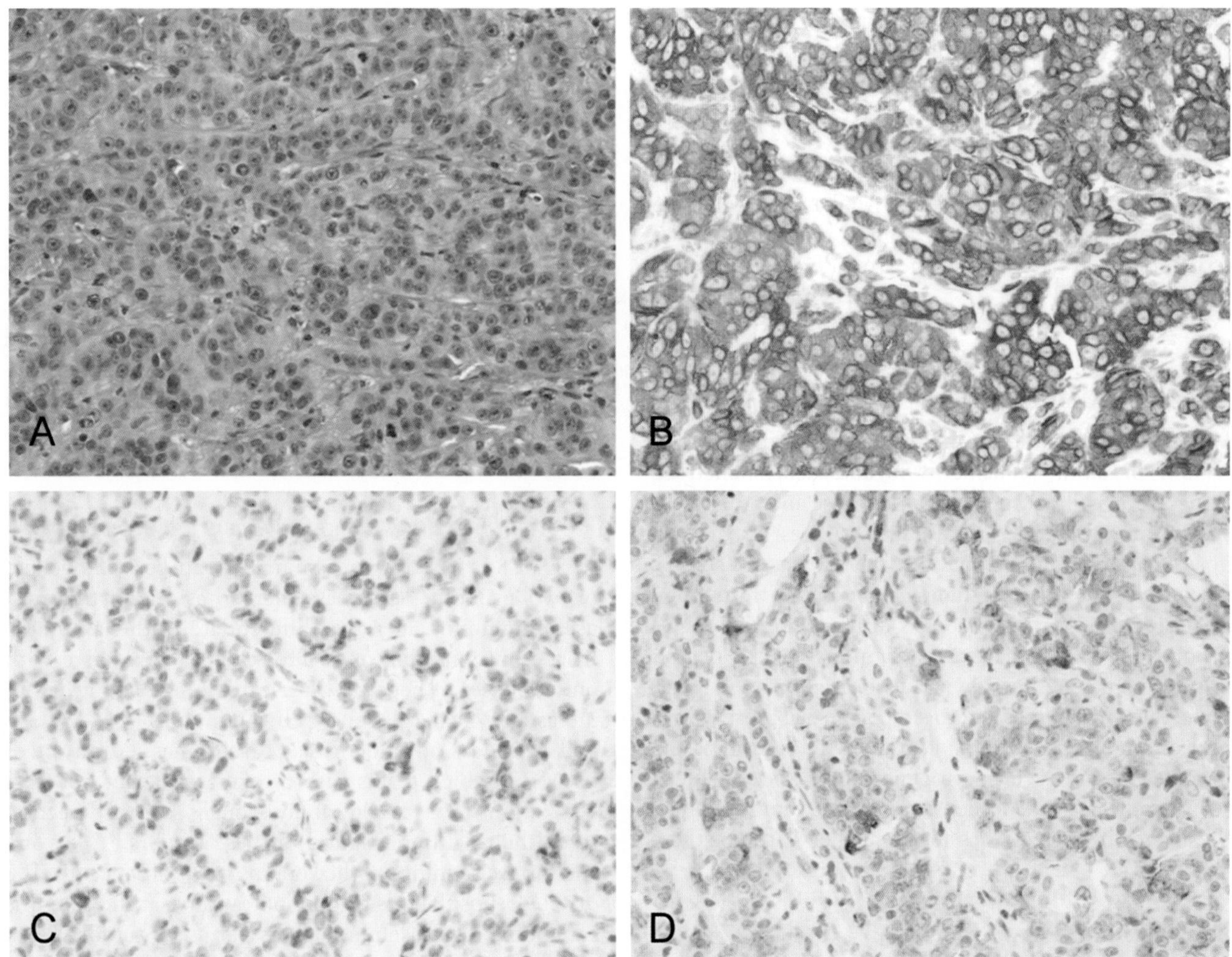

FIGURE 42–1 CUP in a 78-year-old female with excision of a 1.5 cm inguinal lymph node. **A:** A representative hematoxylin and eosin–stained section compatible with features of ductal breast adenocarcinoma. **B–D:** Immunohistochemical staining of sections from the same block as in **(A)**. **B:** Diffuse strong staining for CK7. **C:** Positive staining for ER. **D:** Positive staining for GCFDP-15. Immunostains for CK20, PR, WT1, synaptophysin, chromogranin, and S-100 were negative (not shown). The case was signed out as suggestive of a breast primary. This case also illustrates unusual patterns of metastasis in CUPs, here from a likely breast carcinoma to an inguinal lymph node.

most common sites of metastasis are lymph nodes, liver, bone, lung, pleura, peritoneum, and brain.[8-10] Generally, the patterns of metastatic spread are well established for various tumors and are useful in suggesting a likely primary site. However, metastatic spread of CUPs may be unusual for many of the ultimately proven primary sites. Therefore, location of metastases in a patient with CUP may not be predictive of a primary site and should be interpreted with caution (Fig. 42.1). The primary tumor is identified in only 5% to 15% of patients with CUP during their lifetime.[3,11] However, significantly more primary malignancies are identified at the time of autopsy. In a meta-analysis of three cross-comparable autopsy series covering a study period from 1980 to 2000, a primary tumor was identified in 64% (98 of 153) of patients. The most common primary site was lung (36%) followed by pancreas (12%), colon (11%), kidney (8%), stomach (8%), liver (5%), ovary (4%), gallbladder (3%), bladder/ureter (3%), breast (2%), head and neck (2%), thyroid (2%), pleura (1%), small intestine (1%), and adrenal gland (1%).[12-14] Approximately 50% to 60% of CUPs are well- or moderately differentiated adenocarcinomas, 30% are poorly differentiated carcinomas (with or without glandular features), 5% to 15% are squamous carcinomas, and 5% are neuroendocrine carcinomas.[15,16]

It is important to recognize patients with CUPs of favorable subgroups for whom specific treatments afford better prognosis. They constitute approximately 20% of all patients with CUP and include women with adenocarcinoma involving only axillary lymph nodes (treated as breast carcinoma), women with serous adenocarcinoma of the peritoneum (treated as ovarian carcinoma), patients with squamous cell carcinoma in cervical lymph nodes (treated as head and neck primary), patients with squamous cell carcinoma involving inguinal lymph nodes (treated as carcinoma of the genital or anorectal area), young men with extragonadal germ cell syndrome (treated as germ cell tumor), men with blastic bone metastasis and elevated serum PSA (treated as adenocarcinoma of the prostate), patients with neuroendocrine carcinoma (may have indolent course, if well differentiated, or treated as small cell carcinoma of the lung, if poorly differentiated), and patients with a single potentially resectable metastasis.[3,8] Prognosis of patients with CUP depends on many variables, including age, histologic type, performance status, decision to undergo treatment, and availability of care at a specialized cancer center. Median survival ranges from 3 to 11 months with the highest median survival of 15.5 months in patients with neuroendocrine carcinoma of all types.[9,10,17]

USE OF IMMUNOHISTOCHEMISTRY FOR PREDICTION OF PRIMARY SITE OF CUP

When confronted with a CUP, characteristic morphologic features of tumors on hematoxylin and eosin–stained sections are usually sufficient to diagnose malignancy, to suggest its metastatic origin and to suggest broad categories of carcinoma, lymphoma, melanoma, or sarcoma. However, when a malignancy is poorly differentiated sub-categorization of tumors is difficult on histological grounds only. Also, metastatic origin may not be obvious in some tumors, especially in adenocarcinomas. To overcome these difficulties and to support initial morphologic impressions, stepwise immunohistochemical analysis and, in some cases, molecular, cytogenetic, and electron microscopy studies may be needed to assign the tumor to one of the above broad categories and to further histotype them.

General Principles of Using Immunomarkers for the Prediction of CUPs

1. Few cellular molecules are relatively specific for broad categories of malignancies and even fewer are specific for individual cancers. However, the particular strength of immunomarkers is in differentiating between a small number of defined possibilities for the site of origin. Therefore, an algorithmic stepwise approach has been suggested to evaluate poorly differentiated metastatic tumors of unknown origin.[18-20]
2. Since tumors often have variable expression of immunomarkers, only the most common immunoprofile is usually indicated in the algorithmic framework. Experience and knowledge of variants of expression of a marker are important in the interpretation of immunostains.
3. Sensitivity of markers generally decreases with the increasing grade of tumors.
4. Atypical or aberrant expression of immunomarkers is not rare. To offset it, the use of panels of several immunomarkers with a known cancer characteristic profile is recommended.
5. Determination of the primary site of a metastasis relies on the combination of clinical, morphological, and immunohistochemical data and requires exclusion of a primary cancer at the site of a metastasis, where appropriate.
6. Immunostaining remains an ancillary method and caution should be exercised if the results are discrepant with clinicomorphological findings. Additional support for diagnosis may be sought by using molecular profiling and electron microscopy.

Antibody Panel for Broad Category Screening

To differentiate between broad categories of malignancies, such as carcinoma, melanoma, sarcoma, and hematolymphoid tumors, the suggested initial panel consists of epithelial markers, such as pan-keratin AE1/AE3 and low molecular weight keratin CAM 5.2 (both cytoplasmic staining), melanocytic marker S100 (cytoplasmic and nuclear staining), and hematolymphoid marker CD45 (membranous staining).[19,21]

Keratin Positivity and the Diagnosis of Carcinoma

AE1/AE3 is a broad-spectrum anti-pan-keratin cocktail of two antibodies that has emerged as one of the most useful immunoreagents to differentiate epithelial tumors from non-epithelial ones. However, it is reactive with only a subset of hepatocellular carcinomas, about half of metastatic clear cell renal cell carcinomas (CC-RCCs), and very few adrenocortical carcinomas. Addition of CAM5.2, which reacts with cytokeratin 8, but not with cytokeratin 18, as is commonly thought, allows detection of epithelial differentiation in these tumors.[22-24] Strong and diffuse staining for the keratins in the absence of S100 or CD45 positivity is a good indication that the tumor is carcinoma or nonseminomatous germ cell tumor. Weak and patchy keratin expression has been described in seminoma, various sarcomas, occasionally in melanomas and hematopoietic tumors, such as non-Hodgkin lymphomas, acute leukemia, and plasmacytoma/myeloma. Weak keratin staining may cause diagnostic difficulties and deciding whether the staining is aberrant or is true to the tumor lineage of differentiation is subjective and may need application of ancillary techniques including electron microscopy.

Diffuse and strong keratin expression is also seen in some sarcomas such as synovial sarcoma, sarcomas with epithelioid differentiation, and chordoma. Since sarcomas are rare among tumors that are likely to present as CUPs, the diagnosis needs a high level of suspicion, molecular genetic testing, and/or electron microscopy.

S-100 Positivity and the Diagnosis of Melanoma

The incidence of melanoma of unknown primary site is estimated at 2.7% of all melanomas.[25] Metastatic melanoma may be composed of large cells, spindle cells, and small cells and may contain, or more rarely entirely consist of, clear, signet ring, pseudolipoblastic, rhabdoid, plasmacytoid, or balloon cells, thus closely mimicking poorly differentiated carcinomas, sarcomas, lymphomas, plasmacytomas, and germ cell tumors.[26] Melanin production is helpful diagnostically; however, 7% to 32%

of melanomas of unknown primary site are amelanotic.[27] S100 is the most sensitive melanoma marker and strongly and diffusely stains 95% or more melanomas, including the desmoplastic variant and metastases.[28,29] Therefore, strong and diffuse S100 staining, in the absence of keratin and CD45 positivity, is suggestive of melanoma. However, melanomas with atypical features, such as signet ring cell and rhabdoid melanomas, do not express S100.[26] Specificity of S100 is also less than ideal, because Langerhans cell histiocytosis, some breast and salivary gland carcinomas, and some sarcomas (including poorly differentiated myxoid liposarcoma and malignant peripheral nerve sheath tumor) are variably positive for S100.[28,30] To suggest melanocytic origin of a poorly differentiated or undifferentiated tumor, neoplastic cells should be positive for one or more additional melanocytic markers, such as HMB-45 and MART-1 (clone M2-7C10).[19,21] Both markers are less sensitive (approx 85%), but more specific than S100, show cytoplasmic staining, and are characteristically nonreactive with carcinomas, hematolymphoid tumors, and sarcomas. Melan A (clone A-103) recognizes the same melanoma antigen and has almost the same sensitivity, as MART-1; however, it also recognizes adrenocortical tumors and Leydig cell tumors of the ovary and testes and, thus, has a lower diagnostic value as a first-line marker for a CUP work-up.[31]

One pitfall in evaluating a lymph node is the presence of aggregates of amelanotic nevus cells in the cortical or medullary areas, which can be interpreted as metastatic melanoma or carcinoma.[32] However, finding similar aggregates in the lymph node capsule is reassuring as this is a typical location for nodal nevi. Moreover, although nodal nevi are strongly positive with S100 and MART-1, they are not reactive with HMB-45, show very low Ki-67 index, and do not have cytologic atypia, mitoses, or prominent nucleoli.[32]

CD45 Positivity and the Diagnosis of Hematolymphoid Tumor

CD45, or common leukocyte antigen (predominantly membranous staining), is a very sensitive and specific marker for non-Hodgkin lymphomas and its strong staining is suggestive of a lymphoid tumor in the absence of keratin and S100 reactivity. Lymphoblastic lymphoma and anaplastic large T-cell lymphoma are often negative for CD45 in routinely fixed, paraffin-embedded sections.[33,34] Lymphoblastic lymphoma may be confirmed using immunostaining for TdT (nuclear staining) and anaplastic large T-cell lymphoma—using a combination of ALK1 and CD30 markers (cytoplasmic and membranous staining, respectively). Extramedullary myeloid cell tumor, also known as granulocytic sarcoma, although rare, may enter into the differential diagnosis of a CUP and may be negative for CD45. It can be identified using myeloid markers, such as CD15, CD43, and myeloperoxidase.[35] Spurious reactivity for CD45 has been reported in rare cases of undifferentiated and small cell carcinoma, mostly from the lung.[36]

When the Panel for Broad Category Screening Is Negative

Vimentin Positivity

Sarcomas are usually positive for the intermediate filament vimentin (cytoplasmic staining), which is considered to be the first-line marker for mesenchymal differentiation. Vimentin is also expressed in renal, ovarian, endometrial, thyroid, and sarcomatoid/undifferentiated carcinomas and melanomas and, thus, is not lineage specific.[37] Nonetheless, isolated vimentin positivity in spindle-shaped, poorly differentiated, or undifferentiated CUPs raises a possibility of a sarcoma.

PLAP and OCT4 Positivity

Seminoma is the only germ cell tumor negative for both pan-keratin AE1/AE3 and Cam 5.2 in approximately 70% of cases. In addition, it may also express vimentin. The diagnosis of seminoma is supported by diffuse positivity for PLAP (cytoplasmic staining) and OCT4 (nuclear staining). PLAP is a very sensitive general marker of germ cell tumors, while OCT4 is also positive in the majority of embryonal carcinomas.

CK7/CK20 Antibody Panel for Initial Categorization of Carcinomas

If a sarcoma or a hematolymphoid tumor is strongly suspected after initial screening, further characterization is usually undertaken by a pathologist with a special interest or training in the respective field and will not be discussed here further.

When a likely diagnosis of a carcinoma is established, the keratin profile may further help subclassify the tumor. Among 20 known keratins (cytokeratins) that define an epithelial line of differentiation, coordinate expression of CK7 and CK20 is especially useful in further narrowing the possibilities for the primary site of a CUP.[38] Carcinomas of different organs vary by their CK7/CK20 patterns, which have high fidelity and are usually retained in metastases.[39,40] Many carcinomas have several CK7/CK20 patterns; however, one or two patterns usually predominate. The major (dominant) and the second most common (significant) CK7/CK20 patterns of different carcinomas are presented in Table 42.1. Of all, the CK7–/CK20+ pattern is the most discriminatory, because few tumors, including colorectal carcinomas, some gastric carcinomas, and Merkel cell carcinoma, have it. The CK7+/CK20– pattern is seen in multiple carcinomas originating from the foregut or mullerian epithelium. The CK7+/CK20+ profile is commonly seen in carcinomas from the upper gastrointestinal tract, pancreas, and bladder. Most solid organ carcinomas, squamous cell carcinoma, and small cell carcinoma are CK7–/CK20–.

TABLE 42–1 Patterns of CK7/CK20 Reactivity in Carcinomas Likely to Present as CUPs

Pattern	CK7+/CK20+	CK7+/CK20–	CK7–/CK20+	CK7–/CK20–
Dominant (>50% of cases)	Urothelial Ca Ovarian mucinous ACa Pancreatic ductal ACa	Breast ACa Lung ACa Lung small cell Ca Ovarian non-mucinous ACa Biliary tract ACa Endometrial ACa Endocervical ACa Cervical squamous Ca Esophageal ACa Salivary gland Ca Embryonal CA (GST) Thyroid Ca	Colorectal Ca Merkel cell Ca	Adrenocortical Ca Hepatocellular Ca Prostate ACa Clear cell renal Ca Seminoma Squamous cell Ca Neuroendocrine Ca
Significant (>10%, ≤50% of cases)	Gastric ACa Biliary tract CA Esophageal ACA Appendicial mucinous ACa Small intestinal Ca	Pancreatic ductal ACa Gastric ACa Urothelial Ca Lung squamous Ca Head and neck squamous Ca Small intestinal ACa Neuroendocrine Ca Hepatocellular Ca Seminoma	Gastric Ca	Gastric ACa Cervical squamous Ca Merkel cell Ca Embryonal CA (GST)

ACa, Adenocarcinoma; Ca, Carcinoma; GST, Germ cell tumor.[38-40]

Categorization of Carcinomas Using Site-Restricted Antibodies and Antibody Panel Approach

Pulmonary Adenocarcinoma

According to autopsy studies, the lung is the most common primary site for adenocarcinomas of unknown origin.[15] Common metastatic sites for pulmonary adenocarcinoma are brain, bone, adrenal glands, and liver. Pulmonary adenocarcinoma may have glandular, papillary, or solid histologic patterns and mucinous, signet ring cell, or clear cell features that elicit a broad differential diagnosis at a metastatic site. Lung origin is suspected on the basis of CK7+/CK20– pattern and immunoreactivity to TTF-1, a transcription factor that is involved in the regulation of expression of thyroglobulin and lung surfactant proteins and is present in the vast majority of lung adenocarcinomas and thyroid carcinomas (nuclear staining, Fig. 42.1). TTF-1 is reported to be 95% specific and 73% to 84% sensitive in well/moderately differentiated pulmonary adenocarcinoma. Its sensitivity decreases to about 40% in poorly differentiated and undifferentiated pulmonary adenocarcinomas, thus diminishing the diagnostic value of TTF-1 in poorly differentiated metastases.[41-44] Thyroid papillary or poorly differentiated carcinoma may enter into the differential diagnosis and since both may be TTF-1-positive, additional markers should be used. The co-expression of TTF-1 with thyroglobulin (cytoplasmic staining) or Pax8 (nuclear staining) is diagnostic of thyroid carcinoma and excludes pulmonary adenocarcinoma.[45,46] Expression of TTF-1, more often in a focal manner, can be seen rarely in adenocarcinomas of the colon, kidney, prostate, endometrium, endocervix, and breast (Fig. 42.2).[43,44,47] This rare TTF-1 positivity in gynecological and breast carcinomas is more of a diagnostic problem, since these also exhibit the CK7+/CK20– pattern (see below). Some authors suggested that aberrant expression of TTF-1 is associated with the use of antibody clone SPT24, but not the clone 8G7G3/1; however, this could not be validated in other studies.[44,47,48]

Additional confusion may be caused by a metastasis from a primary lung adenocarcinoma with enteric differentiation which may lose TTF-1 and acquire CK20, CDX2, and MUC2 reactivity mimicking colorectal adenocarcinoma. All seven such adenocarcinomas reported by Inamura et al.[49] retained CK7 expression, allowing separation from colorectal adenocarcinomas. To partially offset difficulties caused by spurious expression of TTF-1, another sensitive marker of lung adenocarcinoma, Napsin A (cytoplasmic staining), can be used.[42] Napsin A is more sensitive than

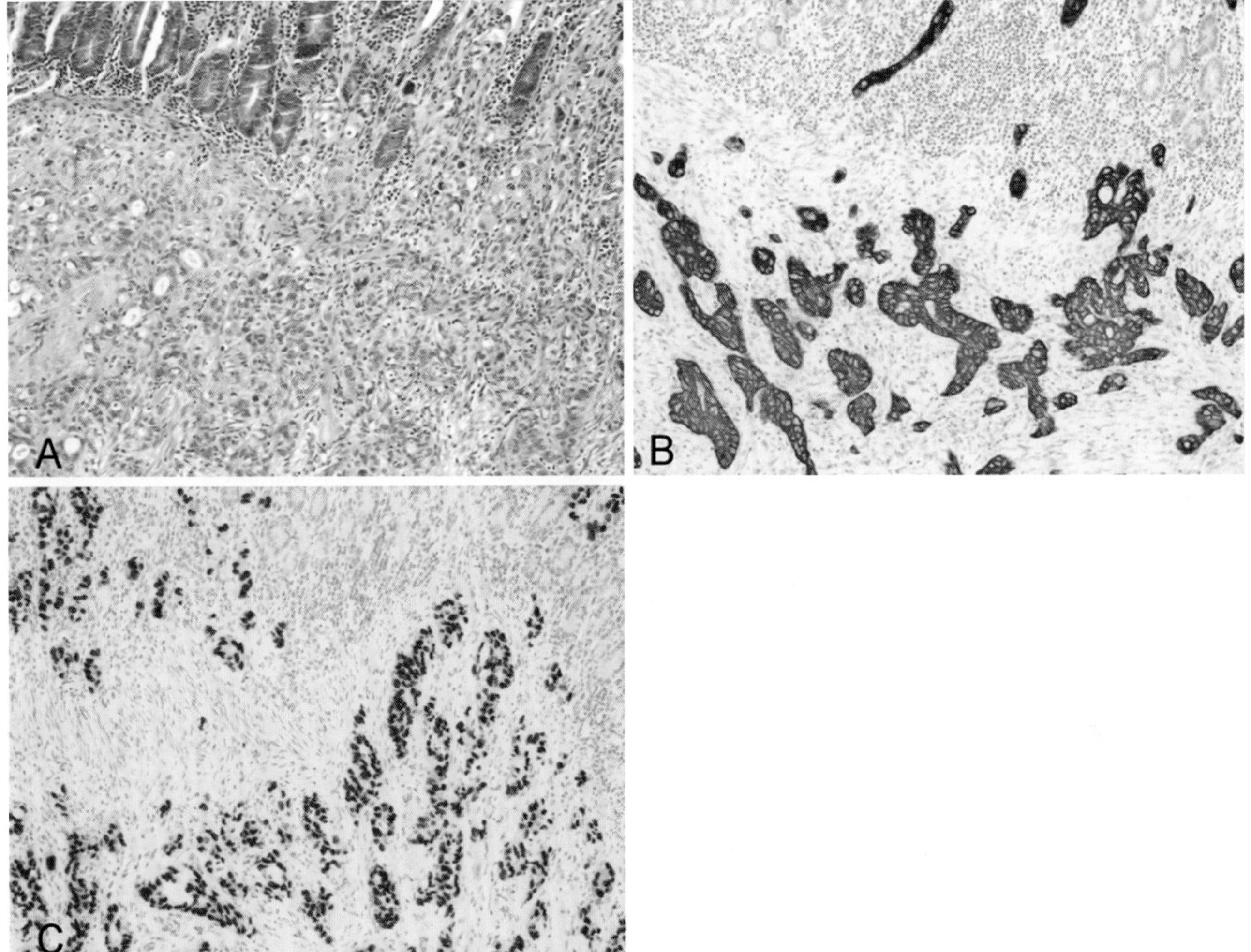

FIGURE 42–2 Poorly differentiated CUP in an 85-year-old male with a small intestine resection. **A:** A representative hematoxylin and eosin–stained section. **B–C:** Immunohistochemical staining of sections from the same block as in **(A)**. **B:** Diffuse strong staining for CK7. **C:** Diffuse strong staining for TTF-1. Immunostains for CK20, CDX2, Hep Par 1, SMAD4, and PSA were negative (not shown). The case was signed out as suggestive of a pulmonary primary.

TTF-1 in recognizing poorly differentiated adenocarcinoma, is positive in some TTF-1–negative cases, and, thus, has additional value in establishing CUP origin from the lung.[42,43] Napsin A is positive in renal cell carcinomas (RCCs) of clear and papillary type and should be used with caution when clear cell or papillary features are present.[42]

Thyroid Carcinomas

Thyroid carcinomas of the papillary type preferentially metastasize to the lymph nodes of the neck, while follicular carcinomas (and also to a lesser degree papillary carcinomas) spread by hematogenous route to lungs, bone, brain, and various other organs. In these tumors, the CK7+/CK20– pattern is dominant. As already mentioned above, 95% to 100% of thyroid carcinomas express TTF-1 and thyroglobulin and 90% express Pax8, a transcription factor crucial for organogenesis of the thyroid gland, kidney, and mullerian system.[41,45,46] A widely metastasizing anaplastic thyroid carcinoma tends to lose TTF-1 and thyroglobulin reactivity; however, 79% of cases retain Pax8 expression, a particularly useful feature in differentiation from poorly differentiated/undifferentiated pulmonary carcinoma.[50] Pax8 is also expressed in renal and mullerian carcinomas and, thus, is best used in panels with other thyroid markers.[45,46]

Breast Adenocarcinoma

Breast adenocarcinoma commonly metastasizes into axillary lymph nodes, bone, lung/pleura, liver, ovary, adrenal glands, and brain. Invasive lobular carcinoma, especially the signet ring cell variant, has a distinctive pattern of metastasizing to the peritoneum, gastrointestinal tract, and ovaries. Although breast cancer only represents approximately 2% of CUPs, in a recent study, breast carcinomas represented 20% of latent primary tumors subsequently identified during life at least 2 months after the initial CUP diagnosis.[51] Approximately 90% of breast cancers are CK7+/CK20– and the remaining are CK7+/CK20+.[38] The most specific immunomarker for breast carcinoma is GCDFP-15, a protein of breast cystic fluid expressed in apocrine glands of various derivation (cytoplasmic stain, Fig. 42.1).[52] GCDFP-15 is 95% specific for breast adenocarcinoma; however its sensitivity is lower, varying from 40% to 75%.[52-54] GCDFP-15 reactivity is also present in a subset of salivary gland and prostate carcinomas and rare skin, ovarian, kidney, and bladder carcinomas.[52] Until recently, GCDFP-15 was thought to reliably distinguish breast carcinoma from pulmonary carcinoma; however, several studies indicate that approximately 5% of pulmonary adenocarcinomas express GCDFP-15.[55] Importantly, half of GCDFP-15-positive lung carcinomas were negative for TTF-1, which may lead to an erroneous diagnosis of breast cancer. Fortunately, none of GCDFP-15–positive lung carcinomas expressed estrogen receptor (ER), progesterone receptor (PR), or mammaglobin (see below). Thus, it is prudent to use additional breast and lung markers, such as ER, mammaglobin, and Napsin A, to confidently differentiate breast and pulmonary carcinomas.[53,55]

Sex hormone receptors, such as ER-α and PR (both nuclear staining), are important group of markers used to predict the origin of a metastasis from the breast or gynecological (GYN) tract. Approximately 75% of metastatic breast cancers are positive for ER (see Fig. 42.1).[56] PR expression is usually heterogeneous in extent and intensity and may be absent altogether. The utility of ER was questioned in reports describing significant ER positivity, sometimes in more than 50% of cases, in pulmonary and gastrointestinal adenocarcinomas.[57] Based on the review of multiple published studies, Wei et al.,[58] have shown that this reactivity is user-dependent and is mostly relevant in the lung with the use of antibody clone 6F11, rather than the clone 1D5. ER reactivity is extremely rare with both antibody clones in gastrointestinal carcinomas. Monoclonal anti-PR antibody reactivity (excluding clone 1A6) is almost 100% specific for carcinomas of the breast or GYN tract origin.[58] Thus, double-positive staining for ER and PR is highly specific for tumors of the breast or mullerian system. It should be noted that ER-β is more widely expressed in different tissues and is not used as a marker for differential diagnostic purposes.

Mammaglobin, a product of the breast-specific gene (cytoplasmic staining), is more sensitive, but less specific marker than GCDFP-15. Its major strength is that it is expressed irrespective of the ER/PR status.[54] It is positive in a subset of endometrioid and salivary gland carcinomas and few melanomas and is best used in a panel with other breast markers.

Hepatocellular Carcinoma

Hepatocellular carcinoma metastasizes most commonly to the adrenal glands and bone. Because of the variants of morphology, including clear cell, pseudo-glandular, and eosinophilic patterns, it may be difficult to distinguish from metastatic adenocarcinoma, RCC, adrenocortical carcinoma, and neuroendocrine carcinoma. Approximately 75% of hepatocellular carcinomas are CK7–/CK20–, which is rarely seen in adenocarcinomas, except prostate adenocarcinoma. Additionally, 20% are CK7+/CK20– and 5% are CK7+/CK20+. Hep Par 1, an antibody to liver mitochondrial enzyme (granular cytoplasmic staining), is strongly positive in benign liver tissue and is considered the most sensitive marker of hepatocellular carcinoma (>90%).[59,60] It is usually negative or sometimes only focally positive in the majority of other carcinomas including intrahepatic cholangiocarcinoma. However, strong staining can be seen in gastric, esophageal, and pulmonary adenocarcinomas and this pitfall should be kept in mind.[59,60] The sensitivity of Hep Par 1 decreases to approximately 50% in poorly differentiated hepatocellular carcinoma.

Another valuable marker is albumin mRNA which is detected by in situ hybridization and is diagnostic of hepatocellular origin. However, this test is not widely available.[61] Additional specific markers are the epithelial markers MOC31 and monoclonal CEA which are uniformly negative in hepatocellular carcinoma and positive in metastatic adenocarcinomas.[62] A metastatic CC-RCC and adrenocortical carcinoma can be generally distinguished from a clear cell hepatocellular carcinoma due to their Hep Par1-/Pax2+/Vimentin+ and Hep Par 1-/Melan A+/Inhibin+ profiles, respectively. Neuroendocrine tumors may have abundant clear or eosinophilic cytoplasm and centrally located nuclei reminiscent of hepatocellular carcinoma; however, they are Hep Par1–/Synaptophysin+/Chromogranin+.

Colorectal Adenocarcinoma

Colorectal adenocarcinoma metastasizes most frequently to the liver, peritoneum, ovaries, and lung. A typical histologic feature that is diagnostically helpful and present in metastases is "dirty necrosis" within glandular lumina consisting of inspissated eosinophilic material intermixed with cellular and nuclear debris. More than 80% of colorectal adenocarcinomas and even higher proportion of metastases exhibit the CK7–/CK20+ pattern, shared only by Merkel cell carcinomas and a subset of gastric carcinomas. However, approximately 10% have the CK7+/CK20+ pattern and another 10% have the CK7–/CK20– pattern; the latter being mostly associated with high levels of microsatellite instability. Importantly, the CK7+/CK20– pattern seen in many types of carcinomas almost never occurs in colorectal cancers. Intestinal origin is supported by usually diffuse and strong nuclear staining for CDX2, a transcription factor controlling intestinal differentiation (nuclear staining, Fig. 42.3). CDX2 staining is positive in 97% to 99% of colorectal adenocarcinomas and their metastases.[63,64] However, it may be absent in some high-grade tumors. For example, the majority of rare colonic medullary carcinomas, also known as undifferentiated carcinomas, do not express CDX2.[64,65] These, as well as some other high-grade tumors, also lose CK20 staining due to their high microsatellite instability

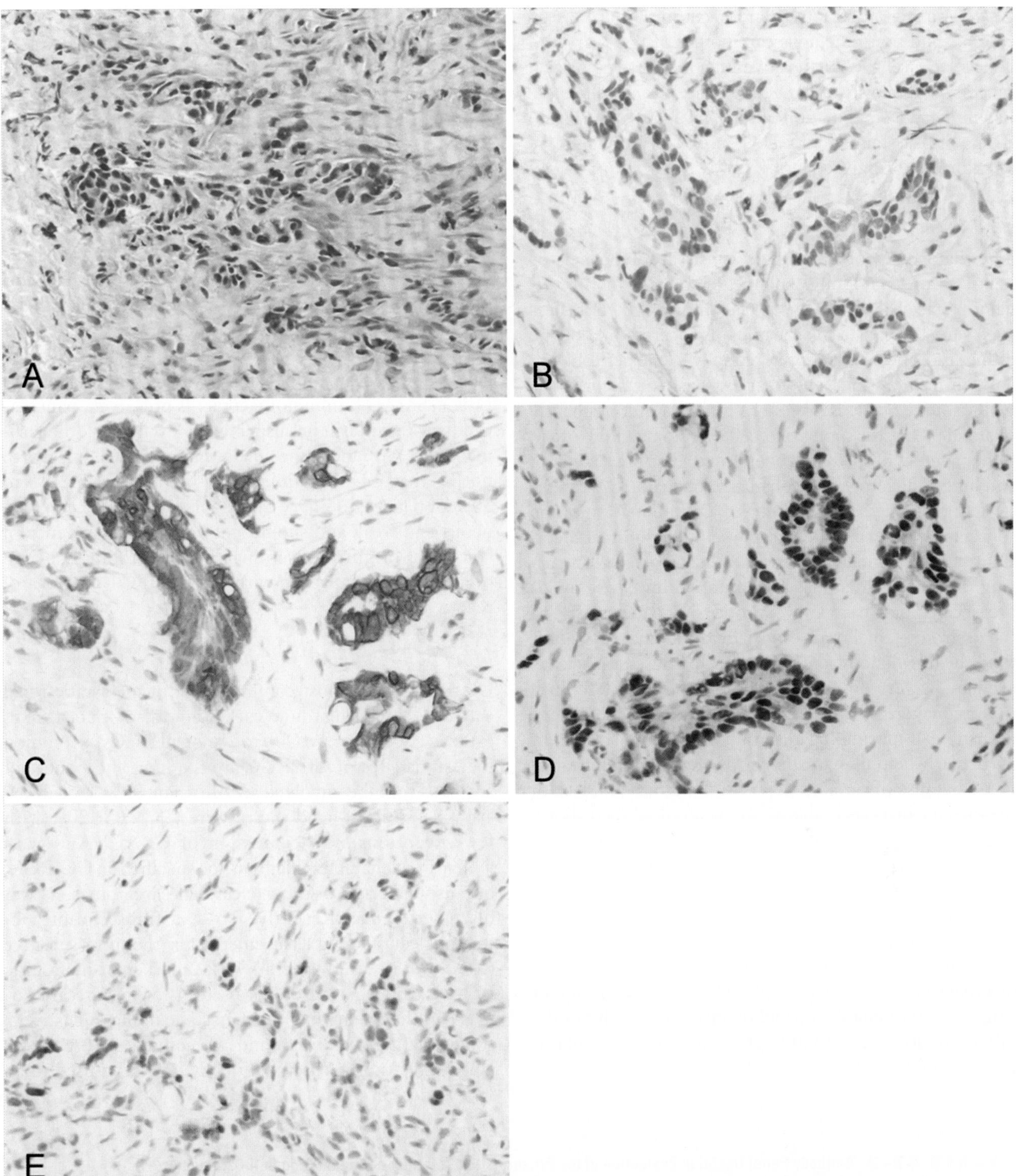

FIGURE 42–3 Poorly differentiated CUP involving the peritoneum, omentum, and liver in a 37-year-old male with pleural effusion. **A:** A hematoxylin and eosin–stained section of a peritoneal nodule. **B–E:** Immunohistochemical staining of sections from the same block as in **(A)**. **B:** Negative staining for CK7. **C:** Diffuse strong staining for CK20. **D:** Diffuse strong staining for CDX2. **E:** Heterogeneous positivity for TTF-1. Immunostains for PSA and PLAP were negative (not shown). The case was signed out as suggestive of a colorectal primary. Focal TTF-1 positivity was considered spurious. Interpretation of Tissue of Origin test from Pathworks Diagnostics also favored colorectal primary with moderate to high confidence.

phenotype and, in a metastatic site, may enter into the differential diagnosis of CK7–/CK20–/CDX2– carcinomas.

Weak, focal, or heterogeneous CDX2 staining is seen in 60% to 70% of gastric and esophageal adenocarcinomas and in 20% to 30% of pancreatic and biliary tract adenocarcinomas.[64] Non-digestive organ tumors with intestinal differentiation, such as bladder adenocarcinoma and mucinous adenocarcinomas of the ovary, are commonly

CDX2-positive. Prostate adenocarcinoma, thyroid carcinoma, and non-mucinous carcinomas of the ovary and uterus are rarely weakly positive. In contrast to colorectal cancers, the majority of these tumors are CK7-positive.[63,66] In summary, a combination of CK7–/CK20+ pattern and strong diffuse staining for CDX2 in a CUP are suggestive of colorectal origin (see Fig. 42.2).

Gastric Adenocarcinoma

The major sites of distant metastasis are liver, peritoneum, ovaries, and lung. Adenocarcinoma of the intestinal type (according to Lauren classification) metastasizes preferentially to the liver, while adenocarcinoma of the diffuse type metastasizes preferentially to the peritoneum, gastrointestinal tract, and ovaries. Gastric cancer is the major source of the Krukenberg tumor, a predominantly bilateral metastatic signet ring cell carcinoma of the ovary. Other sources of the Krukenberg tumor are breast, colon, and lung, which together constitute the majority of metastatic signet ring cell carcinomas.[67] Differentiation of the source of signet ring cell carcinoma in abdominal metastatic sites that include gastrointestinal organs is a recurring diagnostic dilemma. For example, invasive lobular breast carcinoma has a known propensity to metastasize to the gastrointestinal tract, especially the stomach. In addition, the distinction from the primary diffuse gastric cancer may be very difficult morphologically, because both tumors may grow in a single cell pattern and show signet ring cell morphology. Immunohistochemistry is not particularly helpful in the diagnosis of gastric adenocarcinoma because of variable CK7/CK20 pattern and lack of site-specific markers (Table 42.2). As was described above, gastric cancers are positive for CDX2 in approximately two-thirds of cases and the staining is characteristically heterogeneous and weak, but may be strong sometimes. Another relatively helpful marker is Hep Par-1, which is expressed in approximately 50% of gastric carcinomas, including both intestinal and diffuse types.[68] It is also positive in 80% of gastric and 20% of colorectal signet ring cell carcinomas.[67] A panel of antibodies useful in the differentiation of metastatic signet ring cell carcinomas is given in Table 42.2.

Pancreatic and Biliary Tract Carcinomas

The major sites of distant metastases of pancreatic ductal and biliary tract adenocarcinomas are similar to gastric cancer: the liver, peritoneum, bone, and lung. As is true for gastric cancer, immunohistochemistry is not particularly helpful in the diagnosis of pancreatic or biliary tract carcinomas. More than 90% of the tumors are CK7-positive; staining for CK20 is variable (see Table 42.1).[38] One relatively specific, but not sensitive, marker is a transcriptional co-factor DPC4/SMAD4 (cytoplasmic and nuclear staining). Its immunoreactivity is completely lost in approximately 55% of pancreatic ductal carcinomas and distal common bile duct carcinomas.[69,70] It is also lost with lesser frequency in other biliary tract, gallbladder, colon, and ampullary adenocarcinomas.[71] If DPC4/SMAD4 immunoreactivity is preserved, pancreatobiliary origin can be suspected by excluding other primary sites with more specific immunoprofiles. It is worth noting that CDX2 staining may be positive in 20% to 30% of pancreatobiliary cancers but is usually heterogeneous and weak and should not be taken as evidence of colorectal origin.[64] In summary, pancreatobiliary origin of a CUP is compatible with CK7+/DPC4– pattern of reactivity.

Clear Cell Renal Cell Carcinoma

CC-RCC is the most common type of metastatic renal cancer. Collecting duct carcinoma also metastasizes extensively, but is rare (1% to 2% of all RCCs). Common metastatic sites of CC-RCC are the lung and bone, but any site may be involved. More than 90% of tumors are CK7–/CK20– and the rest are CK7+/CK20– (with few exceptions). Co-expression of CKAE1/AE3 with vimentin is characteristic, but not specific for CC-RCC, because it occurs in other clear cell carcinomas, as was discussed above. Recently, Pax-2, a transcription factor (nuclear staining), has emerged as the most sensitive (74% to 85%) and specific (90%) marker of metastatic CC-RCC.[72,73] It is also expressed in few other carcinomas—in the majority of the metastatic mullerian cancers, some parathyroid cancers, and rare colonic and breast carcinomas.[74] Another useful antibody is RCC, raised to an

TABLE 42-2 Antibody Panel Useful in Evaluation of the Primary Site of Metastatic Signet Ring Cell Carcinoma

Antibody	Breast Carcinoma	Gastric Carcinoma	Colorectal Carcinoma	Lung Carcinoma
CK20	–	+/–	+	–
ER	+	–	–	–
Mammaglobin	+	–	–	–
GCDFP-15	+/–	–	–	–
TTF-1	–	–	–	+
Napsin A	–	–	–	+
CDX2	–	+/–, heterogeneous	+, homogeneous	–
Hep Par-1	–	+	–/+	–

antigen of the glycoprotein of the proximal renal tubule (membranous and/or cytoplasmic reactivity). However, Pax-2 is preferable to RCC, because of higher sensitivity in metastatic CC-RCC, lesser problems with specificity, and more straightforward interpretation of staining.[72,73] One drawback of PAX2 is that it is not helpful in distinguishing CC-RCC from clear cell carcinoma of the ovary, which is also positive for PAX-2 (see below). RCC and CD10 can be used to distinguish CC-RCC from clear cell carcinoma of the ovary, which will be negative for these markers. CD10 (membranous and cytoplasmic stain) has high sensitivity for CC-RCC, but low specificity and is best used in a panel.

Ovarian and Uterine Adenocarcinomas

These mullerian (originating from the mullerian ducts) adenocarcinomas metastasize most commonly to the peritoneal cavity, often producing malignant ascites. The majority of CUPs originate from the ovary. Multiple histologic variants including clear cell, mucinous, and high-grade serous carcinomas pose significant problems of differential diagnosis with gastrointestinal and pancreatobiliary tumors, especially in small samples. A related problem is differentiating a primary ovarian carcinoma from a metastasis to the ovary. In this latter respect, conventional pathologic assessment can be helpful even before applying immunohistochemistry. Mounting data suggest that all bilateral mucinous carcinomas and a substantial majority of unilateral mucinous carcinomas measuring less than 10 to 12 cm are of metastatic origin.[75] Metastatic Krukenberg tumor is discussed in the section on gastric adenocarcinoma.

Two-thirds of ovarian mucinous carcinomas are CK7+/CK20+. The remaining ovarian mucinous carcinomas and all other ovarian, endometrial, and endocervical carcinomas are C7+/CK20−. Because an overwhelming majority of these tumors are CK7 positive, a negative CK7 stain nearly completely excludes a mullerian origin.

WT1 is a site-restricted marker helpful in suggesting ovarian/primary peritoneal origin of a CUP. It is a transcription factor (nuclear staining) and a product of Wilms tumor suppressor gene that is important in normal urogenital and mesothelial development and Wilms tumorogenesis. WT1 is positive in greater than 80% of ovarian serous and primary peritoneal carcinomas and a subset of uterine serous carcinomas.[76] It is also positive in a few other cancers, such as mesothelioma, melanoma, acute myeloid and lymphoid leukemias, and various sarcomas. Importantly, and advantageously, WT1 is not expressed in carcinomas of the lung, breast, gastrointestinal tract, pancreas, and biliary tract which commonly enter into the differential diagnosis of CUPs of the peritoneal cavity. In addition to WT1, ER and PR are positive in approximately 70% of ovarian non-mucinous and endometrial adenocarcinomas. ER and PR reactivity supports the interpretation of WT1 positivity as a marker of a serous carcinoma of the GYN tract. It is important to keep in mind that ER and PR are generally negative in the primary ovarian mucinous carcinomas of intestinal type and in endocervical adenocarcinomas.[76,77]

Urothelial Carcinoma

Distant metastases are most commonly seen in the lung, liver, bone, and brain. The majority of urothelial carcinomas express CK7; however, expression of CK20 varies ranging from 22% to 89%. More consistently, CK20 expression was observed in 46% to 58% of tumors, including metastasis.[78,79] Thus, metastatic urothelial carcinoma has both CK7+/CK20+ and CK7+/CK20− patterns.

Uroplakin III is a urothelium-specific protein expressed in differentiated urothelial cells (membranous staining). However, it is positive in only 25% to 50% of metastatic urothelial carcinomas.[78,80] A useful panel consisting of a high molecular weight keratin (also known as CK34betaE12 or keratin 903), thrombomodulin, and CK20 has been proposed.[78] These markers are nonspecific when used in isolation, but their co-expression is not encountered in most non-urothelial carcinomas.[78]

Neuroendocrine Tumors

Both well-differentiated neuroendocrine tumors (WDNETs) and poorly differentiated neuroendocrine carcinomas have CK7−/CK20− and CK7+/CK20− patterns (see Table 42.1). The only exception is Merkel cell carcinoma, which has the CK7−/CK20+ profile and characteristic paranuclear dot-like expression of CK20. In general, neuroendocrine differentiation is supported by diffuse and strong staining with at least one of two general neuroendocrine markers, synaptophysin and chromogranin, which have proved to be highly specific (both cytoplasmic staining). Synaptophysin has better sensitivity than chromogranin and these markers are usually used together.

WDNETs, also known as carcinoids, represent a minority (10%) of neuroendocrine CUPs.[81] They are most often seen in the liver, bone, or lymph nodes and their main primary sources are the gastrointestinal tract, pancreas, and lung. These tumors may have histologic features resembling metastatic adenocarcinoma, RCC, adrenocortical carcinoma, and hepatocellular carcinoma. An indolent course is characteristic. Interestingly, in a recent and largest to date series of 71 patients presenting with liver metastases of WDNET, 15 of 17 patients had an unknown primary site and underwent surgical exploration. In 13 of 15 patients, the primary tumor was found and all 13 originated in the small intestine. The authors concluded that, although the pancreas was the most common primary site overall, an occult WDNET of the pancreas was unlikely to be a source of liver metastases.[82]

Several markers may be helpful in suggesting a primary site of WDNET. TTF-1 is strongly positive in 43% to 80% of metastatic pulmonary WDNET and is absent in WDNET from other locations.[83,84] CDX2 marks metastatic midgut (ileal) WDNET with high sensitivity. Recently, reactivity for PDX1, NESP-55, or Pax8 in the absence of staining for CDX-2 and TTF-1 was suggested as markers for pancreatic WDNET.[85,86] Of note, pancreatic WDNET may show variable, usually weak CDX-2 reactivity in approximately 20% of cases.[86]

Poorly differentiated neuroendocrine tumors include small cell carcinoma, comprising 15% of all neuroendocrine CUPs, and large cell carcinoma, comprising 75% of neuroendocrine CUPs and 10% of all poorly differentiated CUPs.[81] Both subtypes are aggressive tumors arising from the lung and various other organs that respond favorably to platinum-based chemotherapy. The differential diagnosis of small cell carcinoma includes lymphoma, poorly differentiated squamous cell carcinoma, Ewing sarcoma/PNET, and some other small blue cell tumors. Large cell neuroendocrine carcinoma may be very difficult to distinguish from a poorly differentiated/undifferentiated adenocarcinoma on hematoxylin and eosin–stained sections, and although some architectural and cytologic neuroendocrine features may be discernible on close inspection, a high level of suspicion and immunohistochemistry are usually required to make the diagnosis.

Poorly differentiated neuroendocrine carcinoma of the lung, both of small cell and large cell types, is usually positive for TTF-1.[87] However, extrapulmonary neuroendocrine carcinomas are also positive for TTF-1, except Merkel cell carcinoma.[87,88] Therefore, TTF-1 expression by itself should not be used to suggest pulmonary origin of poorly differentiated neuroendocrine carcinoma in extrapulmonary sites.

Squamous Cell Carcinoma

For practical purposes, squamous differentiation in a CUP suggests only a few locations, such as head and neck, lung, esophagus, and the anogenital area (including uterine cervix, vulva, vagina, penis, and anus).[89] Metastasis of squamous cell carcinoma to the upper and mid-cervical lymph nodes is most compatible with the origin from a head and neck primary and portends favorable prognosis. Involvement of lower cervical lymph nodes suggests pulmonary or esophageal origin. Involvement of inguinal nodes is usually due to a primary carcinoma of the anogenital area. The majority of squamous cell carcinomas are CK7–/CK20–, and approximately a quarter is CK7+/CK20–. A high molecular weight keratin CK5 is one of the most sensitive markers of squamous differentiation. Monoclonal antibody against CK5/6 is usually used (cytoplasmic staining) and it is positive in 75% to 100% of squamous cell carcinomas from various organs.[89,90] Its specificity, however, is not perfect because CK5/6 reactivity is observed in the majority of mesotheliomas, urothelial carcinomas, in a subset of pulmonary adenocarcinomas, breast carcinomas of basal/myoepithelial type, ovarian serous and clear cell carcinomas, and rare colonic and other gastrointestinal carcinomas.[89,90] Another useful marker is p63, a transcription factor controlling squamous differentiation (nuclear staining). It is positive in 81% of poorly differentiated squamous cell carcinomas of various locations.[89] It is also positive in the majority of urothelial carcinomas and in a subset of adenocarcinomas of the breast, lung, kidney, ovary, gastrointestinal tract, and pancreas.[89,90] Thus, neither CK5/6 nor p63 is specific for squamous cell carcinoma; however, their coordinated expression was 97% specific in one study.[89] Coordinate expression of CK5/6 and p63 may be present in urothelial carcinoma; thus, additional markers are needed to differentiate urothelial carcinoma from squamous cell carcinoma (see above).

Gene Expression Profiling for Prediction of Primary Site of CUP

An alternative approach to tumor typing is transcriptional profiling based on measuring the levels of differentially expressed mRNAs. Multiple studies have shown that microarray-based and quantitative reverse transcriptase polymerase chain reaction–based (qRT-PCR) gene expression techniques enable accurate prediction of the site of origin of both primary and metastatic tumors.[91-94] When applied to CUPs, the same approaches have shown robust ability to predict the primary site based on indirect correlations with clinicopathologic features (including immunohistochemistry) and response to therapy as "best guess" surrogates for the site of origin.[92,93] Importantly, direct correlation has recently shown 75% accuracy of primary site prediction by a qRT-PCR–based gene expression profiling in 15 of 20 patients with latent primary tumors subsequently identified during life at least 2 months after the initial CUP diagnosis.[51] The main advantage of a microarray-based method is the ability to interrogate thousands of genes, generating massive expression signatures. qRT-PCR may provide broader dynamic range and is more applicable to formalin-fixed paraffin-embedded (FFPE) tissue, features important in the design of a clinical test. Other requirements considered to be important for a clinical test are availability of laser microdissection to enrich the population of malignant cells from small heterogeneous samples and compatibility with a low number of test cells (300 to 500).[95]

More recently, specific cancer types and their metastases were also shown to have consistent patterns of expression of micro-RNAs (miRNAs). miRNAs are small non-coding RNAs that regulate mRNA translation, show highly tissue-specific expression, and are well preserved in FFPE tissue.[96] The feasibility of using miRNA expression profiles to predict the primary site of CUP with high accuracy has been recently demonstrated based on correlations with clinicopathologic features.[97]

Commercialized gene expression tests are currently offered by several reference laboratories clinically to help predict the site of origin of CUP (Table 42.3). Two such tests based on mRNA expression profiling that are available in the United States are the Pathwork Tissue

TABLE 42-3 Clinically Available Molecular Tests for Tissue of Origin Prediction in CUPss

Test	Manufacturer	Sample Type	Test Format	Accuracy	Tissue Type Representation	FDA Cleared	References
Pathwork Tissue of Origin Test	Pathwork Diagnostics, Redwood City, CA	FFPE	2000-Gene microarray	89% (462 FFPE samples)	15 tissue types	Yes	Pillai et al.[98]
CancerTYPE ID	bioTheranostics, Inc., San Diego, CA	FFPE	92-Gene qRT-PCR	83% (187 FFPE samples)	30 tissue types	No	Erlander et al.[99]
ProOnc TumorSource Dx	Prometheus, Inc., San Diego, CA	FFPE	48-miRNA qRT-PCR	84% (74 FFPE samples	25 tissue types	No	Rosenfeld et al.[96] Varadhachary et al.[97]
CupPrint	Agendia, BV, Amsterdam, The Netherlands	FFPE	1900-Gene microarray	83% (84 FFPE samples)	9 tissue types	No, but CE approved	Ma et al.[94]

CE, European conformity marking; FDA, Food and drug administration; FFPE, Formalin-fixed paraffin-embedded tissue; miRNA, microRNA; qRT-PCR, quantitative reverse-transcription polymerase chain reaction.
Adapted from Monzon FA, Medeiros F, Lyons-Weiler M, Henner WD, Identification of tissue of origin in carcinoma of unknown primary with a microarray-based gene expression test. *Diagn Pathol.* 2010;5:3.

of Origin test (Pathwork Diagnostics, Redwood City, CA) and the CancerType ID test (bioTheranostics, San Diego, CA).

The Pathwork Tissue of Origin test has the distinction of being the only FDA-approved test. It was originally developed to analyze the expression of 1,550 genes on an Affymetrix (Santa Clara, CA) microarray using mRNA derived from frozen tumor tissue. More recently, the Pathwork Tissue of Origin test has been adapted to accommodate the variably degraded mRNA extracted from FFPE tissue, making the test more suitable for the clinical setting.[98] Currently, the Tissue of Origin test analyzes the expression of 2,000 genes to create a "similarity score" for each of 15 potential tissues types that were included in the original training set. A validation study using 462 FFPE tissue specimens (25 to 57 specimens for each of 15 tissue types) from metastatic tumors or primary tumors that were either poorly differentiated or undifferentiated was performed and found 88.5% agreement with the clinical diagnoses.[98]

A different approach was taken in the design of the CancerTYPE ID (bioTheranostics, Inc., San Diego, CA) test, which uses qRT-PCR to selectively analyze the expression of only 92 genes allowing differentiation between 30 cancer types and 54 histological subtypes with a sensitivity of 83%.[99] This test was developed using a reference set of 2,206 tumor specimens and tested on a first set of 187 tumors and then a second set of 300 cases submitted for clinical testing. Larger scale validation studies are ongoing, which are analyzing reproducibility across multiple institutions. In addition, patient outcomes are being evaluated in prospective studies in which treatment is directed based on the results of this assay.[99]

One miRNA assay has been patented for clinical testing: the ProOnc TumorSource Dx (Prometheus, Inc., San Diego, CA). This is a 48-miRNA qRT-PCR–based assay which uses a binary decision tree and a K-nearest neighbor analysis to assign 25 tumor diagnoses. In a prospective validation study of 84 FFPE CUP tumor samples, 74 cases were successfully processed and the assay tumor assignment was compatible with the clinicopathologic "working diagnosis" in 84%.[97]

The role of gene expression profiling in the clinical prediction of a CUP primary site is not yet fully defined. Studies comparing the accuracy of predictions by gene expression profiling and by immunohistochemistry are not available, since there is no "gold standard" of a primary site determination in CUP. In the author's limited experience, immunohistochemistry and Pathwork Tissue of Origin test were similarly effective at predicting a primary site. Some aspects of commercial gene expression profiling tests to consider are significant cost (approximate list price $3600 to 4000), centralized testing, proprietary nature, and complexity. Future studies are needed to establish whether molecular profiling tests are useful in situations where immunohistochemical evaluation suggests multiple primary sites or where immunohistochemistry is noncontributory.

REFERENCES

1. Pentheroudakis G, Briasoulis E, Pavlidis N. Cancer of unknown primary site: missing primary or missing biology? *Oncologist.* 2007;12(4):418-425.
2. Varadhachary GR, Abbruzzese JL, Lenzi R. Diagnostic strategies for unknown primary cancer. *Cancer.* 2004;100(9):1776-1785.
3. Greco FA, Hainsworth JD. Cancer of unknown primary site. In: DeVita VTJ, Lawrence TS, Rosenberg SA, eds. *Cancer: Principles and Practice of Oncology.* Philadelphia, PA: Lippincott Williams & Wilkins; 2008:2363-2387.
4. Jemal A, Siegel R, Xu J, Ward E. Cancer statistics, 2010. *CA Cancer J Clin.* 2010;60(5):277-300.

5. Blaszyk H, Hartmann A, Bjornsson J. Cancer of unknown primary: clinicopathologic correlations. *APMIS*. 2003;111(12): 1089-1094.
6. Pavlidis N, Briasoulis E, Pentheroudakis G. Cancers of unknown primary site: ESMO Clinical Practice Guidelines for diagnosis, treatment and follow-up. *Ann Oncol*. 2010;21(suppl 5): v228-v231.
7. Varadhachary GR, Talantov D, Raber MN, et al. Molecular profiling of carcinoma of unknown primary and correlation with clinical evaluation. *J Clin Oncol*. 2008;26(27):4442-4448.
8. Seve P. Clinical presentations of metastatic carcinomas of unknown origin. In: Wick MR, ed. *Metastatic Carcinomas of Unknown Origin*. New York, NY: Demos; 2008:1-26.
9. Abbruzzese JL, Abbruzzese MC, Hess KR, Raber MN, Lenzi R, Frost P. Unknown primary carcinoma: natural history and prognostic factors in 657 consecutive patients. *J Clin Oncol*. 1994;12(6):1272-1280.
10. Seve P, Sawyer M, Hanson J, Broussolle C, Dumontet C, Mackey JR. The influence of comorbidities, age, and performance status on the prognosis and treatment of patients with metastatic carcinomas of unknown primary site: a population-based study. *Cancer*. 2006;106(9):2058-2066.
11. Stewart JF, Tattersall MH, Woods RL, Fox RM. Unknown primary adenocarcinoma: incidence of overinvestigation and natural history. *Br Med J*. 1979;1(6177):1530-1533.
12. Maiche AG. Cancer of unknown primary. A retrospective study based on 109 patients. *Am J Clin Oncol*. 1993;16(1):26-29.
13. Hamilton CS, Langlands AO. ACUPS (adenocarcinoma of unknown primary site): a clinical and cost benefit analysis. *Int J Radiat Oncol Biol Phys*. 1987;13(10):1497-1503.
14. Al-Brahim N, Ross C, Carter B, Chorneyko K. The value of postmortem examination in cases of metastasis of unknown origin-20-year retrospective data from a tertiary care center. *Ann Diagn Pathol*. 2005;9(2):77-80.
15. Pentheroudakis G, Golfinopoulos V, Pavlidis N. Switching benchmarks in cancer of unknown primary: from autopsy to microarray. *Eur J Cancer*. 2007;43(14):2026-2036.
16. van de Wouw AJ, Janssen-Heijnen ML, Coebergh JW, Hillen HF. Epidemiology of unknown primary tumours; incidence and population-based survival of 1285 patients in Southeast Netherlands, 1984-1992. *Eur J Cancer*. 2002;38(3):409-413.
17. Stoyianni A, Pentheroudakis G, Pavlidis N. Neuroendocrine carcinoma of unknown primary: a systematic review of the literature and a comparative study with other neuroendocrine tumors. *Cancer Treat Rev*. 2011;37(5):358-365.
18. DeYoung BR, Wick MR. Immunohistologic evaluation of metastatic carcinomas of unknown origin: an algorithmic approach. *Semin Diagn Pathol*. 2000;17(3):184-193.
19. Oien KA. Pathologic evaluation of unknown primary cancer. *Semin Oncol*. 2009;36(1):8-37.
20. Bhargava R, Dabbs DJ. Immunohistology of metastatic carcinomas of unknown primary. In: Dabbs DJ, ed. *Diagnostic Immunohistochemistry*. 3rd ed. Philadelphia, PA: Saunders; 2010:206-255.
21. Bahrami A, Truong LD, Ro JY. Undifferentiated tumor: true identity by immunohistochemistry. *Arch Pathol Lab Med*. 2008;132(3):326-348.
22. Lau SK, Prakash S, Geller SA, Alsabeh R. Comparative immunohistochemical profile of hepatocellular carcinoma, cholangiocarcinoma, and metastatic adenocarcinoma. *Hum Pathol*. 2002;33(12):1175-1181.
23. Sangoi AR, Fujiwara M, West RB, et al. Immunohistochemical distinction of primary adrenal cortical lesions from metastatic clear cell renal cell carcinoma: a study of 248 cases. *Am J Surg Pathol*. 2011;35(5):678-686.
24. Hsu JD, Han CP. Anti-Cytokeratin CAM 5.2 (Becton Dickinson) is not synonymous with CK8/18 monoclonal antibody. Comment on "Pancreatic-type mixed acinar-endocrine carcinoma with alpha-fetoprotein production arising from the stomach: a report of an extremely rare case. *Med Mol Morphol.* (2009) 42:167-174". *Med Mol Morphol*. 2010;43(1):65.
25. Kamposioras K, Pentheroudakis G, Pectasides D, Pavlidis N. Malignant melanoma of unknown primary site. To make the long story short. A systematic review of the literature. *Crit Rev Oncol Hematol*. 2011;78(2):112-126.
26. Banerjee SS, Harris M. Morphological and immunophenotypic variations in malignant melanoma. *Histopathology*. 2000;36(5):387-402.
27. Chang P, Knapper WH. Metastatic melanoma of unknown primary. *Cancer*. 1982;49(6):1106-1111.
28. Ohsie SJ, Sarantopoulos GP, Cochran AJ, Binder SW. Immunohistochemical characteristics of melanoma. *J Cutan Pathol*. 2008;35(5):433-444.
29. Bishop PW, Menasce LP, Yates AJ, Win NA, Banerjee SS. An immunophenotypic survey of malignant melanomas. *Histopathology*. 1993;23(2):159-166.
30. Herrera GA, Turbat-Herrera EA, Lott RL. S-100 protein expression by primary and metastatic adenocarcinomas. *Am J Clin Pathol*. 1988;89(2):168-176.
31. Busam KJ, Iversen K, Coplan KA, et al. Immunoreactivity for A103, an antibody to melan-A (Mart-1), in adrenocortical and other steroid tumors. *Am J Surg Pathol*. 1998;22(1):57-63.
32. Biddle DA, Evans HL, Kemp BL, et al. Intraparenchymal nevus cell aggregates in lymph nodes: a possible diagnostic pitfall with malignant melanoma and carcinoma. *Am J Surg Pathol*. 2003;27(5):673-681.
33. Ozdemirli M, Fanburg-Smith JC, Hartmann DP, et al. Precursor B-lymphoblastic lymphoma presenting as a solitary bone tumor and mimicking Ewing's sarcoma: a report of four cases and review of the literature. *Am J Surg Pathol*. 1998;22(7): 795-804.
34. Gustafson S, Medeiros LJ, Kalhor N, Bueso-Ramos CE. Anaplastic large cell lymphoma: another entity in the differential diagnosis of small round blue cell tumors. *Ann Diagn Pathol*. 2009;13(6):413-427.
35. Traweek ST, Arber DA, Rappaport H, Brynes RK. Extramedullary myeloid cell tumors. An immunohistochemical and morphologic study of 28 cases. *Am J Surg Pathol*. 1993;17(10):1011-1019.
36. Nandedkar MA, Palazzo J, Abbondanzo SL, Lasota J, Miettinen M. CD45 (leukocyte common antigen) immunoreactivity in metastatic undifferentiated and neuroendocrine carcinoma: a potential diagnostic pitfall. *Mod Pathol*. 1998;11(12):1204-1210.
37. Azumi N, Battifora H. The distribution of vimentin and keratin in epithelial and nonepithelial neoplasms. A comprehensive immunohistochemical study on formalin- and alcohol-fixed tumors. *Am J Clin Pathol*. 1987;88(3):286-296.
38. Chu PG, Weiss LM. Keratin expression in human tissues and neoplasms. *Histopathology*. 2002;40(5):403-439.
39. Wang NP, Zee S, Zarbo RJ, Bacchi CE, Gown AM. Coordinate expression of cytokeratins 7 and 20 defines unique subsets of carcinomas. *Appl Immunohistochem*. 1995;3:99-107.
40. Chu P, Wu E, Weiss LM. Cytokeratin 7 and cytokeratin 20 expression in epithelial neoplasms: a survey of 435 cases. *Mod Pathol*. 2000;13(9):962-972.
41. Kaufmann O, Dietel M. Thyroid transcription factor-1 is the superior immunohistochemical marker for pulmonary adenocarcinomas and large cell carcinomas compared to surfactant proteins A and B. *Histopathology*. 2000;36(1):8-16.
42. Bishop JA, Sharma R, Illei PB. Napsin A and thyroid transcription factor-1 expression in carcinomas of the lung, breast, pancreas, colon, kidney, thyroid, and malignant mesothelioma. *Hum Pathol*. 2010;41(1):20-25.
43. Ye J, Findeis-Hosey JJ, Yang Q, et al. Combination of napsin A and TTF-1 immunohistochemistry helps in differentiating primary lung adenocarcinoma from metastatic carcinoma in the lung. *Appl Immunohistochem Mol Morphol*. 2011;19(4):313-317.
44. Comperat E, Zhang F, Perrotin C, et al. Variable sensitivity and specificity of TTF-1 antibodies in lung metastatic adenocarcinoma of colorectal origin. *Mod Pathol*. 2005;18(10):1371-1376.
45. Laury AR, Perets R, Piao H, et al. A comprehensive analysis of PAX8 expression in human epithelial tumors. *Am J Surg Pathol*. 2011;35(6):816-826.
46. Tacha D, Zhou D, Cheng L. Expression of PAX8 in normal and neoplastic tissues: a comprehensive immunohistochemical study. *Appl Immunohistochem Mol Morphol*. 2011;19(4):293-299.
47. Kubba LA, McCluggage WG, Liu J, et al. Thyroid transcription factor-1 expression in ovarian epithelial neoplasms. *Mod Pathol*. 2008;21(4):485-490.

48. Matoso A, Singh K, Jacob R, et al. Comparison of thyroid transcription factor-1 expression by 2 monoclonal antibodies in pulmonary and nonpulmonary primary tumors. *Appl Immunohistochem Mol Morphol.* 2010;18(2):142-149.
49. Inamura K, Satoh Y, Okumura S, et al. Pulmonary adenocarcinomas with enteric differentiation: histologic and immunohistochemical characteristics compared with metastatic colorectal cancers and usual pulmonary adenocarcinomas. *Am J Surg Pathol.* 2005;29(5):660-665.
50. Nonaka D, Tang Y, Chiriboga L, Rivera M, Ghossein R. Diagnostic utility of thyroid transcription factors Pax8 and TTF-2 (FoxE1) in thyroid epithelial neoplasms. *Mod Pathol.* 2008;21(2):192-200.
51. Greco FA, Spigel DR, Yardley DA, Erlander MG, Ma XJ, Hainsworth JD. Molecular profiling in unknown primary cancer: accuracy of tissue of origin prediction. *Oncologist.* 2010;15(5):500-506.
52. Wick MR, Lillemoe TJ, Copland GT, Swanson PE, Manivel JC, Kiang DT. Gross cystic disease fluid protein-15 as a marker for breast cancer: immunohistochemical analysis of 690 human neoplasms and comparison with alpha-lactalbumin. *Hum Pathol.* 1989;20(3):281-287.
53. Yang M, Nonaka D. A study of immunohistochemical differential expression in pulmonary and mammary carcinomas. *Mod Pathol.* 2010;23(5):654-661.
54. Bhargava R, Beriwal S, Dabbs DJ. Mammaglobin vs GCDFP-15: an immunohistologic validation survey for sensitivity and specificity. *Am J Clin Pathol.* 2007;127(1):103-113.
55. Wang LJ, Greaves WO, Sabo E, et al. GCDFP-15 positive and TTF-1 negative primary lung neoplasms: a tissue microarray study of 381 primary lung tumors. *Appl Immunohistochem Mol Morphol.* 2009;17(6):505-511.
56. O'Connell FP, Wang HH, Odze RD. Utility of immunohistochemistry in distinguishing primary adenocarcinomas from metastatic breast carcinomas in the gastrointestinal tract. *Arch Pathol Lab Med.* 2005;129(3):338-347.
57. Lau SK, Chu PG, Weiss LM. Immunohistochemical expression of estrogen receptor in pulmonary adenocarcinoma. *Appl Immunohistochem Mol Morphol.* 2006;14(1):83-87.
58. Wei S, Said-Al-Naief N, Hameed O. Estrogen and progesterone receptor expression is not always specific for mammary and gynecologic carcinomas: a tissue microarray and pooled literature review study. *Appl Immunohistochem Mol Morphol.* 2009;17(5):393-402.
59. Fan Z, van de Rijn M, Montgomery K, Rouse RV. Hep par 1 antibody stain for the differential diagnosis of hepatocellular carcinoma: 676 tumors tested using tissue microarrays and conventional tissue sections. *Mod Pathol.* 2003;16(2):137-144.
60. Kakar S, Muir T, Murphy LM, Lloyd RV, Burgart LJ. Immunoreactivity of Hep Par 1 in hepatic and extrahepatic tumors and its correlation with albumin in situ hybridization in hepatocellular carcinoma. *Am J Clin Pathol.* 2003;119(3): 361-366.
61. Oliveira AM, Erickson LA, Burgart LJ, Lloyd RV. Differentiation of primary and metastatic clear cell tumors in the liver by in situ hybridization for albumin messenger RNA. *Am J Surg Pathol.* 2000;24(2):177-182.
62. Porcell AI, De Young BR, Proca DM, Frankel WL. Immunohistochemical analysis of hepatocellular and adenocarcinoma in the liver: MOC31 compares favorably with other putative markers. *Mod Pathol.* 2000;13(7):773-778.
63. Werling RW, Yaziji H, Bacchi CE, Gown AM. CDX2, a highly sensitive and specific marker of adenocarcinomas of intestinal origin: an immunohistochemical survey of 476 primary and metastatic carcinomas. *Am J Surg Pathol.* 2003;27(3):303-310.
64. Barbareschi M, Murer B, Colby TV, et al. CDX-2 homeobox gene expression is a reliable marker of colorectal adenocarcinoma metastases to the lungs. *Am J Surg Pathol.* 2003;27(2):141-149.
65. Hinoi T, Tani M, Lucas PC, et al. Loss of CDX2 expression and microsatellite instability are prominent features of large cell minimally differentiated carcinomas of the colon. *Am J Pathol.* 2001;159(6):2239-2248.
66. Kaimaktchiev V, Terracciano L, Tornillo L, et al. The homeobox intestinal differentiation factor CDX2 is selectively expressed in gastrointestinal adenocarcinomas. *Mod Pathol.* 2004;17(11):1392-1399.
67. Chu PG, Weiss LM. Immunohistochemical characterization of signet-ring cell carcinomas of the stomach, breast, and colon. *Am J Clin Pathol.* 2004;121(6):884-892.
68. Fan Z, Li J, Dong B, Huang X. Expression of Cdx2 and hepatocyte antigen in gastric carcinoma: correlation with histologic type and implications for prognosis. *Clin Cancer Res.* 2005;11(17):6162-6170.
69. Wilentz RE, Su GH, Dai JL, et al. Immunohistochemical labeling for dpc4 mirrors genetic status in pancreatic adenocarcinomas: a new marker of DPC4 inactivation. *Am J Pathol.* 2000;156(1):37-43.
70. Argani P, Shaukat A, Kaushal M, et al. Differing rates of loss of DPC4 expression and of p53 overexpression among carcinomas of the proximal and distal bile ducts. *Cancer.* 2001;91(7):1332-1341.
71. Maitra A, Molberg K, Albores-Saavedra J, Lindberg G. Loss of Dpc4 expression in colonic adenocarcinomas correlates with the presence of metastatic disease. *Am J Pathol.* 2000;157(4):1105-1111.
72. Sangoi AR, Karamchandani J, Kim J, Pai RK, McKenney JK. The use of immunohistochemistry in the diagnosis of metastatic clear cell renal cell carcinoma: a review of PAX-8, PAX-2, hKIM-1, RCCma, and CD10. *Adv Anat Pathol.* 2010;17(6):377-393.
73. Gokden N, Gokden M, Phan DC, McKenney JK. The utility of PAX-2 in distinguishing metastatic clear cell renal cell carcinoma from its morphologic mimics: an immunohistochemical study with comparison to renal cell carcinoma marker. *Am J Surg Pathol.* 2008;32(10):1462-1467.
74. Zhai QJ, Ozcan A, Hamilton C, et al. PAX-2 expression in non-neoplastic, primary neoplastic, and metastatic neoplastic tissue: a comprehensive immunohistochemical study. *Appl Immunohistochem Mol Morphol.* 2010;18(4):323-332.
75. Yemelyanova AV, Vang R, Judson K, Wu LS, Ronnett BM. Distinction of primary and metastatic mucinous tumors involving the ovary: analysis of size and laterality data by primary site with reevaluation of an algorithm for tumor classification. *Am J Surg Pathol.* 2008;32(1):128-138.
76. Nofech-Mozes S, Khalifa MA, Ismiil N, et al. Immunophenotyping of serous carcinoma of the female genital tract. *Mod Pathol.* 2008;21(9):1147-1155.
77. Vang R, Gown AM, Barry TS, Wheeler DT, Ronnett BM. Immunohistochemistry for estrogen and progesterone receptors in the distinction of primary and metastatic mucinous tumors in the ovary: an analysis of 124 cases. *Mod Pathol.* 2006;19(1): 97-105.
78. Parker DC, Folpe AL, Bell J, et al. Potential utility of uroplakin III, thrombomodulin, high molecular weight cytokeratin, and cytokeratin 20 in noninvasive, invasive, and metastatic urothelial (transitional cell) carcinomas. *Am J Surg Pathol.* 2003;27(1):1-10.
79. Miettinen M. Keratin 20: immunohistochemical marker for gastrointestinal, urothelial, and Merkel cell carcinomas. *Mod Pathol.* 1995;8(4):384-388.
80. Matsumoto K, Satoh T, Irie A, et al. Loss expression of uroplakin III is associated with clinicopathologic features of aggressive bladder cancer. *Urology.* 2008;72(2):444-449.
81. Spigel DR, Hainsworth JD, Greco FA. Neuroendocrine carcinoma of unknown primary site. *Semin Oncol.* 2009;36(1):52-59.
82. Wang SC, Parekh JR, Zuraek MB, et al. Identification of unknown primary tumors in patients with neuroendocrine liver metastases. *Arch Surg.* 2010;145(3):276-280.
83. Lin X, Saad RS, Luckasevic TM, Silverman JF, Liu Y. Diagnostic value of CDX-2 and TTF-1 expressions in separating metastatic neuroendocrine neoplasms of unknown origin. *Appl Immunohistochem Mol Morphol.* 2007;15(4):407-414.
84. Oliveira AM, Tazelaar HD, Myers JL, Erickson LA, Lloyd RV. Thyroid transcription factor-1 distinguishes metastatic pulmonary from well-differentiated neuroendocrine tumors of other sites. *Am J Surg Pathol.* 2001;25(6):815-819.
85. Long KB, Srivastava A, Hirsch MS, Hornick JL. PAX8 expression in well-differentiated pancreatic endocrine tumors: correlation with clinicopathologic features and comparison with gastrointestinal and pulmonary carcinoid tumors. *Am J Surg Pathol.* 2010;34(5):723-729.
86. Srivastava A, Hornick JL. Immunohistochemical staining for CDX-2, PDX-1, NESP-55, and TTF-1 can help distinguish gastrointestinal carcinoid tumors from pancreatic

endocrine and pulmonary carcinoid tumors. *Am J Surg Pathol.* 2009;33(4):626-632.
87. Kaufmann O, Dietel M. Expression of thyroid transcription factor-1 in pulmonary and extrapulmonary small cell carcinomas and other neuroendocrine carcinomas of various primary sites. *Histopathology.* 2000;36(5):415-420.
88. Agoff SN, Lamps LW, Philip AT, et al. Thyroid transcription factor-1 is expressed in extrapulmonary small cell carcinomas but not in other extrapulmonary neuroendocrine tumors. *Mod Pathol.* 2000;13(3):238-242.
89. Kaufmann O, Fietze E, Mengs J, Dietel M. Value of p63 and cytokeratin 5/6 as immunohistochemical markers for the differential diagnosis of poorly differentiated and undifferentiated carcinomas. *Am J Clin Pathol.* 2001;116(6):823-830.
90. Reis-Filho JS, Simpson PT, Martins A, Preto A, Gartner F, Schmitt FC. Distribution of p63, cytokeratins 5/6 and cytokeratin 14 in 51 normal and 400 neoplastic human tissue samples using TARP-4 multi-tumor tissue microarray. *Virchows Arch.* 2003;443(2):122-132.
91. Ramaswamy S, Tamayo P, Rifkin R, et al. Multiclass cancer diagnosis using tumor gene expression signatures. *Proc Natl Acad Sci U S A.* 2001;98(26):15149-15154.
92. Tothill RW, Kowalczyk A, Rischin D, et al. An expression-based site of origin diagnostic method designed for clinical application to cancer of unknown origin. *Cancer Res.* 2005;65(10):4031-4040.
93. Talantov D, Baden J, Jatkoe T, et al. A quantitative reverse transcriptase-polymerase chain reaction assay to identify metastatic carcinoma tissue of origin. *J Mol Diagn.* 2006;8(3):320-329.
94. Ma XJ, Patel R, Wang X, et al. Molecular classification of human cancers using a 92-gene real-time quantitative polymerase chain reaction assay. *Arch Pathol Lab Med.* 2006;130(4):465-473.
95. Greco FA, Erlander MG. Molecular classification of cancers of unknown primary site. *Mol Diagn Ther.* 2009;13(6):367-373.
96. Rosenfeld N, Aharonov R, Meiri E, et al. MicroRNAs accurately identify cancer tissue origin. *Nat Biotechnol.* 2008;26(4):462-469.
97. Varadhachary GR, Spector Y, Abbruzzese JL, et al. Prospective gene signature study using microRNA to identify the tissue of origin in patients with carcinoma of unknown primary. *Clin Cancer Res.* 2011;17(12):4063-4070.
98. Pillai R, Deeter R, Rigl CT, et al. Validation and reproducibility of a microarray-based gene expression test for tumor identification in formalin-fixed, paraffin-embedded specimens. *J Mol Diagn.* 2011;13(1):48-56.
99. Erlander MG, Ma XJ, Kesty NC, Bao L, Salunga R, Schnabel CA. Performance and clinical evaluation of the 92-gene real-time PCR assay for tumor classification. *J Mol Diagn.* 2011;13(5):493-503.

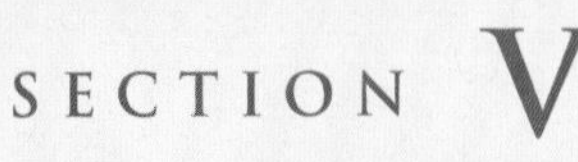

SECTION V

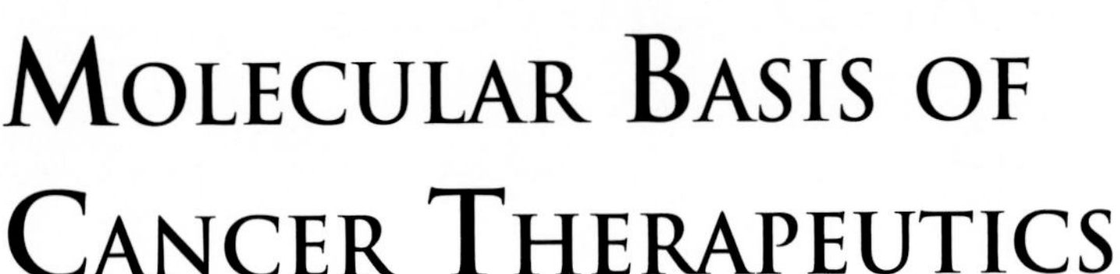

Molecular Basis of Cancer Therapeutics

CHAPTER 43

DNA Repair and Cancer Therapeutics

Mark R. Kelley and Melissa L. Fishel

INTRODUCTION

A cell's genome is its most valuable asset. The information encoded in DNA describes every cellular process, so protecting the genome is essential for ensuring faithful, accurate transmission of information to future generations of cells. However, genomic integrity is constantly challenged by both endogenous and exogenous insults: toxic by-products from normal metabolism and inflammatory responses, environmental xenobiotics, or anticancer treatments.[1] In addition, epigenetics, post-translational modifications, and other factors either help promote or inhibit the production of proteins essential for DNA repair and maintenance.[2] Cancer can deregulate virtually every aspect of DNA repair and derail genomic stability; therefore, the study of DNA repair in its broadest sense seeks to understand (1) mechanistically how repair works on a molecular level, (2) how cancer ambushes and alters DNA repair processes, and (3) how to manipulate those same processes to kill cancer cells.

Many chemotherapeutics and radiotherapeutics work by damaging DNA, so efficient DNA damage response and repair diminish the effectiveness of those treatments. Even though dysfunctional DNA damage recognition and response are cancer hallmarks,[3] cancer has extensive abilities to compensate for such losses, skewing normal levels of repair proteins or recruiting alternate pathways for repair.[4] Intrinsic or acquired resistance of this nature must be overcome, which historically has been achieved by administering a cocktail of chemotherapeutics or a combination of chemotherapy and radiotherapy. However, toxicities and collateral damage increase as more therapeutics are added due to death of normal cells. Treatments that preferentially target cancer cells can alleviate this persistent problem.

One category of new anticancer treatments that fits this bill is small-molecule DNA repair inhibitors, which are showing utility both as a single agent and as adjunctive agents. The most promising molecular targets that are also DNA repair proteins (1) are unique to a repair pathway, (2) are rate-limiting factors, (3) are upregulated due to stimulation from oncogenic pathways, or (4) capitalize on an inherited (germ line) or cancer-induced repair weakness. As each pathway is discussed in this chapter, the reasons for targeting various proteins are described within this framework.

DNA repair inhibitors not only can limit additional toxicities, but they also can produce more than a simple additive effect. These targeted therapeutics often capitalize on a repair weakness to create a synthetic lethality—a situation where mutations of two genes occurring separately can still support cellular viability, but their combined inhibition leads to cell death. Dual inhibition of proteins that results in synthetic lethality is both highly effective and highly selective for cancer killing.[3,5] Poly(ADP-ribose) polymerase (PARP) inhibitors for treating BRCA-deficient breast cancers are the most stunning clinical example to date of exploiting synthetic lethality.

Many inhibitors have caused dose-limiting toxicities when combined with other agents, so a number of strategies are being tested to minimize that problem while maximizing these inhibitors' effectiveness. Strategies include intermittent or alternate scheduling of inhibitors with chemotherapy, using inhibitors as single agents, and pairing inhibitors with localized radiation treatments.[6]

OVERVIEW: HOW DNA REPAIR WORKS

With one exception, DNA repair pathways follow four general steps that can be remembered as "the four Rs": Recognition, Removal, Resynthesis, and Restoration.

In broadest terms, the damage site is *recognized* and made accessible for repairs. Then the damaged base or

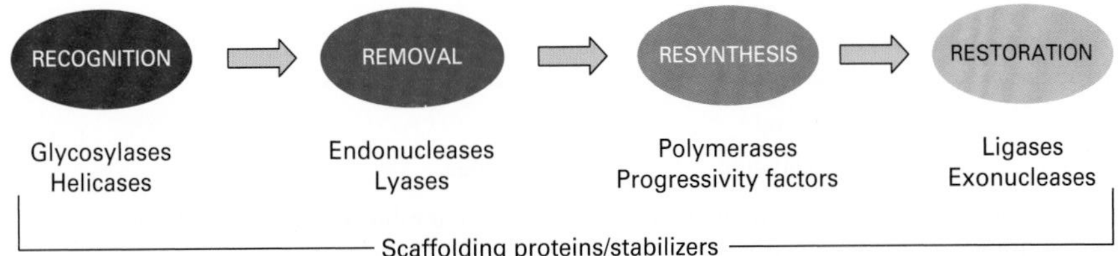

FIGURE 43–1 Broad categories of proteins involved in DNA repair.

bases are *removed* and the site is "prepped" and processed so it can receive the new base(s). This is followed by *resynthesis*: generation of new nucleotide(s) to fill the gap. The final step of *restoring* the DNA helix involves "sealing" the repair site, which may additionally include a "cleanup" process. Figure 43.1 depicts these steps and the repair proteins typically involved in each.

If each repair pathway were a self-contained, rigidly ordered sequence of steps with each repair protein having only one or a few discrete functions, then developing repair inhibitors for clinical use would be fairly straightforward. However, cross talk between pathways occurs, and many proteins directly or indirectly influence other repair pathways. The order in which DNA repair proteins normally assemble to perform their work is unknown and may be altered under oncogenic conditions. In addition, identification of accessory and scaffold proteins involved in the pathways is ongoing. Collectively, this contributes to the complexity of mechanistically understanding DNA repair—and how cancers can alter those pathways for survival purposes. This chapter (1) gives a simplified overview of the steps involved in each DNA repair pathway, (2) describes which proteins in those steps are good targets for inhibition, (3) lists inhibitors that are in development as anticancer agents, and (4) explains the challenges involved in those processes.

While this discussion is limited to DNA repair pathways and their inhibitors, two other categories of related inhibitors need to be mentioned briefly: reduction–oxidation (redox) inhibitors and checkpoint inhibitors.

Redox signaling affects gene expression by making transcription factors bind more or less readily to DNA, which has downstream effects on protein expression.[7-9] Human apurinic/apyrimidinic endonuclease 1 (APE1), a major repair protein of the base excision repair (BER) pathway, exerts redox regulation on a number of transcription factors that affect DNA repair and cell survival and proliferation. Several redox inhibitors are in preclinical development; in vitro studies show that the one specific to APE1 can make tumor cells sensitive to ionizing radiation (IR) and alkylating chemotherapeutics.[10-12]

Checkpoints are a component of the broader scope of DNA damage response. Checkpoints help ensure that DNA reproduction occurs without error, so they are activated at critical phases of the cell cycle when DNA damage is detected. This halts the cell cycle, allowing DNA repairs to take place before progression to the next cell cycle phase is permitted. A hallmark of tumorigenesis is faulty checkpoint activation, which allows damage to go unrepaired.[13] Some checkpoint inhibitors are already clinically available and many more are in development.[14,15]

DIRECT REPAIR (DR)

The DR pathway is the only mode of DNA repair that (1) uses a single protein for its repair, (2) corrects the actual damage without removing the damaged base itself, and (3) is not enzyme driven. The sole protein involved in this simple, efficient repair is O^6-alkylguanine-DNA methyltransferase, also called MGMT or AGT. One molecule of MGMT has the ability to remove only one alkyl group from certain oxygen positions of damaged guanine and thymine bases. When MGMT binds the alkyl group in a stoichiometric reaction, the protein is inactivated and subsequently degraded. Thus, cells need to continually make more MGMT to continue with the repair of these lesions.

MGMT was the first DNA repair gene to be studied at length.[16] It also was the first entity studied for repair inhibition, and it was the target of the first DNA repair inhibitor ever developed—more than 10 years ago.[6] Table 43.1 summarizes research developments to date for MGMT inhibition. More than 20 years of studying of MGMT has revealed many aspects of DNA repair in general, which continue to guide translational research of repair inhibitors overall. Without MGMT repair, alkyl adducts would cause thymine mispairings during replication, leading to erroneous G:C-to-A:T transitions or strand breaks, which would necessitate the involvement of other pathways for DNA repair. Although MGMT is not critical for survival, its influence on other pathways and the multitude of effects its deficiency causes make it an important linchpin in the overall scheme of DNA repair.[6]

BASE EXCISION REPAIR

Pathway Overview

The BER pathway corrects some of the most prevalent forms of DNA damage that occur due to oxidation, alkylation, deamination, and IR. BER repairs single-base (non-helix-distorting) damage that, if left unchecked, would cause incorrect base pairings. If those mispairings were transcribed, the resulting mutations would affect genomic integrity.[8,18] Thus, BER is critical to genome maintenance.

BER repair begins when 1 of 11 damage-specific DNA glycosylases recognizes and removes a damaged base. The glycosylase hydrolyzes the N-glycosidic bond of the

TABLE 43–1 O^6-alkylguanine-DNA methyltransferase Inhibitors in Development and Clinical Use[16,17]

DR Protein	Function(s)	Why It Is a Good Target for Inhibition	Challenges	Compounds Being Investigated
MGMT	• Removes alkyl groups from the O^6 position of guanine and, to a lesser extent, the O^4 position of thymine	• A discrete protein with a highly specialized function in one repair pathway • Methylating *MGMT*'s gene promoter sensitizes cells to alkylating agents and IR	• MGMT inhibition affects both healthy cells and tumor cells • MGMT levels vary greatly among cancers and even within tumor cells • MGMT inhibition does not work if a deficiency exists in the MMR pathway • Other pathways can repair methylating damage in the absence of MGMT	• O^6-BG; first drug developed as a chemosensitizer; still in clinical use today • KU-60019 (cell studies)

O^6-BG, O^6-benzylguanine; DR, direct repair; MGMT, O^6-alkylguanine-DNA methyltransferase; IR, ionizing radiation; MMR, mismatch repair.

damaged nucleotide and flips the damaged base out of the DNA helix into a pocket of the enzyme, leaving an abasic or apyrimidinic/apurinic (AP) site on the helix.[19,20] This AP site is not only the substrate for the next repair step, but it is also a cytotoxic intermediate.[21] To alleviate this potential threat to DNA integrity, repairs need to progress swiftly and accurately without disrupting the cell cycle. Thus, an AP endonuclease needs to process the loose ends left behind from the excision.

In contrast to the plethora of glycosylases that can catalyze the excision step, a single protein called APE1 or APE1/Ref-1 (apurinic/apyrimidinic endonuclease/redox effector factor-1) is responsible for more than 95% of all endonuclease activities.[8] This key activity creates special termini to prep are the abasic site for insertion of the correct resynthesized base.[22] Then a polymerase adds the new base, and a DNA ligase completes the repair by sealing the nick in the single-stranded DNA, restoring the phosphodiester backbone and the helix's integrity.[23,24]

Three other types of proteins also participate in BER. The most ubiquitous type is a scaffolding protein, particularly XRCC1. In general, all scaffolding proteins (1) help stabilize the damaged area during the repair; (2) provide a "base" upon which other proteins attach to perform repairs; (3) increase the helix distortion so that repair proteins can access the damage site more easily; (4) recruit, coordinate, and stimulate other enzymes; and (5) perform additional functions that are still being elucidated.[22,25]

A special protein called PARP1 (poly-ADP ribose polymerase 1) helps assess the extent of the damage and determines whether to signal for repair, apoptosis, or cell cycle arrest. The cell cycle may be halted temporarily to allow sufficient time for the repair to be completed. PARP1 also acts as a scaffold for core BER proteins.[26] Although PARP1 is dispensable to BER, it interacts with other pathways, as noted later in this section regarding its inhibitors (see Fig 43.2 for an overview of the steps involved in BER). Other proteins that perform specialized functions in one BER sub-pathway are discussed in the following paragraphs.

In a class by itself, APE1 performs many other functions, most notably a unique redox function. Numerous transcription factors must stay in a reduced, activated state to bind properly to DNA and thus maintain cellular signaling. APE1 maintains the activity of those transcription factors by reducing them via a thiol/sulfide exchange.[8] Selective inhibition of APE1's redox function is a subject of intense research.

Short- versus Long-Patch BER

BER consists of two sub-pathways: short-patch (SP) and long-patch (LP) BER. These sub-pathways diverge after APE1 performs its endonuclease function. As the pathways' names suggest, the former handles single-base damage that can be repaired quickly, while the latter handles repairs that (1) take longer, (2) involve more repair proteins, and (3) require resynthesis of 2 to 8 nucleotides surrounding the AP site. The structure of the AP site also influences which pathway is induced[8,27] (Fig. 43.2).

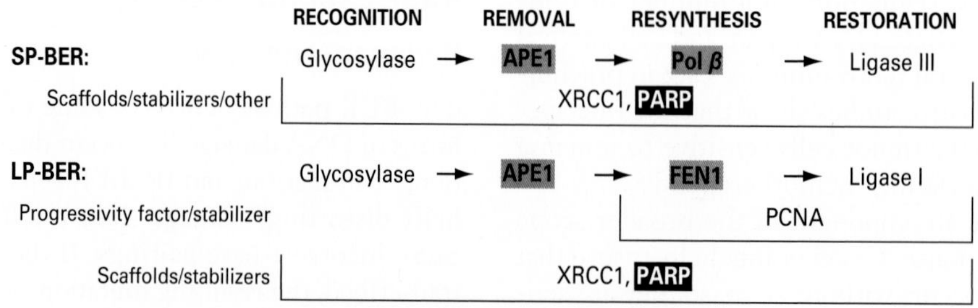

FIGURE 43–2 Overview of base excision repair pathway and targets of inhibitors.

When LP resynthesis occurs, a "flap" of the old nucleotides is left, so the last step of LP-BER before ligation is to cut off that flap, using a special protein called flap endonuclease 1 (FEN1). Other proteins used solely in LP repair include a sliding clamp (PCNA or proliferating cell nuclear antigen), which stabilizes the site and facilitates nucleotide resynthesis, and a replication factor-C (RFC), which inserts the correct nucleotides. The types of polymerases and ligases differ between SP-BER and LP-BER as well.[4]

The mechanisms by which one sub-pathway is chosen over the other are still being investigated; however, numerous factors drive this decision, including (1) the source and type of damage, (2) the type of AP site generated in the first repair step,[8] and (3) the cell cycle phase in progress when the damage occurs.[27]

Small-Molecule Inhibitors in Development

Many chemotherapeutics, including alkylating agents, platinating agents, cytotoxic antibiotics, and taxanes, create DNA lesions that the BER pathway normally repairs.[28-34] From an oncology standpoint, the more impaired BER is, the more effective anticancer agents will be in damaging the DNA of tumor cells and inducing apoptosis. To that end, four BER proteins are being investigated as potential targets for inhibition. Those proteins are FEN1, polymerase β (Pol β), APE1, and PARP. Table 43.2 The first two are still in early stages of preclinical development. Inhibitors of both APE1's repair and redox functions are in various stages of late preclinical development. A number of PARP inhibitors are already in clinical use,

TABLE 43-2 Base Excision Repair Inhibitors in Development and Clinical Use[18]

BER Protein	Function(s)	Why It Is a Good Target for Inhibition	Challenges	Compounds Being Investigated
APE1	• *Repair:* preps AP site to receive new nucleotide(s) • *Redox:* maintains genes in their active, reduced state	• Overexpressed in many cancers • Associated with resistance to alkylating and oxidizing agents • No substitute exists for this protein	• Achieving specificity to solely inhibit the repair or redox function	*Repair:* • Non-specific: • Methoxyamine (binds to the aldehyde in the AP site of DNA) • Lucanthone, miracil D (Top II inhibitors) • Specific: • CRT0044876 • AR03 *Redox:* • E3330 and newer analogs
Pol β	• Resynthesizes nucleotides • Removes certain blocking residues	• A rate-limiting step in BER • Often overexpressed in tumor cells • Associated with resistance to IR, bleomycin, some alkylating agents, and cisplatin	• Difficult to develop an inhibitor specific to the polymerase domain that would not also inhibit polymerases involved in DNA replication • Inhibiting its lyase function may be more lucrative	>60 inhibitors identified; most lacked specificity Most promising so far (cell studies only): • Oleanolic acid • Edgeworin • Betulinic acid • Stigmasterol • NCS-666715
FEN1	• Progressivity factor • Helps polymerases synthesize nucleotides efficiently and accurately	• Elevated in many cancers • Inhibition creates unligatable DNA and makes cells hypersensitive to alkylating agents		• A few hydroxyurea-based FEN1 inhibitors (earliest investigative stages)
PARP1	• Surveillance/damage sensor • Assesses extent of damage; determines whether to signal apoptosisp • Helps decondense chromatin • Recruits repair proteins to the damage site • Facilitates repairs	• Uses NAD^+ to transfer ADP-ribose polymers onto specific acceptor proteins including itself; this modifies the protein's properties • Although not essential to BER, PARP1's absence causes an accumulation of DNA damage that certain cancers cannot repair • Inhibitors potentiate the effects of alkylating agents, platinating agents, topoisomerase I poisons, and IR	• Secondary mutations can correct for this repair deficiency, causing resistance to PARP inhibitors	• PARP inhibitors are already being used to treat familial breast cancers and other cancers with BRCA-like features • >70 clinical trials in progress for second-generation PARP inhibitors and broader use of first-generation inhibitors

BER, base excision repair; APE1, human apurinic/apyrimidinic endonuclease 1; AP, apurinic/apyrimidinic; Pol β, polymerase β; IR, ionizing radiation; FEN1, flap endonuclease 1; PARP1, poly-ADP ribose polymerase 1; NAD^+, nicotinamide adenine dinucleotide ADP, adenosine diphosphate.

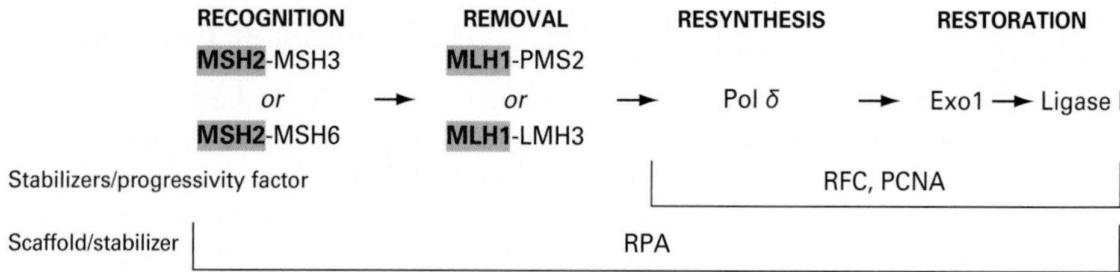

FIGURE 43–3 Overview of mismatch repair pathway and targets of inhibitors.

and trials are ongoing for second-generation PARP inhibitors.[6] Table 43.2 summarizes the roles of these proteins in BER and the challenges involved in creating specific, clinically useful inhibitors to them.

MISMATCH REPAIR (MMR) PATHWAY

MMR prevents mutations from becoming permanent in dividing cells by correcting DNA mismatches generated during DNA replication. A defect or deficiency in MMR greatly increases the spontaneous mutation rate and predisposition to cancer.[35] Not surprisingly, certain inherited cancers such as hereditary non-polyposis colorectal cancer are due to MMR deficiencies. Up to 20% of sporadic cancers are due to MMR defects as well.[36]

Numerous studies have shown that an intact, functioning MMR pathway is essential for proper activation of cell cycle checkpoints; otherwise, DNA damage may proceed unchecked through replication.[35] Such "damage tolerance" creates resistance to a wide variety of chemotherapeutics.

Pathway Overview

MMR corrects single-base-pair mismatches (A–G, T–C) or misaligned short nucleotide repeats (small-loop insertions or deletions) that, if unrepaired, would cause frameshift mutations. Such mismatches occur during the S phase of DNA replication when the errors escape detection by other means.[37]

As with all other pathways, repairs begin when the damage is sensed. In MMR, this is accomplished by a heterodimer of MSH2:MSH6 or MSH2:MSH3. The former recognizes both insertion–deletion mispairs and single-base mismatches, while the latter recognizes only insertion–deletion mispairs. After identifying the type of mismatch, MSH proteins recruit MutL homolog 1 (MLH1) and its binding partners, postmeiotic segregation increased 1 (PMS1) protein and PMS2, to determine the specific strand error. The endonuclease MutL removes the DNA lesion; a DNA polymerase synthesizes a new strand; an exonuclease (Exo1) removes the nucleotides that were replaced; and a DNA ligase completes the repair.[37]

Other proteins are involved as well. RFC helps load PCNA, which functions as a progressivity factor, initiating and facilitating the polymerase's resynthesis work. Replication protein A (RPA) protects the site throughout the repair and functions as a project manager, overseeing all the steps of MMR. Figure 43.3 shows the repair steps of MMR.

Small-Molecule Inhibitors in Development

Manipulating MMR for clinical use presents a unique challenge to researchers seeking to develop new anticancer treatments. In contrast to other pathways where a repair deficiency represents a weakness to exploit, an MMR deficiency causes increased damage tolerance, mutagenicity, and chemoresistance. MMR proficiency increases cells' sensitivity to alkylating agents, antimetabolites, and fluoropyrimidines by 2-fold to 100-fold—so, counterintuitively, the presence of MMR activity triggers other cellular processes that arrest the cell cycle in G2 phase and later trigger cell death pathways.[37] Thus, inhibition of one or more MMR proteins is not a viable treatment approach. Instead, two other avenues are being researched to use MMR aberrations against cancer cells: (1) restoring MMR function and (2) creating a synthetic lethality with MMR[36] Table 43.3.

Hypermethylation of the *hMLH1* gene promoter causes loss of promoter expression in many sporadic cancers, so hypomethylation should be able to restore MMR function, sensitizing cells to various chemotherapeutics. Cell studies of fluoropyrimidine derivative, 5-fluoro-2-deoxycytidine (FdCyd), have demonstrated this potential utility.[36]

A deficiency in MMR can selectively sensitize tumor cells to chemotherapeutic agents. In this manner, methotrexate induces oxidative DNA damage in tumor cells with defects in *MSH2*. The resultant increased accumulation of 8-oxoguanine (8-oxoG) is lethal to cells deficient in MLH1 or MSH2 because they cannot repair that type of damage.[38]

NUCLEOTIDE EXCISION REPAIR (NER) PATHWAY

NER repairs bulky, helix-distorting lesions caused by UV irradiation and chemical mutagens. Chemotherapeutics including cisplatin, carboplatin, and oxaliplatin create these types of bulky adducts by crosslinking adjacent purine bases and forming intrastrand adducts.

TABLE 43-3 Mismatch Repair Inhibitors in Development

MMR Protein	Function(s)	Why It Is a Good Target for Inhibition	Challenges	Compounds Being Investigated
MLH1	• Scaffolding protein • Damage sensor • Helps determine the specific strand error	• Can be hypermethylated to restore functionality	• MMR deficiencies cause or increase chemoresistance • Intact MMR function is crucial for proper cell cycle checkpoint control	• FdCyd
MSH2	• Damage sensor	• Its damage-sensing ability can be bypassed by inducing a synthetic lethality	• Inhibition of MMR proteins is not a viable approach	• Methotrexate[a]

[a]Not a direct MSH2 inhibitor; but, when paired with tumor cells that are MSH2 deficient, it can selectively sensitize those cells.
FdCyd, 5-fluoro-2-deoxycytidine; MMR, mismatch repair; MLH1, MutL homolog 1.

Deficiencies in NER render cells sensitive to platinating agents—which is seen most dramatically in the 95% cure rate of testicular cancer treated with cisplatin.[39] Much of what we know today about NER came from studying NER-deficient autosomal recessive disorders, such as xeroderma pigmentosum (XP) and Cockayne syndrome (CS), which is why many of the proteins in this repair pathway are named starting with the letters "XP" or "CS."

More than 30 proteins participate in the NER pathway, which can be divided into two sub-pathways: global genome repair (GGR) and transcription-coupled repair (TCR).[40] The distinction is predicated on which complex recognizes the helix-distorting damage and which phase of the cell cycle is in progress when the damage is sensed. GGR operates during any phase of the cell cycle; TCR operates only while genes are actively being transcribed.[39]

The proteins involved in NER can distinguish between damaged and undamaged DNA, as well as which strand contains the adduct. When a damage site is identified, DNA repair occurs exclusively on the DNA strand containing the damage.[39,41]

After the initial recognition step, both sub-pathways operate similarly (Fig. 43.4). The initial damage-sensing multi-protein complex recruits a nine-unit complex called transcription factor II H (TFIIH), which includes two helicases (XPB and XPD) that unwind the DNA in opposite directions (3′ and 5′, respectively) at the site of the lesion. Another protein, XPA, helps open the helix and interacts with many of the other core proteins of NER, as noted below. Without XPA, NER cannot occur.[39]

As with other repair pathways, the damage is removed via endonuclease activity. In a carefully regulated manner, XPA and RPA interact with endonucleases XPG and XPF, respectively, to position them correctly so they can perform their precision cutting functions. Each endonuclease makes one incision on one side of the damaged strand, several nucleotides away from the actual damage. Interestingly, XPF also requires ERCC1 to perform its endonuclease activity.[41]

After the lesion is removed, RFC binds to the excision gap and mediates PNCA's activity as a sliding clamp and a progressivity factor to help DNA polymerases δ and ε to synthesize the new nucleotides, using the undamaged DNA strand as a template. XPG removes the flap of original nucleotides that was cut away before resynthesis started. Then a ligase completes the repair. Throughout all these steps, RPA enhances damage sensors' ability to

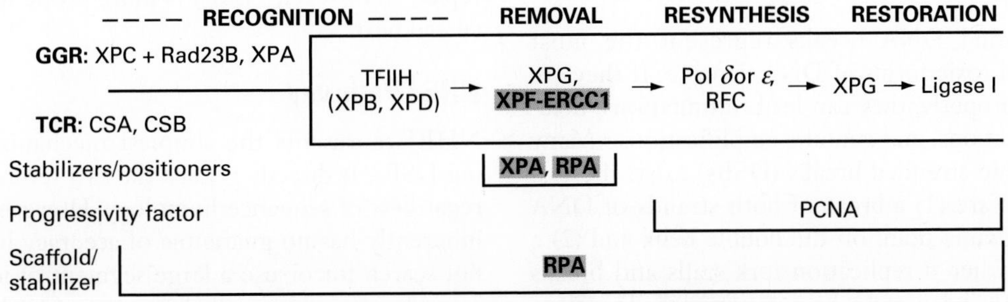

FIGURE 43–4 Overview of nucleotide excision repair pathway and targets of inhibitors.

TABLE 43-4 Nucleotide Excision Repair Inhibitors in Development[39,42-44]

NER Protein	Function(s)	Why It Is a Good Target for Inhibition	Challenges	Compounds Being Investigated
???		• Inhibition decreases the interaction of XPA and ERCC1, as well as other proteins with kinase activity		• UCN-01 is in phases 1 and 2 of clinical trials
XPA	• Stabilizer • Positions endonucleases for excision	• Its only known role is in NER • Not highly expressed; likely a rate-limiting repair factor	• Complexity of the network of protein interactions involved • Chemical similarities in binding pockets of proteins complicate the development of protein-specific inhibitors	• Only in silico models, high-throughput screens, and limited cell studies to date
RPA	• Scaffolding protein • Stabilizer	• Is essential to NER • RPA mutations are linked to development of cancer		
XPF/ERCC1	• Endonuclease	• Its only known role is in NER • Overexpressed in cisplatin-resistant cancers		• RNAi knockdown • Chimeric IgG1 monoclonal antibody (both: cell studies only)

??? = UCN-01 inhibits several proteins, not just one specific protein; non-catalytic aspects of NER (protein–protein and protein-DNA interactions, modulation of transcription regulation) may be more viable targets for inhibition, as seen in the effect of a chimeric IgG1 MAb on reducing XPF/ERCC1 expression.
NER, nucleotide excision repair; RPA, replication protein A.

identify the damage site and stabilizes the damaged DNA complex[41] (see Fig. 43.4).

Small-Molecule Inhibitors in Development

Despite the fact that NER repair requires so many proteins, development of NER inhibitors is a complex process that is in its infancy. One inhibitor called UCN-01 is in phase 2 clinical trials; however, its inhibitory effects are still being characterized and do not seem to be specific to one NER protein.[42] In other research efforts with NER inhibitors, cell studies have shown that decreased ERCC1 expression is associated with better outcomes after cisplatin therapy and inhibition of RPA sensitizes cells to IR as well as cisplatin and etoposide.[39,43] Table 43.4 summarizes research developments to date for NER inhibition.

OVERVIEW: DOUBLE-STRANDED BREAK REPAIR

Double-stranded DNA breaks represent the most dangerous and toxic forms of DNA damage. If they are not repaired properly, they can lead to mutations, deletions, translocations, and genome amplifications.[2] Many forms of double-stranded breaks (DSBs) exist; the two most common are (1) a break of both strands of DNA near or at the same point on the double helix and (2) a DSB formed when a replication fork stalls and breaks upon encountering certain base lesions.[45,46] Transient DSBs also occur when DNA is unwound so it can be transcribed.

DSBs are often challenging to repair, particularly those caused by IR and radiomimetic drugs. Such anticancer treatments can induce multiple kinds of damage simultaneously, including base damage, base loss, and strand breaks within one or two helix turns. Covalent chemical changes can leave "blunt," non-ligatable termini. Such lesions are termed "dirty," "complex," or "difficult."[47]

Two pathways for DSB repair exist in human cells: non-homologous end joining (NHEJ) and homologous recombination repair (HRR). The following two sections of this chapter discuss both pathways. Many factors contribute to which pathway is activated when DSBs are detected, including (1) the cell cycle phase in progress, (2) the DNA damage signaling pathway(s) and checkpoint(s) activated, (3) the "difficulty level" of the repair required, and (4) the structure of the damaged DNA ends.[45]

NHEJ can function during any phase of the cell cycle, and it works faster and simpler than HRR, which is partly why NHEJ is chosen 85% of the time as the means of repair.[47] However, NHEJ is more prone to error, as discussed next.

NHEJ Pathway

NHEJ represents the simplest mechanism for repairing DSBs. It directly rejoins the two severed DNA ends, regardless of sequence homology. However, this process inherently has no guarantee of accuracy because it does not search for or use a large segment of identical DNA as a reference point (called sequence complementarity) to determine which bases were present before the damage occurred. Indeed, typically 1 to 20 nucleotides can be lost from either side of the DSB junction when NHEJ mediates DSB repairs. In addition, sequence alterations can occur at the breakpoint.[45] In this respect, NHEJ paradoxically can contribute to genome protection as well as mutation.

Throughout the entire cell cycle, NHEJ performs "simple" DSB repairs that require minimal end processing before the ends are rejoined. (In contrast, HRR repairs complex damage during and after replication.) NHEJ, like other pathways, follows the four steps, namely recognition, removal, resynthesis, and restoration. However, it also can be thought of in simple terms as (1) detecting and tethering DSB ends together, (2) processing and removing end groups that cannot be ligated, and (3) sealing the break. We have much to learn about NHEJ, including whether the order of its steps is sequential.

Pathway Overview

The core NHEJ proteins and their main functions include the following as shown in Figure 43.5. The Ku heterodimer, comprising Ku70 and Ku80, detects and tethers the broken DNA ends by forming a ring around them and binding them. Ku also attracts other proteins to process the ends.[45] Ku was recently shown to have lyase activity, so it may also contribute to end processing.[48] DNA-dependent protein kinase (DNA-PKcs) in conjunction with Ku juxtaposes and bridges the ends, protects them from nuclease attack, and processes them to make them available for ligation.[45] Collectively, this protein plus the Ku heterodimer are called the DNA–PK complex. This complex also regulates other enzymes that can process the ends. Depending on the type and complexity of the end damage involved, a number of other processing proteins—both endonucleases and exonucleases—are recruited to make the ends ligatable. These proteins include Artemis, PNKP (polynucleotide kinase/phosphatase), WRN (Werner syndrome protein), and TDP1 (tyrosyl DNA phosphodiesterase 1). The MRN (Mre11/Rad50/NBS1) complex has multiple functions as a damage sensor and activator of DNA checkpoints; it also appears to facilitate tethering of the DNA ends and has both endonuclease and exonuclease properties. XRCC4 is a scaffolding protein that stabilizes, positions, and stimulates Ligase IV to seal the ends after processing. Another protein called XLF works cooperatively with XRCC4 and likely helps to position and stimulate Ligase IV as well, but its function is not well characterized.[47] Figure 43.5 depicts the steps of NHEJ.

Several variations of NHEJ repair have been identified; the most well characterized is a specialized form called V(D)J recombination, which occurs only in T and B cells.[47,49] Much less is known about the other NHEJ repair variations.

Small-Molecule Inhibitors in Development

As with MMR, diminished or defective NHEJ functioning results in damage tolerance and chemoresistance. It also leads to increased risk of cancer, particularly lymphoid malignancies.[45] Because of this, therapeutic forays into NHEJ inhibition are moving slowly (Table 43.5). More fruitful efforts related to NHEJ manipulation may come from indirectly modulating NHEJ activity,[47] as noted at the bottom of Table 43.5.

HRR Pathway

HRR is the genome's best guarantee of stability in the face of the most serious and complicated forms of DNA damage. DSBs can occur transiently when topoisomerases uncoil DNA. Breaks to both DNA strands can occur after exposure to IR or certain chemotherapeutics. But perhaps the most common form of DSB occurs when replication forks stall and break at the site of unrepaired DNA lesions.

Replication occurs simultaneously in two directions: 3′ on one DNA strand and 5′ on the other DNA strand. These opposite activities create a "fork" or "Y" shape as replication proceeds. When replication halts on one strand because it encounters an unrepaired lesion or a break, the other strand's replication stalls, which creates another break. In all cases, if such damage were not repaired, it could potentially lead to the loss of enough bases to equal that of losing an entire chromatin arm.[45] Thus, it is imperative that HRR provides error-free DNA repairs.

HRR is aptly named because it finds a large area of homology, usually on a sister chromatid, to use as a template for reproducing the damaged or lost bases. To do this, HRR operates predominantly during the S and G2

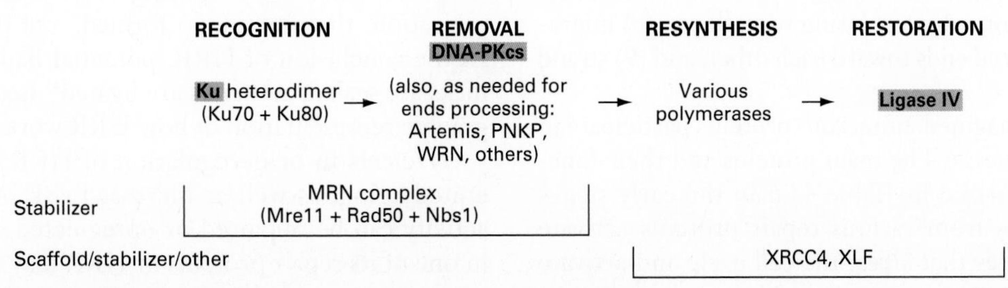

FIGURE 43–5 Overview of non-homologous end joining pathway and targets of inhibitors.

TABLE 43–5 Non-homologous End Joining Inhibitors in Development

NHEJ Protein	Function(s)	Why It Is a Good Target for Inhibition	Challenges	Compounds Being Investigated
DNA-PKcs	• Processes incompatible ends so they can be ligated	• Appears to be unique to NHEJ • Essential for NHEJ activity	Inhibition of NHEJ • Increases DNA damage tolerance • Causes chemoresistance • Predisposes cells to autosomal recessive disorders and malignancies, especially lymphoid cancers	Fairly non-specific: • Wortmannin • Methyl xanthine • Caffeine More specific: • NU7026 • NU7441
PNKP	• Processes incompatible ends so they can be ligated	• Appears to be unique to NHEJ		• A12B4C3 (cell studies only)
Ligase IV	• Seals nicks in final repair step	• A rate-limiting step • Cannot work in the absence of XRCC4		• L189 (in silico screening only)

Indirect ways of modulating NHEJ functionality are being explored as more viable options than direct inhibition. Examples:

- Overexpression of a truncated form of XRCC4 can inhibit NHEJ by interfering with DNA Ligase IV.
- DNA-PKcs can be inhibited indirectly by (1) inhibiting EGFR (epidermal growth factor receptor) or by (2) inhibiting ATM, a DNA checkpoint protein (by using micro-RNA or small-molecule inhibitors).
- Inhibition of topoisomerases that unwind DNA to give NHEJ repair proteins access to the damage is another option.
- Epigenetic factors (methylation of gene promoters) are under investigation as well.

It is yet unknown how or if these findings can translate into future clinical use.

NHEJ, non-homologous end joining; DNA-PKcs, DNA-dependent protein kinases; PNKP, polynucleotide kinase/phosphatase.

phases of the cell cycle—after a cell's DNA has doubled, but before it starts dividing.[45,46]

Pathway Overview

Several sub-pathways of homology-directed repair have been identified,[45] but all forms of HRR follow these general steps: (1) nucleolytic resection of DNA ends to generate an overhanging area of single-stranded DNA, (2) formation of a filament on the end of the resected overhang to search for a large area of homology on the sister chromatid, (3) "invasion" by that filament onto the area of the DNA strand containing the homology, (4) formation of a DNA heteroduplex (called a D-loop), created from displacement by the invading strand, (5) sliding (branch migration) of that D-loop to "read" the area of homology, (6) extension of the overhang as new nucleotides are generated past the original breakpoint, (7) dissolution of the X-shaped structure (called a Holliday junction) that forms as the D-loop pushes along the border between heteroduplex and homoduplex during resynthesis, (8) migration of the repaired ends toward each other, and (9) strand restoration.[2]

As can be imagined, numerous proteins participate in this complex process. The main proteins and their functions are summarized in. Table 43.6 In the early stages of HRR, signals from various repair proteins activate checkpoint kinases that arrest the cell cycle and activate additional DNA repair proteins.[2] Numerous proteins, including those in the MRN complex and others, are recruited to prepare the DNA ends for repair. These proteins include both endonucleases and exonucleases as needed, depending on the structure of the damaged area. Resection of the damage and ends processing leave an overhang that extends beyond the original breakpoint. This structure is critical to the heart of HRR, which is the formation of the Rad51 filament. The proteins comprising the Rad51 filament must be able to attach to the 3′ end of the overhang and create a complex that is able to search for an area of homology.[35] As described in Table 43.6, the Rad51 filament uses a homologous sequence as a template for repairing the DSB. When the Rad51 filament invades the area of homology, it pulls on part of that DNA strand, much like pulling a fabric thread loose in such a way that it creates a loop—hence, the term, D-loop. As already noted, this structure slides along the area of homology during resynthesis, creating an X-shaped junction. Because the two strands of DNA cannot remain connected, HRR has various methods for resolving this crossover connection. Those methods vary according to the direction of branch migration, the junction(s) formed, and other variables. At the conclusion of HRR, potential flaps are removed, nicks are sealed, and ends are ligated[45] (see Fig. 43.6 for a graphic representation of how HRR works).

Defects in or deregulation of HRR leads to accelerated aging, as well as increased risk of cancer. HRR activity can be impaired or upregulated due to a defect in one of its repair proteins or HRR may be upregulated to compensate for an upstream defect in an associated regulatory protein. A stunning example of this is in the loss of both alleles for BRCA1 or BRCA2. This

TABLE 43–6 Main Homologous Recombinant Repair Proteins and Their Functions[35,45,50,51]

Protein	Functions
MRN complex	• Damage sensor • Resects DNA ends
γH2AX	• Recruits repair proteins to damage site • Serves as a docking site for those proteins (including MRN and BRCA1) • Suppresses inappropriate translocations of chromatin fragments
BRCA1	• May participate in signaling response to DNA damage • Interacts indirectly with Rad51
Rad50	• Processes and resects DNA ends
RPA	• Binds to single-stranded DNA • Stimulates recombination
Rad52	• Binds to DNA ends, protecting them from nuclease activity • Overcomes RPA's inhibitory effects on Rad51 • Facilitates Rad51-mediated recombination
BRCA2	• Mediates/facilitates Rad51 formation and its loading onto ssDNA
XRCC2,	• Mediates strand invasion and DNA resynthesis
XRCC3	• Associated with the Rad51 complex
Rad51	• Catalyzes the homology search
filament	• Initiates DNA strand invasion and DNA strand exchange
Rad54	• Stabilizes the Rad51 filament • Stimulates strand invasion and extends the DNA heteroduplex, migrating the branched DNA structures • Later dissociates Rad51 from heteroduplex DNA, allowing DNA polymerases to access the 3′-end
BLM	• Migrates the two junctions toward each other
WRN	• Along with BLM and RecQ, suppresses illegitimate recombination
TOPOIIIα	• Junction resolution: removes the linkages of the two duplexes
Resolvase	• Junction resolution (along with others, like the BLM–TopIIIa–BLAP75 complex)

loss impairs HRR, so cells compensate by using NHEJ to repair DSBs. However, if BRCA-deficient cancers are treated with a PARP inhibitor, the resulting accumulation of DNA damage (from inhibited BER activity) cannot be repaired by NHEJ, which effectively kills BRCA-deficient cancer cells. PARP inhibitors are the most elegant example of efficacious repair inhibition as well as synthetic lethality.[45]

Inhibitors in Development

Despite the success of PARP inhibitors and the great number of proteins specific to HRR, efforts to exploit deficient, proficient, or hyperactive HRR in malignancies are in their infancy. As seen in Figure 43.6, specific HRR inhibitors are notably absent. Instead, efforts to modulate HRR for therapeutic gain are progressing along an indirect route. To this end, three inhibitors are

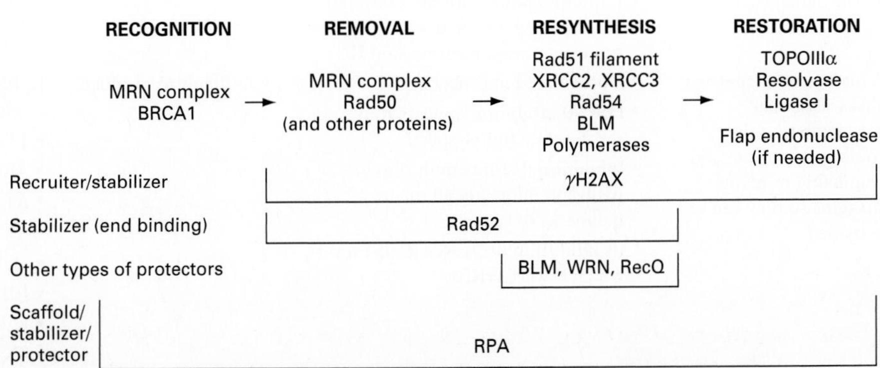

FIGURE 43–6 Overview of homologous recombination repair pathway and potential targets of inhibitors.

in development that have shown promise as potential anticancer agents. PARP has already been discussed in Section *BER*[6]: the other two are heat shock protein 90 (HSP90) and cABL (Abelson murine leukemia viral non-receptor tyrosine kinase).

HSP90 is a molecular chaperone that helps more than 200 proteins fold to their correct conformation, mature, and stabilize so they can be activated; 48 of those proteins are associated directly with oncogenesis.[48] Environmental stress disrupts HSP90's ability to suppress otherwise "silent" genetic variations, such as those in microsatellite repeats[52]; so it is not surprising that HSP90 levels are abnormally high in many cancers. Inhibition of HSP90 decreases Rad51 activity and prevents multiple checkpoint proteins from being activated, both of which derail HRR.[53] These features collectively give HSP90 inhibitors the ability to simultaneously disrupt a wide range of oncogenic pathways, blocking tumors' (1) growth signals, (2) resistance to apoptosis, (3) unregulated replication, (4) neoangiogenesis, and (5) tissue invasion/metastasis.[54] For this reason, a number of HSP90 inhibitors are already in phases 1 and 2 of clinical trials, as noted in. Table 43.7 [55]

cAbl inhibitors have been used with great success against chronic myelogenous leukemia since 2001. In that capacity, they address a problem caused by a gene translocation that fuses part of the *BCR* and *ABR* genes together, which results in accelerated cell division.[56] With respect to HRR, cAbl can disrupt Rad51's ability to bind to DNA; but many other cellular processes are influenced by cAbl as well.[57] It remains to be seen whether a cAbl inhibitor will have clinical utility in treating cancers that exhibit HRR deficiencies (see Table 43.7 for more details about indirect inhibitors of HRR activity).

TABLE 43–7 Homologous Recombinant Repair Small-Molecule Agents in Development

HRR Protein	Function(s)	Why It Is a Good Target for Inhibition	Challenges	Compounds Being Investigated
No direct inhibitors of HRR proteins have been found/developed yet. The following proteins inhibit HRR activity indirectly by modulating (1) DNA damage response mechanisms, (2) protein–protein interactions, or (3) other mechanisms.				
cAbl	• Appears to be a decision maker, determining if damage is too extensive to be repaired	• Inhibits Rad51's DNA strand exchange activity, which stalls HRR • Is activated by IR and alkylating agents • A deletion or translocation on the gene encoding cAbl promotes tumorigenesis	• Also interacts with DNA-PK (in NHEJ pathway) • Participates in many cellular processes • cAbl-deficient cells are resistant to IR and other DNA-damaging agents	• Imatinib (Gleevec) has been available to treat CML since 2001
PARP1	• Surveillance/damage sensor • Assesses extent of damage; determines whether to signal apoptosis • Helps decondense chromatin • Recruits repair proteins to the damage site • Facilitates repairs	• Uses NAD^+ to transfer ADP-ribose polymers onto specific acceptor proteins including itself; this modifies the protein's properties • PARP1 inhibition causes an accumulation of DNA damage and that collapses replication forks; cancers deficient in HRR cannot repair such damage • Inhibitors potentiate the effects of alkylating agents, platinating agents, topoisomerase I poisons, and IR	• Secondary mutations can correct for this repair deficiency, causing a resistance to PARP inhibitors	• PARP inhibitors are already being used to treat familial breast cancers and other cancers with BRCA-like features • >70 clinical trials in progress for second-generation PARP inhibitors and broader use of first-generation inhibitors
HSP90	• A molecular chaperone that is essential for facilitating the folding, maturing, and stabilizing of many proteins so they can be activated	• Upregulated in cancers • HSP90 inhibition appears to be intrinsically tumor specific • Inhibition disrupts multiple pathways, blocking all major hallmarks of cancer • Its inhibition decreases Rad51 levels, which thwart HRR	• Difficult to produce	In Phases 1 and 2 of clinical trials: • 17-DMAG • Alvespimycin • ATI13387 • AUY922 • Debio 0932 • IPI-504 • KW-2478 • SNX-5422 • Synta (STA-9090) Other candidates are in preclinical studies

TABLE 43-8 Summary of Major DNA Repair Pathways

Repair Pathway	Damage Sensors	DNA Access (Helicases; Others)	DNA Incision (Endonucleases)	Scaffolds/ Stabilizing Proteins[a]	New Nucleotide Synthesis (Polymerases; Progressivity Factors)	Flap Excision (Exonucleases)	Ligation
		Activities and Proteins Involved →					
Direct Repair	MGMT	No other proteins involved; direct chemical reversal via stoichiometric reaction					
Base Excision Repair							
Short patch[b]	Damage-specific glycosylases (and PARP1)	(PARP1)	APE1	XRCC1 PARP1 XRCC1	Pol β		Ligase III
Long patch				PCNA PARP1	Pol β, δ, or ε	FEN1	Ligase I
Mismatch Repair	MSH2 + MSH3 or MSH6	N/A	MLH1–PMS2	MLH1	Pol δ or ε RFC + PCNA	ExoI	Ligase I
Nucleotide Excision Repair							
GGR[b]	XPC + Rad23B RPA	XPB and XPD components of TFIIH; also XPA	XPG XPF + ERCC1	XPA RPA	Pol δ or ε RFC	XPG	Ligase I
TCR	CSA, CSB						
Non-homologous end joining (NHEJ)	Ku70, Ku80	MRN complex	DNA-PKcs (Artemis, PNPK, WRN, others as needed)	XRCC4	Various polyases		Ligase IV
Homologous Recombination (HR)	MRN complex	BLM, WRN, others	MRN complex Rad 50 Other proteins	RPA γH2AX BRCA2 Rad52 Rad54	Rad51 filament XRCC2, XRCC3 Polymerases WRN, BLM, RecQ are protectors	If needed	TopoIIIα Resolvase Ligase I

[a]Scaffold proteins and stabilizers may participate in any step or multiple steps of DNA repair. Otherwise, the order in which the enzymes perform their functions is depicted from left to right in this chart.

[b]Predominant sub-pathway.

CONCLUSION

Normal cells possess extensive repair mechanisms to maintain homeostasis (see Table 43.8 for a summary of all DNA repair pathways). Cancerous cells have astonishing abilities to hijack those processes to help them survive. We are still in the early stages of exploring tumor-specific and pathway-specific means of manipulating those survival mechanisms to clinical advantage. The field of DNA repair inhibition shows great promise for developing disruptive forces that can selectively kill cancer cells.

ACKNOWLEDGMENTS

Financial support for this work was provided by the National Institutes of Health NCI CA121168, CA114571, and CA121168S1 (MRK), CA122298 (MLF), the Riley Children's Foundation (MRK), and the Ralph W. and Grace M. Showalter Research Trust Fund (MLF).

REFERENCES

1. Friedberg EC, McDaniel LD, Schultz RA. The role of endogenous and exogenous DNA damage and mutagenesis. *Curr Opin Genet Dev.* February 2004;14(1):5-10.
2. Willers H, Zou L, Pfaffle HN. Targeting homologous recombination repair in cancer. In: Kelley MR, ed. *DNA Repair in Cancer Therapy: Molecular Targets and Clinical Applications.* London: Elsevier; 2012:119-151.
3. Kaelin WG Jr. Synthetic lethality: a framework for the development of wiser cancer therapeutics. *Genome Med.* 2009;1(99):1-6.
4. Bapat A, Fishel ML, Georgiadis M, Kelley MR. Going ape as an approach to cancer therapeutics. *Antioxid Redox Signal.* March 2009;11(3):651-668.
5. Underhill C, Toulmonde M, Bonnefoi H. A review of PARP inhibitors: from bench to bedside. *Ann Oncol.* July 2011;22(2):268-279.

6. Plummer R. Perspective on the pipeline of drugs being developed with modulation of DNA damage as a target. *Clin Cancer Res.* September 2010;16(18):4527-4531.
7. Fan Z, Beresford PJ, Zhang D, et al. Cleaving the oxidative repair protein Ape1 enhances cell death mediated by granzyme A. *Nat Immunol.* February 2003;4(2):145-153.
8. Luo M, He H, Kelley MR, Georgiadis M. Redox regulation of DNA repair: implications for human health and cancer therapeutic development. *Antioxid Redox Signal.* June 2010;12(11):1247-1269.
9. Tell G, Quadrifoglio F, Tiribelli C, Kelley MR. The many functions of APE1/Ref-1: not only a DNA repair enzyme. *Antioxid Redox Signal.* March 2009;11(3):601-620.
10. Luo M, Delaplane S, Jiang A, et al. Role of the multifunctional DNA repair and redox signaling protein Ape1/Ref-1 in cancer and endothelial cells: small molecule inhibition of Ape1's redox function. *Antioxid Redox Signal.* November 2008;10(11):1853-1867.
11. Bapat A, Glass LS, Luo M, et al. Novel small molecule inhibitor of Ape1 endonuclease blocks proliferation and reduces viability of glioblastoma cells. *J Pharmacol Exp Ther.* September 2010;334(3):988-998.
12. Nyland RL, Luo M, Kelley MR, Borch RF. Design and synthesis of novel quinone inhibitors targeted to the redox function of apurinic/apyrimidinic endonuclease 1/redox enhancing factor-1 (Ape1/Ref-1). *J Med Chem.* February 2010;53(3):1200-1210.
13. Wesierska-Gadek J, Maurer M, Zulehner N, Komina O. Whether to target single or multiple CDKs for therapy? That is the question. *J Cell Physiol.* February 2011;226(2):341-349.
14. Tse AN, Carvajal R, Schwartz GK. Targeting checkpoint kinase 1 in cancer therapeutics. *Clin Cancer Res.* April 2007;13(7):1955-1960.
15. Hoeijmakers JH. DNA damage, aging, and cancer. *N Engl J Med.* October 2009;361(15):1475-1485.
16. Gerson SL. MGMT: its role in cancer aetiology and cancer therapeutics. *Nat Rev.* April 2004;4(4):296-307.
17. Vascotto C, Fishel M. Blockade of base excision repair: inhibition of small lesions results in big consequences to cancer cells. In: Kelley M, ed. *DNA Repair in Cancer Therapy: Molecular Targets and Clinical Applications.* London: Academic Press/Elsevier; 2012:29-47.
18. Huffman JL, Sundheim O, Tainer JA. DNA base damage recognition and removal: new twists and grooves. *Mutat Res.* September 2005;577(1-2):55-76.
19. Sancar A, Lindsey-Boltz LA, Unsal-Kacmaz K, Linn S. Molecular mechanisms of mammalian DNA repair and the DNA damage checkpoints. *Annu Rev Biochem.* 2004;73:39-85.
20. Lindahl T. Instability and decay of the primary structure of DNA. *Nature.* April 1993;362(6422):709-715.
21. Hegde ML, Hazra TK, Mitra S. Functions of disordered regions in mammalian early base excision repair proteins. *Cell Mol Life Sci.* November 2010;67(21):3573-3587.
22. Frosina G, Fortini P, Rossi O, et al. Two pathways for base excision repair in mammalian cells. *J Biol Chem.* 1996;271(16):9573-9578.
23. Evans AR, Limp-Foster M, Kelley MR. Going APE over ref-1. *Mutat Res.* 2000;461(2):83-108.
24. Sobol RW. CHIPping away at base excision repair. *Mol Cell.* February 2008;29(4):413-415.
25. Hakme A, Wong HK, Dantzer F, Schreiber V. The expanding field of poly(ADP-ribosyl)ation reactions. 'Protein Modifications: Beyond the Usual Suspects' review series. *EMBO Rep.* November 2008;9(11):1094-1100.
26. Fortini P, Dogliotti E. Base damage and single-strand break repair: mechanisms and functional significance of short- and long-patch repair subpathways. *DNA Rep (Amst).* April 2007;6(4):398-409.
27. Fawcett H, Mader JS, Robichaud M, Giacomantonio C, Hoskin DW. Contribution of reactive oxygen species and caspase-3 to apoptosis and attenuated ICAM-1 expression by paclitaxel-treated MDA-MB-435 breast carcinoma cells. *Int J Oncol.* December 2005;27(6):1717-1726.
28. Alexandre J, Hu Y, Lu W, Pelicano H, Huang P. Novel action of paclitaxel against cancer cells: bystander effect mediated by reactive oxygen species. *Cancer Res.* April 2007;67(8):3512-3517.
29. Meynard D, Le Morvan V, Bonnet J, Robert J. Functional analysis of the gene expression profiles of colorectal cancer cell lines in relation to oxaliplatin and cisplatin cytotoxicity. *Oncol Rep.* May 2007;17(5):1213-1221.
30. Jiang Y, Guo C, Vasko MR, Kelley MR. Implications of apurinic/apyrimidinic endonuclease in reactive oxygen signaling response after cisplatin treatment of dorsal root ganglion neurons. *Cancer Res.* August 2008;68(15):6425-6434.
31. Kelley MR, Fishel ML. DNA repair proteins as molecular targets for cancer therapeutics. *Anticancer Agents Med Chem.* May 2008;8(4):417-425.
32. Burdak-Rothkamm S, Prise KM. New molecular targets in radiotherapy: DNA damage signalling and repair in targeted and non-targeted cells. *Eur J Pharmacol.* December 2009;625(1-3):151-155.
33. American Cancer Society I. What are the different types of chemotherapy drugs? 2011. http://www.cancer.org/Treatment/TreatmentsandSideEffects/TreatmentTypes/Chemotherapy/ChemotherapyPrinciplesAnIn-depthDiscussionoftheTechniquesanditsRoleinTreatment/chemotherapy-principles-types-of-chemo-drugs. Accessed June 17, 2011.
34. Li GM. Mechanisms and functions of DNA mismatch repair. *Cell Res.* January 2008;18(1):85-98.
35. Li L, Wagner M, Meyers M, Boothman D. Defective DNA mismatch repair-dependent c-Abl-p73-GADD45α expression confers cancer chemoresistance. In: Kelley M, ed. *DNA Repair in Cancer Therapy: Molecular Targets and Clinical Applications.* London: Elsevier; 2012:191-204.
36. Kinsella TJ. Coordination of DNA mismatch repair and base excision repair processing of chemotherapy and radiation damage for targeting resistant cancers. *Clin Cancer Res.* March 2009;15(6):1853-1859.
37. Martin SA, McCarthy A, Barber LJ, et al. Methotrexate induces oxidative DNA damage and is selectively lethal to tumour cells with defects in the DNA mismatch repair gene *MSH2*. *EMBO Mol Med.* September 2009;1(6-7):323-337.
38. Shuck SC, Short EA, Turchi JJ. Eukaryotic nucleotide excision repair: from understanding mechanisms to influencing biology. *Cell Res.* January 2008;18(1):64-72.
39. Turchi J, Patrick S. Targeting the nucleotide excision repair pathway for therapeutic applications. In: Kelley M, ed. *DNA Repair in Cancer Therapy: Molecular Targets and Clinical Applications.* London: Elsevier; 2012:109-115.
40. Dip R, Camenisch U, Naegeli H. Mechanisms of DNA damage recognition and strand discrimination in human nucleotide excision repair. *DNA Repair (Amst).* November 2004;3(11):1409-1423.
41. Yamauchi T, Keating MJ, Plunkett W. UCN-01 (7-hydroxystaurosporine) inhibits DNA repair and increases cytotoxicity in normal lymphocytes and chronic lymphocytic leukemia lymphocytes. *Mol Cancer Ther.* February 2002;1(4):287-294.
42. Usanova S, Piee-Staffa A, Sied U, et al. Cisplatin sensitivity of testis tumour cells is due to deficiency in interstrand-crosslink repair and low ERCC1-XPF expression. *Mol Cancer.* 2010;9:248.
43. Helleday T, Lo J, van Gent DC, Engelward BP. DNA double-strand break repair: from mechanistic understanding to cancer treatment. *DNA Repair (Amst).* July 2007;6(7):923-935.
44. Helleday T. Homologous recombination in cancer development, treatment and development of drug resistance. *Carcinogenesis.* June 2010;31(6):955-960.
45. Weinfeld M, Lees-Miller S. DNA double-strand break repair by nonhomologous end joining and its clinical relevance. In: Kelley M, ed. *DNA Repair in Cancer Therapy: Molecular Targets and Clinical Applications.* London: Elsevier; 2012:161-181.
46. Roberts SA, Strande N, Burkhalter MD, et al. Ku is a 5′-dRP/AP lyase that excises nucleotide damage near broken ends. *Nature.* April 2010;464(7292):1214-1217.
47. Mansilla-Soto J, Cortes P. VDJ recombination: artemis and its in vivo role in hairpin opening. *J Exp Med.* March 2003;197(5):543-547.

48. Napierala M, Parniewski P, Pluciennik A, Wells RD. Long CTG.CAG repeat sequences markedly stimulate intramolecular recombination. *J Biol Chem.* September 2002;277(37):34087-34100.
49. Mittelman D, Sykoudis K, Hersh M, Lin Y, Wilson JH. Hsp90 modulates CAG repeat instability in human cells. *Cell Stress Chaperones.* September 2010;15(5):753-759.
50. Messaoudi S, Peyrat JF, Brion JD, Alami M. Recent advances in Hsp90 inhibitors as antitumor agents. *Anticancer Agents Med Chem.* October 2008;8(7):761-782.
51. US National Institutes of Health. Clinical trials of HSP90 inhibitors. http://www.clinicaltrials.gov/ct2/results?term=HSP-90+inhibitor. Accessed October 23, 2011.
52. Shaul Y, Ben-Yehoyada M. Role of c-Abl in the DNA damage stress response. *Cell Res.* January 2005;15(1):33-35.
53. Yuan ZM, Huang Y, Ishiko T, et al. Regulation of Rad51 function by c-Abl in response to DNA damage. *J Biol Chem.* February 1998;273(7):3799-3802.
54. Maxmen A. Beyond PARP inhibitors: agents in pipelines target DNA repair mechanisms. *J Natl Cancer Inst.* August 2010;102(15):1110-1111.
55. US National Institutes of Health. Clinical trials of UNC-01. http://www.clinicaltrials.gov/ct2/results?term=UNC-01. Accessed October 27, 2011.
56. Khanna KK, Jackson SP. DNA double-strand breaks: signaling, repair and the cancer connection. *Nat Genet.* March 2001;27(3):247-254.
57. Podhorecka M, Skladanowski A, Bozko P. H2AX phosphorylation: its role in DNA damage response and cancer therapy. *J Nucleic Acids.* August 2010;Article ID 920161:9 pages.

CHAPTER 44

MONOCLONAL ANTIBODIES FOR THE TREATMENT OF CANCER

Jason C. Steel, Brian J. Morrison, and John C. Morris

INTRODUCTION

Monoclonal antibodies (mAbs) and related immunoconjugates represent one of the fastest expanding areas of pharmaceutical research and development. The estimated 2010 total world market for all mAbs was $15.6 billion. Currently, there are 13 mAbs approved for the treatment of cancer, with another 13 in phase III trials at the present time. For over a hundred years, attempts were made to develop "magic bullets" that would specifically target tumors cells. It was not until the development of hybridoma technology in the 1970s that clinically useful amounts of single specificity antibodies could be generated. The effectiveness of many early mAbs of non-human origin was limited by their immunogenicity and short half-lives. Recombinant DNA methods, transgenic technology, and improved antibody engineering have generated increasing effective mAbs for the treatment of cancer. As a result, a number of newer generation mAbs have affected the natural history of diseases such as diffuse large B-cell lymphoma. As experience has been gained, our ability to better select patients that are more likely to benefit from these often-expensive agents has improved. Examples of this are the recognition of the lack of response of KRAS-mutated colorectal cancers to anti-epidermal growth factor receptor (EGFR) mAbs and the varying benefit obtained in lymphomas from rituximab in patients with different Fc receptor polymorphisms. With an ever-increasing array of new mAbs, many engineered to enhance beneficial functions while deleting undesired effects, or armed with cytotoxins or radioisotopes to enhance tumor cell killing, the future for these "magic bullets" of the 21st century is bright.

ANTIBODY BIOLOGY

Antibody Structure and Function

Antibodies are highly specific glycoproteins of the immunoglobulin superfamily produced by B cells and plasma cells in response to a specific antigen. Immunoglobulins bind to a specific antigenic determinant and neutralize the antigen. The typical valency of a naturally occurring antibody is 2, allowing it to bind to two specific antigenic determinants at a time. However, for certain antibody classes, the valency may be 4 (IgA) or 10 (IgM). The basic structure of all immunoglobulins is a four-chain structure composed of two identical 22-kDa light chains and two identical 55- to 75-kDa heavy chains. Heavy chains (H) are unique for each of the five classes of antibody: γ for IgG, α for IgA, μ for IgM, ε for IgE, and δ for IgD. The light chains (L) for all of the antibody isotypes are either κ or λ types. At the amino-terminal end of both the heavy and light chains is the variable region (V_H or V_L). Within this region lies the antigen-binding site, the diversity of which is based on extensive genomic recombination events of different combinations of >150 variable (V), diversity (D), and joining (J) gene segments that are then further modified by somatic hypermutation. The antigen-binding site is composed of six hypervariable complementarity determining regions (CDRs), three from the V_H and three from the V_L.[1] It is this variability that generates mAbs of unique and differing antigen specificities. Each plasma cell produces a single mAb. The remaining domains comprise the constant regions and are designated C_L in the light chains and C_H1, C_H2, and C_H3 (additionally C_H4 as well for μ and ε) for the heavy chains. Each of these regions exhibits a unique function. The region of the antibody composed of one constant and one variable region from the heavy and light chain that is generated by digestion with the enzyme papain is called the Fab (fragment, antigen binding) region. The divalent version of this fragment is called the F(ab′)2. The Fc fragment consists of the two heavy chains, each with a C_H2 and C_H3 region. The effector functions of an antibody are mediated by this part of the molecule. The Fc region mediates the interaction of an antibody with the Fc receptors (R) of effector cells in antibody-dependent cellular cytotoxicity (ADCC) and with the C1q of the complement system in complement-dependent cytotoxicity (CDC).

There are five classes or isotypes of immunoglobulins based on structural and functional differences: (i) IgM; (ii) IgD; (iii) IgA; (iv) IgE; and (v) IgG. IgM and IgD are the primordial immunoglobulins. IgM typically appears as a complex pentamer with ten antigen-binding sites, but may also exist as a monomer. IgM is the first antibody to be produced by B cells following exposure to an antigen.[2] IgD is a monomer found in very low concentration in the serum where its role is not well understood. IgD is primarily found coexpressed with IgM on the surface of B cells where it functions as a receptor for antigen. IgA, IgE, and IgG are mature antibodies that are found after maturation and class switching. IgA is a monomer that may also appear as a secretory dimer in tears, saliva, mucus, etc. IgA plays a major role in mucosal immunity and can be further divided into two subclasses. IgE is a monomer and is the least abundant immunoglobulin in the serum after IgD. IgE plays a role in responses to parasitic infections and participates in immediate-type hypersensitivity reactions such as anaphylaxis. IgG is the major immunoglobulin in the serum and is involved in humoral immunity predominantly during the secondary immune response, and the presence of antigen-specific IgG generally corresponds to maturation of the antibody response. IgG can be divided into four different subclasses that possess different attributes such as the ability to bind to Fc receptors and activate the complement pathway. The majority of mAbs used clinically are of the IgG isotype. IgG is a versatile antibody as it can carry out all of the functions of immunoglobulin molecules. These functions include but are not limited to (i) activation of complement leading to opsonization of microbes by phagocytes, stimulation of immune cells, or direct lysis of microbes through formation of a complement membrane attack complex; (ii) activation of effector cells; or (iii) direct cytocidal effects on the target cell.

THERAPEUTIC MONOCLONAL ANTIBODIES

History

The quest to produce clinically usable quantities of single specificity or mAbs for therapeutic purposes spanned more than a century. In 1890, von Behring and Kitasato[3] reported that injection of animals with small doses of purified diphtheria toxin (DT) generated neutralizing "antitoxins" in the animals' serum that could protect uninfected animals from a challenge with the organism. Subsequently, similar horse-derived antiserum was successfully used to treat patients with diphtheria and tetanus. In 1895, Hericourt and Richet[4] reported treating cancer patients with antisera obtained from dogs injected with the individual patients' cancer cells. Although it was reported that some tumors "improved" with the injections, no patient was cured, and serum sickness was a common side effect. This approach ultimately lost favor because of inconsistent results and concerns over the specificity and purity of the serum treatments. In the same era, Paul Ehrlich proposed the concept of "magic bullets" that would specifically target cancerous tissue. He described "antikörpers" (antibodies) that might be directed against specific cancers. In his lecture before the Royal Society in 1900, he envisaged that "immunizations such as these which are of great theoretic interest may come to be available for clinical application attacking epithelium new formations, particularly carcinoma by means of specific anti-epithelial sera."[5] Despite early optimism, the potential of mAbs remained elusive for most of the last century until the development of hybridoma technology by Köhler and Milstein in 1975.[6] Since their discovery, the promise of selectively targeting cancers using mAbs has become a reality. Currently, 13 mAbs or antibody conjugates are US FDA-approved for the treatment of cancer (Table 44.1). The first, rituximab (anti-CD20), was approved in 1998 for the treatment of chemotherapy-refractory follicular lymphoma, and more recently in August 2011, the immunotoxin brentuximab vedotin (anti-CD30) was approved for the treatment of relapsed anaplastic large cell lymphoma (ALCL) and Hodgkin lymphoma.

Non-human Monoclonal Antibodies

Early therapeutic mAbs were primarily of murine or rat origin and based on hybridoma technology. These antibodies had an advantage over polyclonal antisera in that they could be produced in much larger amounts and demonstrated greater specificity, as all of the antibody was directed against a single antigenic determinant. The early lack of success of many of these rodent-derived antibodies was due in large part to the dissimilarity between the rodent and human immune systems. These mAbs exhibited short half-lives in vivo, were highly immunogenic in humans, often inducing neutralizing human anti-mouse antibodies (HAMA), and could not adequately recruit immune effector cells because they were unable to interact with human Fc receptors expressed on these cells. Their efficacy was often limited by their inability to act through ADCC, making them relatively weak cytocidal agents. They were also associated with high rates of infusion reactions and anaphylaxis. In addition, many of these early non-human mAbs were not directed against cell surface targets that were accessible to the antibody, limiting their efficacy. Despite these issues, there are a number of non-human

TABLE 44–1 Currently Approved Monoclonal Antibodies and Conjugates for Treatment of Cancer

Agent	Format	Conjugation	Antigen	Indication	Approval
Rituximab (Rituxan)	Chimeric mouse/ human IgG1κ	None	CD20	B-cell NHL	1997
				B-cell CLL	2010
Trastuzumab (Herceptin)	Humanized IgG1κ	None	HER2/*neu* (ErbB2)	Breast cancer	1998
				Gastric cancer	2010
Gemtuzumab ozogamicin (Mylotarg)	Humanized IgG4κ	γ-Calicheamicin	CD33	AML	2000–2010[a]
Alemtuzumab (Campath)	Humanized IgG1κ	None	CD52	B-cell CLL	2001
Ibritumomab tiuxetan (Zevalin)	Murine IgG1κ	^{90}Y	CD20	B-cell NHL	2002
Tositumomab (Bexxar)	Murine IgG2aλ	^{131}I	CD20	B-cell NHL	2003
Cetuximab (Erbitux)	Chimeric mouse/ human IgG1κ	None	EGFR	Colorectal cancer	2004
				Squamous cell carcinoma of the head and neck	2006
Bevacizumab (Avastin)	Humanized IgG1κ	None	VEGF	Colorectal cancer	2004
				Lung cancer	2006
				Breast cancer	2008–2010[b]
				Glioblastoma	2009
				Renal cell cancer	2009
Panitumumab (Vectibix)	Human IgG2κ	None	EGFR	Colorectal cancer	2006
Ofatumumab (Arzerra)	Human IgG1κ	None	CD20	B-cell CLL	2010
Ipilimumab (Yervoy)	Human IgG1κ	None	CTLA-4	Malignant melanoma	2011
Brentuximab vedotin (Adcetris)	Chimeric mouse/ human IgG1κ	MMAE	CD30	Anaplastic large cell lymphoma/Hodgkin lymphoma	2011

NHL, non-Hodgkin lymphoma; CLL, chronic lymphocytic leukemia; AML, acute myeloid leukemia; EGFR, epidermal growth factor receptor; VEGF, vascular endothelial growth factor; CTLA-4, cytotoxic T-lymphocyte antigen 4; MMAE, monomethylauristatin E.

[a]Withdrawn by the manufacturer.

[b]Regulatory approval withdrawn.

mAbs in clinical use, although none as a direct cancer therapy. This includes muromonab-CD3 (Orthoclone OKT3), an anti-CD3 mAb that was the first therapeutic mAb to be approved by the FDA in 1986 for the treatment of allogeneic transplant rejection.[7] It is a murine IgG2a mAb directed against the 20-kDa ζ-subunit of the T-cell receptor complex (CD3) and is approved for the reversal of acute allograft rejection in patients undergoing cardiac, hepatic, and renal transplants. It has also been used for the depletion of T cells from stem cell and bone marrow allografts to treat or reduce the risk of serious graft versus host disease. Muromonab-CD3 has demonstrated modest activity against T-cell lymphoproliferative disorders in a number of small clinical trials. A number of non-human mAbs have been studied for the treatment of various cancers including anti-CD4, anti-CD5, and mAbs against a variety of melanoma and other solid tumor antigens.

Over the last 20 years, the FDA and industry focus has been on developing more human-like mAbs using recombinant DNA technology and transgenic animal systems to overcome the immunogenicity issues with non-human mAbs (Fig. 44.1). Of the 13 mAbs currently approved, 11 are chimeric, humanized, or fully human. Ibritumomab, the murine parent of the chimeric rituximab, and tositumomab, both anti-CD20 mAbs used for radioimmunotherapy of non-Hodgkin lymphoma (NHL), are the only two non-human antibodies approved for the treatment of cancer. This is because they are administered in minute amounts as radioactive conjugates with yttrium-90 and iodine-131, respectively, along with large doses of unlabeled rituximab.

Chimeric, Humanized, and Fully Human Monoclonal Antibodies

As foreign glycoproteins, non-human antibodies are highly immunogenic and almost uniformly result in the induction of HAMA or human anti-rat antibody responses. This results in the rapid removal of the therapeutic non-human mAb from the plasma and an increased risk of systemic inflammatory effects and allergic and infusion reactions. Furthermore, the formation of immune complexes between the non-human mAb and host antibodies neutralizes the therapeutic antibody and may alter its distribution and binding, resulting in undesired side effects. Once initiated, an anti-antibody response severely limits further mAb therapy in a patient. In an effort to overcome the issue of immunogenicity, engineering of non-human mAbs with human constant domains, so-called chimerized or humanized mAbs, or the generation

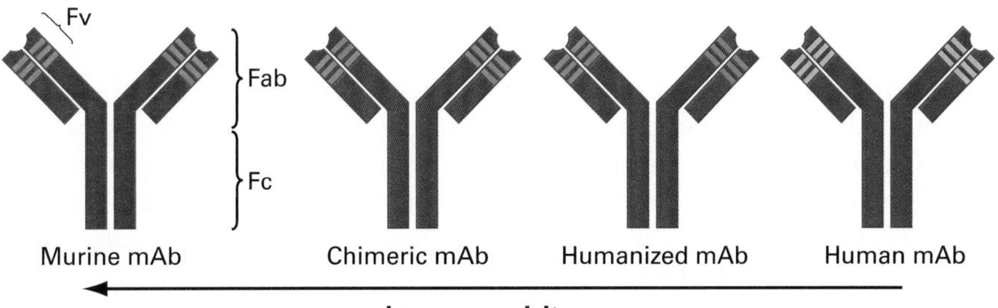

FIGURE 44–1 Structure of murine, chimeric, humanized, and human monoclonal antibodies (mAbs). Murine antibodies are entirely murine and are the most immunogenic and rapidly removed mAb in humans. Chimeric mAbs are made up of rodent variable domains of light and heavy chains (Fv) recombinantly fused to human constant domains, resulting in an mAb which is 65% human and is less immunogenic than murine mAb. Humanized mAbs are 95% of human origin with the remainder made up of six CDRs of the rodent mAb antigen-binding site making it less immunogenic than chimeric mAbs. Human mAbs are 100% human and are the least immunogenic mAb in humans.

of fully human mAbs using transgenic technology has been an active area of research.[8-10]

Chimeric mAbs are generated by linking the rodent light and heavy chain variable domains to the human immunoglobulin constant domains using recombinant DNA technology.[11] This results in an antibody that contains approximately 65% human sequences and that exhibits reduced immunogenicity and an increased serum half-life. Chimeric mAbs used to treat cancer include rituximab approved for the treatment of CD20-expressing NHL and chronic lymphocytic leukemia (CLL), and the anti-EGFR mAb cetuximab approved for the treatment of colorectal cancer and squamous cell carcinoma of the head and neck. Although the immunogenicity of chimeric mAbs is significantly reduced, they are still capable of eliciting a human anti-chimera response in some patients.

Further improvements were achieved in second-generation mAbs by incorporating the six CDRs of the rodent antibody antigen-binding site onto a human IgG antibody framework.[9] Further refinements followed after the recognition that a small number of amino acids in the murine antibody not directly involved in the CDR were still required to maintain the structure of the antigen-binding site and high-affinity binding to the target determinant.[12] This resulted in "humanized" mAbs that contain approximately 95% human sequences. Several clinically approved mAbs are humanized and include trastuzumab (Herceptin) approved for the treatment of HER2/*neu* expressing breast cancer; alemtuzumab (Campath), an anti-CD52 mAb approved for the treatment of B-cell CLL; and bevacizumab (Avastin), an anti-vascular endothelial growth factor (VEGF) mAb approved for the treatment of metastatic colorectal and lung cancer and, until recently, metastatic breast cancer. In general, humanized antibodies bind to their targets more weakly than the murine parent, but the differences between the dissociation constants (K_d) of humanized and the parental mAb are usually small enough to not be significant.[13,14] Although less frequent, humanized mAbs can rarely generate human anti-human antibody responses.[15,16] This is a result of polymorphisms located in the constant regions or anti-idiotypic recognition of the variable domain of the mAb.

In an effort to further improve the performance of mAbs, alternative approaches yielding fully human mAbs have been actively pursued. In one approach, fully human mAbs have been generated using transgenic mice expressing human immunoglobulin genes. Vaccination of these mice using the desired antigen induces fully human antibodies by the mouse.[8] Panitumumab (Vectibix), an anti-EGFR mAb approved for the treatment of metastatic colorectal cancer, and ofatumumab (Arzerra), a directly cytotoxic anti-CD20 mAb approved for the treatment of chemotherapy- and alemtuzumab-refractory CLL, were generated using such a transgenic approach.[17] Alternative approaches include the use of phage display technology. Adalimumab (Humira), a fully human mAb targeting tumor necrosis factor (TNF)-α approved for the treatment of rheumatoid arthritis, was generated using phage display.[18] Phage display techniques have the added benefit of also allowing the enhanced selection of therapeutically relevant features of antibodies.[19]

The antibody Fc region mediates effector function and hence engineering the Fc region to enhance or delete specific functions is an area of active investigation. The Fc region may be altered to augment binding to FcRIII, a stimulatory receptor, and reduce binding to FcRII, an inhibitory receptor, to enhance ADCC. Another strategy to enhance FcRIII binding and improve ADCC is to engineer Fc portions that exhibit reduced fucose glycosylation.[20] Alternatively, the Fc region may be engineered to reduce or enhance CDC by substituting isotypes such as IgG4 that exhibit little complement activation or Fc receptor binding. An additional interaction of the Fc region is with the neonatal receptor FcRn that is involved with immunoglobulin turnover. This receptor is expressed in microvessel endothelial cells, dendritic cells, monocytes, and neonatal intestinal cells of the rat and mouse as well as the human placenta; interacts with IgG Fc in a saturable and pH-dependent manner; and is responsible in part for the extended half-life of IgG in circulation.[21-23] cRn binds to IgG at a slightly acidic pH, but not at neutral or basic pH. This allows FcRn to bind IgG from acidic endosomes generated during pinocytosis and recycle the IgG back to the cell surface where it is released in the slightly basic pH of the blood. This allows for an extended serum half-life. A pharmacokinetic study in rhesus monkeys of two IgG mutants with increased affinity to human FcRn at pH 6.0 demonstrated a twofold increase in the serum half-lives for the mutants compared with wild-type antibody.[22] This approach holds much promise for favorably altering the pharmacokinetics of mAbs, ultimately leading to the potential for less frequent administration of these expensive treatments.

Other Modifications of Monoclonal Antibodies

In addition to the classical bivalent structure, antibody engineering can generate a number of variant molecules to achieve specific effects. Typical bivalent mAbs are limited by their large size and slow penetration of tissue.[24] This is especially problematic when the mAb is designed to deliver a short-lived cytotoxic agent or radioisotope. One approach to improve tissue penetration and pharmacokinetics is single-chain variable fragments (scFv).[8,25,26] These consist of the V_H and V_L chains of an IgG connected by a short linker peptide of 10 to 25 amino acids. These scFv fragments demonstrate improved tissue penetration; however, as a trade-off of being monovalent, they often display fast off-rates for the target antigen. Divalent and trivalent scFv have also been produced by linking two or three scFvs, leading to form tandem scFvs.[27,28] These may be assembled in a number of different formats, such as the formation of diabodies, in which the linker peptides are too short for the two V_L regions to fold together forcing the scFv to dimerize.[29] Diabodies demonstrate a higher affinity for the target compared with the parental scFv due to lower dissociation constants, leading to advantages in dosing and efficacy compared with other mAb formats. Triabodies and tetrabodies have also been produced utilizing still shorter linkers with subsequent increases in target affinity.[30]

A different engineering strategy led to the development of antibody constructs that contain specificities for two different antigens, the so-called bispecific antibodies.[31] Antibody constructs of this nature have been utilized to locally deliver radionuclides, toxins, cytotoxic drugs, and host effector cells to tumor cells.[32-34] One major application of this strategy is to recruit effector cytotoxic T or NK cells to the site of the tumor through combining a tumor-specific antigen specificity with an effector cell receptor, such as CD3 (T cell) or CD16 (NK cell). To be effective, a bispecific antibody must also be capable of appropriately activating the effector cell. Blinatumomab is a bispecific T-cell engager antibody that combines the specificity for CD3 and CD19 in order to redirect T cells to malignant B cells.[35] Problems associated with bispecific antibodies include immunogenicity and manufacturing issues. Catumaxomab is a rat–mouse hybrid IgG2 with dual specificity for CD3 and epithelial cell adhesion molecule (EpCAM) with the Fc-mediated specificity for the FcRIII. It is in phase III clinical trials for epithelial cancers with associated malignant ascites.[36] This molecule can bring together T cells, epithelial tumor cells, and FcRIII-bearing effector cells (NK, macrophages, and dendritic cells) in order to enhance the cellular immune response to tumor. Additional strategies discussed in detail later rely on directly linking mAbs to cytotoxic agents (toxins, chemotherapy, or radionuclides) to selectively target and enhance killing of tumor cells.

MONOCLONAL ANTIBODY ACTION

mAbs may act either in a direct or an indirect manner to kill their target tumor cells. Direct mechanisms refer to the functional outcome of the antibody binding to the target cell and leading to the lysis, apoptosis, or lethal loss of growth stimulation for that cell. Indirect antibody mechanisms are those in which the antibodies are armed with an effector molecule such as an enzyme, radioisotope, cytotoxin, or cytokine to augment their efficacy. mAbs directly kill tumor cells in a variety of ways including (i) induction of apoptosis; (ii) Fc receptor–mediated cytotoxicity through ADCC and CDC; (iii) blockade of receptor–ligand interactions necessary for tumor cell survival; (iv) binding of growth factors; and (v) receptor downmodulation with decreased signaling in pathways critical for survival and growth (Fig. 44.2). Antibodies have a multifunctional nature and these mechanisms are not mutually exclusive. A number of mAbs in clinical use achieve their antitumor effects through multiple mechanisms. Additionally, it is often difficult to demonstrate which mechanisms are at work with a particular mAb in the clinical setting. A greater understanding of the mechanisms through which mAbs exert their activity will allow for improved engineering of future mAbs.

Mechanisms of Action

A common mechanism by which an mAb may affect the killing of a tumor cell is through engagement of surface receptors on the cell and the delivery of an apoptotic signal. Several surface markers including those of the TNF receptor (TNFR) family, Fas, and the receptors for TNF-related apoptosis-inducing ligand (TRAIL) when engaged deliver an apoptotic signal and it is possible for mAbs to mimic the interaction of the native ligand with its receptor. Antibodies that bind agonistically to TRAIL receptor family members are capable of eliciting apoptotic responses.[37] These signals are stimulated by the Fab portion of the antibody and hence strategies such as using scFv can be employed. A number of mAbs are known to induce tumor cell apoptosis at least partially through direct engagement of their target receptor including (i) SGN-30, a chimeric anti-CD30 mAb that has shown clinical activity in Hodgkin lymphoma and ALCL[38]; (ii) lumiliximab, a chimeric macaque–human anti-CD23 mAb[39]; (iii) cetuximab[40]; (iv) rituximab and tositumomab[41,42]; (v) alemtuzumab (anti-CD52)[43]; and (vi) some anti-HER2 mAbs.[44] In addition to direct receptor binding, cross-linking of receptors by the mAb binding to

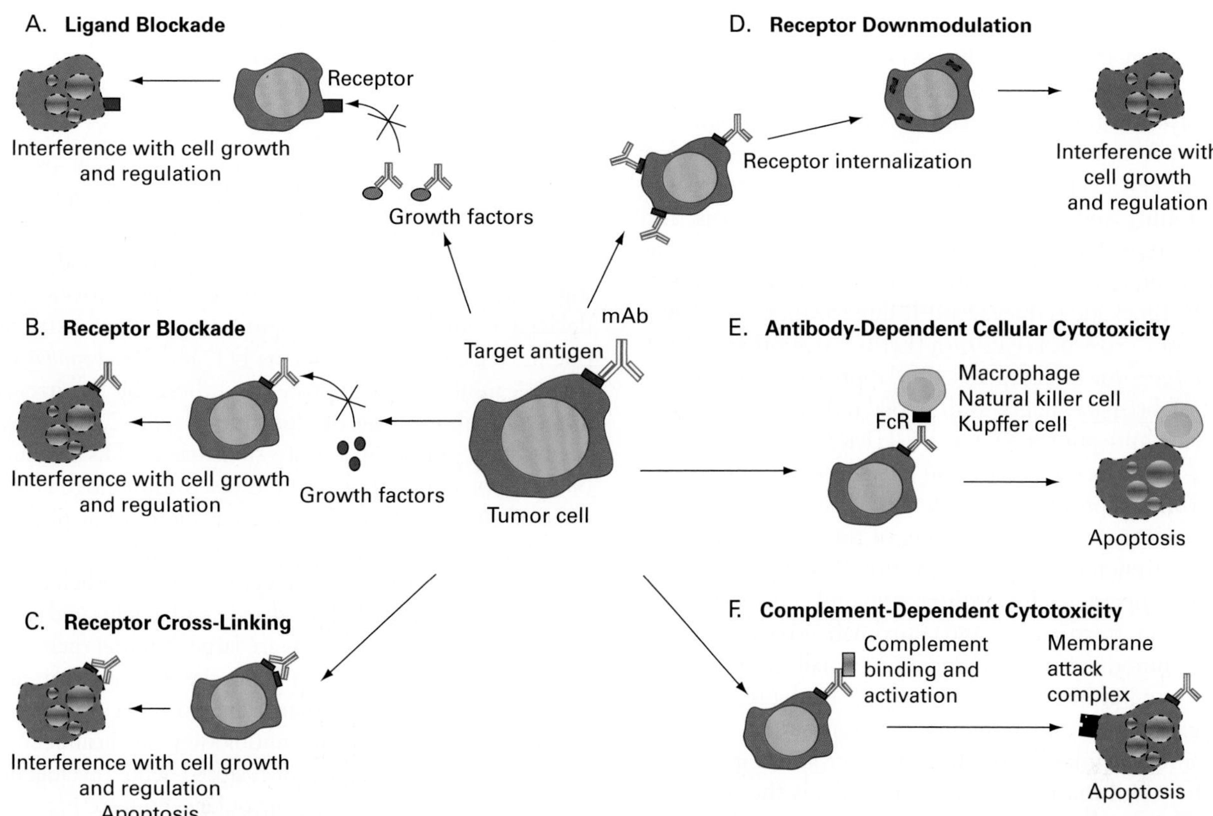

FIGURE 44–2 Monoclonal antibody (mAb) actions on tumor cells. A: Neutralization of tumor-stimulating ligands. mAbs bind to growth factors or other ligands preventing their binding to cellular receptors on tumor or stromal cells inhibiting signaling and stimulation of tumor growth. B: Receptor blockade. mAbs bind directly to the cellular receptor on the surface of the tumor cell preventing the binding of ligands or growth factors to the receptors inhibiting signaling and cell growth. C: Receptor cross-linking and induction of apoptosis. Binding of mAbs can cross-link surface receptors leading to the induction of apoptosis. D: Receptor down-modulation. Antibody binding can induce the internalization of receptors decreasing the number of receptors available on the cell surface for dimerization and signaling. E: Induction of antibody-dependent cellular cytotoxicity. Antibodies bind to cancer cells and recruit macrophages, NK cells, and other phagocytes via Fc receptor interactions to attack the cancer cell. F: Complement-dependant cytotoxicity. Following the binding of mAbs to the cell, complement proteins bind to the antibody Fc region activating the complement cascade and the formation of the membrane attack complex that induces cell lysis.

multiple receptors is believed to be an additional mechanism for inducing apoptosis. mAbs to CD19[45] and CD20[46] have been reported to cause cross-linking–induced apoptosis of B cells. Although the exact function of CD20 is not known, evidence suggests that it acts as a calcium channel to deliver intracellular signals during B-cell activation, growth, and differentiation.[47] Rituximab and tositumomab have been shown to induce apoptosis through CD20 cross-linking.[42,46]

ADCC is a major mechanism for the antitumor activity of many mAbs. ADCC is accomplished by the mAb binding a target and then recruiting the cellular immune system, typically NK cells, neutrophils, and eosinophils that then attack and destroy the tumor cell by various means. Experiments in mouse models have demonstrated that the involvement of ADCC is necessary for the activity of many mAbs including rituximab and trastuzumab.[48] ADCC is Fc-dependent. These mAbs demonstrated decreased efficacy in $FcR^{-/-}$ mice deficient for the expression of FcRIII.[48,49] Clinically, much of the evidence for this mechanism of action comes from studies of rituximab in patients with NHL. It has been found that genetic polymorphisms in the Fc receptors effect the efficacy and clinical outcome of rituximab treatment.[50,51] Patients expressing a phenylalanine at position 158 in FcRIII have a reduced affinity for the Fc binding of IgG1 that correlates with a reduced response to rituximab treatment. These studies provided the justification for mAb engineering to produce one that preferentially binds to FcRIII, a stimulatory receptor compared with the inhibitory FcRII receptor. ADCC has been implicated as an important mechanism for the activity of (i) trastuzumab[52]; (ii) cetuximab[53]; (iii) mAbs against EpCAM[54]; and mAbs against mucin (MUC-1).[55] CDC is another Fc-mediated mechanism of mAb action. In mice deficient for C1q component of the complement system, the protective activity of rituximab was abolished in a syngeneic mouse tumor model.[56] In addition to CDC, complement fixation is also involved in inflammation, chemotaxis, and opsonization, all of which may aid in tumor cell killing.

Another common mechanism of action through which mAbs act is interference with cell growth and regulation often through (i) blocking critical ligand–receptor interactions necessary for tumor survival; (ii) enhancing receptor downmodulation; and (iii) blockade of proangiogenic growth factors. The growth of normal cells and tumor cells is responsive to a number of receptor signaling pathways, although these pathways are often deregulated in tumors. One such receptor pathway is the EGFR that leads to cell cycle progression, proliferation, increased cell motility and migration, inhibition of apoptosis, and angiogenesis.[57] The anti-EGFR mAb cetuximab is a competitive antagonist that inhibits binding of the ligands to EGFR. Blockade reduces EGFR dimerization, signaling, and tumor growth. HER2/*neu* (ErbB2) is another growth factor receptor overexpressed in approximately 20% to 30% of breast cancers and associated with aggressive behavior and poorer survival.[58] HER2 signals through homo- and heterodimerization or with other members of the ErbB receptor family, leading to autophosphorylation and signal transduction. Binding of trastuzumab inhibits dimerization and receptor activation, leading to the loss of signals necessary for proliferation and cell survival.[59,60] In addition, trastuzumab and cetuximab also cause receptor downmodulation by inducing internalization of their respective surface receptors leading to decreased surface expression and reducing the number of receptor monomers available for dimerization and signaling.[14] Another antitumor mechanism of mAbs is the interruption of neoangiogenesis, the formation of new blood vessels necessary for primary tumor growth and metastasis. VEGF is upregulated in many tumors, and its activity is mediated by two primary receptors, VEGFR-1 (Flt-1) and VEGFR-2 (KDR). Inhibition of VEGF signaling by receptor blockade or by neutralization of VEGF has been shown to induce tumor cell apoptosis and growth arrest.[61-63] The humanized anti-VEGF mAb bevacizumab is approved in combination with chemotherapy for the treatment of metastatic colorectal cancer and non–small cell lung cancer.[64] The indication for bevacizumab in metastatic breast cancer was rescinded by the FDA in 2011 because of safety and efficacy concerns.

MODIFIED MONOCLONAL ANTIBODIES

Antibody-Directed Enzyme Prodrug Therapy

As single drugs, many mAbs remain poor direct cytocidal agents. To address this, mAbs have been coupled to a number of cytotoxic agents or radioisotopes to increase tumor killing. One approach to exploit the highly specific targeting of mAbs is antibody-directed enzyme prodrug therapy (ADEPT). In this strategy, an enzyme that activates a non-toxic prodrug to an active cytotoxic agent is coupled to an antibody. This specifically targets the enzyme to tumor cells. Once the excess unbound antibody–enzyme has cleared from the circulation, the prodrug is administered and converted by the enzyme into its active cytotoxic form at the site of the tumor. ADEPT has had some preclinical successes,[65] but the clinical translation of this approach has been difficult, due to immunogenicity of the antibody–enzyme conjugates and limited number of tumor responses.

Immuntotoxins

More widely explored are immunotoxins, which are conjugations of mAbs with toxins that result in highly specific cytotoxicity. In this approach, it is desirable for the target antigen to be internalized upon antibody binding, delivering the toxin into the cell. These toxins, often derived from bacteria or plants sources, are extremely potent. Bacterial toxins such as DT and *Pseudomonas* exotoxin A inhibit cellular protein synthesis by the irreversible ADP ribosylation of elongation factor-2, while plant toxins such as ricin inactivate ribosomes.[66] Disadvantages of this approach include the increased immunogenicity of most of these toxins because of their microbial or plant origins. In addition, many immunotoxin conjugates are nonspecifically taken up by pinocytosis by endothelial cells, resulting in a vascular leak syndrome with edema and weight gain. Also, toxin-armed mAbs are large, limiting their access into solid tumor masses.[67] In 2000, the immunotoxin gemtuzumab ozogamicin (Mylotarg), an anti-CD33 mAb conjugated to the DNA damaging antibiotic γ-calicheamicin, was approved for the treatment of relapsed acute myelogenous leukemia in patients 60 years or older who were not candidates for further chemotherapy.[68] In 2010, it was withdrawn from the market after post-marketing trials raised safety concerns and the drug failed to demonstrate an improvement in patient survival. In 2011, brentuximab vendotin (Adcetris), an immunotoxin composed of an anti-CD30 mAb (SGN-30) and the potent anti-microtubule agent monomethylauristatin E (MMAE), was approved for the treatment of previously treated ALCL and Hodgkin lymphoma. Denileukin diftitox (Ontak) approved for the treatment of cutaneous T-cell lymphoma is often categorized as an immunotoxin; however, this agent is not antibody based, but rather represents a fusion protein between the receptor binding domain of interleukin (IL)-2 and DT linked by a short peptide sequence.[69]

Radioimmunotherapy

Conjugation of mAbs to radioisotopes to deliver radiation to a target cell or tissue also known as radioimmunotherapy is an active area of research.[70-75] Radioimmunotherapy combines the specificity of mAbs with the tumor killing effects of radiation, sparing non-target cells from exposure to high doses of radiation. Several factors need to be weighed when utilizing this therapy including (i) the choice of an antigen that is specific to the tumor, but is not widely expressed on the surface of normal cells; (ii) the method of linking the radionuclide to the mAb; and (iii) the choice of the radionuclide and its half-life. The choice of an appropriate antigen target and hence the specific mAb is critical, as off-target killing needs to be avoided. One consequence of this is the "bystander" or "cross-fire" effect, as radiation can also kill adjacent tumor cells that may not express the target antigen. The greatest clinical experience with radioimmunotherapy is in CD20-expressing lymphomas using radionuclides such as yttrium-90 (^{90}Y)- and iodine-131 (^{131}I)-labeled anti-CD20 mAbs. Tositumomab conjugated to ^{131}I (Bexxar) and ibritumomab tiuxetan conjugated to ^{90}Y (Zevalin) are FDA-approved mAbs.[70,73] Yttrium-90 is an energetic β-emitter and ^{131}I is a mixed β- and γ-emitter. For the treatment of acute and chronic myelogenous leukemia, the humanized anti-CD33 mAb HuM-195 is conjugated to ^{131}I or ^{90}Y.[74] Other β-emitting isotopes being studied include ^{67}Cu, ^{186}Re, and ^{177}Lu. Although there is much less experience, alpha (a) particle emitters such as ^{213}Bi are in early radioimmunotherapy clinical trials.[75] Alpha-emitters have a high energy, with transfer energies ten times greater than β-emitters over a short distance. They have a short half-life compared with β-emitters. Other relevant α-emitters include ^{212}Bi, ^{211}At, and generators based on ^{225}Ac.

Antibody-Linked Cytokines

Immunostimulatory cytokines approved for therapy of cancer include IL-2; interferon-α, -β, and -γ; and hematopoietic growth factors such as granulocyte-macrophage colony-stimulating factor (GM-CSF) and G-CSF. IL-2 is FDA approved for the treatment of metastatic renal cancer and malignant melanoma.[76] A disadvantage associated with administration of these cytokines is systemic toxicity. To address this, a strategy of cytokines genetically linked to mAbs, so-called immunocytokines, has been studied.[77] In preclinical studies, this approach resulted in high intratumoral concentrations of cytokines and increased T- and NK-cell proliferation at the site of the tumor. Treatment of established pulmonary and hepatic metastases in a human melanoma xenograft model by a ganglioside GD2-specific mAb–IL-2 fusion protein resulted in increased survival of treated animals compared with those treated with equivalent doses of IL-2 and antibody alone.[77] Immunocytokine approaches aim to target immune effector cells such as NK and T cells, macrophages, and dendritic cells to the tumor to enhance antitumor immune responses.

TARGETING IMMUNE SYSTEM INHIBITORY CHECKPOINTS

In addition to directly targeting tumors and tumor growth factors such as VEGF, mAbs have been developed that enhance the patient's immune response toward the tumor. These antibodies work by directly inhibiting regulatory cells or interfering with surface receptors and ligands that act to attenuate the immune response. The elimination of immunological checkpoints may permit a more robust immune response to the tumor, although this strategy carries with it the risk of autoimmunity. The removal of immunological checkpoints relies on a pre-established antitumor immune response such as is observed in some patients with malignant melanoma, renal cell tumors, or B-cell malignancies. Alternatively, this immune response may be induced by the administration of an antitumor vaccine in association with these mAbs.

Cytotoxic T-lymphocyte antigen 4 (CTLA-4, CD152), a member of the immunoglobulin superfamily, is the best studied negative regulator of the immune response.[78] CTLA-4 is expressed on the surface of T cells and exhibits immunosuppressive function downmodulating T-cell activation in response to engagement of the T-cell receptor. Blockade of the interaction of CTLA-4 with its ligands CD80 and CD86, using mAbs, has been shown to reverse the inhibition of T-cell activation and stimulate proliferation that leads to enhanced antitumor immunity in both preclinical models and patients.[79,80] Another checkpoint being targeted for immunomodulation is the membrane molecule programmed cell death 1 (PD-1) and its ligand PD-L1.[81-83] PD-1 is a member of the CD28/CTLA-4 family of regulatory T-cell receptors. It is expressed on the surface of activated B and T cells and is involved in the induction of immune tolerance.[81] Its ligand, PD-L1, is constitutively expressed at low levels on hematopoietic cells, including resting T, B, myeloid, and dendritic cells, as well as some non-hematopoietic cells.[84] PD-L1 is upregulated during T-cell activation and it has been shown to interact with PD-1 and CD80. The interaction of PD-1 with its ligands results in an inhibitory signal in activated T cells that promotes their apoptosis and anergy. Similarly, the interaction of PD-L1 and CD80 has also been shown to induce an inhibitory signal to activated T cells.[85] Chronic stimulation of PD-1 may result in T-cell "exhaustion" and attenuation of immune responses.[86] Tumors can exploit these checkpoint controls to inhibit antitumor immune responses. Targeting of PD-1 and it ligands by mAbs represents a promising strategy to remove this checkpoint and thereby augment tumor immunity.

MONOCLONAL ANTIBODIES IN HEMATOLOGICAL MALIGNANCIES

Targeting CD20

CD20 is a 31- to 37-kDa cell surface phosphoprotein found on almost all B cells and B-cell malignancies. It is expressed at all stages of B-cell development except early progenitors, stem cells, plasmablasts, and plasma cells.[87] The presence of CD20 on B-cell malignancies, but not on B-cell progenitors, not only allows this antigen to be targeted, leading to the rapid depletion of B cells, but also allows repopulation of the B-cell niche following treatment. In addition, CD20 is not downmodulated and is not shed from the surface of the B cell, making it an ideal target for mAb cancer therapy.

The first mAb to be approved by the FDA for the treatment of cancer was rituximab (Rituxin) that targets CD20. Rituximab is a chimeric human–mouse IgG1 antibody.[88] It exhibits powerful B-cell-depleting properties through the induction of apoptosis, inhibition of B-cell growth, CDC, sensitization of cells to chemotherapy and radiation, and the induction of ADCC.[89]

Since its approval in 1997, rituximab has revolutionized the treatment of B-cell malignancies, particularly B-cell NHL and B-cell CLL. In a multi-institutional phase II trial of relapsed NHL (Working Formulation grades A-C), 166 patients were treated with rituximab. The overall response rate for this study was 48%, with 6% of patients exhibiting complete response (CR) and the remainder having partial response (PR), a response rate comparable to single-modality chemotherapy. Among those who did not achieve a CR or PR, 56 of 75 patients exhibited reductions in measurable disease. The median response duration was 13 months and toxicity generally mild.[90] Based on these data, rituximab was approved by the FDA for the treatment of relapsed NHL. Further phase III clinical trials comparing chemotherapy (cyclophosphamide, doxorubicin, vincristine, and prednisone; CHOP) with rituximab plus chemotherapy (R-CHOP) showed a higher rate of complete remission in the R-CHOP group (76%, as compared with 63% with CHOP alone). The addition of rituximab to CHOP also showed for the first time a statistically significant prolongation of survival in diffuse large B-cell lymphoma.[91]

Following the success of rituximab, a number of other mAbs targeting CD20 have been developed. Ofatumumab (Arzerra) was approved in 2010 for the treatment of fludarabine- and alemtuzumab-refractory CLL. Ofatumumab is a fully human mAb that binds to both the small and large loops of the CD20 molecule. Binding to both loops of CD20 is thought to bring the antibody in closer proximity to the cell membrane, allowing increased CDC and cell killing. This has been shown in vitro where CDC can be initiated by ofatumumab in cells that are resistant to rituximab.[92] Ofatumumab was shown to be effective in the setting of fludarabine- and alemtuzumab-refractory CLL, with a 43% overall response rate and little serious toxicity.[93] In a retrospective analysis, ofatumumab was equally effective in CLL in terms of overall response rate or median overall survival when comparing patients refractory to rituximab with those who had not been previously treated with rituximab. This is an indication that the killing of CLL cells was maintained with ofatumumab in patients with rituximab-refractory disease.

In addition to rituximab and ofatumumab, which induce their effects by binding to CD20 and require ADCC or CDC for killing, two radiolabeled anti-CD20 antibodies, ibritumomab tiuxetan based on the murine parent mAb of rituximab linked to tiuxetan and conjugated to ^{90}Y (Zevalin) and tositumomab, another murine anti-CD20 mAb labeled with ^{131}I (Bexxar), are approved by the FDA for the treatment of chemotherapy- and rituximab-refractory follicular NHL.[70,73] The radiolabeling of ibritumomab and tositumomab allows these antibodies to kill tumor cells without the need for CDC or ADCC. The radioactive emissions are also effective against cancer cells over a distance of several cell diameters and may therefore kill CD20-negative cells adjacent to CD20-expressing cells through the "bystander effect."[94] This characteristic may be important in cancers refractory to rituximab, which have downmodulated CD20 on the surface of the cells or are resistant to CDC or ADCC.

Ibritumomab tiuxetan and tositumomab have been studied in rituximab-refractory follicular, small B-cell, and mantle cell NHL and have reported overall response rates of 57% to 83%.[94] In a trial in which almost half the patients were deemed to be unresponsive to their immediate prior treatment, ^{90}Y-ibritumomab plus rituximab 250 mg/m^2 × 2 doses was compared with rituximab 375 mg/m^2 weekly × 4 doses.[95] Of those treated with ibritumomab plus rituximab, 80% responded compared with 56% of patients treated with rituximab alone. Thirty percent of the ibritumomab and rituximab group exhibited CR versus 16% in those patients treated with rituximab alone. Adverse events associated with either ibritumomab tiuxetan or tositumomab include infusion-related symptoms, cytokine release syndrome, and tumor lysis syndrome, especially in patients with high circulating B-cell counts. The major toxicity of both radiolabeled antibodies is bone marrow suppression, especially thrombocytopenia and granulocytopenia. Another concern with the murine-derived ibritumomab tiuxetan or tositumomab is the induction of neutralizing HAMA. The frequency of HAMA induction is also related to the amount of prior chemotherapy that a patient has received, occurring less frequently in heavily pretreated patients.

Targeting CD52

CD52 is a glycosylphosphatidylinositol-anchored antigen expressed at high density (>450,000 molecules per cell) on normal and malignant T and B cells, NK cells, monocytes, macrophages, eosinophils, and epithelial cells of the male genital tract. It is not expressed on most granulocytes, erythrocytes, and platelets. CD52 is not expressed on hematopoietic stem cells and plasma cells. The FDA approved alemtuzumab (Campath), a humanized rat mAb that targets CD52 for the treatment of alkylating agent and fludarabine-refractory CLL, in 2001. Alemtuzumab has been shown to initiate CDC and ADCC and induce apoptosis of lymphocytes. In phase II trials in patients with relapsed and resistant low-grade B-cell NHL, alemtuzumab had overall response rates of 14% to 44% with few CR.[96] Alemtuzumab showed significantly greater efficacy in B-cell CLL, with responses reported in 33% to 50% of previously treated, relapsed, or chemotherapy-refractory patients. In 93 patients who failed alkylating agents and fludarabine treated with alemtuzumab 30 mg intravenously three times per week, the overall response rate was 33%. An additional 59% of patients had disease stabilization with resolution or improvement of CLL-related symptoms. It was noted that patients with lymph nodes >5 cm diameter failed to respond to alemtuzumab while the complete resolution of lymphadenopathy was seen in 64% of patients with lymph nodes <2 cm. It is hypothesized that alemtuzumab's lower efficacy in bulky disease is the result of a failure to penetrate the solid tissue, resulting in lower concentrations of the mAb or reduced ADCC at the site of bulky disease. In CLL, the mutation of p53 is correlated to poor response to conventional chemotherapy; however, patients with CLL expressing mutant p53 are twice as likely to respond to alemtuzumab than patients with CLL lacking a p53 mutation.[97]

Targeting CD30

CD30 is a cellular membrane protein of the TNFR family expressed on activated T and B cells. It is also highly expressed on malignant Hodgkin and Reed-Sternberg cells, in ALCL, embryonal carcinomas, and select subtypes of B-cell-derived, NHLs and mature T-cell lymphomas. The immunotoxin brentuximab vedotin (Adcetris, SGN-35) was approved by the FDA in 2011 and became the first new treatment for Hodgkin lymphoma in 30 years. Brentuximab vedotin is an antibody-drug conjugate between the antitubulin agent MMAE and the anti-CD30 mAb cAC10. Clinical studies with unconjugated anti-CD30 antibodies have shown disappointing clinical activity. Objective responses were observed in 6% of patients with Hodgkin lymphoma who were treated with MDX-060[98] and in none of those treated with cAC10 (SGN-30).[99] However, the results of a pivotal phase II study of brentuximab vedotin in relapsed or refractory Hodgkin lymphoma were impressive.[100] In this study, 102 patients with refractory or relapsed classical Hodgkin lymphoma received brentuximab vedotin every 3 weeks for a median of 27 weeks. Of the 102 patients, 97 exhibited a reduction in tumor volume. Of these, 34% had CR and a further 40% had a PR. In a phase II study of relapsed or refractory systemic ALCL, brentuximab vedotin was also shown to be effective. In this single-arm study in 58 patients, the overall response was 86% with CR in 53% of patients. Based on these studies, brentuximab vedotin received accelerated approval for the treatment of Hodgkin lymphoma that has relapsed after autologous stem cell transplant and for the management of relapsed ALCL.

MONOCLONAL ANTIBODIES IN SOLID TUMORS

Targeting the ErbB Receptor Family

The ErbB family of signaling receptor tyrosine kinases includes EGFR (ErbB1), HER2/neu (ErbB2), HER3 (ErbB3), and HER4 (ErbB4). Members of this family are activated by ligand binding and subsequent homo- or heterodimerization of the receptor leading to signal transduction. EGFR overexpression in a variety of tumors is associated with more aggressive behavior and a poorer prognosis.[101] Commonly, HER2 is overexpressed in 20% to 30% of breast cancers and is also associated with poorer prognosis.[58]

Cetuximab (Erbitux) is a chimeric mAb that competitively inhibits the binding of EGF and other ligands to the EGFR on both normal and cancerous tissue, blocking the activation of receptor-associated kinases. Cetuximab has been shown to inhibit cell cycle progression, enhance apoptosis, have anti-angiogenic activity, inhibit metastases, and reduce cellular repair after chemotherapy or radiation injury.[102] Cetuximab is indicated for the treatment of patients with EGFR-expressing, KRAS wild-type metastatic colorectal cancer in combination with chemotherapy and as a single agent in patients who have failed oxaliplatin- and irinotecan-based therapy. It is also approved in combination with radiation therapy for the initial treatment of locally advanced squamous cell carcinoma of the head and neck and in combination with platinum-based therapy with 5-fluorouracil for the first-line treatment of patients with recurrent locoregional disease or metastatic squamous cell carcinoma of the head and neck and as a single agent for the treatment of patients with recurrent or metastatic squamous cell carcinoma of the head and neck who failed prior platinum-based therapy. Adverse reactions include rash, malaise, pulmonary inflammation, and fever. Anaphylaxis appears to be due to host IgE antibodies specific for galactose-α-1, 3-galactose residues expressed on the Fab portion of the cetuximab heavy chain.[103] Panitumumab (Vectibix) is a fully humanized anti-EGFR mAb. Panitumumab is approved for patients with EGFR-expressing metastatic colorectal cancer with progression despite prior treatment. This approval is based on a phase III study of 463 patients with metastatic colorectal cancer randomly assigned to best supportive care compared with best supportive care plus panitumumab.[104] Mean progression-free was survival was longer in patients receiving panitumumab (96 vs. 60 days); however, median times to progression were similar and there was no difference in the overall survival between the two arms. It is important to note that the efficacy of anti-EGFR antibodies is limited to patients with KRAS wild-type tumors and current recommendations are that KRAS status be determined prior to initiating cetuximab or panitumumab therapy.[105]

Trastuzumab (Herceptin) is a humanized mAb directed against the HER2 protein. It is approved for the treatment of patients with metastatic breast cancer whose tumor overexpresses HER2. This includes first-line therapy in combination with paclitaxel and as second-line therapy as a single agent in patients who have failed earlier chemotherapy and in HER2-overexpressing metastatic gastric or gastroesophageal junction adenocarcinoma. Clinical benefit has largely been seen in patients who have 3+ HER2 overexpression by immunohistochemical staining of their tumor. Patients with 2+ HER2 overexpression that may also benefit may be selected based on HER2 gene amplification detected on fluorescence in situ hybridization.

Single-agent trastuzumab response rates range from 12% to 34% for metastatic breast cancer, with improvements in survival rates for HER2-overexpressing patients treated in the adjuvant setting.[106] In a phase III clinical trial of 469 patients with HER2 overexpressing breast cancer who had not previously received chemotherapy, median time to progression, median time to treatment failure, and median overall survival were longer in the treatment arm that received chemotherapy and trastuzumab compared with the arm that received chemotherapy alone.[107] Trastuzumab is believed to have several mechanisms of action. One is through downregulation of cell surface HER2 expression through trastuzumab-mediated endocytosis and degradation of the receptor.[106] The others that contribute to activity include ADCC, in particular a role for the action of tumor-associated NK cells has been described, and suppression of anti-apoptotic pathways.[108] Other studies have shown that trastuzumab can increase DNA strand breaks and cause cell cycle perturbations, inhibition of cell growth, and arrest in the G1 phase of the cell cycle.[109] Adverse reactions include fever, chills, nausea, diarrhea, headache, dizziness, and cardiac failure. The most severe reactions occur in patients with pre-existing pulmonary compromise and in those patients with pre-existing cardiovascular disease. The combination of trastuzumab with anthracyclines results in a higher rate of cardiotoxicity.[110]

Targeting Angiogenesis

VEGF is a 45-kDa glycoprotein and cell-specific mitogen that regulates endothelial cell proliferation, migration, permeability, and survival.[111] VEGF plays a critical role in early tumor vascularization and growth by recruiting bone marrow–derived endothelial stem cells and inducing their differentiation into tumor vessels. In addition, it has been shown to block differentiation of dendritic and other hematopoietic cell lineages and decrease antigen presentation. Elevated levels of VEGF are associated with a poorer prognosis in a variety of tumors.

Bevacizumab (Avastin) is a humanized IgG1 mAb that was approved in 2004 for the first-line treatment of patients with metastatic colorectal carcinoma in combination with fluorouracil-based chemotherapy. It has subsequently been approved for the treatment of metastatic lung cancer, glioblastoma, and metastatic renal cell cancer. Bevacizumab binds with a high affinity and neutralizes all biologically active isoforms of VEGF, thereby preventing the interaction of VEGF with its receptors and inhibiting angiogenesis.

In a trial in metastatic colorectal cancer, 926 patients were randomized to the combination of irinotecan, fluorouracil, and leucovorin (IFL) and bevacizumab or IFL and placebo.[112] The addition of bevacizumab to IFL increased the overall response rate (44.8% vs. 34.8%) and improved progression-free survival (10.6 vs. 6.2 months) and overall survival (20.3 vs. 15.6 months) compared with IFL chemotherapy with placebo. In a trial targeting non–small cell lung cancer, 878 patients with recurrent or advanced non–small cell lung cancer (stage IIIB or IV) were randomized to chemotherapy with paclitaxel and carboplatin alone or paclitaxel and carboplatin plus bevacizumab.[113] The paclitaxel–carboplatin–bevacizumab group had a median overall survival of 12.3 months, compared with 10.3 months in the paclitaxel–carboplatin group. Survival rates were also improved in the paclitaxel–carboplatin–bevacizumab group, with 23% survival at 2 years compared with 15% for the paclitaxel–carboplatin group. The median progression-free survival was also significantly improved in the paclitaxel–carboplatin–bevacizumab arm. After completion of four cycles of chemotherapy, patients are often maintained on bevacizumab until progression. Bevacizumab is also associated with an increased risk of bowel perforation, impaired healing, and wound dehiscence. Less common side effects include hypertension, nephrosis and proteinuria, and thromboembolic events including deep vein thrombosis, pulmonary embolism, pulmonary hemorrhage, and myocardial infarction.

Targeting CTLA-4

CTLA-4 expressed on T cells acts to attenuate the immune response and is a normal homeostatic control to prevent autoimmunity. Due to its strong inhibitory effects on the immune response, CTLA-4 is an attractive target for immunomodulation. Preclinical mouse models using mAbs against CTLA-4 demonstrated significant antitumor efficacy, particularly in immunogenic tumors.

Ipilimumab (Yervoy) is a fully human IgG1 mAb that inhibits CTLA-4-mediated T-cell suppression by blocking its interaction with costimulatory molecules on antigen-presenting cells, leading to enhanced immune responses against tumors. It was approved in 2011 for the treatment of metastatic melanoma. A pivotal gp100 vaccine-controlled phase III trial randomized 676 HLA-A*0201-positive patients with metastatic melanoma, in a 3:1:1 ratio, to receive ipilimumab plus gp100 (403 patients), ipilimumab alone (137 patients), or gp100 alone (136 patients).[80] Ipilimumab was administered at a dose of 3 mg/kg with or without gp100 every 3 weeks for up to four treatments. The median overall survival was 10.0 months among patients receiving ipilimumab plus gp100. This compared with 6.4 months among patients receiving gp100 and 10.1 months for ipilimumab alone. In the ipilimumab-alone group, the overall response rate of 10.9% and a disease control rate (the proportion of patients with PR or CR or stable disease) of 28.5% compared with 1.5% and 11%, respectively, for the gp100 vaccine alone. In the ipilimumab-alone group, 9 of 15 (60.0%) responding patients maintained an objective response for at least 2 years and in the ipilimumab-plus-gp100 group, 4 of 23 patients (17.4%) maintained the response for at least 2 years. Neither of the two patients in the gp100-alone group who had a PR maintained the response for 2 years. There were no differences in the time to progression among treatment arms.

Severe immune-related adverse events occurred in 10% to 15% of patients treated with ipilimumab and in 3% of patients treated with gp100 alone. There were 14 deaths related to ipilimumab (2.1%), 7 associated with immune-related adverse events. In a randomized trial comparing ipilimumab in combination with dacarbazine with dacarbazine plus placebo, ipilimumab improved overall survival in patients with previously untreated metastatic melanoma. Ipilimumab, an mAb, is the first agent to demonstrate an improvement in the survival of patients with metastatic malignant melanoma.

REFERENCES

1. Petersen JG, Dorrington KJ. An in vitro system for studying the kinetics of interchain disulfide bond formation in immunoglobulin G. *J Biol Chem.* 1974;249(17):5633-5641.
2. Burrows PD, Cooper MD. B-cell development in man. *Curr Opin Immunol.* 1993;5(2):201-206.
3. Von Behring E, Kitasato S: Ueber das zustandekommen der diphtherie-immunitat and der tetanus-Immunität bei thieren. *Dtsch Med Wochenschr.* 1890;16:1113-1114.
4. Hericourt J, Richet C. Physologie pathologique'—de la serotherapie dans la traitement du cancer. *C R Hebd Seances Acad Sci.* 1895;121:567.
5. Ehrlich P. On immunity with special reference to cell life: Croonian lecture. In: Himmelweir B, ed. *The Collected Papers of Paul Ehrlich, Vol II: Immunology and Cancer Research.* London: Pergamon; 1956:148-192, 195-196.
6. Köhler G, Milstein C. Continuous cultures of fused cells secreting antibody of predefined specificity. *Nature.* 1975;256(5517):495-497.
7. Goldstein G, Norman DJ, Shield CF 3rd, et al. OKT3 monoclonal antibody reversal of acute renal allograft rejection unresponsive to conventional immunosuppressive treatments. *Prog Clin Biol Res.* 1986;224:239-249.
8. Hudson PJ, Souriau C. Engineered antibodies. *Nat Med.* 2003;9(1):129-134.
9. Riechmann L, Clark M, Waldmann H, Winter G. Reshaping human antibodies for therapy. *Nature.* 1988;332(6162):323-327.
10. Winter G, Milstein C. Man-made antibodies. *Nature.* 1991;349(6307):293-299.
11. Morrison SL, Johnson MJ, Herzenberg LA, Oi VT. Chimeric human antibody molecules: mouse antigen-binding domains with human constant region domains. *Proc Natl Acad Sci U S A.* 1984;81(21):6851-6855.
12. Queen C, Schneider WP, Selick HE, et al. A humanized antibody that binds to the interleukin 2 receptor. *Proc Natl Acad Sci U S A.* 1989;86(24):10029-10033.
13. Presta LG, Lahr SJ, Shields RL, et al. Humanization of an antibody directed against IgE. *J Immunol.* 1993;151(5):2623-2632.
14. Carter P, Presta L, Gorman CM, et al. Humanization of an anti-p185HER2 antibody for human cancer therapy. *Proc Natl Acad Sci U S A.* 1992;89(10):4285-4289.
15. Aarden L, Ruuls SR, Wolbink G. Immunogenicity of anti-tumor necrosis factor antibodies—toward improved methods of anti-antibody measurement. *Curr Opin Immunol.* 2008;20(4):431-435.
16. Ritter G, Cohen LS, Williams C Jr, Richards EC, Old LJ, Welt S. Serological analysis of human anti-human antibody responses in colon cancer patients treated with repeated doses of humanized monoclonal antibody A33. *Cancer Res.* 2001;61(18):6851-6859.
17. Jakobovits A, Amado RG, Yang X, Roskos L, Schwab G. From XenoMouse technology to panitumumab, the first fully human antibody product from transgenic mice. *Nat Biotechnol.* 2007;25(10):1134-1143.
18. Weinblatt ME, Keystone EC, Furst DE, et al. Adalimumab, a fully human anti-tumor necrosis factor alpha monoclonal antibody, for the treatment of rheumatoid arthritis in patients taking concomitant methotrexate: the ARMADA trial. *Arthritis Rheum.* 2003;48(1):35-45.
19. Hoogenboom HR. Selecting and screening recombinant antibody libraries. *Nat Biotechnol.* 2005;23(9):1105-1116.
20. Shinkawa T, Nakamura K, Yamane N, et al. The absence of fucose but not the presence of galactose or bisecting N-acetylglucosamine of human IgG1 complex-type oligosaccharides shows the critical role of enhancing antibody-dependent cellular cytotoxicity. *J Biol Chem.* 2003;278(5):3466-3473.
21. Roopenian DC, Akilesh S. FcRn: the neonatal Fc receptor comes of age. *Nat Rev Immunol.* 2007;7(9):715-725.
22. Hinton PR, Johlfs MG, Xiong JM, et al. Engineered human IgG antibodies with longer serum half-lives in primates. *J Biol Chem.* 2004;279(8):6213-6216.
23. Lee TY, Tjin Tham Sjin RM, Movahedi S, et al. Linking antibody Fc domain to endostatin significantly improves endostatin half-life and efficacy. *Clin Cancer Res.* 2008;14(5):1487-1493.
24. Jain RK. Delivery of molecular and cellular medicine to solid tumors. *Adv Drug Deliv Rev.* 2001;46(1-3):149-168.
25. Adams GP, Schier R, McCall AM, et al. Prolonged in vivo tumour retention of a human diabody targeting the extracellular domain of human HER2/neu. *Br J Cancer.* 1998;77(9):1405-1412.
26. Olafsen T, Tan GJ, Cheung CW, et al. Characterization of engineered anti-p185HER-2 (scFv-CH3)2 antibody fragments (minibodies) for tumor targeting. *Protein Eng Des Sel.* 2004;17(4):315-323.
27. Xiong CY, Natarajan A, Shi XB, Denardo GL, Denardo SJ. Development of tumor targeting anti-MUC-1 multimer: effects of di-scFv unpaired cysteine location on PEGylation and tumor binding. *Protein Eng Des Sel.* 2006;19(8):359-367.
28. Kufer P, Lutterbuse R, Baeuerle PA. A revival of bispecific antibodies. *Trends Biotechnol.* 2004;22(5):238-244.
29. Holliger P, Prospero T, Winter G. "Diabodies": small bivalent and bispecific antibody fragments. *Proc Natl Acad Sci U S A.* 1993;90(14):6444-6448.
30. Le Gall F, Kipriyanov SM, Moldenhauer G, Little M. Di-, tri- and tetrameric single chain Fv antibody fragments against human CD19: effect of valency on cell binding. *FEBS Lett.* 1999;453(1-2):164-168.
31. Chames P, Baty D. Bispecific antibodies for cancer therapy: the light at the end of the tunnel? *mAbs.* 2009;1(6):539-547.
32. Staerz UD, Kanagawa O, Bevan MJ. Hybrid antibodies can target sites for attack by T cells. *Nature.* 1985;314(6012):628-631.
33. Segal DM, Weiner GJ, Weiner LM. Introduction: bispecific antibodies. *J Immunol Methods.* 2001;248(1-2):1-6.
34. Carter P. Improving the efficacy of antibody-based cancer therapies. *Nat Rev Cancer.* 2001;1(2):118-129.
35. Baeuerle PA, Kufer P, Bargou R. BiTE: teaching antibodies to engage T-cells for cancer therapy. *Curr Opin Mol Ther.* 2009;11(1):22-30.
36. Shen J, Zhu Z. Catumaxomab, a rat/murine hybrid trifunctional bispecific monoclonal antibody for the treatment of cancer. *Curr Opin Mol Ther.* 2008;10(3):273-284.
37. Takeda K, Stagg J, Yagita H, Okumura K, Smyth MJ. Targeting death-inducing receptors in cancer therapy. *Oncogene.* 2007;26(25):3745-3757.
38. Wahl AF, Klussman K, Thompson JD, et al. The anti-CD30 monoclonal antibody SGN-30 promotes growth arrest and DNA fragmentation in vitro and affects antitumor activity in models of Hodgkin's disease. *Cancer Res.* 2002;62(13):3736-3742.
39. Pathan NI, Chu P, Hariharan K, Cheney C, Molina A, Byrd J. Mediation of apoptosis by and antitumor activity of lumiliximab in chronic lymphocytic leukemia cells and CD23+ lymphoma cell lines. *Blood.* 2008;111(3):1594-1602.
40. Bianco R, Daniele G, Ciardiello F, Tortora G. Monoclonal antibodies targeting the epidermal growth factor receptor. *Curr Drug Targets.* 2005;6(3):275-287.
41. Shan D, Ledbetter JA, Press OW. Signaling events involved in anti-CD20-induced apoptosis of malignant human B cells. *Cancer Immunol Immunother.* 2000;48(12):673-683.
42. Cardarelli PM, Quinn M, Buckman D, et al. Binding to CD20 by anti-B1 antibody or F(ab')(2) is sufficient for induction of apoptosis in B-cell lines. *Cancer Immunol Immunother.* 2002;51(1):15-24.
43. Rowan W, Tite J, Topley P, Brett SJ. Cross-linking of the CAMPATH-1 antigen (CD52) mediates growth inhibition in human B- and T-lymphoma cell lines, and subsequent emergence of CD52-deficient cells. *Immunology.* 1998;95(3):427-436.
44. Hinoda Y, Sasaki S, Ishida T, Imai K. Monoclonal antibodies as effective therapeutic agents for solid tumors. *Cancer Sci.* 2004;95(8):621-625.
45. Horton HM, Bernett MJ, Pong E, et al. Potent in vitro and in vivo activity of an Fc-engineered anti-CD19 monoclonal antibody against lymphoma and leukemia. *Cancer Res.* 2008;68(19):8049-8057.
46. Shan D, Ledbetter JA, Press OW. Apoptosis of malignant human B cells by ligation of CD20 with monoclonal antibodies. *Blood.* 1998;91(5):1644-1652.
47. Tedder TF, Engel P. CD20: a regulator of cell-cycle progression of B lymphocytes. *Immunol Today.* 1994;15(9):450-454.

48. Clynes RA, Towers TL, Presta LG, Ravetch JV. Inhibitory Fc receptors modulate in vivo cytotoxicity against tumor targets. *Nat Med.* 2000;6(4):443-446.
49. Nimmerjahn F, Bruhns P, Horiuchi K, Ravetch JV. FcgammaRIV: a novel FcR with distinct IgG subclass specificity. *Immunity.* 2005;23(1):41-51.
50. Cartron G, Dacheux L, Salles G, et al. Therapeutic activity of humanized anti-CD20 monoclonal antibody and polymorphism in IgG Fc receptor FcgammaRIIIa gene. *Blood.* 2002;99(3):754-758.
51. Weng WK, Levy R. Two immunoglobulin G fragment C receptor polymorphisms independently predict response to rituximab in patients with follicular lymphoma. *J Clin Oncol.* 2003;21(21):3940-3947.
52. Cooley S, Burns LJ, Repka T, Miller JS. Natural killer cell cytotoxicity of breast cancer targets is enhanced by two distinct mechanisms of antibody-dependent cellular cytotoxicity against LFA-3 and HER2/neu. *Exp Hematol.* 1999;27(10): 1533-1541.
53. Kimura H, Sakai K, Arao T, Shimoyama T, Tamura T, Nishio K. Antibody-dependent cellular cytotoxicity of cetuximab against tumor cells with wild-type or mutant epidermal growth factor receptor. *Cancer Sci.* 2007;98(8):1275-1280.
54. Prang N, Preithner S, Brischwein K, et al. Cellular and complement-dependent cytotoxicity of Ep-CAM-specific monoclonal antibody MT201 against breast cancer cell lines. *Br J Cancer.* 2005;92(2):342-349.
55. Danielczyk A, Stahn R, Faulstich D, et al. PankoMab: a potent new generation anti-tumour MUC1 antibody. *Cancer Immunol Immunother.* 2006;55(11):1337-1347.
56. Di Gaetano N, Cittera E, Nota R, et al. Complement activation determines the therapeutic activity of rituximab in vivo. *J Immunol.* 2003;171(3):1581-1587.
57. Arteaga CL. Epidermal growth factor receptor dependence in human tumors: more than just expression? *Oncologist.* 2002;7(suppl 4):31-39.
58. Slamon DJ, Clark GM, Wong SG, Levin WJ, Ullrich A, McGuire WL. Human breast cancer: correlation of relapse and survival with amplification of the HER-2/neu oncogene. *Science.* 1987;235(4785):177-182.
59. Yakes FM, Chinratanalab W, Ritter CA, King W, Seelig S, Arteaga CL. Herceptin-induced inhibition of phosphatidylinositol-3 kinase and Akt is required for antibody-mediated effects on p27, cyclin D1, and antitumor action. *Cancer Res.* 2002;62(14):4132-4141.
60. Pietras RJ, Poen JC, Gallardo D, Wongvipat PN, Lee HJ, Slamon DJ. Monoclonal antibody to HER-2/neu receptor modulates repair of radiation-induced DNA damage and enhances radiosensitivity of human breast cancer cells overexpressing this oncogene. *Cancer Res.* 1999;59(6):1347-1355.
61. Bruns CJ, Liu W, Davis DW, et al. Vascular endothelial growth factor is an in vivo survival factor for tumor endothelium in a murine model of colorectal carcinoma liver metastases. *Cancer.* 2000;89(3):488-499.
62. Kim KJ, Li B, Winer J, et al. Inhibition of vascular endothelial growth factor-induced angiogenesis suppresses tumour growth in vivo. *Nature.* 1993;362(6423):841-844.
63. Shaheen RM, Tseng WW, Vellagas R, et al. Effects of an antibody to vascular endothelial growth factor receptor-2 on survival, tumor vascularity, and apoptosis in a murine model of colon carcinomatosis. *Int J Oncol.* 2001;18(2):221-226.
64. Presta LG, Chen H, O'Connor SJ, et al. Humanization of an anti-vascular endothelial growth factor monoclonal antibody for the therapy of solid tumors and other disorders. *Cancer Res.* 1997;57(20):4593-4599.
65. Senter PD, Springer CJ. Selective activation of anticancer prodrugs by monoclonal antibody-enzyme conjugates. *Adv Drug Deliv Rev.* 2001;53(3):247-264.
66. Kreitman RJ. Recombinant toxins for the treatment of cancer. *Curr Opin Mol Ther.* 2003;5(1):44-51.
67. Jain RK. Delivery of molecular medicine to solid tumors: lessons from in vivo imaging of gene expression and function. *J Control Release.* 2001;74(1-3):7-25.
68. Sievers EL, Appelbaum FR, Spielberger RT, et al. Selective ablation of acute myeloid leukemia using antibody-targeted chemotherapy: a phase I study of an anti-CD33 calicheamicin immunoconjugate. *Blood.* 1999;93(11):3678-3684.
69. Olsen E, Duvic M, Frankel A, et al. Pivotal phase III trial of two dose levels of denileukin diftitox for the treatment of cutaneous T-cell lymphoma. *J Clin Oncol.* 2001;19(2):376-388.
70. Press OW, Eary JF, Appelbaum FR, et al. Phase II trial of 131I-B1 (anti-CD20) antibody therapy with autologous stem cell transplantation for relapsed B cell lymphomas. *Lancet.* 1995;346(8971):336-340.
71. Axworthy DB, Reno JM, Hylarides MD, et al. Cure of human carcinoma xenografts by a single dose of pretargeted yttrium-90 with negligible toxicity. *Proc Natl Acad Sci U S A.* 2000;97(4):1802-1807.
72. Witzig TE, Gordon LI, Cabanillas F, et al. Randomized controlled trial of yttrium-90-labeled ibritumomab tiuxetan radioimmunotherapy versus rituximab immunotherapy for patients with relapsed or refractory low-grade, follicular, or transformed B-cell non-Hodgkin's lymphoma. *J Clin Oncol.* 2002;20(10):2453-2463.
73. Kaminski MS, Tuck M, Estes J, et al. 131I-tositumomab therapy as initial treatment for follicular lymphoma. *N Engl J Med.* 2005;352(5):441-449.
74. Burke JM, Caron PC, Papadopoulos EB, et al. Cytoreduction with iodine-131-anti-CD33 antibodies before bone marrow transplantation for advanced myeloid leukemias. *Bone Marrow Transplant.* 2003;32(6):549-556.
75. Jurcic JG, Larson SM, Sgouros G, et al. Targeted alpha particle immunotherapy for myeloid leukemia. *Blood.* 2002;100(4):1233-1239.
76. Rosenberg SA, Yang JC, Topalian SL, et al. Treatment of 283 consecutive patients with metastatic melanoma or renal cell cancer using high-dose bolus interleukin 2. *JAMA.* 1994;271(12):907-913.
77. Lode HN, Reisfeld RA. Targeted cytokines for cancer immunotherapy. *Immunol Res.* 2000;21(2-3):279-288.
78. Lenschow DJ, Walunas TL, Bluestone JA. CD28/B7 system of T cells costimulation. *Annu Rev Immunol.* 1996;14:233-258.
79. Quezada SA, Peggs KS, Curran MA, Allison JP. CTLA4 blockade and GM-CSF combination immunotherapy alters the intratumor balance of effector and regulatory T cells. *J Clin Invest.* 2006;116:1935-1945.
80. Hodi FS, O'Day SJ, McDermott DF, et al. Improved survival with ipilimumab in patients with metastatic melanoma. *N Engl J Med.* 2010;363:711-723.
81. Freeman GJ, Long AJ, Iwai Y, et al. Engagement of the PD-1 immunoinhibitory receptor by a novel B7 family member leads to negative regulation of lymphocyte activation. *J Exp Med.* 2000;192:1027-1034.
82. Dong H, Strome SE, Salomao DR, et al. Tumor-associated B7-H1 promotes T-cell apoptosis: a potential mechanism of immune evasion. *Nat Med.* 2002;8:793-800.
83. Iwai Y, Ishida M, Tanaka Y, et al. Involvement of PD-L1 on tumor cells in the escape from host immune system and tumor immunotherapy by PD-L1 blockade. *Proc Natl Acad Sci U S A.* 2002;99:12293-12297.
84. Rodig N, Ryan T, Alie JA, et al. Endothelial expression of PD-L1 and PD-L2 down-regulates CD8+ T cell activation and cytolysis. *Eur J Immunol.* 2003;33:3117–3126.
85. Butte MJ, Keir ME, Phamduy TB, Sharpe AH, Freeman GJ. Programmed death-1 ligand 1 interacts specifically with the B7-1 costimulatory molecule to inhibit T cell responses. *Immunity.* 2007;27:111–122.
86. Shin H, Wherry EJ. CD8 T cell dysfunction during chronic viral infection. *Curr Opin Immunol.* 2007;19:408-415.
87. Stashenko P, Nadler LM, Hardy R, et al. Expression of cell surface markers after human B lymphocyte activation. *Proc Natl Acad Sci U S A.* 1981;78:3848-3852.
88. Reff ME, Carner K, Chambers KS, et al. Depletion of B cells in vivo by a chimeric mouse human monoclonal antibody to CD20. *Blood.* 1994;83:435-445.
89. Smith MR. Rituximab (monoclonal anti-CD20 antibody): mechanisms of action and resistance. *Oncogene.* 2003;22:7359-7368.
90. McLaughlin P, Grillo-Lopez AJ, Link BK, et al. Rituximab chimeric anti-CD20 monoclonal antibody therapy for relapsed indolent lymphoma: half of patients respond to a four-dose treatment program. *J Clin Oncol.* 1998;16:2825-2833.
91. Feugier P, Van Hoof A, Sebban C, et al. Long-term results of the R-CHOP study in the treatment of elderly patients with diffuse large B-cell lymphoma: a study by the Groupe d'Etude des Lymphomes de l'Adulte. *J Clin Oncol.* 2005;23(18):4117-4126.

92. Teeling JL, French RR, Cragg MS, et al. Characterization of new human CD20 monoclonal antibodies with potent cytolytic activity against non-Hodgkin lymphomas. *Blood.* 2004;104(6):1793-1800.
93. Wierda WG, Padmanabhan S, Chan GW, Gupta IV, Lisby S, Osterborg A; for the Hx-CD20-406 Study Investigators. Ofatumumab is active in patients with fludarabine-refractory CLL irrespective of prior rituximab: results from the phase 2 international study. *Blood.* 2011;118(19):5126-5129.
94. Waldmann TA, Morris JC. Development of antibodies and chimeric molecules for cancer immunotherapy. *Adv Immunol.* 2006;90:83-131.
95. Witzig TE, Flinn IW, Gordon LI, et al. Treatment with ibritumomab tiuxetan radioimmunotherapy in patients with rituximab-refractory follicular non-Hodgkin's lymphoma. *J Clin Oncol.* 2002;20:3262-3269.
96. Morris JC, Waldmann TA. Antibody-based therapy of leukaemia. *Expert Rev Mol Med.* September 2009;11:e29.
97. Lozanski G, Heerema NA, Flinn IW, et al. Alemtuzumab is an effective therapy for chronic lymphocytic leukemia with p53 mutations and deletions. *Blood.* 2004;103:3278-3281.
98. Ansell SM, Horwitz SM, Engert A, et al. Phase I/II study of an anti-CD30 monoclonal antibody (MDX-060) in Hodgkin's lymphoma and anaplastic large-cell lymphoma. *J Clin Oncol.* 2007;25:2764-2769.
99. Forero-Torres A, Leonard JP, Younes A, et al. A Phase II study of SGN-30 (anti-CD30 mAb) in Hodgkin lymphoma or systemic anaplastic large cell lymphoma. *Br J Haematol.* 2009;146:171-179.
100. Younes A, Bartlett NL, Leonard JP, et al. Brentuximab vedotin (SGN-35) for relapsed CD30-positive lymphomas. *N Engl J Med.* 2010;363:1812-1821.
101. Mendelsohn J, Baselga J. The EGF receptor family as targets for cancer therapy. *Oncogene.* 2000;19(56):6550-6565.
102. Herbst RS, Kim ES, Harari PM. IMC-C225, an anti-epidermal growth factor receptor monoclonal antibody, for treatment of head and neck cancer. *Expert Opin Biol Ther.* 2001;1(4):719-732.
103. Chung CH, Mirakhur B, Chan E, et al. Cetuximab-induced anaphylaxis and IgE specific for galactose-alpha-1,3-galactose. *N Engl J Med.* 2008;358(11):1109-1117.
104. Van Cutsem E, Peeters M, Siena S, et al. Open-label phase III trial of panitumumab plus best supportive care compared with best supportive care alone in patients with chemotherapy-refractory metastatic colorectal cancer. *J Clin Oncol.* 2007;25(13):1658-1664.
105. Tol J, Punt CJ. Monoclonal antibodies in the treatment of metastatic colorectal cancer: a review. *Clin Ther.* 2010;32(3):437-453.
106. Nahta R, Esteva FJ. Trastuzumab: triumphs and tribulations. *Oncogene.* 2007;26(25):3637-3643.
107. Eiermann W. Trastuzumab combined with chemotherapy for the treatment of HER2-positive metastatic breast cancer: pivotal trial data. *Ann Oncol.* 2001;12(suppl 1):S57-S62.
108. Arnould L, Gelly M, Penault-Llorca F, et al. Trastuzumab-based treatment of HER2-positive breast cancer: an antibody-dependent cellular cytotoxicity mechanism? *Br J Cancer.* 2006;94(2):259-267.
109. Mayfield S, Vaughn JP, Kute TE. DNA strand breaks and cell cycle perturbation in herceptin treated breast cancer cell lines. *Breast Cancer Res Treat.* 2001;70(2):123-129.
110. Slamon DJ, Leyland-Jones B, Shak S, et al. Use of chemotherapy plus a monoclonal antibody against HER2 for metastatic breast cancer that overexpresses HER2. *N Engl J Med.* 2001;344(11):783-792.
111. Hoeben A, Landuyt B, Highley MS, et al. Vascular endothelial growth factor and angiogenesis. *Pharmacol Rev.* 2004;56:549-580.
112. Hurrwitz H, Fehrenbacher L, Novotny W, et al. Bevacizumab plus irinotecan, fluorouracil, and leucovorin for metastatic colorectal cancer. *N Engl J Med.* 2004;350:2335-2342.
113. Sandler A, Gray R, Perry MC, et al. Paclitaxel-carboplatin alone or with bevacizumab for non-small-cell lung cancer. *N Engl J Med.* 2006;355(24):2542-2550.

CHAPTER 45

VACCINES AND CANCER THERAPY

Joseph W. Kim and James L. Gulley

INTRODUCTION

With the advent of sipuleucel-T, the first US Food and Drug Administration (FDA)-approved cancer vaccine, the field of cancer therapeutics entered an era of novel treatments that highlight the success of intense investigations in this field over the last several decades. This chapter will review areas of research in vaccine development, including (a) vaccine targets, (b) vaccine delivery systems, and (c) strategies to improve vaccine efficacy through combination with cytokine adjuvants and other treatment modalities. We will also review important clinical trials in several malignancies, along with issues to consider in designing and conducting clinical research.

TARGETS FOR VACCINE THERAPY

Many potential targets for cancer immunotherapy have been identified, including two major categories of tumor antigens: (a) tumor-specific antigens (TSAs) and (b) tumor-associated antigens (TAAs).

Tumor-Specific Antigens

TSAs are gene products that are uniquely expressed by tumor cells, such as point-mutated *ras* oncogenes,[1] mutated *p53* tumor-suppressor genes, anti-idiotype antibodies,[2] gene translocations, and virally derived products of tumors driven by infectious agents. *Ras* mutations are found in about 20% to 30% of all human tumors, and various vaccine delivery vehicles that target these mutations have been explored. Early clinical trials have shown promising results with *ras*-targeted vaccines in pancreatic, colorectal, and lung adenocarcinomas.[1,3] B-cell lymphomas overexpress a single immunoglobulin variant on their cell surface; therefore, each B-cell lymphoma displays a unique target for immunotherapy.[2]

Tumor-Associated Antigens

TAAs, which are proteins that are overexpressed in tumor cells compared with normal tissues, can be categorized into four major groups: (a) oncofetal antigens, (b) oncogenes and gene products, (c) tissue-lineage antigens (TLAs), and (d) viral antigens. Oncofetal antigens, such as carcinoembryonic antigen (CEA), are normally found during fetal development but are substantially downregulated after birth. The T-box transcription factor brachyury, a protein with an essential role in mesoderm specification during embryonic development, is undetectable in the vast majority of normal tissues but is overexpressed in tumors of the lung, colon, small intestine, stomach, kidney, bladder, uterus, ovary, and testis, as well as in cell lines derived from lung, colon, and prostate carcinoma. Recently, brachyury was described as a driver of epithelial–mesenchymal transition in human carcinoma cells, a process relevant to tumor progression and metastasis.[4] Oncogenes and tumor-suppressor gene products, such as nonmutated HER2/*neu* and *p53*, are analogous to oncofetal antigens in that they can be overexpressed in tumors and may be expressed in some fetal tissues. One of the disadvantages of targeting oncogenes or oncofetal antigens with vaccine is that, because these antigens are expressed in fetal tissue, they may be tolerated by the host immune system, so that vaccine-mediated immunity to these antigens may result in autoimmunity. TLAs such as prostate-specific antigen (PSA), and melanocyte antigens such as MART-1/Melan A, tyrosinase, gp100, and TRP-1 (gp75), are expressed in tumors of a given type and the normal tissue from which they are derived. TLAs are potentially useful targets for immunotherapy if the normal organ/tissue in which they are expressed is not essential, such as the prostate, breast, and melanocyte. Viral antigens, such as the oncoproteins E6 and E7 encoded in human papilloma virus (HPV), are also attractive targets of cancer vaccines.[5] These antigens are implicated in the carcinogenesis of vulvar, cervical, and oropharyngeal malignancies, among others, and are constitutively expressed in preneoplastic lesions as well as invasive carcinomas. HPV$^+$ women with vulvar intraepithelial neoplasia have shown clinical responses following treatment with a synthetic long-peptide vaccine against oncoproteins E6 and E7.[5]

VACCINE DELIVERY SYSTEMS

Vaccine delivery systems can be divided into three basic types (Table 45.1): (a) cell based (autologous whole tumor cells, allogeneic whole tumor cells, and antigen-presenting cells [APCs]), (b) protein/peptide based, and (c) vector based (plasmid DNA, viral vectors, yeast vectors, and bacterial vectors). These vaccine delivery systems have been tested in various stages of preclinical and clinical studies (Fig. 45.1).

Cell-Based Vaccines

Cell-based vaccines include APC and whole tumor cell vaccines, both of which have been extensively studied in preclinical and clinical settings.

TABLE 45–1 Vaccine Delivery Systems

Cell based
APCs loaded with tumor-associated peptide
APCs fused with tumor cells/lysate
APCs transfected with tumor-derived RNA or cDNA
Autologous whole tumor cells
Allogeneic whole tumor cells
Genetically modified tumor cells
Protein/peptide based
Tumor lysates
Heat-shock protein/peptide complex
Tumor-associated antigens
Agonist peptides
Anti-idiotype monoclonal antibody
Monoclonal antibody fusion proteins
Vector based
Plasmid DNA
Bacteria vectors
Listeria
Salmonella
Yeast vectors
Viral vectors
Adenovirus
Vaccinia
Modified vaccinia Ankara
Avipox (fowlpox)

APCs, antigen-presenting cells.

APC-Based Vaccines

The main advantage of APC-based vaccines is that APCs such as dendritic cells (DCs) play an essential role in T-cell activation. Potent tumor antigen-specific T-cell responses can be induced by modifying APCs to bolster their interaction with T cells. There are various ways to load tumor antigens onto vaccines: (a) pulsing with major histocompatibility complex (MHC)-binding peptides, (b) loading with an anti-idiotype antibody, (c) loading with tumor lysates or apoptotic tumor cells, (d) transfection with cDNA or RNA, and (e) transfection with a viral vector.

An example of an APC-based vaccine is sipuleucel-T, which is FDA approved for the treatment of metastatic castration-resistant prostate cancer (mCRPC). Sipuleucel-T is pulsed with the fusion protein PA2024, a recombinant protein of prostatic acid phosphatase (PAP) fused at its C terminus to the N terminus of granulocyte–macrophage colony-stimulating factor (GM-CSF). There is evidence of immune response against PAP in patients treated with sipuleucel-T and, more importantly, prolonged survival in mCRPC patients.

A major disadvantage of sipuleucel-T is that its production involves three costly, labor-intensive steps[6]: (1) collection of peripheral blood mononuclear cells by leukapheresis, (2) further processing of APCs and incubation with PA2024 for activation, and (3) reinfusion of activated APCs into the patient. Each infusion contains a minimum of 50 million CD54$^+$ cells, and the entire process is repeated for each of three infusions of sipuleucel-T.

Whole Tumor Cell Vaccines

Whole tumor cell vaccines are based on two platforms: (a) autologous tumor cells and (b) allogeneic tumor cells. The major advantage of whole tumor cell vaccines is that they provide a broad range of TSAs or TAAs that can be utilized, including antigens that are unidentified as yet. Major disadvantages are costly production and quality control—major considerations for autologous tumor cell vaccines, which involve obtaining fresh tumor cells at surgery, followed by a customized preparation process. OncoVAX, an autologous tumor cell vaccine, has demonstrated survival benefit in stage II colon cancer and is commercially available in Europe.[7,8] Allogeneic tumor cell vaccines, which are usually generated from one or more tumor cell lines, are relatively easy to prepare compared with autologous vaccines.

Several approaches, most involving genetic modification of tumor cells, have been undertaken to enhance the ability of whole tumor cell vaccines to stimulate antitumor immunity. GVAX is derived from irradiated tumor cells genetically modified to secret GM-CSF, an immune stimulant that induces recruitment of DCs. Several GVAX platforms have been produced from autologous or allogeneic tumor cell lines. Prostate GVAX is derived from two prostate cancer cells lines, PC-3 and LNCaP.[9]

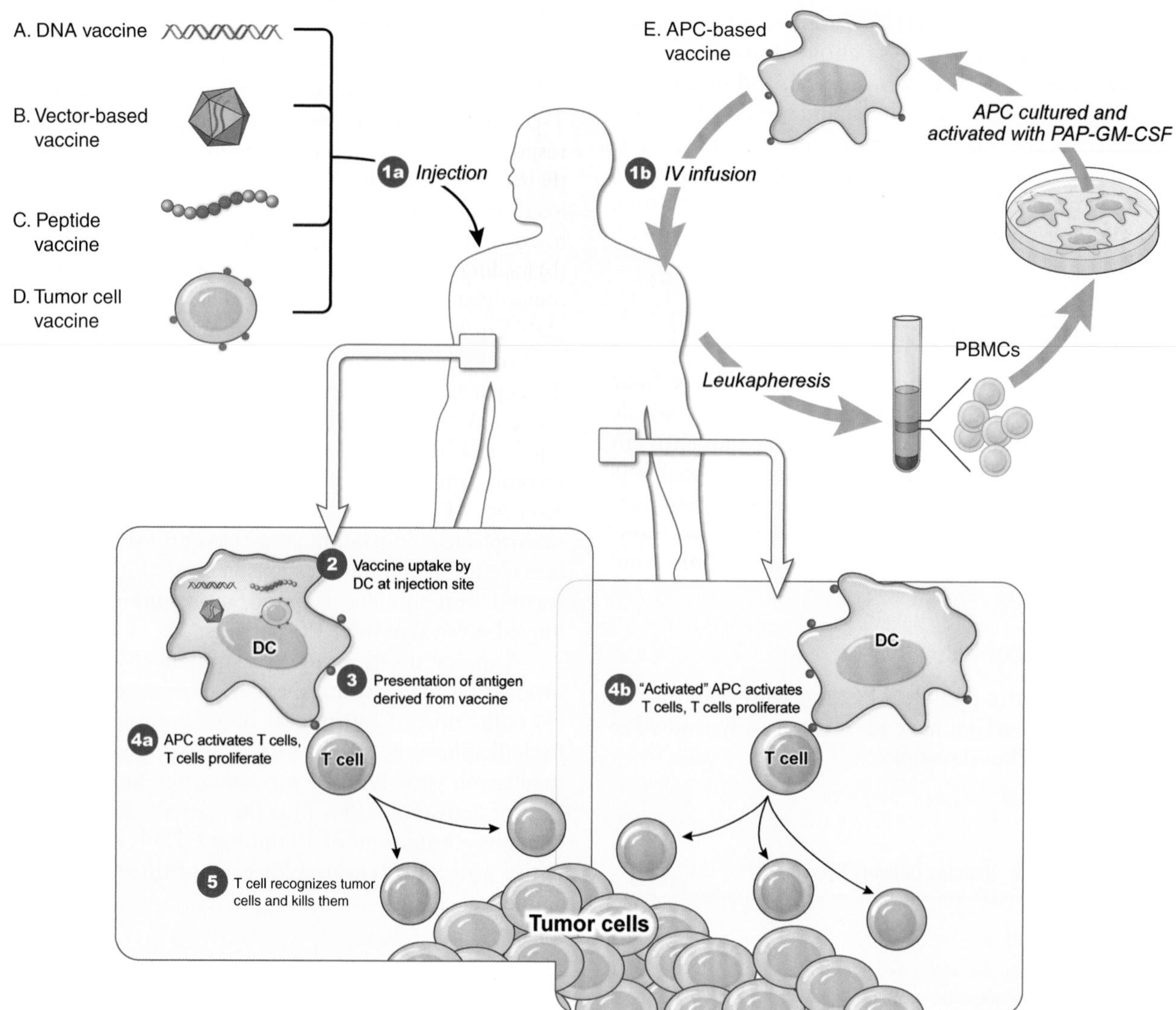

FIGURE 45–1 Vaccine delivery systems. A: DNA vaccine; B: vector-based vaccine; C: peptide vaccine; D: tumor cell-based vaccine; E: antigen-presenting cell-based vaccine. A: DNA vaccines encoding tumor antigens are usually injected subcutaneously. The vaccines are taken up by an antigen presenting cell (APC), such as dendritic cell (DC). APC processes the DNA and expresses the tumor antigens in the context of MHC and costimulatory molecules. APC then activates naive T cells and causes T-cell proliferation. Activated T cells recognize tumor cells that are expressing the antigen and kill them. The steps from the antigen presentation (step 3) to tumor killing (step 5) are shared by other types of vaccines (B, C, and D). B: Vector-based vaccines encoding tumor antigen and costimulatory molecules are usually injected subcutaneously. The vectors infect the APCs at the site of injection. APC expresses the tumor antigen and costimulatory molecules which were encoded in the vaccine. APC presents the antigen in the context of MHC and costimulatory molecules. C: Peptide vaccines are usually the tumor antigens and are usually injected subcutaneously. The vaccines are taken up by APCs. APC processes the peptides and presents the tumor antigens in the context of MHC and costimulatory molecules. D: Tumor cell-based vaccines may be either autologous or allogeneic. Tumor cells carry many tumor antigens. Tumor cells are processed and may be genetically modified to increase its immunogenicity. Tumor cell-based vaccines are usually injected subcutaneously. The vaccines are taken up by APCs. APC processes the tumor cell and presents the tumor antigens in the context of MHC and costimulatory molecules. E: Antigen-presenting cell-based vaccines are prepared through multiple steps: (i) peripheral blood mononuclear cells (PBMCs) are collected via leukapheresis; (ii) PBMCs are then processed and incubated with a tumor antigen, such as PAP-GM-CSF; (iii) PMBCs are then "activated" and express tumor antigen; (iv) "activated" APCs are infused back into the patient. The APC vaccine then activates naive T cells and causes T-cell proliferation. Activated T cells recognize tumor cells that are expressing the antigen and kill them.

In theory, this approach will provoke an immune response to multiple antigens expressed by tumor cells.

Protein/Peptide-Based Vaccines

Peptide vaccines interact with one of two classes of MHC molecules on APCs, depending on their size. Short peptides of 8 to 11 amino acids bind to MHC class I, while peptides of 11 to 15 amino acids bind to MHC class II. Peptide-MHC class I and class II complexes then interact with T-cell receptors (TCRs) on $CD8^+$ and $CD4^+$ T cells, respectively. This interaction, in concert with costimulation, induces T-cell activation. Most peptide vaccines derived from TSAs or TAAs are short peptides that interact with MHC class I. The peptide-MHC class I complexes on an APC activate $CD8^+$ T cells. Theoretically, these MHC-restricted responses are effective only if the appropriate

MHC allele is present. The most studied MHC restriction in humans is HLA-A2, which is found in about 50% of Caucasians. Many clinical trials enroll patients with the HLA-A2 allele to analyze their T-cell responses.

A major advantage of peptide vaccines is that peptides can be modified to strengthen binding with MHC molecules or signal better through the TCR. Both types of agonist peptides can thus induce vigorous T-cell activation. Some peptide vaccines, such as those that target gp100, PSA, and mucin (MUC)-1, have been modified to strengthen and stabilize their binding to MHC molecules. In one study, an agonist peptide derived from human CEA induced a stronger cytotoxic T lymphocyte (CTL) response than the original peptide.[10] Many clinical trials have shown promising results with vaccines derived from various peptides, including gp100, modified MUC-1,[11–13] HSPPC-96, a heat-shock protein,[14] epidermal growth factor (EGF),[15] and HER2/*neu*-related peptides.[16,17]

Vector-Based Vaccines

As platforms for vaccine delivery, vectors have many advantages: (a) the entire tumor antigen gene or parts of that gene can be inserted into the vector; (b) multiple genes, including genes for costimulatory molecules and cytokines, can be inserted into the vector to enhance immune response; (c) many vectors are able to infect APCs so that antigen transgenes can be expressed, processed, and presented to T cells in the context of MHC molecule; (d) the cost of production is relatively low compared with the cost of preparing and purifying whole cell tumor vaccines, APC-based vaccine, or protein-based vaccines.

One of the most studied vectors is vaccinia virus, a poxvirus derived from a benign bovine skin disease, which has been used as a platform for smallpox vaccines. Recombinant vaccinia (rV) viruses have also been studied extensively in human immunodeficiency virus vaccine development. Although rV virus can mount a strong immune response, the response is greatly diminished on subsequent vaccinations due to the development of host neutralizing immunity.[18] To circumvent this problem, preclinical studies found that a strategy of priming with an rV vector followed by boosting with a nonreplicating avipox vector which does not induce host neutralizing response can lead to progressively heightened immune response with each boost.[19] Several clinical trials have since employed this strategy.

Saccharomyces cerevisiae (baker's yeast) has been studied extensively as an attractive vehicle for vaccine delivery. Unlike other immunotherapeutic approaches, *S. cerevisiae* activates DCs via multiple Toll-like receptors, resulting in phagocytosis of the yeast and efficient processing of peptides on both MHC class I and class II.[20] Yeast effectively induces both innate and adaptive cellular immunity.[21] Recombinant *S. cerevisiae* is heat-killed prior to administration. Preliminary results from phase I trials have demonstrated the safety and immunogenicity of heat-killed recombinant *S. cerevisiae*.[22]

STRATEGIES TO IMPROVE VACCINE EFFICACY

Vaccine Adjuvants

Vaccine adjuvants are used to enhance the immunogenicity of an antigen in a vaccine formulation. Several cytokines can enhance the immune response either by (a) promoting the differentiation, activation, or recruitment of APCs, therefore, enhancing antigen presentation and activation of antigen-specific T-cell responses, or (b) by directly acting on T cells.

Immune Adjuvants That Affect APCs

One of the most studied immune adjuvants is the cytokine GM-CSF. Preclinical studies have repeatedly demonstrated that subcutaneous injections of GM-CSF at the vaccination site can significantly increase infiltration of DCs into draining lymph nodes.[23] In other preclinical studies, tumor cells or DCs genetically modified to secrete biologically active GM-CSF have been used to generate a systemic antitumor immune response.[24] Sipuleucel-T, which uses cells enriched for APCs pulsed with a PAP–GM-CSF fusion protein, has demonstrated improved survival in clinical trials. Several clinical trials of PROSTVAC have also employed subcutaneous GM-CSF as a vaccine adjuvant. The definitive role of GM-CSF in combination with PROSTVAC will be evaluated in a phase III trial (NCT01322490). Other agents in this group include CpG oligonucleotides, FLT3 ligand, resiquimod, TLR3 agonist, and poly I:C.[25]

Immune Adjuvants That Affect T Cells

Cytokines such as interleukin (IL)-2, IL-7, IL-15, and IL-12 directly affect T cells by promoting their growth and proliferation, activation, and effector function.[25,26] IL-2, a T-cell growth factor, has been studied most extensively. High-dose IL-2 as a single agent has demonstrated clinical activity in metastatic renal cell carcinoma (RCC) and metastatic melanoma. The disadvantage of IL-2 is its significant systemic toxicity. In preclinical studies, IL-2 has mediated not only proliferation of activated effector T cells and natural killer (NK) cells but also development and homeostasis of regulatory T cells (Tregs).[27] In clinical trials, low-dose IL-2 has been used as an immune adjuvant.[28]

IL-12 is a proinflammatory cytokine that acts directly on cytotoxic effector cells to stimulate their proliferation and increase their cytotoxic function. IL-12 has shown clinical activity against RCC and lymphomas.[29] Like IL-2, it is associated with significant systemic toxicity. A strategy to limit systemic exposure by conjugating IL-12 to an antibody that targets tumor necrosis has been employed in a clinical trial (NCT01417546).

IL-15 is involved in the development and homeostasis of memory CD8$^+$ T cells and NK cells.[26] IL-15 has been shown to play a role in the induction of long-lived, high-avidity CD8$^+$ T cells.[30] An ongoing clinical trial is evaluating autologous DCs manufactured with GM-CSF and IL-15 and loaded with melanoma peptides in resected stage IIIc and IV melanoma (NCT01189383). Another trial is evaluating the safety of recombinant human IL-15 in metastatic melanoma and RCC (NCT01021059).

IL-7, another T-cell growth factor that may have clinical benefit, plays a major role in the expansion of mature T cells. Therapeutic IL-7 was shown to enhance both quantitative and functional immune recovery following T-cell depletion.[31]

Combination Modalities

Vaccines can be combined with other treatment modalities to enhance efficacy.

Tumor cells escape immune recognition by downregulating tumor antigens, MHC expression, or various components of the antigen-processing/presentation mechanism. Several preclinical and clinical studies have shown that radiation, certain chemotherapeutic agents, and hormonal therapies can counteract these escape mechanisms, exert antitumor effects, and facilitate immune-mediated recognition and killing of tumor cells.

Vaccine Plus Radiation

Radiation is a very effective cytotoxic therapy that causes DNA damage either directly or by generating free radicals. It is commonly used to treat many types of cancer as definitive therapy or for palliation of symptoms. It has been reported that local radiation of tumor cells at sublethal doses can modulate numerous classes of genes and consequently alter the phenotype of tumor cells.[32,33] These phenotypic changes make tumor cells more susceptible to killing by CTLs. Some of the genes that are upregulated in human tumor cells post-irradiation are Fas, MHC class 1, intracellular adhesion molecule (ICAM)-1, and TAAs such as CEA, MUC-1, HER2/*neu*, *p53*, and CA125. In preclinical studies, upregulation of Fas expression in tumor cells via sublethal local tumor irradiation with a recombinant anticancer vaccine significantly improved the therapeutic efficacy compared with either modality alone in a murine model.[33] Subsequent studies demonstrated that sublethal irradiation of human colorectal, lung, and prostate cancer cells altered numerous genes and upregulated Fas and other molecules, rendering these tumor cells more susceptible to killing by human CTLs.[32] In a randomized phase II trial in 30 patients with localized prostate cancer, radiotherapy plus PSA vaccine induced a significant increase in PSA-specific T cells and also showed evidence of de novo generation of T cells specific to other prostate-associated antigens not found in the vaccine, a phenomenon known as antigen cascade or epitope spreading.[28] In another clinical study, patients with advanced hepatoma were treated with a single dose of 8 Gy radiation, followed 2 days later by intratumoral injection of autologous immature DCs, followed 3 weeks later by a second vaccination. Of the 14 patients enrolled, 2 had partial responses and 4 had minor responses. Three patients had a >50% decrease in α-fetoprotein (AFP). Of the 10 patients assessed for immunologic response 2 weeks after the second vaccine, 4 had increased NK-cell cytotoxic activity, 7 had AFP-specific immune response by ELISPOT, and 8 had AFP-specific immune response by cytokine release assay.[34]

Vaccine Plus Chemotherapy

For many years, it was generally believed that the cytotoxic properties of chemotherapy would compromise the host immune system. However, emerging evidence suggests that certain chemotherapies are not only compatible with therapeutic cancer vaccines but also enhance their efficacy. Preclinical evidence has shown that certain chemotherapeutic agents upregulate MHC class I and TAAs on the tumor cell surface,[35] deplete Tregs (cyclophosphamide),[36] enhance macrophage antitumor activity and apoptosis (doxorubicin), [37] and increase proinflammatory cytokine production (docetaxel).[38] In a phase II trial, 28 mCRPC patients were randomized to receive either vaccine alone or docetaxel plus vaccine.[39] Patients in the vaccine-alone arm were allowed to cross over to receive docetaxel alone at disease progression. After 3 months of therapy, the median increase in PSA-specific T cells was 3.33-fold in both arms. Interestingly, evidence of antigen cascade was also observed. The study also suggested that those who received docetaxel following progression on vaccine lived longer than the historical control (6.1 vs. 3.7 mo), calling for a prospective randomized trial (NCT01145508). It is unclear whether the immune response potentiated or enhanced the efficacy of the subsequent therapy, leading to enhanced clinical response. An ongoing multicenter, randomized phase II trial of docetaxel with or without pretreatment with PSA-TRICOM vaccine in patients with mCRPC (ECOG E1809) is prospectively evaluating the benefits of vaccine followed by chemotherapy (NCT01145508). In a phase I trial, 17 patients with advanced solid tumors were treated with a plasmid DNA vaccine. Five of 6 patients who developed immunity to the TAA had a marked response to salvage treatment, whereas 10 of 11 patients who did not develop immunity did not respond to subsequent therapy.[40]

Vaccine Plus Hormonal Therapy

Androgen deprivation therapy, long the initial treatment for advanced prostate cancer, has been shown to induce profuse T-cell infiltration of benign glands and tumors in the human prostate. Infiltration by $CD4^+$ T cells and relatively fewer $CD8^+$ T cells is readily apparent after 1–4 weeks of therapy.[41] T cells within a treated prostate show restricted TCR gene usage, consistent with a local oligoclonal response. These findings have implications for the potential use of vaccine in combination with androgen deprivation therapy in prostate cancer and other hormone-sensitive malignancies such as breast cancer. In a phase II trial in nonmetastatic CRPC, 42 patients were randomized to receive either a poxvirus-based PSA vaccine or nilutamide (an FDA-approved androgen receptor antagonist). Patients in either arm who developed rising PSA could cross over to receive the combined therapies. After a median follow-up of 4.4 years, there was a trend toward improved survival in the vaccine arm. A subgroup analysis showed substantial improvement in survival for patients randomized to the vaccine arm who had indolent disease characteristics at baseline (PSA < 20 ng/dL, Gleason score ≤ 7, prior radiotherapy).[42] Another phase II trial randomized 26 patients with nonmetastatic CRPC to receive flutamide alone or with another vector-based PSA vaccine, PSA-TRICOM (PROSTVAC-VF). A preliminary report showed that patients in the combination arm had improved time to progression (TTP) compared with patients who received flutamide alone (223 vs. 85 d, respectively).[43] A randomized phase II trial will examine the sequencing of sipuleucel-T and androgen deprivation therapy in men with nonmetastatic prostate cancer and a rising PSA after primary therapy (NCT01431391).

Vaccine Plus Other Immunotherapies

Other immunotherapies have been tested in combination with vaccine to see if they could enhance or potentiate an immune response. Immunotherapies tested include (a) an immunocytokine fusion protein such as antitumor necrosis antibody conjugated with IL-2 or IL-12 to enhance T-cell activity at the tumor site,[44] (b) immune checkpoint inhibitors such as anti-cytotoxic T lymphocyte antigen (CTLA)-4 antibody[11,45] and anti-PD-1 antibody,[46] and (c) monoclonal antibodies or fusion proteins directed against Tregs.[47] A preliminary report of a phase I trial in 30 patients with mCRPC suggested enhanced clinical benefit with the use of ipilimumab and PROSTVAC.[45] In a phase III trial in advanced melanoma, gp100 combined with ipilimumab did not provide any additional benefit compared with ipilimumab alone.[11] However, when administered prior to high-dose IL-2, gp100 induced improved response rates and progression-free survival (PFS), as well as a trend toward increased overall survival (OS).[48] A randomized, placebo-controlled phase III study in advanced RCC demonstrated that patients with a good prognosis (MSKCC 0) who were treated with a vector-based vaccine (modified vaccinia Ankara-5T4) plus IL-2 had a significant survival advantage compared with patients receiving IL-2 alone (HR 0.54; $P = 0.046$).[49]

Vaccine Plus Small Molecule Inhibitors

Imatinib mesylate, the tyrosine kinase inhibitor that ushered in the era of targeted molecular therapy, has been shown to potentiate an antitumor T-cell response in a murine GIST model.[50] Several vaccines have been studied in clinical trials, administered in combination with imatinib.[51,52] An autologous leukocyte-derived heat-shock protein vaccine in combination with imatinib induced an immunologic response that correlated with clinical response.[52] A tumor cell-based vaccine modified to produce GM-CSF was also evaluated in patients with chronic myelogenous leukemia who had persistent disease while on imatinib. A majority of patients showed a trend toward reduced BCR-ABL by PCR measurement after vaccination, including seven patients whose BCR-ABL level was undetectable by PCR.[51]

Preclinical data from a study of sunitinib in CEA-transgenic mice bearing CEA^+ tumors showed that continuous sunitinib followed by vaccine increased intratumoral infiltration of antigen-specific T lymphocytes, decreased Tregs and myeloid-derived suppressor cells, reduced tumor volumes, and increased survival.[53]

Finally, growing evidence suggests that BRAF kinase inhibitor does not interfere with human lymphocytes across a wide range of concentrations and may enhance T-cell recognition of melanoma without affecting lymphocyte function.[54,55]

VACCINE CLINICAL TRIALS

Tables 45.2 and 45.3 provide an overview of selected clinical trials of cancer vaccines, including primary end points and outcomes, in numerous cancer types.

Prostate Cancer

Several aspects of prostate cancer make it a very attractive target for therapeutic cancer vaccines: (a) its relatively indolent biology allows time for the immune system to generate an immunologic response to vaccine; (b) numerous prostate cancer–associated antigens have been identified, including PSA, PAP, prostate-specific membrane antigen (PSMA), and new gene expressed in prostate (NGEP); (c) because the prostate is a nonessential organ, targeting prostate cancer-associated antigens is unlikely to have significant negative effects.

Recently, there have been landmark developments in immunotherapy for prostate cancer. Sipuleucel-T, the first therapeutic cancer vaccine approved by the FDA, is an autologous DC-based vaccine that is loaded with PA2024, a recombinant fusion protein composed of PAP and GM-CSF. The IMPACT trial demonstrated a 4.1-month absolute benefit in median OS without affecting TTP.[56] These results were consistent with a prior study that showed survival benefit without a change in TTP.[57] Based on the findings from these studies, the FDA approved sipuleucel-T for the treatment of mCRPC.

A vector-based vaccine, PSA-TRICOM (PROSTVAC), is also showing promising results. PSA-TRICOM consists of a poxviral vector engineered with transgenes for PSA and three human T-cell costimulatory molecules (TRICOM): B7.1, lymphocyte function-associated antigen-3, and ICAM-1. In a placebo-controlled, randomized clinical trial in 125 patients with mCRPC, PSA-TRICOM demonstrated a survival benefit of 8.5 months (25.1 vs. 16.6 mo for placebo; $P = 0.0061$).[64] In a separate single-arm study in 32 patients with mCRPC, the median OS was 26.6 months, and enhanced PSA-specific T-cell

TABLE 45–2 Selected Phase III Cancer Vaccine Trials

Cancer Type	Vaccine	ν	Trial Arms	Primary End point	Outcome
Prostate cancer[56]	Sipuleucel-T: APC loaded with PA2024, DC-based vaccine	512	A: sipuleucel-T B: placebo	OS	OS: 25.8 vs. 21.7 mo favoring vaccine (HR 0.78; $P = 0.03$).
Prostate cancer[57]	Sipuleucel-T: APC loaded with PA2024, DC-based vaccine	127	A: sipuleucel-T B: placebo	TTP/OS	No difference in TTP. OS: 25.9 vs. 21.4 mo favoring vaccine ($P = 0.01$)
Prostate cancer[58]	GVAX: allogeneic whole tumor cell vaccine engineered to secrete GM-CSF	626	A: GVAX B: docetaxel + prednisone	OS	No significant difference (20.7 vs. 21.7 mo)
Prostate cancer[59]	GVAX: allogeneic whole tumor cell vaccine engineered to secrete GM-CSF	408	A: docetaxel + GVAX B: docetaxel + prednisone	OS	Terminated early after interim analysis showed OS shorter in docetaxel/vaccine arm vs. docetaxel/prednisone arm (12.2 vs. 14.1 mo; $P = 0.0076$)
Melanoma[60]	Vitespen (HSPPC-96): autologous tumor-derived heat-shock protein (gp96) peptide complex	322	A: vitespen B: standard treatment (physician's choice)	OS	No difference in OS
Melanoma[11]	gp100: peptide vaccine	676	A: gp100 + ipilimumab B: ipilimumab alone C: gp100 alone	OS	A: 10.0 mo (vs. C, HR 0.68; $P < 0.001$) B: 10.1 mo (vs. C, HR 0.66; $P = 0.003$) C: 6.4 mo
Melanoma[48]	gp100: peptide vaccine	185	A: high-dose IL-2 alone B: gp100 with adjuvant Montanide ISA-51, followed by IL-2	RR	RR: 16% vs. 6% ($P = 0.03$ favoring combination arm) PFS: 3.9 vs. 1.6 mo ($P = 0.008$ favoring combination arm) OS: 17.8 vs. 11.1 mo ($P = 0.06$ favoring combination arm)
Metastatic breast cancer[61]	Theratope: peptide vaccine consisting of synthetic sialyl-Tn coupled with protein carrier KLH	1,028	A: Theratope B: KLH control	OS, TTP	TTP: 3.4 vs. 3.0 mo OS: 23.1 vs. 22.3 mo favoring vaccine (P = not significant)
Colon cancer[7,8]	Autologous whole tumor cell vaccine	245	A: Vaccine after surgery B: No adjuvant therapy after surgery	OS	Improved 5-y OS for stage II colon cancer patients (82.5% vs. 72.7%; $P = 0.010$)
Follicular lymphoma[62]	Mitumprotimut-T: peptide vaccine, idiotype protein chemically conjugated to KLH (Id-KLH)	349	A: mitumprotimut-T/ GM-CSF B: placebo/GM-CSF	TTP	A: 9.0 mo B: 12.6 mo (HR 1.384; $P = 0.019$)
Follicular lymphoma[2]	Peptide vaccine, Id-KLH	234	A: Id-KLH + GM-CSF B: KLH + GM-CSF	DFS	For 117 pts who received the assigned protocol treatment, at median follow-up of 56 mo, DFS was 44.2 vs. 30.6 mo (HR 0.62; $P = 0.047$)
RCC post-nephrectomy[63]	Autologous tumor cell vaccine	558	A: vaccine B: observation	DFS	70-mo PFS was 70% vs. 59.3% favoring vaccine (HR 1.59; $P = 0.0204$)
RCC post-nephrectomy[14]	Vitespen (HSPPC-96): autologous tumor-derived heat-shock protein (gp96) peptide complex	818	A: vitespen B: observation alone post-nephrectomy	RFS	A: 37.7% B: 39.8% (HR 0.923; 95% CI 0.729–1.169; $P = 0.506$)
Metastatic RCC[49]	TroVax (MVA-5T4): MVA engineered to deliver tumor antigen 5T4	733	A: SOC + placebo B: SOC + TroVax SOC = sunitinib, IL-2, or IFN-α	OS	A: 19.2 mo B: 20.1 mo ($P = 0.55$; magnitude of 5T4-specific antibody response associated with enhanced survival)

APC, antigen-presenting cell; CI, confidence interval; CR, complete response; CTC, circulating tumor cell; DC, dendritic cell; DFI, disease-free interval; DFS, disease-free survival; EGF, epidermal growth factor; GM-CSF, granulocyte–macrophage colony-stimulating factor; gp, glycoprotein; HR, hazard ratio; KLH, keyhole limpet hemocyanin; MVA, modified vaccinia Ankara; n/a, not available; ORR, overall response rate; OS, overall survival; PR, partial response; pts, patients; RR, response rate; SD, stable disease; SOC, standard of care; TGF, transforming growth factor; TTP, time to progression.

TABLE 45-3 Selected Pilot/Phase I/II Vaccine Trials

Cancer	Vaccine	ν	Primary End point	Outcome
mCRPC[64]	PSA-TRICOM: recombinant poxviral vector encoding PSA and three T-cell costimulatory molecules	125	PFS	No difference in PFS ($P = 0.6$) OS: 25.1 vs. 16.6 mo (HR 0.56; $P = 0.0061$)
mCRPC[65]	PSA-TRICOM: recombinant poxviral vector encoding PSA and three T-cell costimulatory molecules	32	Immune response	Median OS: 26.6 mo (vaccine) vs. 17.4 mo (Halabi-predicted)
Melanoma[66]	OncoVEX$^{GM\text{-}CSF}$: recombinant oncolytic herpesvirus encoding GM-CSF	50	ORR	ORR: 26% (CR = 8; PR = 5) OS: 16+ mo 2-yr OS: 52%
Melanoma[67]	Allovectin-7: bicistronic plasmid encoding HLA-B7 and β2 microglobulin in a cationic lipid system	133	ORR	ORR: 11.8% Median duration of response: 13.8 mo
Surgically resected melanoma[68]	Autologous dinitrophenyl-modified tumor cell mixed with Bacillus Calmette-Guérin	214	OS	5 yr OS: 44%
Stage II breast cancer post-resection[12]	Peptide vaccine: oxidized mannan-MUC-1	31	n/a	Recurrence rate during 5.5 yr follow-up: 27% vs. 0% ($P = 0.0292$ favoring vaccine)
Breast cancer[69]	PANVAC: recombinant poxviral vector	15	PFS	Clinical improvement and immune response
Lung cancer[13,70]	Stimuvax (L-BLP25): liposome-encapsulated synthetic peptide derived from MUC-1	171	Safety/OS	OS: 17.2 vs. 13.0 mo (HR 0.745; 95% CI 0.533–1.042 favoring vaccine) 3-yr OS: 31% vs. 17% ($P = 0.035$) Stage IIIb LR disease subset OS: 30.6 vs. 13.3 mo (HR 0.548; 95% CI 0.301–0.999) 3-yr OS: 49% vs. 27% ($P = 0.070$ favoring vaccine)
Advanced NSCLC[71]	Lucanix (belagenpumatucel-L): TGF-β2 antisense gene-modified allogeneic tumor cell vaccine	21	Safety/efficacy/ correlation with CTCs	OS: 562 d OS: patients with <2 CTCs at baseline vs. patients with ≥2 CTCs: 660 vs. 150 d ($P = 0.025$)
Stage IIIb/IV NSCLC[15]	Peptide vaccine: human recombinant EGF produced in yeast, chemically conjugated to P64K *Neisseria meningitides* recombinant protein, produced in *Escherichia coli*	80	OS	OS: 11.57 vs. 6.77 mo favoring vaccine (not statistically significant) OS: patients < 60 yr: 11 vs. 5.33 mo ($P = 0.0124$)
Stage IIIb/IV NSCLC expressing MUC1[72]	TG4010 (MVA expressing MUC-1 and IL-2)	148	6-mo PFS	6-mo PFS: 43.2% vs 35.1% ($P = 0.307$) favoring vaccine plus chemotherapy RR: 31% vs. 21%, ($P = 0.082$) favoring vaccine plus chemotherapy
Stage Ib and II NSCLC expressing MAGE-A3[73]	Peptide vaccine: MAGE-A3	182	DFI	HR for DFI: 0.74 (95% CI 0.44–1.20, $P = 0.107$) HR for OS: 0.66 (95% CI 0.36–1.20) in favor of the MAGE-A3 group vs. placebo
Pancreatic cancer[74]	HyperAcute-Pancreas: modified allogeneic pancreatic cancer cell vaccine expressing enzyme α-1,3 galactosyl transferase	73	DFS	1 yr OS: 91% vs. 63% (Halabi-predicted) 2-yr OS: 54% vs. 32% (Halabi-predicted) Median DFS: 16 vs. 11 mo (historical control; RTOG 9704)
Pancreatic cancer[75]	GVAX: irradiated allogeneic pancreatic tumor cell vaccine transfected with GM-CSF	60	DFS	DFS: 17.3 mo (95% CI 14.6–22.8) OS: 24.8 mo (95% CI 21.2–31.6)

APC, antigen-presenting cell; CI, confidence interval; CR, complete response; CTC, circulating tumor cell; DC, dendritic cell; DFI, disease-free interval; DFS, disease-free survival; EGF, epidermal growth factor; GM-CSF, granulocyte–macrophage colony-stimulating factor; gp, glycoprotein; HR, hazard ratio; KLH, keyhole limpet hemocyanin; MVA, modified vaccinia Ankara; n/a, not available; ORR, overall response rate; OS, overall survival; PR, partial response; pts, patients; RR, response rate; SD, stable disease; SOC, standard of care; TGF, transforming growth factor; TTP, time to progression.

responses were associated with improved survival.[65] A global phase III trial is underway to evaluate PROSTVAC in asymptomatic to minimally symptomatic mCRPC, with OS as the primary end point (NCT01322490).

Ipilimumab is a fully humanized monoclonal antibody against CTLA-4, an immune checkpoint molecule expressed by CTLs after activation by APCs. Ipilimumab was initially approved by the FDA for treatment of metastatic melanoma. In a phase I trial involving 14 patients with CRPC, 2 patients had PSA declines > 50%, and one patient developed a grade 3 rash/pruritis requiring systemic corticosteroids.[76] Phase III trials of ipilimumab in prostate cancer are ongoing (NCT01057810).

Prostate GVAX is a vaccine derived from irradiated allogeneic prostate cancer cell lines (LNCaP and PC3) that are genetically modified to secrete GM-CSF. Two phase III clinical trials, VITAL-1 and VITAL-2, evaluated GVAX in mCRPC patients, with OS as the primary end point. VITAL-1 compared GVAX as a monotherapy with docetaxel plus prednisone in asymptomatic mCRPC. VITAL-2 compared GVAX plus docetaxel with docetaxel and prednisone in symptomatic mCRPC. After accruing 408 patients, VITAL-2 was terminated in August 2008 because more deaths had occurred in the experimental arm (67 deaths in the vaccine/docetaxel arm vs. 47 deaths in the docetaxel and prednisone arm). Median OS was 12.2 versus 14.1 months favoring the control arm (HR 1.70; $P = 0.0076$).[59] Following the termination of VITAL-2, an unplanned futility analysis conducted on VITAL-1 indicated that the trial had a <30% chance of meeting its predefined primary end point of improved survival, resulting in its early termination as well. Although the vaccine arm had a more favorable toxicity profile, the median survival was 20.7 versus 21.7 months for the docetaxel arm (HR 1.03; $P = 0.78$).[58] A subset of men with Halabi-predicted survival > 18 months showed a trend toward improved survival in the vaccine arm (29.7 vs. 27.1 mo; $P = 0.60$).

A DNA vaccine encoding PAP has shown promising immune responses, as well as PSA doubling times prolonged from a median 6.5 months pretreatment to 8.5 months on treatment ($P = 0.033$) and 9.3 months on one year post-treatment ($P = 0.054$).[77]

Melanoma

Melanoma is considered one of the most immunogenic solid tumors, making it an attractive target for vaccine development. Not surprisingly, standard treatments for melanoma consist of immunotherapy: high-dose interferon (IFN) and pegylated IFN as adjuvant therapy, and high-dose IL-2 and ipilimumab (anti-CTLA-4 monoclonal antibody) for metastatic disease. However, these immunotherapies are relatively nonspecific and significantly toxic.

A phase III trial in stage IV melanoma randomized 322 patients to receive either vitespen (Oncophage; autologous tumor-derived heat-shock protein gp96 peptide complexes) or a standard treatment of the physician's choice.[60] Although an intention-to-treat analysis showed no statistical difference in OS between the arms, an exploratory landmark analysis suggested that patients who received more than 10 doses of vitespen lived longer than patients in the control arm. Another peptide vaccine, gp100, has been studied in phase III trials. In a phase III trial, patients with advanced melanoma who received gp100 followed by high-dose IL-2 showed statistically significant improvements in response rate and PFS than high-dose IL-2 alone, along with a trend toward improved OS (17.8 mo for the combination arm vs. 11.1 mo; $P = 0.06$).[48]

Vector-based vaccines encoding cytokines have also shown promising results. Intratumoral injection of canarypox virus expressing IL-2 induced local infiltration of T cells and led to partial regression of metastatic melanoma lesions.[78] In a phase II trial with 50 advanced melanoma patients, intratumoral injection of oncolytic herpes simplex virus-1 encoding GM-CSF (OncoVEX$^{GM\text{-}CSF}$) led to an overall response rate of 26%, including 8 complete responses, and a 2-year survival rate of 52%.[66] Allovectin-7, a bicistronic plasmid encoding HLA-B7 and a β2 microglobulin formulated with a cationic lipid system, produced durable clinical responses in a phase II trial.[67] Phase III trials of these vaccines are ongoing (NCT00395070 and NCT00769704).

In a trial of an autologous melanoma cellular vaccine, 214 patients with clinical stage III melanoma were treated with multiple intradermal injections of autologous, hapten-modified melanoma vaccines mixed with Bacillus Calmette-Guérin following low-dose cyclophosphamide.[68] The 5-year OS rate was 44%. Patients who had delayed-type hypersensitivity (DTH) responses to the unmodified tumor cells had significantly longer OS than patients with negative DTH (59.3% vs. 29.3%; $P < 0.001$).[68] Interestingly, OS after relapse was also significantly longer in patients who developed positive DTH to unmodified tumor cells (25.2% vs. 12.3 %; $P < 0.0010$). However, the planned phase III trial was suspended for financial reasons (NCT00477906).

A novel approach tested in clinical trials in melanoma is a DC-based vaccine transfected with autologous tumor mRNA.[79] Vaccine-specific immune responses and clinical responses were observed with this approach.

Breast Cancer

Several breast cancer–associated and carcinoma-associated antigens have been studied as targets for vaccine trials in patients with metastatic breast cancer. Sialyl-Tn (STn), a disaccharide carbohydrate associated with MUC-1, is expressed on the cell surface of multiple human carcinomas. An early clinical trial suggested a survival benefit for patients treated with Theratope, a peptide vaccine consisting of synthetic STn coupled with the protein carrier keyhole limpet hemocyanin (KLH), following pretreatment with intravenous cyclophosphamide. A recent update found no significant difference in OS or TTP, despite significant humoral immune responses to the vaccine.[61]

Numerous clinical trials have been carried out using MUC-1 and/or CEA as targets. In a pilot study, 31 patients with stage II breast cancer who were disease free after surgery were randomized to receive subcutaneous injections of either placebo or oxidized mannan-MUC-1. After >5.5 years of follow-up, the recurrence rate was 27% in the placebo arm versus 0% in the immunotherapy arm ($P = 0.0292$).[12] PANVAC, a poxviral vector-based vaccine targeting CEA and MUC-1 in a TRICOM platform, was evaluated in patients with metastatic breast cancer. Preliminary evidence suggested that both vaccine and vaccine plus docetaxel demonstrated some clinical responses, including a >20% reduction in bulky liver metastases and one patient with a prolonged complete remission both on vaccine alone.[69]

HER2/*neu*, another attractive vaccine target that is overexpressed in breast cancers, is a source of immunogenic peptides such as E75 and GP2. In patients with HER2/*neu*$^+$ breast cancer, HER2/*neu* helper peptide vaccine proved safe when administered concurrently with trastuzumab. The vaccine had no additional cardiac toxicity and was able to induce HER2/*neu*-specific immunity in a majority of patients.[80] In a combined report of two clinical trials, vaccination with E75 peptide was associated with a trend toward decreased disease recurrence compared with the control (8.3% vs. 14.8%).[16] GP2 is a peptide derived from the transmembrane portion of HER2/*neu*. In a phase I trial, GP2 peptide vaccine was well tolerated and safe and was able to induce HER2/*neu*-specific immune responses.[17]

Gastrointestinal Cancers

In the MOSAIC trial, the addition of oxaliplatin to leuocovorin/fluorouracil (FOLFOX) improved 6-year OS by 2.5% and 5-year disease-free survival (DFS) by 5.9% in patients with stage II and III colorectal cancer. However, the OS benefit was statistically significant only in stage III disease.[81] Before FOLFOX became the standard adjuvant therapy in colon cancer, OncoVAX, an irradiated autologous colon cancer cell vaccine, was studied extensively. In a prospective randomized trial in 254 patients with stage II and III colon cancer, 3 weekly doses of OncoVAX followed by a booster at 6 months demonstrated a significant reduction in the rate of recurrence (19.5% for vaccine vs. 31.7% without adjuvant therapy; $P = 0.023$).[7] With a median follow-up of 5.8 years, survival benefit with vaccine was statistically significant in stage II colon cancer, with an absolute difference of 9.8% in 5-year survival rate ($P = 0.010$). However, the difference in survival was not statistically significant in stage III patients.[8] OncoVAX was granted fast-track designation by the FDA and will be studied in a phase III randomized controlled trial in patients with stage II colon cancer following surgery.[82]

CEA is overexpressed in the vast majority of human colorectal, gastric, and pancreatic cancers, approximately 70% of non-small cell lung cancers (NSCLCs), 50% of breast cancers, and in cervical, ovarian, prostate, and head and neck cancers.[83] Several clinical trials have been conducted employing CEA-targeted vaccines in various platforms, including rV virus,[18] recombinant avipox virus,[84] and CEA peptide-pulsed DCs.[85] Priming with rV-CEA-TRICOM followed by multiple boosts with avipox-CEA-TRICOM has generated specific immune responses in patients with advanced gastrointestinal carcinomas and other CEA-expressing carcinomas.[86]

A phase II randomized controlled study[87] involved 74 patients with completely resected metastases from colorectal cancer, who had received perioperative chemotherapy. Patients were randomized to receive four vaccinations with either PANVAC, a poxviral vector encoding CEA, MUC-1, and TRICOM, plus GM-CSF, or DCs modified with PANVAC. There was no significant difference in 2-year recurrence-free survival among the DC arm (50%), the PANVAC arm (56%), and a contemporary control arm (55%). However, at a median follow-up of 40 months, the survival rate for vaccinated patients was 81%, which far exceeded that of the unvaccinated controls.

Algenpantucel-L (HyperAcute Pancreas) is a cancer vaccine consisting of irradiated live, allogeneic human pancreatic cancer cells transfected to express murine α-1,3 galactosyl transferase (α-GT). Exposure of α-GT epitope to the human immune system induces rapid activation of antibody-dependent cell-mediated cytotoxicity, and thus hyperacute rejection of α-GT-expressing allogeneic pancreatic cells. As a result, the cellular fragments bound by anti-α-GT antibodies elicit enhanced, multifaceted immune responses to pancreatic TAAs. A preliminary report of a phase II trial showed prolonged survival in 73 patients with resected pancreatic cancer who received adjuvant gemcitabine with algenpantucel-L.[74] A phase III trial is ongoing in patients with surgically resected pancreatic cancers receiving adjuvant therapy with or without algenpantucel-L (NCT01072981).

Allogeneic whole tumor cell vaccines modified to secrete GM-CSF have also been employed in a phase I trial in patients with pancreatic cancer. Evidence of vaccine-induced immune responses was observed, as measured by DTH.[88] A phase II trial in 60 patients with resected pancreatic cancer demonstrated a median DFS of 17.3 months, with a median OS of 24.8 months.[75] A prospective randomized clinical trial is ongoing in patients with surgically resected pancreatic adenocarcinoma, using this type of vaccine either alone or with low-dose cyclophosphamide, with safety, feasibility, and immune response as primary end points (NCT00727441).

Lung Cancer

L-BLP25 (Stimuvax) is a liposome-encapsulated peptide vaccine consisting of a synthetic peptide derived from the MUC-1 antigen. A phase IIb multicenter trial in patients with stage IIIb and IV NSCLC who had received first-line chemotherapy randomized patients to receive vaccine with best supportive care (BSC) versus BSC alone. Patients in the vaccine arm received a single intravenous dose of cyclophosphamide (300 mg/m^2), followed by 8 weekly subcutaneous injections of L-BLP25 (1,000 μg), followed by maintenance immunization at 6-week intervals.[13] In an updated report,[70] median OS for patients in the L-BLP25 arm was 17.2 months versus 13.0 months in the BSC arm (HR 0.745; 95% CI 0.533–1.042). The 3-year survival rate was 31% for patients receiving L-BLP25 plus BSC versus 17% for patients receiving BSC alone ($P = 0.035$). Subsets of patients with stage IIIb locoregional disease showed an even greater survival benefit: median survival was 17.3 months longer in patients receiving L-BLP25 plus BSC than in those receiving BSC alone (30.6 vs. 13.3 mo, respectively; HR 0.548; 95% CI 0.301–0.999). Currently two phase III trials are ongoing in patients with unresectable stage III NSCLC who had response or stable disease after primary chemoradiotherapy with overall survival as primary end points (NCT00409188 and NCT01015443). The result of one of these phase III trials is expected in 2013.

Belagenpumatucel-L, a transforming growth factor (TGF)-β2 antisense gene-modified allogeneic tumor cell vaccine, has shown evidence of clinical benefit. The vaccine is prepared by transfecting allogeneic NSCLC cells with a plasmid containing a TGF-β2 antisense transgene. In a phase II trial, the vaccine showed a response rate of 15% in 61 patients with advanced NSCLC.[89] In another phase II trial in 21 advanced NSCLC patients treated with belagenpumatucel-L, OS was 562 days. Median survival was 660 days for patients with <2 circulating tumor cells (CTCs)/7 mL at baseline, compared with 150 days for patients with ≥2 CTCs at baseline ($P = 0.025$).[71]

Investigators in Cuba have developed an EGF vaccine composed of human recombinant EGF produced in yeast, conjugated to the P64K *Neisseria meningitides* recombinant protein produced in *Escherichia coli*. A randomized phase II study in 80 patients with stage IIIb/IV NSCLC demonstrated that patients who received EGF vaccine following chemotherapy showed a trend toward improved survival.[15] In a subset analysis of patients younger than 60 years, the survival benefit was statistically significant (11.57 vs. 5.33 mo; $P = 0.0124$). The EGF vaccine is currently approved in Cuba.

In a phase IIB trial, addition of TG4010 (a modified vaccinia Ankara vector expressing MUC-1 antigen and IL-2) to first-line chemotherapy in advanced NSCLC showed improved 6-month PFS of 43.2% versus 35.1% in chemotherapy alone.[90] A peptide vaccine, MAGE-A3, has also suggested clinic benefit in a multicentered, randomized phase II trial in 182 patients with completely resected, MAGE-A3 expressing stage pIb or pII NSCLC.[73] These vaccines are being evaluated in phase III trials (NCT01383148 and NCT00480025).

Other Cancers

B lymphoma cells express a unique variable region in the B-cell receptor that forms a specific antigen-binding site unique to each immunoglobulin and contains a molecular signature or idiotype (Id). This Id moiety serves as an excellent target for B-cell lymphoma vaccines. In a phase III trial, patients with treatment-naïve, advanced-stage follicular lymphoma were randomized to receive Id vaccine (Id-KLH plus GM-CSF) or control (KLH plus GM-CSF). Analysis of 117 patients who achieved complete response revealed a statistically significant difference in DFS favoring the vaccine arm (44.2 vs. 30.6 mo; HR 0.62; $P = 0.047$). The benefit appeared to be more pronounced in patients receiving IgM-Id (52.9 vs. 28.7 mo; $P = 0.001$), but not IgG-Id vaccine (35.1 vs. 32.4 mo; $P = 0.807$).[2]

Two large phase III vaccine trials have been conducted in RCC in the adjuvant setting, one with an autologous renal tumor vaccine and another with vitespen, an autologous heat-shock protein (gp96) peptide complex vaccine. The first trial[63] enrolled 558 RCC patients after radical nephrectomy and randomized them to receive either autologous renal tumor cell vaccine (six intradermal injections at 4-week intervals) or no adjuvant therapy. At 70 months, the PFS rate was 70% in the vaccine arm versus 59.3% in the control arm (HR 1.59; $P = 0.0204$). The vitespen trial enrolled 728 RCC patients after nephrectomy and randomized them to receive vaccine (weekly intradermal injection of vitespen for 4 weeks, then every 2 weeks until vaccine depletion) or observation alone.[14] An intent-to-treat analysis showed no statistically significant difference in DFS or OS between the two arms.

A phase III trial in metastatic RCC randomized 733 patients with good or intermediate prognosis and prior nephrectomy to receive standard of care (sunitinib, IL-2, or IFN-α) with or without TroVax (modified vaccinia Ankara delivering 5T4 tumor antigen).[49] No significant difference was observed between the two arms (20.1 mo for vaccine vs. 19.2 mo for control). However, a subset of patients with good prognosis (MSKCC 0) who were treated with vaccine plus IL-2 showed a statistically significant survival advantage over the control arm (HR 0.74; 95% CI, 0.030–0.98; $P = 0.046$). The magnitude of 5T4-specific antibody response was associated with improved survival. Results of phase II trial in RCC patients treated with MVA-5T4 and IL-2 also showed encouraging signs of clinical benefit.[72] Future randomized phase III trial will be necessary to better delineate the potential effectiveness of MVA-5T4 and IL-2. A phase II trial of a vaccine for high-grade glioma, consisting of autologous tumor lysate-pulsed DCs, showed a correlation between immune response and clinical response.[91] Leukemia vaccines have also shown clinical benefit in early-phase trials. Vaccination with RHAMM, PR-1, WT1, and BCR-ABL induced leukemia antigen-specific CD8$^+$ T cells.[92]

ISSUES IN CANCER VACCINE CLINICAL TRIALS

Even with sound science behind their development, many promising vaccines have failed to demonstrate clinical benefit in definitive phase III trials, raising several issues for consideration.

Ideal Candidates for Vaccine Therapy

Appropriate patient selection is particularly crucial in vaccine clinical trials. The majority of clinical trials with positive outcomes have enrolled patients with (a) good performance status, (b) minimally symptomatic disease, (c) intact immune systems, (d) low tumor volume, (e) a limited number of prior chemotherapies, and (f) relatively longer predicted survival.[8,48,56,57] Additionally, contrary to most trials of adjuvant chemotherapy,[81] subgroup analyses of some vaccine trials suggest that clinical benefit is more pronounced in earlier stage disease[7,12,70] than in late-stage or aggressive disease, or in heavily pretreated patients. In several preclinical studies, high tumor burden has been directly correlated with an increased number of Tregs[93] and increased levels of IL-10, TGF-β, and indoleamine-2,3-dioxygenase, all of which have been shown to inhibit T-cell activation.[94]

In a clinical trial conducted in colorectal cancer patients with minimal tumor burden after metastectomy, a PANVAC-based vaccine suggested survival benefit.[87] However, in a phase III trial in patients with advanced, aggressive pancreatic cancer who had failed prior chemotherapies, vaccination with PANVAC showed lack of clinical benefit.[95] In trials that have enrolled only patients with good prognoses, the survival benefit of therapeutic cancer vaccines has repeatedly been proven. The IMPACT trial of sipuleucel-T[56] and the randomized phase II trial of PROSTVAC-VF,[64] both of which limited enrollment to patients with asymptomatic or minimally symptomatic disease, demonstrated a statistically significant survival benefit for vaccine. Another independent phase II trial of PROSTVAC-VF[65] found that those with longer predicted survival (by the validated Halabi nomogram) received more benefit than those with shorter predicted survival. In contrast, phase III trials[58,59] of GVAX, an allogeneic GM-CSF–secreting tumor cell vaccine, enrolled patients who were deemed candidates for chemotherapy. These trials were terminated early when it became clear that they could not meet their primary end points. The predicted survival for patients was only 13 and 16 months for VITAL-2 and VITAL-1 trials, respectively. Retrospective analyses of these data suggest that patients with longer predicted survival showed a significant survival benefit from vaccine compared with the control arm.[59]

Taken together, evidence from preclinical and clinical studies points to the ideal population for vaccine therapy as patients with low disease volume (e.g., after surgical resection of early-stage disease or metastases), minimal exposure to prior therapies, and indolent disease characteristics.

Efficacy Assessment: RECIST/WHO versus irRC

Appropriate efficacy assessment is a crucial component in the design of vaccine clinical trials. The majority of clinical trials in solid tumors have primarily used RECIST and/or WHO response criteria to evaluate tumor response (e.g., a sustained ≥30% reduction in the sum of the longest diameter of target lesions). However, the value of these criteria depends on the type and chemosensitivity of the tumor and on treatment goals. For highly chemosensitive malignancies, such as germ cell tumors or acute leukemias, these criteria are irrelevant.

The value of RECIST or WHO response criteria in immunotherapy trials is questionable. First, the direct target of a cancer vaccine is not the tumor, but the host immune system. Hence, it may take weeks to months to have an effect on tumor size. Second, the dynamic nature of a potentially beneficial immune response to vaccine with tumor infiltrated by immune cells may cause a transient increase in tumor size and/or development of new lesions, which could be identified as progressive disease by traditional criteria.[96] In trials of ipilimumab in melanoma patients, investigators observed several distinct patterns of response: (a) immediate reduction in the size of baseline lesions, (b) stable disease with a slow, steady decline in total tumor volume, (c) delayed response after an initial increase in total tumor volume, and (d) reduction in total tumor burden in the presence of new lesions.[97] To capture these response patterns, Wolchok et al.[97,98] proposed a new set of immune-related response criteria (irRC) for tumor immunotherapy (Table 45.4), which includes immune-related complete response (irCR), immune-related partial response (irPR), immune-related stable disease (irSD), and immune-related progressive disease (irPD). The novelty of these criteria is that they calculate measurable new lesions as part of total tumor burden and compare this calculation with baseline. The appearance of new lesions does not constitute irPD unless the increase in total tumor volume is >25% relative to baseline and is confirmed by a second tumor assessment ≥4 weeks later. Patients with irPR/irSD who had PD by the WHO criteria had survival outcomes similar to those with CR/PR/SD by the WHO criteria. In fact, irRC identified an additional 10% of patients with

TABLE 45-4 Immune-Related Response Criteria

Overall Response by irRC	Measurable Response (Index Lesions and New, Measurable Lesions)[b]	Nonmeasurable Response (Nonindex Lesions And New, Nonmeasurable Lesions)
irCR[a]	100% decrease	None
irPR[a]	≥50% decrease	Any
irSD	<50% decrease to ≤ 25% increase	Any
irPD[a]	>25% increase	Any

[a]Requires confirmation by a second, consecutive assessment ≥ 4 weeks after the first assessment.

[b]Decreases in tumor burden of measurable (>5 × 5 mm) lesions only, relative to baseline.

Adapted from Wolchok et al.[97] *Clin Cancer Res*. 2009;15(23):7412-7420.

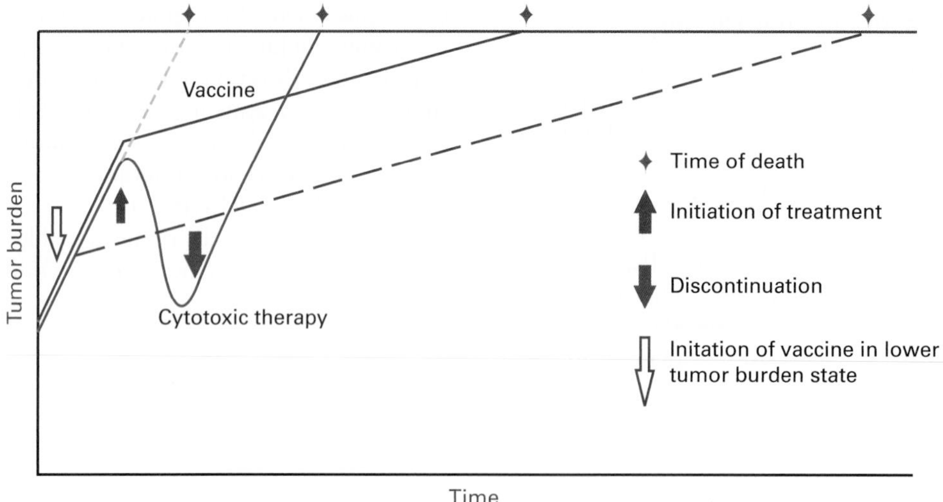

FIGURE 45–2 Tumor growth rate is a dynamic biologic process that is the combined result of cells dying and dividing over time. Cytotoxic therapy reduces tumor burden as long as it is being administered. However, when treatment is terminated, the pretreatment tumor growth rate resumes and the patient succumbs to disease in a predictable manner. A therapeutic cancer vaccine does not decrease tumor burden immediately; however, it can prolong survival by decreasing the tumor growth rate. Initiating vaccine in patients with lower tumor burden can maximize this survival benefit.

favorable survival among those characterized as having PD by the WHO criteria.

Appropriate Primary End Points

Multiple clinical studies suggest that OS should be the primary end point for trials of therapeutic cancer vaccines. Cytotoxic chemotherapies, which have a direct antitumor effect on tumors or their microenvironments, usually produce a positive objective response rate (ORR) and prolonged PFS and occasionally translate into increased OS. On the other hand, a therapeutic cancer vaccine is designed to elicit a lasting host immune response against tumor. It may take weeks to months for the vaccine to have an effect on any tumor shrinkage, but it may have a prolonged effect on tumor growth rate. Hence, ORR and PFS may not be the best criteria for assessing the clinical benefit of a therapeutic cancer vaccine.

The randomized clinical trials of sipuleucel-T highlight the importance of OS as a primary end point. The initial phase III trial of sipuleucel-T failed to meet its primary end point of PFS, but provided evidence of longer OS (25.8 vs. 21.7 mo; $P = 0.032$).[57] When the trial was repeated with OS as the primary end point, it confirmed the survival benefit (25.8 vs. 21.7 mo; HR 0.78; $P = 0.03$) with no improvement in TTP, as seen in the earlier trial. These results led to FDA approval of sipuleucel-T for the treatment of prostate cancer.[56] Similarly, the randomized controlled phase II trial of PROSTVAC-VF failed to meet its primary end point of improved TTP, as determined by new or enlarging tumors or bone metastases, but a survival analysis suggested a clinical benefit for the vaccine.[64] A confirmatory OS end point study is underway (NCT01322490). Likewise, the phase III trial of ipilimumab demonstrated prolonged OS in advanced melanoma patients, with no improvement in median TTP.[11]

Effect on Tumor Growth Rate

The unique patterns of tumor response to immunotherapies and the unprecedented patterns of clinical benefit seen with these agents call for a paradigm shift in cancer therapy and alternative methods of understanding these novel therapeutic agents. This challenge is complicated by the fact that there is no valid biomarker with a demonstrated correlation to clinical benefit. However, a mathematical model of the tumor growth rate constant can potentially account for the long-term survival benefit without a short-term change in disease progression in patients treated with a therapeutic cancer vaccine.[99] This model has been tested in patients treated in several prostate cancer clinical trials at the NCI over the last decade. For patients in chemotherapy trials, there was a very close relationship between PSA kinetics while on treatment and survival. After treatment was discontinued, pretreatment PSA kinetics resumed, and time to death was predictable based on similar pre- and post-treatment PSA trajectories. However, for patients treated with PSA-TRICOM, PSA kinetics did not change immediately while on treatment, but over time, growth rates appeared to decrease and time to death was well beyond what the model predicted (see Fig. 45.2).

CONCLUSIONS

Advancements in the development of therapeutic cancer vaccines are starting to translate into clinical benefit for patients with several types of cancer. Current research is focused on matching vaccine platforms with appropriate targets and on maximizing the efficacy and clinical benefit of cancer vaccines through the use of immune adjuvants and combination treatment modalities.

Over the last decade, clinical trials of therapeutic cancer vaccines have highlighted the need for a new paradigm for clinical trial design that can best translate sound science into clinical practice. Identifying patients who will derive the most benefit from cancer vaccines, improving our understanding of immune-mediated mechanisms, and designing clinical trials with appropriate primary end points will help to move therapeutic cancer vaccines to the forefront of modern cancer treatment.

REFERENCES

1. D'Angelo S, Park B, Krug L, et al. Immunogenicity of GI-4000 vaccine in adjuvant consolidation therapy following definitive treatment in patients with stage I-III adenocarcinoma of the lung with G12C, G12D, or G12V KRAS mutations [abstract]. *J Clin Oncol.* 2011;29:7070.
2. Schuster SJ, Neelapu SS, Gause BL, et al. Vaccination with patient-specific tumor-derived antigen in first remission improves disease-free survival in follicular lymphoma. *J Clin Oncol.* 2011;29(20):2787-2794.
3. Toubaji A, Achtar M, Provenzano M, et al. Pilot study of mutant ras peptide-based vaccine as an adjuvant treatment in pancreatic and colorectal cancers. *Cancer Immunol Immunother.* 2008;57(9):1413-1420.
4. Palena C, Polev DE, Tsang KY, et al. The human T-box mesodermal transcription factor Brachyury is a candidate target for T-cell-mediated cancer immunotherapy. *Clin Cancer Res.* 2007;13(8):2471-2478.
5. Kenter GG, Welters MJ, Valentijn AR, et al. Vaccination against HPV-16 oncoproteins for vulvar intraepithelial neoplasia. *N Engl J Med.* 2009;361(19):1838-1847.
6. Madan RA, Gulley JL. Sipuleucel-T: harbinger of a new age of therapeutics for prostate cancer. *Expert Rev Vaccines.* 2011;10(2):141-150.
7. Vermorken JB, Claessen AM, van Tinteren H, et al. Active specific immunotherapy for stage II and stage III human colon cancer: a randomised trial. *Lancet.* 1999;353(9150):345-350.
8. Uyl-de Groot CA, Vermorken JB, Hanna MG Jr, et al. Immunotherapy with autologous tumor cell-BCG vaccine in patients with colon cancer: a prospective study of medical and economic benefits. *Vaccine.* 2005;23(17–18):2379-2387.
9. Simons JW, Carducci MA, Mikhak B, et al. Phase I/II trial of an allogeneic cellular immunotherapy in hormone-naive prostate cancer. *Clin Cancer Res.* 2006;12(11 pt 1):3394-3401.
10. Salazar E, Zaremba S, Arlen PM, Tsang KY, Schlom J. Agonist peptide from a cytotoxic t-lymphocyte epitope of human carcinoembryonic antigen stimulates production of tc1-type cytokines and increases tyrosine phosphorylation more efficiently than cognate peptide. *Int J Cancer.* 2000;85(6):829-838.
11. Hodi FS, O'Day SJ, McDermott DF, et al. Improved survival with ipilimumab in patients with metastatic melanoma. *N Engl J Med.* 2010;363(8):711-723.
12. Apostolopoulos V, Pietersz GA, Tsibanis A, et al. Pilot phase III immunotherapy study in early-stage breast cancer patients using oxidized mannan-MUC1 [ISRCTN71711835]. *Breast Cancer Res.* 2006;8(3):R27.
13. Butts C, Murray N, Maksymiuk A, et al. Randomized phase IIB trial of BLP25 liposome vaccine in stage IIIB and IV non-small-cell lung cancer. *J Clin Oncol.* 2005;23(27):6674-6681.
14. Wood C, Srivastava P, Bukowski R, et al. An adjuvant autologous therapeutic vaccine (HSPPC-96; vitespen) versus observation alone for patients at high risk of recurrence after nephrectomy for renal cell carcinoma: a multicentre, open-label, randomised phase III trial. *Lancet.* 2008;372(9633):145-154.
15. Neninger Vinageras E, de la Torre A, Osorio Rodriguez M, et al. Phase II randomized controlled trial of an epidermal growth factor vaccine in advanced non-small-cell lung cancer. *J Clin Oncol.* 2008;26(9):1452-1458.
16. Peoples GE, Holmes JP, Hueman MT, et al. Combined clinical trial results of a HER2/neu (E75) vaccine for the prevention of recurrence in high-risk breast cancer patients: U.S. Military Cancer Institute Clinical Trials Group Study I-01 and I-02. *Clin Cancer Res.* 2008;14(3):797-803.
17. Carmichael MG, Benavides LC, Holmes JP, et al. Results of the first phase 1 clinical trial of the HER-2/neu peptide (GP2) vaccine in disease-free breast cancer patients: United States Military Cancer Institute Clinical Trials Group Study I-04. *Cancer.* 2010;116(2):292-301.
18. Tsang KY, Zaremba S, Nieroda CA, Zhu MZ, Hamilton JM, Schlom J. Generation of human cytotoxic T cells specific for human carcinoembryonic antigen epitopes from patients immunized with recombinant vaccinia-CEA vaccine. *J Natl Cancer Inst.* 1995;87(13):982-990.
19. Marshall JL, Hoyer RJ, Toomey MA, et al. Phase I study in advanced cancer patients of a diversified prime-and-boost vaccination protocol using recombinant vaccinia virus and recombinant nonreplicating avipox virus to elicit anti-carcinoembryonic antigen immune responses. *J Clin Oncol.* 2000;18(23):3964-3973.
20. Stubbs AC, Martin KS, Coeshott C, et al. Whole recombinant yeast vaccine activates dendritic cells and elicits protective cell-mediated immunity. *Nat Med.* 2001;7(5):625-629.
21. Haller AA, Lauer GM, King TH, et al. Whole recombinant yeast-based immunotherapy induces potent T cell responses targeting HCV NS3 and Core proteins. *Vaccine.* 2007;25(8):1452-1463.
22. GlobeImmune: targeted molecular immunotherapy [cited October 2011]. http://www.globeimmune.com/technology/publications/.
23. Kass E, Panicali DL, Mazzara G, Schlom J, Greiner JW. Granulocyte/macrophage-colony stimulating factor produced by recombinant avian poxviruses enriches the regional lymph nodes with antigen-presenting cells and acts as an immunoadjuvant. *Cancer Res.* 2001;61(1):206-214.
24. Dranoff G. Coordinated tumor immunity. *J Clin Invest.* 2003;111(8):1116-1118.
25. Cheever MA. Twelve immunotherapy drugs that could cure cancers. *Immunol Rev.* 2008;222:357-368.
26. Waldmann TA. The biology of interleukin-2 and interleukin-15: implications for cancer therapy and vaccine design. *Nat Rev Immunol.* 2006;6(8):595-601.
27. Ahmadzadeh M, Rosenberg SA. IL-2 administration increases CD4+ CD25(hi) Foxp3+ regulatory T cells in cancer patients. *Blood.* 2006;107(6):2409-2414.
28. Gulley JL, Arlen PM, Bastian A, et al. Combining a recombinant cancer vaccine with standard definitive radiotherapy in patients with localized prostate cancer. *Clin Cancer Res.* 2005;11(9):3353-3362.
29. Weiss JM, Subleski JJ, Wigginton JM, Wiltrout RH. Immunotherapy of cancer by IL-12-based cytokine combinations. *Expert Opin Biol Ther.* 2007;7(11):1705-1721.
30. Steel JC, Waldmann TA, Morris JC. Interleukin-15 biology and its therapeutic implications in cancer. *Trends Pharmacol Sci.* 2012;33(1):35-41.
31. Snyder KM, Mackall CL. Fry TJ. IL-7 in allogeneic transplant: clinical promise and potential pitfalls. *Leuk Lymphoma.* 2006;47(7):1222-1228.
32. Garnett CT, Palena C, Chakraborty M, Tsang KY, Schlom J, Hodge JW. Sublethal irradiation of human tumor cells modulates phenotype resulting in enhanced killing by cytotoxic T lymphocytes. *Cancer Res.* 2004;64(21):7985-7994.
33. Chakraborty M, Abrams SI, Coleman CN, Camphausen K, Schlom J, Hodge JW. External beam radiation of tumors alters phenotype of tumor cells to render them susceptible to vaccine-mediated T-cell killing. *Cancer Res.* 2004;64(12):4328-4337.
34. Chi KH, Liu SJ, Li CP, et al. Combination of conformal radiotherapy and intratumoral injection of adoptive dendritic cell immunotherapy in refractory hepatoma. *J Immunother.* 2005;28(2):129-135.
35. Zitvogel L, Apetoh L, Ghiringhelli F, Kroemer G. Immunological aspects of cancer chemotherapy. *Nat Rev Immunol.* 2008;8(1):59-73.
36. Lutsiak ME, Semnani RT, De Pascalis R, Kashmiri SV, Schlom J, Sabzevari H. Inhibition of CD4(+)25+ T regulatory cell function implicated in enhanced immune response by low-dose cyclophosphamide. *Blood.* 2005;105(7):2862-2868.
37. Maccubbin DL, Wing KR, Mace KF, Ho RL, Ehrke MJ, Mihich E. Adriamycin-induced modulation of host defenses in tumor-bearing mice. *Cancer Res.* 1992;52(13):3572-3576.
38. Chan OT, Yang LX. The immunological effects of taxanes. *Cancer Immunol Immunother.* 2000;49(4–5):181-185.

39. Arlen PM, Gulley JL, Parker C, et al. A randomized phase II study of concurrent docetaxel plus vaccine versus vaccine alone in metastatic androgen-independent prostate cancer. *Clin Cancer Res*. 2006;12(4):1260-1269.
40. Gribben JG, Ryan DP, Boyajian R, et al. Unexpected association between induction of immunity to the universal tumor antigen CYP1B1 and response to next therapy. *Clin Cancer Res*. 2005;11(12):4430-4436.
41. Mercader M, Bodner BK, Moser MT, et al. T cell infiltration of the prostate induced by androgen withdrawal in patients with prostate cancer. *Proc Natl Acad Sci U S A*. 2001;98(25):14565-14570.
42. Madan RA, Gulley JL, Schlom J, et al. Analysis of overall survival in patients with nonmetastatic castration-resistant prostate cancer treated with vaccine, nilutamide, and combination therapy. *Clin Cancer Res*. 2008;14(14):4526-4531.
43. Bilusic M, Gulley J, Heery C, et al. A randomized phase II study of flutamide with or without PSA-TRICOM in nonmetastatic castration-resistant prostate cancer (CRPC) [abstract]. *J Clin Oncol*. 2011;29(S7):163.
44. Wen J, Zhu X, Liu B, et al. Targeting activity of a TCR/IL-2 fusion protein against established tumors. *Cancer Immunol Immunother*. 2008;57(12):1781-1794.
45. Madan R, Mohebtash M, Arlen P, et al. Overall survival (OS) analysis of a phase l trial of a vector-based vaccine (PSA-TRICOM) and ipilimumab (Ipi) in the treatment of metastatic castration-resistant prostate cancer (mCRPC) [abstract]. *J Clin Oncol*. 2010;28(S15):2550.
46. Ascierto PA, Simeone E, Sznol M, Fu YX, Melero I. Clinical experiences with anti-CD137 and anti-PD1 therapeutic antibodies. *Semin Oncol*. 2010;37(5):508-516.
47. Dannull J, Su Z, Rizzieri D, et al. Enhancement of vaccine-mediated antitumor immunity in cancer patients after depletion of regulatory T cells. *J Clin Invest*. 2005;115(12):3623-3633.
48. Schwartzentruber DJ, Lawson DH, Richards JM, et al. gp100 peptide vaccine and interleukin-2 in patients with advanced melanoma. *N Engl J Med*. 2011;364(22):2119-2127.
49. Amato RJ, Hawkins RE, Kaufman HL, et al. Vaccination of metastatic renal cancer patients with MVA-5T4: a randomized, double-blind, placebo-controlled phase III study. *Clin Cancer Res*. 2010;16(22):5539-5547.
50. Balachandran VP, Cavnar MJ, Zeng S, et al. Imatinib potentiates antitumor T cell responses in gastrointestinal stromal tumor through the inhibition of Ido. *Nat Med*. 2011;17(9):1094-1100.
51. Smith BD, Kasamon YL, Kowalski J, et al. K562/GM-CSF immunotherapy reduces tumor burden in chronic myeloid leukemia patients with residual disease on imatinib mesylate. *Clin Cancer Res*. 2010;16(1):338-347.
52. Li Z, Qiao Y, Liu B, Laska EJ, et al. Combination of imatinib mesylate with autologous leukocyte-derived heat shock protein and chronic myelogenous leukemia. *Clin Cancer Res*. 2005;11(12):4460-4468.
53. Farsaci B, Higgins JP, Hodge JW. Consequence of dose scheduling of sunitinib on host immune response elements and vaccine combination therapy. *Int J Cancer*. 2012;130(8):1948-1959.
54. Boni A, Cogdill AP, Dang P, et al. Selective BRAFV600E inhibition enhances T-cell recognition of melanoma without affecting lymphocyte function. Cancer Res. 2010;70(13):5213-5219.
55. Comin-Anduix B, Chodon T, Sazegar H, et al. The oncogenic BRAF kinase inhibitor PLX4032/RG7204 does not affect the viability or function of human lymphocytes across a wide range of concentrations. *Clin Cancer Res*. 2010;16(24):6040-6048.
56. Kantoff PW, Higano CS, Shore ND, et al. Sipuleucel-T immunotherapy for castration-resistant prostate cancer. *N Engl J Med*. 2010;363(5):411-422.
57. Small EJ, Schellhammer PF, Higano CS, et al. Placebo-controlled phase III trial of immunologic therapy with sipuleucel-T (APC8015) in patients with metastatic, asymptomatic hormone refractory prostate cancer. *J Clin Oncol*. 2006;24(19):3089-3094.
58. Higano CS, Saad F, Somer B, et al. A phase III trial of GVAX immunotherapy for prostate cancer versus docetaxel plus prednisone in asymptomatic, castration-resistant prostate cancer (CRPC) [abstract]. ASCO Genitourinary Cancers Symposium. 2009:LBA150.
59. Small EJ, Demkow T, Gerritsen W, et al. A phase III trial of GVAX immunotherapy for prostate cancer in combination with docetaxel versus docetaxel plus prednisone in symptomatic, castration-resistant prostate cancer (CRPC) [abstract]. ASCO Genitourinary Cancers Symposium; 2009:7.
60. Testori A, Richards J, Whitman E, et al. Phase III comparison of vitespen, an autologous tumor-derived heat shock protein gp96 peptide complex vaccine, with physician's choice of treatment for stage IV melanoma: the C-100-21 Study Group. *J Clin Oncol*. 2008;26(6):955-962.
61. Miles D, Roche H, Martin M, et al. Phase III multicenter clinical trial of the sialyl-TN (STn)-keyhole limpet hemocyanin (KLH) vaccine for metastatic breast cancer. *Oncologist*. 2011;16(8):1092-1100.
62. Freedman A, Neelapu SS, Nichols C, et al. Placebo-controlled phase III trial of patient-specific immunotherapy with mitumprotimut-T and granulocyte-macrophage colony-stimulating factor after rituximab in patients with follicular lymphoma. *J Clin Oncol*. 2009;27(18):3036-3043.
63. Jocham D, Richter A, Hoffmann L, et al. Adjuvant autologous renal tumour cell vaccine and risk of tumour progression in patients with renal-cell carcinoma after radical nephrectomy: phase III, randomised controlled trial. *Lancet*. 2004;363(9409):594-599.
64. Kantoff PW, Schuetz TJ, Blumenstein BA, et al. Overall survival analysis of a phase II randomized controlled trial of a poxviral-based PSA-targeted immunotherapy in metastatic castration-resistant prostate cancer. *J Clin Oncol*. 2010;28(7):1099-1105.
65. Gulley JL, Arlen PM, Madan RA, et al. Immunologic and prognostic factors associated with overall survival employing a poxviral-based PSA vaccine in metastatic castrate-resistant prostate cancer. *Cancer Immunol Immunother*. 2010;59(5):663-674.
66. Senzer NN, Kaufman HL, Amatruda T, et al. Phase II clinical trial of a granulocyte-macrophage colony-stimulating factor-encoding, second-generation oncolytic herpesvirus in patients with unresectable metastatic melanoma. *J Clin Oncol*. 2009;27(34):5763-5771.
67. Bedikian AY, Richards J, Kharkevitch D, Atkins MB, Whitman E, Gonzalez R. A phase 2 study of high-dose Allovectin-7 in patients with advanced metastatic melanoma. *Melanoma Res*. 2010;20(3):218-226.
68. Berd D, Sato T, Maguire HC Jr, Kairys J, Mastrangelo MJ. Immunopharmacologic analysis of an autologous, hapten-modified human melanoma vaccine. *J Clin Oncol*. 2004;22(3):403-415.
69. Mohebtash M, Madan RA, Gulley J, et al. PANVAC vaccine alone or with docetaxel for patients with metastatic breast cancer [abstract]. *J Clin Oncol*. 2008;26:3035.
70. Butts C, Maksymiuk A, Goss G, et al. Updated survival analysis in patients with stage IIIB or IV non-small-cell lung cancer receiving BLP25 liposome vaccine (L-BLP25): phase IIB randomized, multicenter, open-label trial. *J Cancer Res Clin Oncol*. 2011;137(9):1337-1342.
71. Nemunaitis J, Nemunaitis M, Senzer N, et al. Phase II trial of Belagenpumatucel-L, a TGF-beta2 antisense gene modified allogeneic tumor vaccine in advanced non small cell lung cancer (NSCLC) patients. *Cancer Gene Ther*. 2009;16(8):620-624.
72. Kaufman HL, Taback B, Sherman W, et al. Phase II trial of Modified Vaccinia Ankara (MVA) virus expressing 5T4 and high dose Interleukin-2 (IL-2) in patients with metastatic renal cell carcinoma. *J Transl Med*. 2009;7:2.
73. Vansteenkiste J, Zielinski M, Linder A, et al. Final results of a multi-center, double-blind, randomized, placebo-controlled phase II study to assess the efficacy of MAGE-A3 immunotherapeutic as adjuvant therapy in stage IB/II non-small cell lung cancer (NSCLC) [abstract]. *J Clin Oncol. 2007*;25(18S):7554.
74. Hardacre J, Mulcahy M, Small W, et al. Effect of the addition of algenpantucel-L immunotherapy to standard adjuvant therapy on survival in patients with resected pancreas cancer [abstract]. *J Clin Oncol*. 2011;29:236.
75. Lutz E, Yeo CJ, Lillemoe KD, et al. A lethally irradiated allogeneic granulocyte-macrophage colony stimulating factor-secreting tumor vaccine for pancreatic adenocarcinoma. A phase II trial of safety, efficacy, and immune activation. *Ann Surg*. 2011;253(2):328-335.

76. Small EJ, Tchekmedyian NS, Rini BI, Fong L, Lowy I, Allison JP. A pilot trial of CTLA-4 blockade with human anti-CTLA-4 in patients with hormone-refractory prostate cancer. *Clin Cancer Res*. 2007;13(6):1810-1815.
77. McNeel DG, Dunphy EJ, Davies JG, et al. Safety and immunological efficacy of a DNA vaccine encoding prostatic acid phosphatase in patients with stage D0 prostate cancer. *J Clin Oncol*. 2009;27(25):4047-4054.
78. Hofbauer GF, Baur T, Bonnet MC, et al. Clinical phase I intratumoral administration of two recombinant ALVAC canarypox viruses expressing human granulocyte-macrophage colony-stimulating factor or interleukin-2: the transgene determines the composition of the inflammatory infiltrate. *Melanoma Res*. 2008;18(2):104-111.
79. Kyte JA, Mu L, Aamdal S, et al. Phase I/II trial of melanoma therapy with dendritic cells transfected with autologous tumor-mRNA. *Cancer Gene Ther*. 2006;13(10):905-918.
80. Disis ML, Wallace DR, Gooley TA, et al. Concurrent trastuzumab and HER2/neu-specific vaccination in patients with metastatic breast cancer. *J Clin Oncol*. 2009;27(28): 4685-4692.
81. Andre T, Boni C, Navarro M, et al. Improved overall survival with oxaliplatin, fluorouracil, and leucovorin as adjuvant treatment in stage II or III colon cancer in the MOSAIC trial. *J Clin Oncol*. 2009;27(19):3109-3116.
82. Vaccinogen Clinical Trials: Proof of Efficacy [cited August 2011]. http://www.vaccinogeninc.com/vaccinogen/clinical-trials/.
83. Schlom J. Carcinoembryonic antigen (CEA) peptides and vaccines for carcinoma. In: Kast M, ed. *Peptide-Based Cancer Vaccines*. Austin, TX: Landes Bioscience; 2000:90-105.
84. Marshall JL, Hawkins MJ, Tsang KY, et al. Phase I study in cancer patients of a replication-defective avipox recombinant vaccine that expresses human carcinoembryonic antigen. *J Clin Oncol*. 1999;17(1):332-337.
85. Fong L, Brockstedt D, Benike C, et al. Dendritic cell-based xenoantigen vaccination for prostate cancer immunotherapy. *J Immunol*. 2001;167(12):7150-7156.
86. Marshall JL, Gulley JL, Arlen PM, et al. Phase I study of sequential vaccinations with fowlpox-CEA(6D)-TRICOM alone and sequentially with vaccinia-CEA(6D)-TRICOM, with and without granulocyte-macrophage colony-stimulating factor, in patients with carcinoembryonic antigen-expressing carcinomas. *J Clin Oncol*. 2005;23(4):720-731.
87. Morse M, Niedzwiecki D, Marshall J, et al. Survival rates among patients vaccinated following resection of colorectal cancer metastases in a phase II randomized study compared with contemporary controls [abstract]. *J Clin Oncol*. 2011;29:3557.
88. Jaffee EM, Hruban RH, Biedrzycki B, et al. Novel allogeneic granulocyte-macrophage colony-stimulating factor-secreting tumor vaccine for pancreatic cancer: a phase I trial of safety and immune activation. *J Clin Oncol*. 2001;19(1):145-156.
89. Nemunaitis J, Dillman RO, Schwarzenberger PO, et al. Phase II study of belagenpumatucel-L, a transforming growth factor beta-2 antisense gene-modified allogeneic tumor cell vaccine in non-small-cell lung cancer. *J Clin Oncol*. 2006;24(29):4721-4730.
90. Quoix E, Ramlau R, Westeel V, et al. Therapeutic vaccination with TG4010 and first-line chemotherapy in advanced non-small-cell lung cancer: a controlled phase 2B trial. *Lancet Oncol*. 2011;12(12):1125-1133.
91. Wheeler CJ, Black KL, Liu G, et al. Vaccination elicits correlated immune and clinical responses in glioblastoma multiforme patients. *Cancer Res*. 2008;68(14):5955-5964.
92. Rezvani K, de Lavallade H. Vaccination strategies in lymphomas and leukaemias: recent progress. *Drugs*. 2011;71(13):1659-1674.
93. Ghiringhelli F, Larmonier N, Schmitt E, et al. CD4+CD25+ regulatory T cells suppress tumor immunity but are sensitive to cyclophosphamide which allows immunotherapy of established tumors to be curative. *Eur J Immunol*. 2004;34(2):336-344.
94. Gulley JL, Madan RA, Schlom J. Impact of tumour volume on the potential efficacy of therapeutic vaccines. *Curr Oncol*. 2011;18(3):e150-e157.
95. Madan RA, Arlen PM, Gulley JL. PANVAC-VF: poxviral-based vaccine therapy targeting CEA and MUC1 in carcinoma. *Expert Opin Biol Ther*. 2007;7(4):543-554.
96. Gulley JL, Arlen PM, Tsang KY, et al. Pilot study of vaccination with recombinant CEA-MUC-1-TRICOM poxviral-based vaccines in patients with metastatic carcinoma. *Clin Cancer Res*. 2008;14(10):3060-3069.
97. Wolchok JD, Hoos A, O'Day S, et al. Guidelines for the evaluation of immune therapy activity in solid tumors: immune-related response criteria. *Clin Cancer Res*. 2009;15(23): 7412-7420.
98. Wolchok JD, Neyns B, Linette G, et al. Ipilimumab monotherapy in patients with pretreated advanced melanoma: a randomised, double-blind, multicentre, phase 2, dose-ranging study. *Lancet Oncol*. 2010;11(2):155-164.
99. Stein WD, Gulley JL, Schlom J, et al. Tumor regression and growth rates determined in five intramural NCI prostate cancer trials: the growth rate constant as an indicator of therapeutic efficacy. *Clin Cancer Res*. 2011;17(4):907-917.

CHAPTER 46

CANCER GENE THERAPY: NUCLEIC ACIDS AS THERAPEUTIC AGENTS

Richard A. Morgan and Daniel Abate-Daga

According to the American Society of Gene and Cell Therapy, gene therapy is defined as a set of strategies that modify the expression of an individual's genes or that correct abnormal genes by means of the administration of a specific DNA or RNA.[1] These include modulation of gene expression at genomic or transcriptomic level, attained by a diverse array of techniques, in order to induce the desired therapeutic effect.

The development of recombinant DNA technology in the 1970s laid the foundations for the idea of treating diseases whose primary cause was a genetic alteration by introducing a functional copy of the defective gene in the diseased tissue. This idea evolved to a broader spectrum of approaches, not necessarily involving the modification of the genetic material. In the context of treatment of cancer, for instance, the ultimate goal is to eliminate the diseased cells rather than to establish a long-term correction of an aberrant gene. Therefore, although cancers are essentially caused by genetic alterations, gene therapy for cancer may be based not only on the modulation of genes involved in its etiopathogeny (e.g., overexpression of tumor suppressor genes and oncogene antagonism) but also in the expression of death-inducing genes, suicide genes, or immune modulators.

MANIPULATION OF GENE EXPRESSION

Expression Cassette Design

Different types of nucleic acids can be administered to modulate the expression of endogenous genes or to induce the expression of exogenous genes. Expression of a protein can be achieved by transfer of the coding sequence of a gene in the form of plasmid DNA or an expression cassette embedded in a viral vector. In either case, the basic gene expression unit must contain a promoter region where transcription factors will bind and activate gene expression; the protein-coding region, normally composed of complementary DNA (cDNA), that is, a DNA sequence that does not include intronic regions present in genomic DNA; and a polyadenylation signal that confers stability to the messenger RNA (mRNA). Promoters used to drive gene expression include the natural promoter of the gene to be expressed, constitutively active viral promoters such as cytomegalovirus, inducible promoters that can be switched on/off by the addition of chemical compounds, and promoters that are active in a cell-specific or time-specific fashion (Fig. 46.1A).

Gene expression can also be induced by the transfer of mRNA directly into the target cell, normally by physical methods such as electroporation. The main limitation of this approach is that production of the protein encoded by this mRNA is linked to the stability of the mRNA, as opposed to a DNA-based expression cassette that continuously expresses new mRNA molecules.

Gene Knockdown: Antisense Oligonucleotides and RNA Interference

The complete sequencing of the human genome and a thorough understanding of the multiple mechanisms whereby gene expression is regulated opened the door, in the last two decades, to novel technologies that allow for the manipulation of gene expression at a post-transcriptional level. There are many disease states where repression of gene expression would be desirable. In this regard,

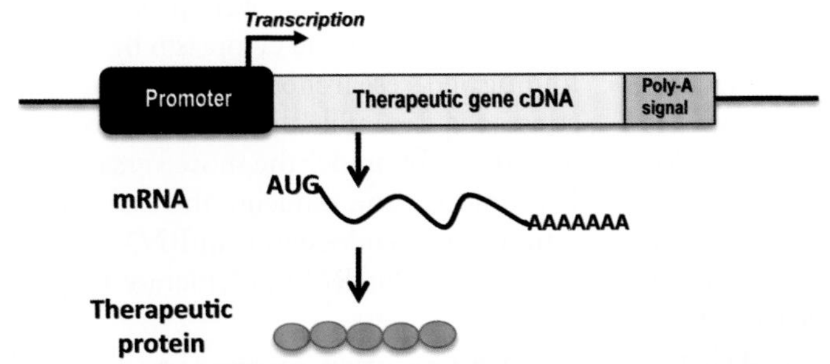

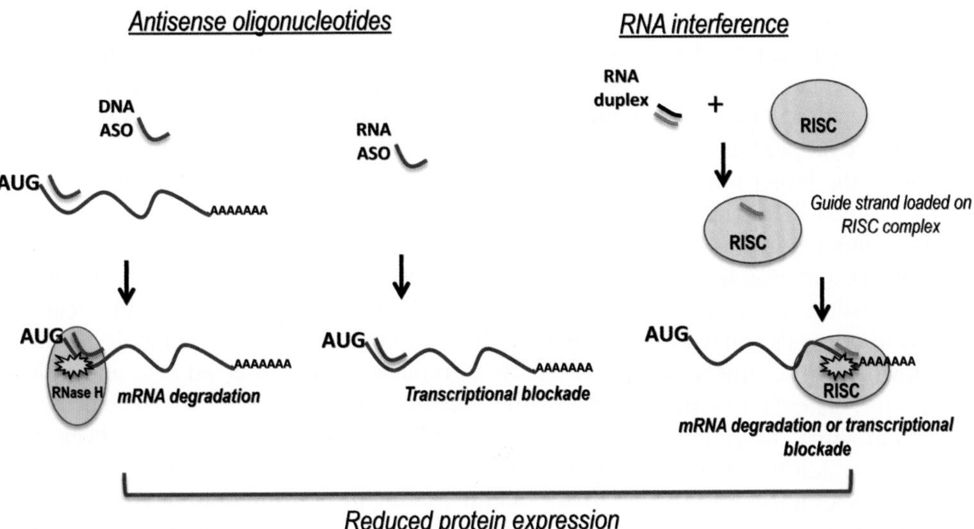

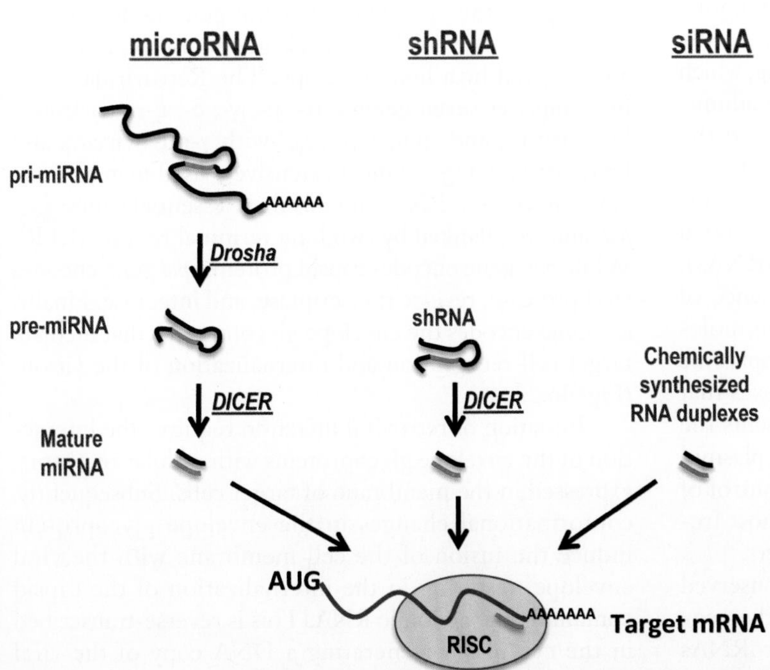

FIGURE 46–1 **(A)** Elements of a basic expression cassette. Transcription of a therapeutic gene cDNA is commanded by an upstream promoter, where transcription factors and RNA polymerase bind. Transcription is terminated by a polyadenylation signal downstream of the coding region. **(B)** Silencing of mRNA expression using ASO is induced by binding of a single-chain DNA oligonucleotides to mRNA leading to its RNase H–mediated digestion, or by a single-chain RNA molecule to the target mRNA, resulting in blockade of protein synthesis. RNAi is induced by RNA duplexes and involves its dissociation and subsequent loading of one strand into the RISC complex. This RNA–protein complex either degrades or blocks the translation of mRNAs with base complementarity to the loaded RNA molecule. **(C)** RNAi is induced by different precursor molecules. The microRNA (miRNA) pathway involves long genomic primary transcripts bearing stem-loop regions (pri-miRNA) that are cleaved by Drosha in the nucleus and further trimmed by DICER in the cytoplasm to generate mature miRNA duplexes. The shRNA pathway involves the transcription of short (≈70 nucleotides) transcripts that form hairpin structures due to intramolecular base pairing. These are trimmed by DICER to generate mature RNA duplexes. Finally, chemically synthesized siRNA molecules are administered directly as RNA duplexes. The final product of either pathway is unwound and loaded into RISC to mediate gene knockdown.

antisense oligonucleotides (ASOs) and RNA interference (RNAi) constitute two analogous yet mechanistically distinct tools for gene silencing.

ASOs are single-stranded DNA or RNA molecules, complementary to a given mRNA. Binding of an ASO to its target mRNA results in inhibition of protein expression by two alternative mechanisms: DNA-based ASOs induce degradation of target RNA by RNase H, whereas RNA-based ASOs block translation of target mRNA without causing its degradation (Fig. 46.1B). In order to increase the stability and silencing capacity of ASO, several chemical alterations to the phosphodiester bonds present in DNA and RNA chains have been investigated, including morpholinos, phosphorothioates, locked nucleic acids, and peptidic nucleic acids.[2]

RNAi is an evolutionarily conserved mechanism of post-transcriptional regulation of gene expression, based on the recognition of target sequences present in mRNA molecules by small RNA molecules. These 21- to 23-nucleotide RNA duplexes can activate either degradation or translational repression of the target mRNA executed by a multiprotein complex named RISC (RNA-induced silencing complex). This phenomenon was initially described in nematodes and plants, and even before its mechanism of action was fully dissected, synthetic RNA molecules were administered to eukaryotic cells and were shown to recapitulate the knockdown of target mRNAs previously described in lower organisms.[3] These synthetic, double-stranded RNAs were termed short interfering RNA (siRNA) (see Fig. 46.1B). Unlike ASOs, siRNAs are administered as double-stranded RNA molecules and degradation of target mRNA or inhibition of its translation occurs in a catalytic rather than stoichiometric fashion. Moreover, while certain ASOs have been reported to induce off-target silencing due to the activation of a type I interferon response, this was not observed with siRNAs.

Although extensively used for functional genomic studies, mainly in vitro, siRNAs need to be repeatedly administered in order to induce long-term silencing, which constitutes a technical obstacle for their in vivo administration for therapeutic purposes. This prompted the development of DNA-encoded RNA molecules that serve as a template for the generation of RNA duplexes similar to siRNA. These approximately 70 nt DNA-encoded RNAs were named short hairpin RNAs (shRNAs), as they fold and self-hybridize due to the presence of palindromic sequences contained in each single molecule. Hairpin-like structures are trimmed by cytoplasmic enzyme DICER to form 21 to 23 nt RNA duplexes that can induce RNAi (Fig. 46.1C). This variant presents the advantage of being amenable for cloning into a plasmid or viral vector and can be expressed under the control of highly active RNA polymerase III promoters, most frequently U6 small nucleolar RNA or H1 promoters.

Further studies established that RNAi was conserved in mammals and that the natural substrates for the generation of RNA-silencing species (called microRNAs [miRNA]) were large genomic transcripts (primary microRNA, pri-miRNA) that were processed in a stepwise fashion in the nucleus and cytoplasm by several enzymes. This finding led researchers to generate longer RNAi substrates that resemble the natural transcripts, thus allowing for expression under the more versatile RNA polymerase II promoters and reducing the toxic effects derived from saturation of endogenous miRNA processing machinery seen using some RNA polymerase III promoter systems.

GENE TRANSFER SYSTEMS

An ideal vector should be able to selectively transduce target cells, resulting in stable expression of the therapeutic gene at levels that are sufficient to induce the desired therapeutic effect. Strategies developed to that end include the use of engineered viruses, artificial particles with membrane fusion properties such as liposomes, and physical methods such as electroporation.

The utilization of viral vectors is based on the ability of certain viruses to introduce genetic material into mammalian cells during their natural infectious cycles. In order to render these viruses capable of delivering the desired genetic material without resulting in the generation of a pathological condition, the genome of naturally occurring viruses needs to be engineered, aiming mainly to ablate their ability to replicate in the infected cells and to load them with exogenous nucleic acids meant to be delivered into the target cell. Several virus species have been used in gene therapy approaches, including DNA and RNA viruses and integrating or non-integrating viruses.

The most frequently used viral vectors are described herein.

Retrovirus

Retroviruses were the first to be developed for their use in gene therapy. The retroviral genome is encoded in two molecules of RNA, packaged in a protein capsid, and covered by a lipid envelope. The Retroviridae family comprises seven genera: α-, β-, γ-, δ-, ε-retroviruses, lentiviruses, and spumaviruses,[4] with γ-retroviruses and lentiviruses being the most extensively used in gene therapy. γ-Retroviral RNA contains three essential genes: *gag*, *pol*, and *env*, flanked by two long terminal repeats (LTR). While *gag* gene encodes capsid proteins, *pol* gene encodes viral protease, reverse transcriptase, and integrase. Finally, *env* gene encodes the envelope glycoproteins that mediate target cell recognition and internalization of the virion[5] (Fig. 46.2A).

Initiation of retroviral infection requires the interaction of the envelope glycoproteins with cellular receptors, expressed in the membrane of target cells. Subsequently, conformational changes in the envelope glycoprotein induce the fusion of the cell membrane with the viral envelope, resulting in the internalization of the capsid containing the genomic RNA. This is reverse-transcribed in the cytoplasm, generating a DNA copy of the viral

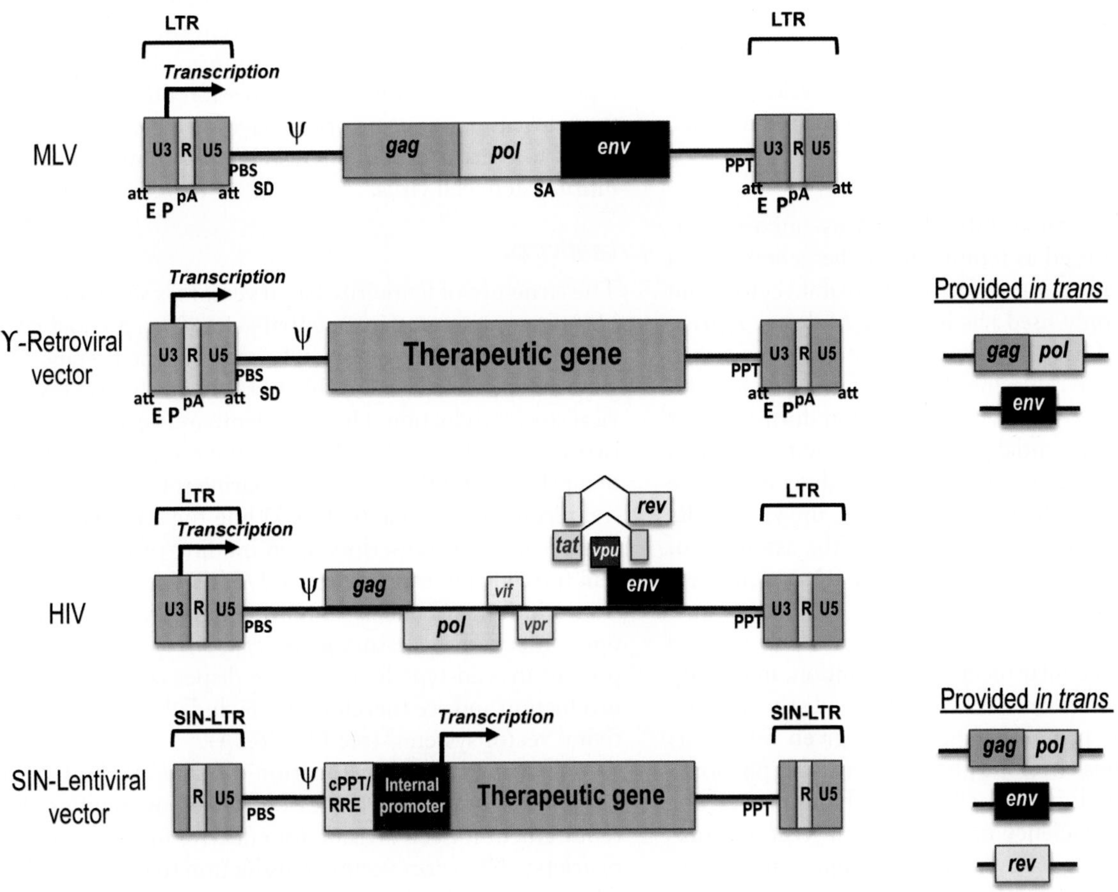

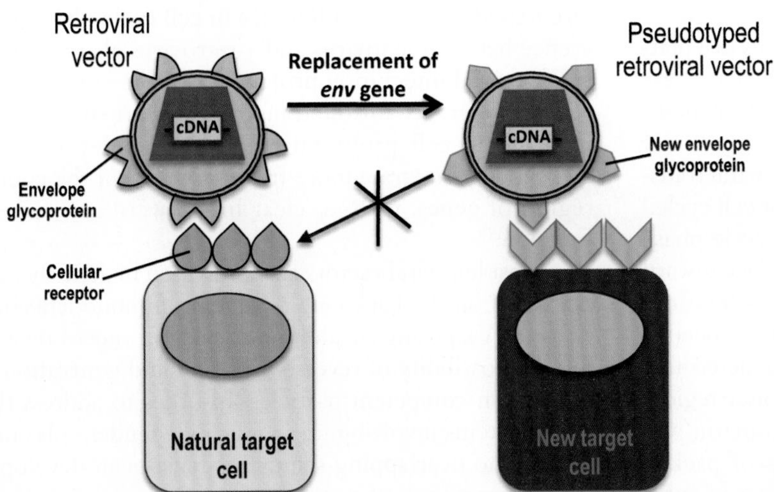

FIGURE 46–2 Retroviral vectors. **(A)** Genomic structure of retroviral vectors. Wild-type MLV γ-retrovirus and MLV-derived vectors are as diagramed. Essential genes *gag, pol,* and *env* are removed from the viral backbone and provided in trans for viral production. Transcription is initiated by the 5′-LTR. Genomic structure of HIV and HIV-derived lentiviral vectors. Essential genes *gag, pol,* and *env* are removed from viral backbone and provided in trans during vector production, along with *rev.* Accessory genes *tat, vpu, vif,* and *vpr* are not included in lentiviral vectors. The U3 regions of the LTRs are partially deleted in the integrated lentiviral vector and lack transcriptional activity; therefore, an internal promoter is included in the design to drive the expression of the therapeutic gene. A *rev*-responsive element (RRE) and central polypurine tract (cPPT) are included to allow for efficient expression. **(B)** Vector pseudotyping. Enveloped viruses can be pseudotyped by replacing envelope glycoproteins with those of another virus or with artificial targeting molecules. This results in modified tropism allowing for transduction of different cell types. ψ, encapsidation signal; E, enhancer; P, promoter; LTR, long terminal repeat; PPT, polypurine tract; pA, polyadenylation signal; att, integration signal; PBS, tRNA primer-binding site; SD, SA, splice donor, splice acceptor.

genome that, upon translocation to the nucleus of the cell, is inserted in the cellular genome by means of the viral integrase. Transcription factors of the host cell will drive the expression of viral genes from the inserted LTRs, giving rise to the RNA and proteins necessary for the assembly of a progeny of viral particles. These are released from the infected cell by budding from the plasma membrane.[5]

γ-Retrovirus Vectors

Different γ-retroviruses (also known as oncoretroviruses) have been used as templates for the generation of recombinant, replication-defective retroviral vectors, but the most commonly used has been the Moloney murine leukemia virus (MLV). The therapeutic gene is inserted in the viral genome replacing the viral genes *gag*, *pol*, and *env*. In order to allow for virus replication during vector production, these essential genes are provided in trans, in cell lines called packaging cells. The recombinant genome contains, apart from the therapeutic gene, the viral LTRs and encapsidation signal that allows for the assembly of viral particles containing recombinant RNA genomes[5] (Fig. 46.2A).

As the envelope glycoprotein encoded by the *env* gene determines cellular receptor recognition, infectivity of retroviral vectors can be tailored by substituting the natural envelope protein encoded by a given retrovirus for a heterogenous envelope glycoprotein. This phenomenon, called pseudotyping, allows for the improvement in transduction efficiency or selectivity in vector transduction. Gibbon ape leukemia virus glycoprotein and the envelope of feline virus RD114, for instance, allow for more efficient transduction of human cells of the hematopoietic lineage than does the broad tropism amphotropic envelope[5] (Fig. 46.2B).

A major limitation in the use of γ-retrovirus as a platform for gene transfer derives from the fact that these require the disassembly of the target cell nuclear membrane to yield complete integration. Therefore, only actively replicating cells are susceptible to retroviral transduction as they transit through the S-phase of cell cycle.[5] Another consequence derived from this cell cycle phase requirement is a bias in integration site preference toward loci encoding for genes involved in cell proliferation. Although retroviral integration is not sequence-specific, it has been described that epigenetic features determine the accessibility of the provirus to a given genomic region. Regions with open, actively transcribed chromatin will be preferentially targeted, whereas regions of packed heterochromatin will have a lower frequency of integration events. Detailed analysis of integration sites by whole-genome sequencing showed that oncoretroviruses integrate most frequently in the vicinity of transcription start sites of actively transcribed genes[6] and it has been postulated that the presence of regulatory elements of the vector might interfere with the expression of such genes.[7]

After integration, epigenetic changes can also condition the expression of retrovirally transduced genes. Silencing of expression cassettes via methylation of retroviral promoters has been shown in murine cells, especially in undifferentiated cells such as hematopoietic stem cells.[8] It is still not clear to what extent this phenomenon applies to cells of human origin, but in an effort to prevent a possible reduction in gene expression efficiency, other γ-retroviruses of murine origin have been assayed as templates for vector development. One such example is the murine stem cell virus.

Lentivirus

The structure of lentivirus-based vectors is similar to that of γ-retroviruses in that essential genes (*gag*, *pol*, and *env*) are replaced by the expression cassette for the therapeutic gene and provided in trans by packaging cells to allow for viral stock production. However, lentiviral vectors contain two additional *cis*-acting elements: the rev-responsive element (RRE) and the central polypurine tract (cPPT)/central termination signal (CTS). While the RRE facilitates nuclear of viral transcripts upon binding of the rev protein (provided in trans), the cPPT/CTS enhances reverse transcription and nuclear import of DNA viral genomes upon infection. Accessory genes *vpu*, *vif*, *vpr*, *tat*, and *nef*, present in wild-type lentivirus are dispensable for vector production and are therefore not included in current lentiviral vector systems[9] (see Fig. 46.2A).

The nuclear translocation ability of lentiviral genomes, granted by the cPPT/CTS, overcomes the requirement for cell division for effective integration that restricts γ-retrovirus vector transduction to dividing cells. This feature makes lentiviral vectors a more versatile gene delivery platform allowing for the transduction of a wide range of cell types, including non-cycling terminally differentiated cells. This difference in cell cycle phase preference between lentivirus and γ-retrovirus also results in a differential integration profile. While the latter display a clear preference for the transcription start site of genes involved in cell proliferation, lentivirus-derived vectors tend to integrate more frequently within the coding region of genes, with no clear bias toward any cellular function.[10]

Most lentiviral vectors currently used in gene therapy are based on the backbone of human immunodeficiency virus (HIV), posing an additional level of concern regarding the possibility of reverse mutation and generation of replication-competent particles. In order to address this issue, systems involving up to four independent plasmids bearing no overlapping sequences have been developed for the expression of *gag*, *pol*, *env*, and *rev* genes in packaging cells.[9]

Initial vector designs used LTR-driven expression, but the HIV LTR has a restricted tropism and is dependent on the tat protein, prompting the development of self-inactivating vectors[11] that use internal promoters to drive gene expression. This modification may also avoid the activation of endogenous genes (for instance, proto-oncogenes) due to the transcriptional activity of LTR.

In addition, this modification prevents the mobilization of integrated lentiviral proviruses in the event of an infection with wild-type HIV.

Lentiviral vectors can also be pseudotyped to express heterogenous envelope glycoproteins in order to change the natural CD4 tropism of HIV and to allow for the transduction of other cell types. Most lentiviral vectors are pseudotyped with vesicular stomatitis virus g-protein, whose cellular receptor is ubiquitously expressed in human cells, thus broadening the spectrum of tissues that can be targeted.[12] Moreover, pseudotyping with the envelope glycoprotein of measles virus has been shown to overcome the blockade of lentiviral transduction of quiescent naïve lymphocytes,[13] suggesting that these manipulations may not only impact on the binding of the vector with its cellular target but also alter the biology of the transduction process at different levels, potentially increasing the versatility of lentivirus-based gene delivery platforms.

For those applications in which high transduction specificity is needed, systems have been developed that ablate the natural tropism of the envelope protein while preserving the capacity of inducing internalization of the viral particle. Tropism is redefined by the expression of a separate protein in the viral envelope that has the ability to bind a membrane protein expressed specifically in the target cells.[14] For example, anti-CD20 single-chain antibodies fused to a membrane-anchoring domain have been used to target lentiviral vectors to tumors of the B-cell lineage, when expressed in conjunction with the Sindbis virus envelope proteins.[15]

Adenovirus

Adenoviruses are non-enveloped viruses of the *Mastadenovirus* genus, Adenoviridae family. A total of 51 serotypes have been described, classified in 6 groups (A–F) displaying variable properties in terms of infectivity and pathogenic potential in humans. Their genome is encoded in a linear, double-stranded DNA molecule of 36 kb, flanked by the inverted terminal repeats (ITR). The 5′-ends are covalently linked to the terminal protein, and viral DNA is also associated with protein VII and μ-peptide, which in turn bind proteins V and VI allowing for the association of viral DNA with the capsid.[16]

The capsid is formed by eight structural proteins: II (that forms the trimeric structures called hexon), III (forming pentamers called penton base), IIIa, IV (that forms the trimeric fiber), IVa2, VI, VIII, and IX. The virion has an icosahedral capsid, with hexon being the faces and penton, the vertexes of the icosahedrons. Fiber protrudes from the vertexes and displays two structurally and functionally distinguishable domains: the shaft and the knob. The shaft domain is involved in the binding to heparan sulfate glucosamine glycans, whereas the knob domain mediates the binding of the virus to its cellular receptor (the coxsackie-adenovirus receptor).[16]

The viral genome encodes for approximately 50 proteins whose transcriptional units overlap along the 36 kb of DNA. RNA alternative splicing allows for the generation of a diverse set of proteins from the relatively small DNA. The adenoviral genome is highly conserved across the spectrum of serotypes, except for the ITRs and fiber protein which is the main antigenic determinant for serotypes.

Adenoviral Infection

Binding of the knob domain to the coxsackie-adenovirus receptor initiates a sequence of events leading to the internalization of the virion into the target cells and delivery of the viral genome into the nucleus. Viral entry into the cell occurs via clathrin-mediated endocytosis. After escaping lysosomal degradation, capsid proteins interact with nuclear pores to inject the viral genome into the nucleoplasm. For the majority of serotypes, the viral genome remains episomal, that is, it does not integrate into the host cell genome. Expression of viral proteins is initiated a few hours after infection.[17]

More than 50 proteins are encoded in the 36 kb adenovirus genome. This compaction is achieved by the use of overlapping open reading frames, which yield multiple transcripts from the same coding DNA, often transcribed in both directions. Alternative splicing of mRNA also contributes to protein diversity. Adenoviral genes can be classified into two categories, based on the timing of their expression: early genes (E1A, E1B, E2, E3, E4, IX, and IVa), for instance, are the first to be transcribed. E1A serves a central function in organizing the expression of genes to coordinate the production and assembly of the viral progeny, activating the expression of the so-called delayed early genes (IX and IVa), ultimately leading to the expression of late genes (L1–L5) in the final phases of viral replication[18] (Fig. 46.3).

In order to produce first-generation adenoviral vectors, the E1 and E3 genes are deleted, thus blocking the transcription of the rest of the adenoviral genes that are necessary for completion of the lytic cycle. The most common design involves insertion of a heterogenous expression cassette in the genomic location of E1. Production of viral vector stocks is achieved by transfection recombinant E1-defective viral genomes into producer cells that provide E1 in trans, such as HEK293 and derivatives. The E3 gene is also deleted in first-generation adenovirus vectors, but unlike E1 genes, E3 does not need to be supplied for in vitro replication. In the latest generation of vector designs, termed "gutless" vectors, only the ITRs and encapsidation signal are retained, which increases the coding capacity of these vectors to more than 30 kb. In this setting, not only E1 genes but the remaining set of adenoviral genes must be provided in trans for vector production[19,20] (see Fig. 46.3).

The widespread expression of the coxsackie-adenovirus receptor in human cells affords the advantage of

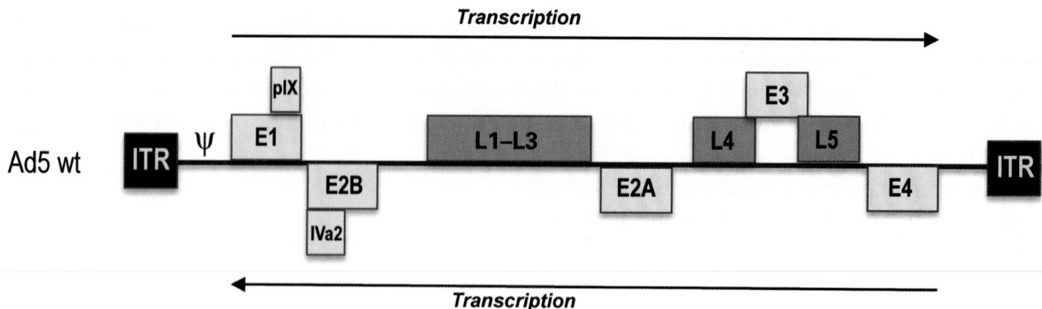

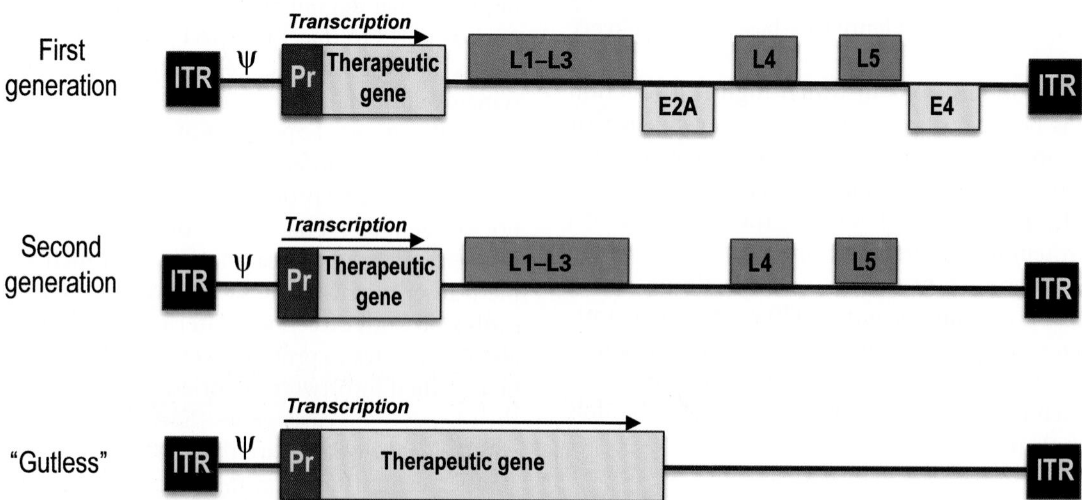

FIGURE 46–3 Adenoviral vectors. Genomic structure of wild-type serotype 5 adenovirus and derived replication-deficient adenoviral vectors. Viral genes are accommodated as overlapping coding sequences represented by boxes. Those in the upper part of the diagram are transcribed rightward whereas those in the bottom are transcribed leftward, by several promoters. In first-generation vectors, E1 region is replaced by the expression cassette of the therapeutic gene including an internal promoter, and E3 region is also eliminated. Transcription of viral genes is not activated due to the deletion of E1. Second-generation vectors also have deletions in E2A and E4 genes. Helper-dependent or gutless adenoviruses consist on the expression cassette flanked by the ITRs and an encapsidation signal (ψ). ITR, inverted terminal repeats; Pr, internal promoter. Early and delayed early genes are represented in light gray; late genes are represented in dark gray.

allowing for transduction of multiple tissues but becomes a hurdle when specific transduction is desired. Moreover, expression of chimeric antigen receptors (CARs) can be reduced in certain tumor cells, negatively impacting on transduction efficiency. Although replacement of determinants of adenovirus tropism is more complicated than in enveloped viruses, efforts to overcome this limitation have been focused on modifying the knob domain of the adenoviral fiber, which acts as a ligand for the coxsackie-adenovirus receptor. Insertion of an RGD tripeptide in the knob domain has been shown to ablate the coxsackie-adenovirus receptor binding and to redirect viral infection toward αvβ integrins.[21] Also, serotype-5 adenoviruses in which the gene encoding for the fiber protein has been replaced for that of a serotype-35 adenovirus (Ad5/F35) has been shown to transduce hematopoietic cells more efficiently than parental serotype-5.[22] This type of "chimerism" between proteins of different serotypes of adenoviruses may help circumvent the action of blocking antibodies commonly present in individuals as a result of previous infections with naturally occurring adenoviruses.

The ability of adenoviral vectors to transduce both dividing and non-dividing cells and their high efficiency of transgene expression along with the technical advantage provided by the high titers achieved in standard viral production protocols have made these vectors the most widely used gene transfer vector in gene therapy clinical trials.

Non-viral Vectors

Gene transfer vehicles not involving the use of viral organisms have been developed, and these have an inherent advantage in terms of biosafety. Some of these vehicles involve biological agents, such as transposons. Transposons were originally described as "mobile" genomic sequences that have the ability to relocate randomly from one chromosomal location to another. Engineering of these elements into gene delivery vectors involves the cloning of the therapeutic gene flanked by inverted repeats (IRs) that mediate recognition of target sequence and ligation and the expression in trans of the enzyme transposase that catalyzes the integration of the IR-flanked genetic material into the host cell chromosomes.[23] Examples of transposons assayed in preclinical models include the Piggybac and Sleeping Beauty systems.[24]

Nucleic acids can also be delivered into cells by means of physical or chemical methods. An example of the former is the use of pulsed electric fields to render plasma membranes transiently permeable to DNA or RNA. This process, called electroporation, can cause significant loss of viability of target cells and is therefore not suitable for many gene transfer applications.[25] Nevertheless, ex vivo electroporation of dendritic cells with nucleic acids encoding tumor antigens has been employed in vaccination studies.[26] Chemical methods involve the formation of complexes between DNA with positively charged polymers or lipids that help neutralize the electrostatic repulsion exerted by membrane phospholipids against negatively charged DNA molecules and also form a particulate suspension that is endocytosed by target cells.[27] Reagents based on diverse chemistries, including glucidic or synthetic polymers (polyethylenimine, dendrimers), have been developed as easily available products, displaying high efficiency of transfection of cell lines. For these reasons, they are widely used for in vitro transfer, mainly in basic research laboratory applications.

CANCER GENE THERAPY STRATEGIES

As mentioned in the beginning of this section, several strategies have been employed to induce the elimination of cancerous cells by targeting different aspects of their biology, including the correction of genetic lesions such as mutated tumor suppressors and the expression of highly active cell death inducers.

Tumor Suppressor Replacement and Oncogene Antagonism

A common trait of cancer cells arising from different tissues is the uncontrolled proliferation that results from deregulation of cell cycle and programmed cell death control mechanisms. Mutations in genes that play a key role in the control of genomic stability and cell proliferation, such as p53, are found in more than 50% of human tumors, providing the rationale for therapeutic strategies aiming at correcting this genetic lesion, thus reverting the malignant phenotype by rendering tumor cells capable of inducing cell death or senescence by endogenous mechanisms.[28]

Preclinical studies showed the feasibility of inducing cell cycle arrest and apoptosis in tumor cells by administration of wild-type p53 using different gene transfer platforms. Tumor suppressor gene replacement was also capable of acting synergistically with chemotherapeutic agents by increasing the sensitivity of tumor cells to DNA damage induced by genotoxic compounds. These results led to the first attempt, reported in 1996, to treat human cancer by restoring p53 function, in which nine patients with non–small cell lung cancer refractory to standard treatments received intratumoral injections of a retrovirus expressing wild-type p53 by the use of a β-actin promoter. Evidence for the induction of apoptosis resulting from in vivo transfer of p53 was provided, in the absence of clinically relevant toxicities, but this was not sufficient to induce any significant clinical responses.[29] In further studies, several groups pursued the p53-replacement strategy using first-generation recombinant adenoviral vectors with the hope of achieving better clinical responses by virtue of the higher transduction efficiency attained with such vectors. Several studies were conducted using Ad-p53, alone or in combination with radiotherapy or chemotherapy, in patients with non–small cell lung cancer, head and neck cancer, and bladder cancer, among others.[30] Results did not meet the efficacy criteria for approval by the US and European agencies, but it did fulfill the requirements of Chinese State Food and Drug Administration who granted Shenzhen SiBiono GeneTech (Shenzhen, China), a license for the commercialization of a serotype 5 recombinant adenovirus expressing p53 for the treatment of head and neck cancer, in 2003.[31] The formulation, available under the brand name Gendicine, became the first gene therapy reagent to become commercially available.

The list of tumor suppressors and regulators of cell cycle progression that have been assayed in preclinical models includes, but is not restricted to, p21, p16, Rb, $p14^{ARF}$, p27, and BRCA1,[32] all of which participate, in normal cells, in the growth suppression induced by environmental stimuli, such as deprivation of nutrients, as well as internal alterations such as DNA damage or alterations to the cell cycle. Proto-oncogenes, in contrast, encode for proteins that participate in signal transduction or execution of mitosis in normal cells. Mutations in their coding sequence or regulatory elements may generate constitutively active variants, termed oncogenes, which drive the uncontrolled proliferation of cells resulting in malignant transformation. Consequently, cancer therapies targeting oncogenes aim at blocking their expression or signaling capacity.

An example of such strategies is the neutralization of epidermal growth factor receptor (EGFR) expression and/or activity. EGFR is a receptor tyrosine kinase involved in the transduction of proliferation and differentiation signals induced by extracellular growth factors. Activating mutations of EGFR can drive malignant transformation and sustain the proliferation of tumor cells. In line with this, multiple small molecule inhibitors and monoclonal antibodies have been shown to inhibit the proliferation of EGFR-expressing cancer cells, providing a proof of principle for EGFR-targeted therapies. In the realm of gene therapy, intratumoral administration of a 39-mer vector-encoded ASO was well tolerated and shown to induce objective responses in 5 of 17 patients with squamous cell carcinoma of head and neck, based on single lesion evaluation. Importantly, responses correlated with baseline expression of EGFR, indicating that the observed biological effects were specific.[33]

Modulation of Pro- and Antiapoptotic Genes

An important limitation of tumor suppressor replacement and oncogene antagonism strategies is that due to the accumulation of multiple mutations, cancer cells may harbor molecular lesions at multiple levels. Thus, insertion of a single effector of a signaling pathway may not be sufficient to restore its functionality. In order to address this issue, many researchers have attempted to activate the normal cellular death program by overexpressing inducers or effectors of the apoptotic cascade. Adenoviral expression of TRAIL death receptor, bax, FAS, or FAS ligand has been tested in vitro and in animal models.[34,35] Conversely, neutralization of antiapoptotic molecules that are often overexpressed in tumor cells has been extensively explored, in some cases as an adjuvant for standard chemotherapeutic agents.

An ASO targeting apoptosis inhibitor BCL2 (Oblimersen) has been extensively tested as sensitizer for chemotherapeutic agents in the treatment of esophageal, gastric, and gastroesophageal carcinoma, chronic lymphocytic leukemia, breast cancer, melanoma, multiple myeloma, and prostate cancer, among others. Although promising results were observed in many phase I clinical trials for Oblimersen in combination with chemotherapy,[36] randomized studies comparing the combination versus chemotherapy alone failed to yield convincing data on the improvement induced by the administration of the ASO.[37]

Suicide Genes

Suicide gene therapy, also known as gene-directed enzyme prodrug therapy, involves the expression of a heterologous enzyme that has the ability to metabolize an otherwise innocuous prodrug into a cytotoxic derivative that can induce cell death. By selectively expressing the activating enzyme in the tumor cells, it is possible to restrict the chemotherapeutic effect of the active drug to these cells, even when the prodrug is administered systemically, thus widening the therapeutic index of the treatment. The paradigmatic Herpes simplex virus thymidine kinase/ganciclovir (HSV-TK/GCV) ensemble is the most extensively studied suicide system. The viral thymidine kinase, when compared with its human counterpart, has a much higher affinity for GCV, which allows it to catalyze the phosphorylation of GCV into its monophosphate form, which is further converted into its di- and triphosphate derivative by cellular kinases. This species acts as a substrate for DNA polymerase due to its homology to 2-deoxy-guanosine and induces cell death by polymerase inhibition and induction of apoptosis. An interesting feature of this system is the so-called by-stander effect, which consists of the induction of cytotoxicity in neighboring cells that were not modified to express the HSV-TK, but that receive phosphorylated metabolites of GCV via gap junction intercellular communication (Fig. 46.4). This

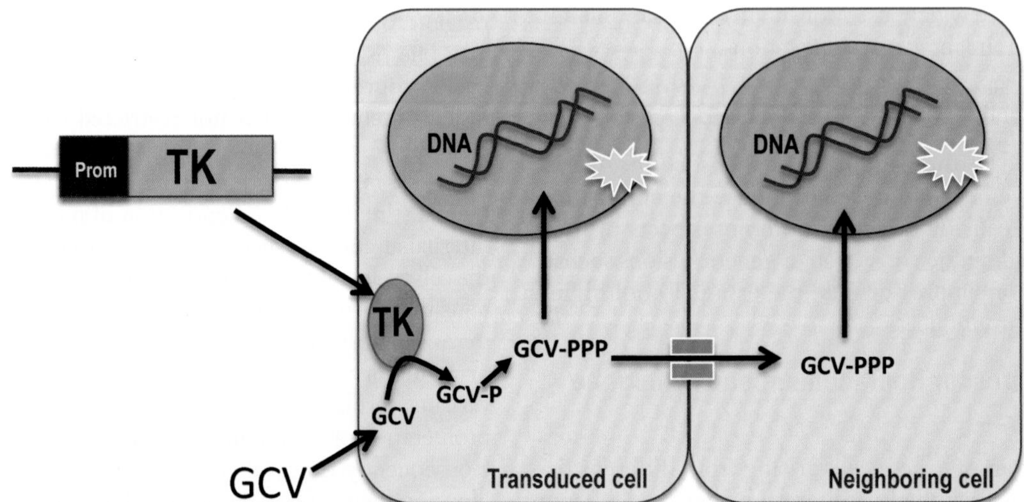

FIGURE 46–4 Suicide gene therapy. Cells engineered to express HSV-TK can metabolize systemically administered GCV into its triphosphorylated form. This species is retained within the cell and incorporated in nascent DNA molecules leading to inhibition of DNA polymerase, genotoxic stress, and apoptosis. Phosphorylated metabolites of GCV can diffuse to neighboring cells through gap junction intracellular communication, causing toxicity in non-transduced neighboring cells. Prom, promoter; GCV, ganciclovir; TK, thymidine kinase.

allows for an amplification of the antitumor effect that may enhance the efficacy of the treatment. The main limitation of this system stems from the fact that it requires active synthesis of DNA to induce cytotoxicity, resulting in reduced efficacy in non-dividing cells.

In the clinical setting, HSV-TK/GCV has been assayed for the treatment of CNS malignancies, malignant melanoma, ovarian cancer, mesothelioma, prostate cancer, colorectal adenocarcinoma, retinoblastoma (RB), EBV-related lymphoid malignancies, head and neck cancer, and hepatocellular carcinoma.[38] Treatments were overall well tolerated with minimal toxicities observed, but only a limited number of objective responses were reported. Other suicide gene systems include cytosine-deaminase/5-fluorocytosine, cytochrome p450/ifosfamide, cytochrome p450/cyclophosphamide, and nitroreductase/5-[aziridin-1-yl]-2,4-dinitrobenzamide.[39]

Although the inducible caspase 9 (iCasp9) cytotoxic gene does not fit the standard definition of a suicide system, as it does not involve the expression of an enzyme that metabolizes a non-toxic prodrug into its cytotoxic derivative, it is often classified as such in the literature. Caspase 9 is a late executor of both intrinsic and extrinsic pathways of apoptosis, whose proteolytic activation leads to DNA fragmentation and cell death. An artificial version of this protein has been created that is expressed as a pair of inactive subunits, and whose coupling and activation can be timely controlled by systemic administration of a small molecule activator. Thus, cells that have incorporated the coding sequence for iCasp9 will undergo apoptosis following dimerization.[40] One of the attractive features of this system relies on the fact that iCasp9 activates one of the last steps in the apoptotic cascades, resulting in cell death as soon as 30 minutes after administration of the activator. To date, this system has been used a safety brake for adoptively transferred lymphocytes that might need to be removed in the event of graft versus host disease,[41] but there are no reports of clinical use as a direct antitumor therapy.

Oncolytic Viruses

The ability of viruses to replicate in and lyse cancer cells was first proposed more than a century ago and served as the foundation for a series of recent attempts to translate this oncolytic potential into more effective alternatives for cancer treatment.

Spontaneous reduction of tumor masses was documented in patients undergoing certain viral infections, especially in young patients diagnosed with hematological malignancies that compromised the immune system.[42] Early attempts to induce such an antitumor effect involved the inoculation of body fluids from clinical isolates into tumoral lesions. Later on, concurrently with the development of techniques for ex vivo culture and amplification, virotherapy gained new impulse in the 1950s and 1960s. Clinical trials utilizing naturally occurring oncolytic viruses or strains selected by prolonged culture in vitro were conducted demonstrating that viral replication occurred in tumor cells, but failed to show induction of clinical benefit. More recently, genetic engineering tools were implemented in the field of virotherapy to restrict replication of viruses, displaying otherwise no natural selectivity for tumor tissue, to cells bearing molecular lesions that are present in transformed but not in normal cells. In 1991, a Herpes simplex virus lacking the thymidine kinase *UL23* gene was reported to selectively propagate in replicating cells and to kill xenografted tumor cells in murine model of glioma.[43] Several viruses were assayed in vitro and in animal models and in clinical trials yielding the first approved therapeutic agent based on viral oncolysis in 2005: E1B 55K gene-deleted adenovirus (H101 (Oncorine); Shanghai Sunway Biotech).[43] Strategies to attain cancer specificity in the different viral platforms, as well as most relevant clinical achievements, are herein summarized.

Modifications to Confer Selectivity

Adenovirus

One of the most common strategies to render a replicative virus tumor selective is the specific deletion of genes responsible for biological functions that are dispensable for replication in tumor cells, but not in normal cells (Fig. 46.5). This approach was utilized to generate the first engineered replicative adenovirus to be tested clinically: dl1520. Adenovirus dl1520 (ONYX-015; Onyx Pharmaceuticals, California) is an oncolytic Ad2/Ad5 hybrid bearing a deletion of E1B 55K and E3B genes. Tumor selectivity was thought to be determined by the lack of E1B 55K which is responsible for inactivation of p53 in the host cell. Such inactivation is instrumental for completion of the lytic cycle in normal cells, as, otherwise, expression of viral genes would trigger a p53-mediated response leading to protein synthesis shut-off and eventually cell death, preventing the production of the viral progeny. As the vast majority of tumor cells present alterations at different levels of the p53 pathway, E1B 55K activity would not be necessary to allow for completion of lytic cycle and amplification of the virus in *trans*formed cells, but these would still be blocked in normal cells with functional p53. Further studies demonstrated, however, that tumor cell selectivity was rather due to differential nuclear export of viral RNAs in tumor and normal cells, caused by the deletion of E1B 55K.[43]

Initial clinical testing in head and neck cancer and pancreatic adenocarcinoma demonstrated the tumor selectivity and safety of ONYX-015 in humans, but failed to show a significant improvement of survival. As a consequence, its utilization as a stand-alone therapy for cancer was not pursued. However, combination of ONYX-015 with chemotherapeutic regimens based on 5-FU and cisplatin systemic administration induced tumor shrinkage in a phase II clinical trial for recurrent head and

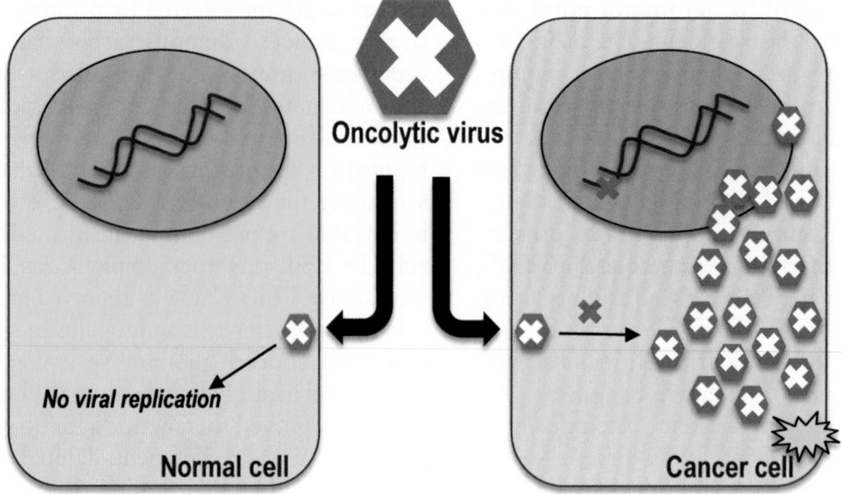

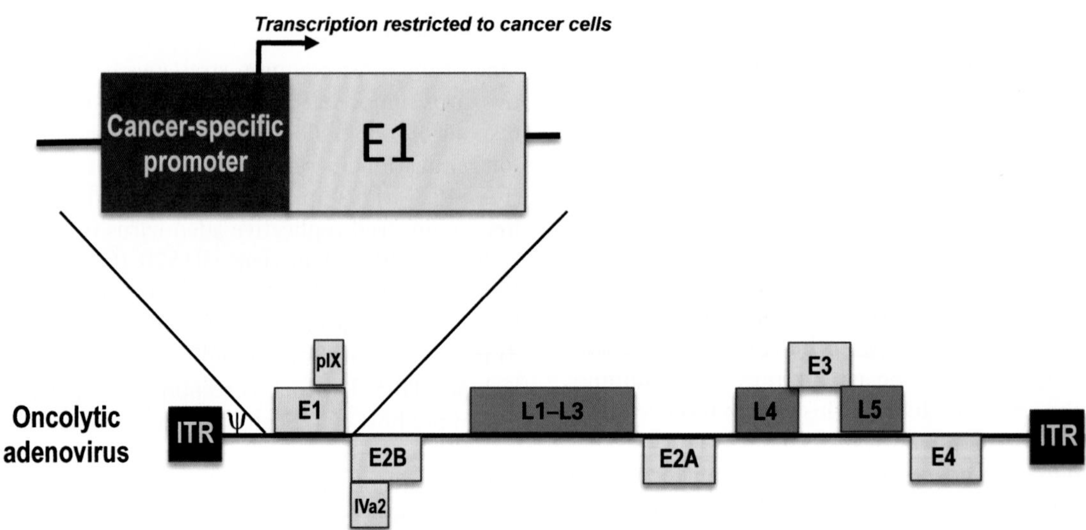

FIGURE 46–5 Oncolytic viruses. Oncolytic viruses are engineered to harbor a mutation that impedes replication in normal cells, but allows for replication in cancer cells where this mutation is complemented by a molecular alteration (red cross) present in transformed but not in normal cells. As a consequence, viral replication leads to cell death and release of viral particles that will be able to restart the cycle. Oncolytic adenoviruses can be generated by replacing the endogenous regulatory elements of E1 by a promoter that is selectively active in cancer cells. As a result, E1 will be expressed in tumor cells, activating the replication of the virus, but will not be expressed in normal cells, resulting in no viral replication.

neck cancer. In addition, H101, an oncolytic adenovirus whose tumor selectivity is based on the same principle as ONYX-015, entered phase III clinical trials for the treatment of squamous cell cancer of the head and neck or esophagus, in China. Statistically significant increase in tumor response rate was reported in this study for the combination of H101 with chemotherapy compared with chemotherapy alone. These results led to the approval of H101 as a therapeutic agent for head and neck cancer in 2005 by the Chinese regulatory agencies.

Modifications of E1A

Being the first viral gene to be expressed shortly after infection, and the master regulator of adenovirus transcription program, E1A has been engineered in different ways to create a checkpoint for viral replication. In addition to its activity as a transcription factor, wild-type E1A protein interacts with components of the host cell to create an appropriate environment for the generation of viral particles. E1A binds to the RB protein–E2F complex, resulting in disruption of the complex and release of free E2F.

Unbound E2F then induces activation of the replication program of the cell, allowing for viral replication. It follows that adenoviruses in which the RB-binding activity of E1A has been ablated will only replicate in cells that are naturally in S-phase, including tumor cells. Ad5-Δ24 expresses a mutated E1A bearing a deletion of 24 amino acids in the domain responsible for RB binding. A recently reported phase I clinical trial using a knob domain–modified version of Ad5-Δ24 expressing the RGD motif demonstrated the safety of intraperitoneal administration of this conditionally replicative adenovirus in patients diagnosed with gynecological malignancies. A total of 22 patients were treated with three daily doses of up to 10^{12} viral particles, resulting in minimal treatment-related toxicity. Although viral replication and generation of humoral immunity against adenovirus was detected, the only evidence of a biological effect was stabilization of disease in 15 (75%) patients. No objective responses were documented in this trial.[44]

An alternative, yet not mutually exclusive, strategy is the transcriptional targeting of E1A expression to cancer cells by replacing E1A endogenous promoter with that of a gene that is transcriptionally active in transformed cells, such as the E2F promoter (see Fig. 46.5). ICOVIR-7 is an oncolytic adenovirus that expresses a mutated E1A bearing the Δ-24 deletion under the control of a modified E2F promoter and displays the RGD modification in its fiber to increase integrin-mediated infection, plus a Kozak consensus sequence for enhanced E1A-Δ24 expression. In a phase I clinical trial of ICOVIR-7, a total of 21 patients with solid tumors from diverse origins were treated with intratumoral injections escalated up to 10^{12} viral particles. Evidences of viral replication were documented in several patients, in the absence of severe toxicity, once more highlighting the safety of viral administration in vivo, but showing suboptimal antitumor activity, with only one partial response reported.[45]

The list promoters tested in experimental settings for the selective expression of E1A includes, but is not restricted to, PSA, COX2, osteocalcin, α-fetoprotein, uPAR, and hTERT. The latter was used to drive the expression of E1A and E1B (linked by an internal ribosome entry site [IRES]) in telomelysin, an oncolytic adenovirus that entered phase I clinical trials for the intratumoral treatment of several types of cancer, resulting in 1 partial response and 11 patients with stable disease in a total of 16. Only mild toxicity was observed, in line with previously reported clinical trials using conditional replicative adenoviruses.[46]

Other Oncolytic Viruses

Herpes Simplex Virus

Herpes simplex virus (HSV-1) is an enveloped non-integrative virus with a DNA genome of more than 150 kb, displaying natural tropism for neural cells. Upon infection, HSV genome remains episomal and can persist in a latent state for long periods of time. Although some naturally occurring HSVs have the ability to replicate in and lyse tumor cells, HSV-based oncolytic viruses have been engineered to ablate their neurotropism and to restrict its replication to tumor cells. This can be attained by deletion of genes that serve replication functions that can be complemented in tumor cells but not in normal tissues.[47,48] An interesting feature of HSV-based oncolytic agents is the presence of thymidine kinase. In those variants where HSV-TK was not removed as tumor specificity modification, it can be used as a molecular probe for non-invasive imaging of viral spread, thanks to its ability to phosphorylate radiolabeled nucleoside analogs, causing their retention in HSV-TK–expressing cells that can be detected by tomographic techniques.[49]

Like oncolytic adenoviruses, HSVs have also been engineered to express genes that may boost their antitumor activity. An example of this is JS1/34.5-/47-/GM-CSF (OncoVEX^{GM-CSF}, BioVex Inc.), a multimutated HSV armed with human granulocyte–monocyte colony forming factor. Tumor selectivity is conferred by deletions in ICP34.5 gene, and additional mutations in ICP47 prevent its blockade of major histocompatibility complex (MHC)-I and MHC-II antigen presentation. Intratumoral injections of OncoVEX^{GM-CSF} in combination with chemoradiotherapy did not increase the toxicity induced by chemoradiotherapy alone, and clinical responses including a complete remission were reported. Conclusions regarding the efficiency of the treatment derived from this study are limited by the fact that surgical resection of tumors was performed in some patients and that the lack of an appropriate control group makes it difficult to dissect the contributions of the diverse components of this combination treatment. Nevertheless, the safety of administration of OncoVEX^{GM-CSF} plus chemoradiotherapy was demonstrated, and the observation of a higher response rate when compared with historical controls led to phase III clinical trials that are in progress.[50]

Measles Virus

Measles is an enveloped RNA virus of the Paramyxoviridae family with a relatively simple genomic structure. Genome encodes six proteins, three of which participate in the formation of the viral envelope. Tumor specificity is determined at a transductional level, by the envelope proteins H (hemagglutinin) and F (Fusion) and by the overexpression of CD46 molecule (the natural cellular receptor of vaccine strains of measles virus) in many tumor types.[51] Two phase I clinical trials have evaluated the feasibility of measles administration in human patients. In both cases, Edmonston vaccine strains were used. In the first trial, six patients diagnosed with cutaneous T-cell lymphoma were locally injected with Edmonston-Zagreb attenuated virus. Regression of injected lesions was documented, although none of the patients met established criteria for objective responses, due to the progression of distant non-injected lesions.[52]

In the second trial, 21 patients diagnosed with gynecological malignancies were treated intraperitoneally with a measles virus engineered to express soluble CEA as a marker gene for monitorization of viral replication. Treatment schedule consisted of injection of different dose levels (10^3 to 10^9 $TCID_{50}$) every 4 weeks for up to six cycles. Although treatment was well tolerated, clinical response was restricted to dose-dependent disease stabilization in 14 of 21 patients with a median duration of 92.5 days (range, 54 to 277 days).[53]

Apart from the intrinsic limitation of the system that stems from poor viral spread within the tumor mass, difficulties in translating preclinical promising results into clinical success can be partially explained by the limitations of the animal models used in experimental studies, which in most cases do not take into account the effects of the host immune response on the system. As suggested by original reports of replicative viruses killing tumors more efficiently in immunosuppressed patients, host's immune system may represent a major hurdle in the efficacy of the treatment. Recent efforts have shifted toward more integrated analyses of viral replication and the resulting immune response. Strategies oriented to masking viruses from host immunity or balancing the induced immune response toward an antitumor rather than antiviral outcome have become a major goal of investigators aiming at building novel therapeutics on the foundations of the old concept of viral oncolysis.

Immune Modulation

Example of cancer gene therapy where the engineered cell is not the cancer cell itself is the use of autologous lymphocytes that are genetically engineered ex vivo to grant them the ability to secrete pro-inflammatory cytokines or to recognize and destroy tumor cells when reinfused into a patient. The feasibility of ex vivo manipulation and reinfusion of hematopoietic cells was first tested in the 1990s when cells "marked" with the neomycin resistance gene were shown to graft in the patients and persist in circulation.[54] Later on, clinical trials involving the transfer of a therapeutic gene followed, showing that gene-modified cells were able not only to persist in circulation but also to revert the phenotype that caused the disease. Tumor recognition properties can be conferred by the expression of T-cell receptors (TCRs) or CARs with known specificity for an antigen that is expressed exclusively or preferentially in tumor cells.

Cytokine Gene Therapy

The concept of adoptive immunotherapy, where activated tumor-targeted immune effector cells are administered, as opposed to active immunotherapy, where an antitumor immune response is triggered in vivo by vaccination, was first successfully demonstrated in metastatic melanoma. In that setting, tumor infiltrating lymphocytes (TILs), obtained by surgical resection of tumoral masses, were expanded ex vivo in the presence of high-dose IL-2 and administered in patients after they had received a preconditioning lymphodepleting treatment. Concomitant administration of TILs with IL-2 resulted in durable clinical responses in an otherwise incurable condition. In order to avoid the toxicity associated with the systemic administration of high doses of IL-2, TILs were genetically engineered to stably produce and secrete IL-2 in a phase I clinical trial for metastatic melanoma. A total of 13 patients were treated with autologous IL-2–transduced TILs in an attempt to provide the necessary cytokine support for TIL engraftment and survival in an autocrine rather than systemic fashion. This resulted in a significant improvement of TIL growth upon cytokine withdrawal ex vivo, but it failed to enhance in vivo proliferation or antitumor efficacy of reinfused TILs. A plausible explanation for this lack of in vivo enhancement is related with the fact that IL-2–transduced TILs had undergone longer ex vivo culture than standard TILs, resulting in an infusion product with shorter telomeres and potentially closer to terminal differentiation.[55]

Another molecule that may improve TIL function in vivo is IL-12, a proinflammatory cytokine that was successfully tested in animal cancer models. Therapies based on systemic administration in humans, however, were hindered by acute toxicity reported in clinical trials,[56] prompting the development of systems to deliver IL-12 to the tumor microenvironment. Such is the case of an oncolytic adenovirus with tumor-specific replication capacity armed with IL-12 that was able to induce antitumor effect in a Syrian hamster model of pancreatic cancer.[57] An alternative strategy consisted in the transduction of tumor-specific T cells with a vector encoding for a single-chain variant of IL-12, resulting in improved functionality of cytotoxic T cells and enhanced engraftment and survival in lymphodepleted mice, in the absence of exogenous cytokines or vaccination.[58] Constitutive expression of IL-12 by T cells, however, negatively impacted on ex vivo expansion of transduced cells due to induction of apoptosis, interfering with the development of clinical grade infusion products. In order to overcome this hurdle, an inducible promoter containing nuclear factor of activated T-cell–responsive elements was utilized to drive the expression of retrovirally transduced IL-12 in tumor-specific cells following encounter of their target antigen. Thus, IL-12 secretion is expected to be restricted to the tumor microenvironment, enhancing T-cell function while minimizing IL-12 toxicity, as was corroborated in a murine model of melanoma.[59]

Tumor-Specific TCRs

The main obstacle to the widespread application of TIL therapy is the ability to grow TILs to clinically relevant amounts in cancer histologies other than melanoma. An alternative to naturally occurring tumor-specific lymphocytes is the generation of tumor-reactive cells using peripheral blood lymphocytes. These are readily accessible and, unlike TILs, do not require surgery. Moreover, they are amenable for ex vivo transduction with retroviral, lentiviral, and non-viral vectors such as transposons and RNA electroporation.

TCRs are heterodimeric membrane proteins that belong to the immunoglobulin superfamily and are composed of two peptides termed α- and β-chains. The TCR is the sole protein determinant of antigen recognition by T cells and does so by the recognition of peptide presented by MHC proteins. Although TCR chains are naturally expressed in an independent fashion, most TCR transfer strategies involve the expression of these chains as a single transcript encoding for both chains separated by a picornavirus 2A ribosomal skip sequence or an IRES (Fig. 46.6). Thus, two poly peptides are synthesized from the same transcriptional unit whose expression can be driven by the LTR, in the case of retrovirally delivered TCR genes. Once these proteins are expressed, they translocate to the plasma membrane and associate with the CD3 complex proteins, containing the signaling domains necessary for signal transduction upon ligation of the relevant antigen (see Fig. 46.6).

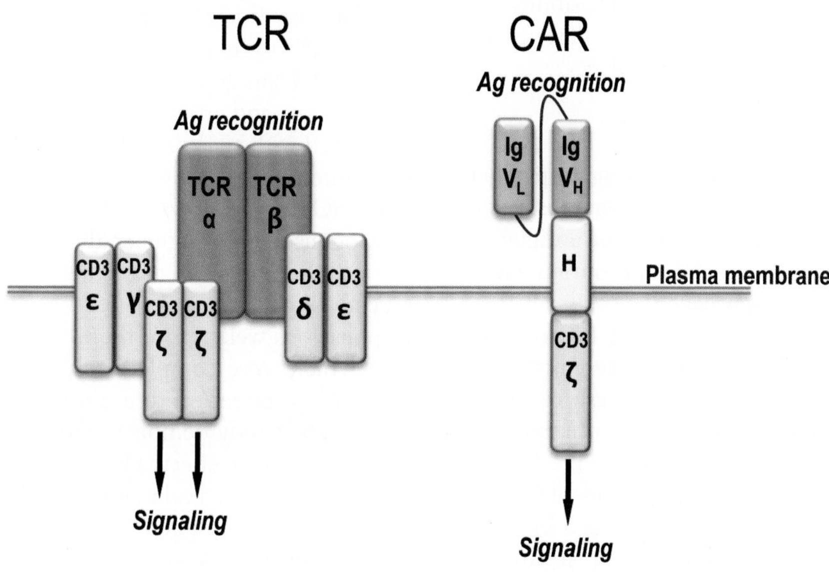

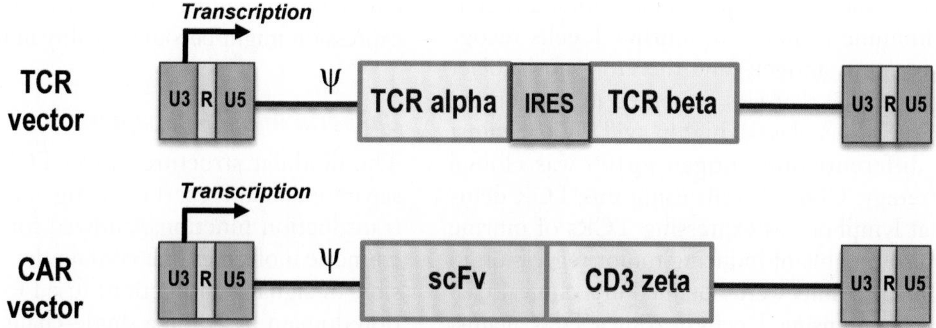

FIGURE 46–6 Engineered immune effector cells. (**A**) Structure of antigen receptors. T-cell receptors (TCRs) are expressed in the plasma membrane as two independent polypeptides (α- and β-chains) that are associated with CD3 complex proteins, containing signaling domains that are activated upon binding of TCR with a cognate antigen peptide. First-generation CARs are expressed in the membrane as a single-chain fusion protein containing an antigen-binding moiety derived from a monoclonal antibody, a hinge region, and the signaling domain of the ζ-chain of the CD3 complex, containing the signaling elements required for activation of the T cell upon antigen binding. (**B**) Retroviral vector for the expression of TCR or CAR molecules. The α- and β-chains of the TCR complex can be expressed from a single transcriptional unit and expressed as independent molecules by placing an internal ribosome entry site (IRES) in between the two coding sequences. CAR molecules are expressed as a single fusion protein.

As TCR-engineered cells still express their endogenous TCRs, some authors have raised the concern that these might associate with the exogenous α- and β-chains to create hybrid TCRs with new specificities. The potential consequence of this pairing would be a reduction in the amount of functional tumor-specific TCRs, resulting in impaired efficiency of the treatment, and the potential generation of reactivity to auto-antigens that might lead to autoimmune toxicity. In order to prevent this, modifications of the natural structure of TCR molecules have been assayed to favor the pairing of the two exogenous chains,[60] as well as the inactivation of the endogenous TCR genes using zinc finger nucleases.[61] Nevertheless, whether the generation of self-reactivity is a theoretical possibility or a clinically relevant phenomenon remains to be determined, but it has not been observed in clinical trials.[62]

Finding Tumor-Specific Targets

Whereas TILs contain a wide variety of antigen specificities, TCR-transduced T cells are administered as a pool of activated lymphocytes directed to the same antigen. As a consequence of this, selection of the appropriate target is a rate-limiting step in this approach.

In early attempts to find tumor-specific antigens, TCRs were cloned from TILs showing high antitumor activity against melanoma. Targets for these receptors were identified, including melanocyte differentiation antigen melan-A (MART-1). After confirming the preferential expression of the antigen in tumor tissue, this TCR was cloned into a γ-retroviral vector and expressed in autologous T cells from patients with malignant melanoma. These efforts led to the first report, in 2006, of TCR-engineered lymphocytes being able to break tolerance and induce tumor regression in humans.[63]

In order to isolate TCR with higher affinity than those derived from human TILs, transgenic mice expressing human leukocyte antigen (HLA)-A2 were generated. Immunization of these mice with human tumor antigens induced an immune response of murine T cells recognizing an exogenous antigen (and therefore not subject to immune tolerance) that was presented in the context of human HLA molecules. A highly avid TCR against melanocyte differentiation antigen gp100 was cloned using this strategy. Clinical trials using this TCR demonstrated that lymphocytes expressing TCRs of murine origin were also capable of inducing tumor regression in humans.[64] Similar results were obtained in a clinical trial for colorectal cancer using T cells bearing a TCR against carcinoembryonic antigen (CEA). This TCR was isolated from a transgenic mouse and subject to further engineering to improve its avidity by including single amino acid substitution in the complementarity-determining region of the α-chain.[65] In both trials on target/off tumor toxicity was observed, due to the expression of these proteins in normal tissue. Despite the transient colitis induced due to the recognition of CEA expression in normal colon epithelium, this trial demonstrated that solid tumors other than melanoma were susceptible of being treated by this approach.

Cancer/Testis Antigens

In the pursuit of the ideal tumor antigen, recent efforts have been focused on cancer/testis (CT) antigens. This category comprises a set of genes that are expressed in several tumors of epithelial origin such as carcinoma of the bladder, liver, and lung, and whose expression in normal adult tissues is restricted to testes, which do not express class I MHC molecules and are therefore not susceptible to attack by cytolytic T cells.

The efficacy and lack of on target/off tumor toxicity of adoptive transfer to T cells expressing anti-CT antigens' TCRs were demonstrated in a clinical trial targeting NY-ESO-1 antigen, which is expressed in 80% synovial cell sarcoma and around 25% of melanomas. Six patients diagnosed with synovial cell sarcoma and 11 patients with melanoma, all of them bearing tumors that expressed NY-ESO-1, were treated in a phase I clinical trial with autologous T cells engineered to express a TCR that recognized that antigen in the context of HLA-A*0201. Of the 6 synovial cell sarcoma patients, 4 experienced objective responses, as well as 5 of the 11 patients with melanoma, 2 of which were complete responders for more than 1 year. No on target/off tumor toxicities were found in this trial.[66] This study demonstrated that cancers other than melanoma can be effectively treated with adoptive transfer of TCR-engineered cells and paves the way to the exploration of other CT antigens as potential therapeutic targets.

The identification of other tumor-specific antigens such as mutated epitopes, now available thanks to the development of high-resolution tumor exome sequencing technologies, will likely expand the possibilities of tumor targeting by adoptive cell transfer therapy (ACT). Furthermore, as high-throughput sequencing platforms become more cost and time efficient, the design of personalized treatments based on individual characterization of tumor antigen expression might become a reality in the near future.

Chimeric Antigen Receptors

The modular structure of the TCR complex, in which separate domains exert the antigen recognition and signal transduction functions, allowed for the development of chimeric molecules that contain the CD3ζ chain (responsible of signal transduction) fused to an antigen recognition domain based on a single-chain antibody (scFv) (see Fig. 46.6). These molecules, termed T-bodies or CARs, can bind proteins expressed in the surface of target cells. Unlike TCRs, CARs can recognize their antigen in the native form, without the requirement of peptide processing by the immune proteasome, and most importantly without HLA restriction. Another interesting feature of antibody-based antigen recognition when compared with TCRs is the possibility of targeting non-peptidic antigens, such as lipids and carbohydrates.

Since the original description of the concept in 1989,[67] CARs have evolved to more complex molecules containing, in addition to CD3ζ chain, the intracellular domains of costimulatory molecules such as CD28, in the so-called second-generation CARs. More recently, third-generation CARs were described to enhance the persistence and effector function of transduced cell by incorporating additional costimulatory molecules such as 41BB and OX40.[68]

In the clinical arena, early phase I trials of first-generation CARs directed to carbonic anhydrase IX receptor in renal cancer, folate receptor in ovarian cancer, and CD171 in neuroblastoma showed limited persistence and no clinical benefits. Nevertheless, second- and third-generation CARs have been recently described to induce long-term biological effects, in some cases resulting in objective clinical responses. Other targets that have been assayed so far include Her2/neu for colon cancer metastasis and disialoganglioside GD2 in neuroblastoma. In the latter, 11 patients were treated, half of which experienced objective responses, including 1 complete remission.[69]

In two independent clinical trials targeting CD19, a marker expressed in hematopoietic cells of the B lineage as well as in malignant B cells, infusion of T cells expressing second-generation CARs resulted in elimination of cancerous and normal cells expressing the antigen. Eradication of B-cell lineage cells was reported in an advanced follicular lymphoma patient treated with autologous T cells transduced to express an anti-CD19 CAR containing a CD28 signaling domain. A partial remission lasting 39 weeks was achieved, along with a selective elimination of B-cell precursors from the bone marrow and depletion of circulating B cells, resulting in hypogammaglobulinemia with normalization of other hematological parameters. Long-term persistence of CAR-expressing lymphocytes was detected, potentially attributable to co-stimulation by the CD28 moiety present in the CAR or due to stimulation by a small subset of reconstituting B-cell precursors.[70] Similarly, a recently published trial using autologous T cells transduced with lentiviral vectors encoding an anti-CD19 CAR, containing a CD137 costimulatory domain, resulted in complete remission of chemotherapy-resistant advanced chronic lymphocytic leukemia in two of three treated patients.[69] Detailed analysis of T-cell growth kinetics in vivo revealed that upon administration of 3×10^8 cells, of which only 5% expressed the CAR, a more than 1,000-fold expansion occurred, remarkably, in the absence of exogenous support cytokines. This was concomitant with elimination of normal B cells and plasma cells, resulting in hypogammaglobulinemia, and a delayed tumor lysis syndrome. Transferred cells lead, ultimately, to the generation of a biologically active, CAR-expressing memory-like population of cells.[71]

Although it remains to be determined whether the increased persistence and activity of these CAR-engineered cells is a consequence of improved design of artificial immune receptors or rather a consequence of intrinsic interactions between host and transferred cells in this particular setting, these reports demonstrate that CAR-based therapies can be safe and efficacious. These qualities, along with the versatility of the system, are likely to foster new series of clinical trials using this technology in the forecoming years.

CONCLUDING REMARKS

A wide array of technologies have been developed since the inception of cancer therapies based on gene transfer, in line with the evolution of the wider field of gene therapy. After two decades of clinical studies, molecular medicine has proved feasible and well tolerated, and recent reports of clinical efficacy indicate that it may have gathered momentum to transition from a promising and intellectually appealing discipline into a clinically relevant alternative for the treatment of human malignancies. This transition will require the development of randomized phase III clinical trials to compare the clinical efficacy of gene therapy protocols with that of standard chemotherapeutic regimens. So far, though, the vast majority of clinical trials have been phase I or II, where small cohorts of heavily pretreated patients with high tumor burden were typically enrolled. Challenges to come also include the adaptation of these protocols to be widely applied in medical institutions other than highly specialized research centers, and this will likely require multiple "bench-to-bed-to-bench" iterations and a close collaboration between basic researchers and medical practitioners.

REFERENCES

1. ASGCT. American Society of Gene and Cell Therapy. www.asgct.org; 2011.
2. Karkare S, Bhatnagar D. Promising nucleic acid analogs and mimics: characteristic features and applications of PNA, LNA, and morpholino. *Appl Microbiol Biotechnol.* 2006;71(5):575-586.
3. Caplen NJ, Parrish S, Imani F, Fire A, Morgan RA. Specific inhibition of gene expression by small double-stranded RNAs in invertebrate and vertebrate systems. *Proc Natl Acad Sci U S A.* 2001;98(17):9742-9747.
4. Knipe DM, Howley PM, Griffin, DE, et al. *Field's Virology.* Philadelphia, PA: Lippincott Williams & Wilkins; 2007.
5. Baum C, Ostertag W, Stocking C, von Laer D. Retroviral vector design for cancer gene therapy. In: Lattime E, Gerson S, eds. *Gene Therapy of Cancer.* San Diego, CA: Academic Press; 2002:3-29.
6. Baum C. Parachuting in the epigenome: the biology of gene vector insertion profiles in the context of clinical trials. *EMBO Mol Med.* 2011;3(2):75-77.
7. Kustikova O, Brugman M, Baum C. The genomic risk of somatic gene therapy. *Semin Cancer Biol.* 2010;20(4):269-278.
8. Ellis J. Silencing and variegation of gammaretrovirus and lentivirus vectors. *Hum Gene Ther.* 2005;16(11):1241-1246.
9. Sadelain M, Riviere I. The advent of lentiviral vectors: prospects for cancer therapy. In: Lattime E, Gerson S, eds. *Gene Therapy of Cancer.* Burlington, MA: Academic Press; 2002:109-124.
10. Biasco L, Ambrosi A, Pellin D, et al. Integration profile of retroviral vector in gene therapy treated patients is cell-specific according to gene expression and chromatin conformation of target cell. *EMBO Mol Med.* 2011;3(2):89-101.
11. Miyoshi H, Blömer U, Takahashi M, Gage FH, Verma IM. Development of a self-inactivating lentivirus vector. *J Virol.* 1998;72(10):8150-8157.

12. Cronin J, Zhang XY, Reiser J. Altering the tropism of lentiviral vectors through pseudotyping. *Curr Gene Ther.* 2005;5(4):387-398.
13. Frecha C, Costa C, Nègre D, et al. Stable transduction of quiescent T cells without induction of cycle progression by a novel lentiviral vector pseudotyped with measles virus glycoproteins. *Blood.* 2008;112(13):4843-4852.
14. Frecha C, Szécsi J, Cosset FL, Verhoeyen E. Strategies for targeting lentiviral vectors. *Curr Gene Ther.* 2008;8(6):449-460.
15. Yang L, Bailey L, Baltimore D, Wang P. Targeting lentiviral vectors to specific cell types in vivo. *Proc Natl Acad Sci U S A.* 2006;103(31):11479-11484.
16. Stewart PL. Adenovirus structure. In: Curiel DT, Douglas JT, eds. *Adenoviral Vectors for Gene Therapy*. San Diego, CA: Academic Press; 2002:1-18.
17. Nemerow GR. Biology of adenovirus cell entry. In: Curiel DT, Douglas JT, eds. *Adenoviral Vectors for Gene Therapy*. San Diego, CA: Academic Press; 2002:19-38.
18. Evans JD, Hearing P. Adenovirus replication. In: Curiel DT, Douglas JT, eds. *Adenoviral Vectors for Gene Therapy*. San Diego, CA: Academic Press; 2002:39-70.
19. Morgan RA. Gene therapy. In: DeVita VTL, Theodore S, Rosenberg SA, eds. *DeVita, Hellman, and Rosenberg's Cancer: Principles and Practice of Oncology*. Philadelphia, PA: Lippincott Williams & Wilkins; 2008:2967-2978.
20. Ng P, Graham FL. Adenoviral vector construction I: mammalian systems. In: Curiel DT, Douglas JT, eds. *Adenoviral Vectors for Gene Therapy*. San Diego, CA: Academic Press; 2002:71-104.
21. Dmitriev I, Krasnykh V, Miller CR, et al. An adenovirus vector with genetically modified fibers demonstrates expanded tropism via utilization of a coxsackievirus and adenovirus receptor-independent cell entry mechanism. *J Virol.* 1998;72(12):9706-9713.
22. Yotnda P, Onishi H, Heslop HE, et al. Efficient infection of primitive hematopoietic stem cells by modified adenovirus. *Gene Ther.* 2001;8(12):930-937.
23. Ivics Z, Izsvak Z. Transposons for gene therapy! *Curr Gene Ther.* 2006;6(5):593-607.
24. Ivics Z, Hackett PB, Plasterk RH, Izsvák Z. Molecular reconstruction of Sleeping Beauty, a Tc1-like transposon from fish, and its transposition in human cells. *Cell.* 1997;91(4):501-510.
25. Gao X, Kim KS, Liu D. Nonviral gene delivery: what we know and what is next. *AAPS J.* 2007;9(1):E92-E104.
26. Gilboa E, Vieweg J. Cancer immunotherapy with mRNA-transfected dendritic cells. *Immunol Rev.* 2004;199:251-263.
27. Tiera MJ, Winnik FO, Fernandes JC. Synthetic and natural polycations for gene therapy: state of the art and new perspectives. *Curr Gene Ther.* 2006;6(1):59-71.
28. Bossi G, Sacchi A. Restoration of wild-type p53 function in human cancer: relevance for tumor therapy. *Head Neck.* 2007;29(3):272-284.
29. Roth JA, Nguyen D, Lawrence DD, et al. Retrovirus-mediated wild-type p53 gene transfer to tumors of patients with lung cancer. *Nat Med.* 1996;2(9):985-991.
30. Meng RD, El-Deiry WS. Clinical applications of tumor-suppressor gene therapy. In: Lattime ECG, Gerson SL, eds. *Gene Therapy of Cancer.* San Diego, CA: Academic Press; 2002:273-278.
31. Peng Z. Current status of gendicine in China: recombinant human Ad-p53 agent for treatment of cancers. *Hum Gene Ther.* 2005;16(9):1016-1127.
32. Meng RD, El-Deiry WS. Cancer gene therapy with tumor suppressor genes involved in cell-cycle control. In: Lattime E, Gerson S, eds. *Gene Therapy of Cancer*. San Diego, CA: Academic Press; 2002:279-297.
33. Lai SY, Koppikar P, Thomas SM, et al. Intratumoral epidermal growth factor receptor antisense DNA therapy in head and neck cancer: first human application and potential antitumor mechanisms. *J Clin Oncol.* 2009;27(8):1235-1242.
34. Norris JS, Hyer ML, Voelkel-Johnson C, Lowe SL, Rubinchik S, Dong JY. The use of Fas Ligand, TRAIL and Bax in gene therapy of prostate cancer. *Curr Gene Ther.* 2001;1(1):123-136.
35. Wack S, Rejiba S, Parmentier C, Aprahamian M, Hajri A. Telomerase transcriptional targeting of inducible Bax/TRAIL gene therapy improves gemcitabine treatment of pancreatic cancer. *Mol Ther.* 2008;16(2):252-260.
36. Moreira JN, Santos A, Simoes S. Bcl-2-targeted antisense therapy (Oblimersen sodium): towards clinical reality. *Rev Recent Clin Trials.* 2006;1(3):217-235.
37. Gjertsen BT, Bredholt T, Anensen N, Vintermyr OK. Bcl-2 antisense in the treatment of human malignancies: a delusion in targeted therapy. *Curr Pharm Biotechnol.* 2007;8(6):373-381.
38. Altaner C. Prodrug cancer gene therapy. *Cancer Lett.* 2008;270(2):191-201.
39. Dachs GU, Hunt MA, Syddall S, Singleton DC, Patterson AV. Bystander or no bystander for gene directed enzyme prodrug therapy. *Molecules.* 2009;14(11):4517-4545.
40. Xie X, Zhao X, Liu Y, et al. Adenovirus-mediated tissue-targeted expression of a caspase-9-based artificial death switch for the treatment of prostate cancer. *Cancer Res.* 2001;61(18):6795-6804.
41. Tey SK, Dotti G, Rooney CM, Heslop HE, Brenner MK. Inducible caspase 9 suicide gene to improve the safety of allodepleted T cells after haploidentical stem cell transplantation. *Biol Blood Marrow Transplant.* 2007;13(8):913-924.
42. Kelly E, Russell SJ. History of oncolytic viruses: genesis to genetic engineering. *Mol Ther.* 2007;15(4):651-659.
43. Wong HH, Lemoine NR, Wang Y. Oncolytic viruses for cancer therapy: overcoming the obstacles. *Viruses.* 2010;2(1):78-106.
44. Kimball KJ, Preuss MA, Barnes MN, et al. A phase I study of a tropism-modified conditionally replicative adenovirus for recurrent malignant gynecologic diseases. *Clin Cancer Res.* 2010;16(21):5277-5287.
45. Nokisalmi P, Pesonen S, Escutenaire S, et al. Oncolytic adenovirus ICOVIR-7 in patients with advanced and refractory solid tumors. *Clin Cancer Res.* 2010;16(11):3035-3043.
46. Nemunaitis J, Tong AW, Nemunaitis M, et al. A phase I study of telomerase-specific replication competent oncolytic adenovirus (telomelysin) for various solid tumors. *Mol Ther.* 2010;18(2):429-434.
47. Todo T. Oncolytic virus therapy using genetically engineered herpes simplex viruses. *Front Biosci.* 2008;13:2060-2064.
48. Kanai R, Wakimoto H, Cheema T, Rabkin SD. Oncolytic herpes simplex virus vectors and chemotherapy: are combinatorial strategies more effective for cancer? *Future Oncol.* 2010;6(4):619-634.
49. Kuruppu D, Dorfman JD, Tanabe KK. HSV-1 viral oncolysis and molecular imaging with PET. *Curr Cancer Drug Targets.* 2007;7(2):175-180.
50. Hu JC, Coffin RS, Davis CJ, et al. A phase I study of OncoVEXGM-CSF, a second-generation oncolytic herpes simplex virus expressing granulocyte macrophage colony-stimulating factor. *Clin Cancer Res.* 2006;12(22):6737-6747.
51. Msaouel P, Iankov ID, Dispenzieri A, Galanis E. Attenuated oncolytic measles virus strains as cancer therapeutics. *Curr Pharm Biotechnol.* 2012;13(9):1732-1741.
52. Heinzerling L, Künzi V, Oberholzer PA, Kündig T, Naim H, Dummer R. Oncolytic measles virus in cutaneous T-cell lymphomas mounts antitumor immune responses in vivo and targets interferon-resistant tumor cells. *Blood.* 2005;106(7):2287-2294.
53. Galanis E, Hartmann LC, Cliby WA, et al. Phase I trial of intraperitoneal administration of an oncolytic measles virus strain engineered to express carcinoembryonic antigen for recurrent ovarian cancer. *Cancer Res.* 2010;70(3):875-882.
54. Rosenberg SA, Aebersold P, Cornetta K, et al. Gene transfer into humans--immunotherapy of patients with advanced melanoma, using tumor-infiltrating lymphocytes modified by retroviral gene transduction. *N Engl J Med.* 1990;323(9):570-578.
55. Heemskerk B, Liu K, Dudley ME, et al. Adoptive cell therapy for patients with melanoma, using tumor-infiltrating lymphocytes genetically engineered to secrete interleukin-2. *Hum Gene Ther.* 2008;19(5):496-510.
56. Cohen J. IL-12 deaths: explanation and a puzzle. *Science.* 1995;270(5238):908.
57. Bortolanza S, Bunuales M, Otano I, et al. Treatment of pancreatic cancer with an oncolytic adenovirus expressing interleukin-12 in Syrian hamsters. *Mol Ther.* 2009;17(4):614-622.
58. Kerkar SP, Muranski P, Kaiser A, et al. Tumor-specific CD8+ T cells expressing interleukin-12 eradicate established cancers in lymphodepleted hosts. *Cancer Res.* 2010;70(17):6725-6734.
59. Zhang L, Kerkar SP, Yu Z, et al. Improving adoptive T cell therapy by targeting and controlling IL-12 expression to the tumor environment. *Mol Ther.* 2011;19(4):751-759.
60. Cohen CJ, Li YF, El-Gamil M, Robbins PF, Rosenberg SA, Morgan RA. Enhanced antitumor activity of T cells engineered to express T-cell receptors with a second disulfide bond. *Cancer Res.* 2007;67(8):3898-9303.

61. Lombardo A, Cesana D, Genovese P, et al. Site-specific integration and tailoring of cassette design for sustainable gene transfer. *Nat Methods*. 2011;8(10):861-869.
62. Rosenberg SA. Of mice, not men: no evidence for graft-versus-host disease in humans receiving T-cell receptor-transduced autologous T cells. *Mol Ther*. 2010;18(10):1744-1745.
63. Morgan RA, Dudley ME, Wunderlich JR, et al. Cancer regression in patients after transfer of genetically engineered lymphocytes. *Science*. 2006;314(5796):126-129.
64. Johnson LA, Morgan RA, Dudley ME, et al. Gene therapy with human and mouse T-cell receptors mediates cancer regression and targets normal tissues expressing cognate antigen. *Blood*. 2009;114(3):535-546.
65. Parkhurst MR, Yang JC, Langan RC, et al. T cells targeting carcinoembryonic antigen can mediate regression of metastatic colorectal cancer but induce severe transient colitis. *Mol Ther*. 2011;19(3):620-626.
66. Robbins PF, Morgan RA, Feldman SA, et al. Tumor regression in patients with metastatic synovial cell sarcoma and melanoma using genetically engineered lymphocytes reactive with NY-ESO-1. *J Clin Oncol*. 2011;29(7):917-924.
67. Gross G, Waks T, Eshhar Z. Expression of immunoglobulin-T-cell receptor chimeric molecules as functional receptors with antibody-type specificity. *Proc Natl Acad Sci U S A*. 1989;86(24): 10024-10028.
68. Park TS, Rosenberg SA, Morgan RA. Treating cancer with genetically engineered T cells. *Trends Biotechnol*. 2011;29(11):550-557.
69. Kalos M, Levine BL, Porter DL, et al. T cells with chimeric antigen receptors have potent antitumor effects and can establish memory in patients with advanced leukemia. *Sci Transl Med*. 2011;3(95):95ra73.
70. Kochenderfer JN, Wilson WH, Janik JE, et al. Eradication of B-lineage cells and regression of lymphoma in a patient treated with autologous T cells genetically engineered to recognize CD19. *Blood*. 2010;116(20):4099-4102.
71. Porter DL, Levine BL, Kalos M, Bagg A, June CH. Chimeric antigen receptor-modified T cells in chronic lymphoid leukemia. *N Engl J Med* 2011;365(8): 725-733.

CHAPTER 47

ANTI-ANGIOGENESIS THERAPY OF CANCER

Kun Guo and Keping Xie

INTRODUCTION

Tumor angiogenesis is the formation of new blood vessels from existing blood vessels and new circulating endothelial progenitor cells from bone marrow.[1] Angiogenesis is essential for tumor growth and is an important component in the metastatic spread of a tumor. The theory that angiogenesis could support tumor growth and therefore could be a target for cancer therapy was explored in publications by Judah Folkman in the 1970s.[2] Since the late 1990s, a novel category of anti-cancer drugs, molecular-targeted drugs, has become available, and angiogenesis has been considered as one of the most important molecular targets for antitumor therapy.[3] The angiogenic process is initiated by growing tumor cells, and sustained angiogenesis is dictated by the biological behavior of the tumor cells, i.e., tumor angiogenesis is tumor growth dependent. Successful induction and maintenance of angiogenesis is in turn important for sustained growth and metastasis of most solid malignancies. Both tumor cells and host cells play important roles in this process, which is often the consequence of an angiogenic imbalance, in which pro-angiogenic factors predominate over anti-angiogenic factors.[1,4-6] Anti-angiogenic therapy inhibits tumor angiogenesis and promotes apoptosis of existing tumor blood vessels, thereby intercepting the supply of oxygen and nutrition essential for tumor growth and metastasis. It was also suggested that anti-angiogenic therapy effectively normalizes abnormal vascular permeability, and thereby decreases the interstitial pressure, which may improve delivery of concomitantly used chemotherapeutic agents to tumor cells.[3] Preclinical studies and early clinical evaluation show promise in the adjunctive use of anti-angiogenesis to overcome the limitations of current therapeutic approaches.[7]

SIGNIFICANCE OF ANGIOGENESIS IN TUMOR PATHOGENESIS

Angiogenesis, the process of forming new blood vessels to support tissue growth, is involved not only with normal and developmental physiological processes that promote embryonic development, tissue repair, and fertility, but also in the development of a number of pathological conditions, including chronic inflammation, tumor growth, and tumor metastasis.[8] Angiogenesis is a complex multistep process comprised of endothelial cell (EC) proliferation, migration, differentiation, and remodeling of the extracellular matrix. It is obvious that tumors need a great bulk of oxygen and nutrients. For the first one million of malignant cells, tumors get their oxygen and nutrients from the host capillaries and extracellular fluid. However, as they outgrow the host supply they start making their own blood vessels.[9] Tumors in particular rely on angiogenesis for their continued growth. In fact, it has been demonstrated that solid tumors cannot grow beyond 2 to 3 mm in diameter without recruitment of their own blood supply and nutrients, and these require angiogenesis to form metastases.

Angiogenesis is a complex multistep process involving ECs, extracellular matrix, and soluble factors in tumor microenvironment, which is genetically more stable than tumor cells (Fig. 47.1).[10] The interaction between tumor cells and their microenvironment is a promising area for the development of novel therapeutic anticancer modalities. The dynamic evolution of angiogenesis is regulated by a number of pro-angiogenic and anti-angiogenic molecules that are necessary for physiologic homeostasis. The formation of new blood vessels has been found to be regulated by inducers and inhibitors. In response to several stimuli, such as oxidative and mechanical stresses and acidosis, cytokines and pro-angiogenic growth factors are released from ECs

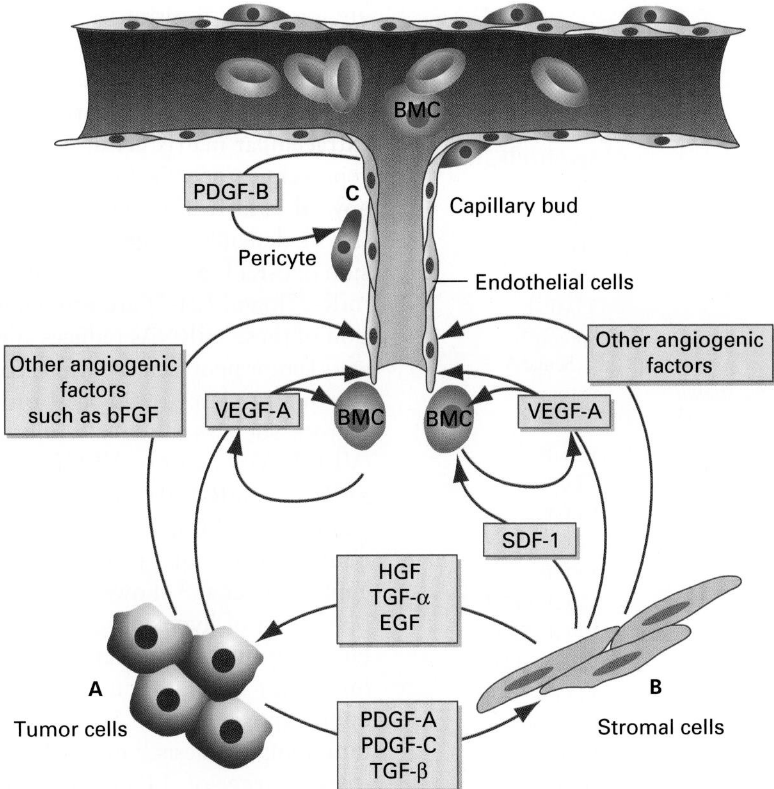

FIGURE 47–1 Molecular and cellular players in the tumor microenvironment. **A:** Tumor cells produce angiogenic factors such as VEGF-A, bFGF, angiopoietins, interleukin-8, PlGF, and VEGF-C. These stimulate resident endothelial cells to proliferate and migrate. **B:** An additional source of angiogenic factors is the stroma, which is a heterogeneous compartment, comprising fibroblastic, inflammatory, and immune cells. Tumor-associated fibroblasts produce chemokines such as SDF-1, which may recruit bone marrow–derived angiogenic cells (BMC). In addition, they produce growth/survival factor for tumor cells such as EGFR ligands, hepatocyte growth factor (HGF), and heregulin. VEGF-A or PlGF may also recruit BMC. Tumor cells may also release stromal cell recruitment factors, such as PDGF-A, PDGF-C, and transforming growth factor (TGF)-β. **C:** Endothelial cells produce PDGF-B, which promotes recruitment of pericytes in the microvasculature after activation of PDGFR-β. (Adapted from Ferrara N, Kerbel RS, *Nature.* 2005;438:967-974.)

and associated stromal cells into the microenvironment.[11] The endogenous angiogenesis inhibitors control tumor cell proliferation, apoptosis, and tumor angiogenesis, which are critical for the growth of primary tumors and metastases.[12] Animal studies suggest that activation of the angiogenesis occurs early in cancer development and is the rate-limiting step for progression. Furthermore, the tumor's ability to activate angiogenesis is a prerequisite for metastatic spread. An angiogenic phenotype has been associated frequently with a poorer prognosis in many cancers.[13]

Several lines of evidence have indicated that the growth, persistence, and metastasis of solid tumors are dependent upon angiogenesis. The process of metastasis formation could be linked to angiogenesis perturbing signaling phenomena. Cancer-associated vessels are different from normal vessels and their ECs could provide useful targets for treatment.[14] Because of this association of angiogenesis with multiple and diverse tumor types, it has long been a goal of clinicians to disrupt angiogenesis as a novel strategy for cancer therapy. The observation of Folkman that tumors are unable to grow more than 2 to 3 mm in the absence of neovascularization laid the foundation for the field of anti-angiogenic cancer therapy.[15] Anti-angiogenic therapy relies on stopping the formation of new capillary vessels around a tumor and breaking up the existing network of abnormal capillaries that feed the growing cancerous mass, thereby both starving it of nutrients and cutting off a pathway for primary metastasis through the endogenous circulatory system.[16] Because anti-angiogenic treatment is cytostatic rather than cytotoxic, patients will need long-term therapy to prevent regrowth of the tumor.[17]

MICRORNAS IN ANTI-ANGIOGENESIS THERAPY

MicroRNAs (miRNAs) are ~20 to 22 nucleotides single-strand, non-coding RNA, which have been recently discovered to control gene expression by acting on target mRNAs for promoting either their degradation or translational repression.[18] Abnormal expression of specific miRNAs has been implicated in various human cancers, and miRNA expression profiles have proved useful in tumor classification, pro gnosis, and predicting response to therapy.[19] The first miRNA profile in ECs was performed by Poliseno et al. in 2006.[20] Working in human umbilical vein endothelial cells (HUVECs), they identified 15 highly expressed miRNAs, which could be predicted to negatively regulate the expression of target genes, including

TABLE 47-1 Angiogenesis Regulatory MicroRNAs[21]

miRNAs	Target Genes
miRNAs that target genes involved in angiogenesis	
miR-126	Spred1/PIK3R2
miR-221/222	c-kit
miR-17-92	Tsp-1
miR-92a	ITGB5
miR-20a	VEGF
miR-17-5p	TIMP-1
miR-23-27	Sprouty2/ Sema6A
miRNAs modulated by angiogenic stimuli	
miR-191	VEGF
miR-155	VEGF
miR-31	VEGF
miR-17-5p	VEGF
miR-18a	VEGF
miR-101	VEGF
miR-130*a*	VEGF, bFGF
miR-296	VEGF, EGF
miR-132	VEGF, bFGF
miR-20a	VEGF
miR-424	Hypoxia
miR-210	Hypoxia
miR-200b	Hypoxia
miRNAs modulated by anti-angiogenic stimuli	
miR-200c	ROS
miR-217	Senescence
miR-34	Senescence
miR-503	High glucose/ diabetes
miR-93	High glucose/ diabetes

miRNAs, microRNAs; VEGF, vascular endothelial growth factor.

receptors for angiogenesis modulating factors.[20] Caporali and Emanueli[21] reported that the relationship between miRNAs and angiogenesis is bidirectional; based on evidence in the literature regarding miRNAs expression and function in ECs, they divided the endothelial miRNAs into two classes: the first class is miRNAs that target genes involved in angiogenesis and the second class is miRNAs whose expression can be modulated by pro-angiogenic or anti-angiogenic stimuli (Table 47.1).

Several reports have represented the great potential application of miRNA-based therapy for the treatment in cancers. Specific endothelial miRNAs have also been indicated to contribute to angiogenic processes. For example, Liu et al.[22] reported that PEGylated LPH (liposome-polycation-hyaluronic acid) nanoparticle effectively delivered anti-miR-296 antisense oligonucleotides to the cytoplasm and downregulated the target miRNA in HUVECs, which further efficiently suppressed blood tube formulation and EC migration, owing to significant upregulation of hepatocyte growth factor–regulated tyrosine kinase substrate (HGS). miR-29b suppresses tumor angiogenesis, invasion, and metastasis of liver cancer.[23] Both gain- and loss-of-function studies showed that miR-29b dramatically suppressed the ability of HCC cells to promote capillary tube formation of ECs and to invade extracellular matrix gel in vitro. Restoration of miR-29b represents a promising new strategy in anti-HCC therapy. Also, miR-221 and miR-222 inhibit stem cell factor (SCF)–dependent angiogenesis by decreasing the expression of c-KIT, a ligand of the SCF receptor.[20] In contrast, miR-27b and Let-7f are pro-angiogenic, because inhibition of these miRNAs reduces angiogenic sprouting.[24]

Tumor neovascularization is partly driven by hypoxia, which stimulates tumor cell production of angiogenic factors such as vascular endothelial growth factor-A (VEGF-A).[25] Most of VEGF-induced miRNAs, such as miR-296, miR-130a, and miR-132, are commonly overexpressed in ECs, and they have been implicated in the control of tumor growth, survival, and angiogenesis. Yamakuchi et al.[26] showed that miR-107 can mediate p53 regulation of hypoxic signaling and tumor angiogenesis targeting hypoxia-inducible factor 1-beta (HIF-1β). An important regulator involved in the cellular response upon hypoxia is TP53, which is associated with increased tumor angiogenesis.[27] miR-107 was identified as a downstream target of TP53 and proved capable of inhibiting the translation of HIF-1β.[26] Moreover, it has been reported that miR-20b plays an important role in the adaptation of tumor cells to oxygen concentration regulating the protein levels of HIF-1α and VEGF-A.[28] Among the angiogenic relevant miRNAs, growth factor–induced miR-296 contributes significantly to angiogenesis by directly targeting the HGS mRNA, leading to decreased levels of HGS and thereby reducing HGS-mediated degradation of the growth factor receptors VEGFR2 and PDGFR.[29] In a mouse model, miR-107 overexpression resulted in decreased vascularity, lower VEGF expression, and smaller tumors. miR-21 targets PTEN enhancing HIF-1α and VEGF-A expression and angiogenesis.[30]

The oncogene c-Myc (MYC) is an important regulator of tumor angiogenesis. MYC is often coactivated with RAS, of which HRAS and KRAS are known to upregulate VEGF.[31] The miR-17-92 cluster was the first oncogenic miRNA cluster to be described in mammals.[32] This cluster, which is upregulated in different cancers, is stimulated by the oncogene myc and targets the secreted factors Tsp1 and connective tissue growth factor, thus promoting angiogenesis.[33] MYC-induced upregulation of the miR-17-92 cluster is directly responsible for activating angiogenesis by downregulation of the anti-angiogenic thrombospondin-1 (THBS1).[33]

IMMUNOTHERAPY IN ANTI-ANGIOGENESIS THERAPY

Angiogenesis, a critical process in the outgrowth and metastasis of tumors, has been described to be involved in the escape of tumors from immune surveillance.[34] Tumors stimulate angiogenesis to meet increasing nutrient and oxygen demands. In addition to their role in vascular remodeling, pro-angiogenic cytokines and effector cells contribute to an immune-inhibitory environment associated with advanced malignancies.[35] Cancer immunotherapy has expanded in the past several years to include therapies utilizing whole cell vaccines, modified antigen-presenting cells, adoptive cell and antibody therapy, live and dead viral vectors, live bacteria, and peptide, protein, and DNA vaccines.[36] Immunotherapy of cancer offers great promise; however, translation into human studies has yielded relatively poor results to date. The concept of combining cancer vaccination with angiogenesis inhibition is appealing, due to favorable safety profile of both approaches, as well as possible biological synergies.[37]

Ongoing angiogenesis has been shown to possess immune suppressive activity through several mechanisms. One of these mechanisms is the suppression of adhesion receptors, such as intercellular adhesion molecule-1 (ICAM-1), vascular cell adhesion molecule-1, and E-selectin on the vascular endothelium.[38] It is reported that tumor ECs have a suppressed expression of adhesion molecules, such as ICAM-1/2, vascular endothelial cell adhesion molecule-1 (VCAM-1), and CD34,[39,40] due to exposure to angiogenic factors such as vascular EC growth factors (VEGFs) and fibroblast growth factors (FGFs).[41] It was also found that ECs isolated from human tumors express significantly lower levels of adhesion molecules that are involved in leukocyte–vessel wall interactions, such as ICAM-1, VCAM-1, E-selectin, and CD34.[38]

Since angiogenesis has this immune suppressive effect, it has been hypothesized that inhibition of angiogenesis may circumvent this problem. Dirkx et al. demonstrated that angiogenesis inhibitors, anginex, endostatin, and angiostatin, and the chemotherapeutic agent paclitaxel increase leukocyte–vessel wall interactions in tumor vessels, which leads to increased leukocyte infiltration into tumor tissue. These results suggest that immunotherapy strategies can be improved by combination with anti-angiogenesis. This antitumor inflammatory effect of angiogenesis inhibitors is mediated by increased expression of adhesion molecules on tumor ECs and not by altered expression of leukocyte adhesion molecules, effects on the amount of circulating leukocytes, or other direct or indirect vascular effects modulating fluid dynamic parameters.[34] Such angiogenesis inhibitors can make tumors more vulnerable for the immune system and may therefore be applied to facilitate immunotherapy approaches for the treatment of cancer.

Targeting tumors using cancer vaccine therapeutics has several advantages, including the induction of long-term immunity, prime boost strategies for additional treatments, and reduced side effects compared with conventional chemotherapeutics.[36] Recent advances in the molecular identification of cancer-specific antigens have given a significant boost to the study of novel vaccines for cancer therapy. Chan et al.[37] reported that combining electroporation-enhanced delivery of pDNA vaccine expressing multiple melanoma antigens and anti-angiogenesis treatment can eradicate established B16F10 tumor in mice. Seavey and Paterson examined the ability of an anti-angiogenesis, *Listeria monocytogenes* (Lm)–based vector to deliver extracellular and intracellular fragments of the mouse VEGFR2/Flk-1 molecule in an autochthonous model for Her-2/neu+ breast cancer. They found that the vaccines could cause epitope spreading to the endogenous tumor protein Her-2/neu and significantly delay tumor onset.[36] Anti-angiogenic immunotherapy offers the possibility to more robustly inhibit tumor angiogenesis and simultaneously impact the immune-inhibitory effects of the pro-angiogenic tumor milieu. Combined or sequential immunization with mismatched vaccines may confer additional therapy and outpace the ability of the tumor to escape by immunoediting. However, these findings warrant further investigation into combination therapies to increase effectiveness of therapeutic vaccines against malignant cancers.

GENE THERAPY IN ANTI-ANGIOGENESIS THERAPY

Angiogenesis is one of the hallmarks of solid tumors. Therefore, to search for more efficient anticancer methods efforts are being made to block tumor angiogenesis. Even though some success has been observed using traditional protein-based inhibitors, alternative strategies and new approaches to inhibit excessive tumor angiogenesis are being developed and tested. Gene therapy represents a powerful tool for therapeutic intervention to angiogenesis.[42] Zhou et al.[43] used the lentivirus vector system to deliver a specially designed small hairpin RNA for human Angiopoietin-2 (Ang2) gene into pancreatic carcinoma cell line and found that the gene therapy exerted anti-angiogenesis effect in vitro and in vivo, and Ang2-targeted gene therapy has the potential to serve as a novel way for pancreatic carcinoma treatment. Hu et al.[44] developed a novel strategy of tumor gene therapy in which bone marrow–derived stromal cells (BMSCs) loaded with recombinant adenoviruses expressing a soluble fragment of VEGF receptor Flt-1 (sFlt-1) could effectively suppress tumor growth through inhibiting angiogenesis and metastases and prolong the lifespan in mouse model, indicating that BMSCs might be employed as an effective carrier for tumor gene therapy. Despite notable successes achieved in studies using oncolytic bacteria for cancer treatment, bacteriolytic therapy in and of itself is often insufficient for complete eradication of experimental tumors.[45] Recent studies indicate that treatments targeting a single molecule/pathway, even if it has pleiotropic effects, are unlikely to be able to completely eradicate tumors; however, if the natural antitumor activity inherent to some anaerobic bacteria strains can be successfully combined with their ability to deliver agents targeting tumor angiogenesis, this will represent a significant step toward reaching this important goal.[46] Gardliket al.[46] discussed four different approaches for using modified bacteria as anticancer therapeutics focus on angiogenesis suppression, which were bactofection, DNA vaccination, alternative gene therapy, and transkingdom RNA interference (RNAi). Kim developed a targeted polymeric gene delivery system, PEI-g-PEG-RGD, which was developed by incorporating the alphanubeta3/alphanubeta5 integrin-binding RGD peptide into the cationic polymer, polyethylenimine (PEI) via a hydrophilic polyethylene glycol (PEG) spacer, and demonstrated that the stable expression of sFlt-1 by EC-targeted non-viral gene delivery inhibited the angiogenesis of ECs. It suggested that the combination of targeted gene carrier and sFlt-1 possesses the potential to be an efficient tool for the anti-angiogenic gene therapy to treat cancer.[47]

Delivery of genes encoding endogenous angiogenesis inhibitors and decoy receptors for pro-angiogenic factors may bear an advantage over classic non-gene therapy in terms of specific targeting, cost-effectiveness, and safety. Zhang et al.[48] showed that DNA vector–based RNAi, in which RNAi sequences targeting murine VEGF isoforms are inserted downstream of an RNA polymerase III promoter, has potential applications in isoform-specific knockdown of VEGF, which may contribute to VEGF isoform-specific treatment in cancer. Gyorffy et al.[49] used intratumor delivery of adenoviral vectors to induce a selective antitumor response by combining the potent angiogenesis inhibitor murine angiostatin with the powerful immune simulator and angiostatic cytokine murine IL-12, and they showed that a short-term course of anti-angiogenic therapy combined with immunotherapy can effectively shrink a solid tumor and vaccinate the animal against rechallenge. Matsuda et al.[50] developed a novel strategy for the tumor angiogenesis–targeted gene therapy by transducing a retroviral vector containing a cDNA for porcine pancreatic elastase 1 to the NIH 3T3 fibroblasts and culturing the fibroblasts in the presence of affinity-purified human plasminogen; they found that the exogenously added plasminogen was digested to generate the angiostatin, a potent angiogenesis inhibitor, which can suppress Lewis lung carcinoma growth in vivo. Modern approaches focused on gene targeting such as RNAi and miRNA will show the future direction in the field of angiogenesis inhibition for cancer treatment.

ANTI-ANGIOGENESIS THERAPY DRUGS

Angiogenesis, the formation of new blood vessels from preexisting vessels, has been shown to be essential for tumor growth, invasion, and development of metastasis. Accumulating evidence indicates that angiogenesis is especially critical for the growth and progression of solid tumors because growth of tumor mass beyond 2 to 3 mm^3 is often preceded by an increase in the formation of new blood vessels essential for the delivery of nutrients and oxygen to and removal of metabolic wastes from the tumor microenvironment.[51] Conventional chemotherapy designed to influence or abolish the ability of cancer cells to replicate does not discriminate effectively between rapidly dividing normal cells and tumor cells, thus leading to several toxic side effects. Since ECs that make up tumor vasculature are genetically stable, cancer treatment targeting tumor ECs exhibits less toxicity and rarely results in drug resistance compared with traditional chemotherapies. Therefore, strategies to block angiogenesis have been studied as a potential therapy for cancer treatment.[52] In recent years, much enthusiasm has been generated about targeted therapies and a number of such target-based anticancer therapies are now experimentally studied. The expanding insight in the process of angiogenesis has resulted in a large number of pharmaceutical agents that have been tested in preclinical studies (Table 47.2) and are currently tested in clinical trials (Table 47.3). Great interest has been taken in targeting the tumor vasculature and many efforts have been directed toward the development of anti-angiogenic agents.[66] In this way, the source of new blood vessels is destroyed, which may prevent further tumor growth, and tumor cells are starved leading to cell death directly.[55] As a proof of principle, human clinical trials in the last few years with anti-angiogenic modalities targeting VEGF and its receptors, especially VEGFR-2 (KDR) using inactivating monoclonal antibodies or kinase inhibitor drugs, as single agents or in combination with chemotherapy, have shown survival benefit in cancer patients of an increasing number of advanced stage malignancies.[62] However, novel and safer agents are needed to complement existing modalities, especially in long-term prevention use.

CONCLUSIONS AND PERSPECTIVES

The process of angiogenesis is complex and involves multiple players.[82,83] Suppression of development of new blood vessels in tumors provides a clear therapeutic benefit in both experimental animals and human patients. Despite the critical role of angiogenesis in tumor growth and dissemination, most anti-angiogenic cancer therapies have had only limited success selectively targeting one of the many factors implicated in this process. The current angiogenesis inhibitors used in clinical trials mostly target single angiogenic proteins and so far show limited effects on tumor growth. In summary, diverse upstream signals, including genetic and epigenetic factors as well as tumor microenvironment factors, use one or more pathways to modulate the expression and function of several transcription factors that are critical to the transcriptional regulation of various genes that are key to tumor angiogenesis.[82] The transcriptional activities of these transcription factors are mainly subject to the Ras/raf/extracellular signal-regulated kinase/p42/p44 mitogen-activated protein kinase (MAPK) and PI3K/Akt signaling pathways and control the expression of their numerous downstream target genes. Searching for the transcription factors critical to angiogenesis and testing them as targets for anti-angiogenic therapy rather than continued targeting of single signal and/or effector factors would be more fruitful (Fig. 47.2).

TABLE 47–2 Experimental/Preclinical Studies of Anti-angiogenesis Therapy Agents in Recent 5 Years

Agents	Description	Targets	Cancer/Cell Type	References
5-Formylhonokiol	Derivative of honokiol	Inactivating the ERK signaling pathway	HUVECs	53,54
Fascaplysin	Isolated from the Fijian sponge *Fascaplysinopsis* Bergquist sp.	CD31, VCAM-1	Sarcoma mice model	55,56
PGA4-3b	The roots of *Platycodon grandiflorum* (Jacq.) A. DC. (Campanulaceae)		HMEC	57
SIM010603	Multi-targeted receptor tyrosine kinase inhibitor	Multi-targeted RTK inhibitor of Kit, VEGFR, PDGFR-b, RET, and FLT3	HT-29, HepG2, A549, NCI-H460, LLC-SW44, BXPC-3	58
LMWH-Endostatin and PG-Endostatin	Endostatin derivatives	Downregulating expression of VEGF and upregulating expression of PEDF	HUVECs	59
The aqueous extract of *Psidium guajava* budding leaves		Inhibit the expressions of VEGF, IL-6, and IL-8 cytokines	Human prostate carcinoma DU-145 cells	60
Concanavalin A	Ca^{2+}/Mn^{2+}-dependent and mannose/glucose-binding legume lectin	IKK-NF-jB-COX-2, SHP-2-MEK-1-ERK, and SHP-2-Ras-ERK anti-angiogenic pathways	PU-1.8, A375, fibroblasts, HepG2, hepatoma, U87 glioblastoma, and p53-null cells	61
Galbanic acid	Isolated from *Ferula assafoetida*	Decreased phosphorylation of p38-MAPK, JNK, and AKT	Mouse Lewis lung cancer	62
Apigenin		Decrease the releasing of VEGF and MMP-8	Human hepatocellular carcinoma cells	63
Terbinafine	An oral antifungal agent		Oral squamous cell carcinoma	64
Curcuma zedoaria	A traditional Chinese herb		HUVECs	65
HM-3	An RGD-modified endostatin-derived polypeptide		Mouse melanoma tumors	66
PEDF	Pigment epithelium–derived factor	Downregulation of VEGF expression in tumor cells through inhibiting HIF-1α	Cervical carcinoma	67
Shallot extract	A heat-stable and flavonoid-rich fraction of shallot extract		HUVECs	68
Curcumin-K30 solid dispersion		CD34 and VEGF	SW480 tumors	69
graveoline derivatives			HUVEC	70
BB	A new synthetic quinazoline derivative, a potent EGFR inhibitor. BB	EGFR	A549 cells	71
Fumagillin	An inhibitor of type 2 methionine aminopeptidase	Cyclin E2, ALCAM, ICAM-1	Colon cancer	72
SCP1	A low-molecular-weight protein isolated from shark cartilage			73
3′-*O*-Acetylhamaudol	Isolated from *Angelica japonica* roots		HUVECs	74
Meisoindigo	An active compound of a Chinese antileukemia medicine		Chronic myelogenous leukemia	75
TSU-68 (SU-6668)	An inhibitor of RTKs	Involved in VEGF, bFGF, and PDGF signaling	Human colon cancer xenografts	76

HUVECs, human umbilical vein endothelial cells; HMECs, human microvascular endothelial cells; MAPK, mitogen-activated protein kinase; JNK, c-jun N-terminal kinase; VEGF, vascular endothelial growth factor.

TABLE 47–3 Clinical Trials of Anti-angiogenesis Therapy Drugs

Drugs	Clinical Trials	Cancer/Cell Type	Reference
Pazopanib	Phase 2 and 3 trials	Solid tumors	52
Bevacizumab, capecitabine, and oxaliplatin	Phase 2 trial	Advanced hepatocellular carcinoma	77
Simvastatin	Phase 2 trial	Metastatic colorectal cancer	78
AG-013736	Phase 2 trial	Acute myeloid leukemia	79
Thalidomide	Phase I clinical trial	Recurrent epithelial ovarian and Peritoneal carcinoma	80
IMC-IC11	Phase I trial	Colorectal carcinoma	81

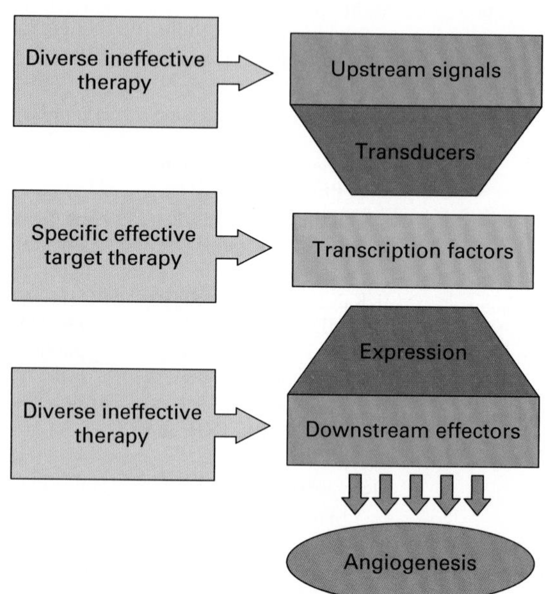

FIGURE 47–2 Effective anti-angiogenesis therapy targeting the transcription factors. Diverse upstream signals, such as tumor genetic, epigenetic, and cellular microenvironment factors, modulate the expression and function of several transcription factors that are critical to the transcriptional regulation of various genes key to tumor angiogenesis. The transcriptional activities of these transcription factors are mainly subject to the Ras/raf/extracellular signal–regulated kinase/p42/p44 MAPK and PI3K/Akt signaling pathways and control the expression of their numerous downstream target genes. Searching for the transcription factors critical to angiogenesis and testing them as targets for anti-angiogenic therapy rather than continued targeting of single signal and/or effector factors would be more fruitful and effective. (Adapted from Xie K, Wei D, Huang S, *Cytokine Growth Factor Rev.* June 2006;17(3):147-156.)

REFERENCES

1. Folkman J. What is the evidence that tumors are angiogenesis dependent? *J Natl Cancer Inst.* 1990;82:4-6.
2. Folkman J. Anti-angiogenesis: new concept for therapy of solid tumors. *Ann Surg.* 1972;175:409-416.
3. Iwasaki J, Nihira S. Anti-angiogenic therapy against gastrointestinal tract cancers. *Jpn J Clin Oncol.* 2009;39: 543-551.
4. Hanahan D, Folkman J. Patterns and emerging mechanisms of the angiogenic switch during tumorigenesis. *Cell.* 1996;86:353-364.
5. Giordano FJ, Johnson RS. Angiogenesis: the role of the microenvironment in flipping the switch. *Curr Opin Genet Dev.* 2001;11:35-40.
6. Udagawa T, Fernandez A, Achilles EG, et al. Persistence of microscopic human cancers in mice: alterations in the angiogenic balance accompanies loss of tumor dormancy. *FASEB J.* 2002;16:1361-1370.
7. Jimenez JA, Kao C, Raikwar S, et al. Current status of anti-angiogenesis therapy for prostate cancer. *Urol Oncol.* 2006;24:260-268.
8. Carmeliet P. Angiogenesis in life, disease and medicine. *Nature.* 2005;438:932-936.
9. Folkman J. Angiogenesis: an organizing principle for drug discovery? *Nat Rev Drug Discov.* 2007;6:273-286.
10. Ferrara N, Kerbel RS. Angiogenesis as a therapeutic target. *Nature.* 2005;438:967-974.
11. Spannuth WA, Sood AK, Coleman RL. Angiogenesis as a strategic target for ovarian cancer therapy. *Nat Clin Pract Oncol.* 2008;5:194-204.
12. Sudhakar A, Boosani CS. Inhibition of tumor angiogenesis by tumstatin: insights into signaling mechanisms and implications in cancer regression. *Pharm Res.* 2008;25:2731-2739.
13. Li Y, Cozzi PJ. Angiogenesis as a strategic target for prostate cancer therapy. *Med Res Rev.* 2010;30:23-66.
14. Napoli C, Giordano A, Casamassimi A, et al. Directed in vivo angiogenesis assay and the study of systemic neoangiogenesis in cancer. *Int J Cancer.* 2011;128:1505-1508.
15. Hwang C, Heath EI. Angiogenesis inhibitors in the treatment of prostate cancer. *J Hematol Oncol.* 2010;3:26.
16. Finney L, Vogt S, Fukai T, et al. Copper and angiogenesis: unravelling a relationship key to cancer progression. *Clin Exp Pharmacol Physiol.* 2009;36:88-94.
17. van Moorselaar RJ, Voest EE. Angiogenesis in prostate cancer: its role in disease progression and possible therapeutic approaches. *Mol Cell Endocrinol.* 2002;197:239-250.
18. Inui M, Martello G, Piccolo S. MicroRNA control of signal transduction. *Nat Rev Mol Cell Biol.* 2010;11:252-263.
19. Kota J, Chivukula RR, O'Donnell KA, et al. Therapeutic microRNA delivery suppresses tumorigenesis in a murine liver cancer model. *Cell.* 2009;137:1005-1017.

20. Poliseno L, Tuccoli A, Mariani L, et al. MicroRNAs modulate the angiogenic properties of HUVECs. *Blood*. 2006;108:3068-3071.
21. Caporali A, Emanueli C. MicroRNA regulation in angiogenesis. *Vascul Pharmacol*. 2011;55(4):79-86.
22. Liu XQ, Song WJ, Sun TM, et al. Targeted delivery of antisense inhibitor of miRNA for antiangiogenesis therapy using cRGD-functionalized nanoparticles. *Mol Pharm*. 2011;8:250-259.
23. Fang JH, Zhou HC, Zeng C, et al. MicroRNA-29b suppresses tumor angiogenesis, invasion and metastasis by regulating MMP-2 expression. *Hepatology*. 2011;54(5):1729-1740.
24. Kuehbacher A, Urbich C, Zeiher AM, et al. Role of Dicer and Drosha for endothelial microRNA expression and angiogenesis. *Circ Res*. 2007;101:59-68.
25. de Krijger I, Mekenkamp LJ, Punt CJ, et al. MicroRNAs in colorectal cancer metastasis. *J Pathol*. 2011;224:438-447.
26. Yamakuchi M, Lotterman CD, Bao C, et al. P53-induced microRNA-107 inhibits HIF-1 and tumor angiogenesis. *Proc Natl Acad Sci U S A*. 2010;107:6334-6339.
27. Yu JL, Rak JW, Coomber BL, et al. Effect of p53 status on tumor response to antiangiogenic therapy. *Science*. 2002;295:1526-1528.
28. Lei Z, Li B, Yang Z, et al. Regulation of HIF-1alpha and VEGF by miR-20b tunes tumor cells to adapt to the alteration of oxygen concentration. *PLoS One*. 2009;4:e7629.
29. Wurdinger T, Tannous BA, Saydam O, et al. miR-296 regulates growth factor receptor overexpression in angiogenic endothelial cells. *Cancer Cell*. 2008;14:382-393.
30. Liu LZ, Li C, Chen Q, et al. MiR-21 induced angiogenesis through AKT and ERK activation and HIF-1alpha expression. *PLoS One*. 2011;6:e19139.
31. Rak J, Yu JL, Kerbel RS, et al. What do oncogenic mutations have to do with angiogenesis/vascular dependence of tumors? *Cancer Res*. 2002;62:1931-1934.
32. Mendell JT. miRiad roles for the miR-17-92 cluster in development and disease. *Cell*. 2008;133:217-222.
33. Dews M, Homayouni A, Yu D, et al. Augmentation of tumor angiogenesis by a Myc-activated microRNA cluster. *Nat Genet*. 2006;38:1060-1065.
34. Dirkx AE, oude Egbrink MG, Castermans K, et al. Anti-angiogenesis therapy can overcome endothelial cell anergy and promote leukocyte-endothelium interactions and infiltration in tumors. *FASEB J*. 2006;20:621-630.
35. Schoenfeld JD, Dranoff G. Anti-angiogenesis immunotherapy. *Hum Vaccin*. 2011;7(9):976-981.
36. Seavey MM, Paterson Y. Anti-angiogenesis immunotherapy induces epitope spreading to Her-2/neu resulting in breast tumor immunoediting. *Breast Cancer (London)*. 2009;1:19-30.
37. Chan RC, Gutierrez B, Ichim TE, et al. Enhancement of DNA cancer vaccine efficacy by combination with anti-angiogenesis in regression of established subcutaneous B16 melanoma. *Oncol Rep*. 2009;22:1197-1203.
38. Griffioen AW. Anti-angiogenesis: making the tumor vulnerable to the immune system. *Cancer Immunol Immunother*. 2008;57:1553-1558.
39. Griffioen AW, Damen CA, Martinotti S, et al. Endothelial intercellular adhesion molecule-1 expression is suppressed in human malignancies: the role of angiogenic factors. *Cancer Res*. 1996;56:1111-1117.
40. Hellwig SM, Damen CA, van Adrichem NP, et al. Endothelial CD34 is suppressed in human malignancies: role of angiogenic factors. *Cancer Lett*. 1997;120:203-211.
41. Tromp SC, oude Egbrink MG, Dings RP, et al. Tumor angiogenesis factors reduce leukocyte adhesion in vivo. *Int Immunol*. 2000;12:671-676.
42. Gardlik R, Celec P, Bernadic M. Targeting angiogenesis for cancer (gene) therapy. *Bratisl Lek Listy*. 2011;112:428-434.
43. Zhou J, Zhang ZX, Zhao H, et al. Anti-angiogenesis by lentivirus-mediated small interfering RNA silencing of angiopoietin-2 gene in pancreatic carcinoma. *Technol Cancer Res Treat*. 2011;10:361-369.
44. Hu M, Yang JL, Teng H, et al. Anti-angiogenesis therapy based on the bone marrow-derived stromal cells genetically engineered to express sFlt-1 in mouse tumor model. *BMC Cancer*. 2008;8: 306.
45. Agrawal N, Bettegowda C, Cheong I, et al. Bacteriolytic therapy can generate a potent immune response against experimental tumors. *Proc Natl Acad Sci U S A*. 2004;101:15172-15177.
46. Gardlik R, Behuliak M, Palffy R, et al. Gene therapy for cancer: bacteria-mediated anti-angiogenesis therapy. *Gene Ther*. 2011;18:425-431.
47. Kim WJ, Yockman JW, Lee M, et al. Soluble Flt-1 gene delivery using PEI-g-PEG-RGD conjugate for anti-angiogenesis. *J Control Release*. 2005;106:224-234.
48. Zhang L, Yang N, Mohamed-Hadley A, et al. Vector-based RNAi, a novel tool for isoform-specific knock-down of VEGF and anti-angiogenesis gene therapy of cancer. *Biochem Biophys Res Commun*. 2003;303:1169-1178.
49. Gyorffy S, Palmer K, Podor TJ, et al. Combined treatment of a murine breast cancer model with type 5 adenovirus vectors expressing murine angiostatin and IL-12: a role for combined anti-angiogenesis and immunotherapy. *J Immunol*. 2001;166:6212-6217.
50. Matsuda KM, Madoiwa S, Hasumi Y, et al. A novel strategy for the tumor angiogenesis-targeted gene therapy: generation of angiostatin from endogenous plasminogen by protease gene transfer. *Cancer Gene Ther*. 2000;7:589-596.
51. Carmeliet P, Jain RK. Angiogenesis in cancer and other diseases. *Nature*. 2000;407:249-257.
52. Schutz FA, Choueiri TK, Sternberg CN. Pazopanib: clinical development of a potent anti-angiogenic drug. *Crit Rev Oncol Hematol*. 2011;77:163-171.
53. Zhu W, Fu A, Hu J, et al. 5-Formylhonokiol exerts anti-angiogenesis activity via inactivating the ERK signaling pathway. *Exp Mol Med*. 2011;43:146-152.
54. Hu J, Chen LJ, Liu L, et al. Liposomal honokiol, a potent anti-angiogenesis agent, in combination with radiotherapy produces a synergistic antitumor efficacy without increasing toxicity. *Exp Mol Med*. 2008;40:617-628.
55. Zheng YL, Lu XL, Lin J, et al. Direct effects of fascaplysin on human umbilical vein endothelial cells attributing the anti-angiogenesis activity. *Biomed Pharmacother*. 2010;64:527-533.
56. Yan X, Chen H, Lu X, et al. Fascaplysin exert anti-tumor effects through apoptotic and anti-angiogenesis pathways in sarcoma mice model. *Eur J Pharm Sci*. 2011;43(4):251-259.
57. Xu Y, Dong Q, Qiu H, et al. A homogalacturonan from the radix of *Platycodon grandiflorum* and the anti-angiogenesis activity of poly-/oligogalacturonic acids derived therefrom. *Carbohydr Res*. 2011;346:1930-1936.
58. Wang D, Tang F, Wang S, et al. Preclinical anti-angiogenesis and anti-tumor activity of SIM010603, an oral, multi-targets receptor tyrosine kinases inhibitor. *Cancer Chemother Pharmacol*. 2011;69(1):173-183.
59. Tan H, Mu G, Zhu W, et al. Down-regulation of vascular endothelial growth factor and up-regulation of pigment epithelium derived factor make low molecular weight heparin-endostatin and polyethylene glycol-endostatin potential candidates for anti-angiogenesis drug. *Biol Pharm Bull*. 2011;34:545-550.
60. Peng CC, Peng CH, Chen KC, et al. The aqueous soluble polyphenolic fraction of *Psidium guajava* leaves exhibits potent anti-angiogenesis and anti-migration actions on DU145 cells. *Evid Based Complement Alternat Med*. 2011;2011:219069.
61. Li WW, Yu JY, Xu HL, et al. Concanavalin A: a potential anti-neoplastic agent targeting apoptosis, autophagy and anti-angiogenesis for cancer therapeutics. *Biochem Biophys Res Commun*. 2011;414(2):282-286.
62. Kim KH, Lee HJ, Jeong SJ, et al. Galbanic acid isolated from *Ferula assafoetida* exerts in vivo anti-tumor activity in association with anti-angiogenesis and anti-proliferation. *Pharm Res*. 2011;28:597-609.
63. Kim BR, Jeon YK, Nam MJ. A mechanism of apigenin-induced apoptosis is potentially related to anti-angiogenesis and anti-migration in human hepatocellular carcinoma cells. *Food Chem Toxicol*. 2011;49:1626-1632.
64. Chien MH, Lee TS, Kao C, et al. Terbinafine inhibits oral squamous cell carcinoma growth through anti-cancer cell proliferation and anti-angiogenesis. *Mol Carcinog*. 2011;51(5):389-399.
65. Chen W, Lu Y, Gao M, et al. Anti-angiogenesis effect of essential oil from *Curcuma zedoaria* in vitro and in vivo. *J Ethnopharmacol*. 2011;133:220-226.
66. Zhu B, Xu HM, Zhao L, et al. Site-specific modification of anti-angiogenesis peptide HM-3 by polyethylene glycol molecular weight of 20 kDa. *J Biochem*. 2010;148:341-347.

67. Yang J, Chen S, Huang X, et al. Growth suppression of cervical carcinoma by pigment epithelium-derived factor via anti-angiogenesis. *Cancer Biol Ther*. 2010;9:967-974.
68. Seyfi P, Mostafaie A, Mansouri K, et al. In vitro and in vivo anti-angiogenesis effect of shallot (*Allium ascalonicum*): a heat-stable and flavonoid-rich fraction of shallot extract potently inhibits angiogenesis. *Toxicol In Vitro*. 2010;24:1655-1661.
69. Chen C, Huang X, Cai H, et al. Anti-proliferation and anti-angiogenesis of curcumin-K30 solid dispersion. *Zhong Nan Da Xue Xue Bao Yi Xue Ban*. 2010;35:1029-1036.
70. An ZY, Yan YY, Peng D, et al. Synthesis and evaluation of graveoline and graveolinine derivatives with potent anti-angiogenesis activities. *Eur J Med Chem*. 2010;45: 3895-3903.
71. Sun QM, Miao ZH, Lin LP, et al. BB, a new EGFR inhibitor, exhibits prominent anti-angiogenesis and antitumor activities. *Cancer Biol Ther*. 2009;8:1640-1647.
72. Hou L, Mori D, Takase Y, et al. Fumagillin inhibits colorectal cancer growth and metastasis in mice: in vivo and in vitro study of anti-angiogenesis. *Pathol Int*. 2009;59:448-461.
73. Rabbani-Chadegani A, Abdossamadi S, Bargahi A, et al. Identification of low-molecular-weight protein (SCP1) from shark cartilage with anti-angiogenesis activity and sequence similarity to parvalbumin. *J Pharm Biomed Anal*. 2008;46: 563-567.
74. Kimura Y, Sumiyoshi M, Baba K. Anti-tumor actions of major component 3'-O-acetylhamaudol of *Angelica japonica* roots through dual actions, anti-angiogenesis and intestinal intraepithelial lymphocyte activation. *Cancer Lett*. 2008;265:84-97.
75. Xiao Z, Wang Y, Lu L, et al. Anti-angiogenesis effects of meisoindigo on chronic myelogenous leukemia in vitro. *Leuk Res*. 2006;30:54-59.
76. Yorozuya K, Kubota T, Watanabe M, et al. TSU-68 (SU6668) inhibits local tumor growth and liver metastasis of human colon cancer xenografts via anti-angiogenesis. *Oncol Rep*. 2005;*14*:677-682.
77. Sun W, Sohal D, Haller DG, et al. Phase 2 trial of bevacizumab, capecitabine, and oxaliplatin in treatment of advanced hepatocellular carcinoma. *Cancer*. 2011;117:3187-3192.
78. Lee J, Jung KH, Park YS, et al. Simvastatin plus irinotecan, 5-fluorouracil, and leucovorin (FOLFIRI) as first-line chemotherapy in metastatic colorectal patients: a multicenter phase II study. *Cancer Chemother Pharmacol*. 2009;64:657-663.
79. Giles FJ, Bellamy WT, Estrov Z, et al. The anti-angiogenesis agent, AG-013736, has minimal activity in elderly patients with poor prognosis acute myeloid leukemia (AML) or myelodysplastic syndrome (MDS). *Leuk Res*. 2006;30:801-811.
80. Chan JK, Manuel MR, Ciaravino G, et al. Safety and efficacy of thalidomide in recurrent epithelial ovarian and peritoneal carcinoma. *Gynecol Oncol*. 2006;103:919-923.
81. Hunt S. Technology evaluation: IMC-1C11, ImClone Systems. *Curr Opin Mol Ther*. 2001:3:418-424.
82. Xie K, Wei D, Huang S. Transcriptional anti-angiogenesis therapy of human pancreatic cancer. *Cytokine Growth Factor Rev*. June 2006;17(3):147-156.
83. Benedito R, Rocha SF, Woeste M, et al. Notch-dependent VEGFR3 upregulation allows angiogenesis without VEGF-VEGFR2 signalling. *Nature*. 2012;484:110-114.

CHAPTER 48

MicroRNAs and Cancer Therapeutics

Maitri Y. Shah and George A. Calin

INTRODUCTION

MicroRNAs (miRNAs) are evolutionarily conserved class of small, regulatory RNAs that negatively regulate gene expression. Extensive research in the last decade has implicated miRNAs as master regulators of cellular processes with essential role in cancer initiation, progression, and metastasis. Widespread deregulation of miRNAs in cancers has identified oncogenic and tumor suppressive roles of these miRNAs. Based on these observations, miRNAs have emerged as promising therapeutic tools for cancer management. In this chapter, we focus on the roles of miRNAs in tumorigenesis, the rationale and strategies for the use of miRNA-based therapy in cancer, and the advantages and current challenges to their use in the clinic.

THE miRNA WORLD

The discovery of miRNAs in the last decade has been one of the most fascinating breakthroughs of recent times. The identification of these regulatory RNAs from the dark matter of the human genome initiated a shift in the paradigms of cancer biology and facilitated a deeper understanding of the human biology. miRNAs are small (19 to 24 nt), endogenous highly conserved non-coding RNAs with imperative regulatory functions.[1] They negatively regulate gene expression by binding to the 3′-untranslated region (3′-UTR) of the target mRNAs and causing mRNA degradation or translational repression. Thus, they are involved in post-transcriptional gene silencing and are predicted to target about 30% of the protein-coding genes.[2] Since its discovery, thousands of miRNAs have been identified in animals, plants, and several viruses. These miRNAs play an important role in multiple biological processes, including developmental timings, embryogenesis, cell differentiation, organogenesis, metabolism, apoptosis, and various diseases, including cancers.[3] miRNA pathways have been implicated as a new layer of gene regulation important in both normal and diseased states, and thus further understanding of the molecular nature and functions of these small regulatory RNAs would help identify novel tools for drug development.

In this chapter, we briefly review the structure, biogenesis, functions, and mechanism of action of these miRNAs, followed by a detailed analysis of the therapeutic potential of these miRNAs. We focus on the strategies presently used for miRNA therapy; discuss their use and drawbacks, and the challenges and future directions for development of miRNA-based therapy for human cancers.

miRNA BIOGENESIS AND MECHANISM OF ACTION

miRNAs are usually transcribed from miRNA genes by RNA polymerase II (RNAPII), as autonomous transcription units, or as clusters from a polycistronic transcription unit, to give a long capped and polyadenylated primary microRNA transcript (pri-miRNA).[4] These can be located in the exonic or intronic regions of non–protein-coding regions or in the intronic region of protein-coding transcription units. This stem-loop structure is then cleaved by a microprocessor complex (composed of RNase III Drosha and double-stranded DNA-binding domain protein DGCR8) to give hairpin-shaped precursors of microRNA (pre-miRNAs).[5] The pre-miRNAs are then exported to the cytoplasm by the nuclear export factor Exportin-5/Ran GTP. Following their export from the nucleus, these pre-miRNAs are further processed to ~22 nt miRNA:miRNA* duplexes by the cytoplasmic RNase III enzyme Dicer and its double-stranded RNA-binding domain protein TRBP. Subsequently, the mature miRNA then gets incorporated into RISC (RNA-induced silencing complex), usually resulting in the repression of target gene expression. RISC usually binds to the 3′-UTR of target mRNAs and brings about cleavage or translational repression of the target mRNAs, depending on the degree of complementarity between miRNA and target mRNA. In humans, miRNAs usually bind to specific sequences with partial complementarity on target RNA transcripts, called "seed sequences" or microRNA response elements (MREs), which then result in translational repression.[1]

Besides the canonical miRNA regulation pathway, several variations have also been reported for the miRNA-mediated regulation. Some miRNAs bind to the 5′-UTR or the open reading frame of the mRNA, resulting in activation rather than suppression of the target genes.[6] A few miRNAs also show decoy activity, by binding directly to the proteins, such as RNA-binding proteins, and thus inhibiting the interaction with their target RNA.[7] Moreover, in certain cases, miRNAs can also regulate gene expression at the transcriptional level,[8] by binding directly to the DNA regulatory elements. Thus, miRNA-mediated regulation of gene expression is a complex science and is still an evolving concept.

miRNAS AS PREFERRED THERAPEUTIC TARGETS FOR CANCER

Cancer represents a complex multistep genetic disorder characterized by deregulation of homeostasis at the genomic, transcriptomic, and proteomic levels.[9] The preferred choice of treatment for most human malignancies for the last century has been surgery and chemotherapy. However, the severe toxicities, adverse side effects, and the poor quality of living associated with the chemotherapeutic treatment emphasize the need for new therapeutic interventions for cancer patients. The major advances in the last decade have focused on designing novel targeted therapy capable of targeting specifically the malignant cells in a more rational way. The advent of miRNAs provides an additional layer of gene regulation on a broad spectrum of biological pathways by fine-tuning protein expression levels. By virtue of their ability to target multiple protein-coding genes and their aberrant perturbations in widespread cancers, miRNAs have emerged to be promising novel therapeutic targets and intervention tools. In the following sections, we briefly discuss the rationale for the use of miRNAs as therapeutic tools in cancer.

Ubiquitous miRNA Alterations in Cancers

Aberrant expression of miRNA levels has been implicated in a broad spectrum of human diseases, including autoimmune, cardiovascular, and psychiatric diseases; diabetes; and cancers.[10] A growing body of evidence suggests that miRNAs play a vital role in cancer predisposition, initiation, maintenance, progression, and metastasis.[11] miRNA expression profiling studies have identified a unique miRNA signature profile that can differentiate normal tissues from cancer tissues and also classify different tumor types and grades.[12] The widespread dysregulation of miRNAs can be explained by their frequent location in cancer-associated hotspots of the human genome, including fragile sites, minimal regions of amplification, loss of heterozygosity sites, and common breakpoint regions.[13] Other mechanisms of this dysregulation include chromosomal deletions or translocations of regions with miRNA genes, epigenetic regulation of miRNA expression, alterations in miRNA promoter activity by oncogenes and tumor suppressor genes (TSGs), alterations in the miRNA processing machinery (such as mutations in Dicer, TRBP2, and Exportin 5), and presence of mutated miRNA structural variants.[14]

miRNAs Function as Oncogenes or TSGs

miRNAs contribute to tumorigenesis by functioning as oncogenes or TSGs.[11,14] miRNAs that target oncogenes and whose expression is lost in most human cancers are classified as tumor suppressor miRNAs (TSmiRs). The loss of TSmiR expression due to somatic alterations or germline mutations can initiate or enhance tumorigenicity. One of the important examples of TSmiRs is miR-15b/miR-16-1 cluster, which is frequently deleted in B-cell chronic lymphocytic leukemia (CLL) and targets several oncogenes such as *BCL2*, *CCND1*, and *WNT3A*.[15] A knockout mouse model targeting the miR-15b/miR-16-1 cluster recapitulated the CLL-associated phenotype, validating the in vivo functionality of these TSmiRs.[16] Other important TSmiRs are the let-7 family members, miR-29, miR-34 family, miR-122, and miR-143/145 cluster.[14] In contrast, overexpressed miRNAs that promote tumorigenicity by targeting TSGs are classified as oncomiRs.[11] One of the most prevalent oncomiR is miR-21, which is overexpressed in almost all human cancers and targets *PTEN* and *PDCD4*.[17] Spontaneous tumorigenesis in transgenic mice overexpressing miR-155 has also established miR-155 as a bona fide oncomiR.[18] Other miRNAs with oncogenic function include miR-17-92 cluster, miR-155, miR-200 family, miR-221/222 cluster, and miR-372/373 cluster.[11]

OncomiR Addiction

The concept of addiction or dependency of tumor cells on activating mutations in certain oncogenic factors for survival and proliferation has been recently demonstrated for oncogenic miRNAs. Medina et al.[19] developed a conditional transgenic mouse overexpressing miR-21 and showed that these mice developed spontaneous pre-B malignant lymphoid-like phenotype. In the absence of miR-21, malignant cells undergo apoptosis and the tumors regress. These in vivo experimental findings from transgenic mice strongly advocate the causative role of miRNAs in carcinogenesis and further support their use for therapeutic intervention.

miRNAs and the Hallmarks of Cancer

Extensive research in the past decade has revealed that miRNAs play an active role in the acquisition of the malignant phenotype by cancer cells. In the context of the hallmarks of cancer, miRNAs have evolved to regulate key cellular processes and tissue architecture, maintaining the fine homeostatic balance in a normal cell. They play important role in cell proliferation, apoptosis, cell cycle regulation, differentiation, and self-renewal.[20] Dysregulation of these miRNA expression levels thus results in disruption of the equilibrium and accumulation of genetic damage, leading to the manifestation of the transformed phenotype. Below we provide a few examples of miRNAs that affect the emerging hallmarks of cancer as described by Hanahan and Weinberg[21,22]: sustaining proliferative signaling (miR-21 and let-7 family)[23]; evading growth receptors (miR-17-92 cluster)[23]; resisting cell death (miR-15/16 and miR-34 cluster)[23]; enabling replicative immortality (miR-34a and miR-372/373 cluster)[23]; inducing angiogenesis (miR-210)[23]; activating invasion and metastasis (miR-10b)[24]; avoiding immune destruction (miR-520d)[25]; deregulating cellular genetics (miR-122 and miR-210)[26,27]; tumor-promoting inflammation (miR-146 and miR-155)[28]; and genome instability and mutation (miR-155).[29]

miRNAs as Biomarkers for Cancer

Because of the widespread dysregulation of miRNAs in all types of tumors, miRNA expression profiling in cancer patients has been a valuable signature classifier.[12] The distinct miRNA expression patterns between the normal and cancer tissues serve as diagnostic, predictive, and prognostic biomarkers. miRNA signatures can classify tumors of different types and grades and also correlate with chemotherapy and incidence of drug resistance patterns. The recent detection of stable miRNAs in serum has opened up new avenues for non-invasive biomarkers in cancer prognosis.[30]

miRNAs and ceRNAs

The recent revolutionary discovery of competing endogenous RNAs (ceRNAs) lend further support to the potential use of miRNAs as therapeutic agents.[31] The ceRNA hypothesis states that the extensive human transcriptome, including transcribed pseudogenes, mRNAs, and long non-coding RNAs interact or crosstalk with each other through the MREs, establishing a comprehensive intricate regulatory network. For example, tumor suppressor *PTEN* is finely regulated by its ceRNAs, PTENP1 pseudogene, and ZEB2 mRNA.[32,33] In the context of miRNA therapy, miRNA modulation may have more profound manifestations in an as-yet-uncharacterized RNA-dependent aspect. miRNAs that form autoregulatory loops with other ceRNAs might undergo analogous genetic alterations in neoplasia via similar underlying mechanisms and pathways. Thus, therapeutic modulation of miRNA levels might shift the balance and set up a cellular cascade enabling a more pronounced biological effect than previously anticipated. This discovery reveals a whole new realm of therapeutic possibilities for human cancers. More research to identify other cancer-associated ceRNA–miRNA networks needs to be done before the full therapeutic potential of such regulatory loops can be exploited.

miRNA-BASED THERAPEUTIC APPROACHES

The ability of miRNAs to regulate cellular processes, their inherent role in carcinogenesis as oncogenes or TSGs, and the aberrant dysregulation of their expression levels in cancer illustrate the potential of miRNA modulation as a viable therapeutic strategy and a powerful intervention tool. The current knowledge available from gene therapy and RNAi technologies can be easily adapted to miRNA therapy. Two strategies could be used for the treatment of cancer using miRNA therapy: first, by targeting multiple molecular defects accumulated in the multistep pathway of a specific cancer—“multiplex RNA inhibition”; second, by using multiple agents to target one specific molecular defect linked with cancer pathogenesis—“sandwich RNA inhibition.”[34]

Current approaches involve either (a) the use of “miRNA-mimics” to substitute for the loss of a TSmiR or (b) the use of “anti-miRNAs” to inhibit the expression of an oncomiR (Table 48.1).

miRNA Mimics—miRNA Replacement Therapy

Alterations or mutations in the TSmiRs impede their inhibitory effect, contributing to oncogenic activation in cancer cells. An effective alternative would be to restore the normal function of these miRNAs by replacing or substituting the lost miRNA using synthetic miRNA-like molecules called “miRNA mimics.” These are small, chemically modified (2′-*O*methoxy) RNA duplexes that can be loaded into RISC and achieve the downstream inhibition of the target mRNAs. Certain modifications to improve the stability and increase the half-life of these mimics include (i) introduction of double-stranded miRNA mimetic and (ii) expression of longer pre–miRNA-like short hairpin RNAs (shRNAs) from plasmid or viral vectors driven by strong promoters.[20] Numerous studies have validated the efficiency of miRNA replacement therapy in in vitro and in vivo models. For example, introduction of miRNA mimics for miR-15a in prostate cancer cell lines induced marked apoptosis and blocked proliferation.[35] Most important in vivo validation of miRNA mimics has been performed for let-7 manipulations in lung cancer models.[36] Intranasal administration of let-7 in a K-ras mutant mouse effectively restrained the growth of the tumors by repression of proliferation and cell cycle pathways.[36,37] Similar in vivo studies have also been performed for miR-34a in a prostate cancer murine model[38] and for miR-26 in an myc-dependent liver cancer model (using adeno-associated virus [AAV]).[39] More recently, a new RNAPII–driven

TABLE 48-1 Advantages and Disadvantages of miRNA-Based Therapeutic Approaches

Method	Definition	Mechanism of Action	Clinical Trial Stage	Advantage	Disadvantage
AMOs	A single-stranded, RNA molecule designed to be complementary to a selected miRNA	Competitive inhibition of mature miRNA	Preclinical studies	Safe, easy to modulate, targeted inhibition	Nuclease sensitivity, poor stability, poor cellular uptake, poor biodistribution
2′-*O*-modified AMOs	Modification of 2′-OH to 2′-*O*methyl and 2′-*O*methoxyethyl groups	Competitive inhibition of mature miRNA	Phase I clinical trial	Nuclease resistance, improved binding affinity, stability, and specificity	Can induce immune system response, few off-target effects, delivery issues
Antagomirs	AMOs modified to have a phosphorothioate backbone and conjugated with cholesterol	Competitive inhibition of mature miRNA	Phase I, II, and III clinical trials	Improved bioavailability, improved stability	Requires high doses, toxic
LNA anti-miRNAs	Addition of an extra methylene bridge connecting the 2′-O atom and the 4′-C atom and "locks" the ribose ring in a C3′-endo or C2′-endo conformation	High-affinity Watson-Crick hybridization with their RNA target molecules—inhibition	Phase I clinical trials	Safe, higher thermal stability, better affinity, improved mismatch discrimination, good biodistribution	Off-target effects, higher toxicity
miRNA sponges	RNA transcripts with multiple tandom repeats of miRNA-binding sites for an endogenous miRNA	Stably interact with corresponding miRNA and prevent its interaction with its target mRNAs	Preclinical studies	More natural-like activity, applicable to silence an entire family of miRNAs	Off-target effects, delivery issues
miRNA masks	Single-stranded 2′-*O*methyl-modified antisense oligonucleotides with entire complementary to the miRNA-binding sites in the 3′-UTR of the target mRNA	"Mask" the target mRNA from the endogenous miRNA and thus prevent its suppression	Preclinical studies	Gene-specific effect, no off-target effects	Limited activity (one target), delivery issues
miRNA mimics	Small, chemically modified (2′-*O*methoxy) RNA duplexes that can be loaded into RISC and achieve the downstream inhibition of the target mRNAs	Assist the miRNA function	Phase I clinical trials	Successfully replace endogenous mature miRNA function	Poor stability, poor biodistribution

AMOs, anti-miRNA oligonucleotides; LNA, locked nucleic acid; 3′-UTR, 3′-untranslated region; RISC, RNA-induced silencing complex.

expression vector for miR-155 has been shown to effectively increase miR-155 expression levels in in vitro and in vivo xenograft models.[40]

Anti-miRs—Antisense Inhibition of Mature miRNA

OncomiRs are frequently overexpressed in cancers, and inhibition of these miRNAs would help restore the normal function of its target tumor suppressive genes. Several miRNA inhibitory agents have been recently tested in preclinical and clinical studies. These models are essentially complementary single-stranded oligonucleotides that can sequester the endogenous miRNA in a conformation that is unable to be processed by the RISC. They include antisense anti-miRNA oligonucleotides (AMOs), locked nucleic acid (LNA) anti-miRNAs, antagomirs, miRNA sponges, miRNA masks, and small molecule inhibitors of miRNAs (Fig. 48.1).

Antisense Oligonucleotides

Inhibition of miRNA activity using synthetic AMOs has been demonstrated in vitro and in vivo. AMOs are single-stranded RNA molecules complementary to the target

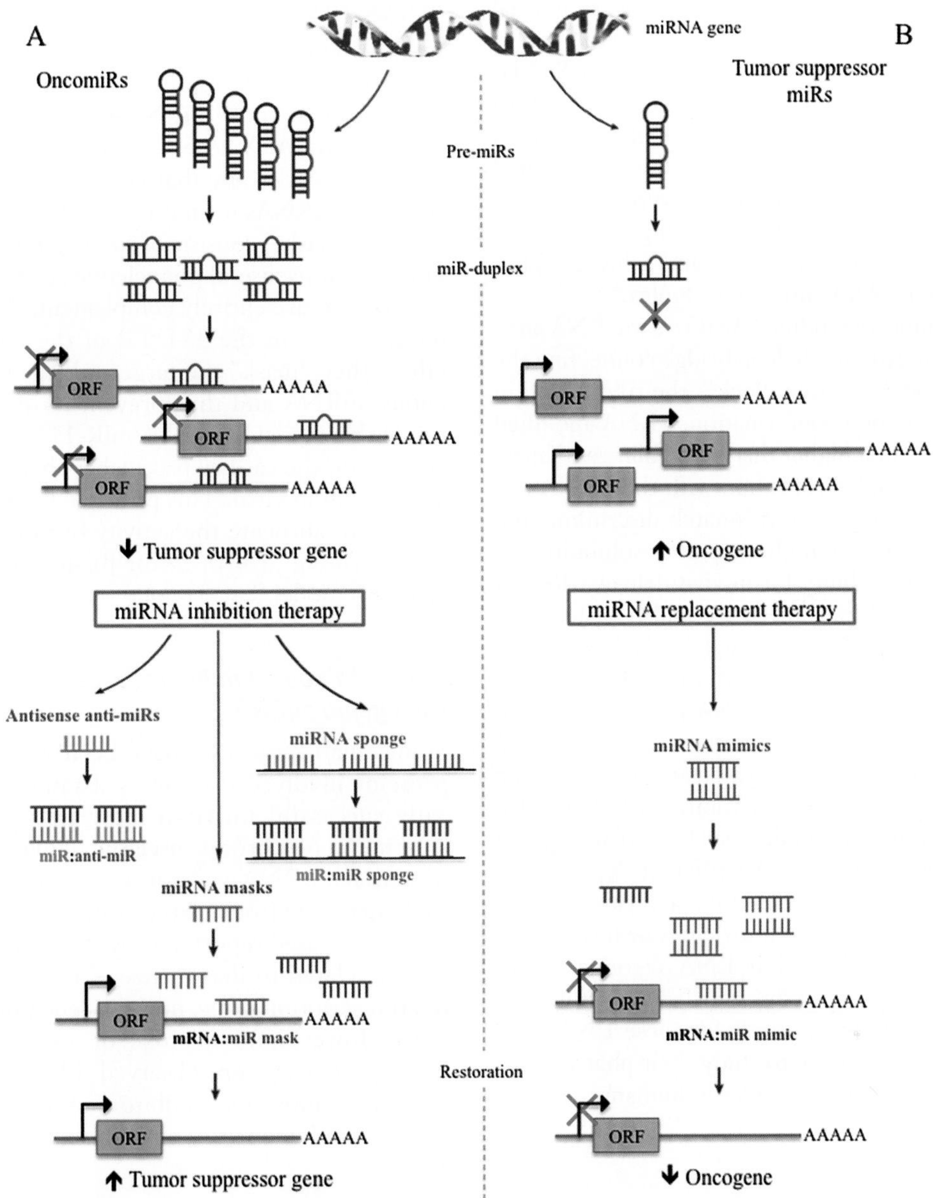

FIGURE 48–1 MicroRNA (miRNA)-based therapy for management of cancer: **(A)** miRNA inhibition therapy for oncomiRs includes antisense anti-miRs (AMOs, modified AMOs, LNA-based AMOs, and antagomirs), miRNA sponges, and miRNA masks; and **(B)** miRNA replacement therapy for tumor suppressive miRs includes miRNA mimics. ORF, open reading frame; anti-miRs, anti-miRNA oligonucleotides; pre-miRNAs, precursors of microRNA.

miRNA.[20,41] They work as competitive inhibitors of miRNAs by annealing to the mature miRNA and inhibiting the interaction of that miRNA with its target mRNAs. Thus, targeted inhibition of a specific miRNA and subsequent upregulation of its target mRNAs can be achieved. The most widely used AMOs are 2′-*O*-methyl AMOs and 2′-*O*-methoxyethyl AMOs. Addition of these different 2′-ribose modifications to AMOs contributes to nuclease resistance and improved binding affinity, stability, and specificity. Addition of a phosphorothioate moiety along with the 2′ modification further enhances the resistance to endonucleases, and better serum stability and cellular uptake.[41] In contrast, unmodified AMOs are unable to inhibit miRNA function in vitro.

Modified AMOs

One of the optimal modifications to AMOs is the addition of cholesterol functionality at the 3′-position of the nucleic acid to generate "antagomirs," modified AMOs complementary to miR-122.[42] Intravenous injection of these antagomirs afforded a marked and specific inhibition of endogenous miR-122 in mice. The effects were long-lasting (up to 23 d) with no noticeable immune response or toxicity. Targeted degradation of the mature miR-122 was observed in the liver and other tissues except the brain, with an upregulation of target mRNAs having the miR-122 interaction sites in their 3′-UTRs. Furthermore, in vivo miR-122 inhibition by antagomirs induced a significant decrease in cholesterol plasma levels in normal as well as diet-induced obese mice, indicating the potential usefulness of antagomirs in metabolic diseases. Similar results were observed when antagomirs against miR-16 were administered in vivo, with efficient silencing in all tissues except the brain. In another study, the same authors reported that longer antagomirs (35 nt) were more effective in vivo, can discriminate between single-nucleotide mismatches of the targeted miRNA, and achieve higher biostability of the miRNA–antagomir duplex.[43]

Another example of modified AMOs is the LNA anti-miRs, in which an extra methylene bridge connecting the 2′-O atom and the 4′-C atom "locks" the ribose ring in a C3′-endo or C2′-endo conformation.[44] LNA-modified oligonucleotides exhibit higher thermal stability and high-affinity Watson-Crick hybridization with their RNA target molecules, with improved mismatch discrimination. Furthermore, they display higher aqueous solubility and increased metabolic stability for in vivo delivery. Recent studies have reported that miR-21 could be effectively silenced in vitro using LNA-modified ASOs, leading to a significant reduction in cell viability.[45] In an in vivo mouse model, intravenous injection of LNA anti-miR showed distinctly superior efficiency in antagonizing miR-122 compared with cholesterol-conjugated antagomirs.[44] The safety and efficacy of these LNA anti-miRs have also been evaluated in primate models, such as African green monkeys[46] and chimpanzees.[47] An efficient depletion of miR-122 in the liver was reported in each case without any evidence of LNA-associated toxicities or histopathologic changes in the animals. Thus, LNA oligonucleotides are uniquely suited for targeting miRNAs both in vivo and in vitro. Phase I clinical trials for these LNA anti-miRs are currently underway to study their pharmacokinetic and pharmacodynamic profiles in humans.

miRNA Sponge

Ebert and colleagues[48] reported a novel system for miRNA antagonism called "miRNA sponges" or "miRNA decoys." These are RNA transcripts with multiple tandom repeats of miRNA-binding sites for an endogenous miRNA. These sponges stably interact with or "soak up" the corresponding miRNA and prevent its interaction with its target mRNAs. The discovery of ceRNAs[31] that function as endogenous miRNA sponges substantiates the mechanism of action and biological relevance of these systems. In order to imitate the miRNA–mRNA binding like in the natural setting, a bulge was introduced at positions 9 to 12, which achieved better activity due to increased miRNA retention. These effects were equivalent to those achieved by modified AMOs. A remarkable attribute of this approach is the ability of miRNA sponge to affect all closely related miRNAs within a family that share overlapping targets. miRNA sponges have also been tested in vivo in mouse models of cardiac hypertrophy research and been proven to be safe and effective.[49]

miRNA Masks

Inhibition of a specific miRNA using the aforementioned strategies causes de-repression of the entire array of target genes that show miRNA-binding sites for that particular miRNA. Xiao et al.[50] developed a gene-specific anti-miRNA therapy that could prevent the repressive action of miRNAs in an mRNA-selective manner. These "miRNA masks" consists of single-stranded 2′-*O*methyl-modified antisense oligonucleotides with locked 5′- and 3′-ends that are entirely complementary to the miRNA-binding sites in the 3′-UTR of the target mRNA. In effect, they "mask" the target mRNA from the endogenous miRNA and thus prevent its suppression. They tested this model on miR-1/miR-133 and its action specifically on the cardiac pacemaker channel genes HCN2 and HCN4 in vitro. This principle has been successfully applied to abrogate the activity of miR-430 on TGF-β (transforming growth factor β) signaling pathway in a zebrafish model.[51]

Small Molecule Inhibitors Targeting Oncogenic miRNAs

Some small molecules have been widely used against proteins involved in cancers. Examples include clinically successful imatinib mesylate (Gleevec) for the treatment of chronic myeloid leukemia.[52] Recently, potential miRNA-specific small molecule inhibitors were identified from a large-scale drug screening using a luciferase-based reporter assay.[53] A hit compound structurally related to diazobenzene 1 was found to reduce the transcription of the miR-21 gene into pri-miR-21 in vitro. However, no cytotoxic or non-specific effects on other processes were observed. Identification of other such small molecule inhibitors of miRNAs might be a useful supplement to conventional chemotherapeutic agents.

THE PROGRESS SO FAR—miRNAS IN PIPELINE

Given the broad range of cancer types affected by miRNAs and their important role as cellular regulators, the field of miRNAs is quickly transitioning from the laboratory bench to the patient bedside. Table 48.2 shows several candidates that have progressed into clinical trials and product development.[54] Among these are mimics of let-7 for lung and non–small cell lung cancers, and miR-34a for liver cancer. Several LNA-based AMOs are still in the preclinical stage for their evaluation in cancers. Other miRNAs currently in clinical trials for non-malignant diseases include miR-208, miR-499, and miR-195 for cardiovascular disorders, and miR-122 for human papilloma virus infections. Clinical trials are also ongoing for testing the effectiveness of miRNA signatures as diagnostic and prognostic markers.

TABLE 48–2 miRNA Therapeutics in Clinical and Preclinical Trials

Target miRNA	Disease Condition	Clinical Trial Stage
	miRNA Inhibition Therapy	
miR-122	HCV	Phase II clinical trials
miR-208 and miR-499	Chronic heart failure	Preclinical animal models
miR-195	Post-myocardial infarction	Preclinical animal models
	miRNA Replacement	
let-7	Lung and non–small-cell lung cancer	Preclinical animal models
miR-34a	Prostate and liver cancer	Preclinical animal models
	Other miRNA Combination Therapies	
miRNAs important in AML	AML	In clinical trials
miR-122 antagomir + HCV	HCV infection, hepatitis	In clinical trials
miRNAs important in AML	AML	In clinical trials
	miRNA Expression Profiling	
miRNAs expressed in the esophagus	Barrett's esophagus, esophageal adenocarcinoma	In clinical trials
miRNAs in renal cell carcinoma	Expression profile of miRNAs in renal cell carcinoma patients	In clinical trials
Circulating miRNAs as biomarkers for sepsis	Sepsis	In clinical trials
Levels of miRNA processing enzymes, Dicer and Drosha	Skin cancer	In clinical trials
miRNAs in inflammatory bowel disease	Inflammatory bowel disease	In clinical trials

HCV, hepatitis C virus; AML, acute myeloid leukemia.

ADVANTAGES OF MIRNA-BASED THERAPY

miRNA-based therapies offer several advantages over the conventional protein-based therapies. The most attractive quality of miRNA as therapeutic agents is their ability to regulate multiple genes, often in the perspective of a common network. Considering that cancer is a heterogeneous disease wherein distinct biological processes often get deregulated and hence cannot be treated by a single-agent therapy, this ability of miRNAs makes them particularly valuable. miRNAs can target multiple genes from the same pathway, and hence targeting of these miRNAs would enable a stronger, more cumulative effect on a set of related target proteins at multiple levels in the same pathway. Moreover, the discovery of more than 1,500 human miRNA adds significantly to the pool of novel druggable targets amenable to pharmacological intervention in cancer management.

The main drawback of protein-based chemotherapy is the adverse side effects experienced due to the off-target effects of these drugs on normal tissues. In contrast, miRNA therapy permits a more effective restoration of the distorted pathway to its normal physiological status. Restoring proteomic homeostasis by modifying miRNA expression in cancer cells may rewire the cell and reverse the cancer phenotype. In addition, since these are natural antisense interactors, their intercellular presence is not detected as non-self by our immune system, thus showing reduced immune response. Furthermore, the small size and low molecular weight of miRNAs render them as attractive options for clinical drug development.

Thus, a unique mechanism of action, an ability to function as master regulators of the human genome, and an apparent lack of adverse effects in normal tissues make miRNAs a promising therapeutic modality for cancer treatment.

THE CHALLENGES AHEAD—PRACTICAL ISSUES WITH MIRNA THERAPY

The major challenges to miRNA-based therapeutics are questions about the mode of delivery, potential off-target effects, and safety concerns.[55] The biological instability of unmodified naked RNAs and AMOs due to rapid degradation by cellular and serum nucleases makes their direct delivery an unfeasible option.[56,57] Additionally, their small size and negative charge could interfere with their ability to cross the cell membranes. Thus, they require some form of targeted delivery vehicle for sufficient tissue specificity and cellular uptake. Both viral and non-viral vehicles have been considered for RNA delivery. Viral options include the use of AAV vectors or lentiviral vectors. Long-lasting and stable knockdown of target transcription can be achieved by the expression of shRNAs from these vectors with either Pol II or Pol III promoters. However, continuous expression of miRNAs can lead to saturation of the endogenous processing machinery and to toxic side effects.[58] Furthermore, immune response induced by these viral vectors may prove to be harmful.

The non-viral delivery options include chemical modifications of the oligonucleotides, lipid complexes with small molecules, liposomes, polymers, antibodies, and nanoparticles.[59] Chemical modifications such as phosphorothioate backbone or cholesterol conjugation show improved stability and availability, but they are frequently associated with impaired function and severe toxicities.[57] The use of liposomes, cationic lipids, and nanoparticles has recently become a popular subject of study due to improved stability, cellular uptake, and biodistribution profile, but it is associated with enhanced immunogenicity.[20] Targeted delivery can also be achieved by tagging of the modified oligonucleotides with antibodies.

Route of administration is another important clinical consideration. Local administration is advantageous since it needs lower RNA doses, causes minor toxic reactions, and achieves better bioavailability of the drug to the target tissue.[34,60] However, local administration can be useful only for solid tumors, since local distribution will be of no use in hematological malignancies like leukemia. Local administration also does not facilitate exposure of metastasizing cancer cells in circulation to the RNA drugs. Systemic delivery is thus a better route of administration since it provides a more effective biodistribution to the target tissues. Nonetheless, barriers to in vivo systemic delivery of miRNAs include renal clearance, failure to cross the capillary endothelium (for RNAs conjugated with large molecules), limited passage through extracellular matrix, and destruction by scavenging macrophages.[60]

Thus, issues concerning stability, toxicity, and immunogenicity of these delivery methods need to be resolved for effective clinical usage of these therapeutic agents.

BEYOND THE BARRIERS—FUTURE DIRECTIONS

The discovery of miRNAs ushered in an era of novel therapeutic modalities for cancer treatment. The importance of these master regulators is evident in their swift adaptation into clinical practice. miRNA-based therapeutics hold great promise, both as novel biomarker and as highly specific, targeted therapies. However, a better understanding of its biogenesis and function will certainly help in the development of these therapies. Identification of all possible mechanisms of gene regulation will help fine-tune our understanding of the miRNA circuitry. Research efforts on improving their chemical designs and developing better delivery options to achieve superior sensitivity and specificity will be of crucial importance. Furthermore, long-term safety of these agents also needs to be evaluated before their transition into clinical use. Finally, more mechanistic studies to identify the interactions of miRNAs with human genome, transcriptome, and proteome will enable us to comprehend the underlying intricate network of molecular regulation. Overall, miRNA-based therapy has the potential to bring an exciting new facet to personalized medicine for cancer treatment; however, a deeper and clearer understanding of its biology is warranted. We are only just beginning to unravel the complexity of the gene regulatory circuitry controlled by miRNAs, with several gaping questions about the large landscape of human miRNome and transcriptome still remaining a mystery.

REFERENCES

1. Ambros V. The functions of animal microRNAs. *Nature*. 2004;431:350-355.
2. Lewis BP, Shih IH, Jones-Rhoades MW, et al. Prediction of mammalian microRNA targets. *Cell*. 2003;115:787-798.
3. He L, Hannon GJ. MicroRNAs: small RNAs with a big role in gene regulation. *Nat Rev Genet*. 2004;5:522-531.
4. Bartel DP. MicroRNAs: genomics, biogenesis, mechanism, and function. *Cell*. 2004;116:281-297.
5. Kim VN. MicroRNA biogenesis: coordinated cropping and dicing. *Nat Rev Mol Cell Biol*. 2005;6:376-385.
6. Vasudevan S, Tong Y, Steitz JA. Switching from repression to activation: microRNAs can up-regulate translation. *Science*. 2007;318:1931-1934.
7. Eiring AM, Harb JG, Neviani P, et al. miR-328 functions as an RNA decoy to modulate hnRNP E2 regulation of mRNA translation in leukemic blasts. *Cell*. 2010;140:652-665.
8. Kim DH, Saetrom P, Snove O Jr, Rossi JJ. MicroRNA-directed transcriptional gene silencing in mammalian cells. *Proc Natl Acad Sci U S A*. 2008;105:16230-16235.
9. Vogelstein B, Kinzler KW. Cancer genes and the pathways they control. *Nat Med*. 2004;10:789-799.
10. Trang P, Weidhaas JB, Slack FJ. MicroRNAs as potential cancer therapeutics. *Oncogene*. 2008;27(suppl 2):S52-S57.
11. Esquela-Kerscher A, Slack FJ. Oncomirs—microRNAs with a role in cancer. *Nat Rev Cancer*. 2006;6:259-269.
12. Calin GA, Croce CM. MicroRNA signatures in human cancers. *Nat Rev Cancer*. 2006;6:857-866.
13. Calin GA, Sevignani C, Dumitru CD, et al. Human microRNA genes are frequently located at fragile sites and genomic regions involved in cancers. *Proc Natl Acad Sci U S A*. 2004;101:2999-3004.
14. Croce CM. Causes and consequences of microRNA dysregulation in cancer. *Nat Rev Genet*. 2009;10:704-714.
15. Calin GA, Cimmino A, Fabbri M, et al. MiR-15a and miR-16-1 cluster functions in human leukemia. *Proc Natl Acad Sci U S A*. 2008;105:5166-5171.
16. Klein U, Lia M, Crespo M, et al. The DLEU2/miR-15a/16-1 cluster controls B cell proliferation and its deletion leads to chronic lymphocytic leukemia. *Cancer Cell*. 2010;17:28-40.
17. Asangani IA, Rasheed SA, Nikolova DA, et al. MicroRNA-21 (miR-21) post-transcriptionally downregulates tumor suppressor Pdcd4 and stimulates invasion, intravasation and metastasis in colorectal cancer. *Oncogene*. 2008;27:2128-2136.
18. Costinean S, Zanesi N, Pekarsky Y, et al. Pre-B cell proliferation and lymphoblastic leukemia/high-grade lymphoma in E(mu)-miR155 transgenic mice. *Proc Natl Acad Sci U S A*. 2006;103:7024-7029.
19. Medina PP, Nolde M, Slack FJ. OncomiR addiction in an in vivo model of microRNA-21-induced pre-B-cell lymphoma. *Nature*. 2010;467:86-90.
20. Garzon R, Marcucci G, Croce CM. Targeting microRNAs in cancer: rationale, strategies and challenges. *Nat Rev Drug Discov*. 2010;9:775-789.
21. Hanahan D, Weinberg RA. The hallmarks of cancer. *Cell*. 2000;100:57-70.
22. Hanahan D, Weinberg RA. Hallmarks of cancer: the next generation. *Cell*. 2011;144:646-674.
23. Dalmay T, Edwards DR. MicroRNAs and the hallmarks of cancer. *Oncogene*. 2006;25:6170-6175.

24. Nicoloso MS, Spizzo R, Shimizu M, et al. MicroRNAs--the micro steering wheel of tumour metastases. *Nat Rev Cancer.* 2009;9:293-302.
25. Stern-Ginossar N, Gur C, Biton M, et al. Human microRNAs regulate stress-induced immune responses mediated by the receptor NKG2D. *Nat Immunol.* 2008;9:1065-1073.
26. Esau C, Davis S, Murray SF, et al. miR-122 regulation of lipid metabolism revealed by in vivo antisense targeting. *Cell Metab.* 2006;3:87-98.
27. Chan SY, Zhang YY, Hemann C, et al. MicroRNA-210 controls mitochondrial metabolism during hypoxia by repressing the iron-sulfur cluster assembly proteins ISCU1/2. *Cell Metab.* 2009;10:273-284.
28. Schetter AJ, Heegaard NH, Harris CC. Inflammation and cancer: interweaving microRNA, free radical, cytokine and p53 pathways. *Carcinogenesis.* 2010;31:37-49.
29. Valeri N, Gasparini P, Fabbri M, et al. Modulation of mismatch repair and genomic stability by miR-155. *Proc Natl Acad Sci U S A.* 2010;107:6982-6987.
30. Cortez MA, Bueso-Ramos C, Ferdin J, et al. MicroRNAs in body fluids--the mix of hormones and biomarkers. *Nat Rev Clin Oncol.* 2011;8:467-477.
31. Salmena L, Poliseno L, Tay Y, et al. A ceRNA hypothesis: the Rosetta Stone of a hidden RNA language? *Cell.* 2011;146:353-358.
32. Karreth FA, Tay Y, Perna D, et al. In vivo identification of tumor-suppressive PTEN ceRNAs in an oncogenic BRAF-induced mouse model of melanoma. *Cell.* 2011;147:382-395.
33. Tay Y, Kats L, Salmena L, et al. Coding-independent regulation of the tumor suppressor PTEN by competing endogenous mRNAs. *Cell.* 2011;147:344-357.
34. Spizzo R, Rushworth D, Guerrero M, Calin GA. RNA inhibition, microRNAs, and new therapeutic agents for cancer treatment. *Clin Lymphoma Myeloma.* 2009;9(suppl 3):S313-S318.
35. Bonci D, Coppola V, Musumeci M, et al. The miR-15a-miR-16-1 cluster controls prostate cancer by targeting multiple oncogenic activities. *Nat Med.* 2008;14:1271-1277.
36. Esquela-Kerscher A, Trang P, Wiggins JF, et al. The let-7 microRNA reduces tumor growth in mouse models of lung cancer. *Cell Cycle.* 2008;7:759-764.
37. Trang P, Medina PP, Wiggins JF, et al. Regression of murine lung tumors by the let-7 microRNA. *Oncogene.* 2010;29:1580-1587.
38. Fujita Y, Kojima K, Hamada N, et al. Effects of miR-34a on cell growth and chemoresistance in prostate cancer PC3 cells. *Biochem Biophys Res Commun.* 2008;377:114-119.
39. Kota J, Chivukula RR, O'Donnell KA, et al. Therapeutic microRNA delivery suppresses tumorigenesis in a murine liver cancer model. *Cell.* 2009;137:1005-1017.
40. Chung KH, Hart CC, Al-Bassam S, et al. Polycistronic RNA polymerase II expression vectors for RNA interference based on BIC/miR-155. *Nucleic Acids Res.* 2006;34:e53.
41. Hutvagner G, Simard MJ, Mello CC, Zamore PD. Sequence-specific inhibition of small RNA function. *PLoS Biol.* 2004;2:E98.
42. Krutzfeldt J, Rajewsky N, Braich R, et al. Silencing of microRNAs in vivo with "antagomirs". *Nature.* 2005;438:685-689.
43. Krutzfeldt J, Kuwajima S, Braich R, et al. Specificity, duplex degradation and subcellular localization of antagomirs. *Nucleic Acids Res.* 2007;35:2885-2892.
44. Vester B, Wengel J. LNA (locked nucleic acid): high-affinity targeting of complementary RNA and DNA. *Biochemistry.* 2004;43:13233-13241.
45. Chan JA, Krichevsky AM, Kosik KS. MicroRNA-21 is an antiapoptotic factor in human glioblastoma cells. *Cancer Res.* 2005;65:6029-6033.
46. Zimmermann TS, Lee AC, Akinc A, et al. RNAi-mediated gene silencing in non-human primates. *Nature.* 2006;441:111-114.
47. Lanford RE, Hildebrandt-Eriksen ES, Petri A, et al. Therapeutic silencing of microRNA-122 in primates with chronic hepatitis C virus infection. *Science.* 2010;327:198-201.
48. Ebert MS, Neilson JR, Sharp PA. MicroRNA sponges: competitive inhibitors of small RNAs in mammalian cells. *Nat Methods.* 2007;4:721-726.
49. Care A, Catalucci D, Felicetti F, et al. MicroRNA-133 controls cardiac hypertrophy. *Nat Med.* 2007;13:613-618.
50. Xiao J, Yang B, Lin H, et al. Novel approaches for gene-specific interference via manipulating actions of microRNAs: examination on the pacemaker channel genes HCN2 and HCN4. *J Cell Physiol.* 2007;212:285-292.
51. Choi WY, Giraldez AJ, Schier AF. Target protectors reveal dampening and balancing of Nodal agonist and antagonist by miR-430. *Science.* 2007;318:271-274.
52. Kantarjian HM, Talpaz M, Giles F, et al. New insights into the pathophysiology of chronic myeloid leukemia and imatinib resistance. *Ann Intern Med.* 2006;145:913-923.
53. Gumireddy K, Young DD, Xiong X, et al. Small-molecule inhibitors of microRNA miR-21 function. *Angew Chem Int Ed Engl.* 2008;47:7482-7484.
54. Wahid F, Shehzad A, Khan T, Kim YY. MicroRNAs: synthesis, mechanism, function, and recent clinical trials. *Biochim Biophys Acta.* 2010;1803:1231-1243.
55. Castanotto D, Rossi JJ. The promises and pitfalls of RNA-interference-based therapeutics. *Nature.* 2009;457:426-433.
56. Aagaard L, Rossi JJ. RNAi therapeutics: principles, prospects and challenges. *Adv Drug Deliv Rev.* 2007;59:75-86.
57. Zhao X, Pan F, Holt CM, et al. Controlled delivery of antisense oligonucleotides: a brief review of current strategies. *Expert Opin Drug Deliv.* 2009;6:673-686.
58. Grimm D, Streetz KL, Jopling CL, et al. Fatality in mice due to oversaturation of cellular microRNA/short hairpin RNA pathways. *Nature.* 2006;441:537-541.
59. Vorhies JS, Nemunaitis J. Nonviral delivery vehicles for use in short hairpin RNA-based cancer therapies. *Expert Rev Anticancer Ther.* 2007;7:373-382.
60. Bader AG, Brown D, Stoudemire J, Lammers P. Developing therapeutic microRNAs for cancer. *Gene Ther.* 2011;18:1121-1126.

CHAPTER 49

Molecular Basis of Cancer Radiation Treatment

Heath Skinner, Amit Deorukhkar, and Sunil Krishnan

Within only a few years following the discovery of x-rays by Roentgen in 1895, this form of ionizing radiation (IR) was applied therapeutically for human malignancy.[1] Since that time, the basis for the action of IR in cancer has transitioned from description of the in vitro and in vivo effects of radiation to a more in-depth understanding of the molecular basis of its therapeutic effect. In this review, we describe the direct effects of IR at the level of the nucleus (primarily DNA damage) as well as the cytoplasm. We then describe some of the key pathways activated by IR and their role in the radiation response. We finally describe some of the key modes of cellular death and arrest induced by IR and conclude with an overview of the bystander effect.

EACH JOURNEY BEGINS WITH A FIRST STEP—EVENTS TRIGGERED BY RADIATION WITHIN A CELL

For many decades, the conceptual underpinning of radiobiology has hinged on the notion that the intrinsic radiosensitivity of tumors is governed by the balance between DNA damage and DNA repair following irradiation. Certainly, there is a large correlation between the extent of radiation-induced DNA damage and the cellular consequences in a tumor cell. At the same time, there has been an increasing recognition that IR not only damages DNA in the cell but also affects several disparate cellular components and these collectively elicit a calibrated and integrated biological response in the irradiated tumor cell. Recent data indicate that both the fate of damaged DNA and the cascade of radiation-induced cytoplasmic signaling events contribute to cellular radiosensitivity.[2] The cellular signaling triggered by therapeutic doses of IR (1 to 5 Gy) occurs at two distinct sites—(i) nuclear signaling events initiated by DNA damage and culminating in blockade of cell cycle progression through G1 and G2/M in an attempt to potentially allow the repair of DNA damage and (ii) cytoplasmic signaling beginning at the receptor level and progressing through ligand-dependent receptor tyrosine kinase (RTK) activation or via reactive oxygen species (ROS)–mediated ligand-independent tyrosine kinase activation.[2,3]

Nuclear Events: Safeguarding the Genetic Code and Machinery

Generally, IR can affect changes in DNA either directly via energy absorption and generation of ion pairs or indirectly via the formation of free radicals in the water surrounding DNA. In either case, the presence of avid ions in proximity to the DNA can lead to (i) alterations in the structure of one or more nitrogenous bases, (ii) a break in the hydrogen bonds between bases, and (iii) a break between one of the deoxyribose sugar and phosphate groups. This damage leads to structural alterations in DNA and, ultimately, chromosomal alteration.

The cell is provided with a number of mechanisms to repair damage to the DNA, which is necessary considering that each day the genome is subjected to thousands of insults that, left unrepaired, could lead to significant abnormality and cellular toxicity or carcinogenesis. Broadly, the cellular response to DNA damage can be divided into two groups: single-stranded and double-stranded DNA repair. Single-stranded breaks (SSBs) in DNA can usually be repaired by the cell, as a template for repair is readily accessible. As such, this type of DNA break is usually nonlethal. Although IR can certainly lead to SSBs, this is not the primary mode of IR-induced lethality and, as such, will not be a focus of this review.

Far more toxic to the cell are double-stranded breaks (DSBs) in the DNA. The frequency of DSBs correlates with in vitro IR-induced toxicity and has been a primary focus of research in examining the effect of IR upon the cancer cell. Unrepaired DSBs can lead to either chromosomal deletion or an aberrant chromosome at the time of mitosis, either of which can result in cell death. The cell has evolved two primary modes of DSB repair: homologous recombination (HR) and non-homologous end joining (NHEJ).

HR involves the use of a sister chromatid as a template for repair; as such, only in the latter portion of S-phase and G2 can this process occur. HR begins by the recognition of the DSB by the Mre11-Rad50-Nbs1 (MRN) complex. This complex aggregates at the site of DSBs and forms foci leading to the eventual synthesis of a new strand of DNA. This involves the generation of a single-stranded region of DNA (ssDNA), invasion of the template strand to create a Holliday junction, DNA synthesis using the sister strand as a template, branch migration, and resolution of the heteroduplex. Rad51, a central player in HR, is loaded onto ssDNA and promotes strand invasion, with Breast Cancer 2 susceptibility protein (BRCA2) having a role in delivering Rad51 to the DNA.[4]

Conversely, NHEJ, which is the major route for DSB repair in the G0/G1 phases of the cell cycle, does not require the presence of a sister chromatid, but instead makes use of microhomologies present in the single-strand overhangs at the end of DSBs. This process frequently results in the loss of nucleotides or translocations. Briefly, the MRN complex is again recruited to DSBs and recognizes microhomologies present within single-strand overhangs. The Ku 70/80 heterodimer also recognizes these DSBs and forms a complex with DNA-dependent protein kinase, catalytic subunit (DNA-PKcs). This complex surrounds the DNA and can serve as a docking site for other proteins involved in NHEJ. Damaged or mismatched nucleotides are then removed via nucleases, the identity of which is not completely known in eukaryotic cells; however, the nuclease Artemis is thought to play a role.[5] The gaps in DNA are then filled by DNA polymerases pol λ and pol μ and the resultant strands are then joined via a complex of XRCC4 (x-ray-complementing Chinese hamster gene 4) and DNA ligase IV[6], which facilitate the final ligation step.

At the level of DSBs, multiple nuclear signaling molecules are involved in sensing the DSBs, recruiting repair proteins to the sites of DNA DSBs,[7,8] arresting the cell cycle to allow repair, and triggering apoptosis if the repair of the damaged DNA is not possible. Two kinases from the phosphatidylinositol-3-kinase (PI3K)–related kinase family, ataxia-telangiectasia mutated (ATM) and ATR (ATM and RAD3 related), orchestrate the cellular response to DSBs. ATM is activated when it is recruited to sites of DSB damage by the MRN complex.[9-12] When activated, ATM phosphorylates a spectrum of proteins, including p53, CHK1 and CHK2 kinases, and histone 2AX (H2AX), which arrest cell cycle progression in preparation for an attempt at DNA repair.[13] ATR phosphorylates CHK1 and the DNA helicase BLM1, which act as "transducers" to modulate apoptosis, DNA repair, and cell cycle arrest. Activation of CHK1 and CHK2 kinases primarily leads to cell cycle arrest at G2/M or S to facilitate the repair process.[14]

Cytoplasmic Events: Taking Stock of Survival Instincts Inside the Cell

Although the effects of IR on DNA can be profound, IR can directly affect other components of the cell, as well. Notably, IR treatment selectively targeting the cytoplasm leads to IR-induced micronuclei formation in surrounding cells.[15] One of the best studied non-nuclear targets of IR is plasma membrane sphingomyelin. Following high-dose IR, sphingomyelin is rapidly hydrolyzed to ceramide via acid sphingomyelinase, a function that may be required for IR-induced apoptosis in some cell types.[16] Ceramide can then activate a variety of downstream pathways to induce apoptosis, including (i) ceramide-activated protein kinases (PKCζ) and kinase suppressor of Ras (KSR), (ii) cathepsin D, and (iii) protein phosphatase 1 and 2.[17] For example, activation of KSR by ceramide leads to the phosphorylation of c-Raf, activation of ERK 1/2 signaling, and, in some cases, apoptosis.[18,19]

Alternatively, ceramide can promote membrane-associated receptor activation by facilitating the clustering of receptors within the lipid rafts.[20] This activation of RTKs (cell surface receptors with intrinsic tyrosine kinase activity) initiates a cascade of proliferative signaling events activating a number of proteins.[21,22] The best characterized among these is signaling through the members of the ErbB/epidermal growth factor receptor (EGFR) family, which often determines the resistance of cells to chemotherapy or radiotherapy.[23-25] Activated ErbBs stimulate many intracellular signaling pathways, and different ErbBs preferentially modulate specific signaling pathways. Two of the main pathways activated by the receptors are the RAS-Raf-MAPK (mitogen-activated protein kinase) and the PI3K/Akt (protein kinase B) pathways. Other important ErbB signaling effectors include (i) the signal transducer and activator of transcription proteins (STATs), (ii) SRC tyrosine kinase, and (iii) the serine/threonine kinase mammalian target of rapamycin (mTOR). These downstream signaling networks play important roles in tumor radiosensitivity by eliciting pro-survival responses and will be discussed in further detail separately.

In contrast to the nuclear signaling, IR-induced cytoplasmic signaling events appear to be much more diverse and intricately hardwired together. In addition to signaling via ceramide, the redox imbalance generated by IR in the cytosol is amplified within the mitochondria and results in sufficient activation of ROS and reactive nitrogen species to inhibit protein tyrosine phosphatases (PTPase).[26] Inhibition of PTPases leads to activation of RTKs and non-RTKs and activation of downstream signaling pathways discussed above.

Convergence of the Nuclear and Cytoplasmic Signaling: Activation of Transcription Factors and Alteration of Gene Expression

Signaling from the cell surface receptors and from the damaged DNA leads to downstream pathways that ultimately result in activation of a variety of transcription factors (TFs) that play a pivotal role in dictating the expression patterns of a diverse set of genes. Among the most important TFs induced by radiation are the nuclear factor kappa B (NF-κB) family of proteins, the STATs, and activator protein-1, which govern various aspects of cellular proliferation, invasion, metastasis, inflammation, and chemoresistance and radioresistance. The first two TFs are especially important as they both are known to be constitutively activated in many cancers and are also linked to chemoresistance and radioresistance.[27-30]

Once activated, these TFs translocate to the nucleus, where they bind to specific DNA sites and engineer an effector response, i.e., trigger the expression of specific genes involved in intricately coordinated regulatory signaling networks. NF-κB alone regulates the expression of genes involved in cell proliferation (cyclin D1), angiogenesis (vascular endothelial growth factor), invasion (matrix metalloproteinases), and a variety of pro-inflammatory genes like tumor necrosis factor (TNF)-α, interleukin (IL)-1, and IL-8, and even chemokine receptors (CXCR4).[30] Activated STAT3 dictates the expression of a multitude of proteins involved in apoptosis, proliferation, and inflammation such as cyclin D1, Bcl-XL, and IL-8. As the cell produces these growth factors and angiogenic factors in response to radiotherapy through the activation of TFs, this also forms one of the underlying mechanisms of inducible radioresistance.[31] Thus, IR-induced signaling within tumor cells leads to converging responses resulting in either of two divergent options—a proliferative pro-survival response or death due to genotoxic/cytotoxic stress.

In the succeeding paragraphs, we provide an overview of the key molecular players that drive these responses and the consequences of a cell going down the road to recovery and resurrection (radiation-induced pro-survival signaling) versus the road to perdition (radiation-induced cell death). We will start with molecular pathways activated in response to a sublethal dose of IR—i.e., those that drive proliferative and pro-survival signals that overcome radiation-induced cell death.

SIGNALING PATHWAYS ALONG THE ROAD TO RECOVERY AND RESURRECTION (RADIATION-INDUCED PRO-SURVIVAL SIGNALING)

Mitogen-Activated Protein Kinases

The MAPKs are a family of kinases comprising at least three members: extracellular signal-regulated kinase (ERK), JNK, and p38-MAPK, which transduce signals from the cell membrane to the nucleus in response to a wide range of stimuli including proliferative signals and cytotoxic stresses.[32] Exposure of cells to physiological stresses such as IR can induce simultaneous activation of multiple MAPK pathways. The mechanism of radiation-induced MAPK pathways varies by cell type and is influenced by the expression of varied growth factor receptors, autocrine factors, and *Ras* mutation status. Activating mutations of K-/N-*Ras* result in constitutively active downstream signaling that, in turn, promotes growth and radiation resistance via the NF-κB, multiple MAPK, or the PI3K pathways, depending on the cell.[33]

In general, the MAPK pathway consists of a series of phosphorylation cascades in which the signal is sequentially transduced from MAPK kinase kinases to MAPK kinases to one of the MAPKs (ERK, JNK, and p38), resulting in the activation of TFs, progression through the cell cycle, and eventual cellular proliferation and survival. The most common extrinsic trigger of this pathway is growth factor/cytokine/mitogen stimulation of the appropriate (cognate) membrane-bound receptor that leads to convergence of signals on the MAPK cascade via the Ras/Raf/mitogen-activated protein kinase (MEK)/ERK proteins. Typically, upon receptor stimulation, an Src homology 2 domain–containing protein (SHC) becomes associated with the C-terminal intracellular domain of the activated receptor. SHC then recruits the growth factor receptor–bound protein 2 and the son of sevenless homolog 1 protein, resulting in activation and membrane localization of Ras via GTP. Ras:GTP then recruits Raf to the membrane where it becomes activated.[34] Raf then transduces the signal downstream, by phosphorylating MEK1, which, in turn, phosphorylates ERK. Activated ERK1 and ERK2 phosphorylate a variety of other substrates which promote cell growth. Exposure to IR induces ERK activation in cells, which is best known to be mediated via radiation-induced EGFR phosphorylation. EGFR is activated in response to clinically relevant doses of 2 to 5 Gy, and this, in turn, can result in activation of ERK in a radiation dose-dependent manner.[33] Apart from radiation-induced RTK phosphorylation, ERbB receptor autocrine ligands also play an important role in ERK activation after radiation exposure; for example, transforming growth factor (TGF)-α is known to mediate secondary activation of the EGFR and downstream activation of the ERK and JNK pathways in a dose-dependent manner.[35,36] Radiation exposure leads to cleavage of pro-TGF-α in the plasma membrane, resulting in its release into the growth media and dose-dependent activation of the ERK and JNK.

JNK (c-Jun N-terminal kinase), also known as stress-activated MAP kinase, a member of the MAP kinase family, also plays a critical role in cell proliferation and apoptosis. JNKs can be activated by a plethora of stimuli, including growth factors, cytokines, and stress (including radiation). The fate of the cell after JNK activation (proliferation vs. cell death) chiefly depends on the type of stimulus and the cell type.[37] There appear to be three distinct mechanisms by which IR activates JNK pathway: (i) IR-induced ceramide generation and the clustering of death receptors on the plasma membrane, (ii) activation of ATM and c-ABL proteins, and (iii) activation via autocrine factors such as TNF-α, EGF, and TGF-β.

PI3K/Akt

The PI3K/Akt signaling pathway is vital to cellular function and is constitutively activated in many cancers.[38] In addition, sublethal doses of IR activate the PI3K/Akt cascade in some cellular contexts—the subsequent stimulation of a cytoprotective response (inhibition of apoptosis and cell cycle arrest) results in increased radioresistance.[39,40] IR-induced PI3K/Akt activation is thought to be mediated at least in part through ERbB tyrosine kinases (such as activation of EGFR). Furthermore, PI3K/Akt can govern intrinsic tumor radiosensitivity via modulation of the DNA repair mechanism, primarily through DNA-PKcs.[41] As stated above, PI3K/Akt activation can also directly influence activation of TF NF-κB, which mediates cytoprotective, inflammatory, and radioresistance responses. PI3K/Akt activation is also vital for the hypoxic response as its activation is essential for hypoxia-inducible factor-1–dependent gene transcription and the subsequent activation of angiogenesis.[42-44] Taken together, radiation-induced activation of the PI3K/Akt pathway elicits diverse cellular responses that govern cell proliferation, DNA repair, and cellular response to hypoxic conditions, all of which contribute to radioresistance.

NF-κB

TF NF-κB regulates inducible gene expression in response to various physiological scenarios via a family of closely related proteins, namely p65 (RelA), RelB, c-Rel, p50/p105 (NF-κB1), and p52 (NF-κB2). Dimers of NF-κB proteins, all of which share an amino-terminal REL homology domain, bind to the κB sites (common sequence motifs in DNA) in promoter or enhancer sequences of target genes and regulate their transcription through the recruitment of transcriptional co-activators and transcriptional co-repressors. NF-κB plays a crucial role in both cancer progression and treatment response as it is constitutively activated in diverse solid malignancies, but not their normal counterparts.[27,45,46] Under normal unstimulated conditions, the NF-κB dimers are sequestered in the cytoplasm by their association with inhibitors of κB (IκBs), which mask the nuclear localization sequence (NLS) of NF-κB. A wide variety of factors such as free radicals, cytokines, IR, growth factors, and multiple cellular stresses are capable of activating these dimers. IR induces NF-κB activation, and consequent tumor radioresistance, through several distinct mechanisms.[47] NF-κB can be activated by signaling through the nucleus, from the cytoplasm, or both.

The activation of NF-κB from nuclear signals is initiated when DNA DSBs transmit a stress signal to the cytoplasm through NEMO (NF-κB essential modulator) and ATM.[48] DNA DSBs activate nuclear ATM kinase which activates ATM which, in turn, phosphorylates SUMO-modified NEMO to remove small ubiquitin-like modifier (SUMO) and facilitate the export of NEMO from the cytoplasm. Cytoplasmic NEMO (still associated with ATM and now associated with ubiquitin) then associates with, and activates, the IKK (IκB kinase) complex, which triggers NF-κB activation.

NF-κB activation signals can also be received from cell membrane via growth factor receptors and other pro-survival proteins upstream of IKK. The PI3K/Akt/PKB pathway is probably the most important pathway known to activate NF-κB, leading to increased antiapoptotic, proliferative, and pro-inflammatory gene expression.[49] Not only growth factor signaling cascades but many cytokine receptors also play an important role in radiation-induced NF-κB activation. For instance, IR activates the TNF-α receptor, which is probably the best described activator of NF-κB. This autocrine secretion of TNF-α is, at least in part, known to play a role in radiation-induced NF-κB activation, as inhibition of this function can lead to tumor radiosensitization.[3]

Essentially, all the NF-κB activation pathways converge upon activation of the IKK complex (IKKα, IKKβ, and IKKγ/NEMO, with IKKβ as the catalytic subunit).[50,51] First, IKK is activated via phosphorylation of IKKβ, which, in turn, phosphorylates IκB, triggering polyubiquitinylation of IκB and its rapid proteasomal degradation. This process exposes the NLS signal on p65 and p50, resulting in nuclear translocation of NF-κB to promote gene transcription. Activated NF-κB can induce gene expression of over 200 genes that are involved in the inhibition of apoptosis, induction of cellular proliferation, enhanced invasive and metastatic phenotype, and inflammation in a wide variety of tumors.[52] IR-induced NF-κB expression in cancer cells is transient, peaking within a few minutes following exposure to IR and returning to baseline levels after a few hours. However, this transiently activated NF-κB can elicit multiple radioresistance signals that can attenuate the lethal effects of radiation.[53]

STATs

The STAT proteins are a family of TFs that play a critical role in inflammation as well as the immune response. These proteins are activated by a wide variety of upstream kinases including Janus kinase, as well as multiple cytokine receptors and growth factor receptors. Once activated, the STATs can then bind DNA and affect the upregulation of pro-inflammatory genes, such as COX-2, IL-6, and IL-8, with the end result being the promotion of cell survival. Furthermore, this pathway exhibits significant cross talk with the NF-κB pathway, which represents yet another level of control of pro-inflammatory and survival signaling. STAT activity, particularly the activity of STAT-3 and STAT-1, has been implicated in IR resistance.[47] Proteomic profiling of radioresistant cells consistently shows upregulation of STAT activity. Furthermore, inhibition of each of these proteins has been shown to increase sensitivity to IR in vitro.

CONSEQUENCES OF TAKING THE ROAD TO PERDITION (RADIATION-INDUCED CELL DEATH)

Apoptosis

Many studies of IR-induced cell death, particularly in hematopoietic cells, initially found a large degree of cell death usually within hours after IR, linked to the induction of apoptosis by IR. Apoptosis is defined as programmed cell death, associated with chromatin condensation, nuclear blebbing, and cell shrinkage and broadly occurs via two mechanisms: the intrinsic and extrinsic pathways. Both pathways require the cleavage of inactive pro-caspase forms to their active forms. The extrinsic pathway is primarily activated via cell surface receptors (e.g., Fas/FasL) and is dependent upon the activation of caspase 8. However, IR-induced apoptosis is thought to primarily occur via activation of the intrinsic pathway and is dependent upon the release of cytochrome c from the mitochondria, leading to the activation of caspase 9. The intrinsic and extrinsic pathways converge primarily on caspase 3, 6, and 7 to initiate apoptosis. These effector caspases in turn cleave and activate a number of substrates, such as poly(ADP-ribose) polymerase (PARP), leading ultimately to cell cycle arrest and dismantling of the cytoskeleton.

Studying the effects of IR-induced apoptosis is complicated by the cell type–specific forms of apoptosis observed. Cells of hematopoietic or lymphocytic lineage undergo rapid apoptosis following IR; however, other cell types may take up to 96 hours to undergo apoptosis following radiation.[54] This effect is further complicated in cancer cells by one of the master regulators of apoptosis, the protein p53. Among other functions, wild-type p53 is stabilized by ATM following IR and leads to cytochrome c release and subsequent apoptosis via the intrinsic pathway. In non-transformed cells, p53 also leads to G1 arrest following IR, allowing for repair of IR-induced DNA damage. However, in cancer cells, p53 is frequently mutated, inhibiting its function in one or both of these responses to IR. This, among other cellular alterations, leads to a diminished apoptotic response in many, if not most, solid tumor cells. Furthermore, when examining sensitivity to IR in vitro, in vivo, or clinically, no measure of apoptosis is reliably correlated with response in cancer cells of epithelial origin.[55] Thus, while IR-induced apoptosis appears to be critical in the case of hematologic or lymphocytic cells, and despite the intense study of IR-induced apoptosis, the case for its importance as a meaningful response to IR in cells derived from solid tumors remains weak.[56]

Mitotic Catastrophe

One of the primary forms of cell death induced by IR in epithelial tumor cells appears to be mitotic death or mitotic catastrophe (MC).[57] This form of cell death occurs after one or several cell divisions following IR and is characterized by aberrant mitosis as well as the formation of multinucleated giant cells or large cells with multiple micronuclei. MC appears to be linked to alterations in the normal functioning of either the G2/M or mitotic spindle checkpoint within the cell cycle, with inhibition of such proteins as chk1 and chk2, cdk1, or Aurora kinase–inducing MC.[58] While certainly important to the cytotoxicity induced by IR, the primary measure of MC in vitro is the microscopic visualization of multinucleated cells or micronuclei, with no real quantitative assay available. Furthermore, the question of cell death after the aforementioned phenotypic changes remains. Several authors have speculated that these cells undergo necrosis, while others have argued that MC represents a special form of delayed apoptosis, particularly in light of some studies showing mitochondrial alteration and caspase activation in MC cells.[59] However, this process is largely p53-independent, in stark contrast to the more common conception of apoptosis as a p53-dependent phenomenon. In fact, it is thought that cells resistant to apoptosis are driven to polyploidy and MC secondary to a dysfunctional checkpoint within the cell cycle. Thus, the exact nature of cell death following MC has yet to be elucidated.

Necrosis

In contrast to other forms of cell death, necrosis is largely a disordered cell death, most often observed after severe stressors or physico-chemical damage to the cell (e.g., severe nutrient deprivation, anoxia, and dramatic changes in temperature or irradiation). Morphologic characteristics of this mode of cell death include swelling of the cytoplasm and organelles with eventual rupture of the cellular membrane. This leads to a brisk immune response within the host, which has been implicated in the modulation of tumor response to radiotherapy.[60] Some element of chromatin condensation and DNA degradation is observed; however, this process is thought to be largely caspase independent and may instead be dependent upon the function of proteases, such as calpains and cathepsins, within the cell.[61-63] At the level of the cell membrane, there is a rapid loss of potential, due to energy depletion in the cell and subsequent loss of function of ATP-dependent ion transport or physical damage of the lipid bilayer. Following this disruption of cellular homeostasis, in particular dramatically increased levels of intracellular Ca^{2+}, mitochondrial dysfunction within the dying cell results in the release of large amounts of ROS, leading to organelle and DNA damage, furthering the process of necrotic cell death. Also, ROS can activate PARP which, although usually associated with apoptosis, can also induce necrosis by depleting the intracellular NAD pool and with a resultant decrease in ATP production.[64]

As mentioned previously, calpains and cathepsins are active in necrosis. Among other functions, these proteases increase lysosome permeability during necrosis, leading to lysosomal rupture and exposure of intracellular structures to enzymatic degradation. Furthermore, the receptor-interacting serine/threonine-protein kinase 1 (RIPK1) has been implicated in the regulation of necrosis in some cellular contexts. Deficiencies in RIPK1 decrease death receptor–mediated necrosis, and RIPK1 has been shown to translocate to the mitochondria in response to cellular stressors and enhance ROS production.[65] However, the exact mechanism of RIPK1 or other cascades involved in the regulation of necrosis has yet to be elucidated.

Autophagy

Another outcome of IR in the cell is autophagy, a process involving the controlled catabolism of intracellular components via lysosomal degradation. Generally, the process of autophagy begins with the production of an autophagosome, which sequesters cytoplasm and intracellular organelles within a bilayer membrane. This autophagosome then fuses with a lysosome, leading to degradation of its contents. Autophagy has historically been associated with nutrient deprivation and represents a cellular adaptation to provide additional energy in extremis. This process is to a large degree controlled by AMP-activated kinase (AMPK) and mTOR. Under normal conditions, AMPK is suppressed and mTOR can inactivate the ULK1 complex (composed of ULK1/2, Atg13, Atg101, and FIP200).[66,67] However, under stress conditions, AMPK inhibits mTOR function; thus ULK1 repression is released, leading to the initiation of the autophagocytic process. Another key signal for initiation of autophagy is the activation of a complex composed of Vps34 and Beclin 1. This complex comprises a functional class 3 PI3K, which produces phosphatidylinositol-3-phosphate and is required for autophagy. The resulting cellular processes are complex and are in the process of being clearly defined; however, two additional proteins, LC-3 and ATG12, appear to be critical for autophagy to continue once initiated.

IR appears to induce autophagy in a number of different cell types; however, it is unclear as to whether this represents a mechanism of cell death to be exploited therapeutically or a mechanism of cellular resistance to IR.[68] In many—but not all—cell types with limited apoptotic potential following IR, induction of autophagy appears to correlate with cell death. Thus, there is speculation that IR-induced autophagy occurs on a spectrum, with a threshold that must be reached before it results in pro-cell death.[58] Below this hypothesized threshold, autophagy could be protective following IR by providing energy for cytoprotective mechanisms within the cell. However, the exact role of autophagy in response to IR is by no means established.

Senescence

A final possible cellular response to IR is the process of cellular senescence, a usually irreversible process of growth arrest resulting in a non-proliferative, but viable cell. Morphologic changes seen in senescent cells include a flattened, "pancake" appearance as well as a granular cytoplasm. Furthermore, these cells can be identified via staining for senescence-associated β-galactosidase, which is active in senescent cells. Replicative senescence was first described in cultured fibroblasts after numerous passages and is due, in large part, to severe telomere shortening and eventual malfunction in the absence of telomerase.[69] This process has been shown to be critical in the process of aging, as well as in several disease states. Furthermore, cytotoxic therapies, including IR, as well as some oncogenic signals (e.g., Ras) can induce a similar process in cells, albeit likely via a different mechanism.[70] In senescent cells, growth arrest is maintained either at G1 or at the G2/M checkpoint largely via the activation of p21 and/or p16, which represent the targets of the two primary mediators of senescence activation, p53 and retinoblastoma protein (Rb). Depending upon the model one or both of these pathways are involved in the induction or maintenance of the senescent phenotype after cytotoxic therapy. However, as IR-induced senescence has also been seen in the absence of either p53 or Rb, other as yet incompletely defined pathways can lead to the senescent phenotype.[70,71] Intracellular ROS levels are also key mediators of IR-induced senescence, in regard to both initiation of senescence and its maintenance.[72-74] Prolonged ROS exposure following IR may lead to chronic DNA damage and upregulation of p21 and p16 necessary for senescence maintenance.

Senescent cells, while non-replicative, may remain viable for prolonged periods of time in vivo, and thus the question remains as to the long-term fate of senescent cells in the body following IR; however, there are some data to suggest that eventually senescent cells become nonviable in vivo.[70] In contrast, some in vitro data suggest that, after exogenous genetic manipulation, senescent cells can reenter the cell cycle, an observation yet to be seen in vivo under non-experimentally manipulated conditions.[70,75]

The question of the relevance of IR-induced senescence to therapeutic response remains unanswered. As this process can occur in a variety of different cellular backgrounds, particularly in the background of absence and at least some forms of mutated p53, it would seem likely that IR-induced senescence would be an important aspect of the clinical response to IR in solid tumors. Preliminary clinical data have linked IR-induced senescence to radiosensitivity; however, it remains to be seen if modulating this mode of response is of therapeutic value.[72]

Traveling Companions—The Bystander Effect

Adding to the complexity of the cellular response to IR, many non-target effects of this treatment have been observed. Specifically, cells that have not been directly treated with IR can be forced to exhibit a response if placed in proximity to cells that have been irradiated, a phenomenon dubbed the "bystander effect." This bystander effect is seen in the context of (i) co-culture experiments with irradiated and non-irradiated cells; (ii) microbeam irradiation, which can be focused at the cellular level; and (iii) incubation of non-irradiated cells with medium from irradiated cells. The phenomenon has also been observed in vivo in multiple studies.[76-79] The mechanism of this phenomenon likely involves the release of cytokines and other factors, including ROS, interleukin 8, TGF-β, Fas ligand, TRAIL, and TNF-α,[80] by the irradiated cell as well as direct cell–cell communication through gap junctions.

At the level of the bystander cell, significant nuclear and mitochondrial DNA damage has been observed, although in a prolonged time frame. This has been linked to intracellular ROS levels either via direct communication between irradiated and non-irradiated cells or in an increase of intracellular ROS production in the non-irradiated bystander cell. Regardless, the bystander effect is substantially inhibited by the presence of antioxidants and potentiated by the manipulations designed to enhance the production of ROS. Furthermore, DNA repair proteins (e.g., γ-H2AX, ATM, and DNA-PKcs) have been shown to be required for the bystander effect to occur in some systems, arguing DNA damage in the bystander cell is affected by irradiated cells. In both oxidative stress and activation of DNA repair, a number of signaling cascades are activated in bystander cells, paralleling many of the pathways activated in directly irradiated cells. For example, the activation of MAPK, ERK 1/2, JNKs, and NF-κB has been observed in bystander cells. Furthermore, in cells with functional p53, levels of this protein, as well as its transcriptional targets, have been shown to be elevated in bystander cells. Downstream of these events, bystander cells have been shown to have increased levels of genetic instability, micronuclei and apoptosis with commiserate decreased clonogenic survival, as well as in vivo viability.

SUMMARY

Early efforts to explain the effects of radiation on cells centered on its effects on DNA at the cellular level. Clonogenic cell survival, and therefore radiosensitivity, was viewed as a function of cellular response to this genotoxic stress. In turn, resistance to radiation was seen as stemming from physiological phenomena occurring to surviving cells between radiation fractions—namely, repopulation, re-assortment of cells to more radioresistant phases of the cell cycle, impaired re-oxygenation of radioresistant hypoxic cells, and repair of radiation-induced DNA strand breaks. While these early phenomenological observations still explain a lot of what transpires within cells and tissues following radiation, a more molecular understanding of these phenomena has opened up the possibility of specifically exploiting these response pathways or interrupting these resistance pathways to achieve greater radiation treatment efficacy. This monograph provides a unified compilation of the multiple events triggered by radiation within a cell, the divergent paths taken by cells that succumb to radiation-induced cell death versus that taken by cells that survive, and the role of unirradiated companions of irradiated cells in modulating the eventual response of tissues to radiation.

REFERENCES

1. Grubbe E. X-rays in the treatment of cancer and other malignant diseases. *Med Rec*. 1902;62(18):692.
2. Szumiel I. Intrinsic radiation sensitivity: cellular signaling is the key. *Radiat Res*. 2008;169(3):249-258.
3. Valerie K, Yacoub A, Hagan MP, et al. Radiation-induced cell signaling: inside-out and outside-in. *Mol Cancer Ther*. 2007;6(3):789-801.
4. O'Driscoll M, Jeggo PA. The role of double-strand break repair—insights from human genetics. *Nat Rev Genet*. 2006;7(1):45-54.
5. Ma Y, Pannicke U, Schwarz K, Lieber MR. Hairpin opening and overhang processing by an Artemis/DNA-dependent protein kinase complex in nonhomologous end joining and V(D)J recombination. *Cell*. 2002;108(6):781-794.
6. Callebaut I, Malivert L, Fischer A, et al. Cernunnos interacts with the XRCC4 x DNA-ligase IV complex and is homologous to the yeast nonhomologous end-joining factor Nej1. *J. Biol. Chem*. 2006;281(20):13857-13860.
7. Su TT. Cellular responses to DNA damage: one signal, multiple choices. *Annu Rev Genet*. 2006;40:187-208.
8. Lord CJ, Garrett MD, Ashworth A. Targeting the double-strand DNA break repair pathway as a therapeutic strategy. *Clin Cancer Res*. 2006;12(15):4463-4468.
9. Bakkenist CJ, Kastan MB. Phosphatases join kinases in DNA-damage response pathways. *Trends Cell Biol*. 2004;14(7):339-341.
10. Falck J, Coates J, Jackson SP. Conserved modes of recruitment of ATM, ATR and DNA-PKcs to sites of DNA damage. *Nature*. 2005;434(7033):605-611.
11. Jazayeri A, Falck J, Lukas C, et al. ATM- and cell cycle-dependent regulation of ATR in response to DNA double-strand breaks. *Nat Cell Biol*. 2006;8(1):37-45.
12. Lee JH, Paull TT. ATM activation by DNA double-strand breaks through the Mre11-Rad50-Nbs1 complex. *Science*. 2005;308(5721):551-554.
13. Andreassen PR, Ho GP, D'Andrea AD. DNA damage responses and their many interactions with the replication fork. *Carcinogenesis*. 2006;27(5):883-892.
14. Zhou BB, Bartek J. Targeting the checkpoint kinases: chemosensitization versus chemoprotection. *Nat Rev Cancer*. 2004;4(3):216-225.
15. Shao C, Folkard M, Michael BD, Prise KM. Targeted cytoplasmic irradiation induces bystander responses. *Proc Natl Acad Sci U S A*. 2004;101(37):13495-13500.
16. Haimovitz-Friedman A, Kan CC, Ehleiter D, et al. Ionizing radiation acts on cellular membranes to generate ceramide and initiate apoptosis. *J Exp Med*. 1994;180(2):525-535.
17. Pettus BJ, Chalfant CE, Hannun YA. Ceramide in apoptosis: an overview and current perspectives. *Biochim Biophys Acta (BBA)—Mol Cell Biol Lipids*. 2002;1585(2-3):114-125.
18. Xing HR, Kolesnick R. Kinase suppressor of RAS signals through Thr269 of c-Raf-1. *J Biol Chem*. 2001;276(13):9733-9741.
19. Blázquez C, Galve-Roperh I, Guzmán M. De novo-synthesized ceramide signals apoptosis in astrocytes via extracellular signal-regulated kinase. *FASEB J*. 2000;14(14):2315-2322.
20. Galabova-Kovacs G, Kolbus A, Matzen D, et al. ERK and beyond: insights from B-Raf and Raf-1 conditional knockouts. *Cell Cycle*. 2006;5(14):1514-1518.
21. Blume-Jensen P, Hunter T. Oncogenic kinase signalling. *Nature*. 2001;411(6835):355-365.
22. Schlessinger J, Lemmon MA. Nuclear signaling by receptor tyrosine kinases: the first robin of spring. *Cell*. 2006;127(1):45-48.
23. Dent P, Yacoub A, Contessa J, et al. Stress and radiation-induced activation of multiple intracellular signaling pathways. *Radiat Res*. 2003;159(3):283-300.
24. Nyati MK, Morgan MA, Feng FY, Lawrence TS. Integration of EGFR inhibitors with radiochemotherapy. *Nat Rev Cancer*. 2006;6(11):876-885.

25. Schmidt-Ullrich RK, Mikkelsen RB, Dent P, et al. Radiation-induced proliferation of the human A431 squamous carcinoma cells is dependent on EGFR tyrosine phosphorylation. *Oncogene.* 1997;15(10):1191-1197.
26. Chiarugi P, Cirri P. Redox regulation of protein tyrosine phosphatases during receptor tyrosine kinase signal transduction. *Trends Biochem Sci.* 2003;28(9):509-514.
27. Pacifico F, Leonardi A. NF-kappaB in solid tumors. *Biochem Pharmacol.* 2006;72(9):1142-1152.
28. Aggarwal BB, Sethi G, Ahn KS, et al. Targeting signal-transducer-and-activator-of-transcription-3 for prevention and therapy of cancer: modern target but ancient solution. *Ann N Y Acad Sci.* 2006;1091:151-169.
29. Ahn KS, Sethi G, Aggarwal BB. Nuclear factor-kappa B: from clone to clinic. *Curr Mol Med.* 2007;7(7):619-637.
30. Aggarwal BB, Vijayalekshmi RV, Sung B. Targeting inflammatory pathways for prevention and therapy of cancer: short-term friend, long-term foe. *Clin Cancer Res.* 2009;15(2):425-430.
31. Tamatani T, Azuma M, Ashida Y, et al. Enhanced radiosensitization and chemosensitization in NF-kappaB-suppressed human oral cancer cells via the inhibition of gamma-irradiation- and 5-FU-induced production of IL-6 and IL-8. *Int J Cancer.* 2004;108(6):912-921.
32. Johnson GL, Lapadat R. Mitogen-activated protein kinase pathways mediated by ERK, JNK, and p38 protein kinases. *Science.* 2002;298(5600):1911-1912.
33. Dent P, Yacoub A, Fisher PB, Hagan MP, Grant S. MAPK pathways in radiation responses. *Oncogene.* 2003;22(37):5885-5896.
34. Marais R, Light Y, Paterson HF, Marshall CJ. Ras recruits Raf-1 to the plasma membrane for activation by tyrosine phosphorylation. *EMBO J.* 1995;14(13):3136-3145.
35. Dent P, Reardon DB, Park JS, et al. Radiation-induced release of transforming growth factor alpha activates the epidermal growth factor receptor and mitogen-activated protein kinase pathway in carcinoma cells, leading to increased proliferation and protection from radiation-induced cell death. *Mol Biol Cell.* 1999;10(8):2493-2506.
36. Hagan M, Wang L, Hanley JR, Park JS, Dent P. Ionizing radiation-induced mitogen-activated protein (MAP) kinase activation in DU145 prostate carcinoma cells: MAP kinase inhibition enhances radiation-induced cell killing and G2/M-phase arrest. *Radiat Res.* 2000;153(4):371-383.
37. Liu J, Lin A. Role of JNK activation in apoptosis: a double-edged sword. *Cell Res.* 2005;15(1):36-42.
38. Chang F, Lee JT, Navolanic PM, et al. Involvement of PI3K/Akt pathway in cell cycle progression, apoptosis, and neoplastic transformation: a target for cancer chemotherapy. *Leukemia.* 2003;17(3):590-603.
39. Bussink J, van der Kogel AJ, Kaanders JH. Activation of the PI3-K/AKT pathway and implications for radioresistance mechanisms in head and neck cancer. *Lancet Oncol.* 2008;9(3):288-296.
40. Zhan M, Han ZC. Phosphatidylinositide 3-kinase/AKT in radiation responses. *Histol Histopathol.* 2004;19(3):915-923.
41. Toulany M, Kasten-Pisula U, Brammer I, et al. Blockage of epidermal growth factor receptor-phosphatidylinositol 3-kinase-AKT signaling increases radiosensitivity of K-RAS mutated human tumor cells in vitro by affecting DNA repair. *Clin Cancer Res.* 2006;12(13):4119-4126.
42. Zhong H, Chiles K, Feldser D, et al. Modulation of hypoxia-inducible factor 1alpha expression by the epidermal growth factor/phosphatidylinositol 3-kinase/PTEN/AKT/FRAP pathway in human prostate cancer cells: implications for tumor angiogenesis and therapeutics. *Cancer Res.* 2000;60(6): 1541-1545.
43. Skinner HD, Zheng JZ, Fang J, Agani F, Jiang B-H. Vascular endothelial growth factor transcriptional activation is mediated by hypoxia-inducible factor 1alpha, HDM2, and p70S6K1 in response to phosphatidylinositol 3-kinase/AKT signaling. *J Biol Chem.* 2004;279(44):45643-45651.
44. Semenza GL. HIF-1: mediator of physiological and pathophysiological responses to hypoxia. *J Appl Physiol.* 2000;88(4):1474-1480.
45. Yu LL, Yu HG, Yu JP, et al. Nuclear factor-kappaB p65 (RelA) transcription factor is constitutively activated in human colorectal carcinoma tissue. *World J Gastroenterol.* 2004;10(22): 3255-3260.
46. Kojima M, Morisaki T, Sasaki N, et al. Increased nuclear factor-kB activation in human colorectal carcinoma and its correlation with tumor progression. *Anticancer Res.* 2004;24(2B):675-681.
47. Deorukhkar A, Krishnan S. Targeting inflammatory pathways for tumor radiosensitization. *Biochem Pharmacol.* 2010;80(12):1904-1914.
48. Hadian K, Krappmann D. Signals from the nucleus: activation of NF-kappaB by cytosolic ATM in the DNA damage response. *Sci Signal.* 2011;4(156):pe2.
49. Kim JH, Lee G, Cho YL, et al. Desmethylanhydroicaritin inhibits NF-kappaB-regulated inflammatory gene expression by modulating the redox-sensitive PI3K/PTEN/Akt pathway. *Eur J Pharmacol.* 2009;602(2-3):422-431.
50. DiDonato JA, Hayakawa M, Rothwarf DM, Zandi E, Karin M. A cytokine-responsive IkappaB kinase that activates the transcription factor NF-kappaB. *Nature.* 1997;388(6642): 548-554.
51. Mercurio F, Zhu H, Murray BW, et al. IKK-1 and IKK-2: cytokine-activated IkappaB kinases essential for NF-kappaB activation. *Science.* 1997;278(5339):860-866.
52. Lin Y, Bai L, Chen W, Xu S. The NF-kappaB activation pathways, emerging molecular targets for cancer prevention and therapy. *Expert Opin Ther Targets.* 2010;14(1):45-55.
53. Wang CY, Mayo MW, Baldwin AS. TNF- and cancer therapy-induced apoptosis: potentiation by inhibition of NF-kappaB. *Science.* 1996;274(5288):784-787.
54. Cohen Jonathan E, Bernhard EJ, McKenna WG. How does radiation kill cells? *Curr Opin Chem Biol.* 1999;3(1):77-83.
55. Brown JM, Wilson G. Apoptosis genes and resistance to cancer therapy: what does the experimental and clinical data tell us? *Cancer Biol Ther.* 2003;2(5):477-490.
56. Brown JM, Attardi LD. The role of apoptosis in cancer development and treatment response. *Nat Rev Cancer.* 2005;5(3):231-237.
57. Dewey WC, Ling CC, Meyn RE. Radiation-induced apoptosis: relevance to radiotherapy. *Int J Radiat Oncol Biol Phys.* 1995;33(4):781-796.
58. de Bruin EC, Medema JP. Apoptosis and non-apoptotic deaths in cancer development and treatment response. *Cancer Treat Rev.* 2008;34(8):737-749.
59. Vakifahmetoglu H, Olsson M, Zhivotovsky B. Death through a tragedy: mitotic catastrophe. *Cell Death Differ.* 2008;15(7):1153-1162.
60. Demaria S, Formenti SC. Sensors of ionizing radiation effects on the immunological microenvironment of cancer. *Int J Radiat Biol.* 2007;83(11-12):819-825.
61. Denecker G, Vercammen D, Declercq W, Vandenabeele P. Apoptotic and necrotic cell death induced by death domain receptors. *Cell Mol Life Sci.* 2001;58(3):356-370.
62. Galluzzi L, Maiuri MC, Vitale I, et al. Cell death modalities: classification and pathophysiological implications. *Cell Death Differ.* 2007;14(7):1237-1243.
63. Golstein P, Kroemer G. Cell death by necrosis: towards a molecular definition. *Trends Biochem Sci.* 2007;32(1):37-43.
64. Decker P, Muller S. Modulating poly (ADP-ribose) polymerase activity: potential for the prevention and therapy of pathogenic situations involving DNA damage and oxidative stress. *Curr Pharm Biotechnol.* 2002;3(3):275-283.
65. Festjens N, Vanden Berghe T, Cornelis S, Vandenabeele P. RIP1, a kinase on the crossroads of a cell's decision to live or die. *Cell Death Differ.* 2007;14(3):400-410.
66. Jung CH, Ro S-H, Cao J, Otto NM, Kim D-H. mTOR regulation of autophagy. *FEBS Lett.* 2010;584(7):1287-1295.
67. Kimmelman AC. The dynamic nature of autophagy in cancer. *Genes Dev.* 2011;25(19):1999-2010.
68. Zois CE, Koukourakis MI. Radiation-induced autophagy in normal and cancer cells: Towards novel cytoprotection and radio-sensitization policies? *Autophagy.* 2009;5(4):442-451.
69. Judith C. Senescent cells, tumor suppression, and organismal aging: good citizens, bad neighbors. *Cell.* 2005;120(4):513-522.
70. Ewald JA, Desotelle JA, Wilding G, Jarrard DF. Therapy-induced senescence in cancer. *J Natl Cancer Inst.* 2010;102(20): 1536-1546.
71. Roninson IB, Broude EV, Chang BD. If not apoptosis, then what? Treatment-induced senescence and mitotic catastrophe in tumor cells. *Drug Resist Updat.* 2001;4(5):303-313.

72. Skinner HD, Sandulache VC, Ow TJ, et al. TP53 disruptive mutations lead to head and neck cancer treatment failure through inhibition of radiation-induced senescence. *Clin Cancer Res.* 2011. http://www.ncbi.nlm.nih.gov/pubmed/22090360. Accessed November 19, 2011.
73. Passos JF, Nelson G, Wang C, et al. Feedback between p21 and reactive oxygen production is necessary for cell senescence. *Mol Syst Biol.* 2010;6:347.
74. Vigneron A, Vousden KH. p53, ROS and senescence in the control of aging. *Aging (Albany NY).* 2010;2(8):471-474.
75. Beauséjour CM, Krtolica A, Galimi F, et al. Reversal of human cellular senescence: roles of the p53 and p16 pathways. *EMBO J.* 2003;22(16):4212-4222.
76. Mancuso M, Pasquali E, Leonardi S, et al. Oncogenic bystander radiation effects in Patched heterozygous mouse cerebellum. *Proc Natl Acad Sci U S A.* 2008;105(34):12445-12450.
77. Singh H, Saroya R, Smith R, et al. Radiation induced bystander effects in mice given low doses of radiation in vivo. *Dose Response.* 2011;9(2):225-242.
78. Burr KL, Robinson JI, Rastogi S, et al. Radiation-induced delayed bystander-type effects mediated by hemopoietic cells. *Radiat Res.* 2010;173(6):760-768.
79. Lorimore SA, Chrystal JA, Robinson JI, Coates PJ, Wright EG. Chromosomal instability in unirradiated hemopoietic cells induced by macrophages exposed in vivo to ionizing radiation. *Cancer Res.* 2008;68(19):8122-8126.
80. Rzeszowska-Wolny J, Przybyszewski WM, Widel M. Ionizing radiation-induced bystander effects, potential targets for modulation of radiotherapy. *Eur J Pharmacol.* 2009;625(1-3):156-164.

CHAPTER 50

NANOTECHNOLOGY AND CANCER THERAPY

Chun Li

INTRODUCTION

Nanotechnology is an applied science that creates and studies assemblies of molecules that have unique physicochemical properties and range in size from 1 to 200 nm range (<1 μm). In the past two decades, tremendous progress has been made in biomedical applications of nanomaterials with new and improved diagnostic and therapeutic efficacy. Oncology is one of the disciplines that have benefited most from nanotechnology. A more broad-based nanotechnology application will come from a better understanding of how nanoparticles interact with biological systems, how multiple functions, including imaging and therapeutic functions, can be built into a single nanoplatform, and how to harness the unique physicochemical properties of nanoparticles that do not otherwise exist in small-molecular-weight molecules for the detection and destruction of cancer cells with high selectivity and efficiency.

Currently, a few nanotechnology-based anticancer therapeutic agents have been successfully introduced into the clinic. Liposomal doxorubicin (Doxil) is the first marketed anticancer nanotherapeutic, approved by the FDA in 2003 for the treatment of advanced ovarian cancer. This was followed by the introduction of human serum albumin–bound paclitaxel (Abraxane) in 2005 for the treatment of metastatic breast cancer. Several dozens more nanotech-based therapeutics are undergoing various stages of clinical trial studies. However, although nanotechnology has shown great promise in many preclinical studies, significant challenges remain, especially in the field of oncology. The major challenges include overcoming biological barriers and successful clinical translation. Most nanoparticles encounter a number of biological barriers after their systemic administration before reaching the disease sites. These biological barriers have to be overcome in order to achieve active targeting, the holy grail of nano-delivery system. The validation in the clinical setting and eventual translation into clinical applications are expected to have significant impact in the treatment of cancer patients. Successful clinical translation requires close partnership between research scientists and clinicians, documentation and better understanding of the toxicity of nanoparticles, and infrastructure for obtaining regulatory approval.

APPLICATIONS OF NANOTECHNOLOGY IN CANCER MEDICINE

On the basis of applications, cancer nanotechnologies can be roughly divided into three categories: drug delivery, harnessing external energy for tumor cell ablation, and surgical guidance. To date, most research activities are in the area of drug delivery. Because most anticancer chemotherapeutic agents are highly toxic, by directing more anticancer drugs into the tumor and protecting them from entering systemic circulation, nanocarriers should provide an opportunity for reduced toxicity and enhanced antitumor efficacy. The net result is an increased therapeutic window.

Drug Delivery

One example of nanotechnology in drug delivery is high-molecular-weight (>50 kDa), water-soluble poly (L-glutamic acid)-paclitaxel (PG-TXL, Opaxio) conjugate. When bound to poly(L-glutamic acid), a biodegradable polyamino acid, the drug is inactive. This reduces the level of the free drug in the blood stream, thus decreasing drug exposure and associated side effects. Unlike blood vessels in healthy tissues, those in tumor tissues have openings and pores large enough to allow preferential accumulation of high-molecular-weight polymer-bound drugs compared with small-molecular-weight free drugs. This phenomenon is termed "enhanced permeability and retention" effect, or EPR effect. Numerous preclinical studies in both ectopic and orthotopic models have shown that PG-TXL has superior antitumor activity against a variety of solid tumors than paclitaxel.[1,2] This is attributed to its prolonged blood circulation time and increased distribution into tumor tissue.[3] PG-TXL is in clinical phase 3 trials. Other polymeric carriers, including dendrimers, poly(glycolic acid–lactic acid) copolymers, and polymeric micelles, are being studied as anticancer drug carriers, and some of them have entered clinical trial studies.

Tumor Cell Ablation

A second application of nanotechnology takes advantage of the unique physicochemical properties of nanoparticles that do not normally exist in small-molecular-weight compounds, namely, their interaction with external energy sources. Various external energy sources have been utilized for both diagnostic and therapeutic purposes (Fig. 50.1). For example, ionizing radiations (x-ray and γ-ray) are used for computed tomography and radiotherapy. Studies on the interaction between radiotherapy and polymeric drug carriers were first reported using PG-TXL as the model system.[4-6] These studies demonstrated remarkable potentiation of response to radiotherapy when a chemotherapeutic agent is administered in the form of polymeric conjugate as compared with when injected as a free drug. Radiofrequency (RF) energy is employed for minimally invasive surgeries, using RF ablation and coagulation. Recent studies have shown that gold nanoparticles can mediate high heating rate with nonionizing RF radiation.[7,8] As a minimally invasive alternative or adjuvant to conventional surgical procedures, photothermal ablation (PTA) treatment has been used successfully for ablation of tumors throughout the body.[9-11] The approach offers the benefit of reduced impact on patient, reduced morbidity, and improved quality of life and is amenable for treatment of non-surgical candidates among others. However, the heating achieved by converting laser energy to thermal energy is nonspecific, meaning that treatment volume and speed are limited by the potential for damage to the surrounding normal tissues. Thus, effective PTA therapy and successful translation of PTA into the clinic will require (1) selective delivery of a sufficient amount of heat-converting nanoparticles to tumor tissue to mediate a photothermal effect, (2) optimal combination of PTA therapy with other treatment modalities, and (3) noninvasive assessment of nanoparticles' accumulation in the tumor to facilitate pretreatment thermal dose calculation, and real-time monitoring of the spatiotemporal heat profile and response to therapy in a given target volume.

The electromagnetic radiation of different energy sources differs in energy level (wavelength) and penetration depth. PTA therapy with near-infrared (NIR, 700 to 900 nm) laser represents a promising therapy. PTA therapy is gaining in popularity because it involves delivery of a specific amount of energy directly into the tumor mass, avoiding systemic effects. Furthermore, PTA therapy may be performed repeatedly without the accumulation of toxic side effects and resistance. NIR light can penetrate through skin and deep into soft tissues (~2 to 5 cm) owing to reduced scattering and tissue absorption.

Image-Guided Surgery

A third area of potential applications of nanotechnology in cancer therapy is image-guided surgery. Tumor-free margin is critical to reduce the rate of recurrence in cancer surgery. Surgeons rely on visual appearance and palpation to assess the extent of resection. Image guidance that helps define tumor margin and detect residual disease is an invaluable tool during surgical operation. Within this field, imaging in the NIR light spectrum offers two essential advantages: increased tissue penetration of light and an increased signal-to-background ratio of contrast agents.[12] Several NIR nanoparticles have been proposed to aid image-guided surgery. Quantum dot nanoparticles are small semiconductor nanoparticles (2 to 10 nm diameter) that possess high quantum yields, tunable fluorescence emission spectra, and high photostability. However, the potential toxicity of quantum dots and safety concerns make it unlikely that they will have clinical applications. A possible exception is sentinel lymph node mapping with quantum dots, in which the nanoparticles are deposited locally in the lymph nodes and are removed during lymphectomy. NIR polymeric nanogel, nanolatex, polymeric

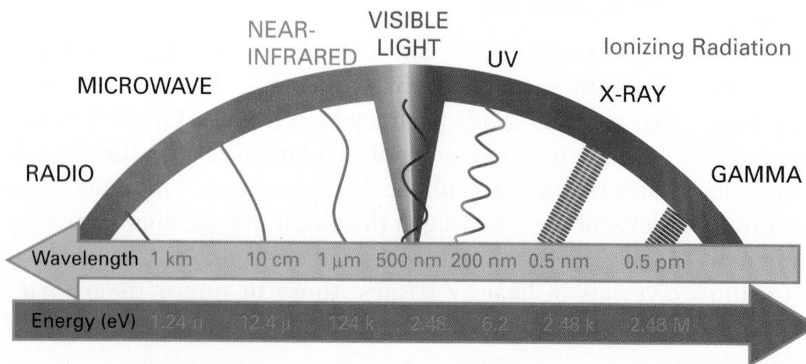

FIGURE 50–1 Electromagnetic spectrum of various energy sources. The approximate wavelengths and energy levels covered in diagnostic/therapeutic applications are shown.

micelles, and silica nanoparticles have been developed as an alternative to quantum dots.[13-15] Interestingly, the tumor uptake of the nanolatex particles correlated well with their blood residence times, but similar correlations were not found between nanogel and nanolatex particles.[13] These results suggest that both the blood circulation time and the extent of hydration of the nanoparticles play an important role in the tumor uptake of nanoparticles. Because particle size, surface charge, and the density of polyethylene glycol coating on the surface of nanoparticles are key factors that influence pharmacokinetics and tumor distribution of nanoparticles after systemic administration,[16] extensive research will have to be performed over the coming years in order to address these issues.

One of the promises of nanotechnology is its ability to provide multiple functions that small molecular compounds cannot, in particular, integrate diagnostic and therapeutic capabilities into a single entity. This allows nanomedicine to be tailored to individual patients on the basis of successful delivery and detection of nanoparticles at the diseased sites. Combining diagnosis and therapy in one process, referred to as cancer theranostics, makes it possible to apply the "see and treat" strategy. Examples of such nanodevices include gold nanoshells encapsulated with superparamagnetic iron oxide for magnetic resonance imaging (MRI)–guided PTA therapy,[17] ^{64}Cu-labeled CuS nanoparticles for positron emission tomography (PET)–guided PTA therapy,[18] and hollow gold nanospheres (HAuNSs) for photoacoustic tomography-guided PTA therapy,[19] among many other nanomaterials. Figure 50.2 shows molecular photoacoustic tomography and micro-PET images of human U87 glioma grown in the brain of a mouse after intravenous injection of Arg–Gly–Glu peptide-coated HAuNSs. Photoacoustic tomography clearly depicted the intravenous delivery of HAuNS targeted to tumor overexpressing integrins $\alpha v\beta 3$. After imaging session, mice were treated with NIR laser, which significantly prolonged the survival of tumor-bearing mice when compared with groups of mice treated with saline, laser alone, targeted HAuNS alone, and non-targeted HAuNS plus laser. These results demonstrate the feasibility of using a single nanostructure for image-guided local tumor PTA therapy using photoacoustic molecular imaging.

Noninvasive imaging can also facilitate elucidation of mechanisms of action for novel nanotherapeutics. For example, poly(L-glutamic acid) was conjugated to Gd-DTPA (an MRI agent) and NIR813 (an NIR dye) to investigate intratumoral distribution of the polymeric carrier.[20,21] The resulting conjugate PG-Gd-NIR813 allowed in vivo MR and/or optical imaging and permitted ex vivo correlation between intratumoral distribution of the polymer and a sub-population of tumor stromal cells. These studies confirmed that PG-Gd-NIR813 has an increased uptake into the tumor tissue; it selectively deposits in the necrotic region of the tumor, and tumor uptake of PG polymer is mediated through infiltrating activated macrophages. With the aid of multimodal imaging approach, it is possible to pinpoint the mechanism by which the polymer is distributed in the tumor in relation to the tumor microenvironment. An in-depth understanding on how polymer therapeutics work will help design future generation of anticancer agents with improved therapeutic window.

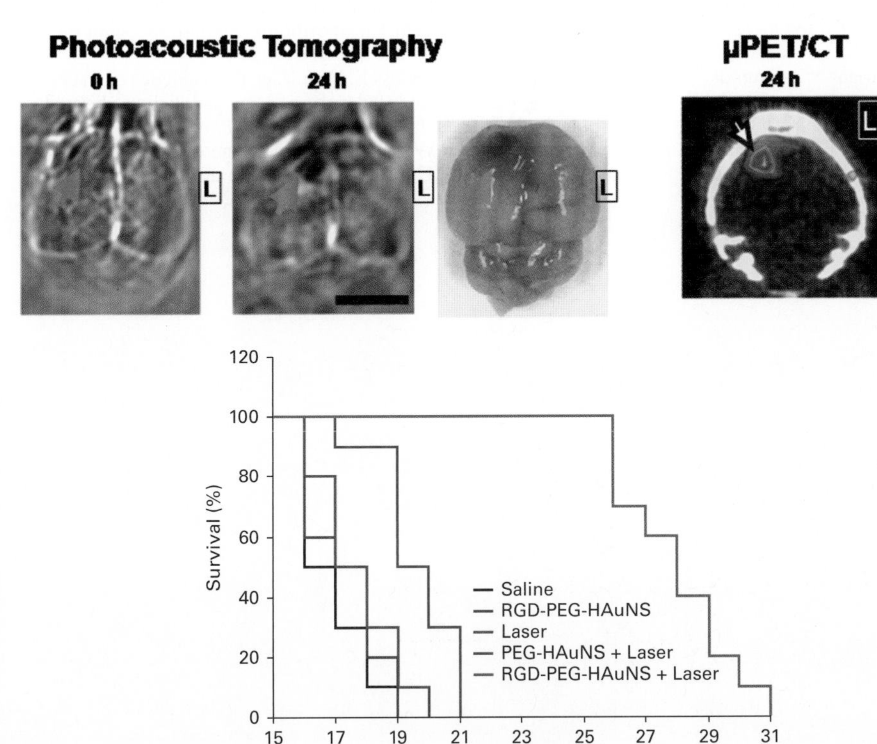

FIGURE 50–2 Photoacoustic tomography and micro-PET images of U87 human glioma in the brains of mice before (0 h) and 24 h after intravenous injection of nanoparticles (top panel; bar, 5 mm). *Arrows*, locations of tumors; L, left. Photothermal ablation of U87 human gliomas in mouse brains (bottom panel). Kaplan-Meier survival curve of tumor-bearing mice with different treatments (n = 10 per group). (Adapted with permission from Lu W, Melancon MP, Xiong C, et al., *Cancer Res.* 2011;71: 6116-6121.)

PERSPECTIVES

Because of enormous challenges in the successful clinical translation of novel nanotechnologies, it is imperative that partnerships are developed at both national and local–regional levels. Nanotechnology research in cancer involves a broad spectrum of disciplines such as engineering, materials, imaging, physical, biological, environmental, and pharmacological sciences. In the United States, the National Cancer Institute has funded 9 multidisciplinary centers that are the primary components for discovery and tool development of nanotechnology in clinical oncology and has awarded 12 partnerships that are designed to promote multidisciplinary research projects in addition to numerous traditional R01/R21-type grants that support a variety of researches focused on applications of nanotechnology in cancer therapy. These programs foster collaboration, promote introduction of innovative nanotechnology in cancer therapy, and address major barriers and fundamental questions in cancer using innovative nanotechnology solutions. It is anticipated that many more nanotechnology-based cancer therapeutics will be introduced into the clinic in the foreseeable future.

REFERENCES

1. Li C, Price JE, Milas L, et al. Antitumor activity of poly (L-glutamic acid)-paclitaxel on syngeneic and xenografted tumors. *Clin Cancer Res.* 1999;5:891-897.
2. Li C, Yu DF, Newman RA, et al. Complete regression of well-established tumors using a novel water-soluble poly(L-glutamic acid)-paclitaxel conjugate. *Cancer Res.* 1998;58:2404-2409.
3. Li C, Newman RA, Wu QP, et al. Biodistribution of paclitaxel and poly(L-glutamic acid)-paclitaxel conjugate in mice with ovarian OCa-1 tumor. *Cancer Chemother Pharmacol.* 2000;46:416-422.
4. Ke S, Milas L, Charnsangavej C, Wallace S, Li C. Potentiation of radioresponse by polymer-drug conjugates. *J Control Release.* 2001;74:237-242.
5. Li C, Ke S, Wu QP, et al. Potentiation of ovarian OCa-1 tumor radioresponse by poly (L-glutamic acid)-paclitaxel conjugate. *Int J Radiat Oncol Biol Phys.* 2000;48:1119-1126.
6. Milas L, Mason KA, Hunter N, Li C, Wallace S. Poly(L-glutamic acid)-paclitaxel conjugate is a potent enhancer of tumor radiocurability. *Int J Radiat Oncol Biol Phys.* 2003;55:707-712.
7. Glazer ES, Zhu C, Massey KL, et al. Noninvasive radiofrequency field destruction of pancreatic adenocarcinoma xenografts treated with targeted gold nanoparticles. *Clin Cancer Res.* 2010;16:5712-5721.
8. Curley SA, Cherukuri P, Briggs K, et al. Noninvasive radiofrequency field-induced hyperthermic cytotoxicity in human cancer cells using cetuximab-targeted gold nanoparticles. *J Exp Ther Oncol.* 2008;7:313-326.
9. Fiedler VU, Schwarzmaier HJ, Eickmeyer F, Muller FP, Schoepp C, Verreet PR. Laser-induced interstitial thermotherapy of liver metastases in an interventional 0.5 Tesla MRI system: technique and first clinical experiences. *J Magn Reson Imaging.* 2001;13:729-737.
10. Vogl TJ, Straub R, Eichler K, Sollner O, Mack MG. Colorectal carcinoma metastases in liver: laser-induced interstitial thermotherapy—local tumor control rate and survival data. *Radiology.* 2004;230:450-458.
11. Vogl TJ, Straub R, Zangos S, Mack MG, Eichler K. MR-guided laser-induced thermotherapy (LITT) of liver tumours: experimental and clinical data. *Int J Hypertherm.* 2004;20:713-724.
12. Keereweer S, Kerrebijn JD, van Driel PB, et al. Optical image-guided surgery—where do we stand? *Mol Imaging Biol.* 2011;13:199-207.
13. Yang Z, Leon J, Martin M, et al. Pharmacokinetics and biodistribution of near-infrared fluorescence polymeric nanoparticles. *Nanotechnology.* 2009;20:165101 (11 pp).
14. Yang Z, Zheng S, Harrison WJ, et al. Long-circulating near-infrared fluorescence core-cross-linked polymeric micelles: synthesis, characterization, and dual nuclear/optical imaging. *Biomacromolecules.* 2007;8:3422-3428.
15. Choi J, Burns AA, Williams RM, et al. Core-shell silica nanoparticles as fluorescent labels for nanomedicine. *J Biomed Opt.* 2007;12:064007.
16. Zhang G, Yang Z, Lu W, et al. Influence of anchoring ligands and particle size on the colloidal stability and in vivo biodistribution of polyethylene glycol-coated gold nanoparticles in tumor-xenografted mice. *Biomaterials.* 2009;30:1928-1936.
17. Melancon M, Lu W, Li C. Gold-based magneto/optical nanostructures: challenges for in vivo applications in cancer diagnostics and therapy. *Mater Res Bull.* 2009;34:415-421.
18. Zhou M, Zhang R, Huang M, et al. A chelator-free multifunctional [64Cu]CuS nanoparticle platform for simultaneous micro-PET/CT imaging and photothermal ablation therapy. *J Am Chem Soc.* 2010;132:15351-15358.
19. Lu W, Melancon MP, Xiong C, et al. Effects of photoacoustic imaging and photothermal ablation therapy mediated by targeted hollow gold nanospheres in an orthotopic mouse xenograft model of glioma. *Cancer Res.* 2011;71:6116-6121.
20. Jackson EF, Esparza-Coss E, Wen X, et al. Magnetic resonance imaging of therapy-induced necrosis using gadolinium-chelated polyglutamic acids. *Int J Radiat Oncol Biol Phys.* 2007;68:830-838.
21. Melancon MP, Lu W, Huang Q, et al. Targeted imaging of tumor-associated M2 macrophages using a macromolecular contrast agent PG-Gd-NIR813. *Biomaterials.* 2010;31:6567-6573.

CHAPTER 51

New Approaches to Integration of Personalized Medicine in Early Cancer Drug Development

Aik-Choon Tan, Stephen Leong, Todd M. Pitts, John J. Tentler, and S. Gail Eckhardt

> Unlike chemo and radiation, which use carpet-bombing tactics that destroy cancer cells and healthy cells alike, these new [targeted] medicines are like a troop of snipers, firing on cancer cells alone and targeting their weakest links.
>
> (Time magazine, 2001)

As we have now entered the era of "targeted" or personalized cancer treatment, the number of therapeutic targets, and hence the number of potential cancer agents, has greatly expanded. Evaluating all of these prospective agents is becoming increasingly difficult with the result that novel approaches are being integrated earlier in drug development, in both the preclinical and clinical setting. The goals of these new approaches are to quickly and effectively identify leading drug candidates, describe the target population, discover a predictive biomarker, and understand pathway changes that may lead to future chemotherapy combinations.

This chapter will review new approaches in the preclinical, bioinformatics, and clinical aspects of early drug development.

THE USE OF PRECLINICAL MODELS IN EARLY DRUG DEVELOPMENT TO IDENTIFY PREDICTIVE BIOMARKERS

In Vitro Cancer Cell Lines

Preclinical evaluation of novel cancer drugs typically begins with efficacy studies in cancer cell lines. In the late 1980s the National Cancer Institute developed the NCI60 panel, consisting of 60 cell lines from numerous cancer types, for the express purpose of providing an in vitro anticancer drug screening platform.[1] Although the NCI60 panel has proven useful, it has limitations in that some cancers are underrepresented or not represented at all. For this reason, many investigators have chosen to create their own cell line panels by acquiring them from large repositories such as the American Type Culture Collection, the Center for Molecular Therapeutics 1000, and other banks at universities and private institutions,[2] often with the intent of achieving greater representation of selected cancer subtypes of interest. The primary advantage of performing initial drug screens in cell lines is that they are relatively inexpensive and high-throughput assays can be performed fairly rapidly, often within 24 to 72 hours. Cell proliferation assays are the most direct way to assess a drug's anticancer activity, examples of which are direct cell counting, colorimetric assays that quantify cell numbers in relation to metabolism of tetrazolium salts (i.e., MTT) by the mitochondria, and cellular protein staining such as the sulforhodamine B (SRB) method. Further assays can be performed to elucidate a drug's mechanism of action, to determine whether it is cytostatic versus cytotoxic, for example. These include colorimetric caspase 3/7 activity assays and annexin V staining to assess apoptosis, propidium iodide staining and flow cytometry for cell cycle analysis, and lysosomal staining of β-galactosidase to assess cellular senescence. All of these assays are applied to enable stratification of cell lines into highly responsive (sensitive) or non-responsive (resistant) to a particular agent. Cancer cell lines are also highly amenable to manipulation through transient and stable transfection of expression vectors encoding gene products as well as small interfering RNAs and reporter constructs, enabling mechanistic studies that confirm the contribution of a particular gene to the responsiveness to a drug. Another advantage of cell lines is that many are well characterized in terms of mutational status and chromosomal aberrations, including amplifications, deletions, and translocations, allowing for molecular and genetic correlations to drug sensitivity. More recently, other annotations, such as gene expression profiles from several gene array platforms, have been made available through publicly accessible databases. Together, this information can provide the basis for predictive biomarker development by comparisons of differences between sensitive and resistant cell lines, which, with appropriate bioinformatics strategies, may potentially be translatable to tumor biology in the clinical setting. Despite the dynamic range afforded by the use of large panels of cancer cell lines, their use as the sole model system for drug efficacy and biomarker development has limited utility. First, cells in monolayer culture do not resemble complex, three-dimensional tumors with respect to exposure to oxygen, nutrients, and drugs as well as interactions with the extracellular matrix (ECM), all of which may influence drug sensitivity. Furthermore, effects of anticancer compounds on tumor angiogenesis cannot be measured in vitro. Three-dimensional spheroid cultures of cell lines grown on a synthetic ECM, such as Matrigel, address some of these shortcomings and, for these reasons, are often used to bridge the gap between drug studies performed on monolayer cultures and in vivo xenografts in mice.[3,4] Second, comparisons of gene expression profiles and cellular pathways between cancer cell lines and tumor cells from the same tissue type have demonstrated some striking differences. For example, Stein and colleagues found that genes belonging to "proliferation" pathways, such as cell cycle, purine and pyrimidine metabolism, and ATP synthesis, were consistently upregulated in cell lines, whereas genes associated with "cell adhesion" pathways such as cell communication, cell adhesion molecules, and ECM–receptor interactions were upregulated in tumors.[5,6] It stands to reason then that these differences in gene expression patterns between cell lines and solid tumors will be reflected in differential responses to anticancer drugs. In summary, cancer cell lines offer a convenient, rapid, and cost-effective platform for initial drug screens, mechanistic studies, and biomarker development. However, caution should be taken when interpreting these results, and complimentary studies using in vivo animal tumor models should be undertaken as further confirmation of a drug's differential effectiveness across a range of in vitro models.

In Vivo Cancer Models

Cell Line Xenografts

The most common in vivo models utilized in early cancer drug development are cell line xenograft tumors in immune compromised mice. Typically, this involves the subcutaneous injection of human cancer cells onto the flank of athymic nude or severe combined immunodeficient mice. Alternatively, orthotopic xenograft models involve the injection of cells within or adjacent to the organ of origin, which may provide a more physiologically relevant model when tissue-specific factors, such as hormones and growth factors, are important for the biology of certain tumors. In either case, these animal models are required for pharmacokinetic studies and are believed to more closely model the anticancer effects of drugs on human tumors as they are propagated in a living organism under the influence of cancer-relevant physiologic processes, such as angiogenesis, invasion, and metastasis, and growth signals from surrounding stroma. Evaluation of drug efficacy is performed by measuring tumors directly with a caliper and calculating tumor volume or through imaging techniques such as dynamic contrast-enhanced magnetic resonance imaging (DCE-MRI) or positron emission tomography (PET).[7] These models can be used to validate the responsiveness of a cell line to a particular agent, although one area of controversy involves selecting the best phenotypic endpoint, with tumor growth inhibition, induction of apoptosis, and tumor regression viewed least to most stringent, respectively.[2] Despite the relative simplicity of these models, there are limitations to the use of cell line xenografts for drug efficacy studies and biomarker development. For one, the host mice are immunocompromised, and the influence of this physiologic state on tumor growth or potential immunomodulatory effects of the drug(s) is difficult or impossible to measure. And while the cell line tumors are supported by stroma, it is of mouse origin, so the effects of an experimental therapy on tumor-stroma signaling may not reflect that on human tumors clinically. Finally, depending on the tissue of origin, some cell lines cannot be placed orthotopically, which limits evaluation of the effects of the tumor microenvironment on drug action. Nonetheless, the fact that one can make adjustments for these differences by comparing the same cell line in vitro versus in vivo supports their use in predictive biomarker development when there is concordance of responsiveness. A lack of concordance obscures the picture but may in fact be informative that microenvironmental factors complicate a purely tumor cell compartment-driven predictive biomarker strategy.[8,9]

Patient-Derived Tumor Explant Models

An advancement over the use of cell line xenografts is the direct implantation of surgical biopsy tumor tissue into immune compromised mice. Although these models have been in existence for over 30 years, only recently they have been consistently applied in early drug development for efficacy and biomarker development studies.[7,10-14] In general, fresh tumor tissue from patients (F0) is sectioned into ~3 mm^3 pieces and subcutaneously implanted into the flank of the mouse, or positioned orthotopically. The tumors are then passaged into consecutive generations

(F1, F2, F3, etc.) until enough material is generated for drug evaluation and biomarker development studies. These patient-derived tumor explants (PDX) hold several advantages over traditional cell line xenograft models. Unlike cell lines, some of which are at very high passage, PDX cells have never been cultured in vitro, and therefore, in theory, maintain the gene expression patterns and mutational status of the tumor in the patient.[6,12,14] They also maintain tumor architecture, including tumor-associated stroma,[10,12] although after a few generations the human cellular stromal components are replaced by mouse components. Together, these features provide a preclinical model system for drug development that more closely recapitulates the clinical scenario. Our group and others have used these models for biomarker discovery either as a training set, when segregated according to responsiveness to a drug, or as near-clinical assessment of the accuracy of a predictive classifier that has been initially developed in traditional cell line models.[7,13,15-17] The limitations of this model are that it requires a clinical protocol and support system for informed consent of patients, tissue collection, and the expense of maintaining a large bank of mice. And as with traditional cell line xenografts, the use of immune compromised mice represents an artificial host environment.

Genetically Engineered Mouse Models

Transgenic models or genetically engineered mouse models (GEMMs) have been used in virtually every area of cancer research, including the elucidation of transformation events and assessing the consequences of activating or inhibiting a specific cellular molecule or pathway.[18] As a model for the evaluation of novel anticancer therapeutics and development of biomarkers, they possess several benefits and also some disadvantages.[19,20] A major advantage is that these tumors can be induced to arise in situ through the defined temporal and tissue-specific activation of an oncogene such as KRAS or myc, thereby providing proof of mechanism and relevant biomarkers, a priori. Transgenic models also have the advantage of arising within the context of an immune competent animal, a limitation of mouse xenograft models. Tumor response to therapy, and therefore response stratification, in these mouse models can be monitored through imaging techniques such as DCE-MRI and PET-CT or by tagging cells with fluorescence and luciferase-based markers that can be engineered into the transgene construct and imaged with an intravital imaging system without having to sacrifice the animal. Disadvantages of GEMMs for drug development and biomarker discovery primarily relate to the fact that they are inherently biased models and thus the complexity of coexisting genetic aberrations that exist in patients are not represented, potentially resulting in overestimation of target and biomarker dependence. Nonetheless, these models have proven invaluable in proving mechanism, which when overlooked can lead to difficulties later on in personalized therapy approaches.

Future Directions

Preclinical models of cancer are an important part of early drug testing and biomarker development. In fact, it is really only in these models that it is feasible to assess and stratify differential responses to a new agent among large panels of cell lines and/or xenografts, thus forming the basis of a predictive classifier. However, as we uncover the complexities of tumor biology, the challenge will be a better utilization of these models to further our understanding of the mechanisms of inherent and acquired drug resistance, the role of factors such as hypoxia, angiogenesis, and the tumor microenvironment in concordantly optimizing both antitumor and predictive biomarker efficacy.

THE CHALLENGES OF SAMPLE ACQUISITION IN EARLY BIOMARKER DEVELOPMENT

Developing biomarkers for patient selection is a key step toward personalized medicine. This requires the acquisition of patient tissue/samples which includes blood (plasma/serum/PBMCs [peripheral blood mononuclear cells]) or tumor tissue (archived formalin-fixed paraffin-embedded [FFPE] and fresh/frozen biopsies or circulating tumor cells [CTCs]) obtained prior to treatment or at the time of disease progression, if assessing resistance biomarkers. Determining the most appropriate tissue to sample is dependent on the type of biomarker one is trying to evaluate (Table 51.1).

Whole blood can be processed to yield plasma (the acellular component of blood remaining after centrifugation), serum (the supernatant remaining after whole blood is permitted to clot), and PBMCs and, while the easiest tissue to obtain, has specific applications. PBMCs are primarily used as a source for normal, germline tissue in performing genomic studies.[21] Using blood-based biomarkers assumes that the tumor releases proteins/enzymes into the systemic circulation and most studies to date have focused on detecting low abundance proteins, which comprise panels of protein biomarkers. For example, in a diagnostic application, combining leptin, prolactin, osteopontin, and insulin-like growth factor II, patients with ovarian cancer could be discriminated over non-diseased patients.[22] Equally as important is the ability to use plasma to detect predictive biomarkers. Kelly et al.[23] demonstrated a panel of three proteins found in plasma that corresponded with response to chemotherapy in esophageal cell line xenografts. In colorectal cancer Halamkova et al,[24] showed that by looking at soluble levels of the plasminogen activator system protein PAI 1 demonstrated a worse response to therapy. Plasma levels of particular proteins during treatment can be prognostic for survival. A phase III study with sorafinib in renal cell carcinoma showed that the levels of VEGF, CAIX,

TABLE 51–1 Types of Biomarker Specimens and Feasible Molecular Tests

	Best Suited for Molecular Test										
Specimen	**DNA (Mutation Detection)**	**DNA (Deep Sequencing)**	**RNA (PCR)**	**RNA (Microarray)**	**RNA (RNA-seq)**	**miRNA (PCR)**	**miRNA (Microarray)**	**miRNA (miRNA-seq)**	**Protein (IHC)**	**Protein (Immunoblotting)**	**Protein (Proteomics)**
Plasma	✓			✓	✓		✓				
Serum	✓										✓
Fresh frozen	✓	✓	✓	✓	✓	✓	✓	✓		✓	✓
Formalin-fixed paraffin-embedded	✓		✓	✓		✓	✓		✓		

PCR, polymerase chain reaction; IHC, immunohistochemical staining.

TIMP-1, and Ras p21 were prognostic for survival. In fact, TIMP-1 has actually emerged as being independently prognostic.[25]

Plasma or serum can also be a useful source of microRNAs (miRNAs). miRNAs are small (~22 nt) regulatory non-coding RNA molecules that can modulate the activity of mRNA targets. They are often dysregulated in cancer, are tissue specific, and can be detected in plasma, serum, and FFPE tissues.[26-28] Like other protein markers, miRNAs to date have been mostly used in the diagnosis or prognosis of cancer and less as predictive biomarkers. For example, miRNA panels, including miR-17-5p, miR-21, miR-106a, and miR-106b, have been shown to be significantly higher in gastric cancer patients than controls.[29] There are also miRNAs that are commonly found in numerous other cancers, including miR-141, miR-200b, and miR-200c, with miR-141 being found most commonly associated with prostate and colon cancer.[30,31] Since miRNAs are stable in both plasma and serum there is an increasing effort to find miRNAs that can predict response to therapy or predict survival. One report demonstrates that miR-let7a and miR-16 levels can predict not only progression-free survival but also overall survival in patients with myelodysplastic syndrome, which can potentially progress to acute myeloid leukemia.[32] There are also reports of miRNAs being used as diagnostic markers of response to chemotherapy. For example, miR-10b has been shown to predict response of pancreatic ductal adenocarcinoma to neoadjuvant therapy.[33] Alternatively, miR-92a-2* has been shown to be a negative marker for response of small cell lung cancer to chemotherapy. This study demonstrated that in addition to gender, patients with tumors that have higher levels of miR-92a-2* did not respond to chemotherapies.[34]

One of the most feasible tumor tissue samples to obtain from cancer patients is FFPE tissue. These samples are versatile and can be used for protein and nucleic acid detection of both tumor and adjacent normal tissues, although quality can be a major concern. Quality is readily impacted by methods of tissue collection, storage, processing, and preparation.[35] Major sources of variability include the duration between tumor removal and processing, procedures for fixation or freezing, and sample storage, all of which can substantially impact the assay being conducted.[29] Some groups, including the Breast International Group and the National Cancer Institute, have developed standard operation procedures for the collection and handling of clinical specimens in breast cancer studies.[36] A couple of groups offer insights into the reporting of biomarker-driven patient studies. Both offer a checklist of sorts that are recommendations on how these data should be presented to reduce inaccurate results. McShane et al.[37] not only describe statistical guidelines for prognostic biomarker studies but also offer guidelines on how to present the data. The Biospecimen Reporting for Improved Study Quality (BRISQ) guidelines break things down into a three-tier system based on importance of being reported. These guidelines go into detail on such things as pre-acquisition of tissue, acquisition of the tissue, stabilization, storage, and quality assurance, all of which should be taken into consideration in order to reduce variability.[38] In terms of use in early drug development, there are numerous examples, some of which have facilitated recent marketing approval, such as crizotinib in anaplastic lymphoma kinase positive (ALK+) NSCLC (non–small cell lung cancer), and vemurafenib in BRAF mutant melanoma.[39,40] Even in scenarios where less well-defined patient populations are known a priori, the assessment of FFPE can be critical in the design of subsequent studies. For example, in the first-in-man study of selumetinib (an MEK inhibitor), a centralized method of biomarker processing and analysis among several sites established phosphorylation of ERK as a reliable downstream effector of MEK inhibition that was necessary but not sufficient for antitumor activity.[41] As personalized medicine increasingly utilizes next-generation sequencing methodologies, the ability to obtain quality DNA from FFPE will become paramount.[42]

Clearly, the gold standard in all assays is the collection of fresh/frozen tumor samples. These are ideal for assessing RNA and DNA for biomarker development. Fresh/frozen samples have many advantages over FFPE for molecular biology work, especially RNA applications, including quantitative real-time polymerase chain reaction (qRT-PCR). RNA extracted from FFPE is often degraded to smaller than 300 bp in length. This is usually due to the long-term room temperature storage of the blocks. The fixation process can lead to further problems because RNA is modified with methylol groups that cross-link with protein resulting in poor yields.[43] Optimization of the RNA extraction procedure and the use of shorter amplicons (<100 bp) for qRT-PCR must be performed to ensure that higher quality RNA is used for such studies. Similar procedures may be used to detect miRNA from FFPE samples and in some cases it has been demonstrated that miRNA is easier to extract because miRNAs are better preserved.[44] Although there are challenges with FFPE samples, when comparisons in gene expression profiles using cDNA-mediated annealing, selection, extension, and ligation from matched FFPE and fresh frozen were performed, after proper normalization, they largely matched,[45] although one should not conclude that full gene array analysis would yield similar results in all cases due to quality of RNA.

Another option for obtaining reliable gene expression data from patient samples is using fine-needle aspirates (FNA). Although the RNA from these samples is usually degraded as well due to bore diameter, reliable and reproducible results can be obtained using shorter amplicons for the RT-PCR.[46] FNA samples can also be reliably used for mutation detection. It has been demonstrated that FNA samples can be stored up to 57 days at room temperature on FTA indicating microcards. The DNA is then isolated and direct sequencing performed to assess for mutations.[47]

Lastly, there has been increasing interest in the collection of CTCs and/or circulating tumor DNA, which are isolated tumor cells/DNA that are identified and measured in the peripheral blood of cancer patients. There is now evidence that CTCs can be used to molecularly characterize tumor cells.[48-50] This provides a simple and convenient method that is far less invasive than a tumor biopsy. Importantly, such an approach enables serial evaluation of the tumor (which may lead to the identification of new mutations), evaluation of pharmacodynamic end points, and in some cases measurement of tumor response. Major challenges with CTCs include their limited supply in the circulation, incomplete biological characterization compared with the primary tumor (in particular concerns over the lack of stromal communication), and the various techniques and platforms available that make comparisons difficult.[51-54] Nonetheless, with advances in the methodology of enrichment and identification of CTCs, their use in clinical trials as a predictive, diagnostic, and prognostic tool may be more prevalent in future clinical trials.

COMPUTATIONAL METHODS FOR THE DEVELOPMENT OF PREDICTIVE BIOMARKERS FROM PRECLINICAL MODELS FOR EARLY DRUG DEVELOPMENT

Cancer is the phenotypic end point of multiple genetic aberrations and epigenetic modifications that have accumulated within its genome. With new and powerful high-throughput technologies, it is now possible to characterize these genetic and epigenetic alterations at high-resolution level across multiple samples. For example, technologies such as genome-wide profiling of mutations by whole-genome sequencing, copy number variations by single nucleotide polymorphisms microarray or deep sequencing, transcriptome by microarray or RNA-seq, miRNA expressions by microarray or miRNA-seq, epigenome by DNA methylation microarray or methylation-based deep sequencing, proteome by protein microarray mass spectrometry (MS), and metabolomics by MS are now not only available but becoming more feasible and cost efficient for researchers. One immediate application of these genome-wide approaches is in cancer drug development, which aims to identify predictive biomarkers that can accurately predict a patient's response to therapy, thereby facilitating individualized treatment. The overarching goal of early pharmacogenomics research is to derive predictive biomarkers in preclinical models that can ultimately be translated into biomarker-driven clinical trials.

The common bottleneck for translating data generated from these genome-wide high-throughput technologies to clinical utility is choosing the appropriate computational and statistical methods to derive accurate predictive biomarkers. The most common computational approach used to develop predictive biomarkers from genome-wide data is known as *machine learning*. The goal of applying machine learning is to derive a classifier from the data. For the development of predictive classifiers, the classifiers must be accurate in classifying new samples (*credibility*) and should be understandable by the human expert (*comprehensibility*). It is important to stress that comprehensibility is an important factor in predictive biomarker development as the features (e.g., genes and proteins) used in the classifier need to be validated by other molecular techniques (e.g., qRT-PCR for gene expression and immunoblotting for protein expression). Therefore, transparent machine learning approaches are preferable over "black box" methods.[55]

We can formulate the predictive biomarker development as a supervised learning problem where the machine learning algorithm is given a set of training data with a p-dimension (e.g., gene expression values) feature vector and its corresponding class label (e.g., sensitive or resistant) in n cell lines. The task of a machine learning algorithm is to construct some function (hypothesis) such that the function approximates the true class label. In machine learning terminology, *training* means synthesizing a hypothesis that best represents the relationship between the inputs and the corresponding outputs (class labels) and the hypothesis performs (predicts) well on future unseen data. All genome-wide high-throughput data are high dimensional (p features) in nature; therefore, strategies to search through the hypothesis space to find the "best" h is crucial for the success of the learning algorithms in this problem. Moreover, the number of training samples, n (<100) is far less than the number of p (>10,000) features; this is known as the "large p small n" problem. Therefore, to avoid over-fitting the classifiers, it is important to only select and include the most informative features in developing the classifiers.

Genomics-Based Predictive Biomarkers

Genome-wide gene expressions profiled by microarray represent the first high-throughput technology widely applied in pharmacogenomics research. Over the past decade, many attempts have been made to develop predictive biomarkers from gene expression profiles of cell lines using different machine learning algorithms. We will describe a strategy to develop predictive biomarkers from preclinical models using genome-wide gene expression profiles in the following section (Fig. 51.1). The described strategy is also applicable to other genome-wide high-throughput data for predictive biomarker development.

The Data Set

Baseline gene expressions profiled by genome-wide microarray from a panel of cell lines (e.g., NCI-60) represent the input data for the classifier. For a typical microarray experiment, the p dimension is about 20,000 gene expressions. However, the n will vary between 10 and 100 cell lines. Investigational drugs will be used to screen the panel of cell lines, and the sensitivity of each cell line will be determined by GI_{50} (50% growth inhibition), IC_{50} (half maximal inhibitory concentration), TGI (total growth inhibition), or LC_{50} (50% lethal concentration). Based on these sensitivity values, a typical approach is to stratify the cell lines into a sensitive or resistant group. To identify informative and robust genes where their expression can be detected as differentially expressed between the sensitive and resistant groups, it is advisable to use at least a fivefold difference in sensitivity as the cutoff for sensitive and resistant groups.[13] Thus, cell lines in the panel will be assigned to the most sensitive or resistant groups according to the established cutoff values, while cell lines falling between the two extremes are classified as intermediate. After the group assignment, the cell lines will be randomly divided into *training*, *validation*, and *test* sets. All data preprocessing steps (e.g., gene expression normalization) should be carried out in each divided set. Examples of challenges in this step are a limited dynamic range of responses to the novel agent, minimal cell lines that fulfill the criteria of sensitive or resistant, and a generalized lack of activity that is reflected by in vitro concentrations that are not clinically achievable. While the former challenges may be ameliorated by working with larger sets of cell lines, the latter requires assessment of issues such as drug stability in culture and the use of a relevant phenotypic end point, among others.[8,56-58]

The Training Set

The definition of the training set is a group of samples that train the learning algorithms to identify a classifier that can distinguish gene expression profiles between sensitive and resistant groups. Of note, a proper sample size

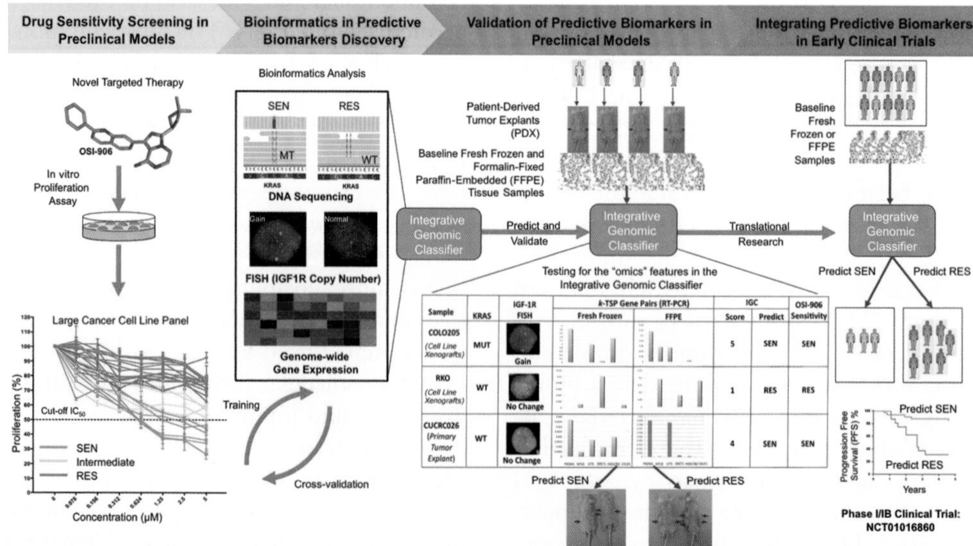

FIGURE 51–1 Overall schema of predictive biomarker development for novel agents. Biomarker development is initiated in preclinical models prior to clinical testing with the intent of performing preliminary feasibility testing in the cohort expansion phase of the initial phase I trial.

for the training set is a critical step in developing a robust and accurate classifier. The objective of having an adequate sample size for the training set is to ensure that the derived classifier has an *expected* accuracy within the range of the *optimal* accuracy. Key factors that determine the number of samples required to train the classifiers are as follows: (i) the largest standardized fold change detectable in the gene expression profiles (i.e., a gene with the largest difference in its average expression between the two classes divided by the within-class standard deviation); (ii) the number of genes on the microarrays; and (iii) the proportion of sensitive and resistant cell lines in the panel. Using these factors, Dobbin et al.[59,60] have developed a computer program to estimate the sample size required to adequately train a classifier. Typically, if the standardized fold change detectable in the gene expression between classes is small, it generally requires more training samples to identify a robust classifier.

The Validation Set

The purpose of the validation set is to optimize the classifier derived from the training set. The cell lines used in the validation set could come from the training set or be independent from the training set. Some algorithms will use the *m*-fold cross-validation of the training set to optimize the classifier. Commonly used *k*-fold includes leave-one-out cross-validation ($m = 1$, also known as the jackknife approach); 3-fold cross-validation ($m = 3$), and 10-fold cross-validation ($m = 10$). If the validation set is independent from the training set, it may provide a more robust set to optimize the classifier. Alternatively, intermediate cell lines not used in training the set could be used as a validation set.[13] The resultant classifier with optimized parameters should be "locked" at the end of validation step. The "locked" classifier will be used to assess its accuracy in an independent test set.

The Test Set

The purpose of the independent test set is to assess the accuracy of the developed classifier from the training set. If a classifier is properly trained and validated, the accuracy of the classifier in discriminating the test set should fall within the estimated accuracy derived from the validation set. The number of test sets required depends upon the proportion of sensitive and resistant cell lines in the population. If the proportion of sensitive and resistant lines is roughly equivalent, five sensitive and five resistant cell lines in the test set will be adequate. However, if the number of sensitive or resistant cell lines is rare in the population, then a larger number of test sets is required.

Model Selection

The next important step in classifier development is the choice of a machine learning algorithm. A complex model will require extensive parameter tuning to find the best classifier, which often involves large numbers of genes in the classifier, which may prove difficult to translate into a clinical test. Conversely, a simple model might be less accurate as fewer genes are involved in the classifier, yet the feasibility of a simple classifier is greater than the complex classifier. Therefore, there is a trade-off between accuracy and interpretability in developing classifiers for predictive biomarkers. Here, we briefly described a simple model (*k-TSP* [*k*-disjoint *T*op *S*coring *P*airs]) and a complex model (COXEN [coexpression extrapolation]) in predictive biomarker development.

The K-TSP Classifier

This novel comparison-based method, *k*-TSP,[61] directly addresses the trade-off between sample size and model complexity in machine learning algorithms as well as "bias–variance" by incorporating simplifying assumptions. This method seeks to discriminate disease classes by finding pairs of genes (or proteins or miRNAs) whose expression levels typically invert from one class to the other. Notably, this algorithm is specifically designed to handle small sample learning problems. Our group has demonstrated that this approach (1) is robust enough to quantify effects, (2) allows direct data integration from multiple sources, (3) is invariant to data preprocessing methods, such as normalization, under very mild assumptions, and (4) achieves or exceeds comparable machine learning methods in classifying high-throughput biomedical data.[61-63] Gene pairs with high scores are viewed as the most informative for classification. Using an internal leave-one-out cross-validation, the final *k*-TSP classifier utilizes the *k disjoint* pairs of genes, which achieve the *k* best scores from the training set. We have employed the *k*-TSP to develop predictive classifiers for novel targeted agents OSI-906, AZD0530, AZD6244, and SKI-606 in colorectal and pancreatic cancers.[13,17,64-66] From our experience,[13,17,64-66] we have found that the number of gene pairs ranges from 1 to 3. For human tumor explants, the *k*-TSP gene classifier will be performed on paraffin tissue blocks as previously described.[13,17,64,65] The gene pair comparisons can be easily interpreted as IF–ELSE decision rules. These gene pairs can be measured by RT-PCR and are thus well suited for clinical applications. Importantly, we continue to revise and refine the integration of *k*-TSP with other predictive biomarkers to facilitate the development of integrated classifiers that may incorporate data from diverse platforms.[13,17]

The COXEN Model

The idea behind the COXEN algorithm[67,68] is to utilize the information-rich data from preclinical models by deriving gene signatures that translate drug sensitivity signatures from one set of cancers (e.g., NCI-60 cell line panel) into another (e.g., bladder cell line panel, BLA-40). As this is a complex model, the COXEN algorithm[67] utilizes several steps and an iteration of multivariate analysis. The algorithm outputs a "COXEN score" that reflects the predicted sensitivity of a particular cell line to the investigational drug being evaluated by the algorithm. The initial step of the COXEN algorithm is to identify a set of genes that are differentially expressed between sensitive and resistant groups in the NCI-60 panel (cell line set 1). The next step of the algorithm is to identify a subset of these genes that demonstrate concordant coexpression relationships between the NCI-60 and BLA-40 cancer cell line panels (cell line set 2). Finally, the last step of the algorithm employs a misclassification-penalized posterior algorithm,[69] a sophisticated learning algorithm based on stepwise incremental classification modeling, to identify the most parsimonious prediction models from the training set. Double cross-validation and multiple iterations (n = 1,000) are implemented in the learning process to determine confidence bounds of the trained classifiers. Based on these confidence bounds, the prediction performance and mean misclassification error rates are obtained for each of the candidate prediction models. The final prediction of a cell line as "sensitive" or "resistant" is determined by the cell's (posterior) classification probability from each prediction model. If classification probability is >0.5 on the basis of the top three to five prediction models, the cell line is considered sensitive; if not, it is considered resistant. The COXEN algorithm has been employed to develop predictive biomarkers for chemotherapies in different cancer types.[67,70,71]

Predictive Biomarkers for OSI-906 in CRC Preclinical Models

Here, we illustrate the described strategy in Figure 51.1, which is based on our experience in developing predictive biomarkers for a selective and orally efficacious dual tyrosine kinase inhibitor (OSI-906) of the insulin growth factor 1 receptor (IGF1R) and insulin receptor in preclinical colorectal cancer models that was translated into a phase I/IB clinical trial.[13,72] To develop predictive biomarkers for OSI-906, we exposed a panel of CRC cell lines to OSI-906 and classified them according to the IC value in vitro as sensitive (<1.5 µmol/L) or resistant (>5 µmol/L).[13] Six cell lines met the criteria as sensitive. Three sensitive and three resistant cell lines were selected as the training set, and their sensitivity was confirmed in in vivo xenograft models. Baseline gene expression for the in vitro and in vivo xenografts (derived from the same sensitive and resistant cell lines in vitro) was profiled and used as the inputs for developing the predictive biomarkers. From cross-validating the training data as well as validating in the left-out cell lines (not used in the training set), the final classifier was a composite of (i) IGF1R copy number by fluorescence in situ hybridization (FISH), (ii) KRAS mutation, and (iii) the three gene pairs identified by the k-TSP classifier; which we call an integrated genomic classifier (IGC). Note that the IGF1R copy number by FISH and KRAS mutational status were incorporated into this classifier based upon their biological relevance and ability to increase the accuracy of the IGC. The k-TSP classifier contains three gene pairs: (*PROM1 > MT1E*), (*LY75 > OXCT1*), and (*HSD17B2 > CALD2*). The first decision rule is interpreted as follows: if the PROM1 expression is higher than MT1E expression, then the patient is predicted as SEN (sensitive), otherwise the patient is predicted as RES (resistant). The second and third gene pairs are interpreted in a similar manner. KRAS wild type predicts for SEN, whereas mutant predicts for RES. Gain of IGF1R as detected by FISH predicts for SEN, and no change or loss of IGF1R as detected by FISH predicts for RES. Within each criterion, a score of 1 indicates a prediction for SEN and a score of 0 indicates a prediction for RES. The final prediction is obtained by summing the equally weighted scores of three gene pairs, the KRAS status, and the IGF1R FISH, where a total predictive score ≥ 4 predicts SEN and a total predictive score < 4 predicts RES. We validated the IGC against 10 direct patient-derived CRC explants and achieved 90% accuracy. To demonstrate that the IGC prediction can be assessed and validated in FFPE samples, we extracted baseline fresh frozen and FFPE DNA and RNA from SEN (COLO205) and RES cell line (RKO) xenograft models. Our data suggest that (1) the k-TSP gene pairs can be detected in FFPE using qRT-PCR, (2) the results are concordant with the fresh frozen samples including the relative expression of the gene pairs, and (3) the predictions were consistent with the IGC utilizing fresh frozen material. We also tested the IGC in all CRC explants, and the predictions of k-TSP gene pairs in both fresh frozen and FFPE were in concordance (Fig. 51.2). This indicates that assessing IGC in FFPE patient samples is a feasible approach. To test this IGC in the clinic, we are currently conducting a predictive biomarker-driven phase I/IB trial (ClinicalTrials.gov#: NCT01016860). While we fully anticipate that further refinement of this IGC will be needed, these are the types of studies that may prove to be important in the initial testing of novel agents where obvious genetic drivers are not present, whereas some type of patient enrichment strategy is needed to ascertain early clinical activity.

Gene expression profiling and other genome-wide high-throughput technologies have advanced our understanding of cancer biology, enabling the discovery of biomarkers or signatures for characterizing and classifying tumor samples. However, due to the inherent differences between preclinical models and patients, only a few of these attempts have been translated into clinical practice. Here, we discuss some of the challenges and lessons learned in developing predictive biomarkers in preclinical models.

Challenges

In vitro sensitivity does not correlate with patient response. Drug screening in cell line panels represents an attractive approach in predictive biomarker development as it is easy to perform and the data can be obtained rapidly when compared with accessing patient samples. The common assays to assess drug activity in vitro are MTT, XTT, SRB, and CyQuant. The common readouts from these assays are GI_{50}, IC_{50}, TGI, and LC_{50}. As these

Sample	KRAS 1 = WT 0 = MUT	IGF1R FISH 1 = Gain 0 = No change/loss	FFPE k-TSP (RT-PCR) 1 = Yes 0 = No			IGC score	Predict	OSI-906 sensitivity
			PROM1 > MT1E	LY75 > OXCT1	HSD17B2 > CALD1			
CUCRC001	0	0	1	1	1	3	RES	RES
CUCRC006	0	0	1	0	1	2	RES	RES
CUCRC007	0	0	0	0	1	1	RES	RES
CUCRC010	1	0	0	1	1	3	RES	RES
CUCRC012	0	0	0	0	0	0	RES	RES
CUCRC021	0	0	1	1	0	2	RES	RES
CUCRC026	1	0	1	1	1	4	SEN	SEN
CUCRC027	0	1	1	1	1	4	SEN	SEN
CUCRC034	1	0	0	0	0	1	RES	RES
CUCRC036	0	0	0	0	1	1	RES	SEN

FIGURE 51–2 Performance of the Integrated Genomic Classifier for OSI-906 in FFPE. All components of the OSI-906 IGC were performed in FFPE (vs. fresh frozen tissue), scored, and compared with the actual human tumor explant response. The accuracy was 90% with 1/10 scores in error. FFPE, formalin-fixed paraffin-embedded tissues; k-TSP, *k*-disjoint *T*op *S*coring *P*airs; RT-PCR, real-time polymerase chain reaction; IGC, integrated genomic classifier.

assays are largely designed to detect differences in cellular proliferation upon drug exposure, it is important to identify the right assay and efficacy end point for a particular class of drugs. An area of controversy is whether in vitro assays should incorporate more stringent end points of response, such as induction of cell death. Moreover, the effective doses used in these assays should correlate with achievable and physiologically relevant drug concentrations in humans.

Established cell lines do not recapitulate the heterogeneity of human tumors. It is well known that some established cell lines that have been cultured for decades have lost the heterogeneity of human tumors and may have undergone significant genetic drift compared with the original tumors from which they were derived.[6,15,73] As some novel anticancer compounds target the stromal components of tumors, established cell lines in vitro will not accurately recapitulate the tumor-stromal microenvironment, potentially resulting in irrelevant effects.

Lessons Learned

Co-developing Predictive Biomarkers in In Vitro and In Vivo Models

As some genes may be expressed differentially in vitro when compared with in vivo, it is important to co-develop the predictive biomarkers from in vitro and in vivo gene expression profiles. One straightforward approach is to develop cell line xenografts as the in vivo models for training the classifier. This also represents a filtering step to remove cell lines that respond discordantly to drugs in in vitro and in vivo models (e.g., a cell line is sensitive to a compound in vitro but failed to show tumor growth inhibition in a mouse xenograft model). Previously, we have shown that training a classifier from in vitro and in vivo models can improve the predictive accuracy in direct patient explant models.[13] Similarly, a recent validation study of the COXEN algorithm in 100 stage I to III breast cancers before preoperative paclitaxel, 5-fluorouracil, doxorubicin, and cyclophosphamide combination chemotherapy demonstrated that a combination of four individual drug sensitivity predictions derived from cell lines in vitro was not accurate (area under the receiver operator characteristic curve [AUC], 0.5; 95% confidence interval (95% CI), 0.41 to 0.59). However, the in vivo COXEN that used informative genes from cell lines but was trained on a separate human data set showed significant predictive value (AUC, 0.67; 95% CI, 0.60 to 0.74). The authors concluded that the genomic predictor that relied solely on a composite of individual drug sensitivity predictions from cell lines did not exhibit any predictive value in patient samples.[70]

Utilizing Direct Patient Explants as an Intermediate Model for Developing and Validating Predictive Biomarkers

Direct patient explants represent an attractive preclinical model to test and develop predictive biomarkers for novel targeted therapy. In contrast to other cell line xenograft models, these specimens have never been cultured in vitro, have not evolved and adapted to those conditions (e.g., hyperoxia, plastic, exogenous media, and serum), and are expected to more accurately model the heterogeneity of human disease. A recent study using direct patient explant models in mice identified a signature of stroma-related gene pathways that predicted poor survival and resistance to gemcitabine in pancreatic cancer patients.[15] We have previously utilized this unique preclinical model to develop predictive biomarkers for erlotinib, SKI-606, OSI-906, AZD6244, AZD0530, and temsirolimus in colorectal and pancreatic cancer.[13,17,65,66,74,75] Although we do not believe that these models will be able to accurately predict which novel agents will be active in a particular disease, we do think that they represent a more stringent scenario for assessing the accuracy of a classifier and making needed revisions prior to clinical application. However, clinical validation of these models for biomarker development is not yet available.

Integrating Multi-layer Biomarkers Can Improve Prediction Accuracy

As the cancer genome has accumulated multiple genetic and epigenetic alterations, it is essential to integrate these changes in the predictive biomarkers to better reflect the state of the cancer. Furthermore, many studies have shown that ensemble approaches often outperform individual classifiers.[76] From our published data, we have demonstrated that integration of the *k*-TSP gene classifier with other molecular biomarkers such as mutation sequencing and FISH data results in a robust and accurate classifier.[13] The final prediction of this integrated predictive classifier can be implemented as majority voting or weighted voting systems, depending on the training and validation data during the biomarker development step. Such a classifier can thus integrate both unbiased and biased biomarker discovery. Clearly, recent drug approvals (e.g., crizotinib[39,77] in NSCLC with *ALK-EML4* as biomarker and vemurafenib[78]) in melanoma with *BRAF* mutation as biomarker have illustrated the utility of markers that identify genetic drivers.[79] However, as several of the projects that comprise the Cancer Genome Atlas are made publicly available, it becomes clear that there are a limited number of true driver mutations in cancer and that cancer drug development will need to increasingly rely upon integrated predictive biomarkers that are either reflective of responsiveness to a drug or identify a complex molecular subset of the disease that is sensitive.[80-87] We think a "bilateral" strategy of agent-directed and molecular subtype–directed predictive biomarker development is likely to be the most successful for agents that are not directed against a driver mutation (Fig. 51.3).

Predictive Biomarkers Should Be Easily Validated in Clinical Samples

The ultimate goal of developing predictive biomarkers from preclinical models is to translate them into biomarker-driven clinical trial selection strategies.[55,88] To facilitate

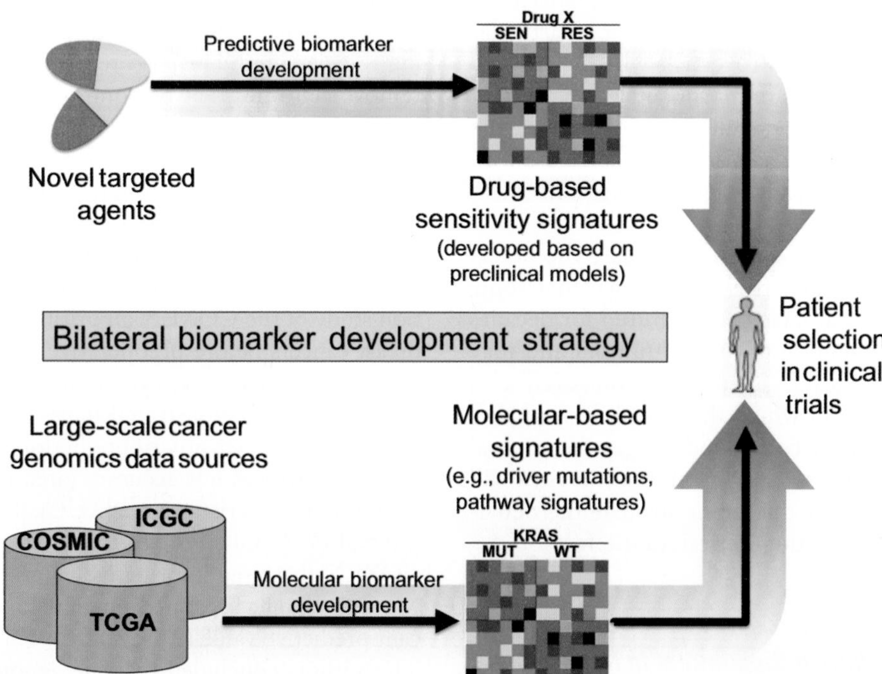

FIGURE 51–3 Bilateral predictive biomarker strategy for novel agents. Both agent-directed and molecular subtype–directed predictive biomarker development are proposed as an optimal approach when a driver mutation is not the basis of a selection marker.

the use of predictive biomarkers in a clinical setting, the ability to generate data from FFPE tissues is essential. Two strategies that could be implemented to achieve this goal are (i) to develop the predictive biomarkers from FFPE samples (e.g., Oncotype Dx[89,90]) which will ensure that the genes embedded in the classifier can be detected in these samples and (ii) to utilize a strategy whereby the number of genes in the predictive classifier is small and easily detectable in FFPE samples by qRT-PCR–based assays.

CHALLENGES OF APPLYING PERSONALIZED THERAPY IN EARLY CLINICAL TRIALS

One of the "best practices" examples of personalized cancer treatment was the development of imatinib (Gleevec) in chronic myelogenous leukemia (CML).[91,92] With the discovery of the BCR-ABL oncoprotein in CML, imatinib, a tyrosine kinase inhibitor of BCR-ABL, began phase I clinical testing in June 1998. The study demonstrated dramatic results in patients with CML leading to rapid Food Drug Administration (FDA) approval in May 2001. Although this clinical trial provided a framework for future targeted agents, the fact that CML is dependent on this "driver event" has made recapitulation of this success difficult until only recently, with the approval of crizotinib for ALK+ patients in NSCLC and vemurafenib for patients with BRAF mutations in advanced melanoma.[40,77] Literally, hundreds of new cancer agents have been evaluated in clinical trials since imatinib's approval with very few successes and at a huge cost in terms of valuable patient resources. After such a promising start, what happened?

We propose several potential challenges:

- Perhaps, there are too many new targets and drugs to evaluate within the proper context of personalized medicine. The Pharmaceutical Research and Manufacturers of America reported that 887 drugs were in clinical trials or awaiting FDA review in 2011 (http://www.phrma.org). This was more than double that of 2005, when fewer than 400 drugs were in development for cancer. With this rising number of competing drugs in clinical development, there has been a concomitant increase in the time it takes to properly evaluate these drugs and a mounting difficulty in the decision process of which drugs to pursue for further development. Likewise, there are numerous examples of "me too" drugs that are similar in structure and target the same pathways in cancer, often without a clearly defined patient selection strategy to "pick the winner." Clearly, collaboration among the pharmaceutical industry and academic centers is needed to develop "centers of expertise" in particular pathways and technologies that can prioritize and streamline these drug candidates for further clinical development.
- The problem of poor accrual to clinical trials. Of over 1.2 million people in the United States with cancer, only 3% to 5% of them will enroll in clinical trials, when up to 20% are actually eligible (www.cancer.org). In a study evaluating the participants of the National Cancer Institute Clinical Trial Cooperative Group's breast, colorectal, lung, and prostate cancer clinical trials between 2000 and 2002, breast cancer patients represented 54.2% of trial participants, although they accounted for only 27.9% of incident cancer cases.[93] In addition, it was reported that racial and ethnic minorities, females, and the elderly were less likely to enroll in cooperative group cancer trials than whites, males, and younger patients, respectively.[93] If this holds true for most clinical trials, the patients enrolling in them are not representative of the general cancer population. New agents, therefore, may not be properly evaluated in their intended population. As we move toward individualized therapy, enhancing the participation of patients in the screening process will become critical, as for many of these agents, the proportion of biomarker positivity is in the range of 5% to 20% and thus to maintain efficiency, large numbers of patients will need to be screened for large numbers of drugs.[77,94] Likewise, adequate representation of women, older patients, and ethic minorities in the early clinical trials is important to ensure that preclinically derived predictive classifiers are valid in those populations as well.
- The majority of cancers are not dependent on "driver" mutations. Unlike CML, where almost all patients harbor the BCR-ABL translocation protein, single "driver" mutations in other cancers are not as prevalent and they often harbor numerous mutations. For example, dozens of mutations have been implicated in the development of colorectal cancer.[95] The more common oncogene mutations, KRAS (40%), PI3K (25%), and BRAF (5% to 10%), are still only present in a subset of colorectal cancer patients and, based upon available data, do not appear to be "drivers" in the classical sense.[96-98] Thus, it is likely that predictive biomarker discovery for many tumor types will require high complexity data, sophisticated discovery algorithms, and multiple platforms. Nonetheless, the risk of not developing such classifiers for targeted agents is that in unselected patient populations they will appear ineffective. With large-scale genomic sequencing projects now starting to be concluded and published, it is also likely that for each tumor type, a number of molecular subtypes will be discovered, leading to the identification of "driver" pathways that can be targeted by single agents or rational combinations.[80,86,98,99] Such a "bilateral" agent-directed and molecular subtype–directed drug development approach may result in a higher success rate of novel agents (see Fig. 51.3).
- The difficulty of integrating putative predictive biomarkers is in early clinical studies. Until

recently, biomarkers in phase I trials were predominantly pharmacodynamic. However, the recent successes of crizotinib and vemurafenib have reinvigorated the incorporation of patient selective markers earlier in development, often during a dose expansion phase. There are still numerous challenges, including the cost and regulatory development of pharmacodiagnostic tests, having to screen large numbers of patients for rare mutations or expression profiles, and the pressure to initiate early clinical trials quickly, before a selection strategy is established due to competitors with similar compounds entering the arena.

In an effort to improve the clinical success of targeted agents, early clinical trials are being designed to overcome some of these obstacles.

Biomarker-Driven Clinical Trials

There has been a shift in integrating biomarkers earlier into clinical trials with new trial designs. In the past, the majority of novel agents in early clinical trials were not developed for a particular patient population, often due to the inability to identify that population or concerns that such selection would be too restrictive early in the development process. Thus, they were generally evaluated using the standard 3+3 dose-escalating phase I study design in an unselected population with advanced cancer. Biomarkers were generally restricted to correlative or exploratory pharmacodynamic studies that were performed with the intent of establishing proof of mechanism. Luckily, recent experience, both positive and negative (below), is clearly supportive of the notion of bilateral agent-directed and tumor molecular subtype–directed patient selection strategies.

Lessons Learned

Positive: Crizotinib

Following the identification of the transforming EMLA-ALK fusion gene in NSCLC,[100] crizotinib, an orally available small molecule inhibitor of the ALK tyrosine kinase, was evaluated in NSCLC.[77] Approximately 1,500 patients with NSCLC were screened, which identified 82 patients with the FISH-positive ALK+ rearrangement. The overall response rate was 57% (47/82): 46 confirmed partial responses and 1 complete response. Another 27 (33%) had stable disease. A majority of the patients were still on study at the time of data-cuff, so no median survival was reported. However, the estimated probability of 6-month progression-free survival was 72%. Crizotinib was approved by the FDA in August 2011. This study demonstrated that proper screening for a biomarker, even a rare mutation, could lead to high response rates and the ability to obtain accelerated marketing approval. It also supported the feasibility of screening a large number of patients even in the phase I setting and established one of the earliest precedents of concordant companion diagnostic and drug marketing approval in oncology.

Negative: EGFR Antibodies

Even when biomarkers are incorporated earlier in clinical studies, they have not always been successful. Cetuximab initially received marketing approval for metastatic colorectal cancer that overexpressed the epidermal growth factor receptor (EGFR) by immunohistochemical staining. In this "selected population," it was still only effective in 10% of patients when used as a single agent. Similar response rates, however, were observed in patients with no EGFR overexpression; therefore, there were patients that were incorrectly prohibited from its use and perhaps from deriving clinical benefit.[101] Conversely, the identification of a negative predictor biomarker (KRAS mutation) was identified 5 years after the approval of cetuximab,[102,103] leading to thousands of patients being treated with the agent and subjected to toxicity with little hope of benefit. This story continues as further work in this area has led to refinement of both agent-based and molecular subtype-based predictive biomarkers for this class of agents.[104-106]

Future Directions

Increasingly, early clinical trials are incorporating tissue biopsies and/or biomarker testing as part of the patient entry criteria.

These criteria are introduced as follows:

1. At the maximum tolerated dose or recommended phase II dose cohorts (dose expansion phase). These cohorts are often disease specific.
2. In all patients and cohorts, when there is sufficient evidence that a predictive biomarker is needed to enrich the patient population.

The main advantage of this approach is to initially test the performance of the biomarker in the intended target population, thereby enhancing the preliminary evidence of antitumor activity and enabling more informed decisions regarding phase II development.

The Challenges

Diagnostic Testing and Validation

Often the testing of novel molecular targets/biomarkers involves novel diagnostic techniques which need to be investigated, validated, and occur in conjunction with the preclinical development of the target agents. The development of these diagnostic tests, however, may not be complete prior to the commencement of phase I trials. There is also the fact that a majority of preclinical compounds will not enter phase I clinical testing. Developing new diagnostics test too early therefore could be futile if the drug does not successfully enter clinical trials.

Treatment Delay

If a biomarker is identified and a reliable test for it exists, there may be issues with treatment delay. Whether a new biopsy or archival tissue is required, it will still take some time to acquire the appropriate tumor sample, send it to a central lab for molecular testing, and then make a decision based upon that result. These findings may take several weeks or more to obtain. Patients and their oncologists may not be willing to wait, especially when there is a chance they may not be eligible for the study. However, with earlier testing, while patients are still receiving treatment and where multiple agents exist in a single protocol, studies like the *Biomarker-Integrated Approaches of Targeted Therapy for Lung Cancer Elimination (BATTLE) program* may be more acceptable to patients and their oncologists.[107]

Cost of Personalized Clinical Trials

Besides the additional cost in the preclinical setting, the cost of biomarker-driven clinical trials is more expensive than standard phase I trials. There will be additional costs in obtaining new biopsies and biomarker analysis. If mutations are rare, more patients are required to be screened for the study, thus driving up the costs. In the crizotinib trial, 1,500 patients with NSCLC had to be screened to identify 82 patients with the FISH-positive ALK+ rearrangement.[77] The time and cost to screen thousands of patients are significant, and, furthermore, a hindrance to trial accrual and drug development. Therefore, more efficient screening methods will need to be employed to ensure that several agents and molecular subtypes are screened for simultaneously.

Multi-arm Patient Selection Trials (Octopus Trials)

Multi-arm (octopus) trials attempt to address the issues of an abundance of agents but restricted patient numbers. These novel studies incorporate multiple arms and multiple drugs, whereby patients are assigned to specific agents (arms) based on their biomarker results. From a patient standpoint, these studies are attractive since they are being evaluated for several drugs at once. For clinicians, multiple mutations can be evaluated simultaneously and thus it is more likely that a potential drug will be identified for the patient.

The main challenge is for the investigator to have access to enough drugs to supply the arms. Rarely will a single pharmaceutical company be able to supply the drugs for all arms, and thus collaboration between several pharmaceutical companies is required. This, obviously, can be a major logistical hurdle. Potential issues may arise with financing these trials, having multiple laboratories carrying out different biomarker testing on the same tissue samples, sharing the intellectual property associated with the study, and collaborating with other companies that have competing agents. Despite these challenges, trials like the BATTLE and the MD Anderson Cancer Center Initiative have demonstrated that these studies may be feasible.[107,108]

CONCLUSIONS

With the ever-expanding knowledge in cancer biology, numerous aberrant pathways are being discovered, and hence many novel targeted agents are being developed. Newer early drug development approaches are therefore needed, and indeed are now being incorporated into phase I clinical development to increase the success of these agents. As we move toward personalized medicine, hopefully more effective treatments will become available to cancer patients that lead to long-term clinical benefit.

REFERENCES

1. Shoemaker RH. The NCI60 human tumour cell line anticancer drug screen. *Nat Rev Cancer*. Oct 2006;6(10):813-823.
2. Sharma SV, Haber DA, Settleman J. Cell line-based platforms to evaluate the therapeutic efficacy of candidate anticancer agents. *Nat Rev Cancer*. Apr 2010;10(4):241-253.
3. Debnath J, Brugge JS. Modelling glandular epithelial cancers in three-dimensional cultures. *Nat Rev Cancer*. Sep 2005;5(9):675-688.
4. Horning JL, Sahoo SK, Vijayaraghavalu S, et al. 3-D tumor model for in vitro evaluation of anticancer drugs. *Mol Pharm*. Sep-Oct 2008;5(5):849-862.
5. Stein WD, Litman T, Fojo T, Bates SE. A Serial Analysis of Gene Expression (SAGE) database analysis of chemosensitivity: comparing solid tumors with cell lines and comparing solid tumors from different tissue origins. *Cancer Res*. Apr 15 2004;64(8):2805-2816.
6. Daniel VC, Marchionni L, Hierman JS, et al. A primary xenograft model of small-cell lung cancer reveals irreversible changes in gene expression imposed by culture in vitro. *Cancer Res*. Apr 15 2009;69(8):3364-3373.
7. Tentler JJ, Tan AC, Weekes CD, et al. Patient-derived tumour xenografts as models for oncology drug development. *Nat Rev Clin Oncol*. June 1 2012;9(6):338-350.
8. Johnson JI, Decker S, Zaharevitz D, et al. Relationships between drug activity in NCI preclinical in vitro and in vivo models and early clinical trials. *Br J Cancer*. May 18 2001;84(10):1424-1431.
9. Tredan O, Galmarini CM, Patel K, Tannock IF. Drug resistance and the solid tumor microenvironment. *J Natl Cancer Inst*. Oct 3 2007;99(19):1441-1454.
10. Bankert RB, Egilmez NK, Hess SD. Human-SCID mouse chimeric models for the evaluation of anti-cancer therapies. *Trends Immunol*. Jul 2001;22(7):386-393.
11. Rubio-Viqueira B, Hidalgo M. Direct in vivo xenograft tumor model for predicting chemotherapeutic drug response in cancer patients. *Clin Pharmacol Ther*. Feb 2009;85(2):217-221.
12. Rubio-Viqueira B, Jimeno A, Cusatis G, et al. An in vivo platform for translational drug development in pancreatic cancer. *Clin Cancer Res*. Aug 1 2006;12(15):4652-4661.
13. Pitts TM, Tan AC, Kulikowski GN, et al. Development of an integrated genomic classifier for a novel agent in colorectal cancer: approach to individualized therapy in early development. *Clin Cancer* Res. Jun 15 2010;16(12):3193-3204.
14. Nemati F, Sastre-Garau X, Laurent C, et al. Establishment and characterization of a panel of human uveal melanoma xenografts derived from primary and/or metastatic tumors. *Clin Cancer Res*. Apr 15 2010;16(8):2352-2362.
15. Garrido-Laguna I, Uson M, Rajeshkumar NV, et al. Tumor engraftment in nude mice and enrichment in stroma- related gene pathways predict poor survival and resistance to gemcitabine in patients with pancreatic cancer. *Clin Cancer Res*. Sep 1 2011;17(17):5793-5800.
16. John T, Kohler D, Pintilie M, et al. The ability to form primary tumor xenografts is predictive of increased risk of disease recurrence in early-stage non-small cell lung cancer. *Clin Cancer Res*. Jan 1 2011;17(1):134-141.
17. Arcaroli JJ, Touban BM, Tan AC, et al. Gene array and fluorescence in situ hybridization biomarkers of activity of saracatinib (AZD0530), a Src inhibitor, in a preclinical model of colorectal cancer. *Clin Cancer Res*. Aug 15 2010;16(16):4165-4177.
18. Politi K, Pao W. How genetically engineered mouse tumor models provide insights into human cancers. *J Clin Oncol*. Jun 1 2011;29(16):2273-2281.
19. Shimizu N, Ando A, Teramoto S, Moritani Y, Nishii K. Outcome of patients with lung cancer detected via mass screening as compared to those presenting with symptoms. *J Surg Oncol*. May 1992;50(1):7-11.
20. Singh M, Johnson L. Using genetically engineered mouse models of cancer to aid drug development: an industry perspective. *Clin Cancer Res*. Sep 15 2006;12(18):5312-5328.

21. Dumeaux V, Olsen KS, Nuel G, Paulssen RH, Borresen-Dale AL, Lund E. Deciphering normal blood gene expression variation—The NOWAC postgenome study. *PLoS Genet*. Mar 2010;6(3):e1000873.
22. Mor G, Visintin I, Lai Y, et al. Serum protein markers for early detection of ovarian cancer. *Proc Natl Acad Sci U S A*. May 24 2005;102(21):7677-7682.
23. Kelly P, Appleyard V, Murray K, et al. Detection of oesophageal cancer biomarkers by plasma proteomic profiling of human cell line xenografts in response to chemotherapy. *Br J Cancer*. Jul 13 2010;103(2):232-238.
24. Halamkova J, Kiss I, Pavlovsky Z, et al. Clinical significance of the plasminogen activator system in relation to grade of tumor and treatment response in colorectal carcinoma patients. *Neoplasma*. 2011;58(5):377-385.
25. Pena C, Lathia C, Shan M, Escudier B, Bukowski RM. Biomarkers predicting outcome in patients with advanced renal cell carcinoma: Results from sorafenib phase III Treatment Approaches in Renal Cancer Global Evaluation Trial. *Clin Cancer Res*. Oct 1 2010;16(19):4853-4863.
26. Esquela-Kerscher A, Slack FJ. Oncomirs - microRNAs with a role in cancer. *Nat Rev Cancer*. Apr 2006;6(4):259-269.
27. Calin GA, Croce CM. MicroRNA signatures in human cancers. *Nat Rev Cancer*. Nov 2006;6(11):857-866.
28. Lu J, Getz G, Miska EA, et al. MicroRNA expression profiles classify human cancers. *Nature*. Jun 9 2005;435(7043): 834-838.
29. Tsujiura M, Ichikawa D, Komatsu S, et al. Circulating microRNAs in plasma of patients with gastric cancers. *Br J Cancer*. Mar 30 2010;102(7):1174-1179.
30. Mitchell PS, Parkin RK, Kroh EM, et al. Circulating microRNAs as stable blood-based markers for cancer detection. *Proc Natl Acad Sci U S A*. Jul 29 2008;105(30):10513-10518.
31. Cheng H, Zhang L, Cogdell DE, et al. Circulating plasma MiR-141 is a novel biomarker for metastatic colon cancer and predicts poor prognosis. *PLoS One*. 2011;6(3):e17745.
32. Zuo Z, Calin GA, de Paula HM, et al. Circulating microRNAs let-7a and miR-16 predict progression-free survival and overall survival in patients with myelodysplastic syndrome. *Blood*. Jul 14 2011;118(2):413-415.
33. Preis M, Gardner TB, Gordon SR, et al. MicroRNA-10b expression correlates with response to neoadjuvant therapy and survival in pancreatic ductal adenocarcinoma. *Clin Cancer Res*. Sep 1 2011;17(17):5812-5821.
34. Ranade AR, Cherba D, Sridhar S, et al. MicroRNA 92a-2*: a biomarker predictive for chemoresistance and prognostic for survival in patients with small cell lung cancer. *J Thorac Oncol*. Aug 2010;5(8):1273-1278.
35. Goldstein NS, Hewitt SM, Taylor CR, Yaziji H, Hicks DG. Recommendations for improved standardization of immunohistochemistry. *Appl Immunohistochem Mol Morphol*. Jun 2007;15(2): 124-133.
36. Leyland-Jones BR, Ambrosone CB, Bartlett J, et al. Recommendations for collection and handling of specimens from group breast cancer clinical trials. *J Clin Oncol*. Dec 1 2008;26(34):5638-5644.
37. McShane LM, Altman DG, Sauerbrei W, Taube SE, Gion M, Clark GM. REporting recommendations for tumor MARKer prognostic studies (REMARK). *Breast Cancer Res Treat*. Nov 2006;100(2):229-235.
38. Moore HM, Kelly AB, Jewell SD, et al. Biospecimen reporting for improved study quality (BRISQ). *Cancer Cytopathol*. Apr 25 2011;119(2):92-101.
39. Shaw AT, Yeap BY, Solomon BJ, et al. Effect of crizotinib on overall survival in patients with advanced non-small-cell lung cancer harbouring ALK gene rearrangement: a retrospective analysis. *Lancet Oncol*. Oct 2011;12(11):1004-1012.
40. Chapman PB, Hauschild A, Robert C, et al. Improved survival with vemurafenib in melanoma with BRAF V600E mutation. *N Engl J Med*. Jun 30 2011;364(26):2507-2516.
41. Adjei AA, Cohen RB, Franklin W, et al. Phase I pharmacokinetic and pharmacodynamic study of the oral, small-molecule mitogen-activated protein kinase kinase 1/2 inhibitor AZD6244 (ARRY-142886) in patients with advanced cancers. *J Clin Oncol*. May 1 2008;26(13):2139-2146.
42. Schweiger MR, Kerick M, Timmermann B, et al. Genome-wide massively parallel sequencing of formaldehyde fixed-paraffin embedded (FFPE) tumor tissues for copy-number- and mutation-analysis. *PLoS One*. 2009;4(5):e5548.
43. Li J, Smyth P, Cahill S, et al. Improved RNA quality and TaqMan Pre-amplification method (PreAmp) to enhance expression analysis from formalin fixed paraffin embedded (FFPE) materials. *BMC Biotechnol*. 2008;8:10.
44. Xi Y, Nakajima G, Gavin E, et al. Systematic analysis of microRNA expression of RNA extracted from fresh frozen and formalin-fixed paraffin-embedded samples. *RNA*. Oct 2007;13(10):1668-1674.
45. Mittempergher L, de Ronde JJ, Nieuwland M, et al. Gene expression profiles from formalin fixed paraffin embedded breast cancer tissue are largely comparable to fresh frozen matched tissue. *PLoS One*. 2011;6(2):e17163.
46. Anderson MA, Brenner DE, Scheiman JM, et al. Reliable gene expression measurements from fine needle aspirates of pancreatic tumors: effect of amplicon length and quality assessment. *J Mol Diagn*. Sep 2010;12(5):566-575.
47. da Cunha Santos G, Liu N, Tsao MS, Kamel-Reid S, Chin K, Geddie WR. Detection of EGFR and KRAS mutations in fine-needle aspirates stored on Whatman FTA cards: is this the tool for biobanking cytological samples in the molecular era? *Cancer Cytopathol*. Dec 25 2010;118(6):450-456.
48. Hauch S, Zimmermann S, Lankiewicz S, Zieglschmid V, Bocher O, Albert WH. The clinical significance of circulating tumour cells in breast cancer and colorectal cancer patients. *Anticancer Res*. May-Jun 2007;27(3A):1337-1341.
49. Zieglschmid V, Hollmann C, Mannel J, et al. Tumor-associated gene expression in disseminated tumor cells correlates with disease progression and tumor stage in colorectal cancer. *Anticancer Res*. Jul-Aug 2007;27(4A):1823-1832.
50. Maheswaran S, Sequist LV, Nagrath S, et al. Detection of mutations in EGFR in circulating lung-cancer cells. *N Engl J Med*. Jul 24 2008;359(4):366-377.
51. Konigsberg R, Gneist M, Jahn-Kuch D, et al. Circulating tumor cells in metastatic colorectal cancer: efficacy and feasibility of different enrichment methods. *Cancer Lett*. Jul 1 2010;293(1):117-123.
52. Sun YF, Yang XR, Zhou J, Qiu SJ, Fan J, Xu Y. Circulating tumor cells: advances in detection methods, biological issues, and clinical relevance. J Cancer Res Clin Oncol. Aug 2011;137(8):1151-1173.
53. Yu M, Stott S, Toner M, Maheswaran S, Haber DA. Circulating tumor cells: approaches to isolation and characterization. *J Cell Biol*. Feb 7 2011;192(3):373-382.
54. Nagrath S, Sequist LV, Maheswaran S, et al. Isolation of rare circulating tumour cells in cancer patients by microchip technology. *Nature*. Dec 20 2007;450(7173):1235-1239.
55. Khleif SN, Doroshow JH, Hait WN. AACR-FDA-NCI Cancer Biomarkers Collaborative consensus report: advancing the use of biomarkers in cancer drug development. *Clin Cancer Res*. Jul 1 2010;16(13):3299-3318.
56. Samson DJ, Seidenfeld J, Ziegler K, Aronson N. Chemotherapy sensitivity and resistance assays: a systematic review. *J Clin Oncol*. Sep 1 2004;22(17):3618-3630.
57. Schrag D, Garewal HS, Burstein HJ, Samson DJ, Von Hoff DD, Somerfield MR. American Society of Clinical Oncology Technology Assessment: chemotherapy sensitivity and resistance assays. *J Clin Oncol*. Sep 1 2004;22(17):3631-3638.
58. Phillips RM, Bibby MC, Double JA. A critical appraisal of the predictive value of in vitro chemosensitivity assays. *J Natl Cancer Inst*. Sep 19 1990;82(18):1457-1468.
59. Dobbin KK, Zhao Y, Simon RM. How large a training set is needed to develop a classifier for microarray data? *Clin Cancer Res*. Jan 1 2008;14(1):108-114.
60. Dobbin KK, Simon RM. Sample size planning for developing classifiers using high-dimensional DNA microarray data. *Biostatistics*. Jan 2007;8(1):101-117.
61. Tan AC, Naiman DQ, Xu L, Winslow RL, Geman D. Simple decision rules for classifying human cancers from gene expression profiles. *Bioinformatics*. Oct 15 2005;21(20):3896-3904.
62. Xu L, Tan AC, Naiman DQ, Geman D, Winslow RL. Robust prostate cancer marker genes emerge from direct integration of inter-study microarray data. *Bioinformatics*. Oct 15 2005;21(20):3905-3911.
63. Xu L, Tan AC, Winslow RL, Geman D. Merging microarray data from separate breast cancer studies provides a robust prognostic test. *BMC Bioinformatics*. 2008;9:125.

64. Messersmith WA, Rajeshkumar NV, Tan AC, et al. Efficacy and pharmacodynamic effects of bosutinib (SKI-606), a Src/Abl inhibitor, in freshly generated human pancreas cancer xenografts. *Mol Cancer Ther*. Jun 2009;8(6):1484-1493.
65. Rajeshkumar NV, Tan AC, De Oliveira E, et al. Antitumor effects and biomarkers of activity of AZD0530, a Src inhibitor, in pancreatic cancer. *Clin Cancer Res*. Jun 15 2009;15(12):4138-4146.
66. Tentler JJ, Nallapareddy S, Tan AC, et al. Identification of predictive markers of response to the MEK1/2 inhibitor selumetinib (AZD6244) in K-ras-mutated colorectal cancer. *Mol Cancer Ther*. Dec 2010;9(12):3351-3362.
67. Lee JK, Havaleshko DM, Cho H, et al. A strategy for predicting the chemosensitivity of human cancers and its application to drug discovery. *Proc Natl Acad Sci U S A*. Aug 7 2007;104(32):13086-13091.
68. Smith SC, Baras AS, Lee JK, Theodorescu D. The COXEN principle: translating signatures of in vitro chemosensitivity into tools for clinical outcome prediction and drug discovery in cancer. *Cancer Res*. Mar 1 2010;70(5):1753-1758.
69. Soukup M, Cho H, Lee JK. Robust classification modeling on microarray data using misclassification penalized posterior. *Bioinformatics*. Jun 2005;21 Suppl 1:i423-430.
70. Lee JK, Coutant C, Kim YC, et al. Prospective comparison of clinical and genomic multivariate predictors of response to neoadjuvant chemotherapy in breast cancer. *Clin Cancer Res*. Jan 15 2010;16(2):711-718.
71. Williams PD, Cheon S, Havaleshko DM, et al. Concordant gene expression signatures predict clinical outcomes of cancer patients undergoing systemic therapy. *Cancer Res*. Nov 1 2009;69(21):8302-8309.
72. Flanigan SA, Pitts TM, Eckhardt SG, et al. The insulin-like growth factor I receptor/insulin receptor tyrosine kinase inhibitor PQIP exhibits enhanced antitumor effects in combination with chemotherapy against colorectal cancer models. *Clin Cancer Res*. Nov 15 2010;16(22):5436-5446.
73. Derose YS, Wang G, Lin YC, et al. Tumor grafts derived from women with breast cancer authentically reflect tumor pathology, growth, metastasis and disease outcomes. *Nat Med*. October 2011;17(11):1514-1520
74. Jimeno A, Tan AC, Coffa J, et al. Coordinated epidermal growth factor receptor pathway gene overexpression predicts epidermal growth factor receptor inhibitor sensitivity in pancreatic cancer. *Cancer Res*. Apr 15 2008;68(8):2841-2849.
75. Garrido-Laguna I, Tan AC, Uson M, et al. Integrated preclinical and clinical development of mTOR inhibitors in pancreatic cancer. *Br J Cancer*. Aug 24 2010;103(5):649-655.
76. Tan AC, Gilbert D. Ensemble machine learning on gene expression data for cancer classification. *Appl Bioinformatics*. 2003;2(3 Suppl):S75-83.
77. Kwak EL, Bang YJ, Camidge DR, et al. Anaplastic lymphoma kinase inhibition in non-small-cell lung cancer. *N Engl J Med*. Oct 28 2010;363(18):1693-1703.
78. Bollag G, Hirth P, Tsai J, et al. Clinical efficacy of a RAF inhibitor needs broad target blockade in BRAF-mutant melanoma. *Nature*. Sep 30 2010;467(7315):596-599.
79. Gerber DE, Minna JD. ALK inhibition for non-small cell lung cancer: from discovery to therapy in record time. *Cancer Cell*. Dec 14 2010;18(6):548-551.
80. Integrated genomic analyses of ovarian carcinoma. *Nature*. Jun 30 2011;474(7353):609-615.
81. Verhaak RG, Hoadley KA, Purdom E, et al. Integrated genomic analysis identifies clinically relevant subtypes of glioblastoma characterized by abnormalities in PDGFRA, IDH1, EGFR, and NF1. *Cancer Cell*. Jan 19 2010;17(1):98-110.
82. Agrawal N, Frederick MJ, Pickering CR, et al. Exome sequencing of head and neck squamous cell carcinoma reveals inactivating mutations in NOTCH1. *Science*. Aug 26 2011;333(6046): 1154-1157.
83. Stransky N, Egloff AM, Tward AD, et al. The mutational landscape of head and neck squamous cell carcinoma. *Science*. Aug 26 2011;333(6046):1157-1160.
84. Wood LD, Parsons DW, Jones S, et al. The genomic landscapes of human breast and colorectal cancers. *Science*. Nov 16 2007;318(5853):1108-1113.
85. Jones S, Zhang X, Parsons DW, et al. Core signaling pathways in human pancreatic cancers revealed by global genomic analyses. *Science*. Sep 26 2008;321(5897):1801-1806.
86. Comprehensive genomic characterization defines human glioblastoma genes and core pathways. *Nature*. Oct 23 2008;455(7216):1061-1068.
87. Weir BA, Woo MS, Getz G, et al. Characterizing the cancer genome in lung adenocarcinoma. *Nature*. Dec 6 2007;450(7171):893-898.
88. Taube SE, Clark GM, Dancey JE, McShane LM, Sigman CC, Gutman SI. A perspective on challenges and issues in biomarker development and drug and biomarker codevelopment. *J Natl Cancer Inst*. Nov 4 2009;101(21):1453-1463.
89. Paik S, Shak S, Tang G, et al. A multigene assay to predict recurrence of tamoxifen-treated, node-negative breast cancer. *N Engl J Med*. Dec 30 2004;351(27):2817-2826.
90. Paik S. Development and clinical utility of a 21-gene recurrence score prognostic assay in patients with early breast cancer treated with tamoxifen. *Oncologist*. Jun 2007;12(6):631-635.
91. Druker BJ, Talpaz M, Resta DJ, et al. Efficacy and safety of a specific inhibitor of the BCR-ABL tyrosine kinase in chronic myeloid leukemia. *N Engl J Med*. Apr 5 2001;344(14):1031-1037.
92. Druker BJ, Guilhot F, O'Brien SG, et al. Five-year follow-up of patients receiving imatinib for chronic myeloid leukemia. *N Engl J Med*. Dec 7 2006;355(23):2408-2417.
93. Murthy VH, Krumholz HM, Gross CP. Participation in cancer clinical trials: race-, sex-, and age-based disparities. *JAMA*. Jun 9 2004;291(22):2720-2726.
94. Slamon DJ, Leyland-Jones B, Shak S, et al. Use of chemotherapy plus a monoclonal antibody against HER2 for metastatic breast cancer that overexpresses HER2. *N Engl J Med*. Mar 15 2001;344(11):783-792.
95. Futreal PA, Coin L, Marshall M, et al. A census of human cancer genes. *Nat Rev Cancer*. Mar 2004;4(3):177-183.
96. Bass A. Impact of KRAS and BRAF gene mutations on targeted therapies in colorectal cancer. *J Clin Oncol*. Jul 1 2011;29(19): 2728-2729.
97. Van Cutsem E, Kohne CH, Lang I, et al. Cetuximab plus irinotecan, fluorouracil, and leucovorin as first-line treatment for metastatic colorectal cancer: updated analysis of overall survival according to tumor KRAS and BRAF mutation status. *J Clin Oncol*. May 20 2011;29(15):2011-2019.
98. De Roock W, Claes B, Bernasconi D, et al. Effects of KRAS, BRAF, NRAS, and PIK3CA mutations on the efficacy of cetuximab plus chemotherapy in chemotherapy-refractory metastatic colorectal cancer: a retrospective consortium analysis. *Lancet Oncol*. Aug 2010;11(8):753-762.
99. Li J, Shen H, Himmel KL, et al. Leukaemia disease genes: large-scale cloning and pathway predictions. *Nat Genet*. Nov 1999;23(3):348-353.
100. Soda M, Choi YL, Enomoto M, et al. Identification of the transforming EML4-ALK fusion gene in non-small-cell lung cancer. *Nature*. Aug 2 2007;448(7153):561-566.
101. Chung KY, Shia J, Kemeny NE, et al. Cetuximab shows activity in colorectal cancer patients with tumors that do not express the epidermal growth factor receptor by immunohistochemistry. *J Clin Oncol*. Mar 20 2005;23(9):1803-1810.
102. Van Cutsem E, Kohne CH, Hitre E, et al. Cetuximab and chemotherapy as initial treatment for metastatic colorectal cancer. *N Engl J Med*. Apr 2 2009;360(14):1408-1417.
103. Tol J, Koopman M, Cats A, et al. Chemotherapy, bevacizumab, and cetuximab in metastatic colorectal cancer. *N Engl J Med*. Feb 5 2009;360(6):563-572.
104. De Roock W, Jonker DJ, Di Nicolantonio F, et al. Association of KRAS p.G13D mutation with outcome in patients with chemotherapy-refractory metastatic colorectal cancer treated with cetuximab. *JAMA*. Oct 27 2010;304(16):1812-1820.
105. Janakiraman M, Vakiani E, Zeng Z, et al. Genomic and biological characterization of exon 4 KRAS mutations in human cancer. *Cancer Res*. Jul 15 2010;70(14):5901-5911.
106. Gazin C, Wajapeyee N, Gobeil S, Virbasius CM, Green MR. An elaborate pathway required for Ras-mediated epigenetic silencing. *Nature*. Oct 25 2007;449(7165):1073-1077.
107. Kim ES, Herbst RS, Wistuba II, et al. The BATTLE Trial: Personalizing Therapy for Lung Cancer. *Cancer Discovery* June 2011 1:44-53.
108. Tsimberidou AM, Iskander NG, Hong DS, et al. Personalized medicine in a phase I clinical trials program: The M. D. Anderson Cancer Center Initiative. J Clin Oncol 29: 2011 (suppl; abstr CRA2500).

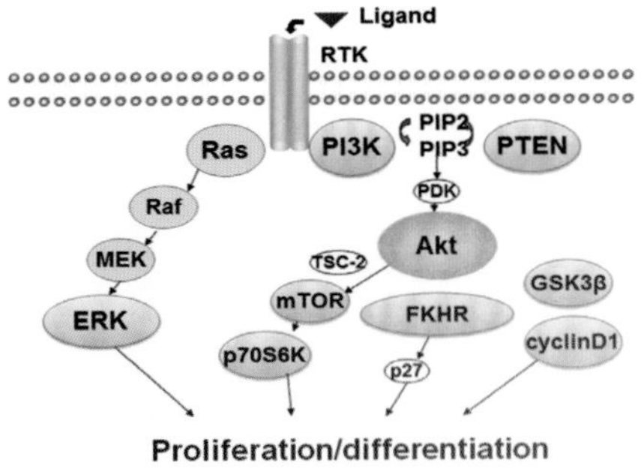

SECTION VI

Personalized Medicine and Targeted Therapy of Cancer

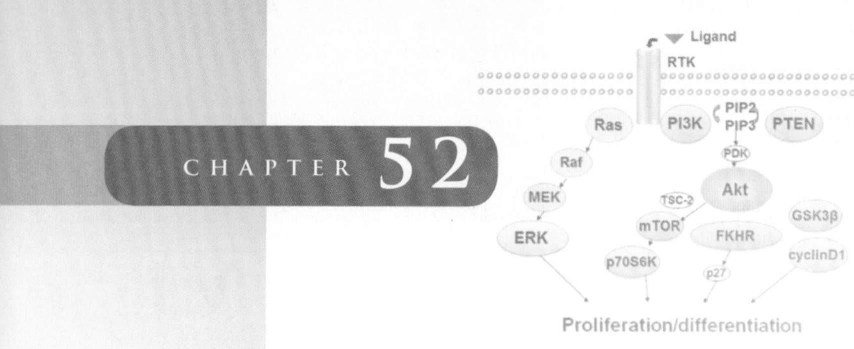

CHAPTER 52

PERSONALIZED MEDICINE AND TARGETED THERAPY OF LUNG CANCER

Mary C. Pinder-Schenck and Scott J. Antonia

INTRODUCTION

Lung cancer is the leading cause of cancer deaths in the United States and worldwide, accounting for over 1 million deaths annually.[1] Non–small cell lung cancers (NSCLCs) represent approximately 80% of all lung cancers. Long-term survival remains low for patients with NSCLC, with only 16% surviving 5 years.[2] This poor survival is in part explained by the large percentage of patients who present with metastatic disease, for whom local therapies such as surgery and radiation play little role. Until the last decade, platinum-based chemotherapy was the mainstay of treatment for patients with advanced NSCLC, resulting in modest improvements in overall survival. Increasingly, however, advances in the molecular characterization of NSCLC have resulted in therapies targeting specific oncogenic pathways or molecular abnormalities. These therapies have resulted in a meaningful survival advantage for subpopulations of NSCLC patients and have ushered in a paradigm shift in the management of this disease. In a relatively short period of time, molecular testing and tailored therapy has become the standard approach in the clinic for patients with advanced NSCLC. Our research focus has also shifted, and clinical trials have moved away from targeting the heterogeneous population of NSCLC patients to trials aimed at specific subpopulations based on molecular testing. In addition to the potential for improved survival, targeted therapies generally offer patients the possibility of milder side-effect profiles and the ability to sustain treatment for longer time periods.

While this rapid shift in our understanding and treatment of NSCLC offers significant promise for the future, the present continues to represent challenges to clinicians and researchers. The need for larger amounts of tumor tissue for clinical decision-making, appropriate clinical trial selection, and translational research will require an increase in invasive procedures for patients with significant attendant risks and will demand changes in clinical training and practice to facilitate adequate and safe tissue procurement and processing. As NSCLC becomes divided into smaller subpopulations based on molecular typing, accrual of patients to clinical trials will require a high level of sophistication on the part of clinicians and the cooperation of multiple researchers and institutions. Although side effects of targeted agents are often considered less severe than those for traditional chemotherapy, their management comes with a new set of challenges. Each new class of targeted agents has brought unique and sometimes unanticipated side effects. The recognition and management of these side effects will continue to evolve and will require rapid assimilation and distribution of knowledge that often has not been a part of traditional oncology training programs.

Although our understanding of the molecular underpinnings of NSCLC has advanced rapidly, a large number of patients are not currently candidates for targeted therapy. The development of targeted therapy for small cell lung cancer has been characterized by multiple promising preclinical targets, which ultimately ended in unsuccessful clinical trials. While some patients with NSCLC may be able to access novel targeted therapies through clinical trials, approximately 50% of NSCLC patients have tumors with no known molecular targets. Finally, for patients who do respond to targeted agents, the eventual development of resistance has been the rule thus far. Identifying mechanisms of targeted therapy resistance and overcoming or preventing them represents another area that is rapidly evolving.

This chapter reviews the development and current evidence for U.S. Food and Drug Administration (FDA)–approved targeted therapies. We outline resistance mechanisms and side effects of these agents as well as ongoing challenges for the implementation of personalized medicine in the clinic. We also review the evidence for biomarkers of chemotherapeutic effectiveness that may allow for improved selection of chemotherapeutic agents for individual patients. Finally, we discuss molecular targets with agents currently in development.

CHEMOTHERAPY IN THE TREATMENT OF NSCLC

While significant advances had been made since the initial use of chemotherapy in the 1940s, as late as the mid-1990s, considerable controversy surrounded the use of chemotherapy in patients with NSCLC. In 1995, the Non-Small Cell Lung Cancer Collaborative Group published a meta-analysis of chemotherapy in NSCLC, using individual patient data from 52 randomized clinical trials.[3] Based on their analysis, the authors concluded that, in advanced NSCLC, cisplatin-based chemotherapy yielded a modest benefit compared with supportive care alone, with a hazard ratio (HR) of 0.73 ($P < 0.0001$) and a 1½ month increase in median survival time. The authors also noted that the addition of chemotherapy to surgery for early-stage NSCLC appeared to improve outcomes, albeit modestly. Even at this early point in the history of lung cancer therapy, the editorial accompanying the meta-analysis foreshadowed the era of personalized medicine, with a call for "molecular biological characteristics" that might help to identify a subset of NSCLC tumors with enhanced chemotherapy responsiveness.[4]

A series of adjuvant trials in patients with surgically resectable NSCLC were launched because of promising early results for platinum-based chemotherapy. Three large, randomized trials demonstrated a statistically significant survival benefit for cisplatin-based adjuvant chemotherapy.[5-7] Several other trials failed to demonstrate a statistically significant survival benefit for adjuvant chemotherapy[8-11]; however, based on the results of the three positive trials, adjuvant chemotherapy became and remains the standard of care for patients with resected stage II or III NSCLC. The fact that the benefit of adjuvant platinum-based chemotherapy was confined to a relatively small population of patients prompted a series of retrospective analyses of adjuvant trials in an attempt to identify markers of chemotherapy responsiveness, as outlined in the next section.

For advanced disease, a variety of platinum-based doublets were tested, eventually culminating in the landmark Eastern Cooperative Oncology Group (ECOG) 1594 trial, which compared four platinum-based doublets in patients with advanced NSCLC.[12] No significant differences were observed in progression-free or overall survival among the four doublets. However, more favorable toxicity profiles were observed for carboplatin/paclitaxel and cisplatin/gemcitabine. After ECOG 1594, one of these two regimens was commonly employed as the control arm in randomized trials of chemotherapy in NSCLC. A series of clinical trials failed to demonstrate any benefit to adding a third chemotherapeutic agent to a platinum-based doublet. Then, in 2006, the results of ECOG 4599 demonstrated a 2-month improvement in median overall survival with the addition of bevacizumab, a monoclonal antibody that inhibits vascular endothelial growth factor (VEGF)-A, to carboplatin and paclitaxel.[13,14] Another monoclonal antibody, cetuximab, which targets the epidermal growth factor receptor (EGFR), demonstrated a 1.2-month improvement in survival when added to cisplatin and vinorelbine compared with the same chemotherapy doublet alone.

The development of pemetrexed, an inhibitor of multiple folate-dependent enzymes involved in DNA synthesis, in the second-line setting in advanced NSCLC led to a randomized phase III clinical trial comparing cisplatin plus gemcitabine to cisplatin plus pemetrexed.[15] While the two regimens were equivalent in response rate, progression-free survival, and overall survival in the intention to treat population, the authors found that patients with nonsquamous histology had improved survival with the pemetrexed doublet while those with squamous histology had improved survival with the gemcitabine doublet.[16] This trial established the importance of histology in predicting pemetrexed efficacy and led to the FDA approval of pemetrexed in conjunction with cisplatin in the first-line treatment of nonsquamous NSCLC. Potential reasons behind the importance of histology in determining response to pemetrexed are explored in the next section.

CHEMOTHERAPY RESPONSE: PROGNOSTIC AND PREDICTIVE MARKERS

A number of clinically relevant prognostic and predictive markers have emerged from retrospective analyses in both early-stage and advanced NSCLC.[6,17-24] The term *prognostic* refers to a marker that is useful for estimating a patient outcome (such as survival) independent of therapeutic decisions. A *predictive* marker is useful in making therapeutic decisions: the effect of treatment is different in marker-positive and marker-negative patients. These markers will be important in designing future trials in NSCLC and are already being incorporated into prospective clinical trials in the adjuvant and metastatic settings.

Excision Repair Cross Complementation Group 1

The mechanism of action of cisplatin involves the formation of cross-links between strands of DNA. Several components of the DNA damage response network have emerged as important predictors of response to platinum-based chemotherapy. The DNA damage response network consists of a series of redundant cell cycle checkpoints and

DNA repair enzymes that are crucial to maintaining the genomic integrity of the cell. Nucleotide excision repair (NER) is a highly conserved DNA repair pathway, which repairs DNA lesions that alter the helical structure of the DNA molecule and interfere with DNA replication and transcription. Excision repair cross complementation group 1 (ERCC1) is a key enzyme in the NER complex. ERCC1 dimerizes with xeroderma pigmentosum complementation group F (XPF), and this complex is required for the excision of damaged DNA. In vitro data have demonstrated the importance of ERCC1 in repairing DNA cross-links induced by platinum.[25-27]

Retrospective studies of advanced NSCLC patients treated with platinum-based chemotherapy have borne out these preclinical findings: low tumoral expression of ERCC1 is associated with improved survival in patients treated with platinum-based chemotherapy.[28-36] The feasibility of prospectively determining chemotherapy based on expression of ERCC1 and ribonucleotide reductase messenger 1 (RRM1) has been demonstrated in a phase II trial in advanced NSCLC, with promising progression-free and overall survival compared with historic controls.[37] A randomized phase III trial prospectively examined the impact of ERCC1 expression in patients with advanced NSCLC and found that the response rate was improved in the group that received customized chemotherapy based on ERCC1 expression, compared with the control group (treated with cisplatin plus docetaxel regardless of ERCC1 expression).[38] There was no difference in overall survival between the two groups. Another randomized phase III trial, Molecular Analysis Directed Individualized Therapy (MADeIT-P3), comparing tailored therapy to standard chemotherapy, is ongoing.

In the adjuvant setting, retrospective data also indicate that low tumoral expression of ERCC1 is associated with a benefit from platinum-based chemotherapy. A retrospective analysis of the International Adjuvant Lung Cancer Trial (IALT) found that, in patients with ERCC1-negative tumors, adjuvant chemotherapy improved survival compared with no therapy. In patients who received no adjuvant chemotherapy, those with ERCC1-positive tumors had improved survival compared with those with ERCC1-negative tumors.[19] Simon and colleagues have confirmed these findings, postulating that improved prognosis in early-stage patients with ERCC1-positive tumors relates to an intact DNA repair mechanism that diminishes the accumulation of genetic aberrations that ultimately result in a more malignant tumor phenotype and progression of disease.[17] ERCC1 is being incorporated as a prospective biomarker in the design of several adjuvant chemotherapy trials.

Ribonucleotide Reductase Messenger 1

RRM1 encodes one of two regulatory subunits of ribonucleotide reductase. The gene has been mapped to chromosome segment 11p15.5, a region with frequent loss of heterozygosity in NSCLC,[39-41] a characteristic that has been associated with poor survival in early-stage patients.[40] The enzyme ribonucleotide reductase is the rate-limiting enzyme in the conversion of ribonucleotide diphosphates to the corresponding deoxyribonucleotides, a process that is crucial for de novo DNA synthesis as well as repair of damaged DNA.[42-44] In lung cancer cell lines, high expression of RRM1 leads to increased expression of phosphatase and tensin homologue (PTEN), thereby decreasing cell migration, invasiveness, and metastatic potential.[45,46] High levels of RRM1 suppressed carcinogen-induced lung tumors in transgenic mice.[47] RRM1 is the target of the nucleoside analogue gemcitabine (2′,2′-difluorodeoxycytidine), and increased RRM1 expression has been associated with resistance to gemcitabine in vitro.[48,49]

Retrospective analyses of lung cancer clinical trials have borne out these preclinical findings. Rosell and colleagues reported that advanced NSCLC patients treated with platinum-gemcitabine combinations on randomized trials had superior overall survival and improved response to gemcitabine-containing regimens when RRM1 was low in tumor tissue.[50,51] Similarly, patients treated with a non-platinum, gemcitabine-containing doublet improved survival if their tumors expressed lower levels of RRM1.[52]

Similar to ERCC1, patients with early-stage lung cancer treated with surgery alone have a more favorable prognosis if RRM1 levels are high in their tumors.[18,20]

Several studies have found a strong correlation between RRM1 and ERCC1 expression.[18,28,34,50] RRM1, along with ERCC1, has been evaluated for feasibility as a means of customizing chemotherapy in the metastatic setting,[37] and an ongoing randomized phase III trial compares customized chemotherapy based on ERCC1 and RRM1 expression to standard platinum-based chemotherapy. The impact of RRM1 levels on outcomes in patients receiving adjuvant chemotherapy has not been evaluated.

Breast Cancer Gene 1

The breast and ovarian cancer susceptibility gene 1 (BRCA1) was identified in 1990. First sequenced in 1994, the 81-kDa gene was localized on chromosome 17q21.[53] Deleterious BRCA1 mutations are also associated with bilateral breast cancer and earlier age at onset compared with sporadic cancers. BRCA1 is a tumor suppressor gene,[54] and the BRCA1 protein plays key roles in DNA damage detection and repair,[55-57] transcriptional regulation,[58,59] cell cycle control,[60] ubiquitination,[61] and chromatin remodeling.[62] Although the number of patients with cancers related to germline mutations in BRCA1/2 is small, there is now ample evidence that a wider group of sporadic tumors may have BRCA-like phenotypes. While triple-negative breast cancer is the best characterized example, varying levels of BRCA expression have been reported in NSCLC.[22,23] BRCA1 is a prognostic marker in NSCLC, with low levels of mRNA expression associated with prolonged survival in patients with surgically resected disease.[22] BRCA1 is also a predictive marker in NSCLC, with low levels of expression indicating a higher likelihood of response to cisplatin.[63] Conversely, high BRCA expression in NSCLC is associated with platinum resistance and taxane sensitivity.[63,64]

Based on its differential impact on response to platinum and taxanes, prospective clinical trials have been designed incorporating BRCA1 as a biomarker for treatment selection. The Spanish Lung Cancer Group recently reported their feasibility study utilizing BRCA mRNA expression to determine adjuvant therapy in patients with resected stage II-III NSCLC.[65] Assignment of patients to customized chemotherapy was shown to be feasible, with no detrimental effect of treating patients with high BRCA1 levels with docetaxel alone. A randomized phase III study utilizing the same design, the Spanish Customized Adjuvant Trial (SCAT) is ongoing. A similar trial in the metastatic setting, the BRCA1 Expression Customization (BREC) study is also ongoing. When completed, these studies are expected to add substantially to our understanding of BRCA1 as a biomarker in NSCLC.

MutS Homologue 2

The gene MutS Homologue 2 (MSH2) encodes a key protein in the mismatch repair (MMR) pathway, another component of the DNA damage response network. MSH2 recognizes and binds to cisplatin-induced DNA interstrand cross-links, facilitating their excision and repair. MSH2 interacts with ERCC1[66] and several other components of the DNA damage response network, including REV1, Fanconi anemia proteins, and homologous repair factors.[67] Diminished expression of MSH2 has been reported in a subset of NSCLC tumor specimens.[68,69] A polymorphism in the MSH2 gene has been associated with poor prognosis in patients with advanced NSCLC.[70] Scartozzi et al.[68] reported an association of low MSH2 expression with response to oxaliplatin- but not cisplatin-based chemotherapy in patients with advanced NSCLC.

In a recent retrospective analysis of MSH2 expression in IALT biospecimens, Kamal and colleagues explored the prognostic and predictive value of MSH2 in patients with resected NSCLC.[71] The authors showed that low MSH2 was predictive of a benefit from chemotherapy, albeit of borderline statistical significance. Patients whose tumors expressed high levels of MSH2 did not benefit from adjuvant chemotherapy. In the control group, high MSH2 was associated with improved overall survival, suggesting that MSH2 may have value as a prognostic marker in NSCLC. The authors also combined MSH2 with the markers ERCC1 and p27 and found that patients in the subgroups with low MSH2/low ERCC1 or low MSH2/low p27 benefited from adjuvant chemotherapy. Although these findings will require additional confirmation, they suggest that MSH2, either alone or in combination with other biomarkers, may have value as a prognostic and predictive biomarker in NSCLC.

Thymidylate Synthase

The enzyme thymidylate synthase (TS) generates thymidine monophosphate, which is subsequently phosphorylated to thymidine triphosphate for use in DNA synthesis and repair. TS is inhibited by a variety of chemotherapeutic agents, including 5-fluorouracil and pemetrexed. Pemetrexed inhibits multiple enzymes involved in purine synthesis, including TS, dihydrofolate reductase, and glycinamide ribonucleotide formyl transferase.[72] In preclinical models, low levels of these enzymes correlate with sensitivity to pemetrexed.[73,74] Differences in TS expression across histological subtypes of NSCLC have been proposed as a molecular explanation for the effect of histology on outcomes in pemetrexed-treated NSCLC patients.[15] Indeed, in tumor specimens from NSCLC patients, TS protein and messenger RNA levels are significantly higher in squamous cell carcinomas compared with those in adenocarcinomas, suggesting that TS expression, rather than histology, may serve as a more reliable marker of pemetrexed sensitivity.[75-77] Providing additional evidence in support of this hypothesis, a phase II trial of neoadjuvant gemcitabine and pemetrexed in resectable NSCLC demonstrated that response to chemotherapy was inversely correlated with tumoral levels of TS.[21] The International TAilored Chemotherapy Adjuvant (ITACA) trial is a randomized trial utilizing TS and ERCC1 expression to customize adjuvant treatment in the experimental arm; the control arm will receive standard platinum-based doublet therapy.

TARGETED THERAPY OF NSCLC: MONOCLONAL ANTIBODIES

Bevacizumab

Angiogenesis has long been recognized as one of the hallmarks of malignant transformation.[78,79] While small tumors (<2 mm) are able to extract oxygen and nutrients via diffusion, larger tumors require the formation of a neovasculature to sustain their growth.[80] Secretion of proangiogenic factors by tumors results in the recruitment of endothelial precursor cells to the tumor site, proliferation of these cells, and capillary tube formation.[81] Increased angiogenic signaling has been associated with poor prognosis in a number of malignancies, including NSCLC.[82] Expression of VEGF and VEGF receptor and other markers of angiogenesis in lung tumors, such as tumor microvessel density, have all been linked to inferior survival in patients with NSCLC.[83-85]

The importance of angiogenesis in tumor progression and metastasis spurred efforts to develop therapies targeting components of angiogenic signaling. Bevacizumab is a humanized monoclonal antibody with a high affinity for VEGF. By binding circulating VEGF, bevacizumab inhibits binding of VEGF to its receptors, interrupting downstream proangiogenic signaling.[13,86] A randomized phase II trial in 99 patients with advanced NSCLC compared carboplatin and paclitaxel with or without bevacizumab (at a dose of 7.5 mg/kg or 15 mg/kg). Bevacizumab in combination with chemotherapy resulted in higher response rates and improved progression-free survival (at the 15 mg/kg dose). Six severe bleeding events (four of which were fatal) occurred on the bevacizumab arm of this trial and were associated with squamous histology, central tumor location, and cavitation.[87]

The promising results of the phase II trial led to the landmark ECOG 4599 trial, which randomized patients to either carboplatin and paclitaxel alone or in combination with bevacizumab at a dose of 15 mg/kg with continuation of bevacizumab until progression. Due to the safety concerns raised in the phase II study, only patients with nonsquamous histologies were included. Significant improvements were observed for response rates (35% vs. 15%), progression-free survival (6.2 vs. 4.5 months), and overall survival (12.3 vs. 10.3 months) in the bevacizumab arm.[14] Subset analyses indicated that the overall survival benefit of bevacizumab was not observed in women and elderly patients.[88] Clinically significant bleeding, hematologic toxicity, febrile neutropenia, hypertension, and proteinuria were all more common in the bevacizumab arm. The ECOG 4599 investigators collected and analyzed a number of potential biomarkers, including VEGF, basic fibroblast growth factor, and intercellular adhesion molecule (ICAM). Low levels of ICAM were associated with a better prognosis and appeared to be predictive of benefit from bevacizumab treatment. Patients with high levels of plasma VEGF were more likely to respond to bevacizumab plus chemotherapy than to chemotherapy alone, but this did not translate into an overall survival benefit in these patients.[89] Clinically, the development of hypertension during treatment was associated with improved outcomes in patients on the bevacizumab arm of ECOG 4599.[90] Based on the results of ECOG 4599, bevacizumab was approved by the FDA in combination with chemotherapy in the first-line setting for patients with nonsquamous NSCLC.

Bevacizumab was also studied in combination with cisplatin and gemcitabine in the randomized phase III AVAstin in Lung Cancer (AVAiL) trial, which was conducted in Europe and Canada. Patients were randomized to chemotherapy alone or chemotherapy plus bevacizumab (at either 7.5 or 15 mg/kg). The bevacizumab-containing arms showed an improvement in progression-free survival, the primary endpoint of the trial. However, overall survival was not improved with the addition of bevacizumab, though a median overall survival greater than 13 months was seen in all groups. The authors speculated that the widespread use of effective later-line therapies may have contributed to the lack of improvement in overall survival in this study.[91]

Bevacizumab combined with chemotherapy is currently being compared with chemotherapy alone in the adjuvant setting in a large, randomized phase III study (ECOG 1505). Numerous studies combining bevacizumab with other agents are underway in advanced NSCLC, and other drugs targeting angiogenesis are also in development in NSCLC. However, initial results with small-molecule tyrosine kinase inhibitors (TKIs) targeting angiogenesis have been disappointing in NSCLC.[92,93]

Cetuximab

EGFR is expressed in 40% to 80% of NSCLC[94,95] and has been associated with increased tumor proliferation, angiogenesis, invasion, metastasis, and evasion of apoptosis.[95-97] Cetuximab, a monoclonal antibody to EGFR, demonstrated activity in combination with cisplatin in preclinical studies.[98] The results of a randomized phase II trial in patients with advanced EGFR-expressing NSCLC demonstrated an increase in response and an improvement in survival in patients given cetuximab combined with cisplatin and vinorelbine compared with chemotherapy alone. On the basis of these results, the randomized phase III FLEX trial was launched. Conducted in Europe and Asia, FLEX randomized chemotherapy-naïve patients with stage IV NSCLC (any histology) and evidence of tumor EGFR expression by immunohistochemistry (IHC) to either cetuximab plus cisplatin and vinorelbine or chemotherapy alone. The addition of cetuximab to chemotherapy resulted in a statistically significant improvement in overall survival compared with that with chemotherapy alone (11.3 vs. 10.1 months).[99] Response rate, but not progression-free survival, was also improved in patients receiving cetuximab.

The FLEX investigators have explored a number of biomarkers in an attempt to identify the subset of patients most likely to benefit from cetuximab. Unlike the EGFR TKIs, gefitinib and erlotinib, the clinical activity of cetuximab is not linked to the presence of EGFR-activating mutations. The presence of KRAS mutations also did not predict for lack of response to cetuximab.[100] Rash after the first cycle was predictive of benefit for cetuximab. Recently, the FLEX investigators reported that high EGFR expression by IHC was predictive of longer survival in patients who received cetuximab. In patients who received chemotherapy alone, EGFR expression did not affect prognosis or predict a benefit from chemotherapy.[101]

DRIVER MUTATIONS WITH SUCCESSFUL TARGETED THERAPIES

EGFR Mutations and the Small-Molecule Inhibitors of EGFR

EGFR belongs to a family of receptor tyrosine kinases that includes EGFR/ERBB1, HER2/ERBB2, HER3/ERBB3, and HER4/ERBB4. Binding of ligands, including epidermal growth factor, phosphorylates EGFR and results in a number of downstream effects including cell growth, proliferation, and survival. These effects are mediated primarily through the phosphatidylinositol

3-kinase (PI3K)-AKT-mTOR and RAS-RAF-MEK-ERK signaling pathways.

The EGFR TKIs gefitinib and erlotinib were first developed in unselected populations of patients with NSCLC.[102-104] In this setting, tumor response rates were typically 10% or less. However, clinical characteristics of patients who responded to therapy rapidly emerged: female gender, Asian ethnicity, adenocarcinoma histology, and never-smoking status.[102,104-106] In 2004, activating mutations in the tyrosine kinase domain of EGFR were identified as the molecular basis for EGFR TKI sensitivity; these mutations were found to be more common in the clinical subgroups previously identified.[107,108] The incidence of EGFR mutations varies across different populations, with a frequency of 10% to 15% in the predominantly Caucasian populations of the United States, Europe, and Australia while the incidence is as high as 36% in Taiwan and other Asian countries.[109] While mutations are more common in women and never-smokers, they do occur at a lower frequency in all populations, including men and smokers, underscoring the importance of performing molecular testing rather than using clinical characteristics to determine the likelihood of response to EGFR TKIs.[110]

Mutations in EGFR occur within exons 18 to 21 of the gene, which encodes a portion of the EGFR kinase domain. Mutations are usually heterozygous, with gene amplification of the mutant allele occurring. The two most common mutations are in-frame deletions in exon 19 and the L858R point mutation in exon 21. These two abnormalities together comprise 90% of EGFR mutations. A variety of other mutations occur at relatively low frequencies.

Recent randomized clinical trials have confirmed prospectively the strong benefit associated with the use of EGFR TKIs in patients with EGFR mutations. The International Pan-Asia Study (IPASS) trial randomized Asian light or never-smokers with advanced NSCLC or adenocarcinoma histology to front-line treatment with either gefitinib or chemotherapy (carboplatin plus paclitaxel).[111] Patients were not selected for the trial on the basis of EGFR mutation status, but 60% of the patients were found to have an EGFR mutation. In patients with EGFR mutations, gefitinib treatment was associated with significantly improved response rates (71.2% vs. 47.3%) and progression-free survival (HR = 0.48, $P < 0.0001$) compared with chemotherapy. In patients who did not have EGFR mutations, gefitinib treatment was associated with significantly worse outcomes compared with chemotherapy. There was no difference in overall survival for EGFR-positive patients who received gefitinib compared with those who received carboplatin/paclitaxel. A high proportion of patients crossing over to gefitinib upon progression likely accounted for the lack of a difference in overall survival.[112] The Spanish Lung Cancer Study Group conducted a single-arm study of erlotinib in patients with EGFR mutations and demonstrated similar overall survival in patients with EGFR mutations regardless of whether erlotinib was received in the first-, second-, or third-line setting.[113] Subsequent randomized trials have confirmed the favorable results with gefitinib in patients with EGFR mutations[114,115] and have identified similar findings with erlotinib,[116] and in a European population.[117]

Erlotinib has been evaluated as a maintenance treatment after front-line chemotherapy in an unselected population and was associated with improvement in progression-free survival and a modest benefit in overall survival when compared with placebo.[118] While the most impressive results were obtained in patients with EGFR mutations, a benefit was also observed in mutation-negative patients.[119] These results are in keeping with results seen in the second-/third-line setting, where, in spite of modest response rates, erlotinib has been associated with a survival benefit in a broader population[103]; the drug is FDA-approved in an unselected population in the maintenance and second-/third-line setting.

In summary, EGFR mutation status is a powerful predictive marker for response to EGFR TKIs in the metastatic setting. The National Comprehensive Cancer Network (NCCN) has recommended testing of all advanced NSCLC adenocarcinomas for EGFR mutations. In EGFR-positive patients, EGFR TKI therapy is recommended in the first-line setting, based on the superior response rates and progression-free survival as well as more favorable toxicity profile observed across multiple clinical trials. In the maintenance or second-line or greater setting, EGFR TKIs may be used in unselected patients. The role of EGFR TKI therapy in the adjuvant setting remains under investigation and several clinical trials incorporating EGFR mutation status into adjuvant treatment assignment are underway.

Acquired Resistance to EGFR TKIs

In spite of the favorable results observed with the use of EGFR TKIs in patients with EGFR mutations, resistance to these drugs invariably develops. The two major mechanisms of acquired resistance to EGFR TKIs are the development of a second site T790M point mutation in exon 20[120,121] and overexpression of components of the hepatocyte growth factor (HGF) receptor or MET pathway.[122,123]

T790M

At least 50% of patients with acquired resistance to EGFR TKIs will have developed a second mutation that coexists with the primary EGFR mutation.[108,124,125] The most common resistance mutation observed involves the substitution of threonine for methionine at position 790 (T790M). While sensitizing EGFR mutations decrease the receptor's affinity for ATP, T790M restores the receptor's affinity for ATP, allowing the cell to overcome the effects of the TKI.[126] In preclinical models, TKI-resistant cells harboring T790M show diminished proliferation compared with TKI-sensitive cells.[127] Similarly, in patients with acquired resistance, T790M has been associated with a more indolent clinical course.[128,129] Discontinuation of EGFR TKIs in patients with acquired resistance has been associated with accelerated progression, both clinically and radiographically.[130,131] A potential mechanism for this flare phenomenon is the reemergence of faster growing TKI-sensitive cells in the absence of the selective pressure (TKI therapy) that led to the emergence of the slower growing T790M population. This mechanism also likely underlies the observation that patients who develop acquired resistance may respond again to EGFR TKIs after a treatment hiatus.[125] Whether to continue an EGFR TKI after progression in patients with acquired resistance remains an area of active investigation, and there are no consensus guidelines at this time.

Targeting resistance due to T790M has become a priority for clinical trial development. In preclinical models, irreversible EGFR TKIs were effective against T790M mutant lung cancer.[132,133] The irreversible inhibitor, afatinib, was evaluated in a randomized phase III clinical trial; patients in the control arm received placebo.[134] To enter the trial, patients were required to have progression after a minimum of 12 weeks on erlotinib or gefitinib. The trial did not require repeat biopsy for entry and the incidence of T790M was unknown. The primary endpoint of the trial, overall survival, did not differ between afatinib and placebo. Progression-free survival was significantly improved in the afatinib arm: a 7% response rate was observed with afatinib. The lack of a benefit in overall survival may have been related to the use of salvage therapy and the prolonged overall survival seen in the placebo arm of the trial. The combination of the irreversible TKI afatinib with the monoclonal antibody cetuximab resulted in significant regression of tumors in a mouse model of T790M resistance while neither agent alone was effective.[135] While the combination of cetuximab and erlotinib has proven ineffective,[136] a recent phase Ib trial of afatinib and cetuximab demonstrated a response rate of 36% in patients with acquired resistance, suggesting that this strategy may prove useful in the clinic.[137]

MET Amplification

Another well-described mechanism of acquired resistance to EGFR TKI therapy involves amplification of the receptor tyrosine kinase, MET, which occurs in up to 20% of patients with acquired resistance.[122] MET amplification results in activation of ERBB3-PI3K-AKT signaling in the presence of EGFR TKI therapy. MET amplification has been shown to be present in a subpopulation of tumor cells prior to EGFR treatment, with clonal selection of MET-amplified cells occurring after EGFR-directed therapy.[138] A number of strategies to target MET-amplified tumors are in development, including monoclonal antibodies against MET and its ligand, HGF, as well as small-molecule MET TKIs. In a randomized phase II trial, the combination of a MET monoclonal antibody and erlotinib was superior to erlotinib alone in patients with overexpression of MET, regardless of EGFR mutation status.[139]

Anaplastic Lymphoma Kinase Fusions and ALK Inhibitors

In 2007, Soda and colleagues identified fusion of anaplastic lymphoma kinase (ALK) and echinoderm microtubule-associated protein-like 4 (EML4) in 6.7% of Japanese lung cancer tumor specimens.[140] Subsequent reports confirmed EML4-ALK translocations in other populations, with an incidence from 1.6% to 11.6%.[141-145] Clinical characteristics associated with the EML4-ALK fusion gene are similar to those associated with EGFR mutations, although the two mutations are mutually exclusive.[143] Patients with EML4-ALK translocations typically have adenocarcinomas and are light or never-smokers. In addition, ALK aberrations have been associated with younger age at onset,[146] acinar[146] or signet ring[147] features on histology, and thyroid transcription factor-1 (TTF-1) positivity on IHC.[146,148] The presence of an EML4-ALK fusion has been associated with prolonged responses to pemetrexed[149] and resistance to EGFR TKIs.[143,148]

The fusion of EML4 (as well as other fusion partners) to ALK results in constitutive ALK kinase activation. In cell lines and mouse models, EML4-ALK is oncogenic and cancers with this fusion protein are sensitive to ALK inhibition.[150,151] Crizotinib is an oral, small-molecule inhibitor of ALK, with proven preclinical and clinical activity in NSCLC harboring ALK fusions. The drug, which also inhibits MET kinase, was evaluated in the phase I setting, with an expansion cohort at the recommended phase II dose for patients with ALK activation. In the 82 NSCLC patients enrolled in the molecular expansion cohort, the overall response rate was 57%, and an additional 33% had stable disease.[145] The U.S. FDA approved crizotinib in 2011 for the treatment of NSCLC, with evidence of ALK translocation as determined by fluorescence in situ hybridization (FISH). Crizotinib is the only ALK inhibitor that is commercially available at this time.

Methods of Detecting ALK Rearrangements

In addition to FISH, other methods being evaluated for the detection of ALK rearrangements include reverse transcriptase polymerase chain reaction (RT-PCR) and IHC. However, in current clinical trials, FISH is employed as the definitive diagnostic test for ALK rearrangements. In the FISH assay, the 5′- and 3′-ends of the ALK gene are labeled with red and green fluorescent probes. When an ALK rearrangement is present, the red and green signals will be separated in space or split. While this assay has been shown to have a high sensitivity and specificity for detection of ALK rearrangements, it is costly to perform and requires expertise and equipment that may not be widely available. Furthermore, if only a small amount of genetic material is inverted, detection of a split signal may be challenging. While RT-PCR can detect the presence of an ALK rearrangement as well as identify the specific ALK fusion partner and fusion variant, it may not be practical due to the difficulty of obtaining high-quality RNA from formalin-fixed, paraffin-embedded tumor samples. In contrast to FISH and RT-PCR, IHC is widely available and cost-effective and has a rapid turnaround, making it an ideal tool for screening large populations for ALK rearrangements. ALK is not normally expressed in the adult lung (or other adult tissues); therefore, ALK expression is indicative of aberrant ALK signaling. Indeed, IHC is routinely used for the diagnosis of anaplastic large cell lymphoma (ALCL) with ALK rearrangement. However, the IHC antibodies used for the diagnosis of ALK rearrangements in ALCL are unable to detect ALK rearrangements in NSCLC due to the lower expression of ALK. Novel, more sensitive antibodies are under development and may eventually provide a more widely available, cost-effective method of detecting ALK rearrangements.

Targeting Resistance to Crizotinib

Similar to the experience with EGFR TKIs, patients with ALK translocations treated with crizotinib eventually develop drug resistance and disease progression. Currently, mechanisms of acquired resistance to crizotinib are under investigation. Secondary mutations that eliminate the inhibitory activity of crizotinib have been identified in patients who have developed acquired resistance to the drug.[152-154] While the mechanisms by which these mutations cause resistance have not been fully elucidated, leading possibilities include impedance of crizotinib binding or promotion of the kinase's affinity for ATP. Crizotinib resistance may also occur through activation of other signaling pathways, such as EGFR[153] or PI3K.[155]

Currently, clinical trials aimed at patients who have developed resistance to crizotinib fall into three categories: heat shock protein 90 (Hsp90) inhibitors, novel ALK inhibitors, and combinations of ALK inhibitors with drugs targeting other signaling pathways. Hsp90 acts as a cellular chaperone to EML4-ALK, among other proteins. Cell lines harboring crizotinib resistance mutations have demonstrated sensitivity to Hsp90 inhibitors.[156] Clinical trials of two Hsp90 inhibitors, retaspimycin (IPI-504) and ganetespib (STA-9090), have shown efficacy in patients with ALK rearrangements; however, these trials did not include patients with prior crizotinib exposure.[157,158] A number of second-generation ALK inhibitors have demonstrated preclinical efficacy and are in clinical development for the treatment of NSCLC with ALK rearrangements. While preclinical models have demonstrated increased potency of these agents, it remains unknown whether this will translate into effective treatment of crizotinib resistance in patients. Finally, two studies are examining simultaneous targeting of ALK and EGFR: a single-agent phase I/II trial of the dual EGFR-ALK inhibitor AP26113 (NCT01449461) and a combination of crizotinib and the pan-HER inhibitor PF299804 (NCT01441128).

OTHER DRIVER MUTATIONS WITH POTENTIAL TARGETED THERAPIES

Recently, the Lung Cancer Mutation Consortium (LCMC) demonstrated the feasibility of testing tumor samples from advanced NSCLC patients (adenocarcinoma histology) for a variety of driver mutations, with the ultimate goal of identifying patients for appropriate clinical trials based on the tumor's molecular profile. The LCMC investigators found that over 50% of adenocarcinomas harbored mutations that could be targeted either with approved therapies or through clinical trials.[159] The recently reported Biomarker-integrated Approaches of Targeted Therapy for Lung Cancer Elimination (BATTLE) trial also demonstrated the feasibility of real-time testing and treatment decisions based on molecular characteristics of tumors.[160]

KRAS

RAS is the most commonly mutated oncogene in NSCLC, occurring in 20% to 25% of cases.[161] The RAS genes encode a family of membrane-bound GTP-binding proteins. RAS proteins acquire oncogenic potential when a point mutation occurs at codon 12, 13, or 61 of the gene. When mutated, RAS proteins lead to constitutive activation of RAS signaling through impaired GTPase activity. Activated RAS results in proliferation and cell survival, mediated through the mitogen-activated protein kinase (MAPK), PI3K, and STAT signaling pathways.[162] In adenocarcinomas of the lung, mutations in KRAS account for 90% of RAS mutations.[163] KRAS mutations are uncommon in squamous cell carcinomas of the lung.[164] KRAS mutations occur in both smokers and never-smokers and are typically mutually exclusive with other driver mutations such as EGFR and ALK.[165]

KRAS has been explored as a prognostic and predictive marker in NSCLC; however, prospective data are sparse. Small retrospective studies have yielded contradictory results with respect to the influence of KRAS mutations on prognosis in NSCLC. Two meta-analyses have associated KRAS mutations with inferior survival in NSCLC.[166,167] However, many of the included studies did not include information on other prognostic factors (such as stage, performance status, and weight loss) that may have influenced these findings. KRAS mutation status was assessed prospectively in the E3590 trial, which randomized patients with stage II-IIIA NSCLC to either postoperative chemotherapy and radiation or radiation alone.[168] The authors did not find a significant impact of KRAS mutation on prognosis. Similarly, the JBR.10 trial of early-stage lung cancer patients, which assessed KRAS mutational status, did not identify a negative impact of KRAS mutations on overall survival in patients.[29]

The role of KRAS as a predictive marker has also been explored in NSCLC, and emerging data suggest that KRAS mutational status may aid clinicians in predicting response to some currently available treatments. In the JBR.10 adjuvant trial, chemotherapy was associated with a survival benefit in KRAS wild-type but not mutant patients. However, the test for interaction between RAS mutations and chemotherapy was not statistically significant. A pooled analysis of KRAS mutations was performed within a meta-analysis of patients who participated in key adjuvant trials. KRAS mutations were associated with a non-significant trend for worse overall survival, but there was no effect of KRAS mutational status on benefit from adjuvant chemotherapy.[169] Based on these results, KRAS mutational status cannot be recommended to exclude patients from adjuvant chemotherapy.

KRAS mutations have been studied in the metastatic setting as a predictive marker, particularly with respect to response to EGFR-targeted therapies. In colorectal cancer, KRAS mutations are associated with a lack of benefit from EGFR monoclonal antibodies.[170] In lung cancer, however, KRAS mutations have not been associated with a lack of benefit from cetuximab.[100,171] Several studies have implicated KRAS mutations in resistance to the EGFR TKIs gefitinib and erlotinib.[172-174] In the phase III TRIBUTE trial, which compared chemotherapy plus placebo to chemotherapy plus erlotinib in advanced NSCLC patients, patients with KRAS-mutant tumors had lower response rates and inferior survival when erlotinib was added to chemotherapy.[175]

While the high prevalence of mutated KRAS makes it an attractive target, efforts to interrupt RAS signaling have lagged behind those directed at other signaling pathways (EGFR and ALK). At this time, there are no proven therapies specifically directed at KRAS. The recently reported BATTLE trial demonstrated a disease control rate of 79% with the multi-kinase inhibitor sorafenib.[160] While these results will require further study, they have generated significant interest in the use of sorafenib and other Raf/MEK/ERK pathway inhibitors in KRAS-mutant NSCLC. Numerous clinical trials of agents targeting this pathway are currently underway.

BRAF

BRAF is a serine–threonine protein kinase that functions in the RAS/MAPK signaling pathway. BRAF is downstream of KRAS and directly phosphorylates MEK. Subsequent phosphorylation of ERK activates genes involved in proliferation and survival. Mutant BRAF proteins have increased kinase activity and are transforming in vitro.[176] BRAF mutations have been described in multiple cancer types, including NSCLC, where 1% to 3% of cancers are affected.[164,176-178] In NSCLC, BRAF mutations are seen almost exclusively in adenocarcinomas and, in contrast to EGFR and ALK, appear to be more common in current and former smokers, although it should be noted that the number of patients described to date is small.[177,178]

In malignant melanoma, BRAF mutations occur in over 50% of patients and the vast majority of mutations occur at valine 600 (v600) within exon 15 of the kinase domain. In lung cancer, several different BRAF mutations, including V600E, have been described. Preclinical work suggests that mutant BRAF plays a role in lung adenocarcinoma initiation and maintenance. Clinically, BRAF inhibitors have been found to be effective in BRAF-mutated melanoma, and the U.S. FDA recently approved the BRAF inhibitor vemurafenib in V600E-mutated melanoma. This drug and a number of other BRAF inhibitors are currently being tested in patients with BRAF mutant NSCLC. Importantly, non-V600E BRAF mutant lung cancer cell lines exhibited resistance to vemurafenib.[179]

PI3K/AKT/PTEN

The PI3K/AKT/mTOR signaling pathway plays an important role in many human cancers, including NSCLC.[180] The PI3K pathway is a downstream target of EGFR, and PI3K is the main upstream regulator of the mTOR pathway. Both mutation and amplification of the PIK3CA gene can occur and are associated with increased PI3K signaling and AKT expression.[181,182] Somatic mutations in PIK3CA occur in 1% to 3% of NSCLC and are found among smokers and never-smokers and in all histologies, but appear to be more common in squamous cell carcinoma.[181,183,184] No other specific clinicopathologic features have been associated with PIK3CA mutations.[181] These mutations typically occur in either exon 9 (the helical domain) or exon 20 (the kinase domain) of PIK3CA, which encodes the p110α subunit of PI3K. Increased gene copy number through amplification or polysomy can also result in oncogene activation. PIK3CA is located on chromosome 3 in a region that is frequently amplified in lung cancer. Increased PIK3CA copy number was detected in 17% of NSCLC tumors and was significantly more frequent in squamous cell carcinomas (33%) compared with adenocarcinomas (6%).[181]

Coexistence of PI3KCA mutations and mutations in KRAS, EGFR, MEK, BRAF, and ALK has been described.[155] The coexistence of EGFR and PIK3CA may account for acquired resistance to EGFR TKIs in some patients and may represent a potential therapeutic target in this population.[125] Although AKT is a key downstream regulator of PI3K, genetic alterations in AKT had not been identified until recently. Recently, a somatic activating mutation of AKT1 was reported in a variety of malignancies.[185] The E17K mutation in AKT1 results in an amino acid change from glutamic acid to lysine at position 17. This mutation activates AKT1 in a PI3K-independent fashion and is transforming in vitro. In NSCLC, the E17K mutation occurs in approximately 1% of tumors.

The tumor suppressor gene, PTEN, antagonizes the PI3K pathway and loss of PTEN results in overactivation of the PI3K pathway. PTEN mutations that result in PTEN activation occur in multiple malignancies, including NSCLC. Germline mutations in PTEN cause Cowden syndrome, which is associated with multiple hamartomas and cancer susceptibility.[186] Somatic mutations in PTEN have been found in 4% to 8% of NSCLC tumors.[187–189] However, other mechanisms of diminished PTEN function (e.g., silencing through methylation) may be more common. Inactivation of PTEN has been associated with a poor prognosis in NSCLC.[190,191]

Drugs with potential activity against PI3K mutations or amplification, AKT mutations, and PTEN-deficient tumors include PI3K inhibitors, mTOR inhibitors, and AKT inhibitors. A number of drugs in each of these categories are in development, though their clinical activity in patients with aberrations in PI3K, AKT, or PTEN is unknown at this time.

MEK1

The MAPK pathway plays a key role in the EGFR signaling cascade. After activation of EGFR, MEK1 and MEK2 are phosphorylated by RAF1 kinase, resulting in subsequent phosphorylation of ERK1/2. MEK1 mutations occur in approximately 1% of NSCLCs. To date, three different mutations in MEK1 have been described in NSCLC; all occur outside of the kinase domain. Mutations are more common in adenocarcinomas than in squamous cell carcinomas, although no other clinical characteristics of patients with MEK1 mutations have been described. Preclinical data have shown increased MEK kinase activity in the presence of MEK1 mutations.[192,193] In vitro, mutations in MEK1 have been associated with resistance to EGFR TKIs.[192] A number of MEK inhibitors are undergoing evaluation in clinical trials. While preclinical data suggest that cancer cells harboring MEK1 mutations are sensitive to MEK inhibitors, clinical responses of patients are unknown at this time.

HER2

HER2 (ERBB2) is a member of the ERBB family of receptor tyrosine kinases that also includes EGFR (ERBB1), HER3 (ERBB3), and HER4 (ERBB4). Growth factor binding results in heterodimerization of HER2 and another member of the ERBB family.[194] Activation of HER2 in this way initiates the PI3K-AKT-mTOR and RAS-RAF-MEK-ERK pathways, promoting cell survival and proliferation. HER2 appears to be the preferred dimerization partner of all members of the ERBB family.[195] Deregulation of HER2 can occur through protein overexpression, gene copy number gain, or somatic mutation. While HER2 overexpression or gene copy number gains are relatively common in NSCLC, HER2 mutations are found in only 2% to 4% of NSCLCs.[196-199] To date, the only mutation described involves an in-frame insertion within exon 20. Clinically, HER2 mutations appear to be more common in women and never-smokers with adenocarcinoma histology.[196-199]

The HER2 monoclonal antibody trastuzumab and the TKI lapatinib have been evaluated in NSCLC patients. Trastuzumab combined with chemotherapy in unselected patients did not result in improved outcomes compared with historical controls treated with chemotherapy alone.[200,201] Similarly, single-agent lapatinib in an unselected population of patients with NSCLC demonstrated an overall response rate of only 1.3%.[202] Individual cases of response to HER2-targeted therapy in patients with HER2 mutations have been reported.[203,204] In the latter report, De Greve and colleagues describe partial responses to the pan-HER inhibitor afatinib in three heavily pretreated patients with HER2 mutations. A number of agents with activity against HER2 are in clinical trials currently, some of which are specifically recruiting patients with HER2 mutations.

Discoidin Death Receptor 2

When activated by the binding of its endogenous ligand, collagen, the Discoidin Death Receptor 2 (DDR2) promotes cell migration, proliferation, and survival. Recently, mutations have been reported in squamous cell carcinoma of the lung, with a frequency of 3.8%.[205] In addition to sequencing DDR2 and describing the mutation rate in squamous cell lung cancer patient specimens, Hammerman and colleagues demonstrated the sensitivity of DDR2 mutant cells to dasatinib in vitro and in vivo. Dasatinib inhibits multiple tyrosine kinases, including DDR2. The authors also performed sequencing on a patient with a squamous cell carcinoma of the lung who exhibited a partial response to dasatinib and erlotinib on a clinical trial. The patient was found to have a DDR2 mutation and no EGFR mutation. While no clinical trials have specifically targeted patients with DDR2 mutations, prospective trials of dasatinib are anticipated in this patient population.

Fibroblast Growth Factor Receptor 1

The fibroblast growth factor receptor 1 (FGFR1) gene encodes one member of the FGFR family of tyrosine kinase receptors. These receptors are active in signaling networks involved in embryonic development, wound healing, angiogenesis, and metabolism. FGFR signaling has been implicated in the development of multiple cancer types, including NSCLC.[206-208] Recently, Weiss and colleagues examined a large series of lung squamous cell carcinomas and showed amplification of FGFR1 in 22% of samples. In contrast, FGFR1 amplification was observed in only 1% of nonsquamous NSCLC. There was no evidence for FGFR1 mutations.[209] In cell lines, the authors demonstrated the importance of FGFR1 in downstream signaling, leading to cell growth and survival. Additionally, treatment of cell lines with amplified FGFR1 with an FGFR inhibitor resulted in growth inhibition. Several FGFR inhibitors are in early clinical development, and these preclinical studies provide a rationale for targeting FGFR in a molecularly selected subset of NSCLCs.

Insulin-Like Growth Factor System

Increased signaling through the insulin-like growth factor (IGF) system has been linked to increased cancer risk as well as a more aggressive cancer phenotype in multiple solid tumors, including NSCLC. The IGF system consists of the IGF ligands (IGF-I, IGF-II, and insulin), cell surface receptors (IGF-IR, IGF-IIR, and the insulin receptor), and a family of IGF-binding proteins (IGFBPs). Preclinical studies have demonstrated that blocking IGF-IR signaling leads to decreased proliferation and survival of multiple cancer cell types, including NSCLC. Increased IGF signaling has been linked to resistance to the EGFR TKIs, gefitinib and erlotinib.[210,211]

A number of compounds targeting the IGF system, including monoclonal antibodies and small-molecule inhibitors, are in development. The largest experience has been with the monoclonal antibody figitumumab, which targets IGF-IR, thereby blocking ligand binding and receptor activation. Figitumumab in combination with carboplatin and paclitaxel was investigated in a randomized phase II study; patients on the control arm received chemotherapy alone.[212] After completion of the randomized portion of the study, patients with nonadenocarcinoma histology were enrolled in a single-arm extension cohort. Promising activity was observed in the figitumumab arm in patients with squamous histology (overall response rate of 78% in the randomized portion of the study and 64% in the extension cohort). Based on these results, a randomized phase III trial of chemotherapy plus or minus figitumumab was launched. The study was discontinued early when the Data Safety Monitoring Committee found that the combination would be unlikely to meet the primary endpoint of improved overall survival. The investigators reported an imbalance in death and serious adverse events in the figitumumab arm compared with chemotherapy alone.[213] While the development of figitumumab was halted, a number of other agents targeting IGF-IR are being evaluated in clinical trials in NSCLC.

CONCLUSION

The landscape of NSCLC therapy is rapidly evolving, primarily as a result of identifying and targeting driver mutations and signaling pathways relevant to the disease. The success of agents targeting EGFR and ALK has translated into meaningful differences in prognosis for these patient subgroups. Molecular subtyping will define future clinical trials in NSCLC, and recent developments have demonstrated the feasibility of performing molecular subtyping and recruiting to clinical trials directed at small subpopulations of patients with NSCLC.

REFERENCES

1. Parkin DM, Bray F, Ferlay J, Pisani P. Global cancer statistics, 2002. *CA Cancer J Clin*. 2005;55(2):74-108.
2. Greenlee RT, Hill-Harmon MB, Murray T, Thun M. Cancer statistics, 2001. *CA Cancer J Clin*. 2001;51(1):15-36.
3. Chemotherapy in non-small cell lung cancer: a meta-analysis using updated data on individual patients from 52 randomised clinical trials. *BMJ*. 1995;311(7010):899-909.
4. Carbone DP, Minna JD. Chemotherapy for non-small cell lung cancer. *BMJ*. 1995;311(7010):889-890.
5. Arriagada R, Bergman B, Dunant A, Le Chevalier T, Pignon J-P, Vansteenkiste J. Cisplatin-based adjuvant chemotherapy in patients with completely resected non-small-cell lung cancer. *N Engl J Med*. 2004;350(4):351-360.
6. Winton T, Livingston R, Johnson D, et al. Vinorelbine plus cisplatin vs. observation in resected non-small-cell lung cancer. *N Engl J Med*. 2005;352(25):2589-2597.
7. Douillard J-Y, Rosell R, De Lena M, et al. Adjuvant vinorelbine plus cisplatin versus observation in patients with completely resected stage IB-IIIA non-small-cell lung cancer (Adjuvant Navelbine International Trialist Association [ANITA]): a randomised controlled trial. *Lancet Oncol*. 2006;7(9):719-727.
8. Keller SM, Adak S, Wagner H, et al. A Randomized trial of postoperative adjuvant therapy in patients with completely resected stage II or IIIa non-small-cell lung cancer. *N Engl J Med*. 2000;343(17):1217-1222.
9. Le Chevalier T, Dunant A, Arriagada R, et al. Long-term results of the international adjuvant lung cancer trial (IALT) evaluating adjuvant cisplatin-based chemotherapy in resected non-small cell lung cancer (NSCLC). *J Clin Oncol*. 2008;26(15S):398s:Abstract 7507.
10. Scagliotti GV, Fossati R, Torri V, et al. Randomized study of adjuvant chemotherapy for completely resected stage I, II, or IIIa non-small-cell lung cancer. *J Natl Cancer Inst*. 2003;95(19):1453-1461.
11. Strauss GM, Herndon JE II, Maddaus MA, et al. Adjuvant paclitaxel plus carboplatin compared with observation in stage IB non-small-cell lung cancer: CALGB 9633 with the cancer and leukemia group b, radiation therapy oncology group, and north central cancer treatment group study groups. *J Clin Oncol*. 2008;26(31):5043-5051.
12. Schiller JH, Harrington D, Belani CP, et al. Comparison of four chemotherapy regimens for advanced non–small-cell lung cancer. *N Engl J Med*. 2002;346(2):92-98.
13. Presta LG, Chen H, O'Connor SJ, et al. Humanization of an anti-vascular endothelial growth factor monoclonal antibody for the therapy of solid tumors and other disorders. *Cancer Res*. 1997;57(20):4593-4599.
14. Sandler A, Gray R, Perry MC, et al. Paclitaxel-carboplatin alone or with bevacizumab for non-small-cell lung cancer. *N Engl J Med*. 2006;355(24):2542-2550.
15. Scagliotti GV, Parikh P, von Pawel J, et al. Phase III study comparing cisplatin plus gemcitabine with cisplatin plus pemetrexed in chemotherapy-naive patients with advanced-stage non–small-cell lung cancer. *J Clin Oncol*. 2008;26(21):3543-3551.
16. Syrigos KN, Vansteenkiste J, Parikh P, et al. Prognostic and predictive factors in a randomized phase III trial comparing cisplatin–pemetrexed versus cisplatin–gemcitabine in advanced non-small-cell lung cancer. *Ann Oncol*. 2010;21(3): 556-561.
17. Simon G, Sharma S, Cantor A, Smith P, Bepler G. ERCC1 expression is a predictor of survival in resected patients with non-small cell lung cancer. *Chest*. 2005;127:978-983.
18. Zheng Z, Chen T, Li X, Haura E, Sharma A, Bepler G. DNA synthesis and repair genes RRM1 and ERCC1 in lung cancer. *N Engl J Med*. 2007;356:800-808.
19. Olaussen KA, Dunant A, Fouret P, et al. DNA repair by ERCC1 in non-small-cell lung cancer and cisplatin-based adjuvant chemotherapy. *N Engl J Med*. 2006;355(10):983-991.
20. Bepler G, Sharma S, Cantor A, et al. RRM1 and PTEN as prognostic parameters for overall and disease-free survival in patients with non-small-cell lung cancer. *J Clin Oncol*. 2004;22(10):1878-1885.
21. Bepler G, Sommers E, Cantor A, et al. Clinical efficacy and predictive molecular markers of neoadjuvant gemcitabine and

pemetrexed in resectable non-small cell lung cancer. *J Thorac Oncol.* 2008;3:1112-1118.
22. Rosell R, Skrzypski M, Jassem E, et al. BRCA1: a novel prognostic factor in resected non-small-cell lung cancer. *PLoS One.* 2007;2(11):e1129.
23. Cobo M, Massutti B, Moran T, et al. Spanish customized adjuvant trial (SCAT) based on BRCA1 mRNA levels. *J Clin Oncol.* 2008;26(suppl 1):Abstract 7533.
24. Shintani Y, Ohta M, Hirabayashi H, et al. New prognostic indicator for non-small-cell lung cancer, quantitation of thymidylate synthase by real-time reverse transcription polymerase chain reaction. *Int J Cancer.* 2003;104(6):790-795.
25. Lee KB, Parker RJ, Bohr V, Cornelison T, Reed E. Cisplatin sensitivity/resistance in UV repair-deficient Chinese hamster ovary cells of complementation groups 1 and 3. *Carcinogenesis.* 1993;14(10):2177-2180.
26. Dabholkar M, Vionnet J, Bostick-Bruton F, Yu JJ, Reed E. Messenger RNA levels of XPAC and ERCC1 in ovarian cancer tissue correlate with response to platinum-based chemotherapy. *J Clin Invest.* 1994;94(2):703-708.
27. Li Q, Yu JJ, Mu C, et al. Association between the level of ERCC-1 expression and the repair of cisplatin-induced DNA damage in human ovarian cancer cells. *Anticancer Res.* 2000;20(2A):645-652.
28. Vilmar AC, Santoni-Rugiu E, Sørensen JB. ERCC1 and histopathology in advanced NSCLC patients randomized in a large multicenter phase III trial. *Ann Oncol.* 2010;21(9):1817-1824.
29. Lord RVN, Brabender J, Gandara D, et al. Low ERCC1 expression correlates with prolonged survival after cisplatin plus gemcitabine chemotherapy in non-small cell lung cancer. *Clin Cancer Res.* 2002;8(7):2286-2291.
30. Lee HW, Choi Y-W, Han JH, et al. Expression of excision repair cross-complementation group 1 protein predicts poor outcome in advanced non-small cell lung cancer patients treated with platinum-based doublet chemotherapy. *Lung Cancer.* 2009;65(3):377-382.
31. Wang X, Zhao J, Yang L, et al. Positive expression of ERCC1 predicts a poorer platinum-based treatment outcome in Chinese patients with advanced non-small-cell lung cancer. *Med Oncol.* 2010;27(2):484-490.
32. Su C, Zhou S, Zhang L, et al. ERCC1, RRM1 and BRCA1 mRNA expression levels and clinical outcome of advanced non-small cell lung cancer. *Med Oncol.* 2011;28(4):1411-1417.
33. Holm B, Mellemgaard A, Skov T, Skov BG. Different impact of excision repair cross-complementation group 1 on survival in male and female patients with inoperable non–small-cell lung cancer treated with carboplatin and gemcitabine. *J Clin Oncol.* 2009;27(26):4254-4259.
34. Ceppi P, Volante M, Novello S, et al. ERCC1 and RRM1 gene expressions but not EGFR are predictive of shorter survival in advanced non-small-cell lung cancer treated with cisplatin and gemcitabine. *Ann Oncol.* 2006;17(12):1818-1825.
35. Azuma K, Komohara Y, Sasada T, et al. Excision repair cross-complementation group 1 predicts progression-free and overall survival in non-small cell lung cancer patients treated with platinum-based chemotherapy. *Cancer Sci.* 2007;98(9):1336-1343.
36. Azuma K, Sasada T, Kawahara A, et al. Expression of ERCC1 and class III β-tubulin in non-small cell lung cancer patients treated with carboplatin and paclitaxel. *Lung Cancer.* 2009;64(3):326-333.
37. Simon G, Sharma A, Li X, et al. Feasibility and efficacy of molecular analysis-directed individualized therapy in advanced non-small-cell lung cancer. *J Clin Oncol.* 2007;25(19):2741-2746.
38. Cobo M, Isla D, Massuti B, et al. Customizing cisplatin based on quantitative excision repair cross-complementing 1 mRNA expression: a phase iii trial in non–small-cell lung cancer. *J Clin Oncol.* 2007;25(19):2747-2754.
39. Bepler G, Garcia-Blanco MA. Three tumor-suppressor regions on chromosome 11p identified by high-resolution deletion mapping in human non-small-cell lung cancer. *Proc Natl Acad Sci U S A.* 1994;91(12):5513-5517.
40. Bepler G, Gautam A, McIntyre LM, et al. Prognostic significance of molecular genetic aberrations on chromosome segment 11p15.5 in non–small-cell lung cancer. *J Clin Oncol.* 2002;20(5):1353-1360.
41. Pitterle DM, Kim Y-C, Jolicoeur EMC, Cao Y, O'Briant KC, Bepler G. Lung cancer and the human gene for ribonucleotide reductase subunit M1 (RRM1). *Mamm Genome.* 1999;10(9):916-922.
42. Reichard P. From RNA to DNA, why so many ribonucleotide reductases? *Science.* 1993;260(5115):1773-1777.
43. Stubbe J. Ribonucleotide reductases in the twenty-first century. *Proc Natl Acad Sci U S A.* 1998;95(6):2723-2724.
44. Elledge SJ, Zhou Z, Allen JB. Ribonucleotide reductase: regulation, regulation, regulation. *Trends Biochem Sci.* 1992;17(3):119-123.
45. Gautam A, Li Z-R, Bepler G. RRM1-induced metastasis suppression through PTEN-regulated pathways. *Oncogene.* 2003;22(14):2135-2142.
46. Fan H, Huang A, Villegas C, Wright JA. The R1 component of mammalian ribonucleotide reductase has malignancy-suppressing activity as demonstrated by gene transfer experiments. *Proc Natl Acad Sci U S A.* 1997;94:13181-13186.
47. Gautam A, Bepler G. Suppression of lung tumor formation by the regulatory subunit of ribonucleotide reductase. *Cancer Res.* 2006;66(13):6497-6502.
48. Davidson JD, Ma L, Flagella M, Geeganage S, Gelbert LM, Slapak CA. An increase in the expression of ribonucleotide reductase large subunit 1 is associated with gemcitabine resistance in non-small cell lung cancer cell lines. *Cancer Res.* 2004;64(11):3761-3766.
49. Bepler G, Kusmartseva I, Sharma S, et al. RRM1 modulated in vitro and in vivo efficacy of gemcitabine and platinum in non–small-cell lung cancer. *J Clin Oncol.* 2006;24(29):4731-4737.
50. Rosell R, Danenberg KD, Alberola V, et al. Ribonucleotide reductase messenger RNA expression and survival in gemcitabine/cisplatin-treated advanced non-small cell lung cancer patients. *Clin Cancer Res.* 2004;10(4):1318-1325.
51. Rosell R, Scagliotti G, Danenberg KD, et al. Transcripts in pretreatment biopsies from a three-arm randomized trial in metastatic non-small-cell lung cancer. *Oncogene.* 2003;22(23):3548-3553.
52. Souglakos J, Boukovinas I, Taron M, et al. Ribonucleotide reductase subunits M1 and M2 mRNA expression levels and clinical outcome of lung adenocarcinoma patients treated with docetaxel/gemcitabine. *Br J Cancer.* 2008;98(10):1710-1715.
53. Miki Y, Swensen J, Shattuck-Eidens D, et al. A strong candidate for the breast and ovarian cancer susceptibility gene BRCA1. *Science.* 1994;266:66-71.
54. Randrianarison V, Marot D, Foray N, et al. BRCA1 carries tumor suppressor activity distinct from that of p53 and p21. *Cancer Gene Ther.* 2001;8(10):759-770.
55. Shrivastav M, De Haro LP, Nickoloff JA. Regulation of DNA double-strand break repair pathway choice. *Cell Res.* 2008;18(1):134-147.
56. Le Page F, Randrianarison V, Marot D, et al. BRCA1 and BRCA2 are necessary for the transcription-coupled repair of the oxidative 8-oxoguanine lesion in human cells. *Cancer Res.* 2000;60(19):5548-5552.
57. Wang Y, Cortez D, Yazdi P, Neff N, Elledge SJ, Qin J. BASC, a super complex of BRCA1-associated proteins involved in the recognition and repair of aberrant DNA structures. *Genes Dev.* 2000;14(8):927-939.
58. Ouchi T, Monteiro ANA, August A, Aaronson SA, Hanafusa H. BRCA1 regulates p53-dependent gene expression. *Proc Natl Acad Sci U S A.* 1998;95(5):2302-2306.
59. Houvras Y, Benezra M, Zhang H, Manfredi JJ, Weber BL, Licht JD. BRCA1 physically and functionally interacts with ATF1. *J Biol Chem.* 2000;275(46):36230-36237.
60. Mullan PB, Quinn JE, Gilmore PM, et al. BRCA1 and GADD45 mediated G2/M cell cycle arrest in response to antimicrotubule agents. *Oncogene.* 2001;20(43):6123-6131.
61. Starita LM, Parvin JD. Substrates of the BRCA1-dependent ubiquitin ligase. *Cancer Biol Ther.* 2006;5(2):137-141.
62. Ye Q, Hu Y-F, Zhong H, Nye AC, Belmont AS, Li R. BRCA1-induced large-scale chromatin unfolding and allele-specific effects of cancer-predisposing mutations. *J Cell Biol.* 2001;155(6):911-922.
63. Rosell R, Perez-Roca L, Sanchez JJ, et al. Customized treatment in non-small-cell lung cancer based on EGFR mutations and BRCA1 mRNA expression. *PLoS One.* 2009;4(5):e5133.

64. Taron M, Rosell R, Felip E, et al. BRCA1 mRNA expression levels as an indicator of chemoresistance in lung cancer. *Hum Mol Genet*. 2004;13(20):2443-2449.
65. Wang L, Wei J, Qian X, et al. ERCC1 and BRCA1 mRNA expression levels in metastatic malignant effusions is associated with chemosensitivity to cisplatin and/or docetaxel. *BMC Cancer*. 2008;8(1):97.
66. Lan L, Hayashi T, Rabeya RM, et al. Functional and physical interactions between ERCC1 and MSH2 complexes for resistance to cis-diamminedichloroplatinum(II) in mammalian cells. *DNA Repair*. 2004;3(2):135-143.
67. Zhang N, Liu X, Li L, Legerski R. Double-strand breaks induce homologous recombinational repair of interstrand cross-links via cooperation of MSH2, ERCC1-XPF, REV3, and the Fanconi anemia pathway. *DNA Repair*. 2007;6(11):1670-1678.
68. Scartozzi M, Franciosi V, Campanini N, et al. Mismatch repair system (MMR) status correlates with response and survival in non-small cell lung cancer (NSCLC) patients. *Lung Cancer*. 2006;53(1):103-109.
69. Cooper WA, Kohonen-Corish MRJ, Chan C, et al. Prognostic significance of DNA repair proteins MLH1, MSH2 and MGMT expression in non-small-cell lung cancer and precursor lesions. *Histopathology*. 2008;52(5):613-622.
70. Hsu H-S, Lee IH, Hsu W-H, Kao W-T, Wang Y-C. Polymorphism in the hMSH2 gene (gISV12-6T > C) is a prognostic factor in non-small cell lung cancer. *Lung Cancer*. 2007;58(1):123-130.
71. Kamal NS, Soria J-C, Mendiboure J, et al. MutS homologue 2 and the long-term benefit of adjuvant chemotherapy in lung cancer. *Clin Cancer Res*. 2010;16(4):1206-1215.
72. McLeod HL, Cassidy J, Powrie RH, et al. Pharmacokinetic and pharmacodynamic evaluation of the glycinamide ribonucleotide formyltransferase inhibitor AG2034. *Clin Cancer Res*. 2000;6(7):2677-2684.
73. Hanauske A-R, Eismann U, Oberschmidt O, et al. In vitro chemosensitivity of freshly explanted tumor cells to pemetrexed is correlated with target gene expression. *Invest New Drugs*. 2007;25(5):417-423.
74. Takezawa K, Okamoto I, Okamoto W, et al. Thymidylate synthase as a determinant of pemetrexed sensitivity in non-small cell lung cancer. *Br J Cancer*. 2011;104(10):1594-1601.
75. Ceppi P, Volante M, Saviozzi S, et al. Squamous cell carcinoma of the lung compared with other histotypes shows higher messenger RNA and protein levels for thymidylate synthase. *Cancer*. 2006;107(7):1589-1596.
76. Kaira K, Ohde Y, Nakagawa K, et al. Thymidylate synthase expression is closely associated with outcome in patients with pulmonary adenocarcinoma. *Med Oncol*. 2011;28:1-10.
77. Monica V, Scagliotti GV, Ceppi P, et al. Differential thymidylate synthase expression in different variants of large-cell carcinoma of the lung. *Clin Cancer Res*. 2009;15(24):7547-7552.
78. Hanahan D, Folkman J. Patterns and emerging mechanisms of the angiogenic switch during tumorigenesis. *Cell*. 1996;86(3):353-364.
79. Folkman J. Tumor angiogenesis: therapeutic implications. *N Engl J Med*. 1971;285:1182-1186.
80. Carmeliet P. Angiogenesis in life, disease, and medicine. *Nature*. 2005;438:932-936.
81. Fidler IJ, Ellis LM. Implications of angiogenesis for the biology and therapy of cancer metastases. *Cell*. 1994;79:185-188.
82. Weidner N, Folkman J. Tumor vascularity as a prognostic factor in cancer. In: De Vita VT, Hellman S, Rosenberg SA, eds. *Important Advances in Oncology 1996*. Philadelphia, PA: Lippincott-Raven; 1996:167-190.
83. Seto T, Higashiyama M, Funai H, et al. Prognostic value of expression of vascular endothelial growth factor and its flt-1 and KDR receptors in stage I non-small-cell lung cancer. *Lung Cancer*. 2006;53(1):91-96.
84. Fontanini G, Vignati S, Boldrini L, et al. Vascular endothelial growth factor is associated with neovascularization and influences progression of non-small cell lung carcinoma. *Clin Cancer Res*. 1997;3(6):861-865.
85. Fontanini G, Vignati S, Basolo F, et al. Angiogenesis as a prognostic indicator of survival in non-small-cell lung carcinoma: a prospective study. *J Natl Cancer Inst*. 1997;89(12):881-886.
86. Ferrara N, Hillan KJ, Gerber H-P, Novotny W. Discovery and development of bevacizumab, an anti-VEGF antibody for treating cancer. *Nat Rev Drug Discov*. 2004;3(5):391-400.
87. Johnson DH, Fehrenbacher L, Novotny WF, et al. Randomized phase II trial comparing bevacizumab plus carboplatin and paclitaxel with carboplatin and paclitaxel alone in previously untreated locally advanced or metastatic non-small-cell lung cancer. *J Clin Oncol*. 2004;22(11):2184-2191.
88. Ramalingam SS, Dahlberg SE, Langer CJ, et al. Outcomes for elderly, advanced-stage non–small-cell lung cancer patients treated with bevacizumab in combination with carboplatin and paclitaxel: analysis of eastern cooperative oncology group trial 4599. *J Clin Oncol*. 2008;26(1):60-65.
89. Dowlati A, Gray R, Sandler AB, Schiller JH, Johnson DH. Cell adhesion molecules, vascular endothelial growth factor, and basic fibroblast growth factor in patients with non–small cell lung cancer treated with chemotherapy with or without bevacizumab—an eastern cooperative oncology group study. *Clin Cancer Res*. 2008;14(5):1407-1412.
90. Dahlberg SE, Sandler AB, Brahmer JR, Schiller JH, Johnson DH. Clinical course of advanced non–small-cell lung cancer patients experiencing hypertension during treatment with bevacizumab in combination with carboplatin and paclitaxel on ECOG 4599. *J Clin Oncol*. 2010;28(6):949-954.
91. Reck M, von Pawel J, Zatloukal P, et al. Overall survival with cisplatin–gemcitabine and bevacizumab or placebo as first-line therapy for nonsquamous non-small-cell lung cancer: results from a randomised phase III trial (AVAiL). *Ann Oncol*. 2010;21(9):1804-1809.
92. Natale RB, Thongprasert S, Greco FA, et al. Phase III trial of vandetanib compared with erlotinib in patients with previously treated advanced non–small-cell lung cancer. *J Clin Oncol*. 2011;29(8):1059-1066.
93. de Boer RH, Arrieta Ó, Yang C-H, et al. Vandetanib plus pemetrexed for the second-line treatment of advanced non–small-cell lung cancer: a randomized, double-blind phase iii trial. *J Clin Oncol*. 2011;29(8):1067-1074.
94. Hirsch FR, Varella-Garcia M, Bunn PA, et al. Epidermal growth factor receptor in non–small-cell lung carcinomas: correlation between gene copy number and protein expression and impact on prognosis. *J Clin Oncol*. 2003;21(20):3798-3807.
95. Herbst RS, Shin DM. Monoclonal antibodies to target epidermal growth factor receptor–positive tumors. *Cancer*. 2002;94(5):1593-1611.
96. Jost M, Kari C, Rodeck U. The EGF receptor—an essential regulator of multiple epidermal functions. *Eur J Dermatol*. 2000;10:505-510.
97. Kari C, Chan TO, Rocha de Quadros M, Rodeck U. Targeting the epidermal growth factor receptor in cancer. *Cancer Res*. 2003;63(1):1-5.
98. Fan Z, Baselga J, Masui H, Mendelsohn J. Antitumor effect of anti-epidermal growth factor receptor monoclonal antibodies plus cis-diamminedichloroplatinum on well established A431 cell xenografts. *Cancer Res*. 1993;53:4637-4642.
99. Pirker R, Pereira JR, Szczesna A, et al. Cetuximab plus chemotherapy in patients with advanced non-small-cell lung cancer (FLEX): an open-label randomised phase III trial. *Lancet*. 2009;373(9674):1525-1531.
100. O'Byrne KJ, Gatzemeier U, Bondarenko I, et al. Molecular biomarkers in non-small-cell lung cancer: a retrospective analysis of data from the phase 3 FLEX study. *Lancet Oncol*. 2011;12(8):795-805.
101. Pirker R, Pereira JR, von Pawel J, et al. EGFR expression as a predictor of survival for first-line chemotherapy plus cetuximab in patients with advanced non-small-cell lung cancer: analysis of data from the phase 3 FLEX study. *Lancet Oncol*. 2012;13:33-42.
102. Kris MG, Natale RB, Herbst RS, et al. Efficacy of gefitinib, an inhibitor of the epidermal growth factor receptor tyrosine kinase, in symptomatic patients with non–small cell lung cancer. *JAMA*. 2003;290(16):2149-2158.
103. Shepherd FA, Rodrigues Pereira J, Ciuleanu T, et al. Erlotinib in previously treated non-small-cell lung cancer. *N Engl J Med*. 2005;353(2):123-132.
104. Thatcher N, Chang A, Parikh P, et al. Gefitinib plus best supportive care in previously treated patients with refractory advanced non-small-cell lung cancer: results from a randomised,

placebo-controlled, multicentre study (Iressa Survival Evaluation in Lung Cancer). *Lancet*. 2005;366(9496):1527-1537.
105. Fukuoka M, Yano S, Giaccone G, et al. Multi-institutional randomized phase ii trial of gefitinib for previously treated patients with advanced non-small-cell lung cancer. *J Clin Oncol.* 2003;21(12):2237-2246.
106. Miller VA, Kris MG, Shah N, et al. Bronchioloalveolar pathologic subtype and smoking history predict sensitivity to gefitinib in advanced non–small-cell lung cancer. *J Clin Oncol.* 2004;22(6):1103-1109.
107. Paez JG, Jänne PA, Lee JC, et al. EGFR mutations in lung cancer: correlation with clinical response to gefitinib therapy. *Science*. 2004;304(5676):1497-1500.
108. Pao W, Miller V, Zakowski M, et al. EGF receptor gene mutations are common in lung cancers from "never smokers" and are associated with sensitivity of tumors to gefitinib and erlotinib. *Proc Natl Acad Sci U S A*. 2004;101(36):13306-13311.
109. Shigematsu H, Lin L, Takahashi T, et al. Clinical and biological features associated with epidermal growth factor receptor gene mutations in lung cancers. *J Natl Cancer Inst*. 2005;97(5): 339-346.
110. D'Angelo SP, Pietanza MC, Johnson ML, et al. Incidence of EGFR exon 19 deletions and L858R in tumor specimens from men and cigarette smokers with lung adenocarcinomas. *J Clin Oncol*. 2011;29(15):2066-2070.
111. Mok TS, Wu Y-L, Thongprasert S, et al. Gefitinib or carboplatin-paclitaxel in pulmonary adenocarcinoma. *N Engl J Med*. 2009;361(10):947-957.
112. Fukuoka M, Wu Y-L, Thongprasert S, et al. Biomarker analyses and final overall survival results from a phase iii, randomized, open-label, first-line study of gefitinib versus carboplatin/paclitaxel in clinically selected patients with advanced non–small-cell lung cancer in Asia (IPASS). *J Clin Oncol.* 2011;29(21):2866-2874.
113. Rosell R. Screening for epidermal growth factor receptor mutations in lung cancer. *N Engl J Med*. 2009;361:958-967.
114. Mitsudomi T. Gefitinib versus cisplatin plus docetaxel in patients with non-small-cell lung cancer harbouring mutations of the epidermal growth factor receptor (WJTOG3405): an open label, randomised phase 3 trial. *Lancet Oncol*. 2010;11:121-128.
115. Maemondo M, Inoue A, Kobayashi K, et al. Gefitinib or chemotherapy for non–small-cell lung cancer with mutated EGFR. *N Engl J Med*. 2010;362(25):2380-2388.
116. Zhou C, Wu Y-L, Chen G, et al. Erlotinib versus chemotherapy as first-line treatment for patients with advanced EGFR mutation-positive non-small-cell lung cancer (OPTIMAL, CTONG-0802): a multicentre, open-label, randomised, phase 3 study. *Lancet Oncol*. 2011;12(8):735-742.
117. Rosell R, Gervais R, Vergnenegre A, et al. Erlotinib versus chemotherapy (CT) in advanced non-small cell lung cancer (NSCLC) patients (p) with epidermal growth factor receptor (EGFR) mutations: interim results of the European erlotinib versus chemotherapy (EURTAC) phase III randomized trial. *J Clin Oncol*. 2011;29(suppl):a7503.
118. Cappuzzo F, Ciuleanu T, Stelmakh L, et al. Erlotinib as maintenance treatment in advanced non-small-cell lung cancer: a multicentre, randomised, placebo-controlled phase 3 study. *Lancet Oncol*. 2010;11(6):521-529.
119. Coudert B, Ciuleanu T, Park K, et al. Survival benefit with erlotinib maintenance therapy in patients with advanced non-small-cell lung cancer (NSCLC) according to response to first-line chemotherapy. *Ann Oncol*. 2012;23:388-394.
120. Kobayashi S, Boggon TJ, Dayaram T, et al. EGFR mutation and resistance of non–small-cell lung cancer to gefitinib. *N Engl J Med*. 2005;352(8):786-792.
121. Pao W, Miller VA, Politi KA, et al. Acquired resistance of lung adenocarcinomas to gefitinib or erlotinib is associated with a second mutation in the EGFR kinase domain. *PLoS Med*. 2005;2(3):e73.
122. Engelman JA, Zejnullahu K, Mitsudomi T, et al. MET amplification leads to gefitinib resistance in lung cancer by activating ERBB3 signaling. *Science*. 2007;316(5827):1039-1043.
123. Bean J, Brennan C, Shih J-Y, et al. MET amplification occurs with or without T790M mutations in EGFR mutant lung tumors with acquired resistance to gefitinib or erlotinib. *Proc Natl Acad Sci U S A*. 2007;104(52):20932-20937.
124. Arcila ME, Oxnard GR, Nafa K, et al. Rebiopsy of lung cancer patients with acquired resistance to EGFR inhibitors and enhanced detection of the T790M mutation using a locked nucleic acid-based assay. *Clin Cancer Res*. 2011;17(5):1169-1180.
125. Sequist LV, Waltman BA, Dias-Santagata D, et al. Genotypic and histological evolution of lung cancers acquiring resistance to EGFR inhibitors. *Sci Transl Med*. 2011;3(75):75ra26.
126. Yun C-H, Mengwasser KE, Toms AV, et al. The T790M mutation in EGFR kinase causes drug resistance by increasing the affinity for ATP. *Proc Natl Acad Sci U S A*. 2008;105(6):2070-2075.
127. Oxnard GR, Arcila ME, Chmielecki J, Ladanyi M, Miller VA, Pao W. New strategies in overcoming acquired resistance to epidermal growth factor receptor tyrosine kinase inhibitors in lung cancer. *Clin Cancer Res*. 2011;17(17):5530-5537.
128. Oxnard GR, Arcila ME, Sima CS, et al. Acquired resistance to EGFR tyrosine kinase inhibitors in EGFR-mutant lung cancer: distinct natural history of patients with tumors harboring the T790M mutation. *Clin Cancer Res*. 2011;17(6):1616-1622.
129. Rosell R, Molina MA, Costa C, et al. Pretreatment EGFR T790M mutation and BRCA1 mRNA expression in erlotinib-treated advanced non–small-cell lung cancer patients with EGFR mutations. *Clin Cancer Res*. 2011;17(5):1160-1168.
130. Riely GJ, Kris MG, Zhao B, et al. Prospective assessment of discontinuation and reinitiation of erlotinib or gefitinib in patients with acquired resistance to erlotinib or gefitinib followed by the addition of everolimus. *Clin Cancer Res*. 2007;13(17):5150-5155.
131. Chaft JE, Oxnard GR, Sima CS, Kris MG, Miller VA, Riely GJ. Disease flare after tyrosine kinase inhibitor discontinuation in patients with EGFR-mutant lung cancer and acquired resistance to erlotinib or gefitinib: implications for clinical trial design. *Clin Cancer Res*. 2011;17(19):6298-6303.
132. Kwak EL, Sordella R, Bell DW, et al. Irreversible inhibitors of the EGF receptor may circumvent acquired resistance to gefitinib. *Proc Natl Acad Sci U S A*. 2005;102(21):7665-7670.
133. Engelman JA, Zejnullahu K, Gale C-M, et al. PF00299804, an irreversible pan-ERBB inhibitor, is effective in lung cancer models with EGFR and ERBB2 mutations that are resistant to gefitinib. *Cancer Res*. 2007;67(24):11924-11932.
134. Miller VA, Hirsh V, Cadranel J, et al. Phase IIb/III trial of afatinib (BIBW 2992) plus best supportive care (BSC) versus placebo plus BSC in patients failing 1-2 lines of chemotherapy and erlotinib/gefitinib (LUX-Lung 1). *Ann Oncol*. 2010;21(suppl 8):Abstract LBA1.
135. Regales L, Gong Y, Shen R, et al. Dual targeting of EGFR can overcome a major drug resistance mutation in mouse models of EGFR mutant lung cancer. *J Clin Invest*. 2009;119(10):3000-3010.
136. Janjigian YY, Azzoli CG, Krug LM, et al. Phase I/II trial of cetuximab and erlotinib in patients with lung adenocarcinoma and acquired resistance to erlotinib. *Clin Cancer Res*. 2011;17(8):2521-2527.
137. Janjigian YY, Groen HJ, Horn L, et al. Activity and tolerability of afatinib (BIBW 2992) and cetuximab in NSCLC patients with acquired resistance to erlotinib or gefitinib. *J Clin Oncol*. 2011;29(suppl):Abstract 7525.
138. Turke AB, Zejnullahu K, Wu Y-L, et al. Preexistence and clonal selection of MET amplification in EGFR mutant NSCLC. *Cancer Cell*. 2010;17(1):77-88.
139. Spigel DR, Ervin TJ, Ramlau R, et al. Final efficacy results from OAM4558G, a randomized phase II study evaluating METMab or placebo in combination with erlotinib in advanced NSCLC. *J Clin Oncol*. 2011;29(suppl):Abstract 7505.
140. Soda M, Choi YL, Enomoto M, et al. Identification of the transforming EML4-ALK fusion gene in non-small-cell lung cancer. *Nature*. 2007;448(7153):561-566.
141. Wong DW-S, Leung EL-H, So KK-T, et al. The EML4-ALK fusion gene is involved in various histologic types of lung cancers from nonsmokers with wild-type EGFR and KRAS. *Cancer*. 2009;115(8):1723-1733.
142. Perner S, Wagner PL, Demichelis F, et al. EML4-ALK fusion lung cancer: a rare acquired event. *Neoplasia*. 2008;10:298-302.
143. Shaw AT, Yeap BY, Mino-Kenudson M, et al. Clinical features and outcome of patients with non–small-cell lung cancer who harbor EML4-ALK. *J Clin Oncol*. 2009;27(26):4247-4253.
144. Zhang X, Zhang S, Yang X, et al. Fusion of EML4 and ALK is associated with development of lung adenocarcinomas lacking EGFR and KRAS mutations and is correlated with ALK expression. *Mol Cancer*. 2010;9(1):188.

145. Kwak EL. Anaplastic lymphoma kinase inhibition in non-small-cell lung cancer. *N Engl J Med*. 2010;363:1693-1703.
146. Inamura K, Takeuchi K, Togashi Y, et al. EML4-ALK lung cancers are characterized by rare other mutations, a TTF-1 cell lineage, an acinar histology, and young onset. *Mod Pathol*. 2009;22(4):508-515.
147. Rodig SJ, Mino-Kenudson M, Dacic S, et al. Unique clinicopathologic features characterize ALK-rearranged lung adenocarcinoma in the western population. *Clin Cancer Res*. 2009;15(16):5216-5223.
148. Koh Y, Kim D-W, Kim TM, et al. Clinicopathologic characteristics and outcomes of patients with anaplastic lymphoma kinase-positive advanced pulmonary adenocarcinoma: suggestion for an effective screening strategy for these tumors. *J Thorac Oncol*. 2011;6(5):905-912. doi:10.1097/JTO.0b013e3182111461.
149. Camidge DR, Kono SA, Lu X, et al. Anaplastic lymphoma kinase gene rearrangements in non-small cell lung cancer are associated with prolonged progression-free survival on pemetrexed. *J Thorac Oncol*. 2011;6(4):774-780. doi:10.1097/JTO.0b013e31820cf053.
150. Mano H. Non-solid oncogenes in solid tumors: EML4–ALK fusion genes in lung cancer. *Cancer Sci*. 2008;99(12):2349-2355.
151. Soda M, Takada S, Takeuchi K, et al. A mouse model for EML4-ALK-positive lung cancer. *Proc Natl Acad Sci U S A*. 2008;105(50):19893-19897.
152. Choi YL, Soda M, Yamashita Y, et al. EML4-ALK mutations in lung cancer that confer resistance to ALK inhibitors. *N Engl J Med*. 2010;363(18):1734-1739.
153. Sasaki T, Koivunen J, Ogino A, et al. A novel ALK secondary mutation and EGFR signaling cause resistance to ALK kinase inhibitors. *Cancer Res*. 2011;71(18):6051-6060.
154. Sasaki T, Okuda K, Zheng W, et al. The neuroblastoma-associated F1174L ALK mutation causes resistance to an ALK kinase inhibitor in ALK-translocated cancers. *Cancer Res*. 2010;70(24):10038-10043.
155. Chaft JE, Arcila ME, Paik PK, et al. Coexistence of PIK3CA and other oncogene mutations in lung adenocarcinoma – rationale for comprehensive mutation profiling. *Mol Cancer Ther*. 2011;11: 485-491.
156. Katayama R, Khan TM, Benes C, et al. Therapeutic strategies to overcome crizotinib resistance in non-small cell lung cancers harboring the fusion oncogene EML4-ALK. *Proc Natl Acad Sci U S A*. 2011;108(18):7535-7540.
157. Sequist LV, Gettinger S, Senzer NN, et al. Activity of IPI-504, a novel heat-shock protein 90 inhibitor, in patients with molecularly defined non–small-cell lung cancer. *J Clin Oncol*. 2010;28(33):4953-4960.
158. Wong K-K, Koczywas M, Goldman JW, et al. An open-label phase II study of the Hsp90 inhibitor ganetespib (STA-9090) as monotherapy in patients with advanced non-small cell lung cancer. *J Clin Oncol*. 2011;29(suppl):Abstract 7500.
159. Kris M, Johnson BE, Kwiatkowski DJ, et al. Identification of driver mutations in tumor specimens from 1,000 patients with lung adenocarcinoma: the NCI lung cancer mutation consortium (LCMC). *J Clin Oncol*. 2011;29(suppl):Abstract CRA7506.
160. Kim ES, Herbst RS, Wistuba II, et al. The BATTLE trial: personalizing therapy for lung cancer. *Cancer Discov*. 2011;1(1):44-53.
161. Riely GJ, Marks J, Pao W. KRAS mutations in non–small cell lung cancer. *Proc Am Thorac Soc*. 2009;6(2):201-205.
162. Vojtek AB, Der CJ. Increasing complexity of the ras signaling pathway. *J Biol Chem*. 1998;273(32):19925-19928.
163. Bamford S, Dawson E, Forbes S, et al. The COSMIC (Catalogue of Somatic Mutations in Cancer) database and website. *Br J Cancer*. 2004;91(2):355-358.
164. Brose MS, Volpe P, Feldman M, et al. BRAF and RAS mutations in human lung cancer and melanoma. *Cancer Res*. 2002;62(23):6997-7000.
165. Riely GJ, Kris MG, Rosenbaum D, et al. Frequency and distinctive spectrum of KRAS mutations in never smokers with lung adenocarcinoma. *Clin Cancer Res*. 2008;14(18):5731-5734.
166. Huncharek M, Muscat J, Geschwind J-F. K-ras oncogene mutation as a prognostic marker in non-small cell lung cancer: a combined analysis of 881 cases. *Carcinogenesis*. 1999;20(8):1507-1510.
167. Mascaux C, Iannino N, Martin B, et al. The role of RAS oncogene in survival of patients with lung cancer: a systematic review of the literature with meta-analysis. *Br J Cancer*. 2004;92(1):131-139.
168. Schiller JH, Adak S, Feins RH, et al. Lack of prognostic significance of p53 and K-ras mutations in primary resected non–small-cell lung cancer on E4592: a laboratory ancillary study on an eastern cooperative oncology group prospective randomized trial of postoperative adjuvant therapy. *J Clin Oncol*. 2001;19(2):448-457.
169. Tsao M-S, Hainaut P, Bourredjem A, et al. LACE-bio pooled analysis of the prognostic and predictive value of KRAS mutation in completely resected non-small cell lung cancer (NSCLC). *Ann Oncol*. 2010;21(viii):Abstract 1560.
170. Qiu L-X, Mao C, Zhang J, et al. Predictive and prognostic value of KRAS mutations in metastatic colorectal cancer patients treated with cetuximab: a meta-analysis of 22 studies. *Eur J Cancer*. 2010;46(15):2781-2787.
171. Khambata-Ford S, Harbison CT, Hart LL, et al. Analysis of potential predictive markers of cetuximab benefit in BMS099, a phase III study of cetuximab and first-line taxane/carboplatin in advanced non–small-cell lung cancer. *J Clin Oncol*. 2010;28(6):918-927.
172. Massarelli E, Varella-Garcia M, Tang X, et al. KRAS mutation is an important predictor of resistance to therapy with epidermal growth factor receptor tyrosine kinase inhibitors in non–small-cell lung cancer. *Clin Cancer Res*. 2007;13(10):2890-2896.
173. Jackman DM, Miller VA, Cioffredi L-A, et al. Impact of epidermal growth factor receptor and KRAS mutations on clinical outcomes in previously untreated non–small cell lung cancer patients: results of an online tumor registry of clinical trials. *Clin Cancer Res*. 2009;15(16):5267-5273.
174. Pao W, Wang TY, Riely GJ, et al. KRAS mutations and primary resistance of lung adenocarcinomas to gefitinib or erlotinib. *PLoS Med*. 2005;2(1):e17.
175. Herbst RS, Prager D, Hermann R, et al. TRIBUTE: a phase III trial of erlotinib hydrochloride (OSI-774) combined with carboplatin and paclitaxel chemotherapy in advanced non–small-cell lung cancer. *J Clin Oncol*. 2005;23(25):5892-5899.
176. Davies H, Bignell GR, Cox C, et al. Mutations of the BRAF gene in human cancer. *Nature*. 2002;417(6892):949-954.
177. Paik PK, Arcila ME, Fara M, et al. Clinical characteristics of patients with lung adenocarcinomas harboring BRAF mutations. *J Clin Oncol*. 2011;29(15):2046-2051.
178. Pratilas CA, Hanrahan AJ, Halilovic E, et al. Genetic predictors of MEK dependence in non–small cell lung cancer. *Cancer Res*. 2008;68(22):9375-9383.
179. Yang H, Higgins B, Kolinsky K, et al. RG7204 (PLX4032), a selective BRAFV600E inhibitor, displays potent antitumor activity in preclinical melanoma models. *Cancer Res*. 2010;70(13):5518-5527.
180. Samuels Y, Velculescu VE. Oncogenic mutations of PIK3CA in human cancers. *Cell Cycle*. 2004;3(10):1221-1224.
181. Yamamoto H, Shigematsu H, Nomura M, et al. PIK3CA mutations and copy number gains in human lung cancers. *Cancer Res*. 2008;68(17):6913-6921.
182. Kang S, Bader AG, Vogt PK. Phosphatidylinositol 3-kinase mutations identified in human cancer are oncogenic. *Proc Natl Acad Sci U S A*. 2005;102(3):802-807.
183. Kawano O, Sasaki H, Endo K, et al. PIK3CA mutation status in Japanese lung cancer patients. *Lung Cancer*. 2006;54(2):209-215.
184. Samuels Y, Wang Z, Bardelli A, Silliman N, Ptak J, Szabo S. High frequency of mutations of the PIK3CA gene in human cancers. *Science*. 2004;304:554.
185. Bleeker FE, Felicioni L, Buttitta F, et al. AKT1E17K in human solid tumours. *Oncogene*. 2008;27(42):5648-5650.
186. Hollander MC, Blumenthal GM, Dennis PA. PTEN loss in the continuum of common cancers, rare syndromes and mouse models. *Nat Rev Cancer*. 2011;11(4):289-301.
187. Jin G, Kim MJ, Jeon H-S, et al. PTEN mutations and relationship to EGFR, ERBB2, KRAS, and TP53 mutations in non-small cell lung cancers. *Lung Cancer*. 2010;69(3):279-283.
188. Kohno T, Takahashi M, Manda R, Yokota J. Inactivation of the PTEN/MMAC1/TEP1 gene in human lung cancers. *Genes Chromosomes Cancer*. 1998;22(2):152-156.
189. Lee SY, Kim MJ, Jin G, et al. Somatic mutations in epidermal growth factor receptor signaling pathway genes in non-small cell lung cancers. *J Thorac Oncol*. 2010;5(11):1734-1740. doi:10.097/JTO.0b013e3181f0beca.

190. Carpten JD, Faber AL, Horn C, Donoho GP, Briggs SL, Robbins CM. A transforming mutation in the pleckstrin homology domain of AKT1 in cancer. *Nature*. 2007;448:439-444.
191. Tang J-M, He Q-Y, Guo R-X, Chang X-J. Phosphorylated Akt overexpression and loss of PTEN expression in non-small cell lung cancer confers poor prognosis. *Lung Cancer*. 2006;51(2):181-191.
192. Marks JL, Gong Y, Chitale D, et al. Novel MEK1 mutation identified by mutational analysis of epidermal growth factor receptor signaling pathway genes in lung adenocarcinoma. *Cancer Res*. 2008;68(14):5524-5528.
193. Estep AL, Palmer C, McCormick F, Rauen KA. Mutation analysis of BRAF, MEK1and MEK2 in 15 ovarian cancer cell lines: implications for therapy. *PLoS One*. 2007;2(12):e1279.
194. Yarden Y, Sliwkowski MX. Untangling the ErbB signalling network. *Nat Rev Mol Cell Biol*. 2001;2(2):127-137.
195. Graus-Porta D, Beerli RR, Daly JM, Hynes NE. ErbB-2, the preferred heterodimerization partner of all ErbB receptors, is a mediator of lateral signaling. *EMBO J*. 1997;16(7): 1647-1655.
196. Buttitta F, Barassi F, Fresu G, et al. Mutational analysis of the HER2 gene in lung tumors from Caucasian patients: mutations are mainly present in adenocarcinomas with bronchioloalveolar features. *Int J Cancer*. 2006;119(11):2586-2591.
197. Shigematsu H, Takahashi T, Nomura M, et al. Somatic mutations of the HER2 kinase domain in lung adenocarcinomas. *Cancer Res*. 2005;65(5):1642-1646.
198. Stephens P, Hunter C, Bignell G, et al. Lung cancer: intragenic ERBB2 kinase mutations in tumours. *Nature*. 2004;431(7008):525-526.
199. Li C, Sun Y, Fang R, et al. Lung adenocarcinomas with HER2-activating mutations are associated with distinct clinical features and HER2/EGFR copy number gains. *J Thorac Oncol*. 2012;7(1):85-89. doi:10.1097/JTO.0b013e318234f0a2.
200. Langer CJ, Stephenson P, Thor A, Vangel M, Johnson DH. Trastuzumab in the treatment of advanced non-small-cell lung cancer: is there a role? Focus on eastern cooperative oncology group study 2598. *J Clin Oncol*. 2004;22(7): 1180-1187.
201. Gatzemeier U, Groth G, Butts C, et al. Randomized phase II trial of gemcitabine–cisplatin with or without trastuzumab in HER2-positive non-small-cell lung cancer. *Ann Oncol*. 2004;15(1):19-27.
202. Ross HJ, Blumenschein, George R, et al. Randomized phase II multicenter trial of two schedules of lapatinib as first- or second-line monotherapy in patients with advanced or metastatic non–small cell lung cancer. *Clin Cancer Res*. 2010;16(6): 1938-1949.
203. Cappuzzo F, Bemis L, Varella-Garcia M. HER2 mutation and response to trastuzumab therapy in non–small-cell lung cancer. *N Engl J Med*. 2006;354(24):2619-2621.
204. De Grève JL, Teugels E, De Mey J, et al. Clinical activity of BIBW 2992, an irreversible inhibitor of EGFR and HER2 in adenocarcinoma of the lung with mutations in the kinase domain of HER2neu. *J Thorac Oncol*. 2009;4(9 suppl 1):S307.
205. Hammerman PS, Sos ML, Ramos AH, et al. Mutations in the DDR2 kinase gene identify a novel therapeutic target in squamous cell lung cancer. *Cancer Discov*. 2011;1:78-89.
206. Turner N, Grose R. Fibroblast growth factor signalling: from development to cancer. *Nat Rev Cancer*. 2010;10(2):116-129.
207. Fischer H, Taylor N, Allerstorfer S, et al. Fibroblast growth factor receptor-mediated signals contribute to the malignant phenotype of non-small cell lung cancer cells: therapeutic implications and synergism with epidermal growth factor receptor inhibition. *Mol Cancer Ther*. 2008;7(10):3408-3419.
208. Marek L, Ware KE, Fritzsche A, et al. Fibroblast growth factor (FGF) and FGF receptor-mediated autocrine signaling in non-small-cell lung cancer cells. *Mol Pharmacol*. 2009;75(1):196-207.
209. Weiss J, Sos ML, Seidel D, et al. Frequent and focal FGFR1 amplification associates with therapeutically tractable FGFR1 dependency in squamous cell lung cancer. *Sci Transl Med*. 2010;2(62):62ra93.
210. Jones HE, Goddard L, Gee JMW, et al. Insulin-like growth factor-I receptor signalling and acquired resistance to gefitinib (ZD1839;Iressa) in human breast and prostate cancer cells. *Endocr Relat Cancer*. 2004;11(4):793-814.
211. Morgillo F, Woo JK, Kim ES, Hong WK, Lee H-Y. Heterodimerization of insulin-like growth factor receptor/epidermal growth factor receptor and induction of survivin expression counteract the antitumor action of erlotinib. *Cancer Res*. 2006;66(20):10100-10111.
212. Karp DD, Paz-Ares LG, Novello S, et al. Phase II study of the anti–insulin-like growth factor type 1 receptor antibody CP-751,871 in combination with paclitaxel and carboplatin in previously untreated, locally advanced, or metastatic non–small-cell lung cancer. *J Clin Oncol*. 2009;27(15):2516-2522.
213. Jassem J, Langer CJ, Karp DD, et al. Randomized, open label, phase III trial of figitumumab in combination with paclitaxel and carboplatin versus paclitaxel and carboplatin in patients with non-small cell lung cancer (NSCLC). *J Clin Oncol*. 2010;28(suppl):Abstract 7500.

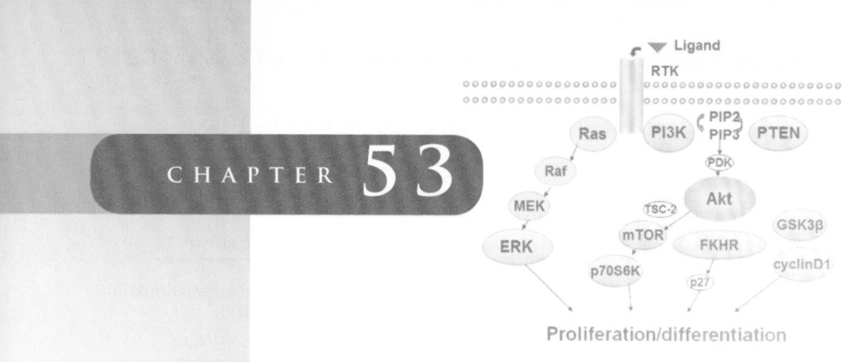

CHAPTER 53

Personalized Medicine and Targeted Therapy of Breast Cancer

Komal Jhaveri, Chau Dang, and Clifford Hudis

INTRODUCTION

Despite significant advances in the adjuvant setting, breast cancer represents a global health problem. In the United States, there are over 230,000 cases of breast cancer with around 40,000 deaths.[1] There has been steady reduction in mortality since 1990, which has been attributed to early detection, more consistent surgery, broad use of radiation therapy, and improved adjuvant treatments.[2] In addition, some risk factors for breast cancer may now be broadly reduced. For example, in 2003, the Women's Health Initiative Study demonstrated that hormone replacement therapy (HRT) was associated with an increased risk of breast cancer.[3] Since their report, there has been a decline in HRT use[4] and a corresponding decrease in the incidence of breast cancer.[3]

Despite these promising trends, the results of therapy are not yet ideal. For example, even for the approximately 1 million women diagnosed annually with early breast cancer worldwide, about one-third will eventually experience distant disease relapse that generally leads to premature death.[5] This is an improvement over the "pre-adjuvant therapy" world of several decades ago, but it clearly indicates that there is progress to be made.

An additional challenge to us as we seek to improve the outcome for breast cancer is the fact that we are not treating just one disease. Instead, we now recognize that breast cancer is a heterogeneous disease that manifests as different molecular subtypes, each of which has a variable response to specific treatments.[6] The most widely accepted classification system divides breast cancer into hormone receptor positives (including the luminal A and luminal B molecular phenotypes), HER2 positive (HER2+), and ER/PR–/HER2– (triple negative). To incorporate personalized medicine, we must recognize this disease's heterogeneity and tailor medical care by addressing the unique biologic profile of each patient's tumor. The entire point of this individualized approach is to enable physicians to recommend the most effective therapy, limit adverse drug reactions, and deliver improved outcomes.

In this chapter, we provide condensed, up-to-date information about prevention strategies and systemic chemotherapy, hormonal therapy, and biologic/targeted therapy of breast cancer in the adjuvant and metastatic settings. We also summarize the efforts utilized to individualize the approach to breast cancer management as we study and incorporate a growing number of novel targeted therapies.

ETIOLOGY AND PREVENTION STRATEGIES

Although numerous risk factors for the development of breast cancer have been established, the etiology of the majority of cases is unknown. Risk factors can be grouped into demographics (increasing age, female gender, ethnicity/race, and higher socioeconomic status), reproductive history (early menarche, late menopause, older age at first live childbirth, and parity), environmental factors (prior thoracic radiation before age 30, HRT, smoking—particularly in premenopausal women, and increased alcohol intake), familial/genetic factors (family history of breast cancer at a young age, inherited breast cancer susceptibility gene such as BRCA1/2, p53, ATM, and phosphatase and tensin homolog [PTEN]), and other factors (proliferative breast disease, previous breast biopsies, and increased body mass index [BMI]).

Except for increasing age, female gender, and increased BMI, these risk factors form a minority of cases.

The Gail model is a breast cancer risk assessment tool that estimates a woman's risk of developing invasive breast cancer.[7] As per the National Comprehensive Cancer Network (NCCN) Breast Cancer Risk Reduction panel, women at increased risk for breast cancer (those with 1.7% or greater 5-year actuarial risk using the Gail model of risk assessment) may consider risk reduction strategies like chemoprevention or prophylactic surgeries. In fact, Gail risk score was one of the eligibility criteria for patients enrolled on the National Surgical Adjuvant Breast and Bowel Project (NSABP) Breast Cancer Prevention Trial (BCPT) and the subsequent Study of Tamoxifen and Raloxifene (STAR) trial.

The BCPT (also known as the P-1 study) marked the beginning of a new paradigm for breast cancer prevention. It showed that tamoxifen, a selective estrogen receptor modulator (SERM), decreased the short-term risk of invasive breast cancer by 49%. The absolute risk reduction was 21.4 cases per 1,000 women over 5 years.[8] However, there was an increased incidence of thromboembolic events and endometrial cancer related to tamoxifen. After 7 years of follow-up, updated results were reported and the reduction in breast cancer incidence was similar to those reported in 1998. The NSABP STAR trial (P-2 study) randomized patients to receive either tamoxifen or another SERM, raloxifene, for 5 years. After a median follow-up of 81 months, raloxifene retained 76% of the effectiveness of tamoxifen in preventing invasive disease, with statistically significant fewer endometrial cancers.[9] Another strategy to interrupt estrogen-driven tumor growth is through aromatase inhibition. When compared with tamoxifen, aromatase inhibitors (AIs) are more effective in reducing breast cancer recurrence and contralateral breast cancer incidence, with minimal toxicity in postmenopausal women with early-stage ER-positive breast cancer.[10,11] Recently, Goss et al. reported the results of the National Cancer Institute of Canada (NCIC) Clinical Trials Group (CTG) MAP.3 trial, where subjects were randomized to receive exemestane, a steroidal AI, versus placebo.[12] At a median follow-up of 35 months, exemestane was associated with a 65% reduction of the annual incidence of invasive breast cancer. Somewhat surprisingly, there were no significant differences in adverse effects in terms of skeletal fractures, cardiovascular events, other cancers, or treatment-related deaths between the two arms.

Risk-reducing surgery may be considered with appropriate genetic counseling in women with a genetic mutation in the BRCA1 or BRCA2 gene. These women have a lifetime risk of 56% to 84% for breast cancer by age 70.[13-15] The estimated lifetime risk for ovarian cancer ranges from 36% to 63% for BRCA1 mutation carriers and 10% to 27% for BRCA2 mutation carriers.[15-18] One of the largest prospective studies published to date on this topic demonstrated that risk-reducing mastectomy was associated with a lower risk of breast cancer, and risk-reducing salpingo-oophorectomy decreased the risk of ovarian cancer, first diagnosis of breast cancer, all-cause mortality, breast cancer–specific mortality, and ovarian cancer–specific mortality.[19]

In summary, breast cancer prevention is possible both surgically and medically. Patients and physicians have three chemoprevention options: tamoxifen, raloxifene, or exemestane. In special circumstances, such as in patients who are carriers of BRCA1/2 gene mutations, risk-reducing surgeries may be considered. However, the risks and benefits associated with these strategies should be evaluated and discussed with the patient as a part of a shared decision-making process.

TREATMENT OF EARLY-STAGE BREAST CANCER

Systemic adjuvant treatment for early-stage breast cancer can be broadly divided into three categories: cytotoxic chemotherapy, hormonal therapy, and biologic/targeted therapy. These therapeutic choices are dependent upon the hormone and HER2 status and represent an example of personalized medicine. Patients with ER and/or PR+ disease are offered adjuvant hormonal therapy and appropriate patients with HER2+ disease are treated with adjuvant trastuzumab therapy (see section "Adjuvant Hormone Therapy"). The use of chemotherapy is currently in some degree of flux.

When to Consider Adjuvant Chemotherapy: Which Tools May Help?

After surgical treatment, adjuvant chemotherapy should be considered for most patients with node-positive or otherwise high-risk disease (i.e., triple-negative breast cancer [TNBC]). Adjuvant systemic chemotherapy is administered in early-stage breast cancer with the intent of eradicating occult micrometastatic disease. However, chemotherapy may not be suitable for all patients with ER+/PR+/HER2– disease and is controversial for some with node-negative disease. Ideally, women who might most benefit from therapy would be identified and those who might not would be spared the deleterious effects of therapy. There are tools that can aid clinicians in objectively assessing the absolute benefits from systemic chemotherapy after local treatment. Adjuvant! Online, developed by Ravdin et al. is a validated computer-based model that determines the risk of recurrence based on age, comorbidities, tumor size and grade, hormone receptor status, and nodal status to estimate the contribution of chemotherapy and/hormonal therapy in risk reduction.[20] However, among the limitations of Adjuvant! Online are that it does not account for HER2 status and it lumps together wide ranges of tumor sizes and numbers of involved nodes. This can introduce some precision. Furthermore, it is based primarily on anatomic spread, rather than molecular biology, and it uses average estimates of treatment effects.

Perhaps the next step in assessing risk and, more importantly, predicting drug effectiveness is genomic analysis. These tools have made it possible to further characterize tumors based on the risk of recurrence after hormonal therapy in defined subsets based on expression profiles. For example, in the NSABP B-14 trial, the OncotypeDX (Genomic Health, Redwood City, CA) assay provides individual, quantitative assessments of the likelihood of breast cancer recurrence after 5 years of treatment with tamoxifen in patients with node-negative disease. It is a reverse transcriptase polymerase chain reaction (RT-PCR) assay that measures the expression of 21 genes consisting of 16 cancer-related genes associated with proliferation, invasion, and ER/PR and HER2 status in addition to the 5 reference genes. The expression of these genes is used to calculate a recurrence score (RS) that predicts the likelihood of recurrence at 10 years.[21] It classifies a patient into three different categories based on the RS, namely low (RS < 18), intermediate (RS 18 to 31), and high (RS ≥ 31), with associated 10-year distant recurrence rates of 6.8%, 14.3%, and 30.5%, respectively. Prediction of treatment effect is more important than pure prognosis. In the NSABP B-20 study, the OncotypeDX also predicted the likelihood of chemotherapy benefit in patients with node-negative ER+ cancer. Those with a low RS derived minimal benefit with adjuvant chemotherapy, whereas those with higher scores evidenced more significant improvements in disease-free survival. Based on this, one would predict that those with low scores would be sufficiently treated with hormonal therapy alone.[22] Similarly, the SouthWest Oncology Group (SWOG)-8814 study demonstrated the effectiveness of anthracycline-based chemotherapy plus tamoxifen when administered sequentially in node-positive, ER+ disease with a high RS.[23] However, a retrospective analysis from this study showed little benefit with the addition of anthracycline-based chemotherapy in women with node-positive disease with a low RS.[24] The Breast Cancer Intergroup of North America has concluded the TAILORx (Trial Assigning Individualized Options for Treatment) trial to evaluate the benefit, or not, of chemotherapy combined with hormonal therapy in patients with intermediate RS. This study has reached its target accrual and the results are awaited.[25] Although the OncotypeDX assay was initially tested among patients with node-negative, ER+ disease treated with tamoxifen, this assay has also been studied in node-positive women as well as women treated with anastrozole.[24,26] In January 2011, SWOG activated a phase III trial similar to the TAILORx study focusing on patients with node-positive disease and low-to-intermediate RS. These patients are randomized to chemotherapy followed by hormone therapy or hormone therapy alone.[27] A recent study has shown that combining RS with clinical and pathological information reduces the number of patients being classified into the intermediate-risk category by 30% at a cost of decreased predictive accuracy for the benefits of chemotherapy.[28]

Other gene expression profiling studies have classified breast cancer into five molecular subtypes: luminal A (ER+/HER2–), luminal B (ER+/HER2–), HER2+, basal-like, and normal-like. Luminal A cancers have the best prognosis, HER2+ and basal-like cancers have the worst prognosis, and the prognosis of luminal B cancers is intermediate.[29] The only Food and Drug Administration (FDA)–approved microarray-based assay, MammaPrint, uses a similar approach to define more limited sets of genes for prognostic purposes. MammaPrint, a 70-gene signature (also referred to as the Amsterdam signature), was developed at the Netherlands Cancer Institute. It categorizes patients into two groups—good prognosis and poor prognosis, irrespective of their ER status. The signature largely consists of genes regulating proliferation, plus those involved in invasion, metastasis, stromal integrity, and angiogenesis. Initial validation studies were done by the Translational Breast International Group (TRANSBIG) and this formed the basis of its use in the ongoing MINDACT (Microarray In Node-negative Disease may Avoid ChemoTherapy) study that evaluates which patients can be spared chemotherapy.[30] However, this test has a few differences from OncotypeDX, such as its clinical utility in ER-negative patients, where 0% to 4% are classified as good prognosis, and HER2+ patients, where up to 22% are classified as having good prognosis and not requiring therapy.

The clinical utility of the five intrinsic molecular subtypes defined by gene profiling studies is not straightforward. For example, there is discordance between tumors identified to have the HER2+ molecular subtype and those identified by immunohistochemistry or fluorescence in situ hybridization (FISH). Other limitations include the requirement for fresh frozen tissue for microarray-based signatures. To address this issue, an intrinsic 50-gene set was used to develop an RT-PCR–based predictor called PAM50.[31] The PAM50 gene assay identifies the five intrinsic subtypes (luminal A and B, HER2-enriched, basal-like, and normal-like) and provides a continuous risk score based on the similarity of an individual sample to prototypic subtypes. Recent data suggest that when OncotypeDX assay and PAM50 were compared, there was a large overlap in the ability of these tests to determine the recurrence risk in ER+ breast cancer.[32] In fact, 51% of the patients classified to have intermediate RS by OncotypeDX were recategorized as low-risk luminal A using PAM50. Although these results are encouraging, the prognostic utility of PAM50 is currently restricted to ER+, node-negative disease and the predictive utility is not established.[31]

Patients with ER/PR+/HER2– disease can be risk-stratified to receive adjuvant chemotherapy based on their risk of recurrence as detailed above. Once the decision to give chemotherapy is made, some clinicians may utilize Adjuvant! Online to help choose a cytotoxic therapy based on its additive contribution. Chemotherapy, when offered, is then followed sequentially by adjuvant endocrine therapy. Regardless of adjuvant chemotherapy, these patients with hormone receptor–positive disease should be treated with adjuvant hormonal therapy (discussed in section "Adjuvant Hormone Therapy"). It should also be noted that the benefits of chemotherapy and hormonal therapy are clinically additive (though mathematically multiplicative in terms of risk reductions). The specific chemotherapeutic regimens are discussed below.

Chemotherapeutic Regimens

The 2000 Early Breast Cancer Trialists' Collaborative Group (EBCTCG) overview of polychemotherapy in breast cancer demonstrated that anthracycline-based regimens are superior to non-anthracycline-based therapies in terms of disease-free survival (DFS) and overall survival (OS).[33] A large meta-analysis showed that the addition of a taxane to an anthracycline-based regimen improves DFS and OS in high-risk patients regardless of age, menopausal status, number of nodes involved, hormone receptor status, and type of taxane.[34] There are several effective anthracycline–taxane combinations traditionally studied in patients with node-positive disease. The regimen TAC (docetaxel + adriamycin [A] + cyclophosphamide [C]) is superior to standard FAC (5-fluorouracil + A + C). The popular treatment AC → P (paclitaxel) has largely replaced AC. Furthermore, AC → P given every 2 weeks (dose dense) has shown superiority over the every three-weekly schedule, demonstrated in Cancer and Leukemia Group B (CALGB 9741).[35] ECOG 1199 compared two schedules of two taxanes after AC (every third week or weekly P vs. every third week or weekly D [docetaxel]). This study demonstrated the superiority of weekly paclitaxel and every third week docetaxel to every third week paclitaxel. Thus, AC → weekly P and AC → D are options. In Europe, both FEC → D and FEC → P have replaced FEC.[34] Thus, the addition of a taxane to an anthracycline (AC → P, AC → D, TAC, FEC → P, FEC → D) regimen has consistently demonstrated improved outcomes. Although anthracyline–taxane regimens were studied in node-positive patients, they are certainly appropriate to use in treating selected high-risk patients with node-negative disease (i.e., triple-negative or HER2+ disease).

Non-anthracycline-based therapy, such as cyclophosphamide + methotrexate + 5-fluorouracil (CMF) and DC, has generally been reserved for the treatment of node-negative breast cancers. For those with intermediate-risk, ER/PR+/HER– disease, when chemotherapy is offered, the physician can consider a range of chemotherapeutic regimens from CMF to DC and even to all the available anthracycline–taxane combinations discussed above. It is important to recognize that OncotypeDX assay provides an estimate of the risk of recurrence and the impact of CMF or similar regimens but does not provide guidance as to the specific choice of chemotherapeutic agents.

There is growing controversy over the use of anthracyclines because of their toxicities and the possibility that their superior efficacy is limited to a specific subset (HER2+) where trastuzumab now changes the relative value of different chemotherapy regimens.[36,37] However, HER2 is not the only known target of drugs in this class and there are other potential molecular predictors of response to anthracyclines, such as topoisomerase II (TOPO II) gene aberrations—TOPO II amplifications and deletions, and TOPO II protein overexpression along with other possibilities.[38] In fact, one of the adjuvant trastuzumab trials, the Breast Cancer International Research Group (BCIRG) 006 study, randomized patients with HER2+ disease with an anthracycline–taxane regimen, the same regimen with trastuzumab (H), or a third non-anthracycline regimen with trastuzumab, using docetaxel and carboplatin as the chemotherapy backbone (DCarboH).[39] In this study, TOPO II gene was evaluated by FISH in breast tissue samples from 2,120 patients. A total of 35% of the patients had HER2 and TOP2A coamplification and this subgroup was most sensitive to the anthracyclines, and the DFS benefit from the trastuzumab arms was the same as that derived from just the chemotherapy-alone (anthracycline–taxane/no trastuzumab) arm. In the HER2-amplified/TOPO II nonamplified group, the DFS was equivalent for both trastuzumab-containing arms (DCarboH and AC-DH), suggesting that an anthracycline may not be needed.[39] However, additional confirmatory studies are needed before TOP2A can be used as a predictive marker.

In summary, until definitive molecular predictors are known, when a patient has high-risk disease, based on biologic and/or pathologic parameters, the full package anthracycline–taxane regimens should be considered.

Adjuvant Hormone Therapy

The treatment of ER/PR+ breast cancer involves either blocking the action of estrogen at the receptor or decreasing the production of estrogen. The importance of estrogen withdrawal was first illustrated by Beatson et al. in 1896 when salpingo-oophorectomy demonstrated tumor regressions among some patients with advanced breast cancer.[40] Jensen et al. isolated the ER in the 1960s[41] and the evaluation of ER and PR has been a standard of care for decades. Tamoxifen, an SERM, was the first targeted therapy for breast cancer and in the forefront of personalized medicine in the late 1970s. In overly simplified terms, it antagonizes the action of estrogen in the breast and mimics its action in the bone and the uterus.[42] More recently, AIs that inhibit the aromatase enzyme and decrease the production of estrogen have emerged as a new class of medications. Currently available AIs are categorized into two classes: steroidal (or type I inhibitors—exemestane, formestane, and atamestane) and nonsteroidal (type II inhibitors—anastrozole and letrozole) agents based on their differential mechanism of interaction with the aromatase enzyme.

TABLE 53-1 DFS and OS with the Use of an AI in Primary, Sequential, or Extended Treatment Strategy

Trial (N)	Arm (N)	Median F/U (Months)	DFS HR (95% CI); *P* Value	OS HR (95% CI); *P* Value
Primary				
ATAC[45]	Anas (3,125) vs. Tam (3,116)	120	0.91 (0.83–0.99); 0.04	0.97 (0.88–1.08); 0.6
BIG 1-98[46]	Let (2,463) vs. Tam (2,459)	76	0.88 (0.78–0.99); 0.03[a]	0.87 (0.75–1.02); 0.08[a]
Sequential				
BIG 1-98	Let/Tam (1,540) vs. Let (1,546)	71	0.96 (0.76–1.21); NR	0.90 (0.65–1.24); NR
	Tam/Let (1,548) vs. Let (1,546)	71	1.05 (0.84–1.32); NR[b]	1.13 (0.83–1.53); NR[b]
TEAM[47]	Tam/Exe (4,868) vs. Exe (4,898)	61	0.97 (0.88–1.08); 0.604	1.00 (0.89–1.14); 0.999
IES[48]	Tam/Tam (2,372) vs. Tam/Exe (2,352)	91	0.82 (0.73–0.92); 0.0009	0.86 (0.75–0.99); 0.04
ABCSG 8[49]	Tam/Anas (1,865) vs. Tam (1,849)	72	0.85 (0.71–1.01); 0.067[c,d]	0.64 (0.36–1.13); NR
Extended				
NCIC CTG MA.17[50]	Let (2,583) vs. placebo (2,587) after 5 y of Tam	64	0.68 (0.55–0.83); <0.001	0.98(0.78–1.22); 0.853

[a]Analysis from monotherapy arms; crossovers not censored.
[b]99% confidence intervals are shown to account for multiple comparisons.
[c]Relapse-free survival includes local and distal recurrence, contralateral breast cancer, and death without recurrence.
[d]Patients were censored at the time of crossover.
AI, aromatase inhibitor; Let, letrozole; Tam, tamoxifen; Anas, anastrozole; Exe, exemestane; DFS, disease-free survival; OS, overall survival; NR, not reached; ATAC, Anastrozole, Tamoxifen, Alone or in Combination; BIG 1-98, Breast International Group 1-98; TEAM, Tamoxifen Exemestane Adjuvant mUltinational; IES, Intergroup Exemestane Study; ABCSG 8, Austrian Breast and Colorectal cancer Study Group 8; NCIC CTG MA.17, National Cancer Institute of Canada Clinical Trials Group MA.17; F/U, follow-up; HR, hazard ratio.

The EBCTCG meta-analysis demonstrated the enduring benefit in 15-year relapse-free survival and OS for 5 years of adjuvant tamoxifen for women with early-stage ER and/PR+ breast cancer.[43] Large randomized trials in postmenopausal women evaluated the advantage of AIs when given upfront (primary), sequentially, or as extended therapy after 5 years of tamoxifen.[10,44] The Anastrozole, Tamoxifen, Alone or in Combination (ATAC) trial and the Breast International Group (BIG) 1-98 were upfront trials comparing tamoxifen with anastrozole in ATAC and letrozole in BIG 1-98. The large switching studies included the (1) Tamoxifen Exemestane Adjuvant Multinational (TEAM) trial that compared tamoxifen × 2.5 years followed by exemestane × 2.5 years to exemestane for 5 years; (2) Intergroup Exemestane Study (IES) that compared tamoxifen × 5 years with tamoxifen × 2 to 3 years followed by exemestane × 2 to 3 years; (3) Austrian Breast and Colorectal Cancer Study Group 8 (ABCSG 8) that compared tamoxifen × 5 years with tamoxifen × 2 years followed by anastrozole for 3 years; and (4) the BIG 1-98 trial that evaluated letrozole × 2 years followed by tamoxifen for 3 years, and vice versa. Other switching studies include the German Adjuvant Breast Cancer Group (Arimidex-Nolvadex or ARNO) 95 trial and the Italian Tamoxifen Arimidex (ITA) trial. The NCIC CTG MA.17 trial asked the question if AIs should be given after 5 years of tamoxifen therapy. Significant results from these selected large randomized trials have been summarized in Table 53.1. In summary, incorporation of an AI for adjuvant therapy resulted in improvement of DFS (see Table 53.1), distant recurrence, loco-regional recurrence, and contralateral breast cancer. The absolute reduction in the risk of recurrence associated with AI therapy compared with tamoxifen is <5% through many years of follow-up.[10,44] The absolute difference between OS with AI and that with tamoxifen was fairly modest and was seen in lymph node–positive disease. These data suggest that when administered sequentially after 2 to 3 years of tamoxifen, total treatment with an AI should not exceed 5 years. The question of whether AIs should be given longer than 5 years after 5 years of tamoxifen is being addressed by the MA.17 R (re-randomization) and the NSABP B-42 trials. Until further follow-up data are available, we cannot rule in or out a benefit for AI use beyond 5 years either as upfront or as extended treatment.

It is not clear if the agents or classes of AIs are meaningfully different. With regard to efficacy, The NCIC MA.27 trial showed no material difference between letrozole and exemestane in terms of benefit or toxicity.[51] Similarly, the American College of Surgeons Oncology Group (ACOSOG) Z1031 neoadjuvant trial is a randomized phase II trial that compared letrozole, anastrozole, and exemestane in 377 patients with early-stage ER and/PR+ breast cancer and showed that these three AIs were biologically and clinically similar.

Tamoxifen for 5 years remains the standard of care for premenopausal women. Tamoxifen can also be considered for postmenopausal women who cannot tolerate AIs. Currently, AIs are not recommended for pre- or perimenopausal women. The question of whether tamoxifen or AIs with ovarian ablation are beneficial in premenopausal women is being addressed by the Suppression of Ovarian Function Trial (SOFT) and the Tamoxifen and Exemestane Trial (TEXT). Tamoxifen is associated with increased gynecological complaints and an increased risk of venous thromboembolic events, while AIs may cause more cardiovascular events, hypercholesterolemia, osteoporosis, and hypertension.[44] Therefore, a careful consideration of side-effect profile, comorbidities, and patient preference is necessary to incorporate appropriate adjuvant endocrine strategy.

CYP2D6 is a highly polymorphic drug-metabolizing enzyme that converts tamoxifen, a relatively weak SERM, to endoxifen (4-hydroxy-*N*-desmethyl-tamoxifen), a much more potent metabolite. Recent research has been focused on genotyping patients for the cytochrome P450 2D6 (CYP2D6) in an attempt to identify patients who are most likely to benefit from tamoxifen therapy. Retrospective data suggested that patients who have polymorphisms in the CYP2D6 allele and/or are taking concomitant CYP2D6 inhibitors have low serum endoxifen concentrations and have increased risk of recurrence after tamoxifen.[52] However, there was no clear association between CYP2D6 testing and outcomes in patients taking tamoxifen in the ATAC and BIG 1-98 trials.[53,54] As per the ASCO 2010 Clinical Practice Guidelines, CYP2D6 testing is not recommended when deciding on the use of tamoxifen. However, CYP2D6 interacting agents should be avoided in combination with tamoxifen if other choices are available.[10] Perhaps the extension of pharmacogenomic analysis to other genes, such as variants of CYP19 (that encodes for the aromatase), will help us move toward individualized hormonal therapies.[55]

Adjuvant and Neoadjuvant Biologics/Targeted Therapies

Adjuvant and Neoadjuvant Trastuzumab

Approximately one-fifth of breast cancer patients demonstrate amplification of the HER2 gene in their tumors. Its overexpression is an independently poor prognostic variable. Trastuzumab (Herceptin, Genentech, South San Francisco, CA) is a humanized murine monoclonal antibody that binds to the HER2 extracellular domain IV and leads to cell cycle arrest and apoptosis. The mechanisms of action of trastuzumab are not completely understood but are likely to include antibody-dependent cellular cytotoxicity,[56] inhibition of cell cycle progression by disruption of downstream proliferating signaling pathways,[57] antiangiogenic effects,[58] and downregulation of the HER2 protein by endocytosis and degradation,[59] although data for the latter are conflicting.[60] Due to improved outcomes noted with the addition of trastuzumab to chemotherapy in the metastatic setting,[61] chemotherapy and trastuzumab combinations were explored in the adjuvant and the neoadjuvant setting.

Four large multicenter randomized trials—NSABP B-31, National Cancer Control Treatment Group (NCCTG) N9831, HERceptin Adjuvant (HERA)/BIG 01-01, and the BCIRG 006[39,62,63]—and two other smaller studies, the Finland Herceptin (FinHER)[64] and the Protocole Adjuvant dans le Cancer du Sein (PACS04),[65] collectively enrolled over 14,000 women. These women were randomized to receive standard chemotherapy versus chemotherapy plus trastuzumab. These trials had differences in patient population and study design, and except for the PACS04 trial, the remaining trials revealed a significant effect of adjuvant trastuzumab with an approximate 40% to 50% reduction in the risk of breast cancer recurrence (Table 53.2). A recent meta-analysis of these six adjuvant trials confirmed improvement in DFS and OS in favor of trastuzumab therapy.[66] Questions remain regarding the timing of trastuzumab with respect to chemotherapy. The only trial that compared concurrent versus sequential trastuzumab therapy was the N9831 trial. Updated results of this trial favored the concurrent trastuzumab arm.[62,67] There were increased cardiovascular events with concurrent therapy, and there was no difference in OS between the concurrent and sequential arms.[68]

Although the FinHER trial reported an improvement in DFS and OS with 9 weeks of trastuzumab therapy prior to chemotherapy, currently, 1 year of adjuvant trastuzumab is recommended. Results from the 2-year trastuzumab arm of HERA trial and two other studies, Protocol of Herceptin Adjuvant with Reduced Exposure (PHARE)[69] and Persephone,[70] examining 6 months versus 1 year of therapy, are awaited to further establish the optimal duration of trastuzumab therapy. When trastuzumab was administered concurrently with anthracyclines, there was an increased incidence of cardiotoxicity (8% in the anthracycline-only group to 27% in the combination group).[61] This led to rigorous cardiac monitoring in these six trastuzumab adjuvant therapy trials. Across all trials, the reported incidence of symptomatic congestive heart failure with trastuzumab therapy ranged from 0.4% to 3.9%. Dang and colleagues reported that trastuzumab added to dose-dense AC and paclitaxel is both well tolerated and safe and allows for the use of a superior chemotherapy regimen in combination with trastuzumab for early-stage HER2-positive disease with a low cardiotoxicity risk.[71] BCIRG 006 study was the only study to compare a non-anthracycline regimen (DCarboH) plus trastuzumab with an anthracycline regimen (AC-DH). At 5 years, patients treated with DCarboH had a DFS and OS of 81% and 91%, respectively, compared with 84% and 92%, respectively, for AC-DH. These results were not statistically significant, but the study was not powered for this comparison. Hence, we cannot assume that DCarboH is equivalent to AC-DH.[39]

Neoadjuvant/preoperative/primary systemic chemotherapy allows downstaging of tumor, particularly in women presenting with large, inoperable, locally advanced breast cancer. It potentially increases the chances of breast

TABLE 53-2 Adjuvant Trastuzumab Trials (Trial Design, Patient Characteristics, and Efficacy Results)

Trial	*N*	Study Design	HER2 Testing	Median F/U (Months)	DFS (95% CI)	OS (95% CI)
NSABP B-31[62]	2,101	AC × 4 — R → T × 4; T × 4 H × 52	Local IHC and/or FISH	48	0.52[a] (0.45–0.60)	0.61[a] (0.50–0.75)
NCCTG N9831[62]	1,944	AC × 4 — R → wT × 12; wT × 12 — H × 52; wT × 12 H × 52	Centralized IHC and/or FISH	48		
HERA/ BIG 01-01[63]	5,081	STANDARD CHEMOTHERAPY — R → No H; H × 1 y; H × 2 y	Centralized IHC and/or FISH	48	0.76 (0.66–0.87)	0.85 (0.70–1.04)
BCIRG 006[39]	3,222	R → AC × 4 — D × 4; AC × 4 — D × 4, H × 52; DCarb × 6, H × 52	Centralized FISH	65	Arm B vs. A 0.64 $P \leq 0.001$ Arm C vs. A 0.75 $P = 0.04$	Arm B vs. A 0.63 $P \leq 0.001$ Arm C vs. A 0.77 $P = 0.04$
FinHER[64]	232	R → D × 9 wk; V × 9 wk; D + H × 9 wk; V + H × 9 wk → FEC × 3	Centralized IHC and/or FISH	36	0.42 (0.21–0.83)	0.41 (0.16–1.08)
PACS04[65]	528	R → FEC100 × 6; ED × 6 → HER2+ — R → H × 1 y; NO H	Centralized IHC and/or FISH	48	0.86 (0.61–1.22)	1.27 (0.68–2.38)

[a]Joint analysis of NSABP B-31 arm B and N9831 arm C vs. arm A of both trials.
AC, doxorubicin 60 mg/m^2 plus cyclophosphamide 600 mg/m^2 every 3 weeks; T, paclitaxel 175 mg/m^2 every 3 wk; H, trastuzumab 4 mg/kg loading dose followed by 2 mg/kg weekly × 51 wk; wT, weekly paclitaxel 80 mg/m^2; D, docetaxel 100 mg/m^2 every 3 wk; DCarb, docetaxel 75 mg/m^2 plus carboplatin AUC6 every 3 wk; V, vinorelbine 25 mg/m^2 day 1, 8, and 15 every 3 wk; FEC, fluorouracil 600 mg/m^2, epirubicin 60 mg/m^2 plus cyclophosphamide 600 mg/m^2 every 3 wk; FEC 10, fluorouracil 500 mg/m^2, epirubicin 100 mg/m^2 plus cyclophosphamide 500 mg/m^2 every 3 wk; ED, epirubicin 75 mg/m^2 plus docetaxel 75 mg/m^2 every 3 wk; DFS, disease-free survival; FISH, fluorescence in situ hybridization; IHC, immunohistochemistry; F/U, follow-up.

conservation surgery. There was no difference in DFS or OS when neoadjuvant chemotherapy was compared with adjuvant chemotherapy using identical drug regimens.[72,73] Additionally, preoperative therapy allows for in vivo testing for tumor response, but this has not been validated as clinically useful, whereas it can be a very efficient research approach.

Trastuzumab and other anti-HER2-directed therapies have also been incorporated in the neoadjuvant setting in women with HER2+ breast cancer in an attempt to assess for pathologic complete response (pCR) rates.[33,74–81] Table 53.3 summarizes the major anti-HER2-directed neoadjuvant trials that are either completed or currently ongoing in patients with early-stage HER2+ disease.

The preoperative or neoadjuvant setting provides an opportunity to rapidly test new agents in smaller numbers of patients than the traditional adjuvant setting. This is of special value in HER2-positive disease where there are many active agents (see section "Other Anti-HER2 Strategies"), including monoclonal antibodies (i.e., pertuzumab), tyrosine kinase inhibitors (TKIs) (i.e., lapatinib and neratinib), and many others. Recently, the NeoAdjuvant Lapatinib and/or Trastuzumab Treatment Optimization (NeoALTTO) and the Neoadjuvant Study of Pertuzumab and Herceptin in an Early Regimen Evaluation (NeoSphere) trials demonstrated a doubling of the pCR rates in favor of the dual anti-HER2 agents (added to trastuzumab with cytotoxic therapy) versus trastuzumab with chemotherapy alone.[78,79] Conversely, the GeparQuinto trial showed that lapatinib was inferior to trastuzumab when each was combined with chemotherapy in terms of pCR.[80] The results of the NeoALTTO trial led to the modification of the CALGB 40601 neoadjuvant study in which accrual to the lapatinib + chemotherapy arm was stopped.[77] A unique feature of these neoadjuvant trials are the embedded biomarker studies that help tailor

TABLE 53-3 Summary of Anti-HER2 Blockade in Neoadjuvant Trials for HER2+ Breast Cancer

Trial	Phase	Treatment	Patients	pCR (%)	*P* Value
TECHNO (Untch et al.[74])	**II**	EC → T+H → H	**217**	39	NR
Buzdar et al.[33]	**III and II**		**64**		
		T → FEC	19	26[a]	
		T → FEC → H	23	65.2[a]	0.016
		T → FEC → H	22	54.5[a]	NR
		(nonrandomized, assigned cohort)			
NOAH (Gianni et al.[75])	**III**		**235**		
		AT → T → CMF → H	117	43[b]	0.00
		AT → T → CMF	118	22[b]	
GeparQuattro (Untch et al.[76])	**III HER2+**		**434**		
		EC → D with H	148	32.9	<0.001
		EC → DX with H	146	31	
		EC → DX with H	140	34	
	HER2–	Chemotherapy only	**987**	15.7	
CALGB 40601 (Carey[77])	**III**	T+H → AC → H	**400**	Ongoing	
		T+L → AC → H			
		T+H+L → AC → H			
NeoALTTO/BIG 1-06 (Baselga et al.[78])	**III**		**455**		
		L → L+T → FEC → L	154	24.7	0.34
		H → H+T → FEC → H	149	29.5	
		L+H → L+H+T → FEC → L+H	152	51.3	0.0001
NeoSphere (Gianni et al.[79])	**II**		**417**		
		D+H → FEC → H	107	29	
		D+H+Per → FEC → H	107	45.8	0.014
		D+Per → FEC → H	96	24	0.03
		Per+H → P → FEC → H	107	16.8	0.031
GeparQuinto (Untch et al.[80])	**II**	EC+H → D+H vs.	620	31	<0.05
		ED+L → D+L		22	
CHERLOB (Guarneri[81])	**IIb**		**121**		NR
		T+H → FEC → H	36	25.7	
		T+L → FEC	39	27.8	
		T+H+L → FEC	46	43.1	

pCR, pathologic complete response; A, doxorubicin; E, epirubicin; C, cyclophosphamide; T, paclitaxel; D, docetaxel; FEC, fluorouracil plus epirubicin plus cyclophosphamide; V, vinorelbine; H, trastuzumab; L, lapatinib; Per, pertuzumab; DX, docetaxel plus capecitabine; CMF, cyclophosphamide plus methotrexate plus 5-fluorouracil.

treatment by identifying was stopped reliable predictors of response and/or resistance. Such markers include markers of cell proliferation, angiogenesis, or signal transduction from tumor biopsy and blood specimens. A limitation of these studies is the fact that investigators have not yet shown that changes in response rates (RRs) in the breast with experimental agents necessarily predict the subsequent long-term adjuvant impact of these regimens. This limits the clinical utility, outside of trials, of these observations at present.

Adjuvant Lapatinib

Despite the significant benefit from trastuzumab in the adjuvant and metastatic setting, de novo and acquired resistance have emerged and led to the development of newer agents targeting this pathway. One such new-generation HER2-targeting drug is lapatinib (Tykerb). It is a reversible, small-molecule, dual HER1/HER2 TKI that targets the intracellular domain of HER2 and blocks kinase activation. It was approved by the FDA in 2007 for the treatment of HER2+ metastatic breast cancer (MBC).

Two pilot studies evaluated lapatinib administration with paclitaxel and trastuzumab in the adjuvant setting. Patients in these trials received AC × 4 cycles followed by trastuzumab in combination with lapatinib at 1,000 mg daily for 1 year.[82,83] In both trials, patients reported grade 3/4 diarrhea (ranging from 27% to 42%) requiring dose reduction to 750 mg daily. This led to modification of the lapatinib dose when given concurrently with trastuzumab in the worldwide phase III ongoing trial—Adjuvant Lapatinib and/or Trastuzumab Treatment Optimization (ALTTO). This trial is ongoing with a target accrual of 8,000 patients to one of the four treatment arms following chemotherapy—lapatinib (arm A), trastuzumab (arm B), trastuzumab followed by lapatinib (arm C), or concurrent treatment with both agents (arm D).[84] Recently, based on the preliminary efficacy analysis by the ALTTO trial independent data monitoring committee, the lapatinib-only arm (arm A) was closed as it crossed the futility margin and as such its non-inferiority to trastuzumab will not be reached. While the overall study continues, the committee recommended that patients on this arm should be offered trastuzumab (Perez et al., Oral presentation—ASCO Breast Cancer Symposium, September 2011).

A multicenter, randomized phase III Tykerb Evaluation After Chemotherapy (TEACH) study tested the efficacy of lapatinib for 3,000 patients who had not received adjuvant trastuzumab therapy after completion of adjuvant chemotherapy (as the antibody was not available at that time) or were unable or unwilling to take adjuvant trastuzumab therapy. Participants were randomized to receive lapatinib 1,500 mg or placebo orally administered once daily. DFS is the primary endpoint and recruitment is completed.[85]

Adjuvant Pertuzumab

Another anti-HER2 agent is pertuzumab, which is a humanized monoclonal antibody that binds to a different epitope distally from trastuzumab and acts as a HER2 dimerization inhibitor.[86] The addition of pertuzumab to chemotherapy plus trastuzumab in first-line metastatic setting in the *CL*inical *E*valuation *Of Pertuzumab And TRA*stuzumab (CLEOPATRA) study demonstrated a significant progression-free survival (PFS) benefit (see section Other Anti-HER2 Strategies). A large randomized study is therefore evaluating the efficacy of pertuzumab with chemotherapy and trastuzumab versus chemotherapy and trastuzumab plus placebo in the adjuvant setting in HER2+ primary breast cancer. This trial is now open for recruitment.[87]

Adjuvant and Neoadjuvant Bevacizumab for HER2-Negative Breast Cancer

Another novel biologic therapy in breast cancer involves targeting the vascular endothelial growth factor (VEGF) pathway. VEGF plays a significant role in new blood vessel formation or angiogenesis. It binds to the VEGF receptor (VEGFR), thus leading to tumor growth, survival, and migration. The VEGF/VEGFR pathway includes several ligands (VEGF-A, VEGF-B, VEGF-C, VEGF-D, VEGF-E, and placental growth factor/PlG-F) and their associated VEGFR tyrosine kinases—VEGFR-1/Flt-1, VEGFR-2/Flk-1/KDR and VEGFR-3/Flt-4, and neuropilin-1 and -2.[88] Bevacizumab is a humanized monoclonal antibody that sequesters VEGF-A, leading to normalization of tumor vasculature and possibly more efficient delivery of cytotoxic chemotherapy.[89] It is FDA-approved in the United States for colorectal and lung cancer. In breast cancer, in the metastatic setting, the addition of bevacizumab to chemotherapy showed improved RRs and PFS, but there was no difference in the OS.[90-93] Genentech's bevacizumab (Avastin) was granted accelerated approval by the FDA in February 2008 for locally recurrent or metastatic HER2– breast cancer. However, due to the adverse events associated with bevacizumab and failure of studies to show an OS benefit or reproduce a significant PFS benefit, the FDA announced its withdrawal of the approval for bevacizumab for MBC in December 2010. Table 53.4 has a list of ongoing and completed trials with bevacizumab in the adjuvant setting.

The value of neoadjuvant bevacizumab is less established compared with neoadjuvant trastuzumab. The addition of bevacizumab to EC→D chemotherapy did not improve pCR rates in unselected HER2– breast cancer.[98] However, when a total of 684 patients with TNBC were randomized to EC→D with or without bevacizumab in the GeparQuinto study, pCR was 36.4% versus 27.8% ($P = 0.021$) in favor of the bevacizumab arm.[99] Table 53.5 summarizes completed and ongoing bevacizumab trials in the neoadjuvant setting. Other antiangiogenic TKIs like pazopanib are also being evaluated in the neoadjuvant setting in both hormone receptor–positive and hormone receptor–negative breast cancers.[102]

TABLE 53-4 Trials with Bevacizumab in the Adjuvant Setting

Trial	Arms	N	Phase	Primary Endpoint	Status	Results	Estimated Completion Date
BETH[94]	Arm A: TCH-H +/– B Arm B: TH-FEC-H +/– B	3,509	III	IDFS	Ongoing	NA	June 2021
E2104[95]	Arm A: dd BAC-BT-B Arm B: dd AC-BT-B	226	II	Clinical CHF	Completed	No prohibitive cardiac toxicity with addition of B	NA
E5103[96]	Arm A: AC-TP Arm B: AC-TB Arm C: AC-TB-B	4,950	III	DFS	Completed	NA	November 2013
BEATRICE[97,a]	Arm A: adjuvant chemo + B Arm B: adjuvant chemo	2,582	III	IDFS	Ongoing	NA	January 2015

[a]For triple-negative breast cancer.

TCH, docetaxel, carboplatin (C), trastuzumab (H); B, bevacizumab; FEC, 5-fluorouracil (F), epirubicin (E), cyclophosphamide (C); IDFS, invasive disease-free survival; dd, dose dense; BAC, bevacizumab (B), adriamycin (A), cyclophosphamide (C); BT, bevacizumab, paclitaxel (T); CHF, congestive heart failure; P, placebo.

TREATMENT OF MBC

The treatment of MBC can also be tailored based on the hormone receptor and HER2 receptor status. Patients with ER/PR+ disease can be treated with hormonal therapy, at least initially. Subsequent lines of hormone therapy may be appropriate based on initial response durations. For patients with hormone receptor negative or hormone refractory disease and/or symptomatic or visceral disease, chemotherapy can be offered. Patients with HER2+ breast cancer can be treated with chemotherapy with anti-HER2 agents (trastuzumab or lapatinib) or combined anti-HER2 agents possibly without chemotherapy. While there have been important additions to the armamentarium of biologic therapies, the optimal permutation and combination of targeted therapies is an area of intense investigation. This section summarizes these therapeutic options in detail.

Chemotherapy in the Metastatic Setting

Chemotherapy for MBC is given with palliative intent and is frequently chronic in nature. Improvement in survival remains an important goal in MBC but it is not clear if it is often or always achieved. The current strategy is to establish goals with the patient, use agents individualized to the patients' comorbidities, and offer chemotherapeutic agents (and even combinations) with the acceptable toxicities. For most patients, this involves sequential single-agent therapies that can lead to reduction or stabilization of disease while maintaining an acceptable quality of life. For patients with bulky or symptomatic visceral disease, the goal is to obtain rapid tumor shrinkage and sometimes combination chemotherapy may be helpful here. Of particular note, there is no compelling evidence that combination therapy is superior to single-agent "sequential" therapy in terms of OS. The NCCN guidelines lists

TABLE 53-5 Bevacizumab in the Neoadjuvant Setting

Trial	Arm	N	Phase	Primary Endpoint	Results	Expected Completion Date
GeparQuinto[99]	Arm A: EC-D Arm B: EC-D+B	684	II	pCR	27.8% vs. 36.4% ($P = 0.021$)	NA
CALGB 40603[100]	Arm A: ddAC-T Arm B: ddAC-T + B Arm C: ddAC-T+ carbo Arm D: ddAC-T+ carbo+ B	362	II	pCR	Ongoing	December 2012
NSABP B-40[101]	Arm A: D-AC Arm B: D+B-AC Arm C: D+X-AC Arm D: D+X+B-AC Arm E: D+G-AC Arm F: D+G+B-AC	1,200	III	pCR	Ongoing	April 2012

pCR, pathologic complete response; CALGB, Cancer And Leukemia Group B; NSABP, National Surgical Adjuvant Breast and Bowel Project.

preferred single agents and chemotherapy combination that have demonstrated efficacy in the treatment of MBC (http://www.nccn.org/professionals/physician_gls/pdf/breast.pdf). To date, we have not definitively determined markers that predict response to a specific chemotherapy. The data on TOPO II as a predictor of response to the anthracyclines are controversial.

Endocrine Therapy in the Metastatic Setting

Endocrine therapy should always be considered for appropriate patients in the metastatic setting. It is usually desirable to avoid cytotoxic chemotherapy for as long as possible in patients with ER+ disease, responding to consecutive endocrine therapies. For pre- and perimenopausal patients, when tamoxifen is used, ablating the ovaries can be important (see section Combined Ovarian Suppression and Endocrine Therapy). AIs are reserved for menopausal patients. Both steroidal (exemestane) and nonsteroidal (anastrozole and letrozole) AIs have been compared head-to-head with tamoxifen in the first-line setting and have shown significant improvements in RR and time to progression (TTP).[103-105] To date, OS benefit has not been demonstrated for an AI over tamoxifen, but due to its favorable side-effect profile, AIs have become the agent of choice in first-line metastatic setting in postmenopausal women who are either AI-naïve or have relapsed more than 1 year after adjuvant endocrine therapy.

Fulvestrant is a steroid-based pure antiestrogen and differs from tamoxifen in that it does not exhibit agonist activity. The Evaluation of Faslodex versus Exemestane Clinical Trial (EFECT) demonstrated equal activity for exemestane and fulvestrant in the second-line setting after disease progression on tamoxifen and a nonsteroidal AI. The COmparisoN of Faslodex In Recurrent or Metastatic breast cancer (CONFIRM) trial was a double-blind, multicenter, parallel-group phase III study that established that the dose of 500 mg monthly (new standard) was superior to the previous dose of 250 mg.[106] The Fulvestrant First-line Study Comparing Endocrine Treatments (FIRST) was a phase II trial comparing fulvestrant at 500 mg monthly with anastrozole as first-line treatment in postmenopausal women and showed improved median TTP (23.4 vs. 13.1 months) in favor of the fulvestrant arm, corresponding to a 35% reduction in risk of progression (hazard ratio [HR] 0.66; 95% CI 0.47–0.92).[107]

Combined Ovarian Suppression and Endocrine Therapy

Ovarian suppression can be performed using luteinizing hormone-releasing hormone (LHRH) agonists. Combined therapy with an LHRH agonist and tamoxifen showed a superior overall response rate (ORR) (39% vs. 30%), PFS (HR 0.70), and OS (HR 0.78) compared with LHRH agonist alone in premenopausal women.[108] A small study that compared LHRH agonist plus AI with LHRH agonist plus tamoxifen showed superiority for the former group with higher RR (80% vs. 53%) and median time to death (18.9 vs. 14.3 months).[109] However, additional follow-up data and validation of these results are warranted.

Endocrine Therapy Combined with HER2-Directed Therapy

Patients with asymptomatic or minimally symptomatic ER/PR+/HER2+ disease may be candidates for combination therapy with hormones and HER2-targeted therapy in first-line metastatic setting. Postmenopausal women treated on the TAnDEM study were randomized to receive anastrozole in combination with trastuzumab compared with anastrozole alone and experienced a superior median PFS (4.8 vs. 2.4 months, $P = 0.0016$) compared with patients treated with anastrozole alone.[110] Of note, 70% of patients treated with anastrozole alone received a trastuzumab-containing regimen upon progression. The OS was the same overall, perhaps due to the high crossover incidence. Similarly, lapatinib combined with letrozole also demonstrated improved median PFS (8.2 vs. 3 months, $P = 0.019$) in the first-line treatment of HER2+ MBC.[111] For asymptomatic patients, combined hormone and anti-HER2 therapy is an option, but as there is no OS gain, hormone therapy alone appears reasonable. For symptomatic patients, the combination of chemotherapy with HER2-targeted therapy is preferred (see section Anti-HER2-Directed Therapy in the Metastatic Setting).

The cross talk between the ER and HER2 signaling pathways formed the basis for CALGB 40302 that evaluated patients with hormone receptor–positive MBC treated with fulvestrant plus lapatinib compared with fulvestrant plus placebo after progressing on prior AI therapy. In this placebo-controlled, double-blinded, randomized phase III study, there was no significant improvement in PFS for the combination treatment arm, with a higher rate of grade 3 adverse events including diarrhea, rash, fatigue, and liver function abnormalities compared with placebo. A planned exploratory subset analysis suggested that there might be benefit for this combination in patients with ER/PR+/HER2+ disease, but unlike the anastrozole/trastuzumab and letrozole/lapatinib studies, it was not statistically significant.[112]

Endocrine Therapy Combined with Antiangiogenic Agents

Unlike the combination of endocrine therapy with HER2-directed therapy, the combination of endocrine therapy with antiangiogenic agents has yet to demonstrate superiority over endocrine therapy alone, but research efforts appear promising.

A phase II study of letrozole with bevacizumab established feasibility for an ongoing phase III efficacy trial of this combination which is almost close to accrual (CALGB 40503).[113] The embedded correlative science studies, which include pharmacogenomic assessments that explore single-nucleotide polymorphisms of the VEGF gene, evaluation of response to therapy based on differing tumor

TABLE 53-6 Trastuzumab in the Front-Line Metastatic Setting

Studies	Slamon et al.[61]	Vogel et al.[116]	Burstein et al.[117]	Marty et al.[115]	Kaufman et al.[110]	Valero et al.[118]
N	469	111	54	186	207	263
Treatment	AC/EC +H or T+H vs. chemo	H	VH	DH vs. D	Anas + H vs. Anas	DCbH vs. DH
RR	50% vs. 32%[a]	35% (IHC 3+) 34% (FISH+)	68%	61% vs. 34%[a]	20.3% vs. 6.8%[a]	72% vs. 72%
Median TTP (months)	7.4 vs. 4.6[a]	3.8 (H at 4 mg/kg) 3.5 (H at 2 mg/kg)	NR	11.7 vs. 6.1[a]	4.8 vs. 2.4[a]	10.3 vs. 11.1
Median PFS (months)	NR	NR	NR	NR	4.8 vs. 2.4[a]	NR
Median OS (months)	25.1 vs. 20.3	24.4	NR	31.2 vs. 22.7	28.5 vs. 23.9	37.1 vs. 37.4
Asymptomatic/ symptomatic cardiac dysfunction or symptomatic CHF	AC/EC +H = 27%/16% AC/EC = 8%/3% T + H = 13%/2% T = 1%/1%	H = 3%/?	VH = 15%/2%	DH = 19%/2% D = 8%/0%	Anas/H = 14%/2% Anas = 2%/0%	DCbH = 15%/0% DH = 12%/0.8%

[a]Statistically significant.
? = Unclear on how many had "symptomatic CHF."
RR, response rate; TTP, time to progression; PFS, progression-free survival; OS, overall survival; CHF, congestive heart failure; A, doxorubicin; E, epirubicin; C, cyclophosphamide; T, paclitaxel; D, docetaxel; Cb, carboplatin; V, vinorelbine; H, trastuzumab; Anas, anastrozole; NR, not reported.

subtype—luminal A versus luminal B, and assessment of impact of phosphatidylinositol 3-kinase (PI3K) mutations on the efficacy of bevacizumab added to letrozole, may help to identify which patients may benefit from this combination. The PI3K mutations are reported to be present in 25% of ER+/HER2− breast cancer and are thought to be one of the mechanisms of endocrine resistance. Therefore, a study was conducted in which patients, pretreated with an AI, were randomized to receive tamoxifen (TAM) alone versus tamoxifen plus everolimus (RAD), an mTOR inhibitor, in a phase II randomized study (TAMRAD study). The study met its primary endpoint with a 61% clinical benefit rate (CBR) (95% CI 46.9–74.1) for the combination arm compared with 42% with tamoxifen alone (95% CI 29.1–55.9). TTP and OS increased with the doublet. Although toxicity (fatigue, stomatitis, rash, etc.) increased with the addition of everolimus, it was manageable.[114] Recently, Baselga et al. reported interim results of the Breast cancer trials of OraL EveROlimus-2 (BOLERO-2) that evaluated everolimus in combination with exemestane and significantly extended PFS compared with exemestane plus placebo (10.6 vs. 4.1 months, HR 0.36; $P < 0.001$), thus putting an early end to the trial. These studies are provocative and biomarkers will be important to identify which patients will benefit from a hormonal agent with an mTOR inhibitor, allowing us to tailor treatment in the future.

Anti-HER2-Directed Therapy in the Metastatic Setting

Slamon et al. presented the results of a pivotal phase III trial of trastuzumab in combination with chemotherapy (an anthracycline-based treatment or paclitaxel) that showed improved outcomes over chemotherapy alone.[61] This led to the approval of this agent with paclitaxel (but not with the anthracycline due to enhanced cardiac toxicity) in front-line metastatic setting. Marty et al. showed similar results.[115] Other front-line trials have shown the benefit of trastuzumab alone or added to an AI or other chemotherapy agents (Table 53.6). Trastuzumab is also effective combined with various other chemotherapies in the second-line setting.[119-122]

The role of continuing trastuzumab beyond progression was controversial until recently when Von Minckwitz and colleagues reported the results of a randomized phase III trial addressing the issue. Patients with HER2+ MBC received capecitabine versus capecitabine with trastuzumab continuation after progressing on this antibody. Despite early closure, there was a significant PFS benefit from 5.6 to 8.2 months in favor of the trastuzumab arm ($P = 0.03$).[123] At a median follow-up of 20.7 months, there was no significant improvement in the OS which was the secondary endpoint: 20.6 and 24.9 months in capecitabine versus the capecitabine and trastuzumab arm, respectively (HR = 0.94 [0.65–1.35]; $P = 0.73$). However, in a post hoc analysis, patients receiving anti-HER2 treatment as third-line therapy showed a better post-progression survival than those not receiving this therapy.[124] Another study by Blackwell et al. also demonstrated improved outcomes with the continuation of trastuzumab beyond progression as discussed in later sections.[125]

Lapatinib in the Metastatic Setting

Geyer et al. reported the results of a randomized phase III trial (EGF100151) of capecitabine compared with capecitabine with lapatinib, the results of which were the basis for the approval of lapatinib by the FDA. The study enrolled patients with HER2+ advanced breast cancer previously treated with anthracyclines, taxanes, and trastuzumab. There was a significant improvement in TTP of 6.2 versus 4.3 months (HR 0.57; 95% CI 0.43–0.77; $P < 0.001$) in favor of the combination arm. The ORR was also higher in favor of the lapatinib arm (24% vs. 14%; $P = 0.017$).[126]

The combination of lapatinib with paclitaxel showed no benefit in patients with HER2-negative disease in a phase III study, but in a subset analysis there was a benefit in the HER2+ group.[127] Blackwell et al. demonstrated a PFS benefit of 12 versus 8.4 weeks ($P = 0.029$) for lapatinib in combination with trastuzumab compared with lapatinib alone in a randomized trial of HER2+ MBC patients refractory to trastuzumab therapy, further confirming the role of continued trastuzumab despite progression.[125] Upon progression on a trastuzumab-based treatment, how do we decide to continue trastuzumab or switch to a lapatinib-based treatment or move forward with a dual anti-HER2 therapy? Biomarker studies to evaluate for markers of response and resistance may aid us to tailor therapy better in the future.

Mechanisms of Trastuzumab Resistance

Trastuzumab has greatly improved outcomes in HER2+ disease, but resistance, even if relative or situational, remains an issue. Several molecular mechanisms that have been proposed include hyperactivation of PI3K/AKT pathway, activation of other receptor tyrosine kinases including insulin-like growth factor receptor 1 (IGF-1 receptor), overexpression of membrane-associated mucin (MUC4) to mask or block the trastuzumab binding site, which can interrupt the interaction between HER-2 receptor and this antibody, expression of a truncated (P95) fragment of HER2 that lacks the trastuzumab-binding epitope, and loss of function of the tumor-suppressor PTEN gene.[128] Research efforts are therefore focused on better understanding these novel molecular mechanisms and identifying novel therapeutic targets that might increase the efficacy and duration of trastuzumab-based therapy.

Other Anti-HER2 Strategies

Novel anti-HER2 agents are under development. The unique mechanism of action of various anti-HER2 strategies are summarized in Table 53.7. Broadly, they can be classified into (a) monoclonal antibodies against the extracellular domain II of the HER2 receptor (pertuzumab), (b) antibody drug conjugates (trastuzumab-DM-1 or "T-DM-1"), (c) agents targeting the PI3K/AKT/mTOR pathway, and (d) heat shock protein 90 (Hsp90) inhibitors (Fig. 53.1). Clinical trials of these novel therapies have yielded promising results using pertuzumab, T-DM-1, and Hsp90 inhibitors and these are briefly discussed below. Collectively, these agents offer the possibility of more available options and perhaps even cures, long-term disease control, or possibly treatments without conventional cytotoxic chemotherapeutics.

Pertuzumab exhibits antitumor effects by disrupting the HER2–HER3 heterodimers, leading to inhibition of the PI3K/AKT/mTOR pathway. Phase II trials of combined HER2 blockade with pertuzumab and trastuzumab in patients with metastatic HER2 + breast cancer refractory to trastuzumab therapy demonstrated an ORR ranging from 18% to 24.2%.[129,130] These encouraging results formed the basis of the CLEOPATRA study, which aimed to compare the efficacy and safety of docetaxel plus trastuzumab with the combination of placebo or pertuzumab in 808 previously untreated HER2-positive breast cancer patients. The primary endpoint was the independently assessed PFS, which was 12.4 versus 18.5 months (HR 0.65; 95% CI 0.51–0.75; $P < 0.001$) in favor of the pertuzumab-containing arm. An interim analysis for OS showed a strong trend in favor of the pertuzumab arm, but these data were premature as only 43% of events had occurred thus far. There was no increased cardiac toxicity with the addition of pertuzumab, and the experimental treatment was well tolerated with a low incidence of grade 3/4 diarrhea of 7.9%. Thus, dual anti-HER2 therapy with trastuzumab and pertuzumab with this taxane may become the new standard of care for front-line treatment of patients with HER2-positive MBC.[131]

T-DM-1 is a novel compound in which trastuzumab is conjugated with the fungal toxin DM-1 (maytansine). In T-DM-1, maytansine/DM-1 acts as a microtubule inhibitor and trastuzumab mainly acts as a carrier of DM-1 to the tumor cells labeled with HER2. A phase II trial of single-agent T-DM-1 administered at 3.6 mg/kg every 3 weeks in patients with metastatic HER2+, trastuzumab refractory disease showed an RR of 25.9%.[132] Another phase II trial of T-DM-1 monotherapy in HER2+ MBC patients previously treated with conventional chemotherapy, lapatinib, and trastuzumab showed an RR of 32.7% and a CBR of 52.6%.[133] Hurvitz et al. presented the results of a randomized phase II study comparing trastuzumab plus docetaxel with T-DM-1 in 137 patients with HER2+ MBC in the first-line setting. The median PFS was 14.2 versus 9.2 months in favor of the T-DM-1 arm (HR 0.594; 95% CI 0.364–0.968; $P = 0.0353$). Although the ORR was similar between the two groups (64.2%), there were more durable responses in the T-DM-1 arm (median duration not reached vs. 9.5 months for the docetaxel arm). Additionally, there was a lower rate of grade ≥ 3 adverse events in the T-DM-1 arm (46.4% vs. 89.4%). The authors concluded that the improved PFS in the T-DM-1 arm may be a result of improved tolerability/duration of treatment/response compared with the docetaxel arm.[134] A completed global randomized phase III study (EMILIA) is evaluating T-DM-1 compared with lapatinib plus capecitabine in the second-line setting. Another phase III trial (MARIANNE) is ongoing and evaluating T-DM-1 versus T-DM-1 with pertuzumab

TABLE 53-7 Various Anti-HER2-Directed Treatment Strategies

Drug	Class of Agent	Mechanism of Action	Route of Administration	Status/Phase
Trastuzumab	Monoclonal antibody against HER extracellular domain IV	• ADCC • Disrupts downstream proliferative signaling pathways • Inhibits cell cycle progression • Antiangiogenic effects • Endocytosis and degradation of HER2	Intravenous	Approved
Lapatinib	Small-molecule TKI of EGFR and HER2	• Inhibits receptors' intrinsic tyrosine kinase activity • Prevents downstream transmission of activation signal	Oral	Approved
Neratinib	Irreversible pan-erbB TKI	• Irreversibly inhibits tyrosine kinase activity of HER1, HER2, and HER4 • Prevents downstream transmission of activation signal	Oral	III
Canertinib	Irreversible TKI of EGFR	• Irreversibly inhibits tyrosine kinase activity of HER2, HER3, and HER4 • Antiangiogenic effects • Apoptosis stimulator	Oral	II
Pertuzumab	Monoclonal antibody against HER2 extracellular domain II	• ADCC • Prevents HER2 heterodimerization	Intravenous	III
Trastuzumab-MCC-DM1	Antibody drug conjugate linking trastuzumab to microtubule cytotoxic agent called maytansine	• Targeted cytotoxic drug delivery	Intravenous	III
Ganetespib/ PU-H71/ AUY922/Hsp990	Small-molecule Hsp90 inhibitors	• Inhibits Hsp90's stabilizing effect on client proteins • Facilitates HER2 degradation	Intravenous/ intravenous/ intravenous/oral	II/I/II/I
BKM120, BEZ235	PI3K inhibitors	• Inhibits cell growth and survival via the PI3K/AKT/mTOR pathway	Oral/oral	II/I
MK-2206	Small-molecule serine–threonine kinase inhibitor of AKT	• Inhibits proliferative signaling pathway downstream of PI3K • Antiapoptotic factor	Oral	II
Temsirolimus/ everolimus	Small-molecule serine–threonine kinase inhibitor of mTOR	• Inhibits proliferative signaling pathway downstream of HER2	Intravenous/oral	II/III
AEE788	HER1/2 and VEGFR TKI	• Inhibits multiple receptor tyrosine kinases • Antiangiogenic agent	Oral	I
Ertumaxomab	Trifunctional bispecific antibody	• Inhibits HER2 on tumor cells and CD3 on T cells • Activates immune cells leading to antitumor immune response	Intravenous	II[a]
Cixutumumab (IMC-A12)	Monoclonal antibody against the IGF-1R pathway	• Inhibits cell proliferation and survival by inhibiting the IGF-1 pathway	Intravenous	II
Vorinostat	HDAC inhibitor	• Induce growth arrest, differentiation, and apoptosis	Oral	II

[a]Studies terminated due to change in development plan and not due to safety concerns.

ADCC, antibody-dependent cell-mediated cytotoxicity; TKI, tyrosine kinase inhibitor; HER, human epidermal growth factor receptor; Hsp90, heat shock protein 90; mTOR, mammalian target of rapamycin; EGFR, epidermal growth factor receptor; VEGFR, vascular endothelial growth factor receptor; PI3K, phosphatidylinositol-3-kinase; IGF-1R, insulin-like growth factor 1 receptor; HDAC, histone deacetylase.

versus the combination of trastuzumab plus a taxane (docetaxel or paclitaxel) in HER2+-untreated MBC.

Hsp90 has emerged in recent years as a promising new target for MBC treatment. Hsp90 inhibition leads to simultaneous degradation of critical oncoproteins (CDK4, Raf-1, AKT, HER2, etc.), making Hsp90 an appealing therapeutic target.[135] Modi et al. demonstrated promising activity for 17-AAG (tanespimycin) plus trastuzumab in patients with HER2+ MBC refractory to trastuzumab therapy.[136] This is consistent with the preclinical data that have shown HER2 to be among the most sensitive client proteins of Hsp90 inhibition. Chandarlapaty et al. identified P95HER2 as an Hsp90 client that is degraded by Hsp90 inhibitors. In trastuzumab-resistant models, high levels of P95HER2 were sensitive to Hsp90 inhibition and with chronic exposure, there was sustained loss of both full-length and truncated HER2 expression combined with AKT inhibition, leading to apoptosis and

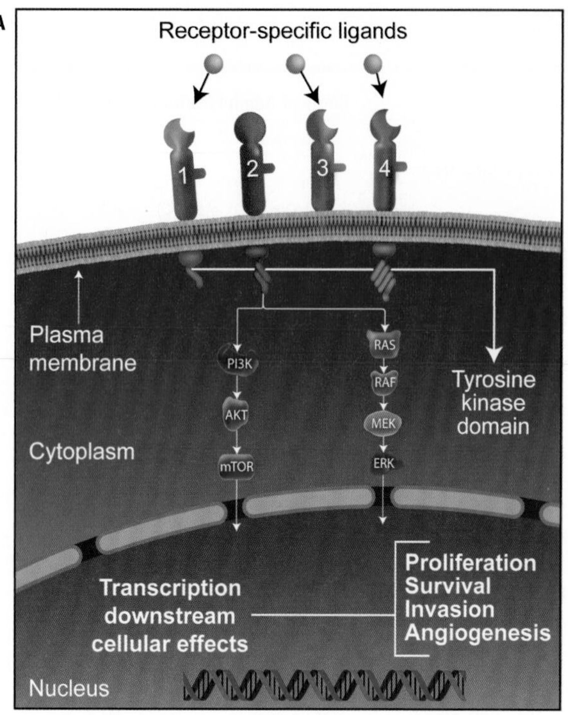

FIGURE 53–1 A: Human epidermal growth factor (EGF) receptors HER1, HER2, HER3, and HER4 are receptor tyrosine kinases that are involved in the signal transduction pathways leading to cell survival and differentiation. Each of these receptors consists of an extracellular binding domain, a transmembrane lipophilic segment, and (except for HER3) a functional intracellular tyrosine kinase domain. When an EGF family ligand binds to the extracellular binding domain, the tyrosine kinase domains are activated by both homodimerization and heterodimerization. Receptor HER2 is an orphan receptor and does not require binding of a ligand for activation. Even in the absence of a ligand, HER2 remains the preferential dimerization partner of other members of the EGF family. Receptor overexpression and mutation can also induce dimerization. **B:** Anti-HER2 strategies: Sites of action of novel agents. (A) Trastuzumab is a monoclonal antibody that binds to the extracellular domain IV of the HER2 receptor. (B) Lapatinib is a tyrosine kinase inhibitor of HER1 and HER2. (C) Neratinib and canertinib are irreversible tyrosine kinase inhibitors of HER1, HER2, and HER4. (D) Hsp90 inhibitors lead to HER2 degradation via the proteasomal pathway by blocking the activity of Hsp90, an ATP-dependent molecular chaperone protein. (E) Pertuzumab is a monoclonal antibody that binds to a distinct epitope of HER2 (extracellular domain II) and prevents ligand-induced homo- and heterodimerization. (F, G, H) Homo- and heterodimerization of the HER family leads to phosphorylation of the tyrosine kinase domain and activation of downstream signaling pathways including the PI3K-AKT-mTOR pathway and the RAF-MEK-MAPK pathway. Downstream effects include cell survival, proliferation, and increased vascular endothelial growth factor (VEGF). Agents directly inhibiting PI3K (BKM120, CEZ235), AKT (MK-2206), and mTOR (temsirolimus, everolimus) are under clinical development. (I) Cixutumumab is a fully human IgG1 monoclonal antibody to the insulin-like growth factor 1 receptor (IGF-1R). It leads to IGF-1R phosphorylation and downstream signaling. It also promotes IGF-1R internalization and degradation. (J) Bevacizumab is a monoclonal antibody targeting VEGF. (K) Pazopanib is a small-molecule tyrosine kinase inhibitor of VEGF and other receptors. (L) Trastuzumab-DM1, an antibody drug conjugate of DM-1/maytansine and trastuzumab, allows for the selective delivery of DM-1, a microtubule inhibitor, to HER2-overexpressing cells.

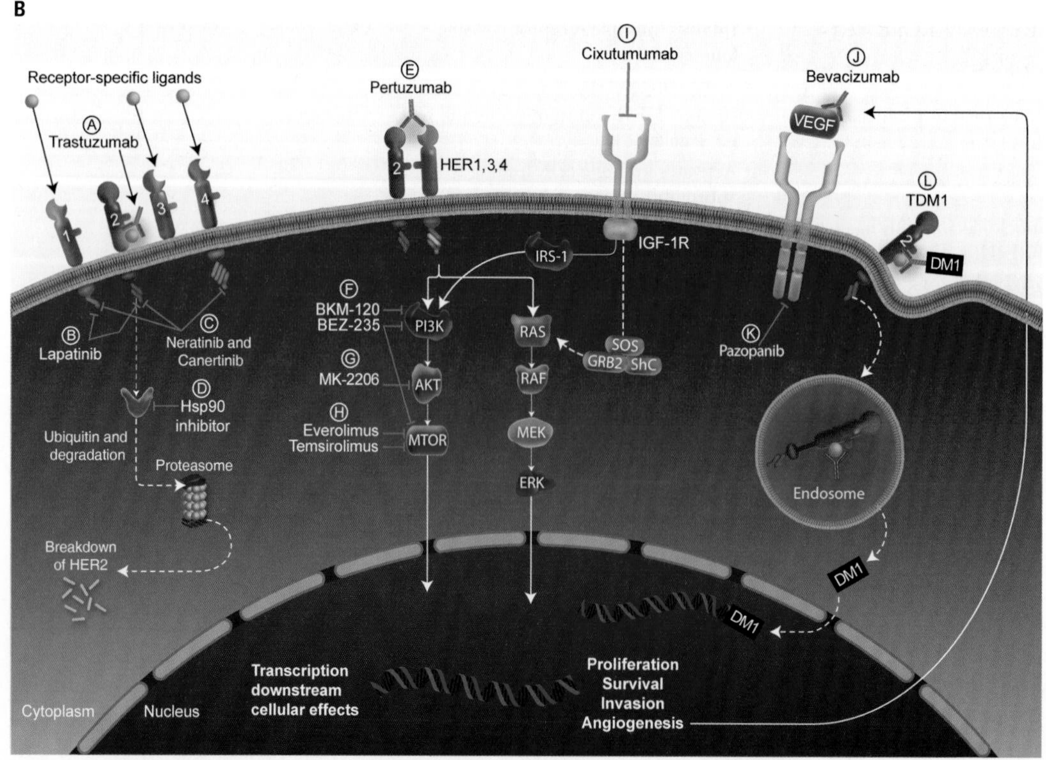

tumor growth inhibition.[137] There are many second-generation, small-molecule Hsp90 inhibitors under clinical evaluation including CNF-2024/BIIB021, AUY922, Ganetespib/STA-9090, and PU-H71.

Approximately 40% and 25% of breast tumors demonstrate PI3K pathway activation through PTEN loss or PIK3CA mutation, respectively.[138,139] Additionally, PI3K pathway activation is suggested as a mechanism of trastuzumab resistance, providing a rational basis for the evaluation of PI3K, AKT, and mTOR inhibitors in HER2-amplified breast cancer.[139] Promising agents such as BKM120 (PI3K inhibitor and mTOR inhibitor), BEZ235 (PI3K inhibitor), MK2206 (AKT inhibitor), and everolimus/temsirolimus (mTOR inhibitors) are being studied in combination with cytotoxic agents and/or other targeted therapies and are under various stages of clinical development (see Fig. 53.1).

Treatment of TNBC in the Metastatic Setting

Chemotherapy

Tumors without both hormone receptor (ER and PR) positivity and HER2 expression are referred to as TNBC. Without these targets, patients do not benefit from endocrine therapy or HER2-directed treatments and are conventionally left with chemotherapy as their only option. Traditional chemotherapeutic agents, like the anthracyclines and taxanes, have higher RRs compared with luminal A or luminal B disease, but the relapse rate remains high and is associated with shorter OS. A meta-analysis of four trials demonstrated a 23% reduction in the risk of disease recurrence with anthracycline-based regimens compared with CMF.[140] On the contrary, the retrospective analysis of the MA.5 trial that compared cyclophosphamide, epirubicin, fluorouracil (CEF) versus CMF in the adjuvant setting suggested no particular benefit with anthracycline-based therapy.[141] Recently, research efforts are focused on those chemotherapeutic agents that target specific molecular defects in TNBC. The TNBC subtype is prevalent among carriers of BRCA1 (and less commonly so in BRCA2) mutations who frequently have a defect in the homologous recombinant DNA repair. The role of platinum salts is well defined in cells that are either BRCA mutants or BRCA-deficient due to their specific mechanism of action in that they cause DNA double-stranded breaks, but these are less defined in the clinic. Platinum agents in the neoadjuvant setting have demonstrated pCR rates of 15% to 83%.[142-145] Although the role of this class of agents is actively being pursued, they are currently not recommended outside of a clinical trial setting for early-stage TNBC. RRs with platinum agents in the metastatic setting have been confounded by addition of other agents. A retrospective study evaluating a taxane–platinum doublet showed no difference in RR between TNBC patients compared with those that did not have TNBC. However, patients with TNBC had a shorter OS, which might reflect their resistance to chemotherapeutic agents including platinum agent or the aggressive biologic behavior of TNBC despite an initial response at the time of treatment.[146] To further validate the RR of TNBC to platinum agent versus other cytotoxic agents, a phase III trial comparing carboplatin with docetaxel in patients with metastatic TNBC is underway (NCT00532727). The p63/73 protein expression seen in 33% of TNBC could be a potential biomarker of platinum sensitivity and is the basis for the Translational Breast Cancer Research Consortium (TBCRC) 009 trial.

Biologic/Targeted Therapies for TNBC

Currently, there is a lack of targeted therapies for this group of patients. Many novel targeted therapies unique to specific signaling pathway are currently being explored in the metastatic setting (Table 53.8). This section briefly reviews the most important potential targeted strategies.

Poly(ADP-ribose) Polymerase Inhibitors

There is a significant overlap between the molecular profiles and clinicopathological features of TNBC and basal-like and BRCA1-associated breast cancers.[147] There is also

TABLE 53-8 Novel Targeted Strategies in TNBC in the Metastatic Setting

Drug	Target/Pathway
BSI-201, olaparib, iniparib, ABT-888	PARP inhibitors/DNA repair pathway
Trabectedin	DNA repair pathway
Bevacizumab	Antiangiogenic agent; monoclonal antibody against VEGF ligand
Sunitinib, sorafenib	Antiangiogenic agent; VEGFR inhibitor
Cetuximab, panitumumab	Monoclonal antibodies against the extracellular domain of EGFR
Gefitinib, erlotinib	TKI targeting the intracellular domain of EGFR
Dasatinib, saracatinib	SRC kinase inhibitor
Bicalutamide	Androgen receptor
Cixutumumab, ganitumab	Monoclonal antibodies against IGF-1R
Everolimus, temsirolimus	mTOR inhibitor
Ganetespib, PU-H71	Small-molecule, non-geldanamycin Hsp90 inhibitors
GC1008, AP 12009, LY2157299	TGF-beta antagonists
Lexatumumab/ tigatuzumab	TRAIL receptor 2 or death receptor 5 agonist
Imatinib	PDGFR, c-KIT

TNBC, triple-negative breast cancer; PARP, poly(ADP-ribose) polymerase; TKI, tyrosine kinase inhibitor; EGFR, epidermal growth factor receptor; VEGFR, vascular endothelial growth factor receptor; IGF-1R, insulin-like growth factor 1 receptor; mTOR, mammalian target of rapamycin; Hsp90, heat shock protein 90; TGF, transforming growth factor; TRAIL, tumor necrosis factor (TNF)–related apoptosis-inducing ligand; PDGFR, platelet-derived growth factor receptor; c-KIT, stem cell growth factor receptor.

evidence that despite the lack of BRCA1 mutation, sporadic TNBC can exhibit BRCA1 protein dysfunction.[148] DNA repair pathways play a significant role in cases of BRCA1 deficiency. One such pathway is the base-excision repair that is partly dependent on poly(ADP-ribose) polymerases (PARPs) (enzymes that catalyze the polymerization of PARP chains in target proteins), particularly PARP1.[149] Another DNA repair pathway, known as homologous recombination, is nonfunctional in BRCA mutants.[150] Therefore when PARP1 is inhibited, there is accumulation of the DNA double-stranded breaks that would have normally been repaired via homologous recombination. Preclinical data suggest that PARP inhibition leads to selective cytotoxicity of BRCA-mutated cells due to a phenomenon known as synthetic lethality. This rapidly translated from preclinical experiments to meaningful clinical advances in BRCA1/2-deficient metastatic breast and ovarian cancer patients.[151]

A phase I trial of olaparib (AZD2281), an oral PARP inhibitor, showed 47% RR in 9 out of 19 patients with confirmed BRCA mutation.[152] There were no responses noted in 37 patients without BRCA mutation. The dose-limiting toxicities were myelosuppression and CNS side effects. Pharmacodynamic effects (increase in γH2AX foci found in plucked eyebrow hair follicles) provided proof of mechanism of synthetic lethality but raised a concern for a risk of accumulation of DNA damage within normal tissue with continuous dosing.[152] A phase II trial of olaparib given at 400 mg twice daily in BRCA-mutant breast cancers produced an ORR of 41%, CBR of 52%, and a median PFS of 6 months.[153]

Another PARP inhibitor, iniparib (BSI-201), that did not appear to have enhanced toxicity in normal tissue was evaluated in combination with carboplatin and gemcitabine (GC) compared with chemotherapy alone in TNBC previously treated with two or more cytotoxic agents. This phase II study showed improved RR, PFS, and OS.[154] These encouraging results led to the phase III trial of this combination, wherein 519 patients were randomized 1:1 to GC alone ($N = 258$) or GC-iniparib ($N = 261$). Crossover to the iniparib arm was allowed upon confirmed disease progression on the GC arm. The primary endpoint was both OS and PFS. However, the phase III trial did not meet the prespecified criteria for significance for the primary endpoints of PFS (4.1 vs. 5.1 months; HR = 0.794 [95% CI 0.646–0.976]) and OS (11.1 vs. 11.8 months; HR = 0.876 [95% CI 0.687–1.116]).[155] A multivariate analysis, comparing first-line patients with second- and third-line patients, showed PFS and OS benefit in the latter group. The toxicity of iniparib plus GC was comparable to that of chemotherapy alone. The lack of survival advantage raised the question about the actual mechanism of action of iniparib. Although iniparib has been listed as a PARP inhibitor, it has 1,000-fold lower PARP inhibitory activity than other agents in this class; it does not have additive toxicity as observed in multiple PARP trials[156]; and despite preclinical data that showed induction of γH2AX foci (a pharmacodynamic readout of DNA damage), it does not appear to do so via PARP1 and 2 inhibition like the other PARP inhibitors (veliparib and olaparib). It does, however, exert an effect on the telomerase pathway on PARP5/6.[157]

Other PARP inhibitors that have confirmed the potential for activity with low toxicity include ABT-888 (veliparib) and MK-4827, and phase I/II trials of these agents are ongoing. Despite the negative phase III study with iniparib, it is still important to pursue studies with other PARP inhibitors in order to assess for a subset of TNBC patients that may benefit from this. This is where BRCA mutational status should be tested and potential predictors of response need to be explored. Many scientific questions remain, such as the role of PARP inhibitors outside of BRCA-deficient tumors, biomarkers that can predict response to treatment, and the choice of the best cytotoxic agent that can be combined with PARP inhibitor. These questions will hopefully be addressed in the near future.

VEGF Pathway Inhibitors

VEGF expression is associated with a shorter survival in TNBC compared with non-TNBC patients and hence targeting it may be a promising treatment strategy.[158] Thus far, in metastatic disease, multiple studies have shown a PFS benefit in subset analyses of TNBC patients. For example, in the E2100 trial comparing paclitaxel with paclitaxel plus bevacizumab, there was a PFS benefit of 10.6 versus 5.3 months in favor of the bevacizumab arm. Similarly, the AVADO trial showed a PFS benefit for docetaxel plus bevacizumab compared with docetaxel alone (8.2 vs. 5.4 months). The RIBBON1 trial showed statistically significant PFS benefit but of a much smaller magnitude compared with the E2100 study.[159] In part, based on these analyses, several randomized trials including the CALGB 40603 and the NSABP B-40 trials are further evaluating the role of bevacizumab in TNBC. However, thus far, there is no OS gain across these front-line studies in metastatic disease. Brufsky et al. showed a trend toward improved OS with the addition of bevacizumab in the TNBC subset in RIBBON2 (12.6 vs. 17.9 months; HR 0.624; $P = 0.0534$) but this should be interpreted with caution as it is exploratory.[160] In late 2010, the FDA began the process of removing the indication for bevacizumab in MBC due to the lack of OS benefit and safety concerns. A 2011 meta-analysis demonstrated that there was an increased risk of fatal adverse events with the addition of bevacizumab, particularly to the taxanes or platinum drugs when compared with chemotherapy alone. The most common adverse events noted in this meta-analysis were hemorrhage (23.5%), neutropenia (12.2%), and gastrointestinal tract perforation (7.1%).[161]

VEGF TKIs have limited activity both as monotherapy and in combination with chemotherapy in the treatment of MBC.[162] For example, sunitinib, a multi-targeted TKI that inhibits VEGFR, c-kit, platelet-derived growth factor receptor, and colony-stimulating factor-1 receptor, has no role in the treatment of breast cancer due to the negative phase III studies.[163,164] Sorafenib, a small-molecule TKI of Raf-1, VEGFR2 and 3, and other targets, has very little single-agent activity as demonstrated in two phase II trials. A phase 2B TIES (Trials to Investigate the Efficacy of Sorafenib) study evaluated the role of chemotherapy (gemcitabine or capecitabine) with or without sorafenib. The results were modestly significant with a median PFS of 3.4 versus 2.7 months in favor of the chemotherapy plus sorafenib arm. The difference in PFS translated into an HR of 0.65, which proved to be statistically significant ($P = 0.01$). The median TTP also favored the sorafenib arm (3.5 vs. 2.7 months, $P = 0.009$).[165] Vandetanib (ZD6474), inhibitor of the VEGFR2, 3, and EGFR, also has no single-agent activity in MBC. An ongoing phase II trial is comparing motesanib with bevacizumab in first-line setting in patients with HER2– MBC. Pazopanib, an inhibitor of the VEGF1, 2, PDGFR-β, and c-kit, is currently being studied in combination with lapatinib in a phase II setting.[162] When axitinib (inhibitor of the VEGF1, 2, PDGFR-β, and c-kit) plus docetaxel was compared with docetaxel plus placebo, there was an increase in the ORR (41.1% vs. 23.6%; $P = 0.011$). Additionally, despite the numerical increase in the TTP, it was not statistically significant (8.1 vs. 7.1 months; HR 1.24; $P = 0.156$) in first-line metastatic setting.[166]

EGFR Inhibitors

EGFR (HER1) is overexpressed in approximately 20% of breast cancers[167] but in up to 60% to 70% of TNBC[168] and 80% of metaplastic carcinomas (a variant of TNBC/basal-like breast cancer),[169] making this a rational experimental target in the treatment of TNBC. Targeted strategies include monoclonal antibodies against the extracellular domain of EGFR (cetuximab or panitumumab) or synthetic TKI targeting the intracellular domain of EGFR (erlotinib and gefitinib). There is a cytotoxic interaction between DNA cross-linking agents such as platinum agents and EGFR inhibitors. Due to the fact that TNBC exhibits both EGFR overexpression and DNA repair defects, the combination of platinums and EGFR inhibitors has been explored in TNBC. The TBCRC study 001 specifically evaluated cetuximab with or without carboplatin. The combination arm yielded an RR of 18% and CBR of 27% versus 10% RR and 10% CBR in the cetuximab alone arm; however, it is undetermined if cetuximab specifically added any value to carboplatin in this study.[170] On the contrary, O'Shaughnessey et al. demonstrated an increased ORR (30% vs. 49%) by adding cetuximab to carboplatin and irinotecan in the TNBC subset of a phase II trial of patients with MBC.[171] Median survival was 12.3 (95% CI 9.7–22.1) versus 15.5 months (95% CI 10.4–19.2). However, diarrhea was exacerbated in the cetuximab arm. The BALI1 trial was a randomized phase II trial that evaluated the role of cisplatin (75 mg/m^2 every 32 weeks for up to six cycles) with or without cetuximab (400 mg/m^2 initial dose followed by 250 mg/m^2 weekly) in metastatic TNBC. The ORR was 20% in the combination arm and 10.3% in the cisplatin arm (odds ratio 2.12; $P = 0.11$) with a median PFS of 3.7 versus 1.5 months, respectively (HR 0.67; $P = 0.032$). However, the difference in the median OS was not statistically significant (12.9 vs. 9.4 months; HR 0.82; $P = 0.031$).[172] Cetuximab has also been effective in combination with a taxane (docetaxel or paclitaxel) with no additional toxicity.[173] Panitumumab is being evaluated in clinical trials. Similar to the experience with monoclonal antibodies against EGFR, the synthetic TKIs against EGFR are thought to be effective only when combined with chemotherapeutic agents (carboplatin and docetaxel).[174]

Androgen Receptor–Targeted Therapy

Doanne and colleagues demonstrated that tumor growth in TNBC cell lines was ER independent and androgen receptor (AR) dependent, supporting AR inhibition as a therapeutic approach.[175] In vitro studies have further demonstrated that AR stimulation in breast cancer cell lines can induce proliferation and promote tumorigenesis.[176] Based on tissue microarray analysis, 20% of TNBC are thought to have AR positivity.[175] A phase II trial is currently underway in the TBCRC with bicalutamide, a nonsteroidal competitive AR inhibitor used in the treatment of advanced prostate cancer, in TNBC. Of the 230 patients who consented for AR testing, 27 were AR+. Sixteen of the planned 27 patients have started treatment and final results are awaited.[177] As noted, the challenge has been the rarity of AR positivity, which in clinical practice has been about 12% among TNBC patients.

Hsp90 Inhibitors

Caldas-Lopes et al. demonstrated impressive tumor regressions and complete response in TNBC xenograft models with a novel Hsp90 inhibitor PU-H71.[178] In TNBC, Hsp90 inhibition leads to (1) downregulation of Ras/Raf/MAPK pathway and G2-M phase that suppresses tumor proliferation; (2) degradation of activated AKT and bcl-XL and induction of apoptosis; (3) inhibition of NF-KB, AKT, ERK2, Tyk2, and PKC and thus reduction of the metastatic potential of TNBC.[178] PU-H71 is being evaluated in a phase I clinical trial in patients with advanced solid tumors, lymphoma, and myeloproliferative disorders.[179]

DISCUSSION

There have been significant innovations both in prevention and treatment strategies for breast cancer management. Patients and physicians have three options for medical prevention of breast cancer: tamoxifen, raloxifene, and exemestane. The actual choice of agent will depend on patient comorbidities and a discussion of the risk–benefit ratio. Anthracycline-taxane–based adjuvant chemotherapy is the established cornerstone of treatment for high-risk breast cancer. The addition of trastuzumab to chemotherapy has significantly improved outcomes for patients with HER2+ disease. There are several other anti-HER2-targeted agents that have been effectively utilized in the metastatic setting and more are being studied. Additionally, novel biologic therapies have been incorporated in treatment strategies for hormone receptor–positive disease and TNBC.

As emphasized in this chapter, we are moving past the era of one-size-fits-all approach to breast cancer management. Ongoing efforts have led to utilization of the personalized approach to breast cancer management in daily practice. However, many challenges and issues remain. We need a better understanding of the molecular biology of breast cancer and tumor microenvironment in order to identify better predictive and prognostic factors. Additionally, we need to identify and validate novel targets and better understand the resistance mechanisms of newer targeted strategies. Ultimately, these efforts have the potential for improved outcomes for the more than 1 million women diagnosed with breast cancer worldwide each year.

REFERENCES

1. NCI. Breast cancer. http://www.cancer.gov/cancertopics/types/breast. 2011.
2. Howlader N, Noone AM, Krapcho M. *Seer Cancer Statistics Review*. Bethesda, MD: National Cancer Institute. http://seer.cancer.gov/csr/1975_2008/, based on November 2010 SEER data submission, posted to the SEER web site, 2011. 1975-2008.
3. Ravdin PM, Cronin KA, Howlader N, et al. The decrease in breast-cancer incidence in 2003 in the United States. *N Engl J Med*. 2007;356:1670-1674.
4. Hersh AL, Stefanick ML, Stafford RS. National use of postmenopausal hormone therapy: annual trends and response to recent evidence. *JAMA*. 2004;291:47-53.
5. World Cancer Report 2008. Boyle P, Levin B, eds. France: International Agency for Research on Cancer (IARC)
6. O'Brien C, Cavet G, Pandita A, et al. Functional genomics identifies ABCC3 as a mediator of taxane resistance in HER2-amplified breast cancer. *Cancer Res*. 2008;68: 5380-5389.
7. NCI. Gail model. http://www.cancer.gov/bcrisktool. Accessed August 2011.
8. Dunn BK, Ford LG. Breast cancer prevention: results of the National Surgical Adjuvant Breast and Bowel Project (NSABP) breast cancer prevention trial (NSABP P-1: BCPT). *Eur J Cancer*. 2000;36:49-50.
9. Vogel VG, Costantino JP, Wickerham DL, et al. Update of the National Surgical Adjuvant Breast and Bowel Project Study of Tamoxifen and Raloxifene (STAR) P-2 trial: preventing breast cancer. *Cancer Prev Res*. 2010;3:696-706.
10. Burstein HJ, Prestrud AA, Seidenfeld J, et al. American Society of Clinical Oncology clinical practice guideline: update on adjuvant endocrine therapy for women with hormone receptor-positive breast cancer. *J Clin Oncol*. 2010;28:3784-3796.
11. Dowsett M, Cuzick J, Ingle J, et al. Meta-analysis of breast cancer outcomes in adjuvant trials of aromatase inhibitors versus tamoxifen. *J Clin Oncol*. 2010;28:509-518.
12. Goss PE, Ingle JN, Alés-Martínez JE, et al. Exemestane for breast-cancer prevention in postmenopausal women. *N Engl J Med*. 2011;364:2381-2391.
13. King MC, Marks JH, Mandell JB. Breast and ovarian cancer risks due to inherited mutations in BRCA1 and BRCA2. *Science*. 2003;302:643-646.
14. Struewing JP, Hartge P, Wacholder S, et al. The risk of cancer associated with specific mutations of BRCA1 and BRCA2 among Ashkenazi Jews. *N Engl J Med*. 1997;336:1401-1408.
15. Chen S, Parmigiani G. Meta-analysis of BRCA1 and BRCA2 penetrance. *J Clin Oncol*. 2007;25:1329-1333.
16. Ford D, Easton DF, Stratton M, et al. Genetic heterogeneity and penetrance analysis of the BRCA1 and BRCA2 genes in breast cancer families. The Breast Cancer Linkage Consortium. *Am J Hum Genet*. 1998;62:676-689.
17. Ponder BAJ, Day NE, Easton DF, et al. Prevalence and penetrance of BRCA1 and BRCA2 mutations in a population-based series of breast cancer cases. *Br J Cancer*. 2000;83:1301-1308.
18. Satagopan JM, Boyd J, Kauff ND, et al. Ovarian cancer risk in Ashkenazi Jewish carriers of BRCA1 and BRCA2 mutations. *Clin Cancer Res*. 2002;8:3776-3781.
19. Domchek SM, Friebel TM, Singer CF, et al. Association of risk-reducing surgery in BRCA1 or BRCA2 mutation carriers with cancer risk and mortality. *JAMA*. 2010;304:967-975.
20. Ravdin PM, Siminoff LA, Davis GJ, et al. Computer program to assist in making decisions about adjuvant therapy for women with early breast cancer. *J Clin Oncol*. 2001;19:980-991.
21. Paik S, Shak S, Tang G, et al. A multigene assay to predict recurrence of tamoxifen-treated, node-negative breast cancer. *N Engl J Med*. 2004;351:2817-2826.
22. Paik S, Tang G, Shak S, et al. Gene expression and benefit of chemotherapy in women with node-negative, estrogen receptor-positive breast cancer. *J Clin Oncol*. 2006;24:3726-3734.
23. Albain KS, Barlow WE, Ravdin PM, et al. Adjuvant chemotherapy and timing of tamoxifen in postmenopausal patients with endocrine-responsive, node-positive breast cancer: a phase 3, open-label, randomised controlled trial. *Lancet*. 2009;374:2055-2063.
24. Albain KS, Barlow WE, Shak S, et al. Prognostic and predictive value of the 21-gene recurrence score assay in postmenopausal women with node-positive, oestrogen-receptor-positive breast cancer on chemotherapy: a retrospective analysis of a randomised trial. *Lancet Oncol*. 2010;11:55-65.
25. NCI. TAILOR RX press release. http://www.cancertrialshelp.org/news_content/TAILORx.aspx. 2010.
26. Dowsett M, Cuzick J, Wale C, et al. Prediction of risk of distant recurrence using the 21-gene recurrence score in node-negative and node-positive postmenopausal patients with breast cancer treated with anastrozole or tamoxifen: a TransATAC study. *J Clin Oncol*. 2010;28:1829-1834.
27. Gonzalez-Angulo AM, Barlow WE, Gralow J. SWOG S1007: a phase III, randomized clinical trial of standard adjuvant endocrine therapy with or without chemotherapy in patients with one to three positive nodes, hormone receptor (HR)-positive, and HER2-negative breast cancer with recurrence score (RS) of 25 or less. *J Clin Oncol*. 2011;29:(suppl). Abstract TPS104.
28. Tang G, Cuzick J, Wale C. Recurrence risk of node-negative and ER-positive early-stage breast cancer patients by combining recurrence score, pathologic, and clinical information: a meta-analysis approach. *J Clin Oncol*. 2010;28(suppl). Abstract 509.
29. Perou CM, Sorlie T, Eisen MB, et al. Molecular portraits of human breast tumours. *Nature*. 2000;406:747-752.
30. Wang Y, Klijn JG, Zhang Y. Gene-expression profiles to predict distant metastasis of lymph-node-negative primary breast cancer. *Lancet*. 2005;365:671-679.
31. Parker JS, Mullins M, Cheang MC, et al. Supervised risk predictor of breast cancer based on intrinsic subtypes. *J Clin Oncol*. 2009;27:1160-1167.
32. Bastien R, Ebbert MTW, Boucher KM. Using the PAM50 breast cancer intrinsic classifier to assess risk in ER+ breast cancers: a direct comparison to oncotype DX. *J Clin Oncol*. 2011;29(suppl). Abstract 503.
33. Buzdar AU, Ibrahim NK, Francis D, et al. Significantly higher pathologic complete remission rate after neoadjuvant therapy with trastuzumab, paclitaxel, and epirubicin chemotherapy: results of a randomized trial in human epidermal growth factor receptor 2–positive operable breast cancer. *J Clin Oncol*. 2005;23:3676-3685.
34. De Laurentiis M, Cancello G, D'Agostino D, et al. Taxane-based combinations as adjuvant chemotherapy of early breast cancer: a meta-analysis of randomized trials. *J Clin Oncol*. 2008; 26:44-53.
35. Hudis C, Citron M, Berry D. Five year follow-up of INTC9741: dose-dense (DD) chemotherapy (CRx) is safe and effective. In: San Antonio Breast Cancer Symposium; December 2005; San Antonio, TX. Abstract.

36. Pritchard KI, Shepherd LE, O'Malley FP, et al. HER2 and responsiveness of breast cancer to adjuvant chemotherapy. *N Engl J Med*. 2006;354:2103-2111.
37. Gennari A, Sormani MP, Pronzato P, et al. HER2 status and efficacy of adjuvant anthracyclines in early breast cancer: a pooled analysis of randomized trials. *J Natl Cancer Inst*. 2008;100:14-20.
38. Dang C, Hudis C. The role of adjuvant anthracyclines for breast cancer treatment: can we use molecular predictors? *Curr Breast Cancer Rep*. 2009;1:5-11.
39. Slamon D, Eiermann W, Robert N, et al. Adjuvant trastuzumab in HER2-positive breast cancer. *N Engl J Med*. 2011;365:1273-1283.
40. Beatson G. On the treatment of inoperable cases of carcinoma of the mamma: suggestions for a new method of treatment, with illustrative cases. *Lancet*. 1896;148:162-165.
41. Jensen EV, Desombre ER, Hurst DJ, Kawashima T, Jungblut PW. Estrogen-receptor interactions in target tissues. *Arch Anat Microsc Morphol Exp*. 1967;56:547-569.
42. Osborne CK. Tamoxifen in the treatment of breast cancer. *N Engl J Med*. 1998;339:1609-1618.
43. Early Breast Cancer Trialists' Collaborative G. Relevance of breast cancer hormone receptors and other factors to the efficacy of adjuvant tamoxifen: patient-level meta-analysis of randomised trials. *Lancet*. 2011;378:771-784.
44. Lao Romera J, Puertolas Hernandez Tde J, Pelaez Fernandez I, et al. Update on adjuvant hormonal treatment of early breast cancer. *Adv Ther*. 2011;28(suppl 6):1-18.
45. Cuzick J, Sestak I, Baum M, et al. Effect of anastrozole and tamoxifen as adjuvant treatment for early-stage breast cancer: 10-year analysis of the ATAC trial. *Lancet Oncol*. 2010;11:1135-1141.
46. Mouridsen H, Giobbie-Hurder A, Goldhirsch A, et al. Letrozole therapy alone or in sequence with tamoxifen in women with breast cancer. *N Engl J Med*. 2009;361:766-776.
47. Rea D, Hasenburg A, Seynaeve C, et al. Five years of exemestane as initial therapy compared to 5 years of tamoxifen followed by exemestane: the TEAM trial, a prospective, randomized, phase III trial in postmenopausal women with hormone-sensitive early breast cancer. *Cancer Res*. 2009;69(9 suppl 3). Abstract II.
48. Coombes R, Kilburn L, Beare S. Survival and safety post study treatment completion: an updated analysis of the Intergroup Exemestane Study (IES)—submitted on behalf of the IES investigators. In: Joint ECCO 15th–34th ESMO Multidisciplinary Congress; September 20-24, 2009; Berlin, Germany. Abstract O-5010.
49. Jakesz R, Gnant M, Griel R, et al. Tamoxifen and anastrozole as a sequencing strategy in postmenopausal women with hormone-responsive early breast cancer: updated data from the Austrian breast and colorectal cancer study group trial 8. In: 31st Annual San Antonio Breast Cancer Symposium; December 10-14, 2008; San Antonio, TX. Abstract 14.
50. Goss PE, Muss HB, Ingle JN, Whelan TJ, Wu M. Extended adjuvant endocrine therapy in breast cancer: current status and future directions. *Clin Breast Cancer*. 2008;8:411-417.
51. Goss PE, Ingle JN, Chapman J-AW, et al. Final analysis of NCIC CTG MA.27: a randomized phase III trial of exemestane versus anastrozole in postmenopausal women with hormone receptor positive primary breast cancer. In: San Antonio Breast Cancer Symposium; December 2010; San Antonio, TX. Abstract.
52. Goetz MP, Rae JM, Suman VJ, et al. Pharmacogenetics of tamoxifen biotransformation is associated with clinical outcomes of efficacy and hot flashes. *J Clin Oncol*. 2005;23:9312-9318.
53. Rae J, Drury S, Hayes DF. Lack of correlation between gene variants in tamoxifen metabolizing enzymes with primary endpoints in the ATAC trial. In: 33rd Annual San Antonio Breast Cancer Symposium; December 9-12, 2010; San Antonio, TX. Abstract S1-7.
54. Leyland-Jones B, Regan M, Bouzyk M, et al. Outcome according toCYP2D6 genotype among postmenopausal women with endocrine-responsive early invasive breast cancer randomized in the BIG 1098 trial. In: 33rd Annual San Antonio Breast Cancer Symposium; December 9-12, 2010; San Antonio, TX. Abstract S1-8.
55. Rae JM. Personalized tamoxifen: what is the best way forward? *J Clin Oncol*. 2011;29:3206-3208.
56. Cooley S, Burns LJ, Repka T, Miller JS. Natural killer cell cytotoxicity of breast cancer targets is enhanced by two distinct mechanisms of antibody-dependent cellular cytotoxicity against LFA-3 and HER2/neu. *Exp Hematol*. 1999;27:1533-1541.
57. Albanell J, Codony J, Rovira A, Mellado B, Gascon P. Mechanism of action of anti-HER2 monoclonal antibodies: scientific update on trastuzumab and 2C4. *Adv Exp Med Biol*. 2003;532:253-268.
58. Izumi Y, Xu L, di Tomaso E, Fukumura D, Jain RK. Tumour biology: herceptin acts as an anti-angiogenic cocktail. *Nature*. 2002;416:279-280.
59. Baselga J, Albanell J, Molina MA, Arribas J. Mechanism of action of trastuzumab and scientific update. *Semin Oncol*. 2001;28:4-11.
60. Austin CD, De Maziere AM, Pisacane PI, et al. Endocytosis and sorting of ErbB2 and the site of action of cancer therapeutics trastuzumab and geldanamycin. *Mol Biol Cell*. 2004;15: 5268-5282.
61. Slamon DJ, Leyland-Jones B, Shak S, et al. Use of chemotherapy plus a monoclonal antibody against HER2 for metastatic breast cancer that overexpresses HER2. *N Engl J Med*. 2001;344:783-792.
62. Perez EA, Romond EH, Suman VJ, et al. Four-year follow-up of trastuzumab plus adjuvant chemotherapy for operable human epidermal growth factor receptor 2-positive breast cancer: joint analysis of data from NCCTG N9831 and NSABP B-31. *J Clin Oncol*. 2011;29(25):3366-3373.
63. Gianni L, Dafni U, Gelber RD, et al. Treatment with trastuzumab for 1 year after adjuvant chemotherapy in patients with HER2-positive early breast cancer: a 4-year follow-up of a randomised controlled trial. *Lancet Oncol*. 2011;12:236-244.
64. Joensuu H, Kellokumpu-Lehtinen PL, Bono P, et al. Adjuvant docetaxel or vinorelbine with or without trastuzumab for breast cancer. *N Engl J Med*. 2006;354:809-820.
65. Spielmann M, Roche H, Delozier T, et al. Trastuzumab for patients with axillary-node-positive breast cancer: results of the FNCLCC-PACS 04 trial. *J Clin Oncol*. 2009;27:6129-6134.
66. Yin W, Jiang Y, Shen Z, Shao Z, Lu J. Trastuzumab in the adjuvant treatment of HER2-positive early breast cancer patients: a meta-analysis of published randomized controlled trials. *PLoS One*. 2011;6(6):e.21030.
67. Perez E, Suman V, Davidson N, et al. Results of chemotherapy alone, with sequential or concurrent addition of 52 weeks of trastuzumab in the NCCTG N9831 HER2-positive adjuvant breast cancer trial. *Cancer Res*. 2009;69(suppl):24. Abstract 701.
68. Azim HA Jr, de Azambuja E, Paesmans M, Piccart-Gebhart MJ. Sequential or concurrent administration of trastuzumab in early breast cancer? Too early to judge. *J Clin Oncol*. 2010;28:e353-e354.
69. Pivot X. Trastuzumab for 6 months or 1 year in treating women with nonmetastatic breast cancer that can be removed by surgery. http://www.clinicaltrials.gov/ct2/show/NCT00381901?term=PHARE&rank=1. Accessed August 29, 2011.
70. Earl H. Trastuzumab in treating women with HER2-positive early breast cancer. http://www.clinicaltrials.gov/ct2/show/NCT00712140?term=Persephone&rank=1. Accessed August 29, 2011.
71. Dang C, Fornier M, Sugarman S, et al. The safety of dose-dense doxorubicin and cyclophosphamide followed by paclitaxel with trastuzumab in HER-2/neu overexpressed/amplified breast cancer. *J Clin Oncol*. 2008;26:1216-1222.
72. Rastogi P, Anderson SJ, Bear HD, et al. Preoperative chemotherapy: updates of National Surgical Adjuvant Breast and Bowel Project Protocols B-18 and B-27. *J Clin Oncol*. 2008;26:778-785.
73. van der Hage JA, van de Velde CJ, Julien JP, Tubiana-Hulin M, Vandervelden C, Duchateau L. Preoperative chemotherapy in primary operable breast cancer: results from the European Organization for Research and Treatment of Cancer trial 10902. *J Clin Oncol*. 2001;19:4224-4237.
74. Untch M, Fasching PA, Konecny GE, et al. Pathologic complete response after neoadjuvant chemotherapy plus trastuzumab predicts favorable survival in human epidermal growth factor receptor 2–overexpressing breast cancer: results from the TECHNO trial of the AGO and GBG study groups. *J Clin Oncol*. 2011;29:3351-3357.
75. Gianni L, Eiermann W, Semiglazov V, et al. Neoadjuvant chemotherapy with trastuzumab followed by adjuvant trastuzumab versus neoadjuvant chemotherapy alone, in patients with HER2-positive locally advanced breast cancer (the NOAH

trial): a randomised controlled superiority trial with a parallel HER2-negative cohort. *Lancet*. 2010;375:377-384.
76. Untch M, Rezai M, Loibl S, et al. Neoadjuvant treatment with trastuzumab in HER2-positive breast cancer: results from the GeparQuattro study. *J Clin Oncol*. 2010;28:2024-2031.
77. Carey L. Paclitaxel and trastuzumab and/or lapatinib in treating patients with stage II or stage III breast cancer that can be removed by surgery. http://clinicaltrials.gov/ct2/show/NCT00770809?term=CALGB+40601&rank=1. Accessed September 3, 2011.
78. Baselga J, Bradbury I, Eidtmann H. First results of the neo-ALTTO trial (BIG 01-06/EGF 106903): a phase III, randomized, open label, neoadjuvant study of lapatinib, trastuzumab, and their combination plus paclitaxel in women with HER2-positive primary breast cancer. In: San Antonio Breast Cancer Symposium; December 2010; San Antonio, TX.
79. Gianni L, Pienkowski T, Im Y-H. Neoadjuvant pertuzumab (P) and trastuzumab (H): antitumor and safety analysis of a randomized phase ii study ('NeoSphere'). In: San Antonio Breast Cancer Symposium; December 2010; San Antonio, TX.
80. Untch M, Loibl S, Bischoff J, et al. Lapatinib vs trastuzumab in combination with neoadjuvant anthracycline-taxane-based chemotherapy: primary efficacy endpoint analysis of the GEPARQUINTO STUDY (GBG 44). In: San Antonio Breast Cancer Symposium; December 2010; San Antonio, TX.
81. Guarneri V. A multicenter phase II study of neoadjuvant lapatinib and trastuzumab in patients with HER2-overexpressing breast cancer. *J Clin Oncol*. 2011;29(suppl).
82. Dang C, Lin N, Moy B, et al. Dose-dense doxorubicin and cyclophosphamide followed by weekly paclitaxel with trastuzumab and lapatinib in HER2/neu-overexpressed/amplified breast cancer is not feasible because of excessive diarrhea. *J Clin Oncol*. 2010;28:2982-2988.
83. Palmieri F, Dueck AC, Johnson DB, et al. Cardiac safety of lapatinib given concurrently with paclitaxel and trastuzumab as part of adjuvant therapy for patients with HER2+ breast cancer: pilot data from the mayo clinic cancer research consortium trial RC0639. *Cancer Res*. 2009;69:24(suppl 3). Abstract.
84. Tomasello G, de Azambuja E, Dinh P, Snoj N, Piccart-Gebhart M. Jumping higher: is it still possible? The ALTTO trial challenge. *Expert Rev Anticancer Ther*. 2008;8:1883-1890.
85. trials Gc. Tykerb evaluation after chemotherapy (TEACH): lapatinib versus placebo in women with early-stage breast cancer. http://clinicaltrials.gov/ct2/show/NCT00374322. Accessed August 29, 2011.
86. Franklin MC, Carey KD, Vajdos FF, Leahy DJ, De Vos AM, Sliwkowski MX. Insights into ErbB signaling from the structure of the ErbB2-pertuzumab complex. *Cancer Cell*. 2004;5: 317-328.
87. Hoffman-La Roche G. A study of pertuzumab in addition to chemotherapy and herceptin (trastuzumab) as adjuvant therapy in patients with HER2-positive primary breast cancer. http://clinicaltrials.gov/ct2/show/NCT01358877?term=adjuvant+pertuzumab&rank=1. Accessed September 2, 2011.
88. Ferrara N, Davis-Smyth T. The biology of vascular endothelial growth factor. *Endocr Rev*. 1997;18:4-25.
89. Kim KJ, Li B, Winer J, et al. Inhibition of vascular endothelial growth factor-induced angiogenesis suppresses tumour growth in vivo. *Nature*. 1993;362:841-844.
90. Miller K, Wang M, Gralow J, et al. Paclitaxel plus bevacizumab versus paclitaxel alone for metastatic breast cancer. *N Engl J Med*. 2007;357:2666-2676.
91. Pivot X, Schneeweiss A, Verma S, et al. Efficacy and safety of bevacizumab in combination with docetaxel for the first-line treatment of elderly patients with locally recurrent or metastatic breast cancer: results from AVADO. *Eur J Cancer*. 2011;47(16):2387-2395.
92. Robert NJ, Dieras V, Glaspy J, et al. RIBBON-1: randomized, double-blind, placebo-controlled, phase III trial of chemotherapy with or without bevacizumab for first-line treatment of human epidermal growth factor receptor 2-negative, locally recurrent or metastatic breast cancer. *J Clin Oncol*. 2011;29:1252-1260.
93. Brufsky A, Bondarenko V, Smirnov S. RIBBON-2: a randomized, double-blind, placebo-controlled, phase III trial evaluating the efficacy and safety of bevacizumab in combination with chemotherapy for second-line treatment of HER2-negative metastatic breast cancer. *Cancer Res*. 2009;69(24 suppl). Abstract no 42.
94. Wolmark N. BETH study: treatment of HER2 positive breast cancer with chemotherapy plus trastuzumab vs chemotherapy plus trastuzumab plus bevacizumab. http://clinicaltrials.gov/ct2/show/NCT00625898. Accessed August 29, 2011.
95. Miller KD, O'Neill A, Perez EA, Seidman AD, Sledge GW. A phase II pilot trial incorporating bevacizumab into dose-dense doxorubicin and cyclophosphamide followed by paclitaxel in patients with lymph node positive breast cancer: a trial coordinated by the Eastern Cooperative Oncology Group. *Ann Oncol*. 2012;23(2):331-333.
96. Miller K. Doxorubicin, cyclophosphamide, and paclitaxel with or without bevacizumab in treating patients with lymph node-positive or high-risk, lymph node-negative breast cancer. http://clinicaltrials.gov/ct2/show/NCT00433511?term=e5103&rank=1. Accessed August 31, 2011.
97. Roche H-L. BEATRICE study: a study of avastin (Bevacizumab) adjuvant therapy in triple negative breast cancer. http://clinicaltrials.gov/ct2/show/NCT00528567. Accessed September 2, 2011.
98. von Minckwitz G, Eidtmann H, Rezai M, et al. Neoadjuvant chemotherapy with or without bevacizumab: primary efficacy endpoint analysis of the GEPARQUINTO study (GBG 44). In: San Antonio Breast Cancer Symposium; December 2010; Abstract (S4-6).
99. Gerber B, Eidtmann H, Rezai M; American Society of Clinical Oncology. Neoadjuvant bevacizumab and anthracycline–taxane-based chemotherapy in 686 triple-negative primary breast cancers: secondary endpoint analysis of the GeparQuinto study (GBG 44). *J Clin Oncol*. 2011;29(15) (May 20 suppl). Abstract 1006.
100. Sikov W. Paclitaxel with or without carboplatin and/or bevacizumab followed by doxorubicin and cyclophosphamide in treating patients with breast cancer that can be removed by surgery. http://clinicaltrials.gov/ct2/show/NCT00861705?term=CALGB+40603&rank=1. Accessed September 3, 2011.
101. Bear HD. Chemotherapy with or without bevacizumab in treating women with stage I, stage II, or stage IIIA breast cancer that can be removed by surgery. http://clinicaltrials.gov/ct2/show/NCT00408408?term=B-40+trial&rank=3. Accessed September 3, 2011.
102. GSK. Treatment with pazopanib for neoadjuvant breast cancer. http://clinicaltrials.gov/ct2/show/NCT00849472?term=pazopanib+neoadjuvant&rank=1. Accessed October 7, 2011.
103. Bonneterre J, Buzdar A, Nabholtz JMA, et al. Anastrozole is superior to tamoxifen as first-line therapy in hormone receptor positive advanced breast carcinoma: results of two randomized trials designed for combined analysis. *Cancer*. 2001;92:2247-2258.
104. Mouridsen H, Gershanovich M, Sun Y, et al. Phase III study of letrozole versus tamoxifen as first-line therapy of advanced breast cancer in postmenopausal women: analysis of survival and update of efficacy from the International Letrozole Breast Cancer Group. *J Clin Oncol*. 2003;21:2101-2109.
105. Paridaens RJ, Dirix LY, Beex LV, et al. Phase III study comparing exemestane with tamoxifen as first-line hormonal treatment of metastatic breast cancer in postmenopausal women: the european organisation for research and treatment of cancer breast cancer cooperative group. *J Clin Oncol*. 2008;26:4883-4890.
106. Di Leo A, Jerusalem G, Petruzelka L, et al. Results of the CONFIRM phase III trial comparing fulvestrant 250 mg with fulvestrant 500 mg in postmenopausal women with estrogen receptor–positive advanced breast cancer. *J Clin Oncol*. 2010;28:4594-4600.
107. Robertson JF, Lindemann JP, Llombart-Cussac A. A comparison of fulvestrant 500 mg with anastrozole as first-line treatment for advanced breast cancer: follow-up analysis from the 'FIRST' Study. In: San Antonio Breast Cancer Symposium; 2010. Abstract S1-S3.
108. Klijn JG, Blamey RW, Boccardo F, Tominaga T, Duchateau L, Sylvester R. Combined tamoxifen and luteinizing hormone-releasing hormone (LHRH) agonist versus LHRH agonist alone in premenopausal advanced breast cancer: a meta-analysis of four randomized trials. *J Clin Oncol*. 2001;19:343-353.
109. Milla-Santos A, Rubagotti A, Perrotta A. A randomized trial of goserelin (Zoladex) + tamoxifen versus goserelin + anastrozole (Arimidex) in pre/perimenopausal patients with hormone dependent advanced breast cancer. *Breast Cancer Res Treat*. 2002;76(suppl 1):S32. Abstract 13.

110. Kaufman B, Mackey JR, Clemens MR, et al. Trastuzumab plus anastrozole versus anastrozole alone for the treatment of postmenopausal women with human epidermal growth factor receptor 2-positive, hormone receptor-positive metastatic breast cancer: results from the randomized phase III TAnDEM study. *J Clin Oncol.* 2009;27:5529-5537.
111. Johnston S, Pippen J Jr, Pivot X, et al. Lapatinib combined with letrozole versus letrozole and placebo as first-line therapy for postmenopausal hormone receptor—positive metastatic breast cancer. *J Clin Oncol.* 2009;27:5538-5546.
112. Burstein H, Barry WT, Cirrincione C. CALGB 40302: fulvestrant with or without lapatinib as therapy for hormone receptor positive advanced breast cancer: a double-blinded, placebo-controlled, randomized phase III study. In: San Antonio Breast Cancer Symposium; December 2010; Abstract.
113. Traina TA, Rugo HS, Caravelli JF, et al. Feasibility trial of letrozole in combination with bevacizumab in patients with metastatic breast cancer. *J Clin Oncol.* 2010;28:628-633.
114. Bachelot T, Bourgier C, Cropet C. TAMRAD: a GINECO randomized phase II trial of everolimus in combination with tamoxifen versus tamoxifen alone in patients (pts) with hormone-receptor positive, HER2 negative metastatic breast cancer (MBC) with prior exposure to aromatase inhibitors (AI). In: San Antonio Breast Cancer Symposium; December 2010; Abstract.
115. Marty M, Cognetti F, Maraninchi D, et al. Randomized phase II trial of the efficacy and safety of trastuzumab combined with docetaxel in patients with human epidermal growth factor receptor 2-positive metastatic breast cancer administered as first-line treatment: the M77001 study group. *J Clin Oncol.* 2005;23:4265-4274.
116. Vogel CL, Cobleigh MA, Tripathy D, et al. Efficacy and safety of trastuzumab as a single agent in first-line treatment of HER2-overexpressing metastatic breast cancer. *J Clin Oncol.* 2002;20:719-726.
117. Burstein HJ, Harris LN, Marcom PK, et al. Trastuzumab and vinorelbine as first-line therapy for HER2-overexpressing metastatic breast cancer: multicenter phase II trial with clinical outcomes, analysis of serum tumor markers as predictive factors, and cardiac surveillance algorithm. *J Clin Oncol.* 2003;21:2889-2895.
118. Valero V, Forbes J, Pegram MD, et al. Multicenter phase III randomized trial comparing docetaxel and trastuzumab with docetaxel, carboplatin, and trastuzumab as first-line chemotherapy for patients with HER2-gene-amplified metastatic breast cancer (BCIRG 007 study): two highly active therapeutic regimens. *J Clin Oncol.* 2011;29:149-156.
119. Esteva FJ, Valero V, Booser D, et al. Phase II study of weekly docetaxel and trastuzumab for patients with HER-2-overexpressing metastatic breast cancer. *J Clin Oncol.* 2002;20:1800-1808.
120. Seidman AD, Fornier MN, Esteva FJ, et al. Weekly trastuzumab and paclitaxel therapy for metastatic breast cancer with analysis of efficacy by HER2 immunophenotype and gene amplification. *J Clin Oncol.* 2001;19:2587-2595.
121. Bartsch R, Wenzel C, Altorjai G, et al. Capecitabine and trastuzumab in heavily pretreated metastatic breast cancer. *J Clin Oncol.* 2007;25:3853-3858.
122. Pegram MD, Pienkowski T, Northfelt DW, et al. Results of two open-label, multicenter phase II studies of docetaxel, platinum salts, and trastuzumab in HER2-positive advanced breast cancer. *J Natl Cancer Inst.* 2004;96:759-769.
123. von Minckwitz G, du Bois A, Schmidt M, et al. Trastuzumab beyond progression in human epidermal growth factor receptor 2-positive advanced breast cancer: a German Breast Group 26/Breast International Group 03-05 study. *J Clin Oncol.* 2009;27:1999-2006.
124. von Minckwitz G, Schwedler K, Schmidt M, et al. Trastuzumab beyond progression: overall survival analysis of the GBG 26/BIG 3-05 phase III study in HER2-positive breast cancer. *Eur J Cancer.* 2011;47(15):2273-2281.
125. Blackwell KL, Burstein HJ, Storniolo AM, et al. Randomized study of Lapatinib alone or in combination with trastuzumab in women with ErbB2-positive, trastuzumab-refractory metastatic breast cancer. *J Clin Oncol.* 2010;28:1124-1130.
126. Geyer CE, Forster J, Lindquist D, et al. Lapatinib plus capecitabine for HER2-positive advanced breast cancer. *N Engl J Med.* 2006;355:2733-2743.
127. Di Leo A, Gomez HL, Aziz Z, et al. Phase III, double-blind, randomized study comparing lapatinib plus paclitaxel with placebo plus paclitaxel as first-line treatment for metastatic breast cancer. *J Clin Oncol.* 2008;26:5544-5552.
128. Nahta R, Esteva FJ. HER2 therapy: molecular mechanisms of trastuzumab resistance. *Breast Cancer Res.* 2006;8:215.
129. Baselga J, Gelmon KA, Verma S, et al. Phase II trial of pertuzumab and trastuzumab in patients with human epidermal growth factor receptor 2-positive metastatic breast cancer that progressed during prior trastuzumab therapy. *J Clin Oncol.* 2010;28:1138-1144.
130. Portera CC, Walshe JM, Rosing DR, et al. Cardiac toxicity and efficacy of trastuzumab combined with pertuzumab in patients with [corrected] human epidermal growth factor receptor 2-positive metastatic breast cancer. *Clin Cancer Res.* 2008;14:2710-2716.
131. Baselga J, Cortés J, Kim S-B, et al. Pertuzumab plus trastuzumab plus docetaxel for metastatic breast cancer. *N Engl J Med.* 2012;366(2):109-110.
132. Burris HA 3rd, Rugo HS, Vukelja SJ, et al. Phase II study of the antibody drug conjugate trastuzumab-DM1 for the treatment of human epidermal growth factor receptor 2 (HER2)-positive breast cancer after prior HER2-directed therapy. *J Clin Oncol.* 2011;29:398-405.
133. Krop I, LoRusso P, Miller K, et al. A phase II study of trastuzumab-DM1 (T-DM1), a novel HER2 antibody–drug conjugate, in HER2+ metastatic breast cancer (MBC) patients previously treated with conventional chemotherapy, lapatinib and trastuzumab. In: San Antonio Breast Cancer Symposium; December 2009; Abstract 710.
134. Hurvitz S, Dirix L, Kocsis L, et al. Trastuzumab emtansine (T-DM1) versus trastuzumab + docetaxel in previously untreated HER2-positive metastatic breast cancer (MBC): primary results of a randomized, multicenter, open-label phase II study (TDM4450g/BO21976). Abstract presented at the European Multidisciplinary Cancer Congress-European Society for Medical Oncology (ESMO) 2011; 2011.
135. Workman P, Burrows F, Neckers L, Rosen N. Drugging the cancer chaperone HSP90: combinatorial therapeutic exploitation of oncogene addiction and tumor stress. *Ann N Y Acad Sci.* 2007;1113:202-216.
136. Modi S, Stopeck A, Linden H, et al. HSP90 inhibition is effective in breast cancer: a phase II trial of tanespimycin (17-AAG) plus trastuzumab in patients with HER2-positive metastatic breast cancer progressing on trastuzumab. *Clin Cancer Res.* 2011;17:5132-5139.
137. Chandarlapaty S, Scaltriti M, Angelini P, et al. Inhibitors of HSP90 block p95-HER2 signaling in Trastuzumab-resistant tumors and suppress their growth. *Oncogene.* 2010;29: 325-334.
138. Nagata Y, Lan KH, Zhou X, et al. PTEN activation contributes to tumor inhibition by trastuzumab, and loss of PTEN predicts trastuzumab resistance in patients. *Cancer Cell.* 2004;6:117-127.
139. Saal LH, Holm K, Maurer M, et al. PIK3CA mutations correlate with hormone receptors, node metastasis, and ERBB2, and are mutually exclusive with PTEN loss in human breast carcinoma. *Cancer Res.* 2005;65:2554-2559.
140. Di Leo A, Isola J, Piette F, et al. A meta-analysis of phase III trials evaluating the predictive value of HER2 and topoisomerase II alpha in early breast cancer patients treated with CMF or anthracycline-based adjuvant therapy. *Breast Cancer Res Treat.* 2008;107. Abstract 705.
141. Cheang MC, Voduc KD, Tu D. Responsiveness of intrinsic subtypes to adjuvant anthracycline substitution in the NCIC.CTG MA.5 randomized trial. *Clin Cancer Res.* 2012;18(8):2402-2412.
142. Chang HR, Glaspy J, Allison MA, et al. Differential response of triple-negative breast cancer to a docetaxel and carboplatin-based neoadjuvant treatment. *Cancer.* 2010;116:4227-4237.
143. Byrski T, Gronwald J, Huzarski T, et al. Pathologic complete response rates in young women with BRCA1-positive breast cancers after neoadjuvant chemotherapy. *J Clin Oncol.* 2010;28:375-379.
144. Silver DP, Richardson AL, Eklund AC, et al. Efficacy of neoadjuvant cisplatin in triple-negative breast cancer. *J Clin Oncol.* 2010;28:1145-1153.
145. Carey LA, Dees EC, Sawyer L, et al. The triple negative paradox: primary tumor chemosensitivity of breast cancer subtypes. *Clin Cancer Res.* 2007;13:2329-2334.

146. Uhm JE, Park YH, Yi SY, et al. Treatment outcomes and clinicopathologic characteristics of triple-negative breast cancer patients who received platinum-containing chemotherapy. *Int J Cancer*. 2009;124:1457-1462.
147. Reis-Filho JS, Tutt AN. Triple negative tumours: a critical review. *Histopathology*. 2008;52:108-118.
148. Turner NC, Reis-Filho JS. Basal-like breast cancer and the BRCA1 phenotype. *Oncogene*. 2006;25:5846-5853.
149. Chalmers AJ. The potential role and application of PARP inhibitors in cancer treatment. *Br Med Bull*. 2009;89:23-40.
150. Au-Yong IT, Evans AJ, Taneja S, et al. Sonographic correlations with the new molecular classification of invasive breast cancer. *Eur Radiol*. 2009;19:2342-2348.
151. Fong PC, Yap TA, Boss DS, et al. Poly(ADP)-ribose polymerase inhibition: frequent durable responses in BRCA carrier ovarian cancer correlating with platinum-free interval. *J Clin Oncol*. 2010;28:2512-2519.
152. Fong PC, Boss DS, Yap TA, et al. Inhibition of poly(ADP-ribose) polymerase in tumors from BRCA mutation carriers. *N Engl J Med*. 2009;361:123-134.
153. Tutt A, Robson M, Garber JE, et al. Oral poly(ADP-ribose) polymerase inhibitor olaparib in patients with BRCA1 or BRCA2 mutations and advanced breast cancer: a proof-of-concept trial. *Lancet*. 2010;376:235-244.
154. O'Shaughnessy J, Osborne C, Pippen JE, et al. Iniparib plus chemotherapy in metastatic triple-negative breast cancer. *N Engl J Med*. 2011;364:205-214.
155. O'Shaughnessey J, Schwartzberg LS, Danso MA. A randomized phase III study of iniparib (BSI-201) in combination with gemcitabine/carboplatin (G/C) in metastatic triple-negative breast cancer (TNBC). *J Clin Oncol*. 2011;29(suppl). Abstract 1007.
156. Carey LA, Sharpless NE. PARP and cancer—if it's broke, don't fix it. *N Engl J Med*. 2011;364:277-279.
157. Ji J, Lee MP, Kadota M, et al. Pharmacodynamic and pathway analysis of three presumed inhibitors of poly (ADP-ribose) polymerase: ABT-888, AZD 2281, and BSI201. In: Proceedings of the 102nd Annual Meeting of the American Association for Cancer Research; 2011; Orlando, FL. Abstract 4527.
158. Linderholm BK, Hellborg H, Johansson U, et al. Significantly higher levels of vascular endothelial growth factor (VEGF) and shorter survival times for patients with primary operable triple-negative breast cancer. *Ann Oncol*. 2009;20:1639-1646.
159. Hudis CA, Gianni L. Triple-negative breast cancer: an unmet medical need. *Oncologist*. 2011;16(suppl 1):1-11.
160. Brufsky AM, Hurvitz S, Perez E, et al. RIBBON-2: A randomized, double-blind, placebo-controlled, phase III trial evaluating the efficacy and safety of bevacizumab in combination with chemotherapy for second-line treatment of human epidermal growth factor receptor 2–negative metastatic breast cancer. *J Clin Oncol*. 2011;29(32):4286-4293.
161. Ranpura V, Hapani S, Wu S. Treatment-related mortality with bevacizumab in cancer patients: a meta-analysis. *JAMA*. 2011;305:487-494.
162. Marty M, Pivot X. The potential of anti-vascular endothelial growth factor therapy in metastatic breast cancer: clinical experience with anti-angiogenic agents, focusing on bevacizumab. *Eur J Cancer*. 2008;44:912-920.
163. Barrios C, Liu M-C, Lee S, et al. Phase III randomized trial of sunitinib versus capecitabine in patients with previously treated HER2-negative advanced breast cancer. *Breast Cancer Res Treat*. 2010;121:121-131.
164. Bergh J, Greil R, Voytko N, et al. Sunitinib (SU) in combination with docetaxel (D) versus D alone for the first-line treatment of advanced breast cancer (ABC). *J Clin Oncol*. 2010;18s(suppl). Abstract LBA1010.
165. Hudis C, Tauer KW, Hermann RC, et al. Sorafenib (SOR) plus chemotherapy (CRx) for patients (pts) with advanced (adv) breast cancer (BC) previously treated with bevacizumab (BEV). Presented at the ASCO 2011 annual meeting. *J Clin Oncol*. 2011;29(15 suppl) (May 20 supplement):1009.
166. Rugo HS, Stopeck AT, Joy AA, et al. Randomized, placebo-controlled, double-blind, phase II study of axitinib plus docetaxel versus docetaxel plus placebo in patients with metastatic breast cancer. *J Clin Oncol*. 2011;29:2459-2465.
167. Kurebayashi J, Okubo S, Yamamoto Y, Sonoo H. Inhibition of HER1 signaling pathway enhances antitumor effect of endocrine therapy in breast cancer. *Breast Cancer*. 2004;11:38-41.
168. Dogu GG, Ozkan M, Ozturk F, Dikilitas M, Er O, Ozturk A. Triple-negative breast cancer: immunohistochemical correlation with basaloid markers and prognostic value of survivin. *Med Oncol*. 2010;27:34-39.
169. Reis-Filho JS, Pinheiro C, Lambros MB, et al. EGFR amplification and lack of activating mutations in metaplastic breast carcinomas. *J Pathol*. 2006;209:445-453.
170. Carey L, Rugo HS, Marcom PK, et al. EGFR inhibition with cetuximab in metastatic triple negative (basal-like) breast cancer. *J Clin Oncol*. 2008;26(suppl 15):43S. Abstract 1009.
171. O'Shaughnessey J, Weckstein DJ, Vukelja SJ, et al. Randomized phase II study of weekly irinotecan/carboplatin with or without cetuximab in patients with metastatic breast cancer. *Br Cancer Res Treat*. 2007;106(suppl 1):S32. Abstract 308.
172. Baselga J. The addition of cetuximab to cisplatin increases overall response rate (ORR) and progression-free survival (PFS) in metastatic triple-negative breast cancer (TNBC): results of a randomized phase II study (BALI-1). ESMO 2010; Program book, page 135; 2010.
173. Nechushtan H, Steinberg H, Peretz T. Preliminary results of a phase I/II of a combination of cetuximab and taxane for triple negative breast cancer patients. *J Clin Oncol*. 2009;27. Abstract 12018.
174. Corkery B, Crown J, Clynes M, O'Donovan N. Epidermal growth factor receptor as a potential therapeutic target in triple-negative breast cancer. *Ann Oncol*. 2009;20:862-867.
175. Doanne AS, Danso M, Lal P, et al. An estrogen receptor-negative breast cancer subset characterized by a hormonally regulated transcriptional program and response to androgen. *Oncogene*. 2006;25:3994-4008.
176. Gucalp A, Traina TA. Triple-negative breast cancer: role of the androgen receptor. *Cancer J*. 2010;16:62-65.
177. Gucalp A, Tolaney SM, Isakoff SJ. Targeting the androgen receptor (AR) for the treatment of AR+/ER-/PR- metastatic breast cancer. TBCRC 011. *J Clin Oncol*. 2012;30(suppl). Abstract 1006.
178. Caldas-Lopes E, Cerchietti L, Ahn JH, et al. Hsp90 inhibitor PU-H71, a multimodal inhibitor of malignancy, induces complete responses in triple-negative breast cancer models. *Proc Natl Acad Sci U S A*. 2009;106:8368-8373.
179. Gerecitano J. The first-in-human phase I trial of PU-H71 in patients with advanced malignancies. http://clinicaltrials.gov/ct2/show/NCT01393509?term=PU-H71&rank=1. Updated July 12, 2011.

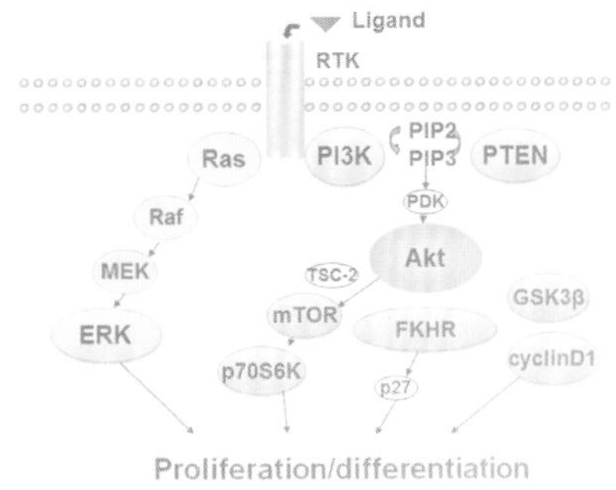

CHAPTER 54

PERSONALIZED MEDICINE AND TARGETED THERAPY FOR COLORECTAL CANCER

Joleen M. Hubbard and Axel Grothey

INTRODUCTION

The treatment of colon cancer has changed dramatically over the past two decades. New therapies have improved survival for patients with both early-stage and advanced diseases. Multiple studies have refined our treatment recommendations in terms of who is appropriate for a particular therapy and how the therapy should be administered. This chapter focuses on how to apply the new standards of care to maximize benefit while minimizing harm for patients with early-stage colon cancer as well as advanced disease. The first portion of the chapter will discuss how to apply both clinical and molecular factors to determine the appropriate care for patients with stage II and III colon cancer. The second portion focuses on how to incorporate targeted therapy into standard cytotoxic regimens for patients with metastatic disease. Finally, the remainder of the chapter provides guidance to tailor treatment for the goals of care of the individual patient.

CURRENT STANDARD OF CARE FOR EARLY-STAGE COLON CANCER

In the early 1990s, Moertel et al.[1] published the results of the pivotal phase III trial, demonstrating a 41% reduction in tumor recurrence with 1 year of adjuvant 5-fluororacil (5-FU) plus levamisole administered to patients when compared with surgery alone. Patients in the treatment arm had a 33% reduction in mortality at 5 years.[2] The benefits of adjuvant therapy were confirmed by the National Surgical Adjuvant Breast and Bowel Project (NSABP) C-03 trial, which administered 1 year of 5-FU plus leucovorin (LV).[3] Subsequent studies demonstrated that the duration of adjuvant therapy with 5-FU/LV could safely be shortened to 6 months, establishing a standard of care for patients with resected stage II and III colon cancer.[4,5]

Since that time, multiple adjuvant colon cancer studies have tested agents that provide survival benefit for patients in the metastatic setting, including bevacizumab, cetuximab, oxaliplatin, and irinotecan. Oxaliplatin was the only new medication that added additional survival benefit when compared with 5-FU/LV alone in the adjuvant setting. The Multicenter International Study of Oxaliplatin/5-Fluorouracil/Leucovorin in the Adjuvant Treatment of Colon Cancer (MOSAIC) trial compared 5-FU/LV plus oxaliplatin (FOLFOX4 regimen) with 5-FU/LV alone as adjuvant therapy for patients with resected high-risk stage II and stage III colon cancer.[6] Three-year disease-free survival (DFS) was 78.2% in the FOLFOX4 arm and 72.9% in the 5-FU/LV arm (72.9%; $P = 0.002$). This translated into an overall survival (OS) benefit at 6 years for stage III patients only (72.9% vs. 68.7% for the FOLFOX4 arm and 5-FU arm, respectively; HR = 0.80; 95% CI, 0.65 to 0.97; $P = 0.023$).[7] With the results of the MOSAIC trial, 6 months of adjuvant FOLFOX chemotherapy became the standard of care for stage III (and selected high-risk stage II) colon cancer patients. Two additional studies, C-07 which investigated another oxaliplatin plus bolus 5-FU regimen (FLOX),[8] and the XELOXA trial, which compared capecitabine and oxaliplatin versus 5-FU/LV, confirmed the DFS benefit of the addition of oxaliplatin to a fluoropyrimidine in the adjuvant setting.[9]

Individualizing Adjuvant Therapy

The aforementioned trials have established a clear benefit of adjuvant oxaliplatin and a fluoropyrimidine for stage III cancers. However, the role of adjuvant therapy for stage II colon cancer remains an area of controversy. The survival for resected stage II colon cancer patients ranges from 75% to 80% at 5 years, and disease recurrence occurs in approximately 20% of patients. Much effort has been dedicated to determine which stage II patients are at the highest risk for recurrence and therefore more likely to benefit from adjuvant therapy. Several pooled analyses specifically evaluating stage II patients in adjuvant therapy trials generally show DFS benefit for stage II patients, but not consistent benefits in OS.

The largest clinical trial designed to address the benefit of adjuvant therapy in stage II colon cancer was the Quick and Simple and Reliable (QUASAR) study.[10] Patients were randomized to receive 5-FU plus folinic acid (n = 1,622) versus observation (n = 1,617). Those patients in the treatment arm had a 5-year OS of 80.3% compared with 77.4% in the observation arm ($P = 0.02$). Patients considered to be at high risk for recurrence (T4 tumors, bowel obstruction or perforation, poorly differentiated tumors, venous invasion, and ≤10 lymph nodes examined) had a greater absolute reduction in mortality than those patients without high-risk features (5.5% vs. 3.6% respectively).

The benefit of oxaliplatin combined with 5-FU has also been evaluated. The MOSAIC trial included 286 patients with high-risk stage II (T4N0M0) tumors. These patients did have a 5.4% improvement in DFS, but this did not translate into an OS benefit.[7] Yothers et al.[11] evaluated the use of oxaliplatin-based regimens among 3,000 patients with stage II colon cancer using data from four adjuvant therapy trials. The investigators found no statistically significant difference in OS, DFS, or time to recurrence (TTR) between patients who received an oxaliplatin-based regimen (n = 2009) and those who received 5-FU/LV (n = 991) alone. The absolute DFS benefit was 3.0% in low-risk and 4.4% in high-risk patients, and the absolute OS gain was 2.5% for low-risk and 3.5% for high-risk stage II patients.

Molecular Markers

Since adjuvant therapy only benefits a small proportion of patients with stage II colon cancer, investigators have been making efforts to develop methods to assess the risk of recurrence. Currently, the molecular markers showing the most promise are microsatellite instability and guanylyl cyclase C.

Deficient Mismatch Repair (Microsatellite Instability)

The loss of mismatch repair (MMR) protein expression results in an inability to consistently replicate repetitive DNA sequences, termed microsatellite instability (MSI-H). This process is involved in approximately 15% of all sporadic colon cancers and 95% of these are due to the loss of the *MLH1* or *MSH2* genes. Patients with deficient mismatch repair tumors (dMMR) are more commonly female, earlier stage, right-sided, and have an overall better prognosis. Tumors with MMR deficiency can be identified by either immunohistochemistry for MMR proteins or polymerase chain reaction assessment of DNA markers for MSI.[12]

In vitro data demonstrated that cells with dMMR are associated with 5-FU resistance.[13] There are also two large clinical studies suggesting patients with dMMR tumors do not benefit from adjuvant 5-FU–based therapy. Ribic et al.[14] investigated 570 samples of stage II and III colon cancers in adjuvant trials investing 5-FU–based therapy versus surgery alone. Patients with microsatellite stable tumors had an OS benefit, with a hazard ratio (HR) for death of 0.72 (95% CI, 0.53 to 0.99; $P = 0.04$). Patients with MSI-H tumors did not obtain an OS benefit, HR for death 1.07 (95% CI; $P = 0.80$). The treatment effect was statistically significantly different between the two groups ($P = 0.01$).

Sargent et al.[15] confirmed this finding in a study examining 457 specimens from patients with stage II and III colon cancer who participated in several adjuvant trials testing 5-FU–based therapy versus observation. Again, patients with proficient mismatch repair (pMMR) did have a DFS and OS benefit; however, those with dMMR did not. In fact, stage II patients with dMMR had a worse OS when treated with 5-FU (HR 2.95; 95% CI, 1.02 to 8.54; $P = 0.04$).

Patients with stage II colon cancer should be tested for MSI, and those with MSI-H tumors should not receive adjuvant 5-FU/LV. Results are awaited from the recently conducted E5202 trial, which randomized patients with stage II colon cancer to receive FOLFOX with or without bevacizumab versus observation based on results of MSI and 18q loss of heterozygosity testing. This trial was closed early due to other adjuvant trials showing lack of benefit for bevacizumab in the adjuvant setting, but hopefully will shed a light on which stage II patients may benefit from adjuvant FOLFOX therapy.

Guanylyl Cyclase 2C

Another molecular marker that may help identify patients with stage II colorectal cancer at risk for recurrence is guanylyl cyclase 2C (GUCY2C), a protein normally only expressed in intestinal cells. Waldman et al.[16] investigated whether GUCY2C could be used for occult metastasis detection using reverse transcriptase-polymerase chain reaction (RT-PCR) on lymph nodes from 257 patients determined to be node negative by standard histopathologic techniques. Those who were GUCY2C negative had a recurrence rate of 6.3% versus 20.9% in the GUCY2C-positive group (P = 0.06). GUCY2C-positive patients had an earlier TTR (HR 4.66; 95% CI, 1.11 to 19.57;

$P = 0.04$) and reduced DFS (HR, 3.27; 95% CI, 1.15 to 9.29; $P = 0.03$) than GUCY2C-negative patients. This study was conducted using fresh frozen tissue, which is a challenge for routine practice. There has been an assay developed for use with paraffin-embedded tissue that is currently being utilized in a prospective study to validate GUCY2C as a predictive marker for recurrence.

Recurrence Risk Assays

OncotypeDx Colon

For patients with stage II colon cancer who do not have clear indications for or against chemotherapy, such as high-risk features or MSI-H tumors, methods to determine the risk of recurrence may aid in decision making for adjuvant treatment. The first study to validate a gene expression assay that can independently predict the risk of recurrence in stage II colon cancer was recently published by Gray et al.[17] Paraffin-embedded tissue samples from 1,436 patients enrolled on the QUASAR study were assessed for 781 candidate genes and 13 cancer-related genes using RT-PCR assays. Ultimately, seven genes were used to determine a recurrence score (RS) and six genes were used to develop a treatment score (TS) to predict treatment benefit. The TS is not validated as a predictor of those who will benefit from 5-FU/LV therapy. However, the RS was validated as a predictor of risk of recurrence in patients treated with surgery alone (HR 1.38; 95% CI, 1.11 to 1.74; $P = 0.004$). This score remained independent of other variables associated with recurrence risk on multivariate analysis (HR 1.43; 95% CI, 1.11 to 1.83; $P = 0.006$). When grouped into low-risk, intermediate-risk, and high-risk scores, the comparison of recurrence risk in the low versus high groups was significant (HR: 1.47; 95% CI, 1.01 to 2.14; $P = 0.046$).

Results investigating another prognostic assay using DNA microarray technology were also recently reported.[18] The assay was developed using 215 patient formalin-fixed paraffin-embedded tissue samples and validated in an additional 144 patient samples. The investigators used a 634-probe assay to categorize patients into low-risk and high-risk groups. The assay was able to predict recurrence of disease for the high-risk patients (HR 2.53; $P < 0.001$) and cancer-related death (HR 2.21; $P = 0.0084$). The prognostic information provided by the assay was independent of other known clinical risk factors. This assay will be validated using previously collected clinical trial samples.

Salazar et al.[19] reported the results of a gene expression signature, known as ColoPrint, to determine prognosis for patients with stage II and III colon cancer. This assay requires fresh frozen tissue to isolate RNA using whole-genome oligonucleotide high-density microarray technology. Those patients classified as high-risk had a 5-year DFS of 67.2% versus 87.6% for low-risk patients (HR 2.5, 95% CI, 1.33 to 4.73; $P = 0.005$). Among stage II patients alone, the signature had an HR of 3.34 for high-risk patients ($P = 0.017$). The signature was an independent prognostic factor on multivariate analysis. However, the use of fresh frozen tissue samples does present a challenge in clinical practice.

The aforementioned assays have the potential to guide treatment in decision making in approximately 70% of patients who do not have clear risk factors for recurrence such as T4 tumors or dMMR by helping to identify patients at higher risk for recurrence in stage II colon cancer. It is important to recognize that these assays predicted the risk of recurrence and/or cancer-related death but did not predict benefit from chemotherapy. The routine use of the OncotypeDx Colon assay is being investigated in a clinical trial to determine how the assay affects oncologists' treatment recommendations as well as patient satisfaction.

ADJUVANT THERAPY FOR ELDERLY PATIENTS WITH COLON CANCER

While several retrospective analyses have demonstrated the survival benefit of adjuvant 5-FU therapy in the elderly,[20-22] the benefit of the addition of oxaliplatin for elderly patients is not clear. A pooled analysis of elderly patients participating in adjuvant and advanced setting clinical trials shows patients ≥70 years can tolerate FOLFOX just as well as younger patients with only neutropenia and thrombocytopenia occurring in significantly higher frequency than younger patients.[23] DFS and OS were similar between younger and older patients as well.

Subset analyses of the adjuvant oxaliplatin trials show conflicting results with regard to whether elderly patients benefit from oxaliplatin-based therapy compared with 5-FU alone. The MOSAIC and C-07 trials did not show benefit for this age group,[7,8] but the XELOXA trial did show a significant improvement in 3-year DFS for elderly patients. (OS results are pending.)[9] Two large pooled data sets also show differing results for the use of oxaliplatin-based therapy in the adjuvant setting. The first was a pooled analysis of 12,669 patients from 6 randomized, adjuvant colon cancer trials which included 2,170 patients ≥70 years.[24] No treatment benefit was seen in those patients treated with oxaliplatin regimens compared with fluoropyrimidine alone. The second study was a SEER-Medicare–based study which involved 8,294 patients >65 years, of which 816 received oxaliplatin-based therapy.[25] When compared with 5-FU/LV alone, it was associated with improved OS and colorectal cancer-specific survival. However, selection bias may have played a role in this population-based study since healthier patients often receive more aggressive treatment.

While the option remains to treat older patients with oxaliplatin-based therapy, it is clear that not all necessarily need doublet therapy. This provides an opportunity for the oncologist to tailor the treatment for the elderly individual. One should feel comfortable treating the elderly with comorbidities with fluoropyrimidine alone, given the lack of data showing a clear benefit from the addition of oxaliplatin in this age group.

CURRENT STANDARDS IN METASTATIC COLORECTAL CANCER

Over the past decade, there have been significant advances in the treatment of metastatic colorectal cancer (mCRC). For many years, 5-FU had been the standard of care and the only option for mCRC. In the mid-1990s, the third-generation platinum compound oxaliplatin and irinotecan, a topoisomerase I inhibitor, were introduced. These agents, in combination with 5-FU/LV, increased OS in patients with mCRC establishing combination chemotherapy as the standard of care in the first-line treatment of mCRC.[26-28] Use of both oxaliplatin and irinotecan in the course of treatment, regardless of sequence order, was shown to improve OS[29] and resulted in OS times in excess of 20 months, nearly double that of 5-FU alone.[30]

More recently, the addition of biologic agents, such as bevacizumab, cetuximab, and panitumumab, to standard cytotoxic chemotherapy has provided an additional survival benefit in mCRC. By binding to vascular endothelial growth factor receptor (VEGF), bevacizumab prevents receptor-mediated intracellular signaling necessary for angiogenesis,[31] thereby suppressing tumor growth and the development of new lesions. The epidermal growth factor receptor (EGFR) is involved in multiple processes that are downregulated in malignancies including cell differentiation, proliferation, migration, angiogenesis and apoptosis.[32] Monoclonal antibodies directed against EGFR (including cetuximab and panitumumab) have been developed with the goal of downstream signal transduction inhibition and modulation of tumor growth.

The development of newer cytotoxic chemotherapeutic agents and biologic therapies has expanded treatment for patients with CRC, in both the adjuvant setting and those with metastatic disease. Combining both cytotoxic chemotherapy and biologic agents has not only led to improved progression-free survival (PFS) and OS in the metastatic setting but also increases the chances of secondary resection for cure in select patients.

Cytotoxic Regimens for mCRC—The Chemotherapy Backbone

FOLFIRI

Two phase III trials have investigated the combination of irinotecan and 5-FU/LV (FOLFIRI) compared with 5-FU/LV, and both demonstrated improved response rate (RR) and PFS for the triple combination regimen.[33,34] The trial by Douillard et al.[33] reported an improved OS 17.4 for the irinotecan-containing regimen versus 14.1 months for the 5-FU/LV arm ($P = 0.031$). Kohne et al.[34] did not report a significant increase in OS for the triple combination regimen when compared with the 5-FU/LV arm, but it was felt that this was due to the availability of second- and third-line therapies. Thus, FOLFIRI became a standard for first-line treatment of mCRC.

FOLFOX

The phase III intergroup trial N9741 comparing FOLFOX, IFL (irinotecan, bolus fluorouracil, and leucovorin), and IROX established the role of FOLFOX in the first-line setting for mCRC.[27] The FOLFOX regimen resulted in a PFS of 8.7 months and OS of 19.5 months, significantly greater than either infusional 5-FU (IFL) or IROX. Results of this trial resulted in the widespread use of FOLFOX in the first-line setting for mCRC across the United States.

Toxicities from oxaliplatin administration include diarrhea, mucositis, neutropenia, and neuropathy. Strategies to minimize these toxicities include removing the second day 5-FU bolus (FOLFOX6) and reducing the biweekly oxaliplatin dose to 85 mg/m^2 (modified FOLFOX6).

Substituting Capecitabine

Trials combining the oral 5-FU prodrug capecitabine with oxaliplatin (in the form of CAPOX or XELOX) have shown efficacy comparable to infusional 5-FU/LV regimens in the treatment of mCRC.[35,36] A pooled analysis of six clinical trials including 3,494 patients investigating oxaliplatin plus capecitabine or infusional 5-FU showed that RRs overall were improved in the 5-FU arms compared with capecitabine, with an odds ratio of 0.85 (95% CI, 0.74 to 0.97; $P = 0.02$).[37] However, the improved RR did not translate into improved PFS or OS for the 5-FU arms. Based on results of the meta-analysis, capecitabine was found to be non-inferior to 5-FU. Regimens using bolus 5-FU had greater incidence of neutropenia, whereas the capecitabine regimens were more likely to cause thrombocytopenia and hand–foot syndrome. Of note, patients in the United States often do not tolerate capecitabine as well as European patients.[38] As a result, the dose of capecitabine is commonly reduced by 20% when used with oxaliplatin regimens, but this does not appear to compromise efficacy.[39]

Incorporating Targeted Therapy in mCRC Regimens

The current standard of care in advanced disease is to combine targeted therapy with cytotoxic chemotherapy, provided there are no contraindications to the specific agents. The following section discusses the evidence to support the use of this combination approach and, in the case of EGFR inhibitors, highlights new molecular markers used to predict which patients will benefit. Table 54.1 lists the advantages and disadvantages for the two classes of targeted therapy.

TABLE 54–1 Bevacizumab versus Endothelial Growth Factor Receptor Antibodies in Advanced Colorectal Cancer

Agent	Strength	Weakness
Bevacizumab	• Delay in tumor progression • Gain in time • Toxicity profile	• Limited single-agent activity • Weak effect on RR (per RECIST)
EGFR antibodies	• Single-agent activity • Consistent increase in RR • Activity independent of line of therapy • Predictive marker	• Gain in time to progression moderate • Toxicity profile

EGFR, endothelial growth factor receptor.

Antiangiogenic Agents

Bevacizumab

The pivotal phase III trial AVF2107 demonstrating benefit of bevacizumab in combination with chemotherapy in the first-line setting for mCRC was reported by Hurwitz et al. in 2004.[40] Patients were randomized to receive irinotecan, bolus fluorouracil, and leucovorin plus bevacizumab versus IFL plus placebo. Combination of IFL plus bevacizumab led to significantly higher RR (44.8% vs. 34.8%, $P = 0.004$), PFS (10.6 vs. 6.2 months, $P < 0.001$), and median survival (20.3 vs. 15.6 months, $P < 0.001$) when compared with IFL plus placebo group (Table 54.2). This trial led to the approval of bevacizumab for the first-line treatment of mCRC and established a new standard in first-line therapy.

The results of the AVF2107 trial prompted amendments of trials ongoing at the time to include bevacizumab. The NO16966 trial, originally designed to compare FOLFOX4 with XELOX as first-line treatment for mCRC, was amended to further randomize patients to receive bevacizumab or placebo in a 2 × 2 design.[41] The addition of bevacizumab significantly improved PFS, but there was no significant difference in OS (see Table 54.2). The authors speculated that the lack of survival benefit may be explained by the lack of bevacizumab therapy until progression, which resulted in shorter duration of bevacizumab therapy than prior studies. In those patients who did continue bevacizumab until progression, the "on-treatment" PFS was 10.4 months in the bevacizumab arm and 7.9 months in the control arms ($P < 0.0001$).

Three additional phase III trials have also demonstrated benefit for the addition of bevacizumab to standard chemotherapy with results as shown in Table 54.1. The Three Regimens of Eloxatin Evaluation (TREE-1) study compared mFOLFOX6, bolus 5-FU/oxaliplatin (bFOL), and capecitabine with oxaliplatin (CapeOx), and TREE-2 added bevacizumab to each arm.[39] There was no significant difference in overall response rate (ORR), time to treatment failure (TTF), or median OS among the oxaliplatin regimens in either the TREE-1 or TREE-2 cohorts. Statistical analysis to compare the TREE-1 and TREE-2 cohorts was not performed since the study was not designed to compare the two groups. However, a median OS of 26.1 months with mFOLFOX plus bevacizumab is among the highest reported in the literature. The addition of bevacizumab to oxaliplatin-based regimens did not significantly alter the toxicity profile.

In the E3200 study, mCRC patients refractory to irinotecan-based therapy were randomized to FOLFOX4, FOLFOX4 plus bevacizumab, or bevacizumab alone.[42] The bevacizumab dose was 10 mg/kg in both arms as opposed to 5 mg/kg used in first-line trials. The bevacizumab-only arm was closed early due to inferior survival found on interim analysis. The addition of bevacizumab to FOLFOX4 significantly extended median OS by 2 months when compared with FOLFOX4 alone.

The Bolus, Infusion, or Capecitabine with Camptosar ± Celecoxib (BICC-C) trial was originally designed to compare three irinotecan regimens as first-line treatment for mCRC: FOLFIRI, irinotecan plus bolus 5-FU/LV (mIFL), and irinotecan plus oral capecitabine (CapeIRI).[43] The trial was modified to compare FOLFIRI plus bevacizumab or mIFL plus bevacizumab. The CapeIRI arm was dropped due to toxicity reasons. In both phases of the BICC-C trial, FOLFIRI offered superior results when compared with alternative irinotecan-based regimens, and the addition of bevacizumab appears to provide additional survival benefit. FOLFIRI plus bevacizumab had a significantly higher median survival time compared with mIFL plus bevacizumab (OS not reached at the time of publication for FOLFIRI plus bevacizumab versus 19.2 months in the mIFL plus bevacizumab arm, $P = 0.007$).

Common side effects associated with bevacizumab include hypertension, epistaxis, headache, rash, chills, and proteinuria. Life-threatening complications such as arterial thrombotic events (ATEs), bleeding, gastrointestinal perforation, and wound healing complications are rare (1% to 2%).[44]

Aflibercept

Aflibercept (also known as VEGF trap) is a soluble fusion protein consisting of portions of the extracellular domains

TABLE 54-2 Phase III Trials Involving Bevacizumab in Advanced Colorectal Cancer

	Regimen	*n*	RR (%)	*P* Value	PFS (Months)	HR	*P* Value	OS (Months)	HR	*P* Value
First line										
AVR2107[41]	IFL + bev	402	44.8	0.004	10.6	0.54	<0.001	20.3	0.66	<0.001
	IFL	411	34.8	—	6.2	—	—	15.6	—	—
NO16966[42]	XELOX/FOLFOX4 + bev	699	49	0.31	9.4	0.83	0.0023	21.3	0.89	0.0769
	XELOX/FOLFOX4	701	47	—	8.0	—	—	19.9	—	—
TREE-1[40]	mFOLFOX6	49	41	—	8.7	—	—	19.2	—	—
	bFOL	50	20	—	6.9	—	—	17.9	—	—
	CapeOx	48	27	—	5.9	—	—	17.2	—	—
TREE-2[40]	mFOLFOX6 + bev	71	52	—	9.9	—	—	26.1	—	—
	bFOL + bev	70	39	—	8.3	—	—	20.4	—	—
	CapeOx + bev	72	46	—	10.3	—	—	24.6	—	—
BICC-C[44]	FOLFIRI	144	47.2	—	7.6	—	—	23.1	—	—
	mIFL	141	43.3	—	5.9	—	—	17.6	—	—
	CapeIri	145	38.6	—	5.8	—	—	18.9	—	—
	FOLFIRI + bev	57	57.9	—	11.2	—	0.28	NR	—	0.007
	mIFL + bev	60	53.3	—	8.3	—	—	19.2	—	—
Second line										
E3200[43]	FOLFOX4 + bev	291	22.7	<0.0001	7.3	0.61	<0.001	12.9	0.75	0.0011
	FOLFOX4	286	8.6	—	4.7	—	—	10.8	—	—
	bev	243	3.3	—	—	—	—	10.2	—	—

RR, response rate; PFS, progression-free survival; HR, hazard ratio; OS, overall survival; NR, not reported.

of human VEGFR1 and VEGFR2 fused to a human IgG1 Fc portion. Aflibercept binds all isoforms of VEGF-A, VEGF-B, and placental growth factor with higher affinity than the native receptors.[45]

Aflibercept combined with cytotoxic chemotherapy was recently studied in a randomized phase III trial involving 1,226 patients with advanced colorectal cancer, the VEGF Trap with Irinotecan in Colorectal cancer after failure of an oxaliplatin-containing regimen (VELOUR) trial.[46] Patients with mCRC who had previously progressed on an oxaliplatin-based regimen were randomized to receive either FOLFIRI + placebo or FOLFIRI + aflibercept. The addition of aflibercept to FOLFIRI in this second-line trial led to a significant improvement in PFS (6.9 vs. 4.7 months for FOLFIRI alone, HR 0.76, $P = 0.00007$), RR (19.8% vs. 11.1%, $P = 0.0001$), and OS (13.5 vs. 12.06 months, HR 0.82, $P = 0.0032$) when compared with FOLFIRI alone. The benefit was attenuated among the 28% of patients who had prior therapy with bevacizumab. When compared with the findings of the E3200 trial, comparing FOLFOX with or without bevacizumab in second-line therapy after failure of IFL, the PFS and OS on the VELOUR trial are remarkably similar, confirming a role for VEGF inhibition in second-line colorectal cancer.

EGFR Inhibitors

Cetuximab

In 2001, Saltz et al.[47] reported results of a phase II study investigating the activity of the EGFR inhibitor cetuximab in patients with EGRF-expressing mCRC refractory to 5-FU and irinotecan. In this trial, 121 patients were treated with weekly cetuximab at 400 mg/m^2 loading dose and 250 mg/m^2 for subsequent weekly doses, plus the same dose of irinotecan they were previously receiving. The addition of cetuximab to irinotecan produced a 17% partial RR and 31% of patients had minor responses or stable disease. A subsequent phase II trial of 57 patients showed activity of cetuximab alone at the same doses in irinotecan-refractory patients.[48] Partial responses were seen in 10.5% of patients and 35% of patients had either a minor response or stable disease.

The activity of cetuximab in chemotherapy-refractory patients was confirmed by a larger trial involving 329 patients with EGFR-expressing mCRC, reported by Cunningham et al. in 2004.[49] Patients were randomized to receive cetuximab plus irinotecan or cetuximab alone in a 2:1 ratio. The ORR was 22.9% (95% CI, 17.5 to 29.1) and 10.8% (95% CI, 5.7 to 18.1), respectively, $P = 0.007$. The median time to tumor progression (TTP) was also significantly longer in the combination therapy group (4.1 months) when compared with the cetuximab alone group (1.5 months) with HR 0.54 (95% CI, 0.42 to 0.71; $P < 0.001$). There was no statistically significant survival difference between the two groups, with a median OS of 8.6 months in the combination therapy arm and 6.9 months in the cetuximab alone arm ($P = 0.48$). The lack of OS benefit was felt due to cross over to receive irinotecan when patients in the cetuximab-only group progressed.

The major toxicities from the aforementioned trials attributable to cetuximab were cutaneous and allergic reactions. In the latter two trials, skin reactions of acne-form rash were seen in 80% to 88% of patients within 1 to 3 weeks after initiating therapy and 5% of patients experienced an allergic reaction. Interestingly, in the latter two studies, the degree of response appeared to correlate with the amount of skin toxicity, and patients with a skin rash had significantly improved survival compared with those who did not develop a rash. Allergic reactions respond to typical treatment, including epinephrine, antihistamines, and corticosteroids. The acne-form rash can be attenuated by the addition of minocycline.[50]

The aforementioned studies were conducted in patients with tumors expressing the EGFR, known to be present in approximately 60% to 80% of colorectal cancers.[48,49,51] However, neither the presence nor degree of EGFR expression appears to correlate with response to EGFR inhibitors; therefore, immunohistochemical testing for EGFR is no longer recommended.[48,49,52,53]

The Erbitux Plus Irinotecan for Metastatic Colorectal Cancer (EPIC) study investigated the use of irinotecan plus cetuximab versus irinotecan alone as second-line therapy for mCRC after oxaliplatin-based chemotherapy.[54] The combination of irinotecan and cetuximab was found to be superior to irinotecan alone in terms of RR, PFS, and quality of life analysis of global health. The two arms did not differ significantly in median OS and were felt to be a result of a large number of patients (46.9%) treated with cetuximab post-trial, with the majority (87.2%) in combination with irinotecan.

Panitumumab

Panitumumab, a human monoclonal antibody targeting the EGFR, also has activity in mCRC. Panitumumab was initially studied in the treatment-refractory setting and demonstrated survival benefit over best supportive care (BSC).[55] The Panitumumab Randomized trial In combination with chemotherapy for Metastatic colorectal cancer to determine Efficacy (PRIME) study used FOLFOX as a chemotherapy backbone for patients in the first-line setting of mCRC.[56] In this study, the addition of panitumumab resulted in a significant increase in PFS for KRAS wild-type (WT) patients (see below), 9.6 versus 8.0 months for FOLFOX alone (HR 0.80; 95% CI 0.66 to 0.97; *P* – 0.02).

Predictive Markers of EGFR Inhibitor Efficacy

KRAS

Recent research has identified a subset of individuals who do not benefit from therapy with EGFR inhibitors. This was first reported by Lievre et al.[57,58] who found patients with the KRAS mutation did not appear to benefit from cetuximab therapy. KRAS is a protein in the downstream intracellular signaling pathway of EGFR involved in cell differentiation, proliferation, and angiogenesis. Mutations in the KRAS gene cause KRAS to be constitutively activated rendering antibodies that target EGFR ineffective. This information led investigators to perform outcome analyses of phase III trials involving EGFR inhibitors according to KRAS status, the results of which are shown in Table 54.3.

Two randomized phase III trials of an EGFR inhibitor versus BSC as last-line therapy confirmed that patients with KRAS mutant tumors do not benefit from EGFR antibody therapy. In two separate trials, both panitumumab and cetuximab significantly improved RR and PFS over BSC alone.[59,60] Among patients who had tissue available for KRAS analysis, the benefit of the EGFR inhibitor over BSC was increased in KRAS WT patients.[55,61] Patients with KRAS mutant tumors had no benefit from the EGFR antibody in either trial. Among the BSC groups, those individuals with KRAS mutations did not fare worse than those without, suggesting this is not a prognostic marker but merely a predictive marker of outcomes.

Similar results were seen with the use of cetuximab in combination with cytotoxic therapy in the first-line setting of mCRC in two phase III trials. The Cetuximab Combined with Irinotecan in First-Line Therapy for Metastatic Colorectal Cancer (CRYSTAL) trial investigated FOLFIRI versus FOLFIRI plus cetuximab in the first line of mCRC.[62] Cetuximab, in combination with FOLFIRI, increased RRs by approximately 8% and significantly prolonged PFS by 0.9 months. Median OS was not statistically different between the two arms. KRAS mutation testing was done on archived tumor tissue of 540 patients (45%). For KRAS WT patients, the addition of cetuximab to FOLFIRI improved median PFS for 9.9 versus 8.7 months and ORR increased by 16%. In patients with KRAS mutations, no improvement in RR or PFS was achieved by adding cetuximab to FOLFIRI.[62] The addition of cetuximab to FOLFIRI did not improve OS in either treatment arm, but two-thirds of patients received subsequent chemotherapy likely confounding the results.

The initial results of the Oxaliplatin and Cetuximab in First-Line Treatment of mCRC (OPUS) trial comparing FOLFOX4 versus FOLFOX4 plus cetuximab in the first-line treatment of mCRC showed the addition of cetuximab did not significantly improve PFS or RR compared with FOLFOX alone.[63] ORR was 46% versus 36% and odds ratio 1.52 (95% CI, 0.98 to 2.36, $P = 0.064$). The investigators also performed a retrospective analysis to evaluate the impact of KRAS mutations on treatment response.[64] In the KRAS WT group, the addition of cetuximab to FOLFOX4 significantly increased RRs (61% vs. 37%, odds ratio = 2.54; 95% CI, 1.24 to 5.23; $P = 0.011$) and median PFS (7.7 vs. 7.2 months, $P = 0.016$) compared with FOLFOX4 alone. In the KRAS mutant group, there was a trend toward worse RRs in the cetuximab plus FOLFOX4 arm versus FOLFOX4 alone (33% vs. 49%, $P = 0.11$) and median PFS significantly worsened (5.5 vs. 8.6 months, $P = 0.019$).

Two recently completed trials evaluating the use of cetuximab with cytotoxic therapy in the first-line setting of mCRC have failed to show a PFS benefit, even among KRAS WT individuals. In the COntinuous chemotherapy

TABLE 54–3 Phase III Endothelial Growth Factor Receptor Inhibitor Trials in Advanced Colorectal Cancer

Trial	Regimen	n	RR (%)	P Value	PFS Months	HR	P Value	OS (Months)	HR	P Value
First line										
CRYSTAL[65]	FOLFIRI + cetuximab	599	46.9	0.004	8.9	0.85	0.048	19.9	0.93	0.31
	FOLFIRI	599	38.7	—	8.0	—	—	18.6	—	—
	WT KRAS FOLFIRI + cetuximab	172	59.3	NR	9.9	0.68	0.02	24.9	0.84	NR
	WT KRAS FOLFIRI	176	43.2	—	8.7	—	—	21.0	—	—
	Mut KRAS FOLFIRI + cetuximab	105	36.2	NR	7.6	1.07	0.75	17.5	1.03	NR
	Mut KRAS FOLFIRI	87	40.2	—	8.1	—	—	17.7	—	—
OPUS[67]	FOLFOX4 + cetuximab	169	46	0.64	7.2	0.931	0.617	NR	NR	NR
	FOLFOX4	168	36	—	7.2	—	—	NR	—	—
	WT KRAS FOLFOX4 + cetuximab	61	61	0.011	7.7	0.570	0.0163	NR	NR	NR
	WT KRAS FOLFOX4	73	37	—	7.2	—	—	NR	—	—
	Mut KRAS FOLFOX4 + cetuximab	52	33	0.106	5.5	1.8	0.0192	NR	NR	NR
	Mut KRAS FOLFOX4	47	49	—	8.6	—	—	NR	—	—
PRIME[58]	*WT KRAS* FOLFOX4 + panitumumab	325	55	0.068	9.6	0.80	0.02	23.9	0.83	0.072
	WT KRAS FOLFOX4	331	48	—	8.0	—	—	19.7	—	—
	Mut KRAS FOLFOX4 + cetuximab	221	40	—	7.3	1.29	0.02	15.5	1.24	0.068
	Mut KRAS FOLFOX4	219	40	—	8.8	—	—	19.3	—	—
COIN[68]	*WT KRAS* oxaliplatin + fluorp + cetuximab	362	64	0.049	8.6	0.96	0.60	17.0	1.04	0.67
	WT KRAS oxaliplatin + fluorp	367	57	—	8.6	—	—	17.9	—	—
	Mut KRAS oxaliplatin + fluorp + cetuximab	297	NR	NR	NR	NR	NR	13.6	0.98	0.80
	Mut KRAS oxaliplatin + fluorp	268	NR	—	NR	—	NR	14.8	—	—
NORDIC VII[69] First line	*WT KRAS* FLOX + cetuximab	303	46	0.87	7.9	1.07	0.66	20.1	1.14	0.66
	WT KRAS FLOX	—	47	—	8.6	—	—	22.0	—	—
	Mut KRAS FLOX + cetuximab	195	49	0.31	9.2	0.71	0.07	21.1	1.03	0.89
	Mut KRAS FLOX	—	40	—	7.8	—	—	20.4	—	—
Second line										
EPIC[56]	Irinotecan + cetuximab	648	16.4	<0.0001	4.0	0.69	<0.0001	10.7	0.9775	0.71
	Irinotecan	650	4.2	—	2.6	—	—	10.0	—	—
181[59]	*WT KRAS* FOLFIRI + panitumumab	303	35	<0.001	5.9	0.73	0.004	14.5	0.85	0.12
	WT KRAS FOLFIRI	294	10	—	3.9	—	—	12.5	—	—
	Mut KRAS FOLFIRI + panitumumab	238	13	—	5.0	0.85	0.14	11.8	0.94	NR
	Mut KRAS FOLFIRI	248	14	—	4.9	—	—	11.1	—	—
Last line										
Cunningham[51]	Irinotecan + cetuximab	218	22.9	0.007	4.1	0.54	<0.001	8.6	0.91	0.48
	Cetuximab	111	10.8	—	1.5	—	—	6.9	—	—
VanCutsem[62]	Panitumumab	231	10	<0.0001	8.0 wk	0.54	<0.0001	ND	1.00	0.81
	BSC	232	0	—	7.3 wk	—	—	—	—	—
Amado[57]	*WT KRAS* panitumumab	124	17	—	12.3 wk	0.45	<0.0001	8.1	0.99	—
KRAS analysis	*WT KRAS* BSC	119	—	—	7.3 wk	—	—	7.6	—	—
	Mut KRAS panitumumab	84	0	—	7.4 wk	0.99	—	4.9	1.02	—
	Mut KRAS BSC	100	0	—	7.4 wk	—	—	4.4	—	—
Jonker[63]	Cetuximab	287	8	<0.001	1.9	0.68	<0.001	6.1	0.77	0.005
	BSC	285	0	—	1.8	—	—	4.6	—	—
Karapetis[64] KRAS analysis	*WT KRAS* cetuximab	—	12.8	—	3.7	0.4	<0.001	9.5	0.55	<0.001
	WT KRAS BSC	—	0	—	1.9	—	—	4.8	—	—
	Mut KRAS cetuximab	—	1.2	—	1.8	0.99	0.96	4.6	0.98	0.89
	Mut KRAS BSC	—	0	—	1.8	—	—	4.5	—	—

RR, response rate; PFS, progression-free survival; HR, hazard ratio; OS, overall survival; WT, wild type; MT, mutant; ND, no difference; NR, not reported; fluorp, fluoropyrimidine; wk, weeks.

plus cetuximab or INtermittent chemotherapy (COIN) study, patients with previously untreated mCRC were randomized to receive an oxaliplatin-based regimen (CAPOX or FOLFOX) with or without cetuximab.[65] Among KRAS WT patients (see below), there was no benefit with the addition of cetuximab, with PFS of 8.6 months in both arms. Likewise, the NORDIC VII trial randomized patients to receive FLOX plus cetuximab versus FLOX.[66] KRAS WT patients had a PFS of 7.9 months in the experimental arm compared with 8.7 months in the control arm (HR 1.07; $P = 0.66$). The reasons for the lack of benefit with addition of cetuximab to first-line therapy in the COIN and NORDIC VII trials, as opposed to the PRIME and CRYSTAL trials (see below), remain unclear. However, multiple trials have consistently shown benefit in later lines of therapy (see Table 54.3).

The above analyses demonstrate that patients with KRAS mutant tumors (approximately 40% of all patients with mCRC) do not derive benefit from treatment with EGFR inhibitors. Tumors should be tested for KRAS status prior to initiation of therapy with cetuximab or panitumumab. This will prevent patients from receiving a costly and potentially harmful medication where benefit is lacking.

BRAF

BRAF is a primary effector of the KRAS signaling. Mutations in the BRAF gene occur most frequently on exon 15 (V600E) and are present in about 4% to 14% of patients with CRC.[67] It is mutually exclusive in the presence of a KRAS mutation. Retrospective data suggest that the BRAF mutation is also a predictive marker of a response to EGFR inhibitors. In a small retrospective analysis, it was shown that patients with KRAS WT but BRAF mutant tumors had an impaired response to EGFR inhibition with either cetuximab or panitumumab.[68] This was confirmed in an analysis of the CRYSTAL study. Patients with KRAS WT/BRAF mutant tumors in the cetuximab arm did not have a statistically significant benefit in RR, PFS, or OS as opposed to those with KRAS WT/BRAF WT tumors.[69]

NRAS and PIK3CA

In addition to KRAS and BRAF, there is also preliminary evidence that mutations in two other components of the signal transduction pathway, NRAS and PI3K, also render tumors unresponsive to EGFR inhibitors.[70] A total of 773 tumor samples from chemotherapy-refractory patients who underwent treatment with cetuximab plus chemotherapy were evaluated for mutations in KRAS, BRAF, NRAS, and PIK3CA. Overall, the RR rate for the unselected population was 24.5%. When selected for KRAS WT, the response increased to 36.3%, and when selected for KRAS, BRAF, NRAS, and PIK3CA WT, the RR was 41.2%. Further validation on the use of these markers as predictors of EGFR inhibitor response is needed, but this study highlights the potential ability to carefully select patients with the highest chance to benefit from EGFR inhibition.

Combined VEGF and EGFR Inhibition

The combination of VEGF and EGFR inhibition has been tested in several clinical trials. Initially, the combination appeared promising based on results of the randomized phase II study BOND2, which evaluated cetuximab and bevacizumab with or without irinotecan in mCRC patients who failed at least one irinotecan-containing regimen.[71] Among the patients randomized to the triple therapy arm, median TTP was 7.3 months, RR was 37%, and OS was 14.5 months. In the cetuximab plus bevacizumab arm, median TTP was 4.9 months, RR was 20%, and the OS was 11.4 months. Toxicities were not greater than what was anticipated with each of the drugs alone.

In contrast to BOND2, the Panitumumab Advanced Colorectal Cancer Evaluation (PACCE) trial comparing FOLFOX or FOLFIRI plus bevacizumab, with or without panitumumab, showed inferior PFS in the panitumumab arm (10.0 months) compared with the control arm (11.4 months; HR, 1.27; 95% CI, 1.06 to 1.52).[72] While RR did not differ among the groups, patients receiving FOLFOX, bevacizumab, plus panitumumab had worse OS compared with FOLFOX and bevacizumab alone (19.4 vs. 24.5 months, respectively; HR, 1.43; 95% CI, 1.11 to 1.83) and did not differ in the FOLFIRI-containing patients. The decrease in OS in the FOLFOX arms was felt to be a result of the increased toxicity in the panitumumab arm, which included grade 3/4 skin, diarrhea infections, and pulmonary embolism.

However, the results of the CAIRO2 study confirmed that combined VEGF and EGFR inhibition is ineffective and potentially harmful.[73] Patients with untreated mCRC were randomized to receive capecitabine, oxaliplatin, and bevacizumab with or without cetuximab. The four-drug regimen resulted in worse PFS (9.4 months) when compared with the control arm (10.7 months; $P = 0.01$). RR and OS did not differ between the two arms, but quality of life was significantly decreased in the cetuximab arm. Based on the results of the PACCE and CAIRO2 studies, dual antibody therapy should not be performed outside of a clinical trial.

STRATEGIES TO MAXIMIZE THERAPEUTIC BENEFIT OF AVAILABLE REGIMENS

The optimal way to manage patients with mCRC should be determined on an individual basis. The first priority is to decide whether the patient has resectable or potentially resectable disease since surgery is the only potential for cure in these patients. For the majority of patients who will not be candidates for surgical resection, the goal is to administer the available agents in a manner that will maximize survival while preserving quality of life.

Resectable or Potentially Resectable Disease

Neoadjuvant Therapy

There is no clear proven benefit for preoperative systemic therapy for those patients whose liver disease is resectable upon presentation. Potential benefits to this approach include gaining information on the biology of the disease, determining sensitivity to chemotherapeutic agents, and treating occult metastases which would theoretically reduce the risk of recurrence.[74] Disadvantages include increased perioperative morbidity and missing a window of opportunity for resection.[75]

There is one European phase III trial comparing perioperative therapy (six cycles of FOLFOX4 before and after surgery) with surgery alone.[76] Eligible patients who received perioperative therapy had an 8.1% improvement in 3-year PFS over patients in the surgery alone arm (HR of 0.77, 95% CI, 0.60 to 1.00; $P = 0.041$). Among the patients who underwent surgery, 3-year PFS was increased to 9.2% (HR 0.73, 95% CI, 0.55 to 0.97, $P = 0.025$). Eight patients had progression of disease that prevented them from undergoing resection. Postoperative complications, including biliary fistula, hepatic failure, intra-abdominal infection, and the need for re-operation, were higher in the perioperative therapy arm (25% vs. 16%, $P = 0.04$), although all of these complications were reversible.

Guidance on whether to administer neoadjuvant therapy to patients with liver-limited metastatic disease is available from a retrospective study of 1,568 patients who underwent hepatectomy reported by Nordlinger et al.[77] This study identified several factors associated with poorer survival, including multiple metastases, lesions > 5 cm, synchronous presentation, high tumor marker levels, and lymph node–positive primary lesions. Therefore, it is reasonable to consider neoadjuvant therapy in patients who have one or more of these factors or in patients who would appear to have a difficult resection without shrinkage of disease.[78]

Conversion Therapy

Approximately 20% to 25% of patients have resectable disease upon presentation and an additional 10% to 15% of patients will achieve a resectable status with systemic therapy, known as conversion therapy.[79,80] Specifically regarding metastases to the liver, eligibility for surgical resection no longer depends upon the number and size of lesions, but rather on the amount of remaining viable liver after resection, generally about 30% of initial liver volume.[80] As a result, a greater number of patients are undergoing resection of their liver metastases. The 5-year survival of these patients now ranges between 45% and 60%.[81,82]

In a retrospective analysis of unresectable liver-limited mCRC, 51% of patients with unresectable liver disease responded well enough to combination 5-FU/LV/oxaliplatin chemotherapy to undergo surgical resection with curative intent.[83] Median survival was improved (48 months; 95% CI, 25 to 71) when compared with those who were unable to undergo resection (15.5 months; 95% CI, 13.5 to 17.5). Two prospective trials have previously documented improved resection rates with therapy containing oxaliplatin when compared with regimens without oxaliplatin,[30,84] and conversion of unresectable to resectable disease has been seen with irinotecan-based regimens as well.[85] Survival benefit with resection of liver metastases whether they are resected initially or down-sized by chemotherapy and then resected has been achieved.[86]

Suggestion from preliminary results of a phase II trial has shown that bevacizumab may add benefit in the neoadjuvant setting.[87] Retrospective data from randomized phase III trials also provide evidence for the fact that bevacizumab increased RR, potentially improving chances for respectability.[39,42,43] In the AVF2107 trial, 8.4% of patients in the bevacizumab arms underwent metastectomy with curative intent versus 6.1% in the chemotherapy alone arms.[40]

Cetuximab has also been shown to increase conversion rates. Results from the CRYSTAL trial show that FOLFIRI plus cetuximab in the neoadjuvant setting led to a greater percentage of patients being able to undergo curative resection (7.0% vs. 3.7%) and improved R0 resection rates (4.8% vs. 1.7%).[62] Similarly, the addition of cetuximab to FOLFOX4, compared with FOLFOX4 alone, improved resection rates (6.5% vs. 3.6%) and R0 resection (4.7% vs. 2.0%), as seen in the OPUS trial.[63] There is also evidence that the addition of cetuximab to FOLFIRI in chemorefractory patients leads to improved resectability rates.[88]

Two additional issues must be considered with any type of preoperative therapy. First, there is potential for hepatotoxicity from the systemic agents themselves. Patients have a greater rate of postoperative complications with increasing cycles of chemotherapy.[89,90] Second, preoperative therapy may produce a radiologic complete response interfering with the intraoperative detection of lesions. This situation limits the ability of achieving an R0 resection since there is a high likelihood of microscopic residual disease.[91] Therefore, it is generally recommended that preoperative chemotherapy be limited to four to six cycles or until patients become resectable.

Adjuvant Therapy

The role of adjuvant therapy after resection of mCRC is not clearly defined. An analysis of pooled data from two randomized phase III trials comparing adjuvant therapy with 5-FU versus observation after R0 resection showed a non-significant improvement in PFS (27.9 vs. 18.8 months; HR = 1.32; 95% CI, 1.00 to 1.76; $P = 0.058$) and median OS (62.2 vs. 47.3 months, HR = 1.32; 95% CI, 0.95 to 1.82; $P = 0.095$) with adjuvant therapy.[92] Additionally, two large international retrospective studies with adjuvant 5-FU did show an OS benefit compared with surgery alone.[93,94]

With the development of more effective therapy, adjuvant therapy likely improves survival after R0 resection. Although an oxaliplatin-based regimen has not formally been tested against surgery alone, it is generally assumed that the benefits of FOLFOX in patients with resected stage II/III disease seen in the MOSAIC trial[6,7] would also apply to resected mCRC. FOLFIRI, after resection of colorectal liver metastases, has not been shown to provide significant benefit over 5-FU alone.[95] Based on the results of the NASBP C-08 trial which showed no OS benefit of adding bevacizumab to FOLFOX for resected stage II/III CRC, the use of bevacizumab as adjuvant therapy cannot be recommended outside of a clinical trial.[96]

Unresectable Disease

The standard of care in the first-line setting of unresectable mCRC is triple-drug cytotoxic chemotherapy in combination with bevacizumab. FOLFOX and FOLFIRI have been shown to have similar efficacy in terms of RR, PFS, and OS.[30,97] The choice between whether to use FOLFOX or FOLFIRI should depend upon the anticipated toxicity profile. Oxaliplatin causes both an acute, cold-sensitivity neuropathy and a long-term peripheral neuropathy, which develop with cumulative doses. The main side effects of irinotecan include diarrhea, myelosuppression, and alopecia.

Special considerations exist for the use of bevacizumab in combination with cytotoxic chemotherapy. There is a 2-fold risk of ATEs with the use of bevacizumab in patients greater than 65 years of age and a 3.6-fold risk in patients with a prior history of ATEs.[98] Analysis of the BRiTE (Bevacizumab regimens: Investigation of treatment side effects and safety) registry confirmed an increased risk of ATEs in patients greater than 75 years.[99] Therefore, caution should be taken when considering bevacizumab in the elderly, and bevacizumab is contraindicated for those with prior ATEs.

As noted above, the use of cetuximab and panitumumab should be restricted to patients with WT KRAS status. Additionally, the rash associated with the use of these agents is a consideration for those who are concerned about cosmesis, such as those who do public speaking.

Stop-and-Go Strategy

In the United States, FOLFOX is most commonly used in first-line therapy for mCRC. In a detailed analysis of N9741, neurotoxicity and myelosuppression were the most frequent dose-limiting toxicities with FOLFOX.[100] In an attempt to minimize oxaliplatin neurotoxicity, the method of stop-and-go oxaliplatin administration was investigated in the optimal duration of oxaliplatin (OPTIMOX) trials.[101,102] In the OPTIMOX1 trial, patients were randomized to arm A, FOLFOX4 until disease progression or unacceptable toxicity, or arm B, FOLFOX7 for six cycles with maintenance 5FU/LV until progression and then reintroduction of FOLFOX7 for six more cycles. The two arms did not differ in RR (58.5% in arm A; 59.2% in arm B; P = NS), PFS (9.0 months in arm A; 8.7 months in arm B; $P = 0.04$), or OS (19.3 months arm A; 21.2 months arm B; HR = 0.93; 95% CI, 0.72 to 1.11; $P = 0.49$). Toxicity profiles did not differ significantly between the two arms. As expected, the risk of developing grade 3 to 4 toxicity, including grade 3 neuropathy, was reduced during the oxaliplatin-free interval in arm B.

Only 40.1% of patients in arm B of the OPTIMOX1 trial received the per-protocol reintroduction of oxaliplatin. This was due to progression (18.5%), toxicity (18.4%), and secondary surgery (5.5%), and no specific reason was given in 17.5% of the patients. Since the majority of patients did not receive oxaliplatin reintroduction and survival rates were similar, it leaves the question of whether the full clinical benefits were achieved with six cycles of FOLFOX7. However, patients who were treated at centers that reintroduced oxaliplatin in greater than 50% of patients had an overall median survival time of 25.5 months. While the authors questioned the feasibility of oxaliplatin reintroduction due to the numerous protocol violations, this improved survival time suggests it could have an impact on survival.

Results from the OPTIMOX2 trial stress the importance of maintenance therapy between intervals of FOLFOX chemotherapy.[101] This phase II trial randomized patients to an OPTIMOX1 regimen with six cycles of FOLFOX7, followed by maintenance of 5-FU/LV until progression and then reintroduction of FOLFOX7. The OPTIMOX2 arm completely stopped chemotherapy after six cycles of FOLFOX7, with reintroduction of FOLFOX7 on progression before tumors reached baseline measurements. There was a trend toward improved PFS (36 weeks in the OPTIMOX1 arm versus 29 weeks in the OPTIMOX2 arm, $P = 0.08$). The median OS was 24.6 months in the OPTIMOX1 arm and 18.9 months in the OPTIMOX2 arm, which was statistically significant ($P = 0.05$). Based on results from this study, chemotherapy-free intervals are not recommended for patients with mCRC.

The intermittent administration of oxaliplatin and the addition of bevacizumab in the first-line treatment of patients with mCRC were investigated in the Combined Oxaliplatin Neurotoxicity Prevention Trial (CONcePT).[103] Patients were randomized to receive continuous or intermittent FOLFOX plus bevacizumab. In the intermittent arm, if patients had at least stable disease after eight 2-weekly cycles of FOLFOX plus bevacizumab, oxaliplatin was stopped and a maintenance therapy with infusional 5-FU/LV plus bevacizumab was started. After another eight cycles, oxaliplatin was re-introduced. TTF, the primary end point of the trial, was significantly longer in patients receiving the intermittent oxaliplatin schedule, 5.6 versus 4.2 months with an HR of 0.58 and a P-value of 0.0025. There was also a strong trend toward longer PFS on the intermittent oxaliplatin arm as well as a more than 50% reduced incidence of severe neurotoxicity (10% vs. 24%) when compared with the continuous oxaliplatin arm.

CONCLUSIONS

Incorporating both clinical and molecular factors is crucial for individualized care of the patient with early-stage colon cancer as well as advanced disease. Deciding on the appropriate therapy for resected stage II and III disease should involve a discussion on the degree of benefit, carefully weighing the long-term risks of oxaliplatin-based therapy.

The optimal approach to the patient with mCRC should be determined on an individual basis, utilizing a multidisciplinary team consisting of surgeons, medical oncologists, radiation oncologists, and radiologists. Patients with resectable or potentially resectable disease may be considered for neoadjuvant and subsequent adjuvant therapy. Targeted therapies, especially when combined with cytotoxic therapy, have improved RRs and survival outcomes for patients with advanced disease, and current predictive markers for the EGFR inhibitors help determine which patients stand to benefit. Strategies such as the intermittent administration of oxaliplatin may enable the clinician to maximize therapeutic benefit while maintaining quality of life for the patient.

REFERENCES

1. Moertel CG, Fleming TR, Macdonald JS, et al. Levamisole and fluorouracil for adjuvant therapy of resected colon carcinoma. *N Engl J Med.* 1990;322:352-358.
2. Moertel CG, Fleming TR, Macdonald JS, et al. Fluorouracil plus levamisole as effective adjuvant therapy after resection of stage III colon carcinoma: a final report. *Ann Intern Med.* 1995;122:321-326.
3. Wolmark N, Rockette H, Fisher B, et al. The benefit of leucovorin-modulated fluorouracil as postoperative adjuvant therapy for primary colon cancer: results from National Surgical Adjuvant Breast and Bowel Project protocol C-03. *J Clin Oncol.* 1993;11:1879-1887.
4. Haller DG, Catalano PJ, Macdonald JS, et al. Phase III study of fluorouracil, leucovorin, and levamisole in high-risk stage II and III colon cancer: final report of Intergroup 0089. *J Clin Oncol.* 2005;23:8671-8678.
5. Efficacy of adjuvant fluorouracil and folinic acid in colon cancer. International Multicentre Pooled Analysis of Colon Cancer Trials (IMPACT) investigators. *Lancet.* 1995;345:939-944.
6. Andre T, Boni C, Mounedji-Boudiaf L, et al. Oxaliplatin, fluorouracil, and leucovorin as adjuvant treatment for colon cancer. *N Engl J Med.* 2004;350:2343-2351.
7. Andre T, Boni C, Navarro M, et al. Improved overall survival with oxaliplatin, fluorouracil, and leucovorin as adjuvant treatment in stage II or III colon cancer in the MOSAIC trial. *J Clin Oncol.* 2009;27:3109-3116.
8. Kuebler JP, Wieand HS, O'Connell MJ, et al. Oxaliplatin combined with weekly bolus fluorouracil and leucovorin as surgical adjuvant chemotherapy for stage II and III colon cancer: results from NSABP C-07. *J Clin Oncol.* 2007;25:2198-2204.
9. Haller DG, Tabernero J, Maroun J, et al. Capecitabine plus oxaliplatin compared with fluorouracil and folinic acid as adjuvant therapy for stage III colon cancer. *J Clin Oncol.* 2011;29:1465-1471.
10. Quasar Collaborative G, Gray R, Barnwell J, et al. Adjuvant chemotherapy versus observation in patients with colorectal cancer: a randomised study. *Lancet.* 2007;370:2020-2029.
11. Yothers GA, Allegra CJ, O'Connell MJ, et al. The efficacy of oxaliplatin (Ox) when added to 5-fluorouracil/leucovorin (FU/L) in stage II colon cancer *J Clin Oncol.* 2011;29(suppl):Abstract 3507.
12. Bertagnolli MM, Niedzwiecki D, Compton CC, et al. Microsatellite instability predicts improved response to adjuvant therapy with irinotecan, fluorouracil, and leucovorin in stage III colon cancer: Cancer and Leukemia Group B Protocol 89803. *J Clin Oncol.* 2009;27:1814-1821.
13. Carethers JM, Chauhan DP, Fink D, et al. Mismatch repair proficiency and in vitro response to 5-fluorouracil. *Gastroenterology.* 1999;117:123-131.
14. Ribic CM, Sargent DJ, Moore MJ, et al. Tumor microsatellite-instability status as a predictor of benefit from fluorouracil-based adjuvant chemotherapy for colon cancer. *N Engl J Med.* 2003;349:247-257.
15. Sargent DJ, Marsoni S, Monges G, et al. Defective mismatch repair as a predictive marker for lack of efficacy of fluorouracil-based adjuvant therapy in colon cancer. *J Clin Oncol.* 2010;28:3219-3226.
16. Waldman SA, Hyslop T, Schulz S, et al. Association of GUCY2C expression in lymph nodes with time to recurrence and disease-free survival in pN0 colorectal cancer. *JAMA.* 2009;301:745-752.
17. Gray RG, Quirke P, Handley K, et al. Validation study of a quantitative multigene reverse transcriptase-polymerase chain reaction assay for assessment of recurrence risk in patients with stage II colon cancer. *J Clin Oncol.* 2011;29(35):4611-4619.
18. Kennedy RD, Bylesjo M, Kerr P, et al. Development and independent validation of a prognostic assay for stage II colon cancer using formalin-fixed paraffin-embedded tissue. *J Clin Oncol.* 2011;29(35):4620-4626.
19. Salazar R, Roepman P, Capella G, et al. Gene expression signature to improve prognosis prediction of stage II and III colorectal cancer. *J Clin Oncol.* 2011;29:17-24.
20. Jessup JM, Stewart A, Greene FL, Minsky BD. Adjuvant chemotherapy for stage III colon cancer: implications of race/ethnicity, age, and differentiation. *JAMA.* 2005;294:2703-2711.
21. Sargent DJ, Goldberg RM, Jacobson SD, et al. A pooled analysis of adjuvant chemotherapy for resected colon cancer in elderly patients. *N Engl J Med.* 2001;345:1091-1097.
22. Sundararajan V, Mitra N, Jacobson JS, Grann VR, Heitjan DF, Neugut AI. Survival associated with 5-fluorouracil-based adjuvant chemotherapy among elderly patients with node-positive colon cancer. *Ann Intern Med.* 2002;136:349-357.
23. Goldberg RM, Tabah-Fisch I, Bleiberg H, et al. Pooled analysis of safety and efficacy of oxaliplatin plus fluorouracil/leucovorin administered bimonthly in elderly patients with colorectal cancer. *J Clin Oncol.* 2006;24:4085-4091.
24. Jackson McCleary NA, Meyerhardt J, Green E, et al. Impact of older age on the efficacy of newer adjuvant therapies in >12,500 patients (pts) with stage II/III colon cancer: findings from the ACCENT database. *J Clin Oncol.* 2009;27(suppl):15s. Abstract 4010.
25. Hsiao FS, Mullins CD, Onukwugha E, Pandya NB, Seal BS, Hanna N. Relative survival of adjuvant chemotherapy using 5-FU/LV alone, oxaliplatin, or irinotecan-based combination regimens among stage III colon cancer patients age 65 and older: an analysis using SEER-Medicare data. 2010 Gastrointestinal Cancers Symposium; 2010. Abstract 360.
26. de Gramont A, Figer A, Seymour M, et al. Leucovorin and fluorouracil with or without oxaliplatin as first-line treatment in advanced colorectal cancer. *J Clin Oncol.* 2000;18:2938-2947.
27. Goldberg RM, Sargent DJ, Morton RF, et al. A randomized controlled trial of fluorouracil plus leucovorin, irinotecan, and oxaliplatin combinations in patients with previously untreated metastatic colorectal cancer. *J Clin Oncol.* 2004;22:23-30.
28. Saltz LB, Cox JV, Blanke C, et al. Irinotecan plus fluorouracil and leucovorin for metastatic colorectal cancer. Irinotecan Study Group. *N Engl J Med.* 2000;343:905-914.
29. Grothey A, Sargent D, Goldberg RM, Schmoll HJ. Survival of patients with advanced colorectal cancer improves with the availability of fluorouracil-leucovorin, irinotecan, and oxaliplatin in the course of treatment. *J Clin Oncol.* 2004;22:1209-1214.
30. Tournigand C, Andre T, Achille E, et al. FOLFIRI followed by FOLFOX6 or the reverse sequence in advanced colorectal cancer: a randomized GERCOR study. *J Clin Oncol.* 2004;22:229-237.
31. Willett CG, Boucher Y, di Tomaso E, et al. Direct evidence that the VEGF-specific antibody bevacizumab has antivascular effects in human rectal cancer. *Nat Med.* 2004;10:145-147.
32. Ciardiello F, Tortora G. A novel approach in the treatment of cancer: targeting the epidermal growth factor receptor. *Clin Cancer Res.* 2001;7:2958-2970.
33. Douillard JY, Cunningham D, Roth AD, et al. Irinotecan combined with fluorouracil compared with fluorouracil alone as first-line treatment for metastatic colorectal cancer: a multicentre randomised trial. *Lancet.* 2000;355:1041-1047.
34. Kohne CH, van Cutsem E, Wils J, et al. Phase III study of weekly high-dose infusional fluorouracil plus folinic acid with or without irinotecan in patients with metastatic colorectal

cancer: European Organisation for Research and Treatment of Cancer Gastrointestinal Group Study 40986. *J Clin Oncol.* 2005;23:4856-4865.
35. Cassidy J, Clarke S, Diaz-Rubio E, et al. Randomized phase III study of capecitabine plus oxaliplatin compared with fluorouracil/folinic acid plus oxaliplatin as first-line therapy for metastatic colorectal cancer. *J Clin Oncol.* 2008;26:2006-2012.
36. Porschen R, Arkenau HT, Kubicka S, et al. Phase III study of capecitabine plus oxaliplatin compared with fluorouracil and leucovorin plus oxaliplatin in metastatic colorectal cancer: a final report of the AIO Colorectal Study Group. *J Clin Oncol.* 2007;25:4217-4223.
37. Arkenau HT, Arnold D, Cassidy J, et al. Efficacy of oxaliplatin plus capecitabine or infusional fluorouracil/leucovorin in patients with metastatic colorectal cancer: a pooled analysis of randomized trials. *J Clin Oncol.* 2008;26:5910-5917.
38. Haller DG, Cassidy J, Clarke SJ, et al. Potential regional differences for the tolerability profiles of fluoropyrimidines. *J Clin Oncol.* 2008;26:2118-2123.
39. Hochster HS, Hart LL, Ramanathan RK, et al. Safety and efficacy of oxaliplatin and fluoropyrimidine regimens with or without bevacizumab as first-line treatment of metastatic colorectal cancer: results of the TREE study. *J Clin Oncol.* 2008;26:3523-3529.
40. Hurwitz H, Fehrenbacher L, Novotny W, et al. Bevacizumab plus irinotecan, fluorouracil, and leucovorin for metastatic colorectal cancer. *N Engl J Med.* 2004;350:2335-2342.
41. Saltz LB, Clarke S, Diaz-Rubio E, et al. Bevacizumab in combination with oxaliplatin-based chemotherapy as first-line therapy in metastatic colorectal cancer: a randomized phase III study. *J Clin Oncol.* 2008;26:2013-2019.
42. Giantonio BJ, Catalano PJ, Meropol NJ, et al. Bevacizumab in combination with oxaliplatin, fluorouracil, and leucovorin (FOLFOX4) for previously treated metastatic colorectal cancer: results from the Eastern Cooperative Oncology Group Study E3200. *J Clin Oncol.* 2007;25:1539-1544.
43. Fuchs CS, Marshall J, Mitchell E, et al. Randomized, controlled trial of irinotecan plus infusional, bolus, or oral fluoropyrimidines in first-line treatment of metastatic colorectal cancer: results from the BICC-C study. *J Clin Oncol.* 2007;25:4779-4786.
44. Hurwitz H. Integrating the anti-VEGF-A humanized monoclonal antibody bevacizumab with chemotherapy in advanced colorectal cancer. *Clin Colorectal Cancer.* 2004;4:S62-S68.
45. Reichert JM. Antibody-based therapeutics to watch in 2011. *MAbs.* 2011;3:76-99.
46. Van Cutsem E, Tabernero J, Lakomy R, et al. Intravenous (IF) aflibercept versus placebo in combination with irinotecan/5-FU (FOLFIRI) for second-line treatment of metastatic colorectal cancer (MCC): results of a multinational phase III trial (EFC10262-VELOUR). *Ann Oncol.* 2011;22(suppl 5) Abstract O-0024 and Oral Presentation at: ESMO 13th World Congress on Gastrointestinal Cancer; June 22-25, 2011; Barcelona, Spain.
47. Saltz L, Rubin M, Hochster HS, et al. Cetuximab (IMC-C225) plus irinotecan (CPT-11) is active in CPT-11-refractory colorectal cancer (CRC) that expresses epidermal growth factor receptor (EGFR). *Proc Am Soc Clin Oncol.* 2001;20. Abstract 7.
48. Saltz LB, Meropol NJ, Loehrer PJ Sr, Needle MN, Kopit J, Mayer RJ. Phase II trial of cetuximab in patients with refractory colorectal cancer that expresses the epidermal growth factor receptor. *J Clin Oncol.* 2004;22:1201-1208.
49. Cunningham D, Humblet Y, Siena S, et al. Cetuximab monotherapy and cetuximab plus irinotecan in irinotecan-refractory metastatic colorectal cancer. *N Engl J Med.* 2004;351:337-345.
50. Scope A, Agero AL, Dusza SW, et al. Randomized double-blind trial of prophylactic oral minocycline and topical tazarotene for cetuximab-associated acne-like eruption. *J Clin Oncol.* 2007;25:5390-5396.
51. Porebska I, Harlozinska A, Bojarowski T. Expression of the tyrosine kinase activity growth factor receptors (EGFR, ERB B2, ERB B3) in colorectal adenocarcinomas and adenomas. *Tumour Biol.* 2000;21:105-115.
52. Chung KY, Shia J, Kemeny NE, et al. Cetuximab shows activity in colorectal cancer patients with tumors that do not express the epidermal growth factor receptor by immunohistochemistry. *J Clin Oncol.* 2005;23:1803-1810.
53. Hebbar M, Wacrenier A, Desauw C, et al. Lack of usefulness of epidermal growth factor receptor expression determination for cetuximab therapy in patients with colorectal cancer. *Anti-Cancer Drugs.* 2006;17:855-857.
54. Sobrero AF, Maurel J, Fehrenbacher L, et al. EPIC: phase III trial of cetuximab plus irinotecan after fluoropyrimidine and oxaliplatin failure in patients with metastatic colorectal cancer. *J Clin Oncol.* 2008;26:2311-2319.
55. Amado RG, Wolf M, Peeters M, et al. Wild-type KRAS is required for panitumumab efficacy in patients with metastatic colorectal cancer. *J Clin Oncol.* 2008;26:1626-1634.
56. Douillard JY, Siena S, Cassidy J, et al. Randomized, phase III trial of panitumumab with infusional fluorouracil, leucovorin, and oxaliplatin (FOLFOX4) versus FOLFOX4 alone as first-line treatment in patients with previously untreated metastatic colorectal cancer: the PRIME study. *J Clin Oncol.* 2010;28:4697-4705.
57. Lievre A, Bachet JB, Le Corre D, et al. KRAS mutation status is predictive of response to cetuximab therapy in colorectal cancer. *Cancer Res.* 2006;66:3992-3995.
58. Lievre A, Bachet JB, Boige V, et al. KRAS mutations as an independent prognostic factor in patients with advanced colorectal cancer treated with cetuximab. *J Clin Oncol.* 2008;26:374-379.
59. Van Cutsem E, Peeters M, Siena S, et al. Open-label phase III trial of panitumumab plus best supportive care compared with best supportive care alone in patients with chemotherapy-refractory metastatic colorectal cancer. *J Clin Oncol.* 2007;25:1658-1664.
60. Jonker DJ, O'Callaghan CJ, Karapetis CS, et al. Cetuximab for the treatment of colorectal cancer. *N Engl J Med.* 2007;357:2040-2048.
61. Karapetis CS, Khambata-Ford S, Jonker DJ, et al. K-ras mutations and benefit from cetuximab in advanced colorectal cancer. *N Engl J Med.* 2008;359:1757-1765.
62. Van Cutsem E, Kohne CH, Hitre E, et al. Cetuximab and chemotherapy as initial treatment for metastatic colorectal cancer. *N Engl J Med.* 2009;360:1408-1417.
63. Bokemeyer C, Bondarenko I, Makhson A, et al. Cetuximab plus 5-FU/FA/oxaliplatin (FOLFOX-4) versus FOLFOX-4 in the first-line treatment of metastatic colorectal cancer (mCRC): OPUS, a randomized phase II study. ASCO Annual Meeting Proceedings. *J Clin Oncol.* 2007;25(18S) (pt I) (June 20 Supplement). Abstract 4035.
64. Bokemeyer C, Bondarenko I, Makhson A, et al. Fluorouracil, leucovorin, and oxaliplatin with and without cetuximab in the first-line treatment of metastatic colorectal cancer. *J Clin Oncol.* 2009;27:663-671.
65. Maughan TS, Adams RA, Smith CG, et al. Addition of cetuximab to oxaliplatin-based first-line combination chemotherapy for treatment of advanced colorectal cancer: results of the randomised phase 3 MRC COIN trial. *Lancet.* 2011;377:2103-2114.
66. Tveit K, Guren T, Glimelius B, et al. Randomized phase III study of 5-fluorouracil/folinate/oxaliplatin given continuously or intermittently with or without cetuximab, as first-line treatment of metastatic colorectal cancer: the NORDIC VII study (NCT00145314), by the NORDIC Colorectal Cancer Biomodulation Group. In: 35th Congress of the European Society for Medical Oncology (ESMO); 2010; Milan, Italy.
67. Artale S, Sartore-Bianchi A, Veronese SM, et al. Mutations of KRAS and BRAF in primary and matched metastatic sites of colorectal cancer. *J Clin Oncol.* 2008;26:4217-4219.
68. Di Nicolantonio F, Martini M, Molinari F, et al. Wild-type BRAF is required for response to panitumumab or cetuximab in metastatic colorectal cancer. *J Clin Oncol.* 2008;26:5705-5712.
69. Van Cutsem E, Lang I, Folprecht G, et al. Cetuximab plus FOLFIRI in the treatment of metastatic colorectal cancer (mCRC): the influence of KRAS and BRAF biomarkers on outcome: Updated data from the CRYSTAL trial. In: 2010 Gastrointestinal Cancers Symposium; 2010; Orlando, FL.
70. De Roock W, Claes B, Bernasconi D, et al. Effects of KRAS, BRAF, NRAS, and PIK3CA mutations on the efficacy of cetuximab plus chemotherapy in chemotherapy-refractory metastatic colorectal cancer: a retrospective consortium analysis. *Lancet Oncol.* 2010;11:753-762.
71. Saltz LB, Lenz HJ, Kindler HL, et al. Randomized phase II trial of cetuximab, bevacizumab, and irinotecan compared

with cetuximab and bevacizumab alone in irinotecan-refractory colorectal cancer: the BOND-2 study. *J Clin Oncol.* 2007;25:4557-4561.
72. Hecht JR, Mitchell E, Chidiac T, et al. A randomized phase IIIB trial of chemotherapy, bevacizumab, and panitumumab compared with chemotherapy and bevacizumab alone for metastatic colorectal cancer. *J Clin Oncol.* 2009;27:672-680.
73. Tol J, Koopman M, Cats A, et al. Chemotherapy, bevacizumab, and cetuximab in metastatic colorectal cancer. *N Engl J Med.* 2009;360:563-572.
74. Blazer DG III, Kishi Y, Maru DM, et al. Pathologic response to preoperative chemotherapy: a new outcome end point after resection of hepatic colorectal metastases. *J Clin Oncol.* 2008;26:5344-5351.
75. Petrelli NJ. Perioperative or adjuvant therapy for resectable colorectal hepatic metastases. *J Clin Oncol.* 2008;26:4862-4863.
76. Nordlinger B, Sorbye H, Glimelius B, et al. Perioperative chemotherapy with FOLFOX4 and surgery versus surgery alone for resectable liver metastases from colorectal cancer (EORTC Intergroup trial 40983): a randomised controlled trial. *Lancet.* 2008;371:1007-1016.
77. Nordlinger B, Guiguet M, Vaillant JC, et al. Surgical resection of colorectal carcinoma metastases to the liver. A prognostic scoring system to improve case selection, based on 1568 patients. Association Francaise de Chirurgie. *Cancer.* 1996;77:1254-1262.
78. Nordlinger B, Van Cutsem E, Gruenberger T, et al. Combination of surgery and chemotherapy and the role of targeted agents in the treatment of patients with colorectal liver metastases: recommendations from an expert panel. *Ann Oncol.* 2009;20:985-992.
79. Abdalla EK, Adam R, Bilchik AJ, Jaeck D, Vauthey JN, Mahvi D. Improving resectability of hepatic colorectal metastases: expert consensus statement. *Ann Surg Oncol.* 2006;13:1271-1280.
80. Poston GJ, Adam R, Alberts S, et al. OncoSurge: a strategy for improving resectability with curative intent in metastatic colorectal cancer. *J Clin Oncol.* 2005;23:7125-7134.
81. Abdalla EK, Vauthey JN, Ellis LM, et al. Recurrence and outcomes following hepatic resection, radiofrequency ablation, and combined resection/ablation for colorectal liver metastases. *Ann Surg.* 2004;239:818-825; discussion 25-27.
82. Pawlik TM, Scoggins CR, Zorzi D, et al. Effect of surgical margin status on survival and site of recurrence after hepatic resection for colorectal metastases. *Ann Surg.* 2005;241:715-722, discussion 22-24.
83. Giacchetti S, Itzhaki M, Gruia G, et al. Long-term survival of patients with unresectable colorectal cancer liver metastases following infusional chemotherapy with 5-fluorouracil, leucovorin, oxaliplatin and surgery. *Ann Oncol.* 1999;10:663-669.
84. Delaunoit T, Alberts SR, Sargent DJ, et al. Chemotherapy permits resection of metastatic colorectal cancer: experience from Intergroup N9741. *Ann Oncol.* 2005;16:425-429.
85. Pozzo C, Basso M, Cassano A, et al. Neoadjuvant treatment of unresectable liver disease with irinotecan and 5-fluorouracil plus folinic acid in colorectal cancer patients. *Ann Oncol.* 2004;15:933-939.
86. Adam R, Avisar E, Ariche A, et al. Five-year survival following hepatic resection after neoadjuvant therapy for nonresectable colorectal. *Ann Surg Oncol.* 2001;8:347-353.
87. Gruenberger T, Kaczirek K, Bergmann M, Zielinski CC, Gruenberger B. Progression-free survival in a phase II study of perioperative bevacizumab plus XELOX in patients with potentially curable metastatic colorectal cancer. *J Clin Oncol.* 2008 ;26(May 20 suppl). Abstract 4073.
88. Adam R, Aloia T, Levi F, et al. Hepatic resection after rescue cetuximab treatment for colorectal liver metastases previously refractory to conventional systemic therapy. *J Clin Oncol.* 2007;25:4593-4602.
89. Aloia T, Sebagh M, Plasse M, et al. Liver histology and surgical outcomes after preoperative chemotherapy with fluorouracil plus oxaliplatin in colorectal cancer liver metastases. *J Clin Oncol.* 2006;24:4983-4990.
90. Karoui M, Penna C, Amin-Hashem M, et al. Influence of preoperative chemotherapy on the risk of major hepatectomy for colorectal liver metastases. *Ann Surg.* 2006;243:1-7.
91. Benoist S, Brouquet A, Penna C, et al. Complete response of colorectal liver metastases after chemotherapy: does it mean cure? *J Clin Oncol.* 2006;24:3939-3945.
92. Mitry E, Fields ALA, Bleiberg H, et al. Adjuvant chemotherapy after potentially curative resection of metastases from colorectal cancer: a pooled analysis of two randomized trials. *J Clin Oncol.* 2008;26:4906-4911.
93. Kornprat P, Jarnagin WR, Gonen M, et al. Outcome after hepatectomy for multiple (four or more) colorectal metastases in the era of effective chemotherapy. *Ann Surg Oncol.* 2007;14:1151-1160.
94. Parks R, Gonen M, Kemeny N, et al. Adjuvant chemotherapy improves survival after resection of hepatic colorectal metastases: analysis of data from two continents. *J Am Coll Surg.* 2007;204:753-761; discussion 61-63.
95. Ychou M, Hohenberger W, Thezenas S, et al. A randomized phase III study comparing adjuvant 5-fluorouracil/folinic acid with FOLFIRI in patients following complete resection of liver metastases from colorectal cancer. *Ann Oncol.* 2009;20:1964-1970.
96. Allegra CJ, Yothers G, O'Connell MJ, et al. Phase III trial assessing bevacizumab in stages II and III carcinoma of the colon: results of NSABP protocol C-08. *J Clin Oncol.* 2011;29:11-16.
97. Colucci G, Gebbia V, Paoletti G, et al. Phase III randomized trial of FOLFIRI versus FOLFOX4 in the treatment of advanced colorectal cancer: a multicenter study of the Gruppo Oncologico Dell'Italia Meridionale. *J Clin Oncol.* 2005;23:4866-4875.
98. Scappaticci FA, Skillings JR, Holden SN, et al. Arterial thromboembolic events in patients with metastatic carcinoma treated with chemotherapy and bevacizumab. *J Natl Cancer Inst.* 2007;99:1232-1239.
99. Kozloff MF, Berlin J, Flynn PJ, et al. Clinical outcomes in elderly patients with metastatic colorectal cancer receiving bevacizumab and chemotherapy: results from the BRiTE observational cohort study. *Oncology.* 2010;78:329-339.
100. Green E, Sargent DJ, Goldberg RM, Grothey A. Detailed analysis of oxaliplatin-associated neurotoxicity in Intergroup trial N9741. In: Program and Abstracts of the American Society of Clinical Oncology 2005 Gastrointestinal Cancers Symposium; January 27-29, 2005; Hollywood, FL. Abstract #182.
101. Chibaudel B, Maindrault-Goebel F, Lledo G, et al. Can chemotherapy be discontinued in unresectable metastatic colorectal cancer? The GERCOR OPTIMOX2 study. *J Clin Oncol.* 2009;27:5727-5733.
102. Tournigand C, Cervantes A, Figer A, et al. OPTIMOX1: a randomized study of FOLFOX4 or FOLFOX7 with oxaliplatin in a stop-and-go fashion in advanced colorectal cancer—a GERCOR study. *J Clin Oncol.* 2006;24:394-400.
103. Grothey A, Nikcevich DA, Sloan JA, et al. Intravenous calcium and magnesium for oxaliplatin-induced sensory neurotoxicity in adjuvant colon cancer: NCCTG N04C7. *J Clin Oncol.* 2011;29:421-427.

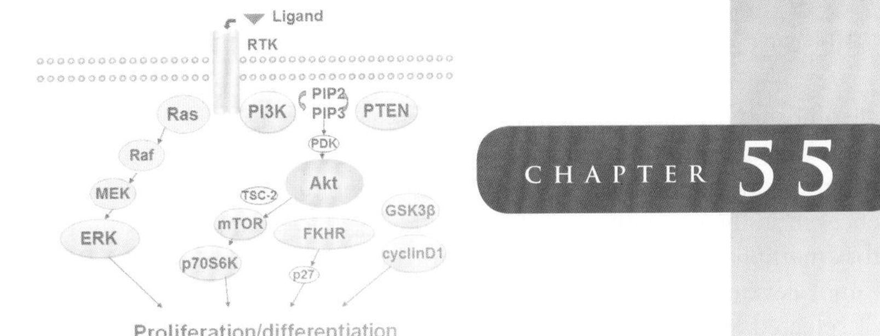

CHAPTER 55

Personalized Medicine and Targeted Therapy of Esophageal Cancer

Harry H. Yoon and Frank A. Sinicrope

INTRODUCTION

Esophageal cancer has an annual incidence of 16,640 cases and is highly fatal with a mortality of 14,500 cases in the United States.[1] While an uncommon cancer, its incidence has risen rapidly in the last 30 years, particularly in Western countries. Two histologic types of cancer arise in the esophagus: squamous cell carcinoma (ESCC), which is associated with chronic smoking and alcohol consumption, and adenocarcinoma (EAC), which frequently arises in a premalignant condition known as Barrett's esophagus (BE). BE represents a replacement of the normal squamous mucosa with metaplastic Barrett's epithelium in which the rate of progression to high-grade dysplasia or adenocarcinoma has been reported as 2.2 to 5.8 cases per 1,000 person-years.[2-4] Major risk factors for the development of BE and EAC include symptomatic gastroesophageal reflux disease, obesity, and tobacco use.[5,6] While ESCC is the most common histologic type in the world, its incidence has been surpassed by EAC in the United States.[7] Among U.S. males, the incidence of adenocarcinoma of the esophagus, gastroesophageal junction (GEJ), and gastric cardia is among the fastest rising of all cancers. This increase appears authentic and unrelated to misclassification or overdiagnosis.[7]

At diagnosis, 28%, 35%, and 37% of patients with esophageal cancer have localized, regional (i.e., T3-4 or node positive), or metastatic disease, respectively.[8] While survival rates appear to have improved since 1973, outcomes remain poor for all non-localized disease, with 3-year overall survival (OS) rates being 45%, 25%, and 4% for localized, regional, and metastatic cancer, respectively.[8] Therapy for local disease primarily consists of en bloc surgical resection of the esophagus and/or GEJ. Survival in locally advanced disease has been improved modestly by the addition in recent years of chemotherapy or chemoradiotherapy before and/or after surgery.[9-12] Therapy for advanced disease remains palliative and consists of systemic chemotherapy that lengthens survival modestly compared with best supportive care alone.[13] While no standard chemotherapy regimen exists for advanced disease, doublet or triplet combinations are often administered and usually include a fluoropyrimidine, platinum (cisplatin, oxaliplatin, carboplatin), taxane, camptothecin (irinotecan), and/or epirubicin.[14,15] Given the incurability and poor prognosis in advanced disease, therapeutic options should be chosen with consideration for quality of life. While SCC and EAC are epidemiologically and biologically distinct, no clear differences in the efficacies of therapies have emerged to date, with the exception that HER2-targeted therapy has received rigorous attention only in EAC. In addition, recent data[16,17] in ESCC have cast doubt as to the necessity of resection following chemoradiotherapy, but definitive neoadjuvant therapy has yet to be adequately tested in EAC patients. Given the predominance of EAC in the United States with most studies of targeted therapy in these patients, this review will focus on the personalized medicine and targeted therapy of EAC.

The great majority of EACs are characterized by chromosomal instability, whereas microsatellite instability is much less common and accounts for only 5% of EACs.[18] Acid and bile reflux cause direct tissue injury and inflammation, which generates reactive oxygen species and nitric oxide. Oxidative damage is a potent mutagen and has been implicated in loss of heterozygosity (LOH) and other chromosomal rearrangements.[19] Studies have identified loss or gain at multiple chromosome arms during disease progression, likely due to genetic heterogeneity, differences in study populations, as well as differences in laboratory methods.[18-23] While neutral mutations not critical for tumor development may "hitchhike" on clonal expansions of selected lesions,[24] several molecular aberrations have been repeatedly detected and have known biological relevance for EAC development. A recent Human Hap300 single-nucleotide polymorphism (SNP) array study of 23 EACs reported an average of 97 copy number changes per cancer (range 23 to 208) that ranged from small homozygous deletions to large chromosome regions.[20,25] All tumors had LOH involving chromosome 17p, and alterations were identified in known tumor suppressor genes and oncogenes such as *CDKN2A*, *TP53*, *FHIT*, and *MYC*, as well as new candidate gene regions. Analysis of chromosome abnormalities in Barrett's epithelium adjacent to EACs has led to the hypothesis that 9p LOH and also methylation and mutation of *CDKN2A* are early events in BE that precede 17p LOH and *TP53* mutation, and subsequent DNA tetraploidy and aneuploidy.[24,26-28]

Molecular pathways relevant to esophageal carcinogenesis have been identified and represent potential therapeutic targets in this malignancy. Significant progress has been made in the preclinical development and clinical evaluation of targeted therapeutic agents in esophageal cancer patients. Data are most mature for agents targeting the HER/epidermal growth factor receptor (EGFR) and angiogenesis pathways, and therefore, we will focus on data relevant to these pathways in this chapter. In addition, we briefly review data in the development and identification of prognostic biomarkers, including the use of gene expression profiling, SNPs, microRNAs, and DNA methylation, in this malignancy.

HER/ErbB PATHWAY

The epidermal growth factor (ErbB) family consists of four closely related transmembrane tyrosine kinase receptors that include EGFR (also known as HER1), ErbB2 (HER2), ErbB3 (HER3), and ErbB4 (HER4). Each receptor comprises an extracellular domain at which ligand binding occurs, an α-helical transmembrane segment, and an intracellular protein tyrosine kinase domain. Small peptide ligands include epidermal growth factor–like molecules, transforming growth factor α (TGF-α), and neuregulins. After ligand binding, homo- or heterodimerization with another ErbB receptor occurs, thereby triggering intracellular signaling through a complex and tightly controlled array of signaling pathways that drive and regulate many cellular functions, including cell proliferation, migration, differentiation, and angiogenesis.[29,30]

Epidermal Growth Factor Receptor

The primary intracellular pathways implicated following phosphorylation of EGFR are the phosphoinositol 3-kinase (PI3K)/Akt and RAS/mitogen-activated protein kinase (MAPK) pathways.[31,32] The PI3K pathway is involved in survival signaling, and downstream of this pathway is the mammalian target of rapamycin (mTOR). The RAS/MAPK pathway is involved in cancer cell cycle progression and cell proliferation.[33]

In esophageal or GEJ adenocarcinoma, overexpression of EGFR proteins was detected in 32% to 59% of tumors by immunohistochemistry (IHC).[34-36] Phosphorylated EGFR was also detected in GEJ/gastric tumors and strongly correlated with total EGFR.[36] *EGFR* gene amplification, detected by fluorescence in situ hybridization (FISH), has been detected in approximately 8% to 50% of EACs,[37-39] though one study of 68 GEJ/gastric cases found no amplification.[40] In some, but not other studies, EGFR expression has been associated with adverse disease characteristics.[34-36] Based on these findings, multiple phase I/II studies of EGFR-targeted therapies have been evaluated in patients with esophageal cancer. Available EGFR inhibitors include two classes of agents, i.e., monoclonal antibodies (mAbs) and small molecule tyrosine kinase inhibitors (TKIs).[41] TKIs bind intracellularly at the tyrosine kinase binding domain, whereas mAbs bind extracellularly, blocking ligand binding and receptor dimerization, and sometimes through antibody-dependent cellular cytotoxicity (ADCC).[42] Due to short half-lives, TKIs such as erlotinib and gefitinib are dosed on a continuous daily basis and are oral agents. By contrast, mAbs such as cetuximab and panitumumab are given intravenously and have an extended half-life of approximately 7 days.[43] mAbs are cleared and recycled by reticuloendothelial cells, mostly in the liver, whereas TKIs are metabolized by the CYP450 system, which creates the potential for adverse interactions with other drugs and food ingredients.

The largest TKI trial in upper gastrointestinal (GI) cancer (Southwest Oncology Group Trial 0127) was a single-arm phase II study in which 70 previously untreated patients with advanced esophagogastric carcinoma received erlotinib 150 mg daily.[40] Patients were stratified by tumor location, as esophageal/GEJ ($N = 44$) versus gastric ($N = 26$). The gastric stratum was closed after the first phase due to lack of activity, whereas the esophageal/GEJ strata completed full accrual. All objective responses (one complete and four partial) were observed in the esophageal/GEJ arm (overall response rate [ORR] 9%; 95% confidence interval [CI] 3% to 22%). Diagnostic archived biopsies in 54 patients were analyzed for EGFR, pAKT, and TGF-α by IHC, but overexpression did not correlate with antitumor activity. There was no evidence of *EGFR* gene amplification or mutations in exons 18, 19, and 21. In two other single-arm studies in advanced esophagogastric cancer, oral gefitinib at a dose of 250 or 500 mg daily yielded partial response rates of 3% to 11%, median duration of progression-free survival (PFS) of 1.9 to 2.0 months, and OS of 4.5 to 5.5 months.[44,45] Mutated *EGFR* was not predictive of response. Lapatinib, an oral inhibitor of EGFR and HER2, was also tested in patients with upper GI malignancies.[46] No objective responses were observed and only 2 of 25 treated patients achieved disease stabilization.

The anti-EGFR mAb, cetuximab, has been evaluated in esophageal cancer, partly based on the low frequency of *KRAS* mutations that negatively predict for cetuximab response. Cetuximab monotherapy was evaluated in 55 patients with previously treated EAC, yielding a median PFS of 1.8 months and median OS of 4 months.[47] Cetuximab administered in combination with chemotherapy (FOLFIRI [fluorouracil (5-FU) plus irinotecan], FOLFOX [5-FU plus oxaliplatin], cisplatin plus docetaxel) has been tested in advanced gastric/GEJ cancer where it was associated with ORRs of 41% to 50%, with a median time to progression of 5.0 to 8.0 months and a median OS of 9 or more months (Table 55.1).[50,51,57] The Cancer and Leukemia Group B (CALGB)[54] led a three-arm trial for chemo-naïve patients with advanced ESCC or EAC including GEJ tumor whereby all patients (N = 245) received cetuximab. The chemotherapy backbones differed among the three groups: (1) ECF (epirubicin, cisplatin, plus continuously infused 5-FU); (2) IC (irinotecan plus cisplatin); or (3) FOLFOX (oxaliplatin plus 5-FU). The ECF and FOLFOX arms with cetuximab had the highest response rates (ORR 58% and 51%, respectively), meeting criteria for further development, whereas the IC arm had the lowest ORR of 38%. The ECF and FOLFOX arms showed median PFS of 5.6 and 5.7 months and OS of 10.0 and 10.0 months, respectively. Compared with ECF, FOLFOX was less toxic and may be a preferred backbone for subsequent trials with targeted agents.

A randomized phase II study of 150 patients with advanced adenocarcinoma of the GEJ or stomach who received chemotherapy with or without cetuximab has been preliminarily reported.[58] Previously untreated patients were administered docetaxel plus oxaliplatin (DOCOX) with or without cetuximab.[58] Slightly more than half the patients had GEJ cancer, and the remainder had gastric cancer. While the combined therapies were well tolerated, ORRs (24% vs. 29%), median PFS (4.7 vs. 5.1 months), and median OS (9.0 vs. 8.5 months) did not differ between the study arms. The potential activity of cetuximab in advanced ESCC was suggested in a randomized phase II study by the Arbeitsgemeinschaft Internistische Onkologie.[53] Among 62 eligible patients, 32 received cetuximab plus cisplatin and 5-FU, and 30 received chemotherapy alone. Cetuximab did not increase grade 3 to 4 toxicity except for rash (6% vs. 0%) and diarrhea (16% vs. 0%). The ORR was 19% vs. 13%, and the disease control rate was 75% versus 57% for the cetuximab-chemotherapy versus chemotherapy-alone arms, respectively. Median PFS was 5.9 versus 3.6 months and OS was 9.5 versus 5.5 months, favoring the cetuximab arm. No *KRAS* codon 12 or 13 tumor mutations were identified in 37 tumors.

Definitive evaluation of whether EGFR-targeted mAbs add clinical benefit to chemotherapy is awaited in two ongoing phase III trials in previously untreated patients with advanced gastric/GEJ carcinoma. Patients receive epirubicin, oxaliplatin, capecitabine [Xeloda] (EOX) chemotherapy with or without panitumumab (REAL-3), or cisplatin plus capecitabine with or without cetuximab (EXPAND). Phase II studies examining the combination of cetuximab with neoadjuvant radiotherapy are also underway.

HER2/ErbB2

The first novel therapeutic agent shown to improve OS in upper GI tumors was trastuzumab. Trastuzumab is a HER2-targeted mAb that induces ADCC, inhibits HER2-mediated signaling, and prevents cleavage of the extracellular domain of HER2. In HER2-positive breast cancer, trastuzumab has shown a survival advantage in early and metastatic disease and is now standard of care.[59-61] In the vast majority of breast cancers, HER2 overexpression is due to gene amplification, and HER2 overexpression and/or gene amplification predicts for better outcomes with trastuzumab.[59] Early studies detected HER2 overexpression or amplification in 7% to 36% of gastric carcinomas, and in preclinical models, trastuzumab showed at least additive antitumor effects when combined with oral 5-FU (capecitabine) or cisplatin, or both.[62]

The Trastuzumab for Gastric Cancer (ToGA) study was an international multicenter open-label phase III randomized clinical trial, which enrolled 594 patients with inoperable, locally advanced or metastatic HER2-overexpressing adenocarcinoma of the stomach or GEJ. Patients were randomly assigned (1:1) to receive either trastuzumab plus chemotherapy or chemotherapy alone. The chemotherapy regimen included cisplatin and a fluoropyrimidine (either capecitabine or continuously infused 5-FU). All tumors were confirmed to be HER2 gene-amplified by FISH or protein overexpression (IHC 3+) using validated assays performed at a central laboratory. Among the 594 patients, 82% had primary gastric cancer, 18% had primary GEJ adenocarcinoma; 97% had metastatic disease. The median age was 60 years (range 21 to 83), and 76% were male. HER2 expression in tumors by IHC showed that 47% of tumors were 3+ (strong), 30% (weak-moderate) were 2+, and 22% were 0 (no expression) or 1+ (faint). All tumors were gene-amplified, except for a small subset of IHC 3+ tumors that were not amplified.

Final analysis demonstrated median OS of 13.8 months for the trastuzumab arm and 11.1 months for the chemotherapy-alone arm (hazard ratio [HR] 0.74; 95% CI 0.60 to 0.91; P = 0.0046). Exploratory analyses in subgroups defined by protein expression suggested that trastuzumab was most effective in prolonging OS in the 294-patient subgroup with HER2 IHC 3+ tumors (HR 0.66; 95% CI 0.50 to 0.87) and less effective in the 160-patient subgroup with IHC 2+ tumors (HR 0.78; 95% CI 0.55 to 1.10). No trastuzumab benefit was apparent in the 133-patient subgroup with HER2 gene-amplified, IHC 0 or 1+ tumors (HR 1.33; 95% CI 0.92 to 1.92). Trastuzumab benefit appeared to be at least as strong in the small 106-patient subgroup with GEJ tumors (HR 0.67; 95% CI 0.42 to 1.08) as compared with the larger

TABLE 55-1 HER/ERBB-Targeted Therapy Trials in Advanced Esophageal Cancer

					Outcomes		
Study	**Agent**	***N***	**Histology**	**Setting**	**ORR**	**Median PFS[a] (months)**	**Median OS (months)**
Tyrosine Kinase Inhibitor							
Dragovich et al.[40]	Erlotinib	68	GEJAC 63% GC 37%	First line	9% GEJ 0% GC	TTF: 2 GEJ 1.6 GC	6.7 GEJ 3.5 GC
Wainberg et al.[48]	Erlotinib + mFOLFOX6	33	EAC 32% GEJAC 68%	First line	51%	5.5	11
Janmaat et al.[45]	Gefitinib	36	EAC 72% ESCC 25%	Second line	3%	2	5.5
Ferry et al.[44]	Gefitinib	27	EAC 100%	Not first line	11%	1.9	4.5
Hecht[46]	Lapatinib	25	EC NOS 48% GEJ 52%	Not first line	0%	NR	NR
Monoclonal Antibody							
Gold et al.[47]	Cetuximab	55	EAC or GEJAC 100%	Second line	5%	1.8	4
Chan et al.[49]	Cetuximab	35	EAC 34% GEJAC 23% GC 43%	Second or third line	3%	1.6	3.1
Pinto et al.[50]	Cetuximab + FOLFIRI	38 EGFR+	GEJAC 10% GC 90%	First line	44%	TTP 8	16
Pinto et al.[51]	Cetuximab + cisplatin/ docetaxel	72	GEJAC 18% GC 82%	First line	41%	TTP 5	9
Lordick et al.[52]	Cetuximab + FUFOX	52	GEJAC 48% GC 52%	First line	65%	TTP 7.6	9.5
Lorenzen et al.[53]	Cetuximab + CF vs. CF	32 vs. 30	ESCC 100%	First line	19% vs. 13%	5.9 vs. 3.6	9.5 vs. 5.5
Enzinger et al.[54]	Cetuximab + ECF vs. Cetuximab + irinotecan/ cisplatin vs. Cetuximab + FOLFOX	82 vs. 83 vs. 80	EAC 52% ESCC 9% GEJAC 39%	First line	58%[b] vs. 38%[b] vs. 51%[b]	5.6 vs. 5.0 vs. 5.7	10 vs. 8.6 vs. 10
Bang et al.[55]	Trastuzumab + CF vs. CF	294 HER2+ vs. 290 HER2+	GEJAC 20% GC 80% vs. GEJAC 17% GC 83%	First line	47% vs. 35%	6.7 vs. 5.5	13.8 vs. 11.1
Rao et al.[56]	Matuzumab + ECX	21	EAC 24% GEJAC 33% GC 43%	First line	65%	5.2	NR

[a]PFS, unless otherwise specified.

[b]EAC and GEJAC only.

GC, gastric adenocarcinoma; GEJAC, gastroesophageal junction adenocarcinoma; G/E, gastroesophageal; EC, esophageal carcinoma; EAC, esophageal adenocarcinoma; ESCC, esophageal squamous cell carcinoma; ASC, adenosquamous carcinoma; NOS, not otherwise specified; CF, cisplatin plus fluorouracil; ECF, epirubicin plus cisplatin plus 5-fluorouracil; ECX, epirubicin plus cisplatin plus capecitabine; ORR, overall response rate; PFS, progression-free survival; OS, overall survival; TTF, time to failure; TTP, time to progression; NR, not reported.

478-patient subgroup with gastric tumors. The combined regimen was well tolerated, with the most common grade 3 and 4 adverse reactions being neutropenia (35%), anemia (12%), diarrhea (9%), nausea (8%), anorexia (7%), and vomiting (6%). Adverse cardiac reactions occurred at the same incidence for patients in both groups; cardiac failure occurred in less than 1%.

Based on this single study, trastuzumab in combination with cisplatin and a fluoropyrimidine was approved by the FDA and the European Commission for the treatment of patients with HER2-overexpressing metastatic gastric/GEJ adenocarcinoma who have not received prior treatment for metastatic disease.

While patients with EAC were not enrolled in ToGA, it is unlikely that a randomized trial limited to EAC will be performed to directly address whether trastuzumab adds survival benefit in HER2-positive EACs. Almost 20% of ToGA subjects had GEJ carcinoma, and trastuzumab benefit was not attenuated in this subgroup. The frequency of HER2 overexpression and/or amplification in esophageal or GEJ adenocarcinoma is at least as high in subcardial gastric tumors and has been reported to be 11% to 40%.[37,63-68] The largest examination of HER2 in EAC was performed at Mayo Clinic, where HER2 protein expression and gene amplification were assessed in 708 EACs. The frequency of HER2 positivity was higher in esophageal versus GEJ tumors (21% vs. 15%, respectively).

HER2 overexpression and gene amplification should be determined using FDA-approved tests. Cases with 3+ or 2+ HER2 expression with gene amplification are eligible for trastuzumab. However, controversy remains on whether cases with 0 to 1+ expression with gene amplification may also derive benefit. In Europe, these patients are not considered eligible for trastuzumab, whereas the FDA has stated that it is "inadvisable to rely on a single method to rule out potential trastuzumab benefit." FDA recommendations are based on the potential intratumoral heterogeneity of HER2 and the post hoc subgroup analysis of ToGA, suggesting that trastuzumab benefit was limited to amplified tumors with 2 to 3+ expression. In contrast to EAC, fewer studies of HER2 expression in ESCC are available. While membrane-associated HER2 overexpression has also been detected, the frequency of overexpression and/or amplification rate varies widely (2% to 19%).[67,69-71] In the largest series with gene amplification data ($N = 144$), the amplification rate was less than 5%.[67] As a result, it is unclear whether HER2 is a viable target in ESCC.

ANGIOGENESIS

Angiogenesis is a critical step in the propagation of malignant tumor growth and metastasis. Multiple proangiogenic factors promote the process of vessel formation, with vascular endothelial growth factor (VEGF) being a central molecule in tumor-mediated angiogenesis. Pivotal trials have shown efficacy for anti-VEGF therapy in selected solid tumors. Accordingly, the VEGF axis has emerged as a key target for various antiangiogenic treatment strategies. The VEGF family comprises six secreted glycoproteins, VEGF-A, VEGF-B, VEGF-C, VEGF-D, VEGF-E, and placental growth factor. The best characterized of the VEGF family members is VEGF-A (commonly referred to as VEGF, also known as vascular permeability factor). VEGF has been shown to promote endothelial cell survival by inhibiting apoptosis related to upregulation of prosurvival proteins such as Bcl-2 and survivin and activating the PI3K/Akt pathway.[72,73] VEGF is a potent endothelial cell mitogen, probably mediated by downstream pathways such as ERK-1/2, JNK/SAPK, and protein kinase C.[74] VEGF also serves as a chemokine for bone marrow–derived endothelial precursors cells, which may contribute cellular components to the growing vascular bed.[75]

VEGF mediates its angiogenic effects via several tyrosine kinase receptors. VEGFR1 (Flt-1) and VEGFR2 (KDR and the murine homologue Flk-1) were originally discovered on vascular endothelial cells.[76] VEGFR3 is primarily associated with lymphangiogenesis.[77] The various members of the VEGF family have differing binding affinities for each of these receptors, which have helped in elucidating their functions. VEGFR1 is critical in developmental angiogenesis, as well as processes including monocyte migration, recruitment of endothelial cell progenitors, and inducing growth factors from endothelial cells.[72,78] VEGFR2 mediates the majority of the downstream effects of VEGF-A, including microvascular permeability, endothelial cell proliferation, and survival.[78,79] VEGFR3 is expressed in the embryonic vasculature and later is limited to lymphatic endothelial cells.[80] Neuropilins (NRP-1 and NRP-2) have been shown to serve as coreceptors for VEGF.[81] NRP-1 and NRP-2 differ from the tyrosine kinase VEGFRs in that they lack an intracellular signaling domain and their activities are mediated, in part, through their function as coreceptors for VEGFR1 and VEGFR2. NRP enhances the binding affinity of ligands to the receptors and affects downstream intracellular signaling.[81]

The progression from normal esophagus to BE and EAC is characterized by neovascularization, with microvessel density doubled in BE and tripled in EAC, as compared with normal esophageal mucosa.[82] Similarly, VEGF expression is increased in EAC as compared with BE, dysplasia, or normal mucosa[83] and has been correlated with adverse pathologic features and adverse clinical outcome.[84-86] In sera or plasma from esophageal cancer patients, VEGF is correlated with increased tumor size, metastases, and poor treatment response and survival.[87-89] VEGFR2 is strongly expressed on vascular endothelial cells within BE,[82] and increased levels of VEGFR2 mRNA have been detected in EACs and ESCCs[90] and correlated with lymph node metastases.[91]

Bevacizumab is an mAb targeting VEGF-A that has been shown to improve patient survival in advanced colorectal cancer patients.[92] Single-arm studies utilizing bevacizumab in combination with chemotherapy have shown ORRs of 27% to 65%, TTP of 8.3 to 12 months, and median OS of 12.3 to 16.8 months (Table 55.2). To date, the only randomized study of this mAb is AVAGAST, a phase III study[93] in which patients with advanced gastric/GEJ cancer ($N = 774$) received bevacizumab 7.5 mg/kg or placebo followed by cisplatin 80 mg/m^2 on day 1 plus capecitabine 1,000 mg/m^2 twice daily for 14 days every 3 weeks. Intravenous fluorouracil was permitted in patients unable to take oral medications. Cisplatin was given for six cycles; capecitabine and bevacizumab were administered until disease progression or unacceptable toxicity. The primary end point was OS. Median OS was 12.1 months in the bevacizumab arm and 10.1 months in the placebo arm (HR 0.87; 95% CI 0.73 to 1.03; $P = 0.1002$). Both median PFS (6.7 vs. 5.3 months; HR 0.80; 95% CI 0.68 to 0.93; $P = 0.0037$) and ORR (46.0% vs. 37.4%; $P = 0.0315$) were significantly improved with bevacizumab versus placebo. The most common grade 3 to 4 adverse events were neutropenia (35%, bevacizumab plus fluoropyrimidine-cisplatin; 37%, placebo plus fluoropyrimidine-cisplatin), anemia (10% vs. 14%), and decreased appetite (8% vs. 11%). While the trial failed to meet the primary end point in the overall study population of patients mostly from Asia and Europe, a preplanned subgroup analysis showed dramatic differences by geographic location. In the Americas, there was improved PFS and OS in the bevacizumab versus control arm (OS: HR 0.63, $P < 0.05$), but not in Asia (HR 0.97). These and other data suggest that upper GI cancers in the United States versus Asia are

TABLE 55-2 Angiogenesis-Targeted Therapy Trials in Advanced Esophageal Cancer

					Outcomes		
Study	**Agent**	***N***	**Histology**	**Setting**	**ORR**	**Median PFS[a] (months)**	**Median OS (months)**
Tyrosine Kinase Inhibitor							
Bang et al.[94]	Sunitinib	78	GEJ 6% GC 94%	Second line	2.6%	2.3	6.8
Ilson et al.[95]	Sorafenib	20	EAC 60% ESCC 10% GEJAC 30%	Not first line	NR	3.7	NR
Sun et al.[96]	Sorafenib + docetaxel/cisplatin	44	GEJAC 74% GC 26%	First line	41%	5.8	13.6
Monoclonal Antibody							
Enzinger et al.[97]	Bevacizumab + docetaxel	20	EAC 50% ESCC 5% GEJAC 20% GC 25%	First or second line	27%	NR	NR
El-Rayes et al.[98]	Bevacizumab + docetaxel/oxaliplatin	23	GC or GEJAC 100%	First line	59%	NR	NR
Enzinger et al.[99]	Bevacizumab + docetaxel/cisplatin/irinotecan	32	EAC 32% ESCC 9% GEJAC 22% GC 37%	First line	63%	NR	NR
Shah et al.[100]	Bevacizumab + DCF	44	EAC 5% GEJAC 45% GC 50%	First line	67%	12	16.8
Shah et al.[101]	Bevacizumab + irinotecan/cisplatin	47	GEJAC 49% GC 51%	First line	65%	TTP 8.3	12.3
Ohtsu et al.[93] (AVAGAST)	Bevacizumab + cisplatin/capecitabine vs. Placebo + cisplatin/capecitabine	387 vs. 387	GEJAC 14% GC 86%	First line	46% vs. 37.4%	6.7 vs. 5.3	12.1 vs. 10.1

[a]PFS, unless otherwise specified.

GC, gastric adenocarcinoma; GEJAC, gastroesophageal junction adenocarcinoma; G/E, gastroesophageal; EC, esophageal carcinoma; EAC, esophageal adenocarcinoma; ESCC, esophageal squamous cell carcinoma; NOS, not otherwise specified; DCF, docetaxel plus cisplatin plus fluorouracil; ORR, overall response rate; PFS, progression-free survival; OS, overall survival; TTP, time to progression; NR, not reported.

biologically distinct, although further study is needed to support this observation. Within AVAGAST, there was no added benefit for bevacizumab in the subgroup of patients with GEJ carcinoma.

The aforementioned data have generated interest in blocking the VEGF axis in upper GI cancers in U.S. patients. Ramucirumab (ImClone, Eli Lilly) is a fully human immunoglobulin G1 mAb that potently binds to the extracellular VEGF-binding domain of VEGFR2. Inhibition of VEGF-stimulated VEGFR2 activation by ramucirumab or its murine version has been shown to confer significant antitumor activity alone or combined with cytotoxic agents in several animal models. In a gastric cancer model, this drug reduced tumor mass and vessel density and increased tumor and endothelial cell apoptosis.[102] An ongoing phase III study is examining ramucirumab versus best supportive care in patients with advanced gastric or GEJ carcinoma in the second-line setting. Other drugs include sunitinib, which is a small molecule inhibitor of receptor tyrosine kinases involved in tumor proliferation and angiogenesis, that targets PDGFR, VEGFR, KIT, FLT-3, and RET. Sorafenib is another multitargeted TKI with activity against the VEGFR receptor. To date, single-arm studies using either agent have shown modest activity (see Table 55.2), but no randomized studies have been reported.

OTHER BIOMARKERS

Other approaches have been undertaken to identify molecular markers that can be used for prognostication or personalization of therapy or to identify dysregulated pathways that could potentially be therapeutically exploited. These approaches have examined molecular aberrations other than those related to mRNA or protein expression alone and include SNPs or microRNA studies. In one of the most rigorous studies reported to identify novel prognostic markers in EAC, gene expression profiling was performed in a training cohort of 75 snap-frozen esophageal and GEJ adenocarcinomas, which found that 199 genes were significantly associated with survival and 270 genes with the number of involved lymph nodes. A short list of 10 genes was analyzed at the protein level using IHC. Of these, only four genes were significantly prognostic (deoxycytidine kinase [DCK], 3′-phosphoadenosine 5′-phosphosulfate synthase 2 [PAPSS2], sirtuin 2 [SIRT2], and tripartite motif-containing 44 [TRIM44]), with TRIM44 having only borderline significance ($P = 0.063$). These four genes were combined to create a molecular prognostic signature, and their protein products were then assessed in 371 independent cases using IHC. This four-gene signature was predictive of survival in the independent cohort, with 5-year survival rates decreasing from 58% to 26% to 14% as the number of dysregulated genes increased from 0 to 1-2 to 3-4, respectively. The four-gene signature was independently prognostic in a multivariable model that included the clinical TNM staging variables ($P = 0.013$). While interesting, the results should be viewed with caution. In the second cohort, when analyzed individually, none of the markers were prognostic except TRIM44 ($P = 0.009$), and only univariate results for TRIM44 were reported. Moreover, it was not clearly reported how the decision was made a priori to assess the four-gene signature, including why two cutpoints were used to categorize the number of dysregulated genes, how those particular cutpoints were selected, and what biologic evidence supported the notion that dysregulation of one gene should be weighted equally with the dysregulation of another. The mechanistic pathobiology of the four genes in this malignancy remains to be elucidated, and the four-gene signature itself has not been validated independently.

SNP

A recent body of work has examined the value of SNPs, particularly in DNA repair and drug-related pathways, in predicting patient outcomes in upper GI cancer. SNPs are single-nucleotide variations between individuals, which have been associated with cancer susceptibility, chemotherapeutic toxicity, and clinical outcome in patients with lung,[103] colon,[104] and head and neck[105] cancer. In one of the largest SNP studies in upper GI cancer, specimens were taken from 210 esophageal cancer patients treated with cisplatin- and 5-FU-based trimodality therapy.[106] Genotyping was performed for pathways involved in cisplatin, 5-FU, and radiation action, including those related to DNA repair and drug detoxification. Variant alleles in the *MTHFR* gene, involved in folate metabolism, were associated with significantly improved survival (HR 0.56; 95% CI 0.35 to 0.89) in patients treated with 5-FU. For patients receiving platinum drugs, the *MDR1 C3435T* variant allele was associated with reduced recurrence risk (HR 0.25; 95% CI 0.10 to 0.64) and improved survival (HR 0.44; 95% CI 0.23 to 0.85). In base excision repair genes, the variant alleles of *XRCC1 Arg399Gln* were associated with the absence of pathologic complete response (pCR) and poor survival. The *XRCC1 Arg399Gln* SNP was analyzed in a separate study of the Eastern Cooperative Oncology Group in 60 treatment-naïve subjects with newly diagnosed resectable EAC who received radiotherapy with concurrent cisplatin-based chemotherapy.[107] The variant allele of the XRCC1 SNP was detected in 52% of subjects and was associated with the absence of a pCR (odds ratio 5.37, $P = 0.062$). Allelic imbalance at this locus was found in only 10% of informative subjects, suggesting that germline genotype may reflect tumor genotype at this locus. These data indicate the potential for germline SNPs to identify responsiveness to radio- and/or chemotherapy, potentially enabling stratification of patients for individualized therapy.

DNA Methylation

Evidence indicates that abnormal DNA methylation is an early event in carcinogenesis.[108] Methylation of the promoter regions of genes including tumor suppressors is commonly found in many human malignancies, including esophageal carcinoma. This hypermethylation leads to the reduced expression of the protein products of tumor suppressor genes that results in unchecked cellular proliferation, tissue invasion, angiogenesis, and metastases. Hypermethylation can be targeted using demethylating agents of which an example is decitabine. These agents, however, affect multiple methylated genes and therefore lack selectivity, yet represent a potential strategy to sensitize tumors to chemotherapy and radiation.

In a retrospective study of patients who received trimodality therapy for EAC or ESCC,[109] promoter methylation patterns of 11 candidate genes were examined in pretreatment tumor specimens ($n = 35$). Genes were selected according to their known ability to predict responsiveness to chemoradiation and/or prognosis, or their role in cell cycle regulation. The number of methylated genes per patient was lower in patients who experienced a pCR than in those who did not (1.4 vs. 2.4 genes per patient; $P = 0.026$). The combined mean level of promoter methylation of *p16*, *Reprimo*, *p57*, *p73*, *RUNX-3*, *CHFR*, *MGMT*, *TIMP-3*, and *HPP1* was also lower in responders than in nonresponders ($P = 0.003$). Similarly, a study of EAC patients who received surgical resection alone found that patients whose tumors had four or more genes methylated in a seven-gene profile (*APC*, *MGMT*, *p16*, *ER*, *E-cadherin*, *TIMP3*, *DAP-kinase*) had earlier tumor recurrence and poorer survival compared with patients who did not.[110]

MicroRNA

Microarray experiments have examined the expression of miRNAs during progression from normal squamous epithelium to Barrett's metaplasia, dysplasia, and adenocarcinoma.[111-113] Results have been inconsistent with each study generating a different set of candidate miRNAs that appear to be differentially expressed. One study found MiR-21, -192, -194, -203, and -223 to be differentially expressed between EAC and normal cells,[112] whereas another study found only MiR-205 to be differentially expressed.[113] In a third study, expression of only MiR-25, -100, -140, and 146a was validated by polymerase chain reaction and shown to differ in tumor versus normal tissues.[111] In terms of prognostic impact, reduced expression of MiR-375 in EAC tissue and MiR-21 in noncancerous tissue from ESCC patients was associated with worse prognosis.[112] Discrepant findings among studies may be related to small study cohorts, differing analysis platforms, and findings in premalignant versus malignant tissues. While miRNAs may be biologically important in esophageal cancers, further study is needed to identify critical miRNAs and establish their clinical relevance and impact.

Tumor Metabolic Activity

Positron emission tomography (PET) measures metabolic activity within tumors and is commonly used to stage patients with esophageal cancer, particularly to detect distant metastases. Emerging data have shown the utility of serial PET scans in determining patient prognosis and in evaluating clinical response to cancer therapy. PET has advantages over CT or MRI that primarily measures anatomical location and tumor size since PET measures metabolic activity within a tumor even when the tumor size is unchanged. PET measures the intensity of fluorodeoxyglucose (FDG) uptake, a glucose analogue that is injected into the patient where it is transported intracellularly and phosphorylated, emitting a positron radiotracer. The phosphorylated form accumulates in tumors and provides a signal of high glycolytic tissue activity. The intensity of FDG uptake is measured as a standardized uptake value (SUV) within specific lesions; SUV is the ratio of mean activity in the region of interest (mCi/mL) over the injected FDG dose per body weight.

Because anticancer therapy (e.g., chemotherapy and radiotherapy) often has substantial toxicity, investigators have sought ways to identify nonresponders earlier, so as to minimize the use of ineffective therapy. In this context, studies have examined the value of obtaining a repeat PET scan during therapy with the idea that metabolic nonresponders can be offered alternative treatment. Accumulating data suggest that assessment of metabolic response may predict for histologic regression after therapy and for OS. Metabolic response is a reduction in FDG uptake between baseline and repeat scans. A study conducted at Memorial Sloan-Kettering in patients with resectable EAC or ESCC showed that metabolic responders, defined as 35% decrease in SUV, after neoadjuvant chemoradiation had an approximately eightfold higher rate of pCR at surgery as compared with nonresponders (32% vs. 4%; $P = 0.009$).[114] Other studies have also shown that metabolic change may predict histologic response.[115-117] An intriguing study examined FDG-PET in patients ($N = 163$ total) who underwent chemoradiation with or without subsequent surgery. While the chemoradiation-alone group showed worse outcomes compared with patients who also underwent surgery, the provocative finding was that patients in the chemoradiation-alone group who had a complete metabolic response had similar OS as did patients who also underwent surgery. Complete metabolic response was associated with a nearly 10-fold improvement in OS. These data suggest that patients who experience a complete PET response after chemoradiation may not derive added benefit from surgical resection.

Two prospective studies attempted to address the question of how patients, identified by PET as nonresponders, should be managed. In both studies, neoadjuvant therapy consisted of chemotherapy without radiation. The first prospective study (MUNICON I) was a randomized phase II trial in which patients with locally advanced gastroesophageal cancer ($N = 119$) underwent PET at baseline and after 2 weeks of chemotherapy.[118] Half of the patients were metabolic responders (using a >35% decrease in SUV as the cutoff) who continued with chemotherapy and then underwent surgery.

Nonresponders discontinued chemotherapy and underwent immediate surgery. The most important finding was that the OS of nonresponders (26 months) who did not receive further chemotherapy was similar to historical controls who received a full course of chemotherapy plus surgery (15 to 18 months).[11,119,120] Nevertheless, the cohort as a whole appeared to have been highly selected, as OS rates exceeded those in other trials. Optimal therapy for nonresponders, or responders for that matter, remains unknown—i.e., whether responders would perform equally well without further chemotherapy, and whether nonresponders would have performed better with further chemotherapy or with a change in preoperative therapy to combined chemoradiation.

To address whether salvage chemoradiation may be an appropriate alternative regimen in nonresponders, a second trial was performed by the same group of investigators (MUNICON II). Fifty-six patients with locally advanced esophageal/GEJ adenocarcinoma underwent FDG-PET at baseline and 2 weeks after initiation of chemotherapy.[121] Whereas responders received further chemotherapy for 3 months prior to surgery, nonresponders received salvage chemoradiation that was followed by surgery. The key analysis in the study was to determine whether nonresponders, by switching to salvage chemoradiation early prior to surgery, could have an R0 resection rate of 94% (predetermined by investigators), which would be improved as compared with the 74% R0 rate in MUNICON I. However, the R0 rate among nonresponders in MUNICON II was only 70%. As a result, the investigators concluded that other approaches, such as alternative chemotherapy agents, should be considered for salvage therapy in metabolic nonresponders. Taken together, these data suggest the promise of utilizing PET for early response determination to guide patient management. However, this strategy is predicated upon the availability of alternative treatments that demonstrate sufficient efficacy against this malignancy.

SUMMARY AND PERSPECTIVE

Therapy for esophageal cancer has improved with recent success in therapeutically targeting the HER/ErbB family. Despite incremental advances, esophagogastric cancers remain among the most treatment-resistant solid tumors for which novel therapeutic strategies are urgently needed. An increased understanding of the biology of these cancers is expected to lead to new molecular targets for drug development. The first biological agent to demonstrate a survival benefit in these malignancies is the anti-HER2 antibody trastuzumab, as shown in a clinical trial that included patients with GEJ carcinoma. Given the similar frequency of HER2 overexpression/amplification and biologic similarities between EAC and GEJ carcinoma, HER2-targeted therapy is likely to have efficacy in EAC. A phase III study by the Radiation Therapy Oncology Group is underway to assess whether trastuzumab, when added to neoadjuvant chemoradiation and surgery, improves outcomes in locally advanced EAC. HER3 expression has been detected in gastric cancer,[122,123] and similar assessments in EAC are ongoing; the mAb pertuzumab that targets the interaction between HER2 and HER3 has recently shown efficacy in breast cancer.[124] Angiogenesis-targeted therapy has been met with initial disappointment, but further study is underway in subpopulations in which efficacy may be improved. Assessing metabolic response within the tumor after an initial course of anticancer therapy shows promise as a means to allow early discontinuation of ineffective therapy and avoidance of unnecessary toxicity. Further identification of molecular subtypes may increase efficacy of a targeted anticancer agent, but assessment of efficacy in smaller subsets will be limited by issues of feasibility. Moving forward, the development of novel trial designs that incorporate molecular testing and productive collaborations will be required to overcome these challenges.

REFERENCES

1. Jemal A, Siegel R, Xu J, et al. Cancer statistics, 2010. *CA: Cancer J Clin.* 2010;60:277-300.
2. Hvid-Jensen F, Pedersen L, Drewes AM, et al. Incidence of adenocarcinoma among patients with Barrett's esophagus. *N Engl J Med.* 2011;365:1375-1383.
3. de Jonge PJ, van Blankenstein M, Looman CW, et al. Risk of malignant progression in patients with Barrett's oesophagus: a Dutch nationwide cohort study. *Gut.* 2010;59:1030-1036.
4. Bhat S, Coleman HG, Yousef F, et al. Risk of malignant progression in Barrett's esophagus patients: results from a large population-based study. *J Natl Cancer Inst.* 2011;103:1049-1057.
5. Lagergren J, Bergstrom R, Lindgren A, et al. Symptomatic gastroesophageal reflux as a risk factor for esophageal adenocarcinoma. *N Engl J Med.* 1999;340:825-831.
6. Vaughan TL, Davis S, Kristal A, et al. Obesity, alcohol, and tobacco as risk factors for cancers of the esophagus and gastric cardia: adenocarcinoma versus squamous cell carcinoma. *Cancer Epidemiol Biomarkers Prev.* 1995;4:85-92.
7. Pohl H, Welch HG. The role of overdiagnosis and reclassification in the marked increase of esophageal adenocarcinoma incidence. *J Natl Cancer Inst.* 2005;97:142-146.
8. Cen P, Banki F, Cheng L, et al. Changes in age, stage distribution, and survival of patients with esophageal adenocarcinoma over three decades in the United States. *Ann Surg Oncol.* 2012;19:1685-1691.
9. Cunningham D, Allum WH, Stenning SP, et al. Perioperative chemotherapy versus surgery alone for resectable gastroesophageal cancer. *N Engl J Med.* 2006;355:11-20.
10. Van Hagen P, Hulshof MC, van Lanschot JJ, et al. Preoperative chemoradiotherapy for esophageal or junctional cancer. New England Journal of Medicine. 2012;366:2074-2084.
11. Medical Research Council Oesophageal Cancer Working Group. Surgical resection with or without preoperative chemotherapy in oesophageal cancer: a randomised controlled trial. *Lancet.* 2002;359:1727-1733.
12. Gebski V, Burmeister B, Smithers BM, et al. Survival benefits from neoadjuvant chemoradiotherapy or chemotherapy in oesophageal carcinoma: a meta-analysis. *Lancet Oncol.* 2007;8:226-234.
13. Wagner AD, Grothe W, Haerting J, et al. Chemotherapy in advanced gastric cancer: a systematic review and meta-analysis based on aggregate data. *J Clin Oncol.* 2006;24:2903-2909.
14. Cunningham D, Starling N, Rao S, et al. Capecitabine and oxaliplatin for advanced esophagogastric cancer. *N Engl J Med.* 2008;358:36-46.
15. Al-Batran SE, Hartmann JT, Probst S, et al. Phase III trial in metastatic gastroesophageal adenocarcinoma with fluorouracil, leucovorin plus either oxaliplatin or cisplatin: a study of the Arbeitsgemeinschaft Internistische Onkologie. *J Clin Oncol.* 2008;26:1435-1442.

16. Stahl M, Stuschke M, Lehmann N, et al. Chemoradiation with and without surgery in patients with locally advanced squamous cell carcinoma of the esophagus. *J Clin Oncol.* 2005;23:2310-2317.
17. Bedenne L, Michel P, Bouche O, et al. Chemoradiation followed by surgery compared with chemoradiation alone in squamous cancer of the esophagus: FFCD 9102. *J Clin Oncol.* 2007;25:1160-1168.
18. Wijnhoven BP, Tilanus HW, Dinjens WN. Molecular biology of Barrett's adenocarcinoma. *Ann Surg.* 2001;233:322-337.
19. Paulson TG, Reid BJ. Focus on Barrett's esophagus and esophageal adenocarcinoma. *Cancer Cell.* 2004;6:11-16.
20. Nancarrow DJ, Handoko HY, Smithers BM, et al. Genome-wide copy number analysis in esophageal adenocarcinoma using high-density single-nucleotide polymorphism arrays. *Cancer Res.* 2008;68:4163-4172.
21. Li X, Galipeau PC, Sanchez CA, et al. Single nucleotide polymorphism-based genome-wide chromosome copy change, loss of heterozygosity, and aneuploidy in Barrett's esophagus neoplastic progression. *Cancer Prev Res (Phila).* 2008;1:413-423.
22. Jenkins GJ, Doak SH, Parry JM, et al. Genetic pathways involved in the progression of Barrett's metaplasia to adenocarcinoma. *Br J Surg.* 2002;89:824-837.
23. Lai LA, Paulson TG, Li X, et al. Increasing genomic instability during premalignant neoplastic progression revealed through high resolution array-CGH. *Genes Chromosomes Cancer.* 2007;46:532-542.
24. Maley CC, Galipeau PC, Li X, et al. Selectively advantageous mutations and hitchhikers in neoplasms: p16 lesions are selected in Barrett's esophagus. *Cancer Res.* 2004;64:3414-3427.
25. Reid BJ, Li X, Galipeau PC, et al. Barrett's oesophagus and oesophageal adenocarcinoma: time for a new synthesis. *Nat Rev Cancer.* 2010;10:87-101.
26. Leedham SJ, Preston SL, McDonald SA, et al. Individual crypt genetic heterogeneity and the origin of metaplastic glandular epithelium in human Barrett's oesophagus. *Gut.* 2008;57:1041-1048.
27. Barrett MT, Sanchez CA, Prevo LJ, et al. Evolution of neoplastic cell lineages in Barrett oesophagus. *Nat Genet.* 1999;22:106-109.
28. Fritcher EG, Brankley SM, Kipp BR, et al. A comparison of conventional cytology, DNA ploidy analysis, and fluorescence in situ hybridization for the detection of dysplasia and adenocarcinoma in patients with Barrett's esophagus. *Hum Pathol.* 2008;39:1128-1135.
29. Ciardiello F, Tortora G. EGFR antagonists in cancer treatment. *N Engl J Med.* 2008;358:1160-1174.
30. Baselga J, Swain SM. Novel anticancer targets: revisiting ERBB2 and discovering ERBB3. *Nat Rev Cancer.* 2009;9:463-475.
31. Toker A, Yoeli-Lerner M. Akt signaling and cancer: surviving but not moving on. *Cancer Res.* 2006;66:3963-3966.
32. Roberts PJ, Der CJ. Targeting the Raf-MEK-ERK mitogen-activated protein kinase cascade for the treatment of cancer. *Oncogene.* 2007;26:3291-3310.
33. Meloche S, Pouyssegur J. The ERK1/2 mitogen-activated protein kinase pathway as a master regulator of the G1- to S-phase transition. *Oncogene.* 2007;26:3227-3239.
34. Wang KL, Wu TT, Choi IS, et al. Expression of epidermal growth factor receptor in esophageal and esophagogastric junction adenocarcinomas: association with poor outcome. *Cancer.* 2007;109:658-667.
35. Langer R, Von Rahden BH, Nahrig J, et al. Prognostic significance of expression patterns of c-erbB-2, p53, p16INK4A, p27KIP1, cyclin D1 and epidermal growth factor receptor in oesophageal adenocarcinoma: a tissue microarray study. *J Clin Pathol.* 2006;59:631-634.
36. Rojo F, Tabernero J, Albanell J, et al. Pharmacodynamic studies of gefitinib in tumor biopsy specimens from patients with advanced gastric carcinoma. *J Clin Oncol.* 2006;24:4309-4316.
37. Miller CT, Moy JR, Lin L, et al. Gene amplification in esophageal adenocarcinomas and Barrett's with high-grade dysplasia. *Clin Cancer Res.* 2003;9:4819-4825.
38. Rygiel AM, Milano F, Ten Kate FJ, et al. Gains and amplifications of c-myc, EGFR, and 20.q13 loci in the no dysplasia-dysplasia-adenocarcinoma sequence of Barrett's esophagus. *Cancer Epidemiol Biomarkers Prev.* 2008;17:1380-1385.
39. al-Kasspooles M, Moore JH, Orringer MB, et al. Amplification and over-expression of the EGFR and erbB-2 genes in human esophageal adenocarcinomas. *Int J Cancer.* 1993;54: 213-219.
40. Dragovich T, McCoy S, Fenoglio-Preiser CM, et al. Phase II trial of erlotinib in gastroesophageal junction and gastric adenocarcinomas: SWOG 0127. *J Clin Oncol.* 2006;24:4922-4927.
41. Dragovich T, Campen C. Anti-EGFR-targeted therapy for esophageal and gastric cancers: an evolving concept. *J Oncol.* 2009;2009:804108.
42. Imai K, Takaoka A. Comparing antibody and small-molecule therapies for cancer. *Nat Rev Cancer.* 2006;6:714-727.
43. Baselga J, Pfister D, Cooper MR, et al. Phase I studies of anti-epidermal growth factor receptor chimeric antibody C225 alone and in combination with cisplatin. *J Clin Oncol.* 2000;18:904-914.
44. Ferry DR, Anderson M, Beddard K, et al. A phase II study of gefitinib monotherapy in advanced esophageal adenocarcinoma: evidence of gene expression, cellular, and clinical response. *Clin Cancer Res.* 2007;13:5869-5875.
45. Janmaat ML, Gallegos-Ruiz MI, Rodriguez JA, et al. Predictive factors for outcome in a phase II study of gefitinib in second-line treatment of advanced esophageal cancer patients. *J Clin Oncol.* 2006;24:1612-1619.
46. Hecht JR. Lapatinib monotherapy in recurrent upper gastrointestinal malignancy: phase II efficacy and biomarker analyses. In: *2008 Gastrointestinal Cancers Symposium.* Orlando, FL; 2008. Abstract 43.
47. Gold PJ, Goldman B, Iqbal S, et al. Cetuximab as second-line therapy in patients with metastatic esophageal adenocarcinoma: a phase II Southwest Oncology Group Study (S0415). *J Thorac Oncol.* 2010;5:1472-1476.
48. Wainberg ZA, Lin LS, DiCarlo B, et al. Phase II trial of modified FOLFOX6 and erlotinib in patients with metastatic or advanced adenocarcinoma of the oesophagus and gastro-oesophageal junction. *Br J Cancer.* 2011;105:760-765.
49. Chan JA, Blaszkowsky LS, Enzinger PC, et al. A multicenter phase II trial of single-agent cetuximab in advanced esophageal and gastric adenocarcinoma. *Ann Oncol.* 2011;22:1367-1373.
50. Pinto C, Di Fabio F, Siena S, et al. Phase II study of cetuximab in combination with FOLFIRI in patients with untreated advanced gastric or gastroesophageal junction adenocarcinoma (FOLCETUX study). *Ann Oncol.* 2007;18:510-517.
51. Pinto C, Di Fabio F, Barone C, et al. Phase II study of cetuximab in combination with cisplatin and docetaxel in patients with untreated advanced gastric or gastro-oesophageal junction adenocarcinoma (DOCETUX study). *Br J Cancer.* 2009;101:1261-1268.
52. Lordick F, Luber B, Lorenzen S, et al. Cetuximab plus oxaliplatin/leucovorin/5-fluorouracil in first-line metastatic gastric cancer: a phase II study of the Arbeitsgemeinschaft Internistische Onkologie (AIO). *Br J Cancer.* 2010;102:500-505.
53. Lorenzen S, Schuster T, Porschen R, et al. Cetuximab plus cisplatin-5-fluorouracil versus cisplatin-5-fluorouracil alone in first-line metastatic squamous cell carcinoma of the esophagus: a randomized phase II study of the Arbeitsgemeinschaft Internistische Onkologie. *Ann Oncol.* 2009;20:1667-1673.
54. Enzinger PC, Burtness B, Hollis D, et al. CALGB 80403/ECOG 1206: a randomized phase II study of three standard chemotherapy regimens (ECF, IC, FOLFOX) plus cetuximab in metastatic esophageal and GE junction cancer. *J Clin Oncol.* 2010;28:Abstract 4006.
55. Bang YJ, Van Cutsem E, Feyereislova A, et al. Trastuzumab in combination with chemotherapy versus chemotherapy alone for treatment of HER2-positive advanced gastric or gastro-oesophageal junction cancer (ToGA): a phase 3, open-label, randomised controlled trial. *Lancet.* 2010;376:687-697.
56. Rao S, Starling N, Cunningham D, et al. Phase I study of epirubicin, cisplatin and capecitabine plus matuzumab in previously untreated patients with advanced oesophagogastric cancer. *Br J Cancer.* 2008;99:868-874.
57. Han SW, Oh DY, Im SA, et al. Phase II study and biomarker analysis of cetuximab combined with modified FOLFOX6 in advanced gastric cancer. *Br J Cancer.* 2009;100:298-304.
58. Richards DA, Kocs DM, Apira AI, et al. Results of docetaxel plus oxaliplatin (DOCOX) with or without cetuximab in patients with metastatic gastric and/or gastroesophageal junction adenocarcinoma: results of a randomized phase II study. *J Clin Oncol.* 2011;29:Abstract 4015.
59. Slamon DJ, Leyland-Jones B, Shak S, et al. Use of chemotherapy plus a monoclonal antibody against HER2 for metastatic

breast cancer that overexpresses HER2. *N Engl J Med.* 2001;344:783-792.
60. Piccart-Gebhart MJ, Procter M, Leyland-Jones B, et al. Trastuzumab after adjuvant chemotherapy in HER2-positive breast cancer. *N Engl J Med.* 2005;353:1659-1672.
61. Smith I, Procter M, Gelber RD, et al. 2-Year follow-up of trastuzumab after adjuvant chemotherapy in HER2-positive breast cancer: a randomised controlled trial. *Lancet.* 2007;369:29-36.
62. Fujimoto-Ouchi K, Sekiguchi F, Yasuno H, et al. Antitumor activity of trastuzumab in combination with chemotherapy in human gastric cancer xenograft models. *Cancer Chemother Pharmacol.* 2007;59:795-805.
63. Schoppmann SF, Jesch B, Friedrich J, et al. Expression of Her-2 in carcinomas of the esophagus. *Am J Surg Pathol.* 2010;34:1868-1873.
64. Hu Y, Bandla S, Godfrey TE, et al. HER2 amplification, overexpression and score criteria in esophageal adenocarcinoma. *Mod Pathol.* 2011;24:899-907.
65. Langer R, Rauser S, Feith M, et al. Assessment of ErbB2 (Her2) in oesophageal adenocarcinomas: summary of a revised immunohistochemical evaluation system, bright field double in situ hybridisation and fluorescence in situ hybridisation. *Mod Pathol.* 2011;24:908-916.
66. Thompson SK, Sullivan TR, Davies R, et al. HER-2/neu gene amplification in esophageal adenocarcinoma and its influence on survival. *Ann Surg Oncol.* 2011;18:2010-2017.
67. Reichelt U, Duesedau P, Tsourlakis M, et al. Frequent homogeneous HER-2 amplification in primary and metastatic adenocarcinoma of the esophagus. *Mod Pathol.* 2007;20: 120-129.
68. Yoon HH, Shi Q, Sukov WR, et al. Association of HER2/ErbB2 expression and gene amplification with pathological features and prognosis in esophageal adenocarcinomas. *Clin Cancer Res.* NIHMS337983, 2011 [Epub ahead of print].
69. Mimura K, Kono K, Hanawa M, et al. Frequencies of HER-2/neu expression and gene amplification in patients with oesophageal squamous cell carcinoma. *Br J Cancer.* 2005;92:1253-1260.
70. Sunpaweravong P, Sunpaweravong S, Puttawibul P, et al. Epidermal growth factor receptor and cyclin D1 are independently amplified and overexpressed in esophageal squamous cell carcinoma. *J Cancer Res Clin Oncol.* 2005;131:111-119.
71. Sato-Kuwabara Y, Neves JI, Fregnani JH, et al. Evaluation of gene amplification and protein expression of HER-2/neu in esophageal squamous cell carcinoma using fluorescence in situ hybridization (FISH) and immunohistochemistry. *BMC Cancer.* 2009;9:6.
72. Ferrara N, Hillan KJ, Gerber HP, et al. Discovery and development of bevacizumab, an anti-VEGF antibody for treating cancer. *Nat Rev Drug Discov.* 2004;3:391-400.
73. Zachary I. Signaling mechanisms mediating vascular protective actions of vascular endothelial growth factor. *Am J Physiol Cell Physiol.* 2001;280:C1375-C1386.
74. Zachary I, Gliki G. Signaling transduction mechanisms mediating biological actions of the vascular endothelial growth factor family. *Cardiovasc Res.* 2001;49:568-581.
75. Rafii S, Lyden D, Benezra R, et al. Vascular and haematopoietic stem cells: novel targets for anti-angiogenesis therapy? *Nat Rev Cancer.* 2002;2:826-835.
76. Plouet J, Moukadiri H. Characterization of the receptor to vasculotropin on bovine adrenal cortex-derived capillary endothelial cells. *J Biol Chem.* 1990;265:22071-22074.
77. Paavonen K, Puolakkainen P, Jussila L, et al. Vascular endothelial growth factor receptor-3 in lymphangiogenesis in wound healing. *Am J Pathol.* 2000;156:1499-1504.
78. Ferrara N, Gerber HP, LeCouter J. The biology of VEGF and its receptors. *Nat Med.* 2003;9:669-676.
79. Dvorak HF. Vascular permeability factor/vascular endothelial growth factor: a critical cytokine in tumor angiogenesis and a potential target for diagnosis and therapy. *J Clin Oncol.* 2002;20:4368-4380.
80. Kaipainen A, Korhonen J, Mustonen T, et al. Expression of the fms-like tyrosine kinase 4 gene becomes restricted to lymphatic endothelium during development. *Proc Natl Acad Sci U S A.* 1995;92:3566-3570.
81. Soker S, Takashima S, Miao HQ, et al. Neuropilin-1 is expressed by endothelial and tumor cells as an isoform-specific receptor for vascular endothelial growth factor. *Cell.* 1998;92:735-745.
82. Auvinen MI, Sihvo EI, Ruohtula T, et al. Incipient angiogenesis in Barrett's epithelium and lymphangiogenesis in Barrett's adenocarcinoma. *J Clin Oncol.* 2002;20:2971-2979.
83. Lord RV, Park JM, Wickramasinghe K, et al. Vascular endothelial growth factor and basic fibroblast growth factor expression in esophageal adenocarcinoma and Barrett esophagus. *J Thorac Cardiovasc Surg.* 2003;125:246-253.
84. Millikan KW, Mall JW, Myers JA, et al. Do angiogenesis and growth factor expression predict prognosis of esophageal cancer? *Am Surg.* 2000;66:401-405; discussion 405-406.
85. Imdahl A, Bognar G, Schulte-Monting J, et al. Predictive factors for response to neoadjuvant therapy in patients with oesophageal cancer. Eur J Cardiothorac Surg. 2002;21:657-663.
86. Kleespies A, Guba M, Jauch KW, et al. Vascular endothelial growth factor in esophageal cancer. *J Surg Oncol.* 2004;87:95-104.
87. Shimada H, Takeda A, Nabeya Y, et al. Clinical significance of serum vascular endothelial growth factor in esophageal squamous cell carcinoma. *Cancer.* 2001;92:663-669.
88. Wallner G, Ciechanski A, Dabrowski A, et al. Vascular endothelial growth factor and basic fibroblast growth factor in patients with squamous cell oesophageal cancer. *Folia* Histochem Cytobiol. 2001;39(suppl 2):122-123.
89. Dreilich M, Wagenius G, Bergstrom S, et al. The role of cystatin C and the angiogenic cytokines VEGF and bFGF in patients with esophageal carcinoma. *Med Oncol.* 2005;22:29-38.
90. Gockel I, Moehler M, Frerichs K, et al. Co-expression of receptor tyrosine kinases in esophageal adenocarcinoma and squamous cell cancer. *Oncol Rep.* 2008;20:845-850.
91. Loges S, Clausen H, Reichelt U, et al. Determination of microvessel density by quantitative real-time PCR in esophageal cancer: correlation with histologic methods, angiogenic growth factor expression, and lymph node metastasis. *Clin Cancer Res.* 2007;13:76-80.
92. Hurwitz H, Fehrenbacher L, Novotny W, et al. Bevacizumab plus irinotecan, fluorouracil, and leucovorin for metastatic colorectal cancer. *N Engl J Med.* 2004;350:2335-2342.
93. Ohtsu A, Shah MA, Van Cutsem E, et al. Bevacizumab in combination with chemotherapy as first-line therapy in advanced gastric cancer: a randomized, double-blind, placebo-controlled phase III study. *J Clin Oncol.* 2011;29:3968-3976.
94. Bang YJ, Kang YK, Kang WK, et al. Phase II study of sunitinib as second-line treatment for advanced gastric cancer. *Invest New Drugs.* 2011;29:1449-1458.
95. Ilson D, Janjigian YY, Shah MA, et al. Phase II trial of sorafenib in esophageal (E) and gastroesophageal junction (GEJ) cancer: response and protracted stable disease observed in adenocarcinoma. *J Clin Oncol.* 2011;29:Abstract 4100.
96. Sun W, Powell M, O'Dwyer PJ, et al. Phase II study of sorafenib in combination with docetaxel and cisplatin in the treatment of metastatic or advanced gastric and gastroesophageal junction adenocarcinoma: ECOG 5203. *J Clin Oncol.* 2010;28: 2947-2951.
97. Enzinger P, Fidias P, Meyerhardt J, et al. Phase II study of bevacizumab and docetaxel in metastatic esophageal and gastric cancer. In: *ASCO Gastrointestinal Cancers Symposium General Poster Session B.* San Francisco, CA; 2006.
98. El-Rayes BF, Zalupski M, Bekai-Saab T, et al. A phase II study of bevacizumab, oxaliplatin, and docetaxel in locally advanced and metastatic gastric and gastroesophageal junction cancers. *Ann Oncol.* 2010;21:1999-2004.
99. Enzinger P, Ryan DP, Regan EM, et al. Phase II trial of docetaxel, cisplatin, irinotecan, and bevacizumab in metastatic esophagogastric cancer. *J Clin Oncol.* 2008;26:Abstract 4552.
100. Shah MA, Jhawer M, Ilson DH, et al. Phase II study of modified docetaxel, cisplatin, and fluorouracil with bevacizumab in patients with metastatic gastroesophageal adenocarcinoma. *J Clin Oncol.* 2011;29:868-874.
101. Shah MA, Ramanathan RK, Ilson DH, et al. Multicenter phase II study of irinotecan, cisplatin, and bevacizumab in patients with metastatic gastric or gastroesophageal junction adenocarcinoma. *J Clin Oncol.* 2006;24:5201-5206.

102. Jung YD, Mansfield PF, Akagi M, et al. Effects of combination anti-vascular endothelial growth factor receptor and anti-epidermal growth factor receptor therapies on the growth of gastric cancer in a nude mouse model. *Eur J Cancer*. 2002;38:1133-1140.
103. Ryu JS, Hong YC, Han HS, et al. Association between polymorphisms of ERCC1 and XPD and survival in non-small-cell lung cancer patients treated with cisplatin combination chemotherapy. *Lung Cancer*. 2004;44:311-316.
104. Stoehlmacher J, Park DJ, Zhang W, et al. A multivariate analysis of genomic polymorphisms: prediction of clinical outcome to 5-FU/oxaliplatin combination chemotherapy in refractory colorectal cancer. *Br J Cancer*. 2004;91:344-354.
105. Quintela-Fandino M, Hitt R, Medina PP, et al. DNA-repair gene polymorphisms predict favorable clinical outcome among patients with advanced squamous cell carcinoma of the head and neck treated with cisplatin-based induction chemotherapy. *J Clin Oncol*. 2006;24:4333-4339.
106. Wu X, Gu J, Wu TT, et al. Genetic variations in radiation and chemotherapy drug action pathways predict clinical outcomes in esophageal cancer. *J Clin Oncol*. 2006;24:3789-3798.
107. Yoon HH, Catalano PJ, Murphy KM, et al. Genetic variation in DNA-repair pathways and response to radiochemotherapy in esophageal adenocarcinoma: a retrospective cohort study of the Eastern Cooperative Oncology Group. *BMC Cancer*. 2011;11:176.
108. Herman JG, Baylin SB. Gene silencing in cancer in association with promoter hypermethylation. *N Engl J Med*. 2003;349:2042-2054.
109. Hamilton JP, Sato F, Greenwald BD, et al. Promoter methylation and response to chemotherapy and radiation in esophageal cancer. *Clin Gastroenterol Hepatol*. 2006;4:701-708.
110. Brock MV, Gou M, Akiyama Y, et al. Prognostic importance of promoter hypermethylation of multiple genes in esophageal adenocarcinoma. *Clin Cancer Res*. 2003;9:2912-2919.
111. Yang H, Gu J, Wang KK, et al. MicroRNA expression signatures in Barrett's esophagus and esophageal adenocarcinoma. *Clin Cancer Res*. 2009;15:5744-5752.
112. Mathe EA, Nguyen GH, Bowman ED, et al. MicroRNA expression in squamous cell carcinoma and adenocarcinoma of the esophagus: associations with survival. *Clin Cancer Res*. 2009;15:6192-6200.
113. Wijnhoven BP, Hussey DJ, Watson DI, et al. MicroRNA profiling of Barrett's oesophagus and oesophageal adenocarcinoma. *Br J Surg*. 2010;97:853-861.
114. Ilson DH, Minsky BD, Ku GY, et al. Phase 2 trial of induction and concurrent chemoradiotherapy with weekly irinotecan and cisplatin followed by surgery for esophageal cancer. *Cancer*. 2012;118:2820-2827.
115. Javeri H, Xiao L, Rohren E, et al. The higher the decrease in the standardized uptake value of positron emission tomography after chemoradiation, the better the survival of patients with gastroesophageal adenocarcinoma. *Cancer*. 2009;115: 5184-5192.
116. van Heijl M, Omloo JM, van Berge Henegouwen MI, et al. Fluorodeoxyglucose positron emission tomography for evaluating early response during neoadjuvant chemoradiotherapy in patients with potentially curable esophageal cancer. *Ann Surg*. 2011;253:56-63.
117. Monjazeb AM, Riedlinger G, Aklilu M, et al. Outcomes of patients with esophageal cancer staged with [1F] fluorodeoxyglucose positron emission tomography (FDG-PET): can postchemoradiotherapy FDG-PET predict the utility of resection? *J Clin Oncol*. 2010;28:4714-4721.
118. Lordick F, Ott K, Krause BJ, et al. PET to assess early metabolic response and to guide treatment of adenocarcinoma of the oesophagogastric junction: the MUNICON phase II trial. *Lancet Oncol*. 2007;8:797-805.
119. Kelsen DP, Ginsberg R, Pajak TF, et al. Chemotherapy followed by surgery compared with surgery alone for localized esophageal cancer. *N Engl J Med*. 1998;339:1979-1984.
120. Ott K, Weber WA, Lordick F, et al. Metabolic imaging predicts response, survival, and recurrence in adenocarcinomas of the esophagogastric junction. *J Clin Oncol*. 2006;24:4692-4698.
121. zum Buschenfelde CM, Herrmann K, Schuster T, et al. (18) F-FDG PET-guided salvage neoadjuvant radiochemotherapy of adenocarcinoma of the esophagogastric junction: the MUNICON II trial. *J Nucl Med*. 2011;52:1189-1196.
122. Begnami MD, Fukuda E, Fregnani JH, et al. Prognostic implications of altered human epidermal growth factor receptors (HERs) in gastric carcinomas: HER2 and HER3 are predictors of poor outcome. *J Clin Oncol*. 2011;29:3030-3036.
123. Hayashi M, Inokuchi M, Takagi Y, et al. High expression of HER3 is associated with a decreased survival in gastric cancer. *Clin Cancer Res*. 2008;14:7843-7849.
124. Baselga J, Cortes J, Kim SB, et al. Pertuzumab plus trastuzumab plus docetaxel for metastatic breast cancer. *N Engl J Med*. 2012;366:109-119.

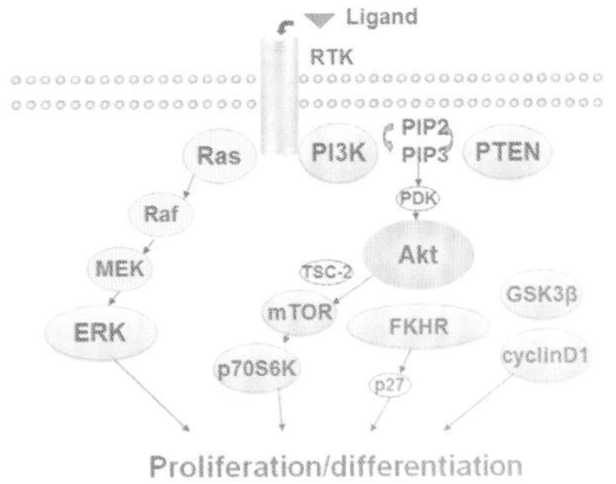

CHAPTER 56

Personalized Medicine and Targeted Therapy of Gastric Cancer

YingWei Xue, XueFeng Yu, and Yanqiao Zhang

Gastric cancer (GC), one of the most common malignant tumors, is the second most common cause of cancer-related death in the world. The management of this common malignancy requires an integrative multidisciplinary approach consisting of surgery, chemoradiation, and targeted therapy.[1,2] Although a detailed description of all treatment modalities of GC is beyond the scope of this chapter, we focus on new developments in individualized managements of GC by minimally invasive surgery and targeted therapy of GC.

INTRODUCTION OF MINIMALLY INVASIVE SURGERY OF GC

For early GC, surgery should be the first choice, and one optimal approach is by minimally invasive surgery. Minimally invasive surgery for GC consists mainly of three types, namely, endoscopic surgery, laparoscopic surgery, and robotic surgery.

Endoscopic Surgery

In recent years, with the rapid development of minimally invasive surgeries and the gradual awareness of the rapid recovery concept, medical professionals began to look for a treatment that could achieve maximal therapeutic effects with minimal invasiveness. Endoscopic mucosal resection (EMR) and endoscopic submucosal dissection (ESD) arose in this setting.

EMR can be used to strip mucosal lesions under endoscopy and achieve complete resection with the use of high-frequency current. This procedure developed from a combination of endoscopic polyp resection, endoscopic mucosal injection technique, titanium clip homeostasis, and other endoscopic techniques, as a new approach to targeting superficial mucosal lesions.[3] The main principle of EMR is injecting saline under the mucous membrane to elevate mucous lesions, which are then removed by a high-frequency electric trap method that eradicates the mucosal layer of early cancer as well as precancerous lesions. This surgery has many advantages over previous procedures, such as a smaller incision, fewer complications, and less pain for the patient; in addition, it is safer and easier to perform than previous procedures. However, EMR generally cannot remove larger lesions with one procedure, which can easily lead to tumor residue and recurrence; having an accurate understanding of the extent of invasion is necessary. An endoscopic ultrasound examination is essential before treatment, which helps not only in determining the extent of disease but also in assessing whether there is gastric lymph node metastasis.

ESD is a highly refined technique compared with EMR. Indications for ESD generally entail early GC. ESD requires specific skill and expertise. The essence of the technique is to dissect the submucosal layer with direct vision and maintain the cutting plane above the underlying muscularis propria.[4] In general, this procedure makes use of an electric knife (IT knife) to insulate the ceramic ball on top to perform a one-time removal of submucosally dissected tissue for early digestive tract cancer.[5] Lesions are first marked by the IT knife, and then the mucosa and submucosa are separated by the IT knife to achieve complete resection. ESD has the advantages of completely removing relatively large lesions at one time with less recurrence of tumor, whereas its disadvantages include higher risk of perforation.

Patients need only 1 day of fasting after ESD and can be discharged 3 days later. Compared with traditional surgery, expense and hospitalization time for ESD are considerably lower, and this procedure is especially suitable for patients who are unwilling to undergo traditional surgery due to age or contraindications. Nevertheless, ESD is still an experimental treatment that should be selected carefully because of a lack of clinical evidence of its efficacy. Furthermore, new ESD devices that render the procedure more safe and efficient are still being developed to improve the overall results from ESD use for early GC.

The specific scope of application for use of EMR and ESD: (1) Tis or T1N0M0 tumors in patients who cannot tolerate laparotomy or laparoscopy. (2) Tis or T1aN0M0 differentiated tumors with a diameter of less than 2 cm, and patient has no ulcer lesions.

Laparoscopic Surgery

In 1994, Kitano, a Japanese scholar, first reported radical gastrectomy by laparoscopy to treat early GC.[6] In 1997, Goh and his colleagues adopted laparoscopy to treat advanced GC.[7] Because of the advantages of laparoscopic surgery (e.g., less bleeding, less postoperative pain, better cosmetic results, rapid recovery of intestinal function, and shorter hospitalization time compared with laparotomy), scholars around the world adopted laparoscopy to treat GC and achieved great success. The laparoscopic technique is now more mature. There are no significant differences between laparotomy (open gastrectomy) and laparoscopy in the number of intraoperative and postoperative complications, and laparoscopy is even superior to laparotomy. Many retrospective comparative trials and randomized controlled trials have confirmed that laparoscopic gastrectomy is safe and feasible and that short-term outcomes are better than those of open gastrectomy in patients with early GC.[8]

As laparoscopic experience has accumulated, the indications for laparoscopic gastrectomy have been broadened to include older and overweight patients and those with advanced GC.[9] Laparoscopy can be applied not only in radical surgery but also in determining preoperative diagnosis and tumor stage and in assisting in percutaneous endoscopic gastrostomy/jejunostomy (PEG/PEJ) with greater superiority. As for treatment principles, laparoscopic GC surgery follows the same principles of laparotomy, including achieving complete resection of the tumor and surrounding tissues, following the tumor non-touch principle, obtaining an adequate cutting margin, and performing complete lymph node dissection. Some studies have confirmed that the 5-year survival rate after laparoscopic surgery was similar to that of laparotomy. Surgical indications and contraindications for laparoscopic surgery are summarized in Table 56.1.

TABLE 56-1 Surgical Indications and Contraindications for Laparoscopic Surgery

Indications

- Invasion depth of GC is within T2
- Other malignant tumors such as malignant mesenchymoma and lymphoma
- Exploration and staging of malignant gastric tumor
- PEG/PEJ of advanced malignant GC

Contraindications

- Gastric serosa is violated, or tumor diameter is no less than 10 cm, or lymph nodes are infused and surround major blood vessels and tumor, with wide invasion of surrounding tissues
- Patients who receive abdominal surgery or GC emergency surgery or have severe adhesions, severe obesity, or cardiopulmonary dysfunction

GC, gastric cancer; PEG/PEJ, percutaneous endoscopic gastrostomy/jejunostomy.

Robotic Surgery (da Vinci)

In recent years, the emerging technology of surgical robots has increased the accuracy and feasibility of surgery to a new level compared with minimally invasive surgery.[10] The da Vinci surgical robot (manufactured by Intuitive Surgical, Sunnyvale, CA) consists of three parts: (i) the main operating console for the surgeon; (ii) the mobile platform near the surgical bed that is composed of a manipulator, camera arm, and surgical instruments; and (iii) the three-dimensional imaging platform for video images. Surgeons do not have direct contact with patients during surgery. With the use of a three-dimensional vision system and motion control calibration system, motions of the arm, wrist, and fingers of surgeons are recorded in computers by sensors and simultaneously transferred to a mechanical arm. All types of special surgical instruments are installed on the anterior part of the mechanical arm to mimic the complex motions the surgeon makes in performing an operation. Currently, surgeries that make use of the da Vinci system in the field of gastrointestinal surgery include gastric reconstruction, stomach reduction surgery, benign tumor resection, bypass operation, radical resection of GC, and complex lymph node dissection. The characteristic features of the da Vinci robotic surgery are summarized in Table 56.2. It is believed that one day da Vinci robotic surgery will replace conventional laparotomy to become the surgeons' preferred technique.

In summary, advanced minimally invasive techniques, such as EMR, ESD, laparoscopy-assisted gastrectomy, and laparoscopy-assisted pylorus-preserving gastrectomy, have been widely performed.[9] In the near future, robotic surgery will become an additional option in minimally invasive surgery for GC. Such developments will be important components of personalized medicine for managing GC and improving the quality of life of patients after GC surgery.

TABLE 56-2 Major Characteristics of da Vinci Robotic Surgery

Unique Advantages:

1. Joint wrist on surgical instrument has more freedom of movement and more flexibility, which expands operational abilities of surgeons, and improves surgical precision.
2. Surgical instruments can eliminate effects of natural vibration of hands during surgery.
3. Surgical instruments on terminal end of system have the functions of traction, cutting, and sewing, et al., which can make surgeons perform precise operations in narrow spaces.
4. Visualized three-dimensional high-definition image with 10–15 times of amplification, which is more clear than the human eyes. Surgeons can adjust the lens on their own to see the vision they want directly, which makes it easy for surgeons to clearly and precisely perform tissue location as well as instrument operation.
5. Surgeons can sit when performing operations, which is beneficial to completion of long-time and complicated surgery.

Disadvantages:

1. Lack of tactile sensation feedback system.
2. The whole equipment is too huge with complicated installation and debugging
3. The system is technically complicated, all types of mechanical failures may occur during surgery, such as halfway crash.
4. Systemic study demands more time, and it takes more time for doctors and system to achieve full cooperation.
5. Preoperative preparation and intraoperative equipment replacement take too much time.
6. The surgical robot is expensive.

MOLECULAR PATHOGENESIS AND TARGETED THERAPY OF GC

Although the diagnostic techniques and surgical skills have improved in recent years, the cure rate of surgical treatment is still very low. The prognosis of patients with advanced cancer is still poor. Chemotherapy also shows some limitations and inefficacy even though the regimens are continuously updated.

Recently, research interest has focused on the root causes of GC and demonstrated that some molecular biomarkers may be associated with postoperative relapse of GC and the response to chemotherapy and targeted therapy. The increasing role of molecular pathology in medical practice and the application of targeted therapy in individualized treatment urgently require a better understanding of the molecular pathology of GC and more knowledge of targeted treatment techniques.

Integrated researches in molecular pathology have shown that GC is a chronic proliferative disease. The pathogenesis of GC involves *Helicobacter pylori* infection, chronic active or atrophic gastritis, and intestinal metaplasia. The development of GC is characterized by multiple genetic and epigenetic alterations. Genetic polymorphism is also an important endogenous cause.

The genetic abnormality during gastric carcinogenesis is a complex and multistep process. The steps include activation of oncogenes, inactivation of tumor suppressor genes, overexpression of growth factors/receptors and abnormal expression of matrix metalloproteinases (MMPs), abnormality of DNA repair genes and cell adhesion molecules, and abnormalities of cell cycle regulators. The epigenetic changes are due to gene silencing of tumor suppressors by CpG island methylation and overexpression of tumor-promoting genes at the transcriptional level. Additionally, genetic polymorphisms predispose an individual to cancer and alter his/her susceptibility to cancer.[11] So a better understanding of the pathogenesis of GC is useful for improving our diagnostic techniques and molecular therapeutic strategies. We will describe the molecular carcinogenesis of GC in the following text.

Activation of Oncogenes and Inactivation of Tumor Suppressor Genes

Activation of proto-oncogenes and inactivation of tumor suppressor genes play a very important role in the development of GC.

Proto-oncogenes are ubiquitous in living organisms, which are highly conservative during evolution. They belong to the house-keeping gene family, including members such as *src*, *ras*, *myc*, *sis*, and *myb*. The proteins encoded by these genes have very important physiological functions, e.g., growth factor, growth factor receptor, intracellular informational molecules, and transcriptional regulators. Therefore, in the complex pathway of signal transduction, the abnormal expression or overexpression of proto-oncogene–encoded proteins will disturb the normal cellular signal transduction pathway, which subsequently leads to the disorder of cell proliferation and differentiation.

Tumor suppressor genes are negative regulatory genes. The coexpression of these genes with oncogenes is important in regulating normal cell growth, proliferation, and differentiation. *P53* and *Rb* are two important tumor suppressor genes. The proteins encoded by tumor suppressor genes can inhibit cell growth and induce terminal cell differentiation or programmed cell death. The deletion or inactivation of tumor suppressor genes will result in carcinogenesis. In gastric tissues, the abnormality of oncogenes and tumor suppressor genes will increase the risk of GC.

P53 is a tumor suppressor gene, which is located in the short arm of chromosome 17. *P53*-encoded protein is involved in cell cycle control and tumorigenesis. Therefore, mutation or allelic deletion of *P53* gene will lead to the inactivation of its function. This gene plays an important role in the development of a number of human tumors. In GC, the abnormality of *P53* gene includes missense mutation, reading frame shift, and loss of heterozygosity. Immunohistochemical analysis showed that the prevalence of *P53* mutation ranged from 13% to 50% in GC.[12]

Rb gene is the first identified tumor suppressor gene. Three key members of *Rb* family are involved in the regulation of cell cycle. They are pRB/p105, pRB2/p130, and p107. Studies have revealed that loss of function or low expression of the members of the RB protein family was present in many tumors. In the tissue of GC, loss of pRB/p105 function is also prevalent. However, the role and mechanism of pRB/p105 in GC are still unknown. The other two proteins also play important roles in the tumorigenesis of GC, which still require further research.[13]

Overexpression of Growth Factor/Receptor and Angiogenic Factor

GC cells produce various growth factors and express their receptors abnormally. These factors have important biological effects. They induce not only cell growth but also extracellular matrix degradation and angiogenesis, which can facilitate tumor invasion and metastasis.

Epidermal Growth Factor

Epidermal growth factor receptor (EGFR) is a transmembrane glycoprotein, including three domains: one extracellular functional domain to bind with EGF, one short transmembrane domain, and one intracellular domain with tyrosine kinase activity. Growth factors such as transforming growth factor α (TGF-α) and EGF are the endogenous ligand of EGFR. EGFR binding with ligand can regulate normal cell growth and differentiation. The biological property of EGFR and its high expression in tumors can increase the invasion of tumor cells, facilitate tumor angiogenesis, and inhibit the apoptosis of tumor cells. Meanwhile, they are also the target of antitumor therapy. Some studies have reported that the level of EGFR mRNA was significantly higher in tumor samples than in normal tissues. EGFR overexpression was identified in 29.6% to 46.6% of GCs.[12] The abnormal expression of EGF, TGF, and their receptors is associated with the depth of tumor infiltration, progression, and adverse outcomes.[14]

ErbB2 (HER-2)

HER-2 proto-oncogene is the encoding gene of EGF receptor 2 (HER-2). ErbB2/HER-2 is a transmembrane tyrosine kinase receptor. It is highly homologous to EGFR. It is a member of the EGFR family. The expression of erbB2-encoded protein can be detected in normal gastric mucosa.[15] However, HER-2 is positive in 21% of the gastric adenocarcinoma tissues.[16] Generally, HER-2 expression is associated with large tumors, lymphatic invasion, metastasis, and serosal invasion. The 5-year survival rate in patients positive for HER-2 expression is much lower than that in patients without HER-2 expression. Therefore, HER-2 is an independent prognostic factor of GC.[17]

Vascular Endothelial Growth Factor and Tumor Angiogenesis

Angiogenesis is a complicated process, including the secretion of metalloproteinases and other matrix-degrading enzymes, cell migration, endothelial cell division and proliferation, as well as vessel formation. Tumor angiogenesis is mediated and controlled by the angiogenic factors secreted by tumor cells and stromal cells. The neovessels of tumor cells not only provide the substances essential for tumor growth but also increase the chance of metastasis of tumor cells via blood vessels. The formation of neovessels is essential for tumor metastasis. As the density of tumor vessels increases, the opportunity for tumor metastasis also increases significantly. This predicts poor outcomes. In GC, there is a positive association between microvessel count, metastatic potential, and poor prognosis.[11] The anti-angiogenic treatment strategy includes the following: (1) intervene the ligand, receptor, and downstream signal system of angiogenesis; (2) upregulate or release the endogenous angiogenesis inhibitors; (3) directly target tumor vasculature system by inhibiting the proliferation of endothelial cells or activating the apoptosis of endothelial cells.[18] Currently, vascular endothelial growth factor (VEGF) is the primary target of anti-angiogenic therapy.

Matrix Metalloproteinases

MMPs are another major factor to facilitate angiogenesis. The main function of these enzymes is to degrade and alter the extracellular matrix surrounding the tumor. Inhibition of MMPs will lead to the inhibition of neovessel formation in tumor tissues. Some studies have confirmed the prognostic value of MMPs in patients with GC. For example, the level of MMP-2 antigen is an independent prognostic marker in GC. Hence, MMP inhibitors may be a good intervention strategy.[19] In addition, high expression of cyclooxygenase (COX)-2, TGF-α, MMP-7, and MMP-9 in GC implies poor prognosis.[20]

DNA Repair Genes

There are numerous DNA repair genes in cells. They are responsible for the repair of specific DNA damage and so play an important role in avoiding gene mutation and keeping genome stability. DNA repair enzymes do not inhibit cell proliferation directly. However, if they lose the gene repair ability, especially the ability to repair the genes controlling cell growth and proliferation, gene mutation will increase. The accumulation of high-frequency DNA misrepair will lead to the inactivation of some key genes associated with cell growth and proliferation and eventually result in carcinogenesis. Dysfunction of mismatch repair gene will lead to microsatellite instability (MSI). The prevalence of MSI is 16% to 36% in GC. It may be the second most important risk factor to predict the development of GC.[21] The occurrence of GC is associated with at least two different types of gene instability, i.e., chromosome instability (loss of heterozygosity pathway) and microsatellite instability (MSI pathway). The GC associated with MSI usually shows lack of hMLH1 expression and high methylation of hMLH1 promoter. MSI frequency is positively correlated to multiple tumors.

MSI frequency is relatively higher in patients with multiple cancers. The detection of MSI in GC patients can predict the risk of another cancer. Meanwhile, a number of studies have demonstrated that MSI is associated with low-level tumor invasion and good prognosis.[11] Recent researches have shown that the progression-free survival (PFS) appeared longer in GC patients with high-level MSI than in those patients with low-level MSI or microsatellite stability.[22]

Cell Adhesion Molecules

Cell adhesion molecules are defined as molecules involved in the cell–cell interaction or the interaction between cell and extracellular matrix. They play an important role in maintaining cellular structure and normal tissue function. All cell adhesion molecules are transmembrane glycoproteins. Their molecular structure is composed of three parts: (1) extracellular domain, N-terminal of the peptide chain, with sugar chain, responsible for recognizing ligand; (2) transmembrane domain, usually crosses the membrane once; and (3) cytoplasmic domain, C-terminal of the peptide chain, usually of small size, or directly connects to the skeleton structure under plasma membrane or the intracellular chemical signal molecule to activate signal transduction pathway. Cell adhesion molecules are generally classified into five types: cadherins, selectin, immunoglobulin superfamily, integrin, and hyaladherin. The most frequently studied cell adhesion molecules in GC tissues are cadherins and hyaladherin.

The effect of cadherin is dependent on Ca^{2+}. Up to now, more than 30 cadherins have been identified. They are widely distributed in various tissues. Cadherins are implicated in cell junction, cell differentiation, and inhibition of cell migration. E-cadherin is a member of the cadherin family. Reduction or loss of E-cadherin on cell surface is reported in many types of cancer tissues, which makes the cancer cell drop off from the tumor easily, and provides an opportunity for cancer invasion and metastasis. For this reason, some authors considered E-cadherin as a metastasis-inhibiting molecule. The degradation product of epithelial E-cadherin is the soluble fragments of epithelial cadherins, which can be detected in the plasma of cancer patients. The soluble fragment of epithelial cadherins is a reliable marker for predicting the prognosis of GC. High-level soluble fragment of epithelial cadherins indicates extensive cancer metastasis.[23] Dysadherin is a tumor-related membrane glycoprotein. It can downregulate the expression of epithelial cadherins, promoting tumor metastasis. The patients have the worst prognosis if they have both positive dysadherin and low expression of epithelial cadherins. But dysadherin is not an independent prognostic factor.[24]

Hyaladherins are a group of molecules that bind to the sugar chain of hyaluronic acid. They have similar amino acid sequences and spatial conformation. CD44 is a member of the hyaladherin family and is a transmembrane glycoprotein that is expressed on the cell surface. It is extensively distributed and can be detected in lymphocytes and fibroblasts. CD44 is a very important hyaluronic acid receptor. It is the main component of extracellular matrix, which can facilitate the cell–cell and cell–matrix interaction. Numerous CD44 cell subtypes can be identified on the surface of tumor cells. Serum CD44 level is correlated to the prognosis of GC. Moreover, CD44 is also involved in the activation and reflux of lymphocytes, adhesion to extracellular matrix, angiogenesis, and cell proliferation and migration. Studies indicated that the survival in patients with low CD44v6 expression was significantly better than that in patients with high expression.[25] Additionally, the serum level of soluble CD44v6 is a prognostic predictor in poorly differentiated GC.[26] CD44v9 expression is associated not only with tumor invasion, metastasis, and advanced stage but also with the tumor recurrence mortality of GC.[27,28]

Abnormality of Cell Cycle Regulation

Cell cycle is regulated by both positive and negative regulators. The disorder of cell cycle regulators will cause gene instability and cell proliferation and finally lead to carcinogenesis. The abnormal expression and gene alteration of cyclins and cyclin-dependent kinase (CDK) are important in the tumorigenesis of GC. Gene amplification of cyclin E is present in 15% to 20% of GC samples.[11] An increased expression of cyclin E correlates with tumor stage, invasion, and proliferation. It may be used as a biomarker of malignant cancer phenotype. P21 protein is a cell cycle regulator, which can cause tumor arrest at G1 phase and lead to DNA repair or apoptosis. *p53* participates in cell cycle regulation in part through p21 induction. Inactivation of p53 is important for carcinogenesis, which occurs in over 60% of all GCs.

Cell cycle checkpoints control cell cycle transitions and ensure DNA replication and chromosome segregation with high fidelity. Checkpoint kinase 1 (Chk1) and checkpoint kinase 2 (Chk2) are DNA damage-activated kinases involved at the G2/M checkpoint. Damaged DNA can activate Chk1 and Chk2 to block cell cycle and have the damaged DNA repaired. Both Chk1 and Chk2 are overexpressed in more than 70% of GCs associated with the *p53* mutation.[11]

Epigenetic Alterations

Both abnormalities of the transcription step and post-translational modifications belong to the epigenetic alterations that occur in GC. The abnormal methylation of CpG islands—usually associated with tumor suppressor genes—leads to transcriptional silencing, inactivation of gene function, and finally carcinogenesis.[29,30] In GC, aberrant methylation occurs in several tumor suppressor genes, such as *p16*, CDH1 (E-cadherin), HMLH1, RAR-beta, RUNX3, MGMT (O^6-methylguanine methyltransferase), and TSP1 (thrombospondin-1), with the incidence of methylation ranging from 10% to 70%.[11]

Several studies found that the epigenetic alterations of tumor-related genes are associated with age. The effect of epigenetic factors on genes also increases with age. Other studies also demonstrated that the methylation level is significantly higher in stage III/IV cancer patients than in stage I/II patients. This further supports the fact that the methylation of tumor-related genes gradually increases as cancer progresses.[31] Therefore, the methylation of some specific genes can be taken as the molecular marker of the transition from precancerous lesion to malignant cancer.

Genetic Polymorphism

Genetic polymorphism is a very important endogenous factor of carcinogenesis, including single-nucleotide polymorphism (SNP), repetitive sequence, gene insertion, deletion, and recombination. SNP is the most common genetic polymorphism in human genome. The most representative genetic polymorphism in GC tissues includes inflammatory factor IL-1B and its antagonistic gene IL-1RN, as well as *N*-acetyltransferase. SNP is present in HER-2 transmembrane domain. SNP is also found in the promoter region of EGF (61 A/G), E-cadherin (–160C/A), MMP-1 (–1607 1G/2G), and MMP-9 (–1562 C/T) genes. The SNPs in the above-described promoter region can affect gene expression. The SNPs of HER-2, EGF, and E-cadherin are associated with the risk of GC. The HER-2, E-cadherin, and MMP-9 genotypes of GC patients are associated with cancer invasion, metastasis, and stages. However, MMP-1 is only associated with histological differentiation. So, the SNPs of HER-2, E-cadherin, and MMP-9 in GC could serve as a predictor of the risk for malignant phenotype of GC. However, contradictory viewpoints are reported in terms of the relation between E-cadherin SNP and GC.[32,33]

INDIVIDUALIZED TREATMENT

Pharmacological therapy is one of the most important approaches to GC. The issue of most concern is how to choose an effective and less toxic drug. However, tumor cells are characteristic of heterogeneity, pleomorphism, various levels of differentiation, and varied susceptibility to different drugs. There is no drug effective for all types of tumor cells. Therefore, for GC patients at an advanced stage, development of more effective, sensitive drugs at adequate dosage and individualized treatment plans are pressing problems to be resolved at present. The drugs currently available for treating GC include 5-fluorouracil, platinum, doxorubicin, taxanes, irinotecan, and molecular targeted drugs.

In the 1990s, several phase III clinical trials confirmed that 5-fluorouracil–based chemotherapy provided survival benefits to patients with advanced stage GC. The subsequently developed three-drug combination chemotherapy, including epirubicin, cisplatin, 5-fluorouracil, showed survival benefits for GC patients. This regimen has become the standard therapy for GC at present. For more than 10 years, the newly developed cytotoxic drugs, such as irinotecan, taxanes, oxaliplatin, and oral fluorouracils (S-1, capecitabine), have shown promising and encouraging efficacy. Currently, 5-fluorouracil can be replaced with capecitabine and cisplatin replaced with oxaliplatin in the typical three-drug regimen. The newly updated regimen has demonstrated good safety and efficacy in GC and gastroesophageal junction adenocarcinoma.

Although current chemotherapy regimens are continuously improving, the prognosis of patients with advanced cancer is still poor. Fortunately, the development of some targeted drugs, which specifically interfere with tumor cell growth, cell cycle, apoptosis, angiogenesis, and invasion, brings new hope to patients with advanced GC. The targeted drugs currently available include EGFR inhibitors, HER-2 inhibitors, anti-angiogenic drugs, cell cycle inhibitors, COX inhibitors, and MMP inhibitors.

EGFR Inhibitors

EGFR is a cell surface receptor. It is the binding site for the members of the EGF family. EGFR is expressed in about 50% to 60% of gastric cells. EGFR has been intensively and extensively studied in basic and clinical trials. Anti-EGFR drugs are the first molecular targeted drugs used to treat solid tumors.[34] Previous studies have confirmed the expression of EGFR in GC. Anti-EGFR drugs such as erlotinib, gefitinib, cetuximab, and panitumumab have been used in clinical studies. Anti-EGFR drugs in combination with cytotoxic agents have achieved encouraging results in treating stage II GC in clinical trials.

Cetuximab and Panitumumab

Cetuximab is one of the most commonly used anti-EGFR monoclonal antibodies. It is a human–mouse chimeric IgG1 anti-EGFR monoclonal antibody. Cetuximab has shown significant efficacy in metastatic colorectal cancer. As an IgG1 antibody, its antitumor mechanism includes competitive inhibition of EGF and its ligand, as well as antibody-dependent cell-mediated cytotoxicity reaction. Several phase II trials have established that cetuximab, particularly with irinotecan, increased response rates to 62% in advanced stage GC.[35] Cetuximab in combination with other various chemotherapy agents is effective in 40.5% to 65.2% of the untreated progressive GCs. Time to progression is 2.1 to 8 months. The overall survival is 5.3 to 16 months. Cetuximab is well tolerated. The main adverse events are acneiform eruptions and diarrhea. The density of skin rash is associated with clinical efficacy. Several ongoing phase III clinical trials are examining which chemotherapy regimen is the best to combine with cetuximab to maximize patient survival.

Panitumumab is a fully humanized IgG2 anti-EGFR monoclonal antibody. Compared with best support care, panitumumab treatment achieved significantly longer PFS in patients with advanced colorectal cancer. Based on such good results, a phase III clinical trial of panitumumab plus epirubicin, oxaliplatin, and capecitabine for advanced and locally advanced esophagogastric cancer (REAL-3) is under way. The result is expected to be released in 2013.

Erlotinib and Gefitinib

Both erlotinib and gefitinib are tyrosine kinase inhibitors. In a phase II clinical study, gefitinib alone was used to treat advanced GC and esophagogastric junction adenocarcinoma. Efficacy was evaluable in 27 patients. Three patients achieved partial response. The efficacy rate was 37%.[36] In another phase II clinical trial, oral erlotinib alone was used to treat advanced GC and esophagogastric junction adenocarcinoma. Of the 70 patients, no objective response was observed in the 26 patients with GC, while the overall efficacy rate was 11% in the patients with esophagogastric junction adenocarcinoma. The median survival was 3.5 months in GC patients and 6.7 months in patients with esophagogastric junction adenocarcinoma.[37] Apparently, the result of tyrosine kinase inhibitor in GC is disappointing. For this reason, phase III clinical trial was not conducted subsequently.

HER-2 Inhibitor

HER-2 proto-oncogene is the gene encoding the human EGF receptor 2. The amplification of HER-2 proto-oncogene causes the overexpression of HER-2 receptor on cell surface. This is important in the regulation of normal cell proliferation.[38] HER-2 overexpression is a predictor of poor patient prognosis and lack of response to chemotherapy or endocrine therapy. HER-2 expression level in GC tissue is an independent predictor of the prognosis of GC. HER-2 overexpression is identified in 20% of the well-differentiated adenocarcinomas.[39]

Trastuzumab

Recently, an open, randomized controlled phase III trial (ToGA study) proved the efficacy of trastuzumab against HER-2–positive GC.[40] A total of 594 patients were randomized to receive trastuzumab plus chemotherapy or chemotherapy alone. The median overall survival was 13.8 months in the patients treated with trastuzumab plus chemotherapy and 11.1 months in the patients treated with chemotherapy alone. The median survival is about 3 months longer by adding trastuzumab. The risk of death was reduced by 26% (hazard ratio, 0.74). The ToGA trial confirmed for the first time that trastuzumab plus chemotherapy can improve survival in advanced stage GC patients. This study also demonstrated for the first time that patients with advanced GC can benefit from the regimen containing targeted drug in terms of survival. This study is a landmark study for the role of trastuzumab in GC. Trastuzumab plus chemotherapy provides a new treatment option for HER-2–positive patients with advanced GC or esophagogastric junction adenocarcinoma.

Lapatinib

Lapatinib is a dual-functional drug targeting both EGFR and HER-2. It has shown potent activity in vivo and in vitro. Lapatinib can lead to growth arrest and/or apoptosis in EGFR-dependent and HER2-dependent tumor cell lines. Lapatinib has been extensively studied in many clinical trials of breast cancer. A phase II clinical study (SWOG) was also conducted in GC. Of the 47 patients receiving lapatinib alone for the first-line treatment of progressive or metastatic GC, 4 were confirmed to have partial response and 10 were evaluated as having stable disease. The time to progression was 1.9 months. The overall survival was 4.8 months. Lapatinib is well tolerated. Lapatinib monotherapy is effective in GC and esophagogastric junction adenocarcinoma.[41] In another phase II clinical trial, lapatinib plus capecitabine was used as the first-line treatment of advanced GC. Efficacy was evaluable in 67 patients. The overall response rate was 22.4%. Stable disease was found in 45% of the patients. The median follow-up period was 26.4 weeks. Follow-up is ongoing for 39% of the patients. The results up to now have shown that the anticipated efficacy has been reached with good tolerability. These favorable results have provided rationale for conducting clinical trial of lapatinib in combination with other chemotherapy agents.

Anti-angiogenic Drugs

The formation of neovessels is a key factor of tumor metastasis. Increased density of blood vessels is associated with tumor metastasis and poor prognosis. In GC, there is a positive association between microvessel count, metastatic potential, and poor prognosis. In clinical practice, the most commonly used anti-angiogenic drugs include the monoclonal antibody bevacizumab and tyrosine kinase inhibitors sunitinib and sorafenib.

Bevacizumab

VEGF can induce angiogenesis in vitro. The main function of VEGF is to facilitate pathological angiogenesis. Anti-VEGF monoclonal antibody and other vascular endothelial inhibitors can block the growth of some tumor cell lines. Bevacizumab can reduce the pathological angiogenesis by inhibiting VEGF and promote the formation of normal blood vessels, which is helpful for the delivery of cytotoxic agents to tumor tissues.[42] At present, the clinical trial of VEGF inhibitor in the management of GC is ongoing. Not long ago, the humanized anti-VEGF monoclonal antibody bevacizumab was approved by the Food and Drug Administration for the first-line treatment of metastatic colorectal cancer in combination with chemotherapy. As for GC, bevacizumab plus chemotherapy has achieved satisfactory results in a phase II clinical trial in GC patients. Bevacizumab in combination with irinotecan and cisplatin was used to treat inoperable or metastatic GC. The efficacy rate was 65% in the 47 patients. The median time to progression was 8.9 months. The overall survival was 12.3 months. The favorable results of phase II clinical trials have justified a phase III clinical trial (AVAGAST), in which bevacizumab in combination with capecitabine and cisplatin was used as the first-line treatment for advanced GC. Bevacizumab-containing regimen significantly increased PFS and objective response rate compared with treatment with chemotherapy alone. Unfortunately, bevacizumab combination therapy did not show significant survival advantage.

Sorafenib and Sunitinib

Sorafenib and sunitinib are orally administered, multi-target tyrosine kinase inhibitors. They can directly inhibit VEGF receptor and other tyrosine kinase receptors. In a phase II clinical trial, 72 advanced GC patients with prior chemotherapy were treated with oral sunitinib monotherapy. Partial response was documented in two patients. Twenty-five patients showed stable disease lasting more than 6 weeks. The median PFS was 2.3 months. The overall survival was 6.8 months.[43] The trial indicates that oral sunitinib monotherapy is unsatisfactory as the second-line treatment of advanced GC. However, sunitinib showed certain antitumor activity. In future clinical trials, it is worthy to further explore the efficacy of sunitinib plus chemotherapy as the first-line treatment of advanced GC. In another phase II clinical study, sorafenib was combined with docetaxel and cisplatin for the treatment of metastatic or inoperable advanced GC or esophagogastric junction adenocarcinoma. The results showed that 18 of the 44 patients achieved partial response. The median PFS was 5.8. Median overall survival was 13.6 months. The main adverse event was neutropenia. The incidence of grade 3 or 4 neutropenia was 64%.

The result of this clinical trial is encouraging. Sorafenib is effective and less toxic, which makes it advantageous in treating GC. Further studies are required to evaluate the efficacy of sorafenib in combination with other chemotherapy regimens in GC.[44]

Cell Cycle Inhibitor

CDKs are members of the protein kinase family. They are named so for their regulatory role in cell cycle. They are also implicated in transcriptional regulation, mRNA processing, and nerve cell differentiation. A CDK inhibitor is a protein that interacts with a cyclin–CDK complex to block kinase activity, usually during G1. Flavopiridol, a semisynthetic flavone, is a CDK inhibitor. A number of relevant reports have demonstrated that flavopiridol can induce tumor apoptosis in chemotherapy-treated gastric cell lines. In a phase I clinical trial, continuous infusion of flavopiridol over 72 hours induced complete clinical response in an advanced GC patient. The time to progression was more than 48 months.[45] However, in the subsequent phase II clinical trial, the same regimen did not result in any objective response. Furthermore, patients experienced serious adverse reactions. Therefore, it is generally considered that no antitumor activity of flavopiridol monotherapy is observed in advanced GC.[46] Now, a phase II clinical trial of flavopiridol in combination with irinotecan is under way.

COX Inhibitor

Research has revealed that COX-2 is overexpressed in GC tissues. Chronic *H. pylori* infection can cause an increase in COX-2. Epidemiological data indicate that long-term treatment with COX inhibitors can reduce the incidence of gastrointestinal tumors, especially GC. Targeted inhibition of COX, especially COX-2 isoforms, can lead to the inhibition of tumor cell growth and apoptosis of GC cells. COX-2 inhibitors play an important role in the prevention and treatment of GC. However, COX-2 inhibitors have not been recommended for the clinical treatment of GC. The dosage and safety of COX-2 inhibitors should be further elucidated.

MMP Inhibitor

MMPs belong to the zinc finger–dependent protein hydrolase family. MMPs mediate the degradation of extracellular matrix and subsequently lead to tumor cell invasion and metastasis. MMP-2, MMP-7, MMP-9, and MMP-14 are overexpressed in GC.[47-49] The expression of MMP-2 is closely related to the progression of GC and metastasis to lymph nodes.[50] MMP-9 expression is associated with poor prognosis of GC.[51] In the past several years, efforts were made to develop MMP inhibitors and conduct clinical trials to examine the effects of MMP inhibitors in GC. But all the results were unsatisfactory. This may be due to the inappropriate study design or the criteria for patient enrollment. Marimastat is a class of brand new antitumor drugs targeting MMPs. Numerous clinical studies have confirmed that marimastat could effectively inhibit tumors and inhibit the growth, invasion, and metastasis of tumor cells. A randomized, double-blind, phase III clinical trial compared marimastat with placebo in patients with advanced GC and gastroesophageal junction adenocarcinoma. Patients ($n = 396$) were randomized to receive oral marimastat or placebo. The median survival was 138 days in the patients receiving placebo and 160 days in the patients treated with oral marimastat. Two-year survival rate was 3% and 9%, respectively. PFS was also significantly longer in the marimastat-treated patients ($P = 0.009$). Oral marimastat provides significant survival benefits. This justifies further studies.

Hereditary Diffuse Gastric Cancer

The incidence of GC shows large geographic differences worldwide, with the lowest rates occurring in most Western industrialized countries including the United States and the United Kingdom; in contrast, relatively high rates of GC occur in Japan, Korea, China, and South America, particularly Chile.

Of the two major diagnostic categories of GC, namely intestinal type, which appears to be causally associated with environmental perturbations, and diffuse GC (DGC) type, the latter is more often ascribed to host factor effects.[52] Lynch et al.[53] note that the incidence of DGC remains stable and possibly may be increasing[54] as compared with the intestinal type, which may be declining in incidence. Hereditary diffuse GC (HDGC) has been described as following an autosomal dominant inheritance pattern attributable to mutations of the type 1 E-cadherin (epithelial) gene referred to as *CDH1* (epithelial cadherin/Online Mendelian Inheritance in Man no. 19,209). The decreased expression of this gene in DGC is noteworthy and may well account for the pathologic differences between intestinal and diffuse variants of GC in a subset of families.[55-57] The diffuse type pathology is characterized by poorly cohesive clusters of cells that infiltrate the gastric wall, leading to its widespread thickening and rigidity, known as *linitis plastica*.[56] The stomachs of *CDH1* mutation carriers who have undergone prophylactic gastrectomy have shown the presence of in situ signet ring carcinomas.[58] Pathology findings indicate that the signet cell phenotype is submucosal (Fig. 56.1), severely limiting the ability of currently available screening procedures to detect early GC.

It is noteworthy that "...*CDH1* germline mutations have been identified in approximately 40% to 50% of well defined HDGC families from low-incidence populations."[56,59,60] "There is also an excess of lobular carcinoma of the breast in women from HDGC families with *CDH1* mutations."[57,61,62] "The clinical advantage of identifying a *CDH1* mutation carrier is its level of certainty of disease expression, limited only by its penetrance, which, in DGC, is estimated to be in the range of 70% ...."[53,56,63] Unfortunately, it is not possible to critically assess the penetrance phenomenon, meaning that it is impossible to determine which *CDH1* carriers of this autosomal dominantly inherited deleterious gene mutation will express DGC; therein, prophylactic total gastrectomy is a reasonable option for the *CDH1* mutation carrier, given the

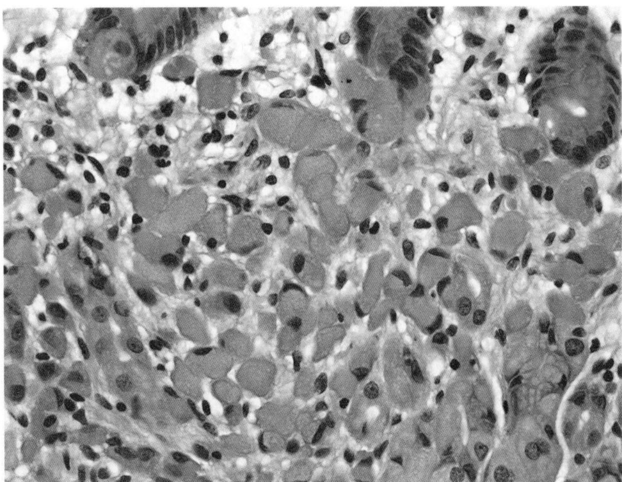

FIGURE 56–1 This is a photomicrograph of a focus of occult diffuse gastric cancer from a member of the family shown in Figure 56.2. The cancer was stage 1A, and the gastrectomy was presumed curative. (Republished with permission from Lynch H, Grady W, Suriano G, Huntsman D. Gastric cancer: new genetic developments. *J Surg Oncol.* 2005;90:114-133. Copyright © 2005 Wiley-Liss Inc., A Wiley Company. All rights reserved.)

extreme difficulty in its early diagnosis and its exceedingly poor prognosis when there is regional or distant spread.[59,64] However, it is extremely important that the carrier of this potentially lethal mutation be sufficiently educated about the pros and cons of all aspects of this disease, including the advantage of prophylactic total gastrectomy versus its sequelae, namely, weight loss, morbidity, and mortality.

Figure 56.2 portrays an HDGC family with multiple germline mutation carriers, each of whom could become a candidate for prophylactic total gastrectomy. Figure 56.3 is a second HDGC family with examples of several

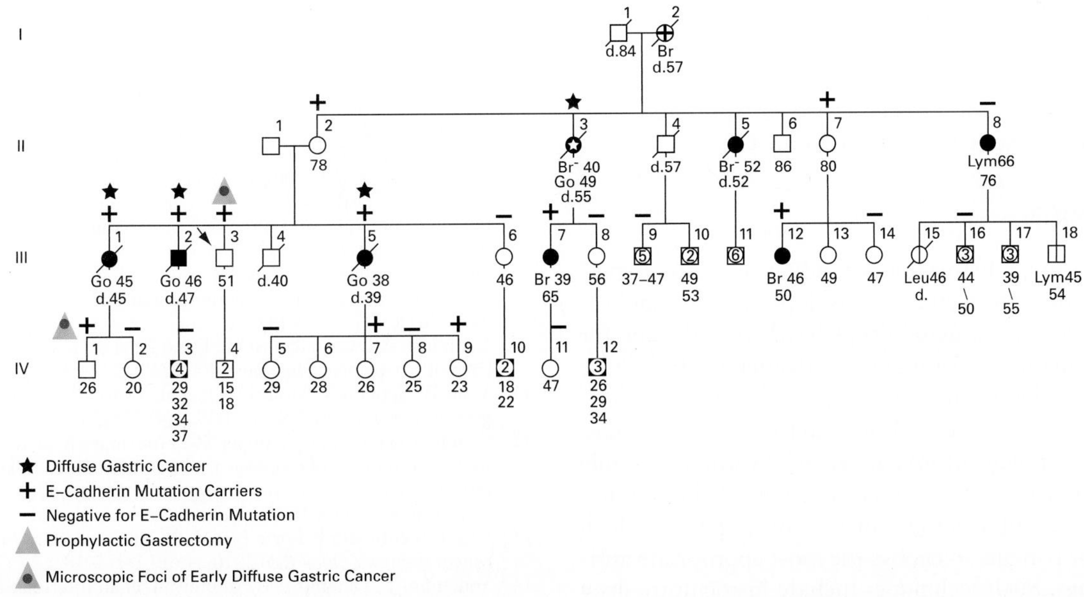

FIGURE 56–2 This pedigree depicts a hereditary diffuse gastric cancer family in which three of the proband's siblings died of diffuse gastric cancer within an 18-mo period. The findings of mutations of the type 1 E-cadherin (epithelial) gene *CDH1* in the mother (individual II-2) of the sibship at age 78 y and in her sister (individual II-7) at age 80 y, both symptom free, indicated reduced penetrance of this mutation. (Republished with permission from Lynch HT, Kaurah P, Wirtzfeld D, et al. Hereditary diffuse gastric cancer: diagnosis, genetic counseling, and prophylactic total gastrectomy. *Cancer.* 2008;112:2655-2663, Copyright © 2008 American Cancer Society, Inc., published by Wiley-Liss, Inc.)

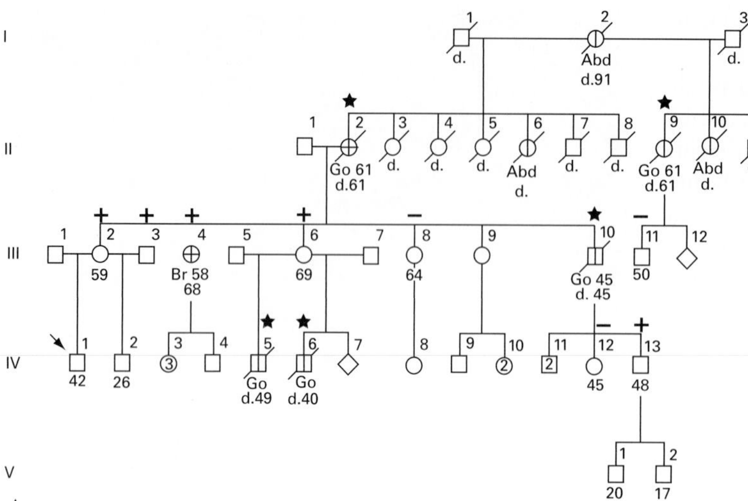

★ Diffuse Gastric Cancer
+ E-Cadherin Mutation Carriers
— Negative for E-Cadherin Mutation

FIGURE 56–3 This is a hereditary diffuse gastric cancer syndrome family in which initial testing was done on individual III-6, who was identified as positive for a type 1 E-cadherin (epithelial) gene *CDH1* mutation. She was selected because, through two marriages, she had sons (individuals IV-5 and IV-6) with diffuse gastric cancer, and her mother (individual II-2) died of gastric cancer. Thus, individual III-6 was considered an obligate germline mutation carrier, which was confirmed by the presence of the deleterious *CDH1* mutation. (Republished with permission from Lynch HT, Kaurah P, Wirtzfeld D, et al. Hereditary diffuse gastric cancer: diagnosis, genetic counseling, and prophylactic total gastrectomy. *Cancer.* 2008;112:2655-2663, Copyright © 2008 American Cancer Society, Inc., published by Wiley-Liss, Inc.)

persons affected with DGC. A single individual, namely III-6, was determined to be an obligate gene carrier by virtue of two HDGC mutation-carrying progeny (IV-5 and IV-6) from two separate matings.[53]

Mutations have been described in more than 40 HDGC families of diverse ethnic backgrounds. It is noteworthy that two-thirds of HDGC families reported to date have proved negative for the *CDH1* germline mutation. A number of candidate genes have been identified through analysis of the molecular biology of E-cadherin. Specifically, the E-cadherin cytoplasmic tail interacts with catenins, assembling the cell adhesion complex involved with E-cadherin–mediated cell–cell adhesion. β-catenin and γ-catenin compete for the same binding site on the E-cadherin cytoplasmic tail, directly linking the adhesion complex to the cytoskeleton through α-catenin. β-Catenin gene (*CTNNB1*) mutations that have been described predominantly in intestinal-type GCs and *CTNNB1* gene amplification and overexpression have recently been described in a mixed-type GC.[56]

CONCLUSION

In recent years, a better understanding of the biological properties of tumors and the development and application of molecular targeted drugs have created hope for the individualized treatment of advanced GC. These advances also lend confidence to health-care professionals to explore new targeted drugs and treatment regimens. In the development of individualized treatment, people pay attention not only to pharmacological therapy but also to the techniques to evaluate drug response, which is useful for patients to choose the most appropriate anticancer drugs. Such techniques include histoculture drug response assay and collagen gel droplet embedded culture drug sensitivity test. At present, these methods have been used to predict the sensitivity to specific type of anticancer drugs. Every effort should be made to provide the most appropriate treatment regimen to the individual patient, avoid unnecessary waste of health-care resources, and reduce the incidence of toxic or adverse effects due to inadequate or delayed treatment. The eventual goal is to maximally increase patient survival time.

REFERENCES

1. Jamal A, Siegel R, Xu J, Ward E. Cancer statistics. *CA Cancer J Clin.* 2010;60:277-300.
2. Wong H, Yau T. Targeted therapy in the management of advanced gastric cancer: are we making progress in the era of personalized medicine? *Oncologist.* February 2012. [Epub ahead of print]
3. Lightdale CJ. Endoscopic mucosal resection: this is our turf. *Endoscopy.* 2004;36(9):808-810.
4. Lee WS, Cho JW, Kim YD, et al. Technical issues and new devices of ESD of early gastric cancer. *World J Gastroenterol.* August 2011;17(31):3585-3590.
5. Soetikno R, Kaltenbach T, Yeh R. Endoscopic mucosal resection for early cancer of the upper gastrointestinal tract. *J Clin Oncol.* 2005;23(20):4490-4498.
6. Kitano S, Iso Y, Moriyama M, et al. Laparoscopy-assisted Billroth gastrectomy. *Surg Laparosc.* 1994;4(2):146.
7. Goh PM, Khan AZ, So JB, et al. Early experience with laparoscopic radical gastrectomy for advanced GC. *Surg Laparosc Endosc Percutan Tech.* 2001;11(2):83.
8. Kitano S, Shiraishi N, Uyama I, et al. A multicenter study on oncologic outcome of laparoscopic gastrectomy for early cancer in Japan. *Ann Surg.* 2007;245(1):68.
9. Koeda K, Nishizuka S, Wakabayashi G. Minimally invasive surgery for gastric cancer: the future standard of care. *World J Surg.* 2011;35(7):1469-1477.
10. Lanfranco AR, Czstellanos AE, Desai JP, et al. Robotic surgery: a current perspective. *Ann Surg.* 2004;239(1):14-21.
11. Yasui W, Sentani K, Motoshita J, et al. Molecular pathobiology of gastric cancer. *Scand J Surg.* 2006;95(4):225-231.
12. Stemmermann G, Heffelfinger SC, Noffsinger A, et al. The molecular biology of esophageal and gastric cancer and their precursors: oncogenes, tumor suppressor genes, and growth factors. *Hum Pathol.* 1994;25(10):968-981.
13. Cito L, Pentimalli F, Forte I, et al. Rb family proteins in gastric cancer (review). *Oncol Rep.* 2010;24(6):1411-1418.
14. Yonemura Y, Takamura H, Ninomiya I, et al. Interrelationship between transforming growth factor-alpha and epidermal growth factor receptor in advanced gastric cancer. *Oncology.* 1992;49(2):157-161.
15. Cohen JA, Weiner DB, More KF, et al. Expression pattern of the neu (NGL) gene-encoded growth factor receptor protein (p185neu) in normal and transformed epithelial tissues of the digestive tract. *Oncogene.* 1989;4(1):81-88.

16. Houldsworth J, Cordon-Cardo C, Ladanyi M, et al. Gene amplification in gastric and esophageal adenocarcinomas. *Cancer Res*. 1990;50(19):6417-6422.
17. Yonemura Y, Ninomiya I, Yamaguchi A, et al. Evaluation of immunoreactivity for erbB-2 protein as a marker of poor short term prognosis in gastric cancer. *Cancer Res*. 1991;51(3):1034-1038.
18. Terman BI, Stoletov KV. VEGF and tumor angiogenesis. *Einstein Quart J Biol Med*. 2001;18:59-66.
19. Kubben FJ, Sier CF, van Duijn W, et al. Matrix metalloproteinase-2 is a consistent prognostic factor in gastric cancer. *Br J Cancer*. 2006;94(7):1035-1040.
20. Fanelli MF, Chinen LT Sr, Begnami MD, et al. The influence of CD44v6, TGF-α, COX-2, MMP-7, and MMP-9 on clinical evolution of patients with gastric cancer. *J Clin Oncol*. 2011;29:(suppl 4; abstract 21).
21. Becker KF, Keller G, Hoefler H. The use of molecular biology in diagnosis and prognosis of gastric cancer. *Surg Oncol*. 2000;9(1):5-11.
22. Cho HJ, Kim J, Im S, et al. Clinicopathologic characteristics of microsatellite instability (MSI) tumors in resected gastric cancer patients. *J Clin Oncol*. 2010;28:15s (suppl; abstract 4040).
23. Chan AO, Lam SK, Chu KM, et al. Soluble E-cadherin is a valid prognostic marker in gastric carcinoma. *Gut*. 2001;48(6):808-811.
24. Shimada Y, Yamasaki S, Hashimoto Y, et al. Clinical significance of dysadherin expression in gastric cancer patients. *Clin Cancer Res*. 2004;10(8):2818-2823.
25. Yamamichi K, Uehara Y, Kitamura N, et al. Increased expression of CD44v6 mRNA significantly correlates with distant metastasis and poor prognosis in gastric cancer. *Int J Cancer*. 1998;79(3):256-262.
26. Saito H, Tsujitani S, Katano K, et al. Serum concentration of CD44 variant 6 and its relation to prognosis in patients with gastric carcinoma. *Cancer*. 1998;83(6):1094-1101.
27. Mayer B, Jauch KW, Günthert U, et al. De-novo expression of CD44 and survival in gastric cancer. *Lancet*. 1993;342(8878):1019-1022.
28. Yokozaki H, Yasui W, Tahara E. Genetic and epigenetic changes in stomach cancer. *Int Rev Cytol*. 2001;204:49-95.
29. Yasui W, Oue N, Ono S, et al. Histone acetylation and gastrointestinal carcinogenesis. *Ann N Y Acad Sci*. 2003;983:220-231.
30. Yasui W, Oue N, Aung PP, et al. Molecular-pathological prognostic factors of gastric cancer: a review. *Gastric Cancer*. 2005;8(2):86-94.
31. Oue N, Mitani Y, Motoshita J, et al. Accumulation of DNA methylation is associated with tumor stage in gastric cancer. *Cancer*. 2006;106(6):1250-1259.
32. Wu MS, Huang SP, Chang YT, et al. Association of the -160 C → a promoter polymorphism of E-cadherin gene with gastric carcinoma risk. *Cancer*. 2002;94(5):1443-1448.
33. Pharoah PD, Oliveira C, Machado JC, et al. CDH1 c-160a promotor polymorphism is not associated with risk of stomach cancer. *Int J Cancer*. 2002;101(2):196-197.
34. Pao W, Chmielecki J. Rational, biologically based treatment of EGFR-mutant non-small-cell lung cancer. *Nat Rev Cancer*. 2010;10(11):760-774.
35. Stein A, Al-Batran SE, Arnold D, et al. Cetuximab with irinotecan as salvage therapy in heavily pretreated patients with metastatic gastric cancer. *Proc Gastrointest Am Soc Clin Oncol Symp*. 2007(abstract 47).
36. Ferry DR, Anderson M, Beddows K, et al. Phase II trial of gefitinib (ZD1839) in advanced adenocarcinoma of the oesophagus incorporating biopsy before and after gefitinib. *Proc Am Soc Clin Oncol*. 2004;23:317(A4021).
37. Dragovich T, McCoy S, Urba SG, et al. SWOG 0127 phase II trial of erlotinib in GEJ and gastric adenocarcinomas. *Proc Gastrointest Am Soc Clin Oncol Symp*. 2005;107:A49.
38. Hynes NE, Lane HA. ERBB receptors and cancer: the complexity of targeted inhibitors. *Nat Rev Cancer*. 2005;5:341-354.
39. Ming SC. Cellular and molecular pathology of gastric carcinoma and precursor lesions: a critical review. *Gastric Cancer*. 1998;1:31-50.
40. Bang YJ, Van Cutsem E, Feyereislova A, et al. Trastuzumab in combination with chemotherapy versus chemotherapy alone for treatment of HER2-positive advanced gastric or gastro-oesophageal junction cancer (ToGA): a phase 3, open-label, randomised controlled trial. *Lancet*. 2010;376:687-697.
41. Shah MA, Ramanathan RK, Ilson DH, et al. Multicenter phase II study of irinotecan, cisplatin, and bevacizumab in patients with metastatic gastric or gastroesophageal junction adenocarcinoma. *J Clin Oncol*. 2006;24(33):5201-5206.
42. Tong RT, Boucher Y, Kozin SV, et al. Vascular normalization by vascular endothelial growth factor receptor 2 blockade induces a pressure gradient across the vasculature and improves drug penetration in tumors. *Cancer Res*. 2004;64(11):3731-3736.
43. Bang YJ, Kang YK, Kang WK, et al. Phase II study of sunitinib as second-line treatment for advanced gastric cancer. *Invest New Drugs*. 2011;29(6):1449-1458.
44. Sun W, Powell M, O'Dwyer PJ, et al. Phase II study of sorafenib in combination with docetaxel and cisplatin in the treatment of metastatic or advanced gastric and gastroesophageal junction adenocarcinoma: ECOG 5203. *J Clin Oncol*. 2010;28(18):2947-2951.
45. Thomas JP, Tutsch KD, Cleary JF, et al. Phase I clinical and pharmacokinetic trial of the cyclin-dependent kinase inhibitor flavopiridol. *Cancer Chemother Pharmacol*. 2002;50(6):465-472.
46. Schwartz GK, Ilson D, Saltz L, et al. Phase II study of the cyclin-dependent kinase inhibitor flavopiridol administered to patients with advanced gastric carcinoma. *J Clin Oncol*. 2001;19(7):1985-1992.
47. Nomura H, Sato H, Seiki M, et al. Expression of membrane-type matrix metalloproteinase in human gastric carcinomas. *Cancer Res*. 1995;55(15):3263-3266.
48. Honda M, Mori M, Ueo H, et al. Matrix metalloproteinase-7 expression in gastric carcinoma. *Gut*. 1996;39(3):444-448.
49. Sier CF, Kubben FJ, Ganesh S, et al. Tissue levels of matrix metalloproteinases MMP-2 and MMP-9 are related to the overall survival of patients with gastric carcinoma. *Br J Cancer*. 1996;74(3):413-417.
50. Mönig SP, Baldus SE, Hennecken JK, et al. Expression of MMP-2 is associated with progression and lymph node metastasis of gastric carcinoma. *Histopathology*. 2001;39(6):597-602.
51. De Mingo M, Morán A, Sánchez-Pernaute A, et al. Expression of MMP-9 and TIMP-1 as prognostic markers in gastric carcinoma. *Hepatogastroenterology*. 2007;54(73):315-319.
52. Lauren P. The two histological main types of gastric carcinoma: diffuse and so-called intestinal-type carcinoma: an attempt at a histo-clinical classification. *Acta Pathol Microbiol Scand*. 1965;64:31-49.
53. Lynch HT, Kaurah P, Wirtzfeld D, et al. Hereditary diffuse gastric cancer: diagnosis, genetic counseling, and prophylactic total gastrectomy. *Cancer*. 2008;112:2655-2663.
54. Crew KD, Neugut AI. Epidemiology of gastric cancer. *World J Gastroenterol*. 2006;12:354-362.
55. Guilford P, Hopkins J, Haraway J, et al. E-cadherin germline mutations in familial gastric cancer. *Nature*. 1998;392:402-405.
56. Lynch HT, Grady W, Suriano G, Huntsman D. Gastric cancer: new genetic developments. *J Surg Oncol*. 2005;90:114-133.
57. Suriano G, Yew S, Ferreira P, et al. Characterization of a recurrent germ line mutation of the *E-cadherin* gene: implications for genetic testing and clinical management. *Clin Cancer Res*. 2005;11:5401-5409.
58. Carneiro F, Huntsman DG, Smyrk TC, et al. Model of the early development of diffuse gastric cancer in E-cadherin mutation carriers and its implications for patient screening. *J Pathol*. 2004;203:681-687.
59. Suriano G, Oliveira C, Ferreira P, et al. Identification of CDH1 germline missense mutations associated with functional inactivation of the E-cadherin protein in young gastric cancer probands. *Hum Mol Genet*. 2003;12:575-582.
60. Kaurah P, MacMillan A, Boyd N, et al. Founder and recurrent *CDH1* mutations in families with hereditary diffuse gastric cancer. *JAMA*. 2007;297:2360-2372.
61. Keller G, Vogelsang H, Becker I, et al. Diffuse type gastric and lobular breast carcinoma in a familial gastric cancer patient with an E-cadherin germline mutation. *Am J Pathol*. 1999;155:337-342.
62. Oliveira C, Seruca R, Caldas C. Genetic screening for hereditary diffuse gastric cancer. *Expert Rev Mol Diagn*. 2003;3:201-215.
63. Caldas C, Carneiro F, Lynch HT, et al. Familial gastric cancer: overview and guidelines for management. *J Med Genet*. 1999;36:873-880.
64. Bacani JT, Soares M, Zwingerman R, et al. CDH1/E-cadherin germline mutations in early onset gastric cancer. *J Med Genet*. 2006;43:867-872.

CHAPTER 57

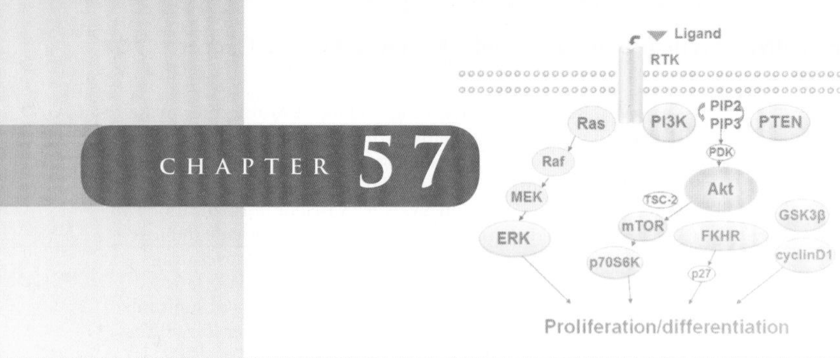

Personalized Medicine and Targeted Therapy for Prostate Cancer

Madhuri Bajaj, Michael A. Carducci, and Elisabeth I. Heath

INTRODUCTION

Prostate cancer is the most common non-skin malignancy in men worldwide. In the United States, there was an estimated 240,890 new diagnoses of prostate cancer and 33,720 prostate cancer deaths in 2011, representing 28% of new cancer cases and 10% of male cancer deaths.[1] Patients diagnosed with localized disease achieve high cure and extended long-term survival rates with standard approaches. Despite definitive therapy, 25% to 30% of patients will develop locoregional recurrence or metastatic disease.[2] The current standard of care for castrate-sensitive metastatic prostate cancer is androgen deprivation therapy via surgical or medical castration. With the use of gonadotropin-releasing hormone (GnRH) analogues, antiandrogens, or both, disease progression typically occurs within 12 to 24 months of initial androgen deprivation, often demonstrated by a rise in prostate-specific antigen (PSA) from treatment nadir.[3] Once prostate cancer progresses in the face of castrate levels of testosterone (<1.73 nmol/L or 50 ng/dL), it is termed castrate-resistant prostate cancer (CRPC). In the past, treatment of CRPC was limited to systemic therapies, such as mitoxantrone, radioactive isotopes, and bisphosphonates, whose goal was to provide symptomatic relief.[4-6] Now, chemotherapeutic agents, docetaxel and cabazitaxel, have shown improved overall survival, but with only a median of approximately 2 to 3 months in comparison to mitoxantrone.[7,8] In addition, sipuleucel-T and abiraterone have also gained Food and Drug Administration (FDA) approval for patients with CRPC.[9,10]

With the expanding options for men with metastatic CRPC, an emerging focus of research is to personalize treatment options for patients as well as to optimize the sequence of available single or combination therapies. As none of the available agents are curative, a significant effort to develop novel therapies with curative intent remains ongoing. Currently, there are two main approaches to categorize the various underlying mechanisms of castration resistance: androgen receptor (AR) dependent and AR independent.[11] Based on current research, the knowledge surrounding the mechanisms underlying malignant proliferation, angiogenesis, and ultimately metastasis has improved. With our increased understanding of therapeutic targets, we are getting closer to being able to eventually provide individualized therapy for men with prostate cancer. This chapter reviews multiple novel and available therapies for men with prostate cancer, focusing on agents that target the androgen-dependent and androgen-independent pathways that have recently entered clinical trials, including their molecular rationale and available clinical data.

ANDROGEN-DEPENDENT PATHWAYS

Androgens are the key regulators of cell growth and proliferation in prostate cancer, which is why androgen deprivation therapy is initially highly effective due to the induction of apoptosis. Persistent AR activation is an important mediator of disease progression in CRPC.[12] There are multiple mechanisms by which this happens, including (1) AR overexpression; (2) AR mutations that increase androgen sensitivity to or activation by other steroids; (3) increased local androgen production by prostate cells via expression of steroidogenic enzymes; (4) AR activation via cross talk of signal transduction pathways (epidermal growth factor, insulin-like growth factor [IGF], and interleukin-6); (5) modulated expression of co-activators or co-repressors of AR; and (6) proteolytic processing of AR to an androgen-independent isoform.[13] Preclinical research has validated these concepts and thus has served as the basis for the translation of novel, potent AR-targeted therapies into clinical trials. Therefore, most CRPCs are not truly castration resistant. A recent study reported novel forms of AR alteration that are prevalent in CRPC. Through sequence analysis and subsequent experimental validation studies, two most abundantly expressed variants, AR-V1 and AR-V7, were discovered. AR-V1 and AR-V7 mRNA showed an average 20-fold higher expression in CRPC ($n = 25$) when compared with castrate-sensitive prostate cancer ($n = 82$; $P < 0.0001$). Among the castrate-sensitive prostate cancer, higher expression of AR-V7 predicted biochemical recurrence following surgical treatment ($P = 0.012$). The results of this study suggest a novel mechanism for the development of CRPC and the possible role of AR variants as biomarkers and therapeutic targets in advanced prostate cancer.[14]

ANDROGEN ANTAGONISTS

AR-targeted approaches include AR antagonists, such as bicalutamide, flutamide, and ketoconazole, agents that block the production of hormones that activate the AR. The advancements in AR-mediated CRPC progression discussed above support the hypothesis that additional hormonal inhibition via the next-generation androgen inhibitors such as MDV3100 and abiraterone is an effective option for treating CRPC (see Table 57.1).

MDV3100 is an AR antagonist with higher affinity than bicalutamide for AR and has no agonist activity in experimental CRPC models.[15] MDV3100 prevents binding of the androgen to the AR, thus preventing nuclear translocation of the AR complex. It also prevents the binding of the AR complex to DNA. This triple action of AR blockade, prevention of nuclear translocation of AR complex, and DNA-binding inhibition results in apoptosis of prostate cancer cells.[16] In a phase I/II study of 140 patients with progressive CRPC treated with MDV3100 (doses 30 to 600 mg/d), 56% had a ≥50% reduction in PSA and 22% of 59 patients with soft tissue disease had partial responses. PSA declines of ≥50% were reported in 62% of the 65 chemotherapy-naïve patients and 51% of 75 patients previously treated with chemotherapy, while stable disease was reported in 74% of patients with measurable soft tissue lesions and in 62% of patients with bone lesions.[17] No additional antitumor benefit to doses greater than 150 mg/d was noted. These results, along with a favorable safety profile (fatigue being the most common but at doses exceeding >240 mg/d), have led to the current phase III trials studying MDV3100.

The AFFIRM (A Multinational Phase 3, Randomized, Double-Blind, Placebo-Controlled Efficacy and Safety Study of Oral MDV3100 in Patients with Progressive Castration Resistant Prostste Cancer Previously Treated with Docetaxel-Based Chemotherapy) trial is a randomized, double-blind, placebo-controlled, multicenter, phase III trial evaluating MDV3100 at 160 mg/d compared with placebo in pretreated docetaxel CRPC patients that was stopped early in November 2011 after a planned interim analysis demonstrated a 4.8-month median overall survival advantage in the MDV3100 arm (NCT00974311). As reported by the Independent Data Safety and Monitoring Committee (IDMC), the estimated median survival for men treated with MDV3100 was 18.4 months compared with 13.6 months for men treated with placebo. MDV3100 provided a 37% reduction in risk of death compared with placebo (hazard ratio = 0.631). The IDMC further determined, considering the observed safety profile, that MDV3100 demonstrated a favorable risk-to-benefit ratio sufficient to stop the study. A full analysis of the results from AFFIRM, including safety data, is expected soon.[14,18] The PREVAIL (A Multinational Phase 3, Randomized, Double-Blind, Placebo-Controlled Efficacy and Safety Study of Oral MDV3100 in Chemotherapy-Naive Patients with Progressive Metastatic Prostate Cancer Who Have Failed Androgen Deprivation Therapy) trial is a different study that is actively recruiting phase III trial evaluating chemotherapy-naïve CRPC patients treated with 160 mg/d of MDV3100 with standard of care compared with placebo with standard of care (NCT01212991). With a target

TABLE 57-1 Antiandrogen Agents

Target	Agent	Patient Population	Phase	Primary End Point	ClinicalTrials.gov Identifier
Androgen biosynthesis inhibitor	Abiraterone	Asymptomatic or mildly symptomatic CRPC	I II	OS, PFS	NCT00887198
Androgen biosynthesis inhibitor	TAK-700	Chemotherapy-naïve, nonmetastatic CRPC	II	PSA	NCT01046916
Antiandrogen	MDV3100	CRPC after docetaxel failure	III	OS	NCT00974311
	MDV3100	Chemotherapy-naïve metastatic CRPC	III	OS, PFS	NCT01212991

CRPC, castrate-resistant prostate cancer; OS, overall survival; PFS, progression-free survival; PSA, prostate-specific antigen.

accrual goal of 1,700 patients, the study is continuing to accrue with the primary end points as overall survival and progression-free survival (PFS) and secondary end points of time to initiation of cytotoxic chemotherapy and time to first skeletal-related event (SRE).[19]

A second-generation antiandrogen, ARN-509, is undergoing clinical evaluation as well. ARN-509 inhibits both AR nuclear translocation and AR binding to androgen response elements in DNA. The compound also does not exhibit agonist activity in prostate cancer cells that overexpress AR. Currently, it is in phase II clinical trials (NCT01171898).

ANDROGEN SYNTHESIS INHIBITORS

Several clinical studies have demonstrated that CRPC cells continue to be under the influence of androgen signaling as evidenced by the high number of AR expression.[20] As a result, these newer agents tend to be more specific targets of enzymes downstream in the hormonal cascade. Abiraterone acetate is more potent than ketoconazole and a selective inhibitor of the 17-α-hydroxylase and the C17,20-lyase function of CYP17A1.[21] In a phase II trial, a total of 47 men with metastatic CRPC deemed refractory to docetaxel-based chemotherapy were given oral abiraterone at 1,000 mg daily. The results were PSA declines of ≥30%, ≥50%, and ≥90% seen in 68% (32 of 47), 51% (24 of 47), and 15% (7 of 47) of patients, respectively.[22] These results, coupled with a favorable safety profile, have laid the foundation for the development of two randomized, double-blind, placebo-controlled, phase III clinical trials. Recently, the first of the phase III trials involving 1,195 metastatic prior docetaxel-treated CRPC patients given abiraterone plus prednisone showed improved overall survival compared with placebo plus prednisone (median overall survival time 14.8 vs. 10.9 mo; hazard ratio [HR] 0.65; $P < 0.0001$). All secondary end points, including time to PSA progression (10.2 vs. 6.6 mo; $P < 0.001$), PFS (5.6 vs. 3.6 mo; $P < 0.001$), and PSA response rate (29% vs. 6%, $P < 0.001$), favored abiraterone.[9] Common side effects with this agent include hypokalemia, hypertension (HTN), and pedal edema. The effects are explained by a syndrome of mineralocorticoid excess, which improves with eplerenone, a mineralocorticoid receptor antagonist. Based on these results, the FDA granted approval in April 2011 of abiraterone for the treatment of metastatic CRPC patients who have progressed on docetaxel-based chemotherapy. The second of the phase III trials investigating abiraterone in asymptomatic or mildly symptomatic men with metastatic CRPC who had not received prior chemotherapy has completed accrual, with final results pending (NCT00887198).

TAK-700 is a novel, selective CYP450c17 inhibitor similar to abiraterone by reducing testosterone and dehydroepiandrosterone levels. In a phase I/II study of this compound in asymptomatic metastatic CRPC patients, the drug was tolerated well at various doses and there was a 50% decline in 12 of 15 patients who were treated with ≥300 mg twice daily for ≥3 months.[23] No dose-limiting toxicity was seen and the most common adverse events (AEs) were fatigue in 16 patients (62%), nausea (38%), constipation (35%), and vomiting (30%). The preliminary phase I/II study results have led to a phase II, ongoing evaluation of TAK-700 at a dose of 400 mg twice daily with prednisone in metastatic CRPC patients.[24] There are now two phase III multicenter, randomized, double-blind trials that are evaluating the TAK-700 plus prednisone compared with placebo plus prednisone in metastatic CRPC patients. One trial will evaluate in the chemotherapy-naïve patients (primary end point: overall survival and radiographic PFS)[25] (NCT01193244), while the other focuses on the post-docetaxel progression patient population (primary end point: overall survival)[26] (NCT01193257). Both trials are actively recruiting with a target accrual of 1,000 to 1,400 patients and results are expected to be available by 2013 to 2014.

Other potent next-generation antiandrogens in development such as TOK001, an orally bioavailable small molecule CYP17,20-lyase inhibitor with additional direct AR antagonist activity, are currently being studied in a phase I/II study of CRPC patients (NCT00959959).

Androstenediol is an adrenal androgen that is thought to promote AR activity and PSA expression. When HE3235, an androstenediol inhibitor, was added to LNCaP cell lines exposed to dihydrotestosterone or androstenediol, there was inhibition of tumor formation/growth, likely through the induction of proapoptotic effect on tumor cells.[27] Currently, phase I/II study has been completed and results have shown HE3235 to be well tolerated across a range of doses (NCT00716794).[28]

Advances in the understanding of androgen signaling in metastatic CRPC have led to the evolution of multiple hormonal therapies, including abiraterone, TAK-700, and MDV3100. This class of agents is extremely useful as patients will often consider treatment with pills rather than systemic chemotherapy. There is also a familiarity of androgen modulators as therapy because patients are continuing to receive androgen deprivation therapy with luteinizing hormone–releasing hormone or GnRH agents and they have most likely been treated with antiandrogens such as flutamide and nilutamide in the past. In addition, agents modulating the androgen signaling axis frequently result in PSA reduction, another familiar signal of treatment effect. Therefore, development and approval of agents targeting the androgen signaling axis remain an extremely important approach in metastatic CRPC.

NON–ANDROGEN-DEPENDENT PATHWAYS

Prostate cancer progression is not only mediated by the androgen axis, as there are multiple other pathways that give rise to disease advancement. The precise mechanisms of the pathways discussed below are less clear, including whether they are truly androgen-independent. Although a prostate cancer stem cell has not yet been elucidated, the progression of prostate cancer from androgen dependence to castration-resistant tumor with features of antiapoptotic, chemotherapy resistance, and non-hormonal dependence pathways appears to be suggestive of a stem cell presence. The pathways include the epidermal growth factor receptor (EGFR), vascular endothelial growth factor receptor (VEGFR), phosphoinositide-3 kinase (PI3K)/protein kinase B (Akt), insulin-like growth factor 1 receptor (IGF-1R), mitogen-activated protein kinase, Src, endothelin receptor, and receptor activator of nuclear factor-κB ligand (RANKL). The interplay between these pathways highlights the importance of the need to develop therapeutic agents that can simultaneously inhibit them so as to produce clinically durable responses. These key pathways that are the current focus of active research with targeted agents are discussed below.

PI3K/Akt/mTOR Pathway

Upregulation of the PI3K/Akt/mammalian target of rapamycin (mTOR) pathway is present in multiple tumors, including prostate cancer. PI3K is activated by several extracellular receptors, such as EGFR, IGF-1R, and oncogenes like RAS.[29] Activated PI3K induces phosphorylated Akt to activate mTOR, which regulates cell growth, proliferation, and angiogenesis.[30] The loss of tumor suppressor gene PTEN occurs in more than 50% of metastatic disease and in approximately 20% of locally advanced disease.[31] PTEN negatively regulates PI3K/Akt survival pathway, leading to high levels of phosphorylated Akt in advanced prostate cancer.[32] Preclinical studies have shown that PTEN function loss and/or the activation of PI3K/Akt/mTOR pathway can result in androgen-independent prostate cancer.[33] Moreover, the deletion of PTEN has been associated with poor early disease progression and cancer-related mortality in CRPC patients through mechanisms including activation of the AR and androgen-responsive genes (see Table 57.2).[34]

There have been several mTOR inhibitors developed, as mTOR is an important downstream effector of the PI3K/Akt pathway. The mTOR inhibitor sirolimus, also known as rapamycin, is an immunosuppressive agent used in solid organ transplants as well as in coronary stents to prevent restenosis due to its anti-proliferative qualities. Single agent activity of mTOR inhibitors in advanced CRPC tumors is low.[35] There are multiple trials that are ongoing evaluating mTOR inhibitors in combination with cytotoxic and/or bisphosphonate therapy. In a phase I dose-escalation trial, everolimus was combined with docetaxel in metastatic CRPC patients that were chemotherapy-naïve, and no dose-limiting toxicities were noted. There were 14 evaluable patients, of which 10 had metabolic stable disease and 4 had a metabolic partial response.[36] Everolimus was also studied in combination with bevacizumab and docetaxel in a phase I trial of chemotherapy-naïve metastatic CRPC patients, and 10 out of the 12 patients experienced a 50% PSA decline.[37] There was also a phase II study of everolimus as a single agent in 19 docetaxel-refractory CRPC patients and the median TTP was 85 days; however, no PSA responses were noted.[38] Other mTOR inhibitors such as temsirolimus have also been shown to inhibit the growth of prostate cancer cells in combination with docetaxel in cell lines and xenografts.[39] Ridaforolimus was evaluated in a phase II, randomized, placebo-controlled trial with bicalutamide in asymptomatic, metastatic, prior docetaxel-refractory CRPC patients, which has completed accrual. The primary end point was PSA response, and dose-limiting toxicities and the results are awaited (NCT00110188). The toxicities of rapamycin analogues are not dose related and thus very predictable, including maculopapular rash, hypertriglyceridemia, hyperglycemia, allergic reactions, pedal edema, mucositis, and thrombocytopenia.[40]

Interestingly, rapamycin itself was administered for 14 days in men prior to radical prostatectomy. In the prostate, rapamycin inhibited prostate cancer S6 phosphorylation and achieved a three- to fourfold higher concentration compared with blood. There was, however, no effect on AKT phosphorylation, tumor proliferation, or apoptosis observed.[41]

It is unclear as to what role mTOR inhibitors will truly play in the treatment of men with CRPC, but upstream pathway targeting of PI3K and Akt directly appears to be an emerging area of interest. PI3K inhibitor BKM120 is in a phase II trial in men with CRPC who progressed after docetaxel-based chemotherapy (NCT01385293). Akt inhibitor MK2206 is being evaluated with bicalutamide in patients with rising PSA at high risk for progression after primary therapy (NCT01251861). MK2206 is also being evaluated in combination with hydroxychloroquine in a

TABLE 57-2 mTOR Targets

Target	Agent	Patient Population	Phase	Primary End Point	ClinicalTrials.gov Identifier
mTOR	Everolimus	Metastatic or locally advanced CRPC that is not progressing rapidly	II	PFS	NCT00976755
	Temsirolimus	Chemotherapy-naïve CRPC	II	Tumor response	NCT00919035
	Ridaforolimus plus bicalutamide	Asymptomatic metastatic CRPC	II	PSA response	NCT00777959

CRPC, castrate-resistant prostate cancer; PFS, progression-free survival; PSA, prostate-specific antigen.

phase I trial (NCT01480154). At this time, it is too early to determine whether this class of inhibitors will impact men with CRPC.

Src Pathway

Src (sarcoma) family kinases play an important role in prostate cancer. They are tyrosine kinases responsible for signal transduction from a range of upstream proteins, including epidermal growth factor, platelet-derived growth factor, and vascular endothelial growth factor (VEGF).[42] There is evidence demonstrating overexpression of Src in prostate cancer cell lines along with reduced tumor proliferation, invasion, and migration.[43] In advanced prostate cancer, Src is involved in androgen-independent growth pathways, such that low androgen activity in prostate cancer cells is associated with high Src activity and thus they are more sensitive to Src blockade.[44] In recent studies of tumor samples of CRPC patients, Src kinase activity was increased in about 30% of cases and this corresponded to a shorter overall survival duration.[45] Src is also required in osteoclast functioning as its inhibition decreases bone turnover.[46]

Dasatinib is an oral tyrosine kinase inhibitor with potent activity against not only the Src family kinases but also BCR-ABL, platelet-derived growth factor receptor (PDGFR), and c-kit. It has been noted to have preclinical activity against prostate cancer cells[47] as well as anti-osteoclast activity.[48] A phase II trial evaluated dasatinib in 47 chemotherapy-naïve CRPC patients, of which 25 patients received a dose of 100 mg twice daily and 22 received a twice-daily dosing of 70 mg. Forty-one (87%) patients had documented bone disease. At 12 weeks, 43% of patients (20/47) did not show progression of disease, while at 24 weeks 19% of patients (9/47) did not show progression of disease as determined by RECIST criteria. In terms of PSA response, only three patients showed ≥50% declines in PSA.[49] Overall, dasatinib was well tolerated, but as noted in the hematologic literature, pleural effusions in 51% of the overall population were present despite dose adjustments from 100 to 70 mg twice daily. Additional side effects include diarrhea (62%), nausea (47%), and fatigue (45%). An expansion of the phase II study to determine tolerability of 100 mg once-daily dosing of dasatinib in men with chemotherapy-naïve CRPC was completed.[50] There was a similar degree of activity with the double dosing and favorable safety profile. Moreover, a confirmed PSA decline of ≥50% from baseline was observed in one patient (2%) with no other signs of clinical or radiographic progression. Future clinical trials with dasatinib evaluating survival, bone biomarkers, and SREs are proceeding with 100 mg once-daily dosing.

Another phase II trial investigated the combination of dasatinib with docetaxel in 31 chemotherapy-naïve men with metastatic CRPC. Twenty-one of the 31 patients had measurable disease by RECIST criteria and 16 of these patients had stable disease after more than 21 weeks. Furthermore, 30 of 31 patients had a best response of improved (32%) or stable disease (65%) after 6 weeks or more, which was objectively evidenced by bone scan. In this study, combining the use of dasatinib 100 mg daily and docetaxel, the incidence of pleural effusions in the entire population study was 7%, much less than the 51% reported in the higher dosing trials previously addressed.[51]

Currently, a randomized, double-blind, phase III trial comparing docetaxel combined with dasatinib (100 mg daily) with docetaxel combined with placebo in chemotherapy-naïve patients with CRPC has been completed (NCT00744497). The primary end point of this trial is overall survival and secondary end points will include the rate of change in urinary N-telopeptide, time to first SRE, rate of change in pain intensity, time to PSA progression, and safety and tolerability of combination therapy. Results are expected to be available in 2013.[52]

Saracatinib (AZD0530) is another oral Src inhibitor that is in clinical development after preclinical studies demonstrated that it inhibits proliferation and migration in a range of prostate cancer cell lines, including in androgen-independent xenografts.[53] Saracatinib has also shown anti-osteoclast activity both in vitro and in vivo. In a phase II single-arm trial of saracatinib monotherapy in advanced CRPC patients, 5 of 28 patients had a slight PSA decline, although not more than 30%. The median PFS interval was 8 weeks.[54] Efforts for additional development of this compound in men with prostate cancer are unknown at this time.

VEGF Pathway

Angiogenesis is a process by which a malignant tumor develops the ability to metastasize in addition to local invasion. VEGF, VEGFR-1, and VEGFR-2 are mediators of angiogenesis, and in human prostate cancer cells, there is increased plasma level of VEGF and overexpression of VEGFR-1 and VEGFR-2[55] which has been correlated with poor prognosis and cancer progression.[56] Similarly, antibodies to VEGF have slowed the progression of prostate xenograft growth rates, especially in combination with chemotherapy.[57] Based on these preclinical data, the rationale for targeting the VEGF pathway is a reasonable approach and three such agents are currently in phase III trials: bevacizumab, aflibercept, and sunitinib (see Table 57.3).

Bevacizumab is a humanized monoclonal antibody directed against VEGF-A and causes potent inhibition of VEGFR signaling and angiogenesis. Bevacizumab is approved for use in combination with chemotherapy for patients with metastatic colorectal, breast, and lung cancers. In prostate cancer, bevacizumab has been evaluated in several clinical trials, such as the Cancer and Leukemia Group B (CALGB) phase II trial of bevacizumab in combination with docetaxel and estramustine in 79 metastatic CRPC patients.[58] PSA decline >50% from baseline occurred in 81% of patients, median time to progression was 9 months, and overall survival was 21 months. These favorable trials led to a recent phase III

TABLE 57–3 Vascular Endothelial Growth Factor Receptor Targeted Agents

Target	Agent	Patient Population	Phase	Primary End Point	ClinicalTrials.gov Identifier
VEGF	Bevacizumab plus lenalidomide plus docetaxel and prednisone	Metastatic chemotherapy-naïve CRPC	II	Safety	NCT00942578
	Aflibercept (VEGF trap) plus docetaxel and prednisone	Metastatic chemotherapy-naïve CRPC	III	OS	NCT00519285
VEGFR	Cediranib	Metastatic chemotherapy-naïve CRPC after docetaxel failure	II	PFS	NCT00436956
	Cediranib plus docetaxel and prednisone	Chemotherapy-naïve CRPC	II	PFS	NCT00527124
VEGFR, PDGFR	Sunitinib plus prednisone	Metastatic CRPC after docetaxel failure	III	OS	NCT00676650

CRPC, castrate-resistant prostate cancer; OS, overall survival; PFS, progression-free survival; VEGF, vascular endothelial growth factor; VEGFR, vascular endothelial growth factor receptor; PDGFR, platelet-derived growth factor receptor.

randomized placebo-controlled trial of docetaxel, prednisone, and bevacizumab versus docetaxel and prednisone in 1,050 chemotherapy-naïve metastatic CRPC patients with primary end point of overall survival. Although there was median PFS in the bevacizumab arm of 9.9 months compared with the 7.5 months of the control arm ($P < 0.0001$), the overall survival time was *not* statistically significant.[59] Bevacizumab has notable toxicities, including HTN, thromboembolism, hemorrhage, gastrointestinal (GI) perforation, and proteinuria. Unfortunately, a negative study with bevacizumab poses a challenge for further development of agents modulating the VEGF signaling axis. Despite the commonality of VEGF modulation, other agents in this class are not all the same. Therefore, there is a rationale, albeit a diminishing one for further development of similar agents in men with CRPC.

Aflibercept (VEGF Trap) is a recombinant fusion protein consisting of human VEGFR extracellular domains fused to the Fc portion of human immunoglobulin G1. It provides inhibition of VEGF-A, VEGF-B, and VEGFR-1 and VEGFR-2 by binding and inactivating these circulating factors.[60] Phase I trials have shown safety of aflibercept in combination with docetaxel,[61] which led to the ongoing phase III, randomized, double-blind, placebo-controlled trial of docetaxel with or without aflibercept in patients with metastatic CRPC (NCT00519285). The toxicity profile of aflibercept resembles bevacizumab as they both share a similar mechanism of action. It remains to be seen whether the results will be similar to bevacizumab as well.

Sunitinib is an oral multi-targeted tyrosine kinase inhibitor of VEGFR, PDGFR, and KIT. A phase II study investigating sunitinib in 36 metastatic prior docetaxel-treated CRPC patients demonstrated a 12-week PFS in 78.9% of patients. Therapy was discontinued in 47% of patients due to toxicity and there were two early deaths.[62] Recently, a phase II study was presented evaluating sunitinib in combination with docetaxel as a first-line treatment in 55 patients with metastatic CRPC. Despite an encouraging PSA response rate in 56% of patients, the combination resulted in a 15% rate of febrile neutropenia and dose reductions were required for sunitinib (26% of patients) and docetaxel (33% of patients).[63] The phase III trial, SUN 1120, evaluating sunitinib with prednisone was terminated early in September 2011 after a planned interim analysis revealed that the combination of sunitinib with prednisone was unlikely to improve overall survival compared with prednisone alone.[41] The early termination is disappointing, but perhaps not unexpected as combination therapy with sunitinib and a variety of cytotoxic chemotherapy has not been shown to be well tolerated.

Sorafenib is an orally administered multitargeted kinase inhibitor and has inhibitory action against Raf kinase, PDGFR, VEGFR-2 and VEGFR-3, and c-kit pathways. In prostate cancer, phase II trials of single-agent sorafenib used in the pre- or post-docetaxel setting have reported modest activity with a low rate of PSA response and a median PFS of 2 to 4 months.[64] However, discordant responses in these trials were seen with increasing PSA levels but improved scans or symptoms, suggesting that PSA may not be reliable as a marker of an antitumor effect with sorafenib. Interest has also been garnered surrounding the hypothesis that sorafenib may potentiate the effects of docetaxel. A phase I dose-escalation study recently reported that the combination of docetaxel and sorafenib was well tolerated with no dose-limiting toxicity observed at the doses tested; the recommended dose of sorafenib was 400 mg twice daily given continuously with standard dose docetaxel 75 mg/m^2 every 3 weeks. There was, however, a high rate of febrile neutropenia (8 of 24 patients) and uncomplicated neutropenia (5 of 24 patients).[65] Preliminary results of a phase II study using docetaxel and sorafenib as first-line treatment in men with CRPC also showed discordant PSA/clinical response.[66] A similar finding was reported recently in a phase II study in which patients who had progressed on docetaxel or mitoxantrone were re-challenged with the same chemotherapy on which they had progressed in addition to sorafenib. Fourteen patients were evaluable at the time of reporting. Of these, 11 (73%) had stable disease radiographically for a median time of 6.7 months. Six of 14 (42%) patients had a decrease in PSA level after adding sorafenib. PSA responses did not correlate with radiographic changes or clinical benefit.

Cediranib is yet another oral small molecule inhibitor of VEGFR tyrosine kinase. A phase II trial of 34 post–docetaxel-treated patients on cediranib was evaluated for PFS as determined by clinical and radiographic criteria (i.e., not PSA level). Of the 23 evaluable patients, 13 showed tumor shrinkage and 4 met the criteria for partial response. As with the previous studies, PSA levels did not correlate well with imaging responses.[67] There are additional combination studies with cediranib, including docetaxel as well as dasatinib.

The challenge that remains with agents impacting the VEGF signaling pathway is an apparent low clinical effect as well as higher than expected side effects particularly in combination with chemotherapy. In the era of effective agents that effectively target the androgen pathway, careful thought must be given to design newer clinical trials evaluating agents that may impact VEGF signaling.

Other Anti-angiogenic Agents

The exact mechanisms by which lenalidomide, an analogue of thalidomide, demonstrates activity in CRPC are unclear. However, the anti-angiogenic and immunomodulatory effects of the drug likely contribute to its efficacy. Evidence also suggests that lenalidomide inhibits the VEGF-induced PI3K–Akt pathway signaling, contributing to enhanced apoptosis.[68] Lenalidomide demonstrated a synergistic effect when paired with paclitaxel in patients with CRPC receiving prior taxanes.[69] The drug went on to be evaluated in combination with docetaxel, which showed efficacy (half of the 31 patients had a >50% PSA decline) in patients with chemotherapy-naïve disease and in chemotherapy failures.[70] These results led to a phase III trial that set out to compare docetaxel and prednisone with and without lenalidomide in CRPC patients. This trial, however, was recently discontinued after the data monitoring committee had determined that the combination of docetaxel and prednisone plus lenalidomide would not demonstrate a statistically significant treatment effect against the primary end point of overall survival versus docetaxel and prednisone plus placebo.[71] Nonetheless, research with lenalidomide is ongoing, particularly in the biochemically recurrent prostate cancer arena. Recently, a retrospective exploration into the immunological parameters of men with PSA relapse disease was presented. Patients were treated with either 5 or 25 mg of lenalidomide in a randomized phase II trial and observed for whether immunological changes correlated with disease progression. Results suggested that the induction of novel anti-prostate antibodies could be a potential mechanism for lenalidomide response while the observed changes in serum IL-8 levels might serve as a potential biomarker in treated patients.[72]

Furthermore, lenalidomide was evaluated in nonmetastatic biochemically relapsed prostate cancer in a recent phase I/II double-blinded, randomized study. Sixty men were randomized to lenalidomide 5 mg/d (n = 26) or 25 mg/d (n = 34) for 3 weeks repeated monthly for 6 months or until dose-limiting toxicity or disease progression. Grade 3/4 toxicity rates were 12% (n = 3) with 5 mg and 29% (n = 10) with 25 mg (P = 0.1), most commonly neutropenia (five patients, all on 25 mg). Two patients per arm had thromboembolic events. The change in PSA slope was greater with 25 versus 5 mg (P = 0.005). With a mean follow-up of 31.4 months (range 14 to 44), five patients on 25 mg and one patient on 5 mg remain on the study. Thus, lenalidomide had demonstrated acceptable toxicity and was associated with long-term disease stabilization and PSA declines. Hence, immunomodulatory agents seem to have a role in prostate cancer, but their optimal utility remains under investigation.

Tasquinimod is an orally administered anti-angiogenic drug that significantly improved PFS compared with placebo in a randomized phase II trial of 201 metastatic CRPC patients (7.6 vs. 3.3 mo; P = 0.0042).[73] Although bone alkaline phosphatase levels were stabilized in the tasquinimod group, PSA kinetics were less affected. Side effects in the experimental arm included GI disorders, fatigue, musculoskeletal pains, and elevations of pancreatic and inflammatory biomarkers. Grade 3 to 4 AEs, including asymptomatic elevations of laboratory parameters, were reported in 40% of patients receiving tasquinimod versus 10% receiving placebo; deep vein thrombosis (4% vs. 0%) was more common in the tasquinimod arm. Currently, a phase III trial comparing tasquinimod and placebo for men with asymptomatic or minimally symptomatic metastatic CRPC prior to chemotherapy is underway (see Table 57.4).[74]

TABLE 57-4 Other Agents

Target	Agent	Patient Population	Phase	Primary End Point	ClinicalTrials.gov Identifier
S100A9	Tasquinimod	Metastatic CRPC prior to chemotherapy	III	PFS	NCT01234311—
IGF-1R	Cixutumumab plus mitoxantrone and prednisone	Metastatic CRPC after failure on docetaxel-based chemotherapy	II	PFS	NCT00683475
	Figitumumab plus docetaxel and prednisone	Chemotherapy-naïve or docetaxel-refractory CRPC	II	PSA, tumor response	NCT00313781

CRPC, castrate-resistant prostate cancer; OS, overall survival; PFS, progression-free survival; PSA, prostate-specific antigen; IGF-1R, insulin-like growth factor 1 receptor.

IGF-1 Pathway

IGF-1R–mediated signaling regulates cellular processes of proliferation, differentiation, and apoptosis; thus, it has been implicated to have a critical role in the development of malignancies.[75] In vitro models have demonstrated that high IGF-1R levels in prostate cancer cells can lead to androgen independence.[76] Various studies in transgenic mice have demonstrated IGF-1R expression to be greater in high-grade, malignant prostate stromal tissue.[77] These findings have led to the rationale to devise several methods to block IGF signaling in preclinical model studies.

In a meta-analysis of clinical studies, elevated circulating concentrations of IGF-1 were associated with a greater risk of prostate cancer.[75] Humanized monoclonal antibodies to IGF-1R have been developed and are currently under clinical investigation. For prostate cancer treatment, there are three IGF-1R–directed antibody therapies, such as cixutumumab (IMC-A12), figitumumab (CP-751,871), and AMG-479. Figitumumab and AMG-479 were found to be tolerable based on phase I and phase II trials.[78,79] Unfortunately, figitumumab is no longer being developed due to reporting of high treatment-related mortality rates in combination with cytotoxic therapy. Cixutumumab has been evaluated in a phase II setting for men with asymptomatic metastatic CRPC. Stable disease was reported in 9 out of 31 patients for 6 months (range, 7.4 to 12.5 mo).[80] Additional studies with cixutumumab include combination study of leuprolide acetate in men with newly diagnosed metastatic prostate cancer (NCT01120236 and SWOG0925). The primary objective of this trial is to determine the undetectable PSA rate at 7 months. Another study is combination of cixutumumab with temsirolimus in men with CRPC (NCT01026623). Results of tolerability and antitumor activity from agents targeting the IGF pathway will be eagerly awaited.

Chaperone Proteins

Heat shock (chaperone) proteins, such as hsp90, are known to have antiapoptotic properties and have thus become a reasonable target for anti-neoplastic therapy. Hsp90 is an essential molecular protein complex for AR stability and maturation; thus, it has become a viable target for CRPC therapy as well.[81] Clusterin, an alternative chaperone protein, is expressed during periods of cellular stress and has an ability to inhibit apoptosis via inhibition of activated Bax, a critical proapoptotic Bcl-2 family member.[82] Clusterin has also been found to activate the PI3K/Akt pathway through cell surface receptor signaling.[83] Clusterin has been associated with androgen-independent progression in preclinical models of prostate cancer, such that its expression increases after castration and with castrate-resistant disease.[84]

Custirsen (OGX-011) is a second-generation phosphorothioate antisense molecule that inhibits clusterin by decreasing mRNA translation of clusterin in tumors of patients with localized prostate cancer.[85] In phase I trials, custirsen delivered with standard chemotherapy doses to docetaxel-refractory prostate cancer patients was found to be feasible and tolerated.[86] A randomized phase II study of docetaxel plus prednisone with or without custirsen in patients with metastatic CRPC (n = 82) demonstrated a median overall survival time in the custirsen arm (23.8 vs. 16.9 mo; HR, 0.61), although rates of PSA and tumor response were similar.[87] Currently, a phase III trial of OGX-011 plus docetaxel and prednisone in patients with metastatic CRPC with a primary end point of overall survival is enrolling.

A phase II trial of STA-9090, a second-generation hsp90 inhibitor, is currently underway in CRPC men who have received prior docetaxel therapy (NCT01270880). Previous first-generation inhibitors (including 17-AAG and 17-DMAG) were difficult to tolerate and had minimal activity in men with CRPC.[88] STA-9090 is a more potent and active agent with a much better tolerated side effect profile. A biomarker study evaluating STA-9090 alone and in combination with dutasteride is also enrolling (NCT01368003). As agents that inhibit hsp90 pathway improve its efficacy and reduce its toxicity profile, this pathway remains one with a robust rationale and preclinical and clinical activity.

BONE-RELATED PATHWAYS

Therapies directed toward bone progression of prostate cancer have sound biologic rationale, given the high propensity of prostate cancer to metastasize to the bone. There is a complex interplay between osteoblasts, osteoclasts, cancer cells, and the bone microenvironment, all of which are mediated by cellular signaling. Prostate cancer cells secrete endothelin-1, which stimulates osteoblast proliferation. Osteoclasts are induced by cytokines to express RANKL, which promotes bone resorption. The release of growth factors by osteoblasts stimulates tumor cells, thus leading to a vicious cycle (see Table 57.5).[89]

RANKL

Until recently, the only standard of care was to administer a bisphosphonate, such as zoledronic acid, to help minimize the bone resorption, which leads to reduction of SREs. Denosumab, a humanized monoclonal antibody with specificity for the RANKL, was shown to be superior to zoledronic acid in a study of 1,901 men with CRPC. Denosumab delayed or prevented SREs more effectively than zoledronic acid.[90] The median time to first on-study SRE, the primary end point, was 20.7 months for denosumab compared with 17.1 months for zoledronic acid (HR 0.82; 95% CI, 0.71 to 0.95; P = 0.0002). There were no differences in PSA time, overall disease progression, or overall survival. The two treatment groups had a similar frequency of serious toxicities; the cumulative incidence of osteonecrosis of the jaw was similar in the two groups (denosumab 2.3% vs. zoledronic acid

TABLE 57-5 Bone Targeted Agents

Target	Agent	Patient Population	Phase	Primary End Point	ClinicalTrials.gov Identifier
Src	Dasatinib or nilutamide	Metastatic CRPC	II	PFS	CT00918385
	Saracatinib	Recurrent or progressive prostate or breast cancer with bone metastases	II	Bone markers	NCT00558272
RANKL	Denosumab	CRPC with bone metastases	III	Time to SRE	NCT00321620
	Denosumab	Nonmetastatic CRPC	III	Time to bone metastases	NCT002860910

CRPC, castrate-resistant prostate cancer; PFS, progression-free survival; SRE, skeletal-related event; RANKL, receptor activator of nuclear factor-κB ligand.

1.3%). These results, combined with two other pivotal phase III trials of the same, led to the FDA approval of denosumab for prevention of skeletal complications in patients with bone metastases from solid tumors, except multiple myeloma.

Denosumab was also found to improve bone metastasis–free survival (29.5 mo) compared with placebo in men with CRPC disease (25.2 mo). There was, however, no survival benefit with denosumab in the phase III trial that was reported at the European Society for Medical Oncology Meeting 2011. In September 2011, denosumab received indication to increase bone mass in patients at high risk for fracture receiving androgen deprivation therapy for nonmetastatic prostate cancer. Fortunately for men with CRPC, there are now two FDA-approved agents to help improve and strengthen metastatic bones. Zoledronic acid requires intravenous infusion and monitoring of renal function. Denosumab is a subcutaneous injection and monitoring of calcium and other electrolytes. Both agents have a role in prostate cancer patients. There are multiple other agents that are being investigated that have targeted activity at the bone interface, which are discussed in detail below.

Endothelin Axis

Endothelin signaling pathway involves the endothelin peptides (endothelin-1, endothelin-2, and endothelin-3) and receptors (ET-A and ET-B), which are involved in the growth and progression of prostate cancer by cell proliferation, angiogenesis, and metastasis.[91] There are currently two agents that are further along the development pipeline in regard to endothelin antagonists, atrasentan and zibotentan.

Atrasentan is an orally bioavailable competitive inhibitor of ET-1 that binds to ET-A with a 1,800-fold selectivity than ET-B.[89] In a double-blind, placebo-controlled phase III study of 809 metastatic CRPC patients, atrasentan did not improve the primary end point of time to progression (TTP) compared with placebo (HR 0.89; 95% CI, 0.76 to 1.04; $P = 0.136$).[92] The most common toxicities in both studies were peripheral edema, nasal congestion, and headache.[93] The SWOG S0421 was a placebo-controlled phase III trial comparing docetaxel plus prednisone with or without atrasentan in metastatic CRPC patients with bone metastases (NCT00134056). Unfortunately, the study was discontinued by the Data and Safety Monitoring Committee after initial results had failed to demonstrate an improvement in overall survival or PFS in the atrasentan arm compared with patients who received a placebo. Despite initial enthusiasm for atrasentan, the results as a single agent and in combination with chemotherapy were a disappointment.

Zibotentan (ZD4054) is an orally bioavailable specific inhibitor of ET-A that is more selective than atrasentan.[94] A phase II double-blind, randomized study tested two doses of zibotentan versus placebo in 312 men with CRPC with bone disease who were asymptomatic or minimally symptomatic and had rising PSA levels. In the mature data analysis, there was a trend toward a 3.6-month improvement in overall survival for patients in the zibotentan 10 mg group compared with placebo (23.5 vs. 19.9 mo, respectively; $P = 0.254$) and a 4.0-month improvement in overall survival for patients in the zibotentan 15 mg group versus placebo (23.9 vs. 19.9 mo, respectively; $P = 0.103$).[95] Unfortunately, multiple recent phase III trials of zibotentan did not show a significant improvement in the primary end point of overall survival, including the ENTHUSE (A Phase III trial of 2D40S4(Z1betentan) (Endothelin A Antagonist) and Doetayel in Metastatic Hormone Resistant Prostate Cancer M0 study comparing zibotentan with placebo in CRPC patients with PSA progression-only disease (NCT00626548).[96] Currently, there is an ongoing multinational phase III trial, ENTHUSE M1C (NCT00617669), comparing docetaxel with or without zibotentan in metastatic CRPC patients. Should this trial not achieve its primary objective, it is possible that perturbation of the endothelin signaling pathway may not be an effective therapeutic strategy.

c-Met Pathway

MET is a receptor tyrosine kinase that has roles in oncogenic signaling, angiogenesis, and metastasis. Androgen deprivation activates MET signaling in prostate cancer cells. Activated MET is particularly highly expressed in bone. Preclinical studies have suggested that MET signaling may promote survival of prostate cancer cells.[97] Cabozantinib (XL184) is a small molecule inhibitor of multiple kinase signaling pathways, including MET, RET, VEGFR2/KDR, and KIT. In a recently presented phase II study, cabozantinib has shown promising activity in men with bone metastases with dramatic improvement in bone scans in most patients.

Metastatic CRPC patients with progressive measurable disease received cabozantinib at 100 mg orally daily over 12 weeks with a primary end point of objective response rates. Accrual was halted at 168 patients based on an observed high rate of clinical activity. Of the 100 evaluable patients with a median age of 68, 86% of patients had complete or partial resolution of lesions on bone scan as early as week 6. About 64% had improved pain and the most commonly related grade 3/4 AEs were fatigue (11%), HTN (7%), and hand–foot syndrome (5%); no related grade 5 AEs were reported. PSA changes were independent of clinical activity and overall, week 12 disease control rate (PR+SD) was 71%.[98] Current studies are proceeding with a lower dose of cabozantinib in order to improve drug tolerability. The relationship between c-met inhibition and metastatic bone disease has yet to be properly elucidated, but multiple research efforts are underway to improve our understanding of this novel finding.

PERSONALIZED THERAPY FOR PROSTATE CANCER

The treatment for prostate cancer, similar to breast cancer, has the potential to become individualized. By focusing on specific molecular pathways, we can use genomic and proteomic analyses to tailor treatment according to individual tumor characteristics and thereby select patients who are more likely to benefit from different therapies. The principle of chemotherapy capitalizes on the fact that tumors are composed of a high proportion of cells that are in the replication process, thus being able to target DNA synthesis. Although cytotoxic therapy is the standard of care for progressive metastatic CRPC, it is not curative and has toxicity associated with it. Fortunately, in prostate cancer, many novel agents are currently being developed with focus in androgen signaling, cell signaling, and bone metastatic signaling pathways.

As previously described, AR gene and protein upregulation during tumor progression is a critical event in the development of CRPC. When prostate cancer progresses despite initial androgen deprivation therapy, there are data suggesting that CRPC tumors with AR gene amplification respond better to combined androgen blockade than those tumors without AR amplification, based on predictive markers of response.[85] The difficulty with the AR, however, lies with its biological heterogeneity and androgen independence; thus, finding a single agent to treat CRPC is likely not possible. Thus, recent studies have focused on a genomic-guided approach. For example, a transcription signature for AR activity was identified by using an androgen-sensitive prostate cancer cell line (LNCaP). In human prostate tumor tissues, AR activity was noted to be high in localized, untreated tumors and lower in tissues following neoadjuvant androgen deprivation therapy and in CRPC. This suggests that AR activity appears to decrease with prostate cancer progression.[86] Interestingly, the level of AR signature expression can be predictive for specific therapies, such as the Src inhibitor dasatinib. Furthermore, a correlation has been established between low AR activity and a sensitivity signal to dasatinib ($P = 0.019$). It appears that those CRPC patients with low AR activity in their tumor specimens may benefit from dasatinib more than an antiandrogen target.

To evaluate this further, a genomic-guided prospective study has been completed in metastatic CRPC patients where either an antiandrogen such as nilutamide or dasatinib will be administered to patients based on high and low levels of AR activity, respectively. Those that progress on either treatment were offered combination therapy (NCT00918385). Although this trial is terminated, the clinical trial design is one to be further explored. As the use of biomarkers becomes more integral in the treatment decision-making process, appropriate steps to comply with necessary regulatory requirements must be taken. Incorporating exciting new markers with novel therapies will move us closer to developing personalized therapy for men with prostate cancer.

Circulating tumor cells (CTCs) represent an exciting area of research enabling the molecular characterization of metastatic prostate cancer tissue without relying on previously obtained tissue specimens, which are usually representative of localized prostate cancer. Based on multiple prospective studies, enumeration of CTCs before and after chemotherapy has shown to be predictive of overall survival in metastatic CRPC patients.[87,99] There is much work ahead in terms of CTC characterization, gene profiling, and, more importantly, the change in these profiles with disease progression. At the current time, CTCs themselves are FDA cleared to use in patients with CRPC for predictive monitoring.

Another area of ongoing research is the role of genetic polymorphisms affecting proteins involved in drug function or metabolism and consequences on response to targeted therapies in prostate cancer. In a study of prostate cancer patients who were treated with androgen deprivation, polymorphisms in three separate genes involved in hormone synthesis (CYP19A1, HSD3B1, and HSD17B4) were significantly ($P = 0.01$) associated with a longer time to progression, with best responses observed in patients with multiple polymorphisms.[90] Furthermore, there is some evidence to suggest a survival correlation in CRPC patients treated with docetaxel with specific genotypes of ABCB1 (encoding a drug efflux protein) and CYP1B1 (encoding an enzyme involved in estrogen metabolism), thus supporting the need for further elucidation of pharmacogenomic factors in future prospective studies in order to provide tailored therapy in metastatic CRPC patients.

CONCLUSION

Multiple novel pathways and therapeutic agents that target them have been identified in prostate cancer. In the past 10 years, significant advances have been made leading to multiple FDA-approved medications to treat patients with CRPC. Despite progress in the field, current treatments are not curative and a definitive prolonged and sustained survival benefit has yet to be established. With several failed phase III clinical trials, it is becoming more clear that there needs to be careful evaluation and perhaps potential change in how early-phase trials are designed. Potential ways are to develop improved biologic markers and imaging studies to assess patient response and extent of disease. A further challenge will be to identify which patients will benefit from particular treatment regimens earlier on in their clinical state, ideally before progression to CRPC. Hence, it is paramount that we continue to improve our understanding and investigate newer agents and technology to help clinicians deliver the best treatment for the patient.

REFERENCES

1. Jemal A, Siegel R, Xu J, Ward E. Cancer statistics, 2011. *CA Cancer J Clin*. July-August 2011;61:212-236.
2. D'Amico AV, Whittington R, Malkowicz SB, et al. Biochemical outcome after radical prostatectomy, external beam radiation therapy, or interstitial radiation therapy for clinically localized prostate cancer. *JAMA*. September 1998;280:969.
3. Hamberg P, Verhagen PC, de Wit R. When to start cytotoxic therapy in asymptomatic patients with hormone refractory prostate cancer? *Eur J Cancer*. June 2008;44:1193.
4. Tannock IF, Osoba D, Stockler MR, et al. Chemotherapy with mitoxantrone plus prednisone or prednisone alone for symptomatic hormone-resistant prostate cancer: a Canadian randomized trial with palliative end points. *J Clin Oncol*. June 1996;14:1756.
5. Oosterhof GO, Roberts JT, de Reijke TM, et al. Strontium(89) chloride versus palliative local field radiotherapy in patients with hormonal escaped prostate cancer: a phase III study of the European Organisation for Research and Treatment of Cancer, Genitourinary Group. *Eur Urol*. November 2003;44:519.
6. Saad F, Gleason DM, Murray R, et al. A randomized, placebo-controlled trial of zoledronic acid in patients with hormone-refractory metastatic prostate carcinoma. *J Natl Cancer Inst*. October 2002;94:1458.
7. Petrylak DP, Tangen CM, Hussain MH, et al. Docetaxel and estramustine compared with mitoxantrone and prednisone for advanced refractory prostate cancer. *N Engl J Med*. October 2004;351:1513.
8. Tannock IF, de Wit R, Berry WR, et al. Docetaxel plus prednisone or mitoxantrone plus prednisone for advanced prostate cancer. *N Engl J Med*. October 2004;351:1502.
9. de Bono JS, Logothetis CJ, Molina A, et al. Abiraterone and increased survival in metastatic prostate cancer. *N Engl J Med*. May 2011;364:1995.
10. Kantoff PW, Higano CS, Shore ND, et al. Sipuleucel-T immunotherapy for castration-resistant prostate cancer. *N Engl J Med*. July 2010;363:411.
11. Attar RM, Takimoto CH, Gottardis MM. Castration-resistant prostate cancer: locking up the molecular escape routes. *Clin Cancer Res*. May 2009;15:3251.
12. Chen Y, Sawyers CL, Scher HI. Targeting the androgen receptor pathway in prostate cancer. *Curr Opin Pharmacol*. August 2008;8:440.
13. Devlin HL, Mudryj M. Progression of prostate cancer: multiple pathways to androgen independence. *Cancer Lett*. February 2009;274:177.
14. Hu R, Dunn TA, Wei S, et al. Ligand-independent androgen receptor variants derived from splicing of cryptic exons signify hormone-refractory prostate cancer. *Cancer Res*. January 2009;69:16.
15. Tran C, Ouk S, Clegg NJ, et al. Development of a second-generation antiandrogen for treatment of advanced prostate cancer. *Science*. May 2009;324:787.
16. Miller K. Words of wisdom. Re: antitumour activity of MDV3100 in castration-resistant prostate cancer: a phase 1-2 study. Scher HI, Beer TM, Higano CS, et al. Prostate Cancer Foundation/Department of Defense Prostate Cancer Clinical Trials Consortium. *Eur Urol*. September 2010;58:464.
17. Scher HI, Beer TM, Higano CS, et al. Antitumour activity of MDV3100 in castration-resistant prostate cancer: a phase 1-2 study. *Lancet*. April 2010;375:1437.
18. AFFIRM: A Multinational Phase 3, Double-Blind, Placebo-Controlled Efficacy and Safety Study of Oral MDV3100 in Patients with Progressive Castration-Resistant Prostate Cancer Previously Treated With Docetaxel-Based Chemotherapy [Clinical Trials.gov identifier NCT00974311]. US National Institutes of Health. http://clinicaltrials.gov. Accessed February 9, 2011.
19. PREVAIL: A Multinational Phase 3, Double-Blind, Placebo-Controlled Efficacy and Safety Study of Oral MDV3100 in Chemotherapy-Naive Patients with Progressive Metastatic Prostate Cancer Who Have Failed Androgen Deprivation Therapy [Clinical Trials.gov identifier NCT01212991]. US National Institutes of Health. http://clinicaltrials.gov. Accessed February 9, 2011.
20. Taplin ME, Regan MM, Ko YJ, et al. Phase II study of androgen synthesis inhibition with ketoconazole, hydrocortisone, and dutasteride in asymptomatic castration-resistant prostate cancer. *Clin Cancer Res*. November 2009;15:7099.
21. Yap TA, Carden CP, Attard G, de Bono JS. Targeting CYP17: established and novel approaches in prostate cancer. *Curr Opin Pharmacol*. August 2008;8:449.
22. Danila DC, Morris MJ, de Bono JS, et al. Phase II multicenter study of abiraterone acetate plus prednisone therapy in patients with docetaxel-treated castration-resistant prostate cancer. *J Clin Oncol*. March 2010;28:1496.
23. Drecier R, Angus DB, MacVicar GR, et al. Safety, pharmacokinetics, and efficacy of TAK-700 in castration-resistant metastatic prostate cancer: a phase I/II open label study. *Genitourin Cancer Symp Proc*. 2010;89. Abstract 103.
24. Safety Study of TAK-700 in Subjects with Prostate Cancer. [Clinical Trials.gov identifier NCT00569153]. US National Institutes of Health. http://clinicaltrials.gov. Accessed December 20, 2011.
25. Study Comparing Orteronel Plus Prednisone in Patients with Chemotherapy-Naive Metastatic Castration-Resistant Prostate Cancer [Clinical Trials.gov identifier NCT01193244]. US National Institutes of Health. http://clinicaltrials.gov. Accessed December 20, 2011.
26. Study Comparing Orteronel Plus Prednisone in Patients with Metastatic Castration-Resistant Prostate Cancer [Clinical Trials.gov identifier NCT01193257]. US National Institutes of Health. http://clinicaltrials.gov. Accessed December 20, 2011.
27. Trauger R, Corey E, Bell D, et al. Inhibition of androstenediol-dependent LNCaP tumour growth by 17alpha-ethynyl-5alpha-androstane-3alpha, 17beta-diol (HE3235). *Br J Cancer*. April 2009;100:1068.
28. Montgomery RB, Morris MJ, Ryan CJ, et al. HE3235, a synthetic adrenal hormone disease-modifying agent, in castrate resistant prostate cancer: results of phase I/II clinical trial. *J Clin Oncol*. 2010;28(15 suppl):385s. Abstract 4674.
29. LoPiccolo J, Blumenthal GM, Bernstein WB, Dennis PA. Targeting the PI3K/Akt/mTOR pathway: effective combinations and clinical considerations. *Drug Resist Updat*. February-April, 2008;11:32.
30. Gera JF, Mellinghoff IK, Shi Y, et al. AKT activity determines sensitivity to mammalian target of rapamycin (mTOR) inhibitors

by regulating cyclin D1 and c-myc expression. *J Biol Chem.* January 2004;279:2737.
31. McMenamin ME, Soung P, Perera S, Kaplan I, Loda M, Sellers WR. Loss of PTEN expression in paraffin-embedded primary prostate cancer correlates with high Gleason score and advanced stage. *Cancer Res.* September 1999;59: 4291.
32. Graff JR. Emerging targets in the AKT pathway for treatment of androgen-independent prostatic adenocarcinoma. *Expert Opin Ther Targets.* February 2002;6:103.
33. Shen MM, Abate-Shen C. PTEN inactivation and the emergence of androgen-independent prostate cancer. *Cancer Res.* July 2007;67:6535.
34. Wang Y, Mikhailova M, Bose S, Pan CX, deVere White RW, Ghosh PM. Regulation of androgen receptor transcriptional activity by rapamycin in prostate cancer cell proliferation and survival. *Oncogene.* November 2008;27:7106.
35. Amato RJ, Jac J, Mohammad T, Saxena S. Pilot study of rapamycin in patients with hormone-refractory prostate cancer. *Clin Genitourin Cancer.* September 2008;6:97.
36. Ross RW, Beer TM, Jacobus S, et al. A phase 2 study of carboplatin plus docetaxel in men with metastatic hormone-refractory prostate cancer who are refractory to docetaxel. *Cancer.* February 2008;112:521.
37. Gross ME, Soscia J, Sakowsky S, et al. Phase I trial of RAD001, bevacizumab, and docetaxel for castration-resistant prostate cancer. *J Clin Oncol.* 2009;27(15 suppl):272s. Abstract 5154.
38. George DJ, Armstrong AJ, Creel P, et al. A phase II study of RAD001 in men with hormone-refractory metastatic prostate cancer (HRPC). Presented at the 2008 American Society of Clinical Oncology Genitourinary Cancers Symposium; February 14-16, 2008; San Francisco, CA. Abstract 181.
39. Fung AS, Wu L, Tannock IF. Concurrent and sequential administration of chemotherapy and the mammalian target of rapamycin inhibitor temsirolimus in human cancer cells and xenografts. *Clin Cancer Res.* September 2009;15:5389.
40. Raymond E, Alexandre J, Faivre S, et al. Safety and pharmacokinetics of escalated doses of weekly intravenous infusion of CCI-779, a novel mTOR inhibitor, in patients with cancer. *J Clin Oncol.* June 2004;22: 2336.
41. Armstrong AJ, Netto GJ, Rudek MA, et al. A pharmacodynamic study of rapamycin in men with intermediate- to high-risk localized prostate cancer. *Clin Cancer Res.* June 2010;16:3057.
42. Fizazi K. The role of Src in prostate cancer. *Ann Oncol.* November 2007;18:1765.
43. Summy JM, Gallick GE. Src family kinases in tumor progression and metastasis. *Cancer Metastasis Rev.* December 2003;22:337.
44. Mendiratta P, Mostaghel E, Guinney J, et al. Genomic strategy for targeting therapy in castration-resistant prostate cancer. *J Clin Oncol.* April 2009;27:2022.
45. Tatarov O, Mitchell TJ, Seywright M, Leung HY, Brunton VG, Edwards J. SRC family kinase activity is up-regulated in hormone-refractory prostate cancer. *Clin Cancer Res.* May 2009; 15:3540.
46. Araujo J, Logothetis C. Targeting Src signaling in metastatic bone disease. *Int J Cancer.* January 2009;124:1.
47. Nam S, Kim D, Cheng JQ, et al. Action of the Src family kinase inhibitor, dasatinib (BMS-354825), on human prostate cancer cells. *Cancer Res.* October 2005;65:9185.
48. Koreckij T, Nguyen H, Brown LG, Yu EY, Vessella RL, Corey E. Dasatinib inhibits the growth of prostate cancer in bone and provides additional protection from osteolysis. *Br J Cancer.* July 2009;101:263.
49. Yu EY, Wilding G, Posadas E, et al. Phase II study of dasatinib in patients with metastatic castration-resistant prostate cancer. *Clin Cancer Res.* December 2009;15:7421.
50. Yu EY, Massard C, Gross ME, et al. Once-daily dasatinib: expansion of phase II study evaluating safety and efficacy of dasatinib in patients with metastatic castration-resistant prostate cancer. *Urology.* May 2011;77:1166.
51. Araujo J, Gallick G, Trudel G, et al. Dasatinib and docetaxel combination treatment for patients with castration-resistant progressive prostate cancer: a phase 1.2 study (CA 180-086). *J Clin Oncol.* 2009;27:15s. Abstract 5061.
52. Randomized Study Comparing Docetaxel Plus Dasatinib to Docetaxel Plus Placebo in Castration-Resistant Prostate Cancer [Clinical Trials.gov identifier NCT00744497]. US National Institutes of Health. http://clinicaltrials.gov. Accessed December 20, 2011.
53. Yang JC, OK JH, Busby JE, Borowsky AD, kung HJ, Evans CP. Aberrant activation of androgen receptor in a new neuropeptide-autocrine model of androgen-insensitive prostate cancer. *Cancer Res.* January 2009;69:151.
54. Lara PN Jr, Longmate J, Evans CP, et al. A phase II trial of the Src-kinase inhibitor AZD0530 in patients with advanced castration-resistant prostate cancer: a California Cancer Consortium study. *Anticancer Drugs.* March 2009;20:179.
55. Huss WJ, Hanrahan CF, Barrios RJ, Simons JW, Greenberg NM. Angiogenesis and prostate cancer: identification of a molecular progression switch. *Cancer Res.* March 2001;61:2736.
56. George DJ,Halabi S, Shepard TF, et al. Prognostic significance of plasma vascular endothelial growth factor levels in patients with hormone-refractory prostate cancer treated on Cancer and Leukemia Group B 9480. *Clin Cancer Res.* July 2001;7:1932.
57. Sweeney P, Karashima T, Kim SJ, et al. Anti-vascular endothelial growth factor receptor 2 antibody reduces tumorigenicity and metastasis in orthotopic prostate cancer xenografts via induction of endothelial cell apoptosis and reduction of endothelial cell matrix metalloproteinase type 9 production. *Clin Cancer Res.* August 2002;8:2714.
58. Picus J, Halabi S, Kelly WK, et al. A phase 2 study of estramustine, docetaxel, and bevacizumab in men with castrate-resistant prostate cancer: results from Cancer and Leukemia Group B Study 90006. *Cancer.* February 2011;117:526.
59. Kelly WK, Halabi S, Carducci MA, et al. A randomized, double-blind, placebo-controlled phase III trial comparing docetaxel and prednisone with or without bevacizumab in men with castration-resistant prostate cancer (CALGB 90401). *J Clin Oncol.* 2010;28(28 suppl): LBA4511.
60. Verheul HM, Hammers H, van Erp K, et al. Vascular endothelial growth factor trap blocks tumor growth, metastasis formation, and vascular leakage in an orthotopic murine renal cell cancer model. *Clin Cancer Res.* July 2007;13:4201.
61. Isambert N, Freyer G, Zanetta S, et al. A phase I dose escalation and pharmacokinetic (PK) study of intravenous aflibercept (VEGF trap) plus docetaxel (D) in patients (pts) with advanced solid tumors: preliminary results. *J Clin Oncol.* 2008;26:3599. Abstract.
62. Periman PO, Sonpavde G, Bernold DM, et al. Sunitinib malate for metastatic castration resistant prostate cancer following docetaxel-based chemotherapy. *J Clin Oncol.* 2008;26:5157. Abstract.
63. Zurita AJ, Liu G, Hutson T, et al. Sunitinib in combination with docetaxel and prednisone in patients with metastatic hormone-refractory prostate cancer. *J Clin Oncol.* 2009;27:5166. Abstract.
64. Aragon-Ching JB, Jain L, Gulley JL, et al. Final analysis of a phase II trial using sorafenib for metastatic castration-resistant prostate cancer. *BJU Int.* June 2009;103:1636.
65. Mardjuadi F, Medioni J, Kerger J, et al. A phase I study of sorafenib in association with docetaxel-prednisone in chemonaive metastatic castration-resistant prostate cancer. *J Clin Oncol.* 2009;27:5153. Abstract.
66. Cetnar JP, Rosen MA, Vaughn DJ, et al. Phase II study of sorafenib and docetaxel in men with metastatic castration resistant prostate cancer. *J Clin Oncol.* 2009;27:e16055. Abstract.
67. Karakunnel JJ, Gulley JL, Arlen P, et al. Cediranib (AZD2171) in docetaxel-resistant, castration-resistant prostate cancer. *J Clin Oncol.* 2009;27:5141. Abstract.
68. Lu L, Payvandi F, Wu L, et al. The anti-cancer drug lenalidomide inhibits angiogenesis and metastasis via multiple inhibitory effects on endothelial cell function in normoxic and hypoxic conditions. *Microvasc Res.* March 2009;77:78.
69. Mathew P, Tannir N, Tu SM, Carter CM, Bekele NB, Pagliaro L. A modular phase I study of lenalidomide and paclitaxel in metastatic castration-resistant prostate cancer following prior taxane therapy. *Cancer Chemother Pharmacol.* March 2010;65:811.
70. Petrylak D, Resto-Garces K, Tibyan M, Mohile S. A phase I open-label study using lenalidomide and docetaxel in castration-resistant prostate cancer. ASCO Annual Meeting Proceedings (Post-Meeting Edition). *J Clin Oncol.* 2009;27. Abstract 5156.
71. Celgene to discontinue docetaxel and prednisone plus lenalidomide phase III trial on CRPC. http://www.news-medical.net/news/20111123/Celgene-to-discontinue-docetaxel-and-prednisone-plus-lenalidomide-Phase-III-trial-on-CRPC.aspx.

Press Release on November 23, 2011. Accessed December 20, 2011.

72. Zabransky DJ, Smith HA, Thoburn CJ, et al. Lenalidomide modulates IL-8 and anti-prostate antibody levels in men with biochemically recurrent prostate cancer. *Prostate*. 2012;72: 487-498.
73. Pili R, Haggman M, Stadler WM, et al. Phase II randomized, double-blind, placebo-controlled study of tasquinimod in men with minimally symptomatic metastatic castrate-resistant prostate cancer. *J Clin Oncol*. October 2011;29:4022.
74. A study of tasquinimod in men with metastatic castrate resistant prostate cancer [identifier NCT01234311]. ClinicalTrials.gov Website. http://clinicaltrials.gov/ct2/show/NCT01234311. Accessed December 20, 2011.
75. Renehan AG, Zwahlen M, Minder C, O'Dwyer ST, Shalet SM, Egger M. Insulin-like growth factor (IGF)-I, IGF binding protein-3, and cancer risk: systematic review and meta-regression analysis. *Lancet*. April 2004;363:1346.
76. Krueckl SL, Sikes RA, Edlund NM, et al. Increased insulin-like growth factor I receptor expression and signaling are components of androgen-independent progression in a lineage-derived prostate cancer progression model. *Cancer Res*. December 2004;64:8620.
77. Ryan CJ, Haqq CM, Simko J, et al. Expression of insulin-like growth factor-1 receptor in local and metastatic prostate cancer. *Urol Oncol*. March-April 2007;25:134.
78. Haluska P, Shaw HM, Batzel GN, et al. Phase I dose escalation study of the anti insulin-like growth factor-I receptor monoclonal antibody CP-751,871 in patients with refractory solid tumors. *Clin Cancer Res*. October 2007;13:5834.
79. Tolcher AW, Sarantopoulos J, Patnaik A, et al. Phase I, pharmacokinetic, and pharmacodynamic study of AMG 479, a fully human monoclonal antibody to insulin-like growth factor receptor 1. *J Clin Oncol*. December 2009;27:5800.
80. Higano C, Alumkal J, Ryan CJ, et al. A phase II study evaluating the efficacy and safety of single agent IMC A12, a monoclonal antibody, against the insulin-like growth factor-1 receptor, as monotherapy in patients with metastatic, asymptomatic castration-resistant prostate cancer. *J Clin Oncol*. 2009;27(27 suppl):269s. Abstract 5142.
81. Banerji U. Heat shock protein 90 as a drug target: some like it hot. *Clin Cancer Res*. January 2009;15:9.
82. Zhang H, Kim JK, Edwards CA, Xu Z, Taichman R, Wang CY. Clusterin inhibits apoptosis by interacting with activated Bax. *Nat Cell Biol*. September 2005;7:909.
83. Ammar H, Closset JL. Clusterin activates survival through the phosphatidylinositol 3-kinase/Akt pathway. *J Biol Chem*. May 2008;283:12851.
84. July LV, Akbari M, Zellweger T, Jones EC, Goldenberg SL, Gleave ME. Clusterin expression is significantly enhanced in prostate cancer cells following androgen withdrawal therapy. *Prostate*. February 2002;50:179.
85. Chi KN, Eisenhauer E, Fazli L, et al. A phase I pharmacokinetic and pharmacodynamic study of OGX-011, a 2′-methoxyethyl antisense oligonucleotide to clusterin, in patients with localized prostate cancer. *J Natl Cancer Inst*. September 2005;97:1287.
86. Chi KN, Siu LL, Hirte H, et al. A phase I study of OGX-011, a 2′-methoxyethyl phosphorothioate antisense to clusterin, in combination with docetaxel in patients with advanced cancer. *Clin Cancer Res*. February 2008;14:833.
87. Chi KN, Hotte SJ, Yu E, et al. Mature results of a randomized phase II study of OGX-011 in combination with docetaxel/prednisone versus docetaxel/prednisone in patients with metastatic castration-resistant prostate cancer. *J Clin Oncol*. 2009;27:5012. Abstract.
88. Heath EI, Hillman DW, Vaishampayan U, et al. A phase II trial of 17-allylamino-17-demethoxygeldanamycin in patients with hormone-refractory metastatic prostate cancer. *Clin Cancer Res*. December 2008;14:7940.
89. Chi KN, Bjartell A, Dearnaley D, et al. Castration-resistant prostate cancer: from new pathophysiology to new treatment targets. *Eur Urol*. October 2009;56:594.
90. Fizazi K, Carducci M, Smith M, et al. Denosumab versus zoledronic acid for treatment of bone metastases in men with castration-resistant prostate cancer: a randomised, double-blind study. *Lancet*. March 2011;377:813.
91. Bagnato A, Rosano L. The endothelin axis in cancer. *Int J Biochem Cell Biol*. 2008;40:1443.
92. Carducci MA, Saad F, Abrahamsson PA, et al. A phase 3 randomized controlled trial of the efficacy and safety of atrasentan in men with metastatic hormone-refractory prostate cancer. *Cancer*. November 2007;110:1959.
93. Nelson JB, Love W, Chin JL, et al. Phase 3, randomized, controlled trial of atrasentan in patients with nonmetastatic, hormone-refractory prostate cancer. *Cancer*. November 2008;113:2478.
94. Warren R, Liu G. ZD4054: a specific endothelin A receptor antagonist with promising activity in metastatic castration-resistant prostate cancer. *Expert Opin Investig Drugs*. August 2008;17:1237.
95. James ND, Caty A, Payne H, et al. Final safety and efficacy analysis of the specific endothelin A receptor antagonist zibotentan (ZD4054) in patients with metastatic castration-resistant prostate cancer and bone metastases who were pain-free or mildly symptomatic for pain: a double-blind, placebo-controlled, randomized phase II trial. *BJU Int*. October 2010;106:966.
96. AstraZeneca halts phase III trial of ZIBOTENTAN in nonmetastatic castrate resistant prostate cancer. http://www.astrazeneca.com/Media/Press-releases/Article/0022011AstraZeneca-halts-phase-III-trial-of-ZIBOTENTAN. Accessed December 20, 2011.
97. Zhang S, Zhau HE, Osunkoya AO, et al. Vascular endothelial growth factor regulates myeloid cell leukemia-1 expression through neuropilin-1-dependent activation of c-MET signaling in human prostate cancer cells. *Mol Cancer*. 2010;9:9.
98. Hussain M, Smith MR, Sweeney CP, et al. Cabozantinib (XL184) in metastatic castration-resistant prostate cancer (mCRPC): results from a phase II randomized discontinuation trial. *J Clin Oncol*. 2011;29(suppl). Abstract 4516.
99. de Bono JS, Scher HI, Montgomery RB, et al. Circulating tumor cells predict survival benefit from treatment in metastatic castration-resistant prostate cancer. *Clin Cancer Res*. October 2008;14:6302.

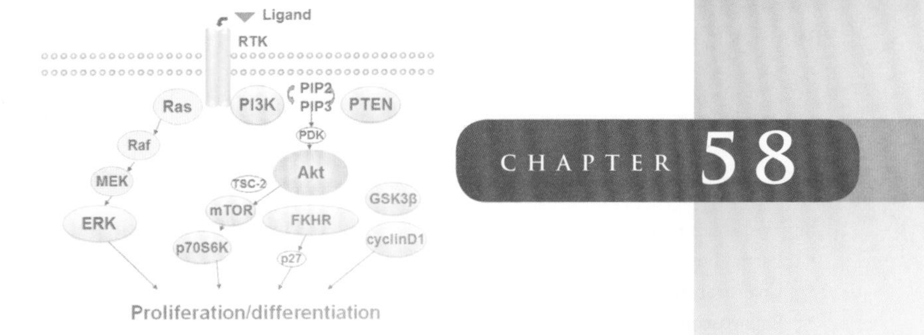

CHAPTER 58

Personalized Medicine and Targeted Therapy of Hepatocellular Carcinoma

Jiang Hongchi, John W. Linford, and Ahmed O. Kaseb

INTRODUCTION

Liver cancer is the fifth most frequently diagnosed cancer in men and the third most frequent cause of cancer death in men worldwide. In 2008, 748,300 new liver cancer cases were diagnosed worldwide, and 695,900 liver cancer–related deaths occurred worldwide; half these cases and deaths were estimated to occur in China.[1] Liver cancer can be classified as primary or metastatic. Hepatocellular carcinoma (HCC) is the most common type of primary liver cancer and accounts for more than 85% of liver cancer cases worldwide. Globally, HCC *incidence* rates are two to eight times *higher* in men than in women in both low- and high-incidence areas. In the United States and Europe, chronic hepatitis C virus infection is the main risk factor for HCC, whereas in Asia and Africa, chronic hepatitis B virus infection is the leading risk factor and might be further enhanced by exposure to aflatoxin B1. In the majority of patients (95% in the West and 60% in Asian countries), HCC results from preexisting liver cirrhosis, which markedly increases the risk of HCC.

In general, the major treatment options for HCC can be categorized as shown in Table 58.1. The treatment plan is usually complex and individualized, which often necessitates the involvement of hepatologists, transplant surgeons, pathologists, medical oncologists, surgical oncologists, cross-sectional radiologists, interventional radiologists, and pathologists, thereby necessitating careful coordination of care.

Several prognostic staging systems have been proposed for HCC, including the Okuda system, the American Joint Commission on Cancer tumor-lymph node-metastasis system, the Cancer of the Liver Italian Program system, the Barcelona Clinic Liver Cancer (BCLC) system, the Chinese University Prognostic Index, the Japanese Integrated Staging system, and the Groupe d'Etude de Traitement du Carcinome Hepatocellulaire system. Recently, there has been much debate regarding which of the existing staging systems for HCC is the best. Results from recent studies have shown that the BCLC staging system, which has been repeatedly validated, provides the best prognostic stratification when compared with other staging systems.[2]

The BCLC staging system was suggested in 1999 as a modification of the Okuda system. According to the BCLC staging system, HCC can be classified into five stages on the basis of tumor-related parameters (i.e., tumor size, number of involved lymph nodes, and vascular invasion), the patient's clinical condition (i.e., Eastern Cooperative Oncology Group performance status), and liver function (i.e., Child-Pugh classification). This information forms the framework for categorizing HCC into very early, early, intermediate, advanced, and terminal (0, A, B, C, and D, respectively) stages. In addition to its use in prognosis, the BCLC concept directly links the stage of disease to respective treatment strategies and was recently updated on the basis of data from patients with advanced disease,[3] as shown in Figure 58.1. It has been endorsed by the American Association for the Study of Liver Diseases (AASLD) and the European Association for the Study of the Liver as a criterion for making decisions in the routine clinical setting. However, the debate persists over which staging system to use, where different centers rely on different staging systems on the basis of the type of practice, patient demographics, underlying causes of liver disease, and proportions of patients

TABLE 58–1 Treatment Options for Hepatocellular Carcinoma

Surgical treatment
- Partial hepatectomy
- Liver transplantation
- Laparoscopic hepatectomy

Ablation techniques
- Percutaneous ethanol injection
- Radiofrequency ablation

Transarterial therapies
- Embolization
- Chemoembolization
- Radioembolization

External beam radiation therapy
- Three-dimensional conformal radiotherapy
- Stereotactic radiotherapy
- Proton and heavy ion radiotherapy

Systemic therapies
- Chemotherapy
- Hormonal therapy
- Immunotherapy
- Targeted therapy

Multimodality approaches

with cirrhosis differing by country. Further studies on the variable predictive value of staging systems, adjusted for the applied therapy, are required to determine the most accurate staging system.

SURGICAL TREATMENT

Partial Hepatectomy

For patients with early-stage HCC, partial hepatectomy is a potentially curative therapy.[4] Recently, partial hepatectomy for selected patients with HCC was shown to result in low-operative morbidity and mortality rates of <5%.[5] Two decades ago, long-term survival was seldom achieved via partial hepatectomy. More recently, however, several retrospective studies have indicated that 5-year survival rates of patients who undergo partial hepatectomy for HCC can exceed 50%,[6] and some studies have shown that in selected patients with early-stage HCC and preserved liver function, partial hepatectomy can result in a 5-year survival rate as high as 70%.[7] The increased long-term survival rates can be attributed to the following major advances: diagnosis of asymptomatic HCC and more accurate staging have facilitated the identification of patients with early-stage disease; meanwhile, more accurate evaluation of underlying liver function has resulted in the exclusion of patients in whom resection would likely cause higher rates of postoperative complications and mortality.

In recent years, surgeons have also refined the selection criteria for partial hepatectomy candidates. In general, tumor-related and patient-dependent factors and institutional experience should be considered before partial hepatectomy is performed. Tumor-related factors include tumor number, size, and location, extrahepatic disease, involvement of major vasculature, and the extent of

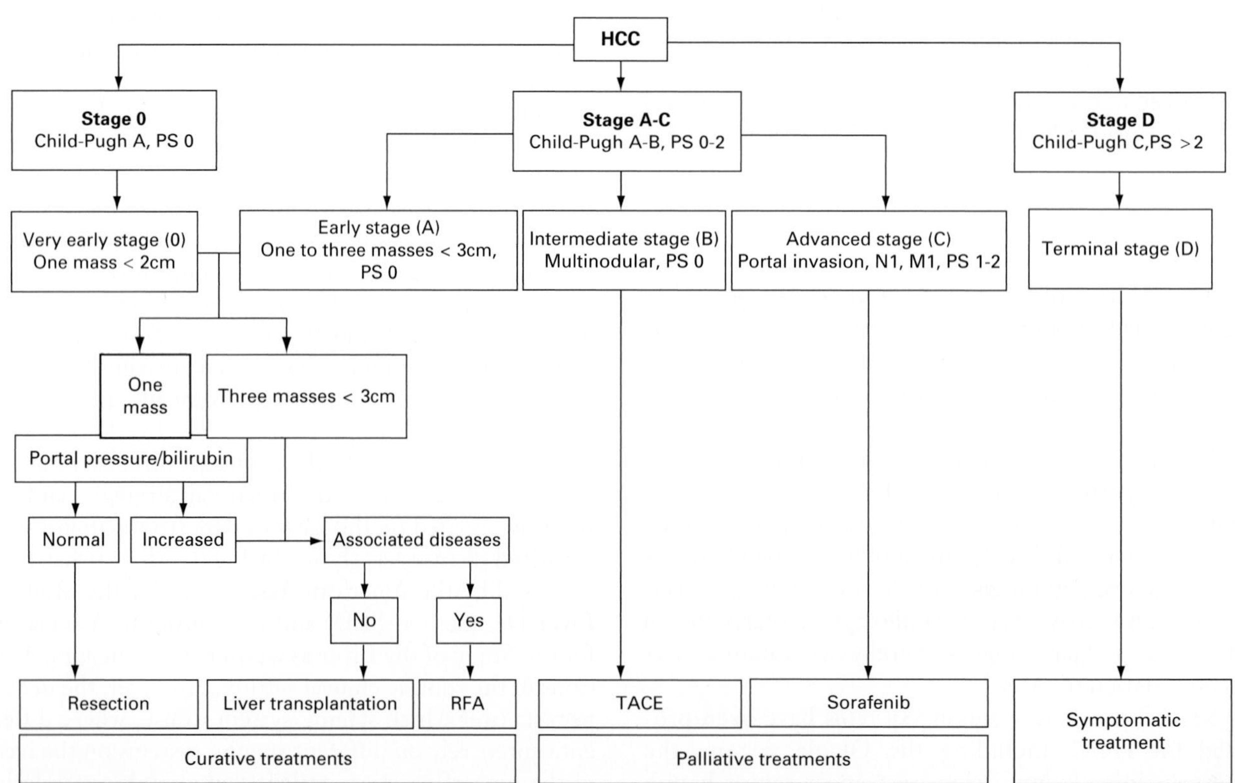

FIGURE 58–1 The BCLC staging system and management of HCC. M, metastasis classification; N, node classification; PS, performance status; RFA, radiofrequency ablation; TACE, transarterial chemoembolization.

resection required to achieve R0; patient-dependent factors include physical condition, liver function, and comorbid conditions. For years, the selection of candidates for partial hepatectomy has been based on the Child-Pugh classification system. However, some patients with Child-Pugh A liver function may already have advanced liver disease, with increased bilirubin levels, significant portal hypertension, or even minor fluid retention requiring diuretic therapy, all of which precludes partial hepatectomy.[8] Thus, a recent study has suggested that the Child-Pugh system is more useful for identifying patients with decompensated liver disease—in other words, for ruling out patients for partial hepatectomy.[9]

According to the BCLC staging system, hepatectomy is restricted to patients with a single HCC mass less than 2 cm and well-preserved liver function (i.e., Child-Pugh A), without clinical evidence of portal hypertension or increased bilirubin levels. Resections in such patients are associated with almost no risk of posthepatectomy liver failure and excellent long-term survival rates.[7] However, a prospective analysis showed acceptable outcomes for patients with BCLC stage B and C disease.[10] Extrahepatic disease and invasion of the portal vein trunk, inferior vena cava, and common hepatic artery are common contraindications to surgical resection; however, tumor size and number do not determine the success of resection. Large but solitary HCC tumors may be resected with good prognosis,[11] and resection can result in survival benefits even for patients with multiple tumors.[6]

In Europe and the United States, an evaluation of significant portal hypertension via clinical examination or hepatic vein catheterization is considered a key part of the presurgical assessment. Studies have indicated that a normal bilirubin concentration in the absence of significant portal hypertension is the best predictor of an excellent outcome after surgery, with almost no risk of postoperative liver failure. Such patients do not have liver decompensation after partial hepatectomy and may achieve a 5-year survival rate of more than 70%.[7] In contrast, other studies have shown that the majority of patients with significant portal hypertension develop postoperative decompensation and have a 5-year survival rate of <50%. The 5-year survival rate of patients with both significant portal hypertension and elevated bilirubin levels and/or multifocal disease is <30%, regardless of their Child-Pugh classification.[6] Nevertheless, other studies have shown that portal hypertension is not an absolute contraindication to resection in patients with HCC and cirrhosis. Using a standardized protocol with preoperative treatment of varices and ascites, extent of resection guided by indocyanine green retention rate at 15 minutes, and aggressive treatment of recurrence, one study reported a 5-year overall survival rate of 60% in 434 patients with HCC and Child-Pugh A liver function who had multiple tumors and/or portal hypertension.[6] An analysis of 241 patients with cirrhosis and HCC indicated similar perioperative outcomes and survival rates in patients with and without portal hypertension who had similar preoperative liver function and intraoperative courses.[12]

Partial hepatectomy for HCC is classified as anatomic or nonanatomic resection. Anatomic resection is the removal of segments of the liver on the basis of segmental anatomy, and nonanatomic resection is the removal of the tumor using negative pathologic margins, as shown in Figure 58.2. Improved preoperative imaging studies, routine use of intraoperative ultrasonography, a thorough understanding of the vascular and segmental anatomy of the liver, the application of new surgical instruments and technology, and improved perioperative anesthesia management have resulted in an increase in the number of patients who successfully undergo hepatic resection. A fundamental understanding of hepatic anatomy is vital for any surgeon to perform hepatic surgery. Mastery of the operative steps, coupled with an understanding of liver anatomy and the common variants thereof, is the foundation for safe hepatic surgery.

Because of so much overlap among the designations for hepatic lobes, sections, sectors, and segments used worldwide, new guidelines for this terminology based on the anatomic descriptions of Couinaud were established in 2000 in Brisbane at the consensus conference of the

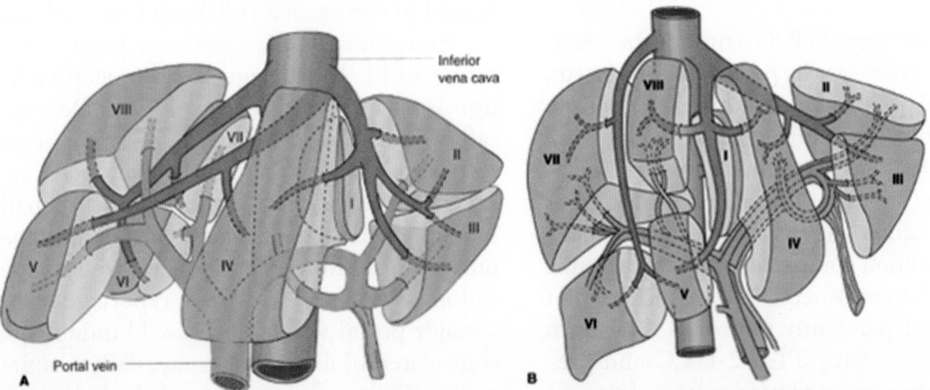

FIGURE 58–2 Segmental anatomy of the liver according to Couinaud's nomenclature as seen at laparotomy in the anatomic position (A) and in the ex vivo position (B). (From Schulick RD. Hepatobiliary anatomy. In: Mulholland MW, Lillemoe KD, Doherty GM, eds. *Greenfield's Surgery: Scientific Principles and Practice*. 4th ed. Baltimore, MD: Lippincott Williams & Wilkins; 2006:893-910.).

TABLE 58-2 Selected Clinical Trials of Systemic Targeted Therapies in Patients with Advanced Hepatocellular Carcinoma

Study	Regimen	Phase	Sample Size	Response Rate%	Median Survival (Months)
Abou-Alfa et al.[13]	Sorafenib	II	137	8	9.2
Llovet et al.[14]	Sorafenib	III	299	2	10.7
Cheng et al.[15]	Sorafenib	III	150	3.3	6.5
Philip et al.[16]	Erlotinib	II	38	7.8	13
Thomas et al.[17]	Erlotinib	II	40	0	6.25
Thomas et al.[18]	Bevacizumab + erlotinib	II	40	20.6	15.6 (PFS 9 mos)
Zhu et al.[19]	Everolimus	I/II	28	4	8.4
Sun et al.[20]	Capecitabine + oxaliplatin + bevacizumab	II	40	20	9.8
Zhu et al.[21]	GEMOX+ bevacizumab	II	33	20	9.6
Louafi et al.[22]	GEMOX + cetuximab	II	43	23	9.2
O'Neil et al.[23]	Capecitabine + oxaliplatin + cetuximab	II	25	11	TTP 4.3
Abou-Alfa et al.[24]	Doxorubicin + sorafenib vs. doxorubicin	II	47/49	4 vs. 2	13.8 vs. 6.5
Hsu et al.[25]	Capecitabine + bevacizumab	II	45	9	5.9

International Hepato-Pancreato-Biliary Association, as shown in Table 58.2.[26] According to these guidelines, the right liver comprises segments V through VIII, and "right hepatectomy" (right hemihepatectomy) is the appropriate term for resection of these segments. "Left hepatectomy" (left hemihepatectomy) is the appropriate term for resection of segments II through IV. A right hepatectomy can be extended farther to the left to include segment IV, and a left hepatectomy can be extended farther to the right to include segments V and VIII. "Extended right/left hepatectomy" and "right/left trisectionectomy" are appropriate terms for resection of these segments. Resection of segments II and III, which is a commonly performed sublobar resection, is referred to as a "left lateral sectionectomy." Resections of segments VI and VII or segments V are referred to as "right posterior sectionectomy" and "right anterior sectionectomy," respectively. Single-segment or bi-segmental resections can always be simply referred to by a numerical description of the segments to be resected.

Because of the propensity of HCC to invade the vascular invasion and metastasize via the portal venous system, studies have suggested performing anatomic resections in which the hepatic segments confined by tumor-bearing portal tributaries are removed to eradicate vascular invasion and intrahepatic metastases.[27] Results of studies conducted at various centers have shown a survival benefit with anatomic resection compared with nonanatomic resection of HCC.[28,29] A retrospective study showed that anatomic resection independently improved long-term survival rates in patients with T1–T2 HCC and presumed that this benefit was attributed to the clearance of venous tumor thrombi within the resected domain.[28] A review of 233 patients who underwent partial hepatectomy showed that anatomic resection diminished the early intrahepatic recurrence rate compared with non-anatomic resection.[29] Although anatomic resection for HCC is associated with improved survival, the extent of hepatectomy should be individualized on the basis of chronic liver damage and hepatic functional reserve.[30] Nonanatomic resection, during which the tumor is removed using negative pathologic margins, preserves the future liver remnant (FLR) for adequate postoperative hepatic function. However, the optimal width of the pathologic margin is unclear and controversial. A prospective randomized trial indicated that a wide resection margin (2 cm) led to a higher 5-year survival rate of 74.9%, compared with a narrow resection margin (1 cm). The benefit of a wide margin was more evident in small HCC tumors (2 cm or smaller), and all recurrences at the resection margins were observed in the narrow margin group.[31] Conversely, data from another study with 465 patients revealed no significant differences between the groups with wide and narrow surgical margins with regard to recurrence and overall survival rates.[32]

Since most HCC cases arise from cirrhosis, preservation of FLR for adequate postoperative hepatic function is an important consideration. Despite the overall safety of extended hepatectomy, complications related to postoperative liver insufficiency, such as coagulopathy, cholestasis, edema, and impaired hepatic synthetic function, persist and can often prolong recovery and hospitalization. Interest in preoperative portal vein embolization (PVE) increased upon reports that thrombosis of a major portal vein branch could induce ipsilateral and contralateral lobe hypertrophy. PVE was first described in the 1980s and was accomplished via a percutaneous, transhepatic route. PVE provides some patients with prohibitively small FLRs the opportunity for resection if they achieve an adequate hypertrophic response.[33] Many studies have confirmed that PVE is effective in inducing hypertrophy of nonembolized hepatic segments. PVE is often performed in the setting of a planned right or left trisectionectomy when the patient's FLR is thought to be too small to support liver function. In general, 4 weeks is needed to achieve an adequate hypertrophic response after PVE.

Advances in imaging techniques have enabled three-dimensional (3D) modeling of the liver with accurate FLR, estimation of the total liver volume, and visualization of the arterial and venous supply and biliary drainage. Liver volumetry is mostly performed using computer-assisted models of contrast-enhanced spiral computed tomography (CT), and the ratio of FLR/total liver volume is then determined. There is no universal agreement on an adequate FLR/total liver volume ratio for avoiding postoperative liver failure. Some studies have suggested that the ratio should be at least 20% in patients without cirrhosis and 30% to 40% in patients with a Child-Pugh A score.[34] In a recent study of 112 patients who underwent PVE, major and liver-related complications, the severity of hepatic dysfunction or insufficiency, the length of hospitalization, and 90-day mortality rates were significantly greater in patients whose FLR was 20% or less or whose degree of hypertrophy was less than 5% compared with patients with higher values.[35] A larger FLR may be necessary in patients who have received preoperative chemotherapy and in patients with fatty liver disease or with normal livers who are undergoing a complex hepatectomy. The combination of PVE and transarterial chemoembolization (TACE) has yielded encouraging results. Sequential TACE and PVE before surgery increased the rate of hypertrophy of the FLR and induced a high rate of complete tumor necrosis associated with longer recurrence-free survival.[36] PVE can also serve as a stress test of the regenerative capacity of the liver, and an inadequate hypertrophic response can be used to identify patients at risk for postoperative hepatic failure.

Liver Transplantation

Theoretically, liver transplantation is an ideal therapeutic option for patients with early-stage HCC.[37] The rationale supporting liver transplantation for HCC includes two aspects. On one hand, HCC tumors are commonly multifocal, and the extent of disease is often underestimated using current CT or magnetic resonance imaging (MRI). On the other hand, more than 80% of HCC cases arise in cirrhotic livers that do not have sufficient FLRs to tolerate formal resection.[38] Liver transplantation can be performed to remove both detectable and undetectable tumors and to treat underlying liver cirrhosis, making it an appealing option for patients with HCC. Five-year posttransplant survival rates have increased dramatically from only 20% to 50% in the 1990s[38] to 70% to 75% currently, according to the Organ Procurement and Transplantation Network/United Network for Organ Sharing database.

In 1996, Mazzaferro et al.[39] reported that survival rates were markedly improved when liver transplantation was restricted to a subgroup of patients with unresectable HCC who met specific selection criteria known as the Milan criteria (MC). The MC posited that excellent results could be achieved in patients with early-stage HCC, either solitary HCC that is 5 cm or smaller or up to three nodules with the largest being 3 cm or smaller, along with the absence of gross vascular invasion or extrahepatic spread.[39] The limited number of available organs for transplantation calls for strict selection criteria that include only patients with early-stage HCC, which means that some patients with slightly more advanced HCC who might also have acceptable survival after transplantation are excluded from the procedure.[40] This has incited controversies about whether and to what extent transplantation criteria for HCC can be expanded. Support for more liberal selection criteria is mainly twofold. First, with the development of imaging techniques, accumulating evidence shows varying degrees of understaging among original diagnoses ranging between 10% and 15%.[41] Second, because of the long waiting time for transplantation, there is a chance that HCC will progress beyond the listing criteria. However, for patients with disease beyond the standard listing criteria (i.e., MC) but with no macrovascular invasion or extrahepatic spread, survival duration after transplantation is comparable to that of patients within the MC. In patients who meet extended criteria and undergo transplantation, most groups report a 5-year survival rate of about 50%, which is the lowest rate acceptable by current standard.[42,43] Considering these results, there is definitely some room to expand the criteria.

In 2001, the University of California, San Francisco, was the first group to propose expanded criteria, and it reported excellent outcomes. According to the University of California, San Francisco, transplant candidates should have a single tumor that is 6.5 cm or smaller, a maximum of three tumors with the largest lesion being 4.5 cm or smaller, and a total tumor burden of 8 cm or less.[44] However, most groups adhere to the more restrictive criteria because of (1) the lack of donor organs, (2) an increased risk of recurrence, and (3) increased rates of tumor progression if patients with advanced disease are included. The shortage of available donor organs is the main limitation to liver transplantation and contributes to prolonged waiting time. Prolonged waiting time is associated with increased dropout rates owing mainly to tumor progression beyond that allowed with the current selection criteria. In an intention-to-treat analysis, a group from the University of California, San Francisco, showed that the implementation of expanded criteria resulted in a 25% dropout rate for 1 year and resulted in a survival rate of only 60% in patients who underwent transplantation.[45]

So far, the majority of studies evaluating expanded criteria have been developed using tumor size and number as the principal markers of tumor aggressiveness and recurrence risk. However, many alternative molecular parameters, such as the degree of differentiation,[46] the gene-expression profile,[47] and the identification of circulating cancer cells,[48] have recently been described. Genotype analysis can potentially further improve the prediction of tumor recurrence. The fractional allelic loss rate of a group of nine microsatellite markers that are located close to or within known tumor suppressor genes has been reported to have a higher predictive value of tumor recurrence than vascular invasion. There is no doubt that future models will incorporate other aspects of tumor biology as evaluation markers.

Since 2002, the Model for End-Stage Liver Disease (MELD) score has been adopted by the Organ Procurement and Transplantation Network/United Network for Organ Sharing to provide an estimate of the risk of death within 3 months for patients on the waiting list for cadaveric liver transplantation and to allocate deceased-donor livers in the United States. The MELD score is a 6- to 40-point scale based on serum total bilirubin levels, creatinine levels, and international normalized ratio. Although it accurately predicts early mortality in chronic viral or alcoholic liver disease, the MELD score cannot predict mortality in HCC. To ensure that patients with HCC have equal opportunities for transplantation, additional points known as "HCC MELD exception" are currently given to HCC patients: 22 points for solitary HCC 2 to 5 cm or 3 nodules each less than 3 cm.[49] In addition, a 10% point increase is given for every 3 months the patient has been on the waiting list. This revision has had a positive effect for HCC liver transplant candidates, as the waiting list dropout rate has decreased, and transplant rates have increased with excellent long-term outcomes. A recent consensus meeting claimed that, despite the exception, posttransplant survival rates in patients with HCC were not as high as that in patients without HCC who had equivalent MELD scores, because some fast progressing tumors were not detected.[50] Therefore, new criteria for allocation points have been proposed. A 3-month waiting time will be adopted in the future to allow for the detection of those fast progressing tumors and the exclusion of those patients from transplantation.

In addition to a priority policy, pretransplant locoregional therapies have been widely adopted by the liver transplant community. Their main function is to prevent disease progression while the candidate is on the waiting list and to prevent waiting list dropout. The most common modalities include TACE, radiofrequency ablation (RFA), and combinations of TACE and RFA.[51] TACE was performed by most groups because it reduces tumor burden and delays tumor progression. However, the possibility of inducing liver failure and death in patients with decompensated disease makes it incapable of being applied in all candidates. Some authors have suggested administering sorafenib as a bridging therapy because it has been shown to delay disease progression, but further data from randomized trials are required to evaluate this indication. Although there are no data from randomized control trials that indicate that pretransplant locoregional therapies[51] prevent dropout or reduce posttransplant tumor recurrence, statistical modeling has shown that such interventions are cost-effective if the expected waiting time is longer than 6 months.[52]

Because cadaveric donor organs are scarce, living-donor liver transplantation (LDLT) was introduced to expand the donor pool and reduce the dropout rate. After the first successful attempt, many studies have demonstrated that LDLT is an appropriate alternative for patients with HCC within the MC[53] and perhaps some patients beyond the MC. A study of 56 patients with HCC treated with LDLT showed that 15 of the 20 patients who did not meet the MC had a median recurrence-free survival duration of 12 months. Because those who had disease recurrence survived for a median of 20 months, the authors suggested applying different selection criteria for LDLT.[54] However, data supporting expanded criteria for LDLT are not yet sufficient. The main risks for LDLT recipients are dropout rate and expected survival, which are 4% per month and 70% at 5 years, respectively. The risks to the healthy live donor are the greatest disadvantage of LDLT. Based on an estimate of 14,000 LDLTs performed worldwide, the donor death rate is 0.1% to 0.3%.[55] Taking all these risks into account, LDLT is considered a cost-effective approach if the waiting time for a traditional transplant exceeds 7 months.[56]

Laparoscopic Hepatectomy

Laparoscopic hepatectomy was first introduced in 1991 for the treatment of benign liver tumors in gynecologic laparoscopic surgery. Since then, large series, meta-analyses, and reviews have illustrated the feasibility and safety of laparoscopic hepatic surgery for benign and malignant tumors, although no randomized controlled trial (RCT) has been reported to compare laparoscopic hepatectomy with open liver resection. An international review of 2,804 patients who underwent laparoscopic hepatic resections showed that both minor and major laparoscopic hepatic resections were safe and rendered acceptable morbidity and mortality rates and that 3- and 5-year survival rates in patients with HCC and colorectal cancer metastases were comparable to those achieved with open hepatic resection.[57] Over half of the 2,804 resections were performed for malignant tumors, 45% for benign lesions, and 2% for live donor hepatectomy. Of the resections, 75% were performed totally laparoscopically, 17% were performed using the hand-assisted approach (i.e., the operation is started laparoscopically to mobilize the liver and perform the initial hilar dissection, then the parenchymal transection is completed via a small open incision or slight extension of the hand-port incision),[58] 2% were performed using a laparoscopic-assisted open hepatic resection (hybrid) technique, and the remaining 5% were performed using other techniques or were converted to open hepatectomies.[57]

The first consensus meeting on laparoscopic liver surgery was held at the University of Louisville in 2008. This meeting resulted in the formulation of consensus statements on laparoscopic liver surgery that incorporated the opinions of international experts in laparoscopic and open liver surgery.[59] The consensus conference used the terms "pure laparoscopy," "hand-assisted laparoscopy," and "hybrid technique" to define laparoscopic liver surgery procedures. Currently acceptable indications for laparoscopic liver resection are solitary lesions that are 5 cm or smaller and located in liver segments 2 to 6. More advanced laparoscopic hepatic resections (e.g., right or left hepatectomies) should be reserved for experienced surgeons. The original wording seems somewhat redundant. For patient safety, laparoscopic hepatic resections should be converted to open surgery in cases that require extended operating time. In emergent situations, efforts should be made to control bleeding before converting to a formal open approach. Utilization of a hand-assisted approach or hybrid technique may be faster, safer, and more efficacious. Laparoscopic live donor hepatectomy remains the most controversial application of laparoscopic liver surgery and should only be carried out after the establishment of a worldwide registry.

The largest matched comparison of laparoscopic (n = 54) and open liver (n = 125) resection for HCC in patients with cirrhosis showed that short-term benefits were greater with laparoscopic liver resection than open liver resection, without compromising the long-term outcomes. Morbidity was significantly lower in the laparoscopic group, and the 3-year overall survival rates and disease-free survival rates of the two groups were not significantly different.[60] These results have been supported by data from other groups.[60,61] In addition, there were no significant differences in margin-free resections between laparoscopic and open liver resections.[62-64] Several studies have shown that blood loss is lower with laparoscopic resection than with open liver resection for HCC.[62-64] Postoperative pain control was also better in laparoscopic cases, as the duration of narcotic administration was shorter and the total amount of pain medication required was smaller.[65] Meanwhile, almost all the studies comparing laparoscopic with open liver resection have consistently shown that hospitalization is significantly shorter after laparoscopic liver resection. Laparoscopic liver resection for HCC has also been shown to facilitate subsequent liver transplantation. Patients who underwent prior laparoscopic liver resection had significantly fewer adhesions, shorter hepatectomy time, shorter total operating room time, lower blood loss, and less need for blood transfusion compared with the open surgery group.[66]

Ablation

Patients who are not medically eligible for resection or transplantation might be candidates for local ablative therapies. Some studies have shown that ablative therapy is most effective in smaller HCC tumors.[67] Destruction of tumor cells can be achieved by injecting chemical substances (e.g., ethanol and acetic acid) or by modifying the temperature at the targeted site (e.g., radiofrequency, microwave, laser, and cryotherapy). Although ablative therapies can be administered using percutaneous, laparoscopic, or open approaches, they are commonly performed percutaneously under ultrasound guidance, as shown in Figure 58.3. The two most commonly used approaches to ablation therapy are percutaneous ethanol injection (PEI) and RFA.

PEI works in two ways: (1) as it diffuses into the neoplastic cells, it leads to coagulation necrosis and causes immediate dehydration of the cytoplasm, and (2) ethanol induces endothelial cell necrosis and platelet aggregation, resulting in small-vessel thrombosis with subsequent ischemia of the tumor tissue. The complete rate of necrosis caused by PEI is 90% to 100% in HCC smaller than

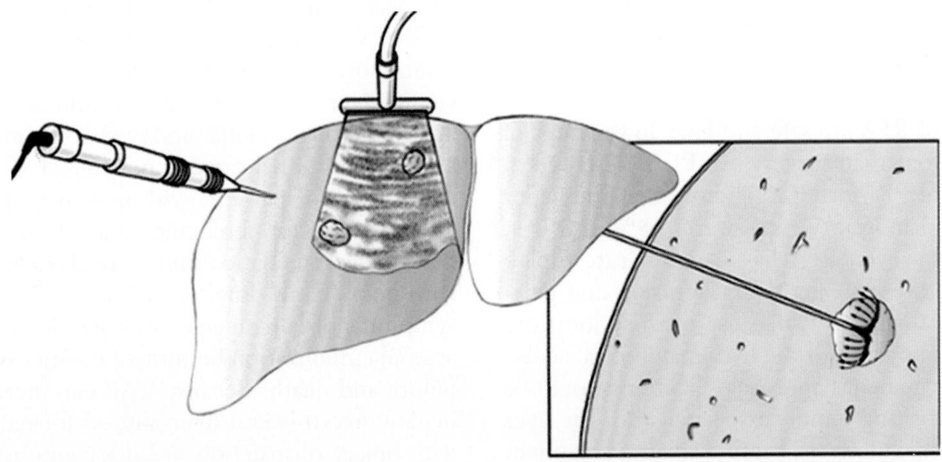

FIGURE 58–3 Technique for ablation. Under ultrasound guidance, the probe is inserted into a lesion and ablation is performed.

2 cm, but is reduced to 70% in tumors between 2 and 3 cm and to 50% in tumors that are 3 to 5 cm.[68] Long term study has shown that patients with Child-Pugh A liver function and complete tumor necrosis may achieve a 5-year survival rate of 42%.[69] To prevent patient drop-out, some centers use PEI to treat small HCC tumors as a bridge to liver transplantation.[70] However, PEI therapy must be administered in repeated injections on separate days and rarely causes complete necrosis in tumors larger than 3 cm. The presence of intratumoral septa impedes the diffusion of the injected ethanol to the entire tumor volume. Some researchers maintain that PEI for large HCC tumors should be facilitated by arterial embolization.

RFA induces a thermal injury to the target tissue by transformation of electromagnetic energy into thermal energy. Single or multiple cooled-tip electrodes or single electrodes with a J-hooked needle delivering heat around the tip are used to induce tumor necrosis in a wide region. The efficacy of RFA in tumors 2 cm or smaller is similar to that of ethanol, whereas in tumors larger than 2 cm, the efficacy of RFA is greater.[71] In addition, fewer treatment sessions are required for RFA than for PEI. According to the BCLC staging system, patients with very early-stage (0) disease and early-stage (A) disease with contraindications for surgery are candidates for RFA.[3]

The technical effectiveness of ablation is commonly assessed using findings on contrast-enhanced CT or MRI 1 month after the completion of therapy. If there are no longer any enhanced regions within the entire tumor during the arterial phase and at least a 0.5 cm margin of apparently normal hepatic tissue surrounding the tumor during the portal phase, the tumor is considered to be successfully ablated.[72] Reported rates of overall survival vary widely across studies of patients with HCC treated with ablation. This likely reflects differences in specific disease characteristics, such as the size and number of tumors. In a prospective study of 50 patients with HCC who underwent RFA while waiting for liver transplantation, the rate of complete tumor necrosis was 55% overall and 63% when only tumors 3 cm or smaller were considered.[73] Therefore, tumor size is a critical factor for determining the effectiveness of ablation therapy for HCC.

Both PEI and RFA are safe and have lower rates of major complications than surgery. An RCT designed to compare RFA and PEI for HCC showed that the major complication and mortality rates were 4.8% and 0%, respectively.[74] However, RFA has a higher rate (up to 10%) of adverse events (e.g., pleural effusion and peritoneal bleeding) than PEI.[75] Because of their location, lesions in certain portions of the liver may not be accessible using a percutaneous approach. Caution should be exercised when treating tumors associated with the liver capsule and near major vessels, because ablative treatment may lead to organ rupture or the exposure of organ to large amounts of heat.

Percutaneous local ablation in patients who are eligible for resection remains controversial. Several RCTs of early-stage HCC have reported equivalent outcomes after surgical resection and local ablation[76,77]; however, because of sample size limitations and the inclusion of a mixture of candidates with various stages of disease, the data showing similar oncological outcomes for the two options do not provide sufficient evidence to draw final conclusions about the value of local ablation as first-line treatment for early-stage HCC. Additional trials of HCC that account for liver function and disease stage and etiology are needed. The combination of resection and RFA has been suggested for patients with multifocal HCC and preserved liver function and may be a valuable option for patients who are not eligible for liver transplantation.

Transarterial Therapies

Transarterial therapy is administered for HCC on the basis of the fact that most of the blood supply to the tumor comes from the hepatic artery, whereas the majority of the blood supply to normal liver tissue comes from the portal vein. In very early-stage disease, blood supply to the tumor comes from the portal vein, and as the tumor grows and progresses, the blood supply progressively comes from the hepatic artery. Transarterial therapy targets the branch of the hepatic artery feeding the portion of the liver in which the tumor is located via selective catheter-based infusion of particles. The three common transarterial therapies are transarterial embolization (TAE), TACE, and transarterial radioembolization.

TAE is performed to obstruct the hepatic artery supplying the tumor during an angiographic procedure, resulting in tumor ischemia followed by tumor necrosis. Gelatin sponge particles, polyvinyl alcohol particles, polyacrylamide microspheres, metallic coils, and even autologous blood clots have been used as emulsifying agents to block arterial flow. When TAE is combined with the prior injection into the hepatic artery of a concentrated dose of chemotherapeutic agents (e.g., doxorubicin and cisplatin), usually mixed with lipiodol, the procedure is known as TACE. To induce minimal injury to the surrounding nontumorous hepatic parenchyma, the procedure necessitates the advancement of the catheter into the hepatic artery and then to lobar and segmental branches, with the aim of being as selective as possible. TAE and TACE are considered for patients with nonsurgical HCC who are also ineligible for percutaneous ablation and have no evidence of extrahepatic tumor spread. In addition, patients with poor (Child-Pugh C) liver function and/or clinical symptoms of end-stage cancer should be excluded from arterial embolization because of the increased risk of liver failure and death. Because TAE can increase the risk of hepatic necrosis and liver abscess formation in patients with biliary obstruction or biliary enteric bypass, a total bilirubin level of <3 mg/mL should be considered as a relative contraindication.[78]

Both TAE and TACE can induce tumor necrosis in more than 50% of treated patients,[79] although fewer than 2% of treated patients achieve a complete response (CR). Besides the reduction in overall tumor size, decreased concentrations of tumor markers and the identification of large intratumoral necrotic areas on dynamic CT or MRI are used to evaluate treatment response. RCTs have indicated that TACE yields a survival benefit in patients with unresectable HCC compared with supportive care. One- and two-year survival rates in patients who received TAE, TACE, or supportive care were 82% and 63%, 75% and 50%, and 63% and 27%, respectively.[80] When clinical studies are designed to evaluate the effectiveness of TAE or TACE, the authors are frequently confounded by a wide range of factors, including the type of embolic particles infused, the type of chemotherapy administered, the type of emulsifying agent used, and the number of treatment sessions scheduled. Thus, robust evidence is urgently needed to determine the best obstructing agents, the optimal chemotherapeutic agents, and the most effective retreatment schedule.

The common complications of TAE and TACE include acute portal vein thrombosis, cholecystitis, bone marrow suppression, and other toxic effects.[81] A postembolization syndrome involving fever, abdominal pain, and a moderate degree of intestinal ileus is associated with acute ischemia induced by hepatic artery obstruction and appears in more than 50% of patients who undergo TAE or TACE. The syndrome is usually self-limited in less than 48 hours. Fasting is required for 24 hours, and prophylactic antibiotics are not routinely used.[81] Fever is induced by tumor necrosis, and only a small proportion of patients develop severe infection such as hepatic abscess or cholecystitis. Reported TAE- and TACE-related mortality rates are <5%.[81]

HCC has traditionally been regarded as a radioresistant tumor because of the limited ability to deliver lethal doses of radiation using external beam techniques and the damage to normal liver parenchyma and surrounding organs. Transarterial radioembolization with yttrium-90 (an emitter of β-radiation) microspheres is a new concept in radiation therapy for HCC. Radiolabeled particles are injected via the hepatic artery, trapped at the precapillary level, and emit lethal internal radiation to the tumor. This mechanism limits exposure to the surrounding normal parenchyma and provides higher dose radiation than external beam radiotherapy.[82] A single-center, prospective, longitudinal cohort study including 291 patients showed a survival benefit of transarterial radioembolization.[83] In this study, the response rate was 42%, which is similar to that reported in another phase II study.[84] The median survival times of patients with Child-Pugh A and B liver function were 17.2 and 7.7 months, respectively. Patients with Child-Pugh B liver function who had portal vein thrombosis had poor outcomes, and the median survival time in this group was 5.6 months.[83] Toxic effects associated with radioembolization included fatigue, pain, nausea, vomiting, and bilirubin toxicity.[83,84] Robust evidence of the efficiency of radioembolization in HCC is lacking and more RCTs are needed.

External Beam Radiotherapy

Because the radiation dose required for controlling local tumor exceeds the radiation tolerance of the whole-liver and some other surrounding organs, large-volume or whole-liver radiotherapy results in high rates of radiation-induced liver disease and poor tumor response rates. Therefore, the role of external beam radiotherapy for HCC has traditionally been limited. Recently, developments in radiotherapy techniques, including 3D-CRT, stereotactic radiotherapy (SRT), and proton and heavy ion radiotherapy, have allowed the focal administration of higher doses of radiation to HCC tumors while sparing surrounding liver parenchyma.[85]

Three-dimensional CRT is a delivery method that incorporates rigid immobilization and 3D computer planning and treatment systems to produce a high-dose area of radiation that conforms to the shape of the target. Some studies have shown the feasibility and efficacy of high-dose 3D-CRT in cirrhotic patients with small HCC and patients with portal venous invasion.[86,87] SRT has been used to deliver highly conformal radiation in high doses to HCC tumors by employing immobilization and stereotactic localization. Using SRT, high doses can be delivered with minimal exposure to surrounding liver tissues, thereby minimizing normal liver damage, when compared with conventional radiotherapy and even 3D-CRT. A prospective study including 31 patients with small and large HCC tumors and Child-Pugh A liver function suggested that six-fraction SRT is safe for unresectable HCC.[88] The ability of SRT to provide local control without serious toxic side effects has also been indicated in several other studies. Protons and heavy ions are heavier than electrons, and their positive charge and unique dose distribution render them favorable for the treatment of deep-seated HCC surrounded by normal liver tissues. A prospective study including 24 patients with HCC and Child-Pugh A or B liver function was designed to evaluate the toxic and antitumor effects of carbon ion radiotherapy for HCC. In this study, no severe adverse effects and no treatment-related deaths were reported, and the overall tumor response rate was 71%.[89] Actuarial data from a phase II trial revealed a 2-year survival rate of 55% and a local tumor control rate of 75% in 34 patients with unresectable HCC who received proton therapy.[90]

New radiotherapy techniques and fractionation schedules make radiotherapy a safer and more effective option for the palliative treatment of HCC. Although several trials have reported excellent local HCC control with sufficient radiation doses, high-quality evidence from RCTs is still needed to support these findings before any of the various modalities of external beam radiotherapy can be included in standard treatment algorithms for HCC.

SYSTEMIC CHEMOTHERAPY

As HCC is often beyond surgical therapy at presentation, systemic therapy is required, and the systemic treatment of HCC is complicated by the variable biologic behavior and morphology of the malignancy and by the likely coexisting chronic liver disease with cirrhosis.

Efforts to treat advanced HCC with systemic chemotherapy have been unsatisfactory. Systemic therapies have primarily used the cytotoxic agent adriamycin as the backbone of treatment regimens, and disease-free survival and overall survival have remained poor, demonstrating a limited impact on the natural history of advanced HCC. Single-agent adriamycin showed an 8.3% response rate and median survival duration of only 10.6 weeks.[91] A randomized phase III study comparing adriamycin with combination chemotherapy consisting of cisplatin, interferon-alpha, doxorubicin, and 5-fluorouracil (PIAF) found a response rate of 20.9% in the PIAF arm. However, the study did not demonstrate a significant difference in overall survival duration, with only 8.67 months in the PIAF arm compared with 6.83 months in the adriamycin arm ($P = 0.83$).[92]

In 1997, a meta-analysis of 37 randomized clinical trials of systemic and regional chemotherapy in 2803 HCC patients concluded that nonsurgical therapies were either ineffective or minimally effective.[93] As a result of these poor outcomes, HCC became regarded as refractory to chemotherapy. Subsequently, molecular characterization of HCC identified aberrant signaling pathways and led to the development of targeted agents as potential therapeutic choices for this chemotherapy-resistant disease; see Table 58.2.

SELECTED MOLECULAR THERAPEUTIC TARGETS IN HCC

The Ras/Raf/mitogen-activated protein kinase (MAPK) kinase (Mek)/extracellular signal-regulated kinase (Erk) pathway, phosphoinositide-3 kinase (PI3K)/protein kinase B (Akt)/mammalian target of rapamycin (mTOR) pathway, epidermal growth factor receptor, platelet-derived growth factor receptor (PDGFR), fibroblast growth factor receptor, and vascular endothelial growth factor receptor (VEGFR) have been recognized as crucial intracellular signaling pathways in HCC. These pathways result in the proliferation, survival, migration, and metastasis of tumor cells. The identification of these pathways has enabled the development of targeted agents (used alone or in combination) as potential treatments for HCC.

Efforts to develop effective molecular targets for HCC therapy involve targeting both the extracellular growth factors and the intracellular signaling pathways; see Figure 58.4. To date, targeting of antiangiogenic pathways carried significant promise given the significance of this pathway in HCC carcinogenesis. In fact, the

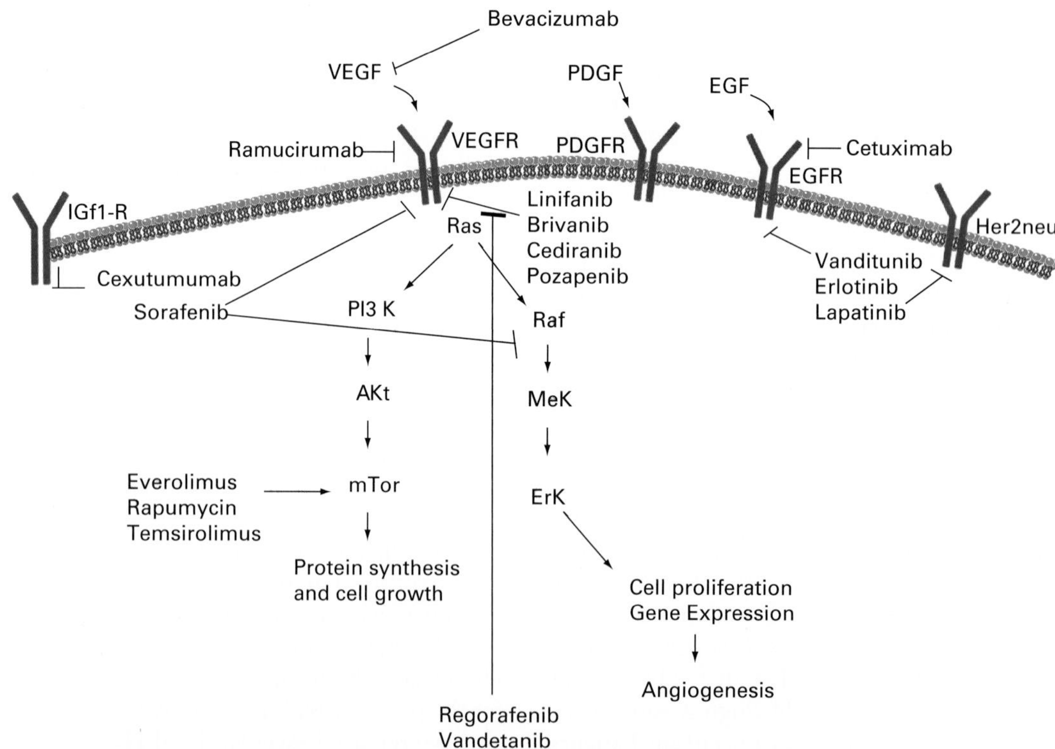

FIGURE 58–4 Select relevant pathways in HCC pathogenesis. EGFR, epidermal growth factor receptor; EGF, epidermal growth factor; VEGF, vascular endothelial growth factor; VEGFR, vascular endothelial growth factor receptor; Her2neu, human epidermal growth factor-2; IGF1-R, insulin-like growth factor 1 receptor; PI3K, phosphoinositide 3 kinase; mTor, mammalian target of rapamycin; Mek, mitogen-activated protein kinase kinase; Erk, extracellular signal-regulated kinase.

hypervascularity of HCC on imaging scans is pathognomonic for HCC diagnosis, even in the absence of pathology confirmation according to the AASLD guidelines.[94]

Ras/Raf/Mek/Erk Pathway

The MAPK pathway includes a cascade of phosphorylation of four major cellular kinases: Ras, Raf, Mek, and Erk. These intermediates are found in high levels in both HCC cell lines and human tissue specimens.[13,95-98] The activation of the MAPK pathway results in increased cellular differentiation and proliferation. Thus, this pathway and its intermediates are viable targets for HCC therapy.

Sorafenib, an Raf kinase inhibitor, has undergone phase I, II, and III trials in patients with advanced HCC. In addition to targeting Raf, sorafenib also targets VEGFR. The initial phase II trial of sorafenib reported a response rate of 2.2%. Despite that, 33.6% of patients were found to have stable disease (SD) for at least 4 months. During the trial, central tumor necrosis was noted in many of the tumors.[13]

This phase II trial reported an overall survival of 9.2 months and led to a placebo-controlled phase III international trial in HCC patients with Child-Pugh A cirrhosis. The median overall survival duration in the sorafenib arm was 10.7 months compared with 7.9 months in the placebo arm, thus demonstrating a 2.8-month improvement in overall survival (HR: 0.69; 95% CI: 0.55 to 0.87; $P = 0.0006$).[14,99,100]

Subsequently, in 2007, the oral anticancer agent sorafenib (Nexavar) was approved for use in both the United States and the European Union to treat patients with HCC. This represented a significant step forward in providing targeted therapy for patients with advanced HCC; see Table 58.2.

Additional studies of sorafenib in conjunction with other treatments are ongoing. Additional studies assessing sorafenib in conjunction with locoregional therapies, specifically TACE, have demonstrated the relative safety of combined antiangiogenic therapy and regional interventions.[101] Notably, in addition to targets in the Ras/Raf/MEK/ERK pathway at the level of the Raf kinase, sorafenib also exhibits antiangiogenic activity by targeting VEGFR and PDGFR tyrosine kinases.

PI3K/AKT/mTOR Pathway

PI3K has also been found to be upregulated in a subset of HCC patients.[102] The action of PI3K leads to the activation of AKT and the phosphorylation and inactivation of pro-apoptotic proteins. The downstream events are responsible for proliferation and apoptosis linked to the cell cycle.[103,104] The inactivation of these pro-apoptotic proteins leads to unregulated cell cycle activity. In addition, mTOR is downstream of AKT and regulates cellular translational activities. Rapamycin, an antibiotic that inhibits mTOR, has been shown to have activity against HCC cell lines[105,106] and is currently being evaluated in a post-liver transplantation setting since it also possesses immunosuppressant activity.

Epigenetic Changes

Epigenetic modifications occur during the process of hepatic carcinogenesis. Hypermethylation and histone deacetylation accumulate during chronic injury of the liver and lead to the inactivation of several tumor suppressor genes in HCC. Epigenetic therapy has been applied in the treatment of hematologic malignancies and solid tumors, and use of epigenetic therapy has been shown to cause chemosensitization in HCC cell lines.[107,108] Preclinical activity of the histone deacetylase inhibitor PXD101 (belinostat) was found to inhibit cell growth in HCC cell lines in a dose-dependent manner and led to apoptosis.[109] In a phase I trial of belinostat, 12 HCC patients were enrolled and maximum tolerated dose was not reached. A phase II trial was subsequently initiated.[110]

Rationale for Antiangiogenic Therapy in HCC

In 1999, assessment of hyperplastic hepatic nodules and varying stages of HCC led to the suggestion that tissue-level VEGF expression increased with the progressive development of HCC. Evidence of increased angiogenesis and unpaired artery formation was also observed.[111]

Further evaluation of serum levels of VEGF in HCC demonstrated that VEGF is frequently expressed in HCC, and quantitative analysis showed significant increased expression in patients with HCC compared with control patients and patients with benign liver lesions.[112,113] Another study reported VEGF tissue expression in 88.8% of HCC tumors assessed by immunohistochemistry.[113]

Pathologic correlation between increased VEGF expression and HCC development led to efforts to identify a correlation between VEGF expression and arterial enhancement on imaging studies. Studies have suggested that the intensity of both the MRI signal and the CT enhancement correlates with the level of VEGF tissue expression in HCC. Subsequently, this correlation between VEGF expression and tumor vascularity has elicited substantial interest in antiangiogenic therapy in HCC.[114-116]

Antiangiogenic Agents in HCC

Bevacizumab

Bevacizumab became a logical choice for study in the treatment of HCC because of the correlation between VEGF and HCC development. Bevacizumab is a recombinant humanized monoclonal antibody that targets circulating VEGF and has been assessed in phase II trials in patients with advanced HCC. One of these studies reported a response rate of 13% and a 6-month progression-free survival (PFS) rate of 65%.[117] In another phase II trial in patients with advanced HCC, bevacizumab was combined with gemcitabine and oxaliplatin and resulted in an overall response rate of 20%.[21]

A phase II trial of bevacizumab combined with capecitabine as first-line therapy for advanced HCC reported a response rate (CR + partial response [PR]) of 16% (95% CI: 4.5% to 36.1%) and a disease control rate (CR + PR + SD) of 60% (95% CI: 38.7% to 78.9%) with a median overall survival of 10.7 months (95% CI: 5.3 to 14.7) and median PFS of 4.1 months.[118] Another phase II study of advanced or unresectable metastatic HCC treated 30 patients with the combination of bevacizumab, oxaliplatin, and capecitabine and reported an 11% response rate with mean PFS of 5.4 months.[119]

After preclinical studies, erlotinib and bevacizumab were combined in a phase II, single-arm, open-label trial. The primary end point was PFS at 16 weeks of continuous therapy. Forty patients were enrolled in the trial, and the primary end point of PFS at 16 weeks was achieved in 62.5% of patients. Median PFS was 39 weeks, and median overall survival was 68 weeks.[18,120,] An ongoing clinical trial is assessing this combination as second-line therapy for patients with advanced HCC who had received sorafenib treatment as a first-line therapy.

Additional ongoing trials are assessing different vascular-targeting agents. In addition, preclinical studies of agents that target other foci that interact with VEGF have shown promising results.[121,122] Minor or low response rates have also been identified in the use of thalidomide and megestrol in advanced HCC.[25,123-125]

Combination Systemic Therapy for HCC

Hepatocarcinogenesis is a complex process resulting in many heterogeneous molecular abnormalities.[126-129] Sorafenib, with its ability to target a variety of pathways, is a rational choice for therapy. Combination therapy will need to build off this baseline with rationally designed treatment regimens. Combination therapy should be based on preclinical data models. Additional efforts in identifying molecular targets and surrogate markers in HCC are necessary to provide methods for assessing clinical efficacy of combined agents.

Antiangiogenic therapy provides a unique base for combined therapy. Tumor neovessels differ from normal vasculature with their irregular and hyperpermeable nature. Irregular blood flow and increased interstitial pressure can impair the delivery of oxygen (a known radiation sensitizer) and drugs to cancer cells. It appears that antiangiogenic therapy normalizes tumor vasculature, resulting in improved delivery of cytotoxic agents. This may result in improved efficacy of cytotoxic agents.[15] This concept of combining antiangiogenic therapy with a cytotoxic agent is currently being assessed in HCC in a randomized trial comparing sorafenib with a combination of sorafenib and doxorubicin.

Finally, in treating patients with HCC, it is challenging to assess response to targeted therapy combinations. Currently, there are no validated biomarkers to utilize during treatment or in clinical trial. In addition, targeted therapies inhibit molecular components of cellular proliferation and angiogenesis, which is more likely to delay disease progression and to stabilize tumor size, rather than tumor shrinkage as an objective response. Therefore, additional efforts at validating surrogate response biomarkers and imaging end points are essential.

REFERENCES

1. Jemal A, Bray F, Center MM, et al. Global cancer statistics. *CA Cancer J Clin*. 2011;61:69-90.
2. Marrero JA, Fontana RJ, Barrat A, et al. Prognosis of hepatocellular carcinoma: comparison of 7 staging systems in an American cohort. *Hepatology*. 2005;41:707-716.
3. Bruix J, Sherman M; American Association for the Study of Liver Diseases. Management of hepatocellular carcinoma: an update. *Hepatology*. 2011;53:1020-1022.
4. Truty MJ, Vauthey JN. Surgical resection of high-risk hepatocellular carcinoma: patient selection, preoperative considerations, and operative technique. *Ann Surg Oncol*. 2010;17:1219-1225.
5. Chok KS, Ng KK, Poon RT, et al. Impact of postoperative complications on long-term outcome of curative resection for hepatocellular carcinoma. *Br J Surg*. 2009;96:81-87.
6. Ishizawa T, Hasegawa K, Aoki T, et al. Neither multiple tumors nor portal hypertension are surgical contraindications for hepatocellular carcinoma. *Gastroenterology*. 2008;134:1908-1916.
7. Llovet JM, Fuster J, Bruix J. Intention-to-treat analysis of surgical treatment for early hepatocellular carcinoma: resection versus transplantation. *Hepatology*. 1999;30(6):1434-1440.
8. D'Amico G, Garcia-Tsao G, Pagliaro L. Natural history and prognostic indicators of survival in cirrhosis: a systematic review of 118 studies. *J Hepatol*. 2006;44:217-231.
9. Ribero D, Curley SA, Imamura H, et al. Selection for resection of hepatocellular carcinoma and surgical strategy: indications for resection, evaluation of liver function, portal vein embolization, and resection. *Ann Surg Oncol*. 2008;15:986-992.
10. Torzilli G, Donadon M, Marconi M, et al. Hepatectomy for stage B and stage C hepatocellular carcinoma in the Barcelona Clinic Liver Cancer classification: results of a prospective analysis. *Arch Surg*. 2008;143:1082-1090.
11. Yang LY, Fang F, Ou DP, et al. Solitary large hepatocellular carcinoma: a specific subtype of hepatocellular carcinoma with good outcome after hepatic resection. *Ann Surg*. 2009;249:118-123.
12. Cucchetti A, Ercolani G, Vivarelli M, et al. Is portal hypertension a contraindication to hepatic resection? *Ann Surg*. 2009;250:922-928.
13. Abou-Alfa GK, Schwartz L, Ricci S, et al. Phase II study of sorafenib in patients with advanced hepatocellular carcinoma. *J Clin Oncol*. 2006;24:4293-4300.
14. Llovet J, Ricci S, Mazzaferro V, et al. Randomized phase III trial of sorafenib versus placebo in patients with advanced hepatocellular carcinoma (HCC) (SHARP Investigators Study Group). *J Clin Oncol*. 2007;25:LBA1.
15. Cheng AL, Kang YK, Guan Z. Efficacy and safety of sorafenib in patients in the Asia-Pacific region with advanced hepatocellular carcinoma: a phase III randomized, double-blind, placebo-controlled trial. *Lancet Oncol*. January 2009;10(1):25-34.
16. Philip PA, Mahoney MR, Allmer C, et al. Phase II study of erlotinib in patients with advanced hepatocellular cancer. *J Clin Oncol*. September 2005;23(27):6657-6663.
17. Thomas MB, Chandha R, Abrruzzes J. Phase 2 Study of erlotinib in patients with unresectable hepatocellular carcinoma. *Cancer*. 2007;110(5):1059-1067.
18. ThomasMB, Morris JS, Chadha R, et al. Phase II trial of the combination of bevacizumab and erlotinib in patients who have advanced hepatocellular carcinoma. *J Clin Oncol*. 2009;27:843-850.
19. Zhu AX, Abrams TA, Ryan DP. Phase 1/2 of everolimus in advanced hepatocellular carcinoma. *Cancer*. 2011;117(22):5094-5102.
20. Sun W, Haller DG, Mykulowycz K, et al. Phase 2 trial of bevacizumab, capecitabine, and oxaliplatin in treatment of advanced hepatocellular carcinoma. *Cancer*. 2011;117(14):3187-3192.

21. Zhu AX, Blaszkowsky LS, Ryan DP, et al. Phase II study of gemcitabine and oxaliplatin in combination with bevacizumab in patients with advanced hepatocellular carcinoma. *J Clin Oncol.* 2006;24:1898-1903.
22. Louafi S, Boige V, Ducreux M, et al. Gemcitabine plus oxaliplatin (GEMOX) in patients with advanced hepatocellular carcinoma (HCC): results of a phase II study. *Cancer.* 2007;109:1384-1390.
23. O'Neil BH, Bernard SA, Goldberg RM, et al. Phase II study of oxaliplatin, capecitabine, and cetuximab in advanced hepatocellular carcinoma. *J Clin Oncol.* 2008 Gastrointestinal Cancers Symposium, 2008, Abstract No. 228.
24. Abou-Alfa GK, Johnson P, Knox JJ, et al. Doxorubicin plus sorafenib vs doxorubicin alone in patients with advanced hepatocellular carcinoma. *JAMA.* 2010;304(19).
25. Villa E, Ferretti I, Grottola A, et al. Hormonal therapy with megestrol in inoperable hepatocellular carcinoma characterized by variant oestrogen receptors. *Br J Cancer.* 2001;84:881-885.
26. Terminology Committee of the International Hepato-Pancreato-Biliary Association: The Brisbane 2000 terminology of liver anatomy and resections. *HPB (Oxford).* 2000;2:333.
27. Hasegawa K, Kokudo N, Imamura H, et al. Prognostic impact of anatomic resection for hepatocellular carcinoma. *Ann Surg.* 2005;242:252-259.
28. Wakai T, Shirai Y, Sakata J, et al. Anatomic resection independently improves long-term survival in patients with T1-T2 hepatocellular carcinoma. *Ann Surg Oncol.* 2007;14:1356-1365.
29. Kobayashi A, Miyagawa S, Miwa S, et al. Prognostic impact of anatomical resection on early and late intrahepatic recurrence in patients with hepatocellular carcinoma. *J Hepatobiliary Pancreat Surg.* 2008;15:515-521.
30. Yamashita Y, Taketomi A, Itoh S, et al. Long term favorable results of limited hepatic resections for patients with hepatocellular carcinoma: 20 years of experience. *J Am Coll Surg.* 2007;205:19-26.
31. Shi M, Guo RP, Lin XJ, et al. Partial hepatectomy with wide versus narrow resection margin for solitary hepatocellular carcinoma: a prospective randomized trial. *Ann Surg.* 2007;245:36-43.
32. Matsui Y, Terakawa N, Satoi S, et al. Postoperative outcomes in patients with hepatocellular carcinomas resected with exposure of the tumor surface: clinical role of the no-margin resection. *Arch Surg.* 2007;142:596-603.
33. Nagino M, Kamiya J, Nishio H, et al. Two hundred forty consecutive portal vein embolizations before extended hepatectomy for biliary cancer: surgical outcome and long-term follow-up. *Ann Surg.* 2006;243:364-372.
34. Shoup M, Gonen M, D'Angelica M, et al. Volumetric analysis predicts hepatic dysfunction in patients undergoing major liver resection. *J Gastrointest Surg.* 2003;7:325-330.
35. Ribero D, Abdalla EK, Madoff DC, et al. Portal vein embolization before major hepatectomy and its effects on regeneration, resectability and outcome. *Br J Surg.* 2007;94:1386-1394.
36. Ogata S, Belghiti J, Farges O, et al. Sequential arterial and portal vein embolizations before right hepatectomy in patients with cirrhosis and hepatocellular carcinoma. *Br J Surg.* 2006;93:1091-1098.
37. Jarangin WR. Management of small hepatocellular carcinoma: a review of transplantation, resection, and ablation. *Ann Surg Oncol.* 2010;17:1226-1233.
38. Marsh JW, Geller DA, Finkelstein SD, et al. Role of liver transplantation for hepatobiliary malignant disorders. *Lancet Oncol.* 2004;5:480-488.
39. Mazzaferro V, Regalia E, Doci R, et al. Liver transplantation for the treatment of small hepatocellular carcinomas in patients with cirrhosis. *N Engl J Med.* 1996;334:693-699.
40. Mazzaferro V, Llovet JM, Miceli R, et al. Predicting survival after liver transplantation in patients with hepatocellular carcinoma beyond the Milan criteria: a retrospective, exploratory analysis. *Lancet Oncol.* 2009;10:35-43.
41. Burrel M, Llovet JM, Ayuso C, et al. MRI angiography is superior to helical CT for detection of HCC prior to liver transplantation: an explant correlation. *Hepatology.* 2003;38:1034-1042.
42. Roayaie S, Frischer JS, Emre SH, et al. Long-term results with multimodal adjuvant therapy and liver transplantation for the treatment of hepatocellular carcinomas larger than 5 centimeters. *Ann Surg.* 2002;235:533-539.
43. Neuberger J. Developments in liver transplantation. *Gut.* 2004;53:759-768.
44. Yao FY, Ferrell L, Bass NM, et al. Liver transplantation for hepatocellular carcinoma: expansion of the tumor size limits does not adversely impact survival. *Hepatology.* 2001;33:1394-1403.
45. Yao FY, Bass NM, Nikolai B, et al. Liver transplantation for hepatocellular carcinoma: analysis of survival according to the intention-to-treat principle and dropout from the waiting list. *Liver Transpl.* 2002;8:873-883.
46. Cillo U, Vitale A, Bassanello M, et al. Liver transplantation for the treatment of moderately or well-differentiated hepatocellular carcinoma. *Ann Surg.* 2004;239:150-159.
47. Hoshida Y, Villanueva A, Kobayashi M, et al. Gene expression in fixed tissues and outcome in hepatocellular carcinoma. *N Engl J Med.* 2008;359:1995-2004.
48. Cheung ST, Fan ST, Lee YT, et al. Albumin mRNA in plasma predicts post-transplant recurrence of patients with hepatocellular carcinoma. *Transplantation.* 2008;85:81-87.
49. Freeman RB, Wiesner RH, Edwards E, et al. Results of the first year of the new liver allocation plan. *Liver Transpl.* 2004;10:7-15.
50. Pomfret EA, Washburn K, Wald C, et al. Report of a national conference on liver allocation in patients with hepatocellular carcinoma in the United States. *Liver Transpl.* 2010;16:262-278.
51. Di Bisceglie AM. Pretransplant treatments for hepatocellular carcinoma: do they improve outcomes? *Liver Transpl.* 2005;(11 suppl 2):S10-S13.
52. Llovet JM, Mas X, Aponte JJ, et al. Cost effectiveness of adjuvant therapy for hepatocellular carcinoma during the waiting list for liver transplantation. *Gut.* 2002;50:123-128.
53. Takada Y, Ueda M, Ito T, et al. Living donor liver transplantation as a second-line therapeutic strategy for patients with hepatocellular carcinoma. *Liver Transpl.* 2006;12:912-919.
54. Kaihara S, Kiuchi T, Ueda M, et al. Living-donor liver transplantation for hepatocellular carcinoma. *Transplantation.* 2003;75: S37-S40.
55. Ringe B, Strong RW. The dilemma of living liver donor death: to report or not to report? *Transplantation.* 2008;85:790-793.
56. Sarasin FP, Majno PE, Llovet JM, et al. Living donor liver transplantation for early hepatocellular carcinoma: A life-expectancy and cost-effectiveness perspective. *Hepatology.* 2001;33: 1073-1079.
57. Nguyen KT, Gamblin TC, Geller DA. World review of laparoscopic liver resection-2,804 patients. *Ann Surg.* 2009;250:831-841.
58. Koffron AJ, Kung RD, Auffenberg GB, et al. Laparoscopic liver surgery for everyone: the hybrid method. *Surgery.* 2007;142:463-468.
59. Buell JF, Cherqui D, Geller DA, O'Rourke N, et al. The international position on laparoscopic liver surgery: The Louisville Statement, 2008. *Ann Surg.* 2009;250:825-830.
60. Belli G, Limongelli P, Fantini C, et al. Laparoscopic and open treatment of hepatocellular carcinoma in patients with cirrhosis. *Br J Surg.* 2009;96:1041-1048.
61. Lee KF, Chong CN, Wong J, et al. Long-term results of laparoscopic hepatectomy versus open hepatectomy for hepatocellular carcinoma: a case-matched analysis. *World J Surg.* 2011. [Epub ahead of print]
62. Belli G, Fantini C, Belli A, et al. Laparoscopic liver resection for hepatocellular carcinoma in cirrhosis: long-term outcomes. *Dig Surg.* 2011;28:134-140.
63. Tranchart H, Di Giuro G, Lainas P, et al. Laparoscopic resection for hepatocellular carcinoma: a matched-pair comparative study. *Surg Endosc.* 2010;24:1170-1176.
64. Cai XJ, Yang J, Yu H, et al. Clinical study of laparoscopic versus open hepatectomy for malignant liver tumors. *Surg Endosc.* 2008;22:2350-2356.
65. Tsinberg M, Tellioglu G, Simpfendorfer CH, et al. Comparison of laparoscopic versus open liver tumor resection: a case-controlled study. *Surg Endosc.* 2009;23:847-853.
66. Laurent A, Tayar C, Andréoletti M, et al. Laparoscopic liver resection facilitates salvage liver transplantation for hepatocellular carcinoma. *J Hepatobiliary Pancreat Surg.* 2009;16:310-314.
67. Livraghi T, Meloni F, Di Stasi M, et al. Sustained complete response and complications rates after radiofrequency ablation of very early hepatocellular carcinoma in cirrhosis: is resection still the treatment of choice? *Hepatology.* 2008;47:82-89.

68. Ishii H, Okada S, Nose H, et al. Local recurrence of hepatocellular carcinoma after percutaneous ethanol injection. *Cancer.* 1996;77:1792-1796.
69. Sala M, Llovet JM, Vilana R, et al. Initial response to percutaneous ablation predicts survival in patients with hepatocellular carcinoma. *Hepatology.* 2004;40:1352-1360.
70. Schwartz M, Roayaie S, Uva P. Treatment of HCC in patients awaiting liver transplantation. *Am J Transplant.* 2007;7:1875-1881.
71. Cho YK, Kim JK, Kim MY, et al. Systematic review of randomized trials for hepatocellular carcinoma treated with percutaneous ablation therapies. *Hepatology.* 2009;49:453-459.
72. Mori K, Fukuda K, Asaoka H, et al. Radiofrequency ablation of the liver: determination of ablative margin at MR imaging with impaired clearance of ferucarbotran-feasibility study. *Radiology.* 2009;251:557-565.
73. Mazzaferro V, Battiston C, Perrone S, et al. Radiofrequency ablation of small hepatocellular carcinoma in cirrhotic patients awaiting liver transplantation: a prospective study. *Ann Surg.* 2004;240:900-909.
74. Lin SM, Lin CJ, Lin CC, et al. Randomised controlled trial comparing percutaneous radiofrequency thermal ablation, percutaneous ethanol injection, and percutaneous acetic acid injection to treat hepatocellular carcinoma of 3 cm or less. *Gut.* 2005;54:1151-1156.
75. Shiina S, Teratani T, Obi S, et al. A randomized controlled trial of radiofrequency ablation with ethanol injection for small hepatocellular carcinoma. *Gastroenterology.* 2005;129:122-130.
76. Huang GT, Lee PH, Tsang YM, et al. Percutaneous ethanol injection versus surgical resection for the treatment of small hepatocellular carcinoma: a prospective study. *Ann Surg.* 2005;242:36-42.
77. Chen MS, Li JQ, Zheng Y, et al. A prospective randomized trial comparing percutaneous local ablative therapy and partial hepatectomy for small hepatocellular carcinoma. *Ann Surg.* 2006;243:321-328.
78. Ramsey DE, Kernagis LY, Soulen MC, et al. Chemoembolization of hepatocellular carcinoma. *J Vasc Interv Radiol.* 2002;13:S211-S221.
79. Llovet JM, Bruix J. Systematic review of randomized trials for unresectable hepatocellular carcinoma: chemoembolization improves survival. *Hepatology.* 2003;37:429-442.
80. Llovet JM, Real MI, Montaña X, et al. Arterial embolisation or chemoembolisation versus symptomatic treatment in patients with unresectable hepatocellular carcinoma: a randomised controlled trial. *Lancet.* 2002;359:1734-1739.
81. El-Serag HB, Marrero JA, Rudolph L, et al. Diagnosis and treatment of hepatocellular carcinoma. *Gastroenterology.* 2008;134:1752-1763.
82. Sato K, Lewandowski RJ, Bui JT, et al. Treatment of unresectable primary and metastatic liver cancer with yttrium-90 microspheres *Cardiovasc Intervent Radiol.* 2006;29:522-529.
83. Salem R, Lewandowski RJ, Mulcahy MF, et al. Radioembolization for hepatocellular carcinoma using Yttrium-90 microspheres: a comprehensive report of long-term outcomes. *Gastroenterology.* 2010;138:52-64.
84. Kulik LM, Carr BI, Mulcahy MF, et al. Safety and efficacy of 90Y radiotherapy for hepatocellular carcinoma with and without portal vein thrombosis. *Hepatology.* 2008;47:71-81.
85. Choi BO, Jang HS, Kang KM, et al. Fractionated stereotactic radiotherapy in patients with primary hepatocellular carcinoma. *Jpn J Clin Oncol.* 2006;36:154-158.
86. Mornex F, Girard N, Beziat C, et al. Feasibility and efficacy of high-dose three-dimensional-conformal radiotherapy in cirrhotic patients with small-size hepatocellular carcinoma non-eligible for curative therapies—mature results of the French Phase II RTF-1 trial. *Int J Radiat Oncol Biol Phys.* 2006;66:1152-1158.
87. Nakagawa K, Yamashita H, Shiraishi K, et al. Radiation therapy for portal venous invasion by hepatocellular carcinoma. *World J Gastroenterol.* 2005;11:7237-7241.
88. Tse RV, Hawkins M, Lockwood G, et al. Phase I study of individualized stereotactic body radiotherapy for hepatocellular carcinoma and intrahepatic cholangiocarcinoma. *J Clin Oncol.* 2008;26:657-664.
89. Kato H, Tsujii H, Miyamoto T, et al. Results of the first prospective study of carbon ion radiotherapy for hepatocellular carcinoma with liver cirrhosis. *Int J Radiat Oncol Biol Phys.* 2004;59:1468-1476.
90. Bush DA, Hillebrand DJ, Slater JM, et al. High-dose proton beam radiotherapy of hepatocellular carcinoma: preliminary results of a phase II trial. *Gastroenterology.* 2004;127:S189-S193.
91. Lai CL, Wu PC, Chan GC, Lok AS, Lin HJ. Doxorubicin versus no antitumor therapy in inoperable hepatocellular carcinoma. *Cancer.* 1988;62:479-483.
92. Yeo W, Mok TS, Zee B, et al. A randomized phase III study of doxorubicin versus PIAF for unresectable hepatocellular carcinoma. *J Natl Cancer Inst.* 2005;97:1532-1538.
93. Simonetti RG, Camma C, Fiorello F, et al. Hepatocellular carcinoma. A worldwide problem and the major risk factors. *Dig Dis Sci.* 1991;36:962-972.
94. Bruix J, Sherman M. Management of hepatocellular carcinoma. *Hepatology,* 2005;42(5):1208-1236.
95. McKillop IH, Schmidt CM, Cahill PA, et al. Altered expression of mitogen-activated protein kinases in a rat model of experimental hepatocellular carcinoma. *Hepatology.* 1997;26:1484-1491.
96. Ito Y, Sasaki Y, Horimoto M, et al. Activation of mitogen-activated protein kinases/extracellular signal-regulated kinases in human hepatocellular carcinoma. *Hepatology.* 1998;27:951-958.
97. Toyoda M, Hashimoto N, Tokita K, et al. Increased activity and expression of MAP kinase in HCC model rats induced by 3′-methyl-4-dimethylamino-azobenzene. *J Hepatol.* 1999;31:725-733.
98. Feng DY, Zheng H, Tan Y, et al. Effect of phosphorylation of MAPK and Stat3 and expression of c-fos and c-jun proteins on hepatocarcinogenesis and their clinical significance. *World J Gastroenterol.* 2001;7:33-36
99. Llovet J RS, Mazzaferro V, et al. Sorafenib improves survival in advanced hepatocellular carcinoma (HCC): results of a phase III randomized placebo-controlled trial (SHARP trial). *J Clin Oncol.* 2007;25(suppl):LBA1.
100. Llovet JM, Ricci S, Mazzaferro V, et al. Sorafenib in advanced hepatocellular carcinoma. *N Engl J Med.* 2008;359:378-390.
101. Pawlik TM, Reyes DK, Cosgrove D, Kamel IR, Bhagat N, Geschwind JF. Phase II trial of sorafenib combined with concurrent TACE with drug-eluting beads for hepatocellular carcinoma. *J Clin Oncol.* 2011;29:3960-3967.
102. Alexia C, Bras M, Fallot G, et al. Pleiotropic effects of PI-3′ kinase/Akt signaling in human hepatoma cell proliferation and drug-induced apoptosis. *Ann N Y Acad Sci.* 2006;1090:1-17.
103. Saxena NK, Sharma D, Ding X, et al. Concomitant activation of the JAK/STAT, PI3K/AKT, and ERK signaling is involved in leptin-mediated promotion of invasion and migration of hepatocellular carcinoma cells. *Cancer Res.* 2007;67:2497-2507.
104. Sahin F, Kannangai R, Adegbola O, et al. mTOR and P70 S6 kinase expression in primary liver neoplasms. *Clin Cancer Res.* 2004;10:8421-8425.
105. Sieghart W, Fuereder T, Schmid K, et al. Mammalian target of rapamycin pathway activity in hepatocellular carcinomas of patients undergoing liver transplantation. *Transplantation.* 2007;83:425-432.
106. Kanda T, Tada M, Imazeki F, et al. 5-Aza-2′-deoxycytidine sensitizes hepatoma and pancreatic cancer cell lines. *Oncol Rep.* 2005;14:975-979.
107. Ocker M, Alajati A, Ganslmayer M, et al. The histone-deacetylase inhibitor SAHA potentiates proapoptotic effects of 5-fluorouracil and irinotecan in hepatoma cells. *J Cancer Res Clin Oncol.* 2005;131:385-394.
108. Ma B, Chan S, Chan A. The preclinical activity of the histone deacetylase inhibitor PXD101 (belinostat) in hepatocellular carcinoma cell lines. *Invest New Drugs.* April 2010;28(2):107-114.
109. Yao DF, Dong ZZ, Yao M. Specific molecular markers in hepatocellular carcinoma. *Hepatobiliary Pancreat Dis Int.* 2007;6:241-247.
110. Yeo W, et al. A phase I/II study of belinostat (PXD101) in patients with unresectable hepatocellular carcinoma. *J Clin Oncol.* ASCO Annual Meeting Proceedings Part I. 2007;25(18S, June 20 suppl): Abstract 15081.
111. Park YN, Kim YB, Yang KM, et al. Increased expression of vascular endothelial growth factor and angiogenesis in the early stage of multistep hepatocarcinogenesis. *Arch Pathol Lab Med.* 2000;124:1061-1065.
112. Zhao J, Hu J, Cai J, et al. Vascular endothelial growth factor expression in serum of patients with hepatocellular carcinoma. *Chin Med J (Engl).* 2003;116:772-776.

113. Huang GW, Yang LY, Lu WQ. Expression of hypoxia-inducible factor 1alpha and vascular endothelial growth factor in hepatocellular carcinoma: impact on neovascularization and survival. *World J Gastroenterol.* 2005;11:1705-1708.
114. Kanematsu M, Osada S, Amaoka N, et al. Expression of vascular endothelial growth factor in hepatocellular carcinoma and the surrounding liver: correlation with angiographically assisted CT. *AJR Am J Roentgenol.* 2004;183:1585-1593.
115. Kanematsu M, Semelka RC, Osada S, et al. Magnetic resonance imaging and expression of vascular endothelial growth factor in hepatocellular nodules in cirrhosis and hepatocellular carcinomas. *Top Magn Reson Imaging.* 2005;16:67-75.
116. Wang B, Gao ZQ, Yan X. Correlative study of angiogenesis and dynamic contrast-enhanced magnetic resonance imaging features of hepatocellular carcinoma. *Acta Radiol.* 2005;46:353-358
117. Malka D, Dromain C, Farace F, et al. Bevacizumab in patients with advanced hepatocellular carcinoma: preliminary results of a phase II study with circulating endothelial cell (CEC) monitoring. *J Clin Oncol.* 2007;25:4570.
118. Hsu C, Yang T, Hsu C, et al. Modified-dose capecitabine + bevacizumab for the treatment of advanced/metastatic hepatocellular carcinoma (HCC): a phase II, single-arm study. *J Clin Oncol.* 2007;25:15190.
119. Sun W, Haller DG, Mykulowycz K, et al. Combination of capecitabine and oxaliplatin with bevacizumab in treatment of advanced hepatocellular carcinoma: a phase II study. *J Clin Oncol.* 2007;25(18S):4574.
120. Thomas MB, Chadha R, Iwasaki M, Glover K, Abbruzzese JL. The combination of bevacizumab and erlotinib shows significant biological activity in patients with advanced hepatocellular carcinoma. *J Clin Oncol.* 2007;25(18S):4567.
121. Okano H, Shiraki K, Yamanaka Y, et al. Functional expression of a proliferation-related ligand in hepatocellular carcinoma and its implications for neovascularization. *World J Gastroenterol.* 2005;11:4650-4654.
122. Zhang Q, Tang X, Lu QY, et al. Resveratrol inhibits hypoxia-induced accumulation of hypoxia-inducible factor-1alpha and VEGF expression in human tongue squamous cell carcinoma and hepatoma cells. *Mol Cancer Ther.* 2005;4:1465-1474.
123. Lin AY, Brophy N, Fisher GA, et al. Phase II study of thalidomide in patients with unresectable hepatocellular carcinoma. *Cancer.* 2005;103:119-125.
124. Patt YZ, Hassan MM, Lozano RD, et al. Thalidomide in the treatment of patients with hepatocellular carcinoma: a phase II trial. *Cancer.* 2005;103:749-755.
125. Chao Y, Chan WK, Wang SS, et al. Phase II study of megestrol acetate in the treatment of hepatocellular carcinoma. *J Gastroenterol Hepatol.* 1997;12:277-281.
126. Marongiu F, Doratiotto S, Montisci S, et al. Liver repopulation and carcinogenesis: two sides of the same coin? *Am J Pathol.* 2008;172:857-864.
127. Varnholt H. The role of microRNAs in primary liver cancer. *Ann Hepatol.* 2008;7:104-113.
128. Pang RW, Poon RT. From molecular biology to targeted therapies for hepatocellular carcinoma: the future is now. *Oncology.* 2007;72(suppl 1):30-44.
129. Jain RK. Antiangiogenic therapy for cancer: current and emerging concepts. *Oncology (Williston Park).* 2005;19:7-16.

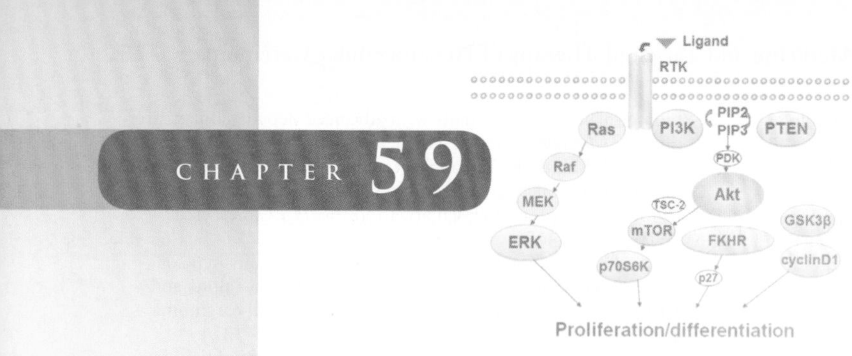

CHAPTER 59

Personalized Medicine and Targeted Therapy of Pancreatic Cancer: Current Status and Proposed Strategies

Milind Javle

INTRODUCTION

The burden of pancreatic cancer continues to be considerable, despite its relatively low incidence rate. At the beginning of the 21st century, the estimated number of cases of pancreatic cancer worldwide was 110,000, with a mortality rate of 98%.[1] The incidence is three to four times higher in the western countries than in Asia or Africa.[1] This geographical variation is likely to change, however, as the incidence of this disease in developing countries is rising, most likely secondary to environmental factors such as smoking and adoption of a western lifestyle.[2] In the United States, 44,030 new cases of pancreatic cancer were diagnosed, with 37,660 estimated deaths in 2011.[3] Surgically resectable pancreatic cancer is considered as potentially curable. Unfortunately, only 20% of patients present at an early, resectable stage of disease and the 5-year survival after surgery remains poor at 20% to 30%. The majority of patients with pancreatic cancer are diagnosed at an advanced stage of disease and their 5-year survival is below 5%.

Gemcitabine was approved for the treatment of advanced pancreatic cancer over a decade ago, based on an improved survival rate and "clinical benefit response" as compared with 5-fluorouracil (5-FU).[4] Since then, a number of gemcitabine-based chemotherapeutic combinations were investigated in the phase II and phase III settings. These included gemcitabine with 5-FU, irinotecan, cisplatin, oxaliplatin, or capecitabine. None proved to be superior to single-agent gemcitabine.[5] Similar disappointing results were noted with gemcitabine-based targeted agent combinations, such as gemcitabine with marimastat, tipifarnib, bevacizumab, and cetuximab.[6-9] The only study to report success with a targeted agent recently was with the epidermal growth factor receptor (EGFR) blocker erlotinib plus gemcitabine. In the clinical trial conducted by the National Cancer Institute of Canada, the gemcitabine plus erlotinib arm resulted in a small but statistically significant survival improvement over gemcitabine alone.[10] An important recent development in this field was the phase III clinical trial conducted by the PRODIGE Intergroup in France of 5-FU, irinotecan, and oxaliplatin (FOLFIRINOX) versus gemcitabine for patients with metastatic pancreatic cancer having a good performance status.[11] This trial demonstrated that aggressive, multi-agent chemotherapy is tolerable in a subset of pancreatic cancer patients and can result in a clinically meaningful survival improvement (11 vs. 7 months in the FOLFIRINOX vs. gemcitabine arms, respectively). Even though this trial represents an important advance in this field, clearly we need to reconsider our approach to this disease and examine the reasons for the limited therapeutic success.

Late detection due to relatively nonspecific presenting symptoms and molecular heterogeneity of pancreatic cancer are believed to account for its poor prognosis. Addressing the former will be challenging; given the relatively low incidence of pancreatic cancer, screening strategies are unlikely to be practical for sporadic cases. Most cases of pancreatic cancer are sporadic or secondary to environmental exposure; genetic predisposition is demonstrable in 5% to 10% of the affected population. It is critical that we explore these genetic syndromes that are associated with pancreatic cancer. An understanding of the genetics of familial colorectal and breast cancer has contributed significantly toward their prevention and therapy. Such an understanding in pancreatic cancer may have important therapeutic implications. An important example in the regard is the familial breast and ovarian cancer syndrome associated with *BRCA2* mutation; the affected families also carry a small risk of pancreatic cancer. Patients with pancreatic cancer and *BRCA2* mutation benefit from synthetic lethal interaction with poly(ADP ribose) polymerase (PARP) inhibitors.[12] PARP inhibition for *BRCA2* mutation–associated pancreatic cancer probably represents the first example of a personalized approach to pancreatic cancer at the molecular level and is discussed later.

MOLECULAR HETEROGENEITY OF PANCREATIC CANCER

Recent successes with targeted therapy have occurred in cancers with identifiable activating mutations. For instance, clear cell renal carcinoma is associated with mutation of the *VHL* tumor-suppressor gene.[13] This results in the accumulation of hypoxia-inducible factors that stimulate angiogenesis through vascular endothelial growth factor and its receptor. Anti-angiogenic agents such as bevacizumab, sorafenib, and sunitinib have therefore been of therapeutic value in this disease. Other examples include crizotinib for non–small cell lung cancers that have anaplastic lymphoma kinase (ALK) gene rearrangements,[14] hedgehog inhibitors for basal cell carcinoma with mutations in the patched homologue 1 (PTCH1)[15] and smoothened homologue (SMO) genes, and vemurafenib (PLX4032) for malignant melanoma with b-raf mutations.[16]

The above encouraging results have not been seen in pancreatic cancer with targeted therapies. The molecular heterogeneity of pancreatic cancer is a significant limitation in this regard. Jones et al. performed a comprehensive genetic analysis of 24 pancreatic cancers. They noted that each cancer contained an average of 63 genetic alterations, most of which were point mutations. These alterations defined a core set of 12 cellular signaling pathways and processes that were each genetically altered in 67% to 100% of the tumors (Table 59.1).[17] Analysis of the tumor transcriptome with next-generation sequencing provided independent evidence for the significance of these pathways.

The importance of targeting oncogenic mutations in cancer has been highlighted with the success of erlotinib therapy in lung cancer.[18] However, these mutations are uncommon and epigenetic changes in cancer appear to be at least as important for therapeutic targeting as somatic mutations. DNA methylation consists of the addition of a methyl (CH3) residue on cytosine preceding a guanosine, known as CpG dinucleotides (p stands for phosphate). This modification is catalyzed by a DNA methyltransferase family (DNMT1, 3a and 3b). Alteration of DNA methylation patterns leads to deregulation of gene expression and functional defects, in the absence of mutations. Thus, epigenetic alterations may have the same therapeutic implications as in the case of functional mutations in cancer. For instance, Drew et al. recently demonstrated that the PARP inhibitor AG014699 was cytotoxic to breast cancer cells with mutated BRCA 1/2 or breast cancer cells with epigenetically silenced *BRCA1*.[19] Epigenetic alterations in pancreatic cancer are currently being explored. Methylation markers may also have a role in early detection; a panel of the same has been proposed using pancreatic juice samples and may help diagnosis of cancer in cases of chronic pancreatitis.

Another novel area is this field is microRNA research. MicroRNAs are short, noncoding segments of RNA that are involved in the regulation of gene expression. Jamieson et al. performed a global microRNA expression analysis in surgically resected pancreatic cancer and identified a high expression of miR-21 and reduced expression of miR-34a and miR-30d as prognostic markers associated with poor survival.[20] Currently, the most promising miRNA targets in pancreatic cancer indicative of gemcitabine resistance are miRNA-15a, miRNA-21, miRNA-34, miRNA-200b, miRNA-200c, miRNA-214, miRNA-221, and members of the Let-7 family.[21-23]

The above data highlight the genetic, epigenetic, and molecular complexity of pancreatic cancer and underscore the reasons for poor outcomes with standard, one-size-fits-all therapy for pancreatic cancer.

PERSONALIZED THERAPIES IN DEVELOPMENT IN PANCREATIC CANCER

While the concept of personalized therapy is being actively promoted in recent times, it is not new. Customization of therapy, based on clinical parameters like performance status, age, stage, or laboratory parameters, is routine in oncology. In the post-genomic era, however, the potential for personalized therapy, directed against specific molecular targets in the cancer tissue, has increased exponentially.

While personalized therapy in pancreatic cancer is still at a nascent stage, several promising leads could make this approach a reality. Our experience in this regard with PARP inhibitors, transforming growth factor beta (TGF-β) pathway, insulin-like growth factor receptor (IGF-1R) pathway, and gemcitabine pharmacokinetics related to pancreatic cancer is discussed below.

Aberrant DNA Repair and PARP Inhibitors

In 2005, two groups independently demonstrated the efficacy of PARP inhibitors in homologous recombination (HR)–defective cell lines and xenograft models.[24,25] PARP is an integral component of single-strand break (SSB) DNA repair. HR is the principal DNA double-strand break (DSB) DNA repair mechanism and may be frequently defective

TABLE 59–1 Comprehensive Genetic Analysis of Pancreatic Cancer Revealed That 12 Processes or Signaling Pathways Were Genetically Altered in the Vast Majority of the Cancers

Regulatory Process or Pathway	Altered Genes Detected	Fraction of Tumors with Genetic Alteration of at Least One of the Genes (%)
Apoptosis	9	100
DNA damage control	9	83
Regulation of G1/S phase transition	19	100
Hedgehog signaling	19	100
Homophilic cell adhesion	30	79
Integrin signaling	24	67
c-Jun N-terminal kinase signaling	9	96
KRAS signaling	5	100
Regulation of invasion	46	92
Small GTPase-dependent signaling (other than KRAS)	33	79
TGF-β signaling	37	100
Wnt/Notch signaling	29	100

TGF-β, transforming growth factor beta.

in some cancers. In the presence of PARP inhibitors, the failure to repair SSB results in collapsed replication forks and DSBs that require HR for repair. In the presence of HR defects that occur in BRCA mutations, these lesions are lethal either because they persist or because they can only be repaired by alternative error-prone pathways including nonhomologous end joining and single-strand annealing, resulting in genomic instability. PARP inhibitors have shown a lot of promise with *BRCA* mutation–associated breast and ovarian cancers and breast cancers with DNA repair defects, such as triple-negative breast cancers. Similarly, preliminary reports suggest clinical responses in *BRCA* mutation–associated pancreatic cancers to PARP inhibition and cisplatin-based therapy; we have seen impressive responses with iniparib for patients with *BRCA2* mutation–associated pancreatic cancer (Figs. 59.1 and 59.2). Although these results are exciting, the incidence of pancreatic cancer with *BRCA2* mutation is low (5%), and therefore strategies to expand the use of DNA repair beyond the narrow scope of *BRCA* mutations need to be explored. Recently, the *PALB2* gene that encodes a BRCA-binding protein has been identified as a pancreatic cancer susceptibility gene.[26] Inactivation of PALB2 as a result of biallelic mutation resulted in long-term responses to mitomycin and represents one of the first documented examples of successful personalized therapy based on genomic sequencing.

Exploiting Synthetic Lethality in Pancreatic Cancer

Synthetic lethality is a term to describe the combined lethal effect of two genetic variations that are otherwise non-lethal when occurring in isolation and PARP inhibitors have reinforced the value of synthetic lethal targeting for cancer therapy. It has been noted for instance that PARP inhibitors may be synthetically lethal in sporadic cancers that bear somatic mutations or epigenetic silencing in the various components of the HR pathway. HR is a complex process with multiple proteins, including ATM, ATR, CHK1, RAD51 and its homologues, the FANC proteins, MRE11/RAD50/NBS1. These proteins are inhibited by the PARP inhibitors KU0058684 and KU0058948.[27] Li et al. reported the significant prognostic importance of polymorphisms of the genes involved in HR in pancreatic cancer.[28] Maacke et al. reported that Rad51, which mediates DNA repair via HR, is overexpressed in 66% of the pancreatic adenocarcinoma cases.[29] *PTEN* is one of the most commonly mutated tumor suppressors in human cancer and its loss is common in pancreatic cancer; PTEN deficiency was associated with defective HR.[30-32] The latter was targeted successfully by the PARP inhibitor olaparib.[33] The above data strongly suggest that (a) DNA repair defects are common in pancreatic cancer and (b) these defects are potentially targetable with PARP and other DNA repair inhibitors.

Targeting Proteins and Protein Kinases

The identification of overexpressed proteins and protein kinases in cancer through tissue array and modern proteomic profiling technologies and their association with carcinogenesis and correlation with poor prognosis has spurred the development of targeted inhibitors to signaling proteins. A good example in regard is the TGF-β signaling pathway.

TGF-β is a multifunctional polypeptide. It has a context-dependent role in carcinogenesis, which can be either tumor suppressive or promoting. During the early phase of carcinogenesis, TGF-β acts as a tumor suppressor by inducing cell cycle arrest and possibly apoptosis. However, in late stages of progression, as tumor cells evade the growth inhibition by TGF-β, the role of TGF-β signaling is often switched from tumor suppression to promotion. SMAD4 plays a key role in TGF-β signal transduction

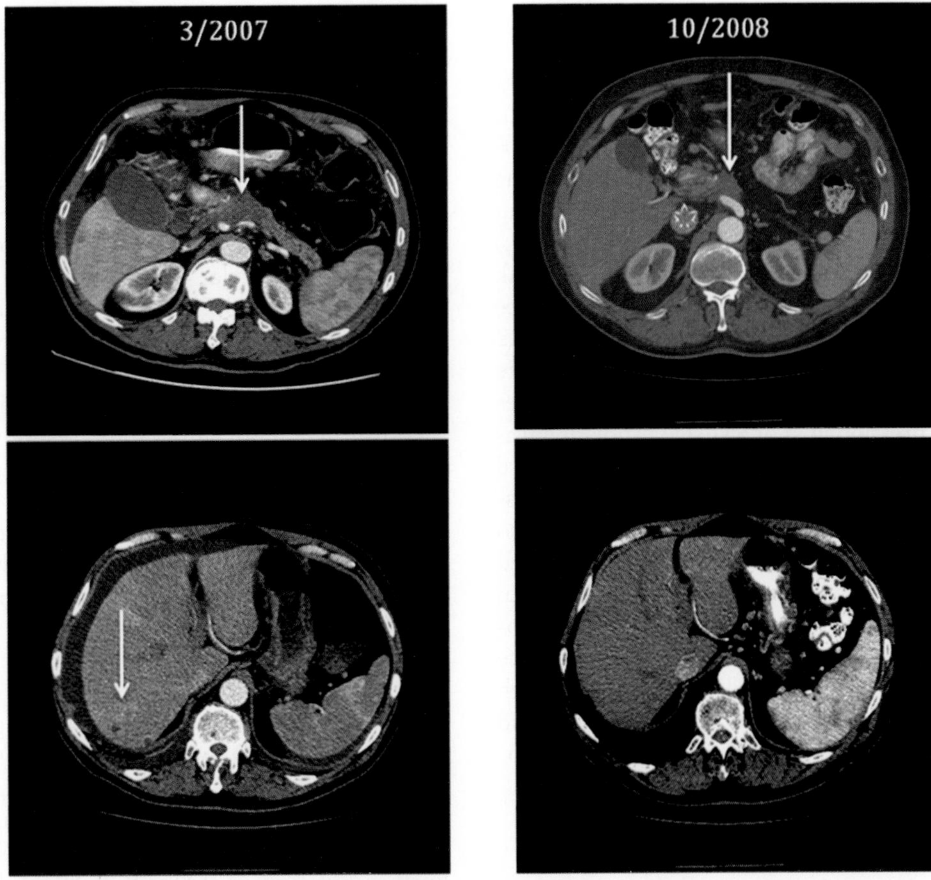

FIGURE 59–1 Computerized tomography scan showing sustained response to cisplatin and poly(ADP ribose) polymerase inhibitor in the presence of the *BRCA2* mutation. Pancreatic adenocarcinoma involving the body and liver.

and gene regulation. SMAD4 loss is common in pancreatic cancer and is in fact utilized as a diagnostic tool for occult cancers so as to confirm their pancreatic origin. Although SMAD4 is a tumor suppressor, it also plays a context-dependent dual role. Inactivation–deletion or point mutations of the tumor-suppressor gene SMAD4/DPC4 are seen in 50% of pancreatic adenocarcinomas.[34,35] Loss of SMAD4/DPC4 is associated with a poor prognosis in pancreatic cancer.[35] Cells expressing Smad4 showed an enhanced epithelial–mesenchymal transition, mainly in the presence of altered SMAD4 protein and normal signal transducer and activator of transcription 3 (STAT-3) activity. A recent hypothesis suggests that loss of SMAD4 leads to aberrant activation of STAT-3, contributing to the switch of TGF-β from a tumor-suppressor to a tumor-promoting pathway in pancreatic cancer.[36]

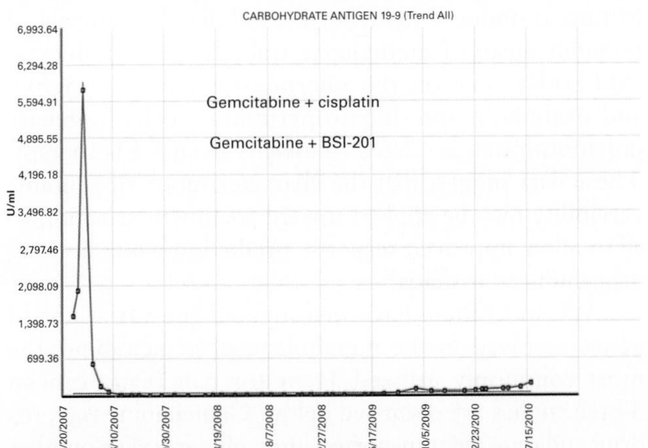

FIGURE 59–2 Sustained CA 19-9 response to cisplatin and poly(ADP ribose) polymerase inhibitor in the presence of *BRCA2* mutation.

TGF-β–targeted therapeutic approaches include antisense oligonucleotides, small molecule inhibitors of the TGF-βRI/II kinase, and TGF-β neutralizing antibodies. Several of these are currently in clinical trials. Inhibitors of TGF-β have shown promising preclinical cytotoxic activity in pancreatic cancer. LY2109761 is an orally active Tβ RI/II kinase dual inhibitor. The efficacy of LY2109761 on tumor growth, survival, and reduction of spontaneous metastasis has been evaluated in an orthotopic murine model of metastatic pancreatic cancer.[37] LY2109761 significantly inhibited tumor growth, suppressed both basal and TGF-β1–induced cell migration and invasion, and induced anoikis. In vivo, LY2109761, in combination with gemcitabine, significantly reduced the tumor burden, prolonged survival, and reduced spontaneous abdominal metastases.

The key questions that need to be addressed with a promising target such as TGF-β, for which inhibitors currently exist, are what group of patients can be selected and how could the tumor-suppressive effect of TGF-β be maintained at the same time?

We recently measured plasma TGF-β1 in 643 advanced pancreatic cancer cases (data unpublished). In patients with locally advanced and metastatic disease (n = 355), there was a significant association between plasma TGF-β1 and survival, with the median survival among those in the top quartile of TGF-β1 levels (>19.05 ng/mL) being 27.7 versus 40 weeks for low levels (log-rank $P = 0.0125$, adjusted for baseline CA 19-9 and performance status). Immunohistochemical (IHC) studies for TGF-βR2 expression were performed in 87 cases. In the multivariate Cox model, after adjusting for clinical prognostic variables and TGF-βR2 expression, loss of SMAD4 expression was significantly associated with lower overall survival (hazard ratio: 1.85; 95% CI: 1.06-3.23; $P = 0.03$). Progressive disease on a first-line gemcitabine-based regimen was also more common in the SMAD4 IHC 0 group as compared with higher scores (46.5% vs. 38.1% progressed; chi square $P = 0.069$). These data suggest that patient subgroups with high TGF-β1 levels in the plasma and tissue could be preselected for the neutralizing antibodies such as LY2109761, which do not affect TGF-β synthesis and thereby maintain its tumor-suppressive role while contributing toward inhibition of established cancers.

IGF-1R Pathway

The IGF pathway is thought to be an important player in the pancreatic carcinogenesis and is being investigated as a target for therapy in several cancer types. The IGF-1R pathway may also play a role in the development and progression of pancreatic cancer.[38,39] A recent study by Dong et al. indicated that genetic variations in the IGF axis pathway have a prognostic role in locally advanced pancreatic cancer.[40] Three clinical trials have been conducted in pancreatic cancer with IGF-1R-targeted therapy. In our institution, the monoclonal antibody MK-0646 (Dalotuzumab) was investigated in a three-arm randomized phase II clinical trial of gemcitabine + MK-0646, gemcitabine + erlotinib + MK-0646, and gemcitabine + erlotinib (control arm). In this trial, 72 patients were enrolled, of whom 20% had sustained partial responses in the study arms receiving MK-0646.[41] Similar results were noted by Kindler et al. in a randomized prospective clinical trial of gemcitabine + AMG479 (IGF-1R-directed monoclonal antibody), gemcitabine + AMG655 (antibody against DR5, death receptor), and gemcitabine + placebo. In a final analysis of this phase II, the 12-month overall survival was 39%, 20%, and 23% in the AMG479, AMG655, and control arms, respectively, with a hazard ratio of 0.65 in favor of the study arms.[42] A phase III clinical trial of gemcitabine and/or AMG479 is currently ongoing. In these trials, myelosuppression including neutropenia and thrombocytopenia was common (10% patients developed grade 3 or 4 hematologic toxicity).

Given the interest in the IGF pathway and the development of potentially efficacious synthetic inhibitors, identification of predictive biomarkers represents a priority area for research. Receptor expression has been correlated with the efficacy of anti-cancer agents including tyrosine kinase inhibitors. However, in a randomized phase II clinical trial of the IGF-1R monoclonal antibody cixutumumab for patients with advanced colorectal cancer, no correlation was demonstrated between high IGF-1R expression and radiologic response.[43] Zha et al. investigated molecular predictors to the IGF-1R monoclonal antibody h10H5 and noted that in breast cancer and colorectal cancer at least 1,300 receptors per cell were needed for the anti-tumor efficacy of h10H5 in vitro.[44] However, in the latter study, receptor expression alone was insufficient for anti-tumor response and IGF-1R expression may have a greater role as a negative predictor. Whether standard immunohistochemistry is adequate for the detection of very low levels of the receptor remains to be proven, however. Activation of IGF axis within the tumor may have the greatest validity for the prediction of anti-tumor effect. For instance, IRS1 is an important component of the IGF signaling pathway and could serve as a biomarker for sensitivity to inhibitors.

Pitts et al. reported an unbalanced gain of IGF-1R based on ploidy in OSI-906–sensitive colorectal cancer cell lines, without an increase in IGF-1R gene amplification.[45] Gualberto et al. reported that the mesenchymal phenotype was least likely to respond to IGF-1R inhibition.[46] Further investigation for the IGF-1R inhibitor susceptible phenotype in the clinical setting will build on the above observations.

Exploiting Gemcitabine Pharmacokinetics to Optimize Therapy

Personalization of anti-cancer therapy based on interindividual genetic differences (pharmacogenetics) is still at a nascent stage in oncology. However, there have been recent successful examples in gastrointestinal oncology with meaningful clinical impact. These include identification of UGT1A1 polymorphism as a predictor for irinotecan-induced neutropenia and diarrhea, impact of polymorphism of methylenetetrahydrofolate reductase (MTHFR) gene on the pharmacodynamics of 5-FU, and oxaliplatin and dihydropyrimidine dehydrogenase polymorphisms as related to toxicity from 5-FU therapy. These data suggest that the characterization of genomic variability may be applied toward treatment selection so as to allow improved response prediction while limiting drug-induced toxicity.[47]

We and others have investigated the variations of genes involved in the metabolism of gemcitabine, the most commonly utilized agent for pancreatic cancer. These studies are discussed below. Gemcitabine is a prodrug and must be transported intracellularly via a number of membrane transport mechanisms and get activated by deoxycytidine kinase to gemcitabine triphosphate for its pharmacologic effect. Gemcitabine deactivation occurs via cytidine deaminase. Ribonucleotide reductase regulatory subunit M1 (RRM1) is a DNA repair enzyme and its overexpression correlates with gemcitabine resistance. Preclinical evaluation in lung cancer demonstrated that RRM1 overexpression may be a marker of poor response to gemcitabine therapy.[48] Human equilibrative nucleoside transporter 1 (HENT1) is the major transporter protein for gemcitabine and its expression may have a predictive value. Farrell et al. retrospectively investigated HENT1 expression in patients treated on the adjuvant RTOG trial 9704.[49] In this study, HENT1 protein expression as measured by immunohistochemistry was associated with increased overall and disease-free survival in patients receiving adjuvant gemcitabine. No such association was noted in those patients receiving adjuvant 5-FU.

Our group has investigated the prognostic significance of single-nucleotide polymorphisms (SNPs) of gemcitabine metabolic genes in patients with surgically resectable and locally advanced pancreatic cancer.[50] Though none of the SNPs affected survival individually, a combined genotype was observed, in which the survival worsened with increasing number of adverse genetic alterations. There was a correlation between adverse genotypes and hematologic toxicity in our study. Ueno et al. have also linked genomic variations with pharmacokinetic changes.[51] The above studies are retrospective and the use of these genetic variations as predictive biomarkers for gemcitabine therapy has not yet been approved by the Food and Drug Administration (FDA). The path forward would include their prospective validation in a clinical trial. Such a proposed trial is particularly relevant today, since a viable alternative to gemcitabine exists in the FOLFIRINOX regimen.

BIOMARKER DEVELOPMENT IN PERSONALIZED THERAPIES

Pharmaceutical sponsors have been impacted by several failed clinical trials in unselected pancreatic cancer populations and are increasingly adopting the biomarker-based approach for further investigation. In pancreatic cancer, tissue-based correlative studies are complicated by the fact that tumor is surrounded by a dense stroma. Furthermore, most biopsies are usually obtained via fine-needle aspiration, thereby limiting the amount of material available for high-throughput technologies, which have considerable tissue requirement for analysis. Molecular heterogeneity within the tumor and between primary and metastatic sites adds further complexity to the field. Academic laboratories have been in the forefront of the discovery stage of biomarker development; unfortunately, most of their work has been in the field of prognostic rather than predictive biomarkers. The resources required for predictive biomarker identification are typically greater and beyond the scope of academic investigators.

Newer technologies including protein and gene arrays allow the investigators to interrogate the whole genome, transcriptome, proteome, and metabolome using tumor and surrogate tissues such as blood and body fluids. There have been successful examples in breast cancer with array-based assays: the treatment of breast cancer has been impacted upon by the Oncotype and MammaPrint systems.[52,53] The identification of driver mutations has had a significant clinical impact in some cancers. Examples of these are EGFR mutations, b-raf mutations, her-2/neu mutations, c-kit mutations, BCR-ABL translocation, and EML4-ALK translocation: these have led to specific targeted therapies for specific cancer subtypes.

In the United States, all predictive biomarker tests have to be compliant with the Clinical Laboratory Improvement Amendment (CLIA) act of 1988.[54] "CLIA" laboratories have to follow FDA guidelines for biomarker assessment. However, most biomarkers are discovered in research laboratories that are not CLIA regulated. For their clinical implementation, they have to undergo a complex and lengthy process of validation and qualification, which are described below. Terms like "biomarker development" and "validation" are being synonymously used in the literature; however, this is incorrect and appropriate nomenclature should be emphasized, as this field is critical toward the development of personalized therapies. The steps involved in biomarker development for personalized therapies are (1) discovery, (2) validation, (3) qualification, and finally (4) clinical implementation.

The biomarker discovery step for predictive biomarkers typically starts with the establishment of a correlative relationship between the biomarker and clinical outcome of interest, such as overall survival. While ideally a causal relationship should also be established, this is often too complex, especially in heterogeneous solid tumors. Ideally, clinical correlative studies should be combined with the analysis of preclinical model systems.

The biomarker validation step is performed to ensure that the analytic techniques are reliable, robust, and reproducible. In general, Good Laboratory Practice techniques are emphasized, but there is flexibility in regard to the rigorousness of the validation procedures: a biomarker used as a research tool in the laboratory setting has lower validation requirements as compared with another used in the clinical setting. The steps involved in validation include the establishment of a detailed validation plan; pre-study validation wherein the parameters like accuracy, reproducibility, precision, and appropriate controls are established; and finally the in-study validation, which includes the analysis of patient samples.

Biomarker qualification is designed to prove its clinical utility and determine the sensitivity and specificity. The process begins with a retrospective analysis of material from clinical studies and correlation with clinical outcome. An alternative is to use archival material from biobanks that have recently emerged at major academic centers. Following this, a prospective evaluation is required, usually as a companion diagnostic in a clinical trial. These trials, however, do not necessarily include biomarker evaluation as their primary endpoint and such a study is essential as a final step of the qualification process. The latter step includes randomizing patients to biomarker-based or non–biomarker-based therapies with targeted therapeutics so as to independently assess both the prognostic and the predictive impact of the biomarker in question. The FDA has a process in place for biomarker qualification, which forms a regulatory guideline, and typically, this process starts with a letter of intent to the FDA.[55] As per this FDA guidance, "qualification is a conclusion that, within the stated context of use, the results of assessment with a biomarker can be relied upon to adequately reflect a biological process, response, or event, and support use of the biomarker during drug or biotechnology product development, ranging from discovery through post-approval."

The final step in the development process is its clinical implementation. This process begins with regulatory approval of the biomarker and depends on clinical acceptance and cost-effectiveness of the impacted therapies. Examples of biomarkers with high clinical acceptance include k-ras mutation in colorectal cancer and her-2/neu mutation in breast cancer. Others such as UGT1A1 polymorphism for the prediction of irinotecan toxicity have not gained wide acceptance, despite their approval.[56] This may be explained by the observation that UGT1A1 polymorphism-related irinotecan toxicity occurs at high doses that are seldom used in practice, whereas its clinical impact with lower doses of irinotecan is less clinically relevant.

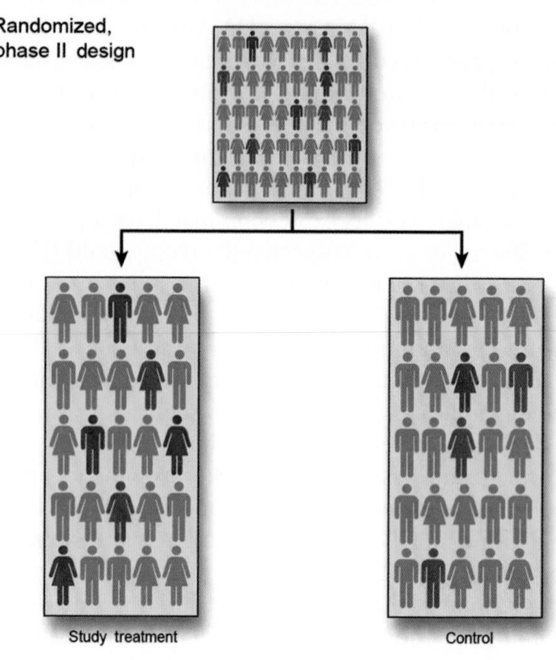

FIGURE 59–3 Randomized, controlled clinical trial. Study subjects are equally randomized between investigational therapy and control. This study design does not account for the disparate prevalence of the predictive biomarker in the two patient groups. This design is relatively inflexible.

CLINICAL TRIAL STRATEGIES: BIOMARKER AND CLINICAL CODEVELOPMENT

A common requirement for clinical trials of personalized therapies is the concurrent development of diagnostics related to predictive biomarkers. This presents challenges for clinical trial design beyond the traditional phase II and III studies. Ideally, if the drug development plan includes a biomarker-driven strategy, exploratory studies for predictive biomarkers should be in the phase I component itself. Predictive power of the candidate biomarker could then be explored in the phase II component. This may require target enrichment rather than blinded, randomized phase II studies. We propose that the frequency of the biomarker may have implications on phase II trial design. For instance, if the biomarker is present in a minority of the population, a blinded, randomized trial where the control arm is either standard-of-care or placebo carries the risk of type I error, depending upon the number of patients with the relevant biomarker in the study arm. This is illustrated in Figure 59.3. Unfortunately, this has been the case for most "screening" randomized phase II trials in pancreatic cancer. In these cases, "target enrichment" strategies will yield better results.

Two possible target enrichment strategies in the phase II setting are the stratification and adaptive designs. The former strategy was utilized in the development of the monoclonal antibody trastuzumab.[57] Patients were enrolled irrespective of their her-2/neu status, but the trial was adequately powered for the biomarker frequency, and the 5% type I error was allocated between the comparison of treatments overall and within biomarker-positive patients. In the stratified designs, while the availability of tissue for biomarker studies is mandated, the actual analysis can be conducted toward the conclusion of the clinical trial and enrollment of patients is not dependent on biopsy results as the population biomarker frequency can be reliably estimated based on existing data. This design is often adequate for the investigation of a single therapeutic and the clinical impact of this strategy is proven (for instance, with trastuzumab).

Adaptive Bayesian designs were used in the Biomarker-Integrated Approaches of Targeted Therapy for Lung Cancer Elimination (BATTLE) trial and the Investigation of Serial Studies to Predict Your Therapeutic Response with Imaging and Molecular Analysis 2 (I-SPY2) trial in breast cancer.[58] Recently, the FDA guidance defined a clinical study using an adaptive design as one that "includes a prospectively planned opportunity for modification of one or more specified aspects of the study design and hypotheses based on analysis of data (usually interim data) from subjects in the study. Analyses of the accumulating study data are carried out at

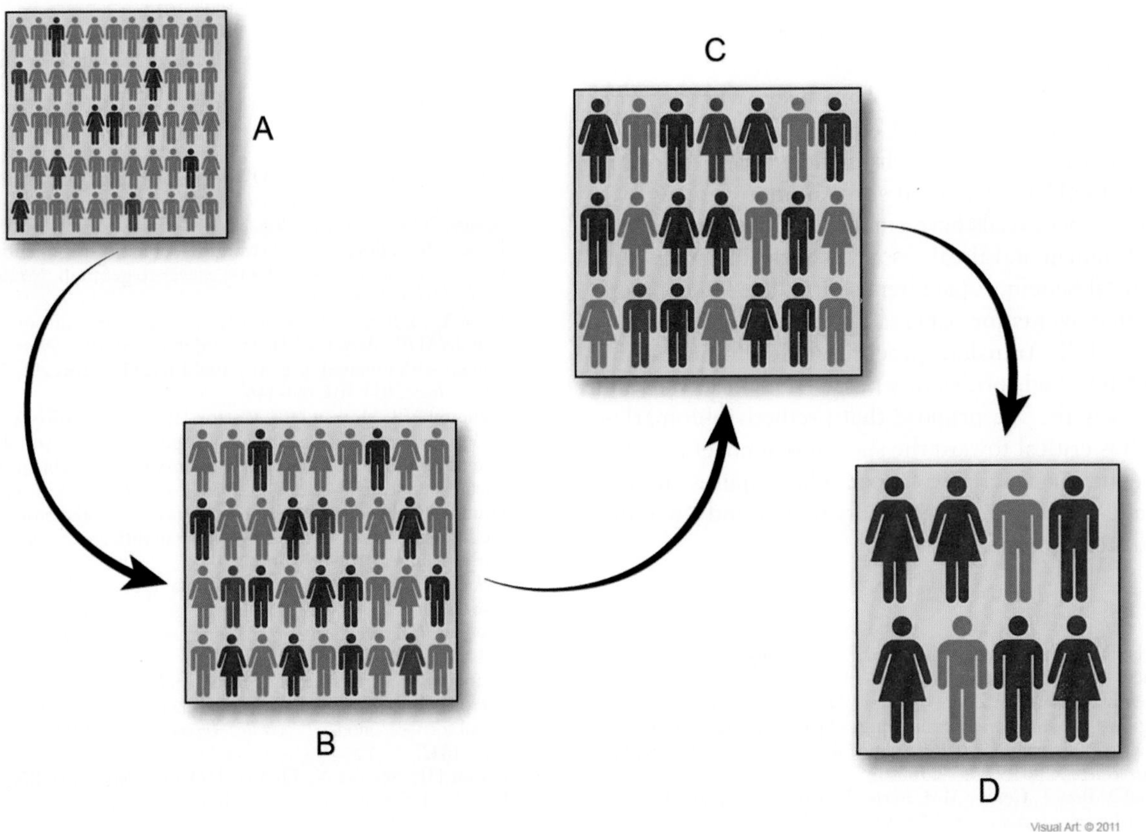

FIGURE 59–4 Bayesian adaptive clinical trial design enriches the study population for the potential predictive biomarker. Enrolled study subjects are not preselected and have two potential biomarkers—marked blue and red (**A**). As the study progresses, the study outcomes are utilized to adaptively enroll subjects with the greatest likelihood of a positive result. Biomarker blue has a positive correlation with clinical outcome on interim analysis (**B**). Study enrollment is "adapted" to include those with the favorable biomarker (**C**). Finally, the study population gets enriched for the blue biomarker (**D**).

prospectively planned time points within the study, can be performed in a fully blinded manner or in an unblended manner, and can occur with or without formal statistical hypothesis testing."[59] This is illustrated in Figure 59.4. These designs are particularly useful when the distribution of the biomarker within the population is not known with a great degree of certainty. Furthermore, more than one therapeutic can be assessed simultaneously in a multi-arm phase II study. Tissue biopsy analysis (either obtained as a part of the trial or through retrospective analysis of archival material) is mandated prior to treatment administration as the results of the same are used to allocate the treatment arm. These trials are intrinsically adaptive in that as the clinical data become more mature, as usually determined on an interim analysis, the study conduct can be modified accordingly. In a multi-arm adaptive phase II trial, several therapeutic agents can be examined and pharmaceutical companies can utilize this information to move the most promising agent to the phase III setting. While the clinical benefit of the stratification design is proven, the adaptive designs are relatively novel and their therapeutic benefit therefore remains to be proven. An interesting new trial design proposed is the adaptive phase III clinical trial, wherein the biomarker development occurs primarily in the phase III setting.[60]

The adaptive phase III trial is based on the hypothesis that the probability of identifying a predictive biomarker is high. Patients in this trial design may be randomized to a hypothetical drug X versus control. All patients included have adequate biopsy sample prior to enrollment and the analysis for predictive biomarkers is performed retrospectively. Following completion of trial accrual, if a log-rank comparison of survival reveals clear superiority in the treatment arm ($P < 0.001$), the study compound will be declared as effective for the entire study cohort. If on the other hand, the survival difference is less striking, then an adaptive signature approach as recommended by Freidlin et al. may be used.[61] In the latter instance, a predictive classifier is created in which a set of biomarkers is individually assessed for their predictive value in a randomly selected training set consisting of 33% of the study population. Subsequent training and validation of the biomarker occur in the remainder (67%) of the population (validation set). This design is further discussed by Scher et al.[60]

To our knowledge, there have been over 14 randomized, controlled phase III clinical trials in advanced pancreatic cancer, 2 of which (gemcitabine + erlotinib and FOLFIRINOX) showed survival improvement over controls.[7] These trials have entailed considerable investment of human and fiscal resources with extremely limited clinical benefit. A paradigm shift in the development of targeted agents for pancreatic cancer is needed so as to successfully translate preclinical development and research into high-probability phase III clinical trials and patient benefit. We propose that predictive biomarker research is critical toward the success of a novel targeted therapeutic for pancreatic cancer. This requires support from industry, academia, regulatory bodies, and advocates so as to result in patient benefit.

REFERENCES

1. Parkin DM, Bray F, Ferlay J, Pisani P. Estimating the world cancer burden: Globocan 2000. *Int J Cancer*. 2001;94:153-156.
2. Chen KX, Wang PP, Zhang SW, Li LD, Lu FZ, Hao XS. Regional variations in mortality rates of pancreatic cancer in China: results from 1990-1992 national mortality survey. *World J Gastroenterol*. 2003;9:2557-2560.
3. Jemal A, Bray F, Center MM, Ferlay J, Ward E, Forman D. Global cancer statistics. *CA Cancer J Clin*. 2011;61:69-90.
4. Burris HA 3rd, Moore MJ, Andersen J, et al. Improvements in survival and clinical benefit with gemcitabine as first-line therapy for patients with advanced pancreas cancer: a randomized trial. *J Clin Oncol*. 1997;15:2403-2413.
5. El-Rayes BF, Philip PA. A review of systemic therapy for advanced pancreatic cancer. *Clin Adv Hematol Oncol*. 2003;1:430-434.
6. Van Cutsem E, van de Velde H, Karasek P, et al. Phase III trial of gemcitabine plus tipifarnib compared with gemcitabine plus placebo in advanced pancreatic cancer. *J Clin Oncol*. 2004;22:1430-1438.
7. Rocha-Lima CM. New directions in the management of advanced pancreatic cancer: a review. *Anticancer Drugs*. 2008;19:435-446.
8. Philip PA, Benedetti J, Corless CL, et al. Phase III study comparing gemcitabine plus cetuximab versus gemcitabine in patients with advanced pancreatic adenocarcinoma: Southwest Oncology Group-directed intergroup trial S0205. *J Clin Oncol*. 2010;28:3605-3610.
9. Kindler HL, Niedzwiecki D, Hollis D, et al. Gemcitabine plus bevacizumab compared with gemcitabine plus placebo in patients with advanced pancreatic cancer: phase III trial of the Cancer and Leukemia Group B (CALGB 80303). *J Clin Oncol*. 2010;28:3617-3622.
10. Moore MJ, Goldstein D, Hamm J, et al. Erlotinib plus gemcitabine compared with gemcitabine alone in patients with advanced pancreatic cancer: a phase III trial of the National Cancer Institute of Canada Clinical Trials Group. *J Clin Oncol*. 2007;25:1960-1966.
11. Conroy T, Desseigne F, Ychou M, et al. FOLFIRINOX versus gemcitabine for metastatic pancreatic cancer. *N Engl J Med*. 2011;364:1817-1825.
12. Fogelman DR, Wolff RA, Kopetz S, et al. Evidence for the efficacy of Iniparib, a PARP-1 inhibitor, in BRCA2-associated pancreatic cancer. *Anticancer Res*. 2011;31:1417-1420.
13. Moore LE, Nickerson ML, Brennan P, et al. Von Hippel-Lindau (VHL) inactivation in sporadic clear cell renal cancer: associations with germline VHL polymorphisms and etiologic risk factors. *PLoS Genet*. 2011;7:e1002312.
14. Shaw AT, Yeap BY, Solomon BJ, et al. Effect of crizotinib on overall survival in patients with advanced non-small-cell lung cancer harbouring ALK gene rearrangement: a retrospective analysis. *Lancet Oncol*. 2011;12:1004-1012.
15. Von Hoff DD, LoRusso PM, Rudin CM, et al. Inhibition of the Hedgehog pathway in advanced basal-cell carcinoma. *N Engl J Med*. 2009;361:1164-1172.
16. Flaherty KT, Puzanov I, Kim KB, et al. Inhibition of mutated, activated BRAF in metastatic melanoma. *N Engl J Med*. 2010;363:809-819.
17. Jones S, Zhang X, Parsons DW, et al. Core signaling pathways in human pancreatic cancers revealed by global genomic analyses. *Science*. 2008;321:1801-1806.
18. Kobayashi S, Boggon TJ, Dayaram T, et al. EGFR mutation and resistance of non-small-cell lung cancer to gefitinib. *N Engl J Med*. 2005;352:786-792.
19. Drew Y, Mulligan EA, Vong WT, et al. Therapeutic potential of poly(ADP-ribose) polymerase inhibitor AG014699 in human cancers with mutated or methylated BRCA1 or BRCA2. *J Natl Cancer Inst*. 2011;103:334-346.
20. Jamieson NB, Morran DC, Morton JP, et al. MicroRNA molecular profiles associated with diagnosis, clinicopathological criteria, and overall survival in patients with resectable pancreatic ductal adenocarcinoma. *Clin Cancer Res*. 2012;8(2):534-545.
21. Hummel R, Hussey DJ, Haier J. MicroRNAs: predictors and modifiers of chemo- and radiotherapy in different tumour types. *Eur J Cancer*. 2010;46:298-311.
22. Ohuchida K, Mizumoto K, Kayashima T, et al. MicroRNA expression as a predictive marker for gemcitabine response after surgical resection of pancreatic cancer. *Ann Surg Oncol*. 2011;18:2381-2387.
23. Frampton AE, Krell J, Jacob J, Stebbing J, Jiao LR, Castellano L. microRNAs as markers of survival and chemoresistance in pancreatic ductal adenocarcinoma. *Expert Rev Anticancer Ther*. 2011;11:1837-1842.
24. Bryant HE, Schultz N, Thomas HD, et al. Specific killing of BRCA2-deficient tumours with inhibitors of poly(ADP-ribose) polymerase. *Nature*. 2005;434:913-917.
25. Farmer H, McCabe N, Lord CJ, et al. Targeting the DNA repair defect in BRCA mutant cells as a therapeutic strategy. *Nature*. 2005;434:917-921.
26. Jones S, Hruban RH, Kamiyama M, et al. Exomic sequencing identifies PALB2 as a pancreatic cancer susceptibility gene. *Science*. 2009;324:217.
27. McCabe N, Turner NC, Lord CJ, et al. Deficiency in the repair of DNA damage by homologous recombination and sensitivity to poly(ADP-ribose) polymerase inhibition. *Cancer Res*. 2006;66:8109-8115.
28. Li D, Liu H, Jiao L, et al. Significant effect of homologous recombination DNA repair gene polymorphisms on pancreatic cancer survival. *Cancer Res*. 2006;66:3323-3330.
29. Maacke H, Jost K, Opitz S, et al. DNA repair and recombination factor Rad51 is over-expressed in human pancreatic adenocarcinoma. *Oncogene*. 2000;19:2791-2795.
30. Hunt CR, Gupta A, Horikoshi N, Pandita TK. Does PTEN loss impair DNA double-strand break repair by homologous recombination? *Clin Cancer Res*. 2011;15;18(4):920-922.
31. Ming M, Feng L, Shea CR, et al. PTEN positively regulates UVB-induced DNA damage repair. *Cancer Res*. 2011;71:5287-5295.
32. Meyn RE. Linking PTEN with genomic instability and DNA repair. *Cell Cycle*. 2009;8:2322-2323.
33. Mendes-Pereira AM, Martin SA, Brough R, et al. Synthetic lethal targeting of PTEN mutant cells with PARP inhibitors. *EMBO Mol Med*. 2009;1:315-322.
34. Tascilar M, Skinner HG, Rosty C, et al. The SMAD4 protein and prognosis of pancreatic ductal adenocarcinoma. *Clin Cancer Res*. 2001;7:4115-4121.
35. Blackford A, Serrano OK, Wolfgang CL, et al. SMAD4 gene mutations are associated with poor prognosis in pancreatic cancer. *Clin Cancer Res*. 2009;15:4674-4679.
36. Zhao S, Venkatasubbarao K, Lazor JW, et al. Inhibition of STAT3 Tyr705 phosphorylation by Smad4 suppresses transforming growth factor beta-mediated invasion and metastasis in pancreatic cancer cells. *Cancer Res*. 2008;68:4221-4228.

37. Melisi D, Ishiyama S, Sclabas GM, et al. LY2109761, a novel transforming growth factor beta receptor type I and type II dual inhibitor, as a therapeutic approach to suppressing pancreatic cancer metastasis. *Mol Cancer Ther*. 2008;7:829-840.
38. Withers DJ, Burks DJ, Towery HH, Altamuro SL, Flint CL, White MF. Irs-2 coordinates Igf-1 receptor-mediated beta-cell development and peripheral insulin signalling. *Nat Genet*. 1999;23:32-40.
39. Golan T, Javle M. Targeting the insulin growth factor pathway in gastrointestinal cancers. *Oncology (Williston Park)*. 2011;25: 518-526, 529.
40. Dong X, Javle M, Hess KR, Shroff R, Abbruzzese JL, Li D. Insulin-like growth factor axis gene polymorphisms and clinical outcomes in pancreatic cancer. *Gastroenterology*. 2010;139:464-473, 473.e1-473.e3.
41. Javle MM, Varadhachary GR, Fogelman DR, et al. Randomized phase II study of gemcitabine (G) plus anti-IGF-1R antibody MK-0646, G plus erlotinib (E) plus MK-0646 and G plus E for advanced pancreatic cancer. ASCO Meeting Abstracts. *J Clin Oncol*. 2011;29(suppl):Abstract 4026.
42. Kindler HL, Richards DA, Stephenson J, et al. A placebo-controlled, randomized phase II study of conatumumab (C) or AMG 479 (A) or placebo (P) plus gemcitabine (G) in patients (pts) with metastatic pancreatic cancer (mPC). ASCO Meeting Abstracts. *J Clin Oncol*. 2010;28(suppl):Abstract 4035.
43. Reidy DL, Vakiani E, Fakih MG, et al. Randomized, phase II study of the insulin-like growth factor-1 receptor inhibitor IMC-A12, with or without cetuximab, in patients with cetuximab- or panitumumab-refractory metastatic colorectal cancer. *J Clin Oncol*. 2010;28:4240-4246.
44. Zha J, O'Brien C, Savage H, et al. Molecular predictors of response to a humanized anti-insulin-like growth factor-I receptor monoclonal antibody in breast and colorectal cancer. *Mol Cancer Ther*. 2009;8:2110-2121.
45. Pitts TM, Tan AC, Kulikowski GN, et al. Development of an integrated genomic classifier for a novel agent in colorectal cancer: approach to individualized therapy in early development. *Clin Cancer Res*. 2010;16:3193-3204.
46. Gualberto A, Dolled-Filhart M, Gustavson M, et al. Molecular analysis of non-small cell lung cancer (NSCLC) identifies subsets with different sensitivity to insulin like growth factor I receptor (IGF-IR) inhibition. *Clin Cancer Res*. 2010;16(18): 4654-4665.
47. Lowery MA, O'Reilly EM. Genomics and pharmacogenomics of pancreatic adenocarcinoma. *Pharmacogenomics J*. 2012;12(1):1-9.
48. Bepler G, Kusmartseva I, Sharma S, et al. RRM1 modulated in vitro and in vivo efficacy of gemcitabine and platinum in non-small-cell lung cancer. *J Clin Oncol*. 2006;24:4731-4737.
49. Farrell JJ, Elsaleh H, Garcia M, et al. Human equilibrative nucleoside transporter 1 levels predict response to gemcitabine in patients with pancreatic cancer. *Gastroenterology*. 2009;136:187-195.
50. Okazaki T, Javle M, Tanaka M, Abbruzzese JL, Li D. Single nucleotide polymorphisms of gemcitabine metabolic genes and pancreatic cancer survival and drug toxicity. *Clin Cancer Res*. 2010;16:320-329.
51. Ueno H, Kiyosawa K, Kaniwa N. Pharmacogenomics of gemcitabine: can genetic studies lead to tailor-made therapy? *Br J Cancer*. 2007;97:145-151.
52. NSABP study confirms oncotype DX predicts chemotherapy benefit in breast cancer patients. *Oncology (Williston Park)*. 2006;20:789-790.
53. Slodkowska EA, Ross JS. MammaPrint 70-gene signature: another milestone in personalized medical care for breast cancer patients. *Expert Rev Mol Diagn*. 2009;9:417-422.
54. Medicare, Medicaid, and Clinical Laboratories Improvement Act (CLIA) patient confidentiality rules; proposed rule. *Fed Regist*. 1988;53:10404-10406.
55. International Conference on Harmonisation; Guidance on E16 Biomarkers Related to Drug or Biotechnology Product Development: Context, Structure, and Format of Qualification Submissions; availability. Notice. *Fed Regist*. 2011;76:49773-49774.
56. Iyer L, Das S, Janisch L, et al. UGT1A1*28 polymorphism as a determinant of irinotecan disposition and toxicity. *Pharmacogenomics J*. 2002;2:43-47.
57. Mandrekar SJ, Sargent DJ. Clinical trial designs for predictive biomarker validation: one size does not fit all. *J Biopharm Stat*. 2009;19:530-542.
58. Gold KA, Kim ES, Lee JJ, Wistuba II, Farhangfar CJ, Hong WK. The BATTLE to personalize lung cancer prevention through reverse migration. *Cancer Prev Res (Phila)*. 2011;4:962-972.
59. Berry DA. Adaptive clinical trials in oncology. *Nat Rev Clin Oncol*. 2011;9(4):199-207.
60. Scher HI, Nasso SF, Rubin EH, Simon R. Adaptive clinical trial designs for simultaneous testing of matched diagnostics and therapeutics. *Clin Cancer Res*. 2011;17:6634-6640.
61. Freidlin B, Jiang W, Simon R. The cross-validated adaptive signature design. *Clin Cancer Res*. 2010;16:691-698.

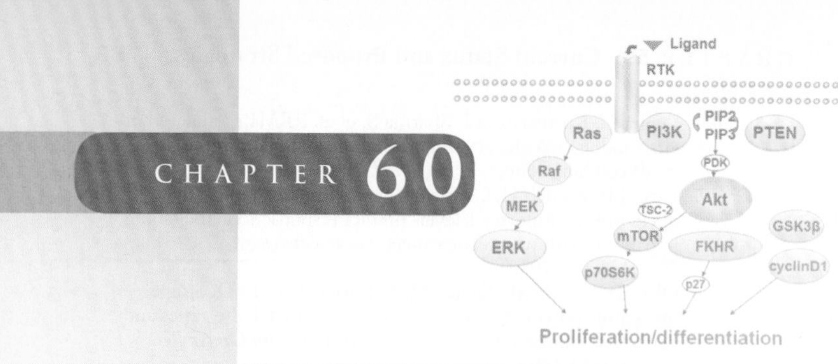

CHAPTER 60

Personalized Medicine and Targeted Therapy of Neuroendocrine Neoplasms

Jeana Garris and James C. Yao

INTRODUCTION

Neuroendocrine tumors (NETs) represent an eclectic group of malignancies that arise from neuroendocrine cells scattered throughout the body. They are subdivided into categories based on the primary site of disease and further classified by a grading system. Outside of a few hereditary cancer syndromes, the environmental and genetic risk factors involved in carcinogenesis are not well understood.[1] Many small NETs can remain silent during the patients' lifetime and are only incidentally found at autopsy.[2] Others can present as symptomatic tumors localized to the organ of origin, have regional spread, or with a variable volume of distant metastatic disease.

NETs may be classified as functional or nonfunctional types based on whether they produce peptides or amines that cause a distinct syndrome. Hormone secreted can include vasoactive intestinal polypeptide, insulin, glucagon, gastrin, adrenocorticotropic hormone, and somatostatin. Classic carcinoid syndrome is a conglomeration of symptoms related to secretion of serotonin into the systemic circulation. It can include flushing, diarrhea, abdominal pain, carcinoid heart disease, telangiectasia, wheezing, and pellagra. Flushing is generally a dry, reddening of the face and upper torso, as opposed to menopausal hot flashes that tend to lead to sweating.

EPIDEMIOLOGY

According to the SEER (The Surveillance, Epidemiology, and End Results) database, there has been a significant increase in the reported annual age-adjusted incidence of NETs from 1973 (1.09/100,000) to 2004 (5.25/100,000).[3] It is also likely underestimated due to the underreporting of what were considered benign tumors in the past but now have been shown to have malignant potential. Approximately 21% of those with well-differentiated tumors and 30% of those with moderately differentiated tumors had synchronous distant metastasis at diagnosis, whereas 50% of those with poorly differentiated tumors or undifferentiated tumors had synchronous distant metastasis at diagnosis.[3] The median survival duration in patients with well- to moderately differentiated NETs was 124 and 64 months, respectively. Patients with poorly differentiated and undifferentiated tumors had identical survival curves; the median survival duration in these patients was 10 months.[3]

PATHOLOGIC CLASSIFICATION AND STAGING OF NETS

Grade and Differentiation

Although grade and differentiation have often been used interchangeably, there are implicit differences in these terms. Differentiation refers to the similarity between the tumor histology and tissue of origin, whereas grade is based on markers of proliferation such as mitotic rate and Ki-67 proliferative index. Both the European Neuroendocrine Tumor Society (ENETs) and American Joint Commission on Cancer (AJCC) have adopted a common grading system based on mitotic rate and Ki-67 (Table 60.1).[4,5] In general, poorly differentiated (high-grade) tumors are characterized by an elevated mitotic rate (>20 mitoses per 10 high-powered fields), a high Ki-67 proliferative index (typically >20%), extensive

TABLE 60-1 Grading Systems for Neuroendocrine Tumors

Grade	Criteria
Low grade (G1)	<2 mitoses/10 hpf and <3% Ki67 index
Intermediate grade (G2)	2–20 mitoses/10 hpf or 3-20% Ki67 index
High grade (G3)	>20 mitoses/10 hpf or >20% Ki67 index

necrosis, and pleomorphism. Well-differentiated tumors are considered low to intermediate grades and are sometimes called carcinoid tumors. It is commonly accepted that low-grade tumors have a Ki-67 of <2% and intermediate grade is considered 3% to 20%. The uniform application of this grading system will be critical for optimal clinical care and future progress in this field.

In general, the principles of therapy for poorly differentiated or high-grade NETs fundamentally differ from those for well-differentiated (low- to intermediate-grade) NETs. High-grade NETs are aggressive, fast growing tumors. The management strategies of these tumors parallel those of small cell lung cancer. While distinction between low- to intermediate-grade tumors offers prognostic value, well-differentiated tumors are generally managed in a similar manner.

Staging

As with grading, ENETs[4,5] and AJCC have proposed TNM staging systems for NETs.[6] While these two staging systems are similar for tumors arising in the luminal gut, they differ for earlier stage tumors arising in the pancreas or appendix. In pancreatic NETs, for example, the ENETs system incorporates tumor diameter in its assessment of T stage, whereas the AJCC system incorporates factors determining tumor resectability. Both systems have been clinically validated and are identical in their definitions of stage IV disease. Whether one system is superior for pancreas in particular continues to be debated. However, with the adoption of AJCC system by the Union for International Cancer Control (UICC), this will likely be the widely used system.

Other Immunohistochemical Studies

In addition to Ki-67 and/or mitotic rate, other immunohistochemical studies often include chromogranin A (CGA), synaptophysin, and cytokeratin. If an unknown primary tumor is found, additional pathology testing may be warranted. TTF-1 (thyroid transcription factor-1) staining often points to thyroid or a thoracic primary site, whereas CDX-2 often points to luminal bowel. Recent studies also suggest that allelic loss of chromosome 18 is characteristic of small bowel carcinoids.[7] Further studies are needed to confirm whether loss of heterozygosity of chromosome 18 can be used to classify unknown primary NETs or direct therapy.

Hereditary Syndromes

There are endocrine-associated autosomal dominant diseases that can manifest in formation of tumors throughout the body system, excluding midgut carcinoid tumors. Multiple endocrine neoplasia type 1 (MEN-1) can affect the parathyroid, endocrine pancreas, and anterior pituitary.[1] There is almost always a reported family history of benign tumors forming in the parathyroid gland causing hypercalcemia and nephrolithiasis at an early age of onset. The pituitary tumors may present with vision changes and should be surgically resected if at all possible. NETs of the pancreas are detected as well and may be functional or non-functional. Carcinoids of the lung and thymus can also occur. In general, NETs of pancreas, lung, and thymus have a greater malignant potential.

MEN-2 is a similar disease characterized most often by medullary thyroid carcinoma, then pheochromocytoma and primary hyperparathyroidism. Hereditary medullary thyroid cancer can occur in 25% to 30% of cases and MEN-2 should be suspected and evaluated by genetic counseling.

Tuberous sclerosis (TSC) is associated with benign hamartomas and low-grade neoplasms of the brain, heart, skin, kidney, lung, and pancreas. The most common clinical signs can be mental retardation and epilepsy. Mutations to TSC1 and TSC2 can lead to high levels of mammalian target of rapamycin (mTOR) signaling causing protein synthesis and cell growth.[8] This pathway has been of particular interest in treating this disease as well as other endocrine neoplasms.

Diagnosis and Workup

Presentation of symptoms can be variable based on the patient's primary site of disease. A locoregional small bowel carcinoid may present with a mass manifesting obstructive type symptoms. Carcinoid syndrome is more likely to occur in patients with advanced disease of the midgut and may also be the first initial sign of concern. This is likely due to the fact that secreted hormones are metabolized in the liver through portal circulation, prior to reaching systemic flow.

Generally, laboratory studies are recommended as well as hormone-related studies including 24-hour urine 5-HIAA (5-hydroxyindoleacetic acid) with strict dietary restrictions prior to collection, serum CGA, neuron-specific enolase (NSE), and other hormones that may be secreted based on presenting symptoms. CGA is present in secretory granules of neuroendocrine cells. It can be falsely elevated with the use of proton pump inhibitors as well in patients with chronic gastritis, kidney dysfunction, or liver dysfunction. The urine 5-HIAA gives a consistent measurement of serotonin metabolism in the body that can correlate to carcinoid syndrome. NSE is a glycolytic isoenzyme located in the cytoplasmic compartment of cells.

Because of the rare nature of NETs, these markers have low positive predictive value and should not be used in screening low-risk patients. They can be helpful among patients with suspected disease and as prognostic markers.

Recently, studies have focused on possible serum biomarkers to evaluate disease response and survival. It has been shown that patients with metastatic pancreatic NETs with a baseline-elevated CGA had a decreased median progression-free survival (PFS) as opposed to baseline non-elevated CGA (8.3 vs. 15.6 mo).[9] The same was true for the baseline-elevated NSE, with a median PFS of 7.6 months when compared with the 12.3 months in non-elevated patients.[9] These markers may also be shown to be prognostic indicators in the future for patients receiving treatment. A study showed that those undergoing treatment with everolimus with early CGA response had statistically significant improvement in median PFS than those that did not show an early CGA response (13.3 vs. 7.5 mo).[9] The same was true for patients with early response in the serum NSE (8.6 vs. 2.9 mo). Median overall survival (OS) in patients with elevated baseline CGA was 16.95 months and had not been reached at the time of reporting for the non-elevated group. Elevated NSE versus non-elevated NSE showed an OS of 14.0 versus 24.9 months.[9]

It is recognized that NETs can sometimes change which hormones and amines they produce. The general principle of biomarker measurement is to evaluate a large panel of a marker at key points of the disease such as at diagnosis or relapse. In doing so, you may identify a few biomarkers that are elevated in the particular patient in question and follow these over time, correlating them to imaging findings. It is generally not necessary to check every biomarker at every visit.

It is recommended that initial workup include a multiphasic computed tomography (CT) or magnetic resonance imaging (MRI) of the abdomen and pelvis as well as an [^{111}In-DTPA^{0}]octreotide scintigraphy. For evaluation of an unknown primary tumor but suspected midgut, a CT with negative bowel contrast may elucidate a primary tumor. [^{111}In-DTPA^{0}]octreotide scintigraphy is helpful to identify areas of unknown disease located throughout the body. Fludeoxyglucose positron emission tomography imaging is usually reserved for poorly differentiated tumors with a higher proliferative rate.

SURGICAL MANAGEMENT

Surgery is the only curative approach for NET patients and should be considered first-line for local–regional disease of any primary site. In patients with carcinoid syndrome, every attempt to have this well controlled prior to surgery is recommended. After complete resection of disease, there is no role for adjuvant therapy. In patients with bulky disease or metastasis, cytoreductive resection should be considered to reduce the risk of future complications or current symptoms. Liver transplantation in the face of metastatic disease to the liver has long been an area of debate. It has traditionally been restricted to individuals with limited tumor bulk, absence of disseminated disease, and biologically favorable features. The UNOS database was analyzed for all patients undergoing transplantation in the United States from October 1, 1988, through January 31, 2008. Data from all patients undergoing liver transplantation for metastatic NETs were captured for analysis, which totaled 150 patients. Overall, 1-, 3-, and 5-year survival rates were 81%, 65%, and 49%, respectively.[10]

Liver-Directed Therapy

Cytoreduction of liver tumor burden can be quite beneficial for patients' quality of life. Techniques can include such things as ablative procedures and hepatic artery embolizations that are bland, chemotherapy based, or with radioactive microspheres. No good comparative studies have been performed to assess OS benefit from one technique to another.

Yttrium-90 is a pure high-energy β-emitter with a mean tissue penetration of 2.5 mm. The principle surrounding the therapy is the preferential tumor-related vascular distribution of the radioactive microspheres, which allows the delivery of high doses of radiation to the tumor with relative sparing of normal liver parenchyma. It is important to recognize that radioembolization has distinct dissimilarities from other hepatic embolization procedures. Although a direct comparison has not been performed within the context of a clinical trial, the acute and subacute toxicities associated with this treatment in patients with hepatocellular carcinoma and colorectal cancer appear to be more tolerable than those associated with other hepatic embolization procedures and have allowed the treatment to be delivered on an outpatient basis. Neuroendocrine hepatic metastases may also be amenable to hepatic artery radioembolization because they share characteristics of hypervascularity and multifocality.[11]

A study of 42 patients was done to evaluate the safety, efficacy, and symptom control of radioembolization in patients with unresectable NET with liver metastases.[12] Contrast-enhanced axial CT and/or MRI images were available in 40 patients. Imaging follow-up using RECIST [Response Evaluation Criteria in Solid Tumors] at 3-month follow-up demonstrated partial response, stable disease, and progressive disease in 22.5%, 75%, and 2.5% of patients, respectively. Thirty-eight of 42 patients showed tumor-related clinical symptoms before treatment. In 36 of 38 patients, a significant improvement or disappearance of clinical symptoms was observed 3 months after treatment.[12]

SYSTEMIC THERAPY FOR PANCREATIC NETS

Chemotherapy for Pancreatic NETs

Pancreatic NETs have long been treated with streptozocin-based therapy. Common streptozocin-based regimens used for pancreatic NETs include streptozocin/

5-fluorouracil, streptozocin/doxorubicin, or a three-drug combination of streptozocin/doxorubicin/5-fluorouracil.[13] The Eastern Cooperative Oncology Group subsequently compared streptozocin plus 5-fluorouracil with streptozocin plus doxorubicin[14] and reported a significantly higher response rate (69% vs. 45%), time to progression (median, 20 vs. 7 mo), and OS (median, 2.2 vs. 1.4 y) for streptozocin plus doxorubicin. Two recent case series using modern response criteria, however, reported only modest response rates of 9%.[15,16] With the controversy regarding the role of chemotherapy in the management of unresectable and metastatic pancreatic NETs, we a review of the M.D. Anderson cancer center experience with a three-drug regimen of 5-flurouracil, doxorubicin, and streptozocin,[13] showed a response rate of 39%, with median response duration of 9.3 months. The 2-year PFS rate was 41% and the 2-year OS rate was 74%.

Temozolomide, an oral analogue of dacarbazine, has been found to be active in pancreatic NETs. Studies in glioma suggest deficient O^6-methylguanine DNA methyltransferase (MGMT) expression may be a predictive marker for benefit to temozolomide. MGMT deficiency was observed in 19 of 37 (51%) pancreatic NETs and 0 of 60 (0%) carcinoid tumors ($P < 0.0001$) in a recent study.[17] In the clinical cohort, 18 of 53 (34%) patients with pancreatic NETs but only 1 of 44 (2%) patients with carcinoid tumors experienced a partial or complete response to temozolomide-based therapy. Clinical outcome strongly correlated with MGMT expression status suggesting MGMT may be used as a predictive biomarker in the future.

In smaller case series, higher response rates have been reported for the combination of capecitabine and temozolomide.[18] However, an adequate prospective controlled study to define the role of temozolomide or combination temozolomide-based combination therapy in pancreatic NET is lacking, and promising activity of this cytotoxic agent awaits confirmation.

mTOR Inhibition in Pancreatic NETs

Everolimus inhibits mTOR, a serine–threonine kinase that stimulates cell growth, proliferation, and angiogenesis. Genetic cancer syndromes (TSC2, NF-1 [neurofibromatosis type 1], and vHL [von Hippel-Landau]), somatic mutations identified using an exome sequencing approach, and expression profiling have consistently implicated a dysfunction of the mTOR pathway as a critical event in pancreatic NETs.[8,19,20]

Both temsirolimus and everolimus have been studied in NETs (Tables 60.1 and 60.2). In the temsirolimus study, 37 patients with progressive NETs received temsirolimus intravenously at 25 mg/wk.[21] The investigators found that temsirolimus had modest clinical activity, with a response rate of 5.6% and median time to progression of 6 months.

Everolimus was studied in a multi-national phase II study (RADIANT-1) enrolling 160 patients with advanced pancreatic NETs and evidence of RECIST-defined progression following chemotherapy. In *stratum 1*, 115 patients were treated with everolimus 10 mg/d; in *stratum 2*, 45 patients were treated with everolimus 10 mg/d plus octreotide LAR ≤ 30 mg every 28 days. In *stratum 1*, 11 (9.6%) patients showed partial response and 78 (67.8%) had stable disease, yielding a clinical benefit of 77.4%. In *stratum 2*, 2 (4.4%) patients achieved partial response and 36 (80.0%) patients had stable disease, yielding a clinical benefit of 84.4%. Median PFS was 9.7 months in patients in *stratum 1*, and 16.7 months in patients in *stratum 2*.[22]

Activity of everolimus was further confirmed in RADIANT-3, a multi-national double-blind placebo-controlled phase III study among patients with progressive advanced pancreatic NETs.[23] The study enrolled 410 patients. Median PFS was 11.0 months (95% confidence interval [CI], 8.4 to 13.9) in the everolimus group, when compared with 4.6 months (95% CI, 3.1 to 5.4) in the placebo group, representing a 65% reduction (Table 60.2; hazard ratio [HR] = 0.35, 95% CI, 0.27 to 0.45; $P <$ 0.0001) in the estimated risk of progression.

TABLE 60-2 Recent Phase III Studies in Advanced Neuroendocrine Tumors

Regimen	*N*	Median PFS/TTP (Months)	*P*
Pancreatic NETs			
Sunitinib	171	11.4 PFS	0.0001[a]
Placebo		5.5	
Everolimus	410	11 PFS	<0.0001
Placebo		4.6	
Carcinoid tumors			
Octreotide LAR	90	14.3 TTP	<0.0001
Placebo		6.0	
Everolimus + octreotide LAR	429	16.4 PFS	0.026[b]
Placebo + octreotide LAR		11.3	

PFS, progression-free survival; TTP, time to progression.
[a]Not statistically significant due to unplanned analyses and early termination.
[b]Not statistically significant. Pre-specified boundary is $P \leq 0.0246$.

VEGF Inhibition in Pancreatic NETs

Another highly investigated target in NETs is the vascular endothelial growth factor (VEGF) signaling pathway. Sunitinib is a tyrosine kinase inhibitor that targets this as well as platelet-derived growth factor receptors (PDGFRs)-α and PDGFR-β, stem-cell factor receptor (c-kit), and VEGF receptor (VEGFR)-2 and VEGFR-3. Sunitinib was evaluated in a large phase II study in NETs.[24] A higher response rate was observed in the pancreatic NET group (16.7%) compared with the carcinoid group (2.4%). This along with a promising median PFS of 7.7 (95% CI, 6.5 to 12.5) months in the pancreatic NET group led to the development of a multinational phase III study. Although the enrollment of 340 patients was originally planned, the study terminated early prior to the first planned interim analysis after enrollment of 171 patients. With 81 events, an improvement in PFS with sunitinib was observed. Median PFS was 11.4 months in the sunitinib arm compared with 5.5 months in the placebo arm (Table 60.2; HR = 0.42, 95% CI, 0.26 to 0.66).[25] Although the study failed to achieve statistical significance due to unplanned interim analyses and early termination, its results are supported by other studies of VEGF inhibitors in pancreatic NET.[24,26,27]

SYSTEMIC THERAPIES FOR CARCINOIDS

The oncologic management of carcinoid tumors remains a challenge. While somatostatin analogues (SSAs) are effective for the control of carcinoid syndrome, there are currently no FDA approved drugs for the control of tumor growth.

SSA in Carcinoid Tumors

Native human somatostatin functions as an inhibitor of endocrine activity but has a very short half-life. In the digestive tract, it decreases portal blood flow, reduces gastrointestinal secretion, inhibits peristalsis, and downregulates the secretion of other gastrointestinal hormones. Somatostatin exerts its effects through interaction with five somatostatin receptors (ssts1–5). Synthetic SSAs, such as octreotide and lanreotide, have been designed with a longer half-life of 2 hours and a higher binding affinity to somatostatin receptors. Both analogues bind avidly to sst2 and moderately to sst5. Octreotide has been FDA approved since 1987 for carcinoid syndrome. In a landmark study, octreotide was tested in 25 patients with malignant carcinoid syndrome.[28] Flushing and diarrhea were substantially palliated in 22 patients (88%), and major reductions in urine 5-HIAA were reported in 18 cases (72%).[28] Pasireotide, a novel SSA, is currently in clinical development. It binds avidly to four of the five somatostatin receptors (sst1, sst2, sst3, and sst5). An open-label trial evaluated the activity of subcutaneous pasireotide in patients with carcinoid syndrome whose symptoms were inadequately controlled on octreotide.[29] Preliminary data indicated activity in this refractory population.

Previously, SSAs have been used to control the symptoms associated with carcinoid syndrome. The Placebo-controlled, double-blind, prospective, Randomized study on the effect of Octreotide LAR in the control of tumor growth in patients with metastatic neuroendocrine MIDgut tumors (PROMID) study showed that long-acting octreotide significantly improved the time to progression in treatment-naïve patients with midgut carcinoids (Table 2; HR = 0.34, 95% CI, 0.2 to 0.59).[30] Median time to tumor progression in the octreotide LAR and placebo groups was 14.3 and 6 months, respectively. Functionally active and inactive tumors responded similarly. The extent of hepatic tumor burden (patients with ≤10% hepatic tumor load) appeared to be a prognostic factor.[30] The utility of SSAs such as octreotide or lanreotide for control of tumor growth in NETs of other primary sites remains undefined.

Chemotherapy in Carcinoid Tumors

In most midgut NETs, there has been no evidence to support the use of chemotherapy. However, streptozocin-based treatments have been shown to be effective in pancreatic NETs with a response rate of 35% to 55%.[13] Low-grade NETs originating outside the pancreas appear generally resistant to the effects of cytotoxic chemotherapy.

Interferon in Carcinoid Tumors

Interferon can exert antitumor effects through a variety of mechanisms such as inhibition of angiogenesis and in NETs, interferon-α can also induce upregulation of somatostatin receptors. Early trials of interferon-α in hormonally functional NETs took place prior to the introduction of SSAs and reported significant palliation of hormonal symptoms such as flushing and diarrhea along with reductions of tumor markers in over 50% of patients.[31] Objective tumor response rates have generally been low.

mTOR Inhibition in Carcinoid Tumors

Everolimus was also evaluated in a separate phase III study among patients with progressive well-differentiated NETs and history of carcinoid syndrome. Four hundred and twenty nine patients were randomized to receive octreotide LAR plus everolimus or matching placebo.[32] The study demonstrated a 5.1 (from 11.3 to 16.4 mo) months of improvement in PFS (Table 60.2; HR = 0.77; 95% CI, 0.59–1.00).[32] The observed P value = 0.026, however, missed the pre-specified boundary 0.0246. Informative censoring may have caused a loss of events and statistical power. Imbalances in randomization may have also placed patients with worse prognosis in the everolimus arm. The efficacy of everolimus in NETs of non-pancreatic origin will need to be confirmed in a future study.

VEGF Inhibition in Carcinoid Tumors

Similar to pNETs, carcinoids are classically vascular with high expression of VEGF. Bevacizumab is a recombinant humanized monoclonal antibody that binds to VEGF-A. In a phase II trial, 44 patients with metastatic carcinoid tumors were randomized to receive 18 weeks of treatment using octreotide in combination with 3-weekly bevacizumab at 15 mg/kg or weekly pegylated interferon α-2b at 0.5 μg/kg.[33] At 18 weeks of disease progression, patients then received a combination of all the three drugs. Those in the bevacizumab arm demonstrated better partial response rate (18% vs. 0%). There was also an improvement in PFS at 18 weeks (95% vs. 68%, $P = 0.02$). The trial also assessed tumor blood flow, tumor blood volume, and permeability using functional CT, reporting a significant reduction in tumor blood flow parameters.[33,34] The efficacy of bevacizumab in carcinoid tumors is being tested in an ongoing phase III study that will compare octreotide LAR and bevacizumab with octreotide LAR and interferon (SWOG [Southwest Oncology Group] 0518).

Peptide Receptor Radiotherapy for NETs

Peptide receptor radiotherapy delivers a high dose of radiation to the tumor by linking radioisotopes to SSAs. Recent studies have focused on ^{90}Y-DOTA-Phe^{1}-Tyr^{3}-Octreotide (^{90}Y-DOTATOC and ^{90}Y-Edotreotide) and ^{177}Lu-DOTA-Tyr^{3}-octreotate (^{177}Lu-DOTATATE). Although two small studies with ^{90}Y-DOTATOC reported response rates of 23% and 24%,[35,36] only a 4% response rate was observed in a larger prospective study with 90 patients.[37] Studies of ^{177}Lu-DOTATATE have also generally reported favorable results. In one large series, authors reported the efficacy results from 310 of 504 patients treated,[38] showing a promising response rate of 30%. These studies also showed that it is essential to demonstrate sufficient tumor targeting using a "tracer" administration of the proposed therapeutic agent or its surrogate. Higher uptake is associated with better response. It is recommended that [^{111}In-DTPA^{0}]octreotide scintigraphy be performed to assess the degree of uptake prior to somatostatin receptor targeted radiotherapy. In general, levels of tumor uptake less than that seen in the normal liver are considered inadequate for therapy.

In general, peptide receptor radiotherapy with ^{90}Y-DOTATOC or ^{177}Lu-DOTATATE has demonstrated promising activity in reported studies. However, these results should be interpreted with caution as many studies have not included intent-to-treat analysis, and randomized controlled studies are lacking.

SYSTEMIC THERAPY FOR HIGH-GRADE NETS

High-grade (or poorly differentiated) NETs appear to be highly sensitive to platinum-based cytotoxic chemotherapy regimens. The clinical characteristics of extra pulmonary poorly differentiated NETs are similar to small cell carcinomas of the lung. In one study investigating cisplatin and etoposide in gastrointestinal NETs, a response rate of 67% was observed in poorly differentiated tumors versus 7% in well-differentiated tumors.[39] Another study of cisplatin and etoposide in poorly differentiated NETs of the gastrointestinal tract demonstrated a response rate of 42%.[40] The durations of response in both studies were short, with median survivals of only 15 to 19 months.[39,40]

SUMMARY

Although much is still unknown about the carcinogenesis of NETs, extensive investigation is being undertaken to discover novel pathways and treatments based on recent studies. The progress of finding therapeutic options has been expedited in recent years with the greater understanding of molecular and genetic components of this group of diverse tumors. The recent completions of phase III studies of octreotide, sunitinib, and everolimus have demonstrated the feasibility of rigorous evaluations of novel antitumor therapies in patients with NETs. The approval of everolimus and sunitinib for pancreatic NET has brought about much needed treatment options for this patient population.

REFERENCES

1. Yao JC, Rindi G, Evans DB. Pancreatic endocrine tumors. In: DeVita VT, Lawrence TS, Rosenberg SA, eds. *Cancer: Principles & Practice of Oncology*. 8th ed. Philadelphia, PA: Wolters Kluwer/Lippincott Williams & Wilkins; 2008:1702-1721.
2. Moertel CG, Sauer WG, Docherty MB, Baggenstoss AH. Life history of the carcinoid tumor of the small intestine. *Cancer*. 1961;14:291-293.
3. Yao JC, Hassan M, Phan A, et al. One hundred years after "carcinoid": epidemiology of and prognostic factors for neuroendocrine tumors in 35,825 cases in the United States. *J Clin Oncol*. June 2008;26(18):3063-3072.
4. Rindi G, Kloppel G, Alhman H, et al. TNM staging of foregut (neuro)endocrine tumors: a consensus proposal including a grading system. *Virchows Arch*. October 2006;449(4):395-401.
5. Rindi G, Kloppel G, Couvelard A, et al. TNM staging of midgut and hindgut (neuro) endocrine tumors: a consensus proposal including a grading system. *Virchows Arch*. October 2007;451(4):757-762.
6. Edge SB, Byrd DR, Compton CC, Fritz AG, Greene FL, Trotti A. *AJCC Cancer Staging Manual*. 7th ed. New York, NY: Springer; 2010.
7. Wang GG, Yao JC, Worah S, et al. Comparison of genetic alterations in neuroendocrine tumors: frequent loss of chromosome 18 in ileal carcinoid tumors. *Mod Pathol*. August 2005;18(8):1079-1087.
8. Yao JC. Molecular targeted therapy for carcinoid and islet-cell carcinoma. *Best Pract Res Clin Endocrinol Metab*. March 2007;21(1):163-172.
9. Yao JC, Pavel M, Phan AT, et al. Chromogranin A and neuron-specific enolase as prognostic markers in patients with advanced pNET treated with everolimus. *J Clin Endocrinol Metab*. December 2001;96(2):3741-3749. Epub October 12, 2011.
10. Gedaly R, Daily MF, Davenport D, et al. Liver transplantation for the treatment of liver metastases from neuroendocrine tumors: an analysis of the UNOS database. *Arch Surg*. August 2011;146(8):953-958.
11. Murthy R, Kamat P, Nunez R, et al. Yttrium-90 microsphere radioembolotherapy of hepatic metastatic neuroendocrine carcinomas after hepatic arterial embolization. *J Vasc Interv Radiol*. January 2008;19(1):145-151.
12. Paprottka PM, Hoffmann RT, Haug A, et al. Radioembolization of symptomatic, unresectable neuroendocrine hepatic metastases using yttrium-90 microspheres. *Cardiovasc Intervent Radiol*. August 2011.
13. Kouvaraki MA, Ajani JA, Hoff P, et al. Fluorouracil, doxorubicin, and streptozocin in the treatment of patients with locally advanced and metastatic pancreatic endocrine carcinomas. *J Clin Oncol*. December 2004;22(23):4762-4771.
14. Feng W, Brown RE, Trung CD, et al. Morphoproteomic profile of mTOR, Ras/Raf kinase/ERK, and NF-kappaB pathways in human gastric adenocarcinoma. *Ann Clin Lab Sci*. Summer 2008;38(3):195-209.
15. Cheng PN, Saltz LB. Failure to confirm major objective antitumor activity for streptozocin and doxorubicin in the treatment of patients with advanced islet cell carcinoma. *Cancer*. September 1999;86(6):944-948.
16. McCollum AD, Kulke MH, Ryan DP, et al. Lack of efficacy of streptozocin and doxorubicin in patients with advanced pancreatic endocrine tumors. *Am J Clin Oncol*. October 2004;27(5):485-488.
17. Kulke M, Hornick J, Frauenhoffer C, et al. O^6-Methylguanine DNA methyltransferase deficiency and response to temozolomide-based therapy in patients with neuroendocrine tumors. *Clin Cancer Res*. 2009;15(1):338-345.

18. Strosberg JR, Fine RL, Choi J, et al. First-line chemotherapy with capecitabine and temozolomide in patients with metastatic pancreatic endocrine carcinomas. *Cancer*. January 2011;117(2):268-275.
19. Jiao Y, Shi C, Edil BH, et al. DAXX/ATRX, MEN1, and mTOR pathway genes are frequently altered in pancreatic neuroendocrine tumors. *Science*. March 2011;331(6021):1199-1203.
20. Missiaglia E, Dalai I, Barbi S, et al. Pancreatic endocrine tumors: expression profiling evidences a role for AKT-mTOR pathway. *J Clin Oncol*. January 2010;28(2):245-255.
21. Duran I, Kortmansky J, Singh D, et al. A phase II clinical and pharmacodynamic study of temsirolimus in advanced neuroendocrine carcinomas. *Br J Cancer*. November 2006;95(9):1148-1154.
22. Yao JC, Lombard-Bohas C, Baudin E, et al. Daily oral everolimus activity in patients with metastatic pancreatic neuroendocrine tumors after failure of cytotoxic chemotherapy: a phase II trial. *J Clin Oncol*. January 2010;28(1):69-76.
23. Yao JC, Shah MH, Ito T, et al. Everolimus for advanced pancreatic neuroendocrine tumors. *N Engl J Med*. February 2011;364(6):514-523.
24. Kulke MH, Lenz HJ, Meropol NJ, et al. Activity of sunitinib in patients with advanced neuroendocrine tumors. *J Clin Oncol*. July 2008;26(20):3403-3410.
25. Raymond E, Dahan L, Raoul JL, et al. Sunitinib malate for the treatment of pancreatic neuroendocrine tumors. *N Engl J Med*. February 2011;364(6):501-513.
26. Hobday TJ, Rubin J, Holen K, et al. MC044h, a phase II trial of sorafenib in patients (pts) with metastatic neuroendocrine tumors (NET): a Phase II Consortium (P2C) study. *J Clin Oncol*. 2007;25(18S):abstr 4504.
27. Phan AT, Yao JC, Fogelman DR, et al. A prospective, multi-institutional phase II study of GW786034 (pazopanib) and depot octreotide (sandostatin LAR) in advanced low-grade neuroendocrine carcinoma (LGNEC). *J Clin Oncol*. 2010;28(7s):abstr 4001.
28. Kvols L, Moertel C, Schutt A, Rubin J. Treatment of the malignant carcinoid syndrome with a long-acting somatostatin analogue (SMS 201-955): preliminary evidence that more is not better (abstract). *Proc Am Soc Clin Oncol*. 1987;6:95.
29. Kvols L, Wiedenmann B, Oberg K, et al. Safety and efficacy of pasireotide (SOM230) in patients with metastatic carcinoid tumors refractory or resistant to octreotide LAR: results of a phase II study. *J Clin Oncol*. 2006;24(18S):198s.
30. Rinke A, Muller HH, Schade-Brittinger C, et al. Placebo-controlled, double-blind, prospective, randomized study on the effect of octreotide LAR in the control of tumor growth in patients with metastatic neuroendocrine midgut tumors: a report from the PROMID Study Group. *J Clin Oncol*. October 2009;27(28):4656-4663.
31. Oberg K, Funa K, Alm G. Effects of leukocyte interferon on clinical symptoms and hormone levels in patients with mid-gut carcinoid tumors and carcinoid syndrome. *N Engl J Med*. 1983;309(3):129-133.
32. Pavel ME, Hainsworth JD, Baudin E, et al. Everolimus plus octreotide long-acting repeatable for the treatment of advanced neuroendocrine tumours associated with carcinoid syndrome (RADIANT-2): a randomised, placebo-controlled, phase 3 study. *Lancet*. December 2011;378(9808):2005-2012.
33. Yao JC, Phan A, Hoff PM, et al. Targeting vascular endothelial growth factor in advanced carcinoid tumor: a random assignment phase II study of depot octreotide with bevacizumab and pegylated interferon alpha-2b. *J Clin Oncol*. March 2008;26(8):1316-1323.
34. Ng CS, Charnsangavej C, Wei W, Yao JC. Perfusion CT findings in patients with metastatic carcinoid tumors undergoing bevacizumab and interferon therapy. *AJR Am J Roentgenol*. March 2011;196(3):569-576.
35. Waldherr C, Pless M, Maecke HR, Haldemann A, Mueller-Brand J. The clinical value of [90Y-DOTA]-D-Phe1-Tyr3-octreotide (90Y-DOTATOC) in the treatment of neuroendocrine tumours: a clinical phase II study. *Ann Oncol*. July 2001;12(7):941-945.
36. Waldherr C, Pless M, Maecke HR, et al. Tumor response and clinical benefit in neuroendocrine tumors after 7.4 GBq (90) Y-DOTATOC. *J Nucl Med*. May 2002;43(5):610-616.
37. Bushnell DL Jr, O'Dorisio TM, O'Dorisio MS, et al. 90Y-edotreotide for metastatic carcinoid refractory to octreotide. *J Clin Oncol*. April 2010;28(10):1652-1659.
38. Kwekkeboom DJ, de Herder WW, Kam BL, et al. Treatment with the radiolabeled somatostatin analog [177 Lu-DOTA 0,Tyr3] octreotate: toxicity, efficacy, and survival. *J Clin Oncol*. May 2008;26(13):2124-2130.
39. Moertel CG, Kvols LK, O'Connell MJ, Rubin J. Treatment of neuroendocrine carcinomas with combined etoposide and cisplatin. Evidence of major therapeutic activity in the anaplastic variants of these neoplasms. *Cancer*. 1991;68(2):227-232.
40. Mitry E, Baudin E, Ducreux M, et al. Treatment of poorly differentiated neuroendocrine tumours with etoposide and cisplatin. *Br J Cancer*. December 1999;81(8):1351-1355.

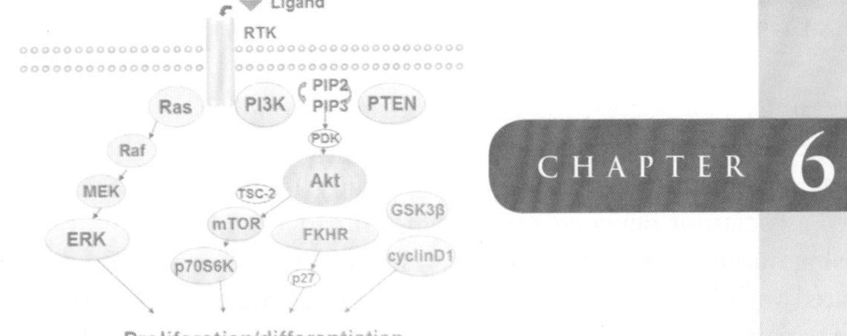

CHAPTER 61

Personalized Medicine and Targeted Therapy of Head and Neck Cancer

Ronald Myint, Kathryn A. Gold, and Edward S. Kim

Head and neck cancer is the fifth most common cancer worldwide.[1] This broad category includes malignancies of the nasal cavity, oral cavity, pharynx, and larynx. Our focus will be on head and neck squamous cell cancer (HNSCC), as this histology accounts for >90% of the tumors in this region. In the United States, there will be 40,250 estimated new cases in 2012. There are approximately 12,000 new cases each in the tongue, mouth, pharynx, and larynx.[2] The major risk factors for HNSCC include smoking, alcohol, and human papilloma virus (HPV). Smoking and alcohol have synergistic effects.

HNSCC is a challenging malignancy to treat. Although most patients with HNSCC present with potentially curable localized or locally advanced disease, treatment can cause significant morbidity. Impairments of speech, swallowing, breathing, and cosmetic appearance can all hamper a patient's quality of life.

About 30% to 40% of patients present with stage I or II disease. They can be treated with surgery or radiation alone and have a 5-year overall survival of 70% to 90%. Locally advanced HNSCC (stages III, IVa, and IVb) is managed with multimodality therapy, potentially including chemotherapy, radiation, and/or surgery. Five-year overall survival for these patients is 30% to 60%.[3] Initial presentation with metastatic disease is uncommon, but many patients may eventually develop recurrent or metastatic disease, and prognosis is poor for these patients.

No improvement in overall survival has been demonstrated with chemotherapy in the metastatic setting. Even active agents such as cisplatin and pemetrexed used in combination have not shown a survival benefit in a randomized phase 3 trial completed in March 2010.[4] A total of 795 patients with recurrent/metastatic HNSCC were randomized to cisplatin plus pemetrexed versus cisplatin monotherapy. The 1-month advantage in overall survival for the doublet arm of 7.3 versus 6.3 months for the monotherapy arm was not statistically significant ($P = 0.082$).

Targeted therapy is a prime focus of current cancer research due to the promise of more effective therapy with less toxicity. Major advances and survival benefits have already been seen with targeted therapy in various cancer types. Examples include trastuzumab in human epidermal growth factor receptor 2 (HER2/neu)–positive breast cancer, erlotinib in epidermal growth factor receptor (EGFR) mutation-positive non–small cell lung cancer, cetuximab in KRAS wild-type colon cancer, and bevacizumab in colon and non–small cell lung cancers. Although HNSCC has only one Food and Drug Administration (FDA)–approved targeted therapy, cetuximab, research is actively being pursued, and we review possible targets with their associated inhibitors.

HPV AS A RISK FACTOR

HPV is emerging as a major etiology of squamous cell carcinoma of the oropharynx, particularly in the base of the tongue and tonsillar regions, and it was found to be etiologically associated with 25% of HNSCC.[5] A landmark study published in 2000 established HPV as a causal agent for HNSCC. Tumor tissue from 253 patients with HNSCC was tested for HPV. About 25% of the tumors were positive for HPV, and the high-risk HPV strain, oral HPV-type 16 (HPV-16), was found in 90% of the HPV tumors.[5]

Although the incidence of HNSCC due to smoking is decreasing as smoking rates decrease in the US population, the incidence of HPV-associated HNSCC is increasing. This increase is thought to be secondary to changes in sexual practice, as HPV is well known to be sexually transmitted. A case–control study found a positive association between oropharyngeal cancer and increasing numbers of sexual partners.[6] HNSCC was also associated with HPV-16. These associations were found in both patients with and without a history of heavy smoking and alcohol use.

Patients with HPV-related HNSCC have a better prognosis compared with HPV-negative HNSCC. This was confirmed in a prospective trial of 96 patients with locally advanced HNSCC of the oropharynx or larynx.[7] All patients received two cycles of neoadjuvant chemotherapy with carboplatin and paclitaxel followed by definitive chemoradiation with weekly paclitaxel. HPV was detected by polymerase chain reaction or fluorescence in situ hybridization. HPV was detected in 40% of the patients. The 2-year overall survival was 95% for patients with HPV-positive tumors and 62% for those with HPV-negative tumors ($P = 0.005$). Response rates after neoadjuvant chemotherapy were 82% versus 55% ($P = 0.01$), and response rates after chemoradiation were 84% versus 57% ($P = 0.007$). Patients with HPV-positive tumors had lower risks of progression and death even after adjustment for age, stage, and performance status.

HPV status was also found to be a strong independent prognostic factor for survival. A retrospective analysis of HPV status and survival among 323 patients with stage III or IV oropharyngeal HNSCC found that the 3-year overall survival for patients with HPV-positive tumors was 82.4% versus 57.1% for those with HPV-negative tumors ($P < 0.001$).[8] After adjusting for age, TNM (tumor/node/metastasis) stage, smoking history, race, and treatment received, patients with HPV-positive tumors had a 58% reduction in the risk of death.

Demographics of patients with HPV-positive HNSCC also appear to be distinct from those with HPV-negative tumors. In a study of 66 patients with locally advanced HNSCC, HPV-positive tumors were associated with younger age (55 vs. 63 y, $P = 0.016$), male sex (73.3% of males had HPV-positive tumors compared with 41.7% for females, $P = 0.08$), and nonsmoking ($P = 0.037$).[9]

In support of the data above, a recent study published in October 2011 determined the HPV status of 271 tissue samples of oropharyngeal HNSCC collected from 1984 to 2004 from the Surveillance, Epidemiology, and End Results (SEER) database.[10] HPV positivity was associated with a median survival of 131 versus 20 months for HPV-negative tumors ($P < 0.001$). In the period 1984 to 1989 compared with 2000 to 2004, HPV prevalence increased from 16.3% to 71.7%. From 1988 to 2004, the incidence of HPV-negative tumors declined by 50%. It was extrapolated that by 2020, the incidence of HPV-positive oropharyngeal cancer would surpass the incidence of cervical cancer.

As HPV-related tumors seem to respond well to both chemotherapy and radiation, the question arises as to whether we are overtreating patients with HPV-related tumors and exposing them to unnecessary treatment-related toxicity. RTOG-1016, which is currently enrolling, randomizes patients with HPV-positive tumors to radiation with either cetuximab or cisplatin. Trials like this will help us determine how to treat these patients with maximal efficacy while limiting treatment-related toxicities.

A vaccine against high-risk subtypes of HPV has been approved for the prevention of precursors to cervical cancer.[11] If the use of this vaccine becomes widespread, we may see decreasing numbers of HPV-related oropharyngeal cancers.

EPIDERMAL GROWTH FACTOR RECEPTOR

Most epithelial cancers are associated with activation of EGFR, and most HNSCCs show overexpression of EGFR.[12] Increased expression of EGFR on tumor cells causes uncontrolled proliferation and cancer progression. Binding of ligand to the transmembrane EGFR causes autophosphorylation and intracellular signaling via tyrosine kinase activity. This intracellular signaling results in increased cell proliferation, activation of angiogenesis, and inhibition of apoptosis.[13]

EGFR expression is also a prognostic marker in head and neck cancer. A correlative study in 2002 analyzed tissue from 155 patients with HNSCC with quantitative EGFR immunohistochemistry.[14] Multivariate analysis showed that increased EGFR expression was significantly associated with decreased overall survival and increased local recurrence. There was a wide variation in EGFR expression in HNSCCs, and there was no association between the amount of EGFR expression and TNM stage. EGFR expression was detected in 95% of the 155 HNSCC specimens analyzed.

A common source of confusion is EGFR overexpression, which occurs in HNSCC, versus EGFR mutation, which occurs in non–small cell lung cancer. In lung cancer, mutation of the EGFR gene causes autophosphorylation of the receptor, unregulated downstream signaling, and uncontrolled proliferation. In contrast, in HNSCC, EGFR is not mutated but overexpressed. In a 2008 study, 91 HNSCC specimens were analyzed for EGFR mutations, of which only 1 specimen had an EGFR mutation and 1 had a KRAS mutation.[15] All 91 tumors expressed EGFR, and 68% had high expression by immunohistochemistry. It was also found that EGFR overexpression was significantly associated with positive nodal stage and poorer tumor differentiation. Thus it was concluded that EGFR overexpression, not mutation, was the cause of abnormal activation of the EGFR pathway in HNSCC. Patients with HNSCC are not routinely tested for EGFR mutations. The majority of HNSCCs express EGFR, so anti-EGFR therapy can be given without further testing.

There are two main types of EGFR antagonists, monoclonal antibodies such as cetuximab and panitumumab versus low molecular weight EGFR tyrosine kinase inhibitors such as erlotinib and gefitinib. The mechanism of action for the monoclonal antibodies is competitive inhibition. They bind to the extracellular domain of EGFR and prevent ligand binding, thereby preventing activation of downstream signaling pathways. Conversely, the low molecular weight tyrosine kinase inhibitors work intracellularly, by preventing ATP binding/activation of the tyrosine kinase domain of EGFR, thus preventing autophosphorylation and downstream signaling of proliferation pathways.[13]

EGFR Monoclonal Antibodies

Since EGFR was found to be overexpressed in the majority of HNSCCs and associated with a worse prognosis, it was a logical target for inhibition with anti-EGFR therapies. In 2006, the FDA approved cetuximab in combination with radiation for locally advanced HNSCC. It is also approved as monotherapy for platinum-refractory disease.

The phase 3 study that led to the FDA approval of cetuximab in 2006 randomized patients with locoregionally advanced HNSCC (stage III or IV without distant metastases) to high-dose radiation alone (50 to 60 Gy) or radiation plus cetuximab.[16] Cetuximab was dosed at 400 mg/m^2 followed by 250 mg/m^2 weekly during radiation. Median overall survival for the concurrent arm was 49 versus 29.3 months for radiation alone ($P = 0.03$). Median duration of locoregional control was 24.4 versus 14.9 months ($P = 0.005$). The addition of cetuximab to radiation did increase acneiform rash and infusion reactions, but the incidence of grade 3 or 4 side effects was not significantly different between the two arms.

Another landmark trial with cetuximab in HNSCC was in first-line treatment for recurrent or metastatic disease. Published in 2008, the Erbitux in First-Line Treatment of Recurrent or Metastatic Head and Neck Cancer ("EXTREME" study) was a two-arm multicenter phase 3 randomized trial of 442 patients.[17] In the control arm, 220 patients received cisplatin or carboplatin plus fluorouracil. In the experimental arm, 222 patients received the same chemotherapy plus cetuximab. All patients received cisplatin 100 mg/m^2 or carboplatin AUC (area under the curve) 5 on day 1 and fluorouracil 1,000 mg/m^2 days 1 to 4 every 3 weeks for a maximum of six cycles. Cetuximab was dosed at 400 mg/m^2 and then 250 mg/m^2 weekly with chemotherapy and continued as maintenance after six cycles if patients had a response or stable disease. Median overall survival was 10.1 months in the cetuximab plus chemotherapy arm and 7.4 months in the chemotherapy-alone arm ($P = 0.04$). Median progression-free survival was 5.6 versus 3.3 months ($P < 0.001$), and response rate was 36% versus 20% ($P < 0.001$), both favoring the cetuximab arm. There were no deaths secondary to cetuximab, but 9% had grade 3 skin reactions and 3% had grade 3 or 4 infusion reactions. Nine patients in the cetuximab arm had sepsis, compared with one patient in the chemo-alone arm ($P = 0.02$).

Another FDA-approved indication for cetuximab in HNSCC is in the recurrent/metastatic setting after progression on platinum-based chemotherapy. There are three large, single-arm phase 2 trials in this setting published from 2005 to 2007.[18-20] A paper published in 2008 combined the data from these three trials and compared the data with a retrospective study of patients who received various second-line treatments after platinum failure.[21] There were a total of 278 patients with recurrent/metastatic HNSCC who progressed on prior platinum therapy. One hundred and three patients received cetuximab monotherapy and the rest received cetuximab plus cisplatin or carboplatin. Efficacy data were compared with a retrospective study of 151 patients (45% received best supportive care, 28% chemotherapy, 17% radiation, and 10% chemotherapy + radiation). Response rates were 13% for patients who received cetuximab only, 10% for cetuximab + platinum, and 3% in the control group who received various second-line treatments. Disease control rate (complete response + partial response + stable disease) was 46% for cetuximab monotherapy, 53% to 56% for cetuximab + platinum, and 15% in the control group. Median survival was 5.9 months for cetuximab monotherapy, 5.2 to 6.1 months for cetuximab + platinum, and 3.4 months for the control group. These results showed that cetuximab is a reasonable option that can provide a modest response in the recurrent/metastatic setting, where there are few good treatment options.

EGFR overexpression may be associated with decreased response to cetuximab. In a phase 3 randomized study of cisplatin plus cetuximab versus cisplatin alone in metastatic HNSCC, investigators measured EGFR expression by immunohistochemistry.[22] Patients with low to moderate expression of EGFR gained a benefit in terms of response rate with combined treatment (41% vs. 12%, $P = 0.03$); patients with high expression of EGFR did not benefit from the combination (response rate 12% vs. 6%, $P = 0.99$). A possible hypothesis is that higher doses of cetuximab are needed for tumors with higher EGFR expression to adequately inhibit all the EGFRs.

Another anti-EGFR monoclonal antibody, panitumumab, is FDA approved for KRAS wild-type metastatic colorectal cancer. It is a fully humanized monoclonal antibody that is thought to cause less infusion reactions than cetuximab, which is a mouse/humanized monoclonal antibody. The two drugs appear to have similar efficacy as monotherapy in metastatic colorectal cancer.[23,24] One ongoing phase 3 trial (NCT00820248) is evaluating radiation with concurrent panitumumab or cisplatin for locally advanced HNSCC.[4] A variable is that the panitumumab arm is getting accelerated fractionation radiation, and the cisplatin arm is getting standard fractionation. The estimated enrollment is 320 patients and the estimated completion date is March 2015. A phase 3 trial (NCT00460265), Study of Efficacy in Patients with Recurrent/Metastatic Head and Neck Cancer or "SPECTRUM" trial, is randomizing patients with recurrent or metastatic disease to receive cisplatin and fluorouracil with or without panitumumab.[4] The estimated enrollment is 658 patients, and the estimated study completion date is September 2012.

EGFR Tyrosine Kinase Inhibitors

In contrast to cetuximab, the EGFR tyrosine kinase inhibitors do not have proven efficacy in HNSCC. A phase 3 randomized trial compared gefitinib with methotrexate in recurrent HNSCC.[25] A total of 486 patients were randomly assigned to gefitinib 250 or 500 mg po daily, or methotrexate 40 mg/m^2 IV weekly. Median overall survival was 5.6, 6, and 6.7 months. Response rates were 2.7%, 7.6%, and 3.9%. Differences in overall survival and response rate were not statistically significant. In a phase 2 study by Kim et al.,[26] 47 patients with recurrent/metastatic HNSCC were treated with erlotinib, cisplatin, and docetaxel. The overall response rate by RECIST criteria was 67% and disease control rate was 95%. After a median follow-up of 19 months, median overall survival was 11 months and progression-free survival was 6 months. The combination was well tolerated. These results were encouraging compared with a study of cisplatin and docetaxel, where the response rate was 40% and median survival was 9.6 months.[27] A randomized study of cisplatin and docetaxel with or without erlotinib is currently accruing patients.[4]

A phase 2 trial of locally advanced HNSCC evaluated the efficacy of adding erlotinib and bevacizumab to concurrent chemoradiation.[28] Sixty untreated patients received neoadjuvant chemotherapy with carboplatin, paclitaxel, 5-fluorouracil, and bevacizumab followed by concurrent chemoradiation with erlotinib, bevacizumab, and paclitaxel. After a median follow-up of 32 months, the estimated 3-year progression-free survival was 71% and 3-year overall survival was 82%. About 95% of patients had complete or partial responses after concurrent therapy. Eighty-eight percent of patients experienced grade 3 or 4 mucositis, but no unexpected side effects occurred from the addition of erlotinib. The authors suggested that the efficacious results warranted future trials adding the targeted agents erlotinib and bevacizumab into first-line treatment for locally advanced HNSCC. This trial was conducted in the community setting (Sarah Cannon Oncology Research Consortium), suggesting the feasibility of this treatment regimen in the community.

Erlotinib was evaluated in the neoadjuvant setting in a phase 1 trial at MD Anderson.[29] Thirty-four patients with resectable HNSCC were randomized to receive erlotinib 150, 200, or 300 mg daily. Erlotinib was generally well tolerated. Median duration on treatment was 19 days, 25% had responses by RECIST criteria, 71% had stable disease, and only 4% had progression.

DUAL EGFR/HER2 INHIBITION

HER2 forms a heterodimer with EGFR, increasing downstream signaling and possibly EGFR resistance. There is an oral targeted therapy that inhibits both these targets, lapatinib, which is approved for breast cancer. A phase 2 study evaluated lapatinib in recurrent/metastatic HNSCC.[30] It was given to patients both naive and refractory to EGFR inhibitor therapy. The toxicity profile was favorable, but no objective responses were seen. An ongoing phase 3 trial (NCT00424255) is a randomized, double-blind, placebo-controlled study of patients with locally advanced HNSCC with high-risk disease after surgery.[4] All patients will receive adjuvant radiation with a concurrent platinum-based chemotherapy regimen with or without lapatinib. The estimated enrollment is 680 patients and the estimated study completion date is June 2012. Other phase 2 trials are studying lapatinib plus capecitabine in recurrent/metastatic HNSCC (NCT01044433), lapatinib plus concurrent radiation for patients with locally advanced disease who cannot tolerate concurrent cytotoxic chemotherapy (NCT00490061), and neoadjuvant lapatinib or placebo followed by concurrent chemoradiation in locally advanced HNSCC (NCT00371566).[4]

ANGIOGENESIS

Angiogenesis is the formation of new blood vessels and is an integral component of tumor growth. Unlike normal blood vessels, tumor blood vessels are irregular and have increased permeability.[31] These "leaky" blood vessels may prevent effective drug delivery to the tumor. Targeting angiogenesis not only inhibits tumor blood vessel formation but also allows increased delivery of chemotherapy to the tumor. The importance of vascular endothelial growth factor receptor (VEGFR) in angiogenesis has made it a target for cancer therapy. VEGFR overexpression is associated with a worse prognosis and more advanced disease in a variety of solid tumors.[32]

Bevacizumab was the first VEGFR inhibitor approved by the FDA. It is a humanized monoclonal antibody against VEGFR. It is FDA approved in combination with chemotherapy in metastatic colon and non–small cell lung cancer. The more common toxicities of bevacizumab include hypertension, proteinuria, bleeding, thrombosis, and delayed wound healing.

In 2008, there was a phase 1 trial combining bevacizumab with fluorouracil, hydrea, and radiation for treatment in poor-risk, localized HNSCC.[33] The treatment was overall well tolerated. The median overall survival for patients who did not receive prior radiation was an impressive 40.1 months, but only 9.2 months for patients who received prior radiation. A phase 2 trial combined bevacizumab with pemetrexed as first-line therapy for recurrent/metastatic HNSCC.[34] Bevacizumab was administered 15 mg/kg IV and pemetrexed 500 mg/m^2 IV every 21 days. Disease control rate was 86%, response rate was

30%, and complete response was seen, where median overall survival was 11.3 months.

In an ongoing phase 3 trial by the Eastern Cooperative Oncology Group (NCT00588770), patients with recurrent/metastatic HNSCC are being randomized to chemotherapy with cisplatin, docetaxel, and fluorouracil with or without bevacizumab.[4] The estimated enrollment is 400 patients, and the estimated completion date is August 2013. Another ongoing phase 2 trial (NCT00409565) is evaluating the combination of bevacizumab and cetuximab in recurrent/metastatic HNSCC.[4]

MULTIKINASE INHIBITORS

Sorafenib is an oral agent that inhibits cell surface receptors, including VEGFR, platelet-derived growth factor receptor (PDGFR), cytokine receptor (c-KIT), and the intracellular RAF kinases. It is approved for metastatic renal cell carcinoma and hepatocellular carcinoma. A phase 2 trial evaluated sorafenib as first-line therapy in 41 patients with recurrent/metastatic HNSCC.[35] The estimated median overall survival was 9 months and progression-free survival was 4 months. An ongoing phase 2 randomized trial (NCT00939627) is comparing cetuximab plus sorafenib versus cetuximab plus placebo for refractory/recurrent/metastatic HNSCC.[4]

Sunitinib is another oral multikinase inhibitor, whose targets include PDGFR and VEGFR, among others. A phase 2 trial evaluated 38 patients with refractory HNSCC treated with sunitinib 37.5 mg po daily.[36] At 6 to 8 weeks after treatment initiation, a disease control rate of 50% was seen. By RECIST criteria, 1 patient had a partial response, 18 had stable disease, and 19 had progressive disease. There were significant toxicities, including 4 patients with fatal bleeding events and 15 patients with local complications (tumor skin ulceration or tumor fistula).

Pazopanib is a newer agent used for metastatic renal cell carcinoma. Its targets include PDGFR, VEGF, c-KIT, and fibroblast growth factor receptor. It has fewer side effects than sunitinib. An ongoing single-arm phase 2 trial (NCT01377298) of pazopanib in cisplatin-refractory recurrent/metastatic HNSCC has an estimated enrollment of 45 patients and the study completion date of May 2014.[4]

INSULIN-LIKE GROWTH FACTOR RECEPTOR

Another potential target in HNSCC is the insulin-like growth factor type-1 receptor (IGF-IR). IGF-IR is a transmembrane tyrosine kinase receptor. The binding of the ligand IGF, activates the receptor via autophosphorylation. This leads to subsequent activation of downstream signaling cascades such as Ras-Raf-mitogen–activated protein kinase and phosphatidylinositol 3-kinase protein kinase.[37] This leads to increased cell proliferation and resistance to apoptosis. IGF-IR was suggested to be integral to tumor transformation and survival, but only minimally involved in normal cell growth.[38] Activation of IGF-IR has been shown to be a vital component of multiple cancers, including breast and colon.[39,40]

In addition to cancer proliferation, IGF-IR has been implicated in resistance to EGFR inhibitors such as erlotinib.[41] IGF-IR can bind to EGFR and form a heterodimer on the cell membrane. This heterodimer formation activates IGF-IR downstream signaling and thus cell proliferation. Treatment with erlotinib increases this heterodimer formation, leading to erlotinib resistance. Erlotinib resistance was overcome in experiments of non–small cell lung cancer cells in vitro and in vivo via IGF-IR inhibition.[41]

IMC-A12 (Cixutumumab, manufactured by ImClone Systems) is a monoclonal antibody that inhibits the IGF-IR. In cell line and xenograft models of HNSCC, IMC-A12 acts as a potent radiosensitizer.[42] An ongoing phase 2 trial (NCT00617734) is studying IMC-A12 with or without cetuximab in platinum-refractory HNSCC.[4] IMC-A12 is dosed at 10 mg/kg IV over 1 hour every 2 weeks. The study enrolled 97 patients and the estimated study end.

Another novel agent is OSI-906 (manufactured by OSI Pharmaceuticals). It is an oral dual inhibitor of IGF-IR and an insulin receptor inhibitor. A phase 2 study (NCT01427205) at MD Anderson is randomizing patients with platinum-refractory recurrent/metastatic HNSCC to OSI-906 plus cetuximab or cetuximab plus placebo.[4] The estimated enrollment is 55 patients.

PROTEASOME

The proteasome is a proteinase complex that breaks down intracellular proteins, including cells that regulate apoptosis. Proteasome inhibitors have been shown to cause apoptosis and act as a sensitizer for both chemotherapy and radiation.[43] Bortezomib is a proteasome inhibitor approved by the FDA for multiple myeloma. In a laboratory study, HNSCC cell lines were treated with bortezomib monotherapy or in combination with cisplatin and docetaxel.[44] Bortezomib monotherapy not only showed significant antitumor activity but also enhanced the effectiveness of cisplatin and docetaxel. Also, the dose of cisplatin and docetaxel could be reduced when bortezomib was added without compromising efficacy, which may limit side effects of the traditional cytotoxic chemotherapy.

In a phase 2 trial (NCT00425750), the combination of bortezomib and docetaxel was studied in 25 patients with recurrent/metastatic HNSCC.[4] This study has completed enrollment and the results are pending. A phase 1 trial enrolled patients with locally advanced or recurrent HNSCC to receive bortezomib and cetuximab with concurrent radiation.[45] There was evidence of early progression with combined therapy. Bortezomib was found to inhibit cetuximab by causing EGFR stabilization and also found to increase HNSCC cytokines. It was concluded that the combination of bortezomib and cetuximab with concurrent radiation should be avoided.

SRC FAMILY KINASES

Increased expression of Src family kinases has been linked to increased invasiveness and progression in HNSCC.[46] C-Src, a member of the Src family, is overexpressed in HNSCC.[47] C-Src is activated downstream of EGFR and leads to increased tumor proliferation.[48] Dasatinib is an oral multikinase inhibitor that inhibits the Src family kinases, c-KIT, PDGFR, and most notably BCR-ABL, for its main indication in chronic myeloid leukemia. In a phase 2 study conducted by MD Anderson, 15 patients with recurrent/metastatic HNSCC after platinum chemotherapy were treated with dasatinib.[49] It was not well tolerated, with four patients hospitalized for toxicity and three patients requiring dose reductions. At 8 weeks, two patients (16.7%) had stable disease and no objective responses were observed. An ongoing phase 1/2 trial (NCT00882583) is treating patients with locally advanced HNSCC with dasatinib, cetuximab, and concurrent radiation with or without cisplatin.[4] The estimated enrollment is 98 and the estimated study end date is January 2014.

JAK-STAT PATHWAY

Lai and Johnson[50] have suggested that the Janus-activated kinase (JAK) inhibitors may have a role in the treatment of HNSCC. The JAK-STAT (signal transducer and activator of transcription) pathway is well described in the myeloproliferative disorders, particularly polycythemia vera, essential thrombocythemia, and primary myelofibrosis. Ligand binding activates the JAKs, which phosphorylate STAT proteins, and internalizes the dimer into the nucleus. Activation of downstream targets leads to increased angiogenesis, immune resistance, and cell proliferation.[51] Increased expression of STAT3 was found in the mucosa of patients with HNSCC, and activated STAT3 was suggested to be an early event in HNSCC carcinogenesis.[52] Independent of JAK, the STAT proteins can also be activated by additional pathways, including c-SRC kinase, EGFR,[48] erythropoietin receptor,[53] and interleukin receptor.[51]

No STAT3-specific inhibitors are in clinical development due to problems with drug delivery and stability.[50] However, there are several JAK inhibitors in active clinical trials. INCB018424 (Ruxolitinib, manufactured by Incyte Corporation) is an oral inhibitor of JAK1 and JAK2 that was shown to benefit patients with myelofibrosis.[54] Ruxolitinib has been studied in prostate (NCT00638378) and pancreatic (NCT01423604) cancers, but none yet in HNSCC.[4] Another JAK2 inhibitor, AZD1480 (manufactured by AstraZeneca), has an ongoing phase 1 study (NCT01219543) in Asian patients with advanced solid tumors refractory to conventional therapies and hepatocellular carcinoma.[4]

p53

p53 is a well-known tumor suppressor gene that has been described as "the guardian of the genome." Li-Fraumeni syndrome is a hereditary disorder due to a mutation in p53 that is associated with multiple cancers. About half of HNSCCs have p53 mutations, and loss of p53 function has been linked to invasiveness.[55] A study found that smoking and alcohol were associated with increased p53 mutations in HNSCC.[56] HPV-positive HNSCC is less likely to have a p53 mutation.[5] Gene therapy targeting p53 has been largely unsuccessful, with a phase 3 trial unable to demonstrate clear benefit.[57]

CONCLUSION

Head and neck cancers are common malignancies that cause significant morbidity and mortality. Most patients present with advanced disease and have a high mortality rate. Due to these facts, it is imperative to advance the field to benefit patients with HNSCC. Targeted or personalized therapy has the potential to improve treatment of these malignancies while limiting the side effects of therapy. Extensive research is being conducted to find molecular targets and therapeutic inhibitors of these targets.

In this chapter, we reviewed some of the more promising molecular targets in HNSCC and their associated inhibitors. These include EGFR and cetuximab and erlotinib, EGFR/HER2 and lapatinib, VEGFR and bevacizumab, IGF-IR and cixutumumab, c-Src and dasatinib, JAK-STAT pathway and JAK2 inhibitors, proteasome and bortezomib, p53, and multikinase targets and pazopanib, sunitinib, and sorafenib. There are numerous phase 2 and 3 trials looking at the efficacy of these agents in HNSCC as monotherapy, combined with traditional cytotoxic chemotherapy, with concurrent radiation, and in the neoadjuvant/adjuvant setting with surgery.

Currently, the only FDA-approved targeted therapy for HNSCC is cetuximab, a monoclonal antibody inhibitor of EGFR. Indications for cetuximab are with concurrent radiation for locally advanced HNSCC and for platinum-refractory recurrent/metastatic HNSCC. The National Comprehensive Cancer Network (NCCN) guidelines category 1 recommendations for cetuximab are with concurrent radiation for locally advanced disease and in combination with cisplatin/carboplatin and fluorouracil for recurrent/unresectable/metastatic non-nasopharyngeal HNSCC. Other NCCN indications for cetuximab are as monotherapy and in combination with cisplatin for recurrent/metastatic non–nasopharyngeal HNSCC.

REFERENCES

1. Siegel R, DeSantis C, Virgo K, et al. Cancer treatment and survivorship statistics, 2012. *CA Cancer J Clin*. 2012;62:220-241.
2. Siegel R, Ward E, Brawley O, et al. Cancer statistics, 2011: the impact of eliminating socioeconomic and racial disparities on premature cancer deaths. *CA Cancer J Clin*. 2011;61:212-236.
3. Stenson K. UpToDate. In: Basow DS, ed. *UpToDate*. Waltham, MA: Wolters Kluwer;2011.
4. National Institutes of Health. Clinical trials registry 2012. http://www.clinicaltrials.gov.
5. Gillison ML, Koch WM, Capone RB, et al. Evidence for a causal association between human papillomavirus and a subset of head and neck cancers. *J Natl Cancer Inst*. 2000;92:709-720.
6. D'Souza G, Kreimer AR, Viscidi R, et al. Case-control study of human papillomavirus and oropharyngeal cancer. *N Engl J Med*. 2007;356:1944-1956.
7. Fakhry C, Westra WH, Li S, et al. Improved survival of patients with human papillomavirus-positive head and neck squamous cell carcinoma in a prospective clinical trial. *J Natl Cancer Inst*. 2008;100:261-269.
8. Ang KK, Harris J, Wheeler R, et al. Human papillomavirus and survival of patients with oropharyngeal cancer. *N Engl J Med*. 2010;363:24-35.
9. Worden FP, Kumar B, Lee JS, et al. Chemoselection as a strategy for organ preservation in advanced oropharynx cancer: response and survival positively associated with HPV16 copy number. *J Clin Oncol*. 2008;26:3138-3146.
10. Chaturvedi AK, Engels EA, Pfeiffer RM, et al. Human papillomavirus and rising oropharyngeal cancer incidence in the United States. *J Clin Oncol*. October 2011; (published online).
11. Kahn JA. HPV vaccination for the prevention of cervical intraepithelial neoplasia. *N Engl J Med*. 2009;361:271-278.
12. Dassonville O, Formento JL, Francoual M, et al. Expression of epidermal growth factor receptor and survival in upper aerodigestive tract cancer. *J Clin Oncol*. 1993;11:1873-1878.
13. Ciardiello F, Tortora G. EGFR antagonists in cancer treatment. *N Engl J Med*. 2008;358:1160-1174.
14. Ang KK, Berkey BA, Tu X, et al. Impact of epidermal growth factor receptor expression on survival and pattern of relapse in patients with advanced head and neck carcinoma. *Cancer Res*. 2002;62:7350-7356.
15. Sheikh Ali MA, Gunduz M, Nagatsuka H, et al. Expression and mutation analysis of epidermal growth factor receptor in head and neck squamous cell carcinoma. *Cancer Sci*. 2008;99:1589-1594.
16. Bonner JA, Harari PM, Giralt J, et al. Radiotherapy plus cetuximab for squamous-cell carcinoma of the head and neck. *N Engl J Med*. 2006;354:567-578.
17. Vermorken JB, Mesia R, Rivera F, et al. Platinum-based chemotherapy plus cetuximab in head and neck cancer. *N Engl J Med*. 2008;359:1116-1127.
18. Baselga J, Trigo JM, Bourhis J, et al. Phase II multicenter study of the antiepidermal growth factor receptor monoclonal antibody cetuximab in combination with platinum-based chemotherapy in patients with platinum-refractory metastatic and/or recurrent squamous cell carcinoma of the head and neck. *J Clin Oncol*. 2005;23:5568-5577.
19. Herbst RS, Arquette M, Shin DM, et al. Phase II multicenter study of the epidermal growth factor receptor antibody cetuximab and cisplatin for recurrent and refractory squamous cell carcinoma of the head and neck. *J Clin Oncol*. 2005;23:5578-5587.
20. Vermorken JB, Trigo J, Hitt R, et al. Open-label, uncontrolled, multicenter phase II study to evaluate the efficacy and toxicity of cetuximab as a single agent in patients with recurrent and/or metastatic squamous cell carcinoma of the head and neck who failed to respond to platinum-based therapy. *J Clin Oncol*. 2007;25:2171-2177.
21. Vermorken JB, Herbst RS, Leon X, et al. Overview of the efficacy of cetuximab in recurrent and/or metastatic squamous cell carcinoma of the head and neck in patients who previously failed platinum-based therapies. *Cancer*. 2008;112:2710-2719.
22. Burtness B, Goldwasser MA, Flood W, et al. Phase III randomized trial of cisplatin plus placebo compared with cisplatin plus cetuximab in metastatic/recurrent head and neck cancer: an Eastern Cooperative Oncology Group study. *J Clin Oncol*. 2005;23:8646-8654.
23. Jonker DJ, O'Callaghan CJ, Karapetis CS, et al. Cetuximab for the treatment of colorectal cancer. *N Engl J Med*. 2007;357:2040-2048.
24. Van Cutsem E, Peeters M, Siena S, et al. Open-label phase III trial of panitumumab plus best supportive care compared with best supportive care alone in patients with chemotherapy-refractory metastatic colorectal cancer. *J Clin Oncol*. 2007;25:1658-1664.
25. Stewart JS, Cohen EE, Licitra L, et al. Phase III study of gefitinib compared with intravenous methotrexate for recurrent squamous cell carcinoma of the head and neck [corrected]. *J Clin Oncol*. 2009;27:1864-1871.
26. Kim ES, Kies MS, Glisson BS, et al. Final results of a phase II study of erlotinib, docetaxel and cisplatin in patients with recurrent/metastatic head and neck cancer [abstract]. *J Clin Oncol*. ASCO Annual Meeting Proceedings Part I. 2007;25(18S, June 20 suppl): Abstract 6013.
27. Glisson BS, Murphy BA, Frenette G, Khuri FR, Forastiere AA. Phase II trial of docetaxel and cisplatin combination chemotherapy in patients with squamous cell carcinoma of the head and neck. *J Clin Oncol*. 2002;20:1593-1599. © 2002 by American Society of Clinical Oncology.
28. Hainsworth JD, Spigel DR, Greco FA, et al. Combined modality treatment with chemotherapy, radiation therapy, bevacizumab, and erlotinib in patients with locally advanced squamous carcinoma of the head and neck: a phase II trial of the Sarah Cannon Oncology Research Consortium. *Cancer J*. 2011;17:267-272.
29. William Junior WN, Weber RS, Lee JJ, et al. Randomized trial of a short course of erlotinib 150 to 300 mg daily prior to surgery for squamous cell carcinomas of the head and neck (SCCHN) in current, former, and never smokers: objective responses and clinical outcomes. . *J Clin Oncol*. 2011;29(suppl):5520.
30. Abidoye OO, Cohen EE, Wong SJ, et al. A phase II study of lapatinib (GW572016) in recurrent/metastatic (R/M) squamous cell carcinoma of the head and neck (SCCHN) [abstract]. *J Clin Oncol*. ASCO Annual Meeting Proceedings (Post-Meeting Edition). 2006;24(18S, June 20 suppl): Abstract 5568. © 2006 American Society of Clinical Oncology.
31. Jain RK. Tumor angiogenesis and accessibility: role of vascular endothelial growth factor. *Semin Oncol*. 2002;29:3-9.
32. Jenab-Wolcott J, Giantonio BJ. Bevacizumab: current indications and future development for management of solid tumors. *Expert Opin Biol Ther*. 2009;9:507-517.
33. Seiwert TY, Haraf DJ, Cohen EE, et al. Phase I study of bevacizumab added to fluorouracil- and hydroxyurea-based concomitant chemoradiotherapy for poor-prognosis head and neck cancer. *J Clin Oncol*. 2008;26:1732-1741.
34. Argiris A, Karamouzis MV, Gooding WE, et al. Phase II trial of pemetrexed and bevacizumab in patients with recurrent or metastatic head and neck cancer. *J Clin Oncol*. 2011;29:1140-1145.
35. Williamson SK, Moon J, Huang CH, et al. Phase II evaluation of sorafenib in advanced and metastatic squamous cell carcinoma of the head and neck: Southwest Oncology Group Study S0420. *J Clin Oncol*. 2010;28:3330-3335.
36. Machiels JP, Henry S, Zanetta S, et al. Phase II study of sunitinib in recurrent or metastatic squamous cell carcinoma of the head and neck: GORTEC 2006-01. *J Clin Oncol*. 2009;28:21-28.
37. Barnes CJ, Ohshiro K, Rayala SK, et al. Insulin-like growth factor receptor as a therapeutic target in head and neck cancer. *Clin Cancer Res*. 2007;13:4291-4299.
38. Larsson O, Girnita A, Girnita L. Role of insulin-like growth factor 1 receptor signalling in cancer. *Br J Cancer*. 2007;96(suppl):R2-R6.
39. Zhang X, Lin M, van Golen KL, et al. Multiple signaling pathways are activated during insulin-like growth factor-I (IGF-I) stimulated breast cancer cell migration. *Breast Cancer Res Treat*. 2005;93:159-168.
40. Reinmuth N, Fan F, Liu W, et al. Impact of insulin-like growth factor receptor-I function on angiogenesis, growth, and metastasis of colon cancer. *Lab Invest*. 2002;82:1377-1389.
41. Morgillo F, Woo JK, Kim ES, et al. Heterodimerization of insulin-like growth factor receptor/epidermal growth factor receptor and induction of survivin expression counteract the antitumor action of erlotinib. *Cancer Res*. 2006;66:10100-10111.
42. Riesterer O, Yang Q, Raju U, et al. Combination of anti-IGF-1R antibody A12 and ionizing radiation in upper respiratory tract cancers. *Int J Radiat Oncol Biol Phys*. 2010;79:1179-1187.

43. Voorhees PM, Dees EC, O'Neil B, et al. The proteasome as a target for cancer therapy. *Clin Cancer Res*. 2003;9:6316-6325.
44. Wagenblast J, Hambek M, Baghi M, et al. Antiproliferative activity of bortezomib alone and in combination with cisplatin or docetaxel in head and neck squamous cell carcinoma cell lines. *J Cancer Res Clin Oncol*. 2008;134:323-330.
45. Argiris A, Duffy AG, Kummar S, et al. Early tumor progression associated with enhanced EGFR signaling with bortezomib, cetuximab, and radiotherapy for head and neck cancer. *Clin Cancer Res*. 2011;17:5755-5764.
46. Koppikar P, Choi SH, Egloff AM, et al. Combined inhibition of c-Src and epidermal growth factor receptor abrogates growth and invasion of head and neck squamous cell carcinoma. *Clin Cancer Res*. 2008;14:4284-4291.
47. van Oijen MG, Rijksen G, ten Broek FW, et al. Overexpression of c-Src in areas of hyperproliferation in head and neck cancer, premalignant lesions and benign mucosal disorders. *J Oral Pathol Med*. 1998;27:147-152.
48. Xi S, Zhang Q, Dyer KF, et al. Src kinases mediate STAT growth pathways in squamous cell carcinoma of the head and neck. *J Biol Chem*. 2003;278:31574-31583.
49. Brooks HD, Glisson BS, Bekele BN, et al. Phase 2 study of dasatinib in the treatment of head and neck squamous cell carcinoma. *Cancer*. 2011;117:2112-2119.
50. Lai SY, Johnson FM. Defining the role of the JAK-STAT pathway in head and neck and thoracic malignancies: implications for future therapeutic approaches. *Drug Resist Updat*. 2010;13:67-78.
51. Sriuranpong V, Park JI, Amornphimoltham P, et al. Epidermal growth factor receptor-independent constitutive activation of STAT3 in head and neck squamous cell carcinoma is mediated by the autocrine/paracrine stimulation of the interleukin 6/gp130 cytokine system. *Cancer Res*. 2003;63:2948-2956.
52. Grandis JR, Drenning SD, Zeng Q, et al. Constitutive activation of Stat3 signaling abrogates apoptosis in squamous cell carcinogenesis in vivo. *Proc Natl Acad Sci U S A*. 2000;97:4227-4232.
53. Lai SY, Childs EE, Xi S, et al. Erythropoietin-mediated activation of JAK-STAT signaling contributes to cellular invasion in head and neck squamous cell carcinoma. *Oncogene*. 2005;24:4442-4449.
54. Verstovsek S, Kantarjian H, Mesa RA, et al. Safety and efficacy of INCB018424, a JAK1 and JAK2 inhibitor, in myelofibrosis. *N Engl J Med*. 2010;363:1117-1127.
55. Forastiere A, Koch W, Trotti A, et al. Head and neck cancer. *N Engl J Med*. 2001;345:1890-1900.
56. Brennan JA, Boyle JO, Koch WM, et al. Association between cigarette smoking and mutation of the p53 gene in squamous-cell carcinoma of the head and neck. *N Engl J Med*. 1995;332:712-717.
57. Nemunaitis J. Head and neck cancer: response to p53-based therapeutics. *Head Neck*. 2010;33:131-134.

CHAPTER 62

PERSONALIZED MEDICINE AND TARGETED THERAPY FOR MELANOMA

Keith T. Flaherty

INTRODUCTION

The elucidation of somatic genetic changes in melanoma has provided a framework for developing targeted therapy that directly opposes activated oncogenes or signal transduction pathways that are apparently active as a consequence of tumor suppressor loss. By far, the best validated therapeutic approach in this area is BRAF inhibition in patients with metastatic melanoma harboring activating BRAF mutations. Single-agent BRAF inhibitor therapy significantly alters the natural history of metastatic melanoma, has established the proof-of-concept for targeted therapy in this disease, and has provided a basis for developing combination targeted therapy. The PI3K (phosphoinositide 3-kinase) and p16/Rb pathways are known to be activated in conjunction with BRAF mutations activating the mitogen-activated protein (MAP) kinase pathway, but can also be implicated in some BRAF wild-type tumors. Developing combination regimens to antagonize primary and secondary oncogenic pathways simultaneously is a current focus of clinical research. Activating NRAS mutations continue to pose a challenge with regard to direct or indirect pharmacologic inhibition and represent a unique subpopulation of advanced melanomas. Finally, uveal melanoma has recently been found to harbor unique somatic changes in G proteins that activate downstream signal transduction and a tumor suppressor gene, the function of which continues to be investigated. This review explores the matrix of genetic alterations identified to date in melanoma for which therapeutic strategies have been or are currently being studied in the clinic.

MAP KINASE PATHWAY

MAP kinase pathway activation has long been associated with melanoma pathophysiology. The molecular underpinnings of this were thought to relate to autocrine or paracrine growth factor receptor signaling. However, it has become clear that it is a consequence of activating mutations in signal transduction molecules in the pathway in the vast majority of cases. This genetic evidence supports the near requirement for MAP kinase pathway activation to drive melanoma progression and dissemination. The most commonly mutated oncogene in melanoma is BRAF.[1] The next most common is NRAS,[2] for which the MAP kinase pathway is one of several effector pathways. Lastly, activating CKIT mutations can constitutively activate the MAP kinase pathway.[3] The fact that these three genetic events appear to be mutually exclusive reinforces the biologically redundant role that each plays in contributing to transformation.[4]

NRAS

Analogous to activating mutations in KRAS in many epithelial cancers, 20% of melanomas harbor activating mutations in NRAS. These mutations are transforming when combined with inactivation of either p53 or p16.[5,6] And a transgenic model replicates the disease process well when NRAS mutations are combined with the p53 loss.[7] NRAS is a GTPase and, in the presence of mutations commonly found in melanoma, the ability of NRAS to hydrolyze GTP to GDP is impaired. As a consequence, NRAS remains GTP bound and is constitutively active.

This type of molecular alteration, in which an element of NRAS activity is lost, creates a unique challenge in terms of developing a pharmacologic approach to inhibit NRAS directly. To directly antagonize NRAS, agents would need to be devised that restore the GTPase activity, induce an allosteric change in NRAS that favors the GDP-bound state, or interfere with the interaction of NRAS with its essential co-factors or substrates. None of these approaches have yet been successful in producing a clinically viable therapeutic approach.

In the absence of pharmacologic inhibitors, preclinical data have been generated showing that knockdown of NRAS RNA decreases the proliferation of NRAS mutant melanoma cell lines, induces apoptosis, and sensitizes cells to the cytotoxic effect of conventional DNA-interacting chemotherapy.[8] Thus, preclinical data support the potential therapeutic relevance of targeting NRAS when it is mutated. Over a decade ago, attempts were made to develop pharmacologic inhibitors of one of the key post-translational modifications that RAS requires to become membrane localized and available for activation. Such farnesyltransferase inhibitors were shown to decrease RAS expression and had both anti-proliferative and pro-apoptotic effects in vitro.[9] In clinical trials, farnesyltransferase inhibitors induced dose-limiting toxicities, but they had minimal evidence of anti-tumor activity in cancers that harbor NRAS mutations. Biochemical evidence of RAS effector pathway inhibition was never robustly demonstrated. Although never definitively shown, the prevailing view of these agents is that concentrations that could be tolerably or safely achieved in patients were limited by inhibition of other farnesylated proteins in normal tissues. Thus, these agents were felt to be incapable of exerting a significant effect on mutated RAS in tumor due to this lack of selectivity. Very little exploration of farnesyltransferase inhibitors has been undertaken in NRAS mutant melanoma, but the lack of validation of these agents in other RAS mutant cancers provided little reason for enthusiasm. In a single-agent clinical trial with one orally available farnesyltransferase inhibitor, no responses were seen in a small cohort of genetically unselected patients and further investigation was terminated.[10] More recently, a farnesyltransferase inhibitor was combined with sorafenib (the broad-spectrum RAF/vascular endothelial growth factor receptor kinase inhibitor) in a clinical trial among patients with metastatic melanoma, but again, significant clinical activity was not observed.[11]

Recent attention has turned to the concept of combining inhibitors that block RAS effector pathway signaling as an indirect approach. While the MAP kinase and PI3K pathways have been well described as important RAS effectors, it is also well known that additional RAS effector pathways exist. Nonetheless, early evidence suggests that in some NRAS the melanomas are sensitive to the effects of MAP kinase kinase (MEK) inhibitors,[12] and it is hoped that in a larger subset of NRAS the tumors will be susceptible to combined MEK and PI3K pathway inhibition.[13] Preclinical studies have not yet defined the optimal point of intervention in the PI3K pathway (PI3K itself, AKT, or further downstream), so it is not possible to determine if the optimal RAS effector pathway blocking strategy is being tested in ongoing clinical trials. It seems plausible that not all NRAS mutated melanomas will signal downstream of RAS in the same way, due to differences in concomitant genetic alterations, and that more than one therapeutic strategy might be needed when targeting downstream of RAS. The field continues to await the development of direct NRAS antagonists, but such an agent would seem to be the most likely approach to have an optimal therapeutic index.

BRAF

BRAF mutations are present in 50% of advanced cases of melanoma.[1] While many mutations have been identified that cluster in two segments of the kinase domain, patients' tumor harbors mutations that alter the valine residue at the 600 position in the amino acid sequence. The most common of these is glutamate substitution that confers constitutive activation of BRAF (V600E), with an 800-fold increase in the ability to phosphorylate the downstream substrate MEK. Like other oncogenes, the introduction of V600E BRAF into normal melanocytes results in senescence. But in melanocytes with preexisting p16 loss, V600E BRAF drives the MAP kinase pathway in an RAS-independent fashion and produces clonogenic growth. While other investigations have suggested that factors other than p16 loss are essential for reversal of senescence,[14] the key finding is that melanoma formation requires at least one tumor suppressor gene to be disabled in conjunction with activating BRAF mutations to result in melanoma. In transgenic mouse models, the most potent combination of oncogene/tumor suppressor gene in spawning melanoma is V600E BRAF combined with PTEN (phosphatase and tensin homolog deleted on chromosome 10) deletion.[15] Of course, with a large burden of additional mutations known to occur in melanoma, the contribution of other secondary or tertiary events in melanoma formation remains to be determined.

In experimental systems, BRAF appears to be an important driver of proliferation and cell survival despite being accompanied by many additional genetic alterations that impact diverse pathways beyond the MAP kinase pathway. In the years before selective, small molecule inhibitors of BRAF were available, RNA knockdown experiments suggested that selective depletion of the BRAF mutant allele would universally inhibit cell proliferation in vitro.[16] More variably, induction of apoptosis was observed, providing the first evidence that heterogeneity in responsiveness may be expected with BRAF antagonists.[17] Selective MEK inhibitors demonstrated MAP kinase pathway inhibition independent of the presence or absence of BRAF mutation.[18] However, these agents demonstrated far greater effect on cell cycle and cell death in cells that harbor BRAF mutation than RAS mutated cell lines for cancer cell lines wild type for BRAF and NRAS/KRAS. Selective BRAF inhibitors have a far more selective effect on biochemical evidence of MAP kinase pathway inhibition as well as suppression of proliferation and induction of apoptosis.[19] In fact, selective BRAF inhibitors with diverse chemical composition have demonstrated either no inhibitory effect on MAP kinase pathway signaling or a stimulatory effect, particularly in cells that harbor activating RAS mutations or constitutively active receptor tyrosine kinase signaling.[20-22] In BRAF mutant cancer cell lines, however, selective BRAF inhibitors have a reproducible, profound inhibitory effect on MAP kinase pathway signaling.[23] The observation of cell death in vitro is limited to BRAF mutant cancer cells, but not all such models are equally sensitive.

Extracellular signal-regulated kinase (ERK) inhibition represents a distinct and potentially advantageous strategy for targeting tumors with upstream activating mutations in the MAP kinase pathway, namely BRAF and NRAS. Preclinical investigations of BRAF and MEK inhibitors in melanoma models harboring BRAF mutations reveal that each effects MAP kinase–regulated gene expression in a similar fashion.[24] Notably, negative regulators of BRAF and MEK are expressed at lower levels after pharmacologic inhibition of BRAF or MEK.[25] Sprouty is a well-described RAF deactivator and the dual-specific phosphatases (DUSP4 and DUSP6) dephosphorylate MEK. While the consequences of this altered expression in these molecules are not fully known, it is anticipated that lowered expression of Sprouty and DUSP4 would tend to counteract the inhibitory effect of either a BRAF or an MEK inhibitor, limiting the ability to extinguish MAP kinase pathway output. ERK has distinct feedback regulators. Thus, it is postulated that ERK inhibition might be associated with differential effects on MAP kinase pathway signaling and the inability of feedback regulators to defeat that effect. This remains to be established in humans and it is possible that the greater degrees of pathway inhibition that are postulated for ERK inhibitors might not be well tolerated in normal tissues. Nonetheless, this approach appears to be worthy of exploring.

CLINICAL INVESTIGATION OF BRAF AND MEK INHIBITORS

In clinical trials, BRAF inhibition has emerged as the single most effective strategy for antagonizing mutated BRAF and as a new treatment standard for patients with metastatic disease (Fig. 62.1). Selective BRAF inhibitors induce tumor regression in approximately 90% of patients treated with metastatic melanoma harboring a V600E BRAF mutation.[26,27] The duration of these responses is highly variable, with some lasting only a few months, while others are durable beyond 1.5 years.[28] The median duration of response is 6 months from the time that initial response was documented (typically 2 mo after the initiation of therapy). Despite the fact that some responses are very short lived, the BRAF has recently demonstrated a significant survival advantage compared with conventional cytotoxic chemotherapy as first-line treatment for metastatic melanoma patients.[27] Understanding the

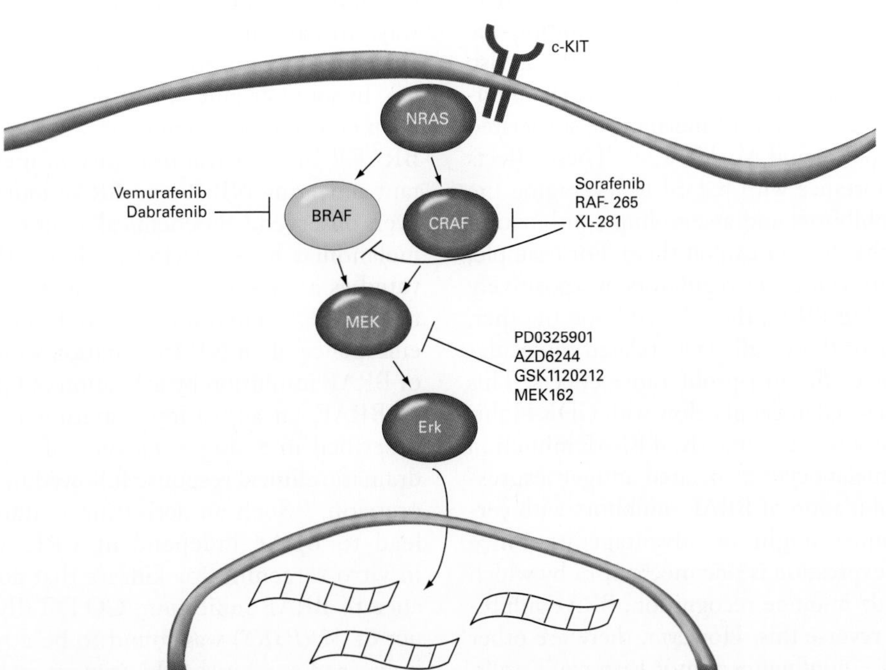

FIGURE 62–1 The MAP kinase pathway and the agents in clinical development targeting RAF and MEK.

mechanisms by which some BRAF mutant melanoma cells within a given patient's tumor survive the initial course of treatment and how cells are able to resume proliferation after being successfully arrested for several to many months is a critical area of investigation currently. This topic is addressed in detail below.

As might be predicted by the fact that BRAF appears to exert its oncogenic effect through MEK activation, selective and allosteric MEK inhibitors have also demonstrated significant activity in patients with metastatic melanoma harboring V600E mutations.[29,30] The results of ongoing clinical trials are needed to determine if MEK inhibition is equally advantageous compared with BRAF inhibition in these patients as a first-line strategy. As mechanisms of resistance to BRAF inhibition are becoming better defined, it is increasingly clear that MEK inhibitors may add value to BRAF inhibition as a way of overcoming some mechanisms of MAP kinase pathway reactivation.[31]

An important line of investigation regarding the molecular pathophysiology of tumors that harbor activating BRAF mutations considers these downstream consequences of this oncogene. As a consequence of MEK and ERK activation, an important set of genes have their expression altered to the presence of mutated BRAF. MITF, the transcription factor described as the master regulator of melanocyte differentiation and itself a potential melanoma oncogene, is suppressed by mutated BRAF.[32,33] This has several key consequences, one of which is the upregulation of cell cycle–related genes, such as CDK2, and decreased expression of melanocyte-associated antigens.[34] Knockdown of mutated BRAF RNA can reverse either of these phenomena. This has the expected consequence of decreased cellular proliferation, which may be, in part, a consequence of direct BRAF inhibition due to increased MITF target gene transcription. It has also become clear that by restoring MITF levels, BRAF inhibition can restore the expression of melanocyte-associated antigens, such as gp-100 and MART-1.[35,36] These effects have potential importance with regard to leveraging the effects of BRAF inhibitors and assembling combination therapy regimens that further exploit them. For example, if some, but not all, cell cycle regulators are positively impacted by inhibiting BRAF, then the addition of other, selective inhibitors of those cell cycle–related molecules might further enhance the anti-proliferative effects. This is a topic that is discussed in detail below with CDK4 inhibition as a potential strategy. Similarly, if BRAF inhibition results in greater melanocyte-associated antigen expression, then the combination of BRAF inhibitors with certain immunotherapies might be advantageous. Since decreased antigen expression is one mechanism by which melanoma can evade immune recognition, BRAF inhibitors could help to reverse this. However, there are other factors that negatively influence tumor reactive T cells, including PD-L1 and IDO expression in the tumor microenvironment, which may need to be directly targeted to take advantage of the positive immunologic effects of BRAF targeted therapy.[37,38]

BRAF INHIBITOR RESISTANCE

Since the first observations of clinical response to selective BRAF inhibitors and subsequent emergence disease progression, describing the molecular basis of acquired resistance has been a very active research area. Two parallel strategies have been pursued: in vitro selection of BRAF mutant cell lines that are able to proliferate after chronic BRAF inhibitor exposure and analysis of patient tumor biopsies procured before therapy and again at the time of disease progression. These investigations have produced several leads with regard to the molecular determinants of acquired resistance, though definitive proof in large, prospectively characterize cohorts is still awaited.

In the context of early phase clinical trials with vemurafenib and dabrafenib, serial tumor biopsies were performed at baseline and after the first few weeks of therapy to determine the effect of BRAF inhibitor therapy on the MAP kinase pathway, as assessed by ERK phosphorylation. Among patients who received the recommended phase II dose of either agent, 80% to 100% decreases in semiquantitative assessments of pERK were observed.[23,39] Thus, it appears that robust pathway inhibition is achieved in all cases. In approximately two-thirds of patients' tumor samples characterized at the time of disease progression there is evidence of reactivation of pERK, while the others continue to demonstrate suppressed levels of ERK activation.[40] This has set the framework for investigating mechanisms that might account for restoration of MAP kinase pathway signaling or those that might be able to circumvent the MAP kinase pathway. To date, novel mutations in the kinase domain of BRAF have not been observed.[41]

In some instances, activating NRAS mutations have been detected in conjunction with persistence of V600E BRAF.[41] In the natural history of melanoma, concomitant activating NRAS and BRAF mutations are rarely, if ever, observed.[4] Biochemical analyses of NRAS mutant melanomas have previously shown that CRAF is activated as a consequence of constitutively active NRAS, not BRAF.[42] Therefore, it would be expected that the emergence of an NRAS mutation would result in bypass of BRAF inhibition by activation of CRAF. Downstream of BRAF, an activating mutation in MEK1 has been described in a single instance of a patient who had a dramatic clinical response followed by rapid disease progression.[43] Such an activating mutation would clearly lead to BRAF-independent ERK activation. In the in vitro screening for kinases that could confer resistance to BRAF inhibition, COT/TPL2 (the gene product of *MAP3K8*) was found to be a particularly potent inducer of resistance.[44] In primary melanoma specimens, COT amplification was detected in a notable subset of melanomas and appears to confer relative resistance to

BRAF inhibition. Among a few patient tumor samples taken before treatment and after several weeks of therapy, COT upregulation was observed. Although it has not been extensively studied in cancer, COT is an MAP kinase downstream of BRAF, known to phosphorylate MEK. Thus, it is quite plausible that increased COT signaling could account for reactivation of the MAP kinase pathway in the setting of ongoing BRAF inhibition. Each of these mechanisms by which the MAP kinase pathway is reactivated must be corroborated in a larger number of patient tumor samples in order to understand the frequency with which they contribute to BRAF inhibitor resistance.

Upregulation of receptor tyrosine kinase signaling has been implicated as a means by which PI3K pathway activation can mediate BRAF inhibitor resistance. Assaying for the expression and activation of a large number of receptor tyrosine kinases, investigators described marked and selective upregulation of platelet-derived growth factor receptor beta in a significant minority of tumor samples taken at the time of disease progression and compared with baseline samples.[41] This appeared to be associated with AKT activation. Similarly, when melanoma cell lines were cultured in the presence of a sublethal dose of a selective BRAF inhibitor, insulin-like growth factor receptor expression was increased in the emerging resistant clones compared with the same cell lines prior to BRAF inhibitor exposure.[45] This also correlated with AKT phosphorylation. Lastly, in a single instance, a progressing tumor lesion was biopsied and found to have homozygous PTEN deletion, whereas at baseline PTEN was intact.[45] Although this represents a single case, the significance of this observation is amplified by the clear role that PTEN loss plays in melanoma biology.

PI3K PATHWAY

As noted above, genetic evidence in sporadic melanoma and the construction of transgenic models that recapitulate the disease reinforce the importance of the PI3K pathway in melanoma pathophysiology (Fig. 62.2). Approximately half of all BRAF mutant melanomas have concomitant loss of expression of PTEN.[46,47] This includes instances of homozygous deletion, missense mutations that alter function, or genetic and epigenetic mechanisms that result in decreased PTEN protein expression. Separately, there appears to be a subset of melanomas that harbor AKT3 amplification, which appears to be an independent mechanism of co-activating the PI3K, a pathway in conjunction with BRAF mutations.[48] The direct consequence of PTEN loss or AKT3 amplification remains to be fully elucidated; however, recent evidence suggests that activation of the PI3K pathway in melanoma is a critical determinant of pro-apoptotic BIM expression. Specifically, PTEN loss suppresses BIM expression and renders the cells more resistant to induction of apoptosis. In in vitro, it is clear that BRAF mutant/PTEN deleted melanoma cell lines do not undergo apoptosis to the same degree that BRAF mutant/PTEN intact cells do.[49,50] This resistance can largely be overcome by concomitant inhibition of BRAF and PI3K. It would be anticipated that AKT inhibition would be similarly effective, and perhaps even more downstream inhibition of mammalian target of rapamycin (mTOR) signaling could suffice.[15] However,

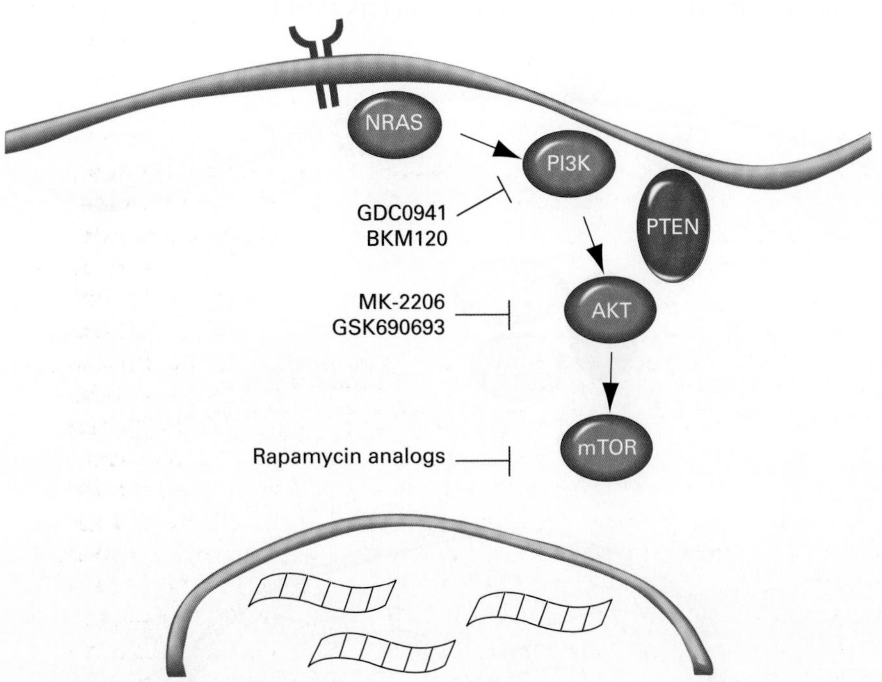

FIGURE 62–2 PI3K pathway.

data are lacking in animal models or in human clinical trials to conclude which of these approaches would maximize efficacy while minimizing toxicity. The lack of efficacy associated with single-agent mTORC1 inhibition with a rapamycin analog in a phase II trial only reinforces the notion that this pathway is a complementary oncogenic pathway in melanoma and not a driver.[51]

Although phosphorylation of S6 kinase and activation of PRAS40 are thought to largely be the consequence of PI3K or AKT activation, it is clear that mutated BRAF can control S6 activation in some circumstances. It has recently been described that AMP kinase is directly regulated by BRAF and hyper-activated in the setting of mutated BRAF.[52] This can result in phosphorylation of S6 kinase in a PI3K pathway-independent fashion. Since S6 is canonically described as downstream of AKT, it was a striking observation that an oncogene in the MAP kinase pathway could exert such a direct influence on it. This relationship underscores the importance of understanding the downstream molecular effects, both positive and negative, of any given targeted therapy in order to develop rationally designed combination therapies. In cancer cells in which S6 activity is downstream of BRAF, it would be hypothesized that greater degrees of cell death would be triggered by BRAF inhibitor monotherapy than in cells where S6 activation is regulated by the PI3K pathway. Only the latter group might stand to benefit from the addition of a PI3K pathway inhibitor to a BRAF inhibitor (though this correlation has yet to be determined in patients). This appears to be an important dichotomy in regard to relative sensitivity or resistance to BRAF targeted therapy and requires further clinical and translational investigation.

Clinical trials will be initiated in the near future investigating combinations of BRAF or MEK inhibitors with PI3K or AKT inhibitors. As there is a large diversity of PI3K inhibitors currently in clinical development with regard to their selectivity for various PI3K isoforms and cross-reactivity with mTOR and DNA-PKs, it remains uncertain which of these combinations will be optimal.[53] Furthermore, there are several AKT inhibitors in clinical development with different potencies and specificities against the three AKT isoforms and ATP-competitive versus non-competitive properties. This area of investigation is certainly of high priority given the existing genetic and experimental evidence; however, a robust and efficient preclinical basis for determining the optimal strategy for combining such agents would significantly accelerate the development of the optimal strategy.

c-KIT

The one receptor tyrosine kinase that has been found to harbor activation mutations in melanoma is c-KIT.[3] Within acral lentiginous and mucosal melanoma, both relatively uncommon subtypes of melanoma in comparison to melanoma arising on the head and neck, trunk, or extremities, approximately 10% of cases are found to have mutation in *CKIT*. Amplification of mutated or wild-type CKIT can also be found in these same melanoma histologies. A subset of these mutations have been described in gastrointestinal stromal tumors (GISTs) and are well defined with regard to their signaling properties as well as their susceptibility to imatinib and other small molecular inhibitors of the KIT tyrosine kinase domain.[54] In phase II clinical trials administering single-agent imatinib to patients with CKIT mutations, objective responses have been observed in the subset of patients whose tumors show well-defined imatinib-responsive mutations in GIST.[55,56] Unfortunately, the majority of patients in this

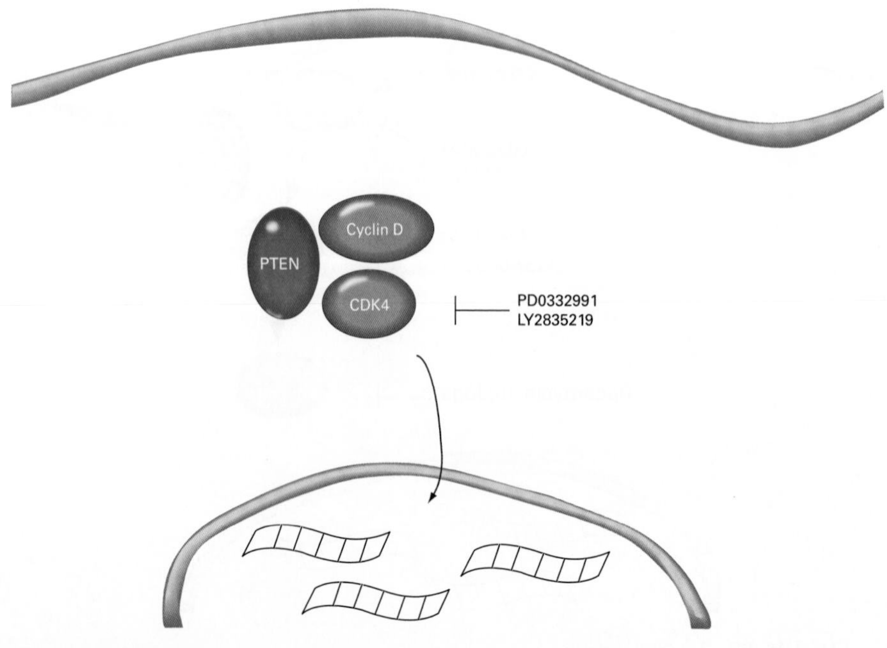

FIGURE 62–3 p16, cyclin D, and CDK4.

small genetically defined subset do not have previously described imatinib-responsive mutations, and novel KIT inhibitors may be needed to test the oncogenic role of these poorly defined KIT mutations. Due to the relative infrequency with which KIT mutations are found, even within the appropriate histologic subtypes, it has taken several years to complete multi-center phase II trial clinical trials in this population.

P16, CYCLIN D, AND CDK4

Extensive genetic evidence suggests that CDK4 is a particularly important regulator of cell cycle in melanoma (Fig. 62.3). Two of the best described melanoma predisposition genes in families with a strong penetrance of melanoma are p16 inactivating mutations and CDK4 activating mutations.[57,58] In sporadic melanomas, p16 mutation or loss, CDK4 mutation or amplification, and cyclin D application are commonly found.[4,47] There is a large degree of overlap between these genetic alterations in BRAF mutation, though incomplete. As cyclin D is a necessary cofactor for CDK4 activity and p16 is the negative regulator of CDK4 activation, any of these genetic events could be expected to upregulate CDK4 activity and contribute to cell cycle progression. Melanoma cells that harbor concomitant BRAF and CDK4 activating mutations are relatively resistant to BRAF inhibitors compared with BRAF mutant/CDK4 wild-type cell lines.[59] Extensive preclinical studies with CDK4 mRNA knockdown or direct pharmacologic inhibition have not been undertaken. Preliminary investigations suggest synergy in target mutant BRAF and CDK4 when p16 is lost or mutated.[60,61] More direct pharmacologic investigations are now increasingly feasible given the emergence of several small molecule selective CDK4/6 inhibitors. In clinical trials, such an agent appears to have single-agent antitumor effects in cyclin D–amplified lymphomas and thus appears to be an attractive candidate therapy for exploration in melanoma, either alone or in combination with BRAF inhibitors.

p53

Unlike in many epithelial cancers, p53 is largely wild type and expressed normal levels in melanoma.[47] However, loss of p53 function is well documented in melanoma and p16 loss of function has been postulated to account for some of this.[62] Also, amplification of hdm2, a negative regulator of p53 function, has been described in a subset of melanomas.[63] These observations provide opportunities for exploring hdm2 antagonists in melanoma. A subpopulation of melanoma cell lines undergoes apoptosis with an hdm2 antagonist in vitro. In many BRAF mutant melanoma cell lines, there is synergistic induction of apoptosis when combining MEK and hdm2 antagonists.[64] Unlike other activated oncogenes and signal transduction pathways in melanoma, this concept takes advantage of the persistence of wild-type p53 in the vast majority of melanoma. This opportunity could play an important role in combination targeted therapy regimens as hdm2 antagonist advance in clinical trials.

UVEAL MELANOMA

Recent discoveries regarding the genetic underpinnings of uveal melanoma have largely accounted for the unique genomic profile of uveal melanoma in comparison to cutaneous and mucosal melanoma. Each of the well-described oncogenes and tumor suppressor genes that play a significant role in cutaneous melanoma is absent in uveal melanoma. However, two recently defined oncogenes and one tumor suppressor gene that are genetically altered in 80% to 90% of all uveal melanomas are found exclusively in that disease entity and not in cutaneous melanoma. Specifically, the vast majority of uveal melanomas harbor activating mutations in either GNAQ or GNA11 in a mutually exclusive fashion.[65,66] Both of these G protein alpha subunits are implicated in the activity of protein kinase C, the MAP kinase pathway, and other signal transduction pathways. Reminiscent of NRAS mutations, these mutations in GNAQ and GNA11 disable the GTPase activity of these enzymes and render them consecutively GTP bound and active. Restoring the diminished GTPase activity will likely be as much of a drug development challenge as direct pharmacologic inhibitors of mutated RAS proteins have been. Intensive effort has been undertaken in preclinical systems to understand which signal transduction pathways are essential for the oncogenic effects of either of these mutated G proteins. Biochemical evidence suggests that the MAP kinase pathway and PKC signaling represent critical nodes of signaling and potential points for therapeutic intervention.[67] The availability of selective MEK inhibitors and, in the near future, ERK inhibitors provides a basis for exploring the MAP kinase dependence of these tumors. Potent and selective PKC inhibitors have recently been developed and provide a basis for exploring this point of intervention.[68] The field of targeted therapy in uveal melanoma is in its infancy. Nonetheless, for the first time, this unique subset of melanomas has bona fide therapeutic targets.

Complementing the discovery of GNAQ/GNA11 activating mutations was the observation that BAP1, which resides on the short arm of chromosome 3, is commonly inactivated through point mutation in uveal melanoma.[69] Chromosome 3p loss has long been known to confer poor prognosis in uveal melanoma and is present in 80% to 90% of metastatic cases.[70] Deep sequencing of the short arm of chromosome 3 revealed frequent mutations in this poorly defined molecule. BAP1 has been implicated in cell cycle regulation through interactions with BRCA1 and BARD1 and histone-modifying complexes.[71] Separately, BAP1 appears to be involved in developmental pathways through an interaction with ASXL1 in a deubiquitinase complex.[72] While mutations have

TABLE 62-1 Oncogene Targeted Drugs in Melanoma Clinical Trials

Oncogene	Pathway	Drug	Phase of Clinical Trial in Melanoma	ClinicalTrials.gov Listing for Ongoing Trials
BRAF	MAP kinase			
Non-selective		Sorafenib	Phase III (completed)[74, 75]	
		XL-281	Phase I (completed)	
		RAF-265	Phase I	NCT00095693
Selective		PLX4032	Phase III (completed)[26,27]	
		GSK2118436	Phase III (completed)	
MEK	MAP kinase	AZD6244	Phase II (completed)	
		PD0325901	Phase I (completed)	
		GSK1120212	Phase III (completed)	
NRAS	MEK	AZD6244	Phase II (completed)[29]	
		PD0325901	Phase I (completed)	
		GSK1120212		
	PI3K/AKT/mTOR	GDC0941 (PI3K)		
		BKM120 (PI3K)		
		MK-2206 (AKT)		
		GSK690693 (AKT)		
		Temsirolimus (mTOR)	Phase II (completed)[51]	
c-KIT	Growth factor receptor	Imatinib	Phase II (completed)	
		Nilotinib	Phase III first-line	NCT01028222
			Phase II second-line	NCT01099514
		Dasatinib	Phase II	NCT00700882
CDK4	p16/cyclin D/CDK4	PD032991		
		LY2835219	Phase I expansion	NCT01394016
GNAQ/GNA11	MAP kinase	AZD6244	Phase II	NCT01143402

MAP, mitogen-activated protein kinase; MEK, MAP kinase kinase; PI3K, phosphoinositide 3-kinase; mTOR, mammalian target of rapamycin.

been identified in several BAP1 domains, the greatest concentrations are found in the BARD1- and BRCA1-binding domains. Lacking pharmacologic strategies for restoring BAP1 function, histone deacetylase inhibitors have been investigated as a means of disrupting the cell cycle dysregulation that results from BAP1 loss of function. Several histone deacetylase inhibitors appear to have potential therapeutic effect in uveal melanoma cell lines harboring BAP1 mutations.[73] Much more experimental investigation is needed in order to determine how best to leverage the discovery of BAP1 mutations with regard to new treatments. As with GNAQ/GNA11 mutations, the discovery of BAP1 mutations clearly sets the agenda for translational research relating to targeted therapies in uveal melanoma.

CONCLUSION

The melanoma field is quite far along in terms of defining the key somatic genetic underpinnings of melanoma formation and dissemination. BRAF, the most frequently mutated oncogenes in melanoma, has now been validated as a therapeutic target in patients with metastatic disease. Responses have also been observed in a small subset of melanoma patients whose tumors harbor activating CKIT mutations and constitutes the next likely new treatment standard with targeted therapy in melanoma. Approximately half of all melanomas do not have a single-agent targeted therapy approach that has been validated. NRAS mutations represent a notable 20% subpopulation, but effective therapeutic strategies to antagonize NRAS itself or RAS effector pathways have been elusive. While the field continues to define a foundation of single-agent targeted therapy for the large proportion of patients for whom this approach does not apply, investigations are accelerating with BRAF inhibitor–based combination targeted therapy (Table 62.1). While many opportunities have emerged based on preclinical studies and analysis of BRAF inhibitor–resistant tumor samples, the major challenge that confronts the field is the prioritization of each combination approach and how best to tailor combination strategies to molecularly defined patient populations. There is clearly significant room for improvement on the efficacy associated with single-agent targeted therapy in metastatic melanoma, and thus, there is a need for a continued focus on clinical trials that seek to expose a new point of vulnerability. It is possible that the most dramatic clinical benefits will be seen in the adjuvant setting for patients with resected, high-risk melanomas. However, metastatic disease remains the venue in which novel therapeutic approaches can be most efficiently studied at a molecular level as well as for clinical efficacy. Now more than ever, the melanoma field has a shared focus on leveraging our molecular understanding of this disease for improvement of treatment outcomes.

REFERENCES

1. Davies H, Bignell GR, Cox C, et al. Mutations of the BRAF gene in human cancer. *Nature*. 2002;417:949-954.
2. Albino AP, Le Strange R, Oliff AI, et al. Transforming ras genes from human melanoma: a manifestation of tumour heterogeneity? *Nature*. 1984;308:69-72.
3. Curtin JA, Busam K, Pinkel D, et al. Somatic activation of KIT in distinct subtypes of melanoma. *J Clin Oncol*. 2006;24: 4340-4346.
4. Curtin JA, Fridlyand J, Kageshita T, et al. Distinct sets of genetic alterations in melanoma. *N Engl J Med*. 2005;353:2135-2147.
5. Milagre C, Dhomen N, Geyer FC, et al. A mouse model of melanoma driven by oncogenic KRAS. *Cancer Res*. 2010; 70:5549-5557.
6. Nogueira C, Kim KH, Sung H, et al. Cooperative interactions of PTEN deficiency and RAS activation in melanoma metastasis. *Oncogene*. November 2010;29(47):6222-6232.
7. Ferguson B, Konrad Muller H, Handoko HY, et al. Differential roles of the pRb and Arf/p53 pathways in murine naevus and melanoma genesis. *Pigment Cell Melanoma Res*. December 2010;23(6):771-780.
8. Smalley KS, Eisen TG. Farnesyl thiosalicylic acid inhibits the growth of melanoma cells through a combination of cytostatic and pro-apoptotic effects. *Int J Cancer*. 2002;98:514-522.
9. Smalley KS, Eisen TG. Farnesyl transferase inhibitor SCH66336 is cytostatic, pro-apoptotic and enhances chemosensitivity to cisplatin in melanoma cells. *Int J Cancer*. 2003;105:165-175.
10. Gajewski TK, Niedzwiecki D, Johnson J, et al. Phase II study of the farnesyltransferase inhibitor R115777 in advanced melanoma: CALGB 500104. *J Clin Oncol*. 2006;24.
11. Margolin KA, Moon J, Flaherty LE, et al. Randomized phase II trial of sorafenib with temsirolimus or tipifarnib in metastatic melanoma: Southwest Oncology Group Trial S0438. *J Clin Oncol*. 2011;28(15s):2010. Abstract 8502.
12. Dry JR, Pavey S, Pratilas CA, et al. Transcriptional pathway signatures predict MEK addiction and response to selumetinib (AZD6244). *Cancer Res*. 2010;70:2264-2273.
13. Jaiswal BS, Janakiraman V, Kljavin NM, et al. Combined targeting of BRAF and CRAF or BRAF and PI3K effector pathways is required for efficacy in NRAS mutant tumors. *PLoS One*. 2009;4:e5717.
14. Dhomen N, Reis-Filho JS, da Rocha Dias S, et al. Oncogenic BRAF induces melanocyte senescence and melanoma in mice. *Cancer Cell*. 2009;15:294-303.
15. Dankort D, Curley DP, Cartlidge RA, et al. BRaf(V600E) cooperates with PTEN loss to induce metastatic melanoma. *Nat Genet*. 2009;41:544-552.
16. Wellbrock C, Ogilvie L, Hedley D, et al. V599EB-RAF is an oncogene in melanocytes. *Cancer Res*. 2004;64:2338-2342.
17. Sumimoto H, Miyagishi M, Miyoshi H, et al. Inhibition of growth and invasive ability of melanoma by inactivation of mutated BRAF with lentivirus-mediated RNA interference. *Oncogene*. 2004;23:6031-6039.
18. Solit DB, Garraway LA, Pratilas CA, et al. BRAF mutation predicts sensitivity to MEK inhibition. *Nature*. 2006;439:358-362.
19. Tsai J, Lee JT, Wang W, et al. Discovery of a selective inhibitor of oncogenic B-Raf kinase with potent antimelanoma activity. *Proc Natl Acad Sci U S A*. 2008;105:3041-3046.
20. Poulikakos PI, Zhang C, Bollag G, et al. RAF inhibitors transactivate RAF dimers and ERK signalling in cells with wild-type BRAF. *Nature*. 2010;464:427-430.
21. Heidorn SJ, Milagre C, Whittaker S, et al. Kinase-dead BRAF and oncogenic RAS cooperate to drive tumor progression through CRAF. *Cell*. 2010;140:209-221.
22. Hatzivassiliou G, Song K, Yen I, et al. RAF inhibitors prime wild-type RAF to activate the MAPK pathway and enhance growth. *Nature*. 2010;464:431-435.
23. Bollag G, Hirth P, Tsai J, et al. Clinical efficacy of a RAF inhibitor needs broad target blockade in BRAF-mutant melanoma. *Nature*. 2010;467:596-599.
24. Packer LM, East P, Reis-Filho JS, et al. Identification of direct transcriptional targets of (V600E)BRAF/MEK signalling in melanoma. *Pigment Cell Melanoma Res*. 2009;22:785-798.
25. Pratilas CA, Taylor BS, Ye Q, et al. (V600E)BRAF is associated with disabled feedback inhibition of RAF-MEK signaling and elevated transcriptional output of the pathway. *Proc Natl Acad Sci U S A*. 2009;106:4519-4524.
26. Flaherty KT, Puzanov I, Kim KB, et al. Inhibition of mutated, activated BRAF in metastatic melanoma. *N Engl J Med*. 2010; 363:809-819.
27. Chapman PB, Hauschild A, Robert C, et al. Improved Survival with Vemurafenib in Melanoma with BRAF V600E Mutation. *N Engl J Med*. 2011.
28. Kim KB, Flaherty KT, Chapman PB, et al. Pattern and outcome of disease progression in phase I study of vemurafenib in patients with metastatic melanoma (MM). *J Clin Oncol*. 2011;29 (suppl). Abstract 8519.
29. Kirkwood JM, Bastholt L, Robert C, et al. Phase II, open-label, randomized trial of the MEK 1/2 inhibitor selumetinib as monotherapy versus temozolomide in patients with advanced melanoma. *Clin Cancer Res*.
30. Infante JR, Fecher LA, Nallapareddy S, et al. Safety and efficacy results from the first-in-human study of the oral MEK 1/2 inhibitor GSK1120212. *J Clin Oncol*. 2010;28(15 suppl):2010. Abstract 2503.
31. Paraiso KH, Fedorenko IV, Cantini LP, et al. Recovery of phospho-ERK activity allows melanoma cells to escape from BRAF inhibitor therapy. *Br J Cancer*. 2010;102:1724-1730.
32. Garraway LA, Widlund HR, Rubin MA, et al. Integrative genomic analyses identify MITF as a lineage survival oncogene amplified in malignant melanoma. *Nature*. 2005;436:117-122.
33. Wellbrock C, Rana S, Paterson H, et al. Oncogenic BRAF regulates melanoma proliferation through the lineage specific factor MITF. *PLoS One*. 2008;3:e2734.
34. Du J, Widlund HR, Horstmann MA, et al. Critical role of CDK2 for melanoma growth linked to its melanocyte-specific transcriptional regulation by MITF. *Cancer Cell*. 2004;6:565-576.
35. Boni A, Cogdill AP, Dang P, et al. Selective BRAFV600E inhibition enhances t-cell recognition of melanoma without affecting lymphocyte function. *Cancer Res*. 2010;70:5213-5219.
36. Kono M, Dunn IS, Durda PJ, et al. Role of the mitogen-activated protein kinase signaling pathway in the regulation of human melanocytic antigen expression. *Mol Cancer Res*. 2006;4:779-792.
37. Fourcade J, Kudela P, Sun Z, et al. PD-1 is a regulator of NY-ESO-1-specific CD8+ T cell expansion in melanoma patients. *J Immunol*. 2009;182:5240-5249.
38. Polak ME, Borthwick NJ, Gabriel FG, et al. Mechanisms of local immunosuppression in cutaneous melanoma. *Br J Cancer*. 2007;96:1879-1887.
39. Kefford R, Arkenau H, Brown MP, et al. Phase I/II study of GSK2118436, a selective inhibitor of oncogenic mutant BRAF kinase, in patients with metastatic melanoma and other solid tumors. *J Clin Oncol*. 2010;28(15s):8503.
40. McArthur GA, Ribas A, Chapman PB, et al. Molecular analyses from a phase I trial of vemurafenib to study mechanism of action and resistance in repeated biopsies from BRAF mutation–positive metastatic melanoma patients. *J Clin Oncol*. 2011;29(suppl):2011. Abstract 8502.
41. Nazarian R, Shi H, Wang Q, et al. Melanomas acquire resistance to B-RAF(V600E) inhibition by RTK or N-RAS upregulation. *Nature*. 2010;468:973-977.
42. Marquette A, Andre J, Bagot M, et al. ERK and PDE4 cooperate to induce RAF isoform switching in melanoma. *Nat Struct Mol Biol*. 2011;18:584-591.
43. Wagle N, Emery C, Berger MF, et al. Dissecting therapeutic resistance to RAF inhibition in melanoma by tumor genomic profiling. *J Clin Oncol*. August 2011;29(22):3085-3096.
44. Johannessen CM, Boehm JS, Kim SY, et al. COT drives resistance to RAF inhibition through MAP kinase pathway reactivation. *Nature*. 2010;468:968-972.
45. Villanueva J, Vultur A, Lee JT, et al. Acquired resistance to BRAF inhibitors mediated by a RAF kinase switch in melanoma can be overcome by cotargeting MEK and IGF-1R/PI3K. *Cancer Cell*. 2010;18:683-695.

46. Tsao H, Goel V, Wu H, et al. Genetic interaction between NRAS and BRAF mutations and PTEN/MMAC1 inactivation in melanoma. *J Invest Dermatol.* 2004;122:337-341.
47. Daniotti M, Oggionni M, Ranzani T, et al. BRAF alterations are associated with complex mutational profiles in malignant melanoma. *Oncogene.* 2004;23:5968-5977.
48. Stahl JM, Sharma A, Cheung M, et al. Deregulated Akt3 activity promotes development of malignant melanoma. *Cancer Res.* 2004;64:7002-7010.
49. Paraiso KH, Xiang Y, Rebecca VW, et al. PTEN loss confers BRAF inhibitor resistance to melanoma cells through the suppression of BIM expression. *Cancer Res.* 71:2750-2760.
50. Xing F, Persaud Y, Pratilas CA, et al. Concurrent loss of the PTEN and RB1 tumor suppressors attenuates RAF dependence in melanomas harboring (V600E)BRAF. *Oncogene.*
51. Margolin K, Longmate J, Baratta T, et al. CCI-779 in metastatic melanoma: a phase II trial of the California Cancer Consortium. *Cancer.* 2005;104:1045-1048.
52. Esteve-Puig R, Canals F, Colome N, et al. Uncoupling of the LKB1-AMPKalpha energy sensor pathway by growth factors and oncogenic BRAF. *PLoS One.* 2009;4:e4771.
53. Courtney KD, Corcoran RB, Engelman JA. The PI3K pathway as drug target in human cancer. *J Clin Oncol.* 2010;28:1075-1083.
54. Heinrich MC, Owzar K, Corless CL, et al. Correlation of kinase genotype and clinical outcome in the North American Intergroup Phase III Trial of imatinib mesylate for treatment of advanced gastrointestinal stromal tumor: CALGB 150105 Study by Cancer and Leukemia Group B and Southwest Oncology Group. *J Clin Oncol.* 2008;26:5360-5367.
55. Guo J, Si L, Kong Y, et al. Phase II, open-label, single-arm trial of imatinib mesylate in patients with metastatic melanoma harboring c-Kit mutation or amplification. *J Clin Oncol.* 2011;29:2904-2909.
56. Carvajal RD, Antonescu CR, Wolchok JD, et al. KIT as a therapeutic target in metastatic melanoma. *JAMA.* 2011;305:2327-2334.
57. Hussussian CJ, Struewing JP, Goldstein AM, et al. Germline p16 mutations in familial melanoma. *Nat Genet.* 1994;8:15-21.
58. FitzGerald MG, Harkin DP, Silva-Arrieta S, et al. Prevalence of germ-line mutations in p16, p19ARF, and CDK4 in familial melanoma: analysis of a clinic-based population. *Proc Natl Acad Sci U S A.* 1996;93:8541-8545.
59. Smalley KS, Lioni M, Dalla Palma M, et al. Increased cyclin D1 expression can mediate BRAF inhibitor resistance in BRAF V600E-mutated melanomas. *Mol Cancer Ther.* 2008;7:2876-2883.
60. Zhao Y, Zhang Y, Yang Z, et al. Simultaneous knockdown of BRAF and expression of INK4A in melanoma cells leads to potent growth inhibition and apoptosis. *Biochem Biophys Res Commun.* 2008;370:509-513.
61. Li J, Xu M, Yang Z, et al. Simultaneous inhibition of MEK and CDK4 leads to potent apoptosis in human melanoma cells. *Cancer Invest.* 28:350-356.
62. Yang G, Rajadurai A, Tsao H. Recurrent patterns of dual RB and p53 pathway inactivation in melanoma. *J Invest Dermatol.* 2005;125:1242-1251.
63. Muthusamy V, Hobbs C, Nogueira C, et al. Amplification of CDK4 and MDM2 in malignant melanoma. *Genes Chromosomes Cancer.* 2006;45:447-454.
64. Ji Z, Njauw CN, Taylor M, et al. p53 rescue through HDM2 antagonism suppresses melanoma growth and potentiates MEK inhibition. *J Invest Dermatol.* February 2012;132(2):356-364.
65. Van Raamsdonk CD, Bezrookove V, Green G, et al. Frequent somatic mutations of GNAQ in uveal melanoma and blue naevi. *Nature.* 2009;457:599-602.
66. Van Raamsdonk CD, Griewank KG, Crosby MB, et al. Mutations in GNA11 in uveal melanoma. *N Engl J Med.* 2010;363:2191-2199.
67. van Biesen T, Hawes BE, Raymond JR, et al. G(o)-protein alpha-subunits activate mitogen-activated protein kinase via a novel protein kinase C-dependent mechanism. *J Biol Chem.* 1996;271:1266-1269.
68. Wagner J, von Matt P, Sedrani R, et al. Discovery of 3-(1H-indol-3-yl)-4-[2-(4-methylpiperazin-1-yl)quinazolin-4-yl]pyrrole-2,5-dione (AEB071), a potent and selective inhibitor of protein kinase C isotypes. *J Med Chem.* 2009;52:6193-6196.
69. Harbour JW, Onken MD, Roberson ED, et al. Frequent mutation of BAP1 in metastasizing uveal melanomas. *Science.* December 2010;330(6009):1410-1413.
70. Tschentscher F, Prescher G, Horsman DE, et al. Partial deletions of the long and short arm of chromosome 3 point to two tumor suppressor genes in uveal melanoma. *Cancer Res.* 2001;61:3439-3442.
71. Jensen DE, Proctor M, Marquis ST, et al. BAP1: a novel ubiquitin hydrolase which binds to the BRCA1 RING finger and enhances BRCA1-mediated cell growth suppression. *Oncogene.* 1998;16:1097-1112.
72. Tse WK, Eisenhaber B, Ho SH, et al. Genome-wide loss-of-function analysis of deubiquitylating enzymes for zebrafish development. *BMC Genomics.* 2009;10:637.
73. Landreville S, Agapova OA, Matatall KA, et al. Histone deacetylase inhibitors induce growth arrest and differentiation in uveal melanoma. *Clin Cancer Res.* January 2012;18(2):408-416.
74. Eisen T, Ahmad T, Flaherty KT, et al. Sorafenib in advanced melanoma: a Phase II randomised discontinuation trial analysis. *Br J Cancer.* 2006;95:581-586.
75. Hauschild A, Agarwala SS, Trefzer U, et al. Results of a phase III, randomized, placebo-controlled study of sorafenib in combination with carboplatin and paclitaxel as second-line treatment in patients with unresectable stage III or stage IV melanoma. *J Clin Oncol.* 2009;27:2823-2830.

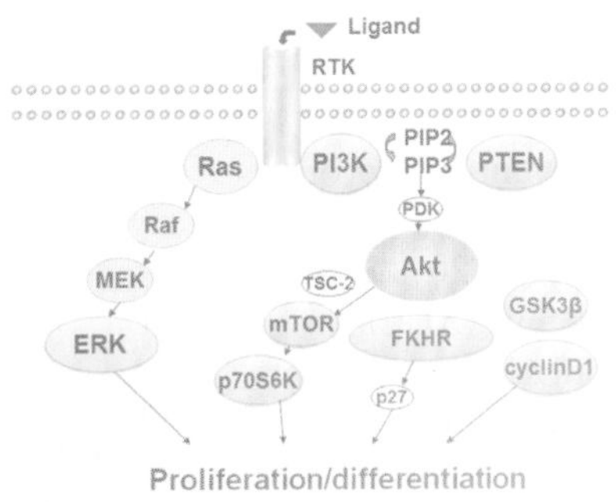

CHAPTER 63

PERSONALIZED MEDICINE AND TARGETED THERAPY OF LEUKEMIA

Pavan Kumar Bhamidipati, Elias Jabbour, and Jorge Cortes

CHRONIC MYELOGENOUS LEUKEMIA

Chronic Myeloid Leukemia History and Epidemiology

Chronic myeloid leukemia (CML) is a myeloproliferative neoplasm with annual incidence of 1 to 2 cases per 100,000 adults and accounts for approximately 15% of newly diagnosed cases of leukemia in adults.[1] The median age of presentation is 67 years, and there is a slight male predominance of 1.3:1.[2] Thirty percent of patients are 60 years or older, with the median age at presentation being 45 to 50 years. Almost a third of the patients (~30%) are ≥ 60 years of age, with the median age at presentation being 45 to 50 years.[3,4] CML in children constitutes 3% of childhood leukemia.

Nowell and Hungerford were the first two scientists who developed techniques to detect a small chromosome in the bone marrow of patients with CML, and it was named "Philadelphia chromosome (Ph)" based on the city where it was first discovered. Rowley discovered that Ph resulted from translocation between chromosomes 9 and 22. Until the 1970s, CML was considered as an incurable disease. Until 10 years ago, the mainstay of treatment for CML included drugs like interferon alpha (IFN-α), hydroxyurea, busulfan, and allogeneic hematopoietic stem cell transplantation (allo-HSCT).[5] IFN-α increased survival but had significant side effects. Allo-HSCT was the only curative treatment, but carried a substantial morbidity and mortality, and was limited to patients with a suitable donor and performance status. However, with the introduction of many tyrosine kinase inhibitors (TKIs), allo-HSCT is used less often in CML treatment.

Etiopathology and Genetics

The pathogenesis of CML involves a characteristic genetic abnormality: the fusion of Abelson murine leukemia (ABL) gene on chromosome 9 with the breakpoint cluster region (BCR) gene on chromosome 22. In 95% of cases, this fusion is the result of a balanced translocation between chromosomes 9 and 22 [t(9;22)(q34;q11)], "Philadelphia chromosome," which is a hallmark of CML. However, in 5% of the cases, an unbalanced translocation occurs, which leads to a break in exon 2a of the ABL gene. The break in BCR could be at e1, b2, b3, or e19. As a result, four kinds of BCR-ABL fusion proteins are described. These are e1a2, b2a2, b3a2, and e19 a2. ABL gene encodes a non-receptor tyrosine kinase and has a vital role in ATP metabolism and thus in cellular functions.

The fused BCR-ABL gene encodes the BCR-ABL oncoprotein, which contains the activated tyrosine kinase region of Abl and is 185 to 230 kDa in size. The most common 210-kDa BCR-ABL fusion protein, p210BCR-ABL is a deregulated, constitutively active tyrosine kinase that promotes growth and replication. This is through causing aberrancies in proliferation, apoptosis resistance, and adhesion through interference with beta-integrin signaling and with multiple downstream pathways, such as the Jak-STAT, PI3K/Akt, JUN kinase, MYC, Wnt-beta-catenin, and Ras-Raf-MAPK signaling routes.

This contributes to leukemogenesis by creating a cytokine-independent cell cycle with aberrant apoptotic signals in response to cytokine withdrawal.[6] Overactive ABL also leads to genetic and epigenetic instability within the clone, which manifests as acquisition of new genetic abnormalities (clonal evolution) that eventually evolves into blast crisis (BC).

BCR-ABL fusion protein is also seen in 20% to 30% of patients with acute lymphocytic leukemia (ALL); prognosis for these patients is poor, with only 10% of patients with "Philadelphia-positive" (Ph+) ALL achieving long-term survival with traditional chemotherapy.[7] In 50% to 80% of cases of adult Ph+ ALL, the nature of the BCR-ABL fusion is different from that in CML; instead of a 210-kDa protein product, a 190-kDa product with higher tyrosine kinase activity is generated. The 210-kDa BCR-ABL protein accounts for the other 20% to 50% of adult patients with Ph+ ALL.[7,8]

The causal role that BCR-ABL plays in leukemogenesis led to the development of TKIs, which target the BCR-ABL oncoprotein and represent the bulk of pharmaceutical research performed in this arena within the past decade. This "targeted therapy" modality not only has changed dramatically the outcome of this disease—from a 10-year overall survival (OS) of 10% to 80-90%—but has also given rise to what others have called a "molecular revolution in cancer therapy."

The disease progresses through three distinct phases: a chronic phase (CML-CP), which lasts 3 to 6 years, followed by an accelerated phase (CML-AP) and then blast phase (CML-BP), which is of a short duration.[9,10] TKIs mitigate the oncogenic activity of the BCR-ABL protein through competitive inhibition at the ATP-binding site, leading to the inhibition of phosphorylation of proteins involved in BCR-ABL–mediated intracellular signal transduction and thereby causing the arrest of growth and apoptosis in CML cells.

Currently, patients with CML-CP can expect a life span of approximately 25 years and beyond, thanks to TKIs for transforming CML from a disease that was once fatal, with a 40% 7-year survival rate, to one that is chronic, with a 90% 7-year survival rate. Introduction of second-generation TKIs has further improved outcomes, giving an extra edge in the treatment of CML.

Management of CML

The current National Comprehensive Cancer Network (NCCN) guidelines for the management of adult patients with CML-CP call for the patient's full medical history and performing a physical evaluation including an assessment of spleen size by palpation. Blood work should include a complete blood count with platelets and a chemistry profile. Human leukocyte antigen tissue typing should also be performed, especially if therapeutic allo-HSCT is being considered. A bone marrow aspirate and biopsy should be performed for a morphologic review (percent blasts and percent basophils) and cytogenetic (CG) analysis with fluorescence in situ hybridization (FISH) and quantitative polymerase chain reaction (qPCR).[2]

Treatment

The core of personalized therapy lies in the patient's age, CG abnormalities, associated molecular abnormalities, and concurrent comorbidities.

Definitions

The European LeukemiaNet (ELN) has set the definitions of what constitutes the treatment response. CML treatment response monitoring parameters are summarized in Table 63.1. These constitute three major groups based on the normalization of either blood counts (hematologic response) or the diminishment of Ph+ chromosome levels (CG remission) or the diminishment of BCR-ABL transcript levels (molecular response). Also note the milestones that constitute the optimal response per ELN's criteria.

TABLE 63–1 Monitoring Treatment Response in chronic myeloid leukemia

Complete Hematologic Remission	Cytogenetic Remission				Molecular Response	
1. Normalization of peripheral counts and differential[a] 2. Disappearance of all signs and symptoms of CML[b]	Karyotype analysis of metaphases				Quantitative PCR	
	MCyR (0–34% Ph+)				CMR	MMR
	CCR	PCyR	Minor cytogenetic response (minor CR/MCyR)	No cytogenetic response	Undetectable BCR-ABL transcripts	BCR-ABL/ABL ratio of <0.1% (International scale)
Optimal response—3 mo	(0% Ph+)	1–35% Ph+	36–95% Ph+	>95% Ph+		
Optimal response	12 mo	6 mo	3 mo	–		18 mo

PCR, polymerase chain reaction; CML, chronic myeloid leukemia; CR, complete remission; MCyR, major cytogenetic response; Ph, Philadelphia chromosome; CMR, complete molecular response; MMR, major molecular response; CCR, complete cytogenetic response; PCyR, partial cytogenetic response.

[a]Normalization of peripheral counts is defined through platelet count less than 450×10^9, WBC less than 10×10^9, the absence of immature granulocytes, and less than 5% basophils on differential.

[b]Includes resolution of splenomegaly.

CML-CP: Frontline Treatment Options—BCR-ABL–Targeted Therapy

Current guidelines recommend any of the three TKIs, imatinib, dasatinib, or nilotinib, as options, with a category 1 recommendation for the initial treatment of CML-CP (except for CML with p190 BCR-ABL).[2] Allo-HSCT or other chemotherapy agents are no longer recommended as upfront treatments for CML-CP, given the excellent outcomes and long-term survival achieved with the TKIs.[11]

Treatment Options

- IFN-α has been used for CML treatment since 1980. Typically, the drug is started at a relatively low dose of approximately 2 to 3 × 10^6 U/m^2 SQ 3 days per week. IFN-α is not a specific therapy for CML. At MD Anderson Cancer Center (MDACC), 80% of patients with Ph+ early CML-CP treated with IFN-α alone or in combinations achieved complete hematologic response (CHR); 55% had a CG response, which was major and durable in 25%. Although IFN-α was associated with significant survival prolongation compared with conventional chemotherapy, the severe side effects particularly fever, chills, and flu-like symptoms, hypothyroidism, and hemolytic anemia with this therapy were associated with very high dropout/discontinuation rate. This drug is out of vogue in the treatment of CML and is not used routinely anymore.
- IFN plus cytarabine (ara-C): The addition of low-dose ara-C to IFN-α has shown improved outcome in some earlier studies. In a study from the MDACC, of 140 patients with Ph+ early CML-CP treated with IFN-α 5 MU/m^2 daily and ara-C 10 mg daily, CHR was achieved in 92% of patients, major cytogenetic response (MCyR) in 50%, and complete cytogenetic response (CCyR) in 31%. With a median follow-up of 42 months, the 4-year estimated survival rate was 70%. The toxicity of the combined treatment of IFN plus ara-C was substantial and included fatigue, muscle aches, nausea, vomiting, diarrhea, and significant thrombocytopenia. The survival and time to blastic transformation were similar to that of IFN-α alone.[12]
- TKIs

First-Generation TKIs

Imatinib

Imatinib mesylate (*Gleevec, Novartis Pharma*) was the first TKI to receive approval by the US Food and Drug Administration (FDA) in 2001 as a second-line agent for the treatment of patients with CML-CP at a dose of 400 mg/d and at a higher dose of 600 mg/d for CML-AP and CML-BP disease. Because of its success, it was subsequently approved as a frontline agent in 2002. It works through competitive inhibition at the ATP-binding site of the BCR-ABL protein, which results in the inhibition of phosphorylation of proteins involved in signal transduction. It inhibits as well the receptor for platelet-derived growth factor (PGDF), and c-kit tyrosine kinases.[13] BCR-ABL inhibition by TKIs results in the arrest of growth or apoptosis in hematopoietic cells that express this translocation without affecting the normal cells.[13,14]

The landmark phase III IRIS trial (International Randomized Study of interferon versus imatinib) was the first to clearly demonstrate the superiority of imatinib treatment in CML-CP compared with IFN-α, the standard of care at that time.[15] One thousand and six individuals were randomized to receive imatinib 400 mg/d or IFN-α plus ara-C. After a median follow-up of 19 months, outcomes in patients receiving imatinib were significantly better than in those treated with IFN-α plus ara-C, including CHR (95% vs. 55%, $P < 0.001$), MCyR (85% vs. 22%, $P < 0.001$), and CCyR (74% vs. 9%, $P < 0.001$) rates. At 18 months, the estimated rate of freedom from progression (FFP) to accelerated phase or BC was 97% in the imatinib group and 92% in the IFN-α plus ara-C group ($P < 0.001$).

The responses to imatinib were also durable; as shown with an 8-year follow-up of the IRIS study,[16] the cumulative CCyR rate was 83% and the estimated OS was 93%. Only 15 patients (3%) exhibiting a CCyR progressed to AP/BP, and none of the patients exhibiting a major molecular response (MMR) at 12 months progressed to AP/BP (Fig. 63.1).

Institutional data from the MDACC demonstrated progressive improvements of survival in patients with early CML-CP that were attributable to imatinib therapy. A 2009 analysis found that there was an 84% survival rate of patients treated with imatinib at 9 years from initial referral compared with less than 60% survival of patients treated from 1990 to 2000, less than 40% survival of those treated from 1982 to 1989, and less than 20% of those treated from 1965 to 1981.

Upfront treatment with higher doses of imatinib (800 mg/d) has not been shown to be superior to imatinib 400 mg/d in terms of both CCyR and MMR.[17,18] Despite the excellent response rates seen with imatinib, the 8-year follow-up data from the IRIS study showed that 37% had discontinued treatment for several reasons, including adverse events (AEs) or unsatisfactory therapeutic outcome.[16]

Also, despite the above-mentioned positive results, many CML patients treated with imatinib do not achieve a CCyR, while others have drug resistance or cannot tolerate drug-related toxicities.[19] Although second-generation TKIs were first developed and approved as second-line treatment for patients who failed or were intolerant to imatinib, their increased potency, tolerance, and safety profiles have made them attractive candidates for use as frontline agents and were finally approved in this setting.

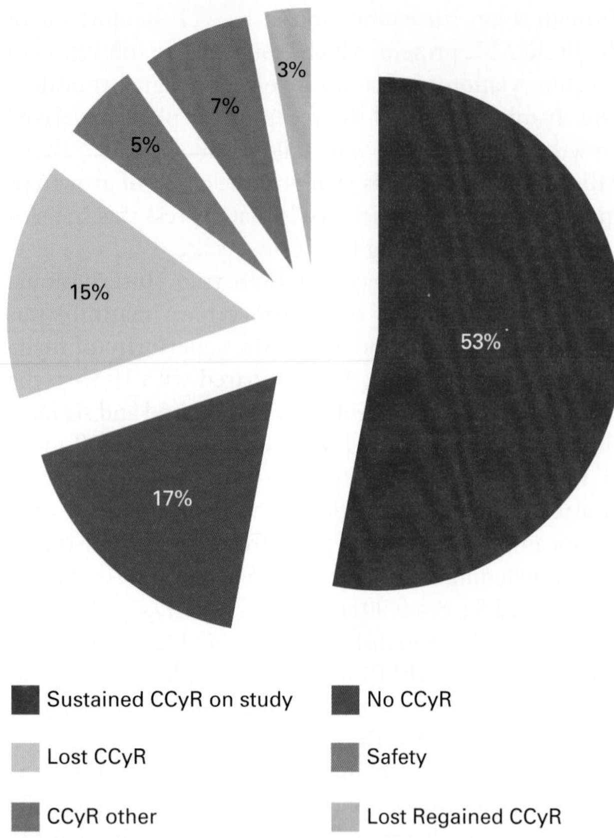

FIGURE 63–1 IRIS 8-year update on sustained CCyR. CCyR, complete cytogenetic response; IRIS, The International Randomized Study of Interferon versus STI571.

Second-Generation TKIS

Dasatinib in the Frontline Setting

Dasatinib (*Sprycel, Bristol-Myers Squibb*) is an oral, second-generation TKI with the advantage of binding to BCR-ABL protein regardless of conformational state (active and inactive). In vitro, it is 350 times more potent than imatinib.[20-22] In addition, dasatinib is a multi-targeted kinase inhibitor with the ability to block the Src family, inhibiting cell proliferation through a separate kinase inhibition.[23]

Cortes et al. at MDACC published a dose optimization study in which 50 patients with newly diagnosed CML-CP were randomized to dasatinib 100 mg once daily or 50 mg twice daily in the frontline setting. Median follow-up was 24 months. Of the 50 patients enrolled in the study, 49 (98%) attained a CCyR and 41 (82%) attained an MMR. Ninety-four percent of patients attained CCyR by 6 months. There was no difference in response rate by treatment arm. There was no significant difference in toxicity between the two arms, and the actual median dose at 12 months was 100 mg (range 20 to 100 mg).[24]

The DASISION was an international, multicenter, randomized phase III trial that compared dasatinib with imatinib for frontline treatment in 519 patients with CML-CP.[25] Patients were randomized to receive dasatinib 100 mg once daily or imatinib 400 mg once daily. After a minimum follow-up of 12 months, the rate of CCyR was higher with dasatinib than with imatinib (77% vs. 66%, $P = 0.007$). The best cumulative MMR rate by 12 months was also significantly higher (46% vs. 28%, $P < 0.0001$). There were also numerically fewer progressions to AP/BP with dasatinib (1.9% vs. 3.5%). Similar results were observed with a minimum of 18 months follow-up[26] showing that dasatinib was superior to imatinib with respect to the primary endpoint, the rate of CCyR. The likelihood of achieving a CCyR at any time was higher with dasatinib versus imatinib (85% vs. 80%; hazard ratio [HR] = 1.5, $P < 0.0001$).[26]

In addition, the secondary endpoint, the rate of MMR, was also significantly improved with dasatinib compared with imatinib. The likelihood of achieving MMR at any time with dasatinib was significantly higher than with imatinib (57% vs. 41%; HR = 1.8, $P < 0.0001$).

In terms of the safety profile, grade 3 to 4 neutropenia occurred at the same frequency with both drugs, whereas grade 3 to 4 thrombocytopenia occurred more frequently with dasatinib.[27] Non-hematologic side-effect rates were lower with dasatinib compared with imatinib, including fluid retention, edema, nausea, vomiting, and myalgia. Rates of grade 3 to 4 non-hematologic side effects were low in both arms (0% to 1%). However, dasatinib was associated with the development of pleural effusions, which occurred in 14% of patients versus 0% in the imatinib arm.

Based on these data, on October 28, 2010, the FDA approved dasatinib as a frontline therapy for the treatment of newly diagnosed adult patients with CML-CP, with a recommended dose of 100 mg/d.

Another study by the Southwest Oncology Group (SO325) compared dasatinib 100 mg with imatinib 400 mg in newly diagnosed CML-CP patients. The study showed that dasatinib was associated with greater MMR compared with imatinib at 12 months. However, the 12-month rates of CHR, CCyR, OS, or progression-free survival (PFS) were comparable between treatment groups. The lack of statistical significance in rates of CCyR was likely due to the fact that patients who were not evaluable were considered non-responders.[28] These results are depicted in Table 63.2.

Nilotinib in the Frontline Setting

Nilotinib (*Tasigna, Novartis Pharma*) has a similar chemical structure to imatinib and binds to the inactive conformation of BCR-ABL. However, due to its improved topographical fit, it has higher affinity and is 10- to 50-fold more potent in vitro.[21,25] It also has increased selectivity for the ABL protein and less cross-reactivity with c-KIT and the PGDF receptor (PDGFR), which may account for the less frequent pleural effusions as seen with dasatinib.

In vitro, nilotinib is 30 times more potent than imatinib and is active against many imatinib-resistant BCR-ABL mutations. In 2007, nilotinib was initially approved in the United States for CML-CP patients who have

TABLE 63-2 Response Rates with Frontline Dasatinib

Study	Number of Patients	CCyR (%)	MMR (%)	PFS (%)	OS (%)
MDACC	62	98	71	–	–
DASISION[a]	259	78	57	94.9 (18 mo)	96 (18 mo)
S0325	123	82	59	99 (12 mo)	100 (12 mo)

CCyR, complete cytogenetic response; MMR, major molecular response; PFS, progression-free survival; OS, overall survival; MDACC, MD Anderson Cancer Center.
[a]cCCyR (confirmed complete cytogenetic response) is reported for DASISION study.

failed or are intolerant of imatinib, as well as for CML-AP patients. But, based on the data below, on June 17, 2010, the FDA granted accelerated approval of nilotinib as a frontline drug for the treatment of adult patients with newly diagnosed CML-CP. The recommended nilotinib dose for this indication is 300 mg orally twice daily.

Cortes et al. at MDACC assessed 51 patients with newly diagnosed CML-CP treated with nilotinib 400 mg twice daily in the frontline setting. Fifty (98%) attained a CCyR and 39 (76%) attained an MMR. Ninety-six percent attained CCyR by 3 months and 98% attained CCyR by 6 months. The projected event-free survival (EFS) at 24 months was 90%. The median dose at 12 months was 800 mg. The results of this study point to nilotinib as being an effective option for frontline treatment of patients with CML-CP.

In the phase II GIMEMA trial, 73 patients were treated with nilotinib at a dose of 400 mg twice daily with a median follow-up of 30 months. Rates of CCyR, MMR, and CMR at 24 months were 92%, 82%, and 12%, respectively. One patient showed progression to advanced disease and was shown to have the T315I mutation. The discontinuation rate due to AEs was 5%. These results confirm that nilotinib is highly efficacious in the frontline setting.[29]

ENESTnd was a phase III, multicenter, randomized study that compared nilotinib with imatinib in patients with newly diagnosed CML, in which 846 patients were randomly assigned to nilotinib 300 mg twice daily, nilotinib 400 mg twice daily, or imatinib 400 mg daily (with dose escalation permitted).[30]

In the analysis of 24-month data, nilotinib at 400 mg twice daily resulted in superior PFS compared with imatinib (97.9% vs. 95.2%, $P = 0.0437$). Nilotinib also significantly improved the rates of CCyR and MMR at 24 months. CCyR at 24 months was 87% with 400 mg twice daily nilotinib compared with 77% with imatinib ($P = 0.0018$). Likewise, MMR at 24 months was 59% with 400 mg nilotinib versus 37% with imatinib ($P < 0.0001$). There were also significantly fewer progressions to AP/BC with nilotinib.

Based on these data, nilotinib has been approved for the frontline therapy of CML. The gap in efficacy in favor of nilotinib has persisted over time, and it appears that nilotinib may improve both short-term and long-term outcomes compared with imatinib. All efficacy endpoints continued to be superior for nilotinib at 24 months of follow-up.[19]

As with dasatinib, the OS of nilotinib versus imatinib was higher but not statistically significant (97.4% and 97.8% vs. 96.3%).[30]

In the ENESTnd trial, nilotinib was also shown to be safe and well tolerated with no increase in side effects compared with imatinib. By contrast, treatment-related gastrointestinal toxicity and fluid retention of all grades were more frequent with imatinib than they were in either nilotinib arm.[19] Nevertheless, nilotinib can prolong the QT interval, and there have been cases of pericardial effusion and arrhythmias reported with this drug.[31] Caution should be taken in patients with a history of cardiac disease. The results of these nilotinib trials are summarized in Table 63.3.

Bosutinib in the Frontline Setting

Bosutinib is an oral, third-generation dual Src/ABL TKI and has been estimated to be 45 to 50 times more potent than imatinib. With minimal inhibition of PDGFR and

TABLE 63-3 Nilotinib for Newly Diagnosed CML-CP

Phase of Study	Number of Patients (*n*)	Dose	CCyR (%)	MMR (%)
II	67	400 mg twice daily	93	81
II (GIMEMA trial)	73	400 mg twice daily	96	85
III (ENESTnd trial)	846	300 mg (nilotinib) ($N = 282$)	80	44
		400 mg (nilotinib) ($N = 281$)	78	43
		400 mg (imatinib) ($N = 283$)	65	22

CML-CP, chronic myeloid leukemia chronic phase; CCyR, complete cytogenetic response; MMR, major molecular response.

c-KIT, compared with other TKIs, bosutinib is more therapeutically specific, potentially resulting in less myelosuppression and fluid retention.[32,33] It is still under investigation and is currently not FDA approved for upfront treatment of patients with newly diagnosed CML-CP.

The phase I study identified a treatment dose of 500 mg daily and showed evidence of clinical efficacy. It was tested in the frontline setting in the BELA study, a phase III, randomized, open-label, multicenter study, that randomly assigned 502 patients with CML-CP to bosutinib 50 mg daily versus imatinib 400 mg/d.[34] CCyR by 12 months was the primary endpoint of the study and was not met. This may be due to the fact that non-evaluable patients were considered non-responders. Best cumulative rates of CCyR by 12 months were not significantly higher for bosutinib compared with imatinib (70% vs. 68%, $P = 0.6$), although MMR rates by 12 months were (39% vs. 26%, $P = 0.002$). There were fewer progressions to AP/BP with bosutinib than with imatinib (2% vs. 4%) but the difference was not statistically significant. In evaluable patients only, bosutinib did induce a significantly higher rate of CCyR compared with imatinib (78% vs. 68%, $P = 0.026$). In addition, there was a significantly higher MMR with bosutinib in both the intent-to-treat and evaluable populations (intent-to-treat patients: 39% vs. 26%, $P = 0.002$; evaluable patients: 43% vs. 27%, $P < 0.001$). Discontinuation of treatment due to drug-related AEs occurred in 19% of patients in the bosutinib arm and 5% of patients in the imatinib arm. The authors suggested that these discontinuations were mostly attributable to the non-hematologic side effects of bosutinib that some centers had not had prior experience with, such as higher rates of diarrhea on bosutinib (68%) compared with imatinib (21%) that have historically been categorized as transient and occurring early. Unfortunately, these issues may have confounded the primary endpoint of the study. And these non-evaluable patients were considered non-responders in this study. More follow-up on these studies is needed to determine whether these responses are sustained and whether bosutinib is truly superior to imatinib.

However, increasing incidence of imatinib resistance and intolerance in the frontline setting necessitated the development of alternative therapies and thus second- and third-generation TKIs came into vogue. Even though third-generation TKIs are reserved for resistant and failed disease, there is a substantial amount of data supporting the improvement in outcome in long-term follow-up of the second-generation TKIs nilotinib and dasatinib in the frontline setting.

Improving Responses in Frontline Therapy

Two studies looked at the benefit of combining imatinib with other agents to improve outcomes of frontline treatment.

The Tyrosine Kinase Inhibitor Optimization and Selectivity (TOPS) phase III trial randomized 476 patients 2:1 to receive high-dose imatinib of 800 mg ($N = 319$) or standard dose of 400 mg ($N = 157$) daily. The study showed that high-dose imatinib of 800 mg improved the rate of responses and eventually showed a trend toward better EFS. However, at 12 months, differences in MMR and CCyR rates were not statistically significant (MMR 46% vs. 40%, $P = 0.2035$; CCyR 70% vs. 66%, $P = 0.3470$).[18]

Early response to imatinib therapy is associated with survival benefit (see below) and may also be related to imatinib dosing. An analysis of 281 patients with CML who received frontline imatinib therapy (73 patients, 400 mg/d; 208 patients, 800 mg/d) reported a suboptimal response at 6 to 12 months in 12% to 17% of patients treated with imatinib 400 mg/d and 1% to 4% of patients treated with imatinib 800 mg/d ($P = 0.002$).[35,36] But the higher dose is associated with substantial side effects and 400 mg is the standard dose exercised.

Imatinib has been tested recently in combination with other chemotherapy drugs. The French study SPIRIT enrolled 636 patients with CML-CP disease to receive imatinib 400 mg or 600 mg, imatinib 400 mg plus pegylated IFN-α-2a, or imatinib 400 mg plus low-dose ara-C.[37] The first interim analysis reported best response in the imatinib plus IFN-α arm, with a 12-month CCyR and MMR of 71% and 61%, respectively, compared with 57% and 40%, respectively, for imatinib 400 mg alone. However, 46% of the patients discontinued IFN-α during the first year of therapy owing to side effects, possibly accounting for the same 4-year EFS found in both arms (92% and 91%).

In these studies, even though better CCyR and MMR rates were seen initially with a high dose or in combination with IFN-α, the side effects were substantial.

Monitoring Treatment Response

The primary goal of therapy for patients with CML is still the achievement of CCyR. Those who achieve this goal have a low probability of eventually progressing. Also, achieving an MMR early is desirable as it further improves the long-term outcome. Thus, following up qPCR for this molecular response at various time points as stated by ELN is important. In the IRIS study, patients who achieved MMR by 12 months had estimated EFS of 99% at 7 years and MMR by 18 months had 100% FFP to AP/BC and 95% EFS at 7 years compared with those with CCyR without MMR by 18 months.[38] Please refer Table 63.1 for treatment response parameters.

Defining Treatment Response and Failure

Based on available evidence and the outcomes of four expert consensus conferences, the ELN has published management recommendations (later adapted by the NCCN), including definitions for treatment failure, suboptimal response, and optimal response, in patients with CML treated with imatinib and other second-generation TKIs. The criteria defining treatment response are summarized in Table 63.4. The ELN has set forth monitoring

TABLE 63-4 European LeukemiaNet's Criteria for Patient Failure and Suboptimal Response to Imatinib Therapy

Time on Therapy (mo)	Treatment Failure	Suboptimal Response	Optimal Response
3	No CHR	No CG response	CHR with <95% Ph+
6	>95% Ph+ (no CyR)	36–95% Ph+ (less partial CyR)	≤35% Ph+ (partial CyR)
12	≥35% Ph+	1–35% Ph+ (partial CyR)	0% Ph+
18	≥1% Ph+	<MMR	MMR
Any	• Loss of CHR • Loss of CCyR • Mutation • CE	• Loss of MMR • Imatinib-sensitive mutation	Stable or improving MMR

CCyR, complete cytogenetic response; CE, clonal evolution; CG, cytogenetic; CHR, complete hematologic response; MMR, major molecular response; Ph, Philadelphia chromosome.

guidelines to identify patients with an inadequate response to therapy and who require a change in treatment[2,39] (see Table 63.4).

An optimal response is defined as a CHR at 3 months, an MCyR at 3 months, partial cytogenetic response at 6 months, a CCyR at 12 months, and an MMR at 18 months. Criteria for failure with imatinib therapy include no CG response at 6 months (Ph 100%), no MCyR at 12 months (Ph > 35%), no CCyR after 18 months of therapy, loss of response to imatinib therapy at any time, and CG or hematologic relapse.[11] A suboptimal CG response is not considered a criterion for treatment failure, even though this is the most commonly cited reason for imatinib dose escalation in clinical practice. The risk of loss of MCyR or CHR or progression to AP or BP is highest in the first 2 to 3 years of therapy, with decreases in rates of failure as therapy continues.[16,36,39,40]

The IRIS trial demonstrated that early response to therapy with imatinib was related to improved long-term outcomes, and it highlighted two major treatment endpoints: CCyR and MMR. In a study by Hughes et al.,[41] overall FFP for those who had attained a CCyR at 12 months was significantly higher when compared with those who did not (95% vs. 85%, $P < 0.001$). Overall FFP in patients who achieved a CCyR and an MMR was 100%, compared with 95% for those with a CCyR and no MMR (although not statistically significant).

A recent study from Jabbour et al.[42] also showed that the achievement of an early CCyR was associated with improved survival regardless of the therapy used. For example, patients with and without CCyR at 6 months had a 3-year EFS of 97% and 72% and OS of 99% and 90%, respectively. Similarly, for patients with and without CCyR at 12 months, the 3-year EFS was 98% and 67% and OS was 99% and 94%, respectively. In this study as well, among patients achieving CCyR at 12 months, the depth of molecular response was not associated with differences in OS or EFS. Similar results were obtained in a recent study by Hehlman et al.,[43] where for patients with CML-CP treated with imatinib 400 mg/d or imatinib 800 mg/d or imatinib plus IFN, MMR at 12 months showed better PFS (99% vs. 94%, $P = 0.0023$) and OS (99% vs. 93%, $P = 0.0011$) at 3 years when compared with those with no MMR (independent of what treatment they had received).

Suboptimal responses are those that do not meet criteria for response, nor those for failure, but represent a slow or inadequate response. Suboptimal response early in therapy is more prognostic than at later time points. Patients classified as suboptimal responders at 6 months have similar outcomes in terms of OS, PFS, and EFS as those with failure to therapy. In contrast, those with suboptimal response at 18 months of therapy have outcomes not statistically different than those classified as having an optimal response.[36,41,44] Patients with suboptimal responses have greater risk of disease progression than optimal responders.[40,45] Due to this reason, NCCN guidelines do recommend therapy change as if in treatment failure.

Defining Inadequate Response to TKI

It is sometimes difficult to determine the sufficient length of primary or secondary TKI therapy before it is decided that the patient has exhibited an inadequate response and treatment alternatives should be sought. To better define inadequate response to secondary TKI therapy, one study analyzed outcomes in 113 patients receiving nilotinib ($N = 43$) or dasatinib ($N = 70$) after imatinib failure. The investigators reported that after 12 months of therapy, patients achieving an MCyR had a significant projected 1-year survival advantage of 97% versus 84% in those with a minor CG response or CHR ($P = 0.02$). They concluded that patients achieving no CG response after 3 to 6 months of secondary TKI therapy should be considered for alternative treatments.[46] Another analysis of patients with CML who are being treated with second-generation TKIs after imatinib failure reported that an absence of CG response to previous imatinib therapy, anemia, and a performance status of 1 or higher were all predictive of poor response to second-generation TKI therapy, as measured by EFS. Patients with 0, 1, or 2 adverse factors had an estimated 18-month EFS of 81%, 54%, and 20%, respectively

($P < 0.001$).[47] In light of these findings, it is reasonable to consider alternatives to second-generation TKI therapy in patients presenting with these prognostic factors.

As the IRIS trial and several independent retrospective reviews have confirmed,[15,16,40,41] CG response is the gold standard for assessing optimal response and long-term outcome. Thus, the bone marrow must be reassessed every 3 months for the first 3 years until a CCyR is achieved and confirmed and at least every 3 to 6 months thereafter. Furthermore, as explained above, MMR with CCyR further improves the FFP and PFS. Also, molecular changes can serve as marker for CG relapse and new mutations. Thus, molecular response should be assessed by real-time polymerase chain reaction (RT-PCR) every 3 months in the peripheral blood until MMR and then every 3 to 6 months.[2,36,44,48] The NCCN guidelines state that patients with a stable MMR can be monitored every 6 months.[2]

It is worth mentioning that the endpoints to assess treatment response proposed by the ELN are based on studies with imatinib. These endpoints may not be applicable for patients who are treated upfront with dasatinib or nilotinib. Jabbour et al. recently published that among patients with newly diagnosed CMP-CP treated with second-generation TKIs, those who did not achieve a CCyR at 3 or 6 months did worse than those who did.[49] Dr. Jabbour proposes defining as an optimal response a CCyR at 3 months when using second-generation TKIs. These data need to be validated in further studies.

Monitoring for Surrogate Endpoints and Milestones

Hematologic response should be monitored by peripheral blood every 2 weeks until a CHR is achieved and confirmed and every 3 months thereafter. CCyR is the gold standard for assessing optimal response and long-term outcome.[50,51] Thus, the bone marrow must be reassessed every 3 months for the first 3 years until a CCyR is achieved and confirmed and at least every 3 to 6 months thereafter. Molecular response should be assessed by RT-PCR in the peripheral blood every 3 to 6 months.[39]

Some patients may appear to have rising levels of BCR-ABL transcripts while maintaining a CCyR. These results should be reviewed cautiously. This may be of no significance or may indicate an increased risk for the development of mutations or failure to therapy. A small increase in BCR-ABL transcript levels does not necessarily indicate treatment failure or loss of response. This is supported by the 3-year follow-up of the IRIS trial in which CCyR, regardless of MMR, was associated with improved OS relative to IFN and ara-C.[50] Also, according to the study published by Kantarjian et al., an increase in qPCR among patients in CCyR is not a criterion for treatment failure. Most patients with increases in qPCR remain in CCyR.[52]

If a patient who has previously achieved an MMR is noted to have a 1 log or fivefold increase in BCR-ABL transcripts, the value should be repeated in 1 to 3 months, and, if confirmed, a bone marrow should be repeated to evaluate for loss of CyR.[52-54] Furthermore, the limitation of using molecular response as an endpoint is the lack of standardization of laboratories that perform this test. Laboratories are required to establish a baseline level that is standardized using the international scale.[55] Variability among centers can be introduced because of methodological differences.

TABLE 63-5 FISH and qPCR Interpretation in Patients with CCyR with TKI Therapy

Fish	qPCR	Interpretation
Negative	<0.1%	Excellent response; F/U in 6 mo
Positive	<0.1%	FISH and qPCR false positive or false negative; F/U in 3 mo
Negative	>1%	
Negative	0.1–1%	F/U in 6 mo; F/U in 3 mo if 1 log increase in qPCR
Positive	>1%	Check marrow cytogenetic studies; possibility of disease relapse

FISH, fluorescence in situ hybridization; qPCR, quantitative polymerase chain reaction; CCyR, complete cytogenetic response; TKI, tyrosine kinase inhibitor; F/U, follow-up.

These analyses are summarized in Table 63.5.

Clonal evolution (new-onset chromosomal abnormalities) has a negative effect on survival and can happen during treatment of CML with TKIs. One study assessed the frequency and clinical impact of the development of chromosomal abnormalities in Ph-negative metaphases in 258 patients with newly diagnosed CML who were being treated with imatinib therapy. Patients were followed for a period of 37 months, during which 21 (9%) developed 23 chromosomal abnormalities in Ph-negative cells. The median time from the initiation of imatinib therapy to the appearance of chromosomal abnormalities was 18 months. The most common chromosomal abnormalities were the loss of chromosome Y ($N = 9$; 43%), trisomy 8 ($N = 3$; 14%), and the loss of the long arm of chromosome 20 ($N = 2$; 10%). One patient with a monosomy 7 abnormality developed secondary acute myeloid leukemia (AML). The estimated 4-year PFS was 63% and 88% in those with and without chromosomal abnormalities, respectively. Estimated 4-year OS was 80% and 96% in patients with and without chromosomal abnormalities, respectively. The authors concluded that CG abnormalities can occur in Ph-negative cells in patients with newly diagnosed CML receiving imatinib therapy. While they supported continued CG analysis to identify these abnormalities, they suggested that no changes in treatment strategy are usually warranted in the absence of additional complications and supported additional studies in larger cohorts to better identify the best treatment strategy for these patients.[56]

Patient compliance should be evaluated and mutation analysis should be considered if the patient has been identified as having a suboptimal response or has had a loss of response at any time.[2] Molecular studies including a combination of FISH and qPCR may be required to ensure concordance and high-quality stability of the CCyR. Importantly, both tests can return false-positive or false-negative results. Bone marrow CG studies are also warranted every 2 to 3 years or more if abnormalities are found in Ph-negative diploid cells (e.g., abnormalities in chromosome 5 or 7).

Monitoring Minimal Residual Disease

Available clinical evidence suggests that CML-CP patients require ongoing monitoring of minimal residual disease (MRD) to detect rising MRD and the possibility of CML progression. In an analysis of the IRIS study, it was shown that patients more likely to survive without progression to CML-AP/BP if they experienced an MCyR at 12 months were more likely to avoid progression to CML-AP/BP if they exhibited a CCyR in the second year of treatment. Moreover, molecular response was also predictive of survival without progression to CML-AP/BP. Patients with BCR-ABL mRNA expression levels of more than 10% had an EFS rate of 53% at 84 months, while those with BCR-ABL mRNA levels of less than 0.1% had an EFS rate of 99%.[57]

In a recent analysis of patients with Ph+ CML who received imatinib therapy for at least 18 months, 116 patients in durable CCyR had increases in qPCR, but 11 (9.5%) of these patients experienced CML progression. Of these 11 patients, 10 had either lost or never achieved an MMR and had more than 1 log increase in qPCR. According to the study authors, patients with these characteristics may need to be more closely monitored. Specifically, they suggested that these patients may be evaluated for BCR-ABL mutations and may likewise be candidates for investigational therapies.[52]

Overall, imatinib therapy has been associated with declining rates of disease events over time including loss of CHR, loss of MCyR, progression to AP/BP, or death during treatment.[58]

Monitoring for AP/BC Transformation

The course of CML in patients achieving CCyR on imatinib therapy is in fact highly stable and predictable. Sudden transformation to CML-AP/BC is still possible with imatinib therapy. The risk of loss of MCyR or CHR or progression to AP or BP is highest in the first 2 to 3 years of therapy, with decreases in rates of failure as therapy continues.[16,36,39,40]

Transformation is usually characterized by lymphoid BP in younger patients and is usually responsive to hyper-fractionated cyclophosphamide, vincristine, adriamycin, and dexamethasone (hyper-CVAD) chemotherapy plus TKI therapy.

Imatinib Resistance/Failure

Exclude TKI Intolerance

Before defining a patient as having imatinib resistance and modifying therapy, treatment compliance and drug–drug interactions should be ruled out. Rates of imatinib adherence have been estimated to range from 75% to 90%, and lower adherence rates correlated to worse outcome.[59-61] In one study of 87 patients with CML-CP treated with imatinib 400 mg daily, adherence rate of 90% or less resulted in MMR in only 28.4% compared with 94.5% in patients with greater than 90% adherence rates ($P < 0.001$).[59] CMR rates were 0% versus 43.8%, respectively ($P = 0.002$), and no molecular responses were observed when adherence rates were 80% or lower. Lower adherence rates have been described in younger patients, those with adverse effects of therapy, and those who have required dose escalations.

The emergence of second-generation TKIs has substantially limited the need to continue imatinib therapy in patients exhibiting intolerance.

In general, there is no standard definition of TKI intolerance. A patient should be categorized as being intolerant to TKI therapy if they meet one or more of the following criteria[62]:

1. Any life-threatening grade 4 non-hematologic toxicity;
2. Any grade 3 or 4 non-hematologic toxicity that has recurred despite dose reduction and treatment of symptoms; any grade 2 non-hematologic toxicity that persists for more than a month despite optimal supportive measures;
3. A grade 3 or 4 hematologic toxicity that does not respond to supportive measures and requires dose reductions below the accepted minimal effective dose.[62]

Common toxicity criteria may be used to grade AEs and identify acute toxicities and likewise may help determine TKI intolerance. With long-term therapies such as TKIs, patient quality of life may be a better tool to gauge therapy intolerance.[63] This is a particularly salient factor in CML since patient adherence is critical to successful long-term disease management.

Patients can now switch from imatinib to another TKI rather than transitioning to other therapeutic options such as allo-HSCT, which is associated with substantial morbidity and mortality, and IFN-α, which is considerably less efficacious than TKI therapy.[62,63] Overall, the available TKIs have been associated with similar rates of discontinuation due to AEs.[62]

Mechanisms and Types of Resistance

Approximately 33% of patients are resistant to imatinib therapy.[64,65] This resistance is classified into two types:

1. Primary resistance (failure to achieve any of the landmark responses as per the ENL or NCCN guidelines). Primary resistance can be further divided into primary hematologic resistance, which occurs in

TABLE 63–6 Mechanisms of Imatinib Resistance

BCR-ABL Dependent	BCR-ABL Independent
1. Point mutations (secondary resistance)	1. Prostaglandin-endoperoxide synthase 1/cyclooxygenase 1 (PTGS1/COX1) (Primary resistance)
2. P-Loop	2. P-glycoprotein efflux pumps
3. T315I, F255K, Y253H	3. Reduced expression of hoct1
	4. Increased serum protein α1-acid glycoprotein
	5. Alternative signaling pathway activation
	6. Ras/Raf/MEK kinase, STAT, Erk2

2% to 4% of cases who fail to normalize peripheral counts within 3 to 6 months of initiation of treatment, or primary CG resistance, which is more common and occurs in approximately 15% to 25% of patients (failure to achieve any level of CyR at 6 months, an MCyR at 12 months, or a CCyR at 18 months).[66]

2. Secondary resistance (those who have previously achieved and subsequently lost their response in accordance to those guidelines).

The mechanisms of resistance to imatinib can be either BCR-ABL dependent (gene amplification or point mutations) or BCR-ABL independent. These are grouped in Table 63.6.

Point mutations in the BCR-ABL oncogene are the most common causes of imatinib resistance, particularly secondary resistance.[21,54,65,67-69] Point mutations can change the conformation of the BCR-ABL oncoprotein to the active form (which imatinib is unable to bind to)[70] and can also eliminate critical molecules required for bonding, thus mitigating its efficacy.[21,65,70,71]

Over 100 different point mutations have been identified so far and important examples of such point mutations include T315I, Y253H, and F255K. T315I and certain mutations occurring in the P-loop are the most frequently identified mutations.[72]

One important noteworthy example is the T315I mutation (aka gatekeeper mutation) seen in 4% to 15% of imatinib-resistant patients, which is due to a single C to T nucleotide substitution at position 944 of the Abl gene, resulting in a threonine to isoleucine substitution at amino acid 315 (Th315 to Ile315). This eliminates a critical oxygen molecule needed for hydrogen bonding between imatinib and the Abl kinase. It confers resistance not only to imatinib but also to nilotinib and dasatinib and has also been associated with decrease in PFS and OS.[68,73] The clinical significance of other mutations, such as the P-loop mutations, is still controversial.[68,74]

BCR-ABL–independent mechanisms of resistance to imatinib include the following:

1. Increased efflux of the drug by increased expression of P-glycoprotein (Pgp) efflux pumps.[65,33,75-77]
2. Decreased drug uptake secondary to decreased expression of the drug uptake transporter, human organic cation transporter 1 (hOCT1).[65,78-80]
3. Sequestration of imatinib by increased serum protein α1-acid glycoprotein (AGP), which binds imatinib and impairs subsequent binding to ABL kinase.[33,81,82]
4. Low serum drug concentration and alternative signaling pathway activation, including Ras/Raf/MEK kinase, STAT, Erk2, and SFK phosphorylation of BCR-ABL.[65]
5. Elevated transcript levels of prostaglandin-endoperoxide synthase 1/cyclooxygenase 1 (PTGS1/COX1), which encodes an enzyme that metabolizes imatinib, have also been associated with primary resistance.[83]

Second-Generation TKI Resistance

The resistance can be TKI specific. A study of specific BCR-ABL kinase domain mutations identified after TKI therapy reported that failure of dasatinib therapy was more commonly associated with mutations at V299L and F317, while nilotinib resistance was associated with mutation in the P-loop, especially at Y253 and E255, or at the F311 or F359 residue.[84-88] Indeed, recently, it was shown that the presence of E255K/V, Y253H, or F359C/V mutations at baseline is an independent predictor of worsened PFS in patients with CML-CP.[85] Therefore, dasatinib therapy may be more appropriate for patients with these common mutations, whereas nilotinib may be better suited for those patients with F317L mutations.[87] Patients with T315I mutations do not appear to respond to therapy with imatinib, dasatinib, or nilotinib.[85-88]

Interestingly, an abstract at ASH 2011 showed that ATP-dependent efflux transporters ABCB1 and ABCG2, which are one of the mechanisms of imatinib resistance, are unlikely to impact the efficacy or mediate resistance to the TKI ponatinib.[89]

Mutation Studies in CML

In general, there is no role for mutation studies prior to a confirmed diagnosis of CML or in patients who exhibit a response to TKI therapy. Per ELN recommendations, mutation analysis is beneficial in cases of imatinib failure, in cases of increased BCR-ABL transcript levels leading to MMR loss as well as in any other case of suboptimal response (for imatinib patients), and in case of hematologic or CG failure during second-line dasatinib or nilotinib therapy.

In cases of CG or hematologic relapse, mutation studies may be helpful in choosing between available TKIs. In vitro studies have determined the inhibitory concentration 50% for different TKIs to inhibit BCR-ABL with specific mutations. This information can be used to predict which drug will be the most effective in cases of CML with available mutation analysis data. For instance, TKI inhibitors are not effective in treating patients with CML who have T315I mutations. Treatment options for these patients include allo-HSCT, hydroxyurea, ara-C, homoharringtonine, or novel agents that specifically target this mutation.[90]

Management of Imatinib Resistance

Imatinib Dose Escalation

Imatinib dose escalation is the first-line strategy to combat CG relapse or resistance.[2,44,48] In a retrospective review of patients who underwent imatinib dose escalations as part of the IRIS trial according to IRIS protocol guidelines from a standard dose of 400 mg daily to doses of 600 or 800 mg daily, statistically significant improvement in responses was noted. IRIS protocol guidelines stipulated the following criteria for dose escalation: lack of CHR by 3 months, lack of minor CyR by 12 months, and loss of response at any time. In those who had not achieved a CHR by 3 months, 86% achieved a CHR 3 months after dose escalation and 29% went on to achieve a CCyR by 12 months. In patients who had not achieved a minor CyR by 12 months, 25% achieved an MCyR by 12 months after imatinib dose escalation and 50% by 24 months. Of these patients, 50% went on to achieve a CCyR by 48 months. In patients with a loss of MCyR, 50% re-achieved an MCyR within 12.5 months, 33% of whom went on to achieve a CCyR. In those patients who exhibited progression of disease, 67% experienced normalization of white blood cell (WBC). Of note, dose escalations were not attempted for those who lost CCyR.[91]

In another study assessing 84 patients over 61 months with failure to standard-dose imatinib, doses were escalated to 600 to 800 mg daily. In 21 patients with hematologic failure, 48% achieved a CHR, with only 14% achieving a CG response. In 63 patients with CG failure, 75% responded with CCyR. Two- and three-year EFS rates were 57% and 47%, respectively, with OS rates of 84% and 76%, respectively.[92] Thus, while dose escalation after failure of standard-dose imatinib is an important and viable treatment option, it is likely to be effective only in the subset of patients with previous CG responses and is not indicated for patients with intolerance to the drug. Thus, clinical consideration should be given to second-generation TKIs in that setting.

An increase in imatinib dosing or transition to a second-generation TKI is warranted in patients with Ph of 35% or more at 12 months, who experience no CCyR in the second year of therapy, who have lost their CyR, or who experience a CG relapse. It is probably not a good option for patients who have lost their hematologic response. A study at MDACC showed that, among those with CG failures, a second CCyR was achieved in 52% with dose escalation, and these responses were durable in 88% after 2 years. In contrast, less than 5% of those who had lost their hematologic response (25%) achieved a CG response, and it was transient.[92] Thus, in patients with Ph 100% at 6 months or hematologic relapse should be transitioned from imatinib to one of the second-generation TKIs.

Increasing the dose of imatinib is associated with significant toxicities and diminished tolerability and adherence of therapy. Current treatment guidelines recommend dose escalation of imatinib to 600 or 800 mg/d in cases of suboptimal response.[21] However, it should be acknowledged that there are minimal data available regarding the effectiveness of this approach.[91,92] For patients with clear failure to imatinib therapy, the current approach is to change therapy to a second-generation TKI, although allogeneic stem cell transplantation is also an option following treatment failure.[31,93]

Switching to Second-Generation TKIS

In an international, multicenter, phase II trial assessing 387 patients with CML-CP who had demonstrated imatinib intolerance or resistance (START-C trial), patients were treated with dasatinib 70 mg twice daily. After 2 years, data showed overall rates of CHR of 91%, CCyR of 53%, and MMR of 47%. Two-year PFS and OS were 80% and 94%, respectively.[94] These data were supported by another study, where dasatinib produced MCyR rates of 45% and CCyR rates of 33% in patients with CML-CP who were imatinib resistant or intolerant.[95]

Dasatinib is approved by the FDA since 2006 for second-line treatment of CML-CP with resistance or intolerance to prior therapy with imatinib.[96] A review of available data of dasatinib treating patients with CML-CP suggests that the optimal dosing strategy after imatinib failure is 100 mg/d, which results in MCyR and CCyR rates comparable to other dosing schedules, improved 24-month PFS, and lower rates of grade 3 or 4 neutropenia, thrombocytopenia, and pleural effusions, as well as lower rates of dosing interruptions or reductions.[96-98]

Further evaluation of dasatinib therapy in imatinib-resistant patients with mutations by meta-analysis of three dasatinib studies, including the START-C, START-R, and CA180-034 dose optimization study, revealed that rates of response with dasatinib are favorable in a variety of genetic mutations including E255K/V (CCyR 38%), L248V (CCyR 40%), and G250E (CCyR 33%). CCyR rates were lower in F317L (7%), Q252H (17%), L384M (0%), and V299L (0%). Patients with T315I mutations did not respond to dasatinib.[88]

Nilotinib has also been investigated as a therapeutic strategy in patients with CML-CP who have exhibited imatinib failure. One study included 321 patients receiving nilotinib 400 mg twice daily after previous imatinib failure. In this population, CCyR was achieved in 46%, and among those 56% achieved MMR. The overall MMR rate was 28% for the entire study population. The 24-month rates of PFS and OS were 64% and 87%, respectively.[99]

Another phase II study evaluated nilotinib in 321 patients with CML-CP who were resistant (71%) or intolerant (29%) of imatinib. Investigators reported rapid and durable hematologic and CG responses, with a median time to CHR of 1 month and a median time to MCyR of 2.8 months. Patients entering the study with CHR at baseline had an MCyR rate of 73% compared with an MCyR rate of 51% in patients without baseline

CHR. Estimated OS rates at 12 and 18 months were 95% and 91%, respectively. Other phase II studies of treatment with nilotinib after imatinib failure have likewise shown promising rates of CCyR in patients with CML-CP, as well as those with CML-AP/BP.[100,101]

Nilotinib was initially approved in the United States for CML-CP patients who have failed or are intolerant of imatinib, as well as for CML-AP patients.[30]

Bosutinib is still under investigation and has not been approved for patients with imatinib resistance. A phase I/II study evaluated efficacy and safety of bosutinib (500 mg once daily) in 288 patients with imatinib-resistant or imatinib-intolerant CML-CP.[34] After a median follow-up of 24.2 months, 86% of patients achieved CHR, 53% had an MCyR (41% with a CCyR). At 2 years, PFS was 79% and OS was 92%. Responses were seen across BCR-ABL mutants, except T315I. These data suggest bosutinib is effective and tolerable in patients with imatinib-resistant or imatinib-intolerant CML-CP.

However, in patients who are resistant to current TKIs (particularly those patients harboring a Thr315Ile point mutation in the kinase domain) or refractory to two lines of TKIs, no US FDA–approved therapy is available. Ponatinib is a pan–BCR-ABL protein inhibitor currently being investigated for this situation that has shown some promising results thus far.

These studies are summarized in Table 63.7.

Allogeneic Hematopoietic Stem Cell Transplantation

The number of patients undergoing allo-HSCT for CML-CP has dropped significantly since TKIs were introduced and has more of an important role when patients evolve into AP/BC (see below). However, allo-HSCT remains an important therapeutic option for CML-CP in the following situations:

1. Patients harboring the T315I mutation.
2. Those who fail second-generation TKIs.[39]
3. Patients with CML harboring the p190 BCR-ABL mutation carry a worse prognosis and many experts recommend referring for transplantation upfront in these cases. Switching to nilotinib when dasatinib fails or vice versa is not recommended, although it is currently under investigation.[103]
4. Patients in CP who are young and have available closely matched donor may also be candidates for an allo-HSCT, especially if they harbor TKI-resistant mutations and had no MCyR after 12 months of therapy with second-generation TKIs. Patients who do not exhibit these factors could reasonably continue TKI therapy until failure. Older patients (those over the age of 70) or those unable to find a well-matched stem cell donor may forgo curative HSCT for several years of controlled CML disease.

Many patients may eventually require an HSCT due to the development of TKI resistance mutations or otherwise progressive disease that does not adequately respond to drug therapy.

However, the effects of prior TKI therapy on outcomes in SCT have not been fully characterized. To better understand the effects of prior TKI therapy in patients undergoing HSCT, an analysis of data from the Center for International Blood and Marrow Transplant Research was conducted in 409 patients treated with imatinib prior to HSCT and 900 patients who were not treated with

TABLE 63-7 Response to Second-Generation Tyrosine Kinase Inhibitors (Dasatinib, Nilotinib, and Bosutinib) in Patients Who Are Imatinib Resistant or Intolerant in CML-CP, CML-AP, and CML-BP (95,102)

	Percent Response										
Response	**Dasatinib**				**Nilotinib**				**Bosutinib**		
	CP (*N* = 387)	AP (*N* = 174)	MyBP (*N* = 109)	LyBP (*N* = 48)	CP (*N* = 321)	AP (*N* = 137)	MyBP (*N* = 105)	LyBP (*N* = 31)	CP (*N* = 146)	AP (*N* = 51)	BP (*N* = 38)
Median follow-up (mo)	15	14	12	12	24	9	3	3	7	6	3
% Resistant to imatinib	74	93	91	88	70	80	82	82	69	NR	NR
% Hematologic response	–	79	50	40	94	56	22	19	85	54	36
CHR	91	45	27	29	76	31	11	13	81	54	36
NEL	–	19	7	6	–	12	1	0	–	0	0
% Cytogenetic response	NR	44	36	52	NR	NR	NR	NR	–	NR	NR
Complete	49	32	26	46	46	20	29	32	34	27	35
Partial	11	7	7	6	15	12	10	16	13	20	18
% Survival (at 12 mo)	96 (15)	82 (12)	50 (12)	50 (5)	87 (24)	67 (24)	42 (12)	42 (12)	98 (12)	60 (12)	50 (10)

CML, chronic myeloid leukemia; CP, chronic phase; AP, accelerated phase; MyBP, myeloid blast phase; LyBP, lymphoid blast phase; CHR, complete hematologic response; NEL, no evidence of leukemia.

imatinib prior to HSCT. In patients with first CML-CP, imatinib therapy prior to HSCT was associated with improved survival, but there were no significant differences in treatment-related mortality, relapse, or leukemia-free survival. The authors concluded that these findings would offer a degree of reassurance to patients having received imatinib therapy and requiring SCT.[99]

The role of TKIs after transplant is being currently evaluated. Accumulating data show that TKIs do not seem to increase transplant-related outcome and, when used after low-intensity conditioning regimens, may delay relapse rates and need for donor lymphocyte infusions.[104-106]

Advanced Stage CML

Though imatinib has revolutionized the management of CML-CP, it is less effective in the advanced phases of CML. As mentioned above, mutations, which occur more frequently in the advanced phases of disease, decrease the response rate to TKI-based therapies.[107]

CML-Accelerated Phase

Both dasatinib and nilotinib are FDA approved for use in patients with progression to CML-AP following TKI therapy. Bosutinib also showed similar results in patients with CML-AP and CML-BP who had failed prior imatinib.[108]

Appropriate dosing of dasatinib in CML-AP was evaluated in a study, in which 317 patients were randomized to receive dasatinib at 140 mg daily or 70 mg BID. The results at 2 years after initiation of treatment demonstrated similar efficacy in rates of hematologic and CG responses, as well as in PFS and OS rates. Dasatinib 140 mg once daily did demonstrate an improved safety profile, with statistically fewer patients experiencing pleural effusions (20% vs. 39%, $P < 0.001$).[109] Pleural effusions are the most common non-hematologic AEs, occurring in up to 35% of patients with 17% of those classified as grade 3 or 4 toxicity. This occurs more commonly in CML-AP or CML-BP and at increased frequency in patients with comorbidities including a cardiac history, hypertension, a smoking history and in those receiving BID dosing. This is thought to be the result of dasatinib's cross-reaction with off-target tyrosine kinases.[110] Platelet dysfunction resulting in bleeding has been described and is a function of PDGFR inhibition.[111]

Nilotinib's efficacy in imatinib-resistant or -intolerant CML-AP patients was also observed in a phase II study of 137 patients. After 1 month, 31% achieved a CHR. After 2.8 months, 32% achieved an MCyR. Among those patients who achieved an MCyR, 20% achieved a CCyR, and a durable CCyR at 24 months was observed in 70%. The 24-month OS rate was 67%.[102]

Allogeneic HSCT should be considered early on for these patients based on response to TKI therapy.

CML-Blast Crisis

Patients who have progressed to CML-BC have a very poor prognosis. The phenotype of CML-BC may be myeloid, lymphoid, or undifferentiated.[112]

Although some patients may respond to a TKI, the percentage is small and the duration of treatment is short-lived. The only curative option for these patients is allo-HSCT. TKIs may serve as a good option for those who are not candidates for transplant or as a bridge to allo-HSCT.

For imatinib-naïve patients with myeloid CML-BC, imatinib monotherapy has been shown to be better or equal to chemotherapy, but with better side-effect profile, with treatment-related mortality 1% versus 25%.[113-115]

For lymphoid CML-BP, the efficacy of imatinib alone is limited, and there is considerably more experience successfully combining imatinib or other TKIs with various ALL regimens, which may be employed in lymphoid BC.[116-120]

Patients with imatinib-resistant CML-BC may be treated with second-generation TKIs. In a phase I trial with dasatinib, 44 patients with imatinib-resistant CML (11 patients with CML-AP, 33 patients with CML-BP) were enrolled.[121] The response rates were significant, with an MCyR achieved in 27% to 35% of patients. Nevertheless, responses were short-lived, and the majority of patients with BC relapsed in less than 6 to 12 months. A larger phase II trial with dasatinib enrolled 74 patients with myeloid CML-BC and 42 patients with lymphoid CML-BC that had failed imatinib.[122] Response rates were similar to those seen in the phase I trial, but again, they were short-lived (PFS rates were 5 months). Nilotinib displayed modest efficacy against imatinib-resistant myeloid and lymphoid CML-BC in a phase I study, although the number of patients was small ($N = 8$).[31]

The combination of TKIs and chemotherapy or the combination of two TKIs has not shown to be better than single-agent second-generation TKI.[123,124]

Preliminary data for response to bosutinib among patients in CP, AP, and BP (myeloid and lymphoid) after imatinib failure are summarized in Table 63.7.

In patients with imatinib failure in CML-AP/BP, a second-generation TKI can be used as a bridge therapy to achieve MRD, after which an allo-HSCT should be performed. Similarly, evidence of the T315I mutation in any CML phase should warrant the use of a specific T315I inhibitor, hydroxyurea, or homoharringtonine as a bridge to MRD, followed by an allo-HSCT.

Prognostic Factors in CML

Various factors play a role in determining the prognosis of CML. These include scoring systems, response to therapy, clonal evolution, BCR-ABL mutations, and adherence to therapy.

A. Prognostic Scoring Systems
 1. The Sokal scoring system is the most used in studies to risk-stratify patients with CML. Based on the patient's age, spleen size, platelet count, and the percentage of blasts in the peripheral blood, patients are stratified into three risk groups: low, intermediate, and high. Its main limitation is that it was developed in the chemotherapy and IFN era.
 2. A new score introduced by Hasford et al.[125] termed the EUTOS score, using the percentage of basophils and spleen size, is a significant tool to predict the probability of achieving 18-month CCyR and PFS in patients treated with imatinib. It classifies the patients into high-risk or low-risk categories and 5-year PFS was significantly better in the low- than in the high-risk group (90% vs. 82%, $P = 0.006$). But its validity has not been proven by other investigators.[126]

B. Response to TKI treatment is also a prognostic factor: those who achieve a CCyR at 12 months have a low probability of eventually progressing to AP/BC[16] and have a higher FFP compared with those who do not (85% vs. 95%; $P < 0.001$).[41] Achievement of an MCyR by 12 months also portends improved 3-year survival rate over those who do not (99% vs. 84%, $P < 0.001$).[50]

C. Mutational data can serve not only as a prognostic factor for disease progression but also as a predictor of response to TKI therapy.[85,87,127] The T315I mutation confers resistance to all three TKIs (imatinib, dasatinib, and nilotinib) and has clearly been associated with decreased PFS and OS.[68,73] In an analysis of 1,043 patients who underwent mutational assessment in phase II/III studies in CML-CP, it was found that patients bearing F317L mutations achieved lower CG response rates (MCyR 14%; CCyR 7%) than patients without these mutations.[88] It has also been shown that the presence of E255K/V, Y253H, or F359C/V mutations at baseline is an independent predictor of worsened PFS in patients with CML-CP.[85]

D. Performance status: A recent study has explored factors that may predict response and outcome in patients receiving second-generation TKIs after failing imatinib.[47] In 123 patients with CML-CP post-imatinib failure, 78 were treated with dasatinib and 45 were treated with nilotinib. Investigators found that EFS in response to a second TKI depends on achieving a prior CyR to imatinib and on the patient's performance status. Patients with both risk factors had a 24-month OS of only 40% compared with 95% for patients with neither risk factor. However, the achievement of MCyR with a second TKI by 12 months may compensate for the presence of unfavorable baseline factors.[47]

E. Adherence is another BCR-ABL independent factor that has been shown to affect outcome as mentioned above. This is an important consideration for treating physicians, as, with advancements in treatment, CML has evolved into a chronic condition requiring lifelong daily oral therapy with efficacy inextricably tied to adherence.

F. Clonal evolution: This is associated with poor survival and clonal evolution happening at any time during therapy is considered treatment failure.

Upcoming Therapeutic Options Targeting TKI Resistance

Despite extraordinary progress, a true cure for CML is not generally achieved by ABL kinase inhibitors. TKIs are potent inhibitors of BCR-ABL kinases (among others), resulting in rapid reduction of the majority of cells carrying the Ph chromosomal marker. However, suppression of ABL-driven hematopoiesis may be insufficient to eradicate quiescent stem cells. Studies assessing the combination of TKIs with promising agents are ongoing. These combinations include TKI and hedgehog inhibitors, omacetaxine, vaccines, and hypomethylating agents. If successful, this strategy could lead to a safe and permanent discontinuation of therapy in patients with a good response. The impact of using more potent agents in the frontline setting on the potential to discontinue TKI therapy remains to be determined. The future of CML therapy may include early use of these potent agents, perhaps in combination with new molecules, to help more patients achieve CMR, which could lead to therapy discontinuation and cure. Patients exhibiting resistance mutations causing an imatinib as well as other second-generation TKIs failure stimulated introduction of novel drugs and multiple TKIs.

Ponatinib

Ponatinib (AP24534) is a potent, oral pan–BCR-ABL TKI, which is under active investigation and is promising for patients with CML and Ph+ ALL who fail imatinib, dasatinib, and nilotinib. Importantly, it is active against T315I and other imatinib-resistant mutants. As a FMS-like tyrosine kinase-3 (FLT3) inhibitor, it also has therapeutic relevance in AML.

In vitro, ponatinib potently inhibited native ABL and also several clinically relevant mutations, including Thr315Ile. In a mouse model of human CML, treatment with ponatinib resulted in complete tumor regression. Ponatinib is currently being investigated in a phase II clinical trial in patients with relapsed or refractory CML and Ph+ ALL and also in a phase I trial for AML. Early results from these trials have been promising. The future of CML and Ph+ ALL therapy may include early use of such agents to help greater numbers of patients achieve molecular remission, with the potential of leading to a cure for CML.

Initial dose escalation data showed efficacy at 30 mg daily, with no dose-limiting toxicities (DLTs). A phase I study of oral ponatinib in patients with refractory CML/ALL or other hematologic malignancies recently reported that 66% and 53% of patients with CML-CP achieved MCyR and CCyR, respectively.[128] DLTs reported were elevated pancreatic enzymes, pancreatitis, and rash. With another phase I trial of patients with refractory CML treated with ponatinib, no DLTs were observed, and a CHR was achieved in 16 of 18 patients with CML-CP (88%), including five who had CHR at study entry. In 12 patients with T135I mutations, CCyR was achieved in 89%, and an MCyR was demonstrated in all patients.[129]

Cortes et al. reported phase I results of ponatinib in 2010.[128] The study was an open-label dose escalation study that evaluated safety and clinical responses in refractory CML patients (CML-CP, CML-AP, and CML-BP), Ph+ ALL, AML, and other hematologic malignancies. Of 67 patients enrolled, 48 Ph+ patients were evaluable for response. These included 32 patients in CML-CP and 16 other patients with CML-AP, CML-BP, or Ph+ ALL; 94% of the CML-CP patients had a CHR and 63% had an MCyR (12 complete and 8 partial). Among 11 CML-CP patients with T315I mutations, 100% had CHR and 82% had MCyR. Among the evaluable patients with CML-AP, CML-BP, and Ph+ ALL, 31% had a major HR, 19% had an MCyR, and 6% had an mCyR. Of 9 CML-AP, CML-BP, or Ph+ ALL patients with T315I mutations, 33% had a MHR and 20% had an MCyR.

Responses were also observed in highly refractory patients with either no mutations or other mutations resistant to approved TKIs (e.g., M351T, F359C, F317L, M244V, and G250E). Early MMRs were observed and occurred in 12 patients who were on treatment for ≤4 months, and 4 patients achieved MMRs within 2 months or less. MMRs were also achieved in patients with M351T, F359C, F317L, M244V, and G250E mutations and 1 patient with no mutation.

Ponatinib is generally well tolerated where patients were treated at doses as high as 60 mg; DLT in 4/14 patients treated at 60 mg were pancreatic enzyme elevations and pancreatitis. One of 22 patients treated at the 45 mg dose had a DLT of grade 3 rash. All DLTs were reversible.[128]

Omacetaxine

Omacetaxine, a subcutaneously administered first-in-class cetaxine agent that has a mechanism of action independent of tyrosine kinase inhibition, has also been evaluated in Ph-positive CML patients who have the T315I mutation and resistance to imatinib therapy. It acts through reversible, transient inhibitor of protein elongation that does not depend on BCR-ABL binding. By blocking ribosomal function, the drug decreases intracellular levels of several anti-apoptotic regulatory proteins, inducing antitumor activity via apoptosis.[130]

Omacetaxine had clinical activity and was well tolerated in two phase II, open-label, multicenter studies, including one in CML patients with T315I mutation who had failed prior imatinib (Cortes et al., EHA 2011 Abstract 1012) and the second in CML patients with resistance or intolerance to ≥2 TKIs.[129]

More phase II/III studies investigating the benefit of omacetaxine in patients with CML status post–failed therapy with multiple TKIs, and a significant proportion with baseline mutations, are ongoing. Preliminary data in patients without T315I mutations demonstrate 80% CHR rates, 20% MCyR rates, and 10% MMR rates in CML-CP patients; 75% hematologic response rates including return to chronic phase (RCP) and CHR and 5% CCyR rates in CML-AP; and 8% hematologic response rate including RCP and CHR in CML-BP. In those with CML-CP with T315I mutations, results show achievement of an 85% CHR rate, 28% CyR rate, 15% MCyR rate, 15% MMR rate, and 57% reduction in the T315I clone. OS was not met in this group of patients. In CML-AP, 37.5% showed hematologic response with OS of 18.8 months. In CML-BP, hematologic response was demonstrated in 30% with OS of 1.8 months.[131]

An update combining the two studies that included omacetaxine in patients with T315I mutation who had failed prior imatinib and in patients with resistance or intolerance to ≥2 TKIs was presented at ASH 2010. Thirty-six of the 93 CP patients had been treated previously with three or more TKIs. Over a median follow-up of 7.5 months, 27/36 (75%) achieved or maintained a CHR and 7 (19%) achieved an MCyR (4 complete and 3 partial) with omacetaxine, with a median duration of at least 4 months. These findings support further investigation of this agent in patients failing other TKI therapies.[129,131,132]

While still under investigation, omacetaxine may represent another option for patients with the T315I mutation and resistance to TKI therapy.

Common AEs Associated with CML Therapy

AEs occurring with various drugs used in CML treatment (Table 63.8) include the following:

- Hematologic
- Non-hematologic
- Cardiac
- Fluid balance

The most common events occurring with TKI therapy are hematologic, i.e., cytopenias. Most cytopenia events occur within the first few months of therapy and are only defined as severity grade 1 or 2. Nevertheless, patients receiving TKI therapy should have blood counts assessed weekly during the first month of treatment, once in both the second and third months of treatment, and every 3 months with long-term treatment.[62]

Both dasatinib and nilotinib have the potential for hematologic cross-intolerance with frontline imatinib therapy, but nilotinib may be more likely to result in hematologic cross-intolerance.[62,133] As such, patients experiencing hematologic AEs with imatinib therapy may be

TABLE 63–8 Common and Specific Adverse Effects Associated with Various Tyrosine Kinase Inhibitor Therapies

TKI	AE	Drug-Specific AE
Imatinib	Neutropenia, thrombocytopenia, anemia, elevated liver enzymes, edema, nausea, muscle cramps, musculoskeletal pains, rash, fatigue, diarrhea, and headache	
Dasatinib	More grade 3–4 thrombocytopenia than nilotinib	
	Fluid retention, edema, nausea, vomiting, and myalgia same as with imatinib	Pleural effusions, gastrointestinal bleeding, arrhythmia, and pneumonia/infection same degree compared with nilotinib
Nilotinib	Thrombocytopenia more than imatinib, anemia, and neutropenia and non-hematologic AE less than imatinib	Elevated direct bilirubin and hyperglycemia, prolonged QT interval, pericardial effusion, arrhythmias, and grade 1–2 pancreatitis
Bosutinib	Gastrointestinal symptoms	
Ponatinib	Thrombocytopenia, headache, nausea, arthralgia, and fatigue	Pancreatic enzyme elevations and pancreatitis (DLT)
Omacetaxine	Thrombocytopenia, neutropenia, anemia, febrile neutropenia, bone marrow failure, pancytopenia, and febrile bone marrow aplasia	

TKI, tyrosine kinase inhibitor; AE, adverse effect; DLT, dose-limiting toxicity.

more likely to develop these same reactions with nilotinib. Non-hematologic cross-intolerance has been infrequent with both dasatinib and nilotinib.[62]

Common non-hematologic AEs associated with TKI therapy include fluid retention events, such as pleural effusion; cardiotoxicity, including the development of congestive heart failure and QT prolongation; hepatotoxicity; pancreatic abnormalities; gastrointestinal symptoms; skin problems, such as rash and pruritus; and musculoskeletal complaints.[62]

Choosing TKI Therapies According to AE Profile

Patient communication and monitoring in anticipation of possible effects may limit the clinical impact of these effects and ensure effective treatment. Safety and tolerability are also important considerations in choosing a TKI. The potential impact of the drug's AE profile on any of the patient's preexisting conditions should be considered in choosing between second-generation BCR-ABL inhibitors. Some AEs occur more frequently with certain TKIs as explained above, which may help guide therapeutic choice for some patients.

Patients are at risk for developing pleural effusions while taking dasatinib, and the associated risk factors are disease stage (BC > AP > CP), prior cardiac history, previous lung problems such as smoking or infections, and those patients maintained on starting doses of dasatinib.[110] Uncontrolled diabetes mellitus with blood glucose elevations and prior severe pancreatitis may also be a concern on nilotinib therapy, and these patients should be closely monitored on nilotinib therapy.

Cardiac events, including congestive heart failure, left ventricular dysfunction, and QT prolongation, have all been reported with dasatinib and nilotinib. Though they occurred in <5% of the patient population, a literature review of clinical trials in CML-CP for dasatinib 70 mg twice daily and nilotinib 400 mg twice daily revealed grade 3/4 non-hematologic AEs, including arrhythmias, with both agents.[134] Pancreatitis is observed with ponatinib as a DLT. Dasatinib may be preferred in these patients. Gastrointestinal bleeds were observed with dasatinib, and caution is advised with previous history.[135]

Importantly, patients experiencing an AE attributable to TKI therapy should first receive treatment that attempts to resolve the AE while maintaining TKI therapy, particularly if the patient is responding well to TKI therapy.[62]

Special Situations

CML in Pregnancy

A frequent question is how to manage patients who have CML on imatinib therapy and become pregnant. In a study by Pye et al., the outcome of 125 out of 180 women exposed to imatinib during pregnancy was available.[136] Fifty percent delivered normal infants and 28% underwent elective terminations, 3 following the identification of abnormalities. Three of 12 infants in whom abnormalities were identified (1% of the total) had strikingly similar complex malformations (exophthalmos, renal and bone malformations). We currently recommend stopping imatinib while pregnant and resuming after delivery.

Conclusion

The management of patients with CML has been revolutionized with the introduction of TKI agents, improving prognosis, and changing the paradigm of patient care. With these clinical improvements comes the need for an effective long-term management plan that takes into account important therapeutic issues, which includes long-term monitoring of MRD. Therapeutic contingency plans are also necessary in the event of evidence of resistance to therapy over time. In CML, imatinib-resistant mutations are a difficult challenge, but the approval of dasatinib and nilotinib provides additional treatment options for CML patients. The introduction of novel therapies may further improve outcomes and address these issues as well. Meanwhile, the available agents for CML are not without important adverse effects that could impact tolerability and patient adherence over time, in turn affecting clinical outcomes. Therefore, in the current environment of managing patients with CML, early identification and treatment of AE associated with TKI therapy is critical to ensure long-term patient compliance and successful treatment. In general, there are distinct disease characteristics that favor different second-generation TKIs in patients with CML. For instance, CML-AP/BP may respond better to dasatinib therapy or combination drug strategies. As previously discussed, data from mutation analysis can also be used to choose therapies. The T315I BCR-ABL mutation is not likely to respond to TKI therapy in general, and there is definitely a role for ponatinib and newer therapies and ultimately allo-HSCT.

ACUTE MYELOID LEUKEMIA

Presentation and Diagnosis

AML occurs at a rate of 2.7 per 100,000, with presentation more common in the population over the age of 60 years.[137-139] An increased incidence of AML is seen in males, populations of European descent, and patients with disorders associated with excessive chromatin fragility such as Bloom syndrome, Fanconi anemia, Kostmann syndrome and with Wiskott-Aldrich syndrome or ataxia telangiectasia. Syndromes like Down's (trisomy of chromosome 21), Klinefelter's (XXY and variants), and Patau (trisomy of chromosome 13) have also been associated with an increased occurrence of AML.[140-142]

The incidence of AML is also increased following therapeutic radiation, particularly if given with alkylating agents. Therapy-related AML may arise following treatment with alkylating agents (e.g., cyclophosphamide, melphalan, nitrogen mustard) following a latency period of 4 to 8 years and tends to be associated with abnormalities of chromosome 5 and/or 7. Secondary AML following exposure to topoisomerase II inhibitors (e.g., etoposide and tenoposide) presents with a latency period of 1 to 3 years and is associated with chromosome 11q23 at the location of the MLL gene and with M4 or M5 morphology.[143] Several drugs (chloramphenicol, phenylbutazone, chloroquine, and methoxypsoralen), exposure to benzene, smoking, and use of dyes, herbicides, and pesticides are also implicated in the development of AML.[141,144] AML may develop secondary to a progression of myelodysplastic syndrome (MDS), polycythemia vera, CML, primary thrombocytosis, or paroxysmal nocturnal hemoglobinuria.

The diagnosis of leukemia is often demonstrated by increased number of blasts in the bone marrow, or peripheral blood. By the French-American-British (FAB) Cooperative Group criteria, acute leukemia is diagnosed when a 200-cell differential reveals the presence of 30% or more blasts in a marrow aspirate.[145] The minimal criterion has recently been changed to 20% by the World Health Organization (WHO).[146] Patients with the CG abnormalities t(8;21)(q22;q22), inversion(16)(p13q22) or t(16;16)(p13;q22), and t(15;17)(q22;q12) should be considered to have AML regardless of the blast percentage. After establishing the diagnosis, the blast lineage (myeloid, lymphoid, or undifferentiated) is determined and dictates specific therapy. Lineage determination is made using cytochemical stains. The WHO classification incorporates molecular, CG, and clinical features (prior hematological disorder) to the morphologic characteristics to better recognize the diversity of the disease and its response to therapy. Several chromosomal abnormalities and mutations have been identified that are considered to be of prognostic importance. The t(8;21), t(16;16), and inv(16) mutations are associated with a better prognosis, while alterations of 11q23, leading to the MLL rearrangement (mixed-lineage leukemia), portend a worse outcome (Table 63.9). The mutation in FLT3 (tyrosine kinase receptor) is the most common mutation in AML and is associated with poor clinical outcome. t(15;17) is always associated with acute promyelocytic leukemia (APL) and leads to a mutation in retinoic acid receptor (RAR) implicated in hematopoietic differentiation.

Treatment

Achievement of a complete remission (CR) significantly improves survival in AML; therefore, the objective of therapy is to produce and maintain CR.[147] Criteria for

TABLE 63-9 Acute Myeloid Leukemia Cytogenetic Risk Groups

Karyotype	Frequency (%)	CR (%)	EFS (%)
Favorable			
t(8;21)	5–10	90	60–70
inv(16)	5–10	90	60–70
T(15;17)	5–10	80–90	70
Intermediate			
Diploid, -Y	40–50	70–80	30–40
Unfavorable			
-5/-7	20–30	50	5–10
+8	10	60	10–20
11q23, 20q-, other	10–20	60	10

CR, complete remission; EFS, event-free survival.

CR include platelet count ≥100 × 10^9/L, neutrophil count ≥ 1 × 10^9/L, and ≤5% blasts present in the bone marrow.[148]

AML therapy consists of remission induction and post-remission therapy and has traditionally included the combination of anthracyclines and ara-C. In the "3+7" regimen, the anthracycline (i.e., idarubicin, daunorubicin) is administered for 3 days and ara-C is given at 100 to 200 mg/m^2 daily for 7 days by continuous infusion. Consolidation therapy generally commences once patients are in remission from the "3+7" regimen and consists of the same drugs administered during induction at monthly intervals for 4 to 12 months. In some situations, maintenance therapy may be considered; however, the benefit of traditional maintenance following 3 to 4 months of consolidation is relatively small, and perhaps nonexistent, with respect to survival.[149,150]

The benefit of high-dose cytarabine (HDAC) (1 to 3 g/m^2) is evident in patients < 60 years when HDAC is given during induction, post-remission therapy, and perhaps both during induction and remission therapy. It increases the cure rates to 70% to 80% in patients with inv(16) or t(8;21) and to 30% to 40% in patients with normal karyotype, but very little in patients with prognostically worse karyotypes.[151-154] The toxicity of HDAC (e.g., cerebellar and cerebral) outweighs the anti-AML effect in patients > 65 years; HDAC could also be considered in younger patients (less than 50 to 60 years) with good performance status and intermediate-risk karyotype. HDAC has minimal or no benefit in those with any antecedent of hematologic disorder (AHD), FLT3 mutation, or multidrug resistance positivity. This led to the development of targeted therapies in the management of AML.

Targeted Therapy

Initial studies with gemtuzumab ozogamicin (GO), a monoclonal antibody targeting the CD33 antigen expressed on myeloid leukemia blasts, in combination with the FLAG regimen, improved EFS compared with iron deficiency anemia–based therapies in patients with core-binding factor AML.[155] Despite the advantage in this subset of AML, GO is no longer commercially available after safety concerns were addressed. A confirmatory, postapproval clinical trial was stopped early when no improvement in clinical benefit was observed, and after a greater number of deaths occurred in the GO arm compared with chemotherapy alone.[156]

Acute Promyelocytic Leukemia Treatment

This distinct subtype of AML accounts for 5% to 15% of cases and displays unique clinical, morphologic, and CG features. The translocations between the RARα locus on chromosome 17 and the "promyelocytic leukemia" protein locus located on chromosome 15 are apparent in 95% to 100% of patients with APL.[157,158] Younger age, Hispanic background, and obesity have been identified as independent risk factors for this subset of AML.[159] Recognition of APL is crucial as appropriate treatment is different than the other subtypes of AML, and the potential for cure is high.[160,161]

The first effective treatment to induce a cure rate of 40% was anthracyclines; however, with the addition of all-trans retinoic acid (ATRA), the rate of cure increased to 70%.[162-164] ATRA acts through the promotion of differentiation in the premature promyelocytes. Potentially fatal leukocytosis, known as "differentiation Syndrome," can occur with the use of ATRA that is characterized by fever and leakage of fluid into the extravascular space leading to fluid retention, effusions, dyspnea, and hypotension. Effective management consists of dexamethasone for differentiation syndrome and frequent transfusions of platelets, cryoprecipitate, and fresh frozen plasma to control the bleeding resulting from both plasmin-dependent fibrinolysis and disseminated intravascular coagulation.[165]

Combination therapy with ATRA and anthracyclines, with or without ara-C, has become standard management for newly diagnosed patients with APL. The benefit of arsenic trioxide (ATO), traditionally reserved for relapsed disease, has been reported in the frontline setting. ATRA in combination with ATO displayed favorable responses in untreated patients with AML compared with monotherapy with ATRA or ATO.[166] Improvements in response rates, molecular remissions, and survival have been noted with the inclusion of ATO to induction and consolidation regimens for newly diagnosed patients.[167-169] While the majority of patients diagnosed with APL experience durable remissions with ATRA therapy, relapses still occur. Second molecular remissions have been reported in patients with molecular and hematologic relapse after treatment with ATO as salvage therapy, but coagulopathy and differentiation syndrome were only reported in patients with hematologic relapse.[170]

Newly diagnosed patients with APL can be stratified according to risk category. Low-risk patients present with WBC count less than 10 × 10^9/L and platelet count above 40 × 10^9/L; a WBC count above 10 × 10^9/L identifies high-risk patients. Others are at intermediate risk. Anticipated cure rates are close to 100%, 90%, and 70%, respectively, for low, intermediate, and high risk. Low-risk patients may only require three to four courses of post-remission therapy, following which PCR tests can be done every 3 months for 1 year. Longer post-remission treatment (e.g., 6 months) may be required for intermediate risk, while high-risk patients may benefit from more intense post-remission therapy as they are associated with higher rates of early death due to hemorrhage and a higher risk of relapse. More frequent PCR testing (e.g., monthly in CR) may also be advisable.

New Approaches to AML Treatment

Nucleoside Analogs

Sapacitabine, a novel nucleoside analog, causes irreparable single-strand breaking leading to cell cycle arrest at the G2 phase. Initial investigations in elderly patients with newly diagnosed or relapsed AML showed that sapacitabine was effective, with the highest CR reported in patients assigned to 400 mg twice daily administered 3 days per week.[171] Synergistic activity has been reported with sapacitabine in combination with histone deacetylase inhibitors (HDACIs), thus further exploration of this combination may offer additional benefit.[172] Toxicities included nausea, diarrhea, fatigue, anemia, thrombocytopenia, febrile neutropenia, and peripheral edema.

FLT3 Inhibitors

Targeted therapy allows for personalized treatment regimens to improve outcomes for patients with AML. The FLT3 gene is expressed on 70% to 100% of myeloid leukemia cells and mutated in approximately 30% of adult patients.[173,174] Mutations involving the FLT3 gene are the largest single-gene prognostic factor for patients with AML, and the presence of the FLT3-internal tandem duplication (ITD) mutation, observed in approximately 25% of patients, has been associated with lower CR rates and shorter DFS and OS.[175-177] Targeted therapy with TKIs blocks signal transduction, which promotes tumor cell development. Several TKIs with the ability of inhibiting both wild-type and FLT3-ITD phosphorylation are currently under investigation (Table 63.10). Sorafenib, a TKI already approved for renal cell and hepatocellular cancer, and AC220 demonstrate higher selectivity. Intermediate selectivity is reported with sunitinib, a TKI approved for gastrointestinal stromal tumor and renal cell cancer, and KW-2449. Lestaurtinib and midostaurin display lower selectivity. In vitro induction of cytotoxicity was not dependent on the degree of selectivity; thus, it has been proposed that the most beneficial utilization of these agents may include less selective agents for newly diagnosed AML and more selective agents for relapsed disease.[180]

Sorafenib, a multikinase inhibitor, initially displayed activity in relapsed or refractory AML in phase 1 studies, but transient responses were limited to patients harboring the FLT3-ITD mutation.[181,182] Sorafenib, in combination with idarubicin and ara-C, during induction and consolidation induced CR in 75% of patients with newly diagnosed AML under the age of 60 years.[183] Conversely, in a randomized study in patients over the age of 60 years, the addition of sorafenib to standard 7+3 did not impact CR, EFS, or OS.[184] *AC220*, a highly selective inhibitor for both FLT3-ITD and FLT3 wild type, induced responses, including several CR, in 30% of patients with relapsed/refractory AML.[185] QTc prolongation is noteworthy from the initial evaluation with the drug; however, concomitant medications known to prolong QTc interval were recognized as confounding factors.

The experience with inhibitors that have intermediate selectivity at FLT3, sunitinib and KW-2449, is as a single-agent therapy in relapsed/refractory patients with AML. Inhibition of FLT3 occurs in 50% of FLT3 wild-type and 100% of FLT3-ITD mutations with sunitinib.[186] DLTs, fatigue and hypertension, occurred with 75 mg administered orally daily, thus the starting dose of 50 mg daily was chosen as the MTD. At the lower dose, toxicity was minimal and included edema of the lower limbs, fatigue, taste disturbance, dry skin, fatigue, and nausea/vomiting. Responses were more common in patients with FLT3-ITD versus FLT3 wild type, but all were of short duration. Seven dose levels were evaluated for KW-2499 in the phase 1 trial; however, the study was terminated early due to lack of adequate drug levels being reached.[179]

Agents with a lower selectivity for FLT3, lestaurtinib and midostaurin, have been evaluated in previously treated as well as newly diagnosed patients. In patients with AML, lestaurtinib, also known as CEP-701, 60 mg twice daily induced responses with acceptable toxicity.[187,188] However,

TABLE 63-10 FLT3 Inhibitor Studies in AML

FLT3 Inhibitor	Phase of Study	Dose	CR (%)	Toxicity
High selectivity				
Sorafenib[178]	1/2	400 mg twice daily	56–75[a]	Diarrhea, fatigue, hypokalemia, hyperbilirubinemia
AC220	1	200 mg daily for 14 days per 28-day course	12	QTc prolongation, peripheral edema, dysgeusia
Intermediate selectivity				
Sunitinib	1/2	50–75 mg daily	0	Fatigue, hypertension (DLT), nausea, jaundice
KW2449[179]	1/2	25–500 mg daily	0	Vomiting
Low selectivity				
Lestaurtinib (CEP701)	2	60–80 mg twice daily	26[a]	Nausea, diarrhea, elevated alkaline phosphatase, transaminitis
Midostaurin (PKC412)	2	50 mg twice daily	80[a]	Nausea, vomiting

FLT3, FMS-like tyrosine kinase-3; AML, acute myeloid leukemia; CR, complete remission; DLT, dose-limiting toxicity.

[a]CR reported is in combination with chemotherapy.

combined with chemotherapy in patients with AML in first relapse, lestaurtinib 80 mg twice daily failed to improve response rates or survival.[189] Midostaurin, also known as PKC412, appeared tolerable in initial studies when dosed at 75 mg orally three times daily in patients with relapsed/refractory AML.[190] After some dose modification to further improve tolerability, CR of 80% was reported for newly diagnosed patients with AML following midostaurin, with similar rates of CR in patients with FLT3-ITD and FLT3 wild type.[191]

Histone Deacetylase Inhibitors

Histone deacetylation leading to the silencing of tumor genes has been identified as a target of therapy for patients with AML.[192] HDACIs have several mechanisms, all of which have not been clearly identified, that inhibit growth and induce cell cycle arrest, differentiation, and apoptosis.[193]

Several HDACIs have been evaluated in clinical trials with moderate response rates of 10% to 20% when used as monotherapy. Valproic acid, an oral anticonvulsant, displayed activity in patients with MDS and AML during initial evaluations; however, in combination with decitabine, VPA did not offer significant improvements in response.[194,195] At an MTD of 50 mg/kg, DLT included somnolence and confusion.[196]

Vorinostat (suberoylanilide hydroxamic acid [SAHA]), an HDACI already approved for cutaneous T-cell lymphoma, appears promising when used in combination with hypomethylating agents and induction chemotherapy.[197-199] In newly diagnosed patients with AML, 80% CR was reached with vorinostat in combination with idarubicin and ara-C.[200] Further investigation will determine the optimal dose of vorinostat as well as the long-term value of the addition to induction chemotherapy.

Several other HDACIs remain under early investigation for AML. MGCD0103, entinostat (MS-275), panobinostat (LBH589), and romidepsin (FK228) are active in AML, but the optimal approach to clinical use has yet to be determined.

Farnesyltransferase Inhibitors

Tipifarnib, an oral inhibitor of farnesyltransferase, underwent investigation as an option for elderly patients unfit to tolerate intensive chemotherapy. By inhibiting the "farnesylation" of proteins, this agent prevents the activation of Ras oncogenes, inhibits cell growth, induces apoptosis, and inhibits angiogenesis. In phase I and II studies, tipifarnib induced CR in 14% of patients with AML.[201,202] However, the response rates were considerably lower in the randomized trial of newly diagnosed patients, perhaps due to an overall older population enrolled.[203] When compared with best supportive care, including hydroxyurea, number of deaths and OS were not different between treatment arms. Myelosuppression, including grade 4 neutropenia and thrombocytopenia, is common with tipifarnib. Additional toxicities, hypokalemia and diarrhea of grade 3 to 4 severities, were more common with tipifarnib versus best supportive care.

AML in the Elderly—Role of Hypomethylating Agents

Elderly patients with AML experience considerably lower rates of CR compared with younger patients. The approximate CR rate in patients over the age of 60 years is 45% resulting from leukemic cells resistant to chemotherapy, comorbid conditions, and decreased marrow reserve. Thus, these patients experience shorter remissions, minimal long-term survival, and considerable treatment-related mortality. Worse outcome is attributed to age greater than 75 years, unfavorable karyotype (mostly complex), poor performance status, organ dysfunction, and longer duration of AHD. Patients with none or at most one adverse factor may be candidates for standard intensive therapy; however, low-intensity therapy should be considered for patients with several adverse factors. Hypomethylating agents, azacitidine and decitabine, offer an alternative to traditional chemotherapy regimens for elderly patients with AML. Azacitidine demonstrated prolonged OS compared with conventional care regimens (CCRs) in a subset of patients with AML.[204] When compared with CCR, defined as best supportive care, low-dose ara-C, or intensive chemotherapy, the median OS for azacitidine was significantly longer than that with CCR ($P = 0.005$). Decitabine has yet to display significant survival benefit in patients with AML. Dosed at 20 mg/m^2 intravenously for 5 consecutive days, decitabine demonstrated CR rates of 24%.[205] Response rates are reportedly higher with extension of the schedule to 10 consecutive days.[206]

ACUTE LYMPHOBLASTIC LEUKEMIA

Presentation and Diagnosis

ALL occurs with an incidence of approximately 1 to 1.5 per 100,000 persons, with an early peak in children 4 to 5 years of age followed by a second peak at approximately 50 years of age. Though only comprising about 20% of adult leukemias, ALL is the most common childhood leukemia. The etiology remains unknown. Suggested causes have included chromosomal translocations occurring in utero during fetal hematopoiesis as well as postnatal genetic events. Possible genetic predisposition has been noted following higher incidence reported in mono- and dizygotic twins of patients with ALL. Patients with trisomy 21, Klinefelter's syndrome, and inherited diseases with excessive chromosomal fragility such as Fanconi anemia, Bloom's syndrome, and ataxia telangiectasia are also at higher risk. Infectious etiologies such as human T-cell lymphotropic virus type 1 (HTLV-1), HIV, and lymphoproliferative disorders, as well as varicella and influenza viruses have been implicated with ALL.[207-209]

Classic "B symptoms" such as fever, night sweats, and weight loss, as well as symptoms reflective of bone marrow failure are common in ALL. Leukemia involving the central nervous system (CNS), abdominal masses, and spontaneous tumor lysis syndrome occur commonly in mature B-cell ALL (Burkitt's leukemia).[210] Chin numbness is suggestive of mature B-cell ALL. Approximately 20% of patients present with lymphadenopathy and hepatosplenomegaly, usually asymptomatic, with a higher incidence in mature B-cell and T-cell ALL.

The FAB Cooperative Group distinguishes three ALL groups (L1 to L3) based on morphologic criteria (cell size, cytoplasm, nucleoli, basophilia, and vacuolation).[145] The morphologic distinction between L1 and L2 has lost its prognostic significance, while L3 morphology is associated with mature B-cell ALL (Burkitt's leukemia). The WHO proposed new guidelines for the diagnosis of neoplastic diseases of hematopoietic and lymphoid tissues or lymphomas.[146] In addition to lowering the blast count to ≥20% as sufficient for an ALL diagnosis, the morphologic distinction of L1, L2, and L3 morphologies is abandoned as no longer relevant. Both FAB and WHO classification systems continue to rely heavily on morphological assessment.[211] Identification of the immunophenotype has become a major part of ALL diagnosis.[212-215] Three broad groups can be distinguished: precursor B-cell, mature B-cell, and T-cell ALL.

Treatment of ALL

The complexity of ALL treatment programs serves to mold multiple drugs into specific sequences of dose and time intensity to reconstitute normal hematopoiesis, prevent emergence of resistant subclones, provide adequate prophylaxis of sanctuary sites (e.g., CNS, testicles), and eliminate MRD through post-remission consolidation and maintenance. Induction, intensified consolidation, maintenance, and CNS prophylaxis represent the components of ALL therapy. Vincristine, corticosteroids, and anthracyclines comprise the backbone of therapy, with CR achieved in 70% to 90% of patients maintained through 18 months duration.[216] The substitution of dexamethasone for prednisone enhances the penetration into the cerebrospinal fluid.[217,218] Asparaginase preparations have become standard in pediatric regimens; however, the role in adult therapy has yet to be determined. The German Multicenter Study Group for adult ALL (GMALL) recently reported that pegylated asparaginase, dosed at 2000 U/m^2 combined with induction chemotherapy, increased OS to 80% at 3 years in patients with standard risk disease, but with increased occurrences of grade 3 to 4 bilirubin elevation.[219] Further evaluation with other induction ALL regimens with asparaginase preparations will provide further insight into efficacy and toxicity. Hematopoietic growth factors have been included to stimulate recovery from myelosuppression.[220] Consolidation represents a repetition of a modified induction schedule, rotational consolidation programs, or stem cell transplantation. Novel strategies try to emphasize subtype- and risk-oriented approaches of consolidation programs.

TABLE 63-11 Modifications to the Hyper-CVAD Regimen to Include Targeted Therapy

Feature	Original	Modification
CD20-positive	Hyper-CVAD	Hyper-CVAD plus rituximab
		Hyper-CVAD plus ofatumumab
Ph-positive	Hyper-CVAD	Hyper-CVAD plus imatinib
		Hyper-CVAD plus dasatinib
T-cell	Hyper-CVAD	Hyper-CVAD plus nelarabine

hyper-CVAD, hyperfractionated cyclophosphamide, vincristine, adriamycin, and dexamethasone.

Maintenance therapy, given over 2 to 3 years, includes 6-mercaptopurine, weekly methotrexate, monthly vincristine, and pulses of corticosteroids. No benefit is evident with extension of therapy beyond 3 years or with omission or shortening of therapy. In mature B-cell ALL, short-term dose-intense regimens induce high cure rates with low likelihood of relapse, thus maintenance therapy is not indicated. The best maintenance therapy for patients with Ph+ ALL remains disputed, but should incorporate TKIs.

Further modifications to the hyper-CVAD regimen incorporated rituximab for CD20 positivity, TKIs for Ph+ ALL, and nelarabine in T-cell ALL (Table 63.11). Activity with nelarabine monotherapy has been demonstrated in relapsed T-cell ALL, as well as in combination with chemotherapy in newly diagnosed patients.[221]

Long-term survival of elderly patients with ALL remains low.[222] Myelosuppression-related AEs following intensive chemotherapy represent the primary cause of failure in patients over the age of 60 to 65 years. Administration of chemotherapy in a protected environment should be considered for patients likely to experience complications following chemotherapy.

Targeted Therapy

Targeted therapy in ALL is aimed at various types of cells (e.g., rituximab against B cells and nelarabine against T cells) and BCR-ABL abnormality in Ph+ ALL. They will be discussed here.

Monoclonal Antibodies

Various monoclonal antibodies implemented and currently being investigated are summarized in Table 63.12.

Lower rates of response and survival have been associated with CD20 positivity in B-cell lineage ALL.[223] Higher expression has been reported in mature B-cell and Ph+ ALL. Antibodies targeted toward a specific antigen have been under evaluation in acute leukemia. In B-cell

TABLE 63-12 Targeted Monoclonal Antibodies—Acute Lymphocytic Leukemia

ALL Type	Monoclonal Antibody	Antibody Against
B-cell ALL	Rituximab	CD20
	Ofatumumab	Enhanced CD20 antibody
	Blinotumomab	CD19/CD3
	Inotuzumab ozogamicin	CD22
T-cell ALL	Alemtuzumab	CD52

ALL, acute lymphocytic leukemia.

ALL, rituximab improves outcome and CD20 targeted agents offer benefit to patients that express CD20 positivity regardless of percentage at diagnosis.[224-226] In newly diagnosed patients that were not candidates for allo-HSCT, greater reduction in tumor burden and improvements in the probability of survival at 5 years were improved with rituximab and chemotherapy compared with chemotherapy alone.[227] Furthermore, patients that received rituximab pre–allo-HSCT experienced a higher occurrence of remissions post-transplant when compared with patients that did not receive rituximab. At MDACC, incorporation of rituximab to the hyper-CVAD regimen sustained CR of 70% and survival of 75% through 3 years.[223]

Modification of therapy with ofatumumab, a CD20-targeted monoclonal antibody with improved binding capacity, in place of rituximab, with the hyper-CVAD regimen is under investigation to further improve responses in patients with any level of CD20 expression.

Several other monoclonal antibodies under evaluation have displayed activity in ALL subsets. Blinatumomab, a CD19/CD3 bispecific antibody successfully eradicated MRD in patients with B-cell ALL, with minimal toxicity.[228] Rapid responses were apparent, all occurring within the first cycle of treatment. Another novel compound, inotuzumab ozogamicin, an anti-CD22 antibody conjugated to calicheamicin, demonstrated efficacy in B-cell lymphomas and is now being evaluated at MDACC in patients with relapsed/refractory ALL. Already approved in chronic lymphocytic leukemia, alemtuzumab, targeted toward the CD52 antigen, also demonstrates activity in T-cell leukemia.[229]

Nelarabine (506U78) is a soluble prodrug of arabinofuranosylguanine (ara-G), a deoxyguanosine derivative that is demethylated by adenosine deaminase. In vitro studies have demonstrated that immature T lymphocytes and T lymphoblasts are sensitive to the cytotoxic effects of deoxyguanosine.[230] The intracellular deoxyguanosine triphosphate accumulation with subsequent inhibition of ribonucleotide reductase, inhibition of DNA synthesis, results in T-cell death. In a phase II study including 26 T-cell ALL patients and 13 T-cell lymphoblastic lymphoma, nelarabine induced CR among 31%, with overall response rate of 41%. The DFS was 20 weeks and median OS was 20 weeks. The 1-year survival was 28%. The principal toxicity was grade 3 or 4 neutropenia and thrombocytopenia.[221] Thus, nelarabine also offers a targeted therapeutic advantage in T-cell ALL patients.

TKIs IN PH + ALL

Approximately 20% to 30% of patients with ALL and over half of ALL patients older than 50 display the Philadelphia chromosome, which is the most common CG abnormality in ALL that confers a poor prognosis.[231,232] Produced by the Philadelphia chromosome, BCR-ABL is a constitutively activated tyrosine kinase and is the therapeutic target of inhibition by BCR-ABL TKIs.[113] In 50% to 80% of cases of adult Ph+ ALL, the nature of the BCR-ABL fusion is different from that in CML; instead of a 210-kDa protein product, a 190-kDa product with higher tyrosine kinase activity is generated. The 210-kDa BCR-ABL protein accounts for the other 20% to 50% of adult patients with Ph+ ALL.[7,8] Although Ph+ ALL is associated with an aggressive disease course and a high risk of CNS invasion, TKIs have significantly improved survival outcomes for patients with Ph+ ALL.[118,119,233] Imatinib was approved in the United States and Europe in 2006 for the treatment of adult patients with relapsed or refractory Ph+ ALL.[234,235]

While imatinib can induce CR in newly diagnosed as well as previously treated patients, the majority of patients do not maintain response.[113,236,237] This may be a feasible option for elderly patients unfit to tolerate intensive chemotherapy; however, the short remission durations will likely not offer any improvements in survival. Combination with imatinib and the hyper-CVAD regimen leads to CR of 93% and improves survival and remission durations at 3 years when compared with the hyper-CVAD regimen alone.[118] In separate evaluations, both the Japan Adult Leukemia Study Group (JALSG) and the Group for Research on Adult Acute Lymphoblastic Leukemia (GRAALL) showed that alternating chemotherapy with imatinib has also proved effective at inducing high rates of CR.[238,239] Despite these excellent results, imatinib does have drawbacks including insufficient CNS penetration and the potential for imatinib resistance.[72]

Dasatinib, a more potent second-generation TKI, offers several advantages over imatinib and may overcome the limitations of the first-generation TKI. Dasatinib, unlike imatinib which binds to BCR-ABL in only the closed conformation, can bind in both open and closed conformations with a much higher affinity. In addition, dasatinib can block the Src family of kinases, which expands the target range of inhibition compared with imatinib. As monotherapy or in combination with low-intensity chemotherapy, dasatinib induces CR of moderate durations.[240] Similar to dose optimization studies in

CML, comparable efficacy and less toxicity occur with once-daily versus twice-daily dosing in Ph+ ALL.[241] Combined with hyper-CVAD during induction for newly diagnosed patients with Ph+ ALL, CR rates of 94% and OS of 64% at 2 years were reported.[119] This combination also proved effective in patients with relapsed refractory ALL, with CR reported in 65% of patients and partial CyR in 26%.

The optimal point in therapy as well as treatment duration with a TKI has also been explored. The early initiation of imatinib has been associated with improvements in survival, but the initiation at any point in therapy improves outcomes in patients with Ph+ ALL.[242] The use of more potent TKIs, such as dasatinib, early in therapy may improve the quality of CR and allow for more patients to proceed to allo-HSCT. Thus, durable remissions and improvements in survival are achievable in the future.

TKIs have improved outcomes; however, allo-HSCT remains the only curative option, and it is recommended that patients with Ph+ ALL proceed to this therapy following first remission. These molecularly targeted agents are effective as monotherapy; however, synergistic activity with traditional chemotherapy regimens has improved response rates.

CONCLUSION

Recent discoveries confirm the complexity in the understanding and treatment of acute leukemia. Targets for therapeutic intervention have been identified in both AML and ALL and further investigation of novel therapies will continue to improve outcomes in patients with acute leukemias. Although considered not as toxic as traditional chemotherapy, targeted therapy will bring new adverse effects to light and management strategies will be necessary. Identifying disease characteristics and determining prognosis will continue to be important for directing treatment. Targeted therapy represents the future of leukemia management. With advancements in personalized therapy aimed at molecular or CG features of disease, long-term survival of patients with leukemia appears promising. TKIs remain an important aspect of treatment. For Ph+ ALL, imatinib combined with chemotherapy has improved survival, but the emergence of drug-resistant mutations is a reality. The additional potency and dual BCR-ABL and Src inhibition of dasatinib, as well as its ability to overcome certain imatinib-resistant mutations, make it appealing for Ph+ ALL, and data suggest it should be established as an appropriate frontline therapy in these patients. Ponatinib, while still under investigation, seems very promising and its ability to overcome T315I mutations is of significant importance for TKI-resistant CML and Ph+ ALL patients. Likewise, FLT-3 inhibition is of particular interest in AML patients with FLT-3 ITD mutations, and this type of targeted therapy continues to be studied.

REFERENCES

1. Jemal A, Siegel R, Xu J, Ward E. Cancer statistics, 2010. *CA Cancer J Clin.* September-October 2010;60(5):277-300.
2. O'Brien S, Berman E, Borghaei H, et al.; NCCN Chronic Myelogenous Leukemia Panel (Internet) MNCCn. NCCN Clinical Practice Guidelines in Oncology: chronic myeloid leukemia. Published February 15, 2011. http://www.nccn.org/professionals/physician_gls/pdf/cml.pdf
3. Faderl S, Kantarjian HM, Talpaz M. Chronic myelogenous leukemia: update on biology and treatment. *Oncology (Williston Park).* February 1999;13(2):169-180; discussion 81, 84.
4. Goldman JM, Melo JV. Chronic myeloid leukemia—advances in biology and new approaches to treatment. *N Engl J Med.* October 2003;349(15):1451-1464.
5. Silver RT, Woolf SH, Hehlmann R, et al. An evidence-based analysis of the effect of busulfan, hydroxyurea, interferon, and allogeneic bone marrow transplantation in treating the chronic phase of chronic myeloid leukemia: developed for the American Society of Hematology. *Blood.* [Review]. September 1999;94(5): 1517-1536.
6. Schiffer CA. BCR-ABL tyrosine kinase inhibitors for chronic myelogenous leukemia. *N Engl J Med.* [Review]. July 2007;357(3):258-265.
7. Lee HJ, Thompson JE, Wang ES, Wetzler M. Philadelphia chromosome-positive acute lymphoblastic leukemia: current treatment and future perspectives. *Cancer.* April 2011;117(8):1583-1594.
8. Sawyers CL. Chronic myeloid leukemia. *N Engl J Med.* April 1999;340(17):1330-1340.
9. Savage DG, Szydlo RM, Goldman JM. Clinical features at diagnosis in 430 patients with chronic myeloid leukaemia seen at a referral centre over a 16-year period. *Br J Haematol.* January 1997;96(1):111-116.
10. Faderl S, Talpaz M, Estrov Z, O'Brien S, Kurzrock R, Kantarjian HM. The biology of chronic myeloid leukemia. *N Engl J Med.* [Review]. July 1999;341(3):164-172.
11. Baccarani M, Dreyling M. Chronic myelogenous leukemia: ESMO clinical recommendations for diagnosis, treatment and follow-up. *Ann Oncol.* May 2009;20(suppl 4):105-107.
12. Kantarjian HM, O'Brien S, Smith TL, et al. Treatment of Philadelphia chromosome-positive early chronic phase chronic myelogenous leukemia with daily doses of interferon alpha and low-dose cytarabine. *J Clin Oncol.* January 1999;17(1):284.
13. Druker BJ, Lydon NB. Lessons learned from the development of an abl tyrosine kinase inhibitor for chronic myelogenous leukemia. *J Clin Invest.* [Review]. January 2000;105(1):3-7.
14. Deininger MW, Goldman JM, Lydon N, Melo JV. The tyrosine kinase inhibitor CGP57148B selectively inhibits the growth of BCR-ABL-positive cells. *Blood.* November 1997;90(9): 3691-3698.
15. O'Brien SG, Guilhot F, Larson RA, et al. Imatinib compared with interferon and low-dose cytarabine for newly diagnosed chronic-phase chronic myeloid leukemia. *N Engl J Med.* March 2003;348(11):994-1004.
16. Deininger M, O'Brien SG, Guilhot F, et al. International randomized study of interferon vs. STI571 (IRIS) 8-year follow up: sustained survival and low risk for progression of events in patients with newly diagnosed chronic myeloid leukemia in chronic phase (CML-CP) treated with imatinib. *Blood.* 2009;114(22):462. Abstract 1126.
17. Baccarani M, Rosti G, Castagnetti F, et al. Comparison of imatinib 400 mg and 800 mg daily in the front-line treatment of high-risk, Philadelphia-positive chronic myeloid leukemia: a European LeukemiaNet Study. *Blood.* May 2009;113(19):4497-4504.
18. Cortes JE, Baccarani M, Guilhot F, et al. Phase III, randomized, open-label study of daily imatinib mesylate 400 mg versus 800 mg in patients with newly diagnosed, previously untreated chronic myeloid leukemia in chronic phase using molecular end points: tyrosine kinase inhibitor optimization and selectivity study. *J Clin Oncol.* January 2010;28(3):424-430.
19. Kantarjian HM, Hochhaus A, Saglio G, et al. Nilotinib versus imatinib for the treatment of patients with newly diagnosed chronic phase, Philadelphia chromosome-positive, chronic myeloid leukaemia: 24-month minimum follow-up of the phase 3 randomised ENESTnd trial. *Lancet Oncol.* September 2011;12(9):841-851.

20. Lombardo LJ, Lee FY, Chen P, et al. Discovery of N-(2-chloro-6-methyl- phenyl)-2-(6-(4-(2-hydroxyethyl)-piperazin-1-yl)-2-methylpyrimidin-4-ylamino)thiazole-5-carboxamide (BMS-354825), a dual Src/Abl kinase inhibitor with potent antitumor activity in preclinical assays. *J Med Chem*. December 2004;47(27):6658-6661.
21. O'Hare T, Walters DK, Stoffregen EP, et al. In vitro activity of Bcr-Abl inhibitors AMN107 and BMS-354825 against clinically relevant imatinib-resistant Abl kinase domain mutants. *Cancer Res*. June 2005;65(11):4500-4505.
22. Tokarski JS, Newitt JA, Chang CY, et al. The structure of dasatinib (BMS-354825) bound to activated ABL kinase domain elucidates its inhibitory activity against imatinib-resistant ABL mutants. *Cancer Res*. June 2006;66(11):5790-5797.
23. Shah NP, Tran C, Lee FY, Chen P, Norris D, Sawyers CL. Overriding imatinib resistance with a novel ABL kinase inhibitor. *Science*. July 2004;305(5682):399-401.
24. Cortes JE, Jones D, O'Brien S, et al. Results of dasatinib therapy in patients with early chronic-phase chronic myeloid leukemia. *J Clin Oncol*. 2009 ASCO Annual Meeting Abstracts; 26:abstract 7009. 2010;28:398-404.
25. Shah N, Kantarjian H, Hochhaus A, et al. Dasatinib versus Imatinib in patients with newly diagnosed chronic myeloid leukemia in chronic phase (CML-CP) in the DASISION trial: 18-month follow-up. *Blood*. 2010;21(94). Abstract 116:3828.
26. Kantarjian H, Shah NP, Hochhaus A, et al. Dasatinib versus imatinib in newly diagnosed chronic-phase chronic myeloid leukemia. *N Engl J Med*. June 2010;362(24):2260-2270.
27. Radich JP, Kopecky KJ, Kamel-Reid S, et al. A randomized phase II trial of dasatinib 100 mg vs imatinib 400 mg in newly diagnosed chronic myeloid leukemia in chronic phase (CML-CP): the SO325 Intergroup Trial. ASH Annual Meeting Abstracts. *Blood*. November 2010;116:LBA-6.
28. Weisberg E, Manley PW, Breitenstein W, et al. Characterization of AMN107, a selective inhibitor of native and mutant Bcr-Abl. *Cancer Cell*. February 2005;7(2):129-141.
29. Rosti G, Castagnetti F, Gugliotta G, et al. Excellent outcomes at 3 years with nilotinib 800 mg daily in early chronic phase, Ph(+) chronic myeloid leukemia (CML): results of a phase 2 GIMEMA CML WP clinical trial. ASH Annual Meeting Abstracts. *Blood*. 2010;116:36:abstract 359.
30. Saglio G, Kim DW, Issaragrisil S, et al. Nilotinib versus imatinib for newly diagnosed chronic myeloid leukemia. *N Engl J Med*. June 2010;362(24):2251-2259.
31. Kantarjian H, Giles F, Wunderle L, et al. Nilotinib in imatinib-resistant CML and Philadelphia chromosome-positive ALL. *N Engl J Med*. June 2006;354(24):2542-2551.
32. Cortes J, Kantarjian HM, Kim D-W, et al. Efficacy and safety of bosutinib (SKI-606) in patients with chronic phase (CP) Ph+ chronic myelogenous leukemia (CML) with resistance or intolerance to imatinib. ASH Annual Meeting Abstracts. *Blood*. November 2008;112(11):1098. Abstract 2008; 112:1101.
33. Jabbour E, Cortes J, Kantarjian H. Chronic myeloid leukemia. In: Popat UR, guest editor. *Emerging Cancer Therapies (ECAT) Leukemia*. New York, NY: Demos Medical Publishing LLC; 2011;2(2):239-258.
34. Gambacorti-Passerini C, Kim D-W, Kantarjian H, et al. An ongoing phase 3 study of bosutinib (SKI-606) versus imatinib in patients with newly diagnosed chronic phase chronic myeloid leukemia. ASH Annual Meeting Abstracts. *Blood*. 2010;116:208.
35. Alvarado Y, Kantarjian H, Faderl S, et al. Significance of suboptimal response to imatinib, as defined by the European LeukemiaNet, in long-term outcome for patients (Pts) with chronic phase (CP) chronic myeloid leukemia (CML). ASH Annual Meeting Abstracts. *Blood*. 2007;110:1932.
36. Alvarado Y, Kantarjian H, O'Brien S, et al. Significance of suboptimal response to imatinib, as defined by the European LeukemiaNet, in the long-term outcome of patients with early chronic myeloid leukemia in chronic phase. *Cancer*. August 2009;115(16):3709-3718.
37. Preudhomme C, Guilhot J, Nicolini FE, et al. Imatinib plus peginterferon alfa-2a in chronic myeloid leukemia. *N Engl J Med*. December 2010;363(26):2511-2521.
38. Hughes TP, Hochhaus A, Branford S, et al. Long-term prognostic significance of early molecular response to imatinib in newly diagnosed chronic myeloid leukemia: an analysis from the International Randomized Study of Interferon and STI571 (IRIS). *Blood*. November 2010;116(19):3758-3765.
39. Baccarani M, Cortes J, Pane F, et al. Chronic myeloid leukemia: an update of concepts and management recommendations of European LeukemiaNet. *J Clin Oncol*. [Practice Guideline Review]. December 2009;27(35):6041-6051.
40. Druker BJ, Guilhot F, O'Brien SG, et al.; IRIS Investigators. Five-year follow-up of patients receiving imatinib for chronic myeloid leukemia. *N Engl J Med*. December 2006;355(23): 2408-2417.
41. Hughes TP, Kaeda J, Branford S, et al. Frequency of major molecular responses to imatinib or interferon alfa plus cytarabine in newly diagnosed chronic myeloid leukemia. *N Engl J Med*. October 2003;349(15):1423-1432.
42. Jabbour E, Kantarjian H, O'Brien S, et al. The achievement of an early complete cytogenetic response is a major determinant for outcome in patients with early chronic phase chronic myeloid leukemia treated with tyrosine kinase inhibitors. *Blood*. July 2011;118(17):4541-4546.
43. Hehlmann R, Lauseker M, Jung-Munkwitz S, et al. Tolerability-adapted imatinib 800 mg/d versus 400 mg/d versus 400 mg/d plus interferon-alpha in newly diagnosed chronic myeloid leukemia. *J Clin Oncol*. April 2011;29(12):1634-1642.
44. Marin D, Milojkovic D, Olavarria E, et al. European LeukemiaNet criteria for failure or suboptimal response reliably identify patients with CML in early chronic phase treated with imatinib whose eventual outcome is poor. *Blood*. December 2008;112(12):4437-4444.
45. Hochhaus A, Druker B, Sawyers C, et al. Favorable long-term follow-up results over 6 years for response, survival, and safety with imatinib mesylate therapy in chronic-phase chronic myeloid leukemia after failure of interferon-alpha treatment. *Blood*. February 2008;111(3):1039-1043.
46. Tam CS, Kantarjian H, Garcia-Manero G, et al. Failure to achieve a major cytogenetic response by 12 months defines inadequate response in patients receiving nilotinib or dasatinib as second or subsequent line therapy for chronic myeloid leukemia. *Blood*. August 2008;112(3):516-518.
47. Jabbour E, Kantarjian H, O'Brien S, et al. Predictive factors for response and outcome in patients (pts) treated with second generation tyrosine kinase inhibitors (2-TKI) for chronic myeloid leukemia in chronic phase (CML-CP) post imatinib failure. *Blood*. 2009;114:210:abstract 509.
48. Baccarani M, Saglio G, Goldman J, et al. Evolving concepts in the management of chronic myeloid leukemia: recommendations from an expert panel on behalf of the European LeukemiaNet. *Blood*. September 2006;108(6):1809-1820.
49. Jabbour E, Kantarjian HM, O'Brien S, et al. Front-line therapy with second-generation tyrosine kinase inhibitors in patients with early chronic phase chronic myeloid leukemia: what is the optimal response? *J Clin Oncol*. October 2011;38(5):682-692.
50. Kantarjian HM, Talpaz M, O'Brien S, et al. Survival benefit with imatinib mesylate versus interferon-alpha-based regimens in newly diagnosed chronic-phase chronic myelogenous leukemia. *Blood*. September 2006;108(6):1835-1840.
51. Roy L, Guilhot J, Krahnke T, et al. Survival advantage from imatinib compared with the combination interferon-alpha plus cytarabine in chronic-phase chronic myelogenous leukemia: historical comparison between two phase 3 trials. *Blood*. September 2006;108(5):1478-1484.
52. Kantarjian HM, Shan J, Jones D, et al. Significance of increasing levels of minimal residual disease in patients with Philadelphia chromosome-positive chronic myelogenous leukemia in complete cytogenetic response. *J Clin Oncol*. August 2009;27(22):3659-3663.
53. Ross DM, Branford S, Moore S, Hughes TP. Limited clinical value of regular bone marrow cytogenetic analysis in imatinib-treated chronic phase CML patients monitored by RQ-PCR for BCR-ABL. *Leukemia*. 2006;20(4):664-670.
54. Branford S, Rudzki Z, Walsh S, et al. Detection of BCR-ABL mutations in patients with CML treated with imatinib is virtually always accompanied by clinical resistance, and mutations in the ATP phosphate-binding loop (P-loop) are associated with a poor prognosis. *Blood*. [Research Support, Non-U.S. Govt]. July 2003;102(1):276-283.

55. Hughes T, Deininger M, Hochhaus A, et al. Monitoring CML patients responding to treatment with tyrosine kinase inhibitors: review and recommendations for harmonizing current methodology for detecting BCR-ABL transcripts and kinase domain mutations and for expressing results. *Blood.* July 2006;108(1):28-37.
56. Jabbour E, Kantarjian HM, Abruzzo LV, et al. Chromosomal abnormalities in Philadelphia chromosome negative metaphases appearing during imatinib mesylate therapy in patients with newly diagnosed chronic myeloid leukemia in chronic phase. *Blood.* October 2007;110(8):2991-2995.
57. Hughes TP, Hochhaus A, Branford S, et al. Reduction of BCR-ABL transcript levels at 6, 12, and 18 months (Mo) correlates with long-term outcomes on imatinib (IM) at 72 Mo: an analysis from the international randomized study of interferon versus STI571 (IRIS) in patients (pts) with chronic phase chronic myeloid leukemia (CML-CP). ASH Annual Meeting Abstracts. *Blood.* 2008;112:334.
58. Hochhaus A, Druker BJ, Larson RA, et al. IRIS 6-year follow-up: sustained survival and declining annual rate of transformation in patients with newly diagnosed chronic myeloid leukemia in chronic phase (CML-CP) Treated with Imatinib). ASH Annual Meeting Abstracts. *Blood.* 2007;110:25.
59. Marin D, Bazeos A, Mahon FX, et al. Adherence is the critical factor for achieving molecular responses in patients with chronic myeloid leukemia who achieve complete cytogenetic responses on imatinib. *J Clin Oncol.* May 2010;28(14):2381-2388.
60. Darkow T, Henk HJ, Thomas SK, et al. Treatment interruptions and non-adherence with imatinib and associated healthcare costs: a retrospective analysis among managed care patients with chronic myelogenous leukaemia. *PharmacoEconomics.* 2007;25(6):481-496.
61. Noens L, van Lierde MA, De Bock R, et al. Prevalence, determinants, and outcomes of nonadherence to imatinib therapy in patients with chronic myeloid leukemia: the ADAGIO study. *Blood.* May 2009;113(22):5401-5411.
62. Jabbour E, Deininger M, Hochhaus A. Management of adverse events associated with tyrosine kinase inhibitors in the treatment of chronic myeloid leukemia. *Leukemia.* February 2011;25(2):201-210.
63. Pinilla-Ibarz J, Cortes J, Mauro MJ. Intolerance to tyrosine kinase inhibitors in chronic myeloid leukemia: definitions and clinical implications. *Cancer.* February 2011;117(4):688-697.
64. Hochhaus A, O'Brien SG, Guilhot F, et al. Six-year follow-up of patients receiving imatinib for the first-line treatment of chronic myeloid leukemia. *Leukemia.* June 2009;23(6):1054-1061.
65. Bixby D, Talpaz M. Mechanisms of resistance to tyrosine kinase inhibitors in chronic myeloid leukemia and recent therapeutic strategies to overcome resistance. *Hematology Am Soc Hematol Educ Program.* [Review]. 2009;461-476.
66. Shah NP. Medical management of CML. *Hematology Am Soc Hematol Educ Program.* 2007:371-375.
67. Lee F, Fandi A, Voi M. Overcoming kinase resistance in chronic myeloid leukemia. *Int J Biochem Cell Biol.* 2008;40(3):334-343.
68. Jabbour E, Kantarjian H, Jones D, et al. Frequency and clinical significance of BCR-ABL mutations in patients with chronic myeloid leukemia treated with imatinib mesylate. *Leukemia.* October 2006;20(10):1767-1773.
69. Hochhaus A, Kreil S, Corbin AS, et al. Molecular and chromosomal mechanisms of resistance to imatinib (STI571) therapy. *Leukemia.* November 2002;16(11):2190-2196.
70. Shah NP. Loss of response to imatinib: mechanisms and management. *Hematology Am Soc Hematol Educ Program.* 2005:183-187.
71. Deininger M, Buchdunger E, Druker BJ. The development of imatinib as a therapeutic agent for chronic myeloid leukemia. *Blood.* [Review]. April 2005;105(7):2640-2653.
72. Ravandi F. Managing Philadelphia chromosome-positive acute lymphoblastic leukemia: role of tyrosine kinase inhibitors. *Clin Lymphoma Myeloma Leuk.* [Review]. April 2011;11(2):198-203.
73. Nicolini FE, Corm S, Le QH, et al. Mutation status and clinical outcome of 89 imatinib mesylate-resistant chronic myelogenous leukemia patients: a retrospective analysis from the French intergroup of CML (Fi(phi)-LMC GROUP). *Leukemia.* June 2006;20(6):1061-1066.
74. Khorashad JS, de Lavallade H, Apperley JF, et al. Finding of kinase domain mutations in patients with chronic phase chronic myeloid leukemia responding to imatinib may identify those at high risk of disease progression. *J Clin Oncol.* October 2008;26(29):4806-4813.
75. Che XF, Nakajima Y, Sumizawa T, et al. Reversal of P-glycoprotein mediated multidrug resistance by a newly synthesized 1,4-benzothiazipine derivative, JTV-519. *Cancer Lett.* December 2002;187(1-2):111-119.
76. Kotaki M, Motoji T, Takanashi M, Wang YH, Mizoguchi H. Anti-proliferative effect of the abl tyrosine kinase inhibitor STI571 on the P-glycoprotein positive K562/ADM cell line. *Cancer Lett.* September 2003;199(1):61-68.
77. Rumpold H, Wolf AM, Gruenewald K, Gastl G, Gunsilius E, Wolf D. RNAi-mediated knockdown of P-glycoprotein using a transposon-based vector system durably restores imatinib sensitivity in imatinib-resistant CML cell lines. *Exp Hematol.* July 2005;33(7): 767-775.
78. Thomas J, Wang L, Clark R, Pirmohamed M. Active transport of imatinib into and out of cells: implications for drug resistance. *Blood.* August 2004;104:3739-3745 [published ahead of print]. doi:101182/blood-2003-12-4276.
79. White DL, Saunders VA, Dang P, et al. OCT-1-mediated influx is a key determinant of the intracellular uptake of imatinib but not nilotinib (AMN107): reduced OCT-1 activity is the cause of low in vitro sensitivity to imatinib. *Blood.* July 2006;108(2):697-704.
80. Wang L, Giannoudis A, Lane S, Williamson P, Pirmohamed M, Clark RE. Expression of the uptake drug transporter hOCT1 is an important clinical determinant of the response to imatinib in chronic myeloid leukemia. *Clin Pharmacol Ther.* February 2008;83(2):258-264.
81. Gambacorti-Passerini C, Barni R, le Coutre P, et al. Role of alpha1 acid glycoprotein in the in vivo resistance of human BCR-ABL(+) leukemic cells to the abl inhibitor STI571. *J Natl Cancer Inst.* October 2000;92(20):1641-1650.
82. Widmer N, Decosterd LA, Csajka C, et al. Population pharmacokinetics of imatinib and the role of alpha-acid glycoprotein. *Br J Clin Pharmacol.* July 2006;62(1):97-112.
83. Zhang WW, Cortes JE, Yao H, et al. Predictors of primary imatinib resistance in chronic myelogenous leukemia are distinct from those in secondary imatinib resistance. *J Clin Oncol.* August 2009;27(22):3642-3649.
84. Hochhaus A, Baccarani M, Deininger M, et al. Dasatinib induces durable cytogenetic responses in patients with chronic myelogenous leukemia in chronic phase with resistance or intolerance to imatinib. *Leukemia.* June 2008;22(6):1200-1206.
85. Jabbour E, Jones D, Kantarjian HM, et al. Long-term outcome of patients with chronic myeloid leukemia treated with second-generation tyrosine kinase inhibitors after imatinib failure is predicted by the in vitro sensitivity of BCR-ABL kinase domain mutations. *Blood.* September 2009;114(10):2037-2043.
86. Soverini S, Martinelli G, Colarossi S, et al. Presence or the emergence of a F317L BCR-ABL mutation may be associated with resistance to dasatinib in Philadelphia chromosome-positive leukemia. *J Clin Oncol.* November 2006;24(33):e51-e52.
87. Jabbour E, Kantarjian H, Jones D, et al. Characteristics and outcomes of patients with chronic myeloid leukemia and T315I mutation following failure of imatinib mesylate therapy. *Blood.* July 2008;112(1):53-55.
88. Muller MC, Cortes JE, Kim DW, et al. Dasatinib treatment of chronic-phase chronic myeloid leukemia: analysis of responses according to preexisting BCR-ABL mutations. *Blood.* December 2009;114(24):4944-4953.
89. White DL, Lu L, Clackson TP, Saunders VA, Hughes TP. ATP dependent efflux transporters ABCB1 and ABCG2 are unlikely to impact the efficacy, or mediate resistance to the tyrosine kinase inhibitor, ponatinib. ASH Annual Meeting Abstracts. November 2011;118(21):2745.
90. Kantarjian H, Schiffer C, Jones D, Cortes J. Monitoring the response and course of chronic myeloid leukemia in the modern era of BCR-ABL tyrosine kinase inhibitors: practical advice on the use and interpretation of monitoring methods. *Blood.* February 2008;111(4):1774-1780.
91. Kantarjian HM, Larson RA, Guilhot F, et al. Efficacy of imatinib dose escalation in patients with chronic myeloid leukemia in chronic phase. *Cancer.* February 2009;115(3):551-560.
92. Jabbour E, Kantarjian HM, Jones D, et al. Imatinib mesylate dose escalation is associated with durable responses in patients with chronic myeloid leukemia after cytogenetic failure on standard-dose imatinib therapy. *Blood.* March 2009;113(10): 2154-2160.

93. Deininger MW. Nilotinib. *Clin Cancer Res*. July 2008;14(13): 4027-4031.
94. Mauro MJ, Baccarani M, Cervantes F, et al. Dasatinib 2-year efficacy in patients with chronic-phase chronic myeloid leukemia with resistance or intolerance to Imatinib (START-C). ASCO Annual Meeting Abstracts. *J Clin Oncol*. 2009;26: abstract 7009.
95. Brave M, Goodman V, Kaminskas E, et al. Sprycel for chronic myeloid leukemia and Philadelphia chromosome-positive acute lymphoblastic leukemia resistant to or intolerant of imatinib mesylate. *Clin Cancer Res*. January 2008;14(2):352-359.
96. Stone RM, Kantarjian HM, Baccarani M, et al. Efficacy of dasatinib in patients with chronic-phase chronic myelogenous leukemia with resistance or intolerance to imatinib: 2-year follow-up data from START-C (CA180-013). ASH Annual Meeting Abstracts. *Blood*. November 2007;110(11):734.
97. Baccarani M, Rosti G, Saglio G, et al. Dasatinib time to and durability of major and complete cytogenetic response (MCyR and CCyR) in patients with chronic myeloid leukemia in chronic phase (CML-CP). ASH Annual Meeting Abstracts. *Blood*. 2008;112:450.
98. Shah NP, Kim DW, Kantarjian HM, et al. Dasatinib dose-optimization in chronic phase chronic myeloid leukemia (CML-CP): two-year data from CA180-034 show equivalent long-term efficacy and improved safety with 100 mg once daily dose. ASH Annual Meeting Abstracts. *Blood*. 2008;112:3225.
99. Lee SJ, Kukreja M, Wang T, et al. Impact of prior imatinib mesylate on the outcome of hematopoietic cell transplantation for chronic myeloid leukemia. *Blood*. October 2008;112(8): 3500-3507.
100. Kantarjian HM, Giles FJ, Bhalla KN, et al. Nilotinib in chronic myeloid leukemia patients in chronic phase (CMLCP) with imatinib resistance or intolerance: 2-year follow-up results of a phase 2 study. ASH Annual Meeting Abstracts. *Blood*. 2008;112:3238.
101. le Coutre PD, Giles FJ, Hochhaus A, et al. Nilotinib in chronic myeloid leukemia patients in accelerated phase (CML-AP) with imatinib resistance or intolerance: 2-year follow-up results of a phase 2 study. ASH Annual Meeting Abstracts. *Blood*. 2008;112:3229.
102. Hochhaus A, Guilhot F, Apperley J, et al. Nilotinib in chronic myeloid leukemia patients in accelerated phase (CML-AP) with imatinib resistance or intolerance: 24-month follow-up results of a phase 2 study. *Haematologica*. 2009;94(suppl 2):256. Abstract 0631.
103. Giles FJ, Abruzzese E, Rosti G, et al. Nilotinib is active in chronic and accelerated phase chronic myeloid leukemia following failure of imatinib and dasatinib therapy. *Leukemia*. July 2010;24(7):1299-1301.
104. Oehler VG, Gooley T, Snyder DS, et al. The effects of imatinib mesylate treatment before allogeneic transplantation for chronic myeloid leukemia. *Blood*. February 2007;109(4):1782-1789.
105. Carpenter PA, Snyder DS, Flowers ME, et al. Prophylactic administration of imatinib after hematopoietic cell transplantation for high-risk Philadelphia chromosome-positive leukemia. *Blood*. April 2007;109(7):2791-2793.
106. Olavarria E, Siddique S, Griffiths MJ, et al. Posttransplantation imatinib as a strategy to postpone the requirement for immunotherapy in patients undergoing reduced-intensity allografts for chronic myeloid leukemia. *Blood*. December 2007;110(13):4614-4617.
107. Soverini S, Colarossi S, Gnani A, et al. Contribution of ABL kinase domain mutations to imatinib resistance in different subsets of Philadelphia-positive patients: by the GIMEMA Working Party on chronic myeloid leukemia. *Clin Cancer Res*. December 2006;12(24):7374-7379.
108. Gambacorti-Passerini C, Kantarjian H, Baccarani M, et al. Bosutinib demonstrates clinical activity and is well-tolerated among patients with AP and BP CML and Ph+ ALL. *J Clin Oncol*. 2008;26:abstract 7049.
109. Kantarjian H, Cortes J, Kim D-W, et al. Phase 3 study of dasatinib 140 mg once daily versus 70 mg twice daily in patients with chronic myeloid leukemia in accelerated phase resistant or intolerant to imatinib: 15-month median follow-up. *Blood*. 2009;113:6322-6329.
110. Quintas-Cardama A, Kantarjian H, O'Brien S, et al. Pleural effusion in patients with chronic myelogenous leukemia treated with dasatinib after imatinib failure. *J Clin Oncol*. September 2007;25(25):3908-3914.
111. Quintas-Cardama A, Han X, Kantarjian H, Cortes J. Tyrosine kinase inhibitor-induced platelet dysfunction in patients with chronic myeloid leukemia. *Blood*. July 2009;114(2):261-263.
112. Kantarjian HM, Keating MJ, Talpaz M, et al. Chronic myelogenous leukemia in blast crisis. Analysis of 242 patients. *Am J Med*. September 1987;83(3):445-454.
113. Druker BJ, Sawyers CL, Kantarjian H, et al. Activity of a specific inhibitor of the BCR-ABL tyrosine kinase in the blast crisis of chronic myeloid leukemia and acute lymphoblastic leukemia with the Philadelphia chromosome. *N Engl J Med*. April 2001;344(14):1038-1042.
114. Kantarjian HM, Cortes J, O'Brien S, et al. Imatinib mesylate (STI571) therapy for Philadelphia chromosome-positive chronic myelogenous leukemia in blast phase. *Blood*. May 2002;99(10):3547-3553.
115. Sawyers CL, Hochhaus A, Feldman E, et al. Imatinib induces hematologic and cytogenetic responses in patients with chronic myelogenous leukemia in myeloid blast crisis: results of a phase II study. *Blood*. May 2002;99(10):3530-3539.
116. de Labarthe A, Rousselot P, Huguet-Rigal F, et al. Imatinib combined with induction or consolidation chemotherapy in patients with de novo Philadelphia chromosome-positive acute lymphoblastic leukemia: results of the GRAAPH-2003 study. *Blood*. February 2007;109(4):1408-1413.
117. Yanada M, Naoe T. Imatinib combined chemotherapy for Philadelphia chromosome-positive acute lymphoblastic leukemia: major challenges in current practice. *Leuk Lymphoma*. [Review]. September 2006;47(9):1747-1753.
118. Thomas DA, Faderl S, Cortes J, et al. Treatment of Philadelphia chromosome-positive acute lymphocytic leukemia with hyper-CVAD and imatinib mesylate. *Blood*. June 2004;103(12):4396-4407.
119. Ravandi F, O'Brien S, Thomas D, et al. First report of phase 2 study of dasatinib with hyper-CVAD for the frontline treatment of patients with Philadelphia chromosome-positive (Ph+) acute lymphoblastic leukemia. *Blood*. September 2010;116(12):2070-2077.
120. Gambacorti-Passerini C, Kantarjian H, Bruemmendorf T, et al. Bosutinib (SKI-606) demonstrates clinical activity and is well tolerated among patients with AP and BP CML and Ph+ ALL. ASH Annual Meeting Abstracts. *Blood*. November 2007; 110(11):473.
121. Talpaz M, Shah NP, Kantarjian H, et al. Dasatinib in imatinib-resistant Philadelphia chromosome-positive leukemias. *N Engl J Med*. June 2006;354(24):2531-2541.
122. Cortes J, Rousselot P, Kim DW, et al. Dasatinib induces complete hematologic and cytogenetic responses in patients with imatinib-resistant or -intolerant chronic myeloid leukemia in blast crisis. *Blood*. April 2007;109(8):3207-3213.
123. Quintas-Cardama A, Kantarjian H, Garcia-Manero G, et al. A pilot study of imatinib, low-dose cytarabine and idarubicin for patients with chronic myeloid leukemia in myeloid blast phase. *Leuk Lymphoma*. February 2007;48(2):283-289.
124. Oki Y, Kantarjian HM, Gharibyan V, et al. Phase II study of low-dose decitabine in combination with imatinib mesylate in patients with accelerated or myeloid blastic phase of chronic myelogenous leukemia. *Cancer*. March 2007;109(5):899-906.
125. Hasford J, Baccarani M, Hoffmann V, et al. Predicting complete cytogenetic response and subsequent progression-free survival in 2060 patients with CML on imatinib treatment: the EUTOS score. *Blood*. July 2011;118(3):686-692.
126. Nazha A, Jabbour E, Cortes JE, et al. EUTOS score is not predictive for survival and outcome in patients (pts) with chronic myeloid leukemia in early chronic phase (CML-CP) treated with tyrosine kinase inhibitors (TKIs) at MD Anderson Cancer Center (MDACC). *Blood*. November 2011;118(21):3769.
127. Cortes J, Jabbour E, Kantarjian H, et al. Dynamics of BCR-ABL kinase domain mutations in chronic myeloid leukemia after sequential treatment with multiple tyrosine kinase inhibitors. *Blood*. December 2007;110(12):4005-4011.

128. Cortes J, Talpaz M, Bixby D, et al. A phase 1 trial of oral ponatinib (AP24534) in patients with refractory chronic myelogenous leukemia (CML) and other hematologic malignancies: emerging safety and clinical response findings. ASH Annual Meeting Abstracts. *Blood.* November 2010;116(21):210.
129. Cortes J, Raghunadharao D, Parikh P, et al. Safety and efficacy of subcutaneous-administered omacetaxine mepesuccinate in chronic myeloid leukemia (CML) patients who are resistant or intolerant to two or more tyrosine kinase inhibitors—results of a multicenter phase 2/3 study. ASH Annual Meeting Abstracts. *Blood.* 2009;114(22):abstract 861.
130. Perez-Galan P, Roue G, Villamor N, Campo E, Colomer D. The BH3-mimetic GX15-070 synergizes with bortezomib in mantle cell lymphoma by enhancing Noxa-mediated activation of Bak. *Blood.* May 2007;109(10):4441-4449.
131. Cortes-Franco J, Khoury HJ, Nicolini FE, et al. Safety and efficacy of subcutaneous-administered omacetaxine mepesuccinate in imatinib-resistant chronic myeloid leukemia (CML) patients who harbor the Bcr-Abl T315I mutation—results of an ongoing multicenter phase 2/3 study. *Blood.* November 2009;114(22):644.
132. Cortes JE, Wetzler M, Lipton J, et al. Subcutaneous omacetaxine (OM) treatment of chronic phase (CP) chronic myeloid leukemia (CML) patients following multiple tyrosine kinase inhibitor (TKI) failure. *Blood.* November 2010;116(21):2290.
133. Tinsley SM. Safety profiles of second-line tyrosine kinase inhibitors in patients with chronic myeloid leukaemia. *J Clin Nurs.* May 2010;19(9-10):1207-1218.
134. Carpiuc KT, Stephens JM, Liou SY, Botteman MF. Incidence of grade 3/4 adverse events in imatinib resistant/intolerant chronic phase CML (CP-CML): a comparison of nilotinib and dasatinib. ASCO Annual Meeting Abstracts. *J Clin Oncol.* 2007; 26:abstract 7009.
135. Mathisen MS, Kantarjian H, Cortes J, Jabbour E. Mutant BCR-ABL clones in chronic myeloid leukemia. *Haematologica.* 2011;96(3):347-349.
136. Pye SM, Cortes J, Ault P, et al. The effects of imatinib on pregnancy outcome. *Blood.* [Research Support, Non-U.S. Govt]. June 2008;111(12):5505-5508.
137. O'Donnell MR. Acute leukemias. In: Pazdur R, Coia LR, Hoskins WJ, Wagman LD, eds. *Cancer Management: A Multidisciplinary Approach.* 8th ed. Manhasset, NY: CMP Healthcare Media, the Oncology Group; 2004:747-772.
138. Foon KA, Casciato DA. Acute leukemia. In: Casciato DA, Lowitz BB, eds. *Manual of Clinical Oncology.* 3rd ed. Boston, MA: Little, Brown and Company; 1995:431-445.
139. Abraham J, Monahan BP. The acute leukemias. In: Abraham J, Allegra CJ, eds. *Bethesda Handbook of Clinical Oncology.* 1st ed. Philadelphia, PA: Lippincott, Williams and Wilkins; 2001 Chapter 22:271-285.
140. Pedersen-Bjergaard J, Christiansen DH, Andersen MK, Skovby F. Causality of myelodysplasia and acute myeloid leukemia and their genetic abnormalities. *Leukemia.* November 2002;16(11):2177-2184.
141. Dong F, Brynes RK, Tidow N, Welte K, Lowenberg B, Touw IP. Mutations in the gene for the granulocyte colony-stimulating-factor receptor in patients with acute myeloid leukemia preceded by severe congenital neutropenia. *N Engl J Med.* August 1995;333(8):487-493.
142. West RR, Stafford DA, White AD, Bowen DT, Padua RA. Cytogenetic abnormalities in the myelodysplastic syndromes and occupational or environmental exposure. *Blood.* March 2000;95(6):2093-2097.
143. Ayton PM, Cleary ML. Transformation of myeloid progenitors by MLL oncoproteins is dependent on Hoxa7 and Hoxa9. *Genes Dev.* September 2003;17(18):2298-2307.
144. Crane MM, Strom SS, Halabi S, et al. Correlation between selected environmental exposures and karyotype in acute myelocytic leukemia. *Cancer Epidemiol Biomarkers Prev.* August 1996;5(8):639-644.
145. Bennett JM, Catovsky D, Daniel MT, et al. Proposals for the classification of the acute leukaemias. French-American-British (FAB) co-operative group. *Br J Haematol.* August 1976;33(4):451-458.
146. Harris NL, Jaffe ES, Diebold J, et al. World Health Organization classification of neoplastic diseases of the hematopoietic and lymphoid tissues: report of the Clinical Advisory Committee meeting-Airlie House, Virginia, November 1997. *J Clin Oncol.* December 1999;17(12):3835-3849.
147. Freireich EJ, Gehan EA, Sulman D, Boggs DR, Frei E 3rd. The effect of chemotherapy on acute leukemia in the human. *J Chronic Dis.* December 1961;14:593-608.
148. Cheson BD, Bennett JM, Kopecky KJ, et al. Revised recommendations of the International Working Group for Diagnosis, Standardization of Response Criteria, Treatment Outcomes, and Reporting Standards for Therapeutic Trials in Acute Myeloid Leukemia. *J Clin Oncol.* December 2003;21(24):4642-4649.
149. Preisler HD, Anderson K, Rai K, et al. The frequency of long-term remission in patients with acute myelogenous leukaemia treated with conventional maintenance chemotherapy: a study of 760 patients with a minimal follow-up time of 6 years. *Br J Haematol.* February 1989;71(2):189-194.
150. Sauter C, Alberto P, Berchtold W, et al. Long-term results of two Swiss AML studies. *Haematol Blood Transfus.* 1987;30:38-44.
151. Mayer RJ, Davis RB, Schiffer CA, et al. Intensive postremission chemotherapy in adults with acute myeloid leukemia. Cancer and Leukemia Group B. *N Engl J Med.* October 1994;331(14):896-903.
152. Cassileth PA, Lynch E, Hines JD, et al. Varying intensity of postremission therapy in acute myeloid leukemia. *Blood.* April 1992;79(8):1924-1930.
153. Weick JK, Kopecky KJ, Appelbaum FR, et al. A randomized investigation of high-dose versus standard-dose cytosine arabinoside with daunorubicin in patients with previously untreated acute myeloid leukemia: a Southwest Oncology Group study. *Blood.* October 1996;88(8):2841-2851.
154. Bishop JF, Matthews JP, Young GA, Bradstock K, Lowenthal RM. Intensified induction chemotherapy with high dose cytarabine and etoposide for acute myeloid leukemia: a review and updated results of the Australian Leukemia Study Group. *Leuk Lymphoma.* January 1998;28(3-4):315-327.
155. Borthakur G, Faderl S, Verstovsek S, et al. Clinical and molecular response in core binding factor acute myelogenous leukemia with fludarabine, cytarabine, G-CSF, and gemtuzumab ozogamicin. *Blood.* 2009;114:abstract 2056.
156. US Food and Drug Administration. Gemtuzumab ozogamicin. Available at http://www.fda.gov/AboutFDA/CentersOffices/CDER/ucm216790htm. Accessed July 22, 2010.
157. Melnick A, Licht JD. Deconstructing a disease: RARalpha, its fusion partners, and their roles in the pathogenesis of acute promyelocytic leukemia. *Blood.* May 1999;93(10):3167-3215.
158. Lo Coco F, Diverio D, Falini B, Biondi A, Nervi C, Pelicci PG. Genetic diagnosis and molecular monitoring in the management of acute promyelocytic leukemia. *Blood.* July 1999;94(1):12-22.
159. Estey E, Thall P, Kantarjian H, Pierce S, Kornblau S, Keating M. Association between increased body mass index and a diagnosis of acute promyelocytic leukemia in patients with acute myeloid leukemia. *Leukemia.* October 1997;11(10):1661-1664.
160. Golomb HM, Rowley JD, Vardiman JW, Testa JR, Butler A. "Microgranular" acute promyelocytic leukemia: a distinct clinical, ultrastructural, and cytogenetic entity. *Blood.* February 1980;55(2):253-259.
161. Dyck JA, Warrell RP Jr, Evans RM, Miller WH Jr. Rapid diagnosis of acute promyelocytic leukemia by immunohistochemical localization of PML/RAR-alpha protein. *Blood.* August 1995;86(3):862-867.
162. Fenaux P, Le Deley MC, Castaigne S, et al. Effect of all transretinoic acid in newly diagnosed acute promyelocytic leukemia. Results of a multicenter randomized trial. European APL 91 Group. *Blood.* December 1993;82(11):3241-3249.
163. Ades L, Sanz MA, Chevret S, et al. Treatment of newly diagnosed acute promyelocytic leukemia (APL): a comparison of French-Belgian-Swiss and PETHEMA results. *Blood.* February 2008;111(3):1078-1084.
164. Tallman MS, Andersen JW, Schiffer CA, et al. All-trans retinoic acid in acute promyelocytic leukemia: long-term outcome and prognostic factor analysis from the North American Intergroup protocol. *Blood.* December 2002;100(13):4298-4302.

165. Tallman MS, Kwaan HC. Reassessing the hemostatic disorder associated with acute promyelocytic leukemia. *Blood*. February 1992;79(3):543-553.
166. Shen ZX, Shi ZZ, Fang J, et al. All-trans retinoic acid/As2O3 combination yields a high quality remission and survival in newly diagnosed acute promyelocytic leukemia. *Proc Natl Acad Sci U S A*. April 2004;101(15):5328-5335.
167. Estey EH, Garcia-Manero G, Ferrajoli A, et al. Use of all-transretinoic acid (ATRA) + arsenic trioxide (ATO) to eliminate or minimize use of chemotherapy (CT) in untreated acute promyelocytic leukemia (APL). *Blood*. 2004;104:abstract 393.
168. Ravandi F, Estey E, Jones D, et al. Effective treatment of acute promyelocytic leukemia with all-trans-retinoic acid, arsenic trioxide, and gemtuzumab ozogamicin. *J Clin Oncol*. February 2009;27(4):504-510.
169. Ghavamzadeh A, Alimoghaddam K, Ghaffari S, et al. Results of new cases of APL treatment by arsenic trioxide and long-term follow-up: Is it time for using arsenic trioxide in first-line treatment. *J Clin Oncol*. 2010;28:abstract 6545.
170. Lengfelder E, Lo-Coco F, Montesinos P, et al. Treatment of molecular and clinical relapse of acute promyelocytic leukemia (APL) with arsenic trioxide: results of the European Registry of relapsed APL. *Blood*. 2010;116:abstract 15.
171. Kantarjian HM, Garcia-Manero G, Luger S, et al. A randomized phase 2 study of sapacitabine, an oral nucleoside analogue, in elderly patients with AML previously untreated or in first relapse. *Blood*. 2009;114:abstract 1061.
172. Green SR, Choudhary AK, Fleming IN. Combination of sapacitabine and HDAC inhibitors stimulates cell death in AML and other tumour types. *Br J Cancer*. October 2010;103(9):1391-1399.
173. Gilliland DG, Griffin JD. The roles of FLT3 in hematopoiesis and leukemia. *Blood*. September 2002;100(5):1532-1542.
174. Levis M, Small D. FLT3 tyrosine kinase inhibitors. *Int J Hematol*. August 2005;82(2):100-107.
175. Thiede C, Steudel C, Mohr B, et al. Analysis of FLT3-activating mutations in 979 patients with acute myelogenous leukemia: association with FAB subtypes and identification of subgroups with poor prognosis. *Blood*. [Research Support, Non-U.S. Govt]. June 2002;99(12):4326-4335.
176. Whitman SP, Archer KJ, Feng L, et al. Absence of the wild-type allele predicts poor prognosis in adult de novo acute myeloid leukemia with normal cytogenetics and the internal tandem duplication of FLT3: a Cancer and Leukemia Group B study. *Cancer Res*. October 2001;61(19):7233-7239.
177. Kottaridis PD, Gale RE, Frew ME, et al. The presence of a FLT3 internal tandem duplication in patients with acute myeloid leukemia (AML) adds important prognostic information to cytogenetic risk group and response to the first cycle of chemotherapy: analysis of 854 patients from the United Kingdom Medical Research Council AML 10 and 12 trials. *Blood*. September 2001;98(6):1752-1759.
178. Borthakur G, Kantarjian H, Ravandi F, et al. Phase I study of sorafenib in patients with refractory or relapsed acute leukemias. *Haematologica*. January 2011;96(1):62-68.
179. Pratz KW, Cortes J, Roboz GJ, et al. A pharmacodynamic study of the FLT3 inhibitor KW-2449 yields insight into the basis for clinical response. *Blood*. April 2009;113(17):3938-3946.
180. Pratz KW, Sato T, Murphy KM, Stine A, Rajkhowa T, Levis M. FLT3-mutant allelic burden and clinical status are predictive of response to FLT3 inhibitors in AML. *Blood*. February 2010;115(7):1425-1432.
181. Quintas-Cardama A, Kantarjian H, Andreef M, et al. Phase 1 trial of intermittent administration of sorafenib (BAY 43-9006) for patients (pts) with refractory/relapsed acute myelogenous leukemia (AML). *J Clin Oncol*. 2007;25:abstract 7018.
182. Pratz KW, Cho E, Karp J, et al. Phase I dose escalation trial of sorafenib as a single agent for adults with relapsed and refractory acute leukemias. *J Clin Oncol*. 2009;27:abstract 7065.
183. Ravandi F, Cortes JE, Jones D, et al. Phase I/II study of combination therapy with sorafenib, idarubicin, and cytarabine in younger patients with acute myeloid leukemia. *J Clin Oncol*. April 2010;28(11):1856-1862.
184. Serve H. Sorafenib in combination with standard induction and consolidation therapy in elderly AML patients: results from a randomized, placebo-controlled phase II trial. *Blood*. 2010;116:abstract 333.
185. Cortes J, Foran J, Ghirdaladze D, et al. AC220, a potent, selective, second generation FLT3 receptor tyrosine kinase (RTK) inhibitor, in a first-in-human (FIH) phase 1 AML study. 2009;*Blood*. 2009;114:abstract 636.
186. O'Farrell AM, Foran JM, Fiedler W, et al. An innovative phase I clinical study demonstrates inhibition of FLT3 phosphorylation by SU11248 in acute myeloid leukemia patients. *Clin Cancer Res*. November 2003;9(15):5465-5476.
187. Smith BD, Levis M, Beran M, et al. Single-agent CEP-701, a novel FLT3 inhibitor, shows biologic and clinical activity in patients with relapsed or refractory acute myeloid leukemia. *Blood*. May 2004;103(10):3669-3676.
188. Knapper S, Burnett AK, Littlewood T, et al. A phase 2 trial of the FLT3 inhibitor lestaurtinib (CEP701) as first-line treatment for older patients with acute myeloid leukemia not considered fit for intensive chemotherapy. *Blood*. November 2006;108(10):3262-3270.
189. Levis M, Ravandi F, Wang ES, et al. Results from a randomized trial of salvage chemotherapy followed by lestaurtinib for FLT3 mutant AML patients in first relapse. *Blood*. 2009;114: abstract 788.
190. Stone RM, DeAngelo DJ, Klimek V, et al. Patients with acute myeloid leukemia and an activating mutation in FLT3 respond to a small-molecule FLT3 tyrosine kinase inhibitor, PKC412. *Blood*. January 2005;105(1):54-60.
191. Stone RM, Fischer T, Paquette R, et al. A phase 1b study of midostaurin (PK412) in combination with daunorubicin and cytarabine induction and high-dose cytarabine consolidation in patients under age 61 with newly diagnosed de novo acute myeloid leukemia: overall survival of patients whose blasts have FLT3 mutation is similar to those with wild-type FLT3. *Blood*. 2009;114:abstract 634.
192. Mehnert JM, Kelly WK. Histone deacetylase inhibitors: biology and mechanism of action. *Cancer J*. January-February 2007;13(1):23-29.
193. Minucci S, Pelicci PG. Histone deacetylase inhibitors and the promise of epigenetic (and more) treatments for cancer. *Nat Rev Cancer*. January 2006;6(1):38-51.
194. Kuendgen A, Strupp C, Aivado M, et al. Treatment of myelodysplastic syndromes with valproic acid alone or in combination with all-trans retinoic acid. *Blood*. September 2004;104(5):1266-1269.
195. Garcia-Manero G, Kantarjian HM, Sanchez-Gonzalez B, et al. Phase 1/2 study of the combination of 5-aza-2′-deoxycytidine with valproic acid in patients with leukemia. *Blood*. November 2006;108(10):3271-3279.
196. Soriano AO, Yang H, Faderl S, et al. Safety and clinical activity of the combination of 5-azacytidine, valproic acid, and all-trans retinoic acid in acute myeloid leukemia and myelodysplastic syndrome. *Blood*. October 2007;110(7):2302-2308.
197. Silverman LR, Verma A, Odchimar-Reissig R, et al. A phase I trial of the epigenetic modulators vorinostat, in combination with azacitidine (azaC) in patients with the myelodysplastic syndrome (MDS) and acute myeloid leukemia (AML): a study of the New York Cancer Consortium. *Blood*. 2008;112:abstract 3656.
198. Kirschbaum M, Gojo I, Goldeberg SL, et al. Vorinostat in combination with decitabine for the treatment of relapsed or newly diagnosed acute myelogenous leukemia (AML) or myelodysplastic syndrome (MDS): a phase I dose-escalation study. *Blood*. 2009;114:abstract 2089.
199. Ravandi F, Faderl S, Thomas D, et al. Phase I study of suberoylanilide hydroxamic acid (SAHA) and decitabine in patients with relapsed, refractory or poor prognosis leukemia. *Blood*. 2007;110:abstract 897.
200. Garcia-Manero G, Tambaro FP, Bekele BN, et al. Phase II study of vorinostat in combination with idarubicin (Ida) and cytarabine (ara-C) as front line therapy in acute myelogenous leukemia (AML) or higher risk myelodysplastic syndrome (MDS). *Blood*. 2009;114:abstract 1055.
201. Karp JE, Lancet JE, Kaufmann SH, et al. Clinical and biologic activity of the farnesyltransferase inhibitor R115777 in adults with refractory and relapsed acute leukemias: a phase 1 clinical-laboratory correlative trial. *Blood*. June 2001;97(11):3361-3369.

202. Lancet JE, Gojo I, Gotlib J, et al. A phase 2 study of the farnesyltransferase inhibitor tipifarnib in poor-risk and elderly patients with previously untreated acute myelogenous leukemia. *Blood.* February 2007;109(4):1387-1394.
203. Harousseau JL, Martinelli G, Jedrzejczak WW, et al. A randomized phase 3 study of tipifarnib compared with best supportive care, including hydroxyurea, in the treatment of newly diagnosed acute myeloid leukemia in patients 70 years or older. *Blood.* August 2009;114(6):1166-1173.
204. Fenaux P, Mufti GJ, Hellstrom-Lindberg E, et al. Azacitidine prolongs overall survival compared with conventional care regimens in elderly patients with low bone marrow blast count acute myeloid leukemia. *J Clin Oncol.* February 2010;28(4):562-569.
205. Cashen AF, Schiller GJ, O'Donnell MR, DiPersio JF. Multicenter, phase II study of decitabine for the first-line treatment of older patients with acute myeloid leukemia. *J Clin Oncol.* February 2010;28(4):556-561.
206. Blum W, Garzon R, Klisovic RB, et al. Clinical response and miR-29b predictive significance in older AML patients treated with a 10-day schedule of decitabine. *Proc Natl Acad Sci U S A.* April 2010;107(16):7473-7478.
207. Mahieux R, Gessain A. HTLV-1 and associated adult T-cell leukemia/lymphoma. *Rev Clin Exp Hematol.* December 2003;7(4):336-361.
208. Lombardi L, Newcomb EW, Dalla-Favera R. Pathogenesis of Burkitt lymphoma: expression of an activated c-myc oncogene causes the tumorigenic conversion of EBV-infected human B lymphoblasts. *Cell.* April 1987;49(2):161-170.
209. Vianna NJ, Polan AK. Childhood lymphatic leukemia: prenatal seasonality and possible association with congenital varicella. *Am J Epidemiol.* March 1976;103(3):321-332.
210. Cortes J. Central nervous system involvement in adult acute lymphocytic leukemia. *Hematol Oncol Clin North Am.* February 2001;15(1):145-162.
211. Foa R, Vitale A. Towards an integrated classification of adult acute lymphoblastic leukemia. *Rev Clin Exp Hematol.* June 2002;6(2):181-199; discussion 200-202.
212. Bene MC, Castoldi G, Knapp W, et al. Proposals for the immunological classification of acute leukemias. European Group for the Immunological Characterization of Leukemias (EGIL). *Leukemia.* October 1995;9(10):1783-1786.
213. Huh YO, Ibrahim S. Immunophenotypes in adult acute lymphocytic leukemia. Role of flow cytometry in diagnosis and monitoring of disease. *Hematol Oncol Clin North Am.* December 2000;14(6):1251-1265.
214. Paredes-Aguilera R, Romero-Guzman L, Lopez-Santiago N, Burbano-Ceron L, Camacho-Del Monte O, Nieto-Martinez S. Flow cytometric analysis of cell-surface and intracellular antigens in the diagnosis of acute leukemia. *Am J Hematol.* October 2001;68(2):69-74.
215. Terstappen LW, Huang S, Picker LJ. Flow cytometric assessment of human T-cell differentiation in thymus and bone marrow. *Blood.* February 1992;79(3):666-677.
216. Kantarjian HM, O'Brien S, Smith T, et al. Acute lymphocytic leukaemia in the elderly: characteristics and outcome with the vincristine-adriamycin-dexamethasone (VAD) regimen. *Br J Haematol.* September 1994;88(1):94-100.
217. Jones B, Freeman AI, Shuster JJ, et al. Lower incidence of meningeal leukemia when prednisone is replaced by dexamethasone in the treatment of acute lymphocytic leukemia. *Med Pediatr Oncol.* 1991;19(4):269-275.
218. Hurwitz CA, Silverman LB, Schorin MA, et al. Substituting dexamethasone for prednisone complicates remission induction in children with acute lymphoblastic leukemia. *Cancer.* April 2000;88(8):1964-1969.
219. Folber F, Salek C, Doubek M, et al. [Treatment of adult acute lymphoblastic leukemia according to GMALL 07/2003 study protocol in the Czech Republic - the first experience]. *Vnitr Lek.* March 2010;56(3):176-182.
220. Ottmann OG, Hoelzer D, Gracien E, et al. Concomitant granulocyte colony-stimulating factor and induction chemoradiotherapy in adult acute lymphoblastic leukemia: a randomized phase III trial. *Blood.* July 1995;86(2):444-450.
221. DeAngelo DJ, Yu D, Johnson JL, et al. Nelarabine induces complete remissions in adults with relapsed or refractory T-lineage acute lymphoblastic leukemia or lymphoblastic lymphoma: Cancer and Leukemia Group B study 19801. *Blood.* June 2007;109(12):5136-5142.
222. Thomas DA, O'Brien S, Jorgensen JL, et al. Prognostic significance of CD20 expression in adults with de novo precursor B-lineage acute lymphoblastic leukemia. *Blood.* June 2009;113(25):6330-6337.
223. Thomas DA, O'Brien S, Faderl S, et al. Chemoimmunotherapy with a modified hyper-CVAD and rituximab regimen improves outcome in de novo Philadelphia chromosome-negative precursor B-lineage acute lymphoblastic leukemia. *J Clin Oncol.* August 2010;28(24):3880-3889.
224. Thomas DA, Faderl S, O'Brien S, et al. Chemoimmunotherapy with hyper-CVAD plus rituximab for the treatment of adult Burkitt and Burkitt-type lymphoma or acute lymphoblastic leukemia. *Cancer.* April 2006;106(7):1569-1580.
225. Thomas DA, O'Brien S, Kantarjian HM. Monoclonal antibody therapy with rituximab for acute lymphoblastic leukemia. *Hematol Oncol Clin North Am.* October 2009;23(5):949-971, v.
226. Dworzak MN, Schumich A, Printz D, et al. CD20 up-regulation in pediatric B-cell precursor acute lymphoblastic leukemia during induction treatment: setting the stage for anti-CD20 directed immunotherapy. *Blood.* November 2008;112(10):3982-3988.
227. Hoelzer D, Huettmann A, Kaul F, et al. Immunochemotherapy with rituximab improves molecular CR rate and outcome in CD20+ B-lineage standard and high risk patients; results of 263 CD20+ patients studied prospectively in GMALL study 07/3003. *Blood.* 2010;116:abstract 170.
228. Topp MS, Zugmaier G, Goekbuget N, et al. CD19/CD3 bispecific antibody blinatumomab (MT-103) is highly effective in treatment of patients with minimal residual disease from chemotherapy-resistant B-precursor acute lymphoblastic leukemia. *Blood.* 2010;116:abstract 174.
229. Ravandi F, Aribi A, O'Brien S, et al. Phase II study of alemtuzumab in combination with pentostatin in patients with T-cell neoplasms. *J Clin Oncol.* November 2009;27(32):5425-5430.
230. Cohen A, Lee JW, Gelfand EW. Selective toxicity of deoxyguanosine and arabinosyl guanine for T-leukemic cells. *Blood.* April 1983;61(4):660-666.
231. Kurzrock R, Gutterman JU, Talpaz M. The molecular genetics of Philadelphia chromosome-positive leukemias. *N Engl J Med.* October 1988;319(15):990-998.
232. Carpiuc KT, Stephens JM, Botteman MF, Feng W, Hay JW. A review of the clinical and economic outcomes of imatinib in Philadelphia chromosome-positive acute lymphoblastic leukemia. *Expert Opin Pharmacother.* November 2007;8(16):2775-2787.
233. Thomas DA, Faderl S, Cortes J, O'Brien S, Kantarjian HM. Update of the hyper-CVAD and imatinib mesylate regimen in Philadelphia (Ph) positive acute lymphocytic leukemia (ALL). ASH Annual Meeting Abstracts. *Blood.* 2004;104:abstract 2738.
234. Glivec. Glivec® receives additional EU approvals for use in treating a rapidly progressive form of leukemia and a hard-to-treat solid cancer tumor Novartis. Press Release. September 19, 2006.
235. Gleevec. Gleevec® approved in the US for five rare life-threatening disorders with limited treatment options. Press Release. October 19, 2006.
236. Ottmann OG, Druker BJ, Sawyers CL, et al. A phase 2 study of imatinib in patients with relapsed or refractory Philadelphia chromosome-positive acute lymphoid leukemias. *Blood.* September 2002;100(6):1965-1971.
237. Ottmann OG, Wassmann B, Pfeifer H, et al. Imatinib compared with chemotherapy as front-line treatment of elderly patients with Philadelphia chromosome-positive acute lymphoblastic leukemia (Ph+ ALL). *Cancer.* May 2007;109(10):2068-2076.
238. Towatari M, Yanada M, Usui N, et al. Combination of intensive chemotherapy and imatinib can rapidly induce high-quality complete remission for a majority of patients with newly diagnosed BCR-ABL-positive acute lymphoblastic leukemia. *Blood.* December 2004;104(12):3507-3512.
239. Delannoy A, Delabesse E, Lheritier V, et al. Imatinib and methylprednisolone alternated with chemotherapy improve the outcome of elderly patients with Philadelphia-positive acute lymphoblastic leukemia: results of the GRAALL AFR09 study. *Leukemia.* September 2006;20(9):1526-1532.

240. Ottmann O, Dombret H, Martinelli G, et al. Dasatinib induces rapid hematologic and cytogenetic responses in adult patients with Philadelphia chromosome positive acute lymphoblastic leukemia with resistance or intolerance to imatinib: interim results of a phase 2 study. *Blood*. October 2007;110(7):2309-2315.
241. Lilly MB, Ottmann OG, Shah NP, et al. Dasatinib 140 mg once daily versus 70 mg twice daily in patients with Ph-positive acute lymphoblastic leukemia who failed imatinib: Results from a phase 3 study. *Am J Hematol*. March 2010;85(3): 164-170.
242. Fielding AK, Buck G, Lazarus HM, et al. Imatinib significantly enhances long-term outcomes in Philadelphia positive acute lymphoblastic leukaemia; final results of the UKALLXII/ ECOG2993 trial. *Blood*. 2010;116:abstract 169.

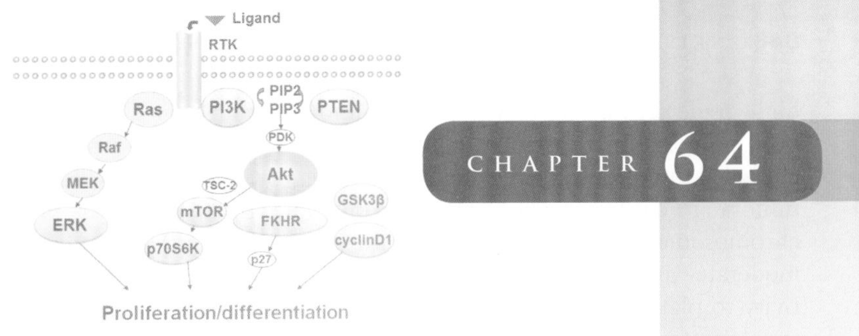

CHAPTER 64

Personalized Medicine and Targeted Therapy of Gynecologic Cancers

Lainie P. Martin and Russell J. Schilder

New molecular tools are more powerful than ever, allowing rapid evaluation of the entire genome of a cell. As we learn more about the genetic makeup of malignant cells and their normal cell counterparts, we will be able to identify mutations that drive pathogenesis of these cancers, and in the era of targeted therapy, the goal will be to customize the treatment of patients with malignant disease. In fact, certain key pathways and mutations in some diseases have already been identified and early approaches to targeting treatment against these pathways and mutations have shown initial signs of benefit. Knowledge of the crucial mutations for a particular patient's cancer is still elusive, and at the molecular level, cancer arising from a gynecologic organ in one patient may be markedly different from that of another patient whose cancer originated and developed at the same site, depending upon the driving mutation(s). At present, most patients with gynecologic cancers receive standard chemotherapy-based regimens that are organ-specific rather than patient-specific. A better understanding of the pathogenesis of disease will help identify subgroups of patients with similar genetic mutations and cellular pathways that drive disease progression, allowing more focused and personalized treatments for these patients.

BIOLOGY AND PATHOGENESIS OF DISEASE

Epithelial Ovarian Cancer

Epithelial ovarian, fallopian tube, and primary peritoneal cancers (hereafter referred to as ovarian cancer due to the very similar biology of these three entities) remain incurable for many women, with the highest case fatality rate of any gynecologic cancer in developed countries. While advances in chemotherapeutic treatment of ovarian cancer have led to prolonged survival in the setting of recurrent disease, most women still ultimately die of their disease.[1] Maximal benefits from novel cytotoxic chemotherapeutic regimens have reached a plateau,[2] and it is expected that the most significant improvements in survival in the future will likely come from integration of novel targeted agents into treatment. Ovarian cancer is not a single disease, and molecular pathways differ for different histologic subtypes. Understanding of membrane receptor expression and function, genetic mutation, epigenetic modification of genes, and the effects of these changes on regulation of certain pathways in tumor cells has improved significantly. Based on this knowledge, efforts have been made to develop therapies that target cellular membrane receptors and their ligands, signaling pathways, and intracellular processes that appear to confer a survival advantage to the cancer cells. Numerous targeted therapies are now available and are being studied in the treatment of ovarian cancer. Given the number of available agents, innovative strategies will be required to evaluate the best ways to use these new drugs, in terms of both disease control and toxicity for patients. It is becoming clear that better ways to characterize ovarian cancer will be needed to optimize the benefit of targeted therapeutics.

Various proposed schemes have been developed to group subtypes within ovarian cancer based on both their observed clinical characteristics and their pathogenesis. Most recently, the disease has been grouped into two types.[3,4] Type I tumors include low-grade serous and endometrioid tumors as well as mucinous carcinomas and clear cell carcinomas (CCCs). Type II tumors include high-grade serous and endometrioid tumors, and it has been proposed that carcinosarcoma and undifferentiated epithelial tumors also be included in this category. Type I tumors are characterized by superior outcome, relative chromosomal stability and fewer genetic alterations than moderate- and high-grade tumors, and relative insensitivity to platinum-based chemotherapy. Type II tumors are characterized by poorer outcome, genomic instability, and, initially, greater sensitivity to chemotherapy. Based on the understanding that distinct histologic subtypes are likely to respond differently to the novel agents that are available to test in ovarian cancer, the Gynecologic Oncology Group (GOG) has developed separate queues and trials for some of these different histological subtypes.

Type II Tumors

The most common subtype of ovarian cancer, high-grade serous carcinoma, has the highest degree of chromosomal instability. Mutations of *p53* have been identified in the majority of high-grade serous carcinomas.[5] Recently, the Cancer Genome Atlas Research Network published data regarding its analysis of 489 cases of high-grade serous carcinoma.[6] Of particular importance was the extremely high prevalence (96%) of *p53* mutation and the finding that the BRCA pathway was dysregulated in approximately half of the specimens evaluated. This analysis also identified 9 mutated genes, 30 somatic copy number mutations, and 4 robust expression phenotypes. While these results demonstrate the significant heterogeneity of this disease, the Atlas may provide a starting point for molecular subtyping high-grade serous carcinoma and evaluating differential responses to some of these new targeted agents.

A recent theory has suggested that the distal fallopian tube may be the site of origin of high-grade serous carcinoma.[7,8] It was noted that women undergoing prophylactic salpingo-oophorectomy often harbored serous tubal intraepithelial carcinomas (STICs) and occult invasive high-grade carcinoma.[9] A later study demonstrated the presence of STICs in more than half of the fallopian tubes of women diagnosed with high-grade serous carcinoma of the peritoneum.[10] Subsequent studies revealed the presence of the same *p53* gene mutations in STICs and high-grade serous carcinomas.[11] This theory is intriguing, as the earliest stages of ovarian cancer pathogenesis have not yet been elucidated and further work looking at the fallopian tubes and ovaries may continue to clarify the early stages of ovarian cancer development.

Type I Tumors

CCCs are the second most common histologic subtype in the United States and are comparatively more prevalent in Asia.[12] While they are grouped with type I tumors because of their relative genetic stability and tendency to present at an earlier stage than type II tumors, they are distinct from other type I ovarian cancers in terms of their developmental pathway.[4] They are often associated with endometriosis, and recent data demonstrate the presence of mutations in *ARID1A*, a tumor suppressor gene, in some patients with ovarian CCC and endometrioid carcinomas arising in association with endometriosis.[13] Interestingly, mutations in *ARID1A* have also been found in areas of endometriosis adjacent to these tumors, suggesting that it is an early oncogenic event. There are also data to suggest alterations in PI3K (phosphoinositide 3-kinase), PTEN (phosphatase and tensin homolog deleted on chromosome 10), and KRAS signaling in some ovarian CCCs.[14] To date, there are no specific targeted agents that have been developed against the mutant *ARID1A*, but of interest, 30% of renal cell carcinomas (RCCs) have been found to have mutations within this gene.[15] Clearly, there are differences between CCC of renal and ovarian origin, but available evidence would suggest more genetic similarity of ovarian CCC to RCC than to ovarian serous cancer,[16] thus supporting the clinical finding that these tumors in general are less sensitive to platinum-based therapy than the more common high-grade serous cancers. These findings suggest that tumor biology–specific trials may be more appropriate when targeted agents are being considered for evaluation. In the last decade, the treatment of RCC has advanced, with the approval of six new therapeutics for treatment of patients with RCC: sorafenib (December 2005), sunitinib (January 2006), temsirolimus (May 2007), everolimus (March 2009), bevacizumab (July 2009), and, most recently, pazopanib (October 2009). Anecdotal reports indicate some activity of sunitinib in ovarian CCC. Trials of tyrosine kinase inhibitors, angiogenesis inhibitors, and mammalian target of rapamycin (mTOR) inhibitors that have demonstrated efficacy in RCC may be the logical first step in the evaluation of targeted therapeutics in ovarian CCC. In support of this premise, recent in vivo work indicates high sensitivity of clear cell ovarian cancer cell lines to sunitinib in comparison to high-grade serous ovarian cancer cell lines.[17]

Ovarian endometrioid cancers have also been linked to endometriosis and high levels of the *ARID1A* mutation have been found, although additional pathways have been noted to be dysregulated, including PTEN, PI3K, and AKT.[18-20]

Low-grade serous carcinomas are molecularly similar to borderline serous tumors and characterized by alterations in *KRAS*, *BRAF*, or *ERBB2*.[21] Ho and colleagues[22] have identified a developmental pathway in which a mutation in *KRAS* or *BRAF* precedes the development of a low-grade serous borderline tumor which can then proceed to an invasive carcinoma. Activation of RAS triggers phosphorylation of the RAF kinase, leading to phosphorylation and activation of MEK1 and MEK2. Activated MEK leads to phosphorylation of ERK1 and ERK2, which results in cellular proliferation. It is known that the RAS/RAF/MEK/ERK signaling pathway can be activated by many extracellular signaling molecules targeting

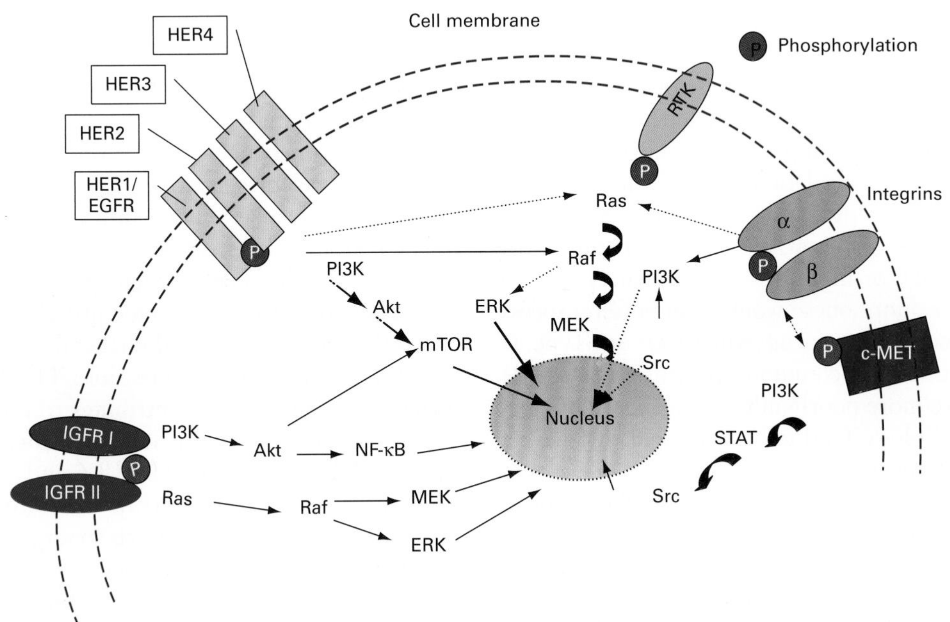

FIGURE 64–1 Pathways of activation through the HER family of receptors, c-Met, Ras/RAF signaling, and the IGF.

various receptors, including the platelet-derived growth factor receptor (PDGFR), the epidermal growth factor receptor (EGFR), and the insulin-like growth factor-1 receptor (IGF-1R). Recent preclinical observations also suggest that the insulin-like growth factor (IGF)-1 pathway may be highly expressed in low-grade serous carcinoma, lending further support to the pivotal role of the RAS/RAF pathway in this histologic subtype.[23]

The RAS/RAF pathway (Fig. 64.1) has been found to be disrupted in multiple types of solid tumors, and there are now several agents under development that may target signaling pathways and proteins along these pathways that may ultimately be found to be critical in maintenance and progression of malignant low-grade serous carcinoma.[21] Studies are aimed toward further elucidation of the key steps in carcinogenesis and maintenance of the malignant phenotype in low-grade serous carcinoma. Agents that inhibit MEK, a downstream target of RAS/RAF, may either enhance efficacy of targeting RAF or obviate the need for specific targeted therapy against the RAF mutation. Efficacy of this approach remains unknown, and clinical trials are needed to evaluate the large number of agents that inhibit upstream and downstream components of this pathway, as well as the various combinations that may be needed to achieve prolonged disease control.

Mucinous carcinomas are the rarest type of advanced ovarian cancer and are often found to have *KRAS* mutations (50%).[24] In light of the rarity of these cancers, they have been harder to study, and no specific therapeutic trials have been completed for women with this subtype, but in light of the high prevalence of *KRAS* mutations, agents targeted to this pathway could be considered.

Research in genomic alterations in the less common subtypes confirms that these subtypes have different genomic patterns and may help provide us with biomarkers of response to some of the new agents becoming available to study in the treatment of ovarian cancer. As the total number of patients with each of these less common subtypes is relatively small in comparison to the total number of patients with ovarian cancers, studies for these subtypes will require collaborations on a national or possibly an international level in order to complete the clinical trials necessary to confirm or refute the efficacy of new regimens. Beyond this limitation, better preclinical models and predictive markers may aid in selecting the best treatments to take to human trials and decrease the number of negative trials performed, thus avoiding unnecessary delays in the discovery and implementation of new, more effective treatments for this disease. A better understanding of the important pathways and networks that drive oncogenesis and malignant progression in the various subtypes of this disease is a first step in developing these tools.

Endometrial Cancer

Endometrial cancer is the most common gynecologic cancer in developed countries; however, most patients (approximately 70%) present with stage I disease and are typically treated surgically.[1] The treatment of more advanced or recurrent endometrial cancer has evolved quite rapidly over the last decade, with the advent of taxane therapy and chemotherapy playing a more important role in the adjuvant setting.[25,26] However, treatment with chemotherapy is limited by the rapid development of resistance, thus stimulating interest in evaluation of newer targeted agents for treatment of this disease. Endometrial cancer has been classified into type I and type II based on whether it developed through an estrogen-dependent mechanism or through an estrogen-independent mechanism.[27,28] Type I tumors comprise the majority of cases, usually present with stage I or II disease, are typically of endometrioid histology and low grade, and have a favorable prognosis. They arise in an environment of unopposed estrogen or high estrogen exposure, tend to occur in younger, more obese women, and often express the estrogen receptor or progestin receptor. Type II endometrial cancers more commonly present with stage III or IV disease, are more poorly differentiated, are of non-endometrioid histology, tend to be aneuploid, and have a less favorable prognosis.

KRAS overexpression is common in both type I and II endometrial cancers, although mutations of *KRAS* have been found primarily in type I cancers.[29] Type I cancers are also more likely to have *PTEN* mutations[30,31] (up to 80%) and microsatellite instability (MSI),[32] while type II tumors are more likely to have mutated *p53*[29,33] or HER2[34] overexpression. Recently, agents targeting the PI3K pathway have become available (see Table 64.3) and are in the early stages of clinical testing. PTEN is a negative regulator of this pathway, and mutations in *PTEN* often lead to activation of the PI3K pathway (see Fig. 64.1), making it an attractive target in endometrial cancer. Further, it has been demonstrated that *PTEN* and *PI3K* mutations can occur simultaneously in endometrial cancer.[35] Of note, loss of PTEN impacts the homologous recombination pathway of DNA repair, limiting the ability of cells to repair double-strand breaks.[36] This has led to interest in the role of synthetic lethality in treating endometrial cancer through the use of poly(ADP-ribose) polymerase (PARP) inhibitors. Preclinical data demonstrate sensitivity of endometrial cells with PTEN deficiency to PARP inhibition.[37]

Recent analysis of *ARID1A* expression and mutation demonstrated somatic mutation in 40% of low-grade endometrial cancers, and loss of expression in 26% in a limited number of samples analyzed, suggesting a possible common developmental pathway with low-grade ovarian endometrioid carcinoma and CCC.[38] While there is no specific targeted therapy linked to this mutation at present, trials that identify effective treatments for cancers with *ARID1A* mutations or overexpression may be of interest in these low-grade endometrial cancers.

Additionally, some endometrial cancers are related to Lynch syndrome and have been found to have MSI, although the therapeutic implications of these alterations are unclear at this time.

Cervical Cancer

Advanced cervical cancer remains a global problem, in spite of available screening technology, which has limited the incidence of this disease in developed countries. The current standard treatments are comprised of chemotherapeutic agents, which have limited efficacy due to early development of chemoresistance. It is well established that the majority of cervical cancers are caused by human papilloma virus (HPV). Beyond the key role of HPV in the oncogenesis of cervical cancer and the development of vaccines against HPV, a limited understanding of the molecular abnormalities of cervical cancer cells that could result in effective targeted approaches has hampered the development of such agents.

The E6 and E7 oncogenic proteins of HPV lead to alterations in cervical epithelial cells that result in cancer development and progression. The E6 oncoprotein inactivates p53 and E7 contributes to the destruction of retinoblastoma protein, resulting in increased oncogenesis.[39,40] Additionally, the HPV E6 and E7 oncoproteins may interact with the EGFR,[41] resulting in increased overexpression, although efforts to target the EGFR have not resulted in effective therapeutic results in this disease.

More recently, efforts to inhibit angiogenesis have had better results. HPV16 has been demonstrated to enhance levels of hypoxia-inducible factor-1 alpha (HIF-1α) protein and vascular endothelial growth factor (VEGF) expression in cervical cancer cells.[42] It has been suggested that the combination of p53 inactivation and increased HIF-1α results in decrease in hypoxia-mediated apoptosis.[43] Further understanding of the role of angiogenesis in cervical cancer may enhance clinical efforts to target this pathway.

TARGETED THERAPY: CURRENT SUCCESSES AND FUTURE DIRECTIONS

Of the targeted therapies evaluated to date, the greatest advances have been in the areas of angiogenesis and PARP inhibition.

Angiogenesis Inhibition

Angiogenesis is a normal physiologic process involving vascular remodeling and new vessel formation. In sequence, angiogenesis occurs through degradation of the basement membrane surrounding capillaries, invasion of the surrounding stroma by endothelial cells in the direction of an angiogenic stimulus, and proliferation of endothelial cells which organize into a network of new blood vessels.[44] "Angiogenesis plays a vital role in tumor formation and metastasis by providing tumors with nutrients and oxygen as well as access to the lymphatic and circulatory systems"? Targeting and inhibiting the process of angiogenesis has led to improvements in the treatment of many solid tumors, including gynecologic cancers. Normal and abnormal angiogenesis is regulated by a balance of proangiogenic and antiangiogenic factors which becomes dysregulated in malignant disease. Many cancers are characterized by increased levels of VEGF,[45] fibroblast growth factor (FGF), angiopoietin (ANG),[46] platelet-derived endothelial cell growth factor (PDGF), as well as other pro-angiogenic cytokines such as tumor necrosis factor-α, interleukin (IL)-6, and IL-8, resulting in sustained angiogenesis.

The VEGF family of proteins and their receptors have been well characterized.[47] There are six known VEGF proteins, VEGF-A, VEGF-B, VEGF-C, VEGF-D, VEGF-E, and placenta-derived growth factor (PlGF)1 and PlGF2,[47] that interact with three known VEGF receptors VEGFR-1 (Flt-1), VEGFR-2 (KDR/Flk-1), and VEGFR-3 (Flt-4). Ligand binding leads to dimerization and activation of signaling cascades, which stimulate angiogenesis within normal and tumor cells. VEGF-A is the most well-characterized member of this family of proteins; it is also known as vascular permeability factor, as it has been found to cause extravasation of fluids and plasma proteins from blood vessels. It is essential for vasculogenesis in the developing embryo and for survival of endothelial cells in newly formed blood vessels.

High levels of VEGF-A expression appear to confer a poor prognosis in patients with ovarian cancer.[48] VEGF has been identified as playing a key role in normal ovarian physiology and mediates ascites formation for some women with ovarian cancer.[49-52] Elevated levels of VEGF have been found in malignant ascites and bevacizumab, a humanized monoclonal antibody that targets angiogenesis by binding to VEGF-A and blocking interaction with its receptor, improves the control of ascites.[51-53] While multiple agents targeting angiogenesis have been explored in ovarian cancer, the most successful has been the monoclonal antibody, bevacizumab (Table 64.1).

Bevacizumab has been evaluated in the setting of both recurrent disease and more recently in combination with front-line chemotherapy. Burger and co-investigators evaluated bevacizumab in a phase II trial (GOG 170D) as a single agent in the second- or third-line setting. The results were notable for an objective response rate (RR) of 21% and a median progression-free survival (PFS) of 4.7 months.[54] Forty percent of patients were progression free at 6 months, as opposed to 16% of historical controls who had received various cytotoxic or other targeted agents. In a phase II trial of bevacizumab combined with low-dose daily oral cyclophosphamide, the RR was 24% with a 6-month PFS of 56%.[55] There are also published data on the use of bevacizumab in combination with taxanes in recurrent ovarian cancer.[56] Recently, data presented from the phase III Ovarian Cancer Education Awareness Network Study (OCEANS) evaluated the combination of carboplatin, gemcitabine, and bevacizumab for six cycles followed by bevacizumab until disease progression versus the chemotherapy alone in 484 women with recurrent disease and demonstrated a PFS of 12.4 versus 8.4 months ($P < 0.0001$).[57]

In light of the activity noted in the setting of recurrent disease, bevacizumab has also been evaluated in combination with carboplatin and paclitaxel in a phase III trial (GOG 218) in front-line treatment in 1,873 women with previously untreated advanced epithelial ovarian, primary peritoneal, or fallopian tube carcinoma.[58] This trial demonstrated that women who received bevacizumab (15 mg/kg every 21 d) in combination with paclitaxel and carboplatin, followed by continued bevacizumab maintenance for a total duration of 15 months, had a median PFS of 14.1 versus 10.3 months in women who received chemotherapy alone (hazard ratio = 0.72, $P < 0.0001$). In a second international phase III study of the International Collaborative Neoplasm Group, ICON 7,[59] of 1,528 women with previously untreated disease, bevacizumab (7.5 mg/kg every 21 d) given in combination with paclitaxel and carboplatin, followed by bevacizumab alone for a total duration of up to 12 months, had a median PFS of 18.3 months compared with 16 months in women who received chemotherapy alone (hazard ratio = 0.79, $P = 0.001$).

Of concern is the risk of bowel perforation, which occurs in 3% to 4% of all patients treated with bevacizumab and in 0% to 11% of patients with ovarian carcinoma.[54,55,60,61] There were no perforations seen in the Burger trial (GOG170D),[54] but a trial of bevacizumab treatment in more heavily pretreated patients[61] was closed early due to a high rate (11%) of perforations. Notably, perforations do not always occur at sites of disease involvement, and it can be difficult to predict who may be at increased risk for perforation, so caution should be

TABLE 64–1 Antiangiogenic Agents Currently in Development in Gynecologic Cancers

Agent	Mechanism	Target	Trials
Bevacizumab	Monoclonal antibody	VEGF-A	Phase III
Aflibercept (VEGF-Trap)	Fusion protein	VEGF-A, VEGF-B, PlGF1, PlGF2	Phase II
Cediranib (AZD 2171)	Tyrosine kinase inhibitor	VEGFR-1-3, PDGFR, c-KIT	Phase III
Vandetanib (ZD 6474)	Tyrosine kinase inhibitor	VEGFR, EGFR	Phase II
Sunitinib (SUO11248)	Tyrosine kinase inhibitor	VEGFR, EGFR, PDGFR, c-KIT	Phase II
Pazopanib	Tyrosine kinase inhibitor	VEGFR1-3, PDGFR-α/β, c-KIT	Phase II
AMG-386	Peptibody	Inhibits Ang1 and Ang2 from binding to Tie2 receptors	Phase III
Vargatef (BIBF 1120)	Triple angiokinase inhibitor	VEGFR, PDGFR, FGFR	Phase III
Brivanib	Tyrosine kinase inhibitor	VEGFR-2, FGFR	Phase II

VEGF, vascular endothelial growth factor; VEGFR, VEGF receptor; PDGFR, platelet-derived growth factor receptor; PlGFR, placenta-derived growth factor receptor; EGFR, epidermal growth factor receptor; FGFR, fibroblast growth factor receptor.

used in determining which patients with recurrent disease should be offered treatment with bevacizumab. In GOG 218, the perforation rate was just under 3%.[58]

Angiogenesis is also important in endometrial cancer,[62,63] and efforts to target angiogenesis are ongoing in this disease. Analysis of bevacizumab (see Table 64.1) in a phase II trial in 52 evaluable patients with endometrial cancer showed that 7 patients (13.5%) responded and 21 (40%) experienced PFS of at least 6 months.[64] No perforations were noted in this trial. Further studies evaluating bevacizumab in patients with endometrial cancer in combination with chemotherapy are ongoing.

In a phase II trial of bevacizumab (see Table 64.1) in 46 patients with advanced cervical cancer, 5 (11%) patients experienced a partial response (PR) and 11 patients (24%) survived without progression for at least 6 months.[65] There were no bowel perforations noted, although one patient developed a fistula.

VEGF-Trap (aflibercept) is a recombinant fusion protein composed of a portion of the extracellular domains of VEGFR-1 and VEGFR-2, fused to the Fc portion of human IgG1.[66] It binds to VEGF-A, VEGF-B, PlGF1, and PlGF2. In a phase I trial of this agent in patients with solid tumors, one patient with ovarian cancer had a PR and improvement in performance status. Preliminary results from a blinded, randomized phase II trial evaluating two different dose levels of VEGF-Trap as a single agent in 162 evaluable patients with recurrent ovarian cancer demonstrated an RR of 10%, with 15% of patients with stable disease at 22 weeks.[67] Aflibercept is now being evaluated in combination with chemotherapy in patients with ovarian cancer[68] and has demonstrated palliation of ascites in patients with ovarian cancer.[69] Results from a trial of VEGF-Trap (see Table 64.1) in patients with recurrent endometrial cancer have not been reported.

Oral agents that work at the intracellular portion of the VEGFR to inhibit signal transduction that triggers angiogenesis have been evaluated in patients with recurrent disease. Examples include sunitinib[70,71] and sorafenib[72,73]; these agents have not demonstrated the degree of efficacy of bevacizumab in the gynecologic cancers, although in many cases, prolonged PFS was noted in comparison to historical controls. In some cases, individual patients have had significant responses to these agents, indicating that the role of angiogenesis is complex, and predictive markers of response are needed to better direct therapy. Sorafenib (see Table 64.1) and sunitinib (see Table 64.1) are undergoing evaluation in combination with other agents in patients with cervical cancer.[74,75] AMG 706 is an oral multikinase inhibitor targeting all known VEGFRs, as well as the PDGFR, c-kit, and the *RET* (rearranged during transfection) protooncogene. In a phase I clinical trial in patients with advanced solid tumors, AMG 706 was well tolerated, with a broad range of activity.[76] It is currently being evaluated in multiple phase I trials in combination with agents known to have activity in ovarian cancer, including paclitaxel, docetaxel, and carboplatin. Cediranib, an oral tyrosine kinase inhibitor of VEGFR-1, VEGFR-2, and VEGFR-3 and c-KIT, has demonstrated RRs of up to 23% in patients with heavily pretreated ovarian cancer.[77] It is currently being evaluated in combination with carboplatin and paclitaxel in patients with platinum-sensitive recurrent ovarian cancer (ICON 6).[78] Pazopanib targets the VEGFR, PDGFR, and c-KIT, and early results in ovarian and cervical cancers have led to additional studies in these diseases.[79-81]

Angiopoietins (ANG-1, ANG-2, and ANG-4) and the TIE-2 receptor tyrosine kinase have been shown to play an important role in tumor angiogenesis. Initially, the TIE-2 receptor, and a closely related TIE-1 receptor with no known ligand or downstream target, was thought mainly to be expressed on endothelial cells; however, recently, it has been shown that the TIE-2 receptor can be expressed on the surface of human tumor cells. TIE-2 on tumor cells may function in a paracrine and/or autocrine manner. In light of this, the ANGs have become a focus of targeted therapy. AMG 386 is a selective ANG-1/2-neutralizing peptibody that inhibits angiogenesis by preventing interaction between ANGs and TIE-2 receptors. The agent was well tolerated as a single agent in a phase I trial, with no dose-limiting toxicity identified.[82] One patient with ovarian cancer remained on treatment for 156 weeks, with a PR. A randomized phase II trial evaluated placebo or two different doses of AMG 386 with weekly paclitaxel and demonstrated improvement in PFS from 5 to 7.3 months with the addition of the AMG-386 to paclitaxel when compared with weekly paclitaxel alone.[83] It is currently being evaluated in an ongoing phase I trial in patients with recurrent ovarian cancer in combination with topotecan or pegylated liposomal doxorubicin[84] and is moving forward to phase III trials in ovarian cancer, as well as early phase trials in endometrial cancer. CVX-060 is a humanized monoclonal antibody that is a fusion of two ANG-2 sequestering peptides bound to an antibody that was developed to target ANG-2 and is currently in evaluation in breast carcinoma and RCC and may be of interest in ovarian cancer.

BIBF 1120 is a triple angiokinase inhibitor, targeting three receptor classes involved in the formation of blood vessels (VEGFR, PDGFR, and FGFR). In a randomized phase II trial in women with recurrent ovarian cancer, 14% of patients who received BIBF 1120 as maintenance therapy after chemotherapy experienced a PFS at 36 weeks compared with 5% of women taking placebo.[85] A phase III trial is ongoing, and additional combinations with this agent are being explored.

There is interest in evaluating combinations of angiogenesis inhibitors, in order to target multiple pathways of angiogenesis simultaneously or a single pathway at multiple steps, in an effort to enhance efficacy. One phase I study combined bevacizumab with continuous daily sorafenib and demonstrated impressive activity in treating recurrent ovarian cancer, with a 46% RR and durable responses lasting up to 22 months. The combination was limited by significant toxicity, requiring dose reductions or cessation of therapy for most patients, leading to extending the phase I study for evaluation of intermittent dosing of sorafenib with bevacizumab.[86] Bevacizumab was evaluated in combination with erlotinib, an EGFR inhibitor, in patients with ovarian cancer, but was closed due to the occurrence of two fatal bowel perforations. Pazopanib (see Table 64.1) was evaluated in combination with lapatinib, an oral agent targeting the EGFR and HER2, but demonstrated no additional benefit over pazopanib monotherapy for patients with recurrent cervical cancer.[81] Many of the more recent monotherapy and combination trials include correlative studies to help identify markers of resistance or response to these treatments. To date, there is no definitive predictive test that has been proven to correlate with response to any of the antiangiogenic agents.

Angiogenesis may be impacted by cellular pathways that modulate the production of known angiogenic factors, or alternatively, by pathways that do not inherently seem to have a direct role in angiogenic signaling. Byzova and colleagues[87] demonstrated that binding of VEGF to VEGF2R on endothelial cells results in activation of signaling through an $\alpha_v\beta_3$ and $\alpha_v\beta_5$ integrin-mediated mechanism. Further, it has been demonstrated in vitro in ovarian cancer cell lines that endothelin-1 signaling leads to upregulation of $\alpha_2\beta_1$ and $\alpha_3\beta_1$ integrins and induction of ILK activation and overexpression resulting in enhanced migration, invasion, and secretion and activation of tumor-associated matrix metalloproteinase (MMP)-2 and MMP-9.[88] A phase II trial of volociximab, a monoclonal antibody against $\alpha_5\beta_1$ integrin, demonstrated little activity in patients with recurrent ovarian cancer, but correlative studies indicate a potential role in the adjuvant setting or in maintenance therapy.[89] Additionally, preclinical data demonstrate that the mTOR inhibitor, everolimus, may impact angiogenesis in addition to its role in inhibiting the mTOR pathway.[90]

PARP Inhibitors

PARP is a key nuclear enzyme involved in the repair of DNA single-strand breaks using base-excision repair. Inhibition of PARP leads to an accumulation of unrepaired DNA single-strand breaks, which leads to double-strand breaks. Activation of BRCA1 and BRCA2 is required for the repair of double-strand DNA breaks. The use of PARP inhibitors in patients with *BRCA* mutations or deficiency is described as synthetic lethality. Synthetic lethality describes a setting in which a cell has a non-lethal mutation in one of two related genes. When the cell carries mutations in both of these genes concurrently, the cell dies. For example, cells with a BRCA mutation are viable, but exposure to a PARP inhibitor results in cell death. PARP inhibitors have been studied as monotherapy in patients with *BRCA* deficiency, whether because of germline mutation or epigenetic modification. Additionally, these agents are being studied in combination with chemotherapeutic agents that cause double-strand breaks, such as alkylating agents, in an effort to enhance the cytotoxicity of such agents. Germline mutation of *RAD51*, a gene important in directing DNA repair through homologous recombination, has also been demonstrated in patients with ovarian cancer, and preclinical data suggest that patients with *RAD51* mutations may be susceptible to PARP inhibition.[91,92] Additionally, the tumor suppressor, PTEN, is important for RAD51expression, and there are data to suggest that *PTEN*-deficient cells are exquisitely sensitive to PARP inhibition.[37] As previously noted, patients with a *BRCA* mutation or deficiency are at risk for developing high-grade serous ovarian carcinoma. In some studies utilizing PARP inhibitors, patients have been selected for a *BRCA* mutation; however, in recognition of the high rate of *BRCA* deficiency among patients with high-grade serous ovarian carcinoma, even in the absence of a BRCA mutation, as noted by Gelmon and colleagues, some trials are selecting on the basis of histology, enrolling patients with high-grade serous carcinoma.[93]

There are currently several PARP inhibitors in various stages of clinical development (Table 64.2). Olaparib (AZD2281), an inhibitor of PARP1 and PARP2, has been studied in patients with *BRCA*-related cancers, including a phase I trial which was enriched for patients with a known *BRCA* mutation.[94] Of the 60 participants, 22 were *BRCA* mutation carriers and 16 had ovarian cancer. Eight of the patients with ovarian cancer experienced a PR and one had stable disease. In a study open to patients with ovarian cancer unselected for *BRCA* status, olaparib was found to have limited toxicity, with a RR of 33% at a dose of

TABLE 64–2 Known Poly(ADP-Ribose) Polymerase Inhibitors Currently in Clinical or Preclinical Development

Agent	Mechanism	Stage of Clinical Development
Olaparib AZD2281 (formerly KU-0059436)	Inhibits PARP1 and PARP2	Phase III
Veliparib ABT-888	Inhibits PARP1 and PARP2	Phase II
Rucaparib AG-014699 (formerly PF-01367338)	Inhibits PARP1	Phase III
CEP-8983/CEP-9722	Inhibits PARP1 and PARP2	Phase II
MK-4287	Inhibits PARP1 and PARP2	Phases I and II
BMN-673	Inhibits PARP—not otherwise specified	Phase I

PARP, poly(ADP-ribose) polymerase.

400 mg twice a day. Patients with ovarian cancer treated at a lower dose of 100 mg twice a day experienced a RR of 13%.[95] An additional study in patients with ovarian and breast cancer included 65 patients with ovarian cancer.[93] Of these patients, 63 had response evaluation criteria in solid tumors (RECIST)–evaluable disease and the overall RR for this group was 29%. The RR for patients with known *BRCA* mutations was 41% (7 of 17) and for those confirmed negative for a known *BRCA* mutation it was 24% (11 of 46). Median PFS for the patients with ovarian cancer was 219 days. RRs in these trials are higher in patients with platinum-sensitive disease than in those with platinum-resistant disease.[93,96] A total of 162 patients with platinum-sensitive recurrent serous ovarian cancer were randomized to receive carboplatin and paclitaxel with or without olaparib, with the patients randomized to the olaparib plus chemotherapy regimen continuing maintenance olaparib after completion of chemotherapy. Patients who received chemotherapy with olaparib and maintenance olaparib experienced a statistically significant improvement in median PFS from 9.6 to 12.2 months.[97] Veliparib (ABT-888) is an oral PARP inhibitor that has primarily been studied in combination with various chemotherapeutic agents, including temozolomide and oral cyclophosphamide, among others. The GOG is currently evaluating multiple regimens that include veliparib.

Folate Receptor Pathway

There are three known isoforms of the folate receptor (FR) in humans, and FR-α has been demonstrated to have a limited distribution in normal adult tissues but is overexpressed on the surface of many solid tumors, including non-mucinous ovarian carcinomas in up to 90% of cases.[98] FR-directed therapeutics have been developed to attempt to target this overexpression of the FR-α, including monoclonal antibodies directly targeted to the receptor, and conjugating drugs or drug carriers to folate. Farletuzumab (MORAb-003) is a humanized monoclonal antibody that targets FR-α.[99] In a phase I trial in patients with heavily pretreated ovarian cancer, this agent was well tolerated, with evidence of stable disease in 9 of 25 patients treated.[99] A phase II trial presented at the European Society for Medical Oncology meeting in 2009 evaluated farletuzumab in combination with carboplatin and paclitaxel in 44 patients with platinum-sensitive recurrent ovarian cancer and demonstrated a high RR, with 20% of responding patients experiencing a longer PFS after this treatment than their first PFS.[100]

c-Met

c-Met is a transmembrane receptor tyrosine kinase (see Fig. 64.1) that is important in tumorigenesis and metastasis across a broad range of human malignancies, including ovarian cancer.[101,102] It is bound by its ligand, hepatocyte growth factor/scatter factor (HGF/SF). Ligand binding results in dimerization and activation of cellular signaling through the RAS/MAPK (mitogen-activated protein kinase) and PI3K pathways.[103] c-Met is overexpressed in human ovarian cancers,[104-106] and high levels of HGF/SF are found in ascites.[107] Additionally, changes in c-Met expression are linked to malignant transformation and high levels of expression correlate with a poor prognosis.[106-109] HGF/SF stimulates endothelial cell proliferation and induction of VEGF, resulting in new blood vessel formation.[110] In addition, HGF stimulates the breakdown of cell–cell adhesions between epithelial cells, allowing the dispersal of cancer cells and possibly increasing their invasiveness as part of the epithelial–mesenchymal transition.[111]

Novel agents targeting the c-Met/HGF pathway, either by binding to the c-Met receptor and inhibiting its activation or by targeting its ligand, HGF, are under evaluation.[112-114] AMG 102 is a monoclonal antibody targeting HGF as monotherapy in patients with RCC and glioma, as well as in combination with cytotoxic chemotherapy and other targeted agents. A trial for patients with recurrent ovarian cancer is ongoing under the auspices of the GOG. TAK-701 is also a humanized monoclonal antibody targeting HGF which is currently undergoing phase I testing.[115] Small molecule inhibitors of c-Met include ARQ197 and PF-02341066 which selectively target c-Met and are being evaluated in early trials. Cabozantinib (XL184), a multikinase inhibitor of RET, c-Met, and VEGFR2,[116] and foretinib (GSK1363089, formerly XL880), which targets c-Met and VEGFR2, are undergoing clinical evaluation. Cabozantinib (XL184) has been shown to be well tolerated with early results of a phase II trial in patients with recurrent ovarian cancer demonstrating an RR of 24%.[117] Phase III trials in thyroid cancer are ongoing as are phase II trials in ovarian and endometrial cancer.

It has been noted that integrins play a role in HGF/SF signaling. Binding of HGF/SF by extracellular matrix molecules, fibronectin and vitronectin, activates $\alpha_v\beta_3$ and $\alpha_5\beta_1$integrins in endothelial cells regulating proliferation through the MAPK and PI3K pathways.[118] c-Met can also associate with $\alpha_6\beta_4$ integrin further modulating c-Met–regulated signaling. Synergism of c-Met with integrins activates FAK and RAS, a point of convergence of integrin and growth factor signaling pathways.[118,119] Additionally, Engelman and co-investigators[120] have shown that c-Met can dimerize with HER-3. Cross-activation of HER pathways may explain resistance to agents such as trastuzumab and pertuzumab. In light of these findings, combined inhibition of c-Met and the HER family of proteins may improve efficacy of molecularly targeted therapy.

HER Family of Growth Factors

The EGFR is one of the ErbB family of four transmembrane signaling receptors: EGFR or HER-1/ErbB1, HER-2/ErbB2, HER-3/ErbB3, and HER-4/ErbB4 (see Fig. 64.1).[121] Each of these receptors has a unique pattern of ligand binding and activation, generally through dimerization with each other to form homodimers or heterodimers. These receptors are important in malignant transformation and disease progression in many epithelial cancers.[122] Multiple investigators have reported associations of overexpression of these receptors and prognosis in ovarian,[123,124] endometrial,[125] and cervical cancer[126] with conflicting prognostic implications.

Efforts to target this pathway with agents that have demonstrated efficacy in other EGFR overexpressing tumors have not demonstrated markedly effective disease control in gynecologic cancers. Cetuximab is a chimeric human–mouse monoclonal antibody that binds to the EGFR and blocks binding of its ligands, EGF and transforming growth factor-alpha, thereby blocking dimerization and activation.[127] Early phase I studies of cetuximab given as a single agent showed stabilization of disease rather than responses. When cetuximab was evaluated in recurrent ovarian cancer as a single agent, efficacy was limited.[128] However, testing in the phase I setting suggested greater efficacy when given in combination with chemotherapy.[127] A trial evaluating cetuximab in the front-line setting in combination with standard chemotherapy for patients with either optimally debulked or suboptimally debulked stage III and IV ovarian cancer showed that there was good tolerance of the regimen, but it did not confer additional benefit over standard chemotherapy.[129] It similarly did not confer additional benefit over platinum alone in recurrent disease.[130] It was also relatively inactive in cervical[131,132] and endometrial cancer.[133]

Gefitinib, an oral TKI, was evaluated in a phase II trial in 26 patients with recurrent ovarian cancer and demonstrated 1 patient with a PR and 8 patients with stable disease.[134] This trial also evaluated the EGFR status of these patients; there was no significant difference based on the level of EGFR expression, although the patient with a response was found to have a mutation in the catalytic domain of the EGFR, which has been previously shown to correlate with improved response to EGFR inhibitors in patients with lung cancer.[135,136] Gefitinib has had minimal activity in cervical[137] and endometrial cancer.[138]

Erlotinib is an oral, reversible, selective inhibitor of the EGFR.[139] In a phase II study in 34 women with recurrent ovarian carcinoma treated with erlotinib, 6% had a PR and 44% had disease stabilization.[140] The median overall survival was 8 months and the 1-year survival was 35.3%. One of the notable side effects was a rash, and there was a positive correlation between the severity of the rash and survival. Erlotinib is being evaluated in combination with chemotherapy in front-line and recurrent disease. Early results have been presented from two front-line phase I studies evaluating erlotinib with standard chemotherapy in patients with advanced disease. While it was well tolerated with carboplatin and paclitaxel,[141] and a phase Ib trial combining erlotinib with docetaxel/carboplatin demonstrated good tolerance of the regimen,[142] a later trial was stopped after accrual of only seven patients due to a high rate of gastrointestinal toxicity.[143] A phase II trial of erlotinib in combination with paclitaxel and carboplatin looked for an end point of pathologic complete response (CR) as evaluated by surgical exploration, but erlotinib was not found to improve the pathologic CR rate in patients with ovarian cancer.[144] Additionally, erlotinib is being evaluated for efficacy as maintenance therapy after completion of front-line therapy in ovarian cancer. It has demonstrated minimal activity in endometrial and cervical cancer.[145,146]

Trastuzumab is a humanized monoclonal antibody that binds to the extracellular domain of HER-2, inhibiting the growth of cancer cells which overexpress this receptor. While this agent has had striking success in treating breast cancers that overexpress HER-2, its utility in ovarian cancer has been limited by a low frequency of overexpression of HER-2. In a phase II GOG trial in patients with recurrent ovarian cancer, only 11% of patients were found to have tumors with HER-2 overexpression, and the overall RR to trastuzumab in this trial was 7%.[147] In a study in patients with HER-2–positive endometrial cancer, unselected for histology, activity was limited.[148]

Pertuzumab is another recombinant humanized monoclonal antibody which binds to the extracellular domain of HER-2, at a different epitope than trastuzumab. It blocks the dimerization site of HER-2 and can block the activity of this receptor even in tumors that do not overexpress HER-2. In preclinical studies, it was shown to inhibit the growth of prostate and breast cancer cell lines that were not inhibited by trastuzumab. A phase I clinical trial of pertuzumab in patients with advanced solid tumors included three patients with ovarian cancer, one of whom experienced disease stabilization and one of whom experienced a PR lasting for at least 11 months at the time of publication.[149] This led to the commencement of a phase II clinical trial of this agent in heavily pretreated patients with advanced resistant ovarian cancer. Preliminary data from 117 evaluable patients in this trial showed a PR rate of 4% and stable disease lasting at least 6 months in 7%.[150] An additional 3% of patients experienced a decline of at least 50% in CA125 levels. In spite of preclinical data suggesting that this agent would have activity in patients whose tumors did not overexpress HER-2,[151] among a subset of 28 patients whose tumor samples were evaluated for HER-2 activation, results indicated greater benefit for those whose tumors demonstrated high levels of activated (phosphorylated) HER-2. Pertuzumab was also evaluated in combination with gemcitabine versus gemcitabine monotherapy in 165 patients with ovarian carcinoma and demonstrated an improvement in RR from 4.6% to 13.8%.[152] In this study, patients found to have a high level of HER-3 mRNA expression had a better overall prognosis. However, patients with a low level of HER-3 mRNA expression seemed more likely to respond to pertuzumab. Preclinical data also suggest efficacy for pertuzumab in combination with other targeted agents, such as trastuzumab[153] and erlotinib,[154] and the trastuzumab/pertuzumab combination is currently being evaluated in patients with breast cancer.

Lapatinib is an oral, reversible dual kinase inhibitor, inhibiting both EGFR and HER-2.[155] Multiple phase I trials demonstrated good tolerance with some efficacy, particularly in the setting of HER-2 overexpression.[156] A phase II trial in patients with recurrent ovarian cancer demonstrated limited efficacy.[157] The GOG tested lapatinib in endometrial cancer, but the study did not go on to second-stage accrual (report pending).

EGFR signaling stimulates FAK-independent activation of the Src, ERK, MAPK, and PI3K pathways and integrin-linked kinase,[158,159] and agents targeting these pathways are also of interest in treating ovarian and endometrial cancer.

IGF Pathway

IGF-1R is a receptor tyrosine kinase that serves as a key positive regulator of the IGF system. Signaling triggers downstream activation of the PI3K-AKT-mTOR and RAF-MEK-ERK signaling pathways (see Fig. 64.1).[160] This pathway includes the IGF-1R, the IGF-2R, the insulin receptor (IR), and hybrid receptors of IGF and insulin which bind to the ligands IGF-1, IGF-2, and insulin. There are also six binding proteins that regulate activity of the IGF pathway, but their function has not yet been defined.

Binding of the IGF-1R leads to recruitment of Src homologous and collagen proteins and insulin receptor substrates (IRS)-1 and IRS-2 to phosphorylation sites on the intracellular domain of the receptor, resulting in downstream activation of the RAF/MEK/ERK and PI3K/AKT/mTOR signaling pathways.[161]

Several agents have been developed to target this pathway and are in early-stage testing (Table 64.3). Monoclonal antibodies include figitumumab, IMC-A12, MK-0646, AVE1642, R1507, BIIB022, and AMG 479. Figitumumab (CP-751,871) is a fully humanized IgG2 monoclonal antibody directed against IGF-1R.[162] In a phase I trial, figitumumab was well tolerated, with no maximum tolerated dose noted, and it is currently under additional clinical evaluation[163] in various cancers in combination with erlotinib, sunitinib, RAD001, and exemestane or various chemotherapy combinations. Cixitumumab (IMC-A12), another anti-IGF-1R monoclonal antibody, is also undergoing phase I and II testing in patients with multiple solid tumors. Ganitumab (AMG-479) is also a fully humanized anti-IGF-1R monoclonal antibody that was well tolerated in a phase I trial in 53 patients with solid tumors[164] and is currently undergoing evaluation in multiple phase I and II trials in combination with other targeted agents or in combination with chemotherapy. There is an ongoing phase III trial in combination with gemcitabine in patients with pancreatic cancer

TABLE 64-3 Agents Targeting the Insulin-Like Growth Factor, PI3K/AKT/mTOR, and RAS/RAF/MEK/ERK Pathways

Figitumumab (CP-751,871)	Monoclonal antibody	IGF-1R
Cixitumumab (IMC-A12)	Monoclonal antibody	IGF-1R
Dalotuzumab (MK0646)	Monoclonal antibody	IGF-1R
Robatumumab (SCH 717454)	Monoclonal antibody	IGF-1R
AVE1642	Monoclonal antibody	IGF-1R
R1507	Monoclonal antibody	IGF-1R
BIIB022	Monoclonal antibody	IGF-1R
Ganitumab (AMG-479)	Monoclonal antibody	IGF-1R
OSI-906	Tyrosine kinase	IGF-1R, IR
XL-228	Tyrosine kinase	IGF-1R, Aurora, Src
NVP-AEW	Tyrosine kinase	IGF-1R kinase
XL147 (SAR245408)	Tyrosine kinase	PI3 kinase
GDC0941	Tyrosine kinase	PI3 kinase
BKM 120	Tyrosine kinase	PI3 kinase
MK2206	Tyrosine kinase	AKT 1, 2, and (minimal) 3
GSK2141795	Tyrosine kinase	AKT (not further specified)
GDC 0068	Tyrosine kinase	AKT 1, 2, and 3
Everolimus (RAD001)	Tyrosine kinase	mTORC1
Temsirolimus (CCI-779)	Tyrosine kinase	mTOR
Ridaforolimus (AP23573, MK-8669)	Tyrosine kinase	mTOR
BEZ235	Tyrosine kinase	PI3 kinase, mTOR
GDC 0980	Tyrosine kinase	PI3 kinase, mTOR
PF04691502	Tyrosine kinase	PI3 kinase, mTOR
Vemurafenib (RG7204, PLX4032)		BRAF
GSK2118436	Tyrosine kinase	BRAF
AZD 6244	Tyrosine kinase	MEK-1 and MEK-2
GSK1120212	Tyrosine kinase	MEK-1 and MEK-2

IGF-1R, insulin-like growth factor-1 receptor; IR, insulin receptor; PI3, phosphoinositide 3; mTOR, mammalian target of rapamycin.

in Japan. Robatumumab (SCH 717454), dalotuzumab (MK0646), AVE1642, and BIIB022 are additional monoclonal antibodies targeting the IGF-1R, which are in early phase testing. Dalotuzumab is being evaluated as a monotherapy and in combination with erlotinib, dasatinib, and other chemotherapeutic regimens in patients with various types of solid tumors, including ovarian cancer.

Small molecule inhibitors of this pathway are also undergoing preclinical and clinical evaluation, although there are potential concerns regarding effects on glucose metabolism due to cross-binding of the IR. OSI-906 has been evaluated in the phase I setting and was well tolerated, with side effects including grade 1 to 2 hyperglycemia, nausea and vomiting, and grade 3 elevated lipase in one patient.[165] This agent also blocks the IR, which may decrease the likelihood of developing resistance to this group of agents targeting the IGF family of receptors. XL-228 was evaluated in a phase I trial in 53 patients and was well tolerated and showed encouraging activity.[166] NVP-AEW 541 is another potent small molecule IGF-1R inhibitor that is being evaluated in the preclinical setting, but has not yet commenced clinical testing.[167]

PI3K/AKT/mTOR

The PI3K/AKT/mTOR pathway is involved in key intracellular responses to stimulation of growth, differentiation, and apoptosis/survival and is known to be dysregulated in a wide spectrum of human cancers (see Fig. 64.1). Dysregulation occurs through loss/mutation of the negative regulator *PTEN*, through *PI3K* mutation/amplification, through AKT/PKB overexpression/overactivation, or through modulation of tuberous sclerosis complex tumor suppressors.[168] Activation of this pathway in tumors is associated with a worse prognosis as they behave more aggressively and have enhanced chemotherapy resistance, possibly because activation of this pathway may prevent apoptosis of cells. Inhibition of the PI3K/AKT/mTOR pathway may enhance the efficacy of conventional chemotherapeutic agents.[169]

The pathway is complex, with numerous downstream effectors and cross talk. Efforts to target upstream activators such as the PI3K and downstream effectors such as mTOR are ongoing (see Table 64.3). There are also efforts to target AKT itself. Recognition of the complexity of the pathway has led to dual inhibitors of PI3K and mTOR in an attempt to provide dual targeting of both upstream activators and downstream effectors, as it is theorized that such dual targeting is less likely to be overcome by the cross talk and redundancy in this pathway. Currently, agents inhibiting PI3K, including XL147, GDC0941, and BKM 120, and agents targeting AKT isoforms 1, 2, and 3 such as MK2206, GSK2141795, and GDC 0068 are in early phase clinical testing in endometrial and ovarian cancer.

mTOR is a ubiquitous protein kinase that plays a central role in cell proliferation. mTOR inhibits eukaryotic initiation factor 4E-binding proteins and activates the 70 kDa ribosomal S6 kinases (i.e., p70S6K1), regulating translation of messages encoding the HIF-1 proteins, c-MYC, and cyclin D1, as well as ribosomal proteins. Additionally, activation of the mTOR pathway leads to the increased production of pro-angiogenic factors (i.e., VEGF) in tumors and to tumor cell, endothelial cell, and smooth muscle cell growth and proliferation.[168] mTOR is comprised of two structurally and functionally distinct multiprotein signaling complexes, mTORC1 (mTOR complex 1, rapamycin sensitive) and mTORC2 (mTOR complex 2, rapamycin insensitive).[170] mTORC1 is primarily activated via the PI3K pathway through AKT, while mTORC2 is activated through an unknown mechanism.[168,170]

Recent data from laboratory models and patient trials show that inhibition of the PI3K/AKT/mTOR pathway may have therapeutic value in the treatment of cancer.[171] AKT may play a role in the resistance of tumor cells to traditional cytotoxic agents by promoting cell survival through antiapoptotic mechanisms, and AKT/mTOR amplification has been demonstrated in human epithelial ovarian cancer.[172,173] Altomare and colleagues[169] used a phospho-specific anti-AKT antibody (SER463) that recognizes all three activated AKT forms (AKT1-3) and showed strong immunohistochemical staining in 68% of ovarian carcinomas. PI3K is activated in more than 60% of cancers with elevated AKT2 activity, thus demonstrating alterations in upstream regulators of catalytic activity.[169] Downstream targets of AKT, including phospho-mTOR, correlated with AKT activation in more than 80% of ovarian carcinomas.[169] The pattern of aberration varies according to the histologic subtype of the disease. Inhibition of downstream targets of the PI3K/AKT/mTOR pathway may kill tumor cells that have a relative dependence on AKT activity for survival. Activation status of the PI3K/AKT/mTOR pathway may be indicative of response to rapamycin analogs such as everolimus (RAD001), a specific inhibitor of mTOR.[168]

This pathway may also be important in chemotherapy resistance. When compared with human ovarian cell lines with low AKT activity, cell lines with high AKT activity exhibit greater resistance to paclitaxel.[169] LY294002, a selective PI3K inhibitor, augmented cisplatin-induced apoptosis in SKOV-3 cells, which exhibit constitutive AKT activation under low serum conditions.[169] Everolimus enhances the ability of cisplatin to inhibit cell proliferation in OVCAR-10 cells, which have elevated AKT/mTOR signaling.[174]

mTORC1-mediated signaling is subject to modulation by the macrocyclic lactone rapamycin and its derivatives (e.g., everolimus, temsirolimus, and ridaforolimus). These agents result in complexes that bind to a specific site near the catalytic domain of mTORC1 and inhibit phosphorylation of mTOR substrates. There were no responses in a phase II trial of everolimus in patients with recurrent endometrial cancer, although 21% of patients experienced disease stabilization at 20 weeks of therapy.[175] Temsirolimus targets and binds to an abundant intracellular protein, FKBP-12, and in this way forms a complex that inhibits mTOR signaling. It has been shown to have modest activity as a single agent in the treatment of patients with persistent or recurrent ovarian cancer.[176] In a phase II trial in endometrial cancer, which included both previously treated and chemotherapy-naïve patients, temsirolimus demonstrated promising activity in the chemo-naive group, with a 14% RR and 69% of patients with stable disease greater than 4 months.[177] Early results were presented in 2011 at the annual meeting of the American Society of Clinical Oncologists (ASCO) of ridaforolimus in patients with recurrent endometrial cancer, with a promising high rate of stable disease and some responses, although the trial is ongoing.[178]

Recently, dual inhibitors of the PI3K pathway and mTOR have been developed, including BEZ235, GDC 0980, and PF04691502. These dual inhibitors may help overcome resistance seen with pure mTOR inhibitors through a positive feedback loop that increases AKT expression.

RAS/RAF/MEK/ERK Pathway Inhibition

RAF are a family of ubiquitous serine/protein kinases (A-RAF, B-RAF, and C-RAF) that promote proliferation and tumorigenesis. The RAS/RAF/MEK/ERK signaling pathway (see Fig. 64.1) plays a central role in the regulation of many cellular processes, including proliferation, survival, differentiation, apoptosis, motility, and metabolism.[179,180] This pathway is one of the most important and best understood MAPK signal transduction pathways, activated by a diverse group of extracellular signals, including ligands for the EGFR, PDGFR, and IGF-1R. Mutations or activation of components of the RAS/RAF signaling pathway can result in cellular proliferation, malignant transformation, and chemotherapeutic resistance. *RAS* genes are among the most frequently mutated oncogenes found in human cancers.[181,182] In addition to being found in almost all pancreatic adenocarcinomas, *RAS* mutations have been found in colorectal carcinoma, in lung adenocarcinomas, and in some breast and ovarian carcinomas. *BRAF* mutations have also been observed in many human cancers, particularly melanoma, thyroid cancer, colorectal carcinoma, and ovarian cancer. These mutations are typically gain-of-function substitutions that render the kinases constitutively active.[182] It has recently been demonstrated that vemurafenib, an oral inhibitor of BRAF, confers clinical benefit, and this agent has been approved for the treatment of patients with metastatic melanoma who have a *BRAF* mutation.[183] Patients participating in this trial had a 48% RR to vemurafenib, but efficacy was limited by later regrowth of cancer; therefore, there is continued interest in identifying additional methods of targeting this pathway. A second agent targeting mutant *BRAF*, GSK2118436, demonstrated activity in patients with metastatic melanoma in a phase I trial and is currently undergoing evaluation in a phase III trial in patients with malignant melanoma.[184] As previously noted, *BRAF* or *KRAS* mutations occur at a high frequency in patients with low-grade serous carcinoma. An alternate approach to direct inhibition of BRAF is targeting this pathway downstream of BRAF, through MEK inhibition. AZD 6244 is a potent, selective, oral small molecule inhibitor of MEK1 and MEK2. The GOG is currently evaluating the use of this agent in patients with recurrent, low-grade serous carcinoma. There is a current phase I trial evaluating the combination of GSK2118436 and GSK1120212, an MEK1/2 inhibitor, to assess the safety and efficacy of dual targeting of BRAF and MEK.[185]

Additionally, K-RAS overexpression is common in both type I and II endometrial cancer, and agents that target downstream activators, such as RAF, MEK, and ERK, are of interest in this disease. Consideration is also being given to concurrently targeting both PI3K/AKT/mTOR and RAS/RAF/MEK/ERK pathways (see Table 64.3).

Aurora Kinase

The aurora kinases (A, B, and C) are a highly conserved family of serine/threonine kinases that play an important role in both normal and aberrant cell division.[186] Aurora A kinase functions primarily in the G2/M phase of cell division and is associated with centrosome maturation, mitotic entry, spindle assembly, and microtubule organization.[186] Amplification and/or overexpression of aurora A kinase is linked to tumor growth and metastases. The aurora A kinase gene (*AURKA*) is located at chromosome 20q13.2, a region that is frequently amplified in malignancies, including melanoma and cancers of the breast, colon, pancreas, ovaries, bladder, liver, and stomach.[186] High levels of aurora A kinase activity are observed in up to 83% of human epithelial ovarian cancers.[187] Aurora A kinase overexpression has been demonstrated to be a negative prognostic marker in cancers such as breast and ovarian cancer.[188] MLN8237 is a second-generation aurora A kinase–selective synthetic small molecule inhibitor that has been shown to cause neutropenia, pancytopenia, stomatitis, somnolence, and alopecia; preliminary results of a phase II monotherapy trial in patients with recurrent, platinum-resistant ovarian cancer were reported last year demonstrating an RR of 10%.[189] Additional trials of this agent in combination with chemotherapy, e.g., weekly paclitaxel, are ongoing in recurrent ovarian cancer.

IMPLICATIONS FOR FUTURE RESEARCH AND CLINICAL PRACTICE

It is expected that understanding of the mechanisms of disease development and progression will help in identification of the targeted therapeutic strategies that are most likely to succeed in advancing treatment for women with gynecologic cancers. While the knowledge of molecular differences between cancer cells and their normal cell counterparts is growing, it is apparent that in many cases, the pathways of importance can vary within a disease. Those outlined above may change in relative importance, and new pathways will be found that have more importance in disease pathogenesis and progression. The preceding paragraphs go into some detail about the differences between the histologic subtypes of ovarian and endometrial cancer, but most trials evaluating targeted agents have been evaluated in a patient population which has been unselected on the basis of histologic or genetic subtype. As we learn more about the different histologic subtypes, we will need to think carefully about how to approach individuals with these cancers. While the traditional approach has been to develop clinical trials geared to a specific disease site, future studies evaluating targeted therapeutic regimens will need to subtype cancers within a disease site, and it is possible that some trials may include patients with multiple disease sites if they share a common dysregulated pathway or gene mutation. Finally, while this chapter focuses on gynecological cancer at the cellular level, knowledge about cancer cell interactions with the tumor milieu and the host immune system will provide additional opportunities for targeting and interfering with disease development and progression in women with gynecological cancers.

REFERENCES

1. Jemal A, Siegel R, Xu J, Ward E. Cancer statistics, 2010. *CA Cancer J Clin*. 2010;60:277-300.
2. Bookman MA, Brady MF, McGuire WP, et al. Evaluation of new platinum-based treatment regimens in advanced-stage ovarian cancer: a phase III trial of the gynecologic cancer intergroup. *J Clin Oncol*. 2009;27:1419-1425.
3. Vang R, Shih Ie M, Kurman RJ. Ovarian low-grade and high-grade serous carcinoma: pathogenesis, clinicopathologic and molecular biologic features, and diagnostic problems. *Adv Anat Pathol*. 2009;16:267-282.
4. Kurman RJ, Shih Ie M. Molecular pathogenesis and extraovarian origin of epithelial ovarian cancer—shifting the paradigm. *Hum Pathol*. 2011;42:918-931.
5. Ahmed AA, Etemadmoghadam D, Temple J, et al. Driver mutations in TP53 are ubiquitous in high grade serous carcinoma of the ovary. *J Pathol*. 2010;221:49-56.
6. Integrated genomic analyses of ovarian carcinoma. *Nature*. 2011;474:609-615.
7. Crum CP. Intercepting pelvic cancer in the distal fallopian tube: theories and realities. *Mol Oncol*. 2009;3:165-170.
8. Piek JM, Kenemans P, Zweemer RP, van Diest PJ, Verheijen RH. Ovarian carcinogenesis, an alternative theory. *Gynecol Oncol*. 2007;107:355.
9. Piek JM, van Diest PJ, Zweemer RP, et al. Dysplastic changes in prophylactically removed Fallopian tubes of women predisposed to developing ovarian cancer. *J Pathol*. 2001;195:451-456.
10. Seidman JD, Zhao P, Yemelyanova A. "Primary peritoneal" high-grade serous carcinoma is very likely metastatic from serous tubal intraepithelial carcinoma: assessing the new paradigm of ovarian and pelvic serous carcinogenesis and its implications for screening for ovarian cancer. *Gynecol Oncol*. 2011;120:470-473.
11. Kindelberger DW, Lee Y, Miron A, et al. Intraepithelial carcinoma of the fimbria and pelvic serous carcinoma: evidence for a causal relationship. *Am J Surg Pathol*. 2007;31:161-169.
12. Anglesio MS, Carey MS, Kobel M, Mackay H, Huntsman DG. Clear cell carcinoma of the ovary: a report from the first Ovarian Clear Cell Symposium, June 24th, 2010. *Gynecol Oncol*. 2011;121: 407-415.
13. Wiegand KC, Shah SP, Al-Agha OM, et al. ARID1A mutations in endometriosis-associated ovarian carcinomas. *N Engl J Med*. 2010;363:1532-1543.
14. Jones S, Wang TL, Shih Ie M, et al. Frequent mutations of chromatin remodeling gene ARID1A in ovarian clear cell carcinoma. *Science*. 2010;330:228-231.
15. Wang X, Nagl NG Jr, Flowers S, Zweitzig D, Dallas PB, Moran E. Expression of p270 (ARID1A), a component of human SWI/SNF complexes, in human tumors. *Int J Cancer*. 2004;112:636.
16. Zorn KK, Bonome T, Gangi L, et al. Gene expression profiles of serous, endometrioid, and clear cell subtypes of ovarian and endometrial cancer. *Clin Cancer Res*. 2005;11:6422-6430.
17. Stany MP, Vathipadiekal V, Ozbun L, et al. Identification of novel therapeutic targets in microdissected clear cell ovarian cancers. *PloS One*. 2011;6:e21121.
18. Campbell IG, Russell SE, Choong DY, et al. Mutation of the PIK3CA gene in ovarian and breast cancer. *Cancer Res*. 2004;64:7678-7681.
19. Obata K, Hoshiai H. Common genetic changes between endometriosis and ovarian cancer. *Gynecol Obstet Invest*. 2000;50(suppl 1):39-43.
20. Cho KR. Ovarian cancer update: lessons from morphology, molecules, and mice. *Arch Pathol Lab Med*. 2009;133:1775-1781.
21. Singer G, Oldt R 3rd, Cohen Y, et al. Mutations in BRAF and KRAS characterize the development of low-grade ovarian serous carcinoma. *J Natl Cancer Inst*. 2003;95:484-486.
22. Ho CL, Kurman RJ, Dehari R, Wang TL, Shih Ie M. Mutations of BRAF and KRAS precede the development of ovarian serous borderline tumors. *Cancer Res*. 2004;64:6915-6918.
23. King ER, Zu Z, Tsang YTM, et al. The insulin-like growth factor 1 pathway is a potential therapeutic target for low-grade serous ovarian carcinoma. *Gynecol Oncol*. 2011;123:13-18.
24. Gemignani ML, Schlaerth AC, Bogomolniy F, et al. Role of KRAS and BRAF gene mutations in mucinous ovarian carcinoma. *Gynecol Oncol*. 2003;90:378-381.
25. Ball HG, Blessing JA, Lentz SS, Mutch DG. A phase II trial of paclitaxel in patients with advanced or recurrent adenocarcinoma of the endometrium: a Gynecologic Oncology Group study. *Gynecol Oncol*. 1996;62:278-281.
26. Fleming GF, Filiaci VL, Bentley RC, et al. Phase III randomized trial of doxorubicin + cisplatin versus doxorubicin + 24-h paclitaxel + filgrastim in endometrial carcinoma: a Gynecologic Oncology Group study. *Ann Oncol*. 2004;15:1173-1178.
27. Bokhman JV. Two pathogenetic types of endometrial carcinoma. *Gynecol Oncol*. 1983;15:10-17.
28. Hecht JL, Mutter GL. Molecular and pathologic aspects of endometrial carcinogenesis. *J Clin Oncol*. 2006;24:4783-4791.
29. Lax SF, Kendall B, Tashiro H, Slebos RJ, Hedrick L. The frequency of p53, K-ras mutations, and microsatellite instability differs in uterine endometrioid and serous carcinoma: evidence of distinct molecular genetic pathways. *Cancer*. 2000;88:814-824.
30. Tashiro H, Blazes MS, Wu R, et al. Mutations in PTEN are frequent in endometrial carcinoma but rare in other common gynecological malignancies. *Cancer Res*. 1997;57:3935-3940.
31. Mutter GL, Lin MC, Fitzgerald JT, et al. Altered PTEN expression as a diagnostic marker for the earliest endometrial precancers. *J Natl Cancer Inst*. 2000;92:924-930.
32. MacDonald ND, Salvesen HB, Ryan A, Iversen OE, Akslen LA, Jacobs IJ. Frequency and prognostic impact of microsatellite instability in a large population-based study of endometrial carcinomas. *Cancer Res*. 2000;60:1750-1752.
33. Kohler MF, Berchuck A, Davidoff AM, et al. Overexpression and mutation of p53 in endometrial carcinoma. *Cancer Res*. 1992;52:1622-1627.
34. Konecny GE, Santos L, Winterhoff B, et al. HER2 gene amplification and EGFR expression in a large cohort of surgically staged patients with nonendometrioid (type II) endometrial cancer. *Br J Cancer*. 2009;100:89-95.
35. Oda K, Stokoe D, Taketani Y, McCormick F. High frequency of coexistent mutations of PIK3CA and PTEN genes in endometrial carcinoma. *Cancer Res*. 2005;65:10669-10673.
36. Mendes-Pereira AM, Martin SA, Brough R, et al. Synthetic lethal targeting of PTEN mutant cells with PARP inhibitors. *EMBO Mol Med*. 2009;1:315-322.
37. Dedes KJ, Wetterskog D, Mendes-Pereira AM, et al. PTEN deficiency in endometrioid endometrial adenocarcinomas predicts sensitivity to PARP inhibitors. *Sci Transl Med*. 2010;2:53ra75.

38. Guan B, Mao TL, Panuganti PK, et al. Mutation and loss of expression of ARID1A in uterine low-grade endometrioid carcinoma. *Am J Surg Path*. 2011;35:625-632.
39. Havre PA, Yuan J, Hedrick L, Cho KR, Glazer PM. p53 inactivation by HPV16 E6 results in increased mutagenesis in human cells. *Cancer Res*. 1995;55:4420-4424.
40. Lechner MS, Laimins LA. Inhibition of p53 DNA binding by human papillomavirus E6 proteins. *J Virol*. 1994;68:4262-4273.
41. Hu G, Liu W, Mendelsohn J, et al. Expression of epidermal growth factor receptor and human papillomavirus E6/E7 proteins in cervical carcinoma cells. *J Natl Cancer Inst*. 1997;89:1271-1276.
42. Tang X, Zhang Q, Nishitani J, Brown J, Shi S, Le AD. Overexpression of human papillomavirus type 16 oncoproteins enhances hypoxia-inducible factor 1 alpha protein accumulation and vascular endothelial growth factor expression in human cervical carcinoma cells. *Clin Cancer Res*. 2007;13:2568-2576.
43. Graeber TG, Osmanian C, Jacks T, et al. Hypoxia-mediated selection of cells with diminished apoptotic potential in solid tumours. *Nature*. 1996;379:88-91.
44. Ausprunk DH, Folkman J. Migration and proliferation of endothelial cells in preformed and newly formed blood vessels during tumor angiogenesis. *Microvasc Res*. 1977;14:53-65.
45. Olson TA, Mohanraj D, Carson LF, Ramakrishnan S. Vascular permeability factor gene expression in normal and neoplastic human ovaries. *Cancer Res*. 1994;54:276-280.
46. Hata K, Nakayama K, Fujiwaki R, Katabuchi H, Okamura H, Miyazaki K. Expression of the angopoietin-1, angopoietin-2, Tie2, and vascular endothelial growth factor gene in epithelial ovarian cancer. *Gynecol Oncol*. 2004;93:215-222.
47. Ferrara N, Gerber HP, LeCouter J. The biology of VEGF and its receptors. *Nat Med*. 2003;9:669-676.
48. Smerdel MP, Waldstrom M, Brandslund I, Steffensen KD, Andersen RF, Jakobsen A. Prognostic importance of vascular endothelial growth factor-A expression and vascular endothelial growth factor polymorphisms in epithelial ovarian cancer. *Int J Gynecol Cancer*. 2009;19:578-584.
49. Martin L, Schilder R. Novel approaches in advancing the treatment of epithelial ovarian cancer: the role of angiogenesis inhibition. *J Clin Oncol*. 2007;25:2894-2901.
50. Verheul HMW, Hoekman K, Jorna AS, Smit EF, Pinedo HM. Targeting vascular endothelial growth factor blockade: ascites and pleural effusion formation. *Oncologist*. 2000;5:45-50.
51. Zebrowski BK, Liu W, Ramirez K, Akagi Y, Mills GB, Ellis LM. Markedly elevated levels of vascular endothelial growth factor in malignant ascites. *Ann Surg Oncol*. 1999;6:373-378.
52. Senger DR, Galli SJ, Dvorak AM, Perruzzi CA, Harvey VS, Dvorak HF. Tumor cells secrete a vascular permeability factor that promotes accumulation of ascites fluid. *Science*. 1983;219:983-985.
53. Numnum TM, Rocconi RP, Whitworth J, Barnes MN. The use of bevacizumab to palliate symptomatic ascites in patients with refractory ovarian carcinoma. *Gynecol Oncol*. 2006;102:425-428.
54. Burger RA, Sill MW, Monk BJ, Greer BE, Sorosky JI. Phase II trial of bevacizumab in persistent or recurrent epithelial ovarian cancer or primary peritoneal cancer: a Gynecologic Oncology Group study. *J Clin Oncol*. 2007;25:5165-5171.
55. Garcia AA, Hirte H, Fleming G, et al. Phase II clinical trial of bevacizumab and low-dose metronomic oral cyclophosphamide in recurrent ovarian cancer: a trial of the California, Chicago, and Princess Margaret Hospital phase II consortia. *J Clin Oncol*. 2008;26:76-82.
56. Cohn DE, Valmadre S, Resnick KE, Eaton LA, Copeland LJ, Fowler JM. Bevacizumab and weekly taxane chemotherapy demonstrates activity in refractory ovarian cancer. *Gynecol Oncol*. 2006;102:134-139.
57. Aghajanian C, Finkler NJ, Rutherford T, et al. OCEANS: a randomized, double-blinded, placebo-controlled phase III trial of chemotherapy with or without bevacizumab (BEV) in patients with platinum-sensitive recurrent epithelial ovarian (EOC), primary peritoneal (PPC), or fallopian tube cancer (FTC). *J Clin Oncol*. 2011;29(suppl). Abstract LBA5007.
58. Burger RA, Brady MF, Bookman MA, et al. Phase III trial of bevacizumab (BEV) in the primary treatment of advanced epithelial ovarian cancer (EOC), primary peritoneal cancer (PPC), or fallopian tube cancer (FTC): a Gynecologic Oncology Group study. *J Clin Oncol*. 2010;28:18s(suppl). Abstract LBA1.
59. Kristensen G, Perren T, Qian W, et al. Result of interim analysis of overall survival in the GCIG ICON7 phase III randomized trial of bevacizumab in women with newly diagnosed ovarian cancer. *J Clin Oncol*. 2011;29(suppl). Abstract LBA 5006.
60. Hochster HS. Bevacizumab in combination with chemotherapy: first-line treatment of patients with metastatic colorectal cancer. *Semin Oncol*. 2006;33:S8-S14.
61. Cannistra SA, Matulonis UA, Penson RT, et al. Phase II study of bevacizumab in patients with platinum-resistant ovarian cancer or peritoneal serous cancer. *J Clin Oncol*. 2007;25:5180-5186.
62. Kamat AA, Merritt WM, Coffey D, et al. Clinical and biological significance of vascular endothelial growth factor in endometrial cancer. *Clin Cancer Res*. 2007;13:7487-7495.
63. Stefansson IM, Salvesen HB, Akslen LA. Vascular proliferation is important for clinical progress of endometrial cancer. *Cancer Res*. 2006;66:3303-3309.
64. Aghajanian C, Sill MW, Darcy KM, et al. Phase II trial of bevacizumab in recurrent or persistent endometrial cancer: a Gynecologic Oncology Group study. *J Clin Oncol*. 2011;29:2259-2265.
65. Monk BJ, Sill MW, Burger RA, Gray HJ, Buekers TE, Roman LD. Phase II trial of bevacizumab in the treatment of persistent or recurrent squamous cell carcinoma of the cervix: a Gynecologic Oncology Group study. *J Clin Oncol*. 2009;27:1069-1074.
66. Dupont J, Rothenberg ML, Spriggs DR, et al. Safety and pharmacokinetics of intravenous VEGF Trap in a phase I clinical trial of patients with advanced solid tumors. *J Clin Oncol*. (Meeting Abstracts) 2005;23:3029.
67. Tew WP, Colombo N, Ray-Coquard I, et al. VEGF-Trap for patients (pts) with recurrent platinum-resistant epithelial ovarian cancer (EOC): preliminary results of a randomized, multicenter phase II study. *J Clin Oncol*. June 20, 2007;25(18S, suppl). Abstract 5508.
68. Coleman RL, Duska LR, Ramirez PT, et al. Phase 1–2 study of docetaxel plus aflibercept in patients with recurrent ovarian, primary peritoneal, or fallopian tube cancer. *Lancet Oncol*. 2011;12:1109-1117.
69. Colombo N, Mangili G, Mammoliti S, et al. A phase II study of aflibercept in patients with advanced epithelial ovarian cancer and symptomatic malignant ascites. *Gynecol Oncol*. April 2012;125(1):42-47.
70. Biagi JJ, Oza AM, Chalchal HI, et al. A phase II study of sunitinib in patients with recurrent epithelial ovarian and primary peritoneal carcinoma: an NCIC clinical trials group study. *Ann Oncol*. 2011;22:335-340.
71. Correa R, Mackay H, Hirte HW, et al. A phase II study of sunitinib in recurrent or metastatic endometrial carcinoma: a trial of the Princess Margaret Hospital, The University of Chicago, and California Cancer Phase II Consortia. *J Clin Oncol*. 2010;28(15S, suppl). Abstract 5038.
72. Matei D, Sill MW, Lankes HA, et al. Activity of sorafenib in recurrent ovarian cancer and primary peritoneal carcinomatosis: a Gynecologic Oncology Group trial. *J Clin Oncol*. 2011;29:69-75.
73. Nimeiri HS, Oza AM, Morgan RJ, et al. Sorafenib (SOR) in patients (pts) with advanced/recurrent uterine carcinoma (UCA) or carcinosarcoma (CS): a phase II trial of the University of Chicago, PMH, and California Phase II Consortia. *J Clin Oncol*. May 20, 2008;26(suppl). Abstract 5585.
74. Kikuchi Y, Takano M, Goto T, et al. Effects of weekly bevacizumab and paclitaxel/carboplatin with or without sorafenib on heavily pretreated patients with recurrent or persistent cervical cancer. *J Clin Oncol*. 2011;29(suppl). Abstract 5085.
75. Townsley CA, Milosevic M, Haider MA, et al. A phase I/II study of cisplatin and radiation in combination with sorafenib in cervical cancer: evaluation of biomarkers. *J Clin Oncol*. 2011;29(suppl). Abstract 5037.
76. Rosen L, Kurzrock R, Jackson E, et al. Safety and pharmacokinetics of AMG 706 in patients with advanced solid tumors. *J Clin Oncol*. June 1, 2005;23(16S Part I of II, suppl):3013.
77. Matulonis UA, Berlin S, Ivy P, et al. Cediranib, an oral inhibitor of vascular endothelial growth factor receptor kinases, is an active drug in recurrent epithelial ovarian, fallopian tube, and peritoneal cancer. *J Clin Oncol*. 2009;27:5601-5606.
78. Raja FA, Griffin CL, Qian W, et al. Initial toxicity assessment of ICON6: a randomised trial of cediranib plus chemotherapy in platinum-sensitive relapsed ovarian cancer. *Br J Cancer*. 2011;105:884-889.

79. Hurwitz HI, Dowlati A, Saini S, et al. Phase I trial of pazopanib in patients with advanced cancer. *Clin Cancer Res*. 2009;15: 4220-4227.
80. Friedlander M, Hancock KC, Rischin D, et al. A phase II, open-label study evaluating pazopanib in patients with recurrent ovarian cancer. *Gynecol Oncol*. 2010;119:32-37.
81. Monk BJ, Mas Lopez L, Zarba JJ, et al. Phase II, open-label study of pazopanib or lapatinib monotherapy compared with pazopanib plus lapatinib combination therapy in patients with advanced and recurrent cervical cancer. *J Clin Oncol*. 2010;28:3562-3569.
82. Herbst RS, Hong D, Chap L, et al. Safety, pharmacokinetics, and antitumor activity of AMG 386, a selective angiopoietin inhibitor, in adult patients with advanced solid tumors. *J Clin Oncol*. 2009;27:3557-3565.
83. Vergote I. A randomized, double-blind, placebo-controlled phase II study of AMG 386 plus weekly paclitaxel in patients (pts) with advanced ovarian cancer. In: Presented at the 35th European Society for Medical Oncology (ESMO) Congress; Milan, Italy. October 8-12, 2010. Abstract 975PD.
84. Wenham RM, Leach JW, Scudder SA, et al. Phase Ib study of AMG 386 combined with either pegylated liposomal doxorubicin (PLD) or topotecan (T) in patients with advanced ovarian cancer. *J Clin Oncol*. 2010;28(15S, suppl). Abstract 5049.
85. Ledermann JA, Hackshaw A, Kaye S, et al. Randomized phase II placebo-controlled trial of maintenance therapy using the oral triple angiokinase inhibitor BIBF 1120 after chemotherapy for relapsed ovarian cancer. *J Clin Oncol*. 2011;29:3798-3804.
86. Azad NS, Posadas EM, Kwitkowski VE, et al. Combination targeted therapy with sorafenib and bevacizumab results in enhanced toxicity and antitumor activity. *J Clin Oncol*. 2008;26:3709-3714.
87. Byzova TV, Goldman CK, Pampori N, et al. A mechanism for modulation of cellular responses to VEGF: activation of the integrins. *Mol Cell*. 2000;6:851-860.
88. Rosano L, Spinella F, Di Castro V, et al. Integrin-linked kinase functions as a downstream mediator of endothelin-1 to promote invasive behavior in ovarian carcinoma. *Mol Cancer Ther*. 2006;5:833-842.
89. Bell-McGuinn KM, Matthews CM, Ho SN, et al. A phase II, single-arm study of the anti-α5β1 integrin antibody volociximab as monotherapy in patients with platinum-resistant advanced epithelial ovarian or primary peritoneal cancer. *Gynecol Oncol*. 2011;121:273-279.
90. Lane HA, Wood JM, McSheehy PMJ, et al. mTOR inhibitor RAD001 (everolimus) has antiangiogenic/vascular properties distinct from a VEGFR tyrosine kinase inhibitor. *Clin Cancer Res*. 2009;15:1612-1622.
91. Meindl A, Hellebrand H, Wiek C, et al. Germline mutations in breast and ovarian cancer pedigrees establish RAD51C as a human cancer susceptibility gene. *Nat Genet*. 2010;42:410-414.
92. Loveday C, Turnbull C, Ramsay E, et al. Germline mutations in RAD51D confer susceptibility to ovarian cancer. *Nat Genet*. 2011;43:879-882.
93. Gelmon K, Tischkowitz M, Mackay H, et al. Olaparib in patients with recurrent high-grade serous or poorly differentiated ovarian carcinoma or triple-negative breast cancer: a phase 2, multicentre, open-label, non-randomised study. *Lancet Oncol*. 2011;12:852-861.
94. Fong PC, Boss DS, Yap TA, et al. Inhibition of poly(ADP-ribose) polymerase in tumors from BRCA mutation carriers. *N Engl J Med*. 2009;361:123-134.
95. Audeh MW, Carmichael J, Penson RT, et al. Oral poly(ADP-ribose) polymerase inhibitor olaparib in patients with BRCA1 or BRCA2 mutations and recurrent ovarian cancer: a proof-of-concept trial. *Lancet*. 2010;376:245-251.
96. Fong PC, Yap TA, Boss DS, et al. Poly(ADP)-ribose polymerase inhibition: frequent durable responses in BRCA carrier ovarian cancer correlating with platinum-free interval. *J Clin Oncol*. 2010;28:2512-2519.
97. Oza AM, Cibula D, Oaknin A, et al. Olaparib plus paclitaxel plus carboplatin (P/C) followed by olaparib maintenance in patients with platinum-sensitive recurrent serous ovarian cancer (PSR SOC): a randomized open label phase II study. *J Clin Oncol*. 2012;30(suppl). Abstract 5001.
98. Toffoli G, Cernigoi C, Russo A, Gallo A, Bagnoli M, Boiocchi M. Overexpression of folate binding protein in ovarian cancers. *Int J Cancer*. 1997;74:193-198.
99. Konner JA, Bell-McGuinn KM, Sabbatini P, et al. Farletuzumab, a humanized monoclonal antibody against folate receptor α, in epithelial ovarian cancer: a phase I study. *Clin Cancer Res*. 2010;16:5288-5295.
100. Armstrong DK, Bicher A, Coleman RL, et al. Exploratory phase II efficacy study of MORAb-003, a monoclonal antibody against folate receptor alpha, in platinum-sensitive ovarian cancer in first relapse. *J Clin Oncol*. May 20, 2008;26(suppl). Abstract 5500.
101. Peruzzi B, Bottaro DP. Targeting the c-Met signaling pathway in cancer. *Clin Cancer Res*. 2006;12:3657-3660.
102. Di Renzo MF, Narsimhan RP, Olivero M, et al. Expression of the Met/HGF receptor in normal and neoplastic human tissues. *Oncogene*. 1991;6:1997-2003.
103. Comoglio PM. Pathway specificity for Met signalling. *Nat Cell Biol*. 2001;3:E161-e162.
104. Di Renzo MF, Olivero M, Katsaros D, et al. Overexpression of the Met/HGF receptor in ovarian cancer. *Int J Cancer*. 1994;58:658-662.
105. Huntsman D, Resau JH, Klineberg E, Auersperg N. Comparison of c-met expression in ovarian epithelial tumors and normal epithelia of the female reproductive tract by quantitative laser scan microscopy. *Am J Pathol*. 1999;155:343-348.
106. Sawada K, Radjabi AR, Shinomiya N, et al. c-Met overexpression is a prognostic factor in ovarian cancer and an effective target for inhibition of peritoneal dissemination and invasion. *Cancer Res*. 2007;67:1670-1679.
107. Corps AN, Sowter HM, Smith SK. Hepatocyte growth factor stimulates motility, chemotaxis and mitogenesis in ovarian carcinoma cells expressing high levels of c-met. *Int J Cancer*. 1997;73:151-155.
108. Wong AS, Leung PC, Auersperg N. Hepatocyte growth factor promotes in vitro scattering and morphogenesis of human cervical carcinoma cells. *Gynecol Oncol*. 2000;78:158-165.
109. Wong AS, Pelech SL, Woo MM, et al. Coexpression of hepatocyte growth factor-Met: an early step in ovarian carcinogenesis? *Oncogene*. 2001;20:1318-1328.
110. Xin X, Yang S, Ingle G, et al. Hepatocyte growth factor enhances vascular endothelial growth factor-induced angiogenesis in vitro and in vivo. *Am J Pathol*. 2001;158:1111-1120.
111. Weidner KM, Sachs M, Birchmeier W. The Met receptor tyrosine kinase transduces motility, proliferation, and morphogenic signals of scatter factor/hepatocyte growth factor in epithelial cells. *J Cell Biol*. 1993;121:145-154.
112. Burgess T, Coxon A, Meyer S, et al. Fully human monoclonal antibodies to hepatocyte growth factor with therapeutic potential against hepatocyte growth factor/c-Met-dependent human tumors. *Cancer Res*. 2006;66:1721-1729.
113. Cao B, Su Y, Oskarsson M, et al. Neutralizing monoclonal antibodies to hepatocyte growth factor/scatter factor (HGF/SF) display antitumor activity in animal models. *Proc Natl Acad Sci U S A*. 2001;98:7443-7448.
114. Jun HT, Sun J, Rex K, et al. AMG 102, a fully human anti-hepatocyte growth factor/scatter factor neutralizing antibody, enhances the efficacy of temozolomide or docetaxel in U-87 MG cells and xenografts. *Clin Cancer Res*. 2007;13:6735-6742.
115. Jones SF, Cohen RB, Bendell JC, et al. Safety, tolerability, and pharmacokinetics of TAK-701, a humanized anti-hepatocyte growth factor (HGF) monoclonal antibody, in patients with advanced nonhematologic malignancies: first-in-human phase I dose-escalation study. *J Clin Oncol*. 2010;28(15S, suppl). Abstract 3081.
116. Yakes FM, Chen J, Tan J, et al. Cabozantinib (XL184), a novel MET and VEGFR2 inhibitor, simultaneously suppresses metastasis, angiogenesis, and tumor growth. *Mol Cancer Ther*. 2011;10:2298-2308.
117. Buckanovich RJ, Berger R, Sella A, et al. Activity of cabozantinib (XL184) in advanced ovarian cancer patients (pts): results from a phase II randomized discontinuation trial (RDT). *J Clin Oncol*. (Meeting Abstract) 2011;29:5008.
118. Rahman S, Patel Y, Murray J, et al. Novel hepatocyte growth factor (HGF) binding domains on fibronectin and vitronectin coordinate a distinct and amplified Met-integrin induced signalling pathway in endothelial cells. *BMC Cell Biol*. 2005;6:8.
119. Trusolino L, Bertotti A, Comoglio PM. A signaling adapter function for alpha6beta4 integrin in the control of HGF-dependent invasive growth. *Cell*. 2001;107:643-654.

120. Engelman JA, Zejnullahu K, Mitsudomi T, et al. MET amplification leads to gefitinib resistance in lung cancer by activating ERBB3 signaling. *Science*. 2007;316:1039-1043.
121. Gross ME, Shazer RL, Agus DB. Targeting the HER-kinase axis in cancer. *Semin Oncol*. 2004;31:9-20.
122. Burgess AW, Cho HS, Eigenbrot C, et al. An open-and-shut case? Recent insights into the activation of EGF/ErbB receptors. *Mol Cell*. 2003;12:541-552.
123. Berchuck A, Rodriguez GC, Kamel A, et al. Epidermal growth factor receptor expression in normal ovarian epithelium and ovarian cancer. I. Correlation of receptor expression with prognostic factors in patients with ovarian cancer. *Am J Obstet Gynecol*. 1991;164:669-674.
124. Bartlett JM, Langdon SP, Simpson BJ, et al. The prognostic value of epidermal growth factor receptor mRNA expression in primary ovarian cancer. *Br J Cancer*. 1996;73:301-306.
125. Khalifa MA, Mannel RS, Haraway SD, Walker J, Min K-W. Expression of EGFR, HER-2/neu, P53, and PCNA in endometrioid, serous papillary, and clear cell endometrial adenocarcinomas. *Gynecol Oncol*. 1994;53:84-92.
126. Kersemaekers A-MF, Fleuren GJ, Kenter GG, et al. Oncogene alterations in carcinomas of the uterine cervix: overexpression of the epidermal growth factor receptor is associated with poor prognosis. *Clin Cancer Res*. 1999;5:577-586.
127. Baselga J, Pfister D, Cooper MR, et al. Phase I studies of anti-epidermal growth factor receptor chimeric antibody C225 alone and in combination with cisplatin. *J Clin Oncol*. 2000;18:904-914.
128. Schilder RJ, Pathak HB, Lokshin AE, et al. Phase II trial of single agent cetuximab in patients with persistent or recurrent epithelial ovarian or primary peritoneal carcinoma with the potential for dose escalation to rash. *Gynecol Oncol*. 2009;113:21-27.
129. Konner J, Schilder RJ, DeRosa FA, et al. A phase II study of cetuximab/paclitaxel/carboplatin for the initial treatment of advanced-stage ovarian, primary peritoneal, or fallopian tube cancer. *Gynecol Oncol*. 2008;110:140-145.
130. Secord AA, Blessing JA, Armstrong DK, et al. Phase II trial of cetuximab and carboplatin in relapsed platinum-sensitive ovarian cancer and evaluation of epidermal growth factor receptor expression: a Gynecologic Oncology Group study. *Gynecol Oncol*. 2008;108:493-499.
131. Santin AD, Sill MW, McMeekin DS, et al. Phase II trial of cetuximab in the treatment of persistent or recurrent squamous or non-squamous cell carcinoma of the cervix: a Gynecologic Oncology Group study. *Gynecol Oncol*. 2011;122:495-500.
132. Farley J, Sill MW, Birrer M, et al. Phase II study of cisplatin plus cetuximab in advanced, recurrent, and previously treated cancers of the cervix and evaluation of epidermal growth factor receptor immunohistochemical expression: a Gynecologic Oncology Group study. *Gynecol Oncol*. 2011;121:303-308.
133. Slomovitz B, Schmeler K, Miller D, et al. Phase II study of cetuximab (erbitux) in patients with progressive or recurrent endometrial cancer. *Gynecol Oncol*. 2010;116(suppl 1). Abstract.
134. Schilder RJ, Sill MW, Chen X, et al. Phase II study of gefitinib in patients with relapsed or persistent ovarian or primary peritoneal carcinoma and evaluation of epidermal growth factor receptor mutations and immunohistochemical expression: a Gynecologic Oncology Group study. *Clin Cancer Res*. 2005;11:5539-5548.
135. Lynch TJ, Bell DW, Sordella R, et al. Activating mutations in the epidermal growth factor receptor underlying responsiveness of non-small-cell lung cancer to gefitinib. *N Engl J Med*. 2004;350:2129-2139.
136. Paez JG, Janne PA, Lee JC, et al. EGFR mutations in lung cancer: correlation with clinical response to gefitinib therapy. *Science*. 2004;304:1497-1500.
137. Goncalves A, Fabbro M, Lhommé C, et al. A phase II trial to evaluate gefitinib as second- or third-line treatment in patients with recurring locoregionally advanced or metastatic cervical cancer. *Gynecol Oncol*. 2008;108:42-46.
138. Leslie KK, Sill MW, Darcy KM, et al. Efficacy and safety of gefitinib and potential prognostic value of soluble EGFR, EGFR mutations, and tumor markers in a Gynecologic Oncology Group phase II trial of persistent or recurrent endometrial cancer. *J Clin Oncol*. 2009;27(suppl). Abstract e16542.
139. Herbst RS, Johnson DH, Mininberg E, et al. Phase I/II trial evaluating the anti-vascular endothelial growth factor monoclonal antibody bevacizumab in combination with the HER-1/epidermal growth factor receptor tyrosine kinase inhibitor erlotinib for patients with recurrent non-small-cell lung cancer. *J Clin Oncol*. 2005;23:2544-2555.
140. Gordon AN, Finkler N, Edwards RP, et al. Efficacy and safety of erlotinib HCl, an epidermal growth factor receptor (HER1/EGFR) tyrosine kinase inhibitor, in patients with advanced ovarian carcinoma: results from a phase II multicenter study. *Int J Gynecol Cancer*. 2005;15:785-792.
141. Blank SV, Curtin JP, Goldman NA, et al. Tolerability of carboplatin, paclitaxel and erlotinib as first-line treatment of ovarian cancer. *J Clin Oncol*. June 1, 2005;23(16S Part I of II, suppl):5052.
142. Vasey PA, Gore M, Wilson R, et al. A phase Ib trial of docetaxel, carboplatin and erlotinib in ovarian, fallopian tube and primary peritoneal cancers. *Br J Cancer*. 2008;98:1774-1780.
143. Holmberg LA, Goff B, Veljovich D. Unexpected gastrointestinal toxicity from Docetaxel/Carboplatin/Erlotinib followed by maintenance erlotinib treatment for newly diagnosed stage III/IV ovarian cancer, primary peritoneal, or fallopian tube cancer. *Gynecol Oncol*. 2011;121:426.
144. Blank SV, Christos P, Curtin JP, et al. Erlotinib added to carboplatin and paclitaxel as first-line treatment of ovarian cancer: a phase II study based on surgical reassessment. *Gynecol Oncol*. 2010;119:451-456.
145. Oza AM, Eisenhauer EA, Elit L, et al. Phase II study of erlotinib in recurrent or metastatic endometrial cancer: NCIC IND-148. *J Clin Oncol*. 2008;26:4319-4325.
146. Schilder RJ, Sill MWP, Lee Y-CM, Mannel RM. A phase II trial of erlotinib in recurrent squamous cell carcinoma of the cervix: a Gynecologic Oncology Group study. *Int J Gynecol Cancer*. 2009;19:929-933.
147. Bookman MA, Darcy KM, Clarke-Pearson D, Boothby RA, Horowitz IR. Evaluation of monoclonal humanized anti-HER2 antibody, trastuzumab, in patients with recurrent or refractory ovarian or primary peritoneal carcinoma with overexpression of HER2: a phase II trial of the Gynecologic Oncology Group. *J Clin Oncol*. 2003;21:283-290.
148. Fleming GF, Sill MW, Darcy KM, et al. Phase II trial of trastuzumab in women with advanced or recurrent, HER2-positive endometrial carcinoma: a Gynecologic Oncology Group study. *Gynecol Oncol*. 2010;116:15-20.
149. Agus DB, Gordon MS, Taylor C, et al. Phase I clinical study of pertuzumab, a novel HER dimerization inhibitor, in patients with advanced cancer. *J Clin Oncol*. 2005;23:2534-2543.
150. Gordon MS, Matei D, Aghajanian C, et al. Clinical activity of pertuzumab (rhuMAb 2C4), a HER dimerization inhibitor, in advanced ovarian cancer: potential predictive relationship with tumor HER2 activation status. *J Clin Oncol*. 2006;24:4324-4332.
151. Agus DB, Akita RW, Fox WD, et al. Targeting ligand-activated ErbB2 signaling inhibits breast and prostate tumor growth. *Cancer Cell*. 2002;2:127-137.
152. Makhija S, Amler LC, Glenn D, et al. Clinical activity of gemcitabine plus pertuzumab in platinum-resistant ovarian cancer, fallopian tube cancer, or primary peritoneal cancer. *J Clin Oncol*. 2010;28:1215-1223.
153. Nahta R, Hung MC, Esteva FJ. The HER-2-targeting antibodies trastuzumab and pertuzumab synergistically inhibit the survival of breast cancer cells. *Cancer Res*. 2004;64:2343-2346.
154. Friess T, Scheuer W, Hasmann M. Combination treatment with erlotinib and pertuzumab against human tumor xenografts is superior to monotherapy. *Clin Cancer Res*. 2005;11:5300-5309.
155. Burris HA III, Hurwitz HI, Dees EC, et al. Phase I safety, pharmacokinetics, and clinical activity study of lapatinib (GW572016), a reversible dual inhibitor of epidermal growth factor receptor tyrosine kinases, in heavily pretreated patients with metastatic carcinomas. *J Clin Oncol*. 2005;23:5305-5313.
156. Dees EC, Burris H, Hurwitz H, et al. Clinical summary of 67 heavily pre-treated patients with metastatic carcinomas treated with GW572016 in a phase Ib study. *J Clin Oncol*. July 15, 2004;22(14S, suppl):3188.

157. Garcia AA, Sill MW, Lankes HA, et al. A phase II evaluation of lapatinib in the treatment of persistent or recurrent epithelial ovarian or primary peritoneal carcinoma: a Gynecologic Oncology Group study. *Gynecol Oncol.*
158. Wells A. Tumor invasion: role of growth factor-induced cell motility. *Adv Cancer Res.* 2000;78:31-101.
159. Ahmed N, Maines-Bandiera S, Quinn MA, Unger WG, Dedhar S, Auersperg N. Molecular pathways regulating EGF-induced epithelio-mesenchymal transition in human ovarian surface epithelium. *Am J Physiol Cell Physiol.* 2006;290: C1532-C1542.
160. Firth SM, Baxter RC. Cellular actions of the insulin-like growth factor binding proteins. *Endocr Rev.* 2002;23:824-854.
161. Chitnis MM, Yuen JS, Protheroe AS, Pollak M, Macaulay VM. The type 1 insulin-like growth factor receptor pathway. *Clin Cancer Res.* 2008;14:6364-6370.
162. Cohen BD, Baker DA, Soderstrom C, et al. Combination therapy enhances the inhibition of tumor growth with the fully human anti-type 1 insulin-like growth factor receptor monoclonal antibody CP-751,871. *Clin Cancer Res.* 2005;11:2063-2073.
163. Haluska P, Shaw HM, Batzel GN, et al. Phase I dose escalation study of the anti insulin-like growth factor-I receptor monoclonal antibody CP-751,871 in patients with refractory solid tumors. *Clin Cancer Res.* 2007;13:5834-5840.
164. Tolcher AW, Sarantopoulos J, Patnaik A, et al. Phase I, pharmacokinetic, and pharmacodynamic study of AMG 479, a fully human monoclonal antibody to insulin-like growth factor receptor 1. *J Clin Oncol.* 2009;27:5800-5807.
165. Lindsay CR, Chan E, Evans TR, et al. Phase I dose escalation study of continuous oral dosing of OSI-906, an insulin like growth factor-1 receptor (IGF-1R) tyrosine kinase inhibitor, in patients with advanced solid tumors. *J Clin Oncol.* 2009;27(suppl). Abstract 2559.
166. Smith DC, Britten C, Garon EB, et al. A phase I study of XL228, a multitargeted protein kinase inhibitor, in patients (pts) with solid tumors or multiple myeloma. *J Clin Oncol.* 2010;28(15S, suppl). Abstract 3105.
167. Esparis-Ogando A, Rodriguez-Barrueco R, Borges J, Ferreira L, Pandiella A, Ocana A. Insulin-like growth factor-I receptor kinase inhibitor NVP-AEW541 is active in breast cancer cells and enhances growth inhibition by herceptin through an increase in cell cycle arrest. *J Clin Oncol.* June 20, 2007;25(18S, suppl): 21077.
168. Bjornsti MA, Houghton PJ. The TOR pathway: a target for cancer therapy. *Nat Rev Cancer.* 2004;4:335-348.
169. Altomare DA, Wang HQ, Skele KL, et al. AKT and mTOR phosphorylation is frequently detected in ovarian cancer and can be targeted to disrupt ovarian tumor cell growth. *Oncogene.* 2004;23:5853-5857.
170. Wullschleger S, Loewith R, Hall MN. TOR signaling in growth and metabolism. *Cell.* 2006;124:471-484.
171. Hidalgo M, Rowinsky EK. The rapamycin-sensitive signal transduction pathway as a target for cancer therapy. *Oncogene.* 2000;19:6680-6686.
172. Bellacosa A, de Feo D, Godwin AK, et al. Molecular alterations of the AKT2 oncogene in ovarian and breast carcinomas. *Int J Cancer.* 1995;64:280-285.
173. Altomare DA, Testa JR. Perturbations of the AKT signaling pathway in human cancer. *Oncogene.* 2005;24:7455-7464.
174. Mabuchi S, Altomare DA, Cheung M, et al. RAD001 inhibits human ovarian cancer cell proliferation, enhances cisplatin-induced apoptosis, and prolongs survival in an ovarian cancer model. *Clin Cancer Res.* 2007;13:4261-4270.
175. Slomovitz BM, Lu KH, Johnston T, et al. A phase 2 study of the oral mammalian target of rapamycin inhibitor, everolimus, in patients with recurrent endometrial carcinoma. *Cancer.* 2010;116:5415-5419.
176. Behbakht K, Sill MW, Darcy KM, et al. Phase II trial of the mTOR inhibitor, temsirolimus and evaluation of circulating tumor cells and tumor biomarkers in persistent and recurrent epithelial ovarian and primary peritoneal malignancies: a Gynecologic Oncology Group study. *Gynecol Oncol.* 2011;123:19-26.
177. Oza AM, Elit L, Tsao M-S, et al. Phase II study of temsirolimus in women with recurrent or metastatic endometrial cancer: a trial of the NCIC clinical trials group. *J Clin Oncol.* 2011;29:3278-3285.
178. Mackay H, Welch S, Tsao MS, et al. Phase II study of oral ridaforolimus in patients with metastatic and/or locally advanced recurrent endometrial cancer: NCIC CTG IND 192. *J Clin Oncol.* 2011;29(suppl). Abstract 5013.
179. Boutros T, Chevet E, Metrakos P. Mitogen-activated protein (MAP) kinase/map kinase phosphatase regulation: roles in cell growth, death, and cancer. *Pharmacol Rev.* 2008;60:261-310.
180. Pearson G, Robinson F, Beers Gibson T, et al. Mitogen-activated protein (MAP) kinase pathways: regulation and physiological functions. *Endocr Rev.* 2001;22:153-183.
181. Schubbert S, Shannon K, Bollag G. Hyperactive Ras in developmental disorders and cancer. *Nat Rev Cancer.* 2007;7:295-308.
182. Davies H, Bignell GR, Cox C, et al. Mutations of the BRAF gene in human cancer. *Nature.* 2002;417:949-954.
183. Chapman PB, Hauschild A, Robert C, et al. Improved survival with vemurafenib in melanoma with BRAF V600E mutation. *N Engl J Med.* 2011;364:2507-2516.
184. Kefford R, Arkenau H, Brown MP, et al. Phase I/II study of GSK2118436, a selective inhibitor of oncogenic mutant BRAF kinase, in patients with metastatic melanoma and other solid tumors. *J Clin Oncol.* 2010;28(15S, suppl). Abstract 8503.
185. Infante JR, Falchook GS, Lawrence DP, et al. Phase I/II study to assess safety, pharmacokinetics, and efficacy of the oral MEK 1/2 inhibitor GSK1120212 (GSK212) dosed in combination with the oral BRAF inhibitor GSK2118436 (GSK436). *J Clin Oncol.* 2011;29(suppl). Abstract CRA8503.
186. Carvajal RD, Tse A, Schwartz GK. Aurora kinases: new targets for cancer therapy. *Clin Cancer Res.* 2006;12:6869-6875.
187. Lin YG, Immaneni A, Merritt WM, et al. Targeting aurora kinase with MK-0457 inhibits ovarian cancer growth. *Clin Cancer Res.* 2008;14:5437-5446.
188. Landen CN Jr, Lin YG, Immaneni A, et al. Overexpression of the centrosomal protein Aurora-A kinase is associated with poor prognosis in epithelial ovarian cancer patients. *Clin Cancer Res.* 2007;13:4098-4104.
189. Matulonis UA, Sharma S, Ghamande S. Single-agent activity and safety of the investigational Aurora A kinase inhibitor MLN8237 in patients with platinum-treated epithelial ovarian, fallopian tube, or primary peritoneal carcinoma. *Ann Oncol.* 2010;2010:viii305. Abstract 974PD.

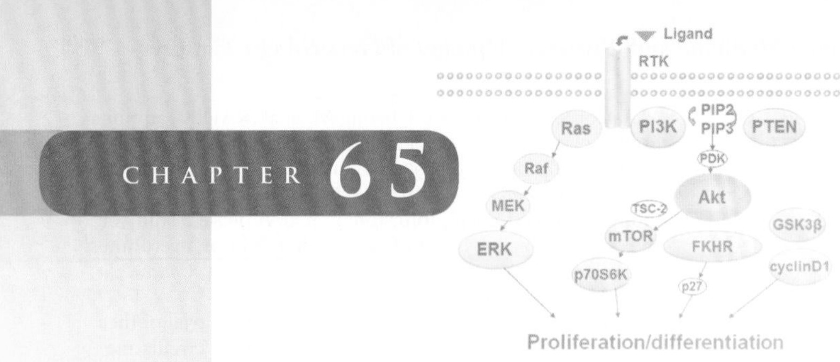

CHAPTER 65

PERSONALIZED MEDICINE AND TARGETED THERAPY OF RENAL CELL CARCINOMA

C. Lance Cowey and Thomas E. Hutson

INTRODUCTION

The therapeutic arsenal for the management of renal cell carcinoma (RCC) has received a surge of new targeted medicines over the last several years, with the Food and Drug Administration (FDA) approval of six new agents and several others in late stages of development. This explosion of therapies has been based on critical advancements in the understanding of RCC molecular biology. With the rapid introduction of new molecularly based agents, clinicians who manage patients with advanced RCC are in great need of sequencing studies and biomarker development to help guide selection among this myriad of treatment options. This chapter will discuss the currently available and upcoming targeted therapies for advanced RCC and the current status of molecular and genetic biomarkers which are being studied and how these markers may impact the field. Additionally, an overview of the current understanding of the molecular biology of RCC will be provided to give the reader the background in which these therapies and markers are being developed.

RCC MOLECULAR BIOLOGY

For United States in 2011, it was predicted that there will be 60,920 numbers of new RCC cases diagnosed and 13,120 numbers of deaths.[1] RCC is a diagnosis that covers a broad group of histologic subtypes, with the most frequent histology being clear cell RCC which occurs in about 75% of cases and the remainder including papillary (~15%), chromophobe (~5%), and oncocytoma (~5%). Over the last 20 years, there have been several major advancements in the understanding of clear cell RCC molecular biology due in a large part to the exploration of hereditary RCC syndrome pathogenesis. von Hippel-Lindau disease is an autosomal dominant hereditary disorder characterized by a constellation of clinical findings, including clear cell RCC, pheochromocytoma, hemangioblastomas, and visceral cysts.[2] Patients with this hereditary syndrome are prone to develop early onset and recurrent clear cell RCCs, which are often bilateral and multifocal in nature. In the early 1990s von Hippel-Lindau disease was found to be the result of a germline mutation in the VHL gene which is located on the short arm of chromosome 3.[3] This gene encodes for a protein that functions as part of an ubiquitin ligase, targeting an important family of transcription factors for degradation known as hypoxia-inducible factors (HIF).[4] The HIF factors, HIF-1 and HIF-2, appear to be the most important in RCC pathogenesis. In normal cellular physiology, the VHL protein recognizes HIF molecules via hydroxylated prolyl residues on the protein, marks them with an ubiquitin tail, and then the polyubiquitinated HIF molecules can be destroyed by the cellular proteasome (Fig. 65.1).[5,6] The prolyl hydroxylation process of HIF is oxygen-dependent, thus creating a cell's oxygen "sensing" capacity. When oxygen levels are low, the prolyl hydroxylase enzyme is unable to act on HIF and therefore HIF levels are allowed to increase which results in the transcription factor being able to bind to its target genes in the nucleus promoting cell survival. Among these HIF target genes are vascular endothelial growth factor (VEGF), platelet-derived growth factor (PDGF), angiopoietin (Ang), epidermal growth factor, carbonic anhydrase IX (CAIX), fibroblast growth factor (FGF), and erythropoietin (EPO).[7,8] These molecular discoveries have shed light on why we observe certain clinical features of clear cell RCC, for example, the marked vascularity of RCC tumors (via activation of VEGF and other pro-angiogenesis genes) and the presence of erythrocytosis (via activation of the EPO gene).

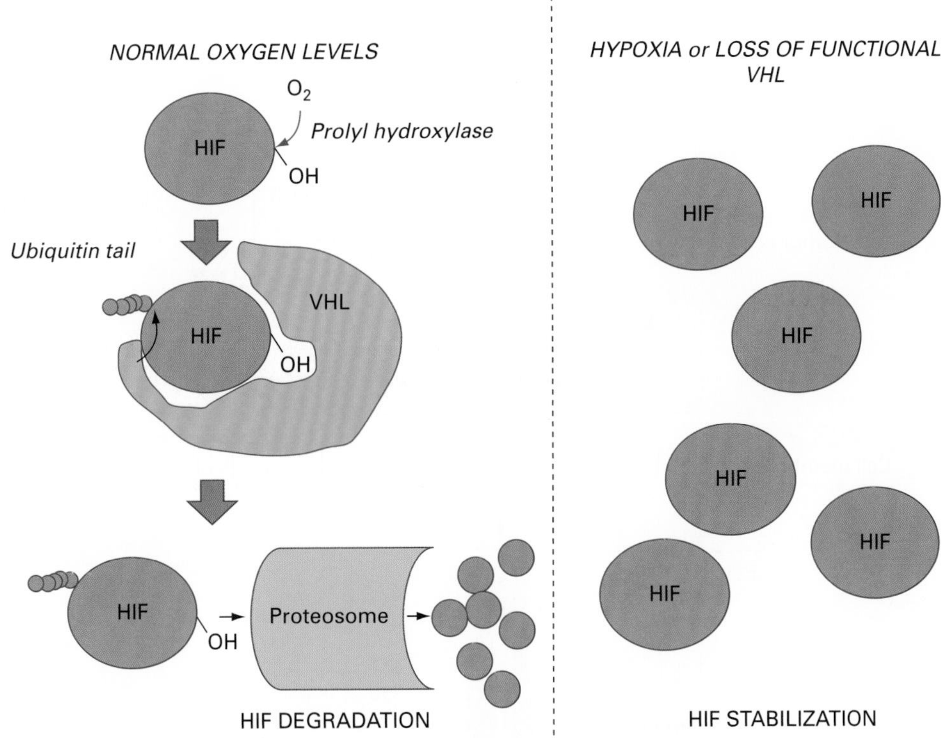

FIGURE 65–1 Regulation of hypoxia-inducible factor (HIF) via von Hippel-Lindau (VHL) ubiquitin ligase activity. Under normal oxygen conditions, the HIF undergoes hydroxylation by the prolyl hydroxylase enzyme. Prolyl hydroxylated HIF is then recognized by the VHL protein ubiquitin ligase complex and a ubiquitin tail is added to the HIF molecule which marks it for degradation by the intracellular proteasome. However, under hypoxic conditions (no prolyl hydroxylase activity) or with lack of functional VHL (via genetic mutation, methylation, etc.), the HIF transcription factor is stabilized and intracellular concentrations increase, allowing for migration to the nucleus and activation of HIF transcriptional gene targets.

In a great majority of sporadic cases of clear cell RCC, an acquired genetic abnormality affecting VHL function has been discovered to be present.[7,9,10] Without functional VHL protein, HIF concentrations are allowed to increase in a non–oxygen-dependent manner within the cell with resultant activation of the wide variety of target genes that can aid in uncontrolled tumor formation, growth, and spread. There are additional other non–oxygen-dependent pathways that play an important role in HIF upregulation, and these pathways can affect tumor cells by augmenting HIF synthesis. Among these growth pathways are the mitogen-activated protein kinase (MAP kinase) pathway[11] and the phosphatidylinositol 3-kinase (PI3K)-Akt-mTOR (mammalian target of rapamycin) pathway. It is based on the increased understanding of this molecular link between VHL and HIF target gene activation that has led to the introduction of a variety of new targeted therapeutics, particularly VEGF and mTOR pathway inhibitors, and will hopefully lead to further therapies and unique molecular biomarker identification (Fig. 65.2).

RCC THERAPEUTIC OVERVIEW

To date, there have been three main classes of drugs approved by the FDA for the treatment of RCC. These classes include immunotherapeutics (the cytokines interferon [IFN] and interleukin-2 [IL-2]), anti-angiogenesis inhibitors (the VEGF pathway inhibitors), and inhibitors of the mTOR complex. For many years, the cytokines, IFN and IL-2, were the only therapeutic options. These drugs demonstrated limited efficacy for the average patient and were approved based on their potential for a durable remission in a small subset of RCC patients.[12] Additionally, these cytokines have widely been criticized for the increased toxicities associated with them, particularly high-dose IL-2. Notably, RCC tumors are resistant to traditional cytotoxic chemotherapeutics for the most part with numerous phase II trials showing little in terms of efficacy.[13]

More recently, a wave of new therapeutics has emerged based on the increased molecular understanding of RCC, in particular many agents that impact the VEGF pathway (Table 65.1). These VEGF inhibitors include several small molecule VEGF tyrosine kinase inhibitors (VEGF TKIs), including sorafenib, sunitinib, pazopanib, and bevacizumab. The other important class of agents that have gained a place in metastatic RCC therapeutics are the mTOR inhibitors. The mTOR complex is a part of the PI3K–AKT signaling pathway and at least part of mTOR's biologic relevance in RCC is that it is an upstream mediator of HIF synthesis.[26] The mTOR inhibitors that have gained the FDA approval for advanced RCC include temsirolimus and everolimus. Despite the approval of several agents in these two different classes of

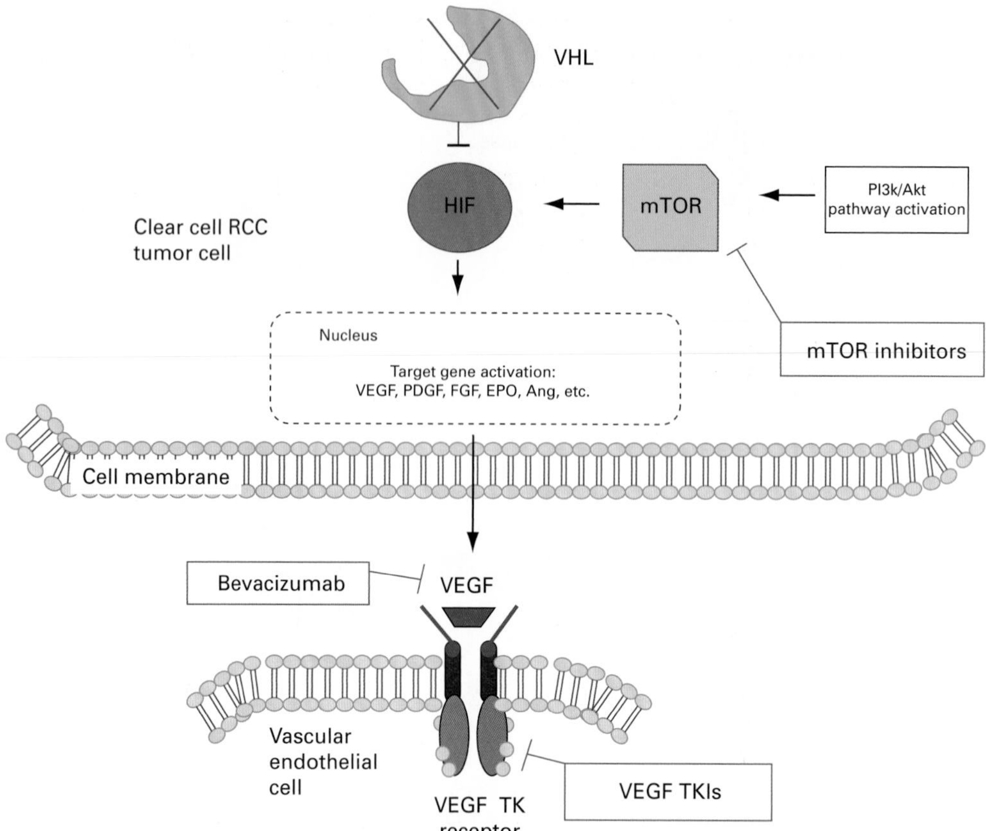

FIGURE 65–2 Molecular biology of RCC and activity of targeted therapies. VHL function is lost in the majority of sporadic clear cell RCC tumors, allowing for HIF-1/2 transcription factor stabilization. The PI3K/Akt/mTOR pathway promotes HIF synthesis. HIF stabilization results in expression of numerous pro-tumorigenic genes, including VEGF which promotes tumor angiogenesis. The currently approved classes of drugs target VEGF (VEGF tyrosine kinase inhibitors [VEGF TKIs] and bevacizumab) and mTOR complex (mTOR inhibitors).

drugs, there is great room for the addition of novel therapeutics which can impact resistance pathways to VEGF or mTOR inhibition or affect other relevant molecular pathways in RCC.

ANGIOGENESIS INHIBITORS

Angiogenesis is one of the well-known hallmarks of cancer. Since Michaelson's[27] early work describing a pro-angiogenic factor which was critical to new blood vessel formation, much has been learned about the VEGF pathway. Via genetic splicing of the VEGF gene, several isoforms of VEGF can be produced which have different roles in angiogenesis and lymphangiogenesis.[28] Perhaps, the most critically important isoform is VEGF-A which binds to VEGF-R1 and VEGF-R2 on the vascular endothelial cell surface and stimulates endothelial cell survival, proliferation, and migration to create new blood vessel sprouting. Given that loss of VHL protein function in RCC tumors augments HIF-induced VEGF gene expression, it is no wonder that these tumors are quite vascular and respond to VEGF pathway inhibition.

In fact, targeting of the VEGF pathway has been a fruitful approach in a variety of cancer types in combination with cytotoxic chemotherapies (for instance, bevacizumab in colon, lung, and breast cancer); however, the benefit of VEGF inhibitors has been even more pronounced in advanced RCC with *single-agent use* of a VEGF inhibitor resulting in dramatic clinical benefit. This is the direct result of the unique dependence of RCC tumors on VEGF-induced angiogenesis that stems from the previously described aberrances in the VHL gene. Of note, as opposed to cytotoxic chemotherapies or other intracellular protein molecularly targeted agents, targeting of the VEGF pathway is a means of disrupting tumor stromal function rather than having direct cytotoxic effects on the cancer cells themselves.

To date, there have been two main approaches in blocking VEGF signaling. One approach is using small molecule inhibitors of the VEGF tyrosine kinase which is present on the vascular endothelial cells within the tumor. The other approach is using a monoclonal antibody to bind the VEGF ligand, thus preventing signaling on the receptor. The FDA-approved VEGF TKIs for RCC are discussed in this chapter, including sorafenib, sunitinib, and pazopanib. The VEGF TKIs, axitinib and tivozanib, are not only currently FDA approved but also worthy of discussion. Also, we review the data on bevacizumab

TABLE 65-1 Currently FDA-Approved Molecularly Targeted Agents for Renal Cell Carcinoma

FDA-Approved Molecularly Targeted Agent	Mechanism of Action	Phase III Trial Patient Population	Clinical Activity	Common Toxicities	References
VEGF pathway inhibitors					
Sorafenib	Oral multi-targeted VEGF TKI	Prior cytokine	Prolonged PFS compared with placebo (5.5 vs. 2.8 mo, $P < 0.000001$)	Diarrhea, rash, fatigue, and hand–foot syndrome	14,15
Sunitinib	Oral multi-targeted VEGF TKI	Treatment-naïve	Prolonged PFS compared with IFN (11 vs. 5 mo, $P < 0.001$)	Diarrhea, rash, fatigue, hand–foot syndrome, and hypertension	16,17
Pazopanib	Oral multi-targeted VEGF TKI	Treatment-naïve or prior cytokine	Prolonged PFS compared with placebo (9.2 vs. 4.2 mo, $P < 0.0001$)	Diarrhea, hypertension, hair color changes, nausea, and anorexia	18
Bevacizumab	Intravenous monoclonal antibody to VEGF-A	Treatment-naïve	Prolonged PFS in combination with IFN compared with IFN alone (AVOREN trial: 10.2 vs. 5.4 mo, $P = 0.0001$; CALGB trial: 8.5 vs. 5.2 mo, $P < 0.0001$)	Fatigue, pyrexia, anorexia, hypertension, and proteinuria	19–22
mTOR inhibitors					
Temsirolimus	Intravenous inhibitor of mTORC1 complex	Treatment-naïve	Prolonged OS compared with IFN (10.9 vs. 7.3 mo, $P = 0.0.008$) and PFS compared with IFN (5.5 vs. 3.1 mo, $P < 0.001$)	Rash, peripheral edema, hyperglycemia, and hypertriglyceridemia	23
Everolimus	Oral inhibitor of mTOR1 complex	Prior VEGF TKI	Prolonged PFS compared with placebo (4.9 vs. 1.9 mo, $P < 0.001$)	Stomatitis, rash, fatigue, and diarrhea	24,25

VEGF, vascular endothelial growth factor; TKI, tyrosine kinase inhibitor; IFN, interferon; PFS, progression-free survival; mTOR, mammalian target of rapamycin; mTORC1, mTOR complex 1; OS, overall survival.

which is a monoclonal antibody directed against VEGF and also FDA approved for use in RCC. Finally, we discuss new angiogenesis targeted therapies which inhibit molecules outside of the VEGF pathway and their potential role in the management of VEGF inhibition escape.

VEGF TKIs

Sorafenib

The first FDA-approved VEGF pathway inhibitor for RCC was sorafenib. This oral agent is a multi-targeted TKI which binds to VEGF-R2–3, PDGF-Rβ, RAF, FLT-3, and c-kit. This drug was first evaluated for its ability as an RAF inhibitor (CRAF >> BRAF) but soon discovered that it was a more potent inhibitor of other tyrosine kinases such as VEGF. Based on its merits as a more potent VEGF TKI, it was further explored in a randomized phase II discontinuation study in patients with advanced RCC.[29] This study included 202 patients with advanced RCC who received treatment with sorafenib for 12 weeks at which time tumor response was assessed. Most of these patients had received some prior systemic therapy (84%), most commonly cytokine therapy (76%). At the 12-week evaluation point, patients who had >25% shrinkage of their tumor burden were allowed to continue sorafenib, patients who had >25% growth of their tumor were discontinued from the study, and patients in between 25% growth and 25% shrinkage were randomized to continue sorafenib or receive placebo. The primary end point of study was 24-week progression-free survival (PFS) of those who were randomized at the 12-week mark. At the 24-week mark, 50% of patients randomized to sorafenib were progression free compared with 18% of those receiving placebo ($P = 0.0077$). The overall PFS for patients treated with sorafenib was 40 weeks.

The striking results of the phase II study led to a large, multicenter randomized placebo-controlled phase III study (TARGET trial) of sorafenib in advanced RCC patients who had received prior cytokine therapy (IL-2 and IFN).[14] This study included 903 patients who were randomized to sorafenib or placebo, and the primary end point was overall survival (OS). Secondary end points included overall response rate (ORR) and PFS. Sorafenib did not improve survival for this group of patients (median survival of 17.8 mo compared with 15.2 mo, $P = 0.146$); however, this may be explained by patient crossover to sorafenib after progression on placebo. When these results were updated, evaluation of patients who did not cross over to sorafenib showed a significant difference between the groups (17.8 mo compared with 14.3 mo, HR 0.78, $P = 0.029$).[15] The secondary end point of PFS was also significant between the two arms (5.5 vs. 2.8 mo, $P < 0.000001$). ORR for sorafenib was 10% compared with 2% for placebo. Common side-effects of sorafenib on the study include diarrhea, rash, fatigue, and hand–foot syndrome. In December 2005, the FDA approval of sorafenib was the first of many molecularly targeted agents to be approved in RCC.

Subsequently, a frontline randomized phase II study comparing sorafenib with IFN has been published. In this trial, patients were randomized 1:1 to receive either 400 mg twice daily or IFN, with a primary end point of PFS.[30] Patients who progressed on IFN were allowed to switch to sorafenib, while patients progressing on sorafenib were allowed to dose escalate to 600 mg twice daily. Interestingly, in the intent-to-treat analysis, the PFS was similar for the two groups (5.7 mo for sorafenib vs. 5.6 mo for IFN, $P = 0.50$). However, patients who received sorafenib had a higher disease control rate (% stable disease + % responders) compared with those who received IFN (sorafenib: 79.4% vs. IFN: 64.1%; $P = 0.006$) and reported an improved quality of life. In terms of patients crossing over to receive sorafenib after IFN progression, these patients had a 76.2% disease control rate and a subsequent PFS of 5.3 months, which are similar to the findings in the large phase III trial previously discussed in this population of patients. Dose escalation to 600 mg twice daily in patients who progressed on initial sorafenib resulted in 41.9% frequency of tumor shrinkage with a median PFS of 3.6 months. The results of this trial reinforce the phase III trial level of evidence of use of sorafenib after cytokines, but do not make an impactful argument for its front line use in unselected RCC patients.

Sunitinib

Sunitinib, a multi-targeted TKI, inhibits VEGF-R1–3, PDGF-Rα, PDGF-Rβ, c-kit, and FLT-3. Two early phase II studies have been performed in metastatic RCC patients who received prior cytokine therapy and demonstrated efficacy with response rates of 33% and 40%.[31,32] These trials led to a pivotal, phase III multicenter study of sunitinib versus IFN in treatment-naïve advanced RCC patients.[16] In this landmark trial, 750 patients were randomized to receive sunitinib or IFN in 1:1 fashion. These patients were required to have clear cell histology and a good performance status. The primary end point of the trial was PFS and secondary end points included ORR, OS, and safety. In terms of the primary end point, there was a significant improvement in median PFS for patients who received sunitinib for 11 months compared with 5 months for the IFN cohort (HR 0.42, $P < 0.001$). Also, a dramatic improvement in response rate was seen with sunitinib, with an ORR of 47% for sunitinib compared with 12% for IFN ($P < 0.001$). In terms of OS, the median OS for the sunitinib group was 26.4 versus 21.8 months for the IFN group (HR 0.821, $P = 0.051$ unstratified log-rank test; $P = 0.013$ unstratified Wilcoxon test).[17] The similarities between these median survival numbers are felt in large part to be due to patients in the IFN arm going on to receive other active targeted agents. The most common toxicities described with sunitinib in this study included diarrhea, rash, fatigue, hand–foot syndrome, and hypertension. Based on the efficacy seen in this study, sunitinib gained FDA approval 1 month after sorafenib in January 2006.

Pazopanib

The last oral multi-targeted TKI to receive FDA approval for advanced RCC is pazopanib. This agent similarly targets the VEGF-R1–3, PDGF-α, PDGF-β, and c-kit tyrosine kinases and has been extensively evaluated in patients with advanced clear cell RCC. After showing tolerability and potential efficacy in a phase I clinical study, pazopanib was explored in a large multicenter phase II study.[33,34] In this study, 225 metastatic RCC patients with predominately clear cell histology, good performance status, and either treatment naïve or had failed one prior cytokine or bevacizumab regimen were enrolled. The study began with plans to perform a randomized discontinuation study similar to the previously discussed sorafenib phase II trial; however, upon analysis of the first 60 patients, a response rate of 38% led the safety and data monitoring committee to recommend making the trial an open-label single-arm phase II trial with a primary end point of response rate. Patients were randomized to placebo ($n = 28$) before the interim change was crossed over to pazopanib. Of the 225 patients enrolled in the trial, most patients were treatment naïve (69%). The ORR observed was 35% and the median duration of response was 68 weeks. The PFS which was a secondary end point was found to be 52 weeks. Pazopanib was tolerated well in this study with the most common adverse events, including fatigue, diarrhea, hair depigmentation, hypertension, and aspartate transferase/alanine transferase elevation.

Based on the promising activity in earlier studies, a multicenter, international randomized phase III trial evaluated the efficacy of pazopanib compared with placebo in metastatic clear cell RCC patients who had progressed on a cytokine therapy or were treatment naïve.[18] In this study, 435 patients were randomized to receive pazopanib or placebo (2:1). The primary end point of the trial was PFS with secondary objectives, including evaluation of RR, OS, and safety. The median PFS for patients receiving pazopanib was 9.2 months (4.2 mo for placebo, HR 0.46, $P < 0.0001$) and the RR was 30%. Patients were stratified in the trial based on whether they were treatment naïve or had a prior cytokine therapy. Patients who were treatment naïve had a median PFS of 11.1 months compared with 2.8 months receiving placebo (HR 0.40, $P < 0.0001$). An update on OS for this study was presented in 2010 at the European Society for Medical Oncology. The median survival for patients receiving pazopanib was 22.5 months compared with 20.5 months in the placebo group ($P = 0.224$), demonstrating the availability of active agents to the placebo group following progressive disease on study. Based on the results of the phase II and phase III studies with pazopanib, this drug received FDA approval in October 2009 for patients with metastatic RCC. Currently, a randomized trial comparing the safety and efficacy of pazopanib and sunitinib in the frontline setting is ongoing (NCT00720941). This trial may aid in selection between these two agents for patients who are treatment naïve.

TABLE 65–2 Activity of Selected Vascular Endothelial Growth Factor (VEGF) Tyrosine Kinase Inhibitors on the VEGF Receptors

Drug	VEGFR1	VEGFR2	VEGF3	References
Sorafenib[a]	—	90	20	35
Sunitinib[a]	2	10	17	36
Pazopanib[a]	10	30	47	37
Axitinib	0.1	0.2	0.1–0.3	38
Tivozanib	0.21	0.16	0.24	39

Values given are the inhibitory concentrations (IC_{50}) in nanomoles. The progression of older agents to new agents demonstrates a clear increase in potency (smaller number=greater potency), particularly at VEGFR-2 which is felt to be most relevant for renal cell carcinoma.
[a]Represents FDA-approved agents.

Axitinib

Axitinib is an investigational agent that potently binds and inhibits VEGFR-1-3, PDGF, and c-kit tyrosine kinases. Similar to the previously discussed drugs this is an orally bioavailable compound; however, the potency at which it binds to the VEGF receptors is much greater than available agents (Table 65.2). This agent has been studied in a couple of phase II trials in metastatic RCC patients who are refractory to prior therapy. Based on prior phase I analysis of safety and pharmacokinetics,[40] a dose of 5 mg twice daily was explored in a phase II study of metastatic RCC patients who were deemed refractory to cytokines.[41] In this single-arm trial, 52 patients were treated with a response rate of 44.2% (primary end point). Other end points in the trial included median time to progression (TTP) which for this cohort was 15.7 months and median survival which was 29.9 months. A subsequent phase II study performed in metastatic RCC patients refractory to sorafenib was performed.[42] Although patients were required to have sorafenib, other therapies could have been administered previously as well and in this study of 62 patients 61.3% had prior cytokines and 22.6% had prior sunitinib. In this trial, patients who were able to tolerate the 5 mg twice daily dose were able to be titrated to higher doses (5→7→10 mg). Approximately half of the patients (53.2%) were able to be titrated up in the study to greater than the starting dose. The primary end point of this study was response rate with secondary end points of PFS, OS, and safety. The ORR was 22.6% for this heavily pretreated population. The median PFS was 7.4 months and OS was 13.6 months. The drug was well tolerated with grade 3/4 adverse events, including hypertension, dysphonia, hand–foot syndrome, fatigue, and diarrhea.

Based on the activity seen in these two second-line phase II trials, a randomized phase III trial comparing axitinib and sorafenib has been performed (AXIS trial).[43] In this trial, 723 patients with metastatic clear cell RCC, who had progressed on a frontline agent which could include sunitinib, bevacizumab plus IFN-α, temsirolimus, or cytokines, were randomized 1:1 to receive axitinib or sorafenib. As in the previously discussed phase II trial, patients who tolerated axitinib were able to have dose escalation. The primary end point of the study was PFS with secondary end points which include response, survival, and duration of response. The median PFS for all patients receiving axitinib was 6.7 months compared with 4.7 months in the sorafenib arm ($P < 0.0001$). Patients who had received cytokines in the first-line setting had a longer PFS with axitinib of 12.1 months compared with 6.5 months with sorafenib (<0.0001). Finally, patients who had prior sunitinib had a shorter PFS of 4.8 months compared with 3.4 months for sorafenib ($P = 0.0107$). The ORR for patients receiving axitinib was 19% compared with 8% for those receiving sorafenib ($P = 0.0001$). The duration of response was 11 months for axitinib and 10.6 months for sorafenib. Insufficient follow-up precluded OS analysis at the time of presentation of this data. Common adverse events seen with axitinib include diarrhea, fatigue, hypertension, dysphonia, and nausea. While this is the first study to show benefit of one targeted therapy directly compared with another in metastatic RCC patients, it remains unclear whether the drug will be FDA approved in the second-line setting. Of note, there is an ongoing phase III randomized trial comparing axitinib to sorafenib in metastatic RCC patients who are treatment naïve and the results of this study are highly anticipated (NCT00920816).

Tivozanib

Tivozanib, similar to axitinib, is a highly potent oral TKI which inhibits VEGF-R1–3, PDGF, and c-kit. Based on phase I clinical study of tivozanib in advanced solid tumors, safety and dosing were established.[44] In a phase II randomized discontinuation trial of tivozanib in metastatic RCC patients, a dose of 1.5 mg once daily 3 weeks on and 1 week off was administered to 272 patients.[39,45] Following a lead-in period on therapy, if patients had more than 25% reduction in target tumor burden, then they continued therapy until progression. Patients who had more than 25% growth of their target tumor burden were discontinued from therapy and patients who had in-between 25% reduction and 25% growth were randomized to receive continued therapy or placebo. The median PFS for all patients was 11.8 months, with the subset of patients having clear cell histology ($n = 225$) and/or prior nephrectomy ($n = 199$) having a median PFS of 14.8 months. The ORR for tivozanib was 25.4%. The promising efficacy results from this study have led to the initiation of an ongoing large multicenter, randomized phase III trial comparing tivozanib with sorafenib in treatment-naïve metastatic clear cell RCC patients (NCT01030783).

Agents That Bind the VEGF Ligand

Bevacizumab

Bevacizumab is a humanized recombinant monoclonal antibody which binds and clears the VEGF-A ligand (all isoforms). Since this agent does not have any other known targets in the body, the side-effect profile of bevacizumab is narrower than that seen with multi-targeted VEGF TKIs. Early development of bevacizumab as an RCC therapeutic included a randomized phase II trial comparing two different doses of bevacizumab in clear cell metastatic RCC patients.[46] This trial included 116 patients who had progressed on IL-2 or were not candidates for IL-2 who were treated with either bevacizumab at 3 or 10 mg/kg or placebo. The study showed a significant improvement in TTP for the higher dose bevacizumab group compared with placebo ($P < 0.001$). The 4-month PFS for the three groups were 64%, 39%, and 20% for the high-dose, low-dose, and placebo groups, respectively. The promise of bevacizumab in the management of RCC led to two large randomized phase III trials.

In the AVOREN trial, 649 patients with treatment-naïve metastatic clear cell RCC were randomized to receive the combination of bevacizumab and IFN to IFN alone.[19] The primary end point was PFS and for the bevacizumab/IFN arm was 10.2 months as opposed to 5.4 months for IFN alone (HR 0.63, $P = 0.0001$). ORR was also found to be higher for the bevacizumab-containing arm (31% vs. 13%). An updated OS analysis did not show a benefit for either group (23.3 for bevacizumab/IFN vs. 21.3 months for IFN, $P = 0.1291$).[20] Common adverse events for the combination arm included fatigue, pyrexia, anorexia, hypertension, and proteinuria. Although they were uncommon, notable adverse events in the bevacizumab-containing arm included gastrointestinal perforation, wound healing complications, and arterial thrombotic events ($n = 5$ for each).

In a similarly designed study by the CALGB cooperative group, a phase III randomized trial of bevacizumab plus IFN versus IFN alone was explored.[21] In this trial 732 patients with treatment-naïve clear cell metastatic RCC were randomized. The primary end point in this study was also PFS; however, secondary end points of response rate, survival, and safety were also evaluated. Similar to the prior study, patients receiving bevacizumab and IFN together had a better median PFS compared with the IFN-alone group (8.5 mo compared with 5.2 mo, $P < 0.0001$). The ORR for the bevacizumab plus IFN group was 25.5% as opposed to 13.1% for the IFN group. Updated OS analysis demonstrated a median OS of 18.3 months for bevacizumab/IFN compared with 17.4 months for IFN alone ($P = 0.097$).[22] Adverse events reported in the study were similar to that of the AVOREN trial. Based on the information obtained from these phase III studies, the FDA approved the combination of bevacizumab and IFN for the management of metastatic RCC in July 2009.

Aflibercept

Similar to bevacizumab, VEGF Trap or aflibercept works by binding and neutralizing circulating VEGF ligand. This molecule is different than bevacizumab in that it is a peptibody, which is a unique molecule made from the Fc portion of human IgG and the extracellular domains of VEGF-R1 and VEGF-R2. This molecule also binds to placental growth factor as well. In a dose-finding phase I clinical study of aflibercept in advanced solid tumor patients, 47 patients were treated with the drug.[47] Of note, two patients with metastatic RCC (total of seven RCC patients included in the trial) had prolonged stable disease (>12 mo). Fatigue, nausea, vomiting, dysphonia, hypertension, and proteinuria were the most common adverse events reported. Aflibercept is currently being evaluated in several phase II trials in several different tumor types, including a phase II cooperative group study in patients with metastatic RCC (NCT00357760).

Other Angiogenesis Inhibitors in Development

Although the VEGF pathway inhibitors discussed thus far have made a large impact in the clinical outcomes of patients with metastatic RCC, this disease remains incurable and all patients over time will have their disease become resistant to these approaches. VEGF inhibitor resistance appears to be a complex process which likely is not due to one particular pathway. In fact, there have been numerous molecular pathways and biologic processes that have been implicated in the development of resistance to VEGF pathway inhibition. The Ang growth factors (Ang-1 and Ang-2) are known to be important regulators of angiogenesis and are also hypoxia-inducible genes which are activated by HIF.[48] Interestingly, serum Ang-2 levels are noted to be elevated in RCC patients upon the development of sunitinib resistance.[49] FGF pathway activation has also been described as a possible resistance mechanism for VEGF inhibition. This growth factor, also a hypoxia-inducible gene target, is produced by many different cells, including endothelial and inflammatory cells, and is an important inducer of angiogenesis via binding to the FGF-R1 and FGF-R2.[50] Similar to Ang-1, increased concentrations of FGF have been demonstrated to be present in preclinical models of VEGF resistance.[51] Additionally, serum FGF levels have been noted to be increased in RCC patients with progression on sunitinib.[52] Finally, several immune factors have been discovered to play a role in VEGF resistance, such as the presence of myeloid-derived suppressor cells within the tumor and the production of pro-inflammatory cytokines (e.g., IL-6, IL-8, and TNF-α).[53,54] Targeting one or more of these possible escape mechanisms may be a fruitful path to overcoming disease resistance and providing further clinical benefit to these patients. This section focuses on several agents that are furthest along in targeting VEGF inhibition escape mechanisms as well as a novel group of anti-angiogenesis inhibitors, the vascular disrupting agents (VDAs), which can result in a mechanical blockage of blood flow to the tumor.

Dovitinib and FGF Inhibition

Dovitinib is a small molecule pan-TKI which potently inhibits VEGF-R1–3, FGF, PDGF-R, Flt-3, and c-kit. The unique feature about this anti-angiogenic agent is its potent binding to the FGF receptor which as previously discussed is a theorized escape mechanism for tumors progressing on VEGF pathway inhibition. This agent has been evaluated in a phase I dose-finding trial in patients with advanced solid tumors.[55] In this trial, 35 patients were treated with dovitinib with dose-limiting toxicities, including hypertension, elevated alkaline phosphatase, and anorexia. There was one response seen (melanoma) and activity seen in gastrointestinal stromal tumors as well. The drug was next explored in a phase I/II study of patients with metastatic clear cell RCC patients who had progressed on other available therapies. An update of this trial was reported at the 2011 Annual Society of Clinical Oncologists (ASCO) national meeting.[56] Based on phase I data, dovitinib was dosed in the phase II portion at 500 mg daily 5 days on, 2 days off with end points, including PFS, OS, and safety. Fifty-one patients were evaluable for efficacy with a partial response rate of 8%, stable disease rate of 37% (SD >4 mo), and 22% progressive disease. At the time of report, the median PFS was 6.1 months and OS of 16 months. Fifty-nine patients were evaluable for safety data and common adverse events, including nausea, vomiting, anorexia, and fatigue. Biomarker analysis demonstrated decreases in soluble VEGF-R2 and increases in serum FGF23, suggesting adequate blockade of both VEGF and FGF pathways. The promise seen in this study has led to the introduction of a randomized phase III study comparing dovitinib with sorafenib in metastatic clear cell RCC patients who have progressed on one VEGF inhibitor (except sorafenib) and one mTOR inhibitor (NCT01223027). This trial should shed light on the benefits of combined VEGF/FGF inhibition in this population compared with continued VEGF inhibition alone.

Angiopoietin Inhibitors

AMG-386

Similar to the previously discussed aflibercept, AMG-386 is a peptibody which binds and neutralizes Ang-1 and Ang-2. This molecule has been shown to have anti-angiogenesis properties in preclinical models and was studied in a phase I clinical study in advanced solid tumors. In this trial 32 patients were treated with the drug.[57] One partial response was seen and 12 patients had stable disease as best response. The common adverse events which were seen included fatigue and peripheral edema. Two phase II trials were subsequently initiated to evaluate the efficacy of the drug in combination with VEGF inhibitors in RCC.

In one phase II trial, exploration of the combination of AMG-386 with sorafenib was performed in patients who were treatment naïve.[58] In this study, two dosing levels were evaluated (10 or 3 mg/kg) in combination with sorafenib versus sorafenib alone. Interestingly, PFS for the three arms was 9 versus 8.5 versus 9 months for high-dose AMG-386/sorafenib, low-dose AMG-386/sorafenib, and sorafenib alone, respectively ($P = 0.523$). An increased ORR was seen with the combination arms compared with sorafenib alone, suggesting some anti-tumor activity of the novel drug (ORRs: 38% high-dose AMG-386, 37% low-dose AMG-386, and 24% for sorafenib alone). Common adverse events seen included diarrhea, hypertension, hand–foot syndrome, and alopecia. Although it is not completely known why this trial did not show an improved PFS for the combination compared with sorafenib, the sorafenib control arm did much better in this trial compared with historical numbers (e.g., 5.7 mo in the frontline placebo-controlled phase II trial). Other reasons may be inadequate dosing of AMG-386 in the study or the lack of relevance of the Ang–Tie pathway for upfront therapy. A second randomized phase II trial is also underway comparing the combination of AMG-386 and sunitinib. This trial is evaluating a higher dose AMG-386 arm (15 mg/kg) plus sunitinib with AMG-386 dosed at 10 mg/kg plus sunitinib (NCT00853372). This study hopefully helps answer the dosing question and combines the agent with a more potent VEGF-R2 inhibitor which may be relevant for Ang–Tie pathway-mediated resistance.

CVX-060

CVX-060 represents another unique peptibody which inhibits the Ang–Tie pathway; however, in this case CVX-060 binds and blocks Ang-2 signaling only. This agent has been evaluated in a phase I trial in advanced solid tumor patients, demonstrating tolerability and potential efficacy.[59] In this study, efficacy data on 30 patients showed that the most common adverse event was fatigue. In a subset of patients, dynamic contrast-enhanced magnetic resonance imaging demonstrated an anti-angiogenic tumor response. A phase I/II clinical study of CVX-060 plus sunitinib is being performed in patients with metastatic RCC already progressed on one treatment (NCT00982657). Additionally, due to the ever-changing landscape of RCC therapeutics, a phase I/II trial of CVX-060 plus axitinib in previously treated patients has also been initiated (NCT01441414). To date, the clinical role for Ang–Tie pathway inhibition for the management of RCC patients has yet to be clarified.

Vascular Disrupting Agents

A novel class of anti-angiogenic agents known as VDAs is in early stages of development. Unlike VEGF, FGF, or other molecularly targeted agents which inhibit growth factor pathways, VDAs induce a mechanical disruption of existing tumoral blood vessels. There are two main classes of VDAs, molecules which impair function of vascular endothelial cell tubulin molecules and the flavonoid VDAs which result in vascular endothelial cell apoptosis. In the first class, endothelial cell tubulin disruption can result in endothelial cell sloughing and subsequent vessel blockage. Although several agents have been in development for a variety of cancers, the agent BNC105 is currently being studied in metastatic RCC. This endothelial tubulin inhibitor is being evaluated in a phase I/II trial in combination with everolimus. The phase I portion of this study has been completed and the phase II portion is currently underway (BNC105 + everolimus vs. everolimus alone) in metastatic RCC patients who have failed prior VEGF inhibitor therapy (NCT01034631).

PI3K/AKT/MTOR PATHWAY INHIBITORS

As previously stated, the PI3K/Akt/mTOR pathway plays an important role in RCC pathogenesis at least in part via stimulation of HIF biosynthesis. However, mTOR, a serine/threonine kinase, is also known to stimulate cellular growth and metabolism which also play an important role. The mTOR complex primarily undergoes activation by Akt which is in turn activated by PI3K. PI3K is regulated by the PTEN molecule which is notably deficient in many aggressive cancers. Critical knowledge regarding the relationship of mTOR and RCC was gained in the study of tuberous sclerosis.[60] In this hereditary disease, the tuberous sclerosis complex gene (TSC1/2) is inactivated which has been linked to RCC development.[61] In cells with TSC loss, HIF-1 protein concentrations are increased which can be reversed with the incorporation of an active TSC gene.[26] It is also important to recognize that there are two mTOR complexes, mTORC1 (a complex of raptor, mLST8, and PRAS40) and mTORC2 (a complex of rictor, proctor, mLST8, and mSINI). The mTOR inhibitors approved for metastatic RCC, temsirolimus and everolimus, are mTORC1 inhibitors, with mTORC2 likely playing a critical role in mTORC1 inhibition resistance. In this section, we discuss the clinical activity of the FDA-approved mTOR inhibitors for RCC and other agents in development relevant to this pathway.

mTORC1 Inhibitors

Temsirolimus

Temsirolimus was the first mTOR inhibitor to obtain FDA approval for the treatment of metastatic RCC. A phase II trial exploring the efficacy and safety of different dose levels of temsirolimus was performed in 111 metastatic RCC patients.[62] Objective response rate (primary end point) was found to be 7% for treated patients. TTP varied from 6.3 to 6.7 to 5.2 months for the different dosing cohorts (25, 75, and 250 mg intravenous weekly). Common side-effects from temsirolimus therapy include rash, mucositis, nausea, hyperglycemia, anemia, and hypertriglyceridemia. Exploration of subsets based on prognostic features demonstrated an improved benefit for patients with a poor-risk grouping. These results led to a large, multicenter randomized phase III trial exploring temsirolimus therapy compared with IFN or the combination of temsirolimus and IFN.[23] In this trial, 626 treatment-naïve patients with at least three poor-risk prognostic factors were randomized. The primary end point for the trial was OS which ended up being 10.9, 8.4, and 7.3 months for the temsirolimus-alone group, the combination temsirolimus and IFN group, and the IFN-alone group, respectively. Common adverse events with temsirolimus include rash, peripheral edema, hyperglycemia, and hypertriglyceridemia. Based on the superior survival seen with temsirolimus compared with IFN, temsirolimus was FDA approved for patients with metastatic RCC. In particular, this therapy is best recommended for poor-risk patients in the treatment-naïve setting. Also of note, this trial did allow non–clear cell RCC patients to enroll and this group also had an improved survival compared with IFN alone (11.6 vs. 4.3 mo, respectively).[63]

Everolimus

Everolimus is an orally bioavailable inhibitor of mTOR which has been explored in patients with metastatic RCC. Based on earlier phase I clinical trials,[64] everolimus given at 10 mg orally daily was evaluated in a phase II trial of metastatic RCC patients who had received at least one prior therapy.[65] In this trial, 37 patients received therapy with everolimus with a primary end point of PFS. The drug was tolerated well with common adverse events, including nausea, anorexia, diarrhea, stomatitis, pneumonitis, and rash. The median PFS from this trial was 11.2 months with a response rate of 14%. The promise of everolimus seen in this trial led to the initiation of a randomized, placebo-controlled phase III trial (RECORD-1 trial).[24,25] In this large multicenter trial, 416 patients with metastatic RCC who had received sunitinib and/or sorafenib were randomized 2:1 to receive everolimus or placebo. The primary end point of this study was PFS with secondary end points of ORR, OS, and safety. The median PFS for patients receiving everolimus was 4.9 months compared with 1.9 months for patients receiving placebo ($P < 0.001$). The OS of patients on the everolimus arm was 14.8 versus 14.4 months for placebo ($P = 0.162$). Common adverse events include stomatitis, rash, fatigue, and diarrhea. Based on the improvement in PFS for patients in the post-TKI setting, everolimus received FDA approval in March 2009.

PI3K/Akt and mTORC2 Inhibitors

As evidenced by the activity of temsirolimus and everolimus, the mTOR pathway is a clinically relevant target in patients with metastatic RCC. Mechanisms of resistance to mTORc1 inhibition remain to be completely elucidated; however, some preclinical evidence suggests that a feedback loop activating Akt via the mTORC2 complex may play some role.[66,67] Evaluation of agents with inhibitory properties on the PI3K/Akt pathway is underway and perhaps these agents may display clinical activity in RCC patients.

The agent that has gone furthest in development is perifosine, which is an indirect inhibitor of the Akt, MAP kinase, and JNK pathways. This drug was studied in a phase II trial of patients with metastatic RCC who had failed one prior VEGF inhibitor or both of one VEGF and one mTOR inhibitor.[68] In a preliminary report of this study, 30 patients who had failed one prior VEGF inhibitor achieved a 3% ORR and 40% stable disease rate. Additionally, 14 patients, who had received both one prior VEGF and one mTOR inhibitor, experienced a 7% ORR and a 50% stable disease rate. The overall PFS for both cohorts was 15 weeks. Adverse effects include nausea, arthralgia, vomiting, fatigue, and cognitive changes. A final update of this study is pending; however, the initial report confirms some single-agent activity of this novel drug class in RCC patients.

BEZ235 is a dual PI3/Akt/mTOR inhibitor which has undergone evaluation in a phase I dose-finding trial.[69] Nausea, vomiting, diarrhea, anorexia, fatigue, and anemia were common adverse events seen in this study. Two partial responses and 16 minor responses were observed (total n = 51 evaluable), demonstrating a broad efficacy signal. Currently, a phase I/II trial in patients with metastatic RCC is ongoing with a planned evaluation of patients who have failed first- or second-line mTOR inhibitors in the phase II population (NCT01453595). A separate phase I trial will evaluate the combination of BEZ235 and everolimus in advanced solid tumor patients, with a subsequent phase II trial including only breast and RCC malignancies (NCT01482156).

BKM-120 is a PI3K inhibitor also in clinical development which has shown early promise. In a phase I dose-escalation trial of BKM120 in solid tumor malignancies, a 58% stable disease rate was observed, with anorexia, diarrhea, nausea, rash, fatigue, hyperglycemia, and depression being common adverse events.[70] A phase I trial of the combination of bevacizumab and BKM-120 in patients with metastatic RCC is planned (NCT01283048).

XL765 is a pan-PI3K/mTORC1/mTORC2 inhibitor which is also in early development. A phase I trial of XL765 has been reported in patients with advanced solid tumors.[71] One patient with metastatic RCC had prolonged stable disease (>3 mo). The agent appeared to be well tolerated with common adverse events, including elevation of liver enzymes, nausea, and diarrhea.

Finally, a potent dual mTORC1 and mTORC2 complex inhibitor, OSI-027, is also in clinical development. This drug has been evaluated in a phase I clinical study in patients with advanced solid tumor malignancies and lymphoma.[72] In this study, the dose-limiting toxicities include fatigue and decrease in left ventricular ejection fraction. Other toxicities noted include fatigue, nausea, diarrhea, and elevated creatinine. In terms of efficacy signal, eight patients (out of total n = 31) experienced prolonged stable disease, including one patient with advanced RCC. At the time of report, the maximum tolerated dose (MTD) had not been identified.

Given the clinical benefits observed with everolimus and temsirolimus, the mTOR pathway is clearly an important target for future investigational drug development. The availability of numerous drugs in the developmental pipeline which block different points in this pathway may make it possible for clinical researchers to tease out parts of the pathway that can be targeted to overcome mTORC1 inhibitor resistance.

SEQUENCING AND COMBINATION TARGETED THERAPY APPROACHES IN RCC

There are many questions that have yet to be answered with the available classes of therapies for RCC that are being addressed in several ongoing trials (Table 65.3). Although the benefits of single targeted agents have been well described, the optimal sequencing of these therapies is unknown. Additionally, single-agent therapies rarely result in complete responses and therefore exploration of combination approaches is underway in an attempt to improve response rates. In this section, we discuss the relevant data that address these key issues.

Sequencing Targeted Therapies in RCC

The results of the RECORD-1 trial (previously discussed) provided rationale for the use of an mTOR inhibitor after VEGF TKI therapy and resulted in the approval of everolimus. The value of sequential use of VEGF inhibitors has also been extensively explored in several studies. Retrospective studies have demonstrated that there is a lack of cross-resistance in sequential use of sorafenib and sunitinib.[73,74] Subsequently, prospective evaluation of sequential VEGF inhibitors has also supported this approach. For example, a phase II trial has showed the benefit of sorafenib sequenced after first-line sunitinib with a TTP of 16 weeks.[75] Additionally, in a separate study, sorafenib has been demonstrated to have efficacy following either bevacizumab or sunitinib.[76] In this trial of 29 evaluable patients, 11 patients had minor responses with a PFS of 3.8 months for the trial. The study of sunitinib in the second line following bevacizumab progression also has demonstrated an ORR of 23% and a median PFS of 7 months.[77] Also of note, recently data have been reported on a phase II trial of pazopanib in metastatic RCC patients who had received either sunitinib or bevacizumab therapy prior to enrollment (patients could have progressed or been intolerant of these therapies).[78] At the time of report, 44 patients had been treated with efficacy information. The response rate for all comers was found to be 20%, with patients having prior bevacizumab having a higher response rate (33%) compared with prior sunitinib (16%). The median PFS for the group as a whole was 9.2 months, with patients in the prior sunitinib category having a 12.06-month median PFS and those in the prior bevacizumab category having a 8.05-month median PFS. This study provides additional information about the potential lack of cross-resistance among some patients receiving sequential VEGF pathway inhibitors. Data regarding activity of second-line axitinib following VEGF inhibitor failure have been discussed earlier and are poised to become the first VEGF TKI to become FDA approved for patient's failing a prior VEGF inhibitor.

The critical question in sequencing is which will be the optimal sequence for the average RCC patient, VEGF inhibitor → VEGF inhibitor or VEGF inhibitor → mTOR inhibitor. There are several ongoing clinical studies that may help answer this question. A key trial

Table 65-3 Summary of Ongoing Clinical Studies Evaluating the Sequencing and Combinations of Currently Approved Targeted Agent

Ongoing Trials Involving Sequencing or Combinations of FDA-Approved Agents	Comparator Arm	Phase of Study	Primary End Point	Reference or NCT Number
Sequencing trials				
Sunitinib → everolimus	Everolimus → sunitinib	2	PFS	RECORD-3 trial (NCT00903175)
Sunitinib → sorafenib	Sorafenib → sunitinib	3	PFS	SWITCH trial (NCT00732914)
Sunitinib → temsirolimus	Sunitinib → sorafenib	3	PFS	Torisel 404 (NCT00474786)
Combination trials				
Bevacizumab + sorafenib	Bevacizumab	2	PFS	BeST trial (NCT00378703)
Bevacizumab + temsirolimus				
Temsirolimus + sorafenib				
Bevacizumab + temsirolimus	Bevacizumab/interferon	3	ORR, PFS	INTORACT trial (NCT00631371)
Everolimus + bevacizumab	Bevacizumab/interferon	2	PFS	RECORD-2 trial (NCT00719264)

FDA, United States Food and Drug Administration; PFS, progression-free survival; ORR, overall response rate.

exploring this question is the phase III Torisel-404 trial which is evaluating the role of sorafenib versus temsirolimus in patients progressing on frontline sunitinib (NCT00474786). The RECORD-3 trial is evaluating the sequence of sunitinib followed by everolimus or everolimus followed by sunitinib (NCT00903175). While this does not have a VEGF inhibitor → VEGF inhibitor arm, it should help shed light on a patient population that benefits from early mTOR inhibition.

Targeted Therapy Combinations in RCC

Attempts to improve on response rates with the use of two targeted agents have been explored in several phase I trials and are currently being evaluated in several randomized phase II studies. Combinations of VEGF pathway inhibitors have been quite challenging due to excess toxicity. In a phase I trial with the combination of bevacizumab and sorafenib, patients were unable to tolerate full doses of both agents (MTD sorafenib 200 mg twice daily and bevacizumab 5 mg/kg every 2 wk).[79] Interestingly, of the 46 patients evaluable for response, 21 patients (46%) had a partial response which is higher than that previously seen for both drugs alone. A phase I trial of bevacizumab and sunitinib demonstrated significant frequencies of cardiovascular toxicity.[80] For example, 60% of patients experienced grade 3/4 hypertension. Forty-eight percent of patients had to discontinue therapy due to toxicity in this study and several patients developed microangiopathic hemolytic anemia and there was one patient death due to myocardial infarction. Although the trial reported a 52% response rate, the potential efficacy was outweighed by the toxicity of the combination.

Efforts to combine VEGF inhibitors and mTOR inhibitors have been somewhat more tolerable, but efficacy signals have been difficult to show in phase II trials. In one study of bevacizumab and everolimus, 80 patients were treated with a response rate of 28% and median PFS of 8.1 months.[81] These results are similar to that seen for bevacizumab and IFN therapy. Additionally, the phase II TORAVA study, reported by Escudier et al.,[82] evaluated the combination of bevacizumab and temsirolimus with sunitinib or bevacizumab/IFN. This study showed no improvement in 48-week PFS (primary end point) for the combination compared with the other arms (30.7% for bevacizumab/temsirolimus compared with 40.5% for sunitinib and 65.9% for bevacizumab/IFN). Toxicities of the bevacizumab and temsirolimus group were higher with three deaths seen as opposed to none in the other treatment arms. There are several studies that should have data reported in the next 1 to 2 years which will provide more insight into the ability to combine available agents. These include the RECORD-2 study (NCT00719264) which is combining everolimus and bevacizumab, the INTORACT trial (NCT00631371) which is comparing bevacizumab and temsirolimus compared with bevacizumab and IFN, and the BeST study (NCT00378703) which is exploring several different combinations, including bevacizumab/sorafenib, temsirolimus/bevacizumab, and temsirolimus/sorafenib.

CLINICAL TOOLS FOR A PERSONALIZED APPROACH IN SELECTING CURRENTLY AVAILABLE TARGETED THERAPIES IN RCC

Currently, there are six targeted agents available for selection by treating oncologists for patients with newly diagnosed metastatic RCC. Having so many treatment options is a luxury compared with other diseases that have limited effective options; however, selection among available agents can be difficult. Choices tailored to patient's comorbid conditions and potential side-effects are commonly done in the community, although there is little prospective evidence that this is the best route. An evidence-based medicine approach can be employed with RCC based on the available clinical trial data (Table 65.4). It is important to understand that the use of prognostic risk factors was employed in patient selection in these pivotal trials. The Memorial Sloan Kettering Cancer Center (MSKCC) and Motzer criteria are the most commonly used prognostic tools which were utilized.[83,84] These prognostic factors were discovered during the cytokine era; however they have been shown to be relevant in today's "targeted therapy age" of RCC treatment as well. These poor risk factors include anemia, elevated lactate dehydrogenase, elevated calcium, poor performance status, and lack of prior nephrectomy. Patients with no risk factors are deemed good risk, one or two risk factors are intermediate risk, and those with three or more risk factors are poor risk. In the original report, these risk factor groups correlate with median survival of 19.9, 10.3, and 3.9 months, respectively. Use of this prognostic factor system is still important in identifying frontline therapy for patients. The frontline selections of sunitinib, pazopanib, or bevacizumab/ IFN would be acceptable choices for good- or intermediate-risk patients based on entry criteria for their respective phase III studies, while temsirolimus is appropriate for patients deemed poor risk by MSKCC criteria. For second-line choices, sorafenib and pazopanib have a high level of evidence supporting the use after cytokine therapies and everolimus has demonstrated benefit after VEGF TKI failure.

In a more recent multicenter retrospective analysis of patients receiving VEGF targeted therapies, several prognostic factors were identified in multivariate analysis.[85] These include anemia, elevated calcium, time from diagnosis to treatment, and poor performance status as poor-risk features, as well as findings of elevated neutrophil count and elevated thrombocyte count (Heng criteria). Notably excluded in these findings are elevated LDH and nephrectomy status. The necessity and timing of primary tumor removal as a part of modern VEGF-directed therapy are being explored in several prospective trials. Other clinically based markers which may be helpful for guiding treatment decisions are being explored. Among these is the understanding that hypertension may be a predictive pharmacodynamic marker for VEGF inhibitor directed therapy. In a large retrospective analysis, including 544 patients receiving sunitinib therapy from 4 prospective trials, Rini et al.[86] showed that patients who developed hypertension (>140/90) as an adverse effect had a higher response rate (ORR for patients with systolic blood pressure > 140 mm Hg was 54.6% compared with 9.7% for patients <140 mm Hg). Additionally, improvements in PFS and OS were seen in those patients who developed hypertension. Currently, an ongoing study of axitinib, which allows for dose increases in the drug in the absence of hypertension, will hopefully expand on our knowledge of this particular clinical marker (NCT00835978).

MOLECULAR BIOMARKERS AND GENETIC PROFILING

With the advent of molecularly targeted therapies for RCC, identification of prognostic and predictive molecular-based biomarkers is currently an important area of basic science and clinical research. There have been several candidate biomarkers identified, but no biomarkers have been prospectively validated in clinical studies. Given the importance of the VHL–HIF gene target pathway in clear cell RCC, different points in this pathway have been explored.

The presence of VHL gene defects has been extensively evaluated as a potential prognostic marker, but studies have shown varying results.[87] One key issue with VHL gene abnormalities is that they are present in the majority, if not all, of sporadic cases of clear cell RCC which make it impractical as a biomarker. Evaluation of HIF expression levels has been something that holds promise as a potential predictive marker in preclinical evaluation. As previously stated, HIF-1 and HIF-2 are the most relevant transcription factors related to VHL loss and these factors

Table 65-4 Options for Therapeutic Selection for Approved Targeted Agents Depending on Clinical Setting based on Level 1 Evidence (Phase III Data)

Approved Molecularly Targeted Agent for RCC	First-Line: Good or Intermediate Risk	First-Line: Poor Risk	Second-Line: Post Cytokine	Second- or Third-Line: Post VEGF TKI
VEGF pathway inhibitors				
Sorafenib			Yes	
Sunitinib	Yes			
Pazopanib	Yes		Yes	
Bevacizumab/IFN	Yes			
mTOR inhibitors				
Temsirolimus		Yes		
Everolimus				Yes

RCC, renal cell carcinoma; VEGF, vascular endothelial growth factor; TKI, tyrosine kinase inhibitor; mTOR, mammalian target of rapamycin.

are known to be differentially expressed.[88] While many of the HIF-1 and HIF-2 gene targets are similar, there are non-overlapping targets which can result in different cancer phenotypes.[89] In an evaluation of the impact of differential HIF factor expression, Gordan et al.[90] demonstrated that there are two distinct VHL-deficient tumor types, those where only HIF-2 is stabilized and those where both HIF-1 and HIF-2 are stabilized. These tumor subsets display different molecular phenotypes which may be exploited as both prognostic and predictive tools. The HIF-1/HIF-2 phenotype tumors appeared to have activation of the Akt/mTOR pathway, while the HIF-2 exhibited more c-myc activation.

Additionally, several HIF target genes have been explored for their biomarker potential. Notable among these are CAIX and VEGF. Similar to VHL loss, presence of CAIX immunohistochemical staining appears to be extremely common in these tumors. Retrospective evaluation of CAIX as a prognostic factor has demonstrated mixed results and to-date this marker has not been validated in a prospective fashion.[91-93] Pharmacodynamic responses of the VEGF ligand and soluble VEGF receptor have been seen with VEGF pathway-directed therapies.[77,94] However, whether measurement of these serum factors is better than utilization of RECIST methods has yet to be proven.

As in many other cancer types, genetic profiling of RCC tumors has taken center stage in the area of identifying unique subsets of patients which may have prognostic and predictive implications. Several different research groups have identified subsets of RCC tumors which may be relevant to clinical practice. One study by Zhao et al.,[95] explored the gene expression profiles of 177 primary clear cell RCC tumors. Using unsupervised hierarchical clustering analysis, a gene set of 259 transcripts was identified, allowing for separation of tumors into five subgroups of tumors. These subgroups could be correlated with survival, independent of other known clinical risk features. In a different analysis, Brannon et al.[96] performed consensus cluster analysis of 48 clear cell RCC tumors and identified 2 subgroups, which were named ccA and ccB. Subsequent analyses of these core arrays were used to generate predictive genes, survival information, and pathway analysis. Interestingly, using the ccA/ccB subsets on the 177 tumors from the Zhao group, survival differences were discovered. At 5 years, the cancer-specific survival for ccA patients was 56%, compared with 29% for ccB patients. Upregulated pathways within each group were also found to differ; for example, ccA tumors having increased angiogenesis and metabolism pathways and ccB tumors having upregulated mitotic cell cycle and epithelial to mesenchymal transition pathways. Finally, the Cleveland Clinic Group recently reported results of a gene expression analysis of 931 tumors with matching clinical data from patients with stage I–III clear cell RCC.[97] The analysis resulted in the discovery of 16 genes which were associated with decreased recurrence risk. Among this favorable prognostic set were genes that include angiogenesis and immune pathway transcripts. The results from these different research groups have demonstrated much promise for application of gene expression sets which may definitely have prognostic implications and also may predict response to targeted therapies. These gene expression sets need to be prospectively evaluated in therapeutic studies to become incorporated into clinical practice.

CONCLUSIONS

An increased understanding of the molecular pathogenesis has led to the discovery and incorporation of several molecularly targeted agents into the clinical management of clear cell RCC patients. Currently, two main classes of targeted agents are in use: the VEGF pathway inhibitors and mTOR inhibitors. These agents have gained their approval by demonstrating survival benefits (PFS or OS) for patients with advanced RCC. The FDA-approved VEGF inhibitors include the VEGF TKIs, sorafenib, sunitinib, and pazopanib, and the monoclonal antibody to the VEGF ligand, bevacizumab. The FDA-approved mTOR inhibitors include everolimus and temsirolimus. Other VEGF TKI agents are currently in late clinical trial development which may also become FDA-approved options, pending the results from these studies. Agents that belong to novel therapeutic classes are also in development and hopefully will provide benefit to patients developing refractoriness to current agents. Choice of initial and subsequent therapies for advanced RCC patient currently involves determination of clinical risk factors; however, there is much room for individualization of selection based on physician experience. Identification and validation of novel molecular biomarker approaches, for example, gene expression array, are needed and this hopefully will aid in appropriate therapy selection for patients based on their individual tumor biology.

REFERENCES

1. Siegel R, Ward E, Brawley O, Jemal A. Cancer Statistics, 2011. *CA Cancer J Clin*. 2011;61(4):212-236.
2. Lonser RR, Glenn GM, Walther M, et al. von Hippel-Lindau disease. *Lancet*. June 2003;361(9374):2059-2067.
3. Latif F, Tory K, Gnarra J, et al. Identification of the von Hippel-Lindau disease tumor suppressor gene. *Science*. May 1993;260(5112):1317-1320.
4. Iwai K, Yamanaka K, Kamura T, et al. Identification of the von Hippel-Lindau tumor-suppressor protein as part of an active E3 ubiquitin ligase complex. *Proc Natl Acad Sci U S A*. October 1999;96(22):12436-12441.
5. Maxwell PH, Wiesener MS, Chang GW, et al. The tumour suppressor protein VHL targets hypoxia-inducible factors for oxygen-dependent proteolysis. *Nature*. May 1999;399(6733):271-275.
6. Ivan M, Kondo K, Yang H, et al. HIFalpha targeted for VHL-mediated destruction by proline hydroxylation: implications for O2 sensing. *Science*. April 2001;292(5516):464-468.
7. Gnarra JR, Tory K, Weng Y, et al. Mutations of the VHL tumour suppressor gene in renal carcinoma. *Nat Genet*. May 1994;7(1):85-90.

8. Iliopoulos O, Levy AP, Jiang C, Kaelin WG Jr, Goldberg MA. Negative regulation of hypoxia-inducible genes by the von Hippel-Lindau protein. *Proc Natl Acad Sci U S A.* October 1996;93(20):10595-10599.
9. Kondo K, Yao M, Yoshida M, et al. Comprehensive mutational analysis of the VHL gene in sporadic renal cell carcinoma: relationship to clinicopathological parameters. *Genes Chromosomes Cancer.* May 2002;34(1):58-68.
10. Shuin T, Kondo K, Torigoe S, et al. Frequent somatic mutations and loss of heterozygosity of the von Hippel-Lindau tumor suppressor gene in primary human renal cell carcinomas. *Cancer Res.* June 1994;54(11):2852-2855.
11. Richard DE, Berra E, Gothie E, Roux D, Pouyssegur J. p42/p44 mitogen-activated protein kinases phosphorylate hypoxia-inducible factor 1alpha (HIF-1alpha) and enhance the transcriptional activity of HIF-1. *J Biol Chem.* November 1999;274(46):32631-32637.
12. Bukowski RM. Cytokine therapy for metastatic renal cell carcinoma. *Semin Urol Oncol.* May 2001;19(2):148-154.
13. Motzer RJ, Russo P. Systemic therapy for renal cell carcinoma. *J Urol.* February 2000;163(2):408-417.
14. Escudier B, Eisen T, Stadler WM, et al. Sorafenib in advanced clear-cell renal-cell carcinoma. *N Engl J Med.* January 2007;356(2):125-134.
15. Escudier B, Eisen T, Stadler WM, et al. Sorafenib for treatment of renal cell carcinoma: final efficacy and safety results of the phase III treatment approaches in renal cancer global evaluation trial. *J Clin Oncol.* July 2009;27(20):3312-3318.
16. Motzer RJ, Hutson TE, Tomczak P, et al. Sunitinib versus interferon alfa in metastatic renal-cell carcinoma. *N Engl J Med.* January 2007;356(2):115-124.
17. Motzer RJ, Hutson TE, Tomczak P, et al. Overall survival and updated results for sunitinib compared with interferon alfa in patients with metastatic renal cell carcinoma. *J Clin Oncol.* August 2009;27(22):3584-3590.
18. Sternberg CN, Davis ID, Mardiak J, et al. Pazopanib in locally advanced or metastatic renal cell carcinoma: results of a randomized phase III trial. *J Clin Oncol.* February 2010;28(6):1061-1068.
19. Escudier B, Pluzanska A, Koralewski P, et al. Bevacizumab plus interferon alfa-2a for treatment of metastatic renal cell carcinoma: a randomised, double-blind phase III trial. *Lancet.* December 2007;370(9605):2103-2111.
20. Escudier B, Bellmunt J, Negrier S, et al. Phase III trial of bevacizumab plus interferon alfa-2a in patients with metastatic renal cell carcinoma (AVOREN): final analysis of overall survival. *J Clin Oncol.* 2010;28(13):2144-2150.
21. Rini BI, Halabi S, Rosenberg JE, et al. Bevacizumab plus interferon alfa compared with interferon alfa monotherapy in patients with metastatic renal cell carcinoma: CALGB 90206. *J Clin Oncol.* November 2008;26(33):5422-5428.
22. Rini BI, Halabi S, Rosenberg JE, et al. Phase III trial of bevacizumab plus interferon alfa versus interferon alfa monotherapy in patients with metastatic renal cell carcinoma: final results of CALGB 90206. *J Clin Oncol.* May 2010;28(13):2137-2143.
23. Hudes G, Carducci M, Tomczak P, et al. Temsirolimus, interferon alfa, or both for advanced renal-cell carcinoma. *N Engl J Med.* May 2007;356(22):2271-2281.
24. Motzer RJ, Escudier B, Oudard S, et al. Efficacy of everolimus in advanced renal cell carcinoma: a double-blind, randomised, placebo-controlled phase III trial. *Lancet.* August 2008;372(9637):449-456.
25. Motzer RJ, Escudier B, Oudard S, et al. Phase 3 trial of everolimus for metastatic renal cell carcinoma: final results and analysis of prognostic factors. *Cancer.* September 2010;116(18):4256-4265.
26. Hudson CC, Liu M, Chiang GG, et al. Regulation of hypoxia-inducible factor 1alpha expression and function by the mammalian target of rapamycin. *Mol Cell Biol.* October 2002;22(20):7004-7014.
27. Michaelson IC. The mode of development of the vascular system of the retina with some observations on its significance for certain retinal disorders. *Trans Ophthalmol Soc UK.* 1948;68:137-180.
28. Tischer E, Mitchell R, Hartman T, et al. The human gene for vascular endothelial growth factor. Multiple protein forms are encoded through alternative exon splicing. *J Biol Chem.* June 1991;266(18):11947-11954.
29. Ratain MJ, Eisen T, Stadler WM, et al. Phase II placebo-controlled randomized discontinuation trial of sorafenib in patients with metastatic renal cell carcinoma. *J Clin Oncol.* June 2006;24(16):2505-2512.
30. Escudier B, Szczylik C, Hutson TE, et al. Randomized phase II trial of first-line treatment with sorafenib versus interferon Alfa-2a in patients with metastatic renal cell carcinoma. *J Clin Oncol.* March 2009;27(8):1280-1289.
31. Motzer RJ, Rini BI, Bukowski RM, et al. Sunitinib in patients with metastatic renal cell carcinoma. *JAMA.* June 2006;295(21):2516-2524.
32. Motzer RJ, Michaelson MD, Redman BG, et al. Activity of SU11248, a multitargeted inhibitor of vascular endothelial growth factor receptor and platelet-derived growth factor receptor, in patients with metastatic renal cell carcinoma. *J Clin Oncol.* January 2006;24(1):16-24.
33. Hurwitz HI, Dowlati A, Saini S, et al. Phase I trial of pazopanib in patients with advanced cancer. *Clin Cancer Res.* June 2009;15(12):4220-4227.
34. Hutson TE, Davis ID, Machiels JP, et al. Efficacy and safety of pazopanib in patients with metastatic renal cell carcinoma. *J Clin Oncol.* December 2009.
35. Wilhelm SM, Carter C, Tang L, et al. BAY 43-9006 exhibits broad spectrum oral antitumor activity and targets the RAF/MEK/ERK pathway and receptor tyrosine kinases involved in tumor progression and angiogenesis. *Cancer Res.* October 2004;64(19):7099-7109.
36. Mendel DB, Laird AD, Xin X, et al. In vivo antitumor activity of SU11248, a novel tyrosine kinase inhibitor targeting vascular endothelial growth factor and platelet-derived growth factor receptors: determination of a pharmacokinetic/pharmacodynamic relationship. *Clin Cancer Res.* January 2003;9(1):327-337.
37. Hurwitz H, Dowlati A, Savage S, et al. Safety, tolerability and pharmacokinetics of oral administration of GW786034 in pts with solid tumors. *J Clin Oncol (Meeting Abstracts).* June 2005;23(16_suppl):Abstract 3012.
38. Hu-Lowe DD, Zou HY, Grazzini ML, et al. Nonclinical antiangiogenesis and antitumor activities of axitinib (AG-013736), an oral, potent, and selective inhibitor of vascular endothelial growth factor receptor tyrosine kinases 1, 2, 3. *Clin Cancer Res.* November 2008;14(22):7272-7283.
39. Bhargava P, Esteves B, Nosov DA, et al. Updated activity and safety results of a phase II randomized discontinuation trial (RDT) of AV-951, a potent and selective VEGFR1, 2, and 3 kinase inhibitor, in patients with renal cell carcinoma (RCC). *J Clin Oncol (Meeting Abstracts).* May 2009;27(15S):Abstract 5032.
40. Rugo HS, Herbst RS, Liu G, et al. Phase I trial of the oral antiangiogenesis agent AG-013736 in patients with advanced solid tumors: pharmacokinetic and clinical results. *J Clin Oncol.* August 2005;23(24):5474-5483.
41. Rixe O, Bukowski RM, Michaelson MD, et al. Axitinib treatment in patients with cytokine-refractory metastatic renal-cell cancer: a phase II study. *Lancet Oncol.* November 2007;8(11):975-984.
42. Rini BI, Wilding G, Hudes G, et al. Phase II study of axitinib in sorafenib-refractory metastatic renal cell carcinoma. *J Clin Oncol.* September 2009;27(27):4462-4468.
43. Rini BI, Escudier B, Tomczak P, et al. Comparative effectiveness of axitinib versus sorafenib in advanced renal cell carcinoma (AXIS): a randomised phase 3 trial. *Lancet.* December 2011;378(9807):1931-1939.
44. Eskens F, de Jonge M, Esteves B, et al. Updated results from a phase I study of AV-951 (KRN951), a potent and selective VEGFR-1, -2 and -3 tyrosine kinase inhibitor, in patients with advanced solid tumors. AACR Meeting Abstracts. *Clin Cancer Res.* April 2008;2008(1_Annual_Meeting):Abstract LB-201.
45. Bhargava P, Esteves B, Al-Adhami M, et al. Activity of tivozanib (AV-951) in patients with renal cell carcinoma (RCC): subgroup analysis from a phase II randomized discontinuation trial (RDT). *J Clin Oncol (Meeting Abstracts).* May 2010;28(15_suppl):Abstract 4599.
46. Yang JC, Haworth L, Sherry RM, et al. A randomized trial of bevacizumab, an anti-vascular endothelial growth factor antibody, for metastatic renal cancer. *N Engl J Med.* July 2003;349(5):427-434.

47. Lockhart AC, Rothenberg ML, Dupont J, et al. Phase I study of intravenous vascular endothelial growth factor trap, aflibercept, in patients with advanced solid tumors. *J Clin Oncol.* January 2010;28(2):207-214.
48. Simon MP, Tournaire R, Pouyssegur J. The angiopoietin-2 gene of endothelial cells is up-regulated in hypoxia by a HIF binding site located in its first intron and by the central factors GATA-2 and Ets-1. *J Cell Physiol.* December 2008;217(3):809-818.
49. Bullock AJ, Zhang L, O'Neill AM, et al. Plasma angiopoietin-2 (ANG2) as an angiogenic biomarker in renal cell carcinoma (RCC). ASCO Meeting Abstracts. June 2010;28(15_suppl): 4630.
50. Beenken A, Mohammadi M. The FGF family: biology, pathophysiology and therapy. *Nat Rev Drug Discov.* March 2009;8(3):235-253.
51. Casanovas O, Hicklin DJ, Bergers G, Hanahan D. Drug resistance by evasion of antiangiogenic targeting of VEGF signaling in late-stage pancreatic islet tumors. *Cancer Cell.* October 2005;8(4):299-309.
52. Tsimafeyeu I, Demidov L, Ta H, Stepanova E, Wynn N. Fibroblast growth factor pathway in renal cell carcinoma. ASCO Meeting Abstracts. *J Clin Oncol.* June 14 2010;28(15_suppl):4621.
53. Finke J, Ko J, Rini B, Rayman P, Ireland J, Cohen P. MDSC as a mechanism of tumor escape from sunitinib mediated anti-angiogenic therapy. *Int Immunopharmacol.* July 2011;11(7):853-858.
54. Konig B, Steinbach F, Janocha B, et al. The differential expression of proinflammatory cytokines IL-6, IL-8 and TNF-alpha in renal cell carcinoma. *Anticancer Res.* March-April 1999;19(2C):1519-1524.
55. Angevin E, Lin C, Pande AU, et al. A phase I/II study of dovitinib (TKI258), a FGFR and VEGFR inhibitor, in patients (pts) with advanced or metastatic renal cell cancer: phase I results. *J Clin Oncol (Meeting Abstracts).* May 2010;28(15_suppl):Abstract 3057.
56. Angevin E, Grunwald V, Ravaud A, et al. A phase II study of dovitinib (TKI258), an FGFR- and VEGFR-inhibitor, in patients with advanced or metastatic renal cell cancer (mRCC). ASCO Meeting Abstracts. June 9, 2011;29(15_suppl):4551.
57. Herbst RS, Hong D, Chap L, et al. Safety, pharmacokinetics, and antitumor activity of AMG 386, a selective angiopoietin inhibitor, in adult patients with advanced solid tumors. *J Clin Oncol.* July 2009;27(21):3557-3565.
58. Rini BI, Szczylik C, Tannir NM, et al. AMG 386 in combination with sorafenib in patients (pts) with metastatic renal cell cancer (mRCC): a randomized, double-blind, placebo-controlled, phase II study. ASCO Meeting Abstracts. *J Clin Oncol.* March 2011;29(7_suppl):309.
59. Rosen LS, Mendelson DS, Cohen RB, et al. First-in-human dose-escalation safety and PK trial of a novel intravenous humanized monoclonal CovX body inhibiting angiopoietin 2. ASCO Meeting Abstracts. *J Clin Oncol.* June 2010;28(15_suppl):2524.
60. Cho D, Signoretti S, Regan M, Mier JW, Atkins MB. The role of mammalian target of rapamycin inhibitors in the treatment of advanced renal cancer. *Clin Cancer Res.* January 2007;13(2 pt 2): 758s-763s.
61. Brugarolas JB, Vazquez F, Reddy A, Sellers WR, Kaelin WG Jr. TSC2 regulates VEGF through mTOR-dependent and -independent pathways. *Cancer Cell.* August 2003;4(2):147-158.
62. Atkins MB, Hidalgo M, Stadler WM, et al. Randomized phase II study of multiple dose levels of CCI-779, a novel mammalian target of rapamycin kinase inhibitor, in patients with advanced refractory renal cell carcinoma. *J Clin Oncol.* March 2004;22(5):909-918.
63. Dutcher JP, de Souza P, McDermott D, et al. Effect of temsirolimus versus interferon-alpha on outcome of patients with advanced renal cell carcinoma of different tumor histologies. *Med Oncol.* 2009;26(2):202-209.
64. Porter LL, Burris HA, Jones SF, et al. Summary of results in patients with metastatic renal cell cancer (RCC) from phase I studies of RAD001 (everolimus). *J Clin Oncol (Meeting Abstracts).* June 2006;24(18_suppl):Abstract 14599.
65. Jac J, Giessinger S, Khan M, Willis J, Chiang S, Amato R. A phase II trial of RAD001 in patients (Pts) with metastatic renal cell carcinoma (MRCC). *J Clin Oncol (Meeting Abstracts).* June 2007;25(18_suppl):Abstract 5107.
66. Breuleux M, Klopfenstein M, Stephan C, et al. Increased AKT S473 phosphorylation after mTORC1 inhibition is rictor dependent and does not predict tumor cell response to PI3K/mTOR inhibition. *Mol Cancer Ther.* April 2009;8(4):742-753.
67. Yu K, Shi C, Toral-Barza L, et al. Beyond rapalog therapy: preclinical pharmacology and antitumor activity of WYE-125132, an ATP-competitive and specific inhibitor of mTORC1 and mTORC2. *Cancer Res.* Jan 15 2010;70(2):621-631.
68. Vogelzang NJ, Hutson TE, Samlowski W, et al. Phase II study of perifosine in metastatic renal cell carcinoma (RCC) progressing after prior therapy (Rx) with a VEGF receptor inhibitor. *J Clin Oncol (Meeting Abstracts).* May 2009;27(15S):Abstract 5034.
69. Burris H, Rodon J, Sharma S, et al. First-in-human phase I study of the oral PI3K inhibitor BEZ235 in patients (pts) with advanced solid tumors. ASCO Meeting Abstracts. June 2010;28(15_suppl):3005.
70. Grana B, Burris HA, Rodon Ahnert J, et al. Oral PI3 kinase inhibitor BKM120 monotherapy in patients (pts) with advanced solid tumors: an update on safety and efficacy. ASCO Meeting Abstracts. June 2011;29(15_suppl):3043.
71. LoRusso P, Markman B, Tabernero J, et al. A phase I dose-escalation study of the safety, pharmacokinetics (PK), and pharmacodynamics of XL765, a PI3K/TORC1/TORC2 inhibitor administered orally to patients (pts) with advanced solid tumors. ASCO Meeting Abstracts. June 2009;27(15S):3502.
72. Tan DS, Dumez H, Olmos D, et al. First-in-human phase I study exploring three schedules of OSI-027, a novel small molecule TORC1/TORC2 inhibitor, in patients with advanced solid tumors and lymphoma. ASCO Meeting Abstracts. June 2010;28(15_suppl):3006.
73. Sablin MP, Negrier S, Ravaud A, et al. Sequential sorafenib and sunitinib for renal cell carcinoma. *J Urol.* July 2009;182(1):29-34; discussion 34.
74. Tamaskar I, Garcia JA, Elson P, et al. Antitumor effects of sunitinib or sorafenib in patients with metastatic renal cell carcinoma who received prior antiangiogenic therapy. *J Urol.* January 2008;179(1):81-86; discussion 86.
75. Di Lorenzo G, Carteni G, Autorino R, et al. Phase II study of sorafenib in patients with sunitinib-refractory metastatic renal cell cancer. *J Clin Oncol.* September 2009;27(27):4469-4474.
76. Shepard DR, Rini BI, Garcia JA, et al. A multicenter prospective trial of sorafenib in patients (pts) with metastatic clear cell renal cell carcinoma (mccRCC) refractory to prior sunitinib or bevacizumab. *J Clin Oncol (Meeting Abstracts).* May 2008;26(15_suppl):Abstract 5123.
77. Rini BI, Michaelson MD, Rosenberg JE, et al. Antitumor activity and biomarker analysis of sunitinib in patients with bevacizumab-refractory metastatic renal cell carcinoma. *J Clin Oncol.* August 2008;26(22):3743-3748.
78. Reeves JA, Spigel DR, Daniel DB, Friedman EK, Burris HA, Hainsworth JD. Pazopanib in patients with metastatic renal cell carcinoma previously treated with sunitinib or bevacizumab: a Sarah Cannon Research Institute phase II trial. *J Clin Oncol (Meeting Abstracts).* 2011;29(15):4659.
79. Sosman JA, Flaherty KT, Atkins MB, et al. Updated results of phase I trial of sorafenib (S) and bevacizumab (B) in patients with metastatic renal cell cancer (mRCC). *J Clin Oncol (Meeting Abstracts).* May 2008 2008;26(15_suppl):Abstract 5011.
80. Feldman DR, Baum MS, Ginsberg MS, et al. Phase I trial of bevacizumab plus escalated doses of sunitinib in patients with metastatic renal cell carcinoma. *J Clin Oncol.* March 2009;27(9):1432-1439.
81. Hainsworth JD, Spigel DR, Burris HA 3rd, Waterhouse D, Clark BL, Whorf R. Phase II trial of bevacizumab and everolimus in patients with advanced renal cell carcinoma. *J Clin Oncol.* May 2010;28(13):2131-2136.
82. Escudier BJ, Negrier S, Gravis G, et al. Can the combination of temsirolimus and bevacizumab improve the treatment of metastatic renal cell carcinoma (mRCC)? Results of the randomized TORAVA phase II trial. *J Clin Oncol (Meeting Abstracts).* May 2010;28(15_suppl):Abstract 4516.
83. Motzer RJ, Mazumdar M, Bacik J, Berg W, Amsterdam A, Ferrara J. Survival and prognostic stratification of 670 patients with advanced renal cell carcinoma. *J Clin Oncol.* August 1999;17(8):2530-2540.

84. Mekhail TM, Abou-Jawde RM, Boumerhi G, et al. Validation and extension of the Memorial Sloan-Kettering prognostic factors model for survival in patients with previously untreated metastatic renal cell carcinoma. *J Clin Oncol.* February 1 2005;23(4):832-841.
85. Heng DY, Xie W, Regan MM, et al. Prognostic factors for overall survival in patients with metastatic renal cell carcinoma treated with vascular endothelial growth factor-targeted agents: results from a large, multicenter study. *J Clin Oncol.* December 2009;27(34):5794-5799.
86. Rini B, Cohen DA, Lu D, et al. Hypertension (HTN) as a biomarker of efficacy in patients (pts) with metastatic renal cell carcinoma (mRCC) treated with sunitinib. *Genitourinary Cancers Symposium-ASCO.* 2010:Abstract 312.
87. Cowey CL, Rathmell WK. VHL gene mutations in renal cell carcinoma: role as a biomarker of disease outcome and drug efficacy. *Curr Oncol Rep.* March 2009;11(2):94-101.
88. Hu CJ, Wang LY, Chodosh LA, Keith B, Simon MC. Differential roles of hypoxia-inducible factor 1alpha (HIF-1alpha) and HIF-2alpha in hypoxic gene regulation. *Mol Cell Biol.* December 2003;23(24):9361-9374.
89. Raval RR, Lau KW, Tran MG, et al. Contrasting properties of hypoxia-inducible factor 1 (HIF-1) and HIF-2 in von Hippel-Lindau-associated renal cell carcinoma. *Mol Cell Biol.* July 2005;25(13):5675-5686.
90. Gordan JD, Lal P, Dondeti VR, et al. HIF-alpha effects on c-Myc distinguish two subtypes of sporadic VHL-deficient clear cell renal carcinoma. *Cancer Cell.* December 2008;14(6):435-446.
91. Sandlund J, Oosterwijk E, Grankvist K, Oosterwijk-Wakka J, Ljungberg B, Rasmuson T. Prognostic impact of carbonic anhydrase IX expression in human renal cell carcinoma. *BJU Int.* September 2007;100(3):556-560.
92. Leibovich BC, Sheinin Y, Lohse CM, et al. Carbonic anhydrase IX is not an independent predictor of outcome for patients with clear cell renal cell carcinoma. *J Clin Oncol.* October 2007;25(30):4757-4764.
93. Li G, Feng G, Gentil-Perret A, Genin C, Tostain J. Serum carbonic anhydrase 9 level is associated with postoperative recurrence of conventional renal cell cancer. *J Urol.* August 2008;180(2):510-513; discussion 513-514.
94. Golshayan AR, Brick AJ, Choueiri TK. Predicting outcome to VEGF-targeted therapy in metastatic clear-cell renal cell carcinoma: data from recent studies. *Future Oncol.* February 2008;4(1):85-92.
95. Zhao H, Ljungberg B, Grankvist K, Rasmuson T, Tibshirani R, Brooks JD. Gene expression profiling predicts survival in conventional renal cell carcinoma. *PLoS Med.* January 2006;3(1):e13.
96. Brannon AR, Reddy A, Seiler M, et al. Molecular stratification of clear cell renal cell carcinoma by consensus clustering reveals distinct subtypes and survival patterns. *Genes Cancer.* 2010;1:152-163.
97. Rini BI, Zhou M, Aydin H, et al. Identification of prognostic genomic markers in patients with localized clear cell renal cell carcinoma (ccRCC). *J Clin Oncol (Meeting Abstracts).* May 2010;28(15_suppl):Abstract 4501.

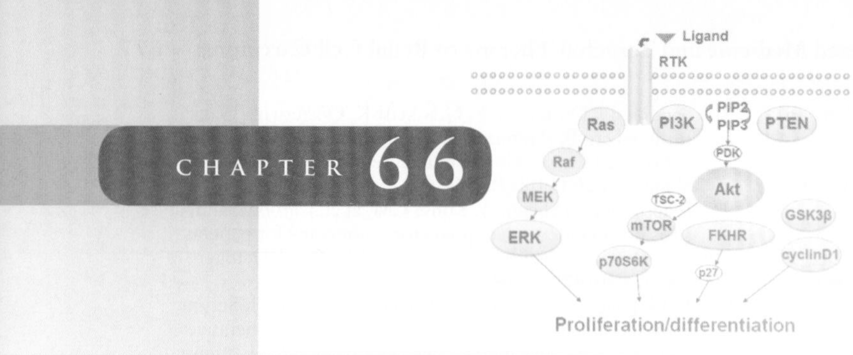

CHAPTER 66

Personalized Medicine and Targeted Therapy of Gliomas

Brett J. Theeler, John De Groot, and W.K. Alfred Yung

INTRODUCTION

The World Health Organization (WHO) classifies tumors of the central nervous system (CNS) into 15 different categories including malignant and non-malignant neoplasms of the brain and cerebral meninges.[1] Included in the WHO classification scheme are glial, neuronal, embryonal, meningeal, hematopoietic, and metastatic tumors of the CNS. Primary CNS neoplasms represent a diverse group of tumors with different biologies, prognoses, and treatments. Glial neoplasms, gliomas, are the most common primary malignant CNS neoplasm in adults. Improved understanding of the molecular biology and underlying pathways driving gliomagenesis will pave the way toward a personalized, targeted approach to treatment of glioma patients.

According to the Central Brain Tumor Registry of the United States, an estimated 62,930 new diagnoses of primary non-malignant and malignant brain and CNS neoplasms were made in 2010. The American Cancer Society estimated that 22,070 patients were diagnosed with malignant CNS in 2009, representing 1.49% of all primary malignant cancers diagnosed that year in the United States.[2] Despite relative rarity, a disproportionate amount of cancer-related morbidity and mortality can be attributed to CNS neoplasms. An estimated 12,920 deaths were expected due to primary CNS malignancies in 2009, and the 5-year relative survival rates after diagnosis were 33.6% for males and 37.0% for females from 1995 to 2006. The survival worsens throughout the life span with 72% of patients aged 0 to 19 surviving 5 years, compared with 5.2% of patients aged 75 or older surviving 5 years during this time period.[2]

Surgical resection and radiotherapy have been the cornerstones of treatment for most types of CNS neoplasms for decades. Save a few exceptions, including medulloblastoma and primary CNS lymphoma, traditional cytotoxic chemotherapies are marginally effective for most primary CNS neoplasms. Exciting new discoveries in basic and translational research have advanced our understanding of tumor genetics and molecular biology. A significant opportunity exists to personalize care using targeted therapeutic approaches in glioma patients with primary CNS tumors.

HIGH-GRADE GLIOMAS

High-grade gliomas (HGGs) account for 80% of malignant CNS neoplasms. HGGs are considered either WHO grade III or IV, with glioblastoma (GB) being the only WHO grade IV glioma.[1] GB accounts for over half of HGGs, the less common grade III (or anaplastic) tumors, including anaplastic astrocytomas (AA), anaplastic oligodendrogliomas (AOs), and anaplastic oligoastrocytomas (AOAs), make up the majority of the remaining HGGs. HGGs are the most common malignant CNS neoplasm in adults. By contrast, HGGs are less common in pediatric patients.[2] Standard therapy for HGGs includes maximal, safe surgical resection followed by postoperative radiotherapy. Retrospective studies strongly support a survival advantage in patients treated with maximal surgical resection.[3] Postoperative, fractionated external beam radiotherapy to a dose of 60 Gy improves overall survival from 3 to 4 months up to 7 to 12 months in HGG patients. The 5-year relative survival rates of HGGs in the United States from 1995 to 2006 (47% for AO, 27% for AA, and 4.4% for GB) highlight the need for better therapeutic strategies.[2]

Conventional chemotherapeutic agents show poor efficacy in newly diagnosed and recurrent HGGs. A meta-analysis of 12 randomized clinical trials demonstrated a modest 6% survival benefit of adjuvant chemotherapy, mainly nitrosoureas, after resection and radiotherapy in patients with HGGs.[4] In recurrent HGGs, a pooled analysis of eight trials demonstrated that 15% and 31% of patients were progression free (PFS [progression-free survival]) at 6 months (PFS6) for GB and AA, respectively, further highlighting the need for better therapeutic approaches.[5]

Glioblastoma

GB is among the most heterogenous of neoplasms. GB has a diverse microscopic appearance with areas of necrosis, hypoxia, ischemia, infiltration, angiogenesis, and varying morphologies. Histomorphologic variants include gemistocyte, epithelioid, small cell, gliosarcoma, giant cell, and GB with an oligodendroglial component.[1,6] Despite unique histomorphologic features, anatomic localization (e.g., gliosarcomas have a predilection for the temporal lobe), radiographic appearance (e.g., giant cell GBs are well circumscribed), and molecular alterations (small cell GBs have high rates of epidermal growth factor receptor [EGFR] amplification and phosphatase and tensin homologue deleted on chromosome 10 [PTEN] deletion, while giant cell GBs have high rates of p53 mutations and PTEN deletion), these variants are not clearly associated with differential outcomes.[1] GBs can be partitioned into primary GBs arising de novo and secondary GBs arising from a grade II or III glial neoplasm. Primary GBs typically occur in patients over the age of 50 years and are characterized by overexpression or mutation of the EGFR, loss of heterozygosity of chromosome 10q, and PTEN mutations. Secondary GBs usually occur in younger patients and are characterized by p53 and IDH1 mutations, overexpression of platelet-derived growth factor receptor (PDGFR), and abnormalities in the retinoblastoma (Rb) pathway.[6]

In the preceding decades, the principal determinant of outcome in patients with GB rested upon pretreatment prognostic factors rather than on the addition of specific therapeutics. Determinants such as age, performance score, and extent of surgical resection were combined to assign patients with HGGs into categories associated with survival. Using recursive partitioning analysis (RPA), Curran et al.[7] developed a classification scheme that helped ensure that homogenous groups of patients were enrolled in clinical trials and provided a more efficient means of comparing results among clinical trials in HGG. The RPA classification remains as a valuable prognostic tool for interpretation of trial results and as a stratification factor for enrolling GB patients in clinical trials.

Prior to 2005, no prospective trials had demonstrated benefit of chemotherapy in patients with newly diagnosed GB. In 2005, a phase III trial conducted by the European Organisation for Research and Treatment of Cancer (EORTC) and the National Cancer Institute of Canada (NCIC) Clinical Trials Group established the current standard of care for patients with newly diagnosed GB. The trial compared standard radiotherapy alone versus radiotherapy plus concurrent temozolomide (TMZ) (75 mg/m^2 of body surface area for 6 wk during radiotherapy). Patients in the combination arm were then treated with adjuvant TMZ (150 to 200 mg/m^2 for 5 d of every 28-d cycle) for six cycles. Radiotherapy combined with TMZ was well tolerated and resulted in a significantly increased median survival from 12.1 to 14.6 months versus radiotherapy alone. The percentage of 2-year survivors had increased from 10.4% in the radiotherapy-only arm to 26.5% in the group given radiotherapy combined with TMZ.[8] A 5-year analysis of the EORTC–NCIC trial reported an improved 5-year survival rate for patients treated with TMZ in addition to radiotherapy compared to radiotherapy alone (9.8% vs. 1.9%).[9] Maximal surgical resection and radiotherapy with concurrent and adjuvant TMZ is now the standard of care for patients with newly diagnosed GB.

A personalized approach combining clinical variables and molecular signatures to assign GB patients to prognostic categories is now possible, and this knowledge is being used for patient stratification in clinical trials. Molecular markers predictive of response to specific therapies have remained elusive in GB. Developing prognostic and predictive biomarkers to move closer to a personalized, targeted approach to GB treatment will be discussed below.

MGMT and Maximizing Alkylator Chemotherapy

While highly statistically significant, the improvement in median OS in the EORTC–NCIC is modest in patients with newly diagnosed GB.[8] There remains a subset of patients who respond poorly to this regimen, and maximizing alkylator chemotherapy is a subject of intense research.

TMZ is an alkylating chemotherapeutic agent, which adds a methyl group to the O^6, N^3, and N^7 positions of guanine on DNA. Alkylation of the O^6 position of guanine results in futile cycling of the mismatch repair system in tumor cells, ultimately inducing apoptosis. O^6-methylguanine-DNA methyltransferase (MGMT) is a DNA repair enzyme that is associated with resistance to alkylator chemotherapy. MGMT removes alkyl groups from the O^6 position on guanine. MGMT is variably expressed in different body tissues with relatively low levels of expression in normal brain. The 5′-promoter region of MGMT contains a CpG island, and methylation of CpG islands in the MGMT promoter region results in epigenetic silencing of gene transcription.[10]

Hegi et al. retrospectively evaluated tumor specimens from the pivotal EORTC–NCIC trial for epigenetic silencing of the MGMT gene. The MGMT gene was noted to be methylated in 45% of cases and these patients had a significantly prolonged OS compared with patients with an unmethylated MGMT promoter region (18.2 vs. 12.2 mo, $P < 0.0001$).[10] MGMT methylation status has since been prospectively evaluated as a prognostic marker in patients treated with radiotherapy and TMZ with completion of RTOG 0525. A total of 833 patients with newly diagnosed GB were randomized to two different regimens (discussed below) of radiotherapy and TMZ with stratification by MGMT status. Patients with MGMT promoter methylation had a statistically significant increase in median OS of 21.2 versus 14 months for patients with an unmethylated MGMT promoter.[11] The results of RTOG 0525 validate the use of MGMT as a prognostic marker both for counseling patients on prognosis and as a necessary stratification factor for clinical trials.

In patients receiving radiotherapy alone in the EORTC–NCIC trial, a survival advantage was also observed in those with methylated versus unmethylated MGMT promoters.[10] In a separate retrospective study of 225 GB patients treated with radiotherapy alone, MGMT promoter methylation status was associated with a statistically significant improvement in PFS and OS.[12] The accumulated results suggest that MGMT promoter methylation is a prognostic molecular marker but is not predictive of outcome. Further, the majority of patients, 50% or more, have an unmethylated MGMT promoter region and an inferior rate of survival with the current standard of care. Patients with an unmethylated MGMT promoter have a survival benefit when treated with TMZ and radiotherapy. In the EORTC–NCIC trial, patients with an unmethylated MGMT promoter had an increased median overall survival (12.7 vs. 11.8 mo) and 2-year survival rate (13.8% vs. <2%), although these results were not statistically significant in a subgroup analysis.[10] While MGMT promoter methylation is associated with improved outcomes in patients treated with the current standard of care, there is no alternative regimen for unmethylated patients. Outside of a clinical trial, the presence or absence of MGMT promoter methylation should not be used as a decision-making tool to justify withholding treatment with the current standard of care.

The lack of evidence supporting MGMT promoter methylation as a predictive marker of response to TMZ seems perplexing given the overlapping DNA repair mechanism of MGMT and cytotoxic mechanism of TMZ. One explanation for this problem is that MGMT promoter methylation, as currently measured, may not correlate with gene function (e.g., protein expression) or may be a marker of overall methylation status. Basic and translational studies have not found a correlation between MGMT promoter methylation and MGMT protein expression in tumor tissue. Immunohistochemical staining of MGMT protein in tumor tissue has not been correlated to promoter methylation status or patient outcome.[13] The pattern of CpG island methylation in the MGMT promoter region is heterogenous in GB and other HGGs, and the specific pattern of methylation necessary to silence the MGMT gene is not known. MGMT promoter methylation is frequently seen in conjunction with other factors associated with improved prognosis, including isocitrate dehydrogenase (IDH) mutations, proneural gene signatures, and the CpG island methylator phenotype, all of which are discussed in later sections. Thus, MGMT promoter methylation may be an epiphenomenon related to these and other prognostic factors.

The putative role of MGMT as a means of chemoresistance to TMZ became the focus of phase II and III clinical trials in newly diagnosed and recurrent GB after the Food and Drug Administration (FDA) approval and widespread use of TMZ. As TMZ is an MGMT substrate, administering dose-intense regimens using frequent, higher, and/or prolonged doses of TMZ was employed to either enhance cytotoxicity in patients with MGMT promoter methylation or overcome resistance in unmethylated patients. The so-called dose-dense (7 d on and 7 d off, at 150 mg/m^2/d) and metronomic TMZ (21 d on and 7 d off, at 100 mg/m^2/d) schedules were tested in initial phase II clinical trials in newly diagnosed and recurrent GB.[14,15] RTOG 0525 randomized 833 patients with newly diagnosed GB to standard versus metronomic dosing of TMZ. Patients were stratified based on MGMT promoter methylation status and RPA classification. The trial did not show a benefit in PFS or OS with metronomic dosing of TMZ overall or in patients with a methylated MGMT promoter.[11] These results suggest that other factors besides the silencing of MGMT in tumor tissue determine benefit from TMZ and that higher doses to overwhelm available MGMT do not improve outcomes. Dose-intense regimens have shown some benefit in recurrent GB with PFS rates improved compared with historical controls treated with other cytotoxic agents.[15] Direct enzymatic inhibition of MGMT and inhibition of PARP (poly(adenosine-diphosphate-ribose) polymerase) are other methods of modulating chemoresistance to TMZ, which are currently being tested in clinical trials.

Another means of optimizing the effects of TMZ includes addition of other chemotherapeutic or targeted agents. Single-arm, phase II clinical trials combining other cytotoxic agents, receptor tyrosine kinase inhibitors (RTKIs), or other targeted agents with TMZ in newly diagnosed GB have all resulted in similar, modest improvements in average OS compared with the results from the EORTC–NCIC and RTOG 0525 clinical trials. Whether the improved survival in single-arm, phase II trials is due to salvage regimens, patient selection, other biases associated with clinical trial enrollment, or actual effects of the targeted agents cannot be easily surmised.[16] The results of these trials emphasize the necessity of conducting randomized phase II trial designs with a control arm using standard TMZ and stratification using molecular prognostic markers, including MGMT methylation, to identify subgroups of patients who may benefit from the addition of additional chemo- and targeted therapies. Ongoing international, randomized phase III clinical trials testing TMZ plus the targeted agents cilengitide and bevacizumab are using MGMT promoter methylation status as a stratification factor in patients with newly diagnosed GB.

MGMT methylation status is controversial as a prognostic factor in recurrent GB. Methylation status is not associated with an improved OS or predictive of response to TMZ in the recurrent setting. According to the studies of initial and recurrent tumor samples, methylation status can change at recurrence.[17] Treatment with TMZ may result in a hypermutation phenotype due to loss of DNA mismatch repair function which is necessary for TMZ-mediated cytotoxicity. This phenotype with impaired DNA repair may be more common in MGMT methylated patients.[18]

Another approach to delivering alkylating chemotherapy involves implanting biodegradable wafers containing BCNU (Gliadel wafers) into the tumor resection cavity. A randomized, placebo-controlled trial yielded a survival benefit of 13.9 months (Gliadel) versus 11.6 months (placebo) in patients with newly diagnosed HGGs including anaplastic tumors; a survival advantage was still observed 2 to 3 years later.[19] BCNU wafers may limit patient eligibility for clinical trials and result in high rates of pseudoprogression after chemoradiation. No prospective studies adding BCNU wafers to radiotherapy and TMZ have been completed to date. BCNU wafers have a diminishing role in the management of patients with GBs given the current standard of care.

MGMT promoter methylation has other important clinical implications besides its role as a prognostic biomarker in newly diagnosed GB. Pseudoprogression, operationally defined as radiographic progression following radiotherapy with subsequent improvement or stabilization on subsequent planned therapy, is seen in 25% to 50% of patients treated with radiotherapy and TMZ. Small retrospective studies suggest that pseudoprogression is seen more frequently in patients with MGMT promoter methylation and may be associated with improved overall survival.[20] It is imperative to recognize pseudoprogression to avoid discontinuing TMZ prematurely or enrolling patients with pseudoprogression in clinical trials potentially leading to falsely optimistic results. MGMT promoter methylation is also associated with higher rates of recurrence outside the initial radiation field, presumably due to enhanced cytocidal activity of radiation combined with TMZ in methylated patients.[21]

Unless enrolled in a clinical trial, all patients with GB should be treated with the current standard of care with concurrent and adjuvant TMZ. Methylation of the MGMT promoter region is prognostic but not predictive of outcome in patients with newly diagnosed GB. MGMT is an important prognostic biomarker for stratification of patients in clinical trials in newly diagnosed GB. As mentioned previously, GBs with an unmethylated MGMT promoter have a relative improvement in OS with the current standard of care, and MGMT promoter methylation status should not be used as a deciding factor on whether or not a patient should be treated with TMZ. Dose-intense regimens of TMZ do not yet have a defined role in newly diagnosed GB, but may have an evolving role in patients with recurrent GB.

IDH Mutations

Metabolic enzymes and metabolites are recently identified candidate oncogenes or tumor suppressors. Using genome-wide sequencing, Parsons et al. first identified IDH1 mutations in 18 of 149 GB samples. These patients were noted to have a prolonged overall survival compared with patients with wild-type IDH.[22] Subsequently, Yan et al. evaluated 445 samples from grade I to IV gliomas and medulloblastomas and 494 non–CNS tumor samples for the presence of IDH1 or IDH2 mutations. No IDH1 or IDH2 mutations were seen in the non–CNS tumor samples. IDH1 or IDH2 mutations were found in over 80% of grade II and III oligodendroglial and astrocytic gliomas and over 80% of secondary GBs.[23] IDH, especially IDH1^{R132H}, mutations appear to be unique to gliomas, although IDH1 mutations were also discovered in a subset of cytogenetically normal acute myelogenous leukemia (AML) with a poor prognosis.[24] The discovery of IDH mutations in gliomas and AML is novel as this metabolic pathway was not previously implicated in oncogenesis.[25]

Five genes encode for three different IDH enzymes: IDH1, IDH2, and IDH3. IDH catalyzes the oxidative decarboxylation of isocitrate to α-ketoglutarate generating NADPH (nicotinamide adenine dinucleotide phosphate). IDH1 is primarily cytoplasmic while IDH2 is a mitochondrial enzyme involved in the tricarboxylic acid cycle. It is noticeable that glial cells have high baseline levels of α-ketoglutarate due to the uptake of glutamate and glutamine which are ultimately metabolized to α-ketoglutarate. IDH1 and IDH2 mutations appear to result in a decrease in enzymatic function with decreased cytoplasmic levels of α-ketoglutarate and NADPH. Decreased cytosolic α-ketoglutarate may result in stabilization of hypoxia-inducible factor-1 alpha (HIF-1α) facilitating cellular proliferation, suggesting wild-type IDH may serve a tumor suppressor function. IDH mutations are heterozygous and may reduce enzymatic function by a dominant negative effect by forming heterodimers of mutant and wild-type IDH resulting in decreased cytosolic α-ketoglutarate. Alternatively, mutant IDH1 may serve as an oncogene by a gain of function; it can convert α-ketoglutarate to d-2-hydroxyglutarate which builds up in the cytoplasm.[25] Suffice it to say, the exact mechanism of tumorigenesis mediated by IDH mutations has yet to be defined.

Primary GB makes up the majority of GBs, with secondary GBs making up 10% or less overall.[6,26] IDH1 mutations are found in over 73% to 88% of secondary GBs and 3 to 7% of primary GBs.[23,26,27] GBs with IDH1 mutations are phenotypically distinct. Over 60% of IDH1 mutant GBs are localized in the frontal lobe and have a peak incidence in the third decade of life. IDH1 mutant GBs often have radiographic features of low-grade gliomas (LGGs) as IDH1 mutant GBs are nonenhancing, are associated with a lesser extent of edema, and have cystic or diffuse components more often than IDH1 wild-type GBs. GBs with IDH1 mutations have a markedly improved overall survival compared with wild-type tumors, overall survival ranging from 24 to 36 months in the setting of an IDH1 mutation versus 9 to 15 months in patients with wild-type tumors.[27-29] IDH2 mutations are found mainly in oligodendroglial tumors and appear to be very rare in astrocytic tumors.[23] There is a higher frequency of MGMT promoter methylation and p53 mutation in IDH1 mutant GBs. The combination of IDH1 mutation and MGMT promoter methylation in patients with GB appears to be associated with improved survival outcomes compared with the presence of either biomarker alone.[28,29] GBs with IDH1 mutations appear to also segregate with tumors with a proneural gene signature and the CpG island methylator phenotype.[29-31] In one study of AAs and GBs, IDH1 mutations were the strongest prognostic factor in a multivariate analysis including the variables age, MGMT methylation, histology, and extent of resection.[27] IDH1 mutations will have an integral role in developing personalized medicine for GB patients as a prognostic biomarker and stratification factor in future clinical trials. Whether IDH mutations will serve as a novel target for future glioma therapeutics will require a greater understanding of mechanisms of tumorigenesis initiated or maintained by these mutations.

Targeting Growth Factor Receptors and Intracellular Signaling

GBs have a complex molecular pathogenesis with loss of function of tumor suppressor genes and oncogene activation within a framework of densely interconnected signaling pathways. As displayed in Figure 66.1, alterations in receptor tyrosine kinase (RTK)/Ras/PI3K (phosphoinositide 3-kinase), p53, and Rb signaling pathways are present in 80% or more of GBs.[32] GBs frequently display amplification or mutations in growth factor receptors, including PDGFR, EGFR, and vascular endothelial growth factor receptor (VEGFR). Other growth factor receptors including ERBB2, MET, and transforming growth factor-beta (TGF-β) are less frequently mutated or overexpressed in GB (see Fig. 66.1). Ligand binding to EGFR, PDGFR, and other growth factor receptors leads to a complex cascade of intracellular signaling activating proliferation, migration, invasion, inhibition of apoptosis, and angiogenesis. The downstream intracellular signaling pathways such as the PI3K/Akt/mammalian target of rapamycin (mTOR) and Ras/Raf/mitogen-activated protein kinase (MAPK) pathways are also dysregulated in GBs.[32]

The EGFR gene is amplified and overexpressed in approximately 50% of GBs, and 20% to 50% of patients with EGFR amplification express the EGFRvIII mutation. The EGFRvIII mutation results in deletion of the extracellular domain of the receptor and a constitutively activated protein.[32,33] EGFR amplification is typically seen in older patients with primary GBs, a classical genetic subtype, and is negatively correlated with IDH1 mutations.[6,30] EGFR amplification has not been consistently associated with inferior survival after controlling for patient age and when comparing with other patients with primary GB. PDGFR receptor subtypes α and β are overexpressed in a smaller proportion of GB patients with a secondary, proneural molecular signature. PDGF signaling may be an early event in gliomagenesis promoting autocrine or paracrine signaling leading to tumor proliferation and angiogenesis.[34]

The PI3K/Akt/mTOR and Ras/Raf/MAPK pathways regulate a diverse array of cellular functions, and activation of these pathways mediates tumor proliferation, migration, invasion, resistance to apoptosis, and angiogenesis in multiple different cancers. Constitutive activation of the PI3K pathway is a hallmark of GBs and is mediated by several different mechanisms. As discussed prior, amplification or mutation of EGFR or other growth receptors (e.g., Erbb2, MET; see Fig. 66.1) is present in over 60% of GBs and preferentially activates the PI3K pathway.[32] PTEN is a tumor suppressor gene and a negative regulator of PI3K. Loss of the PTEN gene on chromosome 10q or mutation of PTEN occurs in 50% or more of GBs.[35] Amplification or mutation of the regulatory subunits of the PI3K gene (e.g., PIK3CA mutations) itself is present in 10% or more of GB patients and provides yet another mechanism of activation of this pathway.[30,36] Ras/Raf/MAPK pathway is activated by inappropriate RTK or integrin activation in gliomas while activating mutations of Ras or BRAF are rare in GBs. However, loss or mutation of the neurofibromatosis type 1 (NF1 gene) occurs in nearly 20% of GBs and leads to constitutive activation of the Ras oncogene and cross-activation of the PI3K pathway.[32]

The signal transducers and activators of transcription (STAT) family of transcription factors have a diverse biologic role by relaying information from the plasma membrane to the nucleus after activation by growth factor and cytokine receptors. STAT3 plays a central role in astrocyte and neural stem cell development. One study of STAT3 in gliomas uncovered a differential role as either a tumor suppressor or oncogene in glioma models. STAT3 appears to act as a tumor suppressor role when PTEN is intact. PTEN-deficient glioma cells have constitutively active Akt, which decrease STAT3 activity resulting in upregulation of interleukin 8 which promotes angiogenesis and invasion. STAT3 acts as an oncogenic switch in the presence of EGFRvIII mutations.[37] STAT3, along with the transcription factor C/EBPβ, is a master regulator of the mesenchymal phenotype in HGGs.[38] STAT3 inhibitors are in early phases of clinical development.

EGFR and PDGFR inhibitors including gefitinib, erlotinib, and imatinib mesylate have been tested in phase II clinical trials. Radiographic responses were rare with no improvement in PFS or OS compared with historical controls in patients with recurrent GB. Analyses from clinical trials using these agents attempted to identify patients with molecular predictors of response to these agents. Theoretically, EGFR inhibitors may be most effective for tumors with EGFR amplification and low levels of phosphorylated Akt or an EGFRvIII mutation and low levels of PTEN expression. Studies retrospectively evaluating for molecular determinants of response in clinical

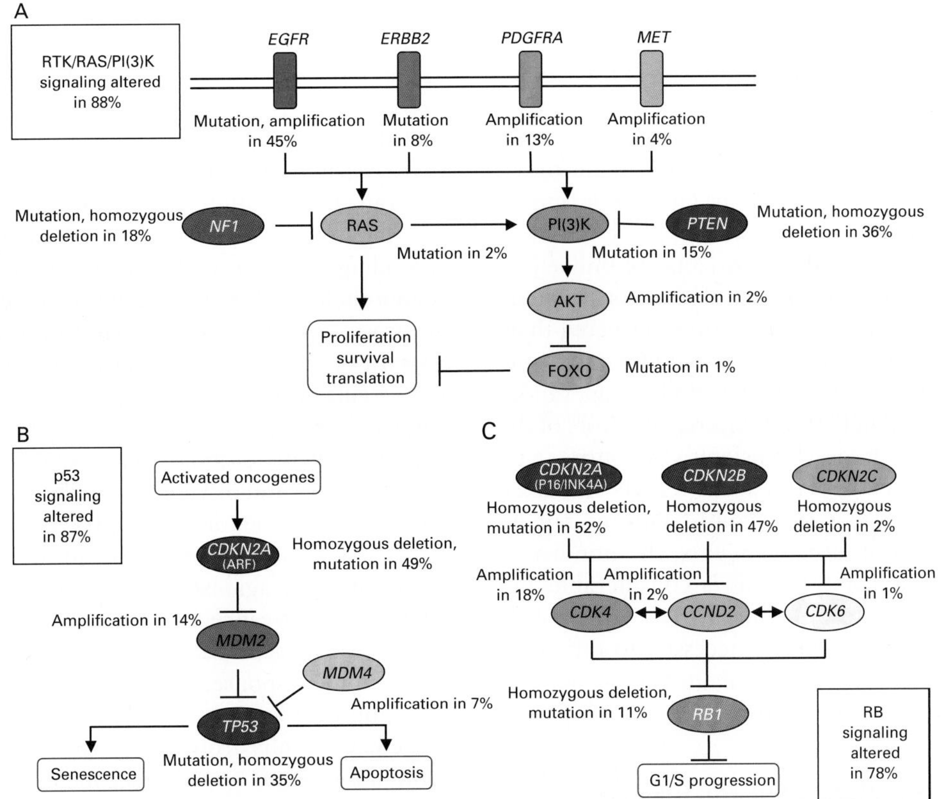

FIGURE 66–1 Frequent genetic alterations in three critical signaling pathways. **A–C.** Primary sequence alterations and significant copy number changes for components of the RTK/RAS/PI3K **(A)**, p53 **(B)**, and RB **(C)** signaling pathways are shown. Red indicates activating genetic alterations, with frequently altered genes showing deeper shades of red. Conversely, blue indicates inactivating alterations, with darker shades corresponding to a higher percentage of alteration. For each altered component of a particular pathway, the nature of the alteration and the percentage of tumors affected are indicated. Boxes contain the final percentages of glioblastomas with alterations in at least one known component gene of the designated pathway. (Reproduced with permission from *Nature* 455:1061-1068 (23 October 2008).)

trials using erlotinib and gefitinib in recurrent GB either yielded conflicting results or have not been replicated in larger, prospective studies.[39,40] A personalized approach using prospective determination of EGFR or other RTK expression, amplification, and dysregulation of downstream pathways to enrich clinical trial populations using RTKIs is a strategy that has not been adequately executed in clinical trials to date.

Trials using the first generation of targeted inhibitors of the PI3K/Akt/mTOR pathway have been unsuccessful. mTOR inhibitors including rapamycin and other analogous drugs have been tested in recurrent GB and have failed to demonstrate efficacy.[41] Combining EGFR and mTOR inhibitors was both ineffective and associated with significant toxicity in recurrent GB trials.[42] Enzastaurin, an inhibitor of protein kinase C and the PI3K/Akt/mTOR pathway, was well tolerated but ineffective in a phase III trial in recurrent GB patients.[43]

The failure of RTK and small molecule inhibitors of intracellular signaling has been disappointing given the frequency of dysregulation of these pathways and their importance in gliomagenesis. While targeted therapy has been unsuccessful in GB to date, important lessons have been learned about the molecular mechanisms that mediate treatment resistance. GBs often display coactivation of multiple RTKs corroborating an approach using multiple RTKIs.[44] RTK switching as seen in EGFR mutant lung cancer may occur in GB which expresses EGFR and other RTKs such as ERBB2 and MET.[45] The PI3K/Akt/mTOR and other downstream intracellular signaling pathways are often redundant. Inhibition of the mTOR pathway may actually lead to pathway activation and more rapid tumor progression due to cross talk between the PI3K and Ras pathways resulting from loss of negative feedback inhibition when blocking only the mTOR pathway.[46]

Another significant question still to be answered is whether targeted agents sufficiently cross the blood–brain barrier (BBB) and achieve adequate intratumoral concentration in order to effect the targeted intracellular signaling pathways. Genotype-enriched, re-biopsy trials may be one method of determining intratumoral concentrations and targeted effects of drugs in patients undergoing a resection for recurrent GB. Alternative dosing regimens used in other cancers such as intermittent, pulsatile dosing regimens of EGFR inhibitors may be a means of overcoming multidrug resistance at the BBB and achieving greater inhibition of targeted pathways in the CNS.[47]

The failure of the targeted therapies tested to date and our expanding knowledge of the complexity and redundancy of intracellular signaling in GB point to the need for a new paradigm for testing targeted agents in clinical trials. Monotherapy trials using single targeted therapeutics in non-selected GB patients are unlikely to be successful or provide adequate information to guide future clinical trials. A new generation of targeted therapeutics is currently being tested, including multiple RTKIs which block EGFR and other RTKs (e.g., vandetanib), dual PI3K and mTOR inhibitors, inhibitors of the Ras pathway such as farnesyltransferase inhibitors (e.g., tipifarnib), and agents that both act as RTKIs and block intracellular signaling (e.g., sorafenib). With the rapidly expanding portfolio of targeted agents, the number of possible therapeutic combinations is considerable and would take decades to test in clinical trials. A personalized approach to trial design is a necessity to rationally test combinations of targeted agents in patient populations enriched with tumors with expression of specific molecular targets.

Targeting Neovascularization and Invasion

The process of acquiring a blood supply to support rapid tumor progression is a hallmark of cancer cells and necessary for development of most cancers. Tissue vascularization and blood vessel growth are mediated by two distinct processes: angiogenesis which involves the sprouting and remodeling of capillaries from pre-existing blood vessels and vasculogenesis which implies the de novo assembly of new blood vessels from bone marrow–derived endothelial cell progenitors. Vascular proliferation is one of the grading criteria and pathologic hallmarks used by the WHO to classify a glioma as WHO grade IV.[1] GBs are among the most highly vascular tumors, and angiogenesis and vasculogenesis play an important role in tumor proliferation, migration, and invasion.

Glioma cells are believed to initially co-opt normal blood vessels and shift toward an angiogenic phenotype in a hypoxic microenvironment.[48] Angiogenesis in response to cellular hypoxia is mediated by HIF-1α. HIF-1α is tightly regulated under normal conditions but under hypoxic conditions is constitutively expressed.[49] Under hypoxic conditions, tumor cells and to a lesser degree endothelial cells secrete vascular endothelial growth factor (VEGF). VEGF-A and its tyrosine kinase receptor, VEGF receptor 2 (VEGFR2), are the principal mediators of angiogenesis in GBs. GBs produce a variety of other proangiogenic proteins, including placental growth factor (PlGF), basic fibroblast growth factor (bFGF), PDGF, hepatocyte growth factor/scatter factor (HGF/SF), and CXCL12.[50,51] Hypoxic conditions and secretion of VEGF by GB cells mobilize and recruit bone marrow–derived progenitors, including endothelial progenitor cells (EPCs), which contribute to angiogenesis and vasculogenesis. Myeloid cells such as monocytes which secrete VEGF are also recruited under hypoxic conditions, incorporate perivascularly, and contribute to neovascularization. VEGFR2 activates the PI3K/Akt/mTOR and Ras/Raf/MAPK pathways involved in glioma proliferation and invasion.[50]

Angiogenesis and vasculogenesis are tightly regulated depending on a delicate balance of various factors involved in endothelial cell proliferation and survival. By contrast, the process of tumor neovascularization is a chaotic process with vessel destabilization, vessel sprouting, necrosis, and vascular thrombosis leading to infarction. The dysregulated angiogenic process with increased expression of proangiogenic proteins and receptors, particularly the increased secretion of VEGF and expression of VEGFR2, provides an avenue for targeted therapeutics.

Bevacizumab, a recombinant humanized monoclonal antibody against VEGF, was originally approved for use in colon cancer and was used initially off-label in patients with recurrent HGGs with impressive rates of radiographic response. Bevacizumab received accelerated FDA approval for recurrent GB in May 2009. Approval hinged on results from two single-arm phase II trials combining intravenous bevacizumab and irinotecan in patients with recurrent HGGs. The FDA's independent review determined response rates of 26% and 35%, PFS6 of 29% in one trial, and a median duration of response of 3.9 months in the other. Steroid doses were reduced by 50% or more in over 50% of the patients enrolled in these trials.[52,53] The safety and efficacy of bevacizumab were confirmed in subsequent clinical trials with response rates of 29% to 35% and PFS6 rates of 43% to 50%.[54] The rates of radiographic response and PFS6 were significantly improved from historical rates with cytotoxic chemotherapy. Despite improved rates of radiographic response, steroid sparing, and PFS, bevacizumab has not resulted in improved survival outcomes compared with historical controls in patients with recurrent GB.

Bevacizumab has been combined with numerous chemotherapeutic and targeted agents in a multitude of clinical trials, mainly in recurrent GB. Combination of bevacizumab with cytotoxic agents including TMZ and irinotecan and targeted agents including tyrosine kinase inhibitors has not resulted in improved rates of PFS or OS compared with bevacizumab alone. Multiple trials combining bevacizumab with other cytotoxic agents, targeted agents, and radiotherapy are currently in progress.

Other agents which inhibit VEGF- and VEGFR-mediated signaling (e.g., sunitinib and pazopanib) have been tested in clinical trials and have not shown single-agent activity in recurrent HGGs. Cediranib, a pan-VEGFR RTKI that also inhibits c-KIT and PDGF, was tested in a phase III clinical trial in recurrent GB after promising results in pre-clinical studies and a phase II study. Cediranib induces rapid vascular normalization which reverses after stopping cediranib. The phase III results were disappointing as cediranib did not produce a statistically significant improvement in PFS or OS compared with CCNU.[55] There are still multiple RTKIs with activity at VEGFR which are being actively tested in clinical trials.

The inability of VEGFR TKIs to thus far produce similar results to bevacizumab has not been explained. It is noticeable that treatment with bevacizumab still offers some benefit in patients first treated with VEGFR TKIs for recurrent GB.[56] Removal of VEGF isoforms from the circulation may have a greater therapeutic index than VEGFR inhibition. VEGF Trap (aflibercept) which sequesters all isoforms of VEGF-A, VEGF-B, and PlGF acting as a soluble, decoy receptor did not show single-agent activity in a trial of recurrent GB and HGGs.[57] The lack of efficacy observed with VEGF Trap suggesting sequestering multiple angiogenic proteins (VEGF-A, VEGF-B, and PlGF) does not improve outcomes compared with inhibiting VEGF-A alone. In one pre-clinical study using a mouse model, bevacizumab, but not sunitinib, inhibited the migration of myeloid cells into orthotopically implanted GBs, perhaps elucidating one mechanism of anti-angiogenic activity unique to bevacizumab.[58]

Bevacizumab has also been tested in newly diagnosed GB patients in combination with radiotherapy and TMZ. Two phase II clinical trials testing TMZ and bevacizumab in newly diagnosed GB patients yielded median overall survivals of 19.6 and 21.2 months, which are similar to the results from other single-arm, phase II clinical trials combining TMZ with other targeted agents. PFS did appear to be improved compared with historical control groups.[59,60] Two ongoing phase III clinical trials which randomized patients to TMZ versus TMZ plus bevacizumab are anxiously awaited to determine whether timing of bevacizumab improves overall survival.

With the approval and widespread use of bevacizumab, resistance to anti-angiogenic therapy is a significant problem in the day-to-day care of patients with GB. Early observations that bevacizumab-treated patients sometimes recur with a diffuse, gliomatosis-like phenotype further heightened concern that bevacizumab may alter the biology of GB by inducing an invasive phenotype.[61] Subsequent retrospective reports from larger groups of patients have not shown a higher rate of distant or diffuse recurrence in bevacizumab-treated patients. Local recurrence is the most common pattern of bevacizumab failure and patients with multifocal or diffuse disease at baseline are more likely to then recur with a multifocal or diffuse pattern.[62] Withdrawal of bevacizumab is difficult after failure, as withdrawal often leads to a rebound in tumor growth and edema. Bevacizumab theoretically increases chemotherapy delivery to tumor cells by vascular normalization, a phenomenon that has been demonstrated in pre-clinical models, although a study using a glioma model and the VEGFR inhibitor vandetanib plus TMZ showed a paradoxical decrease in the efficacy of TMZ when combined with vandetanib.[63] In another study using a glioma model, lower doses of the VEGFR RTKI sunitinib increased intratumoral delivery of TMZ, suggesting the degree of angiogenic inhibition may have important therapeutic implications.[64] Acquired resistance to chemotherapeutic regimens after bevacizumab failure is supported by the observation that salvage regimens are ineffective with rates of PFS6 of 2% or less.[65] An understanding of the mechanisms mediating resistance to anti-angiogenic therapy and a rational, targeted approach to salvage strategies after failure of anti-angiogenic therapy is sorely lacking.

Two models of resistance to anti-angiogenic therapies have been suggested, acquired evasive resistance and intrinsic resistance. Acquired resistance may be due to upregulation of alternative angiogenic signaling pathways (e.g., bFGF, CXCL12, and PlGF), recruitment of vascular progenitor and myeloid cells, or co-option of existing vasculature. Intrinsic resistance implies that redundant and invasive mechanisms are already in place prior to anti-angiogenic treatment and that anti-angiogenic therapy would not be expected to be effective in these patients. Laboratory evidence suggests that VEGF inhibition increases the invasive nature of tumor cells.[66] In a GB mouse model, treatment with anti-angiogenic agents induced an invasive tumor phenotype. Pathologic specimens from GB patients demonstrate tumor invasion despite vascular normalization during bevacizumab therapy.[67] Tumor invasion is an important mechanism of resistance to chemotherapy and targeted therapeutics, including anti-angiogenic therapy.

An invasive phenotype may ultimately lead to treatment failure for all GBs regardless of exposure to anti-angiogenic therapies. Similar to tumor neovascularization, tumor invasion relies on a coordinated series of events at the cellular level. Interactions among cell surface receptors, the extracellular matrix (ECM), and secretion of proteases and growth factors are all necessary to promote tumor cell invasion. The cascade of invasion and metastasis associated with systemic solid malignancies is somewhat different in GB as GBs rarely intravasate into the systemic circulation and metastasize outside of the CNS. But local invasion is a hallmark of GBs and this process is similar mechanistically to that seen in other solid malignancies. Glioma cells have a unique ability to migrate distant from the main bulk of tumor cells and invade along neuronal and vascular ECM structures without remodeling of the ECM; gliomatosis cerebri is an extreme example of this invasive phenotype. Changes in the ECM, altered expression of cell surface receptors, protease expression, and expression and activation of cytoplasmic kinases which promote invasion are all mechanisms exploited by glioma cells to invade normal brain tissue.

GB cells and the surrounding ECM have altered the expression of different glycoproteins and proteoglycans which promote invasion. E-cadherin and N-cadherin which mediate normal cell-to-cell adhesion and activate the β-catenin signaling pathway are expressed in normal levels (N-cadherin) or not expressed at all in glioma cells (E-cadherin).[68] Galectin-1 and SPARC (secreting protein, acidic, and rich in cysteine) are glycoproteins with elevated expression on the surface of gliomas and result in activation of intracellular signaling pathways such as focal adhesion kinase (FAK) which promotes invasiveness.[69] The α_v integrins, $\alpha_v\beta_3$, $\alpha_v\beta_5$, transmembrane receptors which recognize ECM components and activate intracellular signaling, have an altered expression pattern in HGGs promoting tumor invasion.[70] HGF/SF which activates c-MET is overexpressed in gliomas and expression correlates with degree of malignancy and tumor invasion.[71] Proteases, particularly the matrix metalloproteinases (MMPs), degrade the ECM promoting glioma invasion. MMP-2 and MMP-9 are elevated in HGGs and are upregulated after bevacizumab failure.[72] FAK and Src are cytoplasmic tyrosine kinases upregulated in HGGs which activate downstream intracellular signaling pathways, such as the Rho GTPases, which promote invasion.[73]

The regulation and interaction of these pathways are incompletely understood, but agents targeting these pathways have been developed. MMPs were targeted using marimastat. A phase II trial combining marimastat with TMZ in recurrent GB resulted in a PFS6 of 39%, suggesting this may be an attractive target for future clinical trials.[74] MMP inhibitors prolonged the survival of bevacizumab-treated animals, suggesting this may be a target in bevacizumab failure.[72] Cilengitide, an inhibitor of α_v integrins, was inactive as monotherapy in recurrent GB but showed reasonable rates of PFS and OS in newly diagnosed GB when combined with TMZ.[75] A multinational phase III clinical trial evaluating the effectiveness of cilengitide in combination with the standard of care in newly diagnosed GB is currently ongoing. Agents targeting Src (dasatinib) and c-MET (cabozantinib) are being evaluated in early phase clinical trials in recurrent and newly diagnosed GB. Agents targeting HGF/SF and FAK are in the early stages of clinical development. Further study of the biologic mechanisms of invasion and testing of targeted therapeutics with an anti-invasion mechanism will be an important area of future research in neuro-oncology.

Despite widespread clinical use of bevacizumab in recurrent GB, not all patients will achieve a radiographic response or be progression free at 6 months. Developing surrogate markers to predict optimal candidates for anti-angiogenic therapy is needed but these are yet to be identified. The use of conventional magnetic resonance imaging (MRI) in the assessment of GB patients treated with anti-angiogenic therapies is problematic. Bevacizumab therapy results in a marked improvement in contrast-enhanced images on conventional MRI and can occur despite progressive changes on T2/fluid-attenuated inversion recovery (FLAIR) sequences. The Response Assessment in Neuro-Oncology (RANO) criteria take into account qualitative (but not quantitative) changes on T2/FLAIR and two-dimensional measurements of contrast-enhanced images in patients treated with anti-angiogenic agents.[76] The widespread implementation of the RANO criteria in future clinical trials will improve the interpretation of surrogate end points based on conventional MRI.

Due to the effects of anti-angiogenic therapies on blood vessel size and permeability, novel MRI techniques measuring perfusion and permeability have been studied. Apparent diffusion coefficient, a measure of tumor cellularity and water diffusivity, better predicted PFS6 than conventional MRI in one retrospective study of recurrent GB.[77] Studying cediranib in recurrent GB, a so-called vascular normalization index combining K^{trans}, a marker of permeability, generated using dynamic contrast-enhanced MRI, cerebral blood volumes using dynamic susceptibility contrast MRI, and serum collagen IV levels highly correlated with PFS and OS.[78] A retrospective study of patients with recurrent HGG using ^{18}F-fluorothymidine (FLT) PET treated with bevacizumab and irinotecan found that responders on FLT PET had improved survival outcomes compared with non-responders.[79] The cost, lack of widespread availability, and reproducibility of these imaging methodologies currently limit the widespread applicability in the day-to-day care of GB patients. Further development of these and other advanced imaging technologies as surrogate markers of response or failure in clinical trials is an intense area of investigation.

Circulating cells and soluble proteins have been studied as surrogate markers of response to anti-angiogenic therapy. Circulating anti-angiogenic proteins appear to increase during the course of anti-angiogenic therapy. Studying patients with progression while treated with cediranib in recurrent GB, circulating levels of CXCL12, bFGF, and VEGFR2 increased and PlGF decreased. Circulating EPCs are increased in patients with GB and levels of EPCs may be correlated with response to anti-angiogenic therapies.[80] Glioma cells secrete chemokines that recruit proangiogenic myeloid and bone marrow–derived cells to the tumor and contribute to angiogenesis. Elevated baseline levels of monocyte-secreted chemokines were associated with improved response rates while expression of T lymphocyte recruitment and chemotaxis-related genes such as CXCR4 was associated with a decreased time to progression in patients treated with VEGF Trap.[81] Further study of the circulating cells and soluble proteins is needed to determine whether surrogate prognostic or predictive biomarkers of response to anti-angiogenic agents can be found.

Despite widespread use of bevacizumab in patients with recurrent GB, an approach to determine the best candidates for this therapy has not been defined. Bevacizumab may have no effect on overall survival in patients with recurrent GB and patients respond poorly to salvage regimens after treatment failure. Whether bevacizumab improves outcomes in newly diagnosed GB has not been determined and the results of ongoing phase III clinical trials are anxiously awaited. Thus far, results from clinical trials using other anti-angiogenic agents besides bevacizumab in recurrent GB have been disappointing. A better understanding of mechanisms of tumor invasion and therapies targeting these pathways may lead to better outcomes for patients treated with anti-angiogenic agents. A personalized approach combining clinical, neuroimaging, molecular, and circulating factors represents a paradigm to optimize anti-angiogenic therapy in GB patients.

Targeting Glioma Stem Cells

Stem-like cells have been found in different types of cancer including GB and medulloblastoma and may underlie both the pathogenesis and resistance to treatment of different cancer types. Neural stem cells (multipotent and self-renewing) and glial progenitors (self-renewing and capable of producing astrocytes and oligodendrocytes) are found in multiple brain regions, including the subventricular zone and dentate gyrus. Gliomas have stem-like properties including motility, proliferative potential, capacity for self-renewal, and upregulation of pathways important in neuronal and glial development. A population of stem-like cells, herein termed glioma stem cells (GSCs), have been identified in human gliomas.[82,83] GSCs may initiate glioma formation, maintain the neoplastic cell population, and/or promote radioresistance and chemoresistance in GB. Notwithstanding the debate surrounding the existence, identity, and ideal cellular markers (e.g., CD133 and nestin) to identify GSCs, intracellular signaling pathways expressed or upregulated in GSCs are novel targets for cancer therapeutics.

Certain intracellular signaling pathways critical for normal neuronal and glial development are also upregulated in GSCs. The Sonic Hedgehog-Gli (Shh-Gli) pathway is an important pathway in maintenance of neural stem cells; Shh activates the transcriptional regulator Gli which maintains the stem cell populations in the subventricular zone and dentate gyrus. Gli is expressed in GBs, and the Shh-Gli pathway has been implicated in self-renewal and tumorigenesis in GSCs.[84] The canonical, Wnt–β-catenin signaling pathway is also important in the maintenance of stem cell populations. This pathway is aberrantly activated in multiple different cancers, and increased expression of β-catenin has been demonstrated in HGGs.[85] The Notch-delta–like ligand 4 signaling (NOTCH) pathway serves as an important regulator of differentiation and angiogenesis. Stem cell cultures from GB display the expression of NOTCH signaling and this signaling may be differentially activated in grade II to IV gliomas. In one study, NOTCH signaling was inactive in secondary GB, but active in primary GB.[86] Inhibitors of NOTCH (e.g., γ-secretase inhibitors) and Shh-Gli signaling pathways are in early phases of clinical development.

EGFR, PDGFR, and bFGFR (basic fibroblast growth factor receptor) are expressed on neural stem and glial progenitor cell populations and are putative regulators of proliferation, self-renewal, differentiation, and treatment resistance of stem-like cell populations in different cancers. Other signaling pathways downstream from these receptors may also be dysregulated in GSCs, such as activation of the PI3K/Akt/mTOR due to loss of PTEN. TGF-β has pleiotropic effects on glioma proliferation, angiogenesis, invasion, and immune function. TGF-β can increase self-renewal in GSCs and inhibition of TGF-β can decrease the tumor initiation capacity of GSCs.[87] Further understanding of the regulation and interaction of these dysregulated signaling pathways is needed to best utilize targeted therapeutics aimed at GSCs.

GSCs are believed to be maintained in a perivascular niche with endothelial cells secreting soluble factors that maintain GSCs in a stem-like phenotype.[88] Experimentally, disruption of the vascular niche depletes GSCs serving as yet another potential benefit of anti-angiogenic therapy in GB. Regulation of the microenvironment in the perivascular niche, including angiogenesis and vasculogenesis, is important to GSC maintenance. Upregulation of bone morphogenic proteins (BMPs) plays a complex role in differentiation and survival of GSCs. BMP4 may play a role in differentiation and reduction of GSCs; conversely other BMPs may play a proliferative role in GSCs.[89] CD44 which binds to glycoprotein components of the ECM promotes glioma proliferation and invasion and is expressed by a population of GSCs which associate closely with the vasculature.[87] Targeting angiogenesis, NOTCH and TGF-β are potential molecular means of disrupting the perivascular niche thereby targeting GSCs.

Some stem-like cells within GBs have surface characteristics of endothelial cells and anywhere from 20% to 90% of endothelial cells may be tumor derived rather than bone marrow derived. Further, these tumor-derived endothelial cells may be unresponsive to anti-VEGFR–directed therapy and inhibition of VEGFR may lead to an increase in the number of tumor-derived endothelial cells.[90] This may be a potential explanation of innate and/or acquired mechanisms of resistance to anti-angiogenic therapies observed clinically. Anti-angiogenic therapies may have to target tumor-derived and bone marrow–derived endothelium to be effective.

Another therapeutic approach used in other cancers is therapies aimed at inducing differentiation of stem-like cells. Retinoids bind to retinoic acid and retinoid X receptors (RAR and RXR-α, RXR-β, and RXR-γ) and induce differentiation in glioma cells in vitro. 13-*cis*-Retinoic acid has shown modest activity in clinical trials in recurrent HGGs although proponents of this approach argue that retinoids may be more effective if used up front rather than at recurrence.[91] Combining retinoids with other agents targeting differentiation such as NOTCH requires further investigation.

GBs with a mesenchymal genetic signature and inferior survival outcomes also overexpress genes associated with a stem cell phenotype.[92] GSCs are intrinsically resistant to radiotherapy and cytotoxic chemotherapy linking a stem cell–like phenotype to poor outcome and eventual failure of the current standard of care in newly diagnosed GB. Potential mechanisms of resistance include overexpression of MGMT and the expression of the DNA checkpoint proteins CHK1 and CHK2, both of which safeguard the genome by enhancing DNA repair in GSCs.[93] TMZ-treated GSCs behave more aggressively in mouse models compared with untreated tumors and treatment with TMZ may select for cells with stem-like properties further accentuating treatment resistance. GSCs also overexpress ABC transporters responsible for multidrug resistance. ABCG2 (BCRP), which is also expressed at the BBB, is regulated by the PI3K/Akt pathway in GSCs. TMZ is not a substrate for ABCG2 but selects for cells with stem-like properties further propagating a drug-resistant phenotype.[94] Other targeted agents such as imatinib, erlotinib, and gefitinib are substrates for ABC transporters, which may explain the lack of efficacy of these and other targeted agents in GB due to resistance of the GSC population to these targeted agents.

Improving outcomes in GB patients treated with TMZ and targeted agents will require a better understanding of the mechanisms of tumorigenesis and resistance unique to GSCs. As GSCs are resistant to radiotherapy and TMZ, which make up the backbone of the current standard of care, additional targeting of pathways which maintains GSCs may be necessary to further improve survival outcomes in GB patients.

Multigene Sets in GB

GB is a heterogenous disease. The WHO grading scheme allows for separation from grade II and III gliomas with relevance to clinical outcomes but does not explain the range of clinical behavior observed among GB patients. Genetic differences may explain the diverse outcomes and responses to treatments observed in the clinic. Global genomic analysis is a promising approach for developing molecular subtype classifications, multigene clinical predictors, and new targets for therapeutics. The explosion of genomic data sets made available by high-throughput microarray technologies has revolutionized the understanding of different types of cancer. The most well-known project is the Cancer Genome Atlas (TCGA) which profiles DNA, mRNA, microRNA, and epigenetic profiling (DNA methylation).[32] A full discussion of the methods and limitations of evaluating gene expression profiles is beyond the scope of this chapter. Recent gene expression profiling has revealed multiple GB subtypes with different clinical outcomes.

The first study to define multigene sets as a prognostic tool was performed by Phillips et al. Three subgroups were identified as proneural, mesenchymal, and proliferative.[95] A similar analysis of TCGA data set by Verhaak et al. again identified not only proneural and mesenchymal subtypes but also neural and classical subtypes. The proneural subtype was associated with PDGFR amplification, IDH1 mutations, and overexpression of genes related to neural and glial development such as olig2 and SOX. The mesenchymal subtype was associated with increased expression of VEGF, NF1 loss or mutation, and overexpression of genes related to motility, the ECM, and cell adhesion. The TCGA derived classical and neural subtypes were associated with EGFR mutation or amplification, and the classical subtype was associated with PTEN loss.[30]

Tumor grade is clearly associated with the proneural and mesenchymal subtypes. GBs represent a mix of mesenchymal and proneural subtypes. Grade II and III astrocytic, oligodendroglial, and mixed gliomas are almost exclusively proneural.[95] Consistent with these findings, proneural GBs are associated with features of secondary GBs, including younger age at diagnosis, p53 mutations, IDH1 mutations, low rates of EGFR amplification, and PTEN loss.[30] Primary GBs were of the mesenchymal subtype. At recurrence, some proneural tumors develop a mesenchymal genetic signature suggesting that mesenchymal transformation is an important mediator of tumor progression (Fig. 66.2). In the study by Phillips et al., patients with proneural gene signatures had improved patient outcomes compared with patients with mesenchymal signatures.[95] In the analysis by Verhaak et al. from the TCGA, tumor subtype was not associated with patient outcome when grade II and III gliomas were excluded although there was a trend toward improved survival in the proneural GBs.[30]

Further subclassification of neural, classical, or proliferative GB subtypes may be possible, but these other subtypes are not yet well defined biologically or differentiated by clinical outcomes. Colman et al. reported on a 38-gene profile derived from four independent microarray sets consistently associated with patient outcome. This 38-gene profile was refined to a 9-gene set prognostic of outcome in GB after controlling for clinical factors and MGMT methylation status. The 9-gene profile was associated with glioma stem cell–like markers (CD 133 and nestin) in the group of patients with a poor outcome linking stem-like properties and a mesenchymal gene signature.[92] The 9-gene profile can be done on formalin-fixed paraffin-embedded tissue and conceptually represents a multigene tool with broad applicability with further refinement and validation. The 9-gene profile was integrated into the molecular stratification of the ongoing randomized, phase III clinical trial RTOG 0825 in newly diagnosed GB.

A separate study by Noushmehr et al. evaluated epigenetic changes, DNA promoter CpG island methylation patterns in 272 GBs from the TCGA. A distinct CpG hypermethylator phenotype (G-CIMP) was found. G-CIMP tumors were typically found in younger patients

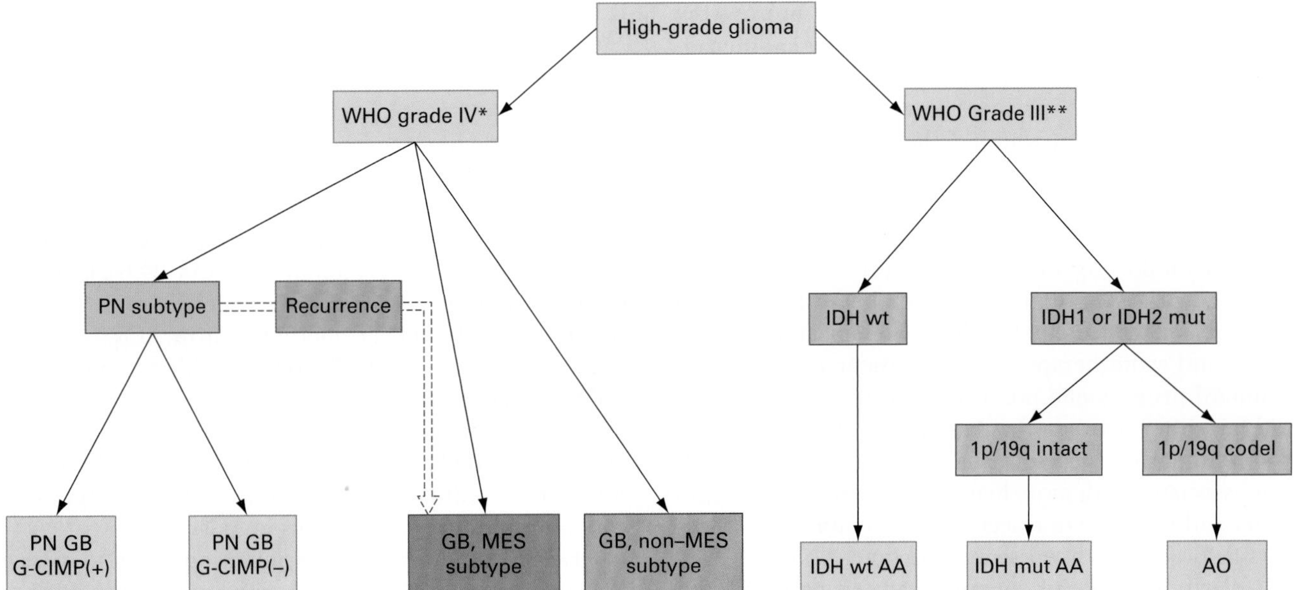

FIGURE 66–2 Proposed molecular classification scheme for high-grade gliomas. Right: Proposed classification scheme for GB including molecular and methylation signature. IDH1 mut is typically found in PN, G-CIMP(+) GBs.[49,51] PN G-CIMP(+) GBs are classified separately from PN G-CIMP(–) GBs due to improved survival with PN G-CIMP(+) tumors.[51] GBs with neurofibromatosis 1 mutations segregate into the MES subtype. The non–PN, non–MES subtypes of GB including the classical and proliferative subtypes[50,138] often have EGFR amplification or overexpression but overall these subtypes are not as well defined. PN GBs may make a PN to MES transformation at recurrence (*red dotted line*). This PN to MES transformation may not occur at recurrence in IDH1 mut, G-CIMP(+) GBs.[49,138] Left: Proposed classification scheme for anaplastic gliomas based on IDH mutation status and 1p/19q chromosomal status (left). IDH wt and IDH mut AAs may represent different subtypes of anaplastic gliomas based on the poor survival outcomes in IDH wt compared with IDH mut AAs.[47] *WHO*, World Health Organization; *PN*, proneural; *MES*, mesenchymal; *GB*, glioblastoma multiforme; *G-CIMP(+)*, CpG hypermethylator phenotype; *IDH1* **or** *IDH2*, isocitrate dehydrogenase 1 or 2 gene; *wt*, wild type; *Mut*, mutation; *Codel*, codeletion; *AA*, anaplastic astrocytoma; *AO*, anaplastic oligodendroglioma.
*Includes GB and all GB variants including gliosarcoma.
**Excludes rare anaplastic glioneuronal tumors and variants.

and also had proneural genetic signatures (see Fig. 66.2). IDH1 and p53 mutations were found primarily within G-CIMP tumors, which also lacked EGFR amplification and loss of PTEN. Patients with G-CIMP tumors experienced significantly improved outcomes compared with non–G-CIMP tumors.[31]

Multigene sets have been shown to be prognostic of outcome in GB. Strong potential exists for using multigene predictors to improve clinical decision-making and as a stratification factor for clinical trials. Figure 66.2 includes a proposed classification scheme for GBs based on genetic and methylation signatures. Balancing proneural and mesenchymal subtypes may be necessary in GB clinical trials to prevent over- or underestimating benefit of a particular agent. Differences in treatment outcomes among different subtypes of gliomas will only be detectable if multigene sets are incorporated into a clinical trial's design. Multigene sets may also prove valuable in the identification of targets for therapeutics. Particular genetic subtypes may respond better to specific targeted agents. For example, mesenchymal tumors may respond better to anti-angiogenic agents while proneural tumors may have a better response to inhibitors of neuronal/glial fate and differentiation when extrapolating from the genes and pathways differentially activated in these tumors.

Anaplastic Gliomas

Anaplastic gliomas (AGs) are classified by the WHO as grade III and the most common AGs are AAs, AOs, and AOAs. Rare astrocytic and mixed glioneuronal tumors such as pilocytic astrocytomas (PAs), gangliogliomas, and pleomorphic xanthoastrocytomas may rarely have anaplastic histology and clinical behavior.[1] AGs are less common than GB, with AAs making up 2.1% and AOs 0.6% of all primary brain tumors in the United States.[2] There is strong evidence that these tumors are separate entities clinically and molecularly with different prognoses and treatment responses. Patients with AAs have a median survival of 2 to 3 years compared to a medial survival of over 5 years in AO patients. AOs tend to have an improved prognosis and response to treatment compared with AAs which are more recalcitrant. Standard treatment for AGs includes maximal, safe surgical resection when feasible and postoperative radiotherapy. The role of chemotherapy, whether before, during, or after radiotherapy, has not been clearly defined.

Two large international clinical trials showed no difference with regard to OS between radiotherapy alone versus radiotherapy before or after PCV (procarbazine, carmustine, and vincristine) chemotherapy in patients with AOs and AOAs. PFS was improved in patients treated with up-front radiotherapy and neoadjuvant PCV plus radiotherapy.[96,97] The lack of symptom and quality of life assessment in these two trials limit the determination of whether the improvements seen in PFS were clinically meaningful or muted by delayed effects of radiotherapy. NOA-04 compared 60 Gy of radiotherapy versus 32 weeks of chemotherapy (PCV or TMZ) following a maximal surgical resection in 318 patients with AGs. Patients in the chemotherapy arm were treated with additional chemotherapy at first recurrence and radiotherapy at second recurrence. A nonstandard primary end point, time to treatment failure, did not differ between the two groups. TMZ and PCV were similarly efficacious in NOA-04 although PCV was associated with more hematologic toxicity. Age ≥ 50 years and incomplete resection were confirmed as factors associated with worsened outcome.[98] NOA-04 did not clarify the role of chemotherapy in patients with AGs. There is an urgent need to develop a personalized, molecular-based approach to supplement the clinical and histopathologic parameters used for managing AGs.

Codeletion on chromosome arms 1p/19q characterizes a subgroup of AGs with an improved prognosis.[99] 1p/19q codeletion is present in approximately 40% of AGs, but this codeletion occurs in 70% or more of AOs.[98,99] AOAs appear to have a rate of 1p/19q codeletion intermediate between AAs and AOs. The histologic classification of oligodendroglial tumors can vary as classification as pure AOs or mixed AOAs may differ among neuropathologists. Due to difficulties with histologic classification, 1p/19q codeletion is often used as a marker of the oligodendroglial lineage (see further discussion in the section Low-Grade Gliomas). In the three trials discussed above, 1p/19q codeletion was associated with significantly longer rates of disease-free and overall survival regardless of initial therapy following surgical resection. A molecular rationale explaining why 1p/19q codeleted AGs have an improved prognosis has yet to be fully elucidated. 1p/19q codeletion is strongly associated with other prognostic biomarkers including IDH mutations and methylation of the MGMT promoter region.[100,101] 1p/19q as determined by fluorescence in situ hybridization has an established role as a prognostic factor in AGs. Internationally, phase III clinical trials testing different combinations of radiotherapy and TMZ in patients with AGs with and without 1p/19q codeletion are ongoing.

AG patients with a methylated MGMT promoter treated with up-front radiotherapy or chemotherapy (either PCV or TMZ) had improved PFS regardless of initial treatment. MGMT promoter methylation is highly correlated to IDH mutations and 1p/19q codeletion in AGs.[98,101] MGMT promoter methylation status is a stratification factor in the ongoing CATNON clinical trial (RTOG 0834) in patients with newly diagnosed AGs with intact 1p and 19q chromosomal arms. Similar to recurrent GB, whether MGMT promoter methylation is prognostic in recurrent AGs is not clear. The role of MGMT promoter methylation as a prognostic biomarker in AGs whether in isolation or in combination with other prognostic biomarkers (e.g., IDH1 or IDH2 mutations or 1p/19q codeletion) requires further analysis.

IDH1 and IDH2 mutations are important prognostic biomarkers in AGs. IDH1 mutations were found to have a stronger impact on prognosis than 1p/19q codeletion or MGMT methylation in the NOA-04 trial. IDH1 or IDH2 mutations are strongly associated with 1p/19q codeletion and MGMT methylation in AOs.[98] When testing a large group of 382 patients with AAs and GBs, IDH1 mutation was the most prominent prognostic factor followed by age, histology (AA or GB), and MGMT promoter methylation status.[27] Determining IDH mutational status will be necessary in order to interpret outcomes from future clinical trials in AGs.

EGFR amplification and mutation, PTEN mutation or loss, and downstream activation of the PI3K/Akt/mTOR are considered hallmarks of primary GBs. AGs display mutation, deletion, or activation of these and other signaling pathways. PI3K activation by PTEN loss or other mechanisms occurs in the majority of AAs. EGFR amplification and PTEN mutation or loss occurs in oligodendroglial tumors but the exact frequency is unknown. AGs with EGFR amplification, PTEN mutation or loss, and constitutive activation of the PI3K/Akt/mTOR pathways are likely to represent a group of tumors with a poor prognosis and may be more likely to be intact on chromosomal arms on 1p/19q, IDH wild type, and unmethylated on MGMT, although this requires further study.

The majority of oligodendroglial tumors with a 1p/19q codeletion have a proneural genetic signature. Oligodendrogliomas with non–proneural genetic signatures have inferior survival outcomes when compared with proneural tumors.[102,103] Likewise, AOs with a G-CIMP hypermethylation signature have improved outcomes compared with non–G-CIMP AOs, and G-CIMP status was strongly correlated with 1p/19q codeletion, IDH mutation, and MGMT methylation.[104] Further evaluation of the genetic signatures and their association with patient outcomes in patients with AGs is needed.

Currently, treatment of AGs varies among neuro-oncologists. Patients with AOs are treated with up-front chemotherapy, postoperative radiotherapy (54 to 60 Gy), or concurrent chemoradiotherapy and adjuvant chemotherapy similar to GBs.[105] AAs are typically treated with postoperative radiotherapy but whether concurrent or adjuvant chemotherapy improves outcomes is uncertain. Using the standard regimen for GB in AGs has not been proven to improve survival outcomes or to have an acceptable rate of treatment-related toxicity. TMZ is rapidly replacing PCV in the long-term management of AGs due to decreased rates of hematologic toxicity. TMZ, and not PCV, is included in the ongoing international phase III clinical trials in patients with and without the 1p/19q codeletion. A retrospective analysis of over 1,000 patients with AOs found a non-significant trend toward improved disease-free survival in a subgroup of patients with AOs with 1p/19q codeletions treated initially with PCV compared with TMZ following surgery.[106] A future comparison of these regimens in AOs with 1p/19q codeletion may be warranted.

AGs have heterogenous outcomes following radiotherapy and chemotherapy. AAs have shorter rates of disease-free and overall survival compared with AOs. 1p/19q codeletion and IDH mutations are prognostic biomarkers which can further separate AGs with regard to outcome. Biomarkers clearly separate subgroups of AGs with different clinical outcomes, for example, IDH mutant versus wild-type AAs, and 1p/19q codeleted versus intact AGs, as discussed above. Figure 66.2 includes a proposed classification scheme for AGs including IDH mutation status and presence or absence of 1p/19q codeletion. The results of ongoing phase III trials are anxiously awaited to help design a next generation of clinical trials in AGs using a biomarker-based, personalized approach.

LOW-GRADE GLIOMAS

Low grade gliomas as classified by the WHO include all grade I and II neoplasms which demonstrate glial differentiation and lack high-grade features. Low grade gliomas include all of the low-grade, diffuse gliomas including astrocytomas, oligoastrocytomas, and oligodendrogliomas, all of which are WHO grade II neoplasms. Other low grade glial neoplasms include pilocytic and pilomyxoid astrocytomas (PMAs), subependymal giant cell astrocytomas, pleomorphic xanthoastrocytomas, and ependymomas. Some neuroepithelial and mixed glial neuronal neoplasms display glial components (e.g., ganglioglioma) but these tumors are classified separately by the WHO.[1] The clinical features, histopathology, and outcomes vary significantly in this group of neoplasms. In general, the WHO grade I gliomas are well circumscribed and potentially surgically curable while the grade II gliomas are diffusely infiltrating and dedifferentiate to HGGs. A current understanding of the molecular pathobiology as it pertains to classification, prognosis, and potential therapeutic approaches will be the focus of the discussion to follow.

Diffuse, Grade II Gliomas

Diffuse, WHO grade II gliomas (LGGs) are relatively rare with approximately 2,000 to 3,000 diagnosed per year in the United States. In adults, low-grade astrocytomas (LGAs) and oligodendrogliomas (LGOs) make up approximately 15% of adult primary brain tumors. These tumors have a peak incidence between ages 35 and 44 and LGGs are more common than GB in young adults.[2] Astrocytic tumors are more likely to be in close proximity to the ventricular system than oligodendroglial tumors which are typically located peripherally near the cortex.[107]

Histologic classification is the mainstay of determining tumor subtype and grade according to the WHO criteria. Cellular neoplasms with oligodendroglial, astrocytic, or mixed histology displaying atypia but lacking mitoses, microvascular proliferation, and necrosis are considered LGGs.[1] Characterization as LGA versus LGO has prognostic value particularly when combined with molecular markers (discussed below). LGOs have a typical range of average survival from 10 to 15 years compared with 5 to 10 years for LGAs. Further, histologic subtypes of astrocytic neoplasms exist including fibrillary, gemistocytic, and protoplasmic although the clinical information gained from these descriptions is unclear. The clinical information gained from fibrillary and protoplasmic descriptions is unclear. Gemistocytic astrocytomas have a more aggressive clinical course than expected for a grade II glioma, suggesting this group may have biologic differences from other LGGs although these differences have not been elucidated.[1]

Prognostication using RPA for LGGs is useful and helps define patients with high-risk versus low-risk clinical features. Age greater than 40, tumor 6 cm or greater in diameter, tumor crossing the midline, neurologic deficit present at diagnosis (excludes seizures), and pure astrocytic histology are all negative prognostic factors. Each of these factors is given a value of 1, with a prognostic score ranging from 0 to 5. Patients stratified as low risk (score 0 to 2) and high risk (score 3 to 5) have a median OS ranging from 3.2 years for high-risk and 7.7 years for low-risk patients.[108] Location in eloquent cerebral cortex may also be a poor prognostic factor incorporated into a separate prognostic scoring system for LGGs.[109] Location near eloquent cortex may significantly contribute to resectability of LGGs negatively impacting survival for sub-totally resected tumors. Most LGGs will undergo a surgical procedure, typically stereotactic biopsy or surgical resection. Stereotactic biopsy can obtain tissue for diagnostic purposes and has low rates of associated morbidity. However, sampling error may result in inaccurate grading in nearly 30% of cases.[110] Stereotactic or open biopsy may be the best option for patients with gliomatosis cerebri or in difficult locations such as the thalamus or brainstem where surgical resection is not feasible.

The accumulated evidence strongly supports a maximal surgical resection for all patients with LGGs when possible. The largest study of extent of resection on survival in LGGs evaluated 216 patients undergoing initial surgical resection and determined volumetric postoperative tumor volumes. Patients with a complete resection had a 10-year survival of nearly 100% in this study with an incremental decrease in survival for incompletely resected tumors.[111] The tumor volume may have impact on tumor dedifferentiation as LGGs with greater preoperative volumes have shorter times to malignant progression than smaller tumors.[109] The extent of resection must be weighed against the risks of functional loss. The use of technologies, including preoperative cortical mapping, intraoperative MRI, and intraoperative cortical stimulation, increases the likelihood of a gross total resection and minimizes postoperative language deficits. Using these techniques, resections of LGGs found in anatomic regions previously considered inoperable can now be performed while minimizing the risks of postoperative morbidity.

Diffuse LGGs extend beyond MRI-defined borders, and surgical management is not curative. Progression and malignant transformation occur at variable intervals depending on histology, prognostic factors, and molecular markers. Which patients to follow closely without adjuvant therapy following surgical resection, the optimal timing of radiotherapy, and the role of chemotherapy are challenging questions in neuro-oncology.

Radiotherapy is the only therapeutic modality which has proven efficacy in a randomized controlled trial in patients with LGG following surgical resection or biopsy. EORTC 22845 evaluated postoperative radiotherapy or radiotherapy at the time of progression, both dosed at 54 Gy. PFS was improved (5.3 vs. 3.4 y) in patients treated with postoperative radiotherapy. However, there was no difference in overall survival between the two groups. Seizure control was improved in patients receiving postoperative radiotherapy.[112] Whether improved PFS and seizure control in EORTC 22845 came at the expense of neurotoxicity related to radiotherapy was not assessed. In a study following LGG patients over an average of 12 years, cognitive deficits were found in 53% of patients with LGGs who received radiotherapy compared with 27% of patients who did not receive radiotherapy.[113] Patients receiving a gross total resection or postoperative chemotherapy may be able to delay or avoid radiotherapy altogether. Thirty-five percent of patients in the delayed radiotherapy arm in EORTC 22845 never required radiotherapy at an average follow-up time exceeding 7 years.[112] Alternatively, outcomes may be improved in patients with high-risk clinical and molecular features when treated with up-front radiotherapy.

Chemotherapy is often used in adjuvant and recurrent settings in patients with LGGs. Cytotoxic chemotherapy, TMZ as a single agent, and PCV are the typical regimens used. The response rate and outcomes in LGG patients treated with chemotherapy appear to be best in patients with favorable prognostic and molecular profiles (e.g., IDH mutation and 1p/19q codeletion, see below). Reduction of seizures may be considered an indication to consider radiotherapy, although TMZ may also improve seizure-related outcomes in LGG patients.[114] TMZ is usually well tolerated with a manageable side effect profile as measured by quality of life and symptom-related outcomes, although prospective comparison of symptom-related outcomes to PCV or radiotherapy has not been done. TMZ has shown efficacy in phase II trials in an adjuvant setting following surgical resection in LGG patients.[115] Whether TMZ can be given up front after surgical resection to delay radiotherapy or whether outcomes can be improved by combining chemotherapy and radiotherapy are questions being addressed in ongoing studies in LGG patients. Ongoing studies have incorporated quality of life and neurocognitive end points to help compare long-term effects of radiotherapy versus chemotherapy.

Molecular markers have become important in the diagnosis and as prognostic markers in LGGs. 1p/19q codeletion occurs due to an unbalanced translocation of chromosomes 1 and 19 with deletions of 1p and 19q. This codeletion confers an improved prognosis in LGG patients.[116] 1p/19q codeletion is rare in LGAs and is found in the majority, 70% or more, of LGOs with mixed oligoastrocytomas having a rate of 1p/19q codeletion intermediate between LGA and LGO. 1p/19q codeletion is often considered a marker of the oligodendroglial lineage, with tumors lacking 1p/19q codeletion considered astrocytic. This is strengthened by the fact that p53 mutations, a marker of astrocytic lineage, and 1p/19q codeletions are nearly always mutually exclusive.[1]

IDH mutations are common in LGGs occurring in approximately 60% to 90% of LGAs and LGOs. The majority of LGAs with p53 mutations and 90% or more of LGOs with 1p/19q codeletion also have IDH mutations. IDH2 mutations are much less common occurring in 5% or fewer of LGGs and are seen mainly in oligodendroglial tumors.[23] Patients with LGGs characterized as LGOs have similar survival to patients with LGGs with IDH mutations and 1p/19q codeletions. Similarly, LGGs characterized as LGAs have similar survival to tumors with IDH and p53 mutations.[117] A molecular classification combining histologic classification with the presence or absence of IDH1 or IDH2 mutations, p53 mutations, and 1p/19q codeletion may provide the most accurate information regarding prognosis (Fig. 66.3A). Appropriate treatment for higher versus lower risk LGGs based on molecular profile has not been established, and combined treatment regimens including radiotherapy and concurrent or adjuvant chemotherapy have not been proven to improve survival or have acceptable rates of toxicity in LGG patients.

Patients with IDH mutations and 1p/19q codeletion have improved outcomes when treated with either chemotherapy or radiotherapy.[118,119] Neither molecular marker appears to be a predictive marker given the improved outcome regardless of postoperative treatment modality. Higher radiographic response rates, mainly manifest as partial responses, are seen in IDH mutated and 1p/19q codeleted LGGs. The molecular rationale for improved prognosis and increase in response rates in 1p/19q codeleted and IDH mutated LGGs has not been explained.

MGMT promoter methylation is a potential prognostic marker in LGGs and has been associated with prolonged rates of PFS and OS in LGG patients.[120] MGMT promoter methylation is usually found in IDH mutated,

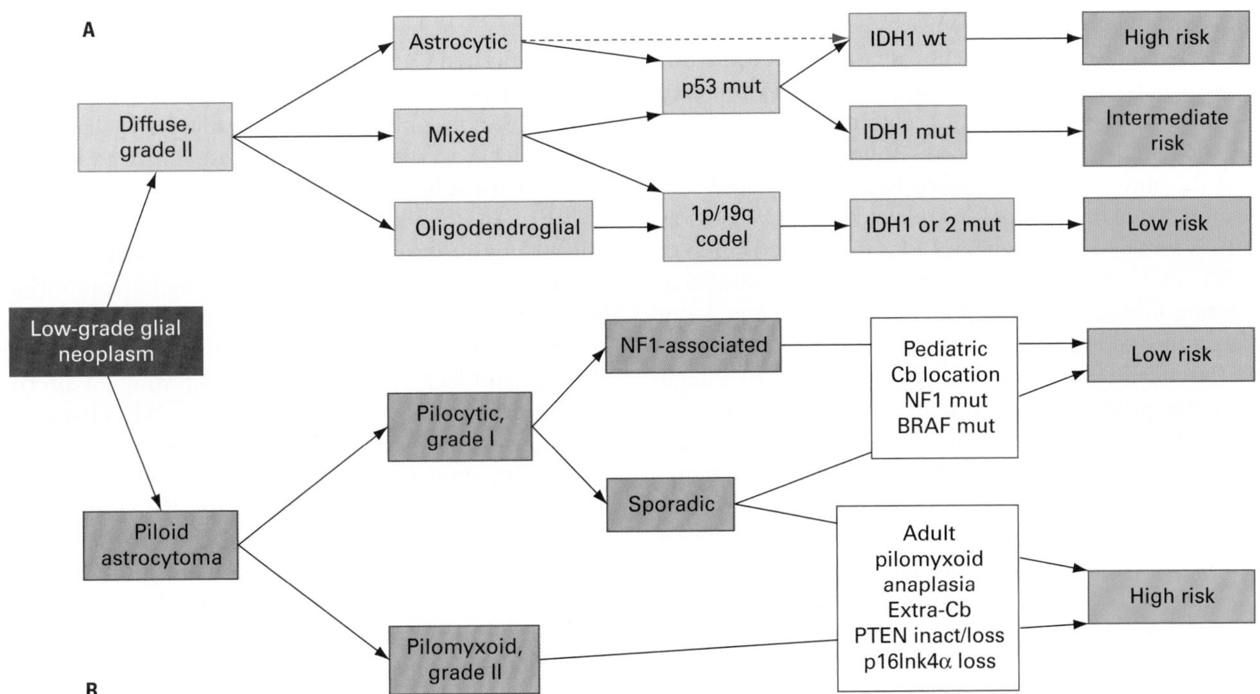

FIGURE 66–3 Proposed algorithm for classification and risk stratification of low-grade gliomas. **A.** High risk indicates a low probability of 5 years of disease-free survival from diagnosis. Intermediate risk indicates an intermediate probability of 5 years of disease-free survival from diagnosis. Low risk indicates a high probability of 5 years of disease-free survival from diagnosis. *Red dotted line* indicates the so-called triple-negative low-grade gliomas (IDH wt, 1p19q intact, p53 wt) which are associated with inferior survival outcomes.[189] **B.** High risk indicates tumors more likely to recur after surgical resection or behave similarly to WHO grade II or III diffuse gliomas. Low risk indicates tumors less likely to recur or progress following surgical resection. *IDH1 or IDH2*, isocitrate dehydrogenase 1 or 2 gene; *Codel*, codeletion; *wt*, wild type; *NF1*, neurofibromatosis 1 gene; *Cb*, cerebellar; *PTEN*, phosphatase and tensin homologue; *Mut*, mutation; *inact*, inactivation.

1p/19q codeleted tumors. IDH mutations appear to have a stronger statistical effect on survival outcomes than MGMT promoter methylation.[119] Similar to HGGs, whether MGMT promoter methylation is predictive of outcomes in TMZ-treated LGG patients or is a marker of improved prognosis irrespective of therapeutic modality has not been established.

Age is an important prognostic factor in LGGs with only 30% to 40% of older LGG patients surviving 5 years. Older patients often have larger tumors, neurologic deficits, and higher rates of astrocytic histology. Differences in treatment patterns may also explain worsened outcomes as older patients in the community may be less likely to have a complete surgical resection and may be more likely to be treated with chemotherapy before radiotherapy.[121] LGGs with p53 mutations have inferior clinical outcomes as likely accounted for by the fact that the majority of these tumors are astrocytic and lack 1p/19q codeletions. While making up a minority of LGGs, IDH wild-type tumors appear to have a significantly worse prognosis than IDH mutated LGGs, with a median PFS of only 1.4 years (vs. 4.7 y) and 14% of patients surviving 5 years (vs. 42%) in one study, and an OS of 150 versus 60 months in IDH1 mutated versus wild-type tumors in another study.[117,122] IDH wild-type LGGs are often "triple-negative" and lack 1p/19q codeletion, p53 mutations, and IDH mutations. The molecular mechanisms of tumor initiation and progression in triple negative LGGs have not been determined.[117,122]

Amplification and mutation of growth factor receptors and constitutive activation of intracellular pathways occur in LGGs but are not as well studied as in GB. PDGFR expression and amplification occurs in gliomas of all grades, appears to increase with grade, but is considered to be an early event in oncogenesis and a putative target in LGGs.[123] PTEN mutation or loss occurs in 30% or more of GBs, but PTEN mutations do not occur frequently in LGGs. However, hypermethylation of the PTEN promoter occurs in approximately 50% or more of LGGs and may serve as an early event in LGG oncogenesis by epigenetic silencing of PTEN expression.[124] Further study and testing of agents targeting growth factor and intracellular signaling in molecularly selected populations of LGG patients is needed.

LGGs with a proneural genetic signature and positive G-CIMP status are associated with improved outcomes. Similar to HGGs, a proneural compared with a mesenchymal genetic signature appears to be associated with an improved prognosis in LGGs.[103] G-CIMP positivity and IDH mutations are strongly associated although the molecular pathways connecting these entities are unknown.[31] The specific genes hypermethylated and downregulated may help delineate the molecular differences between 1p/19q codeleted and IDH mutated LGGs. Analysis of methylation patterns in LGGs with and without 1p/19q codeletions found that two genes (FGFR2 and TNFRS1B) were hypermethylated and downregulated only in 1p/19q codeleted tumors. Pathway analysis revealed that proneural LGGs have activation of the NOTCH and Shh signaling pathways, suggesting that targeting GSCs and developmental pathways may be of interest in LGGs.[125]

Practically, LGG trials can take 10 years or longer given the prolonged survival of some LGG patients. Combining clinical, pathologic, and molecular markers is important in determining the prognosis in patients with LGGs (see Fig. 66.3A). 1p/19q codeletion and IDH mutations are molecular biomarkers associated with an improved prognosis and must be incorporated into future LGG trials. A personalized approach to determining the optimal timing and combination of radiotherapy and chemotherapy in LGGs will likely depend on defining molecular subgroups of LGGs. Defining low-, intermediate-, and high-risk subtypes (see Fig. 66.3A) with specific molecular features may be an efficient method to evaluate targeted therapies in LGG patients.

Pilocytic Astrocytomas

PAs are among the most common pediatric primary brain tumors totaling approximately 15% to 20% of tumors in patients aged 0 to 19. PAs are rare in adults and even rarer in adults over the age of 50.[2] PAs are WHO grade I neoplasms characterized by a biphasic architecture, low proliferative index, and an indolent clinical behavior. PAs can localize throughout the neuraxis in the brain and spinal cord parenchyma.[1] Sporadic PAs are localized primarily in the cerebellum while PAs associated with NF1 are typically located in the optic pathway.

Constitutive activation of the Ras/RAF/MAPK signaling cascade is an important oncogenic event in PAs.[126] About 15% to 20% of PAs occur in the context of NF1. PAs in NF1 are associated with inactivation of the NF1 gene. The gene product of NF1, neurofibromin, binds to Ras acting as a negative regulator of Ras activity. PAs in NF1 appear to have unique patterns of gene expression compared with sporadic PAs in addition to loss of the NF1 gene.[127,128] In general, PAs in NF1 have better clinical outcomes compared with sporadic PAs, particularly when involving the optic pathway.

Optic pathway gliomas (OPGs) are characterized as LGAs which can arise anywhere along the course of the optic pathway. The optic pathway is a unique niche for PAs in NF1 with an overall low rate of histological and clinical progression. OPGs occur in 15% to 20% of patients with NF1, and 40% or more of patients with OPGs have features of NF1.[128] Nearly all OPGs in NF1 are PAs although clinical behavior does not significantly differ by histology in this setting. Sporadic OPGs are more often chiasmal or post-chiasmal compared with NF1-associated OPGs which more often involve the optic nerve. NF1-associated OPGs are more likely to present with precocious puberty while sporadic OPGs have more of a tendency to present with increased intracranial pressure and visual loss. Bilateral OPG is an exclusive feature of NF1. Another interesting feature of NF1-associated OPGs and to a lesser degree PAs in other locations is that spontaneous regression may occur, a phenomenon which has not been explained at the molecular level.[128]

Sporadic PAs are more commonly located in the cerebellum and lack NF1 mutations suggesting an alternative mode of tumorigenesis. Similar to NF1-associated PAs, constitutive activation of the Ras/RAF/MAPK signaling also appears to be an important oncogenic event in sporadic PAs. Abnormalities in the BRAF gene with duplication of chromosome 7q34 and overexpression of the gene product BRAF were detected in LGGs, mainly in sporadic PAs.[129] A novel fusion of the BRAF gene (KIAA1549:BRAF) due to a tandem duplication of 7q34 was found as a genetic signature of sporadic PAs, occurring in over 60% of PAs. The KIAA1549:BRAF fusion is noticeably absent in diffuse astrocytomas and PAs in patients with NF1. The KIAA1549:BRAF fusion is found with higher frequency in posterior fossa, especially cerebellar PAs.[129] The frequency of the KIAA1549:BRAF fusion gene may be lower in adult PAs; it remains to be shown if an alternative mechanism of Ras/RAF/MAPK activation is present in the majority of adult PAs.[130] The BRAF V600E mutation, which is associated with non–cerebellar juvenile PAs, has been reported in a minority of sporadic PAs.[131] IDH mutations, a feature of diffuse LGGs, are absent in PAs. The presence of either the KIAA1549:BRAF fusion gene or IDH1 mutations may be a means of separating PAs and diffuse LGGs, which could be particularly useful in cases difficult to classify on histology alone when only small tumor samples are available (e.g., stereotactic biopsy samples).[132] Supratentorial PAs display a different pattern of gene expression than infratentorial PAs with supratentorial PAs sharing a similar gene expression pattern with supratentorial ependymomas, supporting a region-specific pattern of gene expression and tumorigenesis in PAs.[127]

It is important to differentiate PMAs from PAs. PMAs characteristically have a hypothalamic/chiasmatic localization and are WHO grade II neoplasms with a more aggressive clinical course compared with PAs. PMAs have unique histologic features, such as an angiocentric arrangement of bipolar tumor cells and a myxoid background, and typically lack the Rosenthal fibers and eosinophilic granular bodies characteristic of PAs. Local recurrence and cerebrospinal fluid dissemination occur more often in PMAs than PAs.[1] Due to rarity of this entity, an optimal treatment strategy has not been established.

Despite a grade I designation some PAs display atypical histologic features and an aggressive clinical course.[133] In a day-to-day clinical practice, prediction of behavior of PAs is difficult, and identifying aggressive tumors based on histologic or clinical features alone is not possible with today's current histologic classification scheme. PAs can be mistaken for HGGs on routine brain MRI as aggressive clinical features, including inhomogeneous enhancement, variable thickness of peripheral enhancement, central necrotic areas, and infiltrating margins, can be present in 30% of cases.[134] While aggressive imaging findings do not correlate with histologic evidence of anaplasia, recognizing the spectrum of imaging findings in PAs is important to assure a correct diagnosis is made. PAs with anaplastic histologic features such as high proliferative indices (e.g., MIB-1 labeling index) and necrosis may have rates of PFS survival similar to diffuse, grade II and III gliomas. In contrast to HGGs, microvascular proliferation, VEGF expression, and MGMT promoter methylation are not associated with clinical outcomes in PAs.[135,136] Prior irradiation of PAs is another factor which may be associated with a more aggressive clinical course upon tumor recurrence.

Gene expression profiling was unable to identify genes associated with clinical behavior in PA. Conflicting data exist as to whether presence of the KIAA1549:BRAF fusion gene is associated with improved outcomes in PAs.[137,138] PAs in adults may be more likely to display histologic anaplasia and have higher rates of recurrence or progression than pediatric patients.[139] Whether anatomic location (adult PAs are more often extra-cerebellar), a decreased frequency of BRAF mutations, or other molecular factors dictate a difference in outcomes in adult PAs remains to be determined. Heterozygous loss or decreased expression of PTEN leading to PI3K/Akt activation was seen in over 30% of anaplastic PAs. Loss of p16Ink4α, a regulator of the cell cycle, is associated with anaplastic PAs and worse clinical outcome.[133] In a preclinical model of PA, introducing a BRAF V600E mutation resulted in proliferation followed by oncogene-induced senescence in the presence of p16Ink4α. Oncogene-induced senescence in the presence of a BRAF V600E mutation was subsequently abolished by the loss of p16Ink4α, suggesting p16Ink4α may be an important molecular correlate of recurrence in PAs.[140] Whether BRAF mutations, PTEN loss/inactivation, p16Ink4α, or other molecular alterations can be used routinely as prognostic biomarkers requires further study (Fig. 66.3B).

Sporadic PAs, particularly in a cerebellar location, are typically managed with surgical resection. Up to 100% of patients survive for 5 years and 95% survive 10 years after a surgical procedure.[141] A clear advantage with regard to PFS or OS after gross total resection versus subtotal resection in PAs has not been clearly demonstrated. After a histologic diagnosis of PA is made, observation is typically recommended after a subtotal or gross total resection.

OPGs are considered a separate entity with regard to management, particularly OPGs associated with NF1. Surgery plays minimal, if any, role in the management of these tumors due to their location in the optic pathway. Outside of shunting procedures, surgical resection may be reserved for exceptional cases. For example, surgical debulking may be required to ameliorate hydrocephalus. Large orbital tumors may require surgery for cosmetic purposes when a large degree of proptosis is present in a blind or near-blind eye. Biopsy is rarely needed, especially in the setting of NF1. OPGs should be followed until clear evidence of clinical progression. Radiotherapy is not recommended at the time of first progression in NF1 due to the risk of secondary malignancies, occlusive vasculopathy (moyamoya syndrome), and endocrinopathies. Chemotherapy has been used successfully in OPGs to delay radiotherapy. Carboplatin and vincristine is the most widely accepted chemotherapy regimen. Radiographic responses and visual improvement have been observed but stable disease is the most frequently seen outcome with carboplatin and vincristine.[128,142] Other cytotoxic chemotherapy regimens may be tolerable and result in stable disease in some refractory cases. Radiotherapy should be reserved for cases refractory to chemotherapy with clinical progression. Whether management of sporadic OPGs should be approached differently is not clear although these tumors have a greater risk of progression and appear to be less responsive to chemotherapy.[128] Despite a lack of evidence, an algorithm similar to NF1-associated OPGs is usually followed.

Recurrent or unresectable PAs may be managed with radiotherapy or chemotherapy. In pediatric patients, carboplatin and vincristine are typically used as first-line chemotherapeutic agents for recurrent PAs.[142] Due to the rarity of PA in adults, the efficacy of chemotherapy is unknown. Radiotherapy following surgical resection does not appear to improve OS compared with radiotherapy at recurrence in adult patients.[143] Radiotherapy is typically reserved as a salvage therapy in both adult and pediatric patients. With the recently described mutations in BRAF in PAs, targeted therapy directed at the Ras/RAF/MAPK pathways requires study in pre-clinical and clinical studies. A personalized approach using inhibitors of the Ras/RAF/MAPK signaling cascade may provide an avenue for delivering targeted therapy to selected populations of patients with PA.

The approach to managing patients with PAs depends on many factors, including patient age, anatomic location, and presence or absence of NF1. Figure 66.3B is a proposed classification scheme into higher versus lower risk subgroups, including clinical, pathologic, and molecular factors. The optimal treatment strategy for pilocytic (or pilomyxoid) astrocytomas with a higher versus lower risk profile has not been established.

CONCLUSIONS

Gliomas are a heterogenous group of neoplasms that have traditionally been separated based on pathologic and clinical factors. Our understanding of the molecular events driving glioma initiation and progression is evolving rapidly

(Figs. 66.1 to 66.3). A personalized approach combining multiple clinical and molecular factors will be necessary to optimize clinical trial design and provide our patients with the most up-to-date and accurate prognostic information. A shift toward developing predictive biomarkers of treatment response is necessary to improve outcomes using targeted therapeutics. Predictive biomarkers that can guide treatment decisions for individual patients need to be developed and tested. Rational testing of targeted therapeutics in molecularly defined subgroups of glioma patients will be necessary to achieve the goal of personalized therapy and to ultimately improve survival outcomes.

REFERENCES

1. Louis DN, Ohgaki H, Wiestler OD. *The 2007 WHO Classification of Tumors of the Central Nervous System*. Lyon, France: IARC Press; 2007.
2. CBTRUS. *CBTRUS Statistical Report Primary Brain and Central Nervous System Tumors Diagnosed in the United States in 2004-2006* Central Brain Tumor Registry of the United States, Hinsdale, IL. www.cbtrus.org, 2010.
3. Lacroix M, Abi-Said D, Fourney DR, et al. A multivariate analysis of 416 patients with glioblastoma multiforme: prognosis, extent of resection, and survival. *J Neurosurg*. 2001;95:190-198.
4. Stewart LA. Chemotherapy in adult high-grade glioma: a systematic review and meta-analysis of individual patient data from 12 randomised trials. *Lancet*. 2002;359:1011-1018.
5. Wong ET, Hess KR, Gleason MJ, et al. Outcomes and prognostic factors in recurrent glioma patients enrolled onto phase II clinical trials. *J Clin Oncol*. 1999;17:2572-2578.
6. Ohgaki H, Dessen P, Jourde B, et al. Genetic pathways to glioblastoma: a population-based study. *Cancer Res*. 2004;64:6892-6899.
7. Curan WJ Jr, Scott CB, Horton J, et al. Recursive partitioning analysis of prognostic factors in three Radiation Therapy Oncology Group malignant glioma trials. *J Natl Cancer Inst*. 1993;85:704-710.
8. Stupp R, Mason WP, van den Bent MJ, et al. Radiotherapy plus concomitant and adjuvant temozolomide for glioblastoma. *N Engl J Med*. 2005;352:987-996.
9. Stupp R, Hegi ME, Mason WP, et al. Effects of radiotherapy with concomitant and adjuvant temozolomide versus radiotherapy alone on survival in glioblastoma in a randomised phase III study: 5-year analysis of the EORTC-NCIC trial. *Lancet Oncol*. 2009;10:459-466.
10. Hegi ME, Diserens AC, Gorlia T, et al. MGMT gene silencing and benefit from temozolomide in glioblastoma. *N Engl J Med*. 2005;352:997-1003.
11. Gilbert M, Wang M, Aldape K, al. E. RTOG 0525: A randomized phase III trial comparing standard adjuvant temozolomide (TMZ) with a dose-dense (dd) schedule in newly diagnosed glioblastoma (GBM) *J Clin Ool*. 2011: (suppl 29). Abstract 2006.
12. Rivera AL, Pelloski CE, Gilbert MR, et al. MGMT promoter methylation is predictive of response to radiotherapy and prognostic in the absence of adjuvant alkylating chemotherapy for glioblastoma. *Neuro Oncol*. 2010;12:116-121.
13. Preusser M, Charles Janzer R, Felsberg J, et al. Anti-O6-methylguanine-methyltransferase (MGMT) immunohistochemistry in glioblastoma multiforme: observer variability and lack of association with patient survival impede its use as clinical biomarker. *Brain Pathol*. 2008;18:520-532.
14. Clarke JL, Iwamoto FM, Sul J, et al. Randomized phase II trial of chemoradiotherapy followed by either dose-dense or metronomic temozolomide for newly diagnosed glioblastoma. *J Clin Oncol*. 2009;27:3861-3867.
15. Perry JR, Belanger K, Mason WP, et al. Phase II trial of continuous dose-intense temozolomide in recurrent malignant glioma: RESCUE study. *J Clin Oncol*. 2010;28:2051-2057.
16. Grossman SA, Ye X, Piantadosi S, et al. Survival of patients with newly diagnosed glioblastoma treated with radiation and temozolomide in research studies in the United States. *Clin Cancer Res*. 2010;16:2443-2449.
17. Brandes AA, Franceschi E, Tosoni A, et al. O(6)-methylguanine DNA-methyltransferase methylation status can change between first surgery for newly diagnosed glioblastoma and second surgery for recurrence: clinical implications. *Neuro Oncol*. 2010;12:283-288.
18. Hunter C, Smith R, Cahill DP, et al. A hypermutation phenotype and somatic MSH6 mutations in recurrent human malignant gliomas after alkylator chemotherapy. *Cancer Res*. 2006;66: 3987-3991.
19. Westphal M, Ram Z, Riddle V, Hilt D, Bortey E. Gliadel wafer in initial surgery for malignant glioma: long-term follow-up of a multicenter controlled trial. *Acta Neurochir (Wien)*. 2006;148: 269-275; discussion 275.
20. Brandes AA, Franceschi E, Tosoni A, et al. MGMT promoter methylation status can predict the incidence and outcome of pseudoprogression after concomitant radiochemotherapy in newly diagnosed glioblastoma patients. *J Clin Oncol*. 2008;26:2192-2197.
21. Brandes AA, Tosoni A, Franceschi E, et al. Recurrence pattern after temozolomide concomitant with and adjuvant to radiotherapy in newly diagnosed patients with glioblastoma: correlation With MGMT promoter methylation status. *J Clin Oncol*. 2009;27:1275-1279.
22. Parsons DW, Jones S, Zhang X, et al. An integrated genomic analysis of human glioblastoma multiforme. *Science*. 2008;321: 1807-1812.
23. Yan H, Parsons DW, Jin G, et al. IDH1 and IDH2 mutations in gliomas. *N Engl J Med*. 2009;360:765-773.
24. Marcucci G, Maharry K, Wu YZ, et al. IDH1 and IDH2 gene mutations identify novel molecular subsets within de novo cytogenetically normal acute myeloid leukemia: a Cancer and Leukemia Group B study. *J Clin Oncol*. 2010;28:2348-2355.
25. Thompson CB. Metabolic enzymes as oncogenes or tumor suppressors. *N Engl J Med*. 2009;360:813-815.
26. Nobusawa S, Watanabe T, Kleihues P, Ohgaki H. IDH1 mutations as molecular signature and predictive factor of secondary glioblastomas. *Clin Cancer Res*. 2009;15:6002-6007.
27. Hartmann C, Hentschel B, Wick W, et al. Patients with IDH1 wild type anaplastic astrocytomas exhibit worse prognosis than IDH1-mutated glioblastomas, and IDH1 mutation status accounts for the unfavorable prognostic effect of higher age: implications for classification oomas. *Acta Neuropathol*. 2010;120:707-718.
28. Weller M, Felsberg J, Hartmann C, et al. Molecular predictors of progression-free and overall survival in patients with newly diagnosed glioblastoma: a prospective translational study of the German Glioma Network. *J Clin Oncol*. 2009;27:5743-5750.
29. Lai A, Kharbanda S, Pope WB, et al. Evidene for sequenced molecula evolution of IDH1 mutant globlastom from a distinct cell of origin. *J Clin Oncol*. 2011;29:4482-4490.
30. Verhaak RG, Hoadley KA, Purdom E, et al. Integrated genomic analysis identifies clinically relevant subtypes of glioblastoma characterized by abnormalities in PDGFRA, IDH1, EGFR, and NF1. *Cancer Cell*. 2010;17:98-110.
31. Noushmehr H, Weisenberger DJ, Diefes K, et al. Identification of a CpG island methylator phenotype that defines a distinct subgroup of glioma. *Cancer Cell*. 2010;17:510-522.
32. Comprehensive genomic characterization defines human glioblastoma genes and core pathways. *Nature*. 2008;455: 1061-1068.
33. Frederick L, Wang XY, Eley G, James CD. Diversity and frequency of epidermal growth factor receptor mutations in human glioblastomas. *Cancer Res*. 2000;60:1383-1387.
34. Hermanson M, Funa K, Hartman M, et al. Platelet-derived growth factor and its receptors in human glioma tissue: expression of messenger RNA and protein suggests the presence of autocrine and paracrine loops. *Cancer Res*. 1992;52:3213-3219.
35. Tohma Y, Gratas C, Biernat W, et al. PTEN (MMAC1) mutations are frequent in primary glioblastomas (de novo) but not in secondary glioblastomas. *J Neuropathol Exp Neurol*. 1998;57: 684-689.
36. Kita D, Yonekawa Y, Weller M, Ohgaki H. PIK3CA alterations in primary (de novo) and secondary glioblastomas. *Acta Neuropathol*. 2007;113:295-302.
37. de la Iglesia N, Konopka G, Puram SV, et al. Identification of a PTEN-regulated STAT3 brain tumor suppressor pathway. *Genes Dev*. 2008;22:449-462.

38. Carro MS, Lim WK, Alvarez MJ, et al. The transcriptional network for mesenchymal transformation of brain tumours. *Nature*. 2010;463:318-325.
39. Mellinghoff IK, Wang MY, Vivanco I, et al. Molecular determinants of the response of glioblastomas to EGFR kinase inhibitors. *N Engl J Med*. 2005;353:2012-2024.
40. Haas-Kogan DA, Prados MD, Tihan T, et al. Epidermal growth factor receptor, protein kinase B/Akt, and glioma response to erlotinib. *J Natl Cancer Inst*. 2005;97:880-887.
41. Galanis E, Buckner JC, Maurer MJ, et al. Phase II trial of temsirolimus (CCI-779) in recurrent glioblastoma multiforme: a North Central Cancer Treatment Group Study. *J Clin Oncol*. 2005;23:5294-5304.
42. Kreisl TN, Lassman AB, Mischel PS, et al. A pilot study of everolimus and gefitinib in the treatment of recurrent glioblastoma (GB). *J Neurooncol*. 2009;92:99-105.
43. Wick W, Puduvalli VK, Chamberlain MC, et al. Phase III study of enzastaurin compared with lomustine in the treatment of recurrent intracranial glioblastoma. *J Clin Oncol*. 2010;28:1168-1174.
44. Stommel JM, Kimmelman AC, Ying H, et al. Coactivation of receptor tyrosine kinases affects the response of tumor cells to targeted therapies. *Science*. 2007;318:287-290.
45. Bean J, Brennan C, Shih JY, et al. MET amplification occurs with or without T790M mutations in EGFR mutant lung tumors with acquired resistance to gefitinib or erlotinib. *Proc Natl Acad Sci U S A*. 2007;104:20932-20937.
46. O'Reilly KE, Rojo F, She QB, et al. mTOR inhibition induces upstream receptor tyrosine kinase signaling and activates Akt. *Cancer Res*. 2006;66:1500-150.
47. Gromes C, Oxnard GR, Kris MG, et al. "Pulsatile" high-dose weekly erlotinib for CNS metastases from EGFR mutant non-small cell lung cancer. *Neuro Oncol*. 2011;13:1364-1369.
48. Holash J, Maisonpierre PC, Compton D, et al. Vessel cooption, regression, and growth in tumors mediated by angiopoietins and VEGF. *Science*. 1999;284:1994-1998.
49. Zagzag D, Zhong H, Scalzitti JM, Laughner E, Simons JW, Semenza GL. Expression of hypoxia-inducible factor 1alpha in brain tumors: association with angiogenesis, invasion, and progression. *Cancer*. 2000;88:2606-2618.
50. Kerbel RS. Tumor angiogenesis. *N Engl J Med*. 2008;358: 2039-2049.
51. Zhang YW, Su Y, Volpert OV, Vande Woude GF. Hepatocyte growth factor/scatter factor mediates angiogenesis through positive VEGF and negative thrombospondin 1 regulation. *Proc Natl Acad Sci U S A*. 2003;100:12718-2723.
52. Vredenburgh JJ, Desjardins A, Herndon JE 2nd, et al. Bevacizumab plus irinotecan in recurrent glioblastoma multiforme. *J Clin Oncol*. 2007;254722-4729.
53. Desjardins A, Reardon DA, Herndon JE 2nd, et al. Bevacizumab plus irinotecan in recurrent WHO grade 3 malignant gliomas. *Clin Cancer Res*. 2008;14:7068-7073.
54. Friedman HS, Prados MD, Wen PY, et al. Bevacizumab alone and in combination with irinotecan in recurrent glioblastoma. *J Clin Oncol*. 2009
55. Batchelor T, Mulholland P, Neyns B. A phase III randomized study comparing the efficacy of cediranib as monotherapy, and in combination with lomustine, with lomustine alone in recurrent glioblastoma patients [abstract]. *Ann Oncol*. 2010;21:Abstract LBA7.
56. Scott BJ, Quant EC, McNamara MB, Ryg PA, Batchelor TT, Wen PY. Bevacizumab salvage therapy following progression in high-grade glioma patients treated with VEGF receptor tyrosine kinase inhibitors. *Neuro Oncol*. 2010;12:603-607.
57. de Groot JF, Lamborn KR, Chang SM, et al. Phase II study of aflibercept in recurrent malignant glioma: a North American Brain Tumor Consortium study. *J Clin Oncol*. 2011;29:2689-2695.
58. de Groot, JF, Piao Y. Anti-VEGF but not VEGF receptor inhibitor therapy prolongs survival and blocks myeloid cell recruitment to orthotopic glioblastoma [abstract]. In: *Proceedings of the 97th Annual Meeting of the American Association for Cancer Research 2010*. Washington, DC; Philadelphia, PA: AACR. April 17-21, 2010. Abstract 2279.
59. Lai A, Tran A, Nghiemphu PL, et al. Phase II study of bevacizumab plus temozolomide during and after radiation therapy for patients with newly diagnosed glioblastoma multiforme. *J Clin Oncol*. 2011;29:142-148.
60. Vredenburgh JJ, Desjardins A, Reardon DA, et al. The addition of bevacizumab to standard radiation therapy and temozolomide followed by bevacizumab, temozolomide, and irinotecan for newly diagnosed glioblastoma. *Clin Cancer Res*. 2011;17:4119-4124.
61. Norden AD, Young GS, Setayesh K, et al. Bevacizumab for recurrent malignant gliomas: efficacy, toxicity, and patterns of recurrence. *Neurology*. 2008;70:779-787.
62. Pope WB, Xia Q, Paton VE, et al. Patterns of progression in patients with recurrent glioblastoma treated with bevacizumab. *Neurology*. 2011;76:432-437.
63. Claes A, Wesseling P, Jeuken J, Maass C, Heerschap A, Leenders WP. Antiangiogenic compounds interfere with chemotherapy of brain tumors due to vessel normalization. *Mol Cancer Ther*. 2008;7:71-78.
64. Zhou Q, Gallo JM. Differential effect of sunitinib on the distribution of temozolomide in an orthotopic glioma model. *Neuro Oncol*. 2009;11:301-310.
65. Quant EC, Norden AD, Drappatz J, et al. Role of a second chemotherapy in recurrent malignant glioma patients who progress on bevacizumab. *Neuro Oncol*. 2009;11:550-555.
66. Paez-Ribes M, Allen E, Hudock J, et al. Antiangiogenic therapy elicits malignant progression of tumors to increased local invasion and distant metastasis. *Cancer Cell*. 2009;15:220-231.
67. de Groot JF, Fuller G, Kumar AJ, et al. Tumor invasion after treatment of glioblastoma with bevacizumab: radiographic and pathologic correlation in humans and mice. *Neuro Oncol*. 2010;12:233-242.
68. Utsuki S, Sato Y, Oka H, Tsuchiya B, Suzuki S, Fujii K. Relationship between the expression of E-, N-cadherins and beta-catenin and tumor grade in astrocytomas. *J Neurooncol*. 2002;57:187-192.
69. Shi Q, Bao S, Song L, et al. Targeting SPARC expression decreases glioma cellular survival and invasion associated with reduced activities of FAK and ILK kinases. *Oncogene*. 2007;26:4084-4094.
70. Bello L, Francolini M, Marthyn P, et al. Alpha(v)beta3 and alpha(v)beta5 integrin expression in glioma periphery. *Neurosurgery*. 2001;49:380-389; discussion 390.
71. Abounader R, Laterra J. Scatter factor/hepatocyte growth factor in brain tumor growth and angiogenesis. *Neuro Oncol*. 2005;7:436-451.
72. Lucio-Eterovic AK, Piao Y, de Groot JF. Mediators of glioblastoma resistance and invasion during antivascular endothelial growth factor therapy. *Clin Cancer Res*. 2009;15:4589-4599.
73. Stettner MR, Wang W, Nabors LB, et al. Lyn kinase activity is the predominant cellular SRC kinase activity in glioblastoma tumor cells. *Cancer Res*. 2005;65:5535-5543.
74. Groves MD, Puduvalli VK, Hess KR, et al. Phase II trial of temozolomide plus the matrix metalloproteinase inhibitor, marimastat, in recurrent and progressive glioblastoma multiforme. *J Clin Oncol*. 2002;20:1383-1388.
75. Stupp R, Hegi ME, Neyns B, et al. Phase I/IIa study of cilengitide and temozolomide with concomitant radiotherapy followed by cilengitide and temozolomide maintenance therapy in patients with newly diagnosed glioblastoma. *J Clin Oncol*. 2010;28:2712-2718.
76. Wen PY, Macdonald DR, Reardon DA, et al. Updated response assessment criteria for high-grade gliomas: response assessment in neuro-oncology working group. *J Clin Oncol*. 2010;28:1963-1972.
77. Jain R, Scarpace LM, Ellika S, et al. Imaging response criteria for recurrent gliomas treated with bevacizumab: role of diffusion weighted imaging as an imaging biomarker. *J Neuooncol*. 2010;96:423-431.
78. Sorensen AG, Batchelor TT, Zhang WT, et al. A "vascular normalization index" as potential mechanistic biomarker to predict survival after a single dose of cediranib in recurrent glioblastoma patients. *Cancer Res*. 2009;69:5296-5300.
79. Chen W, Delaloye S, Silverman DH, et al. Predicting treatment response of malignant gliomas to bevacizumab and irinotecan by imaging proliferation with [18F] fluorothymidine positron emission tomography: a pilot study. *J Clin Oncol*. 2007;25:4714-4721.
80. Batchelor TT, Sorensen AG, di Tomaso E, et al. AZD2171, a pan-VEGF receptor tyrosine kinase inhibitor, normalizes tumor vasculature and alleviates edema in glioblastoma patients. *Cancer Cell*. 2007;11:83-95.

81. de Groot JF, Piao Y, Tran H, et al. Myeloid biomarkers associated with glioblastoma response to anti-VEGF therapy with aflibercept. *Clin Cancer Res.* 2011;17:4872-4881.
82. Galli R, Binda E, Orfanelli U, et al. Isolation and characterization of tumorigenic, stem-like neural precursors from human glioblastoma. *Cancer Res.* 2004;64:7011-7021.
83. Singh SK, Hawkins C, Clarke ID, et al. Identification of human brain tumour initiating cells. *Nature.* 2004;432:396-401.
84. Dahmane N, Sanchez P, Gitton Y, et al. The Sonic Hedgehog-Gli pathway regulates dorsal brain growth and tumorigenesis. *Development.* 2001;128:5201-5212.
85. Liu X, Wang L, Zhao S, Ji X, Luo Y, Ling F. beta-Catenin overexpression in malignant glioma and its role in proliferation and apoptosis in glioblastoma cells. *Med Oncol.* 2011;28:608-614.
86. Somasundaram K, Reddy SP, Vinnakota K, et al. Upregulation of ASCL1 and inhibition of Notch signaling pathway characterize progressive astrocytoma. *Oncogene* 2005;24:073-7083.
87. Anido J, Saez-Borderias A, Gonzalez-Junca A, et al. TGF-beta receptor inhibtors target the CD44(high)/Id1(high) glioma-initiating cell population in human glioblastoma. *Cancer Cell.* 2010;18:655-668.
88. Calabrese C, Poppleton H, Kocak M, et al. A perivascular niche for brain tumor stem cells. *Cancer Cell.* 2007;11:69-82.
89. Piccirillo SG, Vescovi AL. Bone morphogenetic proteins regulate tumorigenicity in human glioblastoma stem cells. *Ernst Schering Found Symp Proc.* 2006:59-81.
90. Soda Y, Marumoto T, Friedmann-Morvinski D, et al. Transdifferentiation of glioblastoma cells into vascular endothelial cells. *Proc Natl Acad Sci U S A.* 2011;108:4274-4280.
91. See SJ, Levin VA, Yung WK, Hess KR, Groves MD. 13-cis-retinoic acid in the treatment of recurrent glioblastoma multiforme. *Neuro Oncol.* 2004;6:253-258.
92. Colman H, Zhang L, Sulman EP, et al. A multigene predictor of outcome in glioblastoma. *Neuro Oncol.* 2010;12:49-57.
93. Bao S, Wu Q, McLendon RE, et al. Glioma stem cells promote radioresistance by preferential activation of the DNA damage response. *Nature.* 2006;444:756-760.
94. Bleau AM, Hambardzumyan D, Ozawa T, et al. PTEN/PI3K/Akt pathway regulates the side population phenotype and ABCG2 activity in glioma tumor stem-like cells. *Cell Stem Cell.* 2009;4:226-235.
95. Phillips HS, Kharbanda S, Chen R, et al. Molecular subclasses of high-grade glioma predict prognosis, delineate a pattern of disease progression, and resemble stages in neurogenesis. *Cancer Cell.* 2006;9:157-173.
96. van den Bent MJ, Carpentier AF, Brandes AA, et al. Adjuvant procarbazine, lomustine, and vincristine improves progression-free survival but not overall survival in newly diagnosed anaplastic oligodendrogliomas and oligoastrocytomas: a randomized European Organisation for Research and Treatment of Cancer phase III trial. *J Clin Oncol.* 2006;24:2715-2722.
97. Cairncross G, Berkey B, Shaw E, et al. Phase III trial of chemotherapy plus radiotherapy compared with radiotherapy alone for pure and mixed anaplastic oligodendroglioma: Intergroup Radiation Therapy Oncology Group Trial 9402. *J Clin Oncol.* 2006;24:2707-2714.
98. Wick W, Hartmann C, Engel C, et al. NOA-04 randomized phase III trial of sequential radiochemotherapy of anaplastic glioma with procarbazine, lomustine, and vincristine or temozolomide. *J Clin Oncol.* 2009;27:5874-5880.
99. Cairncross JG, Ueki K, Zlatescu MC, et al. Specific genetic predictors of chemotherapeutic response and survival in patients with anaplastic oligodendrogliomas. *J Natl Cancer Inst.* 1998;90:1473-1479.
100. Labussiere M, Idbaih A, Wang XW, et al. All the 1p19q codeleted gliomas are mutated on IDH1 or IDH2. *Neurology.* 2010;74:1886-1890.
101. van den Bent MJ, Dubbink HJ, Sanson M, et al. MGMT promoter methylation is prognostic but not predictive for outcome to adjuvant PCV chemotherapy in anaplastic oligodendroglial tumors: a report from EORTC Brain Tumor Group Study 26951. *J Clin Oncol.* 2009;27:5881-5886.
102. Ducray F, Idbaih A, de Reynies A, et al. Anaplasti oligodendrogliomas with 1p19q codeletion have a proneural gene expression profile. *Mol Cancer.* 2008;7:41.
103. Cooper LA, Gutman DA, Long Q, et al. The proneural molecular signature is enriched in oligodendrogliomas and predicts improved survival among diffuse gliomas. *PLoS One.* 2010;5:e12548.
104. van den Bent MJ, Gravendeel LA, Gorlia T, et al. A hypermethylated phenotype in anaplastic oligodendroglial brain tumors is a better predictor of survival than MGMT methylation in anaplastic oligodendroglioma: a report from EORTC study 26951. *Clin Cancer Res.* 2011;17:7148-7155.
105. Abrey LE, Louis DN, Paleologos N, et al. Survey of treatment recommendations for anaplastic oligodendroglioma. *Neuro Oncol.* 2007;9:314-318.
106. Lassman AB, Iwamoto FM, Cloughesy TF, et al. International retrospective study of over 1000 adults with anaplastic oligodendroglial tumors. *Neuro Oncol.* 2011;13:649-659.
107. Persson AI, Petritsch C, Swartling FJ, et al. Non-stem cell origin for oligodendroglioma. *Cancer Cell.* 2010;18:669-682.
108. Pignatti F, van den Bent M, Curran D, et al. Prognostic factors for survival in adult patients with cerebral low-grade glioma. *J Clin Oncol.* 2002;20:2076-2084.
109. Chang EF, Smith JS, Chang SM, et al. Preoperative prognostic classification system for hemispheric low-grade gliomas in adults. *J Neurosurg.* 2008;109:817-824.
110. Muragaki Y, Chernov M, Maruyama T, et al. Low-grade glioma on stereotactic biopsy: how often is the diagnosis accurate? *Minim Invasive Neurosurg.* 2008;51:275-279.
111. Smith JS, Chang EF, Lamborn KR, et al. Role of extent of resection in the long-term outcome of low-grade hemispheric gliomas. *J Clin Oncol.* 2008;26:1338-1345.
112. van den Bent MJ, Afra D, de Witte O, et al. Long-term efficacy of early versus delayed radiotherapy for low-grade astrocytoma and oligodendroglioma in adults: the EORTC 22845 randomised trial. *Lancet.* 2005;366:985-990.
113. Douw L, Klein M, Fagel SS, et al. Cognitive and radiological effects of radiotherapy in patients with low-grade glioma: long-term follow-up. *Lancet Neurol.* 2009;8:810-818.
114. Sherman JH, Moldovan K, Yeoh HK, et al. Impact of temozolomide chemotherapy on seizure frequency in patients with low-grade gliomas. *J Neurosurg.* 2011;114:1617-1621.
115. Liu R, Solheim K, Polley MY, et al. Quality of life in low-grade glioma patients receiving temozolomide. *Neuro Oncol.* 2009;11:59-68.
116. Kaloshi G, Benouaich-Amiel A, Diakite F, et al. Temozolomide for low-grade gliomas: predictive impact of 1p/19q loss on response and outcome. *Neurology.* 2007;68:1831-1836.
117. Kim YH, Nobusawa S, Mittelbronn M, et al. Molecular classification of low-grade diffuse gliomas. *Am J Pathol.* 2010;177:2708-2714.
118. Houillier C, Wang X, Kaloshi G, et al. IDH1 or IDH2 mutations predict longer survival and response to temozolomide in low-grade gliomas. *Neurology.* 2010;75:1560-1566.
119. Hartmann C, Hentschel B, Tatagiba M, et al. Molecular markers in low-grade gliomas: predictive or prognostic? *Clin Cancer Res.* 2011;17:4588-4599.
120. Everhard S, Kaloshi G, Criniere E, et al. MGMT methylation: a marker of response to temozolomide in low-grade gliomas. *Ann Neurol.* 2006;60:740-743.
121. Kaloshi G, Psimaras D, Mokhtari K, et al. Supratentorial low-grade gliomas in older patients. *Neurology.* 2009;73:2093-2098.
122. Metellus P, Coulibaly B, Colin C, et al. Absence of IDH mutation identifies a novel radiologic and molecular subtype of WHO grade II gliomas with dismal prognosis. *Acta neuropathologica.* 2010;120:719-729.
123. Varela M, Ranuncolo SM, Morand A, et al. EGF-R and PDGF-R, but not bcl-2, overexpression predict overall survival in patients with low-grade astrocytomas. *J Surg Oncol.* 2004;86:34-40.
124. Wiencke JK, Zheng S, Jelluma N, et al. Methylation of the PTEN promoter defines low-grade gliomas and secondary glioblastoma. *Neuro Oncol.* 2007;9:271-279.
125. Laffaire J, Everhard S, Idbaih A, et al. Methylation profiling identifies 2 groups of gliomas according to their tumorigenesis. *Neuro Oncol.* 2011;13:84-98.
126. Pfister S, Janzarik WG, Remke M, et al. BRAF gene duplication constitutes a mechanism of MAPK pathway activation in low-grade astrocytomas. *J Clin Invest.* 2008;118:1739-1749.

127. Sharma MK, Mansur DB, Reifenberger G, et al. Distinct genetic signatures among pilocytic astrocytomas relate to their brain region origin. *Cancer Res*. 2007;67:890-900.
128. Listernick R, Ferner RE, Liu GT, Gutmann DH. Optic pathway gliomas in neurofibromatosis-1: controversies and recommendations. *Ann Neurol*. 2007;61:189-198.
129. Jones DT, Kocialkowski S, Liu L, et al. Tandem duplication producing a novel oncogenic BRAF fusion gene defines the majority of pilocytic astrocytomas. *Cancer Res*. 2008;68:8673-8677.
130. Hasselblatt M, Riesmeier B, Lechtape B, et al. BRAF-KIAA1549 fusion transcripts are less frequent in pilocytic astrocytomas diagnosed in adults. *Neuropathol Appl Neurobiol*. 2011;37:803-806.
131. Schindler G, Capper D, Meyer J, et al. Analysis of BRAF V600E mutation in 1,320 nervous system tumors reveals high mutation frequencies in pleomorphic xanthoastrocytoma, ganglioglioma and extra-cerebellar pilocytic astoma. *Acta Neuropathol*. 2011;121:397-405.
132. Korshunov A, Meyer J, Capper D, et al. Combined molecular analysis of BRAF and IDH1 distinguishes pilocytic astrocytoma from diffuse astoma. *Acta Neuropathol*. 2009;118:401-405.
133. Rodriguez EF, Scheithauer BW, Giannini C, et al. PI3K/AKT pathway alterations are associated with clinically aggressive and histologically anaplastic subsets of pilocytic aytoma. *Acta Neuropathol*. 2011;121:407-420.
134. Kumar AJ, Leeds NE, Kumar VA, et al. Magnetic resonance imaging features of pilocytic astrocytoma of the brain mimicking high-grade gliomas. *J Comput Assist Tomogr*. 2010;34:601-611.
135. Horbinski C, Hamilton RL, Lovell C, Burnham J, Pollack IF. Impact of morphology, MIB-1, p53 and MGMT on outcome in pilocytic astrocytomas. *Brain Pathol*. 2010;20:581-588.
136. Kurwale NS, Suri V, Suri A, et al. Predictive factors for early symptomatic recurrence in pilocytic astrocytoma: does angiogenesis have a role to play? *J Clin Neurosci*. 2011;18:472-477.
137. Horbinski C, Hamilton RL, Nikiforov Y, Pollack IF. Association of molecular alterations, including BRAF, with biology and outcome in pilocytirocytomas. *Acta Neuropathol*. 2010;119:641-649.
138. Hawkins C, Walker E, Mohamed N, et al. BRAF-KIAA1549 fusion predicts better clinical outcome in pediatric low-grade astrocytoma. *Clin Cancer Res*. 2011;17:4790-4798.
139. Stuer C, Vilz B, Majores M, Becker A, Schramm J, Simon M. Frequent recurrence and progression in pilocytic astrocytoma in adults. *Cancer*. 2007;110:2799-2808.
140. Jacob K, Quang-Khuong DA, Jones DT, et al. Genetic aberrations leading to MAPK pathway activation mediate oncogene-induced senescence in sporadic pilocytic astrocytomas. *Clin Cancer Res*. 2011;17:4650-4660.
141. Burkhard C, Di Patre PL, Schuler D, et al. A population-based study of the incidence and survival rates in patients with pilocytic astrocytoma. *J Neurosurg*. 2003;98:1170-1174.
142. Packer RJ, Ater J, Allen J, et al. Carboplatin and vincristine chemotherapy for children with newly diagnosed progressive low-grade gliomas. *J Neurosurg*. 1997;86:747-754.
143. Ishkanian A, Laperriere NJ, Xu W, et al. Upfront observation versus radiation for adult pilocytic asocytoma. *Cancer*. 2011;117:4070-4079.

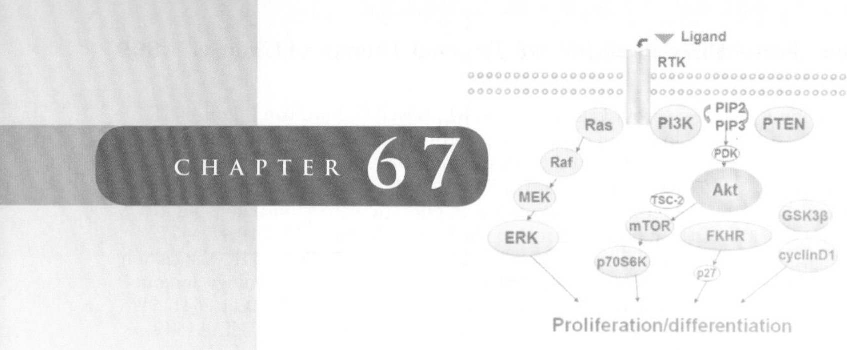

CHAPTER 67

Personalized Medicine and Targeted Therapy for Osteosarcoma

Jonathan Gill, David Geller, and Richard Gorlick

BACKGROUND

Osteosarcoma is the most common malignant bone tumor of children and young adults. It comprises approximately 55% of all malignant bone tumors in this age group. Ewing sarcoma is the next most common at 36%.[1] Most cases of osteosarcoma occur in the proximity of the knee joint involving the distal femur or the proximal tibia. The proximal humerus is the next most common site of disease. As the peak incidence occurs contemporaneously with the peak in growth velocity during adolescence, girls have an earlier age of onset than boys, mirroring the relative timing of the onset of puberty.[2] Within the bone, osteosarcomas generally localize to the metaphysis of long bones, which is the region of the bone involved with growth and elongation. This suggests that stimulation of bone growth and rapid cell turnover play integral roles for malignant transformation and development of osteosarcoma.

Osteosarcomas have tremendous heterogeneity between patients and within cells of the same tumor. The majority of osteosarcomas have complex chromosomal abnormalities marked by aneuploidy. Different degrees of ploidy can be seen within the cells of the same tumor. Chromosomal abnormalities include chromosome loss, chromosome gain, partial deletion, amplification, and marker chromosomes. Marker chromosomes are structurally abnormal chromosomes that cannot be identified.[3] The complex genetic heterogeneity seen in osteosarcomas is fueled by dysregulation of cellular mechanisms necessary for the maintenance of DNA integrity. Approximately one-third of tumors have mutations in p53 and 40% have mutations in the locus of the retinoblastoma gene.[4,5] Tumors that do not have mutations in p53 have been shown to have amplification in *HDM2*, a known suppressor of p53, or alteration in the p16INK4a/p19(ARF) locus.[4] Given the genetic complexity, among other unidentified factors, osteosarcoma has proven to be highly chemoresistant, with very few therapeutic options available for treating clinicians and their patients.

Nevertheless, the use of chemotherapy has been integral to improving outcomes and survival for patients diagnosed with osteosarcoma. Prior to the era of modern chemotherapy, patients with nonmetastatic osteosarcoma were treated by amputation. Greater than 80% of those patients ultimately developed metastases within a median time of 6 months.[6,7] In the early 1980s, a major randomized controlled trial was conducted comparing adjuvant chemotherapy versus observation for patients with newly diagnosed, nonmetastatic osteosarcoma. This trial demonstrated a disease-free survival of 55% to 61% in patients receiving chemotherapy when compared with 11% to 20% in the observation group.[8] Over the ensuing three decades, chemotherapy for osteosarcoma has been varied between three and five agents with limited additional improvement in overall survival. Given current chemotherapy protocols, the expected 5-year overall survival for patients with newly diagnosed osteosarcoma remains 66%.[9]

TRADITIONAL CHEMOTHERAPY

The most important determinant of prognosis for patients with newly diagnosed osteosarcoma is the presence of detectable metastases at presentation. The most recent multinational randomized trial for patients with newly diagnosed osteosarcoma revealed a 5-year event-free survival of 63%.[10] For patients with metastatic disease, on the same protocol, the 5-year event-free survival was 34%.[11] Another variable that has been consistently shown to be important in defining survival is histologic response to neoadjuvant chemotherapy, which may represent among the earliest efforts at personalized chemotherapy.

In the late 1970s and leading up to the early 1980s, the technology for endoprostheses made dramatic improvements. Patients awaiting custom-made endoprostheses were administered neoadjuvant chemotherapy so as to minimize treatment delay while awaiting limb-sparing surgery. A randomized trial comparing immediate surgery versus neoadjuvant chemotherapy demonstrated no difference in event-free or overall survival.[12] A by-product of neoadjuvant chemotherapy was the observation, during pathologic review, that resected tumors displayed varying degrees of treatment effect from the administered chemotherapy. This led to the development of the Huvos grading system for tumor response to neoadjuvant chemotherapy.

The Huvos grading system divides tumor response into four grades. Grade I is viable tumor with little or no effect of chemotherapy identified. Grade II describes a moderate chemotherapeutic effect with areas of acellular tumor osteoid and necrosis consistent with the effect of chemotherapy, with other areas showing histologically viable tumor. Grade III is defined by predominant areas of acellular tumor osteoid and necrosis, with only scattered areas of histologically viable tumor. Grade IV has no areas of viable tumor identified.[13] Grade III is often interpreted as >90% necrosis and grade IV as >95% or >98% necrosis.

In short order, it became clear that patients who exhibited a greater degree of tumor necrosis following neoadjuvant chemotherapy also demonstrated an improved overall survival. Patients with nonmetastatic osteosarcoma with Huvos grades I, II, III, and IV were found to have a disease-free survival of 50%, 66%, 72%, and 91%, respectively.[14] Patients with Huvos grade III or IV treatment effect, or >90% necrosis, are often described as "good responders," while patients with lower Huvos grades, or <90% necrosis, are described as "poor or standard responders." A large retrospective review, including multiple different chemotherapeutic regimens, demonstrated that histologic response is an important determinant of overall survival. Good responders had an overall survival of 68% as compared with poor responders with a 51% overall survival.[15] Once this relationship became apparent, many attempts have been made to improve outcome for children with osteosarcoma by manipulating treatment according to histologic response: increasing preoperative chemotherapy to improve the percentage of patients who are good responders, intensifying chemotherapy for poor responders, and decreasing chemotherapy for good responders.

The net effect has been disappointing. Increasing the number of neoplastic agents administered in the neoadjuvant period has been demonstrated to increase the percentage of patients with tumor necrosis consistent with a "good response". [16] Secondarily, increasing the duration of preoperative chemotherapy also increases the number of patients with "good response."[17] Unfortunately, as the intensity or duration of preoperative chemotherapy is increased, the correlation between "good response" and survival is lost, with the net effect that the patient's overall outcome remains unchanged.[16,17] These results suggest that intensification of preoperative chemotherapy does not change tumor biology or chemoresistance. The Huvos grading system is bifactorial, involving the chemosensitivity of the patient's osteosarcoma and the intensity of the treatment to which it has been exposed. Patients who ordinarily would not be considered good responders but are pushed into the good response group with intensification of chemotherapy, are ultimately relegated to the risk of relapse defined by the intrinsic tumor chemoresistance.

Another approach to the dichotomy of therapies between good and poor responses has been to attempt to "rescue" the poor responders by changing their chemotherapy. Initially, this strategy seemed very promising when Rosen et al.[18,19] reported that patients who had their therapy intensified after having a poor response to neoadjuvant chemotherapy had a disease-free survival of 77%. However, when other groups attempted to reproduce these findings, they reported disappointing results, with relapse-free survival for poor responders of 48% to 53%.[20,21] Before the active agents for osteosarcoma were clearly defined, a randomized trial comparing two treatment regimens crossed over the poor responders to the opposite treatment arm. The event-free survival for the poor responders was worse at 44%, presumably because some of the patients had been taken off of agents active against osteosarcoma.[22] In a review of the results of five trials conducted at the Rizzoli Institute in Italy in which chemotherapy was changed, the same regimen was maintained, or cycles of the same agents were added for poor responders; poor responders who had their treatment regimen changed had a disease-free survival of 46% compared with 59% for patients who continued with the initial chemotherapy. [15] Despite efforts to tailor therapy according to histologic response, unfortunately only three-drug regimens have consistently and conclusively been shown to demonstrate optimal antitumor activity. The selection of methotrexate, doxorubicin, and cisplatin (MAP) is based on efficacy as well as toxicity considerations. Attempts to improve the outcome for poor responders by changing their treatment from this standard three-drug regimen do not lead to increased survival.

Only one trial has attempted to define a low-risk population to reduce chemotherapy to minimize toxicity. COSS-86 was a product of the cooperative German-Austrian-Swiss Osteosarcoma Study Group. Tumors were defined as low risk if none of the trial's defined risk factors were present: tumor length >1/3 of the involved bone; >20% chondroid ground substance in the biopsy specimen; and <20% reduction of early and/or late phase activity in sequential bone scans. If patients had poor response after neoadjuvant chemotherapy, they were upstaged to the high-risk protocol. All patients received two cycles of MAP therapy prior to surgery, but low-risk patients received only two cycles after surgery, when compared with their high-risk cohorts who received four cycles or more. Unexpectedly, the low-risk patients had a disease-free survival of 66%, similar to the high-risk patients.[23] Patients who are good responders to neoadjuvant chemotherapy would be expected to have the best outcomes. These results raised a concern that reducing the duration of therapy for patients expected to do best may compromise their probability of survival. Even the most favorable patient populations cannot have a reduction in their planned therapy.

In an effort to improve survival, ifosfamide has been added to standard MAP therapy. The addition of ifosfamide to neoadjuvant chemotherapy increased the percentage of patients with good response. However, there were no reports of improvement in overall survival.[23-26] A multicentered, randomized trial found no benefit from the addition of ifosfamide to standard MAP therapy.[10,27] Goorin et al.[28] treated newly diagnosed patients with metastatic osteosarcoma with ifosfamide and etoposide in addition to standard MAP therapy and reported an overall survival >40%. This encouraging result led to a multinational trial randomizing patients with poor histologic response to the addition of ifosfamide and etoposide to standard MAP therapy. This trial has completed accrual in 2011. There is hope that this trial will provide a definitive answer to whether or not chemotherapy can be personalized according to histologic response.

NOVEL TARGETS

Human Epidermal Growth Factor Receptor 2

In addition to adjusting patients' therapy according to tumor response to neoadjuvant therapy, in recent years, there has been excitement over adjusting treatment according to the biology of the disease. A novel target and potential prognostic factor in patients with osteosarcoma is human epidermal growth factor receptor 2 (HER2). HER2 is a transmembrane glycoprotein with tyrosine kinase activity that has been implicated in tumorigenesis. HER2 was found to be expressed in 42% of patients with osteosarcoma and its expression was significantly correlated with early pulmonary metastases and worse survival, corroborating an earlier Japanese study.[29,30] However, the importance of HER2 in the biology of osteosarcoma remains controversial, with several reports suggesting that HER2 expression is not a significant determinant in the pathogenesis of osteosarcoma.[31,32] Some of the discrepancy in these results can be explained by the different techniques used in handling the tumor samples and measuring HER2 expression. In 2001, the Children's Oncology Group initiated a phase II trial in patients with metastatic osteosarcoma assessing the benefit of the addition of monoclonal antibody to HER2 (trastuzumab) to the treatment of patients whose tumors overexpress HER2. The results of this trial are greatly anticipated.

Vascular Endothelial Growth Factor

The family of vascular endothelial growth factor receptors (VEGFRs) has also been implicated as important in the prognosis in osteosarcoma. VEGFR-3 has been demonstrated to be overexpressed in osteosarcoma cell lines.[33] Patients whose tumors express VEGFR-3 have been shown to have a decrease in event-free survival and overall survival. However, this effect was not recapitulated with the other VEGFRs.[34] Sorafenib is a nonspecific tyrosine kinase inhibitor that has inhibitory effects on VEGFRs. In a xenograft model of osteosarcoma, sorafenib reduced the tumor growth and increased the overall survival.[35] A single-arm phase II trial of sorafenib in relapsed and unresectable high-grade osteosarcoma demonstrated that single-agent sorafenib led to partial response in 9% of patients with a median progression-free survival of 4 months.[36] The authors note that 6 of 35 patients had partial response or stable disease for greater than 6 months. However, given that sorafenib may target multiple tyrosine kinases, this effect cannot be defined as VEGF specific. Also, the authors did not evaluate tumor VEGFR expression to confirm susceptibility. Other VEGF inhibitors with mixed specificity, such as sunitinib and cediranib, have also been shown to have activity against osteosarcoma in xenograft models.[37,38] Pazopanib is another multitargeted tyrosine kinase inhibitor with anti-VEGF activity. It is currently being studied in a phase I trial in children with relapsed and refractory solid tumors.[37]

Platelet-Derived Growth Factor

Platelet-derived growth factor (PDGF) receptors are also transmembrane tyrosine kinases. The majority of samples from osteosarcoma biopsies express PDGF-A in varying degrees. However, there is still some controversy whether tumors that express elevated levels of PDGF-A portend a worse prognosis.[39,40] Imatinib is a tyrosine kinase inhibitor known to inhibit PDGF receptors. A phase II study using imatinib in children with relapsed or refractory solid tumors found none of the 10 evaluable patients with osteosarcomas had a response to imatinib.[41] Again, criteria for inclusion in this trial did not depend on PDGF receptor expression. The lack of response from inhibition of PDGF receptors in osteosarcoma is hypothesized to be secondary to downstream activation via an alternative pathway.

Insulin-Like Growth Factor

Another transmembrane receptor target that has sparked interest is the insulin-like growth factor receptor (IGF-R). IGF-R is structurally related to the insulin receptor but preferentially binds to IGF. IGF-Rs have been shown to be overexpressed in osteosarcoma cell lines as well as in patient samples.[33,42] Inhibition of the IGF-R in vitro as well as in xenograft models of osteosarcoma has been demonstrated to decrease tumor growth.[43,44] Currently, there are several monoclonal antibodies targeting IGF-R that are being tested in phase I and II trials in patients with osteosarcoma. In a recent trial administering a monoclonal antibody to IGF-R in patients with Ewing sarcoma, elevated levels of circulating IGF were significantly correlated to response to treatment.[45] It will be interesting to delineate if this relationship is also uncovered in patients with osteosarcoma. A significant concern is the uncertainty regarding the clinical development of these agents.

Mammalian Target of Rapamycin

The mammalian target of rapamycin (mTOR) is a serine–threonine protein kinase that regulates protein synthesis by stimulating the translation of proteins required to progress through the G1 to S phase of the cell cycle. Rapamycin-treated osteosarcoma cells in vitro exhibit G1 growth arrest. However, inhibition of mTOR increases the activation of Akt, a serine/threonine protein kinase upstream of mTOR. Akt has been implicated in tumorigenesis by causing resistance to apoptosis and increased cell growth. The Akt activation in response to mTOR inhibition is IGF-1R dependent.[46] The anti-tumor effect of mTOR inhibition is synergistic with IGF-R blockade, even when used in cell lines resistant to IGF-1R antibodies. In xenograft models, the combination of mTOR and IGF-1R inhibition led to an enhanced activity in comparison to each of these agents used individually.[47] These agents make an attractive combination therapy for patients with osteosarcomas that exhibit activation of this pathway. A phase I study examining the safety of this combination in children with relapsed and refractory solid tumors is currently underway.

MET

MET encodes for a transmembrane tyrosine kinase receptor that in the process of tumorigenesis has been implicated in cell transformation, invasive growth, and tumor progression. *MET* overexpression by lentiviral transfection transforms human osteoblasts into osteosarcomas.[48] Met inhibition in human osteosarcoma cell lines inhibits growth and invasion.[49] In pretreatment tumor biopsy specimens, alterations in *MET* were seen in 50% of samples: 41% had deletions and 9% had amplifications. Patients with *MET*-amplified tumors would expect to have a 5-year event-free survival of 28%.[50] Currently, there is a phase I/II study of an Met inhibitor in children with relapsed/refractory solid tumors.

Bone Metabolism

Bisphosphonates stabilize the bone by inhibiting its resorption. In human osteosarcoma cell lines, they have been shown to inhibit the expression of metalloproteinases and invasion.[51] In a xenograft model, zoledronic acid inhibits tumor growth and development of metastasis.[52] A single-arm pilot study of pamidronate in children with newly diagnosed osteosarcoma demonstrated that it can be safely administered without increased toxicity, treatment delay, or diminished function of local reconstruction.[53] The receptor activator of nuclear factor kappa B (RANK) is another target involved with bone metabolism. Increased RANK ligand in initial biopsy specimens is associated with a poor event-free survival of 17.8%.[54] Denosumab is a monoclonal antibody which selectively inhibits RANK ligand. It has been well studied for bone metastases associated with malignancy. In France, zoledronic acid with combination chemotherapy is being studied in a randomized phase III trial in patients with newly diagnosed osteosarcoma. The Children's Oncology Group is conducting a randomized phase II trial of the addition of zoledronic to standard chemotherapy in children with newly diagnosed metastatic osteosarcoma.

In contrast to the medical management of osteosarcoma, the surgical management of osteosarcoma has made major inroads over the past three decades, with personalized options available based on the needs for local control and the age and potential growth of the patient.

SURGERY

The surgical management of osteosarcoma is, by definition, personalized. This is largely a function of the tumor's variability with regard to size, location, and extent. In addition, however, patient variables play a large part in defining surgical challenges and reconstructive options. For example, the surgical management for a high-demand athletic skeletally mature male will typically vary from that of a slight-framed and skeletally immature female. Even this generality may be, on occasion, an incorrect assumption, underscoring the need for individualized care. Management ideally offers the best oncologic and reconstructive procedures in keeping with a patient's hopes, goals, and expectations. In truth, the multitude and variety of surgical options that currently exist bear witness to the need and the benefit of personalized care for the surgical management of osteosarcoma.

Despite improvements in the systemic therapy for osteosarcoma, poor results persist in the absence of surgical treatment,[55] and surgery remains an essential component of care. Surgical management of osteosarcoma dictates complete extirpation of the tumor and, in most cases, the appropriate ensuing reconstruction. Historically, treatment consisted of mutilating surgery such as an amputation or a disarticulation.[56] However, with the realization of vastly improved outcomes, a result of improved systemic therapy, limb-salvage surgery has largely replaced these ablative procedures.[57] Regardless, complete resection of all gross disease remains the cornerstone to oncologic success, and it is generally accepted that functional outcome, while important, is of secondary concern.

Osteosarcoma requires a wide or complete excision, which by definition includes the tumor, its adjacent pseudocapsule, as well as a normal surrounding envelope of tissue. While quantitative values defining a "wide" surgical margin remain controversial, it is generally realized that more margin is safer. Frequently, bone margins of 2 to 3 cm and soft-tissue margins of 1 cm are sought; however, these margins need to be weighed against their cost and the morbidity that they exact, further underscoring the importance of individualized patient planning and personalized treatment approach. With the advent of navigation-guided surgery and robotic-mediated techniques, operative planning opportunities and surgical accuracy have never been greater. There is a renewed interest in obtaining even smaller, albeit negative, margins with the hope of minimizing surgical morbidity and restoring better function while maintaining oncologic standards. Currently, navigation technology can be grouped into preoperative image acquisition and intraoperative image acquisition. Preoperative image acquisition offers the benefit of preoperative planning, which includes measuring, localizing, and positioning of operative osteotomies. Intraoperative image acquisition precludes the need for image registration while offering a phenomenal degree of accuracy. Imaging modalities include computed tomography (CT), magnetic resonance imaging (MRI), CT/MRI combination, as well as fusion techniques that also utilize intraoperative fluoroscopy. Future development of oncologic navigation software and oncology-related navigated instrumentation will greatly aid in surgical accuracy.

While wide excisions have been reported to result in a minimally higher rate of local recurrence when compared with amputations,[58-60] other reports have shown no difference.[61,62] Regardless, similar overall and disease-free survival has been reported and as a result limb-salvage surgery is universally regarded as being oncologically equivalent so long as it is properly indicated.[56,58,62]

Successful surgical management of osteosarcoma is measured primarily by rendering the patient free of all gross disease and secondarily by the longevity and functionality of the reconstruction. Function and aesthetics should not supplant the primary oncologic goal and although limb-salvage surgery is currently indicated in up to 90% of cases, a primary amputation is occasionally required. Amputation is particularly relevant in cases where the patient hopes to participate in athletic, high-demand, and high-impact activities. In such instances, function and longevity are far superior following an amputation, especially considering prosthetic limb evolution and improvement. Once again, the importance of personalizing treatment cannot be overstated and successful treatment often rests not merely on the technical aspects of the surgery, but the indication to proceed at the start.

Reconstruction

Surgical reconstruction is not always necessary and bones such as the proximal fibula, distal ulna, patella, and ribs can be resected, resulting in arguably little to no functional deficit. Typically, however, reconstruction is necessary to achieve limb salvage and to restore limb function. Skeletal reconstruction can be accomplished through a variety of means, including autograft bone, allograft bone, endoprosthetic implants, or allograft prosthetic composites. Autograft bone has limited application but can be used, for example, following an intercalary diaphyseal resection of the tibia. Reconstruction using fibular autograft will initially be undersized and incapable of bearing full weight. Its benefits, however, are realized over time as the graft more reliably heals at the osteotomy sites, hypertrophies, and maintains the ability to heal in the event of future fracture. In the setting of osteosarcoma, the indication for bulk autograft reconstruction is somewhat narrow, however, since the majority of extremity tumors are metaphyseal and joint reconstruction is typically required.

Reconstruction using bulk or structural allograft offers a number of benefits. It remains, to date, the best means with which to reattach essential tendons and ligaments around a joint. This is particularly relevant in the proximal tibia and the proximal humerus where the patellar ligament and the rotator cuff tendons are essential to stability and function. Additionally, allograft bone restores bone-stock, allowing for future surgical options which, in and of them, are frequently more bone sparing. The value in allograft use is that it offers more options to a young patient for whom reconstructive longevity and future reconstructive options are of high import. Osteoarticular allograft reconstruction, typically applied to the knee, spares the opposing articular surface as well as the opposing physis. In addition to allowing for continued growth on the opposing side of the joint, it more accurately recreates a patient's native joint, which may allow for more normal joint dynamics and kinematics compared with those of endoprostheses.[63-65]

Despite its many benefits, bulk allografts have widely recognized and well-characterized limitations, including nonunion, infection, and fracture. Nonunion rates have been reported ranging from 17% to 34%[66-68] and are affected by a variety of factors, most notably the delayed healing effects of chemotherapy.[69] Union rates typically extend beyond 6 months and frequently may exceed 12 months. Infection rates range between 11% and 16%[66,68,70,71] of cases, with most infections occurring within the first month of the index surgery. Fracture rates reportedly range between 10% and 45%[66-68] and frequently require one or more surgical procedures. The successful use of vascularized fibular grafts for failed bulk allograft reconstructions has been reported and, regardless of failure mechanism, this approach merits consideration.[72]

Although allograft bone use has inherent limitations, it remains an important tool in the limb-salvage surgeon's armamentarium. Future improvement will likely be incremental and will undoubtedly work toward decreasing nonunion, infection, and fracture-related complications through technique modification and biologic augmentation.

Currently, many surgeons consider endoprosthetic reconstruction as their preferred reconstructive choice as this is reliable, reproducible, and modular, which permits for accurate reconstruction of the surgical defect while also matching patient size and anatomy. In addition, they permit immediate to early weight bearing, early range of motion, and earlier return to some independent activities. By definition, these joint replacements preclude the development of arthritis, a limitation of osteoarticular allografts. Historically, endoprosthetic replacements were custom-made, requiring 8 to 10 weeks to design and manufacture. However, currently, a plethora of off-the-shelf systems are commercially available.

Limitations of endoprostheses have been well documented and mostly include hardware failure, infection, aseptic loosening, and dislocation, with an overall complication rate, excluding local tumor recurrence, typically ranging from 16% to 22%.[73-75] Implant failure due to mechanical causes such as stem fracture or implant dislocation has been reported to range from approximately 2% to 6%.[73,75-79] Aseptic loosening appears to vary widely in the literature ranging from approximately 2% to over 40%,[73,74,76,77,80] though this has been reduced substantially by using the rotating-hinge style implant.[80] Rates of implant infection range from approximately 2% to 20%[73-80] and are largely recognized to be more frequent in cases of proximal tibial reconstructions. This has been ascribed to the limited soft-tissue coverage over the anterior leg and has prompted the routine use of a gastrocnemius flap with good results. Silver has been recently recognized as having valuable antimicrobial properties, and silver-coated prostheses are becoming commercially available with encouraging early results.

Growing prostheses continue to evolve and currently can be lengthened through noninvasive means. They are particularly relevant for a patient seeking a limb-salvage procedure who is expected to have a 5 cm or greater leg length inequality at skeletal maturity. Unfortunately, these implants are custom-made and command a high cost. Failure of the expansion mechanism has been reported in all commercially available designs to date and some designs require revision to an adult-style implant at skeletal maturity. Despite these challenges, this technology stands on the cutting edge of limb-salvage surgery. It offers the real benefit of fewer surgeries, which most surgeons agree will translate into fewer infections. As these devices become more reliable and less expensive, they will likely play an increasingly important role within a subset of patients.

Despite the limitations noted, endoprosthetic reconstruction offers many benefits to both the patient and the surgeon. Improving current outcomes will likely focus on decreasing mechanical complications such as bearing wear and aseptic loosening as well as minimizing infection.

Allograft prosthetic composite reconstructions blend the techniques of bulk allograft and endoprosthetic reconstructions, incorporating the benefits of both. They are of particular relevance in tumors involving the proximal humerus and proximal tibia for the same reasons noted previously. The technique involves implanting an endoprosthesis within a bulk allograft, resurfacing the articular cartilage, and securing the allograft to the host bone, for example, using internal fixation. Limitations of allograft prosthetic composite reconstructions have been published and to some extent overlap with those previously mentioned for allografts and endoprostheses. In general, they include infection, aseptic loosening, dislocation, fracture, nonunion, hardware failure, and graft resorption.[63,81-89] Reviewing overall complication rates may be somewhat misleading, as not all complications require intervention and not all complications are of equal impact. In certain anatomic regions, the allograft prosthetic composite reconstruction can yield excellent functional outcomes and remains an important reconstructive option.

Rotationplasty is a technique most frequently applied to tumor resections that involve the knee and has been likened to an intercalary resection of the joint. The technique involves resection of the tumor along with the joint, rotation of the distal limb, and reattachment of the tibia to the femur. This effectively converts the ankle functionally and anatomically into the knee and offers a patient who would otherwise require an above-knee amputation to undergo the equivalent of a below-knee amputation. As with many surgeries, proper patient selection is essential for a successful outcome. The typical candidate is a thin skeletally immature patient with significant remaining growth potential who presents with a very large tumor that would otherwise require an above-knee amputation. It is indicated in cases with intra-articular extension, gross contamination of the surrounding soft-tissue structures, or concomitant infection. The involvement of the vascular bundle does not preclude a rotationplasty as it may be re-anastomosed at the time of the resection. Additionally, it is appropriate for a patient who would prefer a biologic reconstruction that would grant them the ability to participate in a high level of impact activities. It has the added benefit of avoiding phantom limb pain and sensation and is not considered by many an amputation of any sort for this reason.

In summary, surgical management of osteosarcoma serves as one of the best examples of personalized management. Success hinges not only on the specifics defined by the tumor but also on the patient's anatomic constraints, growth potential, rehabilitation compliance, expectations, as well as a multitude of related social and personal concerns. Choosing the correct procedure is as much about the patient as it is about the anatomy or the technology at hand. Balancing what can be done with what should be done requires a frank discussion during which time the patient and their family need to understand not only what the immediate proposed surgical procedure entails but also what future complication, challenges, and revisions may be encountered.

CONCLUSION

Traditionally, the medical management of osteosarcoma has hinged upon delineating the differences between patients with good versus poor response to chemotherapy at the time of tumor resection. Intensification of chemotherapy for patients with a poor histologic response has, to this date, not been proven to improve their overall survival. The recently completed randomized multinational trial comparing the addition of ifosfamide and etoposide in patients with poor response will again attempt to address this issue. Additional targeted therapies are being recognized as possible avenues to improve outcomes for children with osteosarcoma. A major difficulty in actively pursuing these targets is the small number of patients. Multi-institutional trials are necessary to achieve accrual for randomized trials. Molecular profiling of tumor samples has been shown to be possible and effective.[90] To further refine personalized treatment for osteosarcoma, hurdles need to be overcome. Randomized trials need to be defined for patients whose tumors exhibit susceptibility to the targeted agent being studied. However, given the small number of patients diagnosed each year, these trials will be technically challenging.

REFERENCES

1. Mirabello L, Troisi RJ, Savage SA. Osteosarcoma incidence and survival rates from 1973 to 2004: data from the Surveillance, Epidemiology, and End Results Program. *Cancer*. 2009;115:1531-1543.
2. Price CH. Primary bone-forming tumours and their relationship to skeletal growth. *J Bone Joint Surg Br.* 1958;40-B:574-593.
3. Bridge JA, Nelson M, McComb E, et al. Cytogenetic findings in 73 osteosarcoma specimens and a review of the literature. *Cancer Genet Cytogenet*. 1997;95:74-87.
4. Overholtzer M, Rao PH, Favis R, et al. The presence of p53 mutations in human osteosarcomas correlates with high levels of genomic instability. *Proc Natl Acad Sci U S A*. 2003;100:11547-11552.
5. Toguchida J, Ishizaki K, Sasaki MS, et al. Chromosomal reorganization for the expression of recessive mutation of retinoblastoma susceptibility gene in the development of osteosarcoma. *Cancer Res*. 1988;48:3939-3943.
6. Marcove RC, Mike V, Hajek JV, Levin AG, Hutter RV. Osteogenic sarcoma under the age of twenty-one. A review of one hundred and forty-five operative cases. *J Bone Joint Surg Am*. 1970;52:411-423.
7. Dahlin DC, Coventry MB. Osteogenic sarcoma. A study of six hundred cases. *J Bone Joint Surg Am*. 1967;49:101-110.
8. Link MP, Goorin AM, Horowitz M, et al. Adjuvant chemotherapy of high-grade osteosarcoma of the extremity. Updated results of the Multi-Institutional Osteosarcoma Study. *Clin Orthop Relat Res*. 1991;270:8-14.
9. Smith MA, Seibel NL, Altekruse SF, et al. Outcomes for children and adolescents with cancer: challenges for the twenty-first century. *J Clin Oncol*. 2010;28:2625-2634.
10. Meyers PA, Schwartz CL, Krailo M, et al. Osteosarcoma: a randomized, prospective trial of the addition of ifosfamide and/or muramyl tripeptide to cisplatin, doxorubicin, and high-dose methotrexate. *J Clin Oncol*. 2005;23:2004-2011.
11. Chou AJ, Kleinerman ES, Krailo MD, et al. Addition of muramyl tripeptide to chemotherapy for patients with newly diagnosed metastatic osteosarcoma: a report from the Children's Oncology Group. *Cancer*. 2009;115:5339-5348.
12. Goorin AM, Schwartzentruber DJ, Devidas M, et al. Presurgical chemotherapy compared with immediate surgery and adjuvant chemotherapy for nonmetastatic osteosarcoma: Pediatric Oncology Group Study POG-8651. *J Clin Oncol*. 2003;21:1574-1580.
13. Rosen G, Marcove RC, Huvos AG, et al. Primary osteogenic sarcoma: eight-year experience with adjuvant chemotherapy. *J Cancer Res Clin Oncol*. 1983;106(suppl):55-67.
14. Meyers PA, Heller G, Healey J, et al. Chemotherapy for nonmetastatic osteogenic sarcoma: the Memorial Sloan-Kettering experience. *J Clin Oncol*. 1992;10:5-15.
15. Bacci G, Mercuri M, Longhi A, et al. Grade of chemotherapy-induced necrosis as a predictor of local and systemic control in 881 patients with non-metastatic osteosarcoma of the extremities treated with neoadjuvant chemotherapy in a single institution. *Eur J Cancer*. 2005;41:2079-2085.
16. Bacci G, Forni C, Ferrari S, et al. Neoadjuvant chemotherapy for osteosarcoma of the extremity: intensification of preoperative treatment does not increase the rate of good histologic response to the primary tumor or improve the final outcome. *J Pediatr Hematol Oncol*. 2003;25:845-853.
17. Meyers PA, Gorlick R, Heller G, et al. Intensification of preoperative chemotherapy for osteogenic sarcoma: results of the Memorial Sloan-Kettering (T12) protocol. *J Clin Oncol*. 1998;16:2452-2458.
18. Rosen G, Caparros B, Huvos AG, et al. Preoperative chemotherapy for osteogenic sarcoma: selection of postoperative adjuvant chemotherapy based on the response of the primary tumor to preoperative chemotherapy. *Cancer*. 1982;49:1221-1230.
19. Rosen G, Nirenberg A. Neoadjuvant chemotherapy for osteogenic sarcoma: a five year follow-up (T-10) and preliminary report of new studies (T-12). *Prog Clin Biol Res*. 1985;201:39-51.
20. Saeter G, Alvegard TA, Elomaa I, Stenwig AE, Holmstrom T, Solheim OP. Treatment of osteosarcoma of the extremities with the T-10 protocol, with emphasis on the effects of preoperative chemotherapy with single-agent high-dose methotrexate: a Scandinavian Sarcoma Group study. *J Clin Oncol*. 1991;9:1766-1775.
21. Provisor AJ, Ettinger LJ, Nachman JB, et al. Treatment of nonmetastatic osteosarcoma of the extremity with preoperative and postoperative chemotherapy: a report from the Children's Cancer Group. *J Clin Oncol*. 1997;15:76-84.
22. Winkler K, Beron G, Delling G, et al. Neoadjuvant chemotherapy of osteosarcoma: results of a randomized cooperative trial (COSS-82) with salvage chemotherapy based on histological tumor response. *J Clin Oncol*. 1988;6:329-337.
23. Fuchs N, Bielack SS, Epler D, et al. Long-term results of the co-operative German-Austrian-Swiss osteosarcoma study group's protocol COSS-86 of intensive multidrug chemotherapy and surgery for osteosarcoma of the limbs. *Ann Oncol*. 1998;9:893-899.
24. Winkler K, Bielack S, Delling G, et al. Effect of intraarterial versus intravenous cisplatin in addition to systemic doxorubicin, high-dose methotrexate, and ifosfamide on histologic tumor response in osteosarcoma (study COSS-86). *Cancer*. 1990;66:1703-1710.
25. Ferrari S, Mercuri M, Picci P, et al. Nonmetastatic osteosarcoma of the extremity: results of a neoadjuvant chemotherapy protocol (IOR/OS-3) with high-dose methotrexate, intraarterial or intravenous cisplatin, doxorubicin, and salvage chemotherapy based on histologic tumor response. *Tumori*. 1999;85:458-464.
26. Bacci G, Briccoli A, Ferrari S, et al. Neoadjuvant chemotherapy for osteosarcoma of the extremity: long-term results of the Rizzoli's 4th protocol. *Eur J Cancer*. 2001;37:2030-2039.
27. Meyers PA, Schwartz CL, Krailo MD, et al. Osteosarcoma: the addition of muramyl tripeptide to chemotherapy improves overall survival—a report from the Children's Oncology Group. *J Clin Oncol*. 2008;26:633-638.

28. Goorin AM, Harris MB, Bernstein M, et al. Phase II/III trial of etoposide and high-dose ifosfamide in newly diagnosed metastatic osteosarcoma: a pediatric oncology group trial. *J Clin Oncol.* 2002;20:426-433.
29. Onda M, Matsuda S, Higaki S, et al. ErbB-2 expression is correlated with poor prognosis for patients with osteosarcoma. *Cancer.* 1996;77:71-78.
30. Gorlick R, Huvos AG, Heller G, et al. Expression of HER2/erbB-2 correlates with survival in osteosarcoma. *J Clin Oncol.* 1999;17:2781-2788.
31. Kilpatrick SE, Geisinger KR, King TS, et al. Clinicopathologic analysis of HER-2/neu immunoexpression among various histologic subtypes and grades of osteosarcoma. *Mod Pathol.* 2001;14:1277-1283.
32. Thomas DG, Giordano TJ, Sanders D, Biermann JS, Baker L. Absence of HER2/neu gene expression in osteosarcoma and skeletal Ewing's sarcoma. *Clin Cancer Res.* 2002;8:788-793.
33. Hassan SE, Bekarev M, Kim MY, et al. Cell surface receptor expression patterns in osteosarcoma. *Cancer.* February 2012; 118(3):740-749.
34. Abdeen A, Chou AJ, Healey JH, et al. Correlation between clinical outcome and growth factor pathway expression in osteogenic sarcoma. *Cancer.* 2009;115:5243-5250.
35. Pignochino Y, Grignani G, Cavalloni G, et al. Sorafenib blocks tumour growth, angiogenesis and metastatic potential in preclinical models of osteosarcoma through a mechanism potentially involving the inhibition of ERK1/2, MCL-1 and ezrin pathways. *Mol Cancer.* 2009;8:118.
36. Grignani G, Palmerini E, Dileo P, et al. A phase II trial of sorafenib in relapsed and unresectable high-grade osteosarcoma after failure of standard multimodal therapy: an Italian Sarcoma Group study. *Ann Oncol.* February 201223(2):508-516.
37. Maris JM, Courtright J, Houghton PJ, et al. Initial testing (stage 1) of sunitinib by the pediatric preclinical testing program. *Pediatr Blood Cancer.* 2008;51:42-48.
38. Maris JM, Courtright J, Houghton PJ, et al. Initial testing of the VEGFR inhibitor AZD2171 by the pediatric preclinical testing program. *Pediatr Blood Cancer.* 2008;50:581-587.
39. Kubo T, Piperdi S, Rosenblum J, et al. Platelet-derived growth factor receptor as a prognostic marker and a therapeutic target for imatinib mesylate therapy in osteosarcoma. *Cancer.* 2008;112:2119-2129.
40. Sulzbacher I, Birner P, Dominkus M, Pichlhofer B, Mazal PR. Expression of platelet-derived growth factor-alpha receptor in human osteosarcoma is not a predictor of outcome. *Pathology.* 2010;42:664-668.
41. Bond M, Bernstein ML, Pappo A, et al. A phase II study of imatinib mesylate in children with refractory or relapsed solid tumors: a Children's Oncology Group study. *Pediatr Blood Cancer.* 2008;50:254-258.
42. Burrow S, Andrulis IL, Pollak M, Bell RS. Expression of insulin-like growth factor receptor, IGF-1, and IGF-2 in primary and metastatic osteosarcoma. *J Surg Oncol.* 1998;69:21-27.
43. Kappel CC, Velez-Yanguas MC, Hirschfeld S, Helman LJ. Human osteosarcoma cell lines are dependent on insulin-like growth factor I for in vitro growth. *Cancer Res.* 1994;54:2803-2807.
44. Houghton PJ, Morton CL, Gorlick R, et al. Initial testing of a monoclonal antibody (IMC-A12) against IGF-1R by the Pediatric Preclinical Testing Program. *Pediatr Blood Cancer.* 2010;54:921-926.
45. Pappo AS, Patel SR, Crowley J, et al. R1507, a monoclonal antibody to the insulin-like growth factor 1 receptor in patients with recurrent or refractory Ewing sarcoma family of tumors: results of a phase II sarcoma alliance for research through collaboration study. *J Clin Oncol.* December 2011;29(34):4541-4547.
46. Wan X, Harkavy B, Shen N, Grohar P, Helman LJ. Rapamycin induces feedback activation of Akt signaling through an IGF-1R-dependent mechanism. *Oncogene.* 2007;26:1932-1940.
47. Kolb EA, Kamara D, Zhang W, et al. R1507, a fully human monoclonal antibody targeting IGF-1R, is effective alone and in combination with rapamycin in inhibiting growth of osteosarcoma xenografts. *Pediatr Blood Cancer.* 2010;55:67-75.
48. Patane S, Avnet S, Coltella N, et al. MET overexpression turns human primary osteoblasts into osteosarcomas. *Cancer Res.* 2006;66:4750-4757.
49. Sampson ER, Martin BA, Morris AE, et al. The orally bioavailable met inhibitor PF-2341066 inhibits osteosarcoma growth and osteolysis/matrix production in a xenograft model. *J Bone Miner Res.* 2011;26:1283-1294.
50. Entz-Werle N, Lavaux T, Metzger N, et al. Involvement of MET/TWIST/APC combination or the potential role of ossification factors in pediatric high-grade osteosarcoma oncogenesis. *Neoplasia.* 2007;9:678-688.
51. Cheng YY, Huang L, Lee KM, Li K, Kumta SM. Alendronate regulates cell invasion and MMP-2 secretion in human osteosarcoma cell lines. *Pediatr Blood Cancer.* 2004;42:410-415.
52. Dass CR, Choong PF. Zoledronic acid inhibits osteosarcoma growth in an orthotopic model. *Mol Cancer Ther.* 2007;6:3263-3270.
53. Meyers PA, Healey JH, Chou AJ, et al. Addition of pamidronate to chemotherapy for the treatment of osteosarcoma. *Cancer.* 2011;117:1736-1744.
54. Lee JA, Jung JS, Kim DH, et al. RANKL expression is related to treatment outcome of patients with localized, high-grade osteosarcoma. *Pediatr Blood Cancer.* May 2011;56(5):738-743.
55. Jaffe N, Carrasco H, Raymond K, Ayala A, Eftekhari F. Can cure in patients with osteosarcoma be achieved exclusively with chemotherapy and abrogation of surgery? *Cancer.* 2002;95:2202-2210.
56. Enneking WF, Dunham W, Gebhardt MC, Malawar M, Pritchard DJ. A system for the functional evaluation of reconstructive procedures after surgical treatment of tumors of the musculoskeletal system. *Clin Orthop Relat Res.* 1993;286:241-246.
57. Bielack S, Jurgens H, Jundt G, et al. Osteosarcoma: the COSS experience. *Cancer Treat Res.* 2010;152:289-308.
58. Rougraff BT, Simon MA, Kneisl JS, Greenberg DB, Mankin HJ. Limb salvage compared with amputation for osteosarcoma of the distal end of the femur. A long-term oncological, functional, and quality-of-life study. *J Bone Joint Surg Am.* 1994;76:649-656.
59. Weeden S, Grimer RJ, Cannon SR, Taminiau AH, Uscinska BM. The effect of local recurrence on survival in resected osteosarcoma. *Eur J Cancer.* 2001;37:39-46.
60. Picci P, Sangiorgi L, Rougraff BT, Neff JR, Casadei R, Campanacci M. Relationship of chemotherapy-induced necrosis and surgical margins to local recurrence in osteosarcoma. *J Clin Oncol.* 1994;12:2699-2705.
61. Lindner NJ, Ramm O, Hillmann A, et al. Limb salvage and outcome of osteosarcoma. The University of Muenster experience. *Clin Orthop Relat Res.* 1999:83-89.
62. Simon MA, Aschliman MA, Thomas N, Mankin HJ. Limb-salvage treatment versus amputation for osteosarcoma of the distal end of the femur. *J Bone Joint Surg Am.* 1986;68:1331-1337.
63. Biau DJ, Dumaine V, Babinet A, Tomeno B, Anract P. Allograft-prosthesis composites after bone tumor resection at the proximal tibia. *Clin Orthop Relat Res.* 2007;456:211-217.
64. Brien EW, Terek RM, Healey JH, Lane JM. Allograft reconstruction after proximal tibial resection for bone tumors. An analysis of function and outcome comparing allograft and prosthetic reconstructions. *Clin Orthop Relat Res.* 1994;303:116-127.
65. Clatworthy MG, Gross AE. The allograft prosthetic composite: when and how. *Orthopedics.* 2001;24:897-898.
66. Mankin HJ, Gebhardt MC, Jennings LC, Springfield DS, Tomford WW. Long-term results of allograft replacement in the management of bone tumors. *Clin Orthop Relat Res.* 1996;324:86-97.
67. Ortiz-Cruz E, Gebhardt MC, Jennings LC, Springfield DS, Mankin HJ. The results of transplantation of intercalary allografts after resection of tumors. A long-term follow-up study. *J Bone Joint Surg Am.* 1997;79:97-106.
68. Brigman BE, Hornicek FJ, Gebhardt MC, Mankin HJ. Allografts about the knee in young patients with high-grade sarcoma. *Clin Orthop Relat Res.* 2004;421:232-239.
69. Hornicek FJ, Gebhardt MC, Tomford WW, et al. Factors affecting nonunion of the allograft-host junction. *Clin Orthop Relat Res.* 2001;382:87-98.
70. Lord CF, Gebhardt MC, Tomford WW, Mankin HJ. Infection in bone allografts. Incidence, nature, and treatment. *J Bone Joint Surg Am.* 1988;70:369-376.
71. Dick HM, Strauch RJ. Infection of massive bone allografts. *Clin Orthop Relat Res.* 1994;306:46-53.
72. Friedrich JB, Moran SL, Bishop AT, Wood CM, Shin AY. Free vascularized fibular graft salvage of complications of long-bone

allograft after tumor reconstruction. *J Bone Joint Surg Am.* 2008;90:93-100.

73. Bickels J, Wittig JC, Kollender Y, et al. Distal femur resection with endoprosthetic reconstruction: a long-term followup study. *Clin Orthop Relat Res.* 2002;400:225-235.
74. Kawai A, Muschler GF, Lane JM, Otis JC, Healey JH. Prosthetic knee replacement after resection of a malignant tumor of the distal part of the femur. Medium to long-term results. *J Bone Joint Surg Am.* 1998;80:636-647.
75. Myers GJ, Abudu AT, Carter SR, Tillman RM, Grimer RJ. Endoprosthetic replacement of the distal femur for bone tumours: long-term results. *J Bone Joint Surg Br.* 2007;89:521-526.
76. Ahlmann ER, Menendez LR, Kermani C, Gotha H. Survivorship and clinical outcome of modular endoprosthetic reconstruction for neoplastic disease of the lower limb. *J Bone Joint Surg Br.* 2006;88:790-795.
77. Torbert JT, Fox EJ, Hosalkar HS, Ogilvie CM, Lackman RD. Endoprosthetic reconstructions: results of long-term followup of 139 patients. *Clin Orthop Relat Res.* 2005;438:51-59.
78. Capanna R, Morris HG, Campanacci D, Del Ben M, Campanacci M. Modular uncemented prosthetic reconstruction after resection of tumours of the distal femur. *J Bone Joint Surg Br.* 1994;76:178-186.
79. Malawer MM, Chou LB. Prosthetic survival and clinical results with use of large-segment replacements in the treatment of high-grade bone sarcomas. *J Bone Joint Surg Am.* 1995;77:1154-1165.
80. Myers GJ, Abudu AT, Carter SR, Tillman RM, Grimer RJ. The long-term results of endoprosthetic replacement of the proximal tibia for bone tumours. *J Bone Joint Surg Br.* 2007;89:1632-1637.
81. Abdeen A, Hoang BH, Athanasian EA, Morris CD, Boland PJ, Healey JH. Allograft-prosthesis composite reconstruction of the proximal part of the humerus: functional outcome and survivorship. *J Bone Joint Surg Am.* 2009;91:2406-2415.
82. Potter BK, Adams SC, Pitcher JD Jr, Malinin TI, Temple HT. Proximal humerus reconstructions for tumors. *Clin Orthop Relat Res.* 2009;467:1035-1041.
83. Gitelis S, Piasecki P. Allograft prosthetic composite arthroplasty for osteosarcoma and other aggressive bone tumors. *Clin Orthop Relat Res.* 1991;270:197-201.
84. Gilbert NF, Yasko AW, Oates SD, Lewis VO, Cannon CP, Lin PP. Allograft-prosthetic composite reconstruction of the proximal part of the tibia. An analysis of the early results. *J Bone Joint Surg Am.* 2009;91:1646-1656.
85. Zehr RJ, Enneking WF, Scarborough MT. Allograft-prosthesis composite versus megaprosthesis in proximal femoral reconstruction. *Clin Orthop Relat Res.* 1996;322:207-223.
86. Farid Y, Lin PP, Lewis VO, Yasko AW. Endoprosthetic and allograft-prosthetic composite reconstruction of the proximal femur for bone neoplasms. *Clin Orthop Relat Res.* 2006;442:223-229.
87. Biau DJ, Larousserie F, Thevenin F, Piperno-Neumann S, Anract P. Results of 32 allograft-prosthesis composite reconstructions of the proximal femur. *Clin Orthop Relat Res.* March 2010;468:834-845.
88. Donati D, Giacomini S, Gozzi E, Mercuri M. Proximal femur reconstruction by an allograft prosthesis composite. *Clin Orthop Relat Res.* 2002;394:192-200.
89. Langlais F, Lambotte JC, Collin P, Thomazeau H. Long-term results of allograft composite total hip prostheses for tumors. *Clin Orthop Relat Res.* 2003;414:197-211.
90. Von Hoff DD, Stephenson JJ Jr, Rosen P, et al. Pilot study using molecular profiling of patients' tumors to find potential targets and select treatments for their refractory cancers. *J Clin Oncol.* 2010;28:4877-4883.

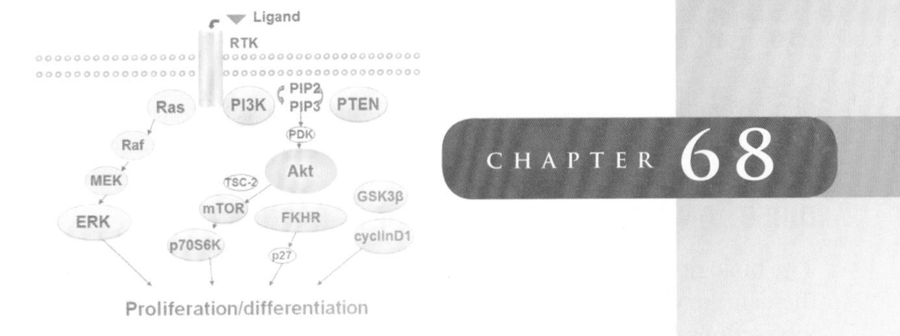

Molecular Basis of Chemoradiotherapy and High-Precision Radiotherapy

Michio Yoshimura, Masahiro Hiraoka, and Hiroshi Harada

INTRODUCTION

Radiation therapy is the medical use of ionizing radiation to control malignant tumor cells. The history of radiation therapy originated from the discovery of X-rays in the field of physics. The therapy has developed dramatically through the integration of latest technologies and knowledge of physics with information for chemistry, engineering, biology, and medical science. It has grown to be one of the three major treatments for cancer. This chapter focuses on the molecular basis by which radiation damages cells and how conventional radiation therapy specifically affects cancer cells. In addition, this chapter introduces the latest innovations and applications in the fields of radiation therapy.

HISTORY OF RADIATION THERAPY FOR CANCER

The history of radiation therapy for cancer started at the end of the 19th century as a result of epoch-making discoveries in physics. Wilhelm Conrad Röntgen discovered X-rays in 1895,[1] Antoine Henri Becquerel found radioactivity emitted by uranium compounds in 1896, and Pierre and Marie Curie isolated the radioactive elements polonium and radium in 1898. Because radiation can penetrate the human body and eventually kills cells, its medical applications were recognized as early as in 1896, just one year after the discovery of X-rays. However, many people unfortunately suffered in those early days because of inadequate knowledge about the risks of radiation. In 1913, William D. Coolidge invented the Coolidge tube, which permits continuous production of X-rays, and is still in use today. Radiation therapy for cancer has continued to improve through the integration of latest technologies and knowledge for various fields and through collaboration between scientists and clinicians.

TYPES OF RADIATION

Radiation can be categorized as "ionizing" or "non-ionizing." "Ionizing radiation" has enough energy to eject electrons from atoms or molecules. Although both ionizing and non-ionizing radiation are injurious, the former is much more toxic. So, ionizing radiation has been mainly used to kill cancer cells.

X-rays and γ-rays are widely used in conventional radiation treatment for cancer. Although both are categorized as electromagnetic radiation and their characteristics do not differ, they are produced in different ways. X-rays are produced in an electrical device which accelerates electrons to high speed; stops them suddenly by using a target made of, for example tungsten; and generates the so-called bremsstrahlung. γ-Rays, by contrast, are emitted from radioactive isotopes, such as ^{60}Co.

Another type of radiation widely used in cancer therapy is particle radiation, using beams of protons and heavy charged ions. Compared with electromagnetic radiation which is thought of as waves of electrical and magnetic energies, these beams transfer particles in addition to energy. Protons are particles with a both positive charge and certain mass. Heavy charged particles are nuclei of elements, such as carbon, neon, argon, and iron, which also have a positive charge because of the dissociation of a negatively charged electron. Relatively complex and expensive equipment is needed to generate and utilize particle beams for cancer therapy. But because of a favorable dose distribution, the number of facilities is increasing.

DIRECT AND INDIRECT EFFECTS OF RADIATION

The biological effects of radiation are largely attributed to the damage of genomic DNA which contains all genetic instructions for development and function. When radiation is absorbed by intracellular biological molecules, it directly binds to DNA in cells. Then, the atoms in the DNA become ionized and damaged. This is the so-called direct effect of radiation. Moreover, radiation can also interact with other atoms and/or molecules (such as water) in cells and produce free radicals. Because free radicals are highly reactive, they can introduce damage to genomic DNA, resulting in cell death. This is the so-called indirect effect of radiation.

Whether radiation acts directly or indirectly on cellular macromolecules is dependent on linear energy transfer (LET), the energy transferred per unit length of track. Direct action is dominant in the case of protons and heavy charged ions whose LET is high. Conversely, about two-thirds of the biological damage from X- and γ-rays are caused by indirect effects because of a low LET.

FACTORS INFLUENCING BIOLOGICAL EFFECT OF IONIZING RADIATION

DNA Repair Pathways

Radiation causes various kinds of DNA lesions, including base damage, single-strand breaks (SSBs), double-strand breaks (DSBs), and DNA–DNA crosslinks. Mammalian cells have developed excellent systems to sense, respond to, and repair these lesions. But once cells fail to repair the damage, they suffer from mutation, carcinogenesis, and death. DNA repair pathways in cancer cells have long been recognized as targets to sensitize the therapeutic effect of radiation. Repair pathways for DSBs, the most lethal form of damage caused by ionizing radiation, are particularly important.[2] In eukaryotic cells, DSBs are repaired via two fundamental mechanisms: homologous recombination repair (HRR) and nonhomologous end-joining (NHEJ)[2] (Table 68.1).

The immediate response of cells to DSBs is the activation of sensor proteins, ATM (ataxia telangiectasia mutated) and ATR (ATM and Rad 3–related) and so on.[3] These factors are recruited to sites of damage and function in both the promotion of DNA repair and prevention of cell cycle progression until the lesions are repaired.[3] The 53BP1 protein functions, at least in part, in the next step and determines the most suitable pathway, HRR or NHEJ, for repair of the DNA damage. HRR is an error-free mechanism because the undamaged homologous chromatid can be used as a template for repair.[2] Representative factors functioning in HRR are RAD51, RAD52, BRCA1, and BRCA2. NHEJ is a relatively error-prone pathway because the activity of this system is just to mediate end-to-end joining.[2] Representative factors in NHEJ are Ku70, Ku80, DNA protein kinase (DNA-PK), and XRCC4. Because the repair of DSBs after radiation therapy is critical to the survival of cancer cells, inhibiting the repair pathways should enhance the therapeutic effect of radiation.[4]

Hypoxia

The presence of molecular oxygen influences the biological effect of low LET ionizing radiation, including X-rays and γ-rays.[5,6] The so-called oxygen effect was first recognized in 1912 by Swartz et al. who noticed that biological reactions to a radium applicator dramatically decreased when it was tightly pushed onto the target skin and the blood flow around it was reduced. Extensive research in the fields of radiation biology and oncology has revealed that cells are approximately two to three times more radioresistant under hypoxic conditions than normoxic conditions.

A milestone study linking the oxygen effect with radioresistance of cancer cells was published by Thomlinson and Gray in 1955,[6] who proposed that oxygen levels decrease in a solid tumor through successive layers of cancer cells distal to blood vessels (Fig. 68.1). Also, it has been reported that cancer cells at a distance of about 10 cell diameters from vessels are viable but highly radioresistant.

The mechanism behind the oxygen effect has not been fully elucidated. However, it is widely believed that oxygen acts to generate free radicals.[5,9] Ionizing radiation literally induces the ionization of target genomic DNA or intracellular molecules such as water and produces highly reactive radicals. Oxygen oxidizes the DNA radicals and is known to make the damage permanent. Conversely, in the absence of oxygen, the DNA radicals are reduced by compounds containing sulfhydryl groups (SH groups), which restore/repair the DNA to its intact form. Thus, irreparable DSBs are significantly less serious in the absence of oxygen, leading to hypoxia-related radioresistance of cells.

TABLE 68–1 Representative Repair Pathways for Double-Strand Breaks

Repair Pathways for DSBs	Fidelity	Representative Factors Involved	Dominant Cell Cycle Status
Homologous recombination repair	Error-free	RAD51, RAD52, BRCA1/2,	Late S, G_2 phases
Nonhomologous end-joining	Error-prone	Ku70, Ku80, DNA protein kinase, XRCC4	Every status

DSBs, double-strand breaks.

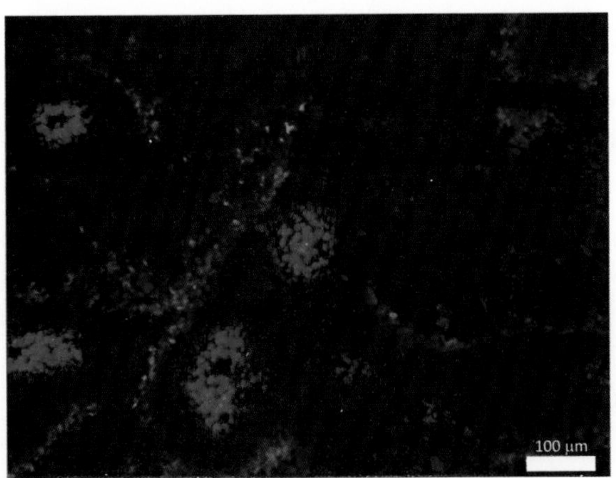

FIGURE 68–1 Tumor hypoxia. A frozen section of a HeLa tumor xenograft was stained with a hypoxic marker, pimonidazole (green).[7,8] Functional tumor blood vessels can be seen as the blue fluorescence of a perfusion marker, Hoechst 33342.

In addition to radiochemical mechanisms, radiobiological mechanisms are also important. Hypoxic stimuli trigger changes in both DNA damage repair pathways[10] and cell death/survival signaling pathways, leading to an increase in the radioresistant phenotype. Moreover, accumulated evidence revealed an important role of a transcription factor, hypoxia-inducible factor 1 (HIF-1).[11-15] Radiation upregulates HIF-1 activity in solid tumors as a result of the increase in oxidative stress[13,14] and improvement in glucose and oxygen availability.[7,8,11,12] HIF-1, then, induces vascular endothelial growth factor (VEGF) expression, protects endothelial cells from cytotoxic effects of radiation, and accelerates postirradiation tumor growth by assuring the delivery of oxygen and nutrients there.[8,12-14,16,17]

Expression of the alpha subunit of the HIF-1 (HIF-1α) protein as well as the intratumor hypoxic fraction has been reported to correlate with a poor prognosis, local tumor recurrence, and distant tumor metastases after radiation therapy.[18-20]

Cell Cycle

The proliferation of cells is strictly regulated as a cycle of four distinct phases: M phase (mitosis), G_1 phase (gap 1), S phase (synthesis), and G_2 phase (gap 2), after which mitosis starts again[21] (Fig. 68.2). Research using various organisms from yeast to mammals has demonstrated that the activity of repair pathways for DSBs is dependent on the status of the cell cycle.[22,23] HRR, an error-free mechanism, occurs predominantly in the late S/G_2 phase, when the intact sister chromatid can be used as a template for repair. NHEJ, an error-prone mechanism, dominantly functions in the G_1 phase during which a template does not exist (see Fig. 68.2). This difference is one of the

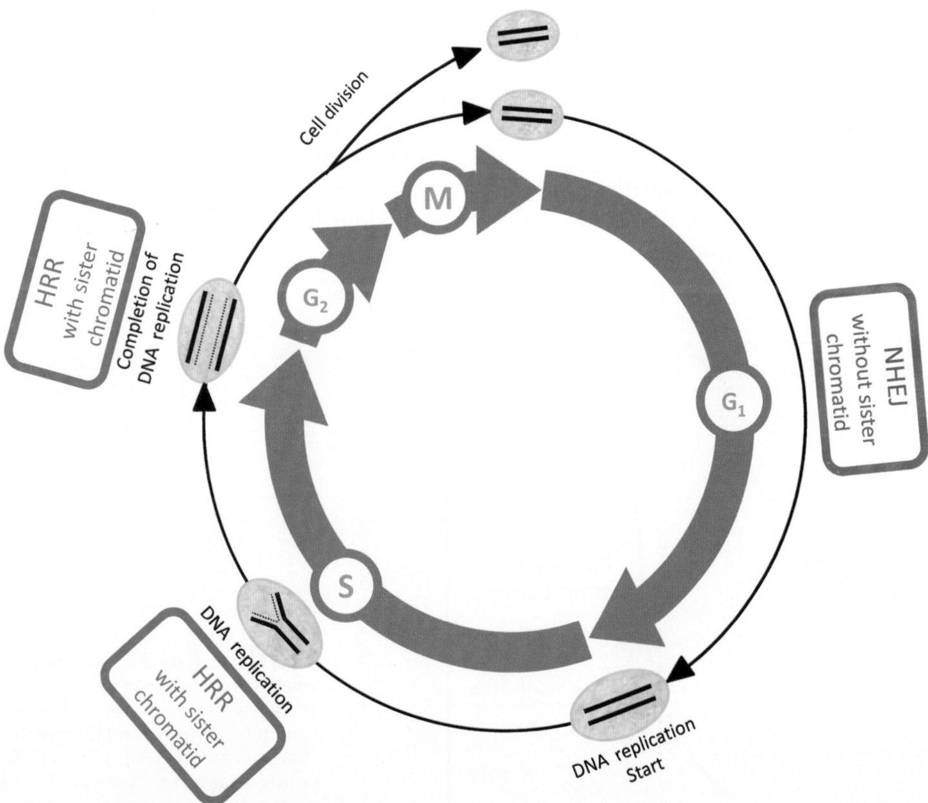

FIGURE 68–2 Cell cycle and DNA repair pathways. Error-free HRR occurs predominantly in the late S/G_2 phase, when the intact sister chromatid can be used as a template for repair. Meanwhile, although error-prone NHEJ functions in every cell cycle status, it is responsible for DNA repair especially in the G_1 phase when no template exists.

reasons for the relative radioresistance of cells in the late S/G_2 phase.

APPLICATIONS OF RADIATION TO CANCER THERAPY

Whether the growth of tumor cells can be controlled with radiation therapy is dependent on whether an effective dose of radiation can be delivered to the target. However, because malignant tumor tissue is usually surrounded by functional normal tissue, excess radiation will lead to side effects and carcinogenesis. Thus, a balance between the damaging of tumor cells and preservation of the surrounding normal tissue is important in radiation therapy.

The Law of Bergonie and Tribondeau

Based on an early observation about the difference in radiosensitivity of cells in rats' testes, Bergonie and Tribondeau proposed the "Law of Bergonie and Tribondeau" in 1906. They stated that "the radiosensitivity of a tissue is directly proportional to the reproductive activity and inversely proportional to the degree of differentiation," and "tissues consisting of rapidly dividing stem cells are quite sensitive to radiation whereas cells that do not divide or only rarely divide are considerably more resistant." Although this law is not necessarily true of every cell in various organs, it is still useful in the prediction of radiosensitivity and side effects in normal tissues during radiation therapy. The radiosensitivity of various normal tissues is briefly summarized in Table 68.2.

Therapeutic Ratio

In order to decrease the side effects of radiation therapy, we have to consider the "therapeutic ratio (TR)," the ratio of the tolerable dose of radiation for normal tissue (tissue tolerance dose) to the dose of radiation required to control tumor growth (tumor lethal dose). Every devised method in radiation therapy so far has aimed to increase the TR, shifting the curve of tumor control and that of the incidence of normal tissue damage to the right and left, respectively (Fig. 68.3).

TABLE 68–2 Relative Radiosensitivity of Cells, Tissues, and Organs

Biological Response	Type
Extremely radiosensitive	Blood-forming organs lymph nodes, thymus, spleen, bone marrow
Moderately radiosensitive	Reproductive organs
Radiosensitive	Digestive organs small intestine, lower intestine, pharynx, esophagus
Moderately radioresistant	Vascular system arteries (lg and sm), capillaries, veins
Radioresistant	Skin
Relatively radioresistant	Respiratory system, and urinary system
Very radioresistant	Muscle, bone and teeth, and connective tissues
Extremely radioresistant	Nervous tissue

Fractionated Radiation Therapy

Multifraction regimens are widely used in conventional radiation therapy for various forms of cancer. This method is largely attributed to accumulated knowledge about tumor pathophysiological responses to ionizing radiation, which potentially affect the radioresistance/radiosensitivity of tumor cells. These factors are known as the four Rs (4Rs) in the fields of radiation biology and oncology.[24]

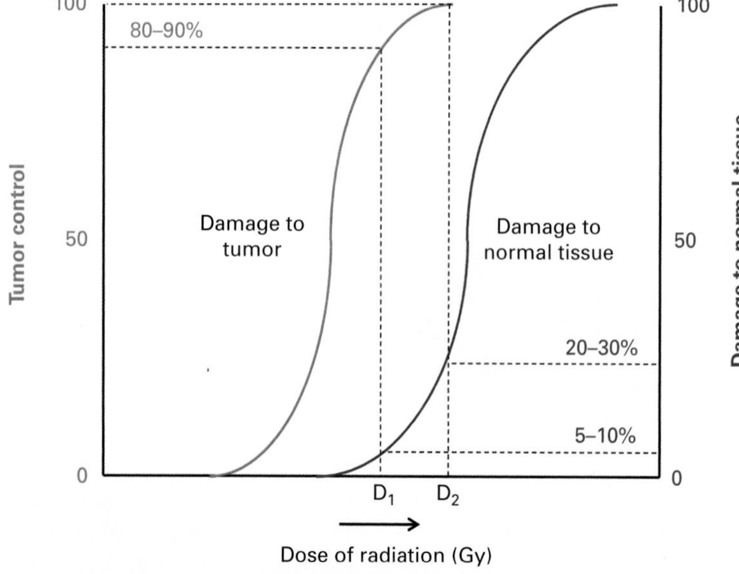

FIGURE 68–3 Therapeutic ratio. The relationship between the dose of radiation and response of cells is generally sigmoid in shape for both tumor control and normal tissue damage. The therapeutic ratio (TR) is the percentage of tumor control that can be achieved for a given level of normal tissue damage. For example, about 80% to 90% tumor control can be achieved by D_1 Gy of radiation which causes 5% to 10% normal tissue damage. If normal tissue can tolerate 20% to 30% damage, tumors can be cured by D_2 Gy of radiation.

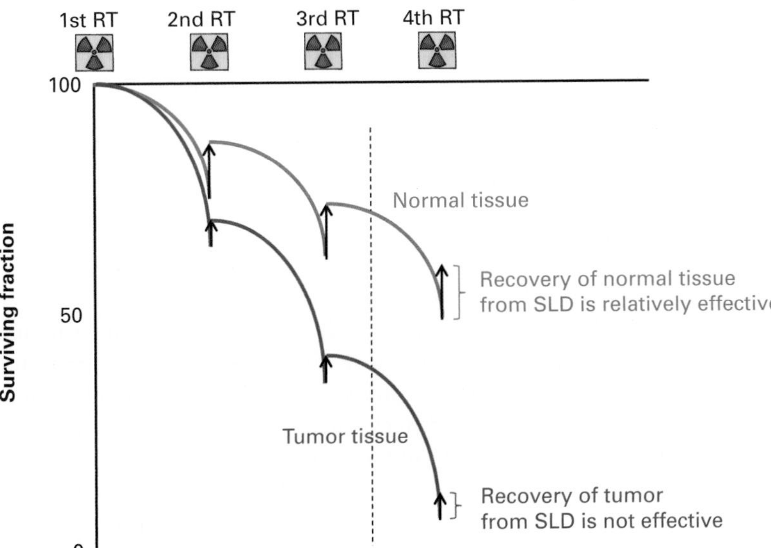

FIGURE 68–4 Enlargement of difference in surviving fraction between tumor tissues and normal tissues after fractionated radiation. The recovery of cancer cells from radiation-induced sublethal damage is less effective than that in normal tissue. So, the difference in the surviving fraction between tumor and normal tissues can be enlarged by repeatedly giving fractionated radiation.

Recovery/Repair of Sublethal Damage

The first R is "recovery/repair."[9] The recovery of cancer cells from radiation-induced sublethal damage is less effective than that in normal tissue. So, by repeatedly administering fractionated radiation to the target, damage can be concentrated in tumor tissues rather than the surrounding areas (Fig. 68.4). Although the biological effects of low LET radiation are generally small with a fractionated compared with non-fractionated (single radiation) protocol, fractionated radiation has the benefit of reducing side effects in normal tissue.

Reoxygenation of Tumor Hypoxia after Radiation Therapy

The second R is "reoxygenation."[9,12] Fractionated radiation therapy has been used to overcome hypoxia-related tumor radioresistance. It has been repeatedly confirmed that the distribution of oxygen from tumor blood vessels to hypoxic tumor cells is dramatically improved after radiotherapy as a result of the death of well-oxygenated tumor cells and a subsequent decrease in oxygen consumption there.[25,26] This phenomenon is recognized as reoxygenation. It has been assumed that, by delivering fractionated radiation just at the timing of the reoxygenation, one can efficiently damage ex-hypoxic cells.[9]

Redistribution/Reassortment of Cells Within the Cell Cycle

The third R is "redistribution/reassortment of cells within the cell cycle."[9,22,23] After radiation damages genomic DNA, cells actively arrest at the G_2/M checkpoint to allow time for repairs (Fig. 68.5). This arrest causes a synchronization of the cell cycle, a phenomenon known as redistribution/reassortment. Because cells are most radiosensitive in these phases, it has been assumed that, by administering second fractionated radiation to cells at this time, one can gain larger therapeutic effects.

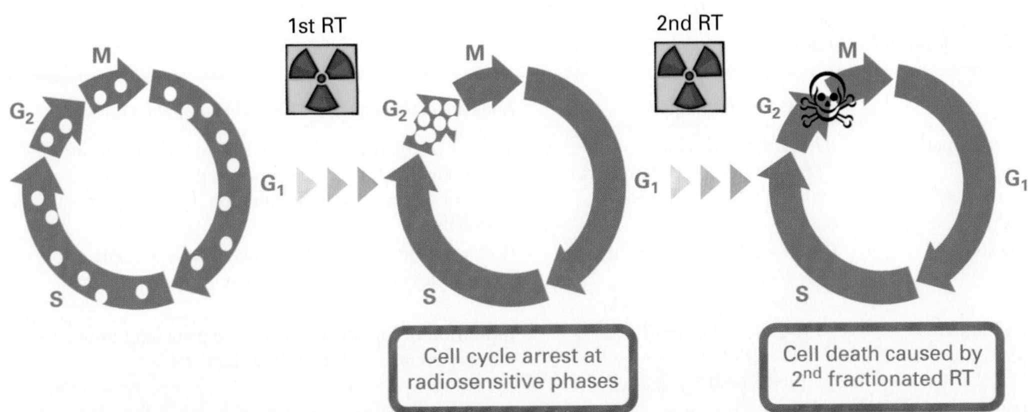

FIGURE 68–5 Redistribution/reassortment of cells within the cell cycle. Radiation causes cell cycle arrest at the G_2/M checkpoint and results in synchronization of the cell cycle. By administering second fractionated radiation to the cells in relatively radiosensitive phases, one can achieve a greater therapeutic effect.

Regeneration/Repopulation

The fourth R is "regeneration/repopulation."[9] After being exposed to radiation, both normal and tumor tissues repopulate to compensate for the damaged regions. The repopulation in normal tissues takes place prior to that in tumor tissues in general. Also, the velocity of the repopulation is faster than that in tumor tissues. With fractionating radiation, one can effectively damage tumor tissues.

CLINICAL APPLICATIONS OF RADIATION AND MOLECULAR BIOLOGY

Increased understanding of the mechanisms behind the biological response to radiation, the development of cytotoxic agents and molecular targeting, and technological innovations in radiation machinery have led to improvements in radiation treatment.

Altered Fractionation

Altered fractionation regimens have attracted considerable attention since the 1970s, with several clinical trials conducted in the 1990s. Representative regimens are hyperfractionation (HF), accelerated fractionation (AF), and accelerated hyperfractionation (AHF) (Table 68.3). HF is a strategy with multiple fractions per day within the same total treatment duration as the conventional regimen. Its aim is to reduce the late effects and achieve the same or better tumor control with acceptable early and late toxicity in normal tissues. AF delivers the same or a slightly reduced dose per fraction to inhibit the repopulation of rapidly growing tumors by reducing the total duration of treatment. AHF is a combination of HF and AF. Various clinical trials on HF, AF, and AHF have been conducted and some of the schemes have become the standard radiotherapy options.[27,29,30]

Chemoradiotherapy

Chemoradiotherapy has progressed rapidly in the past quarter of a century. Its original aim was to target different anatomical sites. Whereas the aim of radiotherapy is local tumor control, that of chemotherapy is the suppression of distant metastasis. This concept is known as "spatial cooperation". However, improved local tumor control has also been recognized. Furthermore, the increased local control reduces the risk of secondary metastasis. These findings support the clinical use of chemoradiotherapy.

Conventional Cytotoxic Drugs

Platinum Compounds

Platinum compounds such as cisplatin, carboplatin, and oxaliplatin are the most important cytotoxic drugs for chemoradiotherapy in a variety of cancers, including lung cancer, head and neck cancer, and uterine cervical cancer. Cisplatin was initially discovered for its bacteriostatic effects,[31] and its anticancer effect was confirmed later.[32] Platinum compounds react with intracellular macromolecules, such as DNA and proteins, and induce intramolecular and/or intermolecular crosslinks, which interfere with replication and repair of DNA and directly contribute to their radiosensitizing effect[33] (Table 68.4). The radiosensitizing effect of platinum compounds has been confirmed in meta-analyses and clinical randomized trials of concurrent chemoradiotherapy for various cancers[34,35,44] as well as in numerous preclinical studies.[45-47]

Antimetabolites

Antimetabolites have antitumor activity, because they are similar in structure to the normal metabolites required for cell function. Antimetabolites show cytotoxic effects by occupying the catalytic sites of essential enzymes and competing with normal metabolites. The antimetabolites used as anticancer agents are categorized into three groups: pyrimidine analogs (5-FU [5-fluorouracil] and gemcitabine), purine analogs (6-mercaptopurine), and folic acid analogs (methotrexate and pemetrexed). Additionally, the prodrugs of 5-FU, including UFT (uracil plus tegafur), capecitabine, and S-1, are also clinically used in the treatment of various cancers. The radiosensitizing effect of antimetabolites is attributed to modulation of the metabolism of deoxynucleotides,

TABLE 68-3 Altered Fractionation

Category	Representative Regimen	Aims and/or Mechanisms Behind Therapeutic Effects	References
Conventional fractionation	([2 Gy/d] × 5 d/wk) × 6 wk = (total 60 Gy in 6 wk)	4Rs (recovery/repair, reoxygenation, redistribution/reassortment, regeneration/repopulation; *see* Section "Fractionated Radiation Therapy" for details)	
Hyperfractionation	(["1.1–1.2 Gy" × 2 times/d] × 5 d/wk) × 6 wk = (total 66–72 Gy in 6 wk)	Better tumor control with reduced early and late toxicities compared with conventional regimens	27
Accelerated fractionation	([1.8–2 Gy × 2 times/d] × 5 d/wk) × 3 wk = (total 54–60 Gy in 3 wk)	Inhibition of repopulation of rapid growing tumors by reducing total treatment duration	27,28
Accelerated hyperfractionation	([1.5 Gy × 2 times/d] × 5 d/wk) × 3–4 wk = (total 45–60 Gy in [4 wk + 1–2 wk interval])	Reduced overall treatment time, improved local control, feasible toxicity	29

TABLE 68-4 Chemoradiotherapy Using Conventional Cytotoxic Agents

Category	Representative Drugs	Mechanisms Behind Radiosensitization	References
Platinum compounds	Cisplatin, carboplatin, oxaliplatin	Intra/intermolecular cross-linking of DNA strands and proteins; interference with replication and DNA repair	34,35,36
Antimetabolites	5-FU, gemcitabine, pemetrexed	Modulation of deoxynucleotide metabolism; modulation of cell cycle distribution and p53 activity; Induction of apoptosis	37–40
Taxanes	Docetaxel, paclitaxel	Inhibition of microtubule function; cell cycle arrest at radiosensitive G_2/M phases; tumor oxygenation; antiangiogenic effects	36,41
Topoisomerase inhibitors	Camptothecin, etoposide	DSBs and replication fork arrest by cleavable complex	29,42,43

alteration of the cell cycle distribution, modulation of the role of the tumor suppressor protein p53, and the induction of apoptosis[48] (see Table 68.4). Chemoradiotherapy combined with antimetabolites is a common treatment option for a variety of tumors, including esophageal, lung, and pancreatic cancer.[37-40]

Taxanes

Taxanes (paclitaxel and docetaxel) are newer anticancer agents compared with the classical drugs such as cisplatin and 5-FU. Taxanes are reported to show radiosensitizing effects through the inhibition of microtubule function, cell cycle arrest at the most radiosensitive G_2/M phases, tumor oxygenation, and inhibition of angiogenesis (see Table 68.4).[49-55] Taxanes are commonly used concurrently or sequentially with radiotherapy in the treatment of malignant tumors such as lung cancers and head and neck cancers.[36,41]

Topoisomerase Inhibitors

DNA topoisomerase I and II are essential nuclear enzymes for DNA replication. Targeting these enzymes with DNA topoisomerase I inhibitors (irinotecan and topotecan) and II inhibitors (etoposide) plays major roles in the treatment of various cancers. Topoisomerase inhibitors are important cytotoxic agents in concurrent radiotherapy for lung cancer (see Table 68.4). The exact mechanism of the radiosensitizing effect is not fully understood, but the involvement of a so-called cleavable complex, which is composed of topoisomerase, DNA, and topoisomerase inhibitors, has been suggested because it causes DSBs, replication fork arrest, and an aborted cleavable complex.[56-60]

Molecular Targeting Drugs in Combination with Radiotherapy

Based on recent advances in our knowledge about the molecular mechanisms behind the cell cycle, cell survival, etc., molecular targeting has been used to enhance the therapeutic effect of ionizing radiation with minimal side effects in normal tissue (Table 68.5).

EGFR Inhibitors

The epidermal growth factor receptor (EGFR) is a transmembrane protein that is abnormally activated in various malignant tumors. Since EGFR plays important roles in proliferation, DNA repair, and apoptosis in cancer cells, it was proposed as a promising target for cancer therapy more than 20 years ago.[84] Given that tumor cell lines with EGFR overexpression showed radioresistance,[85] tyrosine kinase inhibitor (TKI) and EGFR monoclonal antibodies have been expected to enhance the antitumor activity of ionizing radiation[86] (see Table 68.5). Preclinical studies showed that C225 (cetuximab), an anti-EGFR antibody, sensitizes tumor cells to the effects of radiation in both in vitro and in vivo settings.[87,88] Anti-EGFR therapies increase and decrease the proportions of cells in the radiosensitive G_1 phase and radioresistant S phase, respectively. The blockade of EGFR signaling promotes apoptosis, has antiangiogenic effects, and inhibits DNA repair activity through the inactivation of DNA-PK.[86,89-94] Bonner et al.[61,62] conducted a randomized phase III trial comparing radiotherapy alone with radiotherapy plus cetuximab in the treatment of locoregionally advanced squamous cell carcinoma of the head and neck and found that radiotherapy with cetuximab significantly improves 5-year overall survival compared with radiotherapy alone. Cetuximab was approved by the Food and Drug Administration in 2006 for clinical use in combination with radiotherapy for the treatment of head and neck cancers. Many clinical trials are ongoing regarding the combination of radiotherapy with cetuximab or other EGFR inhibitors (e.g., panitumumab and erlotinib) ± cytotoxic agents (http://www.clinicaltrials.gov/).

Inhibitors of Ras-Raf-Map Kinase and PI3K-AKT-Mtor Pathways

Mutation and overexpression of genes constituting the RAS-Raf-MAP (mitogen-activated protein) kinase and PI3K (phosphoinositide 3-kinase)/Akt/mTOR (mammalian target of rapamycin) pathways are responsible for malignant phenotypes of many types of tumor cells. Because these pathways are suggested to increase cellular radioresistance, they have been recognized as

TABLE 68–5 Chemoradiotherapy Using Molecular Targeting Drugs

Category	Representative Drugs	Representative Drugs	Mechanisms Behind Radiosensitization	References
Signaling targets	EGFR inhibitors	Cetuximab, panitumumab, erlotinib	Modulation of cell cycle distribution; induction of apoptosis; inhibition of DNA-PK activity; antiangiogenic effects	61,62
	Inhibitors of the Ras-Raf-MAP kinase pathway	Tipifarnib, AZD6244	Impairment of DNA repair; increase in perfusion; reduced hypoxia	63,64,65
	Inhibitors of the PI3K-Akt-mTOR pathway	Everolimus, BEZ235		66,67
DNA damage response	Inhibitors of DNA repair pathways	Olaparib, veliparib, NU7441	Impairment of DNA repair	68,69,70
	Cell cycle inhibitors	Barasertib	Modulation of cell cycle distribution	71
Epigenetic targets	HDAC inhibitors	Vorinostat, valproic acid	Delay of DSBs repair	72,73
Inflammatory signaling pathways	COX-2 inhibitors	Celecoxib	Cell cycle arrest at radiosensitive G_2/M phases; inhibition of DNA-PK activity	74
Anti-microenvironment targets	Antiangiogenic agents	Bevacizumab	Normalization of tumor vasculature; increase in perfusion; increase in tumor oxygen levels	16,75
	Hypoxia-targeted agents	Tirapazamine	Production of hydroxyl radical and oxidizing radical under hypoxia; HIF-1 inhibitor	5,76–81
	HIF-1 inhibitors	YC-1	Increased radiosensitivity of tumor vasculature through the inhibition of VEGF expression	8,13,82,83

EGFR, epidermal growth factor receptor; DNA-PK, DNA protein kinase; HDAC, histone deacetyltransferase; COX-2, cyclooxygenase-2; DSBs, double-strand breaks; HIF-1, hypoxia-inducible factor 1; VEGF, vascular endothelial growth factor.

excellent targets to enhance the biological effect of radiation (see Table 68.5). Actually, many inhibitors of these pathways have been shown to enhance tumor radiosensitivity at clinically relevant doses in preclinical experiments.[63-66,95-100] The mechanisms of radiosensitization by these inhibitors are not clearly understood, but the inhibition of these pathways may be related to the effects on DNA repair and additionally were found to increase perfusion and to reduce hypoxia.[64,101] Several clinical trials with radiotherapy in combination with these inhibitors are now underway.[67]

Inhibitors of DNA Repair Pathways

Because the cytotoxic effects of radiation are mainly caused by DNA damage, treatment strategies targeting DNA repair pathways are potentially efficacious for tumor radiosensitization (see Table 68.5). Poly(ADP-ribose) polymerase (PARP) is a nuclear protein involved in DNA repair, especially SSB repair. Many PARP inhibitors, e.g., olaparib and veliparib, have been developed for the treatment of cancers with BRCA-1 or BRCA-2 mutations.[102,103] Although SSBs themselves are generally not lethal, SSBs accumulated by PARP inhibition can be converted to lethal DSBs during DNA replication, resulting in radiosensitizing effects.[68,69,104] A few clinical trials with PARP inhibitors in combination with radiotherapy are ongoing.

DNA-dependent protein kinase (DNA-PK) is a key factor in NHEJ. Inhibition of DNA-PK by Wortmannin, NU7441, and IC87361 increased radiosensitization in vitro or in vivo in various tumor cells.[70,105,106] Many types of inhibitors for DNA repair pathways are now being developed. We can expect a radiosensitizing effect, but we should worry about the toxicity to normal tissues.

Cell Cycle Inhibitors

Cell cycle status influences the radiosensitivity of cells as mentioned above; therefore, drugs that induce cell cycle arrest at a radiosensitive phase potentially have radiosensitizing effects. Thus, cell cycle kinase inhibitors could be an attractive target. ATM plays a pivotal role in maintaining genome integrity and in activating cell cycle checkpoints, and ATM inhibitors have actually showed radiosensitizing effects[107,108] (see Table 68.5). Chk1 kinase is an important downstream effector of ATM/ATR pathways and an important molecule for the ionizing irradiation–induced S and G_2 checkpoints. Preclinical data showed that a CHK1 inhibitor can act as a potent radiosensitizer of tumor cells both in vitro and in vivo.[109] The aurora kinases are key regulators of mitosis and are maximally expressed during the G_2/M phases. Several aurora kinase inhibitors have been confirmed to radiosensitize tumor cells in preclinical experiments.[71,110]

HDAC Inhibitors

Histones and DNA constitute the nucleosome, a basic structural unit of chromatin which is essential for DNA packaging in eukaryotic cells. The acetylation status of the former, which is modulated by histone acetyltransferases

(HATs) and histone deacetyltransferases (HDACs), is associated with the regulation of transcriptional initiation.[111] The status of HDACs and HATs has been found to be altered in various tumors and is postulated to be important in carcinogenesis. HDAC inhibitors demonstrate significant biological effects in preclinical tumor models and clinical HDAC inhibitors have been developed rapidly in recent years. Several preclinical studies have shown that HDAC inhibitors, such as vorinostat (SAHA, suberoylanilide hydroxamic acid) and VA (valproic acid), radiosensitize human tumor cells[72,73,112-114] (see Table 68.5). The mechanisms through which they enhance radiosensitivity are not fully understood, but HDAC inhibitors have been suggested to delay the repair of DSBs and therefore prolong radiation-induced γ-H2AX foci in various tumor cells.[72,113] Also, they are reported to attenuate radiation-induced expression of Rad51 and DNA-PK.[113] Several clinical trials combining vorinostat or VA with radiotherapy are now underway.

COX-2 Inhibitors

Cyclooxygenase-2 (COX-2) is a key enzyme required for the synthesis of prostaglandins from arachidonic acid. COX-2 is overexpressed in various tumors and associated with tumor aggressiveness and a poor prognosis.[115-119] Preclinical studies showed that COX-2 inhibitors (e.g., celecoxib) increased the radiosensitivity of a variety of cancer cells[74,120] (see Table 68.5). A possible mechanism of the radiosensitizing effect is that the Cox-2 inhibitors arrest tumor cells at radiosensitive G_2/M phases and inhibit DNA-PK activity.[74,121] Although therapeutic effects have yet to be confirmed in any clinical studies, trials in combination with radiotherapy are ongoing.

Antiangiogenic Agents

Angiogenesis is necessary for tumor growth because it allows tumors to obtain enough oxygen and nutrients for their survival. Inhibition of angiogenesis has been used to suppress tumor growth. Several antiangiogenic agents including an anti-VEGF antibody and TKIs are available for the treatment of various cancers. In combination with radiation therapy, antiangiogenic treatment has been reported to normalize the tumor vasculature, improve perfusion, increase tumor oxygen levels, and eventually enhance the therapeutic effect (see Table 68.5). Moreover, prolonged antiangiogenic treatment can theoretically decrease microvessel density and increase tumor hypoxia, resulting in a decrease in the biological effect of radiotherapy. Thus, the multifactorial mechanisms behind the radiosensitizing effect of antiangiogenic agents remain largely unknown, but preclinical studies have confirmed a positive impact on radiation therapy.[16,75,122] Several phase I–II trials are currently underway in patients with pancreatic, rectal, and head and neck tumors,[123-125] but the therapeutic effects of these combinations have yet to be confirmed. Further investigation is needed.

Hypoxia-Targeting Agents

To overcome hypoxia-related radioresistance, radiosensitizers for hypoxic cells, hypoxic cytotoxins, and HIF-1 inhibitors have been tried (see Table 68.5).

In the 1970s, nitroimidazole derivatives such as misonidazole were found to mimic the effect of oxygen and enhance the cytotoxic effect of ionizing radiation under hypoxic conditions.[126,127] Their clinical benefit, however, remains controversial[128-131] because of the dose-limiting toxicity attributed to their low solubility. Other derivatives with improved solubility have been developed[132] and shown positive therapeutic effects in patients with early nodal disease.

A representative hypoxia-activated prodrug is tirapazamine,[5,76] whose selectivity is attributed to its one-electron reduction to a radical anion and subsequent conversion to a hydroxyl radical or to an oxidizing radical under hypoxia.[77] These radicals are highly reactive and cause DNA damage. Clinical trials with tirapazamine in combination with radiation have demonstrated effects in patients with lung cancer or head and neck cancer,[78,79] but the efficacy of the combination is still controversial.[80,81]

HIF-1 has been recognized as an excellent molecular target for sensitization of the therapeutic effect of radiation.[9-12,15,133] It was confirmed that administration of a representative HIF-1 inhibitor, YC-1,[82,83] to inhibit the radiation-induced activation of HIF-1 significantly delays tumor growth compared with radiation therapy alone.[13,8] It has also been reported that radiosensitizing effects of PI3K inhibitors, mTOR inhibitors, and HSP90 inhibitors were obtained at least in part through the suppression of HIF-1 activity.

HIGH-PRECISION RADIATION THERAPY, INTENSITY-MODULATED RADIATION THERAPY, AND STEREOTACTIC BODY RADIATION THERAPY

Intensity-modulated radiotherapy (IMRT) is a new type of conformal radiotherapy based on the use of non-uniform beam intensities optimized by inverse planning (Table 68.6).[134] This technique can achieve optimal dose distributions and allow the delivery of lower doses of radiation to normal tissue while maintaining or increasing the tumor dose. Furthermore, simultaneous integrated boost (SIB)-IMRT has been developed recently, which allows the simultaneous delivery of different doses of radiation to different target volumes within a single treatment fraction. For example, higher doses of radiation could be delivered to radioresistant hypoxic regions which could be detected by imaging probes for hypoxia, CuATSM, and 18F-MISO. Stereotactic body radiation therapy (SBRT) is a new treatment modality to deliver ablative doses of radiation to a target under various degrees of image guidance while sparing the adjacent normal tissue with high accuracy, using a stereotactic body frame to attain accurate

TABLE 68-6 High-Precision Radiation Therapy

Radiation	Type of Beam	Aim, Characteristics, and/or Advantages	References
Ionizing radiation	IMRT and SBRT	Irradiation to radioresistant fractions with molecular imaging techniques	134,135
Particle therapy	Proton and carbon ions	Unique dose distribution (Bragg peak)	136

IMRT, intensity-modulated radiotherapy; SBRT, stereotactic body radiation therapy.

and precise patient positioning and immobilization (see Table 68.6). SBRT was first introduced in the 1990s and originally derived from techniques of stereotactic radiosurgery used to treat small lesions in the brain and spine. With encouraging results regarding efficacy and safety in retrospective studies at various sites, especially the lungs, SBRT has been adopted as a standard treatment option for early-stage non–small cell lung cancer mainly in medically inoperable patients.[135] Like SIB-IMRT, SBRT can be used to irradiate small radioresistant fractions in tumor as a boost, if the radioresistant areas can be detected by biological imaging.

PARTICLE THERAPY

Particle therapy is a new modality using beams of protons, neutrons, and positive ions (see Table 68.6). The major difference between photon and ion beams (proton and carbon ions) is the distribution of physical dose. The maximum dose of photons is deposited close to the surface of the body, whereas ions enter the body at a low dose and the maximum dose, the so-called Bragg peak, occurs at a certain depth near the end of their range. Additionally, heavy particles like carbon ions have shown increased biological effectiveness characterized by enhanced ionization density in individual tracks, where DNA damage becomes clustered and therefore more difficult to repair.[137] Particle therapy has been in therapeutic use since the 1960s with more than 30 facilities currently in operation worldwide, where skull base tumors, head and neck tumors, hepatocellular carcinomas, soft-tissue sarcomas, and prostate cancers are treated.[136]

SUMMARY

The integration of knowledge from physics, chemistry, biology, and medical science has contributed to the development of cancer radiotherapy ever since X-rays were first discovered in 1895. Recent advances in our understanding of tumor biology and technological innovations have accelerated the development. However, cancer patients can still suffer from tumor recurrence even after the most innovative treatments. Further integration with novel molecular targeting agents or functional (not morphological) imaging techniques for radioresistant cells will be key to further improving the therapeutic effect of radiation.

REFERENCES

1. Rontgen WC. On a new kind of rays. *Science.* 1896;3:227-231.
2. Hartlerode AJ, Scully R. Mechanisms of double-strand break repair in somatic mammalian cells. *Biochem J.* 2009;423:157-168.
3. Durocher D, Jackson SP. DNA-PK, ATM and ATR as sensors of DNA damage: variations on a theme? *Curr Opin Cell Biol.* 2001;13:225-231.
4. Thoms J, Bristow RG. DNA repair targeting and radiotherapy: a focus on the therapeutic ratio. *Semin Radiat Oncol.* 2010;20: 217-222.
5. Brown JM, Wilson WR. Exploiting tumour hypoxia in cancer treatment. *Nat Rev Cancer.* 2004;4:437-447.
6. Thomlinson RH, Gray LH. The histological structure of some human lung cancers and the possible implications for radiotherapy. *Br J Cancer.* 1955;9:539-549.
7. Harada H, Itasaka S, Kizaka-Kondoh S, et al. The Akt/mTOR pathway assures the synthesis of HIF-1alpha protein in a glucose- and reoxygenation-dependent manner in irradiated tumors. *J Biol Chem.* 2009;284:5332-5342.
8. Harada H, Itasaka S, Zhu Y, et al. Treatment regimen determines whether an HIF-1 inhibitor enhances or inhibits the effect of radiation therapy. *Br J Cancer.* 2009;100:747-757.
9. Hall EJ (ed.) *Radiobiology for the Radiologists.* 4th ed. Philadelphia, PA: J.B. Lippincott Company; 1994.
10. Bindra RS, Crosby ME, Glazer PM. Regulation of DNA repair in hypoxic cancer cells. *Cancer Metastasis Rev.* 2007;26:249-260.
11. Harada H. How can we overcome tumor hypoxia in radiation therapy? *J Radiat Res (Tokyo).* 2011;52:545-556.
12. Harada H, Hiraoka M. Hypoxia-inducible factor 1 in tumor radioresistance. *Curr Signal Transduct Ther.* 2010;5:188-196.
13. Moeller BJ, Cao Y, Li CY, Dewhirst MW. Radiation activates HIF-1 to regulate vascular radiosensitivity in tumors: role of reoxygenation, free radicals, and stress granules. *Cancer Cell.* 2004;5:429-441.
14. Moeller BJ, Dewhirst MW. HIF-1 and tumour radiosensitivity. *Br J Cancer.* 2006;95:1-5.
15. Moeller BJ, Dreher MR, Rabbani ZN, et al. Pleiotropic effects of HIF-1 blockade on tumor radiosensitivity. *Cancer Cell.* 2005;8:99-110.
16. Gorski DH, Beckett MA, Jaskowiak NT, et al. Blockage of the vascular endothelial growth factor stress response increases the antitumor effects of ionizing radiation. *Cancer Res.* 1999;59:3374-3378.
17. Zeng L, Ou G, Itasaka S, et al. TS-1 enhances the effect of radiotherapy by suppressing radiation-induced hypoxia-inducible factor-1 activation and inducing endothelial cell apoptosis. *Cancer Sci.* 2008;99:2327-2335.
18. Aebersold DM, Burri P, Beer KT, et al. Expression of hypoxia-inducible factor-1alpha: a novel predictive and prognostic parameter in the radiotherapy of oropharyngeal cancer. *Cancer Res.* 2001;61:2911-2916.
19. Irie N, Matsuo T, Nagata I. Protocol of radiotherapy for glioblastoma according to the expression of HIF-1. *Brain Tumor Pathol.* 2004;21:1-6.
20. Ishikawa H, Sakurai H, Hasegawa M, et al. Expression of hypoxic-inducible factor 1alpha predicts metastasis-free survival after radiation therapy alone in stage IIIB cervical squamous cell carcinoma. *Int J Radiat Oncol Biol Phys.* 2004;60:513-521.
21. Marston AL, Amon A. Meiosis: cell-cycle controls shuffle and deal. *Nat Rev Mol Cell Biol.* 2004;5:983-997.
22. Branzei D, Foiani M. Regulation of DNA repair throughout the cell cycle. *Nat Rev Mol Cell Biol.* 2008;9:297-308.

23. Pawlik TM, Keyomarsi K. Role of cell cycle in mediating sensitivity to radiotherapy. *Int J Radiat Oncol Biol Phys.* 2004;59:928-942.
24. Trott KR. Experimental results and clinical implications of the four R's in fractionated radiotherapy. *Radiat Environ Biophys.* 1982;20:159-170.
25. Dorie MJ, Kallman RF. Reoxygenation in the RIF-1 tumor. *Int J Radiat Oncol Biol Phys.* 1984;10:687-693.
26. Murata R, Shibamoto Y, Sasai K, et al. Reoxygenation after single irradiation in rodent tumors of different types and sizes. *Int J Radiat Oncol Biol Phys.* 1996;34:859-865.
27. Fu KK, Pajak TF, Trotti A, et al. A Radiation Therapy Oncology Group (RTOG) phase III randomized study to compare hyperfractionation and two variants of accelerated fractionation to standard fractionation radiotherapy for head and neck squamous cell carcinomas: first report of RTOG 9003. *Int J Radiat Oncol Biol Phys.* 2000;48:7-16.
28. Poulsen MG, Denham JW, Peters LJ, et al. A randomised trial of accelerated and conventional radiotherapy for stage III and IV squamous carcinoma of the head and neck: a Trans-Tasman Radiation Oncology Group Study. *Radiother Oncol.* 2001;60:113-122.
29. Turrisi AT 3rd, Kim K, Blum R, et al. Twice-daily compared with once-daily thoracic radiotherapy in limited small-cell lung cancer treated concurrently with cisplatin and etoposide. *N Engl J Med.* 1999;340:265-271.
30. Horiot JC, Le Fur R, N'Guyen T, et al. Hyperfractionation versus conventional fractionation in oropharyngeal carcinoma: final analysis of a randomized trial of the EORTC cooperative group of radiotherapy. *Radiother Oncol.* 1992;25:231-241.
31. Rosenberg B, Vancamp L, Krigas T. Inhibition of cell division in *Escherichia coli* by electrolysis products from a platinum electrode. *Nature.* 1965;205:698-699.
32. Rosenberg B, VanCamp L, Trosko JE, Mansour VH. Platinum compounds: a new class of potent antitumour agents. *Nature.* 1969;222:385-386.
33. Eastman A. The formation, isolation and characterization of DNA adducts produced by anticancer platinum complexes. *Pharmacol Ther.* 1987;34:155-166.
34. Chan AT, Leung SF, Ngan RK, et al. Overall survival after concurrent cisplatin-radiotherapy compared with radiotherapy alone in locoregionally advanced nasopharyngeal carcinoma. *J Natl Cancer Inst.* 2005;97:536-539.
35. Rose PG, Bundy BN, Watkins EB, et al. Concurrent cisplatin-based radiotherapy and chemotherapy for locally advanced cervical cancer. *N Engl J Med.* 1999;340:1144-1153.
36. Belani CP, Choy H, Bonomi P, et al. Combined chemoradiotherapy regimens of paclitaxel and carboplatin for locally advanced non-small-cell lung cancer: a randomized phase II locally advanced multi-modality protocol. *J Clin Oncol.* 2005;23:5883-5891.
37. Cooper JS, Guo MD, Herskovic A, et al. Chemoradiotherapy of locally advanced esophageal cancer: long-term follow-up of a prospective randomized trial (RTOG 85-01). Radiation Therapy Oncology Group. *JAMA.* 1999;281:1623-1627.
38. Govindan R, Bogart J, Stinchcombe T, et al. Randomized phase II study of pemetrexed, carboplatin, and thoracic radiation with or without cetuximab in patients with locally advanced unresectable non-small-cell lung cancer: Cancer and Leukemia Group B trial 30407. *J Clin Oncol.* 2011;29:3120-3125.
39. Huguet F, Girard N, Guerche CS, Hennequin C, Mornex F, Azria D. Chemoradiotherapy in the management of locally advanced pancreatic carcinoma: a qualitative systematic review. *J Clin Oncol.* 2009;27:2269-2277.
40. Loehrer PJ Sr, Feng Y, Cardenes H, et al. Gemcitabine alone versus gemcitabine plus radiotherapy in patients with locally advanced pancreatic cancer: an eastern cooperative oncology group trial. *J Clin Oncol.* 2011;29:4105-4112.
41. Vermorken JB, Remenar E, van Herpen C, et al. Cisplatin, fluorouracil, and docetaxel in unresectable head and neck cancer. *N Engl J Med.* 2007;357:1695-1704.
42. Clamon G, Herndon J, Cooper R, Chang AY, Rosenman J, Green MR. Radiosensitization with carboplatin for patients with unresectable stage III non-small-cell lung cancer: a phase III trial of the Cancer and Leukemia Group B and the Eastern Cooperative Oncology Group. *J Clin Oncol.* 1999;17:4-11.
43. Takada M, Fukuoka M, Kawahara M, et al. Phase III study of concurrent versus sequential thoracic radiotherapy in combination with cisplatin and etoposide for limited-stage small-cell lung cancer: results of the Japan Clinical Oncology Group Study 9104. *J Clin Oncol.* 2002;20:3054-3060.
44. Chemotherapy in non-small cell lung cancer: a meta-analysis using updated data on individual patients from 52 randomised clinical trials. Non-small Cell Lung Cancer Collaborative Group. *BMJ.* 1995;311:899-909.
45. Bartelink H, Kallman RF, Rapacchietta D, Hart GA. Therapeutic enhancement in mice by clinically relevant dose and fractionation schedules of cis-diamminedichloroplatinum (II) and irradiation. *Radiother Oncol.* 1986;6:61-74.
46. Carde P, Laval F. Effect of cis-dichlorodiammine platinum II and X rays on mammalian cell survival. *Int J Radiat Oncol Biol Phys.* 1981;7:929-933.
47. Tanabe M, Godat D, Kallman RF. Effects of fractionated schedules of irradiation combined with cis-diamminedichloroplatinum II on the SCCVII/St tumor and normal tissues of the C3H/KM mouse. *Int J Radiat Oncol Biol Phys.* 1987;13:1523-1532.
48. Harada H, Shibuya K, Hiraoka M. Combinations of antimetabolites and ionizing radiation. In: Brown JM, Mehta MP, Nieder C, eds. *Multimodal Concepts for Integration of Cytotoxic Drugs and Radiation Treatment.* Berlin: Springer; 2006:19–34.
49. Mason KA, Kishi K, Hunter N, et al. Effect of docetaxel on the therapeutic ratio of fractionated radiotherapy in vivo. *Clin Cancer Res.* 1999;5:4191-4198.
50. Milas L, Hunter NR, Kurdoglu B, et al. Kinetics of mitotic arrest and apoptosis in murine mammary and ovarian tumors treated with taxol. *Cancer Chemother Pharmacol.* 1995;35:297-303.
51. Milas L, Hunter NR, Mason KA, Kurdoglu B, Peters LJ. Enhancement of tumor radioresponse of a murine mammary carcinoma by paclitaxel. *Cancer Res.* 1994;54:3506-3510.
52. Milross CG, Mason KA, Hunter NR, et al. Enhanced radioresponse of paclitaxel-sensitive and -resistant tumours in vivo. *Eur J Cancer.* 1997;33:1299-1308.
53. Schimming R, Hunter NR, Mason KA, Milas L. Inhibition of tumor neo-angiogenesis and induction of apoptosis as properties of docetaxel (taxotere). *Mund Kiefer Gesichtschir.* 1999;3:210-212.
54. Sweeney CJ, Miller KD, Sissons SE, et al. The antiangiogenic property of docetaxel is synergistic with a recombinant humanized monoclonal antibody against vascular endothelial growth factor or 2-methoxyestradiol but antagonized by endothelial growth factors. *Cancer Res.* 2001;61:3369-3372.
55. Tishler RB, Schiff PB, Geard CR, Hall EJ. Taxol: a novel radiation sensitizer. *Int J Radiat Oncol Biol Phys.* 1992;22: 613-617.
56. Chen AY, Chou R, Shih SJ, Lau D, Gandara D. Enhancement of radiotherapy with DNA topoisomerase I-targeted drugs. *Crit Rev Oncol Hematol.* 2004;50:111-119.
57. Iwata T, Kanematsu T. Etoposide enhances the lethal effect of radiation on breast cancer cells with less damage to mammary gland cells. *Cancer Chemother Pharmacol.* 1999;43:284-286.
58. Kim JH, Kim SH, Kolozsvary A, Khil MS. Potentiation of radiation response in human carcinoma cells in vitro and murine fibrosarcoma in vivo by topotecan, an inhibitor of DNA topoisomerase I. *Int J Radiat Oncol Biol Phys.* 1992;22:515-518.
59. Kirichenko AV, Rich TA, Newman RA, Travis EL. Potentiation of murine MCa-4 carcinoma radioresponse by 9-amino-20(S)-camptothecin. *Cancer Res.* 1997;57:1929-1933.
60. Larsen AK, Escargueil AE, Skladanowski A. Catalytic topoisomerase II inhibitors in cancer therapy. *Pharmacol Ther.* 2003;99:167-181.
61. Bonner JA, Harari PM, Giralt J, et al. Radiotherapy plus cetuximab for squamous-cell carcinoma of the head and neck. *N Engl J Med.* 2006;354:567-578.
62. Bonner JA, Harari PM, Giralt J, et al. Radiotherapy plus cetuximab for locoregionally advanced head and neck cancer: 5-year survival data from a phase 3 randomised trial, and relation between cetuximab-induced rash and survival. *Lancet Oncol.* 2010;11:21-28.
63. Nghiemphu PL, Wen PY, Lamborn KR, et al. A phase I trial of tipifarnib with radiation therapy, with and without temozolomide, for patients with newly diagnosed glioblastoma. *Int J Radiat Oncol Biol Phys.* 2011;81(5):1422–1427.

64. Shannon AM, Telfer BA, Smith PD, et al. The mitogen-activated protein/extracellular signal-regulated kinase kinase 1/2 inhibitor AZD6244 (ARRY-142886) enhances the radiation responsiveness of lung and colorectal tumor xenografts. *Clin Cancer Res.* 2009;15: 6619-6629.
65. Chung EJ, Brown AP, Asano H, et al. In vitro and in vivo radiosensitization with AZD6244 (ARRY-142886), an inhibitor of mitogen-activated protein kinase/extracellular signal-regulated kinase 1/2 kinase. *Clin Cancer Res.* 2009;15:3050-3057.
66. Konstantinidou G, Bey EA, Rabellino A, et al. Dual phosphoinositide 3-kinase/mammalian target of rapamycin blockade is an effective radiosensitizing strategy for the treatment of non-small cell lung cancer harboring K-RAS mutations. *Cancer Res.* 2009;69:7644-7652.
67. Sarkaria JN, Galanis E, Wu W, et al. North Central Cancer Treatment Group Phase I trial N057K of everolimus (RAD001) and temozolomide in combination with radiation therapy in patients with newly diagnosed glioblastoma multiforme. *Int J Radiat Oncol Biol Phys.* 2011;81:468-475.
68. Liu SK, Coackley C, Krause M, Jalali F, Chan N, Bristow RG. A novel poly(ADP-ribose) polymerase inhibitor, ABT-888, radiosensitizes malignant human cell lines under hypoxia. *Radiother Oncol.* 2008;88:258-268.
69. Senra JM, Telfer BA, Cherry KE, et al. Inhibition of PARP-1 by olaparib (AZD2281) increases the radiosensitivity of a lung tumor xenograft. *Mol Cancer Ther.* 2011;10:1949-1958.
70. Zhao Y, Thomas HD, Batey MA, et al. Preclinical evaluation of a potent novel DNA-dependent protein kinase inhibitor NU7441. *Cancer Res.* 2006;66:5354-5362.
71. Tao Y, Zhang P, Girdler F, et al. Enhancement of radiation response in p53-deficient cancer cells by the Aurora-B kinase inhibitor AZD1152. *Oncogene.* 2008;27:3244-3255.
72. Camphausen K, Cerna D, Scott T, et al. Enhancement of in vitro and in vivo tumor cell radiosensitivity by valproic acid. *Int J Cancer.* 2005;114:380-386.
73. Munshi A, Tanaka T, Hobbs ML, Tucker SL, Richon VM, Meyn RE. Vorinostat, a histone deacetylase inhibitor, enhances the response of human tumor cells to ionizing radiation through prolongation of gamma-H2AX foci. *Mol Cancer Ther.* 2006;5:1967-1974.
74. Raju U, Nakata E, Yang P, Newman RA, Ang KK, Milas L. In vitro enhancement of tumor cell radiosensitivity by a selective inhibitor of cyclooxygenase-2 enzyme: mechanistic considerations. *Int J Radiat Oncol Biol Phys.* 2002;54:886-894.
75. Kozin SV, Boucher Y, Hicklin DJ, Bohlen P, Jain RK, Suit HD. Vascular endothelial growth factor receptor-2-blocking antibody potentiates radiation-induced long-term control of human tumor xenografts. *Cancer Res.* 2001;61:39-44.
76. Zeman EM, Brown JM, Lemmon MJ, Hirst VK, Lee WW. SR-4233: a new bioreductive agent with high selective toxicity for hypoxic mammalian cells. *Int J Radiat Oncol Biol Phys.* 1986;12:1239-1242.
77. Baker MA, Zeman EM, Hirst VK, Brown JM. Metabolism of SR 4233 by Chinese hamster ovary cells: basis of selective hypoxic cytotoxicity. *Cancer Res.* 1988;48:5947-5952.
78. Rischin D, Peters L, Fisher R, et al. Tirapazamine, Cisplatin, and Radiation versus Fluorouracil, Cisplatin, and Radiation in patients with locally advanced head and neck cancer: a randomized phase II trial of the Trans-Tasman Radiation Oncology Group (TROG 98.02). *J Clin Oncol.* 2005;23:79-87.
79. von Pawel J, von Roemeling R, Gatzemeier U, et al. Tirapazamine plus cisplatin versus cisplatin in advanced non-small-cell lung cancer: A report of the international CATAPULT I study group. Cisplatin and tirapazamine in subjects with advanced previously untreated non-small-cell lung tumors. *J Clin Oncol.* 2000;18:1351-1359.
80. Williamson SK, Crowley JJ, Lara PN Jr, et al. Phase III trial of paclitaxel plus carboplatin with or without tirapazamine in advanced non-small-cell lung cancer: Southwest Oncology Group Trial S0003. *J Clin Oncol.* 2005;23:9097-9104.
81. Rischin D, Peters LJ, O'Sullivan B, et al. Tirapazamine, cisplatin, and radiation versus cisplatin and radiation for advanced squamous cell carcinoma of the head and neck (TROG 02.02, HeadSTART): a phase III trial of the Trans-Tasman Radiation Oncology Group. *J Clin Oncol.* 2010;28:2989-2995.
82. Shin DH, Kim JH, Jung YJ, et al. Preclinical evaluation of YC-1, a HIF inhibitor, for the prevention of tumor spreading. *Cancer Lett.* 2007;255:107-116.
83. Yeo EJ, Chun YS, Cho YS, et al. YC-1: a potential anticancer drug targeting hypoxia-inducible factor 1. *J Natl Cancer Inst.* 2003;95:516-525.
84. Mendelsohn J, Baselga J. Epidermal growth factor receptor targeting in cancer. *Semin Oncol.* 2006;33:369-385.
85. Akimoto T, Hunter NR, Buchmiller L, Mason K, Ang KK, Milas L. Inverse relationship between epidermal growth factor receptor expression and radiocurability of murine carcinomas. *Clin Cancer Res.* 1999;5:2884-2890.
86. Baumann M, Krause M, Dikomey E, et al. EGFR-targeted anti-cancer drugs in radiotherapy: preclinical evaluation of mechanisms. *Radiother Oncol.* 2007;83:238-248.
87. Huang SM, Bock JM, Harari PM. Epidermal growth factor receptor blockade with C225 modulates proliferation, apoptosis, and radiosensitivity in squamous cell carcinomas of the head and neck. *Cancer Res.* 1999;59:1935-1940.
88. Milas L, Mason K, Hunter N, et al. In vivo enhancement of tumor radioresponse by C225 antiepidermal growth factor receptor antibody. *Clin Cancer Res.* 2000;6:701-708.
89. Huang SM, Harari PM. Modulation of radiation response after epidermal growth factor receptor blockade in squamous cell carcinomas: inhibition of damage repair, cell cycle kinetics, and tumor angiogenesis. *Clin Cancer Res.* 2000;6:2166-2174.
90. Ciardiello F, Caputo R, Troiani T, et al. Antisense oligonucleotides targeting the epidermal growth factor receptor inhibit proliferation, induce apoptosis, and cooperate with cytotoxic drugs in human cancer cell lines. *Int J Cancer.* 2001;93:172-178.
91. Milano G, Magne N. Anti-EGFR and radiotherapy. *Cancer Radiother.* 2004;8:380-382.
92. Dittmann K, Mayer C, Rodemann HP. Inhibition of radiation-induced EGFR nuclear import by C225 (cetuximab) suppresses DNA-PK activity. *Radiother Oncol.* 2005;76:157-161.
93. Friedmann BJ, Caplin M, Savic B, et al. Interaction of the epidermal growth factor receptor and the DNA-dependent protein kinase pathway following gefitinib treatment. *Mol Cancer Ther.* 2006;5:209-218.
94. Toulany M, Kasten-Pisula U, Brammer I, et al. Blockage of epidermal growth factor receptor-phosphatidylinositol 3-kinase-AKT signaling increases radiosensitivity of K-RAS mutated human tumor cells in vitro by affecting DNA repair. *Clin Cancer Res.* 2006;12:4119-4126.
95. Bernhard EJ, McKenna WG, Hamilton AD, et al. Inhibiting Ras prenylation increases the radiosensitivity of human tumor cell lines with activating mutations of ras oncogenes. *Cancer Res.* 1998;58:1754-1761.
96. McKenna WG, Muschel RJ, Gupta AK, Hahn SM, Bernhard EJ. Farnesyltransferase inhibitors as radiation sensitizers. *Semin Radiat Oncol.* 2002;12:27-32.
97. Rudner J, Ruiner CE, Handrick R, Eibl HJ, Belka C, Jendrossek V. The Akt-inhibitor erufosine induces apoptotic cell death in prostate cancer cells and increases the short term effects of ionizing radiation. *Radiat Oncol.* 2010;5:108.
98. Prevo R, Deutsch E, Sampson O, et al. Class I PI3 kinase inhibition by the pyridinylfuranopyrimidine inhibitor PI-103 enhances tumor radiosensitivity. *Cancer Res.* 2008;68:5915-5923.
99. Kim IA, Bae SS, Fernandes A, et al. Selective inhibition of Ras, phosphoinositide 3 kinase, and Akt isoforms increases the radiosensitivity of human carcinoma cell lines. *Cancer Res.* 2005;65:7902-7910.
100. Albert JM, Kim KW, Cao C, Lu B. Targeting the Akt/mammalian target of rapamycin pathway for radiosensitization of breast cancer. *Mol Cancer Ther.* 2006;5:1183-1189.
101. Qayum N, Muschel RJ, Im JH, et al. Tumor vascular changes mediated by inhibition of oncogenic signaling. *Cancer Res.* 2009;69:6347-6354.
102. Bryant HE, Schultz N, Thomas HD, et al. Specific killing of BRCA2-deficient tumours with inhibitors of poly(ADP-ribose) polymerase. *Nature.* 2005;434:913-917.
103. Fong PC, Boss DS, Yap TA, et al. Inhibition of poly(ADP-ribose) polymerase in tumors from BRCA mutation carriers. *N Engl J Med.* 2009;361:123-134.
104. Schreiber V, Dantzer F, Ame JC, de Murcia G. Poly(ADP-ribose): novel functions for an old molecule. *Nat Rev Mol Cell Biol.* 2006;7:517-528.
105. Ortiz T, Lopez S, Burguillos MA, Edreira A, Pinero J. Radiosensitizer effect of Wortmannin in radioresistant bladder tumoral cell lines. *Int J Oncol.* 2004;24:169-175.

106. Shinohara ET, Geng L, Tan J, et al. DNA-dependent protein kinase is a molecular target for the development of noncytotoxic radiation-sensitizing drugs. *Cancer Res.* 2005;65:4987-4992.
107. Hickson I, Zhao Y, Richardson CJ, et al. Identification and characterization of a novel and specific inhibitor of the ataxia-telangiectasia mutated kinase ATM. *Cancer Res.* 2004;64: 9152-9159.
108. Rainey MD, Charlton ME, Stanton RV, Kastan MB. Transient inhibition of ATM kinase is sufficient to enhance cellular sensitivity to ionizing radiation. *Cancer Res.* 2008;68:7466-7474.
109. Syljuasen RG, Sorensen CS, Nylandsted J, Lukas C, Lukas J, Bartek J. Inhibition of Chk1 by CEP-3891 accelerates mitotic nuclear fragmentation in response to ionizing Radiation. *Cancer Res.* 2004;64:9035-9040.
110. Moretti L, Niermann K, Schleicher S, et al. MLN8054, a small molecule inhibitor of aurora kinase a, sensitizes androgen-resistant prostate cancer to radiation. *Int J Radiat Oncol Biol Phys.* 2011;80:1189-1197.
111. Marks P, Rifkind RA, Richon VM, Breslow R, Miller T, Kelly WK. Histone deacetylases and cancer: causes and therapies. *Nat Rev Cancer.* 2001;1:194-202.
112. Baschnagel A, Russo A, Burgan WE, et al. Vorinostat enhances the radiosensitivity of a breast cancer brain metastatic cell line grown in vitro and as intracranial xenografts. *Mol Cancer Ther.* 2009;8:1589-1595.
113. Chinnaiyan P, Vallabhaneni G, Armstrong E, Huang SM, Harari PM. Modulation of radiation response by histone deacetylase inhibition. *Int J Radiat Oncol Biol Phys.* 2005;62:223-239.
114. Entin-Meer M, Rephaeli A, Yang X, Nudelman A, VandenBerg SR, Haas-Kogan DA. Butyric acid prodrugs are histone deacetylase inhibitors that show antineoplastic activity and radiosensitizing capacity in the treatment of malignant gliomas. *Mol Cancer Ther.* 2005;4:1952-1961.
115. Gupta S, Srivastava M, Ahmad N, Bostwick DG, Mukhtar H. Over-expression of cyclooxygenase-2 in human prostate adenocarcinoma. *Prostate.* 2000;42:73-78.
116. Hida T, Yatabe Y, Achiwa H, et al. Increased expression of cyclooxygenase 2 occurs frequently in human lung cancers, specifically in adenocarcinomas. *Cancer Res.* 1998;58:3761-3764.
117. Parrett M, Harris R, Joarder F, Ross M, Clausen K, Robertson F. Cyclooxygenase-2 gene expression in human breast cancer. *Int J Oncol.* 1997;10:503-507.
118. Tucker ON, Dannenberg AJ, Yang EK, et al. Cyclooxygenase-2 expression is up-regulated in human pancreatic cancer. *Cancer Res.* 1999;59:987-990.
119. Zimmermann KC, Sarbia M, Weber AA, Borchard F, Gabbert HE, Schror K. Cyclooxygenase-2 expression in human esophageal carcinoma. *Cancer Res.* 1999;59:198-204.
120. Kishi K, Petersen S, Petersen C, et al. Preferential enhancement of tumor radioresponse by a cyclooxygenase-2 inhibitor. *Cancer Res.* 2000;60:1326-1331.
121. Raju U, Ariga H, Dittmann K, Nakata E, Ang KK, Milas L. Inhibition of DNA repair as a mechanism of enhanced radioresponse of head and neck carcinoma cells by a selective cyclooxygenase-2 inhibitor, celecoxib. *Int J Radiat Oncol Biol Phys.* 2005;63:520-528.
122. Lee CG, Heijn M, di Tomaso E, et al. Anti-vascular endothelial growth factor treatment augments tumor radiation response under normoxic or hypoxic conditions. *Cancer Res.* 2000;60:5565-5570.
123. Crane CH, Winter K, Regine WF, et al. Phase II study of bevacizumab with concurrent capecitabine and radiation followed by maintenance gemcitabine and bevacizumab for locally advanced pancreatic cancer: Radiation Therapy Oncology Group RTOG 0411. *J Clin Oncol.* 2009;27:4096-4102.
124. Czito BG, Bendell JC, Willett CG, et al. Bevacizumab, oxaliplatin, and capecitabine with radiation therapy in rectal cancer: phase I trial results. *Int J Radiat Oncol Biol Phys.* 2007;68:472-478.
125. Seiwert TY, Haraf DJ, Cohen EE, et al. Phase I study of bevacizumab added to fluorouracil- and hydroxyurea-based concomitant chemoradiotherapy for poor-prognosis head and neck cancer. *J Clin Oncol.* 2008;26:1732-1741.
126. Coleman CN. Hypoxic cell radiosensitizers: expectations and progress in drug development. *Int J Radiat Oncol Biol Phys.* 1985;11:323-329.
127. Stratford IJ. Mechanisms of hypoxic cell radiosensitization and the development of new sensitizers. *Int J Radiat Oncol Biol Phys.* 1982;8:391-398.
128. Baillet F, Housset M, Dessard-Diana B, Boisserie G. Positive clinical experience with misonidazole in brachytherapy and external radiotherapy. *Int J Radiat Oncol Biol Phys.* 1989;16:1073-1075.
129. Minsky BD, Leibel SA. The treatment of hepatic metastases from colorectal cancer with radiation therapy alone or combined with chemotherapy or misonidazole. *Cancer Treat Rev.* 1989;16:213-219.
130. Overgaard J, Hansen HS, Overgaard M, et al. A randomized double-blind phase III study of nimorazole as a hypoxic radiosensitizer of primary radiotherapy in supraglottic larynx and pharynx carcinoma. Results of the Danish Head and Neck Cancer Study (DAHANCA) Protocol 5-85. *Radiother Oncol.* 1998;46:135-146.
131. Simpson JR, Bauer M, Perez CA, et al. Radiation therapy alone or combined with misonidazole in the treatment of locally advanced non-oat cell lung cancer: report of an RTOG prospective randomized trial. *Int J Radiat Oncol Biol Phys.* 1989;16:1483-1491.
132. Yahiro T, Masui S, Kubota N, Yamada K, Kobayashi A, Kishii K. Effects of hypoxic cell radiosensitizer doranidazole (PR-350) on the radioresponse of murine and human tumor cells in vitro and in vivo. *J Radiat Res (Tokyo).* 2005;46:363-372.
133. Moeller BJ, Dewhirst MW. Raising the bar: how HIF-1 helps determine tumor radiosensitivity. *Cell Cycle.* 2004;3:1107-1110.
134. Staffurth J. A review of the clinical evidence for intensity-modulated radiotherapy. *Clin Oncol (R Coll Radiol).* 2010;22: 643-657.
135. Lo SS, Fakiris AJ, Chang EL, et al. Stereotactic body radiation therapy: a novel treatment modality. *Nat Rev Clin Oncol.* 2010;7:44-54.
136. Schulz-Ertner D, Tsujii H. Particle radiation therapy using proton and heavier ion beams. *J Clin Oncol.* 2007;25:953-964.
137. Fokas E, Kraft G, An H, Engenhart-Cabillic R. Ion beam radiobiology and cancer: time to update ourselves. *Biochim Biophys Acta.* 2009;1796:216-229.

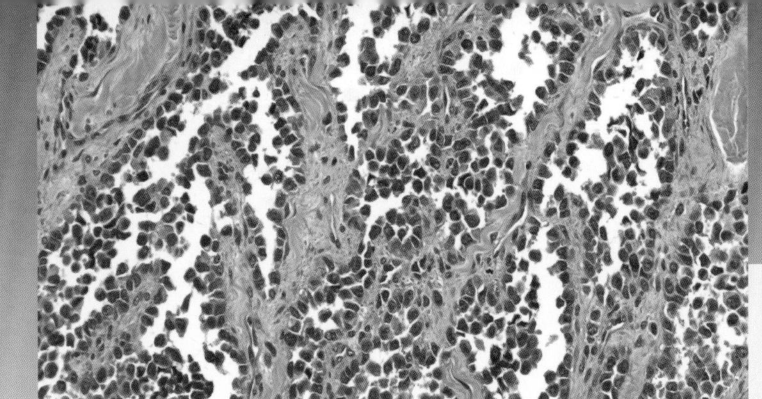

SECTION VII

Future of Molecular Diagnostics and Personalized Cancer Medicine

CHAPTER 69

NEW APPROACHES TO PERSONALIZED MEDICINE AND TARGETED DRUG DISCOVERY

Garrett M. Dancik and Dan Theodorescu

INTRODUCTION

Personalized Medicine relies on two pillars: (1) identification of drivers and/or biomarkers of the malignant phenotype that can be selectively targeted by rationally designed drugs and (2) marker-driven selection of patients that are responsive to such therapies. The personalized drug discovery pipeline has emerged from an increased understanding of cancer as a genetic disease, exponential advances in biotechnology that enable high-throughput data collection of genomic, transcriptomic, proteomic, and epigenetic profiles, and by increases in computational power that enable the cost-effective management and analysis of these large data sets. After biomarkers indicative of cancer-promoting genomic alterations are identified from molecular profiles, effective drugs are identified or developed that target these drivers or biomarkers. In addition, although not all patients treated with targeted agents respond to such therapies despite blockade of the target, it has been recently shown that biomarkers can identify patients that benefit from new targeted therapies as well as already existing therapies, including chemotherapy and radiation. When administered alone or in combination with conventional therapies, targeted agents have shown effectiveness in several cancers, an approach validated by the development and Food and Drug Administration (FDA) approval of several high-profile targeted therapies. FDA-approved targeted therapies include the monoclonal antibody trastuzumab which targets the human epidermal growth factor receptor 2 (HER-2) in breast cancer patients and the ABL tyrosine kinase inhibitor imatinib mesylate for patients with chronic myelogenous leukemia (CML). A selected list of FDA-approved targeted therapies in cancer is provided in Table 69.1.

ENABLING TECHNOLOGIES FOR BIOMARKER DISCOVERY

Cancer is a genetic disease, harboring somatically acquired driver mutations that can manifest at many molecular levels. A genetic mutation is a blueprint for the expression of a protein or functional RNA such as microRNA (miRNA). However, gene expression is often regulated at the epigenetic level, messenger RNA (mRNA) may be post-transcriptionally regulated by an miRNA, and proteins are subject to post-translational modifications. A molecular profile obtained at any of these levels provides a snapshot of the tumor which includes biomarkers that can be exploited for all aspects of personalized medicine, including risk assessment, patient prognosis, prediction of therapeutic response, and targeted therapy if they are drivers of the malignant process.

Advances in biotechnology over the past two decades have yielded high-throughput technologies for profiling patients at the genomic, transcriptomic, epigenetic, and proteomic levels (Table 69.2). Each technology characterizes a tumor at a specific molecular level and has dramatically increased our understanding of cancer risk, development, progression, and therapeutic response, in addition to identifying potential therapeutic targets. More detailed descriptions of the various molecular technologies are described below. Although the different technologies have generally been utilized independently, integration of the various approaches will be required to gain a thorough understanding of tumorigenesis and to realize the full potential of targeted therapy.

TABLE 69–1 Selected FDA-Approved Targeted Therapies in Cancer

Agent (Brand Name)	Target	Current Disease Indication	Year Approved (Last Updated)
Anastrozole (Arimidex)	ER	ER-positive breast cancer	1996
Bevacizumab (Avastin)	VEGF	Metastatic HER-2–negative breast cancer (under review); metastatic renal cell carcinoma; second-line treatment for glioblastoma; unresectable, locally advanced, recurrent, or metastatic, non–squamous, non–small cell lung cancer; metastatic colorectal cancer	2004 (2011)
Bortezomib (Velcade)	Proteasome	Multiple myeloma; mantle cell lymphoma (at least one prior therapy)	2005 (2008)
Cetuximab (Erbitux)	EGFR	Metastatic colorectal cancer; locally or regionally advanced squamous cell carcinoma of the head and neck	2004 (2006)
Crizotinib (Xalkori)	ALK	Locally advanced or metastatic ALK-positive non–small cell lung cancer	2011
Erlotinib hydrochloride (Tarceva)	EGFR	Locally advanced or metastatic non–small cell lung cancer; locally advanced, unresectable or metastatic pancreatic carcinoma	2004 (2010)
Gefitinib (Iressa)	EGFR	Non–small cell lung cancer patients currently or previously benefitting from gefitinib treatment	2003 (2005)
Imatinib mesylate (Gleevec)	BCR–ABL	BCR-ABL–positive chronic myeloid leukemia; BCR-ABL–positive recurrent acute lymphoblastic leukemia; chronic eosinophilic leukemia; gastrointestinal stromal tumor	2006 (2008)
Lapatinib ditosylate (Tykerb)	HER-2	HER-2–positive breast cancer	2007 (2010)
Nilotinib (Tasigna)	BCR–ABL, c-KIT, PDGFR	BCR-ABL–positive chronic myeloid leukemia	2007 (2010)
Sorafenib (Nexavar)	Raf, VEGF, KIT, FLT3	Advanced renal carcinoma; unresectable hepatocellular carcinoma	2005 (2007)
Tamoxifen (Novadex)	ER	ER-positive breast cancer	1977 (1998)
Trastuzumab (Herceptin)	HER-2 (ERBB2)	HER-2–positive breast cancer; HER-2–positive metastatic gastric or gastroesophageal junction adenocarcinoma without prior treatment	2006 (2010)
Vandetanib (Zactima)	EGFR, VEGF, RET	Unresectable, locally advanced, or metastatic medullary thyroid cancer	2011
Vemurafenib (Zelboraf)	BRAF	Metastatic or unresectable melanoma	2011

ER, Estrogen receptor; VEGF, Vascular endothelial growth factor; EGFR, Epidermal growth factor receptor; ALK, Anaplastic lymphoma kinase; PDGFR, platelet-derived growth factor receptor; FLT3, Fms-like tyrosine kinase 3; HER-2, human epidermal growth factor receptor 2.

Gene Expression Profiling

Gene expression profiling is currently the most common way to identify molecular targets in a high-throughput fashion. Gene expression profiling is commonly executed using DNA microarrays, which simultaneously measure the expression level of thousands of genes. The mRNA from a tumor sample is isolated, converted to complementary DNA (cDNA), fluorescently labeled, and allowed to hybridize to known DNA probes that are embedded on a glass or silicon slide (Affymetrix, Agilent Arrays) or attached to silica beads that are randomly arranged on the array (Illumina Arrays). In both cases, the microarray is scanned, and the resulting intensity value of each DNA probe is a measure of mRNA expression for the corresponding gene. In a single-channel or one-color microarray, a single intensity is calculated for each probe and this intensity measures the gene expression level of that probe relative to its gene expression level in the other samples on the array. In two-channel or two-color microarrays, two samples (e.g., a cancer and normal tissue) are labeled with different color dyes (typically Cy3 and Cy5), then allowed to simultaneously hybridize to the DNA probes. A probe's intensity value is a measure of the relative expression of the gene with respect to each paired sample.

The first DNA microarray was developed by researchers at Stanford in 1996. Their two-color microarray utilized robots to spot cDNA on glass slides and was used to identify differentially expressed genes in *Arabidopsis thaliana* under various conditions.[1] Microarrays were quickly applied to cancer, where they were used to identify differentially expressed genes between a human melanoma cell line and its tumor-suppressed counterpart later that year.[2] In a seminal paper describing the first demonstration of molecular classification in cancer, Golub and colleagues[3] used

TABLE 69–2 Molecular Technologies for Biomarker Identification

Molecular Level	Technology	Description	Strengths	Limitations
Transcriptomic	Microarray profiling of gene expression and microRNA	Quantifies mRNA or microRNA levels	Well-established protocol for RNA extraction and hybridization; established methods for data processing and analysis	Cannot detect post-translational modifications such as phosphorylation or novel molecules
Proteomic	Protein microarrays	Quantifies protein levels or protein interactions with proteins, nucleic acids, lipids, drugs, and other small molecules	Can quantify and detect post-translational modifications such as phosphorylation	Cannot detect novel molecules; not all proteins are known; lacking robust detection of proteins across very large concentration range
Genomic	Next (second)-generation sequencing	Sequencing-by-synthesis methods sequence genomic or RNA sequences in real time in a parallel fashion	Can detect novel molecules	Relatively expensive, though costs are rapidly decreasing
Epigenetic	Methylation profiling	Detection of methylated cytosine residues	Epigenetic characterization	Relies on microarrays, sequencing, or bisulfite conversion and is limited by those technologies

DNA microarrays to classify acute leukemias on the basis of gene expression data. Since then, microarrays have been widely used in cancer to identify molecular profiles that correlate with prognosis and response to therapy.

Arrays can also be used to evaluate the expression of miRNA in tumor samples. Genomic miRNAs are between 18 and 24 nucleotides long and regulate gene expression by binding to the 3′-untranslated region of an mRNA in order to prevent transcription or inhibit degradation.[4] Although discovered relatively recently, in 1993,[5] it is clear that miRNAs play important roles in tumorigenesis and can influence drug sensitivity. For example, the miRNA miR-34a, which is deleted in many human cancers, is directly regulated by p53.[6] Microarray studies have identified miRNA biomarkers in bladder cancer[7] and breast cancer,[8] among others.

Proteomics

Protein microarrays are the counterpart to DNA microarrays for the analysis of proteins. A protein microarray allows for the quantification of both a protein in a sample and its interaction with nucleic acids, lipids, drugs, and other small molecules. Importantly, protein microarrays can quantify post-translational modifications such as glycosylation, acetylation, and phosphorylation which are undetectable at the gene expression level. Although a newer technology than DNA microarrays, many protein microarrays are commercially available and have been used for the discovery of diagnostic and prognostic biomarkers in cancer.

Protein microarrays consist of spots of immobilized "bait" or "capture" molecules which may consist of antibodies, proteins, or DNA.[9] In a forward-phase protein microarray (FPPM), the array is queried (i.e., incubated) with a sample of interest, such as a tumor sample. The analytes in the sample are labeled, a subset of the analytes binds to the capture molecules, the array is scanned, and analyte intensity measures the extent of the interaction between the analytes in the sample and the capture molecules. Antibody arrays, which use antibodies as capture molecules, are a common class of FPPM and have been used to identify proteins differentially expressed between tumor and normal samples.[10] In reverse-phase protein microarrays (RPPM), analytes from a biological sample of interest are immobilized on the array, and then queried with antibodies to identify the proteins that are present in the sample.

Several studies illustrate the ability of protein microarrays to characterize protein networks in cancer and their potential for advancing personalized medicine. In particular, an early RPPM study in 2001 identified increased Akt phosphorylation and decreased extracellular signal-regulated kinase (ERK) phosphorylation as prognostic markers for tumor progression in prostate cancer.[11] More recently, Petricoin et al.[12] used an RPPM to probe laser capture microdissected breast cancer tissues with 90 phospho-specific antibodies and identified subgroups of patients that differed in epidermal growth factor receptor (EGFR) family signaling, AKT/mTOR (mammalian target of rapamycin) pathway activation, c-kit/able growth factor signaling, and ERK pathway activation. Conceivably, these patients can be stratified according to these subtypes for the purpose of targeted therapy.

The ability of protein microarrays to quantify post-translational modifications, and phosphorylation specifically, is perhaps its biggest strength. However, several challenges must be met for protein microarrays to realize their full potential. High affinity and highly specific antibodies must be identified that can accurately detect low abundance proteins that exist in the presence of cross-reactive proteins at potentially much greater concentrations. These antibodies must also be able to accommodate the extremely broad range of protein levels that exist in tissue samples (on the order of 10^{10}). Lastly, as with gene expression profiling, protein microarrays can only detect molecules that are known. However, the exact number of polypeptides present in a tissue is not clear.

Next-Generation Gene Sequencing

The completion of the Human Genome Project (HGP) in 2003 ushered in a new era in genomics and personalized medicine. The HGP was sequenced using the Sanger sequencing method, a time-consuming and expensive process compared with current technologies. At a cost of $2.7 billion and a time period of 13 years, the completion of the HGP using Sanger sequencing was not amenable to high-throughput genome analyses. However, next-generation (or second-generation) approaches would be described as early as 2 years later.[13] In contrast to Sanger sequencing, next-generation sequencing utilizes novel chemical approaches to sequence DNA (or RNA) molecules in real time as the DNA is synthesized from an immobile DNA template.[14] Pyrosequencing methods, for example, emit a burst of light whenever a new base is incorporated into the growing DNA strand, while other methods use reversible terminators that result in a short pause when a specific nucleotide is incorporated. These sequencing-by-synthesis approaches are simultaneously applied to multiple DNA templates on a plate and can sequence hundreds of thousands of templates in parallel. As a result, next-generation sequencing technologies can sequence an exponentially greater number of nucleotides than Sanger sequencing for a fraction of the cost. Currently, whole genome sequencing using next-generation technologies costs as low as $5,000 and takes approximately 1 month to complete.

The application of next-generation sequencing technologies to cancer genetics has identified new driver mutations and potential therapeutic targets. In addition to whole cancer genome sequencing, targeted sequencing of known exons (exomes), transcriptomes, and miRNAs may be performed.[15] Following a pilot study that detected mutations from high-throughput sequencing of exonic DNA from acute myeloid leukemia cells in 2003,[16] the first complete cancer genome was sequenced in 2008, when acute myeloid leukemia DNA was compared with DNA from normal skin cells from the same patient.[17] This study identified eight new non-synonymous somatic mutations that occurred in almost all tumors sampled. Other cancer genomes that have been completely sequenced include prostate cancer,[18] breast cancer,[19] melanoma,[20] and lung.[21]

Methylation Screening

DNA methylation involves the addition of a methyl group to a cytosine nucleotide, which usually represses gene expression when methylation occurs in a promoter region. Proper DNA methylation is required for gene regulation during development. Methylation biomarkers have been identified for tumorigenesis and prognosis in various cancers and can be therapeutically targeted.[22] Several methylation screening approaches exist, including gel-based, array-based, and sequence-based methods. Most methods involve DNA digestion with methylation-sensitive and methylation-resistant restriction endonucleases and the comparison between resulting DNA fragments. In addition, methylated regions can be detected by antibodies specific for methylated cytosine, or by bisulfate conversion, where bisulfate treatment of a DNA sequence converts unmethylated cytosines to uracil in a sample that is then sequenced.[23]

DNA methylation has implications for cancer development, prognosis, and treatment. Many studies have found an association between tumorigenesis and either the hypermethylation of tumor suppressor gene promoters[24] or the hypomethylation of oncogene promoters.[25] Furthermore, the recent discovery that the methylation of two tumor suppressor gene promoters is sufficient for oncogenesis suggests that driver mutations may be present at the epigenetic level.[26] DNA methylation is also an avenue for anticancer therapy. The non-specific hypomethylating agent azacytidine was approved by the FDA in 2004 for the treatment of myelodysplastic syndrome, which often progresses to acute myeloid leukemia.[27] Targeted DNA methylation is also possible, as evidenced by the targeted DNA methylation and downregulation of the membrane glycoprotein EpCAM, an approach with clear therapeutic potential.[28] EpCAM is a biomarker in a variety of cancers, including breast, pancreatic, and colon, and is a therapeutic target in several ongoing clinical trials.

IDENTIFICATION OF CANDIDATE BIOMARKERS FOR GUIDING AND DEVELOPING THERAPY

The generation of molecular profiles using the technologies described previously is the basis for biomarker identification in personalized medicine. In the context of drug discovery, biomarkers can be exploited as therapeutic targets and can also identify patients likely to respond to a particular therapy. As mentioned previously, the discovery of a dysregulated tyrosine kinase in CML and the subsequent development of the kinase inhibitor imatinib mesylate is a classic example of the targeted therapy paradigm.[29] Importantly, biomarkers that correlate with prognosis are useful for guiding clinical decisions by assessing the necessity of specific treatments as are biomarkers that predict response to targeted agents.

In general, therapeutic targets can be identified from any kind of molecular profile as long as the biomarkers are accessible to therapeutic agents and are drivers of a cancer-related phenotype. Here, we provide brief descriptions and select examples of the types of biomarkers relevant to personalized cancer care. These include biomarkers for tumor classification, for patient prognosis, and for predicting therapeutic responses from in vivo and from in vitro data.

Biomarkers for Tumor Classification

Tumor subtypes can correlate with prognosis and response to therapy and therefore have relevance to personalized therapy. Tumors may be classified according to subtypes traditionally identified by histopathological presentation, such as the subtypes of non–small cell lung cancer (adenocarcinoma, squamous cell carcinoma, and large cell),[30] or according to previously unknown subtypes with unique molecular profiles.[31] There are many examples of molecular profiling studies for tumor classification. The first use of a gene signature for predictive or classification purposes was described in a landmark paper that described the development of a gene signature that distinguishes acute myeloid leukemia from acute lymphoblastic leukemia.[3] This is highly relevant since the therapy and genetics of these two diseases are very different. Among many other examples, DNA microarrays have been used to identify subtypes in breast cancer,[32] prostate cancer,[33] and bladder cancer.[34]. Kidney cancer subtypes have been identified on the basis of miRNA expression.[35] Protein microarrays have been used to identify and characterize basal-like and luminal breast cancer subtypes based on the phosphorylation status of 100 proteins.[36]

Biomarkers for Patient Prognosis and Response to Therapy

A patient's prognosis reflects the likelihood that a cancer recurs, progresses, or metastasizes and is therefore useful for determining the aggressiveness of treatment directed at reducing these risks. Onco*type* DX is a widely used, commercially available prognostic tool for breast cancer patients. The test predicts the likelihood of recurrence within 10 years, based on the expression levels of 21 genes measured by real-time polymerase chain reaction, and is used to guide clinical decisions regarding the appropriateness of chemotherapy.[37] Examples of prognostic and gene expression signatures developed and validated using microarrays include a 70-gene signature, later developed into the FDA-approved MammaPrint assay, that predicts metastasis in breast cancer patients[38]; a 20-gene signature that predicts nodal metastasis in bladder cancer[39]; and a 6-gene signature that predicts recurrence in non–small cell lung cancer patients.[40] Protein microarrays are now beginning to be used to identify biomarkers whose expression or activation correlates with progression.[41]

Biomarkers predictive of patient response to therapy are both potential therapeutic targets and tools for the selection of patients likely to benefit from current treatments. Appropriate patient selection will lead to the approval of therapeutic agents that have low response rates at the population level but have strong efficacy in specific patient populations and will involve discovering new uses of already existing compounds. A recent example is the FDA approval of the anaplastic lymphoma kinase (ALK) inhibitor crizotinib (Xalkori) in 2011 for the treatment of ALK-positive non–small cell lung cancer patients, along with a companion diagnostic test. The rapid development and approval of this targeted agent was facilitated by the selection of patients responsive to crizotinib in clinical trials. In 2010, a clinical trial for ALK-positive patients was initiated following evidence that crizotinib had clinical activity in two ALK-positive patients in a dose activity study.[42] The FDA approved crizotinib less than 2 years later, only 7 years after lead discovery, and 5 years after the initiation of phase I clinical trials.

Gene expression profiling studies have identified and validated many predictive biomarkers. Examples include gene expression biomarkers that predict response to neoadjuvant paclitaxel and doxorubicin chemotherapy in breast cancer patients,[43] and response to adjuvant cisplatin/vinorelbine chemotherapy in early-stage non–small lung cancer,[44] and a combination of gene expression and protein phosphorylation biomarkers that predict lapatinib sensitivity in bladder cancer.[45]

Drug sensitivity is a function of both how a drug interacts with a patient and how the patient processes the drug. *Pharmacogenomics* is the study of how a patient's genetic variability influences drug metabolism, absorption, and processing of therapeutic compounds. Pharmacogenomic biomarkers are therefore relevant for patient selection and optimizing the dose of the therapeutic agent. A widely cited example of pharmacogenomics is the single nucleotide polymorphisms (SNPs) in the genes *CYP2C9* and *VKORC1*, which influence the metabolism of and patient response to the anticoagulant warfarin.[46] Examples of pharmacogenomics in cancer include the association between polymorphisms in the DNA repair genes *ERCC2* and *XRCC1* and response to platinum chemotherapies,[47] and in thiopurine methyltransferase (*TPMT*) and mercaptopurine sensitivity.[48]

Novel Approaches That Predict Patient Response from In Vitro Assays

The process of identifying drug sensitivity biomarkers in in vitro cell line models has many advantages over biomarker identification in treated patients. In addition to being less time-consuming and less costly, cell line models can easily incorporate newly discovered drugs and combination therapies that have not been examined in clinical trials. Furthermore, the National Cancer Institute (NCI)-60 human tumor cell line screen, which contains publicly available data for thousands of compounds, is a rich resource of information that can be mined for drug sensitivity biomarkers since these lines have been profiled by many of the assays described above such as gene expression, SNP profiling, and DNA copy number information (http://dtp.cancer.gov/mtargets/mt_index.html). The NCI-60 panel consists of 60 human tumors from 9 tissues of origin: breast, central nervous system, colon, leukemia, melanoma, non–small cell lung, ovarian, prostate, and renal. Since 1990, over 100,000 compounds and 50,000 natural products have been screened. Drug sensitivity data are publicly available for more than 45,000, including 93 FDA-approved anticancer agents.[49] The Developmental Therapeutics Program oversees the NCI in vitro drug screening of NCI-60.[50]

This approach naturally raises two questions: first, can in vitro cell line models discover new drugs, and second, are biomarkers that predict therapeutic response in vitro relevant in selecting responsive patients in clinical studies. The answers to both of these would be a qualified "yes." Below are some examples of tools that can accomplish these tasks.

The COMPARE algorithm is a web-based program available for identifying compounds whose NCI-60 drug sensitivities correlate with a selected compound or a molecular target (i.e., a biomarker) of interest.[51] Therefore, COMPARE can identify potential compounds for treating patients expressing a biomarker of interest and for identifying the mechanism of action of a compound based on its similarity with other known compounds. The mechanism of action of the naturally occurring compound halichondrin B was identified through a COMPARE analysis, where it was found to have a COMPARE profile similar to known microtubule polymerization inhibitors. Its interaction with tubulin was subsequently confirmed experimentally,[52] and the synthetic analogue eribulin mesylate (Halaven) was recently approved by the FDA in 2010 for treatment of metastatic breast cancer. Interest in the drug bortezomib increased when a COMPARE analysis found its sensitivity profile to be distinct from other compounds in the database, suggesting a unique mechanism of action. Intensive follow-up studies revealed bortezomib to be a proteasome inhibitor. Only 8 years after initial testing, bortezomib was approved by the FDA in 2003 for the treatment of myeloma.

The connectivity map (CMAP) characterizes the functional relationships between drugs, genes, and disease and is an additional resource for drug discovery.[53] Underlying the CMAP is a database of gene expression profiles of human cell lines that are perturbed by chemicals or genetic reagents (referred to as perturbagens). The CMAP is queried with a list of biomarkers and compounds are identified that have perturbagen profiles correlating with the query, suggesting that the biomarkers are targeted by the compound. An intriguing use of the CMAP is the identification of combination therapies for overcoming drug resistance. When biomarkers for glucocorticoid dexamethasone resistance in acute lymphoblastic leukemia patients were submitted, the CMAP identified the FDA-approved immunosuppressant sirolimus (rapamycin), an mTOR inhibitor.[54] Validation studies found that sirolimus induces glucocorticoid sensitivity in malignant lymphoid cell lines.

COXEN (coexpression extrapolation) is an innovative strategy for drug discovery and for identifying in vivo biomarkers for drug sensitivity based on in vitro drug response data (Fig. 69.1).[55] COXEN uses gene expression profiles as a "Rosetta Stone" for translating drug activity in cell lines to drug activity in patients, by identifying predictive biomarkers that are concordantly expressed between cell lines and patients. COXEN has been used to identify chemosensitivity biomarkers for cisplatin and paclitaxel in bladder cancer, biomarkers for docetaxel and tamoxifen in breast cancer, and as a drug screening tool which identified the promising new agent C1311 in bladder cancer.[56] Using NCI-60 drug sensitivity data, COXEN has also been used to predict overall survival of breast cancer patients treated with 5-fluorouracil, doxorubicin, and cyclophosphamide; survival in bladder cancer patients treated with neoadjuvant methotrexate, vinblastine, doxorubicin, and cisplatin; and survival in ovarian cancer patients treated with platinum-based chemotherapy.[57]

Bioinformatics Tools for Identifying Therapeutic Targets from Biomarkers

Molecular profiles generated from genomic, transcriptomic, proteomic, and epigenetic profiling have been used to identify biomarkers (or gene signatures) that correlate with risk, prognosis, and response to therapy. Biomarkers for response to therapy are directly relevant to drug discovery because they identify patient populations likely to benefit from treatment. Importantly, drugs that have a low efficacy rate at the population level may be very effective in patient populations selected on the basis of response to therapy biomarkers. In addition, all biomarkers, including tumor classification and prognostic biomarkers, can be exploited in two ways: to identify potential therapeutic targets and to identify known compounds that are effective in patients selected on the basis of those biomarkers. The intuitive approach of identifying therapeutic targets from biomarkers is supported by studies where biomarkers predictive or indicative of pathway deregulation correlate with the sensitivity of agents targeting those pathways.[58] Specific well-known examples include the findings that trastuzumab sensitivity correlates with the expression of its target HER-2[59] and gefitinib sensitivity correlates with the mutation status of its target EGFR.[60] Many public databases of molecular profiles, drug sensitivity profiles, and software for their analysis are available to aid in the biomarker identification and drug discovery process (Table 69.3).

Biomarkers are generally identified by analyzing genes or proteins for differential expression using standard statistical tests such as a Student's *t*-test or the nonparametric Wilcoxon rank-sum test, or more advanced models such as empirical Bayes[61] and permutation-based methods.[62] When mining high-dimensional molecular

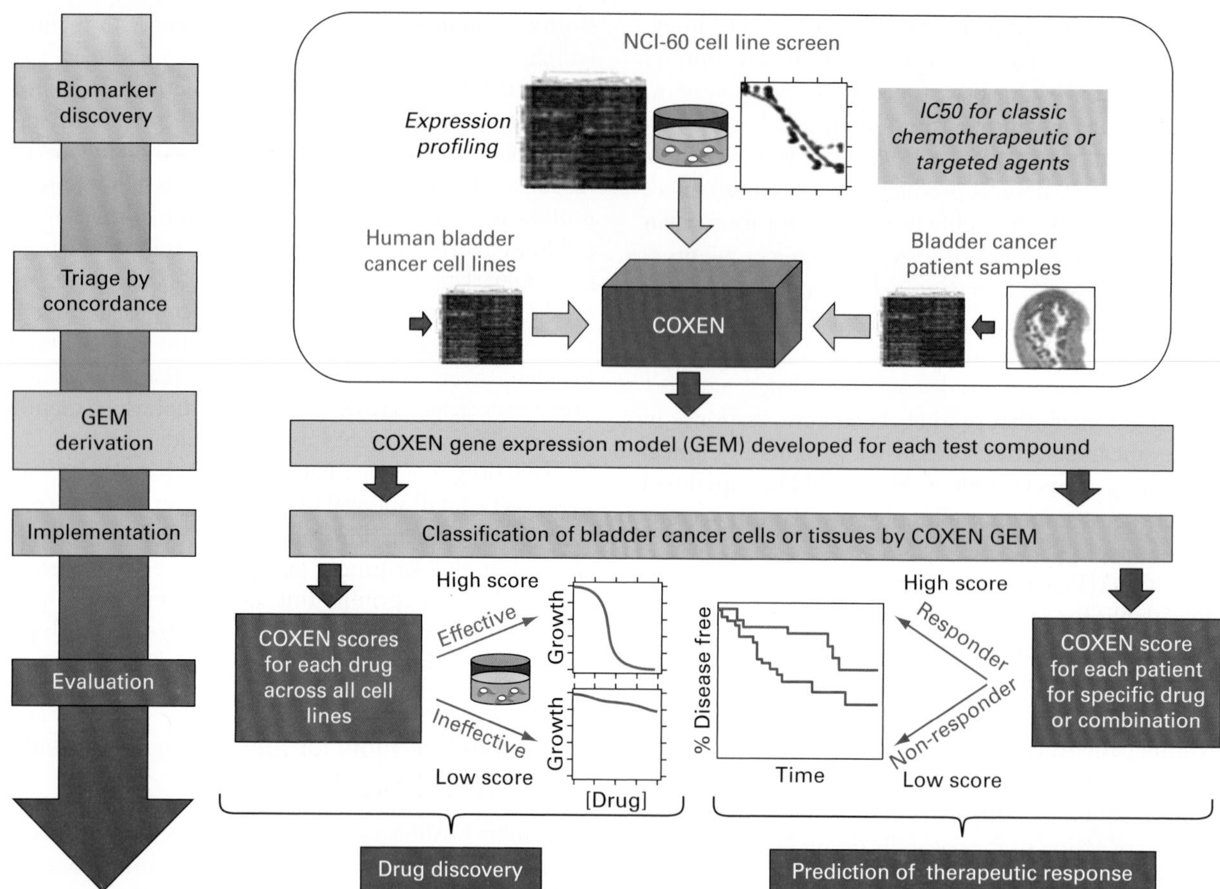

FIGURE 69–1 The COXEN system for drug discovery and prediction of therapeutic responses. Biomarkers for drug sensitivity are identified from molecular (i.e., expression profiling) technologies and drug sensitivity data from NCI-60. Biomarkers are then triaged by concordance which selects only those drug sensitivity biomarkers that are concordantly expressed between cell lines and patients (e.g., in bladder cancer). Concordant biomarkers are used to derive gene expression models (GEMs) which predict single- or multi-agent drug responses in cell lines or in patients in the form of COXEN scores. The COXEN system is then validated using either in vitro data or clinical trial outcomes. For drug discovery, thousands of therapeutic agents are ranked by their COXEN scores in a target population and the most promising agents are selected for further study. Prediction of a patient's therapeutic response to various agents is the basis for personalized therapy and for the selection of likely responders in clinical trials. (Reproduced from Smith SC, Baras AS, Lee JK, et al., *Cancer Res.* 2010;70:1753-1758.)

profiles for differentially expressed genes or proteins, *P*-values from statistical tests are adjusted to account for the large number of genes or proteins under investigation. This is because, for example, the use of standard statistical tests and a *P*-value cutoff of 0.05 would identify 500 genes as being differentially expressed in a microarray study examining 10,000 genes, even if none of the genes were actually differentially expressed. Typically, differentially expressed genes are identified based on a false discovery rate, which is an estimate of the expected proportion of false positives among the selected genes.[63]

Once a list of biomarkers is obtained, several tools are available for identifying common pathways and biological functions associated with the identified biomarkers. In general, each biomarker is assigned to one or more functional categories, for example, based on its Gene Ontology[64] or KEGG pathway assignment.[65] An enrichment analysis then identifies the functional categories overrepresented in the list of genes. A seminal paper in this area, which coined the method of gene set enrichment analysis (GSEA), performs the analysis on a ranked list of biomarkers.[66] Other functional annotation tools include the Database for Annotation, Visualization, and Integrated Discovery[67] and the Gene Ontology enRIchment anaLysis and visuaLizAtion tool (GORILLA).[68] Analyses such as GSEA identify biological pathways involved in tumorigenesis and potential drug targets. For example, a GSEA analysis identified the cell cycle pathway as being enriched in primary and metastatic melanomas compared with benign melanocytic nevi. The most differentially expressed gene in this pathway, polo-like kinase 1 (Plk-1), was found to be overexpressed in melanomas. Targeted knockdown of Plk-1 induces apoptosis in melanoma cell lines, establishing the potential of Plk-1 as a therapeutic target.[69]

In addition to identifying therapeutic targets, one can also identify previously screened compounds that are efficacious in patients with specific biomarker profiles. As described above, the NCI-60 human tumor cell line screen has produced information that can be mined to identify therapeutic agents with drug sensitivities that

TABLE 69-3 Selected Databases and Tools for Therapeutic Targeting and Drug Discovery

Category	Resource	Description	Online Reference
Cancer genome analysis	Catalogue of somatic mutations in cancer (COSMIC)	Database of cancer mutations (literature derived)	http://www.sanger.ac.uk/genetics/CGP/cosmic/
	The Cancer Genome Atlas	Database of cancer mutations (ex vivo derived)	http://cancergenome.nih.gov/
Gene expression analysis	Oncomine	Compendium of gene expression data with analysis tools	https://www.oncomine.org/resource/login.html
	Gene expression omnibus (GEO)	Repository of gene expression data with a curated data set browser and analysis tool. Hosted by NCBI	http://www.ncbi.nlm.nih.gov/geo/
	Array express	Gene expression database hosted by the European Bioinformatics Institute (EBI)	http://www.ebi.ac.uk/arrayexpress/
Functional analyses	Gene ontology (GO)	Controlled vocabulary of genes by biological process, function, and cellular component	http://www.geneontology.org/
	KEGG: Kyoto encyclopedia of genes and genomes	Systems-level organization of genes, including by pathway and disease association	http://www.genome.jp/kegg/
	Database for *A*nnotation, *V*isualization and *I*ntegrated *D*iscovery (DAVID)	Identifies enriched biological themes	http://david.abcc.ncifcrf.gov/
Drug sensitivity	NCI-60 Drug Therapeutic Program (DTP) Human Tumor Cell Line Screen and COMPARE	Drug sensitivities of >45,000 compounds and natural products in NCI-60 cancer cell line panel	http://dtp.nci.nih.gov/branches/btb/ivclsp.html
	Connectivity map	Database of gene expression profiles of perturbed cell lines	http://www.broadinstitute.org/cmap/

correlate with a biomarker or biomarkers of interest. The COMPARE algorithm automates this process when interest is in single biomarkers. The CMAP identifies compounds that target entire biomarker signatures by identifying compounds whose perturbation profiles correlate with a biomarker query.

TARGETED THERAPIES

Identifying the genomic alterations that drive the cancer phenotype is the basis for personalized medicine and this underlies current approaches to drug discovery and targeted therapy. A driver mutation results in the aberrant expression of gene products which become biomarkers for cancer cells and targets for therapy. The targeted therapy paradigm is based on the concept of *oncogene addiction*, the phenomenon by which cancer cells depend on the activity of a single gene for survival; inactivation of the gene results in cell death.[70] Conceptually, appropriate targeting of these aberrantly expressed gene products should efficaciously eliminate cancer cells while minimally injuring non–cancerous cells, thereby minimizing toxic risks for the patient. A large number of molecular targets have been identified, and many targeted agents have been FDA approved and are in routine clinical use (see Table 69.1). Importantly, these therapies serve as a proof of principle that targeted agents are an effective means of combating cancer.

Modern Examples of Targeted Therapies

One of the first modern examples of targeted therapy is the development of the kinase inhibitor imatinib mesylate (Gleevec), which targets a dysregulated ABL kinase in CML. Approximately 95% of CML cases contain a *Bcr–abl* fusion gene arising from a translocation between chromosomes 9 and 22 (the "Philadelphia chromosome"). The *Abl* gene encodes the tyrosine kinase ABL and the fusion protein has enhanced kinase activity that results in increased cell proliferation. The results from the first phase III clinical trial of imatinib mesylate were striking. After 18 months of treatment, 92% of patients receiving imatinib mesylate had no disease progression, compared with 73.5% of patients receiving conventional therapy. Patients in the latter group were therefore allowed to "cross over" to the imatinib mesylate treatment group. Following 5 years of treatment, the survival rate for patients receiving the targeted therapy was 89%, significantly better than previous therapies against CML.[71]

The success of imatinib mesylate has been attributed to the fact that *Bcr–abl* is present in nearly all CML patients, and in patients with this mutation the fusion gene is likely the sole oncogenic driver. However, many examples of targeted therapies validate the approach while also demonstrating the importance of proper patient selection, which matches a patient with the appropriate drug, based on relevant biomarkers. For example, trastuzumab (Herceptin) is a monoclonal antibody that targets HER-2, which is overexpressed in up to 34% of patients with invasive breast cancer. Trastuzumab has a response rate of only 10% at the population level, but a response rate of 35% to 50% when administered to individuals overexpressing HER-2.[59] Other examples of targeted therapies include gefitinib (Iressa), a small molecule EGFR inhibitor for non–small cell lung cancer, and vemurafenib (Zelboraf), which inhibits a specific BRAF mutant present in approximately 50% of melanoma patients.

Novel Approaches to Targeted Therapy

The examples above describe therapeutic targeting of protein products derived from mutated proto-oncogenes. However, approximately 10% of the known somatic mutations in cancer occur in tumor suppressor genes which are inactivated by mutation and therefore cannot be targeted directly. An alternative approach that indirectly targets tumor suppressor genes is based on the concept of *synthetic lethality*. Two genes are considered synthetic lethal if a cell can survive following mutation of either gene alone, but a mutation in both genes is fatal.[72] If two genes within a cell are synthetic lethal, and one of the genes is mutated in cancer, then targeted inactivation of the second gene will selectively kill the cancer cell while leaving non–cancer cells (which do not harbor the first mutation) unharmed.

Although the use of synthetic lethal screens for drug discovery is in its infancy, it is becoming apparent that several known drugs act through synthetic lethal mechanisms. For example, poly(ADP-ribose) polymerase (PARP) inhibitors, which are in clinical trials for several cancers, are synthetic lethal to the DNA repair genes BRCA1 and BRCA2, which are mutated in up to 10% of breast cancers and 15% of ovarian cancers. When PARP detects single-stranded DNA breaks, it functions as a signal for the recruitment of DNA repair proteins. Inhibition of PARP prevents single-stranded DNA break repair, which results in stalled replication forks that eventually experience double-stranded breaks. Without functional BRCA1 and BRCA2 genes, the cell's ability to repair double-stranded DNA breaks is compromised, and apoptosis results. Cancers with BRCA1 and BRCA2 mutations are therefore sensitive to PARP inhibition.[73]

Furthermore, a novel and conceptually robust framework for drug discovery and patient selection emerges from the molecular and bioinformatics technologies described above (Fig. 69.2).[74] First, a biomarker

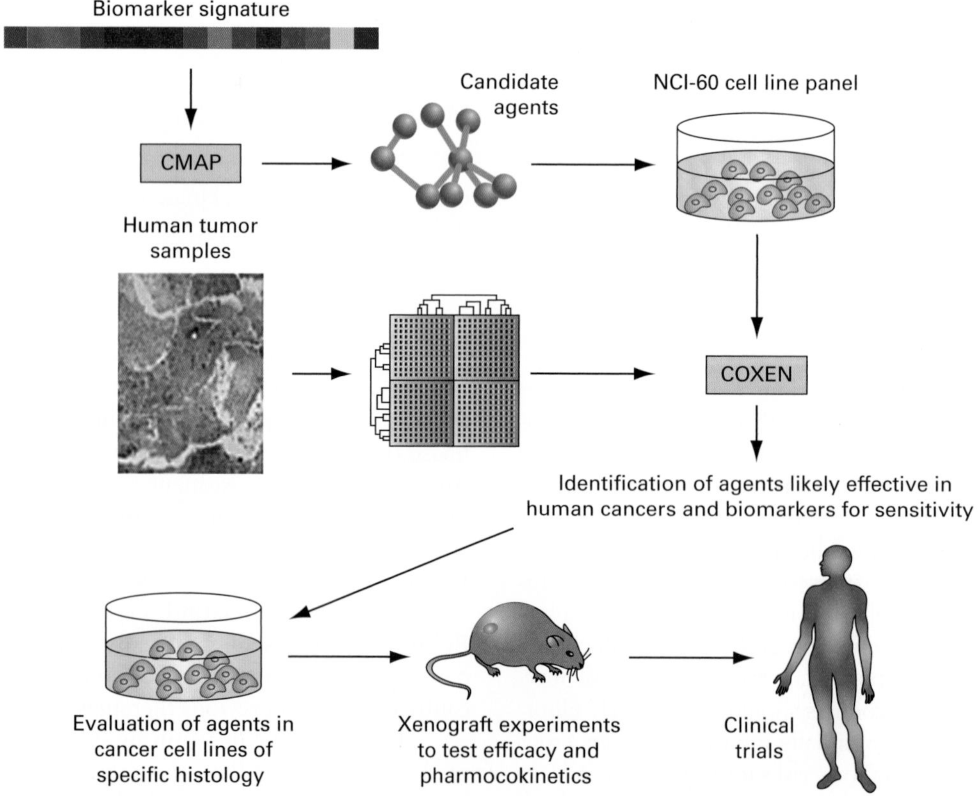

FIGURE 69–2 Novel integrated framework for drug discovery and patient selection using molecular and bioinformatics technologies. The connectivity map (CMAP) identifies candidate therapeutic agents that target a biomarker signature of interest. The COXEN system simultaneously identifies agents that are both efficacious in the NCI-60 cell line panel and likely efficacious in specific populations, and biomarkers predictive of in vivo therapeutic response. The integrated approach could increase the likelihood that targeted therapies succeed in clinical trials and gain FDA approval. (Modified from Smith SC, Theodorescu D. *Nat Rev Cancer*. 2009;9:253-264.)

signature is obtained for a patient population of interest. Second, the CMAP is used to identify candidate therapeutic agents that target the biomarker signature. Third, COXEN is used in conjunction with NCI-60 drug sensitivity data and molecular profiles from a relevant patient population to limit the candidate therapeutic agents to those that are efficacious in the NCI-60 cell line panel and, crucially, are likely to be efficacious in specific patient populations. For each candidate therapy, COXEN also identifies a biomarker signature predictive of patient response. Candidate drugs are then investigated in xenograft experiments and, if promising, analyzed in clinical trials. This integrated approach allows for side-by-side drug discovery and biomarker identification for patient selection and will increase the likelihood that targeted therapies will be successful in clinical trials and gain FDA approval.

In addition, the identification of therapeutic agents in this integrated manner, and the use of the COXEN system specifically, offers the important and intriguing possibility for drug discovery in situations where clinical trials are generally not feasible and current treatments are limited. For example, methods such as COXEN can be used to identify therapeutic compounds for rare "orphan" tumors, for patients who experience second- or third-line treatment failures, and individuals with cancers of unknown primary origin, based on their molecular profiles. COXEN also allows for the prediction of patient response to combination therapies based on in vitro single-agent drug sensitivities[75] and could presumably be used as a drug screening tool to identify novel combination therapies for patients. Before predictive technologies such as COXEN can be used in the clinic, however, important issues need to be addressed, such as what requirements are necessary for predictive technologies themselves to gain FDA approval and under what situations they may be used.

CURRENT CHALLENGES IN DRUG DISCOVERY

The large number of FDA-approved targeted therapies and the clinical benefit they provide are a testament to the targeted therapy paradigm and the clinical importance of understanding cancer at the molecular level. As biotechnologies continue to advance, and in particular as next-generation sequencing becomes cheaper, we expect to see a large increase in the number of targeted therapies as more and more driver mutations are identified. Despite the success stories, however, therapies seldom lead to complete remission of disease. This is due, in part, to an inability to properly select patients who will respond to targeted and conventional treatments, highlighting the importance of drug sensitivity biomarkers and diagnostics for patient selection. In addition, there remain important limitations in our clinical understanding of cancer biology as it relates to tumor heterogeneity, drug resistance, and metastasis. Tumor heterogeneity and genomic instability are a hallmark of cancer. Consequently, not all cells within a tumor may be sensitive to a particular therapeutic agent, and sensitive cells can escape their dependence on therapeutic targets. Furthermore, primary tumors and metastatic tumors can have different drug sensitivities.[76] Within a tumor, cancer stem cells may enter a dormant or quiescent state where they will be more resistant to chemotherapy. However, these quiescent cells can be targeted.[77] In general, combination therapy is a promising solution to some of these challenges.[78] Conceptually, rationally selected combinations of therapeutic agents will destroy the clonal populations of cells within a tumor that may be resistant to individual therapies, both quiescent and rapidly dividing cells, and primary and metastatic tumors that differ in their drug sensitivities. A major challenge moving forward, therefore, is to decipher tumor heterogeneity from molecular profiles in order to identify appropriate combination therapies.

REFERENCES

1. Schena M, Shalon D, Davis RW, et al. Quantitative monitoring of gene-expression patterns with a complementary-DNA microarray. *Science*. 1995;270:467-470.
2. DeRisi J, Penland L, Brown PO, et al. Use of a cDNA microarray to analyse gene expression patterns in human cancer. *Nat Genet*. 1996;14:457-460.
3. Golub TR, Slonim DK, Tamayo P, et al. Molecular classification of cancer: class discovery and class prediction by gene expression monitoring. *Science*. 1999;286:531-537.
4. Munker R, Calin GA. MicroRNA profiling in cancer. *Clin Sci*. 2011;121:141-158.
5. Lee RC, Feinbaum RL, Ambros V. The C-elegans heterochronic gene lin-4 encodes small RNAs with antisense complementarity to lin-14. *Cell*. 1993;75:843-854.
6. Chang TC, Wentzel EA, Kent OA, et al. Transactivation of miR-34a by p53 broadly influences gene expression and promotes apoptosis. *Mol Cell*. 2007;26:745-752.
7. Dyrskjot L, Ostenfeld MS, Bramsen JB, et al. Genomic profiling of microRNAs in bladder cancer: miR-129 is associated with poor outcome and promotes cell death in vitro. *Cancer Res*. 2009;69:4851-4860.
8. Iorio MV, Ferracin M, Liu CG, et al. MicroRNA gene expression deregulation in human breast cancer. *Cancer Res*. 2005;65:7065-7070.
9. Liotta LA, Espina V, Mehta AI, et al. Protein microarrays: meeting analytical challenges for clinical applications. *Cancer Cell*. 2003;3:317-325.
10. Kopf E, Zharhary D. Antibody arrays—an emerging tool in cancer proteomics. *Int J Biochem Cell Biol*. 2007;39:1305-1317.
11. Liotta LA, Paweletz CP, Charboneau L, et al. Reverse phase protein microarrays which capture disease progression show activation of pro-survival pathways at the cancer invasion front. *Oncogene*. 2001;20:1981-1989.
12. Petricoin EF, Wulfkuhle JD, Speer R, et al. Multiplexed cell signaling analysis of human breast cancer applications for personalized therapy. *J Proteome Res*. 2008;7:1508-1517.
13. Schuster SC. Next-generation sequencing transforms today's biology. *Nat Methods*. 2008;5:16-18.
14. Mardis ER. Next-generation DNA sequencing methods. *Annu Rev Genomics Hum Genet*. 2008;9:387-402.
15. Meyerson M, Gabriel S, Getz G. Advances in understanding cancer genomes through second-generation sequencing. *Nat Rev Genet*. 2010;11:685-696.
16. Ley TJ, Minx PJ, Walter MJ, et al. A pilot study of high-throughput, sequence-based mutational profiling of primary human acute myeloid leukemia cell genomes. *Proc Natl Acad Sci U S A*. 2003;100:14275-14280.
17. Mardis ER, Ley TJ, Ding L, et al. DNA sequencing of a cytogenetically normal acute myeloid leukaemia genome. *Nature*. 2008;456:66-72.

18. Berger MF, Lawrence MS, Demichelis F, et al. The genomic complexity of primary human prostate cancer. *Nature*. 2011;470:214-220.
19. Stephens PJ, McBride DJ, Lin ML, et al. Complex landscapes of somatic rearrangement in human breast cancer genomes. *Nature*. 2009;462:1005-1010.
20. Pleasance ED, Cheetham RK, Stephens PJ, et al. A comprehensive catalogue of somatic mutations from a human cancer genome. *Nature*. 2010;463:191-196.
21. Lee W, Jiang ZS, Liu JF, et al. The mutation spectrum revealed by paired genome sequences from a lung cancer patient. *Nature*. 2010;465:473-477.
22. Bartoszek A, Lewandowska J. DNA methylation in cancer development, diagnosis and therapy-multiple opportunities for genotoxic agents to act as methylome disruptors or remediators. *Mutagenesis*. 2011;26:475-487.
23. Laird PW. Principles and challenges of genome-wide DNA methylation analysis. *Nat Rev Genet*. 2010;11:191-203.
24. Hatada I, Fukasawa M, Kimura M, et al. Genome-wide profiling of promoter methylation in human. *Oncogene*. 2006;25:3059-3064.
25. Ehrlich M. DNA hypomethylation, cancer, the immunodeficiency, centromeric region instability, facial anomalies syndrome and chromosomal rearrangements. *J Nutr*. 2002;132:2424s-2429s.
26. Hsiao SH, Teng IW, Hou PC, et al. Targeted methylation of two tumor suppressor genes is sufficient to transform mesenchymal stem cells into cancer stem/initiating cells. *Cancer Res*. 2011;71:4653-4663.
27. Issa JPJ, Kantarjian HM, Kirkpatrick P. Azacitidine. *Nat Rev Drug Discov*. 2005;4:275-276.
28. Rots MG, van der Gun BTF, Maluszynska-Hoffman M, et al. Targeted DNA methylation by a DNA methyltransferase coupled to a triple helix forming oligonucleotide to down-regulate the epithelial cell adhesion molecule. *Bioconjug Chem*. 2010;21:1239-1245.
29. Lydon NB, Druker BJ. Lessons learned from the development of an Abl tyrosine kinase inhibitor for chronic myelogenous leukemia. *J Clin Invest*. 2000;105:3-7.
30. Hou J, Aerts J, den Hamer B, et al. Gene expression-based classification of non-small cell lung carcinomas and survival prediction. *PLoS One*. 2010;5:e10312.
31. Verhaak RG, Hoadley KA, Purdom E, et al. Integrated genomic analysis identifies clinically relevant subtypes of glioblastoma characterized by abnormalities in PDGFRA, IDH1, EGFR, and NF1. *Cancer Cell*. 2010;17:98-110.
32. Kao KJ, Chang KM, Hsu HC, et al. Correlation of microarray-based breast cancer molecular subtypes and clinical outcomes: implications for treatment optimization. *BMC Cancer*. 2011;11:143.
33. Brooks JD, Lapointe J, Li C, et al. Gene expression profiling identifies clinically relevant subtypes of prostate cancer. *Proc Natl Acad Sci U S A*. 2004;101:811-816.
34. Hoglund M, Lindgren D, Frigyesi A, et al. Combined gene expression and genomic profiling define two intrinsic molecular subtypes of urothelial carcinoma and gene signatures for molecular grading and outcome. *Cancer Res*. 2010;70:3463-3472.
35. Yousef GM, Youssef YM, White NMA, et al. Accurate molecular classification of kidney cancer subtypes using microRNA signature. *Eur Urol*. 2011;59:721-730.
36. Lackner MR, Boyd ZS, Wu QJ, et al. Proteomic analysis of breast cancer molecular subtypes and biomarkers of response to targeted kinase inhibitors using reverse-phase protein microarrays. *Mol Cancer Ther*. 2008;7:3695-3706.
37. Allison M. Is personalized medicine finally arriving? *Nat Biotechnol*. 2008;26:509-517.
38. Friend SH, van't Veer LJ, Dai HY, et al. Gene expression profiling predicts clinical outcome of breast cancer. *Nature*. 2002;415:530-536.
39. Theodorescu D, Smith SC, Baras AS, et al. A 20-gene model for molecular nodal staging of bladder cancer: development and prospective assessment. *Lancet Oncol*. 2011;12:137-143.
40. Kim J, Lee ES, Son DS, et al. Prediction of recurrence-free survival in postoperative non-small cell lung cancer patients by using an integrated model of clinical information and gene expression. *Clin Cancer Res*. 2008;14:7397-7404.
41. Aldea M, Clofent J, Nunez de Arenas C, et al. Reverse phase protein microarrays quantify and validate the bioenergetic signature as biomarker in colorectal cancer. *Cancer Lett*. 2011;311:210-218.
42. Kwak EL, Bang YJ, Camidge DR, et al. Anaplastic lymphoma kinase inhibition in non-small-cell lung cancer. *N Engl J Med*. 2010;363:1693-1703.
43. Gianni L, Zambetti M, Clark K, et al. Gene expression profiles in paraffin-embedded core biopsy tissue predict response to chemotherapy in women with locally advanced breast cancer. *J Clin Oncol*. 2005;23:7265-7277.
44. Zhu CQ. Prognostic and predictive gene signature for adjuvant chemotherapy in resected non-small-cell lung cancer. *J Clin Oncol*. 2010;28:4417-24.
45. Theodorescu D, Havaleshko DM, Smith SC, et al. Comparison of global versus epidermal growth factor receptor pathway profiling for prediction of lapatinib sensitivity in bladder cancer. *Neoplasia*. 2009;11:1185-U101.
46. Gulseth MP, Grice GR, Dager WE. Pharmacogenomics of warfarin: uncovering a piece of the warfarin mystery. *Am J Health-Syst Pharm*. 2009;66:123-133.
47. Watters JW, McLeod HL. Cancer pharmacogenomics: current and future applications. *Biochim Biophys Acta-Rev Cancer*. 2003;1603:99-111.
48. Cheok MH, Evans WE. Acute lymphoblastic leukaemia: a model for the pharmacogenomics of cancer therapy (vol 6, pg 117, 2006). *Nat Rev Cancer*. 2006;6:249-249.
49. Holbeck SL, Collins JM, Doroshow JH. Analysis of Food and Drug Administration-approved anticancer agents in the NCI60 panel of human tumor cell lines. *Mol Cancer Ther*. 2010;9:1451-1460.
50. Shoemaker RH. The NCI60 human tumour cell line anticancer drug screen. *Nat Rev Cancer*. 2006;6:813-823.
51. Paull KD, Shoemaker RH, Hodes L, et al. Display and analysis of patterns of differential activity of drugs against human tumor cell lines: development of mean graph and COMPARE algorithm. *J Natl Cancer Inst*. 1989;81:1088-1092.
52. Bai R, Paull KD, Herald CL, et al. Halichondrin-B and homohalichondrin-B, marine natural-products binding in the vinca domain of tubulin—discovery of tubulin-based mechanism of action by analysis of differential cytotoxicity data. *J Biol Chem*. 1991;266:15882-15889.
53. Lamb J, Crawford ED, Peck D, et al. The connectivity map: using gene-expression signatures to connect small molecules, genes, and disease. *Science*. 2006;313:1929-1935.
54. Wei G, Twomey D, Lamb J, et al. Gene expression-based chemical genomics identifies rapamycin as a modulator of MCL1 and glucocorticoid resistance. *Cancer Cell*. 2006;10:331-342.
55. Smith SC, Baras AS, Lee JK, et al. The COXEN principle: translating signatures of in vitro chemosensitivity into tools for clinical outcome prediction and drug discovery in cancer. *Cancer Res*. 2010;70:1753-1758.
56. Lee JK, Havaleshko DM, Cho HJ, et al. A strategy for predicting the chemosensitivity of human cancers and its application to drug discovery. *Proc Natl Acad Sci U S A*. 2007;104:13086-13091.
57. Williams PD, Cheon S, Havaleshko DM, et al. Concordant gene expression signatures predict clinical outcomes of cancer patients undergoing systemic therapy. *Cancer Res*. 2009;69:8302-8309.
58. Bild AH, Potti A, Nevins JR. Linking oncogenic pathways with therapeutic opportunities. *Nat Rev Cancer*. 2006;6:735-U13.
59. Vogel CL, Cobleigh MA, Tripathy D, et al. Efficacy and safety of trastuzumab as a single agent in first-line treatment of HER2-overexpressing metastatic breast cancer. *J Clin Oncol*. 2002;20:719-726.
60. Mitsudomi T, Kosaka T, Endoh H, et al. Mutations of the epidermal growth factor receptor gene predict prolonged survival after gefitinib treatment in patients with non-small-cell lung cancer with postoperative recurrence. *J Clin Oncol*. 2005;23:2513-2520.
61. Smyth GK. Linear models and empirical Bayes methods for assessing differential expression in microarray experiments. *Stat Appl Genet Mol Biol*. 2004;3:Article 3.
62. Chu G, Tusher VG, Tibshirani R. Significance analysis of microarrays applied to the ionizing radiation response. *Proc Natl Acad Sci U S A*. 2001;98:5116-5121.
63. Benjamini Y, Yekutieli D. The control of the false discovery rate in multiple testing under dependency. *Ann Stat*. 2001;29:1165-1188.
64. Botstein D, Ashburner M, Ball CA, et al. Gene ontology: tool for the unification of biology. *Nat Genet*. 2000;25:25-29.

65. Kanehisa M, Ogata H, Goto S, et al. KEGG: Kyoto encyclopedia of genes and genomes. *Nucleic Acids Res*. 1999;27:29-34.
66. Lander ES, Subramanian A, Tamayo P, et al. Gene set enrichment analysis: a knowledge-based approach for interpreting genome-wide expression profiles. *Proc Natl Acad Sci U S A*. 2005;102:15545-15550.
67. Huang DW, Sherman BT, Lempicki RA. Systematic and integrative analysis of large gene lists using DAVID bioinformatics resources. *Nat Protoc*. 2009;4:44-57.
68. Eden E, Navon R, Steinfeld I, et al. GOrilla: a tool for discovery and visualization of enriched GO terms in ranked gene lists. *BMC Bioinformatics*. 2009;10:48.
69. Jalili A, Moser A, Pashenkov M, et al. Polo-like kinase 1 is a potential therapeutic target in human melanoma. *J Invest Dermatol*. 2011;131:1886-1895.
70. Weinstein IB, Joe A. Oncogene addiction. *Cancer Res*. 2008;68: 3077-3080; discussion 3080.
71. Druker BJ, Guilhot F, O'Brien SG, et al. Five-year follow-up of patients receiving imatinib for chronic myeloid leukemia. *N Engl J Med*. 2006;355:2408-2417.
72. Kaelin WG. The concept of synthetic lethality in the context of anticancer therapy. *Nat RevCancer*. 2005;5:689-698.
73. Ashworth A. A synthetic lethal therapeutic approach: poly(ADP) ribose polymerase inhibitors for the treatment of cancers deficient in DNA double-strand break repair. *J Clin Oncol*. 2008;26:3785-3790.
74. Smith SC, Theodorescu D. Learning therapeutic lessons from metastasis suppressor proteins. *Nat Rev Cancer*. 2009;9:253-264.
75. Havaleshko DM, Cho H, Conaway M, et al. Prediction of drug combination chemosensitivity in human bladder cancer. *Mol Cancer Ther*. 2007;6:578-586.
76. Maniwa Y, Yoshimura M, Hashimoto S, et al. Chemosensitivity of lung cancer: differences between the primary lesion and lymph node metastasis. *Oncol Lett*. 2010;1:345-349.
77. Ito K, Bernardi R, Morotti A, et al. PML targeting eradicates quiescent leukaemia-initiating cells. *Nature*. 2008;453: 1072-1078.
78. Loeb LA. Human cancers express mutator phenotypes: origin, consequences and targeting. *Nat Rev Cancer*. 2011;11:450-457.

CHAPTER 70

The Future of Molecular Diagnostics in Oncology

Michael C. Dugan and Dongfeng Tan

Although the future of molecular diagnostics is likely to be shaped by current trends and technologies, this field is evolving rapidly in ways that we can hardly predict with accuracy beyond a few years. One certainty is that the use of molecular diagnostics will become far more routinely established in clinical practice. This will be particularly true for tests using technologies or platforms that have established robust performance characteristics identifying molecular alterations directly paired with targeted therapeutics forming companion diagnostics. We can forecast the changing landscape in terms of evolving newer techniques or methods, paradigm shifts in the use of targeted therapies and companion diagnostics, and other ancillary viewpoints such as how enhancing the assessment of quality, clinical utility, and health economic effects may bear upon decisions related to clinical practice guidelines, regulatory approval, and reimbursement for these tests. From each of these perspectives, a broader view of novel molecular therapeutics emerges in which we are continually adapting new technology, improving clinical utility, and evaluating costs versus benefits for the patient, laboratory, and healthcare systems.

EVOLVING TARGETS AND TECHNIQUES IN CANCER DIAGNOSTICS

Molecular diagnostic assays in oncology have expanded rapidly in the last decade following the earlier development of diagnostic assays based on immunohistochemistry (IHC), cytogenetics, flow cytometry, fluorescent in situ hybridization (FISH), polymerase chain reaction (PCR), and more recently reverse transcriptase PCR, quantitative real-time PCR, dideoxy (Sanger) sequencing, and other techniques.[1-5] Many of these techniques have been incorporated into assays that are routinely ordered in the workup of various hematolymphoid disorders and some solid tumors. In many cases, they are used to determine prognosis, monitor response to treatment, identify recurrence, and for other purposes.[6-9] Newer technologies such as massively parallel next-generation sequencing, competitive genomic hybridization single-nucleotide polymorphism (SNP) arrays, methylation or gene expression assays, microRNA expression levels, and mass spectrometry–based proteomic analysis offer tantalizing glimpses into what might be used in future diagnostic assays and what challenges these tools might present.[10-16]

Examples of novel applications today include dual in situ hybridization assays for HER2 that merge chromogenic in situ hybridization with IHC to better identify gene amplification and genetic heterogeneity in breast, gastric, and ovarian carcinomas and help avoid false-negative results on small biopsies.[17-19] High-resolution SNP arrays pinpoint copy number changes such as small deletions or gains as well as features of allelic imbalance (loss of heterozygosity [LOH]) or uniparental disomy associated with Beckwith-Wiedemann syndrome and cancer predisposition.[20-24]

Both FISH and SNP arrays can detect chromosomal alterations not visible by conventional karyotyping. They have also been used to identify the origins of chromosomal fragments such as double minutes, homozygous staining regions, and others, which can provide clues to gene amplification or deletion that are important to tumorigenesis and tumor behavior.[12,25] SNP arrays have identified deleted tumor-suppressor or regulatory genes associated with aggressive forms of hepatocellular carcinoma and genes associated with key oncologic drivers such as MYCN amplification.[26,27] They have also been used to distinguish neoplasms that are morphologically similar but have different prognoses (e.g., renal tumors or brain tumors) or to distinguish tumor from reactive tissue as in the case of glioma versus gliosis.[28,31] A significant topic of interest for SNP microarrays is small copy number variations, which are common but may have no known or established clinical relevance.[32,33] Interpreting such findings requires considerable experience to put them into proper context.

SEQUENCING THE CANCER GENOME

Dideoxy (Sanger) sequencing was initially introduced into the clinical laboratory for the determination of HIV genotypes associated with drug resistance. More recently, Sanger sequencing has become commonly used for the determination of epidermal growth factor receptor (*EGFR*) mutations, *KRAS* mutations, and other single base pair substitutions and frameshift deletions, such as those responsible for the loss of p53 function in Li-Fraumeni syndrome–related sarcomas.[34] However, major limitations of Sanger sequencing relate to sensitivity in detecting minority allelic variants, and there is a possible error of interpretation requiring a high degree of training and experience for the proper use of this technique.[35]

Massively parallel high-throughput pyrosequencing (454 sequencing) and bead-based microarrays have proven to be highly accurate, sensitive, and reproducible methods that create opportunities to perform high-resolution DNA analysis, to evaluate gene expression and methylation, to analyze exome sequences, and to sequence very complex and polymorphic gene structures such as human leukocyte antigen (HLA).[10,11] High-throughput sequencing also provides a powerful way to evaluate amplified disease-specific regions from mononuclear cell subclones to quantify minimal residual chronic lymphocytic leukemia after therapy.[36]

Various direct gene sequencing assays have generated a paradox similar to that for SNP microarrays: is the information gained useful or is it unnecessary information that may be misleading or without benefit? Despite promises of a new era of personalized medicine based on whole-genome sequencing, there are lingering concerns about how to generate truly useful clinically "actionable" reports with such techniques based on the results of "expected" potential mutations and "unexpected" genetic abnormalities. In the cancer genome, passenger alterations may vastly outnumber the driver events, leading to considerable confusion at best and to unnecessary worry and concern for patients or liability for physicians at worst.

Most of these neoplastic genetic changes are somatic, but answers to uncertainties about inherited colon cancer, prostate cancer, and breast cancer risk will also lie in better understanding of germline variations. Individualized care of patients will rely on the use of high-throughput sequencing to initially identify panels of known target genes in both normal and cancer cells, followed by advanced bioinformatics to rapidly evaluate small changes or SNPs and compare them with established clinical laboratory databases, similar to what is currently practiced in HIV genotyping, but vastly expanded with the use of genome-wide association studies (GWAS).[37-39] These relational databases of genomic information will grow substantially over the next decade. As disease markers and their associations are refined, management of patient care and outcomes will improve. These technologies introduce new levels of data complexity and cost that will have to be optimized to bring them into routine use in the clinical laboratory.

COMBINING TECHNOLOGIES IN ONCOLOGY REPORTING

Despite rapid advances, it remains likely that traditional and novel diagnostics will be combined and used in a complementary way for the foreseeable future. Hematopathology reports currently feature morphologic descriptions, flow cytometry, cytogenetics, and molecular genetics on a single summary report. We can imagine future oncology reports combining many different DNA targets and assay modalities. For instance, PathFinderTG integrates LOH analysis near tumor-suppressor genes, KRAS mutations, cytology, DNA quantity and quality, and protein markers to identify pancreatic cysts as mucinous or non-mucinous and to evaluate the risk of malignancy.[40] Reports can or soon could also define hepatitis B virus (HBV) mutants (HBx) associated with hepatocellular carcinoma, HLA subtypes associated with ovarian cancer prognosis, and human papillomavirus genotypes associated with highest risk of cervical cancer, among others.[41-44] Imagine a report predicting recurrence of HBV-related hepatocellular carcinoma after liver transplant based on evaluation of plasma DNA for allelic variants matched to the original tumor DNA. This has already been described using matrix-assisted laser desorption ionization–time of flight mass spectrometry (on plasma DNA) paired with SNP microarray profiling of tumor DNA extracted from formalin-fixed, paraffin-embedded (FFPE) tissues.[14]

FROM TISSUE TO BLOOD

Various diagnostic needs require the use of many sample types: nasal, cervical, and buccal mucosal swabs; fine needle aspiration cytology; liquid-based cytology media (for cervical cancer screening); and FFPE tissue.[45] Whereas infectious or germline disorder assays are usually performed using fresh tissue DNA sources such as whole-blood lymphocytes, the vast majority of oncology-related defects are acquired or somatic changes seen only in tumor cells. For laboratories, this presents challenges as they need to work with FFPE or limited sample sizes of rather precious tumor procured from computed tomography–guided needle biopsies, aspirates, and other techniques.[45,46] One approach to minimize tissue requirements has been to use laser microdissection to isolate cancer cells of interest from surrounding stroma and non-neoplastic cells in order to perform a molecular cancer classifier based on real-time PCR for expression of 92 genes.[47] With this technique, as few as 300 to 500 cells from a single tissue section can provide as much information as a large battery of immunohistochemistry stains requiring a dozen or more tissue sections.[47] More recent whole-genome amplification techniques such as multiple displacement amplification have enabled genomic characterization of single cells from early-stage embryos for preimplantation genetic diagnosis of fragile X syndrome and other disorders, prefacing techniques aimed at the cancer genome using very limited sample sources such as circulating DNA or tumor cells.[48]

With innovative technologies and continuing improvements, the molecular diagnosis of cancer will perhaps become routine like many blood tests. Larger high-throughput instruments with integrated software and optimized reagents will reduce laborious steps, run failures, and report variations, driving "costs per test" lower over time. At the opposite end of the spectrum, point-of-care testing (POCT) has the potential to reduce turnaround time and eliminate some of the preanalytic costs such as sample packaging, handling, and shipping.[49-51] POCT devices today can assay a few analytes in a short period of time, usually within an hour, and recent advances in lab-on-a-chip technologies could make POCT for nucleic acids practical in settings such as the physician office clinic or even a patient's home.[50,52] These uses and necessary performance characteristics are still to be fully defined but might first encompass recurrence monitoring for established malignancies (e.g., restaging) or other targeted clinical applications.

Determining whether a specific molecular drug target is present in metastatic tumor cells could influence future cancer care and have predictive value; however, it has yet to be established whether molecular analysis of circulating tumor cells (CTCs) or circulating cell-free tumor DNA would predict drug response more accurately than analysis of a primary tumor biopsy specimen. Monitoring genetic variation over time is a potential application. Illustrating this point, there are reports of HER2-positive CTCs in patients with a HER2-negative primary tumor, which might affect the selection of trastuzumab (Herceptin) in advanced disease.[53] There are also descriptions of discordant *PIK3CA* mutations in metastatic breast cancer; *EGFR* mutations detected in plasma DNA; *BRAF* mutations found in circulating melanoma cells; and ERG, androgen receptor, and *PTEN* alterations found in circulating prostate cancer cells in patients nonresponsive to castration.[54-58] Whether or not treatment is initiated or changed with this information, such assays have potential value as a noninvasive means of identifying and confirming recurrent or metastatic disease when biopsy is not possible.

COMPANION DIAGNOSTICS: PREDICTING RESPONSE TO SPECIFIC THERAPIES

The last few years have seen growing recognition that nearly all future therapeutic targets will derive from specific molecular defects that can be identified with companion diagnostic tests, predicting response to those therapies. Pathologists and other diagnostic experts recognize that it is no longer sufficient to classify tumors as to origin and subtype. Today we must consider a plethora of commonly altered epithelial membrane receptors, cell cycle regulatory proteins, signal transaction pathways, and non-random chromosomal alterations. In nearly all tumors, deletions, gains, inversions, translocations, and mutations affecting key cellular components and pathways are driving oncogenesis. Understanding these pathway alterations has become critical to novel pharmaceutical development and will soon become our major diagnostic focus.

Following notable examples such as HER2, bcr-abl, and PML/RARA, in 2008, key evidence from several studies presented at the American Society of Clinical Oncology (ASCO) showed that resistance to cetuximab therapy in metastatic colorectal cancer could be predicted by the presence of activating *KRAS* mutations. These mutations have been identified in codons 12, 13, and 61 in varying frequencies, leading to important differences between tumors and between methods for *KRAS* assays.[59-63] In the last few years, several other single-gene targets in non–small cell lung cancer (NSCLC—*EGFR*, *ALK*) and malignant melanoma (*BRAF*) have become important companion diagnostic targets, with results of assays closely linked to success or failure of particular targeted therapies.[64-67] More recent clinical trials for established targeted therapies, initially used for relapsed or refractory metastatic disease, are demonstrating their value as first-line agents, such as erlotinib (Tarceva) in *EGFR*-mutated NSCLC.[68] Furthermore, well-established assays such as HER2 have found expanded use in advanced gastric and GE junctional adenocarcinoma to predict response to targeted therapy with trastuzumab (Herceptin).[18,69] Hundreds of compounds are now being investigated in various preclinical and clinical trials, most of them in conjunction with a molecular diagnostic assay for a specific target.

Studies of multiple genes in panels, such as Genomic Health's Oncotype Dx, have been evaluated in relation to breast cancer for prognostic and predictive use in making decisions about chemotherapy or in relation to stage II colon cancer where such a panel was shown to be prognostic (for recurrence risk) but not predictive of chemotherapy benefit.[70-73] For some patient populations, germline rather than somatic defects have been evaluated to identify patients predisposed to cancer or more likely to respond to a particular cancer therapy. Examples include the evaluation of mismatch repair protein defects (microsatellite instability high or MSI-H) in suspected hereditary nonpolyposis colorectal cancer (or Lynch syndrome), germline p53 defects (Li-Fraumeni syndrome), hereditary medullary thyroid cancer, and *BRCA1/BRCA2* for breast cancer and ovarian cancer patients and their families.[74-78] Of note, MSI-H colorectal cancer, which can occur in either inherited or sporadic forms, has been characterized as clinically and genetically distinct from other forms of colorectal cancer with chromosome instability or microsatellite and chromosome stability.[75] MSI-H colorectal cancer shows better stage-specific prognosis despite a propensity to less well-differentiated subtypes, higher stage at diagnosis, and lack of 5-fluorouracil monotherapy benefit compared with microsatellite-stable tumors.[75-77] *BRCA1/2* mutation carriers with ovarian carcinoma frequently show durable responses to PEGylated liposomal doxorubicin (Doxil) and poly(ADP)-ribose polymerase inhibitor therapy owing to defective homologous recombination DNA repair.[78,79]

TARGET PROFILES: MOLECULAR TESTING IN AN INFORMATION AGE

The versatility of gene sequencing has offered a broader glimpse of SNPs and other small molecular changes (indels) associated with cancer risk, treatment sensitivity or resistance, and identification of genes not previously known to be associated with cancer. New techniques such as allele-specific PCR, high-resolution melting curve analysis, and high-throughput next-generation sequencing (e.g., 454 sequencing) not only have been used to determine the status of *EGFR*, *KRAS*, and *BRAF* genes (for example, as a reference method for a targeted PCR assay) but can also simultaneously evaluate multiple gene targets for tumor profiling.[59-62,80] Increasingly, attention in clinical research has turned from single targets as first-line choices to entire signal transduction pathways, profiling large numbers of potential targets and assessing molecular pathways in terms of likely pharmacological response or resistance to various agents. Combination therapies in clinical trials are looking to overcome pathways of pharmacological resistance, similar to current triple therapy approaches to HIV infection.[81,82]

In such a treatment paradigm, the value of molecular diagnostics has significantly increased and a premium is placed on diagnostic accuracy and turnaround time. Until recently, the high cost of certain molecular assays and other conventional cytogenetic or FISH techniques favored the use of a sequential algorithmic approach. As targeted therapies move from being used primarily in the metastatic setting into a more prominent role as first-line adjuvant therapies, similar to the role for trastuzumab (Herceptin), the assays will also evolve from ancillary or adjunct tests into a more prominent role as an essential part of the initial diagnostic workup.[83] In this role, the expense of molecular assays is offset by the clinical advantage of more effective therapeutic choice, reduced complications, and collectively reduced pharmaceutical and medical care expenses.

Piloting such a personalized medicine approach, Dr. Daniel Von Hoff of the Translational Genomics Research Institute (TGen) in Phoenix, Arizona, has used advanced diagnostic test panels in oncology trials and clinical practice, while colleagues at the University of Texas MD Anderson Cancer Center in Houston, Texas, have established complex diagnostic panels as part of a treatment triage strategy for clinical trial selection in the BATTLE program.[84,85] Other centers around the world have quickly moved to establish similar studies using molecular diagnostic tests to qualify patients for various trials. In this research setting, unique or novel assays such as high-throughput sequencing can be used, but for most patients once a histologic diagnosis of malignancy is established, the use of specific in vitro diagnostic tests proven to be predictive of response to a particular agent is required for optimizing safety and efficacy and for reducing unnecessary complications or expenses related to noneffective therapy choices.[86,87]

ESTABLISHING SAFETY AND EFFICACY

Wide use of a targeted therapeutic for any malignancy brings considerable need for standardization and optimization of patient selection to ensure safety and efficacy of the therapy. Even small variations in a large tested group can affect many hundreds or thousands of patients.[88] It is important to recognize the value that laboratories have added in developing tests to meet investigational needs or novel and evolving clinical needs. Laboratories have a certain degree of flexibility and response time that an assay or instrument manufacturer does not have. Development of biological therapies and companion diagnostics has matured considerably, however. Rather than a post hoc approach, pharmaceutical development requires standardization of method(s) and quality assurance measures in very early phases, so that the clinical utility of a companion diagnostic can be well established in later phase III and postlaunch phase IV clinical trials.

For *KRAS* and *EGFR* mutation analyses, several testing methods are available but significant differences exist in the limit of detection (sensitivity), mutation coverage, or demonstrated clinical utility.[59,62] Different results may also occur due to tumor sampling, operator training, operator experience, and interpretation for certain methods such as FISH or Sanger sequencing that introduce additional variables. Examples from tests such as BRAF, HER2, and ER/PR testing have demonstrated that as many as 10% to 40% of patients could receive the wrong therapy due to variation in test selection or performance.[86,88-90]

In response to concerns about breast cancer markers, the College of American Pathologists (CAP) and ASCO have worked to establish guidelines for preanalytic handling, testing, and reporting of estrogen receptor, progesterone receptor, and HER2 (gene and protein).[89,90] CAP guidelines for NSCLC specimen handling for *EGFR* and *ALK* testing are currently being drafted. The U.S. Food and Drug Administration (FDA) has established draft guidelines for in vitro companion diagnostics considering more broadly both analytical and clinical validation requirements.[91] For a large number of companion diagnostic tests, this is a work in progress, but CAP has significantly improved its proficiency testing surveys and laboratory accreditation program and developed advanced pathology training programs concerned with these topics (www.cap.org).

In August 2011, the FDA approved a companion diagnostic test, the cobas 4800 *BRAF* V600 Mutation Test, concurrent with the approval of the first-in-class selective BRAF inhibitor, vemurafenib (Zelboraf), for the treatment of *BRAF*^{V600E}-mutant metastatic melanoma.[92] This fast-tracked approval was based on pivotal data from a 675-patient phase III trial (BRIM3)[93] following very promising therapeutic response and safety observed in the more limited phase I and phase II (BRIM2) trials.[94,95] A companion diagnostic test for *ALK* translocations selecting NSCLC patients eligible for crizotinib was approved less than 2 weeks later on the basis of similarly promising results of a targeted therapy.[96] Although difficult to design and execute for such a large clinical study, a disciplined evidence-based approach provides essential details about the potential safety and efficacy of a novel therapy and its companion diagnostic test. With such large investments and high stakes, a complication of therapy anecdotally encountered could derail plans for use of the product. Clinical data derived from controlled studies put complications and outcomes in context and allow a relative risk versus benefit assessment. The trials leading to approval of the Roche cobas BRAF test and Abbott Vysis ALK test are prototypic examples of how companion diagnostics will be evaluated by public health agencies, regulatory agencies, and healthcare plans (payers) for years to come.[97]

ESTABLISHING REIMBURSEMENT FOR CONTINUED IMPROVEMENT

A maturing field highlights the need for appropriate reimbursement for established tests to encourage and maintain continued development and quality improvement at all levels. Novel molecular assays require significant technical and financial investment starting years before the introduction of the test. Cooperation is needed amongst all stakeholders, including national health plans (such as Medicare and the National Health Service), commercial diagnostic test manufacturers, pharmaceutical companies, noncommercial agencies, and academic institutions, to ensure future access to new diagnostic products.[98]

Laboratories in the United States have historically enjoyed considerable leeway in reimbursement due to a system of method or common procedure terminology–based codes (CPT codes), but this has not been of much use in properly valuing companion diagnostics. New molecular CPT codes may partially address this issue but at the risk of simplifying reimbursement to the lowest common denominator, such as a test name, independent of considerations of method, safety, or efficacy. Inadequate reimbursement for molecular testing services stifles quality improvement efforts for existing tests and may severely limit investment in new tests. This could negatively affect patient access to personalized therapies and raise the costs of providing the most effective tests and therapies to patients likely to benefit. In the future, we may have to more carefully distinguish companion diagnostic tests and consider alternate codes for established tests with proven efficacy versus generic tests for which the benefit or predictive value for selecting therapy is less well established. This is a subject of current and likely future consideration as advances in molecular oncology diagnostics continue.

THE PATH FORWARD

Cancer is a molecularly heterogeneous disease. Recent studies have shown the importance of clonal evolution in tumor progression and development of metastasis.[98,99] No doubt, comprehensive genome-wide efforts to catalog somatically altered pathways will improve our understanding of the molecular cancer genetics and will identify novel potential therapeutic targets.

One recent study of the Cancer Genome Atlas Network analyzed 825 primary breast cancers and integrated information across six platforms, namely exome sequencing, DNA methylation, genomic DNA copy number arrays, messenger RNA arrays, microRNA sequencing, and reverse-phase protein arrays.[100] The study provided key insights into previously defined gene expression subtypes and demonstrated the existence of four main breast cancer classes, each of which displays significant molecular heterogeneity. Only three somatic mutations (TP53, PIK3CA, and GATA3) occurred at >10% incidence across all breast cancers, while there were numerous less frequent subtype-associated and novel gene mutations in all breast cancer subtypes, indicating a number of potential therapeutic opportunities.[100] Similarly, an integrated analysis of the genome and transcriptome of deep sequencing of somatic mutations in lung cancers revealed that lung adenocarcinoma often consists of founder clone and subclonal populations, which contain novel point mutations and novel fusions that are possibly targetable for therapy.[99]

Clearly, future studies will need to focus on cancer therapeutics affecting critical genes or key pathways not only in the dominant clone but also in the subclones. Current therapies that focus mainly on the dominant clones would unlikely produce lasting remission or cure in advanced cancer unless dominant genetic alterations in the founder clone as well as emerging secondary clones are targeted specifically for therapy. A systematic approach to procure tumor samples-not only at the time of diagnosis but also serially at the times of relapse to chronicle the dynamic clonal evolution that occurs over time-is essential to make major breakthroughs in personalized cancer therapy.[99]

Advances in molecular oncology diagnostics promise many new avenues for future care improvement, some of which likely will remain investigational, while others may become well-established standards of care. Realizing the dream of targeted therapies and companion diagnostics in oncology will require a concerted long-term effort by commercial manufacturers, healthcare providers, federal agencies, professional societies, and academic institutions to achieve objective improvements in care. These parties have a shared interest in working together to advance the quality of care for unmet medical needs. Recognizing valuable contributions of each party is essential to building dialogue and forming strategies that will pave the way for the future development of effective molecular diagnostic assays.

REFERENCES

1. Montillo M, Schinkoethe T, Elter T. Eradication of minimal residual disease with alemtuzumab in B-cell chronic lymphocytic leukemia (B-CLL) patients: the need for a standard method of detection and the potential impact of bone marrow clearance on disease outcome. *Cancer Invest.* 2005;23(6):488-496.
2. Rudzki Z, Sacha T, Stój A, et al. The gain-of-function JAK2 V617F mutation shifts the phenotype of essential thrombocythemia and chronic idiopathic myelofibrosis to more "erythremic" and less "thrombocythemic": a molecular, histologic, and clinical study. *Int J Hematol.* August 2007;86(2):130-136.
3. Luthra R, Sanchez-Vega B, Medeiros LJ. TaqMan RT-PCR assay coupled with capillary electrophoresis for quantification and identification of bcr-abl transcript type. *Mod Pathol.* January 2004;17(1):96-103.
4. Polampalli S, Choughule A, Prabhash K, et al. Role of RT-PCR and FISH in diagnosis and monitoring of acute promyelocytic leukemia. *Indian J Cancer.* January-March 2011;48(1):60-67.
5. Tubbs RR, Hicks DG, Cook J, et al. Fluorescence in situ hybridization (FISH) as primary methodology for the assessment of HER2 status in adenocarcinoma of the breast: a single institution experience. *Diagn Mol Pathol.* December 2007;16(4):207-210.
6. Morris CM. Chronic myeloid leukemia: cytogenetic methods and applications for diagnosis and treatment. *Methods Mol Biol.* 2011;730:33-61.
7. Tam CS, Shanafelt TD, Wierda WG, et al. De novo deletion 17p13.1 chronic lymphocytic leukemia shows significant clinical heterogeneity: the M. D. Anderson and Mayo Clinic experience. *Blood.* July 2009;114(5):957-964. [Epub May 4, 2009]
8. Zenz T, Benner A, Döhner H, Stilgenbauer S. Chronic lymphocytic leukemia and treatment resistance in cancer: the role of the p53 pathway. *Cell Cycle.* December 2008;7(24):3810-3814. [Epub December 21, 2008]
9. Fritsche HM, Burger M, Dietmaier W, et al. Multicolor FISH (UroVysion) facilitates follow-up of patients with high-grade urothelial carcinoma of the bladder. *Am J Clin Pathol.* October 2010;134(4):597-603.
10. Su Z, Ning B, Fang H, et al. Next-generation sequencing and its applications in molecular diagnostics. *Expert Rev Mol Diagn.* April 2011;11(3):333-343.
11. Fan JB, Hu S, Craumer W, Barker D. BeadArray-based solutions for enabling the promise of pharmacogenomics. *Biotechniques.* October 2005;39(10 suppl):S583-S588.
12. Shao L, Kang SH, Li J, et al. Array comparative genomic hybridization detects chromosomal abnormalities in hematological cancers that are not detected by conventional cytogenetics. *J Mol Diagn.* September 2010;12(5):670-679. [Epub August 19, 2010]
13. Miyake T, Nakayama T, Naoi Y, et al. GSTP1 expression predicts poor pathological complete response to neoadjuvant chemotherapy in ER-negative breast cancer. *Cancer Sci.* February 2012. doi:10.1111/j.1349-7006.2012.02231.x. [Epub ahead of print]
14. Hu J, Wang Z, Fan J, et al. Genetic variations in plasma circulating DNA of HBV-related hepatocellular carcinoma patients predict recurrence after liver transplantation. *PLoS One.* 2011;6(10):e26003. [Epub October 5, 2011]
15. Zen K, Zhang CY. Circulating microRNAs: a novel class of biomarkers to diagnose and monitor human cancers. *Med Res Rev.* March 2012;32(2):326-348. doi:10.1002/med.20215. [Epub November 9, 2010]
16. van Schooneveld E, Wouters MC, Van der Auwera I, et al. Expression profiling of cancerous and normal breast tissues identifies microRNAs that are differentially expressed in serum from patients with (metastatic) breast cancer and healthy volunteers. *Breast Cancer Res.* February 2012;14(1):R34. [Epub ahead of print]
17. Koh YW, Lee HJ, Lee JW, et al. Dual-color silver-enhanced in situ hybridization for assessing HER2 gene amplification in breast cancer. *Mod Pathol.* June 2011;24(6):794-800. [Epub February 11, 2011]
18. Yan B, Yau EX, Choo SN, et al. Dual-colour HER2/chromosome 17 chromogenic in situ hybridisation assay enables accurate assessment of HER2 genomic status in gastric cancer and has potential utility in HER2 testing of biopsy samples. *J Clin Pathol.* October 2011;64(10):880-883. [Epub July 14, 2011]
19. Yan B, Choo SN, Mulyadi P, et al. Dual-colour HER2/chromosome 17 chromogenic in situ hybridisation enables accurate assessment of HER2 genomic status in ovarian tumours. *J Clin Pathol.* December 2011;64(12):1097-1101. [Epub September 6, 2011]
20. Schaaf CP, Wiszniewska J, Beaudet AL. Copy number and SNP arrays in clinical diagnostics. *Annu Rev Genomics Hum Genet.* September 2011;12:25-51.
21. van Essen HF, Ylstra B. High-resolution copy number profiling by array CGH using DNA isolated from formalin-fixed, paraffin-embedded tissues. *Methods Mol Biol.* 2012;838:329-341.
22. Tuna M, Knuutila S, Mills GB. Uniparental disomy in cancer. *Trends Mol Med.* March 2009;15(3):120-128. [Epub February 25, 2009]
23. Romanelli V, Nevado J, Fraga M, et al. Constitutional mosaic genome-wide uniparental disomy due to diploidisation: an unusual cancer-predisposing mechanism. *J Med Genet.* March 2011;48(3):212-216. [Epub November 19, 2010]
24. Cooper WN, Curley R, Macdonald F, Maher ER. Mitotic recombination and uniparental disomy in Beckwith-Wiedemann syndrome. *Genomics.* May 2007;89(5):613-617. [Epub Mar 6, 2007]
25. Lopez-Gines C, Gil-Benso R, Ferrer-Luna R, et al. New pattern of EGFR amplification in glioblastoma and the relationship of gene copy number with gene expression profile. *Mod Pathol.* June 2010;23(6):856-865. [Epub March 19, 2010]
26. Roessler S, Long EL, Budhu A, et al. Integrative genomic identification of genes on 8p associated with hepatocellular carcinoma progression and patient survival. *Gastroenterology.* April 2012;142(4):957-966.e12. [Epub December 24, 2011]
27. Pandita A, Bayani J, Paderova J, et al. Integrated cytogenetic and high-resolution array CGH analysis of genomic alterations associated with MYCN amplification. *Cytogenet Genome Res.* 2011;134:27-39.
28. Hagenkord JM, Parwani AV, Lyons-Weiler MA, et al. Virtual karyotyping with SNP microarrays reduces uncertainty in the diagnosis of renal epithelial tumors. *Diagn Pathol.* November 2008;3:44.
29. Kim HJ, Shen SS, Ayala AG, et al. Virtual-karyotyping with SNP microarrays in morphologically challenging renal cell neoplasms: a practical and useful diagnostic modality. *Am J Surg Pathol.* September 2009;33(9):1276-1286.
30. Abel F, Dalevi D, Nethander M, et al. A 6-gene signature identifies four molecular subgroups of neuroblastoma. *Cancer Cell Int.* April 2011;11:9.

31. Sharma S, Free A, Mei Y, Peiper SC, Wang Z, Cowell JK. Distinct molecular signatures in pediatric infratentorial glioblastomas defined by aCGH. *Exp Mol Pathol.* October 2010;89(2):169-174. [Epub July 16, 2010]
32. Heinrichs S, Kulkarni RV, Bueso-Ramos CE, et al. Accurate detection of uniparental disomy and microdeletions by SNP array analysis in myelodysplastic syndromes with normal cytogenetics. *Leukemia.* September 2009;23(9):1605-1613. [Epub April 23, 2009]
33. Vercauteren SM, Sung S, Starczynowski DT, et al. Array comparative genomic hybridization of peripheral blood granulocytes of patients with myelodysplastic syndrome detects karyotypic abnormalities. *Am J Clin Pathol.* July 2010;134(1): 119-126.
34. Ognjanovic S, Olivier M, Bergemann TL, Hainaut P. Sarcomas in TP53 germline mutation carriers: a review of the IARC TP53 database. *Cancer.* August 2011. doi: 10.1002/cncr.26390. [Epub ahead of print]
35. Rohlin A, Wernersson J, Engwall Y, et al. Parallel sequencing used in detection of mosaic mutations: comparison with four diagnostic DNA screening techniques. *Hum Mutat.* June 2009; 30(6):1012-1020.
36. Logan AC, Gao H, Wang C, et al. High-throughput VDJ sequencing for quantification of minimal residual disease in chronic lymphocytic leukemia and immune reconstitution assessment. *Proc Natl Acad Sci U S A.* December 2011;108(52):21194-21199. [Epub December 12, 2011]
37. Bakir-Gungor B, Sezerman OU. A new methodology to associate SNPs with human diseases according to their pathway related context. *PLoS One.* 2011;6(10):e26277. [Epub October 25, 2011]
38. Daley D. The identification of colon cancer susceptibility genes by using genome-wide scans. *Methods Mol Biol.* 2010;653:3-21.
39. Lascorz J, Försti A, Chen B, et al. Genome-wide association study for colorectal cancer identifies risk polymorphisms in German familial cases and implicates MAPK signalling pathways in disease susceptibility. *Carcinogenesis.* September 2010;31(9):1612-1619. [Epub July 7, 2010]
40. Lapkus O, Gologan O, Liu Y, et al. Determination of sequential mutational accumulation in pancreas and bile duct brushing cytology. *Mod Pathol.* 2006;19:907-913.
41. Wang Q, Zhang T, Ye L, Wang W, Zhang X. Analysis of hepatitis B virus X gene (HBx) mutants in tissues of patients suffered from hepatocellular carcinoma in China. *Cancer Epidemiol.* August 2012;36(4):369-374. [Epub December 16, 2011]
42. Liu Y, Zhong Y, Zou Z, et al. Features and clinical implications of hepatitis B virus genotypes and mutations in basal core promoter/ precore region in 507 Chinese patients with acute and chronic hepatitis B. *J Clin Virol.* March 2010;47(3):243-247. [Epub January 15, 2010]
43. Andersson E, Villabona L, Bergfeldt K, et al. Correlation of HLA-A02* genotype and HLA class I antigen down-regulation with the prognosis of epithelial ovarian cancer. *Cancer Immunol Immunother.* August 2012;61(8):1243-1253. [Epub January 19, 2012]
44. Castle PE, Stoler MH, Wright TC Jr, et al. Performance of carcinogenic human papillomavirus (HPV) testing and HPV16 or HPV18 genotyping for cervical cancer screening of women aged 25 years and older: a subanalysis of the ATHENA study. *Lancet Oncol.* September 2011;12(9):880-890. [Epub August 22, 2011]
45. Klopfleisch R, Weiss AT, Gruber AD. Excavation of a buried treasure—DNA, mRNA, miRNA and protein analysis in formalin fixed, paraffin embedded tissues. *Histol Histopathol.* June 2011;26(6):797-810.
46. Thunnissen E, Kerr KM, Herth FJ, et al. The challenge of NSCLC diagnosis and predictive analysis on small samples. Practical approach of a working group. *Lung Cancer.* April 2012;76(1):1-18. [Epub December 3, 2011. Review]
47. Kerr SE, Schnabel CA, Sullivan PS, et al. Multisite validation study to determine performance characteristics of a 92-gene molecular cancer classifier. *Clin Cancer Res.* July 2012;18(14): 3952-60. [Epub May 30, 2012]
48. Lee HS, Kim MJ, Lim CK, et al. Multiple displacement amplification for preimplantation genetic diagnosis of fragile X syndrome. *Genet Mol Res.* November 2011;10(4):2851-2859.
49. Lee-Lewandrowski E, Lewandrowski K. Perspectives on cost and outcomes for point-of-care testing. *Clin Lab Med.* 2009;29:479-489.
50. Goozner M. From gene testing to the bedside: workshop focuses on future strategies. *J Natl Cancer Inst.* August 2011;103(15):1150-1151.
51. Wang S, Zhao X, Khimji I, et al. Integration of cell phone imaging with microchip ELISA to detect ovarian cancer HE4 biomarker in urine at the point-of-care. *Lab Chip.* October 2011;11(20):3411-3418.
52. Derveaux S, Stubbe BG, Braeckmans K, et al. Synergism between particle-based multiplexing and microfluidics technologies may bring diagnostics closer to the patient. *Anal Bioanal Chem.* 2008;391:2453-2467.
53. Pestrin M, Bessi S, Galardi F, et al. Correlation of HER2 status between primary tumors and corresponding circulating tumor cells in advanced breast cancer patients. *Breast Cancer Res Treat.* December 2009;118(3):523-530. [Epub July 12, 2009]
54. Fehm T, Müller V, Aktas B, et al. HER2 status of circulating tumor cells in patients with metastatic breast cancer: a prospective, multicenter trial. *Breast Cancer Res Treat.* 2010;124:403-412.
55. Dupont Jensen J, Laenkholm AV, Knoop A, et al. PIK3CA mutations may be discordant between primary and corresponding metastatic disease in breast cancer. *Clin Cancer Res.* 2011;17: 667-677.
56. Yung TKF, Chan KCA, Mok TSK, Tong J, To K, Lo YMD. Single-molecule detection of epidermal growth factor receptor mutations in plasma by microfluidics digital PCR in non-small cell lung cancer patients. *Clin Cancer Res.* 2009;15:2076-2084.
57. Fusi A, Berdel R, Havemann S, et al. Enhanced detection of BRAF-mutants by pre-PCR cleavage of wild-type sequences revealed circulating melanoma cells heterogeneity. *Eur J Cancer.* September 2011;47(13):1971-1976. [Epub May 12, 2011]
58. Attard G, Swennenhuis JF, Olmos D, et al. Characterization of ERG, AR and PTEN status in circulating tumor cells from patients with castration-resistant prostate cancer. *Cancer Res.* 2009;69:2912-2918.
59. Tsiatis AC, Norris-Kirby A, Rich RG, et al. Comparison of Sanger sequencing, pyrosequencing, and melting curve analysis for the detection of KRAS mutations: diagnostic and clinical implications. *J Mol Diagn.* July 2010;12(4):425-432. [Epub April 29, 2010]
60. Do H, Krypuy M, Mitchell PL, Fox SB, Dobrovic A. High resolution melting analysis for rapid and sensitive EGFR and KRAS mutation detection in formalin fixed paraffin embedded biopsies. *BMC Cancer.* May 2008;8:142.
61. Borràs E, Jurado I, Hernan I, et al. Clinical pharmacogenomic testing of KRAS, BRAF and EGFR mutations by high resolution melting analysis and ultra-deep pyrosequencing. *BMC Cancer.* September 2011;11:406.
62. Lee S, Brophy VH, Cao J, et al. Analytical performance of a PCR assay for the detection of KRAS mutations (codons 12/13 and 61) in formalin-fixed paraffin-embedded tissue samples of colorectal carcinoma. *Virchows Arch.* February 2012;460(2):141-149. [Epub December 16, 2011]
63. Vaughn CP, Zobell SD, Furtado LV, et al. Frequency of KRAS, BRAF, and NRAS mutations in colorectal cancer. *Genes Chromosomes Cancer.* May 2011;50(5):307-312. doi: 10.1002/ gcc.20854. [Epub February 8, 2011]
64. Pirker R, Herth FJ, Kerr KM, et al. European EGFR Workshop Group. Consensus for EGFR mutation testing in non-small cell lung cancer: results from a European workshop. *J Thorac Oncol.* October 2010;5(10):1706-1713.
65. Gerber DE. EGFR inhibition in the treatment of non-small cell lung cancer. *Drug Dev Res.* December 2008;69(6):359-372.
66. Gerber DE, Minna JD. ALK inhibition for non-small cell lung cancer: from discovery to therapy in record time. *Cancer Cell.* December 2010;18(6):548-551.
67. Halait H, Demartin K, Shah S, et al. Analytical performance of a real-time PCR-based assay for V600 mutations in the BRAF Gene, used as the companion diagnostic test for the novel BRAF inhibitor vemurafenib in metastatic melanoma. *Diagn Mol Pathol.* March 2012;21(1):1-8. [Epub February 2012]

68. Rosell R, Carcereny E, Gervais R, et al. Erlotinib versus standard chemotherapy as first-line treatment for European patients with advanced EGFR mutation-positive non-small-cell lung cancer (EURTAC): a multicentre, open-label, randomised phase 3 trial. *Lancet Oncol*. March 2012;13(3):239-246. [Epub January 26, 2012]
69. Bang YJ, Van Cutsem E, Feyereislova A, et al. Trastuzumab in combination with chemotherapy versus chemotherapy alone for treatment of HER2-positive advanced gastric or gastro-oesophageal junction cancer (ToGA): a phase 3, open-label, randomised controlled trial. *Lancet*. August 2010;376(9742): 687-697. [Epub August 19, 2010]
70. Paik S, Shak S, Tang G, et al. A multigene assay to predict recurrence of tamoxifen treated node negative breast cancer. *N Engl J Med*. 2004;351(27):2817-2826.
71. Lyman GH, Cosler LE, Kuderer NM, Hornberger J. Impact of a 21-gene RT-PCR assay on treatment decisions in early-stage breast cancer: an economic analysis based on prognostic and predictive validation studies. *Cancer*. March 2007;109(6):1011-1018.
72. Partin JF, Mamounas EP. Impact of the 21-gene recurrence score assay compared with standard clinicopathologic guidelines in adjuvant therapy selection for node-negative, estrogen receptor-positive breast cancer. *Ann Surg Oncol*. November 2011;18(12):3399-3406. [Epub May 3, 2011]
73. Gray RG, Quirke P, Handley K, et al. Validation study of a quantitative multigene reverse transcriptase-polymerase chain reaction assay for assessment of recurrence risk in patients with stage II colon cancer. *J Clin Oncol*. December 2011;29(35): 4611-4619. [Epub November 7, 2011]
74. Imyanitov EN, Moiseyenko VM. Drug therapy for hereditary cancers. *Hered Cancer Clin Pract*. August 2011;9(1):5.
75. Cai G, Xu Y, Lu H, et al. Clinicopathologic and molecular features of sporadic microsatellite- and chromosomal-stable colorectal cancers. *Int J Colorectal Dis*. April 2008;23(4):365-373.
76. Guastadisegni C, Colafranceschi M, Ottini L, Dogliotti E. Microsatellite instability as a marker of prognosis and response to therapy: a meta-analysis of colorectal cancer survival data. *Eur J Cancer*. October 2010;46(15):2788-2798. [Epub June 4, 2010]
77. Sinicrope FA, Foster NR, Thibodeau SN, et al. DNA mismatch repair status and colon cancer recurrence and survival in clinical trials of 5-fluorouracil-based adjuvant therapy. *J Natl Cancer Inst*. June 2011;103(11):863-875. [Epub May 19, 2011]
78. Adams SF, Marsh EB, Elmasri W, et al. A high response rate to liposomal doxorubicin is seen among women with BRCA mutations treated for recurrent epithelial ovarian cancer. *Gynecol Oncol*. December 2011;123(3):486-491. [Epub September 25, 2011]
79. Fong PC, Yap TA, Boss DS, et al. Poly(ADP)-ribose polymerase inhibition: frequent durable responses in BRCA carrier ovarian cancer correlating with platinum-free interval. *J Clin Oncol*. May 2010;28(15):2512-2519. [Epub April 20, 2010]
80. Timmermann B, Kerick M, Roehr C, et al. Somatic mutation profiles of MSI and MSS colorectal cancer identified by whole exome next generation sequencing and bioinformatics analysis. *PLoS One*. December 2010;5(12):e15661.
81. Martini M, Vecchione L, Siena S, et al. Targeted therapies: how personal should we go? *Nat Rev Clin Oncol*. November 2011;9(2):87-97. doi: 10.1038/nrclinonc.2011.164.
82. Cortez KJ, Maldarelli F. Clinical management of HIV drug resistance. *Viruses*. April 2011;3(4):347-378. [Epub April 14, 2011]
83. Keedy VL, Temin S, Somerfield MR, et al. American Society of Clinical Oncology provisional clinical opinion: epidermal growth factor receptor (EGFR) mutation testing for patients with advanced non-small-cell lung cancer considering first-line EGFR tyrosine kinase inhibitor therapy. *J Clin Oncol*. May 2011;29(15):2121-2127. [Epub April 11, 2011]
84. Von Hoff DD, Stephenson JJ Jr, Rosen P, et al. Pilot study using molecular profiling of patients' tumors to find potential targets and select treatments for their refractory cancers. *J Clin Oncol*. November 2010;28(33):4877-4883. [Epub October 4, 2010]
85. Gold KA, Kim ES, Lee JJ, et al. The BATTLE to personalize lung cancer prevention through reverse migration. *Cancer Prev Res (Phila)*. July 2011;4(7):962-972.
86. Anderson S, Bloom K, Vallera D, et al. Multi-site analytical performance studies of a real-time polymerase chain reaction assay for the detection of BRAF V600E mutations in formalin-fixed, paraffin-embedded tissue specimens of malignant melanoma. *Arch Pathol Lab Med*. doi: 10.5858/arpa.2011-0505-OA. [Epub February 14, 2012]
87. Dugan M, Lawrence J. Cobas BRAF V600 mutation test and Zelboraf (letter). *CAP Today*. February 2012;8-11.
88. Gregory DM, Parfrey PS. The breast cancer hormone receptor retesting controversy in Newfoundland and Labrador, Canada: lessons for the health system. *Health Manage Forum*. Autumn 2010;23(3):114-118.
89. Hammond ME, Hayes DF, Wolff AC, et al. American Society of Clinical Oncology/College of American Pathologists guideline recommendations for immunohistochemical testing of estrogen and progesterone receptors in breast cancer. *J Oncol Pract*. July 2010;6(4):195-197. [Epub June 23, 2010]
90. Wolff AC, Hammond ME, Schwartz JN, et al. American Society of Clinical Oncology/College of American Pathologists guideline recommendations for human epidermal growth factor receptor 2 testing in breast cancer. *Arch Pathol Lab Med*. 2007;131(1):18-43.
91. Philip R, Carrington L, Chan M. US FDA perspective on challenges in co-developing in vitro companion diagnostics and targeted cancer therapeutics. *Bioanalysis*. February 2011;3(4): 383-389.
92. FDA approves Zelboraf and companion diagnostic test for late-stage skin cancer. http://www.fda.gov/NewsEvents/Newsroom/PressAnnouncements/ucm268241.htm. Accessed August 17, 2011.
93. Chapman PB, Hauschild A, Robert C, et al. Improved survival with vemurafenib in melanoma with BRAF V600E mutation. *N Engl J Med*. June 2011;364(26):2507-2516. [Epub June 5, 2011]
94. Flaherty KT, Puzanov I, Kim KB, et al. Inhibition of mutated, activated BRAF in metastatic melanoma. *N Engl J Med*. August 2010;363(9):809-819.
95. Sosman JA, Kim KB, Schuchter L, et al. Survival in BRAF V600-mutant advanced melanoma treated with vemurafenib. *N Engl J Med*. February 2012;366(8):707-714.
96. Camidge DR, Theodoro M, Maxson DA, et al. Correlations between the percentage of tumor cells showing an ALK (anaplastic lymphoma kinase) gene rearrangement, ALK signal copy number, and response to crizotinib therapy in ALK fluorescence in situ hybridization-positive nonsmall cell lung cancer. *Cancer*. January 2012. doi: 10.1002/cncr.27411. [Epub ahead of print]
97. Cheng S. Koch W, Wu L. Co-development of a companion diagnostic for targeted cancer therapy. *N Biotechnol*. September 2012;29(6):682-688. [Epub February 25, 2012]
98. Gerlinger M, Rowan AJ, Horswell S, et al. Intratumor heterogeneity and branched evolution revealed by multiregion sequencing. *N Engl J Med*. March 2012;366(10):883-892.
99. Cancer Genome Atlas Network. Comprehensive molecular portraits of human breast tumors. *Nature*. September 2012;490(7418):61-70.
100. Govindan R, Ding L, Griffith M, et al. Genomic landscape of non-small cell lung cancer in smokers and never-smokers. *Cell*. September 2012;150(6):1121-1134.

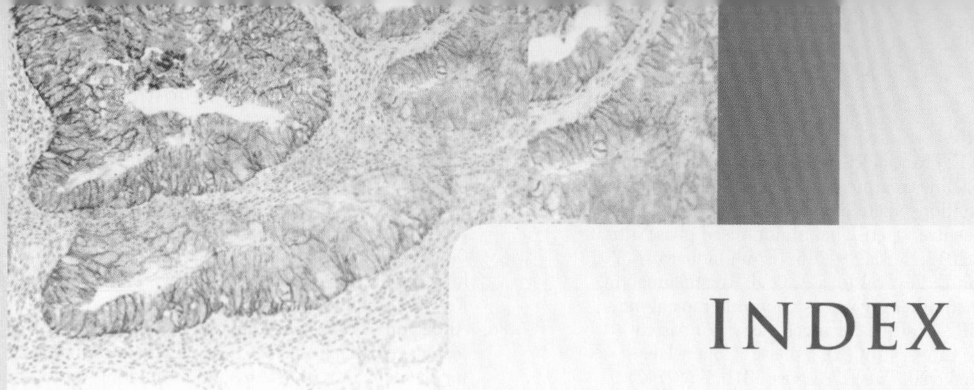

INDEX

Note: Locators followed by 'f' and 't' refer to figures and tables respectively.

A

B

C

D

E

H

I

J

K

M

N

O

P

Q

R

S

T

U

V

W

X

Y

Z